W9-BUN-266

THE WORLD BOOK

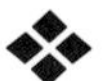

RUSH-PRESBYTERIAN-ST. LUKE'S MEDICAL CENTER

MEDICAL ENCYCLOPEDIA

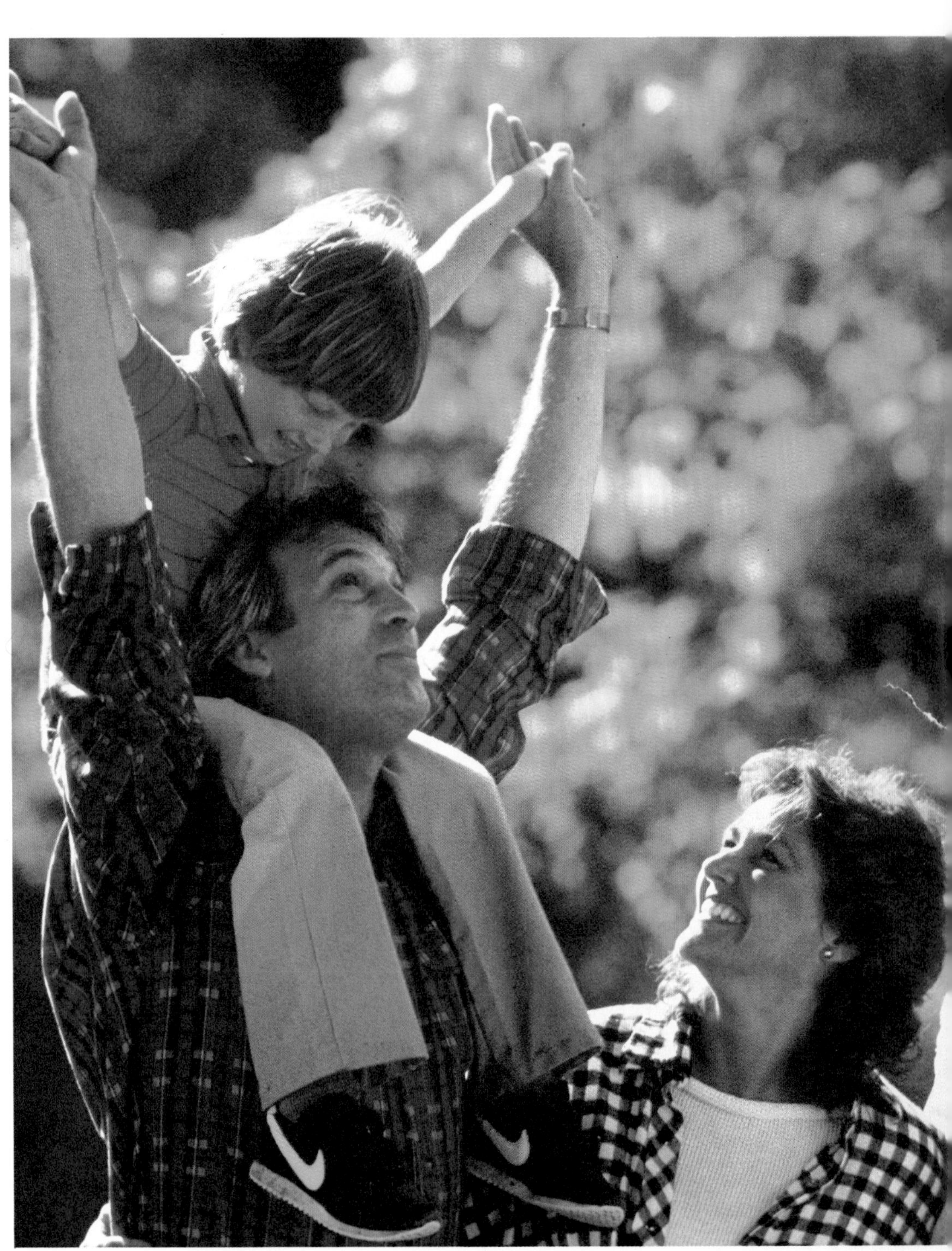

THE WORLD BOOK

RUSH-PRESBYTERIAN-ST. LUKE'S MEDICAL CENTER

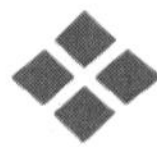

MEDICAL ENCYCLOPEDIA

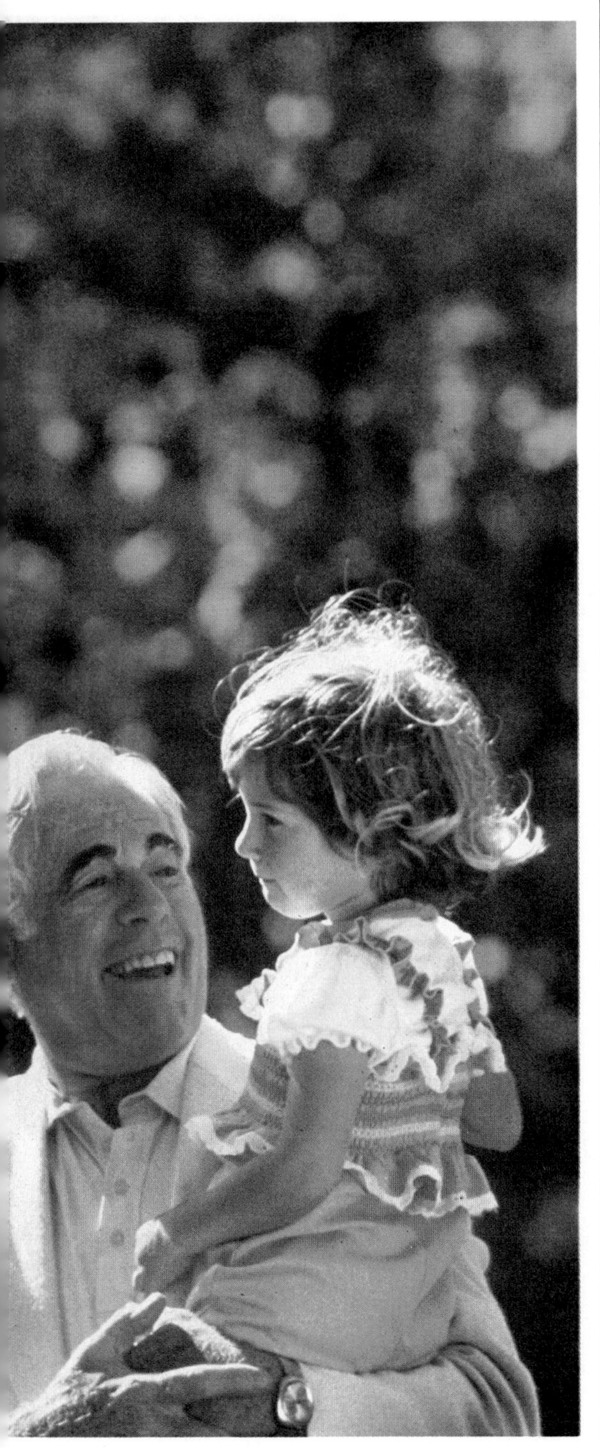

Your Guide to Good Health

World Book, Inc.
a Scott Fetzer company
Chicago London Sydney Toronto

Board of Consultants

The World Book/Rush-Presbyterian-St. Luke's Medical Center Medical Encyclopedia was prepared with the assistance of faculty members of **Rush Medical College, Rush-Presbyterian-St. Luke's Medical Center** of Chicago.

Medical Editor

Erich E. Brueschke, M.D., FAAFP
Professor and Chairman of Family Practice and Senior Attending Physician

Associate Medical Editors

William A. Schwer, M.D.
Associate Professor and Associate Chairman of Family Practice and Associate Attending Physician

Susan Vanderberg-Dent, M.D.
Associate Professor of Family Practice and Associate Attending Physician

Steven K. Rothschild, M.D.
Assistant Professor and Assistant Chairman for Clinical Programs for Family Practice and Assistant Attending Physician

Diane Homan, M.D.
Assistant Professor of Family Practice and Assistant Attending Physician

Thomas Dent, M.D.
Associate Professor of Family Practice

Assistant Medical Editors

Brady Welsh, M.D.
Assistant Professor of Family Practice and Assistant Attending Physician

Carolyn Lopez, M.D.
Assistant Professor of Family Practice and Assistant Attending Physician

Dora Dixie Bell, M.D.
Assistant Professor of Family Practice and Assistant Attending Physician

Wanda Elliott-Pearson, M.D.
Instructor of Family Practice and Adjunct Attending Physician

Consultants

Emergency Medicine
Robert C. Harwood, M.D., M.P.H.
Assistant Professor, Section of Emergency Medicine of the Department of Family Practice

Exercise and Fitness
Keith Berndtson, M.D.
Assistant Professor of Family Practice and Assistant Attending Physician

Family Medicine Surgery
Martin Shobris, M.D., Ph.D.
Associate Professor of Family Practice

General Dentistry
Leon R. Kelleher, D.D.S.
Assistant Professor, Director of the Section of Dentistry, and Senior Attending

Immunology
Henry Gewurz, M.D.
Professor and Chairman of the Department of Immunology/Microbiology and Senior Attending Physician

Infectious Disease
Stuart Levin, M.D.
Professor, Associate Chairman, and Program Director, Department of Internal Medicine, Director, Section of Infectious Disease, and Senior Attending Physician

Nursing
Frances Bryan Brueschke, R.N.
Consultant in Family Medicine Nursing

Nutrition
Susie W. Rockway, Ph.D.
Assistant Professor, Department of Clinical Nutrition

Obstetrics and Gynecology
George D. Wilbanks, M.D.
Professor and Chairman and Senior Attending Physician

Pediatrics
Samuel P. Gotoff, M.D.
Professor and Chairman and Senior Attending Physician

Periodontics
Paul Delaney, D.D.S.
Instructor, Section of Dentistry, and Adjunct Attending

Pharmacology
Donald R. Bennett, M.D., Ph.D.
Associate Professor of Pharmacology and of Family Practice

Physical Medicine and Rehabilitation
Richard F. Harvey, M.D.
Professor and Chairman and Senior Attending Physician

Psychiatry
Jan Fawcett, M.D.
Professor and Chairman and Senior Attending Physician

Psychology
Robert E. Zitter, Ph.D.
Assistant Professor of Family Practice and of Psychology and Social Sciences

Veterinary Medicine
Thomas J. Welsh, D.V.M., Ph.D.
Assistant Professor of Immunology/Microbiology and Director, Comparative Research Center

---

World Book, Inc.
525 West Monroe
Chicago, IL 60606

ISBN 0-7166-3236-5
Library of Congress Catalog Card No. 90-71232

Printed in the United States of America

c/ia

The publisher would also like to thank The American National Red Cross and the National Safety Council, without whose help completion of portions of this publication would not have been possible.

Staff

World Book Publishing

President
Peter Mollman

Publisher
William H. Nault

Editorial

Editor in Chief
Robert O. Zeleny

Executive Editor
Dominic J. Miccolis

Associate Editor
Anne M. O'Malley

Senior Editor
Katie John Sharp

Contributing Editors
Mary Banas
Waldemar Bojczuk
Terry Fertig
Denise Guyer
Susan Lorant
Lori Maxim
Mark F. Toch

Research Editor
Suzanne B. Aschoff

Production Editor
June Huitt

Permissions Editor
Janet T. Peterson

Art

Art Director
Roberta Dimmer

Assistant Art Director
Joe Gound

Photography Director
John S. Marshall

Cover
Shepard Design

Product Production

Manufacturing Director
Henry Koval

Manufacturing Manager
Sandra Van den Broucke

Manufacturing Assistant Manager
Eva Bostedor

Pre-press Director
Jerry Stack

Product Managers
Randi Park
Joann Seastrom

Proofreaders
Anne Dillon
Marguerite Hoye
Daniel Marotta

Contents

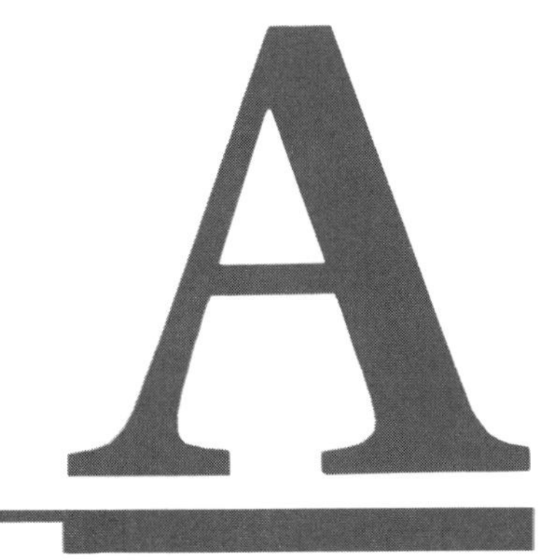

Abdomen (ab′də mən) is the [illegible] cavity below the chest. It is often called the gut, stomach, solar plexus, or belly. The abdomen is bordered by the diaphragm above, the pelvis below, and the back muscles and spine behind. The abdomen contains various major organs, including the liver, spleen, pancreas, gall bladder, stomach, small and large intestines, kidneys, adrenal glands, and bladder. In a woman, the abdomen also encloses the uterus and ovaries. In a man, the abdomen contains the prostate gland.

All the abdominal organs are surrounded by a membrane called the peritoneum. The abdominal cavity is also lined by peritoneum. The front and sides of the abdomen are covered by three layers of abdominal muscles. The abdominal aorta (a major artery that carries blood from the heart) and the major veins lie on the back wall of the abdomen.

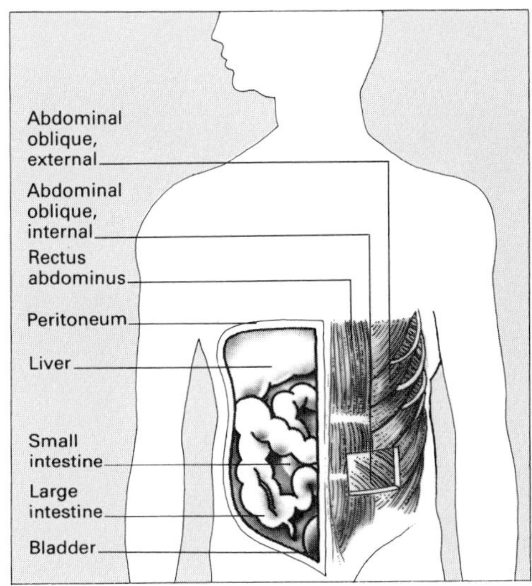

The **abdomen,** the cavity below the chest, contains the liver, spleen, pancreas, stomach, intestines, kidneys, and bladder.

See also ABDOMINAL PAIN.

Abdomen, burst or eviscerated: first aid (ab′də mən, i vis′ə rāt id). An abdominal evisceration or "burst abdomen" is a very rare injury. It is extremely serious because the exposed part of the intestine may become infected, as well as the peritoneum. Both infections can be fatal.

The condition is most commonly caused by the tearing of stitches following surgery or, more rarely, by the rupture of a surgical scar. It also may result from a deep knife wound.

Lay the victim down and keep the intestines clean, moist, and warm. Do not cover with material that clings or loses its structure when wet, for example, toilet paper, paper towels, or absorbent cotton. If sterile dressings and sterile water are available, moisten the dressings and cover. Otherwise, cover the entire abdomen with clean plastic wrap and/or clean aluminum foil, followed by a clean sheet or towel. Do not give the victim anything to eat or drink. Summon medical help immediately.

Abdominal pain can be classified by onset, type, and location: the onset of pain can be either sudden or gradual; the type of pain can be either constant or crampy; the location can be either localized or diffuse. Using a thermometer, check anyone suffering from abdominal pain for a fever.

Q: *What are minor causes of abdominal pain?*

A: *Indigestion* is the most common cause of abdominal distress in both adults and children. Indigestion results from eating too much or eating unsuitable food. It is often accompanied by belching, and a sensation of fullness or nausea. In most cases, indigestion ceases gradually and within a few hours. Antacids may help. Indigestion does not trigger a fever.

Heartburn due to acid rising from the stomach and hiatus hernia, where a part of the stomach protrudes upward through the diaphragm, are other common causes. Persons with persistent heartburn should see a physician.

Gastroenteritis is an inflammation of the lining of the stomach and intestinal tract. It is another common cause of abdominal pain. It can be caused by food poisoning, food allergies, or infections, for example, "stomach flu." The pain is crampy, diffuse, and may come on suddenly. There is nausea, vomiting, and diarrhea. If the cause is infectious, there may be a fever.

Constipation is difficulty in emptying the bowels. The pain is often sudden and may be either constant or crampy. Although the pain is usually diffuse, it can be localized to the left side of the abdomen. Constipation does not cause a fever. The pain is relieved by either passing gas and/or stool.

Irritable colon, which is also known as spastic colon or mucous colitis, is a disturbance of large intestine function. The condition is made worse by periods of emotional stress. The pain is crampy. There can be either constipation, diarrhea, or mucous stools, as well as a loss of appetite. A fever is not a symptom.

Menstrual cramps or painful menstrual periods (dysmenorrhea) are experienced by many women. Pain at ovulation or *mittelschmerz* (middle pain) occurs midway between periods. It can be severe; it is localized to the right or to the left lower abdomen. There is no vomiting, diarrhea, or fever. The pain usually passes in a day or two.

Q: *What are the more serious causes of abdominal pain?*

A: Sudden sharp pain that comes in waves (a condition known medically as colic) may be accompanied by vomiting, sweating, and the need to double up. Colic can be caused by several potentially serious disorders, such as intestinal obstruction; stones in the gall bladder system (biliary colic); or stones in the kidney system (renal colic). *See also* CALCULUS; COLIC.

Continuous pain, together with slight fever, tenderness of the abdomen when touched, and sometimes vomiting may be caused by inflammation of the appendix (appendicitis), colon (colitis), colon pouches (diverticulitis), or gall bladder (cholecystitis). An inflamed pancreas (pancreatitis) causes continuous pain, vomiting, and tenderness to the touch. An inflamed fallopian tube (salpingitis) causes continuous pain, lower abdominal pain, fever, and tenderness to the touch.

Continuous pain that comes on suddenly, producing tenderness of the abdomen when touched, may be caused by a perforated ulcer, an ectopic (tubal) pregnancy, or a leaking abdominal, aortic aneurysm. An abdominal aneurysm may also cause pain in the back.

Q: *What other disorders include abdominal pain as a symptom?*

A: Abdominal pain with backache and frequent, painful passing of urine suggests inflammation of the kidney (pyelonephritis) or of the bladder (cystitis). There may also be a fever. Recurrent abdominal pain may be caused by a peptic ulcer. Abdominal pain is also a symptom of inflammation of the stomach lining (gastritis) or an inflammation of the liver (hepatitis).

Q: *Are children especially subject to abdominal pain?*

A: No. But a child with infection of the middle ear (otitis media) or inflammation of the tonsils (tonsillitis) may complain of a stomachache. There may be two reasons for this: a child's nonabdominal illness may make him or her feel queasy or nauseated; also, a child's vocabulary may be limited to ache or pain associated in the past with abdominal pain or a stomachache.

Abortion (ə bôr′shən) is the termination of a pregnancy before the fetus can survive outside the uterus. Popularly, the term abortion refers to the deliberate or induced termination of a pregnancy, whereas the spontaneous termination of a pregnancy is commonly called a miscarriage or spontaneous abortion. *See also* ABORTION, SPONTANEOUS.

Q: *Why might a woman choose to have an abortion?*

A: A physician might recommend an abortion if tests (for example, amniocentesis) show that the fetus is developing with such a severe abnormality as spina bifida or another genetic defect. A pregnancy is often deliberately terminated if the woman's health is seriously at risk. But the primary reason for voluntary abortion in the U.S. is the woman's decision that having a child at this time is not right for her. The laws regarding abortion are different from state to state. *See also* ABORTION LAW; AMNIOCENTESIS; GENETIC COUNSELING.

Q: ***How is a medically induced abortion performed?***

A: In early pregnancy, an abortion is generally performed using either minor surgery, such as dilatation and curettage, or a suction apparatus. In a pregnancy of four months or more, labor is induced. A prostaglandin gel can be placed into the vagina to begin contractions. The fetus is then delivered vaginally. *See also* DILATATION AND CURETTAGE.

Q: ***Is an induced abortion dangerous to the woman?***

A: A medical abortion in early pregnancy, properly conducted, is a safe and minor operation. It can be performed in a clinic or with brief hospitalization.

An abortion performed by an unskilled person and without sterile conditions exposes the patient to the risk of infection, hemorrhage, future infertility, or even death.

See also PREGNANCY AND CHILDBIRTH.

Abortion law. In some countries, the deliberate termination of a pregnancy is viewed as a criminal act. Many countries, however, have legalized abortion. Restrictions on abortion may differ from country to country and, in the U.S., from state to state. In 1973 the Supreme Court of the U.S. ruled that women have the right to have an abortion. In 1989, the court limited women's access to abortion declaring that states may require physicians to perform tests to determine whether a fetus is viable before performing an abortion on a woman pregnant for 20 or more weeks. The court also ruled that states may outlaw abortion in public hospitals and clinics and prohibit public employees from assisting in abortions. Many states have already begun to make changes to their abortion laws.

The laws regulating abortion after the twelfth week vary from state to state. All states allow abortion when the mother's life is in danger, for example, when an embryo develops in the fallopian tube instead of in the womb. Some states permit abortion if it is likely that the fetus will be born with serious abnormalities, for example, when a woman contracts rubella during early pregnancy.

See also ABORTION; PREGNANCY, ECTOPIC; RUBELLA.

Abortion, spontaneous. A spontaneous abortion is the accidental termination of pregnancy under 20 weeks of gestation. The usual reason for a spontaneous abortion is a defect in the embryo or fetus that prevents its natural development. This defect may be inherited, caused by exposure of the mother to medications or radiation, or result from infectious illness. The first symptom of a threatened spontaneous abortion is vaginal bleeding; this requires immediate medical attention. A spontaneous abortion is most likely to occur in the second or third month of pregnancy. Delivery of a fetus after approximately the twentieth week of pregnancy is known as a stillbirth, if the fetus is dead, or as a premature birth, if the fetus is alive.

See also ABORTION; PREGNANCY AND CHILDBIRTH.

Abortus fever. *See* BRUCELLOSIS.

Abrasion (ə brā′zhən) is a minor injury in which the skin is scraped or grazed hard enough to cause bleeding.

To treat an abrasion, clean the wound immediately with soap and water, using sterilized tweezers to remove any pieces of loose grit in the wound. Rinse thoroughly and dry gently; antiseptics, such as alcohol, are usually not necessary, as they may cause tissue damage. Bandage the area if the wound is still bleeding, if clothing might rub against it, or if dirt could enter. In adults, the wound, if minor, may be left unbandaged. In children, as a rule,

An **abrasion** is an injury to the surface layers of the skin, exposing blood capillaries and nerves. Thoroughly rinse and gently dry an abrasion before bandaging the area.

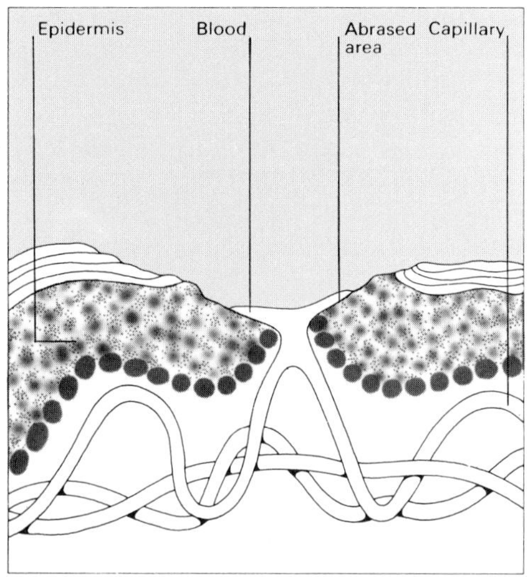

bandaged wounds tend to heal more quickly because they are protected from dirt and, thus, infection. Do not remove scabs that may form over the abrasion; these will fall off during healing. Seek medical attention if there is evidence of infection (redness, swelling, drainage of pus).

Abscess (ab'ses) is a collection of pus usually caused by bacterial infection. Bacteria that invade the body are attacked by white blood cells, and pus is formed, which is discharged through the skin. Boils are surface abscesses. An abscess commonly occurs under the skin and may be caused by an infection of any small gland in the skin (folliculitis), a minor abrasion, or a cut. Abscesses often occur in moist areas of the body, such as the groin or armpit, and are more frequent in persons with diabetes.

Q: *What are some of the symptoms of an abscess?*

A: Pus forms and the surrounding tissues become red, swollen, and painful as the abscess stretches the area and tries to burst through the skin. The pain is due to pressure the pus puts upon nerve endings. Discomfort is relieved when the abscess bursts or is lanced.

Q: *What is the treatment for an external type of abscess?*

A: The aim is to encourage the infection to reach the surface of the skin. The customary home treatment is a warm, moist compress. A medical objection to such treatment is that such a compress makes the surrounding tissue more prone to infection. Painkilling drugs, such as acetaminophen, may be used. The area may be rested, for example, by putting an arm in a sling when there is an abscess in the armpit. A dry dressing should be applied when an abscess comes to a head and discharges.

The abscess may need to be lanced by a physician if there is fever or pain or if the surrounding skin becomes increasingly red and tender.

Q: *What other kinds of abscesses are there?*

A: There are internal abscesses, usually accompanied by fever, local pain, and a tired, rundown feeling. Such abscesses can occur around a tooth (gumboil), in the breast, in bone (in mastoiditis and osteomyelitis), in the liver (in amebic dysentery), in the vagina (Bartholin's cyst), in the appendix (appendicitis), or in the anal area, between the rectum and the ischium (ischiorectal abscess). In all such cases, a physician must be consulted.

Another kind of abscess is the cold abscess, which may be caused by tuberculosis. A cold abscess is so called because it is slow-forming and without pain, redness, or heat.

See also ABSCESS, COLD; BOIL; DIABETES.

Abscess, cold (ab'ses). A cold abscess is an abscess that commonly accompanies tuberculosis. It develops so slowly that there is little inflammation, and it becomes painful only when there is pressure on the surrounding area. This type of abscess may appear anywhere on the body, but it is most commonly found on the spine, hips, lymph nodes, or in the genital region.

See also ABSCESS; TUBERCULOSIS.

Abscess, ischiorectal (ab'ses, is ke o rek'tal). Ischiorectal abscess is an infection between the ischium bone of the pelvis (part of the hipbone) and the adjacent area of the intestine, more usually the anus rather than the rectum. The abscess is painful, with local swelling and extreme tenderness. An ischiorectal abscess requires surgical treatment.

Abscess, parapharyngeal (ab'ses, par ə fah rin'je al). Parapharyngeal abscess is the formation of pus on the lymph nodes located in the pharynx region (part of the throat). Abscess formation usually follows the onset of pharyngitis or tonsillitis and may occur at any age.

See also PHARYNGITIS; TONSILLITIS.

Abscess, peritonsillar (ab′ses, per i ton′si lar). Peritonsillar abscess is an infection of the tissue around the tonsils. It is usually caused by the spread of infection from tonsillitis.

Q: *What are the symptoms of peritonsillar abscess?*

A: The symptoms include fever, severe pain on swallowing, and difficulty in opening the mouth (trismus). The patient's breath may also smell foul, and there may be earache (otalgia).

Q: *How is peritonsillar abscess treated?*

A: Treatment with antibiotics is usually effective in the early stages. However, if the symptoms are severe, a surgical incision of the abscess may be necessary. This allows the pus to drain and usually gives immediate relief. Peritonsillar abscess tends to recur; a physician may advise a tonsillectomy.

See also TONSILLECTOMY; TONSILLITIS.

Abscess, retropharyngeal (ab′ses, re tro fah rin′je al). Retropharyngeal abscess is an inflammation of the lymph nodes in the back walls of the pharynx (part of the throat). The swelling is caused by the formation or discharge of pus. If not treated, the swelling can be significant and can cause acute obstruction and respiratory distress. Treatment involves incision and drainage and appropriate antibiotics.

See also PHARYNX.

Abscess, throat. *See* ABSCESS, PARAPHARYNGEAL; ABSCESS, RETROPHARYNGEAL.

Accident prevention. *See* HOME SAFETY.

Accommodation (ə kom ə dā′shən) is the adjustment made by the lens of the eye, by means of eye muscles, that enables a person to see objects at various distances. The ability of the lens to focus in this way decreases with age, resulting in the condition called presbyopia (farsightedness). Eyeglasses usually correct this condition.

See also EYE; PRESBYOPIA.

ACE inhibitor. *See* ANGIOTENSIN-CONVERTING ENZYME INHIBITOR.

Acetabulum (as ə tab′yə ləm) is the cup-shaped socket at the base of the pelvis into which the ball-shaped top of the thighbone (femur) fits.

Acetaminophen (as ə tə min′ə fən) is a commonly used drug that relieves pain and reduces fever. Acetaminophen is often taken instead of aspirin in order to avoid stomach irritation and allergy to aspirin. It should be given to children in place of aspirin, to avoid the possibility of Reye's syndrome. Acetaminophen, unlike aspirin, does not irritate the stomach or interfere with blood clotting. However, it cannot reduce inflammation as effectively as aspirin. Therefore, it is not as useful in treating such inflammatory conditions as arthritis or rheumatic fever.

When taken in normal doses, acetaminophen seldom causes side effects. In rare cases, however, it may produce allergic reactions. A heavy overdose can cause liver or kidney damage. Acetaminophen is probably best known under the trade name Tylenol®.

See also ASPIRIN; REYE'S SYNDROME.

Acetone (as′ə tōn) is a colorless liquid that is normally produced in the body in very small amounts. Larger quantities are produced if there is a lack of insulin in the body, as may occur with diabetes, starvation, or some severe illnesses. Acetone can be detected in urine and blood tests; it also produces a characteristic fruity smell on the breath.

See also DIABETES; STARVATION.

Acetylcholine (ə sē təl kō′lēn) is a chemical that is produced in nerve endings. It is essential for the transmission of nerve impulses.

See also NERVE.

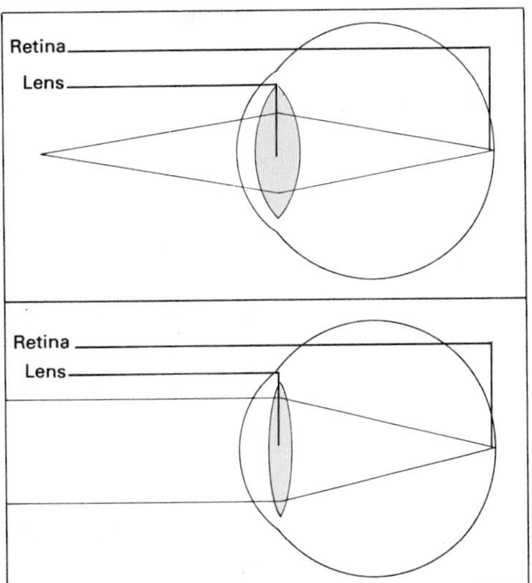

Accommodation is the adjustment made by the lens of the eye that enables one to see objects at various distances.

Acetylsalicylic acid (as ə təl sal ə sil'ik) is the chemical name for the painkilling drug aspirin.

See also ASPIRIN.

Achalasia (ak ə lā'zhə) is a condition in which a nonorganic obstruction of the upper part of the stomach prevents the normal passage of food from the esophagus to the stomach. Difficulty in swallowing results; food may be held in the esophagus and cause it to expand. Vomiting then brings up the food. Pneumonia may follow if food spills into the lungs.

Q: *How is achalasia treated?*

A: The condition is treated with mechanical dilatation of the stomach. Muscle relaxant drugs may be helpful in early cases. Severe cases, however, may require surgery.

Achilles tendon. *See* TENDON.

Achlorhydria (ā klôr hī'drē ə) is the absence of free hydrochloric acid in the gastric juices of the stomach. Hydrochloric acid provides a necessary acidity in the stomach and aids the digestion of proteins. There are rarely any symptoms, and specific treatment for achlorhydria is not necessary.

Achlorhydria may be associated with pernicious anemia and/or with a gastric ulcer. When associated with a gastric ulcer, there is an increased chance of cancer of the stomach.

See also ANEMIA, PERNICIOUS; ULCER, GASTRIC.

Achondroplasia (ā kon drə plā'zhə) is a hereditary, congenital disorder that causes inadequate bone formation in such long bones as the thighbone (femur) and upper armbone (humerus). The disorder is caused by a malfunction in the process that converts cartilage into bone. Achondroplasia can usually be detected at birth.

The condition results in a peculiar form of dwarfism, characterized by short limbs, normal trunk, and a large head. Intelligence is not affected. There is no treatment.

See also DWARFISM.

Acidosis (as ə dō'sis) is a serious condition in which the body's acid-alkali balance is disturbed, and the blood is more acidic than normal. It results from a build-up of carbon dioxide in the blood, often associated with diabetes, a kidney disorder, or starvation. Treatment is determined by addressing the underlying cause of the illness.

Q: *Is acidosis associated with heartburn or indigestion?*

A: No, not in the medical definition of the term. In popular usage, however, some people use acidosis to describe any minor stomach disorder, such as indigestion.

Acne (ak'nē) is a skin disorder that usually affects the face. The neck, shoulders, chest, and back may also be affected. Acne begins under the skin in glands next to the hair follicles. During puberty, these sebaceous glands enlarge and secrete an oily substance—sebum, a lubricant that keeps skin from drying out. If pores near these glands become clogged with dead skin cells or oily cosmetics, the sebum accumulates underneath, causing inflammation in the surrounding skin. The acne is further aggravated when bacteria multiply in the sebum and add to the inflammation and swelling. Repeated infection can cause a more serious condition, and scarring may result.

Q: *Why are young people specifically prone to acne?*

A: The exact cause of the correlation between acne and adolescence is unknown. Contributing factors, however, may include the hormonal changes that normally take place at puberty, as well as emotional stress. Diet and cleanliness are now thought by many physicians to be minor factors.

Q: *What precautions may minimize acne?*

A: Although some physicians recommend the avoidance of foods with a high sugar content and such greasy foods as peanut butter, chocolate, and fried foods, others now feel that dietary restrictions are unwarranted. Most experts agree that greasy or oily cosmetics should be avoided, and the affected areas should be gently cleansed to avoid causing irritation. Acne should not be picked or squeezed; this may lead to severe infection.

Q: *What specific therapies are effective?*

A: Moderate cases of acne may respond to topical use of antibiotics or to small doses of antibiotics administered orally over long periods of time. Other therapies that have been found effective include the topical use of vitamin A acid or benzoyl peroxide.

In 1983 the Food and Drug Administration approved the use of Accutane®, a synthetic chemical related to vitamin A, which is given orally and has been found to be effective in clearing up serious cases of acne.

Q: *Do people other than teenagers suffer from acne?*

A: Adults do not get acne as often as do teenagers. But the condition may affect many women before a menstrual period. Oral contraceptives may help some young women. Simple exposure to sunlight in some cases may also be helpful. Untreated acne often remits spontaneously. To prevent scarring from more serious cases, a physician should be consulted.

Acquired immune deficiency syndrome (AIDS) is a weakening of the body's immune system; it is caused by a virus called HTLV-III (human T-cell lymphotropic virus) or HIV (human immunodeficiency virus). The virus establishes itself inside a T-cell lymphocyte, a major component of the body's immune system. The virus is distinguished from other viruses because of its ability to use the host cell's reproductive system to replicate itself many times; in this way, the AIDS virus eventually destroys the host cell and moves on to infect other T cells. The body is thus left vulnerable to opportunistic infections, which are easily fought off by a normally functioning immune system. The diseases, however, become highly disabling and eventually fatal if the immune system is compromised by AIDS.

The virus may incubate for a period of up to several years, before symptoms start appearing. Initially, the diagnosis is difficult to make. AIDS is characterized by unexplained fever, chills, or night sweats lasting many weeks; a general and persistent feeling of fatigue; an unexplained weight loss over 10 pounds; swollen glands; a dry cough accompanied by a shortness of breath; recurring diarrhea; and pink to purple blotches occurring anywhere on or under the skin, at first resembling bruises, but growing harder than the skin around them and lasting longer than bruises. These symptoms may all be found in other more common illnesses as well.

As the illness progresses, the person with AIDS becomes susceptible to various opportunistic infections. These include pneumonia, shingles, herpes simplex, meningitis, and encephalitis. The most common infection is pneumocystis carinii pneumonia (PCP). Kaposi's sarcoma (KS), a rare tumor, is also common in AIDS victims. Sometimes the onset of one of these infections is the first sign of the presence of AIDS, the patient having never developed any of the warning signs. Eventually the virus can even infect the brain, causing various mental disorders. *See also* KAPOSI'S SARCOMA; PNEUMOCYSTIS CARINII PNEUMONIA.

Q: *How is AIDS passed from person to person?*

A: AIDS is not a casually transmitted disease. It is not passed on via doorknobs, toilet seats, eating utensils, or even by hugging and dry kissing. A person will not get AIDS by sitting in a chair just vacated by a person with AIDS or from breathing the same air or from eating in a restaurant with employees who have AIDS. The skin is an effective barrier against the AIDS virus. As such, quarantine has no role to play in the control of AIDS.

Transmission of the virus occurs almost exclusively by the exchange of certain infected bodily fluids, which are primarily semen and blood, secondarily urine and feces, and possibly also saliva and vaginal secretions. This means unprotected intercourse and the shared use of needles by drug addicts are both conducive to spreading AIDS. The virus is now rarely transmitted via blood transfusions, due to the widespread use by hospitals and blood banks of an AIDS antibody test. Infected mothers can give the disease to their children before or during birth. Finally, it should be noted that low concentrations of the AIDS virus have been found in saliva. Deep, wet kissing may therefore have some risks. However, spitting or salivating on unbroken skin poses no possibility of contagion.

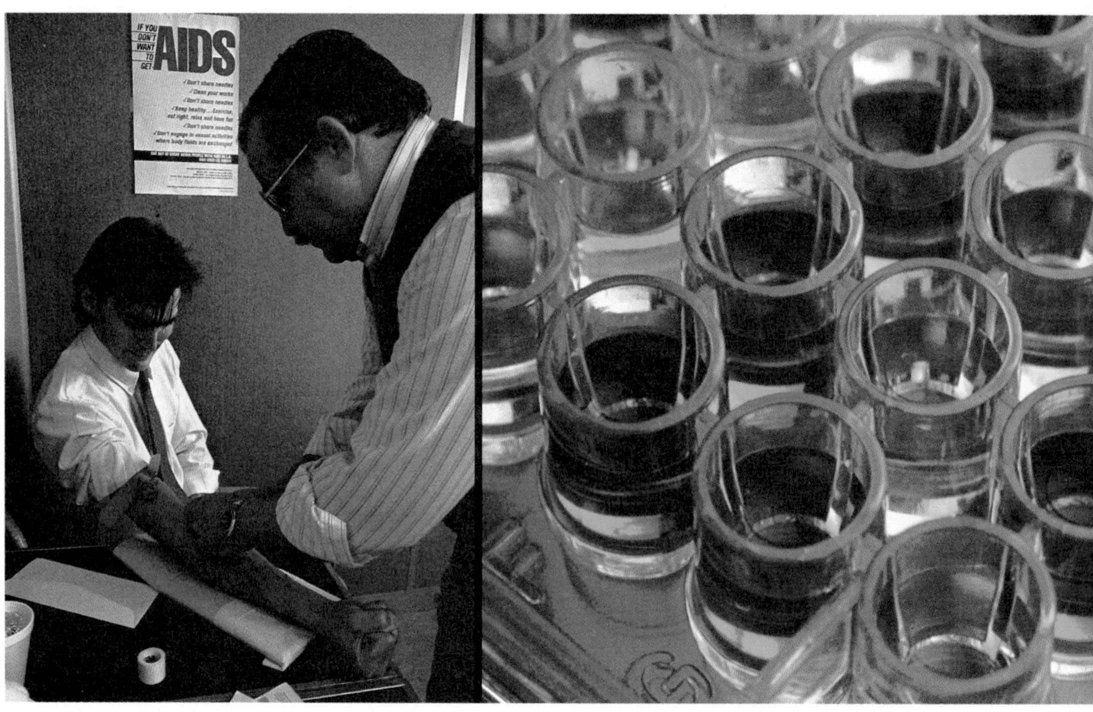

AIDS screening is a procedure used to determine if a person has been exposed to the AIDS virus. Blood is drawn and then tested for the presence of antibodies to the AIDS virus. Antibodies are proteins produced by the body to fight off infection. If a person has been exposed to the AIDS virus, his or her body will produce a particular kind of antibody to fight the virus. If these antibodies are present, the blood serum will turn blue-green, proving that the person has been exposed to the virus. A positive result to the test usually triggers a second and third test to verify the finding.

Q: *How can the spread of AIDS be prevented?*

A: The most obvious prevention is simply abstaining from sex. However, if two people have been in a mutually faithful, monogamous sexual relationship since 1981 and remain so, they need not worry about getting AIDS. Otherwise, preventive knowledge and safe sexual practices are the best alternatives.

A person should be careful never to permit the above-mentioned bodily fluids to enter his or her body. Condoms should be used for all types of intercourse. Hypodermic needles, razors, and toothbrushes should never be shared. Excessive use of alcohol or recreational drugs, which weakens the body's resistance to disease, should also be avoided. The practice of shooting up drugs has always been dangerous; in light of the AIDS crisis, it is much more so.

In the absence of a vaccine and effective treatment, these are the only means of preventing the spread of AIDS.

Q: *Who is at risk for AIDS?*

A: Since 1981, when the first cases of AIDS were diagnosed among homosexual men and intravenous drug users, AIDS has been gradually spreading through other high risk groups and into the general population. Sexual partners and children of both the initial groups are also at high risk. This includes women who have sex with bisexual men.

The risk of contracting AIDS, however, increases for any member of the population who is also a victim of other sexually transmitted diseases, who abuses drugs, who has multiple sex partners, or who has sex with prostitutes. Many infected prostitutes, male and female, are also IV drug users. All these factors compromise the immune system or increase the chances of coming in contact with a person infected with AIDS.

It is repeated exposure to the AIDS virus and compromising one's immune system by the practices noted above, that place an individual at high risk for contracting AIDS.

Q: *What happens to people with AIDS?*

A: After the initial presentation of the illness, patients may have a relatively symptom-free period. Ultimately, they will undergo a repetitive series of opportunistic infections, either with or without associated Kaposi's sarcoma. AIDS itself can directly involve other systems besides the immune system. These include the nervous system, the gastrointestinal tract, and the kidneys. In most cases, patients will die within two to three years, usually from one of the infectious complications.

This unremitting course is often made more tragic by the stigmatization of AIDS patients. Frequently, they may become socially isolated, as they may be avoided by friends and family and prevented from returning to work. In some cases, patients have been ostracized even by hospital personnel. It is to be hoped that this complication of AIDS can be cured by educating the public about the disease.

Q: *Can AIDS be treated?*

A: Approximately half of the people who have developed AIDS are already dead. Very few AIDS victims survive longer than three years. Most experts think that effective therapy will have to include both an antiviral drug and an immune system stimulant. Research into a possible vaccine is also being pursued on several fronts.

Q: *What is the overall impact of an epidemic of such proportions?*

A: AIDS has already had far-reaching effects in areas as diverse as education, sexual mores, substance abuse, health care, medical research, and the economy.

Sex education has in some cases been pushed back to as early as the third grade; instruction has included information on the role of sex in both homosexual and heterosexual relationships, with an emphasis on the prevention of AIDS and other sexually transmitted diseases. Sexual mores and use of drugs and alcohol seem to be undergoing a gradual change, as more people become aware of the role of multiple sex partners and substance abuse in the spread of AIDS.

Hospitals and clinics are learning to share responsibility for the care of AIDS patients with hospices, nursing homes, and other medical facilities. AIDS research may lead to a cure and a vaccine and will surely increase our knowledge in the fields of immunology, virology, and drug therapy.

The costs for all this education, health care, and research have been estimated to reach between 10 and 15 billion dollars annually by 1991. The price tag will have to be met by private insurance companies, government, health care facilities, and the individual.

See also DRUG ABUSE; LYMPHOCYTE; OPPORTUNISTIC INFECTION.

Acrocyanosis (ak rō sī ə nō′sis) is a painless condition in which the fingers and, less commonly, the toes are persistently blue and sweaty. More common among women than men, it is caused either by insufficient blood flow or by low temperatures. The result, in either case, is an extreme sensation of cold for the patient. The treatment is to wear sufficient clothing to keep warm. Smoking may worsen the condition.

Acromegaly (ak rō meg′ə lē) is a disorder in which the bones in the arms and legs get thicker and longer, as do those of the hands, feet, jaw, and skull. Facial features become coarser, and the voice may become deeper. The disorder is caused by an excessive production of growth hormone by the pituitary gland, possibly because of a tumor after puberty. (A related disorder, gigantism, results from overproduction of the growth hormone before puberty.)

In its early stages, acromegaly is almost undetectable. Advanced cases are often accompanied by joint pain, enlarged heart and kidneys, headaches, impairment of vision, and reduced sexual desire.

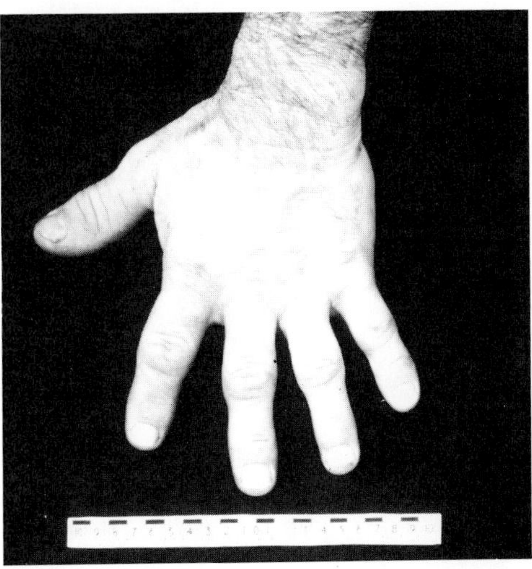

Acromegaly causes the bone structure of the head, hands, and feet to become longer and larger.

Q: *Can any treatment halt the condition?*

A: Skilled medical and surgical care is necessary before too many of the changes become irreversible. X-ray therapy or surgery on the pituitary gland may be recommended.

See also GIGANTISM.

Acrophobia (ak rə fō'bē ə) is an abnormal fear of heights. Occasionally it can be extremely severe and, if a symptom of depression, may require professional treatment.

See also PHOBIA.

ACTH. *See* ADRENOCORTICOTROPIC HORMONE.

Actinomycosis (ak tə nə mī kō'sis) is a long-lasting disease caused by a microorganism *(Actinomyces israelii)* that is normally present in the mouth and throat. Infection occurs most commonly in the jaw or neck, usually following dental trauma, and sometimes in the abdominal membrane or lungs. Hard, very slow-growing swellings form and eventually turn into abscesses. When the abscesses break down, pus is discharged through several openings in the skin. Treatment with penicillin is usually effective.

Acupuncture (ak'yə pungk chər) is an ancient Chinese method of relieving pain and treating disease. The procedure involves the insertion of needles into various parts of the body. Acupuncture has been used to treat conditions such as asthma, deafness, migraines, ulcers, eye diseases, and some types of mental illness.

Acupuncture is a method of relieving pain and treating disease through the insertion of needles into nerve pathways.

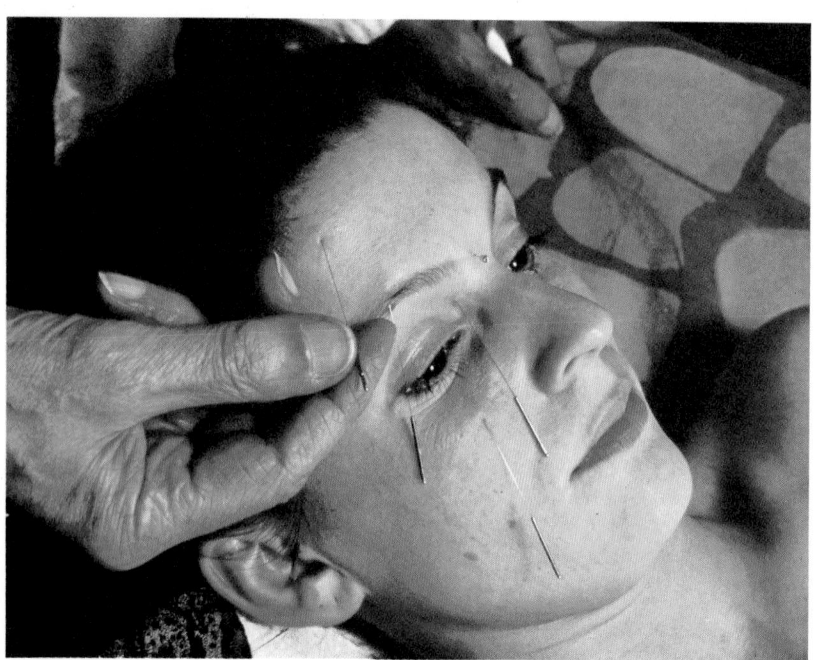

According to Chinese philosophy, disease and pain occur because of an imbalance between two principal forces of nature—Yin and Yang. Acupuncture is thought to restore this balance. Many Chinese and other people believe acupuncture influences a life force that flows along 12 paired and 2 unpaired meridians, channels of energy that run longitudinally in the body. Therapists called acupuncturists insert sharp needles at one or more of hundreds of specific points along the meridian. Insertion of the needles produces a sharp pinching feeling. This feeling quickly disappears and is replaced by an occasional tingling or a sense of numbness, heaviness, or soreness while the needles are in place. The patient is conscious throughout treatment.

Scientists have proposed three major theories of how acupuncture works. One theory suggests that the meridians actually exist and connect the body's organs in a special manner. According to this theory, acupuncture increases activity along the meridians and thus influences organ function. Scientists have also theorized that acupuncture works, at least in part, by increasing the brain's production of natural painkillers called endorphins. These substances are morphine-like chemicals that influence the body's awareness of pain. Scientists also theorize that acupuncture may work through the nervous system by triggering signals that interrupt pain messages sent to the brain. This hypothesis is known as the "gate theory" of pain.

Since the late 1950's, Chinese doctors have performed surgery using acupuncture as a local anesthetic; the patient remains fully conscious during the operation. Acupuncture's practitioners say the anesthetic is effective for complicated operations on the stomach, chest, neck, and head.

Acupuncture is frequently used in the Far East and Southeast Asia. In the United States and other Western countries, it has not yet been totally accepted as a form of medical treatment.

See also ENDORPHIN.

Acute yellow atrophy. See HEPATITIS.

Adam's apple is the cartilaginous structure in the front of the neck. It is part of the voice box (larynx) and is usually larger in men than in women. It grows larger in boys during puberty due to the male sex hormone testosterone. As a result, male vocal cords become longer, and the voice becomes deeper.

See also TESTOSTERONE.

Addiction. *See* ALCOHOLISM; DRUG ADDICTION; SMOKING OF TOBACCO.

Addison's anemia. *See* ANEMIA, PERNICIOUS.

Addison's disease is a rare condition that results from insufficient production by the adrenal gland of several vital hormones. It is caused by a disorder of the adrenal glands themselves or by the failure of the part of the pituitary gland that produces ACTH, the hormone that stimulates the adrenal glands. Addison's disease is most common during middle age. Stopping steroid medications suddenly and without medical supervision can produce a life-threatening Addisonian crisis.

Q: *What are the symptoms of Addison's disease?*

A: Common symptoms may include weakness and dizziness caused by low blood pressure, vomiting, diarrhea, anemia, loss of weight, and a brownish color of the skin and the membranes lining the mouth. It is difficult to diagnose the condition because it is slow to develop and because there may be occasional, temporary improvements in the patient. Tests can reveal the low amount of adrenal hormones in the blood and a disturbance in the balance of salts in the body fluids.

Q: *What is the usual treatment?*

A: Treatment following a correct, early diagnosis can be highly effective. The missing hormones are replaced and recovery is generally speedy.

See also ADRENAL GLAND.

Adenitis (ad ə nī'tis) is an inflammation of a lymph node or gland. Mumps is one example of adenitis.

See also MUMPS.

Adenocarcinoma (ad ə nō kär sə nō'mə) is a cancerous tumor that arises from cells that excrete mucous or other substances. The gastrointestinal tract is the most common site for adenocarcinomas, of which colon cancer is the most prevalent form.

See also CANCER.

Adenoidectomy (ad ə noi dek'tə mē) is an operation for removal of the adenoids.

See also ADENOIDS.

Adenoids (ad'ə noids) are pads of tissue, resembling tonsil tissue, that form a raised surface at the back of the nasal passage. They trap and destroy bacteria that enter the body through the nose, but are not essential for the body's defense against bacteria. They also help the body to build up resistance (immunity) to future infections.

Q: *What can go wrong with the adenoids?*

A: In young children the adenoids are proportionally larger than at any other age. This sometimes causes the nasal passage to become partially blocked, which may result in snoring, breathing through the mouth (because breathing through the nose is difficult), or the build-up of mucus (catarrh or postnasal drip) in the nasal passage. This mucus build-up could cause a runny nose during the day or a cough when the child lies down. The swelling or mucus may also block the tubes that lead from the nasal passage to the middle ears (the eustachian tubes), causing hearing loss. Ear infection may follow.

Q: *What treatment may be prescribed for such conditions?*

A: Antihistamine tablets and nasal drops can reduce congestion, but nasal drops should not be used for more than four days at a time. They may cause irritation and excessive dryness in the nose and make the condition worse. If deafness or infection in the middle ear persists after antibiotic therapy, a physician may recommend surgical

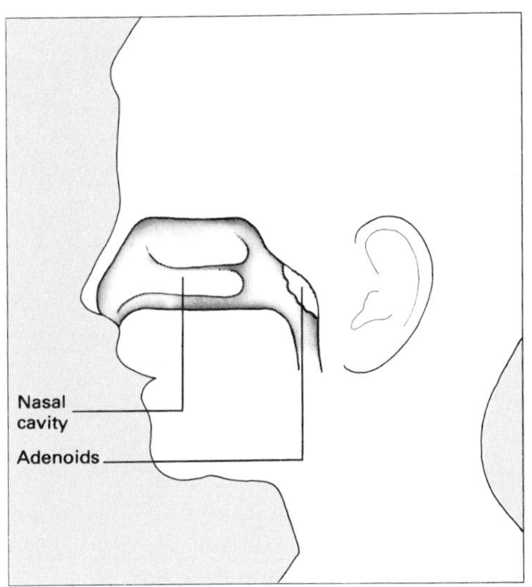

Adenoids, lymphatic tissue at the back of the nasal passage, trap and destroy bacteria that enter the body.

removal of the adenoids (adenoidectomy). The operation is relatively simple.

Q: *Do the adenoids grow again after removal?*

A: Yes, but seldom to the original size.

Adenoma (ad ə nō'mə) is usually a noncancerous (benign) tumor in or resembling glandular tissue. By itself, an adenoma causes no symptoms. Various disorders may result if the adenoma presses on a nearby part of the body.

Adenopathy (ad ə nop'ə thē) is the swelling or enlargement of glands, particularly the lymphatic glands.

See also GLAND; LYMPH NODE.

Adenovirus (ad ə nō vī'rəs) is a group of viruses. Adenovirus infections are frequent and include common colds and various minor feverish respiratory illnesses.

ADH. *See* VASOPRESSIN.

Adhesion (ad hē'zhən) is the growing together of body tissues that are normally separate. Adhesions (protective bands) form in some disorders, following injuries, or following surgery. The sticky healing fluid produced by the damaged internal tissue can solidify to form a band. This band then joins the injured tissue to any body structure or organ with which it comes in contact. Often this is a cavity wall, particularly in the abdomen. Usually this type of adhesion produces no problems. But if the structure so attached is normally free-moving, serious problems may result. The problem may require surgery. Abdominal adhesions of the bowel, for example, can produce pain and obstruction, which may demand surgical correction.

Adolescence (ad ə les'əns) is the period of body growth and mental development that takes place between the onset of puberty and the attainment of physical and emotional maturity. Although girls undergo greater physical change during puberty than do boys, they tend to reach puberty earlier and take less time to reach maturity. Adolescence in young women begins around age 11 and continues through about age 16. In young men, the corresponding period begins about age 13 and continues through about age 18. After about age 14, males are, on the average, heavier and taller than females.

Q: *What physical changes take place during adolescence?*

A: In boys, the genitals increase in size; pubic hair appears, then armpit and facial hair; the voice becomes deeper. In girls, the breasts develop; armpit and pubic hair appears; and menstruation begins.

Q: *What emotional and behavioral changes accompany these physical changes?*

A: Hormonal changes awaken sexual feelings, and many adolescents have some sexual experience. Dating normally begins during mid-adolescence.

Hormonal changes also account for the moodiness for which adolescents are well known. Adolescents who have difficulty adjusting to physical changes may become depressed or apathetic. Alternately, there are times when intense physical energy leads adolescents to unbounded enthusiasm for particular activities or causes.

There may also be a reaction against authority. The individual young person at this time often experiences the desire to express his or her own personality, form a definite character, and experience as many new sensations as possible. Most adolescents welcome the opportunity to take on more responsibility and become more independent. However, they may have difficulty at first in handling the challenge. They may, thus, at one time act independently and at other times want to be more dependent. These natural changes in attitude cause stress for the adolescent. This stress should be recognized by the adolescent and by his or her parents.

Some of the experimentation with activities such as smoking, using drugs, and drinking alcohol that is common among many adolescents, also may represent a form of determined independence, as well as peer pressure. But the desire for new experiences may, in some cases, lead to problems.

Q: *What are important topics to discuss with adolescents?*

A: Children should be told frankly about the upcoming changes in their body. Adolescents need someone to confide in openly and honestly about their relationships with parents and peers. They should also be advised on cigarette smoking, automobile safety, alcohol use, illicit drug use, and sexuality. This information is best supplied by a parent or someone with whom the adolescent has an emotionally stable relationship.

Q: *How can parents help an adolescent child?*

A: Adolescents come under considerable pressure from their own group, which encourages them to conform. The bodily processes leading to physical maturity may also cause discomfort or embarrassment. Parents and others can help by providing understanding, sympathy, advice, and discussion on all the physiological and psychological problems that accompany this time. Late-maturing adolescents, especially boys, tend to have a poorer opinion of themselves than do those who mature early or at an average rate.

See also AGE-BY-AGE CHARTS, APPENDICES.

Adolescent medicine is the branch of medicine that primarily deals with the diagnosis and treatment of diseases of adolescents.

Adolescent suicide is the taking of one's own life when between the ages of 11 and 18. The suicide rate among adolescents has tripled over the last few decades. It is the third leading cause of death for adolescents, second only to accidents and homicides. An increase in the use of alcohol and illicit drugs by this age group is thought to be one reason for the rise.

There are predictors that an adolescent may be considering suicide. If an adolescent: (1) gives away prized possessions; (2) is depressed, in the form of a loss of appetite, weight loss, a change in sleeping habits, or a change in personality; (3) has a low self-esteem; (4) withdraws from regular activities with family and friends; (5) talks about suicide; (6) slips in school performance; professional help should be sought.

See also SUICIDE.

Adrenal gland (ə drē'nəl gland) is one of two small glands that lie one above each kidney. They are also called suprarenal glands. Each is about 2 inches (5cm) in diameter. There are two main sections of the gland: the outer layer, known as the cortex, and the central part, the medulla. The gland acts as a hormone-producing center. The medulla produces epinephrine and norepinephrine. The cortex, stimulated by another hormone (ACTH) from the pituitary gland, supplies the body with three types of hormones: aldosterone; cortisol; and some of the sex hormones, androgen, and progesterone.

Illnesses associated with disorders in the hormone production of the adrenal gland include Addison's disease; Cushing's syndrome; pheochromocytoma.

Adrenaline (ə dren'ə lin), or epinephrine, is a hormone secreted by the central part (medulla) of the adrenal glands. It is the hormone that increases the heartbeat and blood pressure in response to stress or anxiety. The flow of blood to the muscles increases, the skin becomes paler, the pupils of the eyes dilate, and energy-producing glucose is released from the liver. These changes prepare the body for immediate action.

Q: *Is adrenaline used as a drug?*

A: Yes. Natural or chemically produced adrenaline is injected to treat shock, acute allergy attacks, and asthma. It is also used to slow the absorption and thus prolong the effect of local anesthetics, as well as to decrease bleeding during some skin surgeries.

See also ADRENAL GLAND.

Adrenocorticotropic hormone (ə drē nō kôr tə kō trop'ik hôr'mōn), also known as ACTH or corticotropin, is secreted by the pituitary gland at the base of the brain and is responsible for the stimulation of the cortex (outer layer) of the adrenal glands. It causes the adrenal cortex to produce the hormones cortisol, corticosterone, and cortisone. Natural or synthetic preparations of the adrenocorticotropic hormone have been used to treat various disorders, such as asthma, multiple sclerosis, and Bell's palsy. It is also used in a test of adrenal gland function.

Adult is a person who has attained full growth or maturity. Generally speaking, adulthood begins where adolescence and puberty leave off. Full height has been attained, and the development of sex organs is complete.

Humans have been maturing progressively earlier over the years. Among girls in the United States, for example, the onset of menstruation has been occurring approximately three to four months earlier in the last several decades. Many authorities credit the earlier maturation to improvements in living conditions, nutrition, and overall health. In girls, the familiar "growth spurt" usually ends at about age 13.5; in boys, the "growth spurt" ends at about 15.5 years. By the age of 18, growth is almost complete in both sexes, though additional growth is slightly higher in boys.

Full sexual maturity normally does not occur until the late teens or early 20's. Among boys, for example, mature spermatozoa develop between the ages of 14 and 16, but maximum fertility does not take place for several more years. Similarly, a girl can become pregnant and give birth as a teenager, but statistics show that teenage mothers have a high incidence of problem pregnancies.

During adulthood, a person becomes more aware of the inexorable process of aging. Vision and hearing gradually become less acute; organs such as the heart, lungs, and bowels perform less efficiently; and endurance begins to wane. Nevertheless, people are living longer than ever, and many adults remain active and healthy well into their 80's.

See also AGE-BY-AGE CHARTS, APPENDICES.

Adult disorders. See AGE-BY-CHARTS, APPENDICES.

Adult respiratory distress syndrome. See RESPIRATORY DISTRESS SYNDROME, ADULT.

Aerophagia (ār ə fa′jē ə) is the nervous habit of swallowing excessive amounts of air. The habit may be due to poorly fitting dentures or to rapid eating or drinking. This may result in belching and a swelling of the stomach. The habit is unconscious, and it must be made known to a person before the nervous tension causing it can be reduced. The tendency toward aerophagia is reduced when something hard, such as a pipe, is clenched between the teeth.

Aerotitis. See BAROTITIS.

Affective disorder is a pattern of troubled behavior characterized by exaggerated emotional responses and disturbance of mood.

The three common moods of sadness, grief, and elation—when expanded beyond a normal duration, so as to become so entrenched that a normal day's activity is disturbed, or when inappropriate to the stimulus, or when triggered without a stressful life event—become anxiety, depression, and excessive elation. These can grow into clinical disorders if untreated by psychological counseling.

There are two major affective disorders that can expand into chronic melancholia or psychosis. The conditions are either unipolar (depressive only) or bipolar (manic-depressive). Of the two, depression is the more common.

It is estimated that 20 percent of the population suffer from some form of affective disorder during their lifetimes. However, only 15 percent of those affected become chronically ill with a clinical disorder.

Treatment always involves either psychotherapy or drug therapy or a combination of both.

See also ANXIETY; DEPRESSION; ELATION; MANIC-DEPRESSIVE ILLNESS.

Afterbirth is the common name for the placenta and associated membranes that are expelled from the uterus (womb) through the vagina, shortly after childbirth. Expulsion of the afterbirth, the third stage of labor, normally occurs within eight to ten minutes of the delivery of the baby. This is followed by a certain amount of bleeding from the uterus.

See also PREGNANCY AND CHILDBIRTH.

Afterpain may occur following childbirth. The pains are cramp-like contractions of the uterus (womb) as it returns to its normal size; they are more common in second or subsequent births. Pains are normally confined to the first 48 hours after childbirth and may increase during breast feeding. If the womb fails to contract and remains soft, prompt medical attention is needed, as excessive blood loss may occur.

Agammaglobulinemia (ā gam ə glob yə lə nē′mēə), also called hypogammaglobulinemia, is a rare deficiency or virtual absence in the blood of the antibody protein called gamma globulin. When the amount of these proteins is low, the body's natural ability to resist infection is weakened. Treatment is effected by injecting gamma globulin into the bloodstream.

See also GAMMA GLOBULIN.

Age-by-age charts. *See* APPENDICES.

Agent Orange is the American military term for the defoliant sprayed across Southeast Asia during the Vietnam War to destroy crops. The effects of Agent Orange, which contain the highly toxic substance dioxin, are only now being understood. Some veterans have developed cancer or skin conditions as a result of contact with dioxin; others, exposed to this chemical, have had children born with birth defects.

Agglutination (ə glü tə nā′shən) is the clumping together of cells, bacteria, or particles within a fluid. For example, red blood cells clump together if they are mixed with other blood of an incompatible type. This kind of agglutination is used in identifying blood groups.

Agnosia (ag nō′sē ə) is loss of the ability to interpret nerve messages from the senses. It accompanies such brain disorders as brain damage from a stroke or a tumor. The sensory organs themselves, such as those in the nose or ears, continue to function normally, but the brain cannot process the messages properly.

Agoraphobia (ag ər ə fō′be ə) is the irrational fear of leaving the familiar setting of the house. Due to the experience of anxiety attacks in multiple settings, such as stores, church, expressways, and/or open spaces, the individual develops a fear of leaving the house. In its extreme form, the individual may be a virtual prisoner in his or her home environment.

Agoraphobia is diagnosed more often in women than in men. The age of onset is typically the late teens or 20's. Psychiatric intervention usually includes medications to block the anxiety attacks and behavioral therapies to assist the patient in returning to his or her previous life style. This is accomplished by reducing the anticipatory anxiety of leaving the house. A thorough evaluation is necessary to rule out other disorders, for example, depression.

Agranulocytosis (ā gran yə lō sī tō′sis), or granulocytopenia, is an absence of, or deficiency in, white blood cells. It is a serious disorder because the body, lacking white blood cells, can no longer resist infection. The cause of agranulocytosis is not always known, but it most often follows the taking of certain drugs used to treat forms of cancer (such as leukemia). It may also be an early symptom of leukemia itself. The first signs of agranulocytosis may be infected ulcers on the mouth, throat, rectum, or vagina, accompanied by fever. The patient needs isolation in a hospital and may require transfusions of white blood cells.

AIDS. *See* ACQUIRED IMMUNE DEFICIENCY SYNDROME.

Air sickness. *See* MOTION SICKNESS.

Airway is a natural passage in the respiratory tract through which air passes in and out of the lungs during breathing. The principal airways are the windpipe (trachea) and the two main stem bronchi, one going to each lung. The term is also used for an artificial tube used to keep the natural breathing passage open, especially when anesthetics are administered. Such a device is used during surgery on the windpipe (tracheotomy) to correct an obstruction to breathing.

Albino (al bī′nō) is a person whose body tissues lack the coloring matter (pigment) called melanin. Someone who has this relatively rare, congenital condition (albinism) has white hair, milky-white skin, and pinkish irises. Albinism is usually caused by the absence of a specific enzyme resulting from a change in the genes; there is no treatment. Because of the absence of melanin, the skin and eyes of albinos are extra sensitive to the sun's rays. Such individuals are advised to avoid direct sunlight and to wear dark glasses.

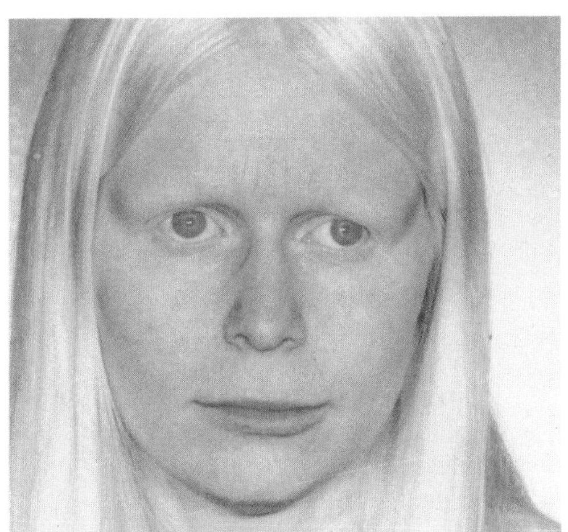

Albino persons lack melanin, the pigment that produces skin color and hair color.

Albumin (al byü'mən) is a simple protein found in almost all animal tissues. Different types of albumin are found in blood, muscle, bone, and other organs and systems. Measurement of the amounts and kinds of albumin in various tissues is part of many diagnostic tests. Albumin in the urine (proteinuria) is usually a symptom of a disorder.

See also PROTEINURIA.

Albuminuria. See PROTEINURIA.

Alcohol (al'kə hôl) is one of a group of liquid organic chemicals of similar structure. Three alcohols only are of medical interest: ethyl alcohol (ethanol), the basic constituent of alcoholic drinks; methyl alcohol (methanol); and isopropyl alcohol (isopropanol). All alcohols are poisonous, but ethyl alcohol is less poisonous than others.

Q: *What are the medical uses of alcohol?*

A: Ethyl alcohol hardens, cleanses, and cools the skin.

Methyl alcohol is used as a cooling lotion to the skin, but it is extremely poisonous when inhaled or drunk and can cause blindness, nerve inflammation (neuritis), and death due to respiratory muscle paralysis.

Isopropyl alcohol is also used as a rubbing alcohol, but it has caused acute intoxication, convulsion, coma, and death in children due to prolonged exposure to vapors during sponging for fevers.

Q: *Are alcoholic beverages dangerous?*

A: Alcoholic drinks are the most commonly abused drug in the U.S. Alcohol is addictive, and its repeated use often results in the need to drink more and more to produce intoxication. Other symptoms of alcohol abuse are impaired coordination and often aggressive actions. Inflammation of the stomach lining (gastritis), vomiting, and "hangover" are almost inevitable. It is also one of the most common causes of hypertension (high blood pressure).

Alcohol acts as a depressant and reduces self-criticism and anxiety. The prolonged use of alcohol can cause damage to nerves (neuritis), the liver (cirrhosis), and the heart muscle (cardiomyopathy). It can also produce mental deterioration (dementia) and increase a tendency toward inflammation of the pancreas (pancreatitis). Chronic gastritis may cause a loss of appetite (anorexia), leading to malnutrition. Alcoholic drinks are high in calories and low in other nutrients. For this reason, heavy drinkers often have a weight problem.

Q: *Is it safe to drink while taking medicines?*

A: No. The effects of alcohol increase the power of drugs contained in, for example, some cough mixtures and sedative drugs, such as sleeping pills, antihistamines, tranquilizers, and muscle relaxants. As a result, one drink may have the effect of several and can cause drowsiness and drunkenness. This is dangerous and can be fatal.

Q: *When should alcohol be avoided?*

A: Alcohol should not be taken by epileptics because it may bring on convulsions. It should be avoided during pregnancy, by diabetics, and by persons with complaints such as gastritis. Consumption of alcohol is illegal for minors.

See also ALCOHOL ABUSE; ALCOHOLISM; CIRRHOSIS.

Alcohol abuse is the improper use of alcohol, a misapplication that can lead to alcoholism. An alcohol abuser is one who drinks beyond sobriety or who mixes alcohol with other chemical substances, but who does not yet have a chemical dependency on alcohol.

The immediate effects of alcohol abuse are the same as those of drunkenness: reduction of motor coordination and decision-making skills, disorientation, sometimes a loss of memory, and physical dehydration. As bouts of drunkenness become habitual and more frequent and when the aftereffects begin interfering with normal living patterns, such as work, family life, etc., then a person is in danger of crossing over from alcohol abuse to alcoholism.

See also ALCOHOLISM.

Alcoholism (al'kə hô liz əm) is a chronic, progressive, and potentially fatal disease. Once it has developed, the victim loses control over his or her drinking habits, and family and social relationships are greatly disrupted. The cause of alcoholism seems to be the interaction between a possible hereditary predisposition, the effects of ethyl alco-

Number and percent of alcohol-related traffic fatalities

Age group of fatality	*Total number of fatalities*	*Percent with driver having .00% blood alcohol concentration*	*Percent with driver with 0.01-0.09% blood alcohol concentration*	*Percent with driver with greater than 0.10% blood alcohol concentration*	*Number of alcohol-related fatalities*
0-14	3,124	76	7	17	745
15-19	6,077	49	15	36	3,115
20-24	7,768	34	13	53	5,140
25-64	20,995	43	9	48	11,985
65 and older	5,555	78	7	15	1,195
Unknown	276	36	11	53	180
Total	43,795	49	10	41	22,360

Source: National Highway Traffic Administration, U.S. Department of Transportation, 1985.

hol (the basic ingredient in alcoholic drinks), and the use of alcohol as a means of coping with life. There are over 10 million Americans who suffer from alcoholism. Approximately 55 million family members and friends are directly affected by these people. Many health professionals now consider alcoholism to be the largest single medical problem in the U.S.

Q: *What are some of the danger signs of alcoholism?*

A: There may be few outward signs during the early stages of alcoholism. The victim may be able to function fairly normally. Some personality changes may be apparent, for example, increasing conflict with family members and an inability to handle stress. Another early symptom is an increase in the amount of alcohol a person needs to drink in order to get the same effect a lesser amount produced in the past. The alcoholic may also experience lapses in memory ("blackouts") and a feeling that a drinking pattern is getting out of control. In the final stages of alcoholism, the victim, while rarely deriving pleasure from alcohol, is unable to go for very long without a drink. One of the prime symptoms of alcoholism, and the symptom that makes the disease so hard to treat, is denial. The alcoholic is unlikely to admit, either to himself or herself or to others, that a problem with alcohol exists. The chronic drinker will probably attribute alcohol-related problems to some other cause. Family members and friends may also deny the problem by looking the other way when destructive behavior is exhibited. This denial can lead to a worsening physical and mental condition. For indicators that might suggest a tendency toward alcoholism refer to the Michigan Alcoholism Screening Test, page 24.

Q: *What are some of the problems associated with alcoholism?*

A: Alcoholism is physically destructive, giving rise to many other forms of disease, for example, cancer of the liver, esophagus, colon, stomach, and breast. Chronic alcohol abuse can also lead to hypertension, stroke, heart attack, and brain damage. Pancreas and kidney disease, along with a host of other physical disorders—hepatitis, cirrhosis, esophageal bleeding, blood disorders—may also result from alcoholism.

Alcoholism can also trigger a host of personal problems. Alcoholics may become less productive at work and may eventually lose their jobs. Marriages may not endure the strain, and children may suffer emotionally and sometimes physically from a parent who is an alcoholic. An alcoholic abuser may feel a general sense of loss of control over his or her life.

Q: *What about alcoholism treatment programs?*

A: In the past, one of the barriers to

successful treatment of alcoholics was the social stigma attached to the disease. People were not only reluctant to admit they had an alcohol problem, they were even less likely to risk social embarrassment by seeking help. In recent years the social stigma has greatly relaxed due in large part to the realization by many Americans that alcoholism is a disease like any other, afflicting millions of people of all ages and all walks of life.

Today, many new and innovative treatment techniques are being used to counteract alcoholism. Some alcoholics may benefit from outpatient or inpatient treatment programs. Occasionally, alcoholics may benefit from pharmacological intervention to treat depression or help maintain sobriety. Medical supervision is usually advisable to treat coincidental medical problems. Advancements in biochemistry are being applied to treat patients through nutritional therapy. This means that vitamins can be used to repair the liver and other damaged body parts. Experimental research is underway to try and diagnose early stage alcoholism, and work is being done to unlock the key to hereditary predisposition to alcoholism.

Alcoholics Anonymous (A.A.), which is now over 50 years old, has been instrumental in providing the long-term, therapeutic treatment recognized as vital in rehabilitating alcoholics. A.A. is an international fellowship of alcoholics and recovered alcoholics that meets regularly to provide support to members and to share experiences with alcohol. A.A. facilities are listed in local telephone directories, as are numerous self-help support groups that have been set up to help family members of alcoholics, for example, Alanon.

Educational programs are seen by many as crucial to any satisfactory solution to the problem of alcoholism. Many schools and community organizations have set up programs to alert people (especially young people) to the dangers of alcohol. Legal remedies, like the raising of the drinking age to 21 and the increased enforcement of drunk-driving laws, have also been undertaken in an attempt to limit access to alcohol.

Michigan alcoholism screening test

(Including point values per various responses)	Yes	No
1. Do you enjoy a drink now and then?	(0)	(0)
2. Do you feel you are a normal drinker? (By normal we mean you drink less than or as much as most other people).	( )	(2)
3. Have you ever awakened the morning after some drinking the night before and found that you could not remember a part of the evening?	(2)	( )
4. Does your wife, husband, a parent, or other near relative ever worry or complain about your drinking?	(1)	( )
5. Can you stop drinking without a struggle after one or two drinks?	( )	(2)
6. Do you ever feel guilty about your drinking?	(1)	( )
7. Do friends or relatives think you are a normal drinker?	( )	(2)
8. Are you able to stop drinking when you want to?	( )	(2)
9. Have you ever attended a meeting of Alcoholics Anonymous (AA) for yourself?	(5)	( )
10. Have you gotten into physical fights when drinking?	(1)	( )
11. Has your drinking ever created problems between you and your wife, husband, a parent, or other relative?	(2)	( )
12. Has your wife or husband (or other family members) ever gone to anyone for help about your drinking?	(2)	( )
13. Have you ever lost friends because of your drinking?	(2)	( )
14. Have you ever gotten into trouble at work or school because of drinking?	(2)	( )
15. Have you ever lost a job because of drinking?	(2)	( )
16. Have you ever neglected your obligations, your family, or your work for two or more days in a row because you were drinking?	(2)	( )

17.	Do you drink before noon fairly often?	(1)	( )
18.	Have you ever been told you have liver trouble? Cirrhosis?	(2)	( )
**19.	After heavy drinking have you ever had delirium tremens (D.T.'s) or severe shaking, or heard voices or seen things that really weren't there?	(2)	( )
20.	Have you ever gone to anyone for help about your drinking?	(5)	( )
21.	Have you ever been in a hospital because of drinking?	(5)	( )
22.	Have you ever been a patient in a psychiatric hospital or on a psychiatric ward of a general hospital where drinking was a part of the problem that resulted in hospitalization?	(2)	( )
23.	Have you ever been at a psychiatric or mental health clinic or gone to any doctor, social worker, or clergyman for help with any emotional problem, where drinking was part of the problem?	(2)	( )
***24.	Have you been arrested for drunk driving, driving while intoxicated or driving under the influence of alcoholic beverages? (If YES, how many times? ________.)	( )	( )
***25.	Have you ever been arrested or taken into custody, even for a few hours, because of other drunk behavior? (If YES, how many times? ________.)	( )	( )

**5 points for delirium tremens
***2 points for *each* arrest
Scoring System: In general, five points or more would place the subject in an "alcoholic" category. Four points would be suggestive of alcoholism, three points or less would indicate the subject was not alcoholic.

Programs using the above scoring system find it very sensitive at the five point level, and it tends to find more people alcoholic than anticipated. However, it is a screening test and should be sensitive at lower levels.

Selzer, M.L., The Michigan Alcoholism Screening Test (MAST): The quest for a new diagnostic instrument. *American Journal of Psychiatry,* Volume 127, p. 1653, 1971. Copyright © 1971. Reprinted by permission.

Aldosterone (al dos'tə rōn) is a hormone released into the bloodstream by the adrenal glands. It helps control the balance of salts in the body. Excessive production causes hypertension (high blood pressure) due to retention of salt (Conn's syndrome).

See also ADDISON'S DISEASE; ADRENAL GLAND.

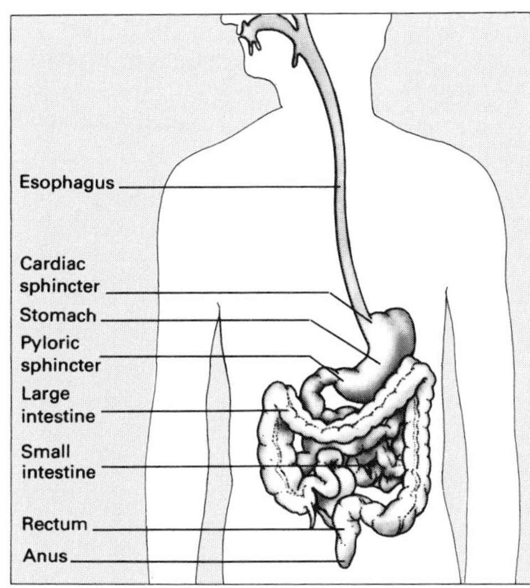

The **alimentary canal,** or the digestive tract, extends from the mouth to the anus.

Alimentary canal (al ə men'tər ē) is the digestive tract, running from the mouth to the anus. It includes the mouth, pharynx (throat), esophagus (gullet), stomach, small intestine, large intestine (colon), and rectum.

Alkali (al'kə lī) is a type of substance that neutralizes an acid. Most medicines used to relieve heartburn and indigestion contain some amounts of alkalis.

For information on alkali burns, *see* POISONING: FIRST AID.

Alkaloid (al'kə loid) is any one of a group of biologically active substances that contain nitrogen. Alkaloids are found in many plants and include such drugs as digitalis (from foxglove), atropine (from belladonna), morphine (from the opium poppy), and caffeine (from coffee and tea). Most alkaloids have a bitter taste and may be highly poisonous if used incorrectly.

Allergic rhinitis. *See* HAY FEVER.

Allergy (al'ər jē) is a condition in which the body reacts with unusual sensitivity to a certain substance or substances. These substances, which are usually proteins, are called antigens. They stimulate the body to produce antibodies, which weaken or destroy the invading antigens. In some cases, when

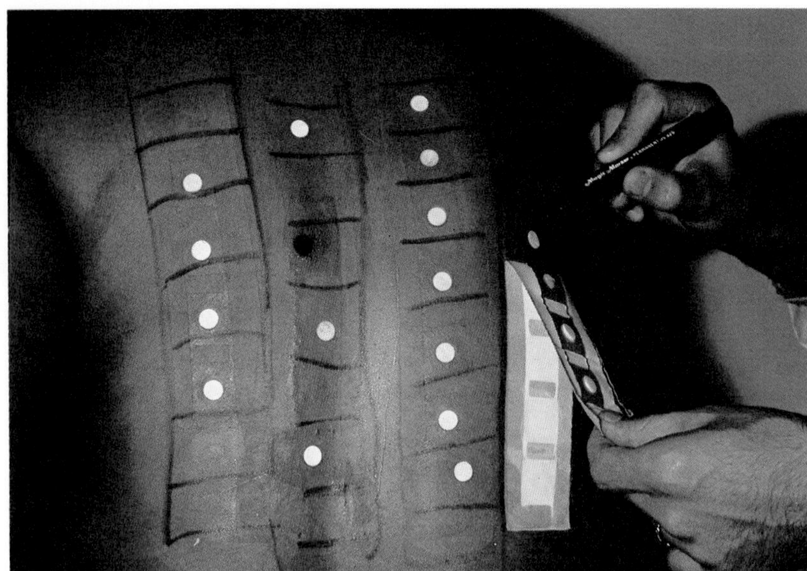

Allergy tests can be done by taping suspected allergens to the surface of the skin and noting reactions.

an antibody reacts with an antigen, the organic compound histamine is released from special body cells called mast cells. It is an excess of histamine that results in allergy symptoms.

Q: *What are the common allergy symptoms?*

A: A runny nose and watering or itching eyes are common to many persons who suffer each year from hay fever. In asthma, there is wheezing; with eczema and hives there is itching, redness, and lumps. An inflammation of the skin (contact dermatitis) may occur from wearing rubber gloves or touching a certain chemical, such as some kinds of soap. A reaction to antibiotics, particularly penicillin, may take the form of a rash. *See also* HAY FEVER.

Q: *Why are some people allergic to certain substances and others not?*

A: This is due partly to hereditary factors; some families seem to be more susceptible to allergies than others, although particular allergies are not necessarily inherited. Emotional disturbances can also set off allergic conditions, and many physicians believe that an emotional factor may be the main factor that triggers an asthma attack.

Q: *How does a physician determine the cause of an allergy?*

A: The physician usually gets a detailed history from the patient to find the most likely source of the problem and may then carry out a skin test. A weak solution of the substances that are suspected is injected into the skin. A red reaction indicates an allergy to that particular substance. Sometimes a patch test is done for the same reason.

Q: *What treatment can be given for an allergic reaction?*

A: If the cause of the allergic reaction is not known, a physician may prescribe antihistamine pills or corticosteroid nasal and lung sprays to control the symptoms. Various medications, including theophylline, are used to treat asthma. *See also* ASTHMA.

When the cause of an allergy is known, the patient can undergo desensitization with injections of the allergen known to cause the symptoms. Beginning with a weak solution, the dose is gradually increased over a period of weeks until a strong solution is reached and the patient is possibly immune to its effects. This process is not always successful; it is considered by some to be potentially dangerous.

Q: *Are there any dangerous allergic reactions?*

A: An allergic reaction to an insect sting or antibiotic drug, such as penicillin, is potentially dangerous and can even be fatal. A mild reaction usually causes a rash. In a violent reaction, which is called anaphylactic shock, the patient finds breathing increasingly difficult. This is an emergency condition, and a physician should be consulted immediately. Fortunately, the condition is rare.

See also HISTAMINE; PATCH TEST; RASH; SHOCK, ANAPHYLACTIC.

Alopecia (al ə pē′shē ə) is the medical term for baldness. Common male pattern alopecia occurs naturally in many men as they grow older. A tendency to go bald is inherited and usually begins at the temples or the crown of the head. In rare cases, baldness is due to an abnormal reaction to the hair substance itself. This could result in a total loss of hair. Alopecia is also a temporary side effect of many cancer chemotherapy drugs. *See also* BALDNESS.

Minoxidil, a recently developed drug, is proving effective as one mode of treating male pattern baldness in certain individuals.

Altitude sickness is the condition that some people experience after ascending rapidly to heights of more than about 6,500 feet (2,000m). Others do not suffer until they reach an altitude of more than 10,000 feet (3,000m). The condition occurs because air at such altitudes contains less oxygen than at lower altitudes. Individual susceptibility varies greatly; it is most severe in the elderly and those with heart or respiratory problems.

Q: *What are the symptoms of altitude sickness?*

A: The symptoms include severe headache, shortness of breath, rapid heartbeat, dizziness, and nausea with diarrhea. Because not enough oxygen reaches the brain, the patient experiences mental confusion and suffers from poor coordination and insomnia. No one with heart or lung disease should consider trips to high altitudes without first consulting a physician.

Q: *What are the remedies for altitude sickness?*

A: In time the body gradually adjusts to the lower oxygen concentration. Physical exertion should be avoided. For severe symptoms, breathing a mixture of pure oxygen and air offers relief.

Alveolus (al vē'ə ləs) is a small sac-like body cavity. The term is usually used to describe the millions of microscopic air sacs (alveoli) of the lung tissue.

See also RESPIRATORY SYSTEM.

Alzheimer's disease (ôlts'hī mərz) is a condition affecting the brain, resulting in a rapid and severe deterioration of mental capacities. It was first recorded in the early part of the 20th century by a German scientist, Dr. Alois Alzheimer. He noted its presence in the autopsy of a middle-aged patient suffering from an acute form of dementia (mental degeneration). Because Alzheimer's disease has often struck both men and women in the 40 to 60 age bracket, it has sometimes been referred to as presenile dementia, a forerunner of senility, detected occasionally in the elderly. This term, however, may be a misnomer, since doctors are now finding that Alzheimer's afflicts older individuals as frequently as it does middle-aged ones. Some research indicates that Alzheimer's may be hereditary, which would help explain its occurrence in the middle-aged as well as in the elderly. *See also* DEMENTIA; SENILITY.

Q: *What are the signs and symptoms associated with Alzheimer's disease?*

A: Doctors have discovered that the nerve cells in the brains of Alzheimer's patients show certain distinct abnormalities. They have cited, for example, the existence of a tangle of nerve fibers, not observed in the brains of normal, healthy adults. They have also located a structure called the neuritic plaque, which is made up of deteriorating nerve endings.

In the early stages of Alzheimer's disease, a person's social skills are well-preserved; there may only be occasional and subtle impairments in memory, calculation, speech, or judgement. It is often difficult to determine a time of onset for the disease. Only after several years do most people with Alzheimer's begin to suffer from severe memory loss. At the later stages, they can no longer recall important events in their lives or recognize such significant people as spouses, children, and siblings. They frequently experience utter confusion and are unable to speak clearly or move with ease. Many patients exhibit a form of paranoia, having fears of things that do not exist. Some are incontinent. *See also* INCONTINENCE.

Q: *What is the precise cause of Alzheimer's disease?*

A: Researchers have not been able to discover the cause. Some feel that Alzheimer's may be related to a chemical deficiency. Others speculate that the source may be a virus. Still, some research has hinted at an excessive accumulation of aluminum in the brain as the cause. Recent research has also indicated the presence of an abnormal protein in Alzheimer's patients, A-68, that is absent in non-Alzheimer's patients. Development of a simple laboratory test could mean better diagnosis, the correction of misdiagnosed Alzheimer's patients, and better treatment at an earlier stage of the disease. A definitive explanation as to the cause of the disease has not yet been reached.

Q: *What is the treatment for Alzheimer's disease?*

A: There is, unfortunately, no effective treatment for preventing or stopping the ravages of the disease. Numerous medications are in the experimental stages and show some promise. The best therapy at present is to keep the patient in his or her most familiar surroundings. The more active the person, the slower the progression of the disease. Studies suggest that a good diet may also help to slow the progression of the illness. Still, most Alzheimer's patients are eventually hospitalized or placed in nursing homes, since family members find it increasingly difficult to provide the constant, around-the-clock care and attention needed. Recently, support groups have been started around the country to help relatives of Alzheimer's victims cope with their own feelings and make adjustments in their lives.

Amalgam (ə mal'gəm) is an alloy of mercury and one or more other metals. Dentists use an amalgam to fill a cavity in a tooth.

Amaurosis (am ô rō'sis) is the medical term for the type of blindness in which the eye itself is undamaged. It is usually caused by a disorder of the optic nerve, spine, or brain; the condition may also result from a disturbance in the circulation of the eye, as in diabetes, or from kidney disorder.

See also AMBLYOPIA; BLINDNESS.

Amblyomma (am blē om'ə) is a family of ticks that infests dogs, cattle, and sheep in the southeastern United States, the tropics of Central and South America, and some parts of Africa. One species, *Amblyomma americanum*, is capable of transmitting Rocky Mountain spotted fever.

See also ROCKY MOUNTAIN SPOTTED FEVER.

Amblyopia (am blē ō'pē ə) is a loss of visual acuity, although the affected eye appears to be normal. The condition results from a variety of causes that generally affect both eyes: alcohol; tobacco; lead poisoning, as well as other poisoning; a deficiency of the B-complex vitamins; and strabismus (lazy eye or crossed eyes).

When amblyopia is due to strabismus, the condition is usually corrected by wearing a patch over the stronger eye, thus strengthening the weaker one.

If the condition is triggered by toxins (toxic amblyopia), treatment involves the removal of the toxin or such specific treatment as chelation in lead poisoning.

If the condition is not corrected, the weak eye can become blind. A physician should always be consulted for such problems.

See also STRABISMUS.

Ameba (ə mē'bə), also spelled amoeba, is a single-celled protozoan, consisting of a shapeless mass of protoplasm enclosed by a flexible membrane and containing one or more nuclei. Under a microscope it appears as a shapeless bit of jelly with one or more dark spots (the nuclei) inside it. The ameba is constantly changing shape by forming temporary extensions of itself called pseudopodia, or false feet, by which it can move or take in food. It reproduces by simply dividing itself in half to form two amebas. Certain forms of a parasitic ameba, entamoeba, exist in the human digestive tract. Some are beneficial, while others may cause amebic dysentery or tropical liver abscess.

See also PROTOZOA.

Amebiasis (am ə bī'ə sis) is an infection of the intestine or liver caused by *Entamoeba histolytica*. It may be transmitted through food or water contaminated with infected feces. Mild amebiasis may have no symptoms, but severe cases may cause sharp abdominal pains, profuse diarrhea, and weight loss. It is most serious in young children and the elderly.

See also AMEBA.

Amebic dysentery. *See* DYSENTERY, AMEBIC.

Amelia (ə mē'lya) is the congenital absence of one or more limbs. Complete amelia refers to the congenital absence of both arms and both legs.

Amelogenesis (am ə lō jen'ə sis) is the formation and development of teeth enamel.

Amenorrhea (ā men ə rē'ə) is the absence or abnormal stoppage of menstruation. Pregnancy is the most common reason for periods to stop. But emotional stress or depression can cause amenorrhea, as can sudden weight loss or the intense physical training of an athlete. There are also other physical causes, including endocrine disorders and diseases that affect the ovaries or uterus. Certain medications can also cause amenorrhea.

With any unexplained stoppage in the menstrual cycle, a physician should be consulted.

See also ANOREXIA NERVOSA; MENSTRUATION.

Ametropia (am ə trō′pē ə) is the condition characterized by an optical defect that prevents images from being properly focused on the retina. The most common refractive error is hyperopia (farsightedness). Nearsightedness (myopia) is also an example of ametropia.

See also HYPEROPIA; MYOPIA.

Amino acid (ə mē′nō) is one of the basic nitrogen-containing substances that go into the making of proteins in living matter. There are more than 20 amino acids required for normal good health, but the human body is not able to make the 8 essential ones. These are taken into the body in proteins from foods, such as milk, meat, fish, eggs, and cheese.

See also PROTEIN.

Amnesia (am nē′zhə) is the complete or partial loss of memory. General (complete) amnesia may be caused by a defect, disease, or injury to the head. It can also be caused by hysteria following a traumatic event. If the cause is emotional, the forgotten memory can be recalled when the sufferer is feeling secure. Professional help may be sought.

Partial amnesia may be caused by certain disorders, for example, alcoholism or a thyroid deficiency. The memory is more likely to forget recent events than those from the past. The term partial amnesia is not used when referring to the random forgetfulness due to Alzheimer's disease or aging.

See also HYSTERIA.

Amniocentesis (am nē ō sen tē′sis) is a procedure recommended for some pregnant women in which a small amount of amniotic fluid is removed for analysis. It is usually performed between the fifteenth and eighteenth week of pregnancy to diagnose specific chromosomal abnormalities or metabolic disorders which can be inherited.

Amniocentesis has been helpful in the diagnosis of Down Syndrome and Tay-Sachs disease. It may also be recommended later in pregnancy to assess fetal lung maturity. The procedure includes both ultrasound scanning, to determine the location of the fetus, and the insertion of a needle attached to a syringe into a part of the uterus. The fluid is then tested for specific defects.

Complications and failures are rare, but amniocentesis is not without hazards. Premature labor or trauma to the fetus or umbilical cord can occur.

See also CHORIONIC VILLUS BIOPSY; HEMOLYTIC DISEASE OF THE NEWBORN; RH FACTOR.

Amnion (am′nē ən) is the membrane lining the womb in which a fetus floats during pregnancy. It is made up of a tough layer of cells.

Amoeba. *See* AMEBA.

Amphetamine (am fet′ə mēn) is a drug that stimulates the central nervous system. It causes a rise in blood pressure, a racing pulse, wakefulness, euphoria, and a loss of appetite. Amphetamines are prescribed by physicians in the treatment of intermittent or cyclic drowsiness (narcolepsy) and excessive muscular and physical activity in children (hyperactivity).

The stimulative effects of amphetamines have led to abuse and addiction. Abuse can lead to compulsive behavior and paranoia. Physicians now prescribe amphetamines with great caution, and supplies are regulated through federal and state laws. Amphetamines have several "street names" including *pep pills* and *speed.*

See also DRUG ABUSE.

Ampicillin (am pə sil′in) is a semisynthetic antibiotic drug that is used to treat infections of the urinary tract, the respiratory tract, and gastrointestinal tract. It can also be used to treat enteric fevers, gonorrhea, and infections in the ear, nose, and throat.

Ampicillin may cause diarrhea, nausea, and vomiting. Allergic reactions may also occur; a person allergic to penicillin will probably also be allergic to ampicillin. If a skin rash develops, a patient should consult a physician immediately. Also, patients suffering from infectious mononucleosis (a viral glandular fever) often show a specific rash with ampicillin use. Rarely, allergic reactions occur in the blood and liver, but these stop when ampicillin therapy is discontinued. There is a possibility that ampicillin may reduce the effectiveness of oral contraceptives.

Ampule (am'pyül) is a small, sealed, glass or plastic container that is used to keep doses of medication sterile.

Amputation (am pyə tā'shən) is the surgical removal of a limb or other part of the body. The reasons for amputation are either damage or disease. When damage is so serious that repair or healing is impossible, amputation may be a physician's only choice.

Q: *What problems face a patient after the amputation of a limb?*

A: Emotional stress is a serious problem after an amputation. Also, a patient may experience sensations as if the limb were still there. This can cause confusion and distress and may persist for several months. A good rehabilitation program therefore includes both physical and psychotherapeutic treatment.

Q: *What about artificial limbs?*

A: When performing an amputation, a surgeon normally tries to leave a stump of bone onto which an artificial limb can be attached. Such a limb can be controlled by brain impulses that remain even after amputation.

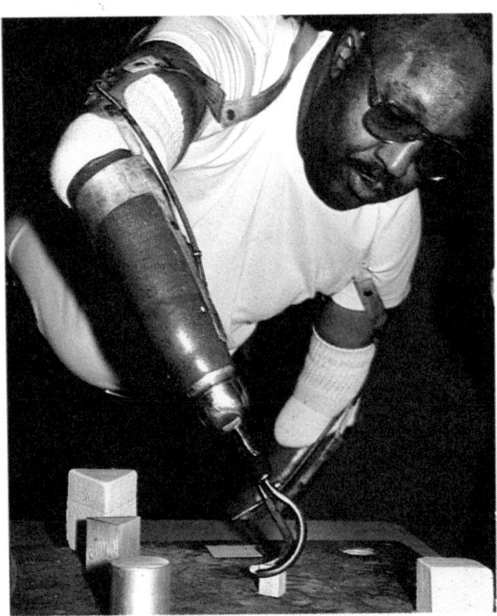

Amputation: the effects of losing a limb can be minimized by the use of an artificial limb, also called a prosthesis.

Amputation, accidental: first aid. Accidental amputation is the severance of a limb or part of a limb due to sudden trauma. It occurs most commonly as a result of an automobile accident or as a result of a limb being trapped in moving machinery. The main danger of an accidental amputation is that the victim may bleed to death.

Treatment. Summon emergency medical aid. Lay the victim down and support the stump in a raised position. (*See* illustrations, page 31.) Try to stop the bleeding by applying direct pressure over the end of the damaged limb. Cover the stump with a thick bandage or a clean towel. Apply continuous pressure over the bandage until the bleeding has stopped. If pressure alone does not stop the bleeding and another person is available, one person should continue to apply pressure over the stump while the other person tries to control the bleeding by pressing over an artery at a pressure point. Release the pressure every 20 minutes for a period of 30 seconds. If bleeding persists apply more padding and maintain the pressure. Do not remove the original bandage.

If possible, the severed limb should be kept, as it may be possible for a surgeon to reattach it. Place the severed limb in a clean, plastic bag and pack ice around the exterior of the bag.

Amyloid (am'ə loid) is an abnormal and complex protein material, of which the exact biochemical structure has not been discovered. Amyloid resembles starch and may accumulate in tissues and organs. This condition is called Amyloidosis.

See also AMYLOIDOSIS.

Amyloidosis (am ə loi dō'sis) is a disorder marked by deposits of a waxy, clear substance (amyloid) in the tissues of the liver, spleen, kidneys, heart, or tongue. The deposits may be associated with chronic infections, inflammations, or some forms of cancer. The cause, however, is often unknown. Amyloidosis interferes with the normal functioning of the organ in which it is present. There is no known cure for the condition, and death results if its presence is not discovered. The only treatment is aimed at curing the diseased organ.

Amyotrophic lateral sclerosis (ə mī ə trof'ik lat'ər əl skli rō'sis) is a motor neuron disease characterized by progressive degeneration of the cerebral cortex and spinal column. Symptoms of the disease include muscular weak-

Accidental amputation: first aid

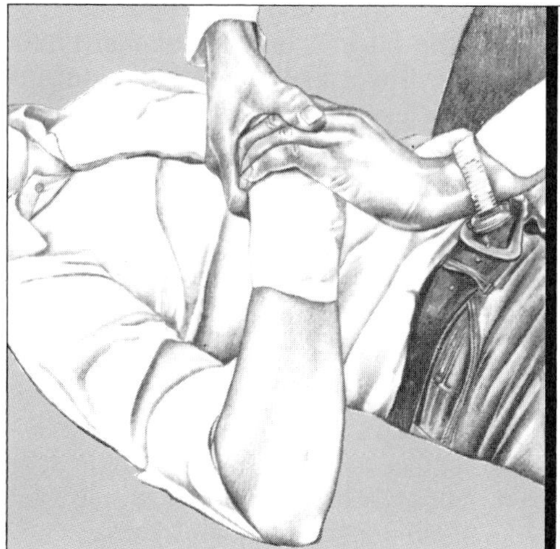

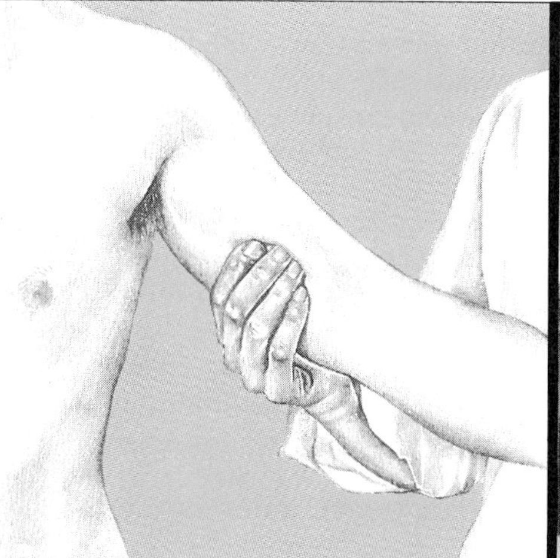

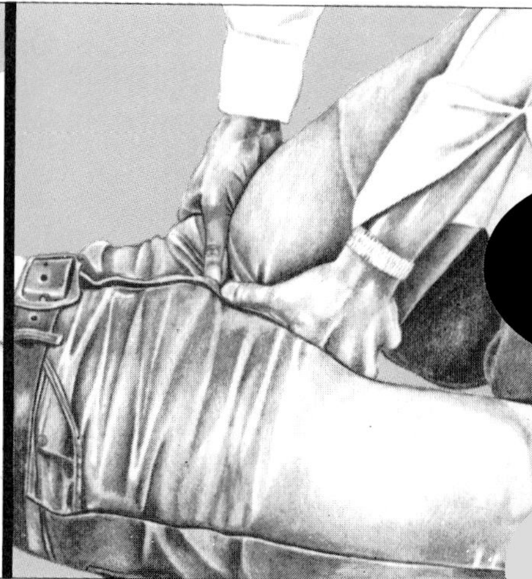

1 Lay the victim down and support the stump in a raised position. Cover the stump with a thick bandage or a clean towel. Apply continuous pressure over the bandage until the bleeding stops. If pressure alone does not stop the bleeding, try to control bleeding by pressing over an artery at a pressure point.

2 The brachial artery—*pressure point for arms*—runs along the inner side of each upper arm. The course of the artery is approximately indicated by the inner seam of a coat sleeve. To apply pressure to the brachial pressure point, put your fingers on the inner side of the victim's upper arm above the artery and press against the underlying bone. *Every 20 minutes, release the pressure over a pressure point for 30 seconds.*

3 The femoral artery—*pressure point for legs*—passes into each leg at a point that corresponds to the center of the fold of the groin. To apply pressure, grasp the victim's thigh with both hands and press directly downward in the center of the groin. Use both thumbs, one on top of the other, and press firmly against the edge of the pelvis. *Every 20 minutes, release the pressure over a pressure point for 30 seconds.*

ness and spasm. An increase in tendon reflexes and spasticity may precede atrophy in the hands, forearms, and legs. The onset of amyotrophic lateral sclerosis generally begins in middle age and progresses rapidly. Death usually occurs within two to five years. The incidence of the disease is greater among males. There is no known cure. Amyotrophic lateral sclerosis is often abbreviated to ALS and is also referred to as Lou Gehrig's disease.

Anabolic steroid. *See* STEROID, ANABOLIC.

Anabolism (ə nab′ə liz əm) is the constructive metabolic process by which simple substances are converted into the more complex compounds of living matter. This requires energy.

Anagen (an′ə jən) is the phase of the hair cycle during which growth takes place.

Anal fissure (ā′nəl fish′ər) is a linear tear in the skin on the edge of the anus. It may be caused by diarrhea, the passing of large bowel movements, or childbirth trauma. It may also be a side effect of medical treatment. Chronic fissures may show an external skin growth at their upper ends. Fissures are common in newborns and children with constipation.

Normally the application of a local anesthetic ointment and the use of stool softeners are sufficient treatment. Occasionally in chronic cases, surgery may be required and is usually curative.

Analgesic (an əl jē′zik) is a type of drug that alleviates pain without loss of consciousness. Analgesics work by reducing the patient's ability to perceive pain. The oldest of the common analgesic drugs is aspirin. A more recent aspirin substitute is acetaminophen (best known under the trade name Tylenol®), which is less irritating to the stomach.

Q: *Are aspirin and acetaminophen regarded as safe drugs?*

A: The two drugs are safe enough to be readily available without prescription. But physicians advise against excessive or prolonged use of these or any other nonprescription analgesics without prior medical consultation.

Q: *What types of pain need stronger analgesics?*

A: With acute or persistent pain, a physician's advice may well be essential. Physicians prescribe strong analgesics with caution, and dosages are carefully regulated because some analgesics can be addictive.

See also ACETAMINOPHEN; ASPIRIN.

Analysis (ə nal′ə sis) is an informal term for psychoanalysis.

See also PSYCHOANALYSIS.

Anaphylactic shock. See SHOCK, ANAPHYLACTIC.

Anasarca (an ə sär′kə) is a generalized swelling (edema) of the body, especially in the legs and abdomen. It results from the accumulation of fluid in body tissues, often accompanying a kidney disorder. The condition was once known as dropsy.

Anastomosis (ə nas tə mō′sis) is the surgical connecting of two tubes in the body. For example, an anastomosis may be created when open ends of the intestine are joined together after the removal of a diseased section between them.

Anatomy (ə nat′ə mē) is the study, classification, and description of the organs and structure of animals and plants. The study is usually based upon dissection and microscopic observation. Human anatomy includes the study of the various components of the human body.

Androgen (an′drə jən) is a substance, usually a hormone, that increases male sex characteristics. Testosterone, the sex hormone produced by the testicles, is an androgen.

See also TESTOSTERONE.

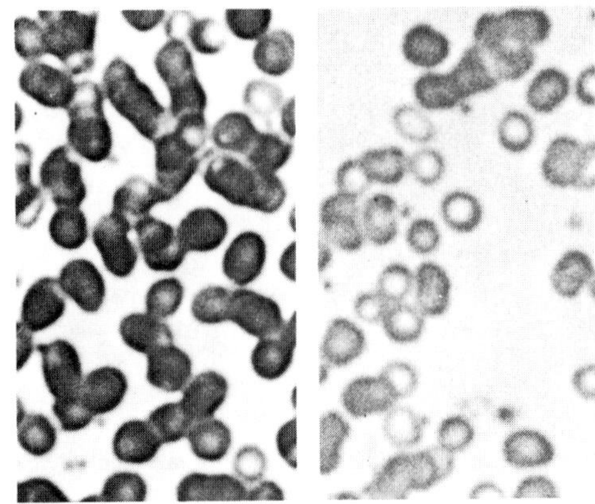

Anemia is a condition in which the blood has fewer red blood cells, *right,* than normal, *left.* Anemia can also be caused by a deficiency of hemoglobin in red blood cells.

Anemia (ə nē′mē ə) is any one of the disorders in which the blood has fewer than the normal number of red blood cells or the red blood cells are deficient in hemoglobin-carrying capacity. Hemoglobin carries oxygen to the tissues. *See also* BLOOD CELL, RED; HEMOGLOBIN.

Q: *What are the symptoms of anemia?*

A: Hemoglobin gives blood its red color, and a person with anemia may be noticeably pale, although various other disorders can also cause paleness. Other symptoms of anemia include tiredness, headaches, dizziness, shortness of breath, and palpitations after only slight exertion.

Q: *Is anemia serious?*

A: There are various types of anemia. It may be only minor and give little cause for concern, or it may be a warning sign of a more serious condition. For this reason, a person should not ignore the symptoms, but should seek advice from a physician.

Q: *How is anemia diagnosed?*

A: Physicians diagnose anemia by obtaining a blood count. They take a small sample of blood from the patient and count the number of red blood cells in it. In a healthy person, each cubic millimeter of blood contains between four and six million red blood cells, which have a normal life of about three to four months and are replaced continually.

Q: *What are the causes of anemia?*

A: Anemia has three chief causes: (1) loss of blood through bleeding (hemorrhage); (2) failure of the body to make enough new or normal red blood cells; or (3) hemolysis, the rapid destruction of the red blood cells in the blood.

Q: *What can prevent the body from making red cells?*

A: Failure of red blood cell production can be caused by faulty diet. Lack of sufficient iron in the food a person eats leads to insufficient hemoglobin in his or her red blood cells. Lack of vitamin C (ascorbic acid) leads to the anemia that accompanies scurvy. Lack of two essential B vitamins, folic acid and vitamin B_{12}, results in the production of fewer but larger than normal red blood cells (macrocytic anemia). Pernicious anemia is due to a vitamin B_{12} deficiency. This deficiency, however, is the result of an absorption defect, rather than a dietary lack. Small amounts of some elements in the diet, such as copper and manganese, are needed for correct red blood cell formation. Lack of these elements may cause anemia; treatment is to add the missing factor to the diet. In severe cases, a physician may prescribe tablets or injections containing the missing factor. *See also* ANEMIA, PERNICIOUS.

Manufacture of red blood cells by the red bone marrow can also be slowed by the suppressing effect of an infection, by poisons such as lead, or by cancer. The anemia is made worse if the cancer invades the bone marrow or begins there, as in leukemia and myeloma. Treatment is to try to remove the cause, to prescribe a diet with additional vitamins, and to give blood transfusions if necessary. *See also* LEUKEMIA; MYELOMA.

Rapid destruction of red blood cells, called hemolytic anemia, occurs in malaria and a few other diseases. It can also arise as a reaction to certain drugs and in sickle cell anemia, thalassemia, and some other inherited disorders, which result in abnormal red cells. Hemolytic anemia can also arise from a blood transfusion with blood of the wrong type or incompatibility of Rh factor between a newborn child and its mother. Treatment is aimed at finding the cause, and blood transfusions may be given. *See also* SICKLE CELL ANEMIA; THALASSEMIA.

Complete failure to produce red blood cells, the disorder called aplastic anemia, may occur suddenly for no apparent reason. Or it may be caused by sensitivity to a drug that results in destruction of bone marrow cells. Treatment is with corticosteroid drugs, blood transfusions, or sometimes bone marrow transplants. *See also* ANEMIA, APLASTIC.

Q: *Should women routinely take iron tablets?*

A: A well-balanced diet provides sufficient iron for a woman with normal menstrual periods. Such a woman needs about 18 mg of iron per day. If her periods are particularly heavy, or if she is pregnant, her iron intake may not keep pace with her loss, and a physician may prescribe additional iron. A pregnant or lactating woman needs 15 to 30 mg of iron daily.

Anemia, aplastic (ə nē′mē ə, ā plas′ tik). Aplastic anemia is a disease that strikes the bone marrow and produces a deficiency of red blood cells, white blood cells, and platelets. Aplastic anemia may be caused by the use of chemical agents, such as benzene, radiation, or sometimes antibiotics or other drugs. Hemorrhages and other life-threatening disorders may accompany aplastic anemia; a bone marrow transplant is the only current effective treatment.

See also BONE MARROW TRANSPLANT.

Anemia, Cooley's. *See* THALASSEMIA.

Anemia, iron deficiency. Iron deficiency anemia is a blood disorder characterized by the body's production of red blood cells, in which the oxygen-carrying component (erythrocyte) is dysfunctional. It is caused by a nutritional deficiency of iron, by excessive iron loss due to gastrointestinal bleeding, or by excessive menstruation.

Anemia, pernicious (ə nē′mē ə, pər nish′əs). Pernicious anemia may cause a severe reduction in the number of red blood cells in the body. It is accompanied by paleness, fatigue, and digestive nervous system disturbances. Pernicious anemia is caused by a deficiency

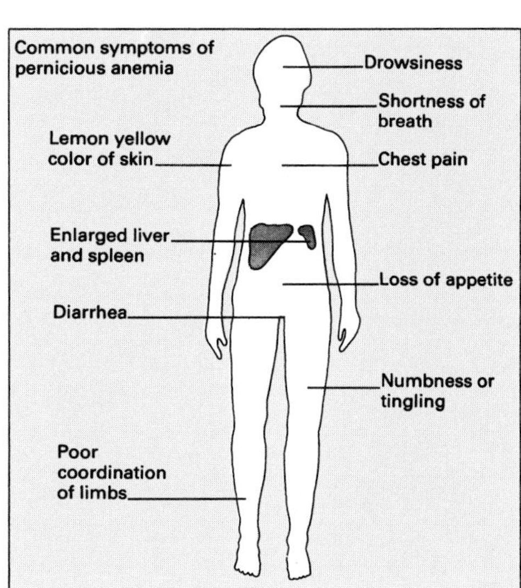

Pernicious anemia, which is caused by a deficiency of a substance called the intrinsic factor, can result in a variety of symptoms that affect the whole body.

of a substance, called an intrinsic factor, normally secreted by the stomach. The intrinsic factor normally combines with the extrinsic factor, vitamin B_{12}, to form a substance that can be absorbed by the body. Vitamin B_{12} is needed for normal division of red blood cells. If not available in sufficient amounts, the red blood cells fail to divide. The red blood cells thus become abnormally large (megaloblastic) and contain higher than normal quantities of hemoglobin (hyperchromic).

Pernicious anemia is a chronic, progressive condition that most frequently strikes older adults, but it can also affect those under 30 years old.

Treatment is usually in the form of injectable vitamin B_{12}. Administration of vitamin B_{12} will result in a relief from symptoms and an improvement in the red blood cell count. Pernicious anemia is also known as Addison's anemia.

Anesthesiology (an əs thē zē ol′ə jē) is the branch of medical science that deals with the administration of general and local anesthetics so that surgery can be performed without pain.

Anesthetic (an əs thet′ik) is any of a group of drugs that cause a loss of sensation. They are given before medical treatment, such as surgery, that would otherwise cause pain. There are many anesthetic drugs, and they can be grouped according to the effect they produce in the patient.

Q: *What are the main types of anesthetics?*

A: A general anesthetic, causing loss of consciousness as well as loss of sensation, is given in most surgical operations. Another group, called local anesthetics, causes loss of sensation only in the area to be treated. Dentists often use a local anesthetic during the filling or extraction of a tooth. A third group is the topical anesthetics, which remove sensation from a surface area such as an eye or the nose. They make possible medical examinations without pain to the patient.

Q: *On what basis are different general anesthetics given?*

A: It is the task of an anesthesiologist to decide which general anesthetic is best for the patient. The anesthesiologist reviews the patient's medical history and may order tests to help select the anesthetic.

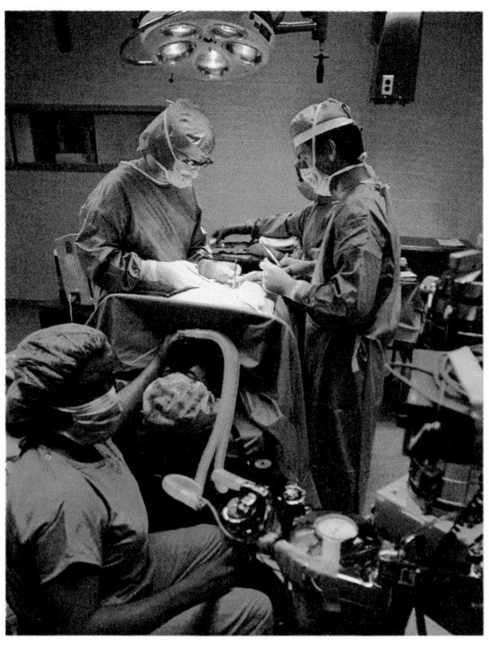

Administered by specialists in **anesthesiology, anesthetics** are given to prevent pain during surgery.

Q: *Are the injections a patient receives when awake part of the anesthetic?*

A: To make the patient relaxed and drowsy, and to dry the mouth and lungs, a sedative injection is given one hour before the operation. Later, immediately before the general anesthetic, an injection of a short-period sleeping drug is given in a vein. This takes effect extremely quickly.

Q: *How is a general anesthetic given?*

A: When the patient is asleep after the intravenous injection, a small dose of a drug that relaxes the muscles is generally given. The drugs that continue the general anesthesia are injected or given as gases either through a face mask or a tube inserted through the mouth or nose into the windpipe. The tube is attached to an anesthesia machine, which ensures maximum control over the quantity and composition of the mixture of anesthetic and oxygen.

Q: *What precautions are taken before the anesthetic is administered and after consciousness has been regained?*

A: The patient is not allowed anything to eat or drink for at least four hours before the operation. This reduces the chances of vomiting and inhaling fluid into the lungs when the anesthetic is being given.

After the operation, the anesthesiologist should remain with the patient until consciousness is regained.

Q: *How do local anesthetics differ from general anesthetics?*

A: A local anesthetic is injected either into the tissues surrounding the area to be treated or next to the nerves serving the area. Adrenaline is sometimes added to the injection to increase the time for which the anesthetic is effective and to reduce bleeding.

Q: *What are the various types of local anesthetic?*

A: There are four types of local anesthetic. (1) The most common form of local anesthetic is the type used for a dental injection, in which the loss of sensation affects only a limited area. (2) A local anesthetic that affects a whole section of the body, such as an arm or a leg, produces what is called regional anesthesia. The injection is given close to where the nerves leave the spinal cord. (3) When an injection is given around the spinal cord (epidural anesthesia) or into the cerebrospinal fluid of the spinal cord (spinal anesthesia), the body is anesthetized below the site of injection. Epidural anesthesia is sometimes used during childbirth. (4) Drugs may be injected to produce partial anesthesia combined with amnesia. The patient then becomes peaceful and relaxed.

Anesthetic, epidural (an əs thet′ik, ep ə dür′əl). Epidural anesthetic is the process by which anesthesia of the pelvic, abdominal, or genital region is achieved. It is a local anesthetic injected into the epidural space of the spinal column. Epidural anesthetic is sometimes used in childbirth.

Aneurysm (an′yə riz əm) is a swelling or ballooning at a weakened point of an artery, a vein, or the heart. More commonly, however, the term aneurysm is used to describe such a swelling in an arterial wall. The weakening of the arterial wall is often a result of hardening of the arteries (arteriosclerosis). Aneurysms may also be caused by hypertension, infection, or a congenital weakness to the vessel wall.

Q: *Can an aneurysm be serious?*

A: Yes. If an aneurysm bursts (ruptures), it is extremely dangerous. An aneurysm in the aorta, the major blood vessel leading from the heart, may partly rupture (dissecting aneurysm). It usually causes enough pain to act as a warning of impending complete rupture. If an aortic aneurysm ruptures completely, death may result. If the burst occurs in the brain, there is a stroke or brain hemorrhage (subarachnoid hemorrhage).

Q: *Can a ruptured aneurysm be treated successfully?*

A: If treatment can be provided promptly, damage from the rupture may be brought under control. A suspected rupture must be confirmed by an X ray of the artery (arteriogram). A surgical operation is then usually required.

Angiitis (an jē i′tis), or angitis, is an inflammation of a blood vessel or lymph gland. It may be caused by an infection or by trauma.

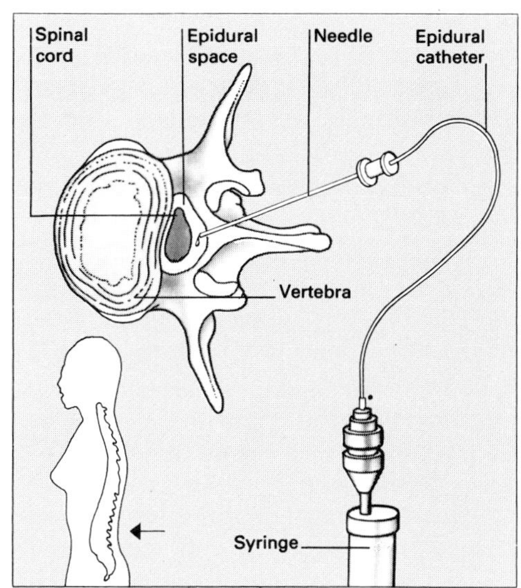

Epidural anesthetic is a process by which the feeling in the pelvic, abdominal, or genital regions can be deadened by the introduction of anesthesia into the epidural space (the space outside the dura mater) of the spinal column.

Angina pectoris (an jī′nə pek′tər is) refers to a specific condition that involves pain from the heart. The pain occurs because not enough oxygen reaches the heart muscle, especially following exercise or excitement. There is a tight feeling across the chest, which may later spread into the neck, jaw, shoulders, and to one or both arms as far as the hands. Occasionally, it may also spread to the upper abdomen. An attack is often accompanied by a feeling of suffocation and impending death.

Q: *What disorders might be associated with angina pectoris?*

A: Coronary heart disease (arteriosclerosis) and coronary spasm are the cause of angina pectoris. The condition is not in itself a heart attack, but may be a warning that one could occur. *See also* ARTERIOSCLEROSIS.

Q: *How is angina pectoris treated?*

A: Overweight people must lose excess fat to reduce strain on the heart. Hypertension must also be controlled. Smoking must be discontinued. Regular moderate exercise improves blood circulation to the heart. Medication, such as nitroglycerine, can help as well. Newer drugs called beta blockers help to prevent pain by reducing the amount of oxygen that the heart muscle needs; they also help to govern the heart rate. A new class of drugs, calcium channel-blockers, are also useful in treatment. *See also* BETA BLOCKER; CALCIUM CHANNEL BLOCKER; NITROGLYCERINE.

Q: *Should a person with angina pectoris become less active?*

A: A person is usually encouraged to lead a normal life. However, a person should learn to recognize how much exercise or excitement he or she can tolerate without bringing on the pain.

Angioblast (an′jē ō blast) is the embryonic tissue from which the blood cells and blood vessels are formed.

Angioblastoma (an jē ō blas tō′mə) is a term given to certain vascular tumors in the brain.

Angiogram (an′jē ō gram) is a series of X-ray visualizations of the heart and blood vessels. A radiopaque substance, that is, a material that does not allow the passage of X rays through it, is injected into a vein or artery, and X-ray pictures are then taken in rapid succession. The series of pictures reveals the size and shape of veins or arteries in organs and tissues. An angiogram is used as a diagnostic tool with certain diseases; arteriosclerosis is an example.

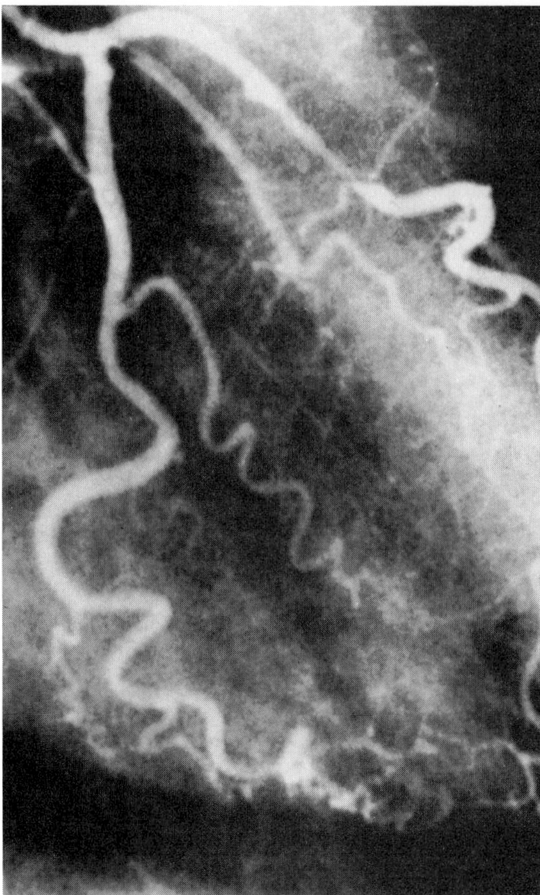

An **angiogram** is a series of X-ray pictures of blood vessels and the internal anatomy of the heart.

Because some people may have an allergic reaction to the radiopaque substance, a careful history of any prior such reactions is taken by the angiographer prior to performing the procedure.

Angiography, digital subtraction (an jē og′rə fē, dij′ə təl səb trak′shən). Digital subtraction angiography (DSA) is a procedure in which a computerized technique is used to observe arterial blood circulation. In DSA, X-ray images of arterial blood vessels are taken both before and after the introduction of a radiopaque dye. These images are converted into digital data; and a computer "subtracts" one set of data from another with the resulting image showing only the dye and, therefore, the shape of the artery through which the blood is flowing. Arterial shape is important in the determination of possible circulatory problems; DSA is therefore an aid in the diagnosis of heart disease and other circulatory disorders.

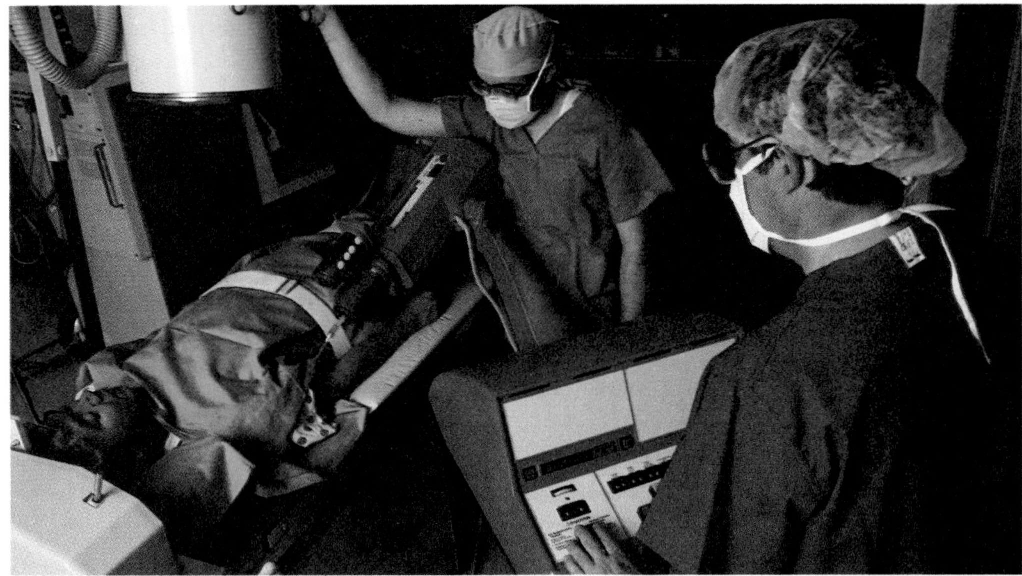

Digital subtraction angiography, *left,* is a procedure, employing both X rays and modern computer techniques, which aids in diagnosing heart disease and other circulatory disorders. After the injection of radiopaque dyes, X-ray visualizations are taken and then converted into digital data. This is "subtracted" by a computer into a single image, which reveals the shape of blood vessels in the heart.

Angioma (an jē ō'mə) is an abnormal growth of tissue formed by a group of small blood vessels. It may be present on the surface of the skin or internally and is not usually malignant (cancerous). On the skin one type of an angioma is a soft, purplish mark called a strawberry nevus. If an angioma occurs in the brain, it can lead to serious conditions such as bleeding (subarachnoid hemorrhage) or a stroke. An angioma that bleeds in the intestine may cause black stools (melena), the vomiting of blood (hematemesis), or anemia.

Q: *What is the treatment for an angioma?*

A: A small angioma in the skin may be burned or corroded away (cauterized), but larger ones need plastic surgery. Sometimes it is not advisable to treat an angioma; disfigurement may be hidden by cosmetics.

Angioneurotic edema (an jē ō nů rot' ik i dē'mə) is a form of giant hives (urticaria) in which large, irritating swellings occur and recur anywhere on or near the surface of the skin. The sporadic type is thought to be caused by an allergy to a specific food or drug or from emotional stress. In the inherited type there is no specific cause of an attack. The condition is not thought to be serious unless it affects the mouth, throat, or larynx, where it may obstruct breathing. In severe attacks treatment may include immediate injection of adrenaline followed by antihistamines and, possibly, steroids. Prevention depends on identifying and eliminating causative factors.

See also HIVES.

Angioplasty (an'jē ō plas tē) is surgical reconstruction of blood vessels, usually damaged by atherosclerosis. If the arteries in question are in the heart, a coronary bypass operation is often recommended.

However, the nonsurgical method of balloon angioplasty is often employed, especially when only one vessel is blocked.

Laser angioplasty is also being developed as a therapy for atherosclerotic plaque build-up. A major problem has long been the extremely high temperatures given out by laser beams, which can burn healthy tissue. The recent invention of a low-heat excimer laser seems to offer some hope for wider future application.

See also ARTERIOSCLEROSIS; ANGIOPLASTY, BALLOON; ANGIOPLASTY, PERCUTANEOUS LASER.

Angioplasty, balloon (an'jē ō plas tē). Balloon angioplasty is a nonsurgical method of clearing coronary and other arteries, blocked by atherosclerotic plaque, fibrous and fatty deposits on the walls of arteries.

A catheter with a balloon-like tip is threaded up from the arm or groin through the artery until it reaches the blocked area. The balloon is then inflated, flattening the plaque and increasing the diameter of the blood vessel opening. The arterial passage is thus widened.

There are limitations, however, to this technique's application, depending on the extent of the disease, the blood flow through the artery, and the part of the anatomy and the particular vessels involved. Thus arteries can be so blocked by plaque build-up or twist and turn so much, that they are impenetrable. Furthermore, the still unknown underlying causes remain unaffected, and plaque build-up recurs within 6 months in up to 30 percent of those treated.

See also ANGIOPLASTY; ARTERIOSCLEROSIS.

Angioplasty, percutaneous laser (an′ jē ō plas tē, pėr kyü tā′nē əs lā′zər). Percutaneous laser angioplasty combines the sciences of fiber optics and excimer laser beam technology. It is potentially safer, more effective, and less expensive than other types of angioplasty.

A catheter is threaded up from the arm or groin to the coronary arteries of the heart. This catheter carries on its tip a lens connected to an outside camera, enabling the physician to see on a monitor the plaque build-up. As the catheter tip moves through the arteries, the physician triggers short bursts from the excimer laser, also mounted on the tip. These bursts, at a temperature of 40°C (104°F), destroy the molecular and chemical bonds of the atherosclerotic plaque instead of burning it, thus avoiding the possibility of damaging surrounding tissue.

This new form of angioplasty is still being developed. How well tissue heals itself after being lased, whether there is danger of a blood clot forming later on, and how long before plaque build-up starts up again are three questions yet to be answered.

Until the underlying causes of atherosclerosis are identified and preventive therapy developed, excimer laser angioplasty should prove far safer and more effective than any other means devised for the treatment of atherosclerosis.

See also ANGIOPLASTY; ARTERIOSCLEROSIS.

Angiotensin-converting enzyme inhibitor (an jē ō ten′sin), usually referred to simply as ACE inhibitor, belongs to a class of drugs that blocks the formation of angiotensin, a naturally-occurring substance produced by the body to constrict blood vessels. ACE inhibitor drugs are used to treat hypertension (high blood pressure) and to reduce the retention of salt and water in the body. Since drugs do not cure high blood pressure, those who require them may have to take them for life.

Side effects of ACE inhibitors may include loss of taste, rashes, gastrointestinal disturbances, and protein in the urine. These can usually be minimized by adjusting the dosage or substituting other drugs.

See also HYPERTENSION.

Animals and disease is a topic of special importance to persons who own or have frequent contact with pets. One of the most popular misconceptions about human and animal diseases is that they are mutually exclusive. They are not. Transmission of animal diseases to humans (zoonosis) can occur through direct contact with the infected animal; contact with the animal's feces or urine; ingestion of undercooked meat or fish; or through insect bites, particularly mosquitoes and ticks.

Zoonoses, or diseases that can be transmitted from animals to humans, may be bacterial, viral, rickettsial, fungal, or parasitic. Among the bacterial diseases are anthrax, brucellosis, campylobacteriosis, cat scratch fever, leptospirosis, Lyme disease, plague, psittacosis, rat bite fever, salmonellosis, and tularemia.

Many animals and animal products can be a source of salmonellosis in humans, including turtles and shellfish. After handling uncooked meat, particularly poultry, hands should be washed before handling other food. All pets should be examined by a veterinarian.

Among the important viral zoonoses are rabies, equine encephalomyelitis, lymphocytic choriomeningitis, and St. Louis encephalitis. In consideration of rabies, animal bites should always be reported to a physician. If possible, the animal should be restrained and confined until it can be determined that it does not have rabies. This is particularly important for wild animals. Children should neither play with them nor keep them as pets.

Ringworm is the most common fungal disease of animals that can be transmitted from animals to humans and back to animals. Contrary to the name, the disease is not caused by a worm. Although the domestic dog and cat are perhaps the most common sources of this disease, other animals may also be sources of infection.

Parasitic diseases constitute a large group of zoonotic diseases and may be caused by worms, protozoa, or mites. Toxoplasmosis is one such protozoan disease. Although the cat is the primary source of this disease for humans, raw or improperly cooked meat may also be a source of infection.

Cats and dogs can also be a source of roundworms to humans. Children who play barefoot in dirt and sandboxes that are contaminated with dog feces can become infected with roundworms or dog hookworms. Sandboxes should be kept covered as cats use them for litter boxes. Young children should not play in areas where pets defecate, and the animal feces should be collected and disposed of promptly.

Contrary to popular belief, animals cannot serve as a source of human pinworms. In addition, pinworms of animals do not infect humans.

There are several tapeworm infections that humans share with animals. These are transmitted by eating infected beef, pork, or fish that has been improperly cooked. Among the parasitic infections that may occur with improperly cooked meat is trichinosis. Meat and fish should be thoroughly cooked to reduce the chances of parasitic infection.

To further reduce the chances of transmission of animal diseases to humans, good personal hygiene should be practiced at all times. Children should be instructed to avoid intimate contact with animals—for example, kissing—and hands should be washed after playing with pets. Pets should be taken in for regular veterinary checkups and vaccinations. Discourage children from making pets of wild animals, as they tend to bite and may carry disease. Pregnant women should avoid exposure to cat litter boxes as toxoplasmosis can cause severe infection of the unborn fetus.

See also ALLERGY; ASTHMA; ENCEPHALITIS; HEPATITIS; MEASLES; PSITTACOSIS; RABIES; RINGWORM; ROUNDWORM; SALMONELLA; SCABIES; TAPEWORM; TOXOCARIASIS; TOXOPLASMOSIS; TUBERCULOSIS; YELLOW FEVER.

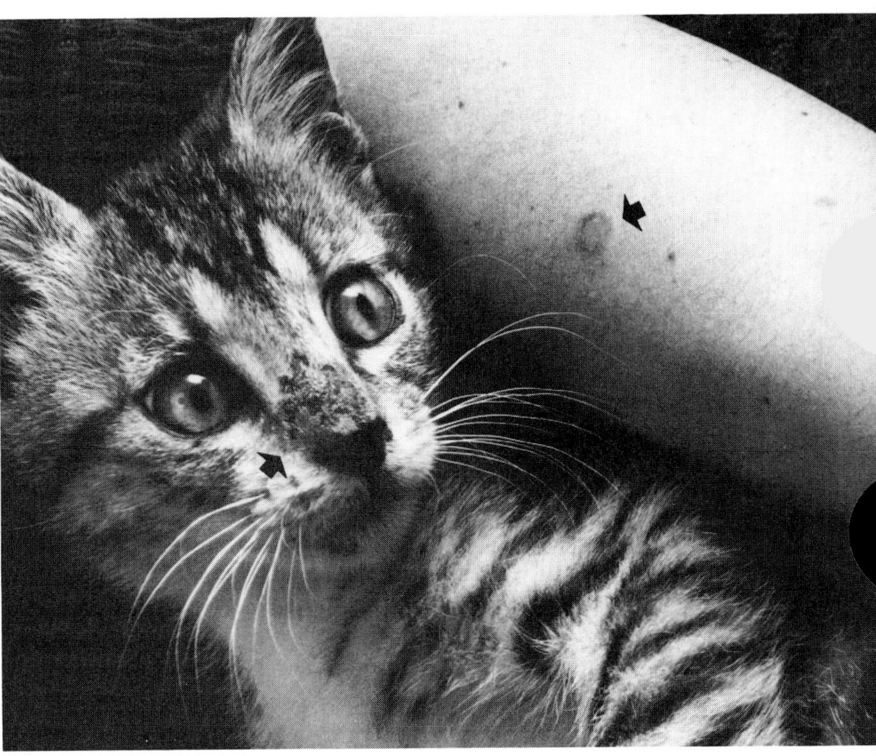

Some **diseases** and infections can be **spread from animals** to human beings. The kitten's nose, *above,* is infected with ringworm, which has been transmitted to the pet owner's arm.

Aniseikonia (an ī sī kō′nē ə) is an abnormal eye condition in which one eye perceives the size and shape of an image differently than the other eye. A serious form of the condition may be correctable through the use of special lenses.

Ankle is the joint between the leg and the foot that joins the shinbone (tibia) and the calfbone (fibula) with the talus bone. The outer side of the ankle is supported by the slender fibula bone and several strong ligaments, which are bands of fibrous tissue that connect bone to bone. The ankle joint allows the foot to move up and down.

Q: *What can go wrong with the ankle?*

A: The most frequent injury is a sprained ankle. A very mild sprain from a twisted ankle entails no torn ligaments. A brief rest with the ankle elevated should eliminate any mild pain or swelling. A severe sprain entails the tearing of ligaments, such as between the fibula and the side of the heel bone (calcaneus). It is accompanied by pain, swelling, and tenderness. Walking is painful with this type of sprain. Treatment includes elevating the ankle and applying an ice pack or cold compress for several minutes at a time, on and off for several hours. This should ease the pain and reduce the swelling. Bandaging the ankle for a few days will help it heal. In severe cases a cast may be required.

A fracture of the ankle may include a break of the fibula or tibia alone or a break of both the fibula and tibia. An X ray will generally reveal such a fracture. A cast is used to hold the broken bones in place until they mend. Treatment may include surgery to place the ends of the broken bones in their proper positions.

Ankles frequently swell because of excessive fluid in the tissues (edema). Such swelling often occurs in hot weather after a person has been standing for a long time. Swelling may also occur during pregnancy and as a result of heart disease. Ankle sprains, varicose veins, obesity, osteoarthritis, rheumatoid arthritis, gout, and local infection may also cause ankle swelling. Resting with feet upraised generally reduces such swelling. Special stockings may also be of help.

See also FRACTURES: FIRST AID.

Ankle fractures: first aid. *See* FRACTURES: FIRST AID.

Ankylosing spondylitis. *See* SPONDYLITIS, ANKYLOSING.

Ankylosis (ang kə lō′sis) is the stiffening or fixation of a joint due to disease, injury, or surgery. The fixation of the joint may occur because of destruction of the joint cartilage. Rheumatoid arthritis triggers this kind of ankylosis. Ankylotic conditions, such as ankylosing spondylitis, may also be inherited. Artificial ankylosis (arthrodesis) is a surgical method of relieving joint pain.

See also ARTHRITIS, RHEUMATOID; ARTHRODESIS; SPONDYLITIS, ANKYLOSING.

Ankylostomiasis (ang kə los tə mī′ə sis), also known as hookworm disease, is the infestation of the small intestine by small worms (*Ancylostoma duodenale* or *Necator americanus*). These worms, which grow up to 0.5 inches (12mm) long, enter the body through the skin, sometimes leaving an itching rash, travel to the lung via the blood and lymph systems, ascend the respiratory tract, are swallowed, and reach the intestine about a week after entering the skin. They attach themselves to the inside of the small intestine and suck blood, which can lead to severe iron deficiency anemia, particularly in malnourished individuals. Their eggs are excreted in the feces and end up living in soil as larvae until they can reenter human skin.

Q: *What are the symptoms of ankylostomiasis?*

A: Symptoms of ankylostomiasis may be pain, diarrhea, nausea, or colic. A long infection can lead to anemia with all the symptoms that accompany that disorder. If the disease is undiscovered in children, it may retard growth and mental development. *See also* ANEMIA.

Ankylostomiasis is diagnosed by testing the feces for eggs.

Q: *In what parts of the world is ankylostomiasis most likely to occur?*

A: It is more common where a hot climate and damp earth are favorable conditions for larvae to thrive, especially if there is poor sanitation as well. The worms usually enter the skin through bare feet that come into contact with larva-den soil. The disorder occurs in tropical areas and in the southern states of the United States.

Anodontia (an ō don′she ə) is the congenital absence of one or more teeth. The absence of such teeth as third molars is fairly common.

Anomaly (ə nom′ə lē) is an irregularity, a deviation from the normal standard. In medicine, the major concern is with congenital anomalies (birth defects), such as blindness, bone disorders, Down's syndrome, heart disease, and spina bifida. These defects arise from the faulty development of the fetus as a result of genetic disorders or other factors, such as a pregnant woman being injured, becoming sick, or taking drugs.

Many anomalies can be treated; others cannot. Some are clinically unimportant. In Aristotle's anomaly, for example, a pencil placed between the crossed first and second fingers feels like two pencils.

See also CONGENITAL ANOMALY.

Anorectic (an ə rek′tik) is a type of drug that reduces the appetite. Most anorectics are amphetamines or related compounds that, because of their addictive properties, are now used only to treat extreme, life-endangering obesity. As a general rule, drugs should not be used to reduce weight.

See also AMPHETAMINE.

Anorexia nervosa (an ə rek′sē ə nėr vō′sə) is a psychiatric disorder characterized by a reduction in food intake due to an extreme anxiety over weight gain. Individuals may also engage in prolonged exercise, exhibit peculiar patterns of handling and preparing food, and show severely disturbed body images.

Anorexia nervosa is often associated with the emotional upheaval that may accompany a significant change in a person's life. Making new friends or maturing sexually may be factors in this emotional disturbance. Family dynamics are becoming increasingly recognized as an important factor in this disorder; patients tend to be "model children."

The condition may be mild, but anorexia nervosa can also be acute and even life-threatening. If forced to eat, a person may vomit after the meal. Loss of food intake leads to a loss of weight, and in women menstruation ceases. The anorexic body, which is starved for calories, starts feeding on its own muscle protein, leading to irregularities in heart rhythm or even to congestive heart failure.

Q: *Can anorexia be detected in its early stages?*

A: Early diagnosis is difficult. The person, especially if adolescent, commonly denies anything is wrong and continues to be cheerful and active. He or she may be deceptive about the quantity of food eaten, and while continuing to express fear of being fat, may deny that he or she is wasting away.

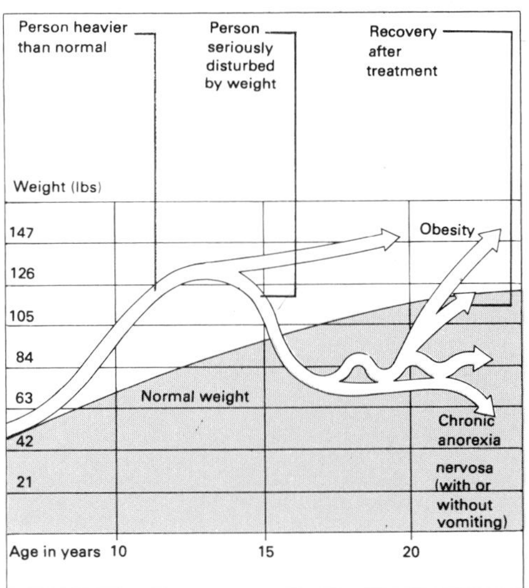

Anorexia nervosa is a psychiatric disorder in which food intake is severely reduced due to anxiety over weight gain.

Q: *How is anorexia nervosa treated?*

A: Treatment begins with measures to improve eating habits and to increase the patient's weight. This is followed by therapy to overcome the emotional basis of the disorder. In severe cases, hospitalization may be needed to save the person's life. Treatment typically includes individual, group, and family therapy and is usually long-term. Antidepressants may also be helpful. Careful evaluation is necessary to rule out other psychiatric disorders, such as depression.

See also BULIMIA.

Anosmia (an oz′mē ə) is the loss or lack of the sense of smell. It may be temporary, from a head cold or other obstruction of the nasal passages; or it may be permanent, resulting from disease of the olfactory nerve, from tumors, from certain kinds of skull fractures, or from psychological factors.

The aging process also diminishes the sense of smell.

Anoxia (an ok′sē ə) is the lack of sufficient oxygen in the body tissues. It occurs when the blood flowing through the lungs does not absorb enough oxygen, when the blood cannot carry its full load of oxygen as in anemia, or when the blood flow slows.

See also HYPOXIA.

Antabuse® (ant′ə byüs) is the registered name for disulfiram, a drug occasionally used for the treatment of alcohol-related problems. Antabuse, taken orally, disrupts the metabolism and produces the chemical, acetaldehyde. Acetaldehyde causes the alcohol consumer to experience headaches, stomach pains, vomiting, vertigo, and/or difficulty in breathing, therefore acting as a deterrent to drinking. Experts stress that Antabuse, which must be taken daily to work effectively, works best for those who drink impulsively rather than regularly.

See also ALCOHOLISM.

Antacid (ant as′id) is a drug or other substance that neutralizes acids; it is usually prescribed to remedy excess acidity in the stomach. Baking soda and calcium carbonate are examples. Antacids may relieve stomach pain, but some may have unpleasant side effects, including constipation (from antacids containing aluminum and calcium) and diarrhea (from antacids containing magnesium). Prolonged use of an antacid should be avoided unless prescribed by a physician.

Antenatal (an tē nā'təl) is another term for prenatal, meaning happening or existing before birth.

Anthracosis (an thrə kō'sis), also known as black lung, is a chronic lung disease caused by the inhalation of coal dust. Symptoms may include progressive shortness of breath and a productive cough, especially after many years of exposure. The condition is aggravated by cigarette smoking. Anthracosis may be halted by stopping further exposure to coal dust.

See also BLACK LUNG; PNEUMOCONIOSIS.

Anthrax (an'thraks) is a rare, infectious disease that is transmitted to humans most commonly by farm animals. The disease is caused by the bacterium *Bacillus anthracis*. Humans most often contract the disease when an opening in the skin comes into contact with an infected hide of an animal. Anthrax may also be spread through the inhalation of bacterium spores. If not properly treated, the disease may be fatal.

Q: *What are the symptoms of anthrax?*

A: Symptoms include nausea, fever, and the occurrence of a skin boil that forms a dark scab. The boil forms slowly and may spread to form other boils. Anyone working with animals or animal products who develops an unusual boil should contact a physician immediately.

Q: *What is the treatment for anthrax?*

A: Immediate treatment with penicillin or tetracycline is usually effective. Unfortunately, anthrax spores are extremely difficult to destroy. Everything that comes in contact with a person who has contracted anthrax must be sterilized. All contaminated animals and animal products must also be destroyed.

Antibiotic (an tē bī ot'ik) is an agent that weakens or destroys bacteria; antibiotics are medicinally used to treat various types of bacterial infections. The various types of antibiotics work either by preventing an infection from growing or by destroying an existing infection. Antibiotics are produced either from a mold or a fungus or are produced synthetically.

Q: *What are the various types of antibiotics and what do they do?*

A: Common forms of antibiotics include aminoglycosides, macrolides, penicillins, tetracyclines, and cephalosporins.

Aminoglycosides work by interfering with the protein formation of bacteria. Aminoglycosides include *gentamicin*, *amikacin*, and *tobramycin*. Side effects can include damage to the nerves of hearing and balance, as well as kidney injury.

Macrolide antibiotics interfere with the protein formation of bacteria during multiplication. *Erythromycin* is a macrolide. Side effects include gastrointestinal discomfort.

Penicillins (discovered by Sir Alexander Fleming in 1928) work by damaging the cell walls of the invading bacteria as the bacteria reproduce. *Penicillin G* and *V* are widely used for streptococcal and other bacterial infections. Broad-spectrum penicillins, such as *ampicillin* and *amoxicillin*, are used on a variety of infections caused by gram-negative organisms. Hypersensitivity reactions, for example, a fever or a rash, are fairly common side effects of penicillin use. Severe allergic reactions (anaphylaxis) rarely occur, but can be life-threatening.

Tetracyclines, which are active against a wide range of bacteria and other organisms, are thought to prevent production of proteins in the invading bacterial cells. The tetracyclines include *tetracycline* and *doxycycline*. Side effects of therapy may include gastrointestinal irritation, sensitivity of the skin to sunlight, and liver and kidney injury. This group of drugs should not be administered during the last four to five months of pregnancy, nor should it be given to children before the age of eight

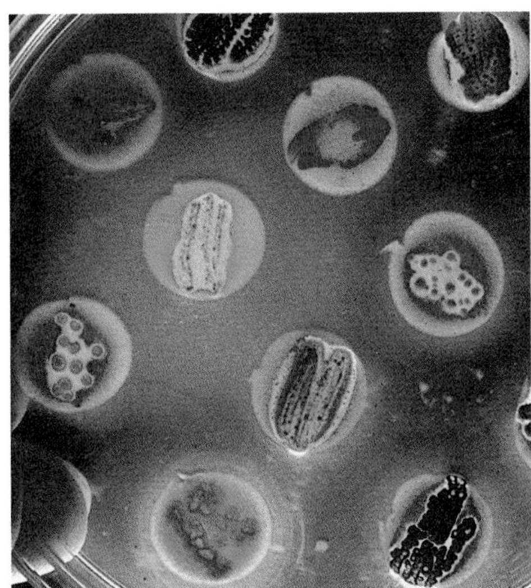

Antibiotics, which destroy or suppress the growth of bacteria, are pictured here growing in a culture medium under laboratory control.

years. Permanent discoloration of developing teeth may result.

Cephalosporins are relatively new antibiotics active against a wide range of bacteria. Like penicillins, they interfere with bacterial cell wall formation. A frequently used cephalosporin is *cefaclor.* Side effects include rashes and fever. Sometimes, persons allergic to penicillins will also be allergic to cephalosporins.

Q: *Should antibiotics be used to fight all infections?*

A: Antibiotics can safely save lives when prescribed appropriately. However, indiscriminate use of these drugs can have serious consequences and can counteract their usefulness. In the approximately 50 years since antibiotics were first administered, a number of bacterial strains that cause disease have become resistant to the antibiotics that were once able to control or destroy them.

Although literally thousands of antibiotic substances have been found in nature or have been produced chemically, relatively few have been proven safe and effective. Certain antibiotics can become toxic when outdated.

Persons who know they are allergic to an antibiotic drug should tell the physician before being treated for any condition. An allergic reaction could lead to anaphylactic shock, which can be life-threatening. Even a lesser reaction can be quite serious and should be monitored by a physician.

See also AMPICILLIN; ERYTHROMYCIN; PENICILLIN; ANAPHYLACTIC SHOCK; TETRACYCLINE.

Antibody (an′tē bod ē) is a substance produced by the body in response to an infection. It combines with an antigen (the foreign substance, such as a virus, that activated it) and neutralizes it. Antibodies are part of the development of natural immunity. They can be produced artificially by immunization.

See also ALLERGY; ANTIGEN; IMMUNITY; IMMUNIZATION.

Anticholinergic (an tē kō lə nėr′jik) usually pertains to a drug that blocks acetylcholine receptors, which results in an inhibition of the transmission of nerve impulses. The drugs are used to treat bladder and intestine smooth muscle spasms and certain neurological disorders (Parkinson's disease, for example). Side effects may include blurred vision, dry mouth, dizziness, and rapid heartbeat. Anticholinergic drugs should not be taken by people with glaucoma and by those who may be subject to urinary retention.

See also GLAUCOMA; PARKINSON'S DISEASE.

Anticoagulant (an tē kō ag′yə lənt) is a drug that interferes with the normal clotting of blood. There are two main groups: direct-action, such as heparin, which is injected into a vein; and indirect-action, such as Coumadin® (warfarin), which is taken by mouth. Heparin acts quickly, but the indirect-acting drugs take up to three days to become effective.

Q: *When are anticoagulants prescribed?*

A: They are prescribed to prevent blood clots that may occur in a coronary artery (myocardial infarction) or in a leg vein (thrombophlebitis). They may also be given with certain surgical operations on the female reproductive system to prevent clotting in leg veins, which tends to occur more frequently with those operations.

Q: *Should a patient who uses anticoagulants observe special precautions?*

A: Patients taking anticoagulants require blood tests to ensure that the correct dosage is maintained. They should also carry a card naming the anticoagulant drug and stating the dosage, in case they are involved in an accident. A patient should also wear a medical identification bracelet or necklace stating that he or she is on anticoagulant therapy. Certain medications should be avoided to ensure that the medication does not alter the anticoagulant effect. Aspirin must be avoided when a patient takes warfarin.

Q: *What are the signs of an overdose of anticoagulants?*

A: Common indications include the appearance of bruising, nosebleeds, excessive menstrual bleeding, and blood in the urine.

Anticonvulsant (an tē kən vul′sənt) is a drug used to treat epilepsy or other disorders that cause convulsions or seizures. Since drowsiness and dizziness may occur, patients are advised not to drink alcohol and to exercise caution in driving. Many anticonvulsant medications have the potential to cause birth defects when taken by pregnant women; however, uncontrolled seizures during pregnancy may also endanger the unborn infant. With some anticonvulsants, patients must take regular blood tests to monitor the level of medication in the body.

See also CONVULSION; EPILEPSY.

Antidepressant (an tē di pres′ənt) is a drug that alleviates depression. These medications work by correcting a biochemical imbalance in the brain that produces depression. There are two main categories of antidepressants: the monoamine-oxidase (MAO) inhibitor group and the tricyclics. The tricyclics are more frequently prescribed because they are generally safer and are often as effective as the MAO inhibitors, although they act more gradually. If MAO inhibitors are prescribed, a person should avoid such foods as cheese, certain meats, alcohol, and some yeast extracts because the chemical properties of these substances interact in a dangerous way with the inhibitors.

Antidepressants should be taken only under professional supervision, as they often produce side effects. Some patients are unable to tolerate certain of these drugs.

See also ANTIDEPRESSANT, TRICYCLIC; DEPRESSION; MAO INHIBITOR.

Antidepressant, tricyclic (an tē di pres′ənt, trī sī′klik). Tricyclic antidepressant is a type of drug that is widely prescribed to reduce mental depression. Tricyclics are usually administered by mouth. The average dosage in most Western countries is between 75 and 300 mg a day. Side effects may include sedation, blurred vision, sweating, constipation, and urinary hesitancy. Seizures and hallucinations are possible, especially in elderly patients with organic brain disease. Side effects are most acute during the first 10 to 15 days of treatment. Taking the full dosage near bedtime minimizes side effects in adults, but not in elderly patients. Patients with a tendency toward seizures, glaucoma, or heart disease may be unable to use tricyclic therapy.

See also DEPRESSION.

Antidiarrheal (an tē dī ə rē′əl) is a drug or other substance, such as paregoric and diphenoxylate, that has the property of correcting diarrhea.

See also DIARRHEA.

Antidiuretic hormone. *See* VASOPRESSIN.

Antidote (an′tē dōt) is a medicine that counteracts the harmful effects of a poison. Antidotes work in a variety of ways: some bind up the poison, preventing absorption of it into the system; others counteract the toxin.

See also POISONING: FIRST AID.

Antiemetic (an tē i met′ik), or antinauseant, is a drug used to prevent or relieve nausea and vomiting. There are three main kinds of antiemetics: phenothiazines (antidopaminergic agents); antihistamines; and anticholinergics. All should be taken with extreme care.

Phenothiazines and other antidopaminergic agents that depress the central nervous system are the most potent drugs to treat nausea and vomiting, but are not useful in treating motion sickness. Side effects of phenothiazine may include drowsiness, hypotension (low blood pressure), and abnormal movement disorders.

Antihistamines, which have a depressant effect on the neural pathways, may also be useful in treating nausea, including that associated with motion sickness and pregnancy. Antihistamines produce drowsiness; people who take them should not drive automobiles, operate dangerous machinery, or drink alcoholic beverages.

Anticholinergics relieve nausea by inhibiting nerve impulse transmissions. They are especially useful in the relief of nausea and vomiting associated with vertigo and motion sickness. Their side effects—blurred vision, dry mouth, and fast heart rate—may limit their prolonged use. Anticholinergic drugs should not be given to people suffering from glaucoma or to people with a tendency toward urine retention problems.

See also ANTICHOLINERGIC; ANTIHISTAMINE; MOTION SICKNESS.

Antigen (an'tə jən) is any foreign protein substance that stimulates the body to produce antibodies, which attempt to counteract that foreign substance. Bacteria, viruses, and such physical agents as pollen may act as antigens.

See also ANTIBODY.

Antihistamine (an tē his'tə mēn) is a medicine that is used to counteract histamine, the chemical released from certain cells during an allergic reaction. Antihistamines suppress the symptoms associated with histamine, but they do not alter the original cause of the reaction. They are used especially in the treatment of hay fever and certain other allergies. Antihistamines, even those available over-the-counter, should be taken with caution.

Q: *In what forms are antihistamines prescribed?*

A: They can be obtained in many forms: for example, as tablets, liquids, by injection, via nose and eye preparations, and in skin creams.

Q: *Do antihistamines have unpleasant or dangerous side effects?*

A: Antihistamines should be used with caution. Many cause drowsiness, and users are warned to avoid taking them before driving an automobile, operating dangerous machinery, or drinking alcohol. Antihistamines often cause dry mouth, may cause a fast heart rate, or may, unless taken with food, irritate the stomach.

Q: *Are antihistamines effective in the treatment of the common cold?*

A: Although antihistamines do not cure the common cold, they may be effective in alleviating some of the symptoms of the disorder.

See also ALLERGY; HAY FEVER; HISTAMINE.

Antiperspirant (an tē pėr'spər ənt) is any of a number of preparations that reduce sweating. They are commonly used to avoid the odor associated with perspiration by reducing skin secretions.

Antipruritic (an tē prů rit'ik) is a drug or other substance that reduces or alleviates itching. Topical anesthetics and antihistamines are used as antipruritics.

See also ANESTHETIC; ANTIHISTAMINE.

Antipyretic (an tē pī ret'ik) is an agent, such as acetaminophen or aspirin, that reduces or prevents fever.

See also ACETAMINOPHEN; ASPIRIN.

Antiseptic (an tə sep'tik) is a substance that kills or prevents the growth of germs on environmental surfaces and on the skin. Hydrogen peroxide, iodine-containing compounds, and alcohol are widely used antiseptics.

See also ALCOHOL; HYDROGEN PEROXIDE; IODINE.

Antiserum (an tē sir'əm) is a clear fluid, derived from blood (serum) taken from a human or animal immunized against a specific infection. This serum contains antibodies that can be injected to give temporary protection against a specific disease (tetanus or diphtheria, for example) to someone who has no immunity to that disease. Antibiotic drugs have largely replaced some types of antiserum. Antiserums can cause allergic reactions, hepatitis, or even severe or fatal shock (anaphylactic shock). Antiserums are, thus, used with great caution.

See also ANTIBODY; IMMUNIZATION; SERUM; VACCINE.

Antisocial personality. See MENTAL ILLNESS.

Antispasmodic (an tē spaz mod'ik) is a type of drug that prevents involuntary muscle contractions. Antispasmodics are used to treat a variety of conditions, including spastic colon and bladder disorders.

Antitoxin (an tē tok'sin) is an antibody formed in the body that acts against a specific bacterial toxin (poison) by combining with it and neutralizing it.

See also ANTIBODY; IMMUNIZATION; VACCINE.

Antitussive (an tē tus'iv) is a drug used to stop coughing. There are two groups of such drugs, narcotic and nonnarcotic. The narcotic drugs depress the so-called cough centers in the brain, but the patient may become dependent on them if they are used for a long period. Codeine is the preparation most commonly used in prescription cough suppressants.

There are many nonnarcotic cough suppressants available. Many of these contain dextromethorphan.

See also CODEINE; COUGH.

Antivenin (an tē ven'in) is a fluid administered intravenously or intramuscularly to treat poisoning caused by the bite of a venomous animal, for example, a snake. Antivenin contains a high concentration of antibodies that are directed against the venom.

See also ANTIBODY.

Antivenom. *See* ANTIVENIN.

Anuria (ə nyůr'ē ə) is a serious malfunction of the kidney in which little or no urine is produced. Without immediate treatment, anuria can be fatal. The kidney failure can be caused by (1) blockage by a stone (calculus) or tumor; (2) disease, such as acute nephritis; or (3) a decrease in blood pressure during shock.

Treatment is urgent and requires skilled care. Fluids in the diet are restricted, except in cases caused by shock, and are given intravenously. Sometimes, renal dialysis is used to allow the patient to get rid of the waste products and toxins produced by the body. In the case of renal failure caused by shock, treatment involves the use of drugs and intravenous fluids to raise the blood pressure. If bleeding has occurred, blood transfusion may be needed.

See also KIDNEY DIALYSIS; KIDNEY DISEASE.

Anus (ā'nəs) is the opening of the lower end of the digestive tract through which solid waste material and undigested food pass out of the body. It is kept closed by a ring of circular muscle called the sphincter. The anus is subject to three common disorders: (1) fissure, a small crack in the skin of the anus; (2) hemorrhoids (piles), varicose veins inside or outside the anus; (3) *pruritus ani* (itching), sometimes caused by a neurosis, but often caused by a minor disorder of the anal skin (for example, as a result of worms).

The first two complaints may be treated medically or, as a last resort, with minor surgery. Pruritus is often treated with a suitable ointment prescribed by a physician. Worms are treated with orally administered medication.

Anvil. *See* INCUS.

Anxiety (ang zī'ə tē) is a feeling of apprehension, uncertainty, and fear in anticipation of or in response to some real or imagined danger. Mild forms of anxiety caused by emotional conflict or life stress are fairly common and are not usually a clinical problem. Exaggerated fear may lead to an anxiety attack. If anxiety at this level is persistent, some form of professional intervention may be necessary. Anxiety can be associated with a specific object or place or may manifest itself as generalized apprehension about most situations. Less common anxiety may be accompanied by repetitive, intensive thoughts that cannot be controlled. *See also* OBSESSION; PANIC ATTACK; PHOBIA.

Q: ***What are symptoms of anxiety?***

A: Subjective symptoms include feelings of inadequacy, persistent feelings of helplessness, and worry. Objective symptoms include restlessness, insomnia, rapid heart rate, light headedness, and diarrhea. Sufferers may verbalize uneasiness regarding life changes. They may avoid situations in which they feel nervous. Children may regress to wetting the bed or have bouts of vomiting and stomach pains.

Q: ***How should anxiety be treated?***

A: In many cases, anxiety associated with recent stress is time limited. If it persists, brief, supportive counseling and/or short-term use of medication may be helpful. Chronic, generalized anxiety can usually be treated through psychotherapy and relaxation techniques. Medication, for example, minor tranquilizers, may help control the symptoms of anxiety. If medication is used, it should be used along with and not as a substitute for any appropriate therapy or relaxation techniques. If troublesome anxiety attacks, phobias, or obsessions are present, psychiatric intervention combining medication and behavioral techniques is usually necessary. A thorough evaluation should be done to rule out other emotional problems, such as depression, as well as medical disorders, such as thyroid dysfunction, that can cause anxiety.

Anxiety attack. See PANIC ATTACK.

Aorta (ā ôr′tə) is the largest artery in the body, supplying blood to the organs alongside its course. It starts at the left ventricle of the heart, then arches upward and backward, giving off branch arteries to the heart muscles, head, and arms. The aorta then runs down the back of the chest, in front of the spine and esophagus (gullet), to reach the abdomen. Just above the pelvis, the aorta divides into the common iliac arteries to the legs.

See also ARTERY. p. 8.

Aortogram (ā ôr′tə gram) is an X-ray picture of the aorta taken after the injection of a special radiopaque dye into the blood vessels or heart. It is a type of arteriogram.

See also AORTA; ARTERIOGRAM.

Apgar score (äp′gar) is a rating system that evaluates a newborn infant's vital functions at one minute and again at five minutes after birth. The baby's heart rate, respiratory effort, muscle tone, reflex response, and color are scored from a low value of zero to a normal value of 2 at the one minute and five minute mark. A maximum score of 10 is rarely achieved at the one minute mark. Babies with a score of 7 to 10 are given routine postnatal care. The lower the rating under 7 the greater the evidence of distress. Infants with low Apgar scores (under 4 or 5) are more likely than those with higher scores to have some serious problems, for example, neurologic damage. Many of these infants, however, will be normal. The rating system was developed by Virginia Apgar, M.D.

APGAR score, family (äp′gar). The family APGAR is a questionnaire that measures satisfaction with the structure and function of a patient's family. It

Family APGAR questionnaire

	Almost always	*Some of the time*	*Hardly ever*
I am satisfied with the help that I receive from my family* when something is troubling me.	______	______	______
I am satisfied with the way my family* discusses items of common interest and shares problem solving with me.	______	______	______
I find that my family* accepts my wishes to take on new activities or make changes in my life style.	______	______	______
I am satisfied with the way my family* expresses affection and responds to my feelings such as anger, sorrow, and love.	______	______	______
I am satisfied with the amount of time my family* and I spend together.	______	______	______

Scoring: The patient checks one of three choices which are scored as follows: 'Almost always' (2 points), 'Some of the time' (1) point, or 'Hardly ever' (0). The scores for each of the five questions are then totaled. A score of 7 to 10 suggests a highly functional family. A score of 4 to 6 suggests a moderately dysfunctional family. A score of 0 to 3 suggests a severely dysfunctional family.

*According to which member of the family is being interviewed, the physician may substitute for the word 'family' either spouse, significant other, parents, or children.

Adapted from Smilkstein, G.: *J Family Practice* 6(6):1231–1234, 1979. © 1979. Reprinted by permission of Appleton and Lange.

has been administered most often as a screening test to study the families of children with chronic physical disorders. Some health professionals feel that the test helps identify chronically ill children likely to experience psychological difficulties because of family adaptation problems.

The acronym APGAR has been used to describe the functional components of Adaptability, Partnership, Growth, Affection, and Resolve. Five closed-end questions are used to gauge a family member's satisfaction with these basic components of family function (*see table, page 47*).

A physician or other health professional may recommend family therapy as a result of low APGAR scores.

Aphakia (ə fā'kē ə) is the condition of an eye in which the lens is absent. In rare cases, aphakia may occur as a congenital abnormality. More commonly, however, aphakia results from an eye injury or following a cataract operation.

See also CATARACT.

Aphasia (ə fā'zhə) is a neurologic condition in which an individual loses the ability to produce and/or understand spoken, written, or symbolic forms of communication. The condition may follow a stroke, concussion, prolonged hypoxia, or heart disease. Sometimes the condition is partial (dysphasia), and the person retains some ability to communicate and to understand communication. Aphasia may be temporary, as when the swelling in the brain goes down following a stroke. Intensive speech therapy is often successful in helping to restore the language function.

See also HEART DISEASE; HYPOXIA.

Aphonia (ə fō'nē ə) is the loss of the ability to produce normal speech sounds; it is sometimes only a temporary condition. Aphonia may be the result of an inflammation of the larynx (laryngitis); interference caused by muscular spasm; occasionally willful silence; or hysteria.

Aphrodisiac (af rə diz'ē ak) is a food, drug, or other substance that arouses sexual desire (libido). There are many substances that are said to have this property, but most are ineffectual. The results of an aphrodisiac are often dependent on how strongly the individual taking the substance believes in it (placebo effect). Many so-called aphrodisiacs are harmless, but some, such as cantharides (dried Spanish fly), may be poisonous, especially when taken in large amounts.

Aphthous ulcer. *See* ULCER, APHTHOUS.

Aplasia (ə plā'zhə) is the defective development or absence at birth of an organ or tissue. Aplasia may occur in the blood system and result in abnormal cell generation and development.

See also ANEMIA, APLASTIC; HYPERPLASIA.

Aplastic anemia. *See* ANEMIA, APLASTIC.

Apnea (ap nē'ə) is the temporary cessation of breathing. The condition may be induced during general anesthesia, or it may be caused by several neurologic disorders. Sleep apnea usually occurs because of airway obstruction; in such cases the sufferer wakes up gasping and may experience drowsiness and headache. Premature infants may experience episodes of apnea due to immaturity of the portion of the nervous system that regulates breathing.

Aponeurosis (ap ə nů rō'sis) is a broad, iridescent, often striated sheet of fiber or tissue that serves as an attachment between muscles and other portions of the anatomy. An aponeurosis is found in the skull, where it brings together the two muscles that hold the nerves of the face. It is also located in the abdomen, atop the rectus abdominis muscles. Often, aponeuroses appear in other parts of the body, as points of origin for certain muscles or as supports for holding muscles together. Sometimes, the aponeurosis stems directly from a bone.

Appendectomy (ap ən dek'tə mē) is the surgical removal of the vermiform appendix, the appendage to the upper part of the large intestine. The operation is generally performed after diagnosis of acute appendicitis, a painful inflammation of the appendix.

Q: *How is the appendectomy performed?*

A: The appendix is removed under general anesthesia, usually through a small incision in the lower, right-hand side of the abdomen. With acute appendicitis, the appendix may burst, and there is the slight risk that the operation itself may cause it to do so. If the appendix bursts and infection spreads to the lining of the abdomen (causing peritonitis), the surgeon leaves a tube in the wound to drain the infection to the surface; after about 48 hours the drain usually can be removed.

Q: *How long does recovery normally take after an appendectomy?*

A: After the operation, recovery is rapid. The stitches are removed after about five days, and the patient is able to leave the hospital within a week. But convalescence may take about a month or more while the various layers of tissue in the abdominal wall heal. In the past an appendectomy was considered a difficult and risky operation, but today the success rate is nearly 100 percent.

See also APPENDICITIS; APPENDIX.

Appendicitis (ə pen də sī′tis) is an inflammation of the vermiform appendix, an appendage to the cecum, the first part of the large intestine. The inflammation results from a bacterial infection that causes the appendix to swell and fill with pus. An early symptom of appendicitis is intermittent pain in the navel region. This becomes more severe and, within hours, localizes to the lower, right-hand corner of the abdomen. The abdominal muscles tighten, and the person loses his or her appetite and becomes nauseated. A slight fever is usual, as is constipation. (The inflammation, however, may on occasion trigger diarrhea.) The lower abdomen is tender. Touching increases the pain.

Q: *If appendicitis is suspected what should be done?*

A: Do not give a laxative. A physician should be consulted immediately. Failure to seek prompt medical attention could result in a burst appendix, causing peritonitis (a critical infection of the abdominal lining). With acute appendicitis, the patient usually is immediately taken to the hospital for an appendectomy, that is, an operation to remove the vermiform appendix. In mild cases of appendicitis, the inflammation may subside by itself.

Q: *Does appendicitis affect certain age groups more than others?*

A: Appendicitis is a common condition (1 to 2 cases per 1000 people annually). The condition can occur at any age. However, males between ages 10 and 30 are affected most commonly.

See also APPENDIX; CECUM; PERITONITIS.

Appendix (ə pen′diks) is any structure attached to a larger more important part. In medical terminology, however, the word appendix usually refers to the vermiform appendix, which is a worm-shaped growth attached to the cecum, or first part, of the large intestine.

In the human being, the vermiform appendix lies at the lower right of the abdomen. Some animals, for example, the higher apes, also have a vermiform appendix. In human beings, the vermiform appendix has no known function.

Inflammation of the appendix causes appendicitis.

See also APPENDICITIS.

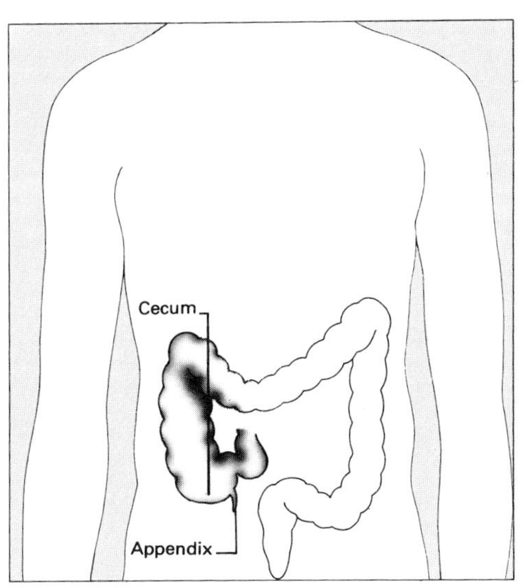

The vermiform **appendix** is a worm-shaped growth attached to the cecum (the first part of the large intestine). In human beings, the appendix has no known function.

Appetite (ap′ə tīt) is a healthy and natural desire for food. It should not be confused with hunger, the unpleasant, sometimes painful sensation caused by the body's need for food.

Many stomach disorders and other illnesses result in or are accompanied by a loss of appetite, which is known medically as anorexia. Some physical dysfunctions, such as an overactivity of the thyroid gland, increase the body's energy requirements and stimulate the appetite.

Such psychological conditions as depression may cause either compulsive eating or near loss of appetite. Anorexia nervosa is a psychological disorder characterized by an unwillingness to eat due to an intense fear of gaining weight. Bulimia, on the other hand, is characterized by uncontrollable binges, which may be followed by vomiting.

It is possible to control appetite with the use of medication; this can, however, be problematic due to dangerous side effects, as well as the potential for addiction. Appetite suppressants are only a short-term solution for the treatment of obesity. They should be used in conjunction with a sensible dietary regimen.

See also ANOREXIA NERVOSA; BULIMIA; DEPRESSION; THYROID GLAND.

Apraxia (ə prak'sē ə) is the inability to execute purposeful acts or to manipulate objects despite the physical ability to do so. The defect is due to disorders of the brain or neural pathways and results in an inability to conceptualize necessary movements and translate these movements into action. Certain types of apraxia may affect specific acts; for example, the inability to determine the use or purpose for such common items as pencils and toothbrushes.

Aqueous humor (ā'kwē əs hyü'mər) is the clear, watery fluid in the eye, just in front of the lens.

See also HUMOR.

Areola (ə rē'ə lə) is any small circular area of a different color. The term is usually used in reference to the area surrounding the nipple of the breast.

See also BREAST.

Argyll Robertson pupil (ar gīl' rob'ert son pyü'pəl) is a disorder in which the process of focusing the eye (accommodation) works normally, although the reflex response to light is absent. The pupil is usually contracted and so may appear smaller than normal. The condition is generally a sign of neurosyphilis, a late manifestation of the sexually transmitted disease syphilis.

See also ACCOMMODATION; SYPHILIS.

Arm is that portion of the upper limb of the body located between the shoulder and elbow. The portion below the elbow is the forearm. The arm contains one large bone, the humerus. The muscles of the arm include the *biceps brachii, brachialis, triceps brachii,* and the *anconeus.* Blood is supplied to the arm by several arteries, including the *brachial artery* and the *radial collateral artery.*

The forearm contains two bones, the radius and ulna. Attached to these bones are 19 muscles that move the wrist and fingers.

See also HUMERUS; RADIUS; ULNA.

Arm fracture: first aid. *See* FRACTURE: FIRST AID.

Armpit, or axilla, is the hollow place under the arm at the shoulder. Strong muscles attached to the chest and shoulder blade form the front and back walls and help to move the arm. The armpit contains arteries and veins, a network of nerves for the arm, sweat glands, lymph glands, and, in adults, hair.

Armpit abscesses may be caused by heavy sweating, infrequent washing, obstructed sweat glands, or too frequent shaving of the hair. Abscesses appear more often in people who have diabetes.

Pain in the armpit may be caused by boils, allergic skin problems, or swollen lymph glands. Painless swelling in the armpit may be a symptom of Hodgkin's disease.

See also ABSCESS; DIABETES; HODGKIN'S DISEASE.

Arrhythmia (ə rith'mē ə) is an irregularity in the heartbeat that produces a variation in pulse rate. In sinus arrhythmia, a normal occurrence in children, the pulse rate increases or decreases with breathing. Breathing alters the activity of the vagus nerve, and this changes the pulse rate. Sinus arrhythmia usually does not require treatment.

Other arrythmias, such as atrial fibrillation, bradycardia (a pulse that is too slow), and tachycardia (a pulse that is too rapid), may be more serious and often require medical evaluation and treatment.

If a physician detects an arrythmia during an exam, an electrocardiogram (EKG) is frequently performed to determine the type of arrythmia.

See also BRADYCARDIA; FIBRILLATION; TACHYCARDIA.

Arsenic (är'sə nik) is a nonmetallic chemical element that occurs chiefly in combination with other elements in the earth's crust. Its oxide, a grayish white powder, is extremely poisonous and may cause death. Accumulation of arsenic in the body causes nerve damage, weakness, headache, indigestion, diarrhea, discoloration and peeling of the skin, thickening of the skin on the palms and soles, white lines crosswise on the fingernails, and mental disorders.

Arteries, hardening of. *See* ARTERIOSCLEROSIS.

Arteriogram (är tir'ē ə gram) is an X-ray photograph of an artery. Before taking the X ray, the radiologist injects a radiopaque dye into the artery.

See also ANGIOGRAM; ARTERY.

Arteriole (är tir'ē ōl) is a blood vessel in a small arterial branch that feeds into capillaries. The muscular walls of arterioles play a major role in the regulation of blood pressure.

See also ARTERY; CAPILLARY; HYPERTENSION.

Arteriosclerosis (är tir ē ō sklə rō'sis) often called "hardening of the arteries," is an arterial disorder characterized by a progressive thickening and hardening of the walls of the arteries. This causes a decrease in or loss of blood circulation. The most common form of arteriosclerosis is atherosclerosis, which is characterized by the deposition of fatty substances in large and medium-sized arteries, such as the arteries that lead to the heart and brain. Atherosclerosis and its complications are a major cause of death in the United States. Heart and brain disease are often the direct result of this accumulation of fatty substances that impair the arteries' ability to nourish vital body organs.

Q: *What causes atherosclerosis?*

A: Hardening of the arteries is thought to be part of the aging process. However, other factors increase the likelihood of atherosclerosis: hypertension (high blood pressure); cigarette smoking; diabetes; obesity; and elevated levels of cholesterol and other fatty substances in the blood. Other factors that probably influence atherosclerosis include physical inactivity and a family predisposition.

Men, especially white men, are more prone to the condition than women. The rate of coronary heart disease is roughly six times greater for white males between the ages of 35 and 44 than it is for women. *See also* CHOLESTEROL; DIABETES; HYPERTENSION; OBESITY; SMOKING OF TOBACCO.

Q: *Is arteriosclerosis always serious?*

A: The seriousness of the condition depends upon which arteries are most affected. A narrowed artery to the heart can cause severe chest pains (angina pectoris) or a heart attack (myocardial infarction). *See also* ANGINA PECTORIS; HEART ATTACK.

A decrease of the blood leading to the brain can cause dizziness, numbness, slurred speech, loss of consciousness (fainting), or a stroke. If the arteries to the legs are affected, the person may feel pain in the calves when walking (intermittent claudication). Blockage in the arteries supplying blood to the kidneys can result in kidney damage. *See also* CLAUDICATION.

Blood clots in combination with arteriosclerosis can pose another serious situation. A blood clot (thrombus) that has formed in a blood vessel or in the heart can break free and travel through the bloodstream. If the clot reaches a vessel that leads to the brain and which is narrowed due to atherosclerosis, the clot may block the flow of blood completely, causing a stroke. If a limb is affected, such an obstruction can cause gangrene (tissue death). Prompt medical attention is mandatory if the limb is to be saved. *See also* BLOOD CLOT; GANGRENE.

Q: *What is the treatment for atherosclerosis?*

A: Although there is no known cure for atherosclerosis, therapeutic agents, such as nitroglycerin or beta-adrenergic blockers employed to increase oxygen levels in the blood supply, have been successful. Coronary-artery bypass surgery

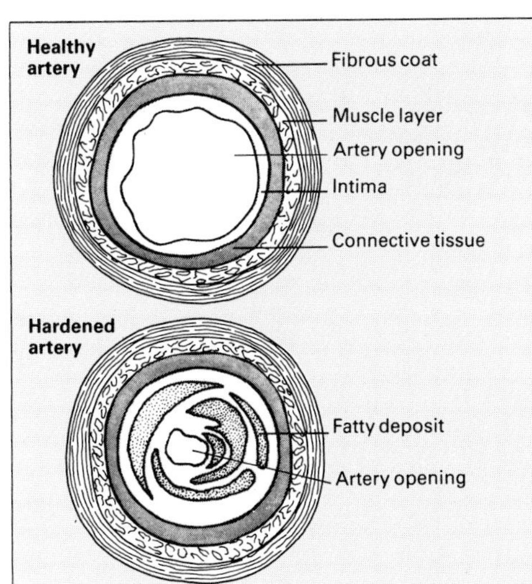

Arteriosclerosis is a disorder characterized by a thickening and hardening of the walls of arteries due to deposits of fatty substances.

may be used as a method of circumventing obstructed arteries. Treatment should also include preventive measures to keep the condition from getting worse. A patient should stop smoking, reduce his or her weight to a normal level, reduce the amount of cholesterol in the diet, keep diabetes under control, and exercise regularly.

See also ANGIOPLASTY; CORONARY-ARTERY BYPASS SURGERY.

Arteritis (är tə rī′tis) is an inflammation of the wall of an artery.

See also ARTERITIS, TEMPORAL; POLYARTERITIS NODOSA.

Arteritis, temporal (är tə rī′tis, tem′pər əl). Temporal arteritis is a progressive inflammation of the cranial blood vessels, especially those vessels in the forehead region. It is now known to be only part of generalized arteritis. Many other arteries may be inflamed at the same time. The disorder occurs most frequently in elderly women. Symptoms include severe headaches and pain with chewing. Diagnosis is made by biopsy of the affected artery. Steroids are the treatment of choice. Temporal arteritis, if untreated, may result in the loss of vision.

See also POLYARTERITIS NODOSA.

Artery (är′tər ē) is one of the tube-shaped blood vessels that carries blood away from the heart to the body's tissues and organs. Arteries are thick-walled, flexible, and muscular. The blood carried by most arteries is bright red because it has picked up oxygen while passing through the lungs. The blood that flows through the pulmonary arteries connecting the right side of the heart with the lungs has not yet picked up oxygen, so this blood has a dark bluish color. Blood flow is assisted by the contraction of the arterial muscles and the impetus given by the heart. This "push" from the heart can be felt where large arteries run near the body surface. *See also* PULSE, TAKING OF.

The largest artery is the aorta, which stems directly from the heart. Two small branches of the aorta, the *coronary* arteries, supply the blood that nourishes the heart muscle itself. The right and left *carotid* arteries carry blood to the two sides of the neck and head. Blood flows to the shoulders and arms through the right and left *subclavian* arteries.

In the abdominal region, the aorta divides into two large branches, the left and right *iliac,* that supply blood to the pelvic region. The iliac arteries then continue into the legs, where they are referred to as the *femoral* arteries.

The blood passes from the arteries into the very small capillaries. In the capillaries, oxygen and nourishment pass into the body's tissues; in exchange, impurities produced by the body's metabolic processes enter the blood. The blood then goes from the capillaries to the veins and returns to the heart. The heart pumps this blood through the pulmonary artery to the lungs, where it receives new oxygen. The blood is then returned to the heart, where it is once again pumped out through the aorta.

If arterial walls become hardened due to the accumulation of fatty substances, then blood flow can be diminished. Hardening of the arteries, arteriosclerosis, may result in heart or brain disease. It is a major cause of death in the U.S.

See also ARTERIOSCLEROSIS; CAPILLARY; HEART; VEIN.

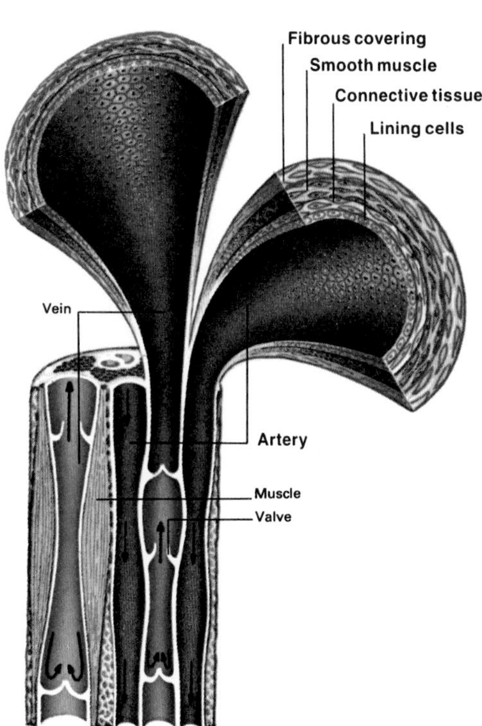

An **artery** is made up of tissue, muscle, and thin, smooth cells. Unlike veins, which carry dull-colored blood toward the heart, most arteries transport bright red, oxygen-rich blood away from the heart to various parts of the body.

Arthritis (är thrī′tis) is any of more than 100 inflammatory joint disorders characterized by pain, swelling, and limited movement. Arthritis may be caused by inflammation or infection in a joint, by degeneration of a joint as a person becomes older, or by a disorder of which arthritis is a symptom. More than 31 million people of all ages suffer from various degrees of the disease in the United States. The three most common forms of arthritis are *osteoarthritis*, *rheumatoid arthritis*, and *gout*.

Q: *What is osteoarthritis?*

A: Osteoarthritis, also called degenerative joint disease, occurs when a joint wears out. It is the type of arthritis most common in the elderly. The connecting surfaces of a joint become rougher as the cartilage lining the joint deteriorates. Osteoarthritis most commonly affects those joints that support weight, for example, the knees, the hips, and the spine. For this reason, the condition can be worse for overweight people. The effects of the aging process can be hastened if joints have been damaged earlier in life by an accident or by injury. Osteoarthritis can not be cured.

Q: *How is osteoarthritis treated?*

A: Treatment for osteoarthritis is constantly improving due to new, highly effective, pain-reducing, and anti-inflammatory drugs. Naproxen, sulindac, ibuprofen, piroxicam, and indomethacin have emerged as useful aspirin substitutes, although aspirin is still very effective. The major advantage of these aspirin substitutes is that they do not need to be taken as frequently as aspirin.

Care should be taken when walking or with other movements. A cane, a walker, or rubber heeled shoes may help alleviate some joint distress. If necessary, a person should lose weight. A living area can be modified to assist an arthritic person: handles near showers, toilets, and beds are useful aids. A straight-backed chair is easiest to use. In severe cases of osteoarthritis, joint replacement via surgery may be effective.

Q: *Can a person become crippled with osteoarthritis?*

A: Patients with osteoarthritis rarely become bedridden or crippled. The bulbous knobs that may develop on the fingers or toes can be painful and stiff, but serious crippling does not result. Pain flares up with sudden activity after rest, and a bad attack may last for several days. Osteoarthritis of a hip or a knee may prevent a patient from walking normally. If the joints in both legs are affected, the patient may become chairbound.

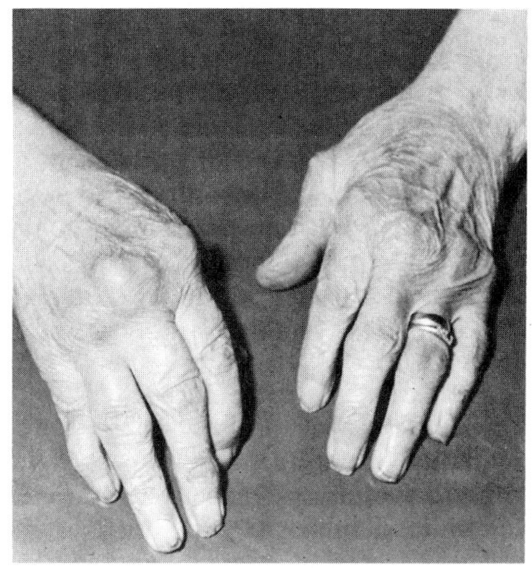

Q: *What is rheumatoid arthritis?*

A: Rheumatoid arthritis is painful swelling, usually of the smaller joints, together with the destruction of tissue around them. It most often begins in early adult life, between the ages of 30 and 40, and, although an attack may subside, it usually flares up again. The cause of this affliction remains unknown. There is a risk with rheumatoid arthritis of crippling or other physical deformity. In children, the condition is known as juvenile rheumatoid arthritis or Still's disease.

Q: *What is the treatment for rheumatoid arthritis?*

A: Treatment is aimed at providing relief from the symptoms and control of the inflammatory process. Damage to the joints that accompanies the disorder cannot, however, be repaired. Heat, in the form of shortwave diathermy, whirlpool baths, and wax baths, can give short-term relief. Physiotherapy may ease the pain and keep the joints mobile. Salicylate drugs (a category that includes aspirin) or other anti-inflammatory drugs may be prescribed. Some deformities resulting from the disease can be remedied by surgical techniques.

Arthritis, any one of more than 100 inflammatory diseases, characteristically produces pain, swelling, and limited movement in joints.

Q: *What is gout?*

A: Gout is a disorder in which the body can not rid itself of all the uric acid it produces. This is caused either by overproduction of uric acid or by an impairment of the removal of uric acid by the kidney. Excessive quantities of uric acid build up in the joints, as well as in various soft tissues. This can cause extremely painful attacks of arthritis. A blood test reveals a high concentration of uric acid in the bloodstream; study of fluid from an affected joint shows uric acid crystals. If diagnosis is made early, future attacks may be prevented by the regular use of drugs, such as probenecid or allopurinol.

Q: *What other disorders cause arthritic symptoms?*

A: Joints may become infected as part of a generalized disease, often accompanied by a fever and a feeling of general illness. Bacterial arthritis is the invasion of joint areas by bacteria, causing swelling and inflammation. It occurs with tuberculosis and gonorrhea. In children, rheumatic fever causes painful joints that become better, then worse over a period of weeks. This is an allergic reaction to streptococcus bacteria. Virus infections, such as rubella (German measles), mumps, and hepatitis, may produce inflamed joints. Arthritis may also be associated with the spinal disorder ankylosing spondylitis, with ulcers in the colon (colitis), or with inflammation of the urethra (Reiter's disease).

Q: *How effective are hydrocortisone or other steroid injections for treating arthritis?*

A: Hydrocortisone can not cure arthritis. Its effect is to reduce the inflammation in a joint and, thereby, relieve the pain. Treatment is highly effective for as long as the drug is present, but when the effect wears off, the pain may return. Too many injections are dangerous, because they may damage the joint.

Q: *How can surgery help patients with arthritis?*

A: A method of stopping pain in a stiff joint (such as the ankle) is the fusing together of bones via an operation (arthrodesis or artificial ankylosis). Another operation is the replacement of the affected joint by an artificial one made of steel or plastic. This is highly effective for arthritic fingers or a hip, but is less successful for knee or ankle joints.

See also ARTHRITIS, RHEUMATOID; GOUT; OSTEOARTHRITIS.

Arthritis, rheumatoid (är thrī′tis, rü′mə toid). Rheumatoid arthritis is a chronic and destructive form of joint inflammation. It is characterized by symmetrical swelling and often afflicts small joints in the wrist, hand, and ankle. Any joint, however, may be affected. The cause is not known, but rheumatoid arthritis is more common in women and usually first affects people between the ages of 30 and 40.

Q: *What are the symptoms of rheumatoid arthritis?*

A: Onset may be sudden, with inflammation in different joints. More often, however, the onset is gradual with more and more joints becoming inflamed. Tenderness in the affected joints is the most telling physical manifestation. Joints become stiff and swollen; corresponding joints on both sides of the body are often affected. The stiffness and swelling tend to be worse in the morning or after exercise. Nodules are frequently felt over joints or bones where they are near the skin surface. A person frequently feels unwell and easily becomes fatigued. Rashes and fevers can occur.

Joints often become deformed because of damage to the surrounding tissue and because of shortening of tendons. Persons with an acute onset of the disorder display obvious symptoms—fever and considerable joint pain. Those with a milder form of rheumatoid arthritis complain more of stiffness and lethargy.

Q: *How is rheumatoid arthritis treated?*

A: Bed rest is often prescribed for short periods during the most acute stages of the disease. Anti-inflammatory drugs are an integral part of any long-term treatment. Drug treatment usually consists of adequate dosages of aspirin or aspirin-like, anti-inflammatory drugs, such as indomethacin or sulindac. Other forms of drug treatment include injections of gold salts, D-penicillamine, and chloroquine.

Use of corticosteroid drugs results in dramatic improvement in the symptoms of rheumatoid arthritis. Their use has to be closely controlled because they may have to be taken for many years, with an increasing likelihood of adverse effects, without preventing the gradual progress of the underlying disorder.

Diet should be normal, and the patient should have frequent nutritious meals and take additional vitamins. Splints may be worn during the day or only at night if one or two joints are more severely affected than the others. Physiotherapy using gentle movements and exercises helps to maintain a full range of movement of the joints.

Q: *Do many patients become disabled?*

A: Most patients with rheumatoid arthritis maintain complete function of the joints. About 30 percent are left with some disability; despite appropriate treatment, 5 to 10 percent are eventually severely disabled.

Q: *What other forms of treatment are there for rheumatoid arthritis?*

A: Various forms of orthopedic surgery may be performed on joints that have become seriously deformed, but in which the active disease has ceased. Minor operations to relieve adhesions or to remove the inflamed synovial membrane (which lines the capsule of a joint and secretes lubricating fluid) may produce considerable improvement. Dramatic progress in replacement surgery now enables surgeons to insert plastic joints in fingers and to carry out total joint replacement in the hips and knees.

However, many patients cannot benefit from these procedures and may have to rely on specially designed appliances and equipment that can make everyday life simpler. These may include modified eating utensils and walking aids.

See also GOLD SALTS TREATMENT; OSTEOARTHRITIS.

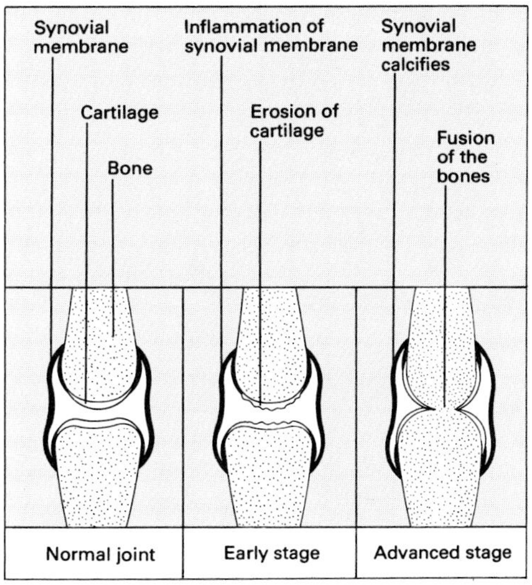

Rheumatoid arthritis is an inflammatory disease that leads to the calcification of joints.

Arthrodesis (är throd′ə sis) is the surgically induced fusing of the bones of a joint (artificial ankylosis). It is used to relieve such painful conditions as severe osteoarthritis; it is also performed to provide support to a joint injured in an accident.

See also ANKYLOSIS; OSTEOARTHRITIS.

Arthrography (är throg′rä fē) is a series of X-ray photographs taken of a joint after the injection of a radiopaque dye material.

Arthroplasty (är′thrə plas tē) is the surgical replacement or restoration of a joint. The surgery is done to reduce pain, restore mobility, or correct a congenital deformity.

See also ARTHRITIS, RHEUMATOID; OSTEOARTHRITIS.

Arthroscopy (är thros′kə pē) is the technique of using an arthroscope, a tube of optical fibers and lenses, to examine a joint or to perform some types of joint surgery. It is mainly employed in connection with knee injuries. Arthroscopy offers the advantage of a very small incision; the joint thus heals more quickly.

Arthroscopy is often performed in an outpatient setting, requiring no overnight hospital stay.

Artificial heart. *See* HEART, ARTIFICIAL.

Artificial insemination. *See* INSEMINATION, ARTIFICIAL.

Artificial kidney. *See* KIDNEY, ARTIFICIAL.

Artificial limb. *See* PROSTHESIS.

Artificial respiration (är tə fish′əl res pə rā′shən) is a lifesaving method used to restore breathing to a person whose breathing has stopped. It is often used to revive a person who has nearly drowned or whose heart has stopped beating. Other emergencies in which artificial respiration may be used are poisoning, stroke, smoke inhalation, electrocution, suffocation, and coma of any cause.

If breathing has stopped, the victim will soon be unconscious. There will be no chest movement, and the skin will be pale or a slightly bluish color. When a person stops breathing, oxygenation of the blood ceases, and irreversible brain damage or death may occur in four to six minutes. Therefore, artificial respiration techniques should be started as quickly as possible and continued until the patient recovers or emergency professional medical aid arrives. If resuscitated, the victim should be carefully observed until medical attention is received.

The most common and most efficient method of artificial respiration is either mouth-to-mouth or mouth-to-nose resuscitation. Barring an accident involving bad facial injuries, mouth-to-mouth resuscitation techniques are the safest and most efficient. Everyone is encouraged to learn these rescue techniques by taking a basic six-hour cardiopulmonary resuscitation (CPR) course.

Mouth-to-Mouth Resuscitation

(1) *Determine Unresponsiveness.* The rescuer should gently shake the victim and shout "Are you OK?" This precaution will prevent injury from attempted resuscitation of a person who is not truly unconscious.

(2) *Call for Help.*

(3) *Position the Victim.* Remove the victim from any immediately dangerous locations, that is, away from fire, smoke, downed electrical power lines, etc. Mouth-to-mouth can be started in water, if the victim is floating with his or her face out of the water. However, it is best to have the victim faceup on a firm surface, such as the floor or the ground.

(4) *Open the Airway.* The most important action for successful resuscitation is to immediately open the airway. In the unconscious victim, the tongue is commonly lax and blocking breathing. Since the tongue is attached to the lower jaw, moving the lower jaw forward will lift the tongue away from the back of the throat and open the airway. In some victims, breathing will now start. To open the airway, put one hand on the victim's forehead and apply firm, backward pressure with the palm to tilt the head back. (If, however, a neck injury is suspected, do not move the head unless absolutely necessary to open the airway.) Place the fingers of the other hand just under the chin and lift to bring the chin forward. (This position will almost close the upper and lower teeth.)

If vomit or foreign material is visible in the mouth, it should be removed. Excessive time must not be taken. Liquids should be wiped out with fingers covered by a piece of cloth. Solids should be "hooked-out" (not pushed in) by the index finger.

(5) *Determine Breathlessness.* With the airway open, look at the chest for signs of breathing. Put your ear next to the nose and mouth and listen for breathing. Feel for the flow of air. If there is no breathing, begin artificial respiration.

(6) *Mouth-to-Mouth Rescue Breathing.* Keep calm. Your breathing should be regular. The hand on the victim's forehead should be used to pinch the victim's nose closed. Take a deep breath and place your mouth tightly over the victim's mouth. Blow until the victim's chest rises. Listen for air being passively exhaled. Repeat with full breaths 12 times a minute. Children get smaller breaths, repeated at 20 times per minute.

(7) *Mouth-to-Nose Rescue Breathing.* This technique is more effective in some cases than mouth-to-mouth. It is recommended when it is impossible to ventilate through the victim's mouth, when the mouth cannot be opened, or when the mouth is seriously injured. Mouth-to-nose is the same as mouth-to-mouth, except the fingers on the chin lift and close the mouth completely. Air is blown into the victim's nose. The mouth may need to be dropped open to allow the victim to passively exhale. A combined mouth and nose resuscitation is used for infants. Here, the rescuer's mouth is placed over the infant's mouth and nose.

(8) *Airway Obstruction.* If the victim does not exhale passively, or his or her chest does not rise, the rescuer should assume the air passage is still blocked. Reposition the head and airway. Try

Mouth-to-mouth resuscitation

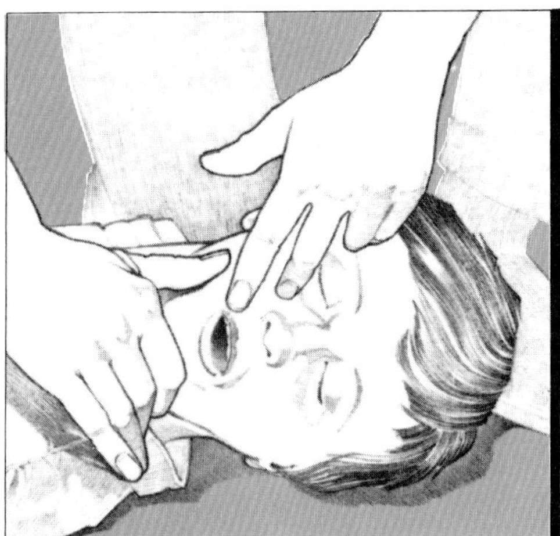

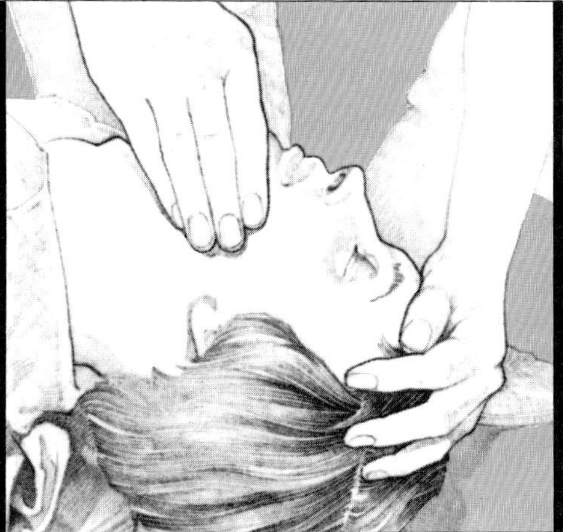

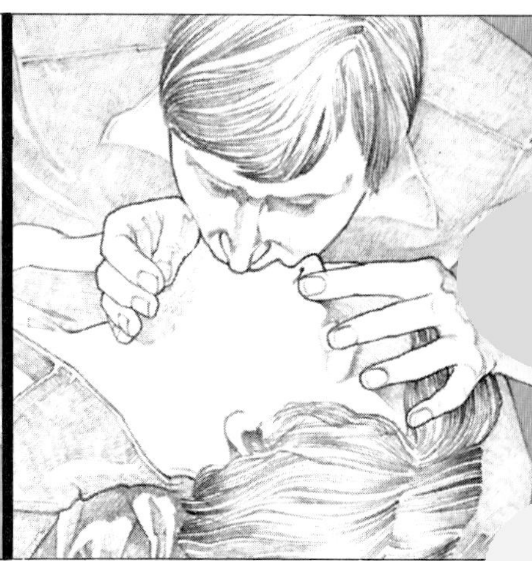

The airway must be opened as soon as possible. In the unconscious victim, the tongue is usually slack and is blocking the airway. Since the tongue is attached to the lower jaw, move the jaw forward; this will lift the tongue and open the airway.
If vomit or foreign material is visible in the mouth, it should be removed. Liquids should be wiped out with fingers (covered, when possible, with a piece of cloth). Solids should be hooked-out (not pushed in) by the index finger.

To open the airway, put one hand on the victim's forehead and apply firm, backward pressure to tilt the head back. (If a neck injury is suspected, do not move the head unless it is essential to open the airway.) Place the fingers of the other hand under the chin and lift to bring the chin forward; the teeth will be almost closed.

Remain calm. Your breathing should be regular. The hand on the victim's forehead should be used to pinch the victim's nose closed. Take a deep breath and place your mouth tightly over the victim's mouth. Blow until the victim's chest rises.

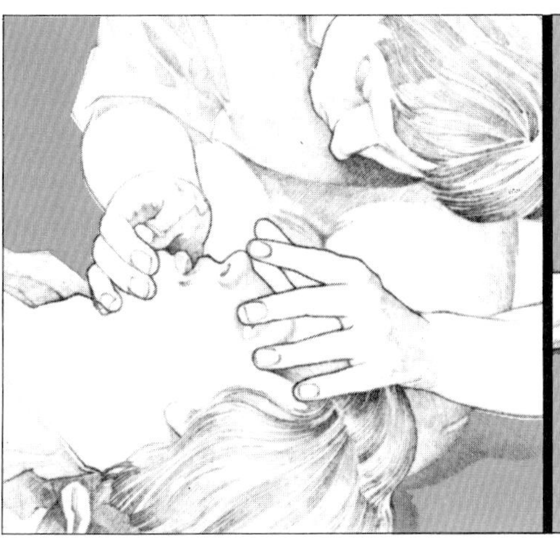

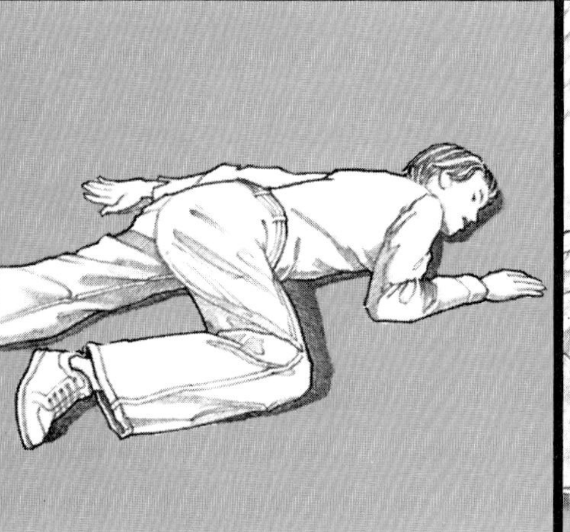

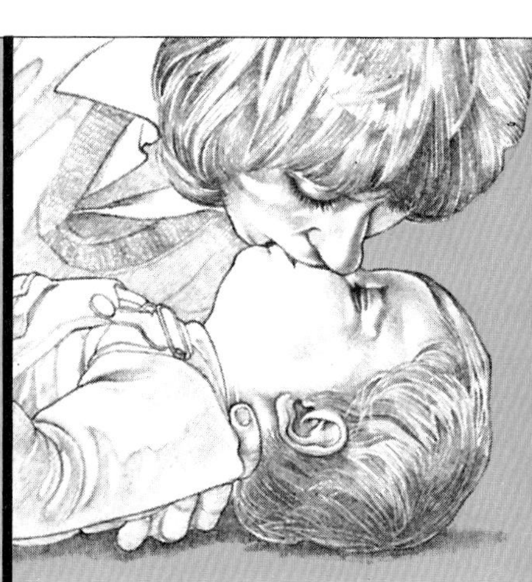

When you have filled the victim's lungs, remove your mouth and watch the chest deflate as you take another deep breath. Repeat the action with full breaths 12 times a minute. (With children, repeat the action 20 times per minute, but with smaller breaths.)

When breathing has been restored, turn the victim over to the recovery position illustrated above. Observe the victim's breathing and take his or her pulse until medical help arrives.

A combined mouth and nose resuscitation is used for infants. Here, the rescuer's mouth is placed over the infant's mouth and nose. Breathe in through your nose, fill your cheeks with air, and puff the air gently into the child. Finish exhaling through your nose. Repeat the action 20 times per minute.

breathing again. If this fails, try wiping or hooking-out the mouth again. If this does not relieve the obstruction, perform a type of Heimlich maneuver. Face the victim and kneel straddling the victim's thighs. Place one of your hands over the other, with the heel of the bottom hand on the victim's abdomen, slightly above the navel, but below the rib cage. Press into the victim's abdomen with a quick upward thrust. Care should be exercised to direct the thrust upward in the midline and not to either side of the abdomen. Do not go too high and push on the ribs. Several thrusts may be necessary to expel an object. In small children, this maneuver must be applied gently. *See also* CHOKING AND COUGHING: FIRST AID.

For infants under one year, avoid the abdominal thrust and the Heimlich maneuver. Instead, the infant should be straddled over your forearm, with the head down and supported by holding the infant's jaw. Rest the same forearm on your thigh and, with the heel of the other hand between the infant's shoulder blades, forcefully deliver four back blows.

If all attempts to dislodge material fail, then a surgical operation to make a hole in the windpipe (cricothyrotomy or tracheotomy) is the last resort.

Asbestosis (as bes tō′sis) is a chronic lung disease caused by the inhalation of asbestos fibers. Progressive shortness of breath and a dry cough are the most common symptoms. People who work with asbestos minerals are most often affected, but the disease may also occur in those casually exposed to asbestos building materials.

Asbestosis may trigger the development of mesothelioma, a rare malignant tumor of the pleura, the tissue covering the lungs. Tobacco smoking greatly increases the risk of such a tumor developing. Because of the long delay between exposure to asbestos and the onset of a mesothelioma, exposure that occurred even decades ago (for example, among World War II shipyard workers) may place a person at risk.

See also PNEUMOCONIOSIS.

Ascariasis (as kə rī′ə sis) is an infection of the stomach and intestinal region by roundworms *(Ascaris lumbricoides)*. The worm eggs are passed in human feces and transmitted through contaminated hands, food, or water. Early symptoms of the infection include coughing and a fever. Abdominal pain and diarrhea can accompany the worms' passage into the intestinal region. Migration of the adult worms into the liver or gall bladder can be fatal. The disease can be avoided through such sanitation habits as handwashing.

See also WORM.

Ascites (ə sī′tēz) is an abnormal accumulation of fluid in the abdominal cavity. Symptoms may include abdominal swelling and lowered urinary output. Ascites may itself be a complication of cirrhosis of the liver or various infectious diseases. Treatment, if possible, should target the underlying cause. Abstinence from alcohol is essential in alcohol-induced cirrhosis. Infective causes should be treated with antibiotics. If the ascites does not improve, treatment should include nutrition therapy (sodium and water restriction) and drugs that help promote urinary output.

See also CIRRHOSIS; EDEMA.

Ascorbic acid (ā skôr′bik) is the chemical name for vitamin C. Principal sources include citrus fruits, potatoes, and such green, leafy vegetables as broccoli. Vitamin C helps build teeth and bones. A lack of sufficient vitamin C causes the disease scurvy.

While it is a commonly held belief that vitamin C prevents or helps to fight the common cold, there is no clear scientific evidence for this.

See also SCURVY; VITAMIN.

Asepsis (ə sep′sis) is the condition of an environment that is free from infecting organisms. In operating rooms, for example, it is most desirable that there be no airborne infection. To achieve asepsis, the air is filtered and kept at a higher pressure than the outside air pressure, so that the aseptic air can not be contaminated by unfiltered air. Operating instruments, surgical clothes, and gloves are all sterilized beforehand, and surgeons scrub their hands and forearms before dressing. Complete asepsis is not possible in a situation where humans are present. In the pharmaceutical industry many drugs are prepared and packaged in closed chambers to ensure sterility of the products.

Aspartame (as par′tām) is a substance obtained from aspartic acid and phenylalanine and often used as an artificial sweetener. It is about 200 times as sweet as sucrose and is used as a sugar substitute. One brand of aspartame is NutraSweet®.

Aspergillosis (as pėr jə lō′sis) is an infection that usually begins in the lungs and is caused by any member of the genus of fungi *Aspergillus*. Although the infection is fairly uncommon, it can be dangerous if it occurs in patients with inadequate immune defenses, such as cancer chemotherapy patients.

Asphyxia (as fik′sē ə) is a condition in which an interference with the breathing process has seriously affected or even stopped the action of the heart and lungs. Irreversible brain damage or death may result unless the victim's breathing (oxygen supply) is restored within four to six minutes.

Asphyxia is most often caused by suffocation (choking or obstruction of the air passages). Other causes include drowning, electric shock, and inhalation of toxic smoke.

See also ARTIFICIAL RESPIRATION; SUFFOCATION.

Aspirin (as′pər in), also known as acetylsalicylic acid, is one of the most commonly used pain-reducing drugs (analgesics) in the world. It is also used as an antipyretic to reduce fever and is beneficial as an anti-inflammatory drug in the treatment of the symptoms of such diseases of the joints as rheumatoid arthritis, osteoarthritis, and rheumatic fever. In addition, aspirin interferes with blood clotting. Research has suggested that it may also be useful in preventing strokes and other disorders that involve blood clots. Heart attack and stroke patients are generally prescribed one aspirin tablet a day to reduce the risk of recurrence.

The usual dosage of aspirin is effective for about three to four hours. Aspirin does not actually cure diseases, but merely relieves symptoms.

Q: *Is aspirin a harmless drug?*

A: Aspirin is a relatively safe drug when taken at recommended dosage levels. However, it can irritate the lining of the stomach and cause small amounts of stomach bleeding. Continued use of large doses of aspirin may cause blood clotting defects and liver and kidney disorders. Continued use of aspirin may also lead to anemia, due to blood loss from the digestive tract. Aspirin should not be given to children who have chicken pox or influenza, as the dangerous condition, Reye's syndrome, may result. It should not be taken by pregnant women, and it should be given with caution to infants.

Q: *Which disorders indicate caution with aspirin?*

A: Persons who have peptic ulcers should not use aspirin without medical advice; internal bleeding may occur, and blood may be vomited (hematemesis). People who suffer from persistent indigestion and patients taking anticoagulant drugs are also advised against taking aspirin. Mild sensitivity to aspirin may cause an itchy skin irritation (urticaria) or allergic asthma. Acetaminophens, such as Tylenol®, are often taken instead of aspirin.

See also ACETAMINOPHEN; REYE'S SYNDROME.

Asthenia (as thē′nē ə) is a condition of weakness, usually arising from muscular or psychological disorders.

Asthma (az′mə) is a chronic respiratory disorder in which a person experiences difficulty in breathing, accompanied by wheezing and a "tight" chest. Additional symptoms can be a dry cough and vomiting (usually in children). An asthma attack may start suddenly; the fear and worry that this causes can prolong the attack.

Q: *What causes asthma attacks?*

A: Asthma attacks are caused by a narrowing of the small bronchial tubes in the lungs. The most common kind of asthma (allergic bronchial asthma) is caused by an allergic reaction. Many pollens, molds, dusts (especially dust containing the house mite), and ani-

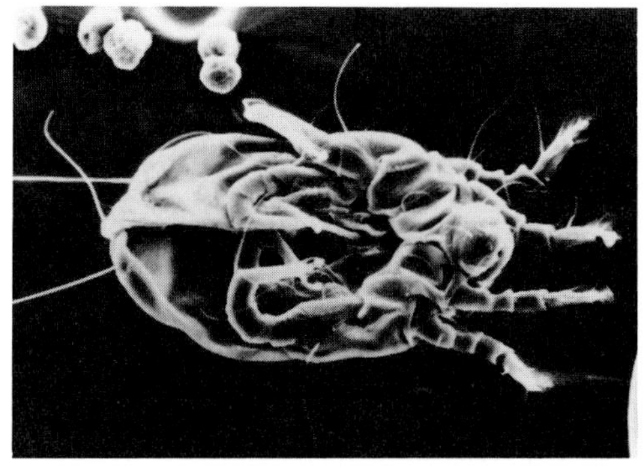

The house mite, commonly found in ordinary house dust, can, in some victims, trigger an allergic reaction that causes an attack of allergic bronchial asthma, the most common type of **asthma.**

mal hair and dander can cause allergic-type asthma attacks. Asthmatic symptoms are sometimes associated with hay fever. Infection in the respiratory system, exposure to cold, exercise, fatigue, irritating fumes, and certain emotional and psychological states can all trigger an asthma attack. These conditions may also serve as secondary factors that increase the severity or frequency of attacks. Asthma from these causes may occur in people who have no history of allergic reactions, as well as in those who do.

Q: *How does asthma interfere with breathing?*

A: Air passes through the lungs via tubes (called bronchi) and smaller vessels (bronchioles). With asthma, the smaller bronchi and bronchioles become swollen and clogged with mucus, and the muscles surrounding the bronchioles contract so that the air that should pass through is unable to do so. The body reacts to the lack of oxygen, and the patient forces more and more air into the lungs. But, because of the blockages, there is difficulty in exhaling it. The wheezing noise is caused by air being forcibly exhaled through the narrowed bronchi. *See also* BRONCHIOLE; BRONCHUS.

Q: *How long does an asthma attack last?*

A: An attack of asthma may last for a few minutes, but most go on for several hours. A severe, prolonged attack (a form of asthma known as status asthmaticus) may last for a number of hours or even days. A person with status asthmaticus requires hospitalization.

Q: *What immediate help can be given to a person suffering from asthma?*

A: With more severe attacks it is important that the patient sit upright, either in a chair or in bed, propped up by pillows. A table in front of the patient is useful; this can be grasped and the arm muscles used to assist breathing. A patient is rarely hungry, but should be encouraged to drink large amounts of liquids. Bronchial dilator inhalants from aerosol cans may be helpful in relaxing the muscles of the bronchioles. These are available by prescription and must be used according to a physician's direction. Severe episodes of asthma require immediate medical attention.

Q: *How does a physician treat asthma between attacks?*

A: The goal is to prevent an attack by keeping the bronchi and bronchioles from becoming narrowed. Theophylline, or such adrenergic drugs as epinephrine and isoproterenol, can relieve bronchospasms and, thus, help to prevent bronchial obstruction. (These drugs can also be used during an asthma attack.) Corticosteroids may be useful for short-term relief in severe cases. A new type of inhalant drug, cromolyn sodium (disodium cromoglycate or DSCG), has also proven successful in preventing asthmatic attacks in some persons. The proper drug or combination of drugs will depend upon the prescribing physician as well as the course of the disorder.

Q: *What is the treatment for severe asthma (status asthmaticus)?*

A: An attack of status asthmaticus requires hospitalization and urgent treatment. Some drug treatments are best administered as a mist through a breathing apparatus. Strong bronchodilators can relieve the attack by relaxing the spasms in the bronchioles. In this situation the patient may be attached to a mechanical respirator to aid breathing.

Q: *Apart from taking the appropriate drugs, what other precautions can be taken to prevent an asthma attack?*

A: Several simple measures can reduce the risk of attack. The appropriate medication should be taken prior to events known to trigger an episode—before exercise, for example. A person with allergic asthma should sleep in a room without carpets or rugs. Blankets and pillows of synthetic fiber reduce the risk of house dust and mites. In dry climates, a humidifier can be used to increase the moisture content of the air in the room.

For patients in whom asthma is caused by respiratory infection, breathing exercises may be of value. A respiratory therapist can teach the patient the most appropriate ones. These exercises are not only a psychological help in preventing an attack, but when minor respiratory infection does occur, the lungs should function more efficiently. An asthmatic patient should seek medical advice promptly when suffering from a respiratory infection.

Q: *Are there any complications involved with chronic asthma?*

A: Because so much air is held in the lungs during an asthma attack, the air sacs (alveoli) can become so stretched that the cell walls may tear. This damage causes a gradual loss of elasticity in the lungs and can lead to the condition known as emphysema. If the patient coughs too much, the surface of a lung may burst, causing the air to escape into the cavity that encloses the lung (pleural cavity). This condition is known as a pneumothorax. *See also* ALVEOLUS.

Other complications can arise from the mucous secretions that do not drain properly during an asthma attack. This can lead to bronchitis and sometimes bronchial pneumonia. Frequent attacks may result in chronic bronchitis.

Q: *What other disorders might be confused with asthma?*

A: A disorder mistakenly known as cardiac asthma has symptoms similar to asthma (gasping for breath, a "tight" chest), but is actually a type of heart disease. Immediate medical attention is required. *See also* ASTHMA, CARDIAC.

Q: *Can asthma be cured completely?*

A: Asthma cannot be cured. The possibility of future attacks can, however, be minimized by drugs and other preventives, but if a person is disposed to asthma, there is always a chance that an attack will occur.

Q: *Is asthma common in children?*

A: Asthma is fairly common in childhood, usually first occurring between the ages of three and eight. Most attacks are an allergic reaction to airborne pollen, certain foods, animal hair, and some other substances. The majority of children with asthma are from families with a history of the illness. Before puberty, asthma occurs more often among boys than girls; after puberty, the incidence is fairly equal between the sexes. Medical treatment includes teaching a child and his or her parents how to detect symptoms of an attack and how to use prescribed medications. Emotional stress can often trigger an asthma attack; children with emotional problems may thus require some form of psychological support.

See also EMPHYSEMA; HAY FEVER; PNEUMOTHORAX.

Asthma, cardiac (az′mə, kär′dē ak). Cardiac asthma is an asthma-like attack that accompanies congestive heart failure. The condition is marked by bronchospasms and wheezing, as well as rapid, shallow breathing, increased blood pressure and heart rate, and a feeling of apprehension. Cardiac asthma is a life-threatening disorder that is caused by body fluids being pushed back through the pulmonary (lung) capillaries. The fluids then quickly enter the bronchioles and alveoli, triggering the symptoms. The

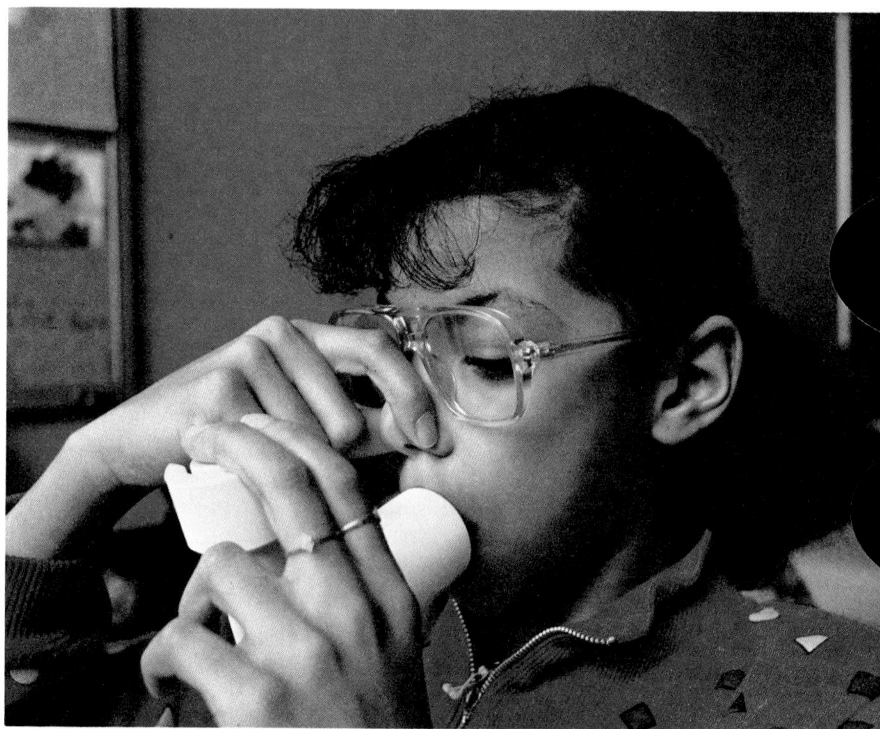

The **asthma** victim experiences wheezing, the sensation of a "tight" chest, and difficulty in breathing. Bronchial dilator inhalants, available by prescription, can be helpful in relaxing the muscles of the bronchioles, airways that connect the bronchi and the lobes of the lung. The relaxation of these muscles aids in the relief of asthmatic symptoms.

condition is sometimes called cardiasthma.

See also PULMONARY DISEASE, CHRONIC, OBSTRUCTIVE.

Astigmatism (ə stig′mə tiz əm) is a distortion in vision caused by an irregularity in the curvature of either the outer layer (cornea) of the eye or the lens. Light rays passing through are not accurately focused on the retina at the back of the eye; the result is a blurring of vision. More serious cases can be compensated for by the use of eyeglasses or contact lenses.

Astringent (ə strin′jənt) is a substance that helps to stop the outflow of internal body fluids, especially of blood or mucus. Astringents may work in a number of ways: (1) by making the blood vessels smaller; (2) by helping the blood to coagulate; or (3) by removing the water that is essential to the formation of mucus. They are important in treating bleeding from the nose and throat, bleeding from surface wounds, and surface ulcers. The most common astringents are metallic astringents (for example, copper sulfate, silver nitrate, or calcium carbonate); epinephrine, natural and synthetic; vegetable astringents (such as witch hazel); and substances containing alcohol (for example, cologne).

Ataxia (ə tak′sē ə) is a condition chararcterized by the loss or impairment of normal coordination, especially the coordination of voluntary movements of the muscles. Ataxia is caused by a lesion in the spinal cord or cerebellum, the part of the brain that helps to control balance. It may be caused by a birth defect, head injury, infection, drug or alcohol overdose, brain tumor, or other disorder.

Atelectasis (at′ə lek′tə sis) is either complete or partial collapse of a lung. The term refers to two distinct conditions. The first is the failure of the lungs to expand at birth, and the second is the collapsed (airless) condition of a segment of a lung. This collapse is generally caused by an obstruction in the tube (bronchus) leading to the lung, or by excessive secretion of mucus in the airway. Such a condition can occur in several respiratory disorders, particularly in pneumonia but also in bronchitis. Pressure from outside the lungs from a tumor or an expanded blood vessel (aneurysm), for example, can also press on part of a lung and cause a collapse.

Q: *What is the treatment for atelectasis?*

A: If the cause of the collapse is a blocked bronchus, such an obstruction may be removed by using a special instrument called a bronchoscope. Atelectasis from other causes can often be corrected by breathing exercises and respiratory therapy treatments.

Q: *Are there any possible complications of atelectasis?*

A: If excessive amounts of mucus are the cause of the collapse, the mucus build-up can become infected. Atelectasis following surgery may cause a fever.

Atheroma (ath ə rō′mə) is an abnormal condition of the large arteries in which areas of the arterial walls become clogged with fatty tissue. It is part of the disease arteriosclerosis.

See also ARTERIOSCLEROSIS; LIPID.

Atherosclerosis. *See* ARTERIOSCLEROSIS.

Athlete's foot, or tinea pedis, is a chronic surface infection of the foot caused by any of a number of fungi. It is characterized by itching, cracking, and small blisters between the toes. Pain and irritation may accompany the infection. The fungus grows on moist skin and is usually transmitted in places where people walk barefoot, such as communal showers and swimming pools. The wearing of confining footwear, such as sneakers, may also induce the infection. The disorder is more prevalent among adults.

Q: *How is athlete's foot treated?*

A: Athlete's foot is usually treated with antifungal lotions, ointments, or powders available without prescription. Finding the most suitable treatment is largely a matter of trial and error. It is important that the infected area be kept dry. Care should be taken to wipe off all moisture after bathing or swimming. If home treatment fails, or if an abscess forms, a health professional should be consulted.

Q: *Can similar infections occur elsewhere on the body?*

A: Yes. Similar infections can appear between the legs (tinea cruris), on the face, under the arms, in the

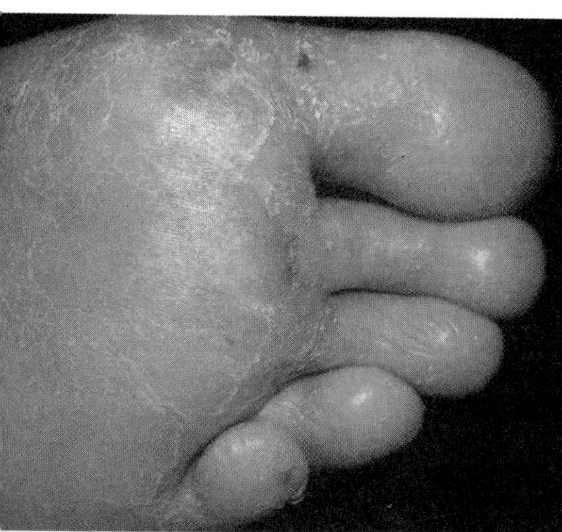

Athlete's foot, a chronic fungal infection, causes itching, cracking, and small blisters between the toes. The condition is treated with nonprescription antifungal medications.

scalp (tinea capitis), and in the beard area (tinea barbae).

Atopic (ə top′ik) refers to a hereditary tendency toward allergic reaction. Asthma, hay fever, and eczema are believed to be atopic allergies. Only a tendency toward an allergic reaction, not a specific disorder, is hereditary.

See also ALLERGY; ASTHMA; ECZEMA; HAY FEVER.

Atrial fibrillation. *See* FIBRILLATION.

Atrium (ā′trē əm) is the medical term for a cavity or chamber. It is used most often to describe each of the two blood-collecting chambers in the heart.

See also HEART.

Atrophy (at′rə fē) is the wasting away of tissue, of an organ, or of the entire body. It may be caused by disease, lack of physical exercise, or poor nutrition.

Atrophy, acute yellow. *See* HEPATITIS.

Atropine (at′rə pēn) is an anticholinergic, alkaloid drug that is extracted from several plants, including the belladonna plant. The actions of atropine result from its blocking of the neurotransmitter acetylcholine. Its effect of stopping the flow of salivary secretions in the mouth makes it valuable as a preanesthetic drug to maintain a clear pathway when the anesthetic is to be inhaled. A weak solution of atropine is often applied to the eye to make the pupil dilate. This makes various eye examinations easier for the physician to do. Atropine is also used to treat involuntary muscle spasms in the intestine and bladder. The drug should not be used by persons suffering from various diseases including glaucoma and urinary tract obstruction. Side effects include facial flushing, dry mouth, accelerated heart beat, and constipation.

See also ACETYLCHOLINE.

Attention deficit disorder is a condition that usually affects school-aged children and is characterized by inattention, impulsivity, or hyperactivity. These disorders are occasionally a result of environmental stress. Most cases, however, are felt to have a biological basis.

Attention deficit disorders should be differentiated from mental retardation, schizophrenia, or a manic-depressive state. The onset is before the age of 7 years, and an estimated 5 percent of school-aged children exhibit characteristics of some form of learning disorder. I.Q. tests taken by these children are normal, and there are no neurologic abnormalities. Attention deficit disorders may result in poor school performance. In some cases, there are specific learning disabilities, such as visual-motor or speech defects. Treatment is complex and should be coordinated with specific educators. There is no proof that dietary changes are beneficial.

See also HYPERACTIVITY.

Audiogram (ô′dē ə gram) is a chart showing the results of a hearing ability test as recorded by a delicate instrument called an audiometer. The test is based upon the human ability to hear sounds of different frequencies and loudness.

See also DEAFNESS.

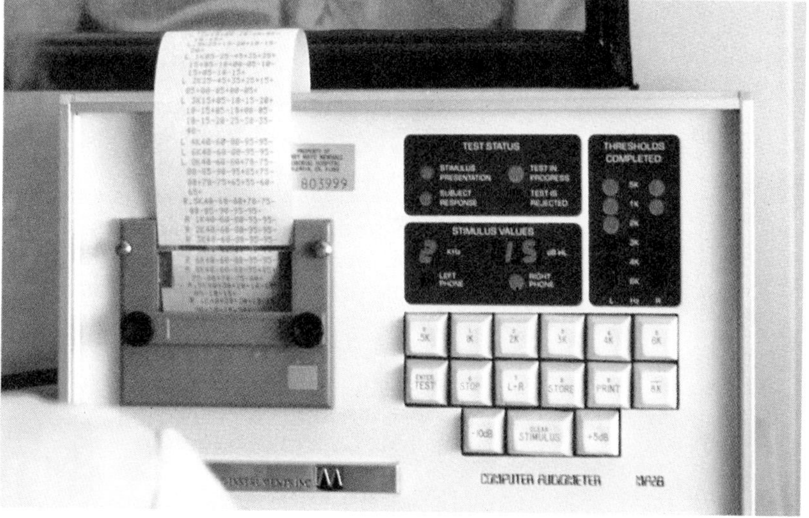

An **audiogram** is a chart that shows the results of a hearing test based upon sounds of different frequencies and loudness.

Auditory nerve. *See* NERVE.

Aura (ôr′ə) is a subjective sensation of awareness that may precede an approaching attack of such disorders as epilepsy or migraine.

Auricle (ôr′ə kəl) is a term that is used to refer to two separate and distinct parts of the body. It can be either (1) the external projecting part of the ear (also called the pinna); or (2) one of the ear-shaped appendages projecting from each atrium of the heart.

See also ATRIUM.

Autism (ô′tiz əm) is a condition characterized by an inability to relate to people. The incidence of the condition is approximately 2 in every 10,000 live births.

Autistic infants do not cuddle and do not like to be picked up. They prefer to be left alone and are intolerant of change in their environment. Autistic children may respond with tantrums to such changes as the rearrangement of furniture or toys. Many autistic children are mute; in others, the development of speech is severely restricted to a repetition of a few words. Physical development is normal.

Q: *Can autism be successfully treated?*

A: Some autistic children improve spontaneously. Others respond to a specialized plan of treatment. However, less than 25 percent of autistic children get better. Over half of all autistic children require residential placement by the end of adolescence.

Autoimmune disease (ô tō i myün′) is any disorder in which the body treats its own tissues or cells as if they were foreign substances and produces antibodies and/or lymphocytes to destroy those tissues or cells. Autoimmunity is known to be the cause of certain types of blood disorders. It is also a suspected factor in such diseases as chronic lymphocytic thyroiditis, multiple sclerosis, ulcerative colitis, and rheumatoid arthritis, although proof of this has not yet been established. In diseases definitely established as autoimmune, treatment includes drugs that suppress the production of antibodies. In a severe case, a patient may require hospitalization.

See also ANTIBODY; LYMPHOCYTE.

Automatism (ô tom′ə tiz əm) is a condition in which a person performs acts without conscious knowledge or later memory of what he or she is doing. Although the person appears to be functioning normally, he or she does not manifest personality, and behavior may be abnormal. The condition commonly represents an hysterical trance. It may also follow some severe trauma or an attack of certain forms of epilepsy. Sleepwalking is one example of automatism.

See also EPILEPSY; SLEEPWALKING.

Automobile, escape from. *See* AUTOMOBILE SAFETY.

Automobile safety. Motor vehicle accidents are the leading cause of accidental deaths. Anyone who drives a car or other vehicle is exposing himself or herself to unavoidable dangers, but it is important to realize that many accidents can be prevented by taking simple safety precautions.

When choosing a car, consider carefully the number of safety factors incorporated into the car's design. Safety regulations now demand that cars be designed in accordance with certain specifications, but above these minimum legal requirements there are wide variations in design.

If you already own a car, there are a number of items of equipment that can improve its safety and for which you, as the owner or driver, are responsible. Some of the items are illustrated in this article. They are not just attractive accessories; they might actually save your life. The National Safety Council recently calculated that if safety belts were worn at all times by all car drivers and passengers, at least 12,000 to 15,000 lives would be saved each year. Many states in the United States now have laws requiring drivers and front-seat passengers to wear safety belts.

Of course, it is important not just to equip your car with these accessories but to use them every time you drive. You should wear your safety belt for every journey, no matter how short. Every time you travel with young children, make sure that they are placed securely in their child seats or harnesses in the center of the back seat. This not only protects children in the event of an accident, but also prevents them from distracting the driver. Child restraints are also required by law in all states. Make sure that the doors are locked. If there is a dog or other animal in the car, it should travel behind a grid in the back of the car.

You should carry a first-aid kit, a fire extinguisher, and a reflective warning device in your car. The warning device can be placed on the road and used as a warning sign in the event of an accident or a breakdown. Also carry a tool box, a tire gauge, and a jack designed for your car.

Your mirrors should be aligned to allow the best possible vision of the traffic behind you. A simple wide driving mirror is safer than a convex mirror, which distorts distances and thereby makes judgment of speeds more difficult. You should have your car regularly serviced, and you yourself should be able to check the condition of the tires, shock absorbers, oil, brakes, windshield wipers, and lights. By caring for the running condition of your car, you minimize the dangers of accident or breakdown.

Emergencies

A responsible driver is aware that at any time he or she may be expected to deal with emergencies. The lives of passengers and others may depend on the driver's knowledge and skill, and the driver should take all possible precautions to minimize the risks of accident or breakdown.

Planning Ahead

Before starting any journey the driver should ensure that his or her car is in good condition. Check the engine oil level, the tire pressures (including the spare tire), the brakes, the headlights, the water level in the cooling system, the battery, and the gasoline. Take a plastic bottle or can in which to carry an emergency supply of water in case you run out. Check the car's equipment; make sure that the jack and the tool box are in the car and that all movable objects in the trunk are secure.

For longer journeys, work out your intended route carefully before setting out, and take maps with you. If possible, find out the weather forecasts for the areas through which you intend to travel. Tell a reliable person details of the route to be taken and your estimated time of arrival.

Safety devices

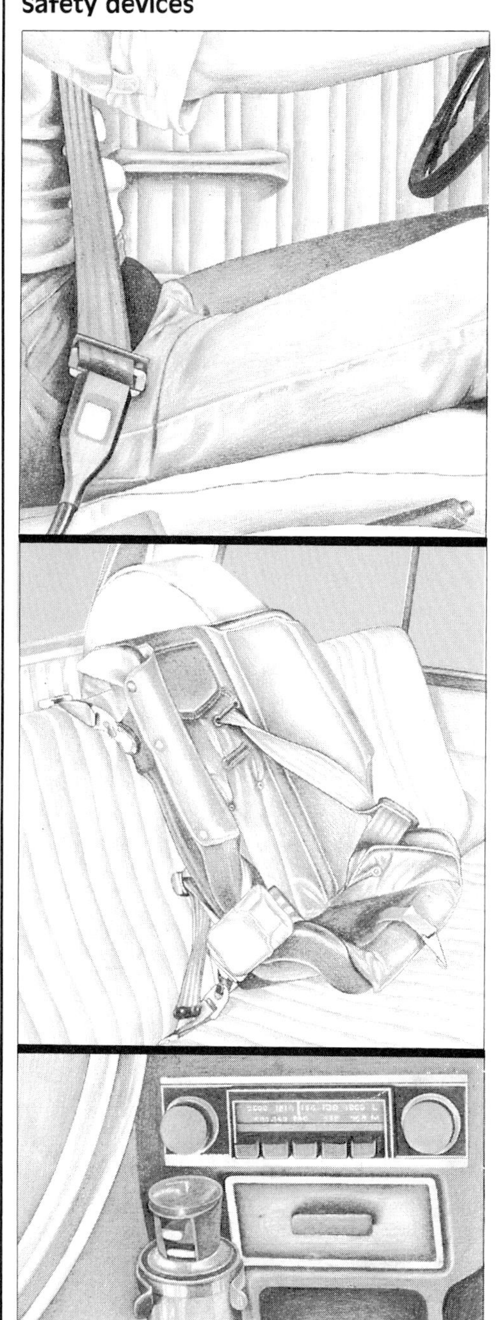

Safety belts
Safety belts with shoulder and lap straps should be worn by the driver and front-seat passengers during every journey. Back-seat passengers should wear their lap belts. Check that safety belts are fitted securely and that they are easily accessible to passengers.

Child seats
Children under the age of five should travel in crash-tested child safety seats that are secured to existing adult seat belts. If a child seat is equipped with a top strap, it must be properly anchored to the car seat. The back center seat position is the safest location in the car. Children over five years should use adult safety belts.

Fire extinguisher
A fire extinguisher should be fitted securely to the interior of the car. The extinguisher can be of the dry powder, liquid, or gas-filled type, but must be capable of extinguishing fuel and electrical fires. Check the pressure regularly. If a fire does start in the car, get all the passengers out of the vehicle.

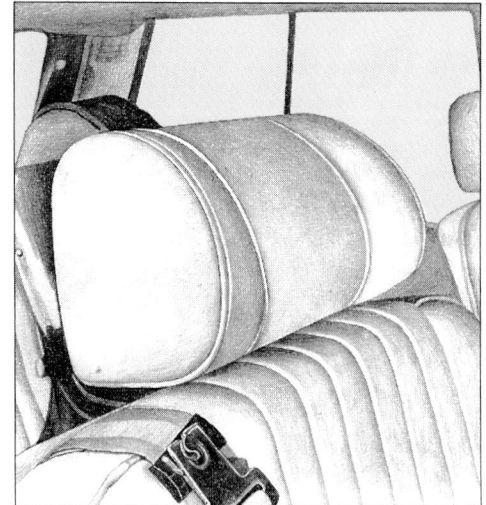

Head restraints

A head restraint prevents whiplash in the event of a collision from behind. Head restraints should be an integral part of the seat or anchored securely to it. They should not obstruct the driver's rear vision. Head restraints that clip onto the seat merely provide a head rest; they do not give enough protection to prevent whiplash injury.

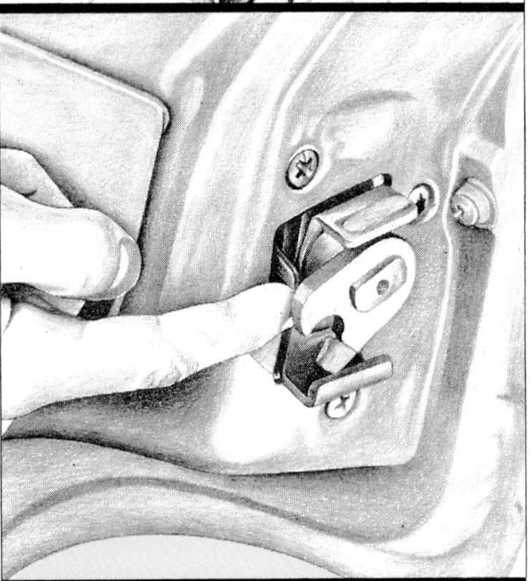

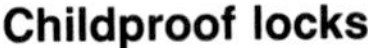

Childproof locks

Any car in which children travel regularly should be fitted with childproof locks. These make it impossible for a child to open the door accidentally. Similar locking devices can be fitted to windows to prevent a child from opening the window beyond a certain level. Children should travel in the back seat of a car, never in the front.

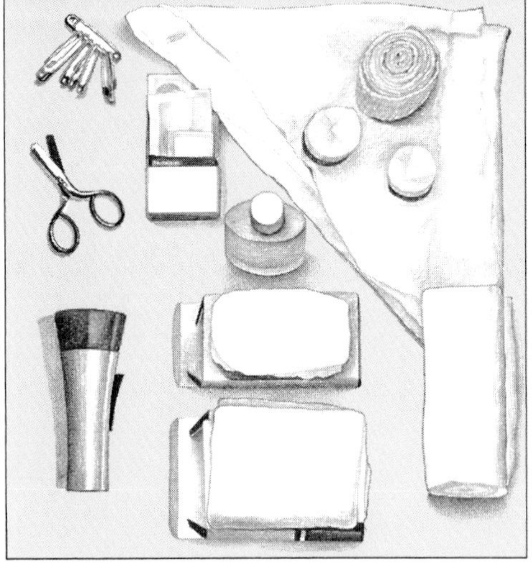

First-aid kit

A first-aid kit should be carried in the car at all times. It should contain bandages, adhesive tape, gauze pads, antiseptic, acetaminophen or aspirin, scissors, and a first-aid handbook. The kit must be closed with a childproof catch, but not locked. Check the supplies before beginning a long journey. It is also useful to keep tissues or cleansing wipes in the car.

Check the supplies in your first-aid box, which should be carried in the car at all times. For long journeys, you should also take emergency supplies of energy-giving food. Chocolate, nuts, raisins, and glucose or dextrose tablets are especially nourishing.

Also take some means of warmth, light, and shelter. If waterproof sleeping bags are not available, take plenty of woolen blankets for every person. For warmth, take a small solid-fuel burner. Candles and matches can also be useful, and a flashlight and flares should be carried in the car.

If your car breaks down in a remote area, you may need to attract rescuers by using some kind of signaling device. This can be done by using, for example, flashing lights, fires, a whistle, or the car's horn. The letters SOS are an internationally recognized distress signal. In the international Morse code these letters are represented by three dots, three dashes, and three dots (··· — — — ···). This pattern can be formed by flashes of light, blasts on a whistle or the car's horn, or sticks or strips of light-colored clothing placed on the ground. Another international distress symbol is a triangular pattern of three fires.

Careful planning of a journey can minimize fatigue, which reduces a driver's concentration and judgment and so increases the chances of an accident. There should be no long, uninterrupted periods of driving, and it is often sensible to share the driving with a person with whom you are traveling. Plan your journey to avoid rush hours in big cities, and stop the car at least once every two hours for physical exercise or light refreshment.

In Case of Accident

If you are involved in a road accident or arrive at the scene of one, you must act promptly and efficiently to help any injured persons and to protect them from further danger. The following actions should be carried out:

(1) To prevent a gasoline explosion or any other form of fire, instruct all drivers present to switch off the ignition in their cars. Spread earth or sand on any gasoline that may have spilled on the road. Allow nobody to smoke. If

Escape from a sinking car

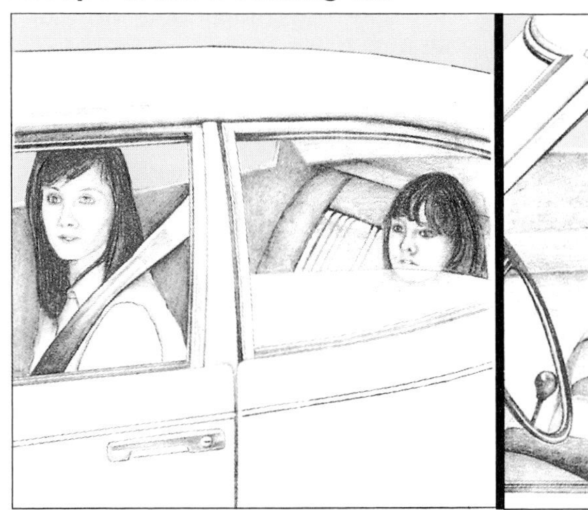

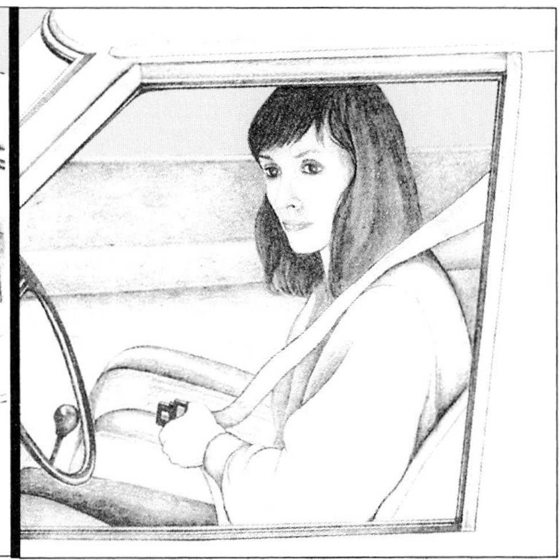

1 If the car floats for a short time, try to escape immediately. If the car starts to sink quickly, close the windows to prevent the water from rushing in. The water enters the car through the many holes in the floor, such as around the handbrake cables and pedals. It is not possible to open the doors until the inside and outside pressures are equal.

2 As the water rises, release the seat belts. Make sure that all passengers are free from restraints. Check that the doors are not locked. Keep a hand on the door handle. Shut off the car's engine, but keep the lights on to aid rescuers. Do not panic.

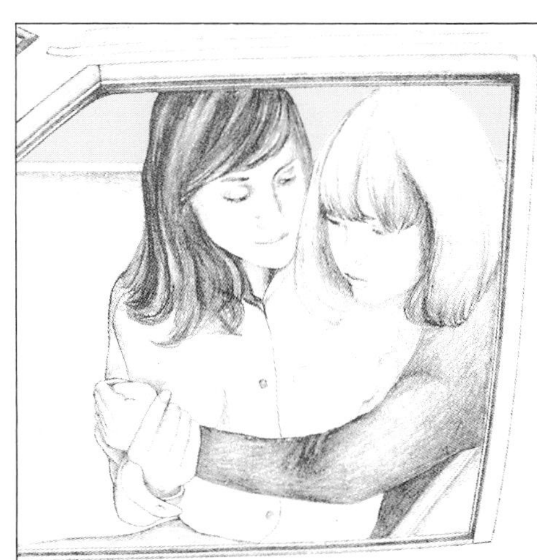

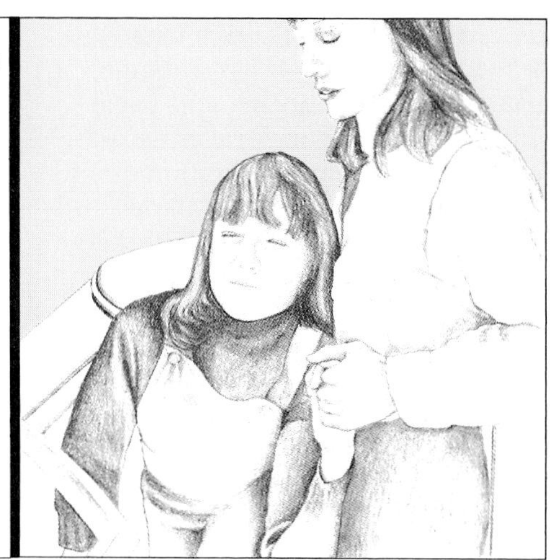

3 Make sure that the heads of all passengers, particularly children or injured persons, are above the water level as it rises. Wait until the water has reached chin level and try to open the doors. They may need several hard pushes.

4 The moment the doors are open, the car begins to sink rapidly. With nonswimmers, form a human chain by holding tightly onto the other passengers. Still holding tightly onto the other passengers, swim strongly and swiftly to the surface.

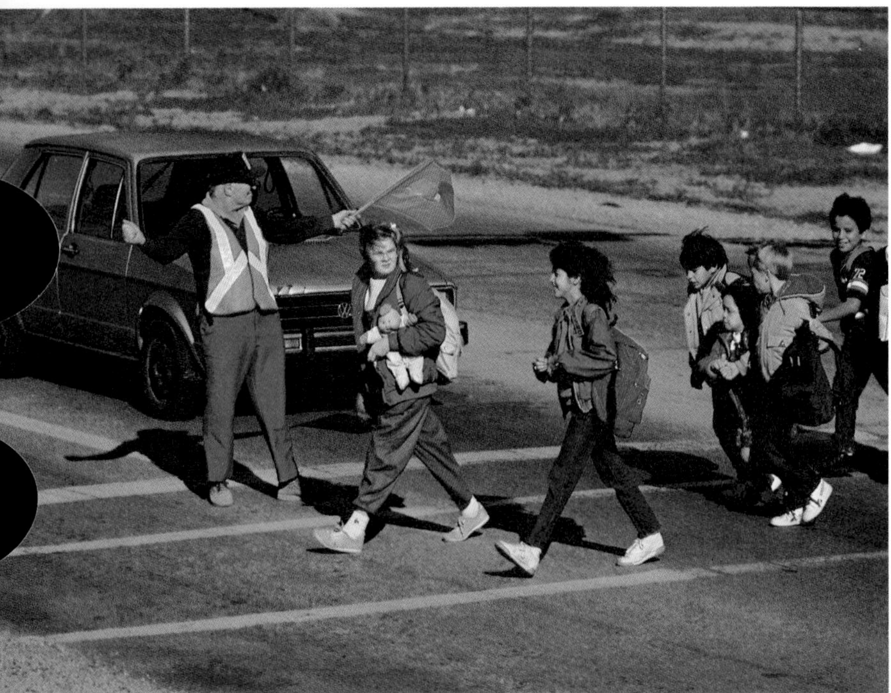

Automobile safety and alertness is particularly important near school crossings.

a fire does start, use an extinguisher, a blanket, or a coat to put it out.

(2) To prevent further collisions, warn oncoming traffic by displaying warning signs at least 50 yards (or meters) from the accident (at least 150 yards at night). Use reflective triangles, if these are available, or ask another person to give the warning and wave the traffic past. If your car is fitted with hazard warning lights, switch them on.

(3) Make sure that an ambulance and the police are summoned immediately. Use the emergency telephone number and give the exact location of the accident and the number of persons injured.

(4) Examine all injured persons and look for any who may have been thrown clear of the accident. Do not move the victims unless they are in immediate danger. Undo safety belts and cautiously remove any safety helmets. If a victim's heart has stopped, give immediate cardiac compression. Then give first aid to all injured parties in order of priority. If an injury is bleeding, apply firm but gentle pressure to the wound with some clean material and fasten a pad over it with a bandage or strip of cloth. If a limb is not broken, it may be raised to lessen bleeding. Do not wipe blood from eyes in case broken glass shards are present. See also ARTIFICIAL RESPIRATION; HEART ATTACK.

(5) Stay with the victims until an ambulance and the police arrive. Reassure them about their condition and keep them warm. Do not give them anything to drink or eat.

If the accident involves a vehicle containing flammable or dangerous chemicals or other goods, make sure that the fire department and police are informed immediately.

Make sure that others present are aware of the danger and keep them away from the vehicle.

Fitness to Drive

The degree of concentration demanded by driving is greater than that demanded by almost any other routine activity. The driver must be able to deal capably and confidently with the changing traffic conditions and must be prepared at all times for unexpected dangers. In an emergency situation, the lives of the driver and the passengers may depend on the speed of the driver's reactions.

To sustain this degree of concentration, the driver must be mentally alert and physically fit. The most common threat to a driver's mental alertness is fatigue, especially on long journeys. To avoid fatigue, the following measures can be taken:

(1) The driver should be seated comfortably, be able to see everything around, and be able to reach all the controls without difficulty.

(2) The car should be well ventilated, with a continuous current of fresh air.

(3) If there is a radio or tape player in the car, the driver must take care that his or her alertness is not dulled by music that is too loud or too soothing.

(4) The driver should avoid eating heavy meals either before or during a journey. He or she should *never* drink alcohol before or while driving.

(5) On long journeys the driver should stop the car at least once every two hours in order to exercise the muscles by walking around or doing physical exercises.

The harmful effects of alcohol on a driver's concentration and judgment are well known, but still need to be emphasized. The particular danger of alcohol is that it may increase the driver's subjective feeling of self-confidence, while at the same time decreasing the actual powers of judgment. Drugs also may have similar effects, and a driver who has been prescribed drugs or who is taking any medicines regularly should consult the physician about the possible effects on his or her driving. *See also* ALCOHOL; ALCOHOL ABUSE.

A less obvious factor that may affect a driver's concentration is nervous tension and stress. One cause of tension may be worries about the car itself. These can be reduced by ensuring that the car is regularly serviced and in good condition and by repairing or replacing faulty parts as soon as the fault becomes apparent. A driver can also suffer from nervous tension if he or she is unnecessarily distracted by other passengers in the car. Children especially become bored and restless on long journeys, and another adult in the car can help the driver by keeping them amused with games of observation. Such games are preferable to reading, which not only is difficult to do in a car, but also may induce sickness.

It is impossible to eliminate all stress from driving, but careful planning before every journey to allow enough time for different road conditions does produce a more relaxed, and, therefore, a more alert driver. If at any time during a journey you feel yourself becoming tense, draw to the side of the road, leave the car, and walk around.

Travel Sickness

Travel sickness is more likely to affect children than adults. It is often preceded by yawning, a general loss of interest, sweating, a cold and shivery feeling, and pallor of the face. If any of these signs are present, stop the car and let the person walk around for awhile. Give the person a sip of water, and when getting back into the car let the person sit in front.

Attacks of travel sickness may be prevented by driving smoothly, cornering and braking gently, and maintaining a flow of fresh air through the car. Make sure that all persons in the car are seated comfortably and that seat belts are worn. Any dangling object, such as a soft toy, should be taken down. Make frequent stops for a little exercise and perhaps some light refreshment, such as a picnic lunch.

There are a number of commercial preparations available for the prevention of travel sickness. No driver should take travel sickness pills without first checking with a physician that it is safe to do so; most of these preparations cause drowsiness.

Body Exercises

Here are a few simple exercises that a driver can do during stops to relieve body tension.

Neck. Relax the shoulders and lean the head back as far as possible for two seconds. Let the head fall forward so that the chin rests on the chest. Relax and repeat.

Shoulders. Rotate the shoulders in a forward motion, one at a time then both together, with the arms dangling loose. Relax and repeat.

Arms and Hands. Clench the fists, bring them to the shoulders, and flex the biceps. Relax and repeat. Alternatively clasp the hands together with the fingers interlocked and try to separate the hands without breaking their grip. Count to ten and relax.

Stomach. Take a deep breath and brace the stomach muscles. Hold to a slow count of 10 and breathe out slowly. Repeat several times.

Legs. Squeeze the thighs together and press the hands against the outside of the legs near the knees. Maintain hand pressure and separate the legs. Count to 10 and relax.

Autonomic nerve. *See* NERVE.

Autonomic nervous system. *See* NERVOUS SYSTEM, AUTONOMIC.

Autoplasty (ô'tə plas tē) is the reconstruction or replacement of an injured or diseased body part by transplanting or grafting tissue from another portion of the patient's own body.

Autopsy (ô'top sē), or post-mortem, is the detailed examination and dissection of a body after death. In no way does this technique violate the body; it is performed in a manner similar to a surgical procedure.

An autopsy can be done for medical or educational reasons at the request of or with the permission of the family and attending physician. This can give the deceased's family the satisfaction of knowing that their loved one has contributed to medical science even in death.

An autopsy can help establish family tendencies to disease and also identify the cause of death. Corneal or organ transplants can help others to lead normal lives.

An autopsy may also be ordered by legal authorities to gather information for use as evidence in any legal proceedings. It may be ordered to establish the cause of death for insurance purposes or to aid in the investigation of contagious diseases or industrial hazards that may pose a danger to public health.

Autosomal (ô tə sō′məl) is a term that pertains to any chromosomes except the sex chromosome. There are 22 pairs of autosomes in the human cell.

See also CHROMOSOME.

Autosuggestion (ô tō səg jes′ chən) is a thought or belief that is repeated to oneself (either mentally or verbally) often as a means of affecting one's behavior. A chant may be a form of autosuggestion.

Axilla (ak sil′ə) is the armpit.

See also ARMPIT.

Axon (ak′son) is the extension of a nerve cell that carries nerve impulses away from the neuron cell body and transmits those impulses to other nerve cells or to body organs.

Azoospermia (ā zō ə spėr′mē ə) is the absence of spermatozoa in the semen. Azoospermia is associated with infertility, but not impotence. It may be caused by a vasectomy or by a dysfunction of the testes.

See also IMPOTENCE; INFERTILITY; VASECTOMY.

Azotemia (az o te′mē ə) is an excess of nitrogenous compounds in the blood. This condition is characteristic of uremia and is caused by the inability of the kidneys to remove urea from the blood.

See also UREMIA.

B

Babinski's reflex (bə bin′skēz rē′fleks) is a condition in which the big toe turns upward instead of curling under when the sole of the foot is stroked. The reflex is normal in infants, but abnormal in children and adults, where it indicates such damage to the nervous system as occurs with a stroke. The condition, also called Babinski's sign, is named after the neurologist who first noted it, Joseph Babinski.

Baby, or infant, is a child from birth to about the age of 18 months. Newborn babies are completely helpless. They cannot sit up, move from one place to another, feed themselves, or talk. With good care, babies gradually learn to do certain things for themselves. By about 18 months of age, most children can walk and run without help, feed themselves, play simple games, and say a few words and phrases. They are then no longer considered to be infants.

Growth and Development

Heredity and environment influence a baby's growth and development. Heredity refers to the characteristics that babies inherit from their parents through the chromosomes. Environment consists of everything with which a baby comes in contact, including the kind of care the baby receives. Environment especially affects the formation of a baby's personality. A few other factors besides heredity and environment can also influence a baby's growth and development. These factors include accidents and illnesses over which parents have little control.

A baby's personality begins to develop soon after birth. The development continues throughout childhood and even throughout life. Most experts believe that a person's very early experiences have a very strong influence on later personality development. For example, infants who never have their needs met when they cry will learn not to cry. They will lie in bed quietly, causing little disturbance. In time, however, their emotional, mental, and social growth will fall behind that of other children. Babies who are cared for lovingly—that is, in close and understanding contact with their parents or other caretakers—have the best chances of developing a normal, healthy personality.

Babies differ in the rate and manner of their growth and development. For example, many infants begin to crawl at about 9 to 10 months of age, but some begin to crawl earlier and others later. Still other babies learn to walk without ever crawling.

The First Month. A baby is considered a *newborn* for about a month after birth. Newborn babies spend much of their time sleeping.

Characteristics of Newborn Babies. Most white children have grayish-blue eyes and pink skin at birth. The color of the eyes may change by the fifth or sixth month. This color then becomes permanent. Most black children have brown eyes and relatively light, pinkish skin at birth. The eyes remain brown. The skin begins to darken a few days after birth.

A newborn baby's head makes up about a fourth of the total body length and is bigger around than the chest. The arms are longer than the legs. These proportions change as a child becomes an adult. The head, for example, grows less than the rest of the body and makes up about one-eighth of an adult's height.

A newborn baby's skull has six soft spots (fontanels) where the bone is not yet completely joined. These areas become completely covered with bone by about the eighteenth month. The other bones in a baby's body are only partly calcified (hardened with calcium) at

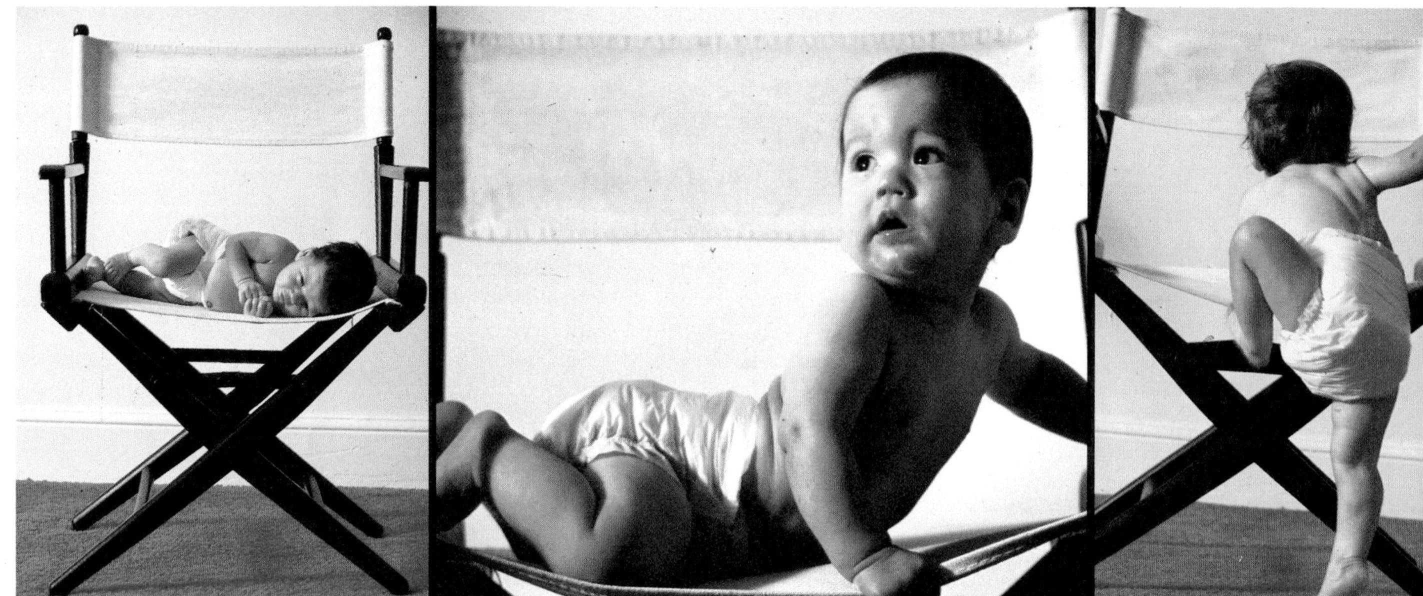

A **baby** is a child up to the age of 18 months. Babies differ in the rate of their growth and development. *Above,* the same baby is pictured at 2 weeks, 29 weeks, and 52 weeks of age. (These photos were taken to show this baby's growth. Never leave a baby alone in a high place or allow a child to climb on a folding chair.)

birth. These bones calcify gradually throughout childhood.

A newborn baby's actions are all reflex actions—that is, they are completely automatic. Newborn infants can suck and swallow, move their arms and legs, and cry to make their needs known. When lying in bed, they often curl up in a position like the one they had in the uterus. If startled by a loud noise or sudden jolt, they jerk their arms and legs outward in a reflex action called the startle, or Moro, reflex. For several months, the baby's neck muscles will not be strong enough to hold the head erect. A person must therefore be careful to support the head while picking up or holding the baby.

Newborn babies can not control the movements of their eyes, but they can tell darkness from light and see objects directly in front of them. They also can hear well. The sense of hearing may be dulled for a few days after birth by fluid in the ear. But as the fluid drains, the baby's hearing becomes normal.

Feeding and Rate of Growth. Newborn babies can swallow only liquids. They therefore get their nourishment by sucking milk from their mothers' breasts or from bottles. Mothers may begin to nurse their babies—that is, feed them milk at the breast—within a few minutes after birth. In most cases, the breasts do not produce a full supply of milk until several days after birth, but the early milk, or colostrum, contains protective antibodies that help the baby avoid infections. Babies who are not breast-fed are given a special formula prepared from cow's milk. This formula resembles mothers' milk and is fed from a bottle.

Newborn babies can digest only small amounts of mothers' milk or formula at a time. As a result, they must be fed often—in most cases, every two to three hours, day and night. Babies lose weight for a few days after birth because their food intake does not yet meet their needs, but most babies regain the lost weight by about the tenth day after birth. They then begin to gain about one ounce (28g) a day.

From One to Six Months. A baby's growth rate slows after the third month. By the seventh month, the rate will have dropped to about one-half ounce (14g) a day.

By the second month, babies have begun to develop various motor skills. Motor skills are controlled movements rather than reflex actions. They depend largely on the development of the brain and nerves.

The development of motor skills begins with the head and progresses downward through other parts of the body. Thus, babies learn to move their heads and eyes before they can control their arms and legs. By the second month, most infants can turn their heads and eyes to follow the movements of people and large objects. By the age of five or six months, most babies can hold their heads erect, grasp objects with their hands, turn themselves over in bed, and sit erect if propped up.

Babies begin to relate to people and things around them at about three months of age. To develop normal human relationships, children need a feeling of trust and security. Parents help develop such a feeling if they treat a baby with love and understanding.

From Six to Twelve Months. Babies achieve a number of "firsts" between six and twelve months of age. The first tooth usually appears about the sixth or seventh month. The teeth then continue to grow out at the rate of about one a month until a child has a complete set of twenty primary, or baby, teeth. Most children have all of their primary teeth by about two-and-one-half years of age. After they are about six months old, babies learn to pick up small objects and pieces of food by clasping them between their fingers and palms. Many babies sit unsupported for the first time at about seven months. By about nine months, they may pull themselves to their feet and stand with support.

At about six months of age, most babies develop a degree of independence. Their personalities then begin to show in various ways. For example, they may want to hold their bottles instead of having them held for them. Gradually, all babies develop characteristic ways of doing things, which differ from the ways other babies do the same things. Such differences in behavior indicate the growth of individuality.

From Twelve to Eighteen Months. Babies learn how to do many things by imitating older persons. Their ability to imitate improves after the twelfth month, because of a sudden advance in brain and nerve development.

Most infants start to walk with support about the twelfth or thirteenth month. They take their first unaided steps by about fifteen months and can run by eighteen months. Babies also start to play with blocks, balls, and other objects about the twelfth month. At first, they may simply throw the objects or put them in their mouths. By the eighteenth month, many infants have learned to pile a few blocks on top of one another and to push objects along the floor with their hands.

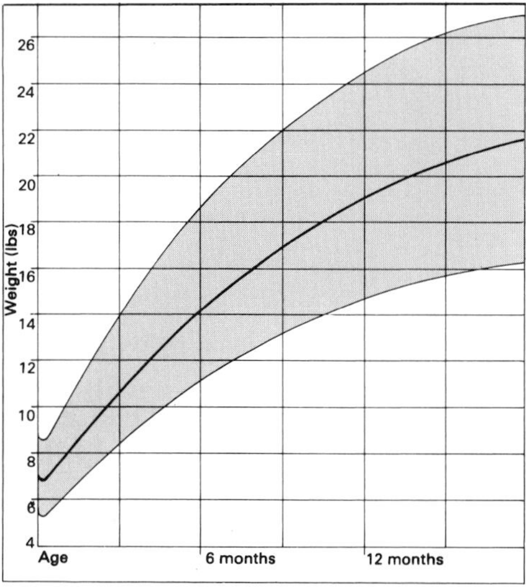

This chart shows the average (as well as normal maximum and minimum) **weight gain** of a baby at 3, 6, 9, 12, 15, and 18 months.

Most babies can say a few words in addition to "Mama" and "Dada" by the age of 12 months. At 15 months, they may "talk" energetically, but they still know few real words. At 18 months, children's vocabularies may consist of about 10 to 20 words. Many children also can combine words into phrases at this age.

Babies understand many more words than they use. By 8 or 9 months, most babies respond to the sound of their names. A one-year-old recognizes the names of a variety of objects and understands "no" and certain other commands. By the age of 15 to 18 months, most babies enjoy listening to simple songs and nursery rhymes. They also may enjoy hearing a story, though the story itself probably means little to them. Most babies at this age like to watch television and look at pictures in books and magazines.

Sometime after 18 months of age, a child may be ready for toilet training—that is, learning to control the bowels and bladder. The age when such control becomes possible varies greatly among children. Parents should not force toilet training, but wait until a child shows readiness for it.

See also AGE-BY-AGE CHARTS, Appendices; BABY CARE.

Baby care is best approached in an organized way. The key to this organization is to correctly equip and arrange the baby's room. Bathing, changing, and feeding the baby also should follow an organized routine whenever possible. Common sense is also essen-

Feeding equipment

A nursing mother should have on her table a bowl of clean water and cotton swabs for washing nipples; a clock to time the baby at the breast; ointment for preventing cracked nipples; and a glass of fresh water for drinking halfway through the feeding.

The parent of the bottle-fed baby should have a thermostatically controlled bottle warmer. A pitcher of water should stand ready to replenish the water in the bottle warmer.

A smooth and shallow weaning spoon, made of bone or plastic, should be available for a baby that is learning to eat solids.

There should also be a box of paper tissues and a cotton diaper folded into a triangle to serve as a bib.

Toilet articles

The toilet items shown here are those most often used. They include baby soap, shampoo, baby oil or lotion, talcum powder or cornstarch, an ointment to protect against diaper rash, a supply of cotton swabs, a real sponge and two rubber sponges, a finetooth comb for treating cradle cap, and a soft hairbrush.

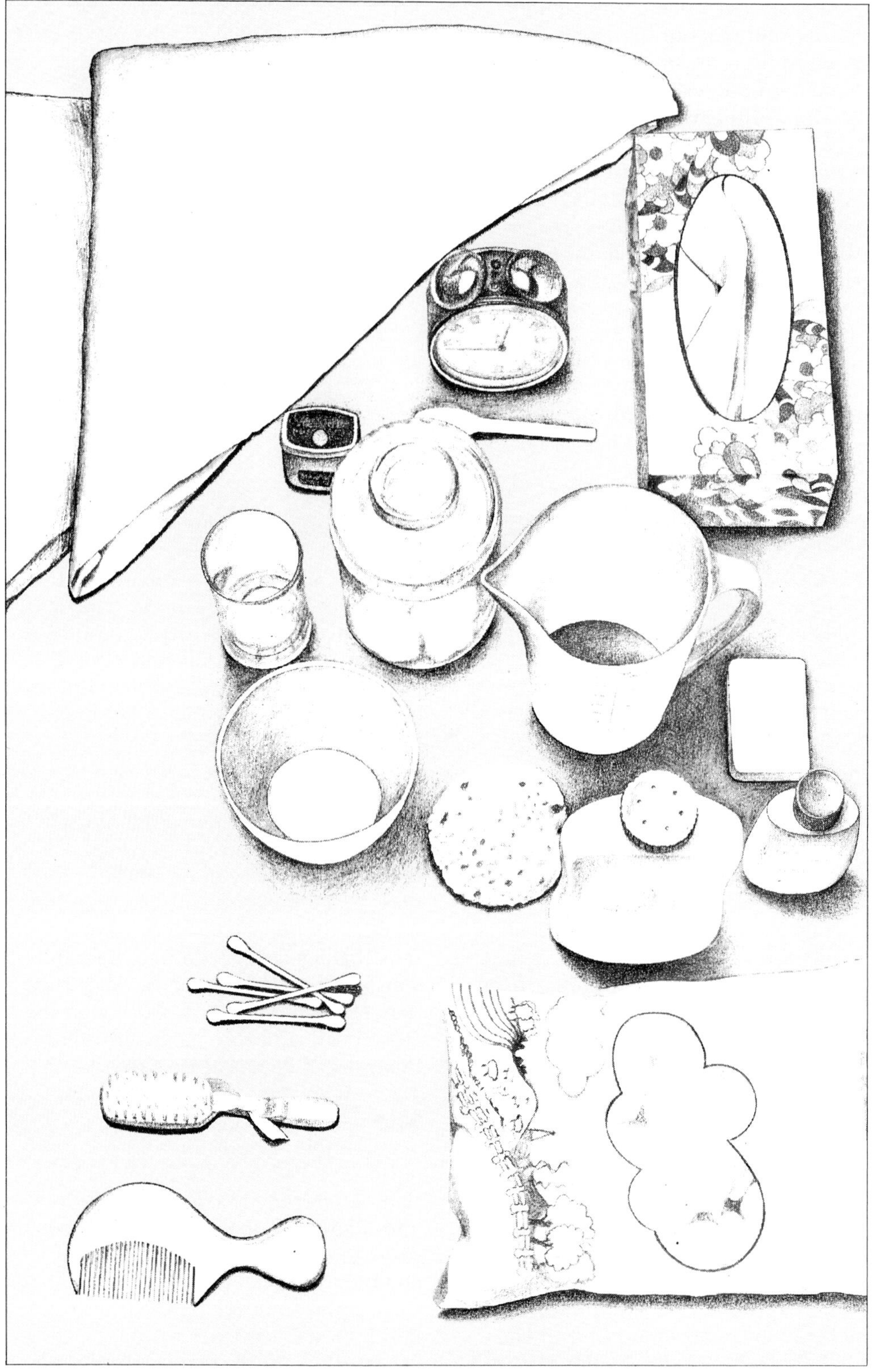

tial, especially concerning the safety of the child. Members of the family with illnesses should be kept out of the baby's room, as should any type of pet.

Parents should remember that general advice of the type offered in this article often refers to the average baby. No individual baby is "average" in every aspect. Slight variations can be discussed with a physician.

The Proper Environment

The Baby's Room. A newborn infant may share the parents' bedroom for the first few months, but even if this is the case, a separate room should be planned and equipped so that everything is conveniently at hand for the main activities in the baby's life: nursing, body hygiene, and diaper changing.

The room itself should be warm and well ventilated. A constant temperature of 68° to 72°F (20° to 22°C) is advisable for any baby who weighs less than 8 pounds (3.6kg), but as the baby grows and puts on weight, the nighttime temperature may be allowed to drop slightly. (*See also* the section in this article on the Baby's Temperature, page 99.) It is important that the air in the room is not dry. If possible, place a humidifier in the room to keep the air warm and moist.

Every baby needs fresh air but should be protected from drafts, so make sure that the crib is not next to an open window when the baby is asleep. In cold weather, the room should be aired when the baby is not occupying it.

Lighting. For the convenience of the parents, the room should be well lighted, but newborn infants are unable to adjust their eyes to a bright light. A ceiling light therefore should have a low-power bulb or a dimmer attachment on the light switch. A small table lamp is useful, particularly when placed on the dresser to illuminate the contents of the drawers.

Even a small baby becomes quickly bored by having nothing to look at. A mobile above the bassinet or crib may hold the infant's attention, as will brightly colored pictures fixed within the baby's field of vision.

Furniture and Equipment. The most important piece of furniture in the baby's room is the bed. The most suitable first bed for a newborn infant is a bassinet, straw basket, or portable crib because a tiny baby feels more secure in a fairly small space. If the baby is going to sleep in a crib, be sure the slats of the crib are no more than 2⅝" (6.6 cm) apart. Any larger and the baby's head could get entrapped between the slats. Put bumper pads around the edge of the crib.

The mattress must be firm and smooth and should fit the bed snugly. Never use a pillow instead of a mattress, and make sure that a waterproof cover fits tightly over the mattress. If you are using a straw or cane bassinet, line the inside with material to prevent the baby from catching or scratching the fingers or face on a rough edge. This also helps to prevent drafts. A baby under the age of one year should never be given a pillow for the head, as it may pose a risk for suffocation.

A low, comfortable chair with armrests and a straight back is another important item in the baby's room. The chair can be used for feeding with the bottle or nursing at the breast. A rocking chair is especially useful for comforting a fussy baby.

All the equipment needed during a diaper change should be within reach so that the parent does not have to leave an infant unattended on the changing surface. A shelf attached to the side of the changing table is useful for storing cream, powder, cotton, and diapers. If this is not possible, make sure that there is a working surface at the correct height next to the changing area. Overhead shelves are convenient, but can be dangerous since a jar or bottle could fall on the baby.

Place two buckets with lids for dirty diapers and clothes by the side of the changing area. A wastebasket also should be beside the changing area for used pieces of cotton.

There should be a plastic bathtub on a sturdy stand in the room and a rack on which to hang towels and a facecloth. It is more suitable to bathe a small baby in his or her room because the temperature is more easily maintained than in an adult bathroom. Even if the room is centrally heated, it may be necessary to boost the room temperature with a heater before bath time. The heater can be either of the radiator type or an electrical heater placed high on the wall.

If parents intend always to feed the baby in his or her own room, a separate low table or cart should be set aside for nursing and feeding articles.

A dresser is useful for storing sheets, blankets, towels, diapers, and clean clothing. As the baby grows out of clothes, they should be stored elsewhere to ensure that the dresser does not become overfull.

Safety. When planning and equipping a baby's room, safety factors should always be kept in mind. Babies quickly become mobile; it is often not until a near-accident occurs that the parents realize how active the baby is.

All the furniture in the room should be strong and stable so that a crawling infant is not able to overturn it. The windows should have safety stops on them so that they cannot be opened wide enough for the child to crawl out of. As an alternative, parents can fix bars (vertical ones) over the window. If there are electrical outlets at ground level, cover them with outlet covers (which are available at hardware or department stores) or place a piece of heavy furniture in front of them because the crawling child will soon try poking something into the plug.

Cribs should be selected carefully. Bars should be no more than 2⅝″ (6.6cm) apart, so that the child cannot get stuck or choke. There must be no peeling paint. Once the crib is set up, do not tie to the bars anything in which the child might become entangled.

Never use an unguarded space heater in a baby's room. Liquid fuel heaters are also dangerous and should not be used.

The Layette (clothing and accessories). A mother-to-be derives great enjoyment out of getting the layette ready. But, pleasant as it is, the monetary cost, the laundering time, and the effort of actually putting clothes on the baby must also be kept in mind.

Diapers are the only form of clothing that need to be bought in quantity. Babies grow quickly in the first months, and their needs constantly change. When shopping for the layette, keep the following in mind: (1) clothing should have growing space; (2) garments should be easy to launder; (3) all items should be safe and comfortable for the baby to wear or use; and (4) garments should be simple enough to take a minimum of time to dress and undress the infant.

Trendy clothes for tots may look cute on dolls, but are often impractical for real, live babies, who loathe being dressed and undressed and express their exasperation by crying loudly and angrily. A crying baby is rigid and uncooperative, as the parent fumbling with buttons and ribbons soon discovers. It is well worth searching for clothing that is secured with snap fasteners rather than that which must be pulled and tugged over the baby's head. Infant clothes should be loose and easy to slip on and off. In addition, older babies will try to chew on buttons, so snaps are much safer.

The newborn baby's tender skin is easily irritated by the starchy substance in new materials. It is wise to launder all clothing, diapers, wrapping blankets, or similar articles that will touch the baby's skin before they are used. Use mild soapsuds in warm water for washing clothes the first time and make sure that all the soap is thoroughly rinsed. Follow the manufacturer's recommendation for laundering sleepwear so as to retain the flame retardant properties.

It is also wise to remove all labels from inside the garments. Labels can irritate a baby's sensitive skin.

The most important article in the baby's layette is the diaper. The choice is wide. A new parent should consider the following:

(1) If a diaper service is available, does it also provide the diapers? Is the price reasonable?

(2) Disposables are of course convenient, but they are costly. Is there enough storage room for the large quantities needed?

(3) Is there time enough for a parent to launder diapers?

When laundering diapers, do not use harsh detergents; many parents prefer to use mild soapsuds. Even more important, it is essential to rinse diapers thoroughly after laundering to prevent irritation of the baby's skin.

Feeding Procedures

Breast-feeding the Baby. In the first two to three days after birth the moth-

Baby garments

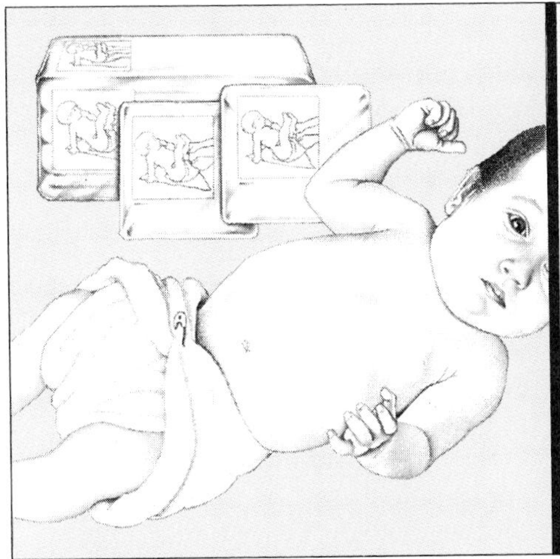

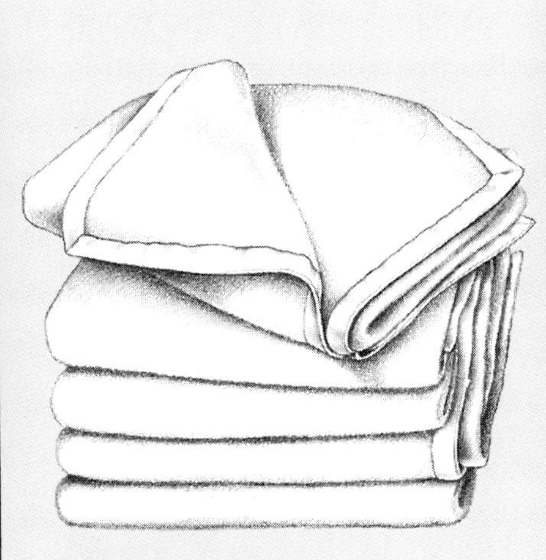

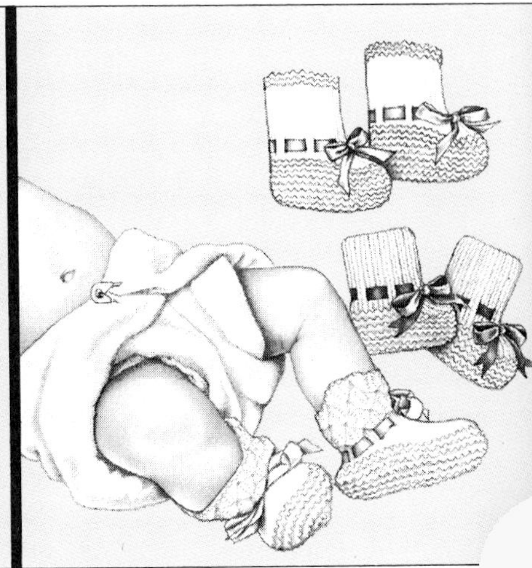

Diapers

If traditional cotton diapers are preferred, it would be wise to buy at least two dozen.

Other essentials are six diaper pins with locking heads, disposable liners, three cotton knit soakers, three small and three medium-sized soft plastic or plastic-lined panties.

Receiving blankets

Four to six receiving blankets, or wrappers, are useful additions to the layette. They should be made of a soft material, such as cotton knit or flannelette.

Being wrapped in a receiving blanket has a calming effect on a newborn baby, whose tendency is to kick and wave. A snugly-wrapped baby will nurse and sleep better.

Booties

Four pairs of plain booties, of the simplest kind, are essential for a baby born during the winter months. An infant's circulation cannot always adjust to changes in temperature. If a baby's feet feel cold, they should be protected by booties. There should be no need for mittens or a cap unless the baby has to go outdoors in cold weather.

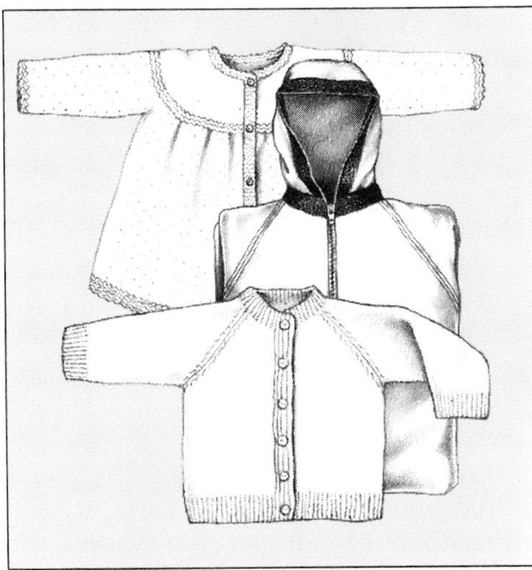

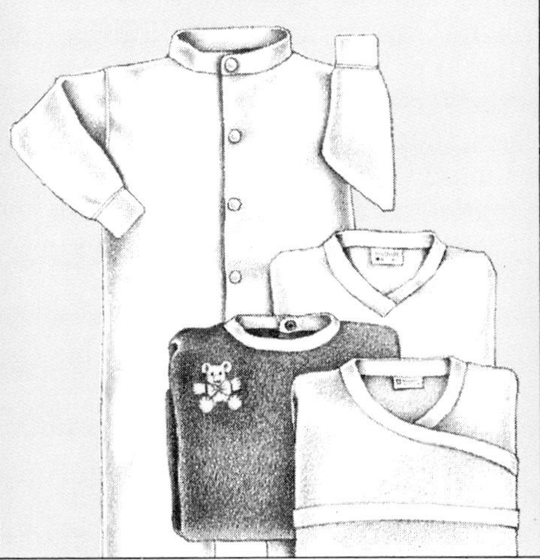

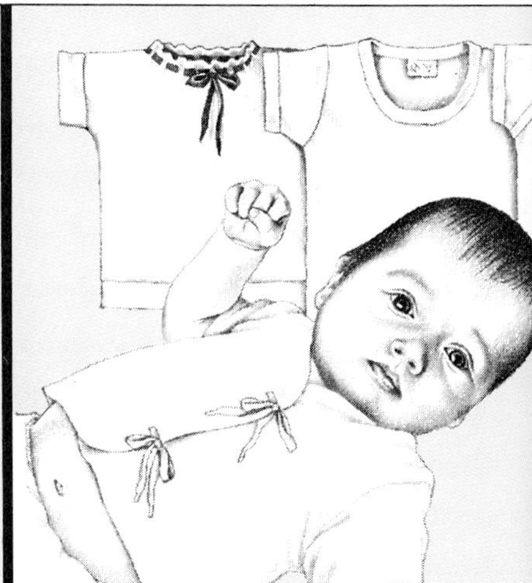

Sweaters or sacks

Two light-knit sweaters or sacks and two heavier-knit ones should be adequate for a newborn baby. The yarn may be of cotton or of synthetic fibers other than nylon, which is not recommended because it does not let the skin "breathe."

Garments with button or snap fasteners are advisable; ribbon ties can get pulled too tight around the neck.

Nightgowns and sleep suits

Nightgowns and sleep suits made of cotton or flannelette keep a baby warm. Sleep and play suits are preferable to gowns as they are more comfortable for the baby.

Later, a parent may choose to switch to a one- or a two-piece stretch suit. It is important to make sure the baby has enough foot room as he or she grows.

Short-sleeved shirts

Four cotton shirts, with short sleeves and a front opening, are essential. It is easier to put this kind on the baby than the type that goes on over the head. Buy the size corresponding to age six months, certainly not smaller.

If the shirts chosen have ribbon ties at the front, make sure that the ribbons are securely sewn on. A baby may swallow a ribbon if it comes off.

er's breasts produce a substance called colostrum. Colostrum resembles melted butter, is high in protein, and contains antibodies that protect the baby. It helps to clear the bowels easily of meconium, a substance in the bowels of all newborn babies. There is no artificial substitute for colostrum.

Breast Milk. Breast milk is easily processed by the infant's digestive system and helps to prevent allergies. Unlike cow's milk, breast milk leaves an acid residue in the bowel and prevents the growth of harmful bacteria. Breastfed babies usually do not suffer from constipation, provided there is an adequate supply of milk. For the first few weeks, bowel movements may be frequent, but these may decrease to two dirty diapers a day.

Although initially some women may experience discomfort, most women find breast-feeding a pleasure once it is established. Emotionally, it ensures a closer bond with the baby; physically, it helps the womb to return more quickly to its normal size. Successful breast-feeding depends on the mother's attitude; prenatal preparation of the breasts and nipples and their postnatal care; a good, balanced diet, with plenty of fluids; rest; and patience.

Prenatal Breast Care. A well-fitting bra should be worn both day and night from the seventh month of pregnancy onward. Starting at that time the nipples should be washed well each day and gently rubbed with a towel after a bath. Some physicians advise applying a bland ointment.

Flat nipples should be drawn out and rolled between thumb and forefinger. At about the eighth month, the breasts should be gently massaged, and a little colostrum should be pressed from each nipple. This helps to open the milk ducts.

Women with inverted nipples can wear devices popularly known as "shells" inside their bras during the last three months of pregnancy. If no improvement takes place, a natural nursing nipple shield is helpful when nursing.

Breast-feeding. Before putting the baby to the breast, clean the breast with a cotton swab dipped in warm water to remove any ointment. Start each feeding on the side opposite the last.

After the feeding, wipe the nipples with cotton dipped in warm water and apply an ointment or spray. Try to avoid using plastic-backed, milk-retaining pads inside the bra because they can make the nipples sore.

The First Week. Patience and perseverance are needed during the first week of breast-feeding when difficulties may arise. Nursing mothers should be aware that it may require a few weeks to establish a steady milk supply.

In the first two to three days the baby sucks colostrum. At this stage the mother does not experience much change in her breasts. Usually between the third and fifth day milk comes in and, as the breasts enlarge, there may be some discomfort or even pain. Should the milk come in with a rush, the baby should be allowed to nurse frequently; this will prevent engorged breasts. Different babies have different needs, and you will have to work out the best schedule for your baby by trial and error.

Breast-feeding Problems. Some women do not produce much milk while in the hospital, but produce more when they return home. Substituting a bottle for breast feeding will actually prevent the development of a steady milk supply since the baby's sucking stimulates the breasts to produce more milk. Frequent nursing, therefore, helps to increase the supply.

It is useful to know before the baby's birth how to press out (express) milk from the breasts. Have a sterilized cup ready. Wash your hands and make sure that they are warm. Sit comfortably at a low table with the cup on the table just under your breast. Massage the whole breast with both hands. Then, with thumb and forefinger of one hand, squeeze the milk reservoir deep behind the areola. Slide thumb and forefinger through 90 degrees round the areola and squeeze again, making sure that all the milk sacs are emptied. Meanwhile, with the other hand, massage the breast gently from top, side, and bottom toward the areola. In the hospital, a hand pump may be supplied with instruc-

Breast-feeding the baby

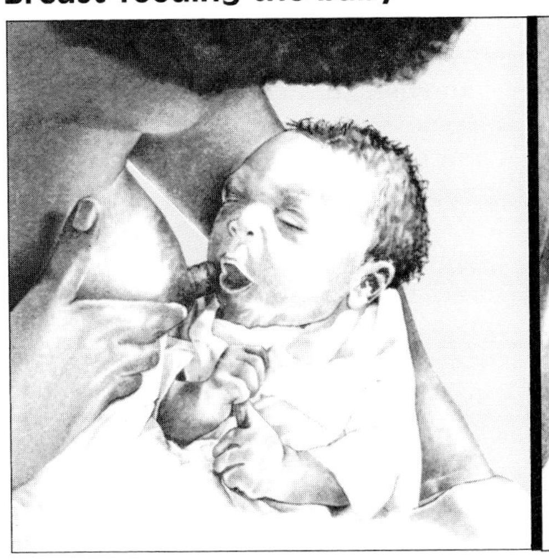

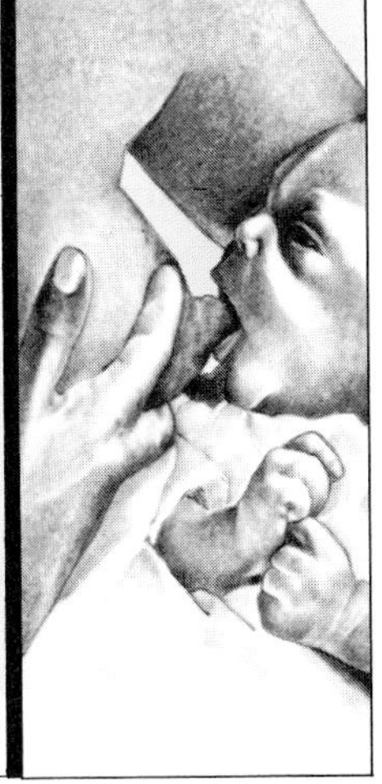

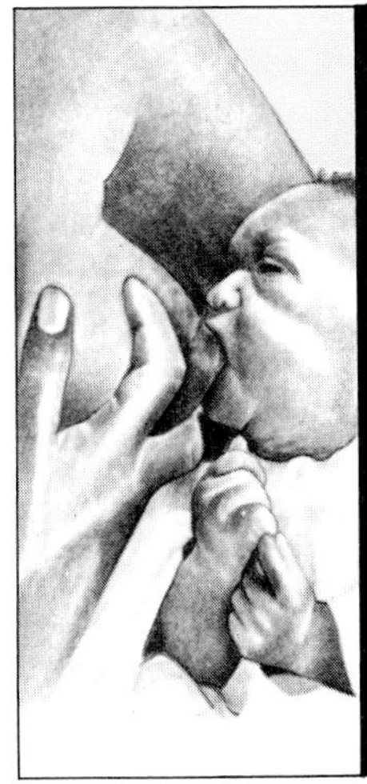

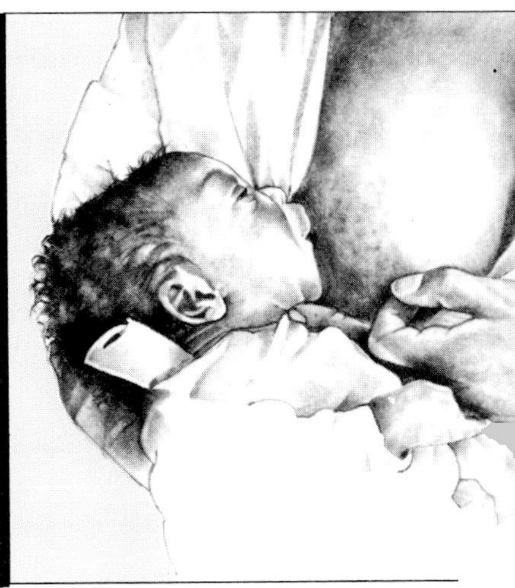

The first time

The newborn's mother should support her breast from underneath and gently guide the nipple toward the baby's mouth.

Although babies nurse better if they are not overdressed, agitated babies benefit from being wrapped with only one arm left free.

On the breast

The nipple and areola are now in the baby's mouth, and the baby's head is resting in the crook of the mother's elbow. The mother can depress the breast above the nipple so as not to smother the baby during nursing.

The baby's hands are clenched at the start of nursing. Satisfied by the milk, the baby relaxes and may touch and pat the breast.

Asleep on the breast

Often a baby falls asleep on the breast in contentment from the warmth and closeness to the mother. Delightful as this may be, it is better to encourage the baby to continue feeding. To do this, the mother should slip her middle finger under the baby's chin and close the mouth.

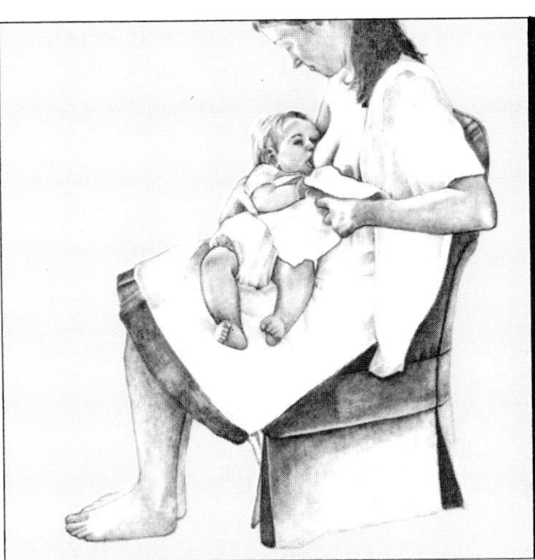

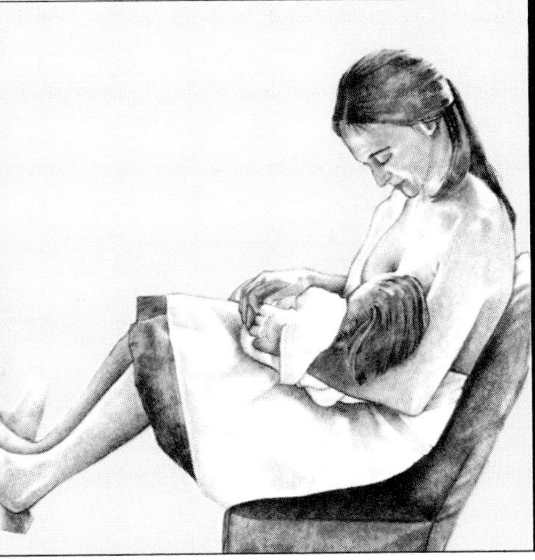

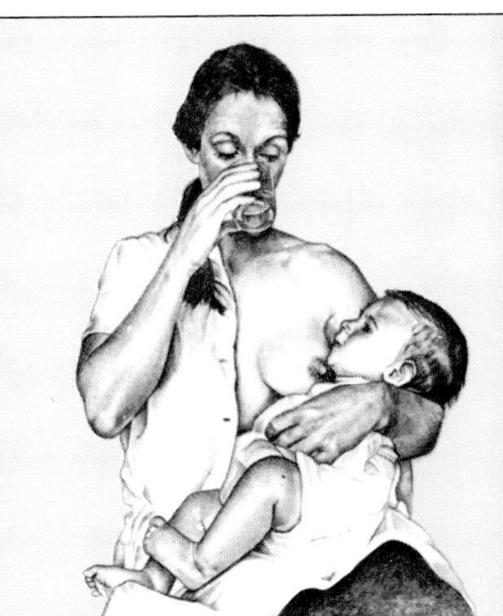

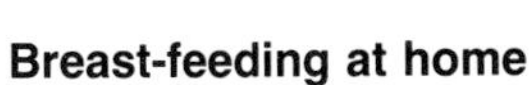

Breast-feeding at home

Once home from the hospital, the mother's early discomfort after the birth should quickly wear off. She can now sit well back in a low chair, feet on the floor to nurse the baby.

When the baby starts to suck, the other breast may leak. This can be controlled by firmly pressing paper tissues against the nipple.

Nursing position

The nursing mother should be relaxed and comfortable.

Another excellent position for nursing is sitting in a low chair, facing the side of a bed, and resting the feet between the mattress and the base of the bed. The thighs should be raised slightly to prevent the baby from slipping off the lap. The shoulders should not be hunched.

The importance of fluids

One-half-hour before nursing the baby, the mother should drink a glass of liquid, such as milk, water, tea, or weak coffee.

The mother should always have a glass of water on the feeding tray. (The water should not be hot; it could spill on the baby.) A nursing mother's fluid intake should increase by two pints a day.

tions on how to use it. Some hospitals use electric pumps. A close-fitting funnel is placed over the nipple, areola, and breast tissue, and the milk is withdrawn by gentle suction produced by the pump. An experienced nurse can provide useful suggestions on the use of the breast pump after the birth of the baby. Such pumps are well worth learning about as they allow the nursing mother increased flexibility, especially if she plans to return to work shortly after the birth of the child. The breast milk may be stored frozen and then warmed and fed to the baby while the mother is away.

Engorgement may occur at the beginning of the milk-producing cycle. The milk-making cells enlarge following hormonal stimulus and an increase in the blood supply. The process lasts for two to three days and in many women causes the breasts to swell painfully. Cold compresses and a mild painkiller should relieve the condition. Nurse the baby frequently, applying warm compresses before feeding. Put a little oil on the breast and express gently.

A relaxed attitude is important to correct any insufficiency in the supply of milk. Follow a sensible diet and eat a little more than was necessary during pregnancy. Drink plenty of liquids, about five pints a day, especially before and during nursing. It is very important to drink at least a quart (four 8oz glasses) of milk a day. Get enough sleep and rest whenever possible. Let the baby nurse frequently, emptying the breasts at every feeding. Consult your physician if you have any questions or problems with breast-feeding.

To prevent excess milk from gushing out, splash the breasts with cold water before nursing, then express a little milk before putting the baby on the breast. Slow the flow of milk to the baby by pressing against the areola with your forefinger and middle finger. The more milk the baby takes, the more the milk supply is stimulated.

The milk may begin to "let down" when you hear your baby crying or when you are out and think about the baby. Fold your arms and press your fists firmly against the nipple and areola area until the tingling sensation stops. Lack of muscle firmness can also cause leaking. Make sure your bra fits firmly and always wear it. Soft cloth pads may be placed in the bra cups to absorb leakage.

Soreness, or even cracks that bleed, may develop if a baby sucks hard or chews the nipple. If this happens, nursing must stop temporarily, and milk from the breasts must be pressed out (expressed) by hand or with a breast pump into a sterile container at regular intervals. The milk should then be offered to the baby from a bottle with a small-hole nipple. A mother's sore nipples heal quickly if the baby does not nurse for about 48 hours. Expose the nipples to the air when possible or sit close to an ordinary light for a few minutes. Take a mild painkiller and use an ointment or spray as recommended by the physician. When the cracks have healed, the baby may be nursed again, but only for short periods at the beginning. Express a little milk first so that the baby finds it easier to mouth the nipple.

Consult the physician if a hard area persists in the breast after nursing and massaging; when a red, painful area, like a boil in the early stages, appears; or if your temperature rises suddenly and you start shivering. Physicians do not agree on whether a nursing mother taking antibiotics should continue to breast-feed. Each situation is different so it would be wise to follow your physician's instructions.

Bottle-feeding a Baby. There are many different reasons for a mother to choose not to breast-feed her baby. Having decided to bottle-feed, a mother should not feel guilty about her decision. Millions of infants reared on formula have grown up healthy.

Combination Feeding. It is helpful that from birth breast-fed babies learn to drink from a bottle. The breast-fed baby can be offered plain, boiled water from a small bottle to pacify him or her between nursing times. A baby of three or four months who has never had a bottle may obstinately refuse one when the mother decides to wean. For this reason, weaning to the bottle should be a gradual, patient process.

A woman who wishes to breast-feed and to return to work outside the home generally finds this no problem if the baby has had experience with a bottle. She can then leave a bottle of formula

Breast-feeding the baby, *continued*

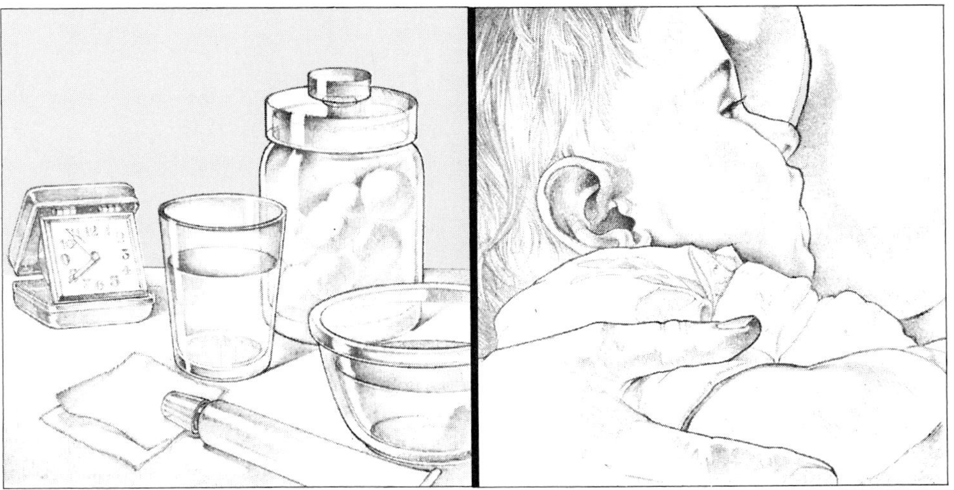

1 Before settling down to feed the baby, the mother should prepare a nursing tray. It should contain warm water and cotton balls for cleaning the breast before and after nursing; a clock; ointment or spray; clean breast pads; and a glass of water. Nursing should be 2 to 3 minutes on each breast the first day; gradually increasing to 10 minutes.

2 The position illustrated is comfortable for both the baby and the mother. Held like this, the baby is able to empty the milk sacs that lie at the top of the breast. Note how much of the nipple and areola is taken into the baby's mouth.

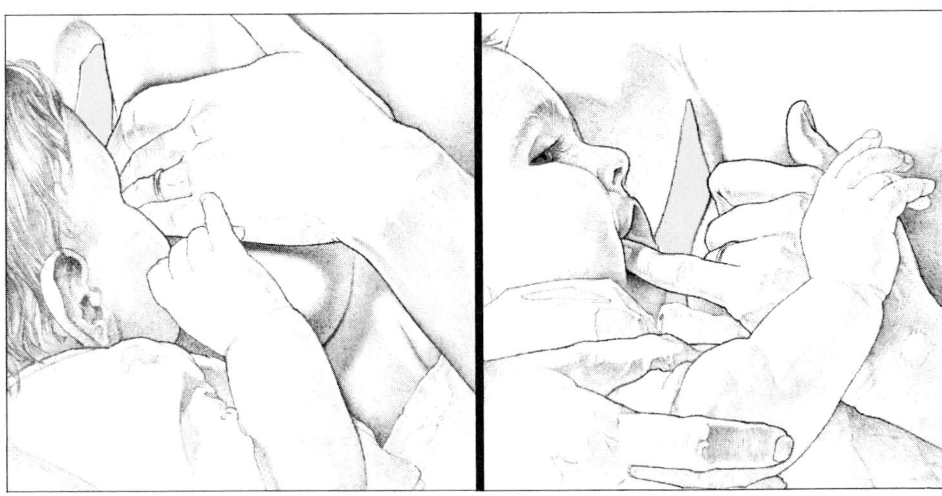

3 When the baby has emptied the forward part of the breast, it is important to massage gently the underarm area of the breast itself, directing the milk toward the nipple. If any lump is felt, the mother should use a circular massage movement; this helps to disperse congested milk and prevent abscesses.

4 To remove the baby from the breast without hurting the nipple, the mother should slip the little finger of her free hand into the corner of the baby's mouth. Newborn babies become sleepy on the breast. Many specialists recommend leaving the baby a shorter time on the first side, so that he or she is still interested in feeding when put on the second side.

Bottle-feeding the baby

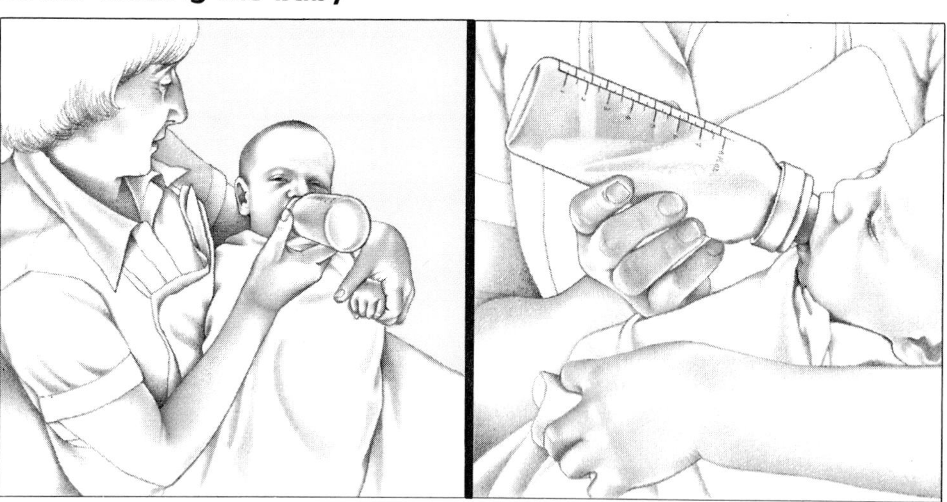

Position of the baby

The parent or baby sitter should sit well back in the chair, in a relaxed position, holding the baby close to the body at an angle of about 45 degrees. The bottle should be held from underneath and tilted so that the nipple is always filled with milk.

It is important to concentrate on the nursing. If the feeder's attention wanders, the bottle may slip and the nipple fill with air.

Giving the bottle

The feeder should make sure that all of the items needed for giving the formula are on hand, so that the baby's nursing time is not interrupted. The following should be on hand: the bottle, a bottle warmer, a box of tissues, and a soft diaper to cover the baby's arms and front. Tucking in the arms stops the baby from grabbing the bottle.

The formula should be given to the baby at body temperature.

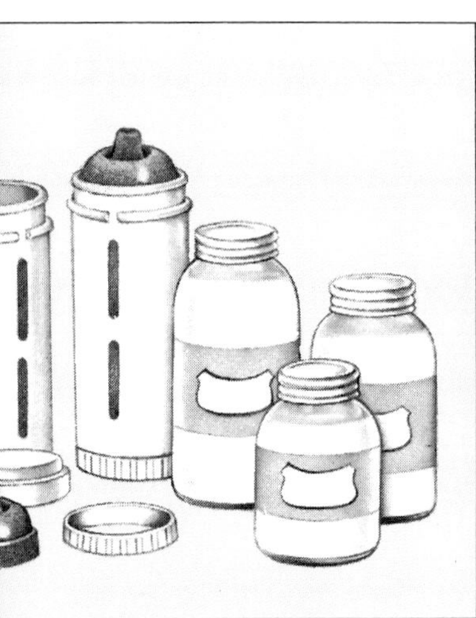

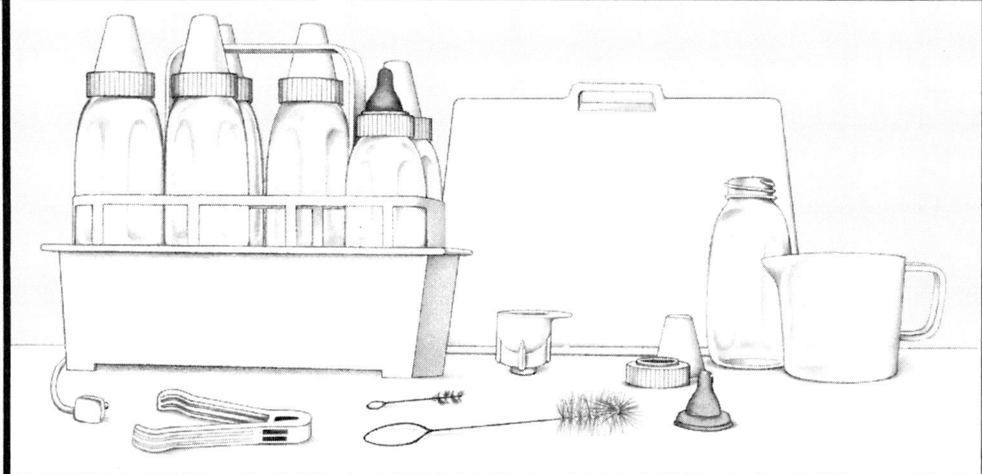

Disposable bottles

There are two kinds of disposable bottles on the market: one is available complete with formula and is thrown away after the feeding; the other is a presterilized plastic sac to which formula is added. The sac fits inside a special holder and is held in place by a retainer ring.

Sterilizing nursing equipment

Bottles, holders, and items of feeding equipment that come in contact with the formula or the baby's mouth can be sterilized.

If the traditional, heat-resistant bottles are used, they should be scrubbed with a bottle brush and detergent and then rinsed well. Nipples should be washed with detergent, rinsed, rubbed with ordinary salt, and rinsed again. The mixing pitcher should be washed thoroughly.

The equipment can be sterilized in boiling water in a large kettle or pail that has a lid. Or, an electric or nonelectric sterilizer kit can be used.

with the baby sitter to give to the baby as a lunchtime substitute for the breast.

A mother's breasts soon adjust to a new schedule, as does the baby. It is important that the bottle is offered at the same time each day. The working mother should eat a nutritious lunch and drink plenty of liquids. She may wish to express and store her milk using a breast pump while she's at work. The baby can then have this milk while the mother is away. *See also* BREAST PUMP.

Choice of Formula. There are many types of formulas available on the market. Some require the addition of water; others are ready for use directly from the can. A mother may continue using the same type that the baby first received in the hospital, or a physician may suggest an alternative.

Condensed milk is not suitable for babies. Pasteurized cow's milk should be introduced only after the baby is six to twelve months old. The milk should then be diluted according to a physician's instructions.

As an aid to the baby's digestive system, it is sometimes necessary to add slightly more water to the formula than the instructions suggest.

How Much Fluid Does a Baby Need? A baby whose birth weight was from six to nine pounds (2.7kg–4.1kg) must be fed every three or four hours round the clock in the first few weeks. Usually after three weeks, a four-hour schedule of five feedings and an eight-hour sleeping gap can be established. Demand feeding, or feeding the baby when he or she is happy rather than by the clock, is desirable.

The amount of milk or formula that a baby should be given each day can be estimated on body weight. In general, for every pound (0.45kg) of weight, the baby should be given 2.5 fluid ounces (75ml). The baby should be allowed to consume as much milk or formula as desired. Obesity is rare in infants that are not yet eating solid foods.

Preparing the Bottles. Either glass bottles or plastic bottles with sterile collapsible liners can be used for nursing. Plastic bottles with collapsible liners are, however, particularly beneficial because the baby does not swallow as much air as is possible with the glass type.

If you have chosen to use the traditional glass bottles, you will need eight 8-ounce (240ml) bottles, at least two 4-ounce (120ml) bottles, and various nipples, caps, and hoods.

Sterilizing the bottles is not necessary. Prompt cleaning with hot soapy water and storing them in a clean, dry place will suffice. Some parents do, however, choose to sterilize the bottles and there is equipment available to do so.

Formula can be made up in bulk in a clean pitcher, or one bottle at a time can be prepared by measuring the ingredients directly into the bottle. For storing in the refrigerator, invert the nipples in the bottle. Cans of prepared formula are also available. Once a can of this formula is opened it must be kept refrigerated and any left unused for 48 hours should be discarded.

Burping a Baby. All babies swallow air when they suck, whether nursed at the breast or on the bottle. The air collects as a bubble in the baby's stomach, causing discomfort and sometimes pain. The baby stops nursing and begins to cry. Many physicians advise a pause about halfway through the feeding in order to burp the baby. Some babies may need to be burped more frequently.

The amount of air a baby swallows depends on both the flow of milk from breast or bottle and on the baby's sucking ability.

It is important that all air bubbles are expelled at the end of the feeding as well, or the baby will cry soon afterward.

There are many different kinds of nipples available for baby bottles. Some are long, some short; some are made of hard rubber, some of soft. The nipples can have a small, medium, or large hole. Buying a selection allows a mother to find the one that is most comfortable and most effective in her baby's mouth. The ability to suck also varies according to the baby's age and whether he or she is hungry. A one-week-old baby, for example, needs a medium-hole or large-hole nipple. A baby sucking through a small hole swallows a lot of air in an effort to get

Burping the baby

Burping the newborn baby

The baby should be sat up in the caregiver's lap. The caregiver's forearm should cross the baby's chest and stomach. The baby should tilt forward diagonally away from the caregiver. His or her forearm should slide up the baby's chest until the baby's head lies in the palm. The other hand should apply gentle pressure to the back.

Burping the "older" baby

An older baby needs to be supported only by one hand under his or her armpit. Again the baby's head should be tilted slightly to the side and the body tilted forward. It is useless to continue to burb the baby, however, if air has not come up by the end of nursing. Some babies do not need burping or may release gas through the rectum.

Burping halfway through nursing

The baby should be sat up in the caregiver's lap. The caregiver should then place one arm across the baby's chest, with the hand under his or her armpit. With the other hand, the caregiver should stroke the baby's back using upward movements only.

The over-the-shoulder position

A caregiver can also hold the baby against his or her body and apply slight palm pressure to the middle of the infant's back. The baby's chin should rest on the caregiver's shoulder. This position is recommended for a baby who is crying. The caregiver can walk around the room carrying the baby and speaking softly.

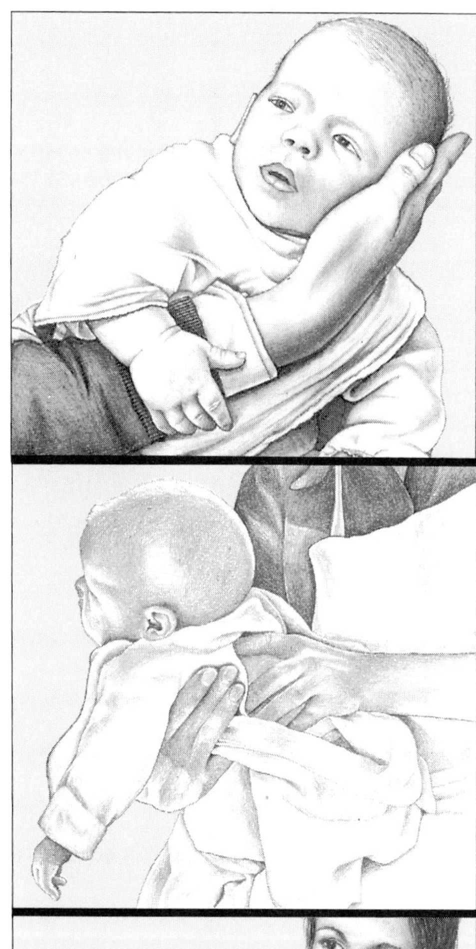

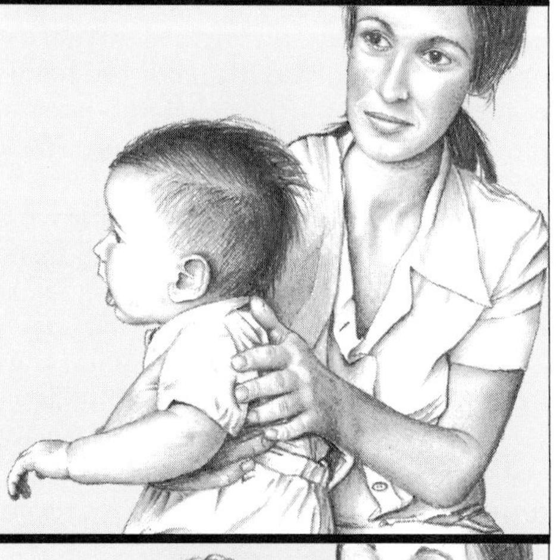

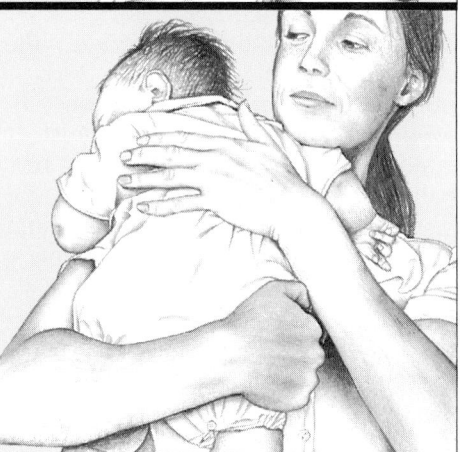

the milk, then falls asleep exhausted and uncomfortable. But if the hole is too large, the milk gushes through so fast that the baby may choke immediately or vomit afterward.

Spitting. A baby who nurses too quickly may vomit slightly after the feeding. Throwing up a small amount of milk is often called spitting and is nothing to worry about. Even if the baby occasionally throws up the entire feeding, there is no need for alarm. If the vomiting occurs repeatedly, however, consult a physician.

When burping a baby in the upright position, rest the baby's chin on your shoulder and be sure to protect your clothing in case the baby should spit or vomit.

Gas Pains. A baby who has swallowed too much air may be unable to expel the bubbles by burping immediately after being fed. The resulting discomfort can last for a few days and demands a great deal of patience. Be aware of a reliable sign that indicates gas: the baby may take two or three gulps of milk, draw away from the breast or bottle, and arch the back.

Nurse the baby slowly and try to relax. Walking slowly round the room with the baby in your arms sometimes helps to start him or her nursing again. Another method is to change the baby to a different nursing position, so that he or she sits more upright. When the condition improves, return the baby to the usual feeding position.

Inexperienced parents or baby sitters commonly try to bring up a baby's gas by striking him or her sharply on the back. But this only makes the baby tense and even less able to release the bubbles. Sometimes such patting may actually cause the baby to throw up some milk.

The illustrations on these pages show some of the best ways to help the baby during the process of nursing, but if no success is achieved within a few minutes, continue with nursing anyway, following the usual routine.

Reluctant Nursers. Because the liver does not work at full capacity for some time after birth, some babies may become slightly jaundiced. It is important that a jaundiced baby drink enough fluids. To encourage a baby to nurse, push gently and rhythmically with the forefinger under the baby's chin. But be patient, because the baby may fall asleep again.

Restless Nursers. Older babies may for one reason or another tend to be restless at nursing time. They wave their arms about, scratching at the bottle or hitting the breast. Such a baby should be held close to the body and wrapped in a blanket from the waist down. The baby's arms may be left free if they are kept out of the way. One arm can be tucked behind the feeder's back, while the other hand can be held. Hold the baby firmly, but not roughly, because this may make the baby struggle even more.

Feeding Solids. There is no set time for introducing solid foods into a baby's diet. Some parents start offering their baby cereal as early as six weeks, but this can place considerable strain on a baby's digestive system. Generally, a baby thrives on a diet of breast milk or formula, supplemented with vitamins, for the first six months. Depending on the individual baby, any time between four and six months may be suitable for the introduction of solids.

Remember that solids given to a baby represent a replacement for milk and are an addition to the baby's previous total consumption. Milk is easy to digest and goes through a baby's system fairly rapidly; solids take longer. The result is that the number of feedings per day can probably be reduced by one, once the baby is on solids. A parent usually chooses the least convenient feeding time as the one to be dropped—generally the A.M. feeding.

There are many signs to tell a parent when a baby needs more than merely milk. A baby is ready for solids when he or she:

- wakes during the night demanding to be fed, having previously for some time slept right through every night without complaint;
- gains only one or two ounces (30 or 60 grams), or nothing at all, during a week;
- seems restless between feedings during the day and wakes up crying too soon before each feeding;
- is no longer satisfied by an eight-ounce (240ml) bottle, or, if breast-fed, interrupts nursing and plucks at the mother's clothing, trying to chew it;
- shows a readiness to chew by picking up objects and trying to put them in the mouth.

A baby's first solid food should consist of a single cereal. Rice is preferred as it is unlikely to cause allergy. Begin with only one teaspoonful of the new food at one mealtime, gradually introducing new foods and flavors over a period of weeks. The chart on page 86 suggests how to do this. In subsequent weeks, single pureed fruits and vegetables may be added.

Any change in feeding pattern can result in the baby's showing no weight gain during that week or even a weight loss. But such a holdup or loss will be made up for by the baby's increased appetite the following week. A cold, an upset stomach, or the process of teething can have the same temporary effect.

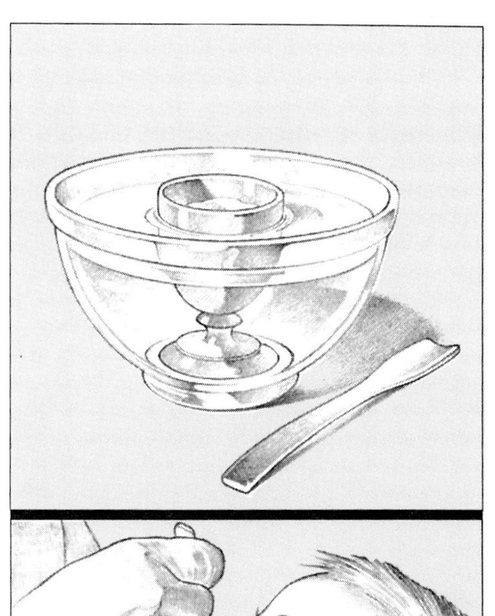

Feeding the baby

Small quantities of food should be kept warm and can be served from an eggcup that has been placed in a bowl of hot water. Babies are puzzled by their first experience with solid foods, and some may reject the first spoonfuls. A little milk should be offered before a taste of the new food.

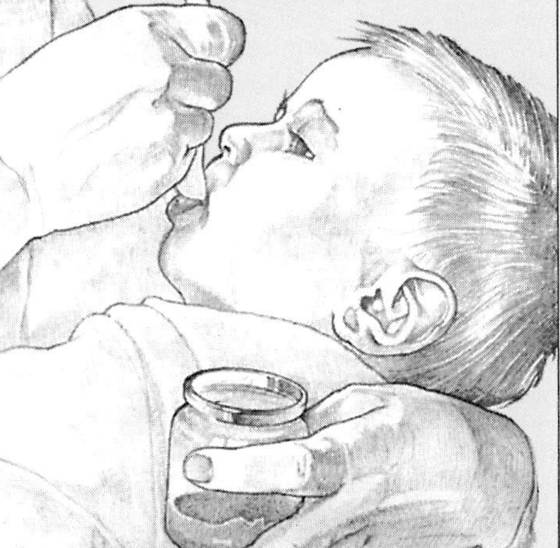

The baby should be held firmly in one arm. A bib or folded diaper tucked under his or her chin can catch dribbles. An almost flat, rounded plastic spoon should be used. It should be placed just inside the baby's mouth, resting on the lower lip. The baby sucks the strained food into his or her mouth.

It is easy to judge the amount of solid food to give a previously bottle-fed baby; the milk in the bottle can be measured. But for a breast-fed baby it may be more difficult.

Any increase in the amount of food given to a baby must be gradual. One teaspoonful more at selected times (see the chart below) is the maximum advisable, especially of fruit and vegetables, for one week at a time. If the baby seems to be gaining weight too rapidly, cereals should be increased even more slowly.

When the baby has reached the stage of having five or six teaspoonfuls of pure vegetables at lunchtime, some meat, poultry, fish, or cheese may be added. The baby's milk consumption may decrease as the consumption of solid foods increases.

Having started on solids at age four months, for example, a six- to seven-month-old infant generally has three main mealtimes plus an afternoon snack of a teething biscuit and a bottle of fruit juice.

Food should be pureed for a baby up to age seven months; the puree should be of sufficiently thick consistency for the baby to be able to eat it from a spoon. Mince or grind food for a baby of age seven to ten months. After this age, a baby can eat food that has simply been cut up into small pieces.

A sample day's menu for a baby at this stage might consist of:

8-9 A.M.	8oz (225g) milk; 4-5oz (113-142g) fruit, possibly with a little cereal. (On alternate days, egg yolk, beginning with a very small quantity.)
12-1 P.M.	5-6oz (142-170g) milk; 4-6oz (113-170g) total of meat, poultry, fish, or cheese, plus vegetables.
afternoon	Juice; teething biscuit;
5:30-6 P.M.	8oz (225g) milk; 4-5oz (113-142g) total of cereal, fruit.
9 P.M.	8oz (225g) milk.

Schedule for introduction of solid foods

Suggested Feeding Times	*Feedings, with additional solids* 1st week	*2nd week*	*3rd week*	*4th week*
6 A.M.*	Milk			
10 A.M.	Milk	Milk 1 teaspoonful strained fruit	Milk 2 teaspoonfuls strained fruit	Milk 3 teaspoonfuls strained fruit
2 P.M.	Milk 1 teaspoonful strained vegetables	Milk 2 teaspoonfuls strained vegetables	Milk 3 teaspoonfuls strained vegetables	Milk 4 teaspoonfuls strained vegetables
3:30-4:30 P.M.	Juice	Juice	Juice	Juice 1 teaspoonful plain yogurt or 1 teaspoonful mashed banana
6 P.M.	Milk	Milk	Milk $\frac{1}{2}$-1 teaspoon unmixed cereal but not wheat	Milk 1-$1\frac{1}{2}$ teaspoonful another cereal
10-11 P.M.*	Milk	Milk	Milk	Milk

*This feeding may have been dropped.

Swaddling the baby

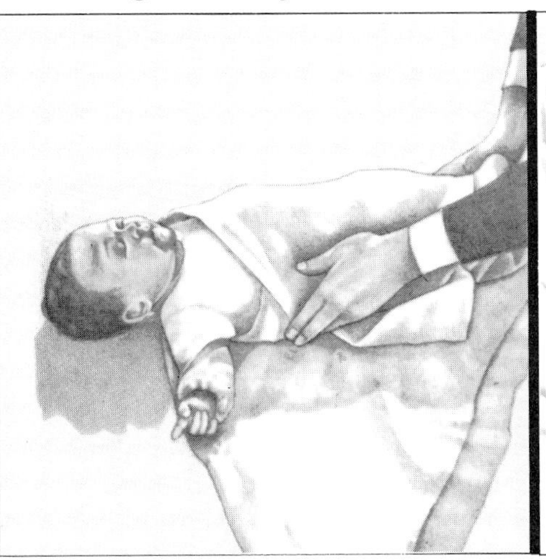

Wrapping the baby
The baby should lie on a receiving blanket folded in a triangle shape. The fold should be under the baby's neck and shoulders. The arms should be placed across the chest at a 45 degree angle. A blanket corner should cover one arm and the chest, and then be tucked smoothly under the body. This should be repeated with the other corner.

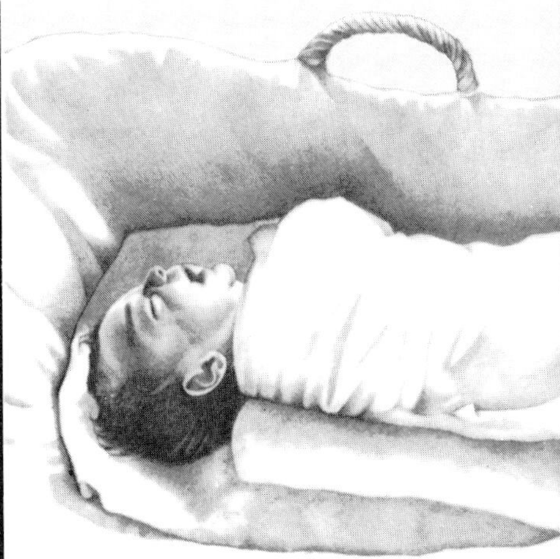

All tucked in
The baby should be wrapped in an overblanket that has been folded in a triangle. The corners should be drawn snugly over the baby's shoulders and tucked under the mattress. After each feeding, the side on which the baby sleeps should be alternated.

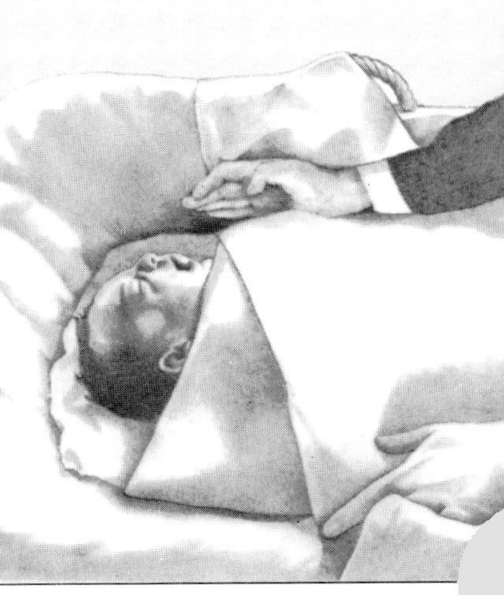

Bassinet position
The newborn baby should not sleep on his or her back. If the baby brings up milk with gas, he or she could choke. The baby should be put on his or her side. A bolster firmly placed against the baby's back, just below the head, will prevent him or her from rolling over.

Sleeping Conditions

Babies may sleep up to 23 hours a day during the first month after birth. Their need for sleep then gradually decreases.

For safety and comfort, a baby should sleep in a specially designed crib. Most cribs have sides with bars that can be lowered and raised by an adult. The slats of the crib should be no more than 2⅝″ (6.6cm) apart. Any wider and the baby's head could become entrapped. Babies should be kept covered in their cribs to avoid chills.

Most infants like to lie on their stomachs or backs with their heads turned toward the lightest part of the room. But a baby's head may become flattened on one side if it is always turned in the same direction. To avoid this problem, babies should be turned head to foot at every other bedtime. They will then have to turn their heads in the opposite direction in order to face the light. If the baby still prefers keeping its head turned in one direction, there is no real cause for alarm; the child normally will outgrow any head flattening by one year of age.

Swaddling the Baby. A newborn baby is much happier if he or she is wrapped up snugly. This custom, called swaddling, is considered old-fashioned and even unkind by some people, but modern research has shown that it is a practical way to help a baby to sleep peacefully.

Remember that the infant is not used to unlimited space, having been confined for months to the restricted space of the womb. Swaddling makes the baby feel more secure and helps him or her to adjust to the world, little by little.

Newborn babies have little or no control over their limbs so they often wake themselves with the jerky movements of their own arms and legs. The well wrapped-up baby is not bothered by this.

How long a parent continues to swaddle a baby depends on whether the baby is of a calm or excitable disposition. But up to six weeks is usually beneficial. At three to six weeks, however, the baby's hands should be al-

Washing the baby

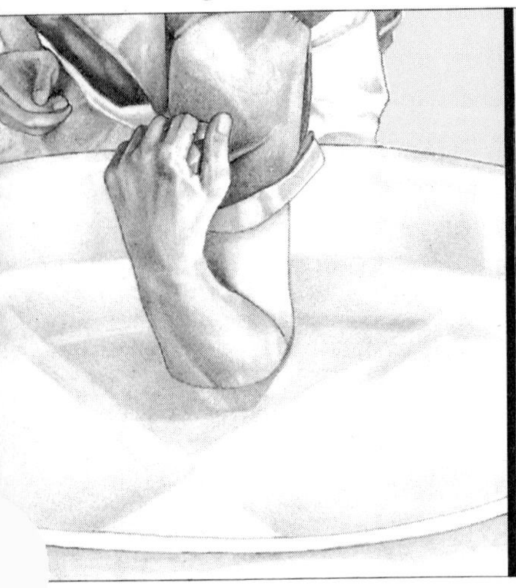

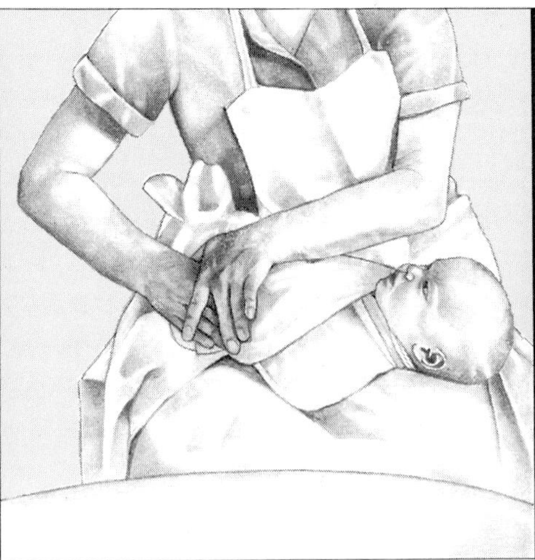

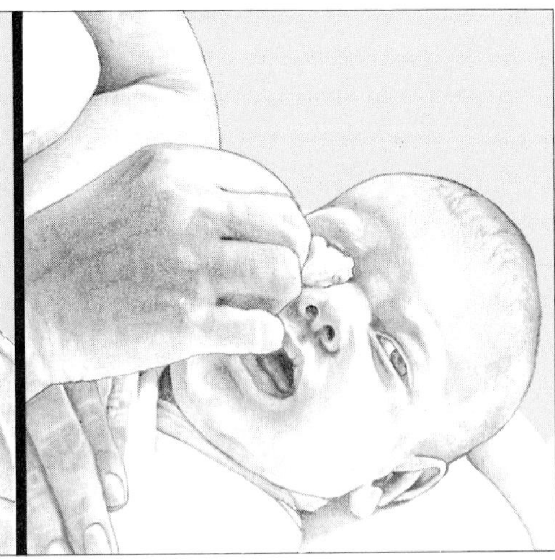

Bath and temperature

The bath water should not be so deep as to cover the baby when he or she is held in it.

The caregiver should dip his or her elbow into the bathwater to test its temperature. The water should be at body temperature.

Lap or changing mat

The difference between dressing and undressing a baby on the caregiver's lap and doing so on a changing mat is largely a matter of convenience. But babies prefer the lap, and it does save the effort of standing up to change a diaper. If a mat is used, it should have padded edges and be covered with a towel.

Washing the face

Before beginning to wash the baby's face, the caregiver should wrap the infant in a towel folded into a triangle. The baby's head should be held in the caregiver's hand.

A fresh cotton ball dipped in water can be used to wipe each eye. The outside of the mouth should also be washed with a clean swab. Then the rest of the face can be washed.

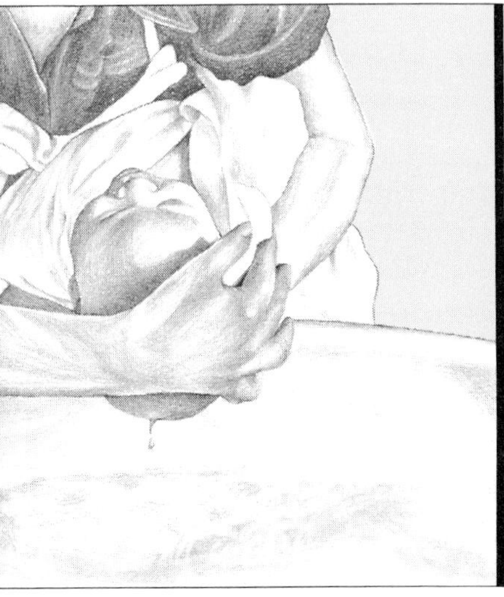

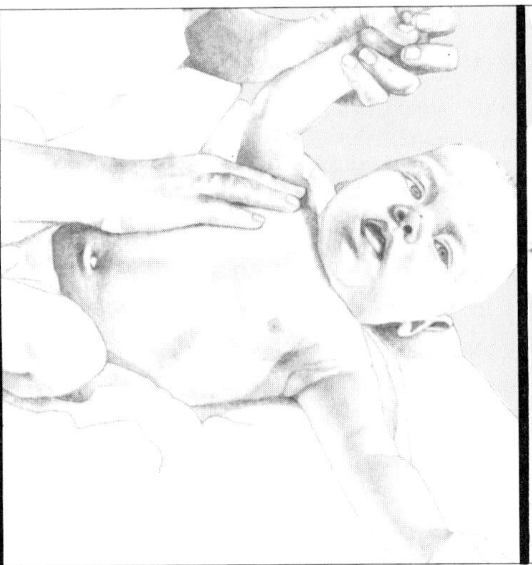

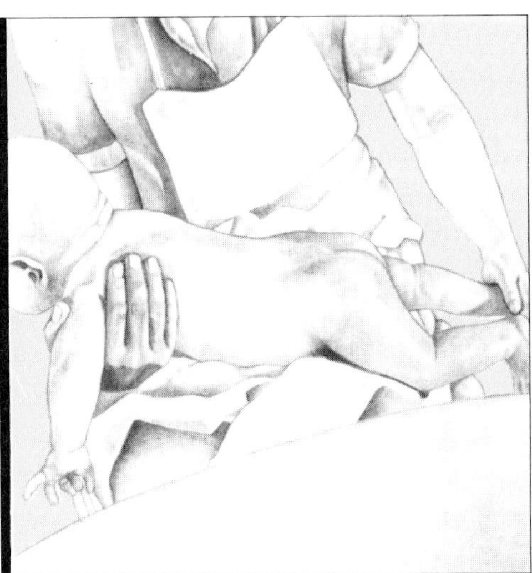

Soaping the head

The baby should be held firmly with one arm, the hand supporting the infant's head. The caregiver's other hand can soap the baby's head. The hair and scalp should be massaged. The caregiver should not be afraid to soap the soft spot on the baby's head.

Baby soap or shampoo should be rinsed off before the next stage of the bath.

Soaping the baby's front

The baby's front should be soaped all over. The folds of the neck under the chin are deep, and milk and moisture can become trapped there. The baby's chin should be lifted gently, and a soapy finger slid along the creases. If this area is not washed and rinsed carefully, it can become inflamed and painful.

Soaping the baby's back

To soap the baby's back, the infant must be turned over. To do so, the caregiver can use one arm to support the baby from the front. The caregiver holds his or her hand around the baby's armpit. Once the baby is facedown on the caregiver's lap, the infant's back can be soaped. After a soapy massage, the infant must be rinsed.

lowed to reach high enough so that he or she can suck the fist or fingers.

Even a newborn baby can lie on the stomach without risk of smothering. Swaddle from the waist down, with the arms free, so that the baby cannot wriggle up the crib or cradle.

Bathing a Baby

Have all the things needed before starting to undress the baby. Each mother establishes her own routine for bathing the baby. Here are some suggestions.

An infant quickly loses body heat, so it is important that the room is warm and that there are no drafts from open windows or doors. A wall thermometer is useful. A bathinette or a plastic tub three-quarters full of lukewarm water should be placed within arm's length. Also needed are a small bowl of warm water in which there is a squirt of liquid bath soap; two small sponges; cotton balls; cotton swabs; disposable wipes; baby oil; soap; shampoo; lotion; talcum powder; a fine-toothed comb; a bristle hairbrush; and a baby comb. A waterproof apron is also required, preferably one with a turkish toweling surface, together with several soft, absorbent towels for patting the baby dry; a fresh diaper; diaper pins; plastic pants; and a set of clean clothes.

Newborn babies heartily dislike facecloths. Until the baby is one month old, use moistened cotton balls to wash his or her face. Afterward, use one of the sponges for the face and the second sponge for the buttocks area when a soiled diaper is removed.

Most babies have diaper rash at one time or another, usually caused by prolonged contact with stools and urine. A physician will recommend an ointment to get rid of the rash. Diaper rash can usually be prevented by spreading on a little petroleum jelly in the diaper region after the baby's bath, and by checking the baby's diapers often and changing them when needed to avoid prolonged contact with urine and stool.

Dry skin is common among newborn babies. Baby oil, gently massaged into the skin, can relieve the condition. But test the oil first on the baby's ankle to make sure that there is not an allergic reaction. Plain petroleum jelly is also useful.

Cradle cap, a patch of yellowish, greasy crusting on the baby's head, should be treated at bath time. After the baby is nursed, massage some oil into the scalp and leave it for several hours until the next meal. By then the scaling should be easy to lift with a fine-toothed comb. At bath time, shampoo and rinse the baby's scalp and dry carefully. Brush the baby's hair.

Throughout bath time reassure the infant by speaking softly. A newborn infant is frightened by loud noises and quick, jerky movements and responds by crying.

Handle the baby gently when dressing him or her. Clothing should be simple to slip on and take off because the baby may be crying and perhaps stiff and rigid from exertion. Loose clothes with snap fasteners are preferable to clothing that has to be pulled over the head.

The Bath. In the early weeks, bathtime may take longer than anticipated because both parent and baby do not know quite what to expect. As soon as a routine is established, the baby will feel more secure and tolerant of handling. The baby should not be immersed in a tub until the umbilical stump has fallen off.

Make sure in these early days that the room and bath temperatures are kept constant throughout the bathtime. The bathwater should be kept at 100–104°F (37–40°C), slightly higher than normal body temperature. Keep a pitcher of warm water near the bath to top off the bathwater should it cool down too much.

Be kind to the baby; handle him or her with warm hands; speak softly in a soothing voice.

Most babies love being in the water, but hate coming out of it; they cry, showing signs of insecurity and shivering. The baby should be wrapped immediately in a towel and held tightly for a moment. This helps a baby to relax again. Now slowly start to dry the baby, either on your lap or on a changing mat. Be sure that a soft, absorbent towel covers the plastic mat before you lay the baby on it. Now gently open the towel in which the baby is wrapped and pat dry with a second towel. Always try to keep covered the parts of the body that are not actually being dried.

Washing the baby, *continued*

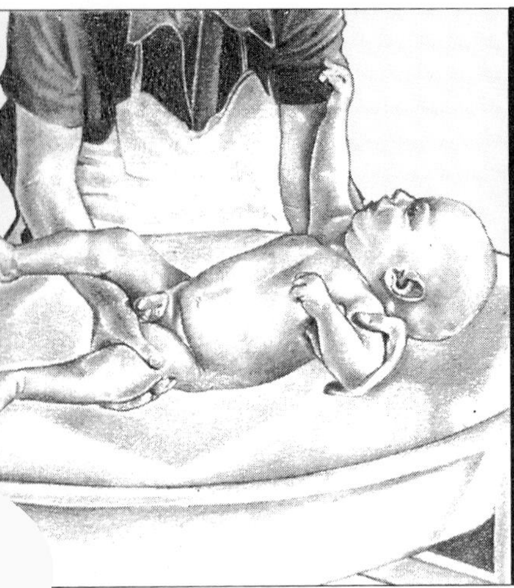

Holding a slippery baby

The baby should be held face-up, the head supported from behind the neck. The caregiver should wrap a thumb over one of the baby's shoulders and wrap fingers around the baby's arm. The caregiver's other hand should be under the baby's buttocks and nearest leg, and be holding the baby's other leg. The baby should be lowered into the water.

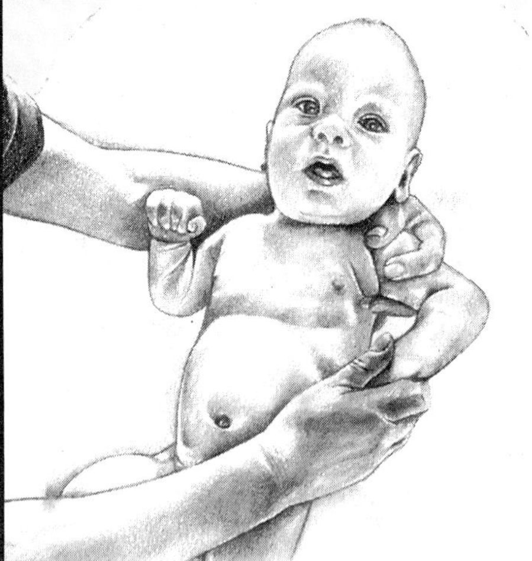

Rinsing off the soap

The caregiver should release his or her grip on the baby's leg once the infant is in the water. With the caregiver's free hand, he or she should sponge and rinse off the baby's armpits and the areas under the neck and between the fingers. In the warm water, the baby's tightly clenched fist will probably open.

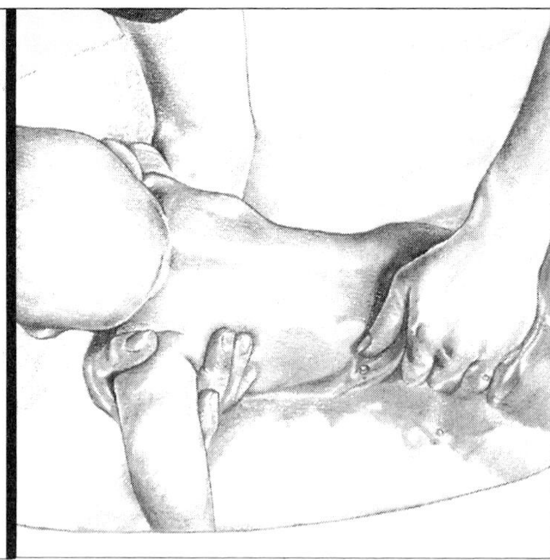

Swimming position

The baby should be held over the caregiver's forearm. The caregiver should put his or her other thumb on the baby's farthest shoulder and use fingers to encircle the baby's arm. The baby's head will then stay clear of the water.

When the baby is lifted out of the tub, a caregiver should have his or her hand on the infant's lower abdomen.

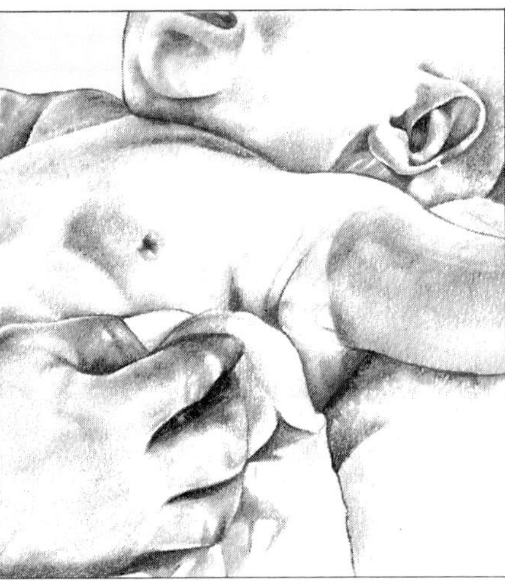

Armpit hygiene

Newborn babies, especially chubby ones, sweat a lot. Consequently, in the first few weeks parents may discover sticky substances in the baby's armpits. The armpits should be soaped gently and then rinsed in the bath. They should be patted dry.

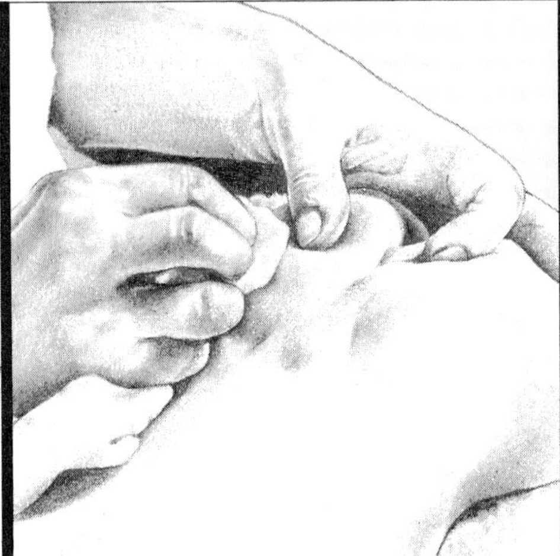

Drying in the creases

It is easy for a parent to overlook some of the baby's folds and creases when drying the infant. The buttocks, which are almost always damp or dirty in the early months, are areas that require special attention. Great care should be taken to dry the deep crease at the top of the buttocks, where irritation can occur.

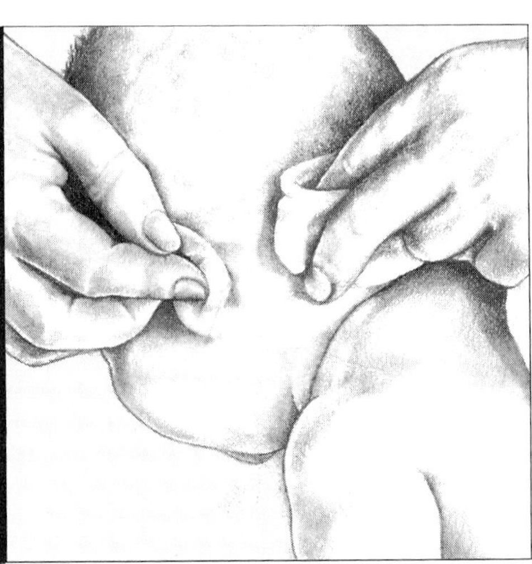

Cleaning around the ears

Cracked skin behind the ears can be painful, but it is not serious. Daily washing behind, below, and above the ears is important. Petroleum jelly should be applied when these areas are clean and dry.

Crust may develop either as an extension of cradle cap or as the result of milk trickling down the cheek and behind the ear when the baby is sleeping sideways.

When the baby is dry, you may apply ointment to the diaper area if you wish, and then begin to dress the baby. Put on the undershirt first to keep the body warm, then the diaper, and finally the sleeper or pajamas.

Changing a Diaper

Ideally, a baby's diaper should be changed both before and after nursing. But until the age of about six weeks, most babies protest loudly and tearfully against anything that delays nursing time. So, provided that the baby has not had a bowel movement, it is better not to insist on a pre-feeding diaper change in the interest of a peaceful nursing session. After the baby has nursed, he or she is generally more cooperative.

Some parents, especially mothers, like to change a newborn baby on their laps; others prefer to use a waterproof changing mat on a bed or a dresser top. The mat should be covered with a soft towel so that the baby is not placed on a cold plastic surface.

No matter how clean the baby is kept, the skin in the diaper area may still become sore and red. When the first signs of diaper rash appear, add extra absorbency by folding a cloth diaper in half and wrapping it round the baby's waist over the clean ordinary diaper. Secure the extra diaper with a diaper pin, like a skirt. During a bout with diaper rash, plastic pants are no longer suitable.

To prevent a cloth diaper from becoming stained, rinse the stools off the diaper as soon as possible. Hold the diaper under running water in the toilet bowl. It should then be put to soak in a sterilizing solution, in the receptacle provided by the diaper service, or in a household bucket.

The parent's hands should be washed thoroughly after a diaper change. It is not appropriate to leave the child unattended for this because some infants will begin to roll over as early as two months. Here again, careful planning is the key in baby care.

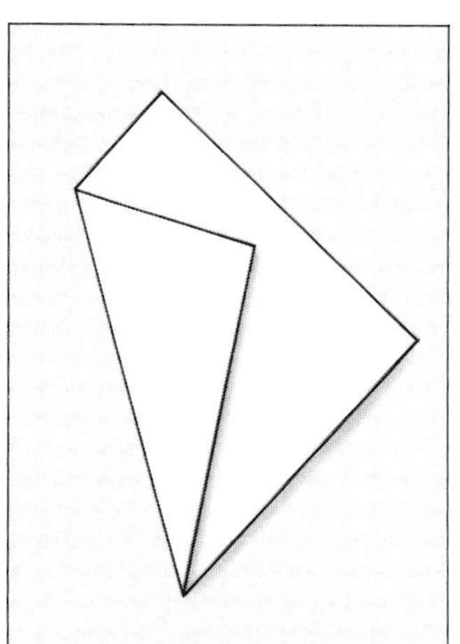

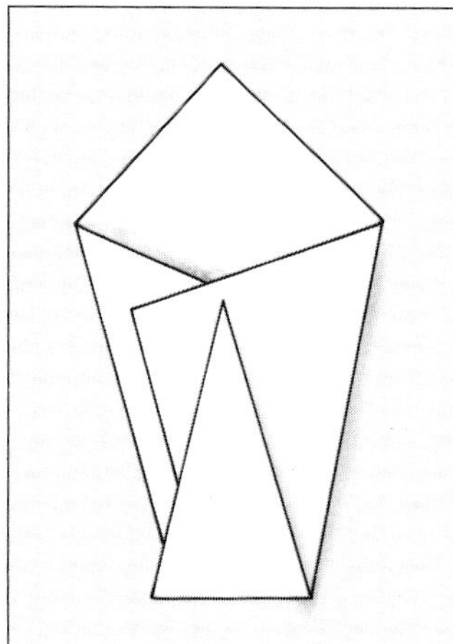

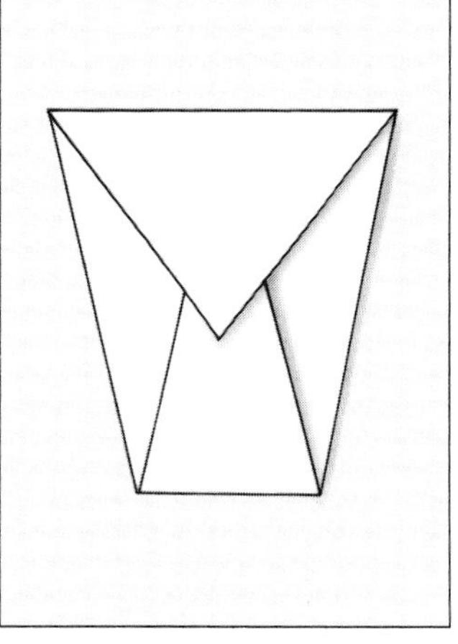

Folding the baby's diapers

To fold the kite-shaped diaper, the diaper should be laid flat in a diamond shape, with a point at the top and bottom. Then each of the side points should be folded toward the center.

Now the narrow, "tail" end of the diaper should be drawn up toward the center. It must be folded at about a third of the way from the bottom. This gives a diaper of about the correct size for a young baby.

Finally, the remaining top flap should be folded toward the center. The wide end should go around the baby's waist.

The diaper can be lined with a muslin diaper folded in thirds. Or, it can be lined with a one-way diaper in which the fabric is treated so that the wetness passes through to the ordinary diaper and keeps the baby's skin dry. A disposable diaper liner can also be used.

Diapering the baby

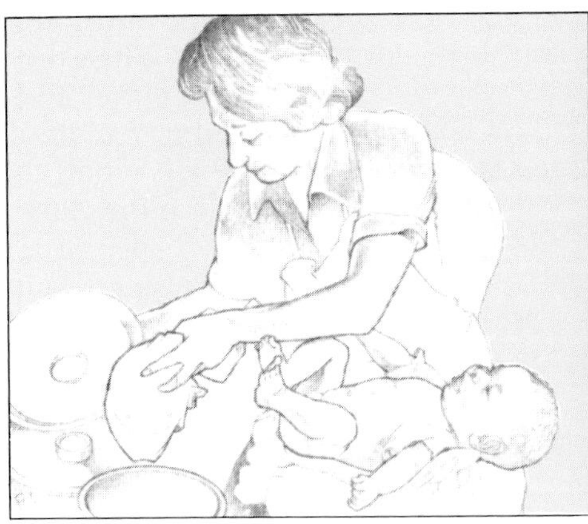

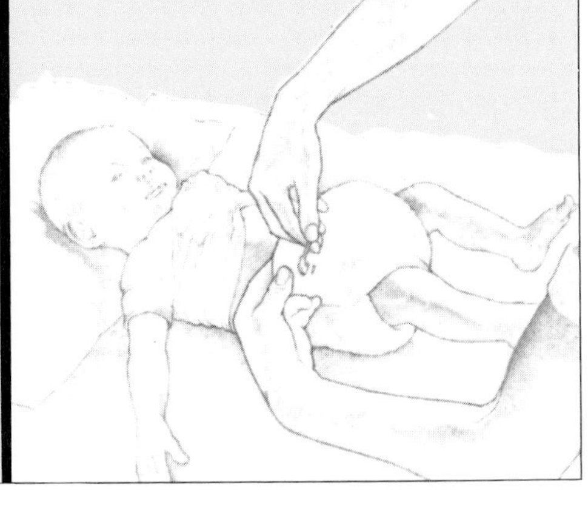

1 The old diaper should be removed and immediately put in an empty household bucket that has a lid. Leaving a dirty diaper on the floor or elsewhere risks infection. Stool should be removed with paper tissues or cotton. The diaper area should be soaped, rinsed, and patted dry. Ointment should be applied.

2 For the first few weeks, an average 7-pound (3kg) baby will need a muslin diaper, folded double and then into a triangle, which can be lined. As the baby grows, the kite-shaped diaper, *above*, is generally more practical because its thickness and size can be adjusted. It also ensures that the baby has less bulk between the legs.

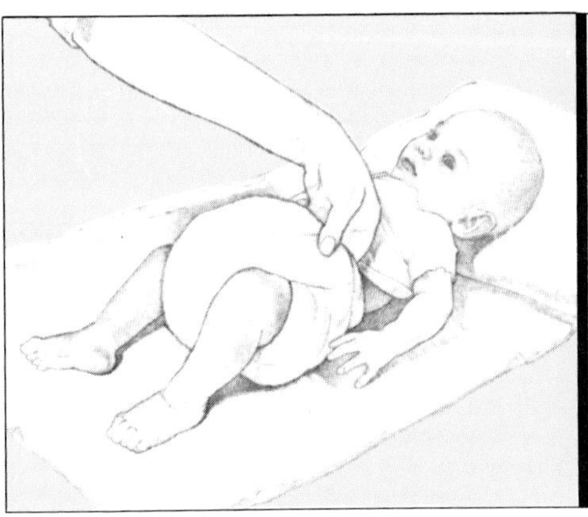

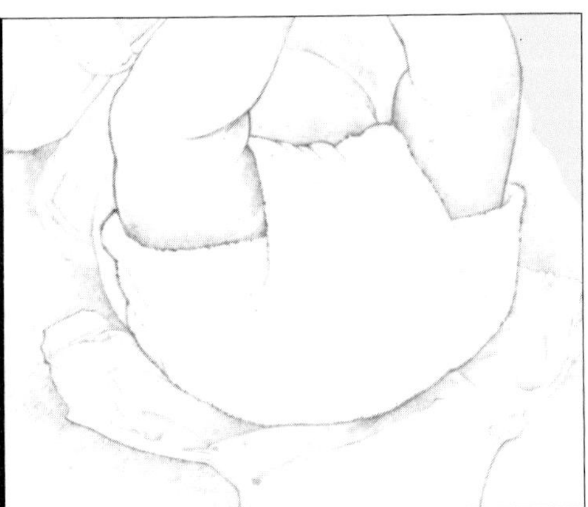

3 The baby should be laid on the diaper with the widest end of the fabric at the baby's waist. The narrow "tail" should be drawn up between the baby's legs, and the inside edges of the flap nipped to reduce bulkiness. The flap should be drawn up over the baby's stomach, and the diaper pinned. Care should be taken that the baby's skin is not pricked.

4 Correct diapering with a kite-shaped diaper results in a pair of neat, well-fitting pants. The shape makes for a good fit around the top of the baby's legs, so that leaks are prevented. A pair of soft plastic pants should not fit too tightly over the abdomen or around the thighs. Air should circulate in the diaper area.

Handling the baby

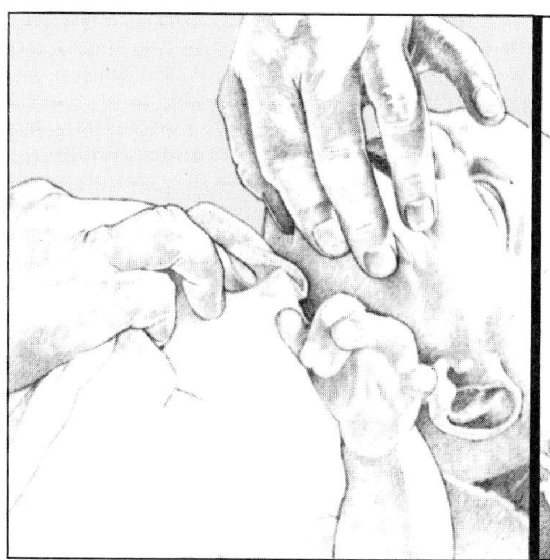

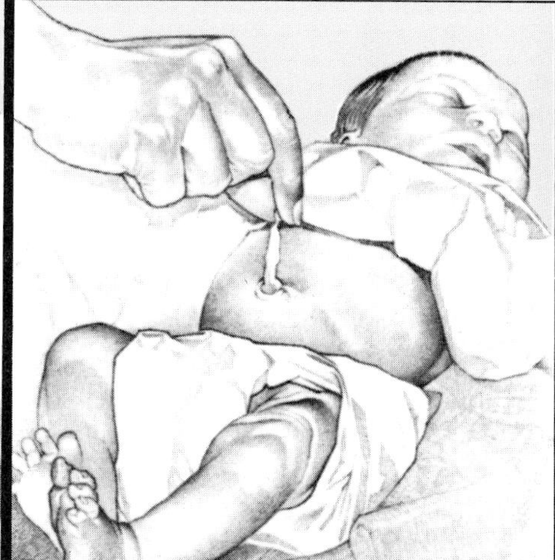

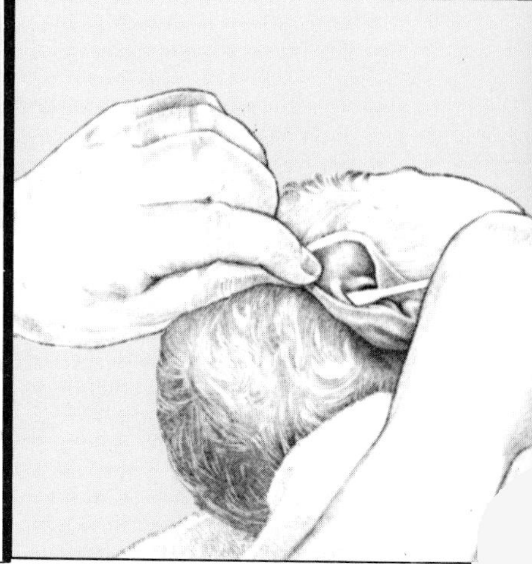

Soreness under the chin

The newborn has a short neck with a great many creases. The area becomes hot and must be soaped and well rinsed.

After the baby is taken out of the bath, his or her head should be gently tilted back, and the chin should be carefully dried.

Care of the navel

The umbilical cord usually falls off one to three weeks after birth.

A slight discharge under the cord is normal. Carefully clean the stump at the base with cotton dipped in rubbing alcohol. Powder should then be applied. Plastic pants should not be worn over the navel during this time.

Cleaning the ears

A newborn's ears frequently collect all kinds of matter: tears, milk, fluff, and wax. The ears should be cleaned with a moistened cotton swab. A fresh swab should be used for each ear. The ears' outer shell-like folds should be carefully wiped. The swab should never be inserted into the baby's ear canal.

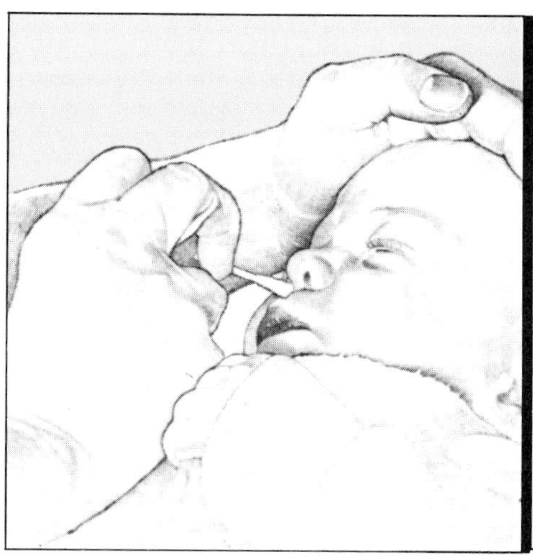

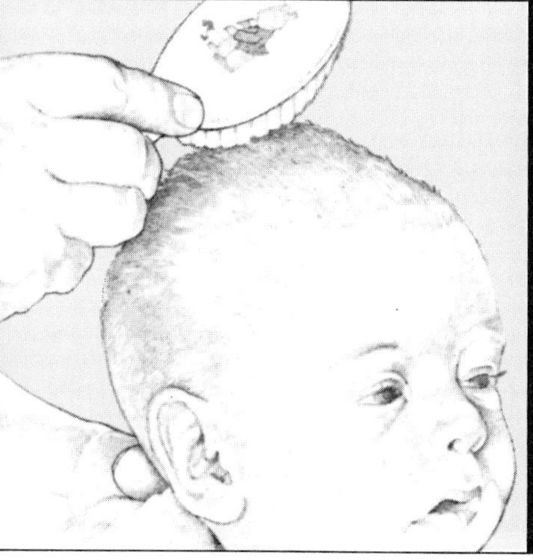

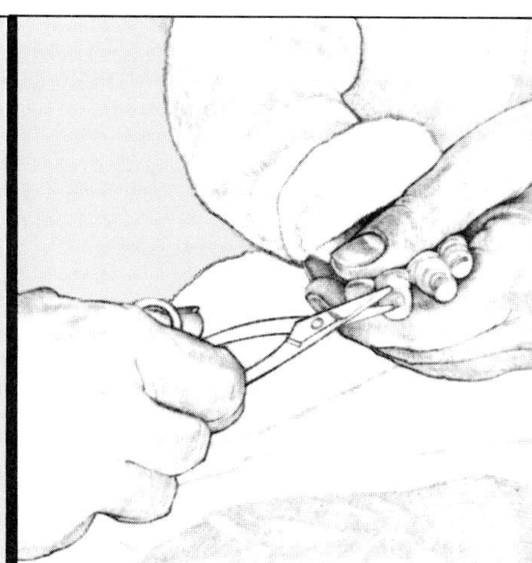

Cleaning the nose

It is important to check daily that there is no obstruction in the nose.

If there is an obstruction, such as mucus or crusts, the caregiver should use a cotton swab to wipe around the entrance to each nostril. The swab should never be inserted into the baby's nostril.

Brushing the hair

The hair should be washed two or three times a week with gentle shampoo and rinsed with warm clean water. For details, see page 89.

Brushing is also excellent for the circulation to the scalp, and it helps prevent cradle cap. Do not be afraid to brush the soft spot on the baby's head.

Cutting the nails

A baby's fingernails are soft but sharp. In the first few weeks, a baby may scratch his or her own face.

When baby's fingernails are cut, his or her hand should be held firmly. Nails should be cut straight across.

A baby's toenails do not usually require cutting for the first four to six months.

The Older Baby. A baby who sleeps through the night may, during that time, soak through an ordinarily folded diaper. Soaking can be prevented to a certain extent by folding the skirt-shaped diaper around the baby's waist. But if the baby moves around the crib during the night (as happens when a baby is about nine months old), the skirt diaper rides up out of position.

To provide a diaper that stays in position and also has plenty of absorbency, fold one diaper lengthways until there are three folds; turn up one end of the diaper to create six thicknesses, and lay the folded diaper inside the kite-folded diaper (see p. 92). This puts eight layers of diaper where it is most needed. Because the diaper is bulky, this method should only be used during the night, not when the baby is awake and active.

Body Care

Most parents are nervous at first about handling tiny and apparently fragile newborn babies. As a mother or father becomes more confident, routine baby care is easier.

To maintain the health of a newborn baby, a basic rule is to keep the baby clean, safe, and well groomed. In the early weeks this means daily attention to the following areas.

Care of the Genitals. Hospitals and visiting nurses are sometimes reluctant to explain how to clean a baby's genitals and often recommend not touching them. But such inaction can lead to infections that might otherwise have been prevented.

The genitals of a baby girl must be kept clean. It is not necessary to wash inside the lips of the vulva during the first week after birth, but the parent should thereafter from time to time wipe the genitals from the front toward the anus with a cotton swab dipped in warm water or baby oil. It is important to do this especially after the baby has passed stools. Any stool or vaginal discharge left on the skin, which can even happen after a bath, can cause a vaginal infection or urinary tract infection if it is not cleaned away.

With a baby boy, never attempt to pull back the foreskin of the penis. The foreskin and the tip of the penis are united at birth and only gradually separate. It is unnecessary to pull back the foreskin in order to wash the penis until the child is about four years old.

Circumcision. Medical opinion is divided about the value of circumcision. If for social or religious reasons a baby is to be circumcised, the operation should be performed before the tenth day after birth. There are two common methods: (1) cutting the foreskin after a mechanical device called a Gomco has severed the tissues to prevent bleeding (the traditional method); or (2) applying a plastic cone to the penis inside the foreskin, stitching round it, and

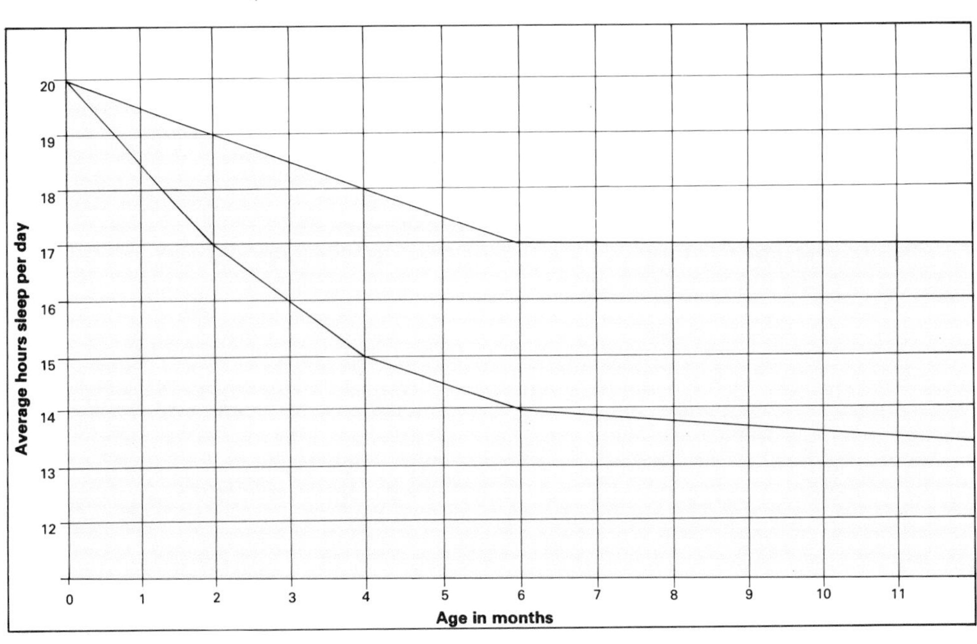

Patterns of sleep

Babies' sleep patterns vary enormously. The amount of sleep a baby needs depends on his or her individual temperament. It is not possible to make a baby sleep if he or she is not tired. However, sleep requirement does tend to decrease as the baby grows older, and by school age the child needs to sleep only at night.

then cutting. The foreskin and the cone fall off together within two or three days.

After a baby is circumcised, a gauze bandage with petroleum jelly is usually applied for 12 to 24 hours. After the bandage has been gently removed, apply a sterile piece of gauze impregnated with petroleum jelly to prevent diapers from sticking to the skin. Similar dressings should be used for at least two more days. After that time, the skin should have healed.

Normal Functions

Sleeping. The number of hours of sleep required each day is not the same for every baby. It depends on the individual baby and on environmental circumstances. Not all babies require the same amount of sleep, and parents should be aware that each baby establishes his or her own sleeping pattern.

The chart on page 94 shows the average number of hours of sleep a baby may take from birth to one year of age during any twenty-four hour period. It is immediately noticeable that, as the baby's age increases, there is also an increasing divergence in the average number of hours of sleep each individual baby requires.

Although newborn babies generally sleep for a total of about twenty hours a day, it is usually for three or four hours at a time, between one nursing and the next. By about six weeks of age, a baby usually begins to sleep for longer periods during the night.

At about six weeks of age a baby begins to need less sleep and to enjoy staying awake for a while after being nursed. At such times, lying on a bed, the baby can be encouraged to use his or her eyes. A colorful mobile is useful for this purpose and can also promote movement and exercise.

Crying. It is important to remember that a baby always has a reason for crying and never does so just to be a nuisance. Crying is a baby's means of communication, generally signifying discontent. A parent or baby sitter soon learns to recognize the sounds and to interpret the reasons: hunger; colic pains; wet or dirty diaper; lack of attention; teething; sudden bright lights; being picked up or looked at by a stranger; and others.

Crying patterns vary as much as do sleeping patterns, and some babies cry more—or less—than others. Most babies up to the age of two or three months have a crying period each day. Parents should not allow themselves to become angry. One method commonly successful in soothing a baby is to walk around slowly, holding the baby upright and speaking gently.

Teething. All babies have to go through the process of teething, but some find it less disturbing or painful than others. The primary teeth, or baby teeth, are already present in the jaw at

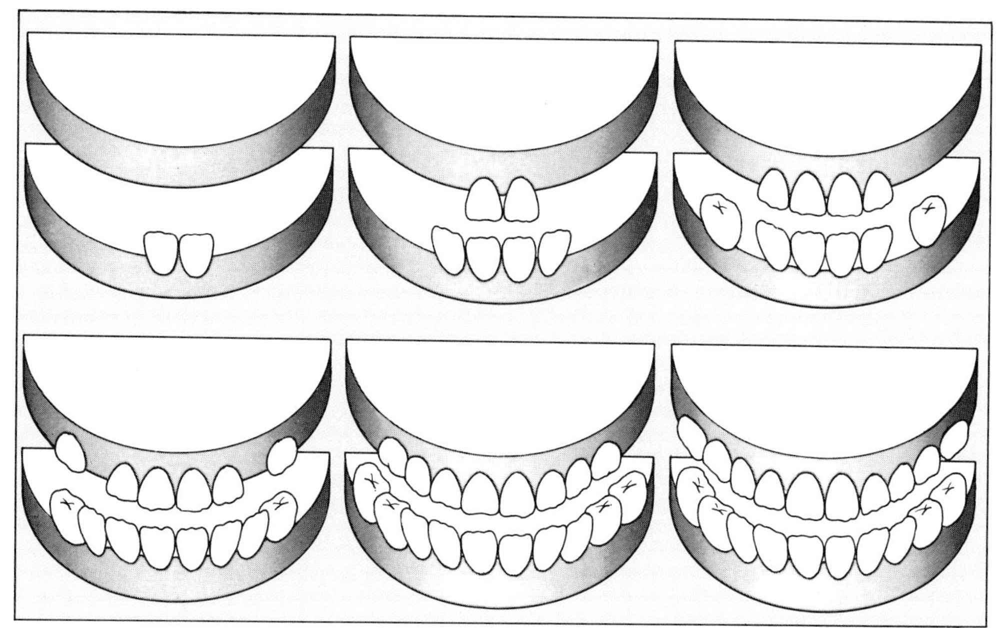

The emergence of teeth

Teeth emerge at an age that varies from baby to baby. Some babies are born with a tooth already cut, others do not begin teething until after the age of 18 months. The plan to the left shows the order in which the 20 primary teeth usually emerge, each taking about 3 weeks to do so.

the time of birth and begin pushing their way through the gums at about age six to eight months. There are 20 primary teeth.

The 32 permanent teeth start to develop when the baby is born. Eventually they begin coming through at age five to six years.

There are many signs by which a parent can know that a baby is teething: the cheeks may become red and blotchy; the gums may swell; the baby may frantically suck the fingers or anything else that is close at hand. Alternatively, the baby may have difficulty sucking; drooling will develop because of the extra saliva produced when a tooth is erupting; there may be earache, a referred pain from the gums; the baby may pull or rub the ears; and dry or sore patches of skin may appear on the face, especially if the baby sleeps on his or her stomach on a sheet damp with saliva.

A baby who is teething may wake up crying several times each night and may cry persistently even when soothed. At such a time, offer the baby a drink of cool water or diluted fruit juice. Special preparations of acetaminophen suitable for babies also are available from most drugstores and may be helpful. During the day the baby's gums may be rubbed with a teething salve to give temporary relief.

To prevent soreness on the baby's mouth and face, apply a barrier cream and do not allow the baby to lie on a damp sheet.

Care of the Teeth. Vitamins A, C, and D and calcium (all in milk) are important for healthy teeth.

To keep the baby teeth healthy, parents should not permit certain eating habits. The baby should never be given undiluted sugary juices, nor a pacifier dipped in honey. Sweet drinks and foods are harmful to teeth, destroying the enamel. Once the baby can chew food, meals should be finished off with a piece of apple or some water. When the baby's teeth erupt, clean the teeth after each meal with a soft, small brush, brushing the teeth up and down and making a game of it so that it becomes a pleasurable part of the daily routine. Use a very small amount of toothpaste containing fluoride. Many babies are given additional protection with fluoride drops from the age of one month if the fluoride content of the local water supply is insufficient.

Toilet Training

Voluntary control over the bladder and the bowels begins at about 18 months to 2 years of age. Accordingly, it seems a waste of time to most parents and physicians to start toilet training an infant before that age.

In time, a baby can train himself or herself. Parents who allow their baby to carry out such natural training should be aware, however, that as with parent-trained babies, one infant can be toilet trained within a few weeks while another may take a year or more. Encouragement should be given as well as praise and even some reward when due.

But most parents prefer to take a more active part in toilet training their child. It is important that parents always appear relaxed about the training program. If the project makes a parent visibly anxious or if it is discussed too earnestly in front of the baby, the baby can become nervous and object to the whole idea.

Toilet Training Method. Start the training program in the morning. Put a fresh diaper on the baby before he or she has breakfast. At the end of the meal, if the baby is still dry and clean, sit him or her on the infant toilet seat. It is a good idea to reserve some favorite toy or toys just for the session.

Each toilet training session should last no longer than five minutes. Stay with the baby during the first few times, but only as company. Do not play with him or her.

At the end of five minutes, the baby should be lifted from the seat. If there is anything in the toilet, the parent should express approval. If not, the parent should merely say something casual like, "We'll try again tomorrow." Parents must avoid showing displeasure at such a time.

This routine can gradually be carried out more than once a day, but not so often that the baby gets the impression that he or she is spending a large part of the day on the toilet.

If the baby cries and obviously objects to sitting on the seat, abandon the toilet training for about a month, then try again.

Eventually, the baby's toilet habits may become so regular that a parent can chart them and use this as an aid to toilet training. However, a toddler should not be allowed to get into the habit of calling for a toilet session at 6 A.M., for example, if a parent resents getting up at that hour.

The parent can adjust the baby's mealtimes and diet to encourage the bowel and bladder to empty at socially convenient hours.

Choice of Toilet Seat. The toilet seat should sit firmly on the floor so that the baby cannot tip over and become frightened. The circumference of the top should fit the baby's bottom. A toilet seat that can be fitted to the ordinary adult toilet may be too high for a baby to relax on. It may be dangerous and is certainly not suitable for a baby that is starting to toilet train. It is much easier for an infant to relax when his or her feet are supported and comfortably resting on the floor.

Perhaps the best time to start training a baby to use a toilet is halfway through the second year. By then a baby has some control over bowel movements and may be aware of a full bladder in time to tell a parent.

Transporting a Baby

Choosing a Baby Carriage. The baby carriage is one of the most expensive pieces of equipment parents have to buy, and it should be chosen with care.

A carriage with large wheels is smoother in motion than one with small wheels. However, a carriage with small wheels at the front and large ones at the back is easier to push over the edge of a sidewalk.

Parents living in a city apartment often find the most convenient kind of carriage is one that can be detached from a foldable frame. The only disadvantage with this kind of carriage is that the lighter structure becomes unsafe when the baby reaches one year of age and is able to rock the carriage.

Be sure that the carriage has safety straps or attachment points for straps. When a baby can sit up in the carriage, he or she must wear straps at all times. The carriage must have good brakes, preferably on each wheel.

The interior of the baby carriage should be easy to clean. There should be an attachable hood and cover and a thick mattress. If the carriage is for outside use, attach a net over the front while the baby sleeps.

For the comfort and convenience of the parents, a carriage should have adjustable handles and a shopping tray or basket under the chassis (and not at either end).

The Bassinet. The travel bassinet should have a wipeable interior and exterior. The sides should be padded and smooth so that the baby can not be hurt. The handles must be strong and located toward the head end of the bassinet. A travel bassinet is lightweight and convenient when traveling, but can be used only for babies under the age of nine months. It is very important that a bassinet never be used to transport a baby in the car.

Some travel bassinets have tubular steel legs and carrying handles with a safety locking device. This type of bassinet folds flat for easy storage in the car trunk.

The Car Seat. All states have laws mandating the use of car seats for children.

A car seat should be of a lightweight, durable material fitted with its own seat belt. Padded "wings" should extend forward from the back rest of the car seat. These should be at head height in order to keep the child's head from snapping too far to the left or the right in case of an accident.

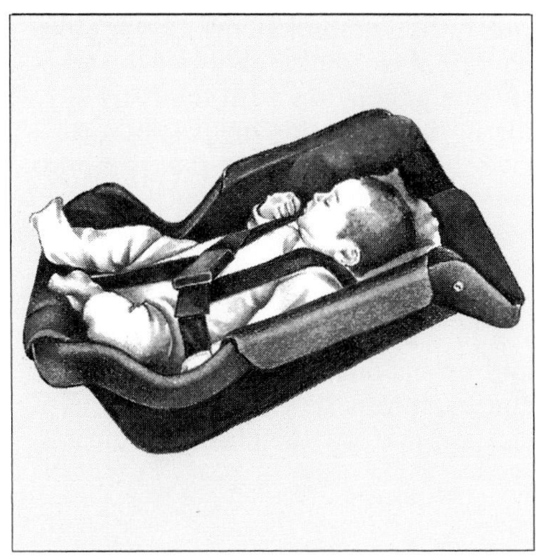

The baby must be strapped in whenever traveling by car. The **car seat** shown is suitable for small babies and should be used with the car seat belt. As the baby grows, he or she can sit up in a seat with a "parachute" harness that can be clipped on whenever needed.

Many parents use a **sling carrier** because it leaves both hands free, and the baby usually sleeps in the sling, soothed by the warmth of close bodily contact. It is usually advisable to wait until the infant is 4 months old before using this type of carrier. However, some carriers have a built-in neck support which makes them appropriate for newborns.

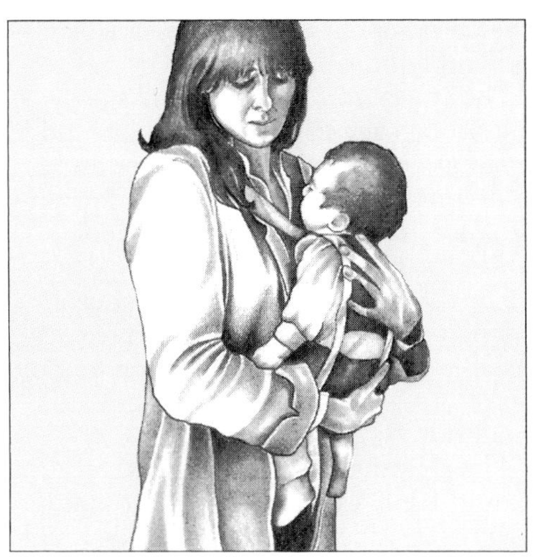

The car seat should also be anchored down with the automobile seat belt in the back seat of the automobile. Passengers in the back seat are at less risk for injury than those in the front seat. For children up to 12 months of age, or 20 pounds (9 kilograms), the car seat should face backward. For older children the car seat can face forward. The child should be placed in the car seat *every* time the car is used for travel, even for short trips in the neighborhood.

The Backpack. A backpack is a useful alternative to the carriage. The baby must be able to support his or her own head before sitting in a backpack, usually around the age of four months. The pack should have adjustable shoulder straps for the parent. It also should be equipped with safety straps for the baby, or attachment points for a harness.

Some backpacks have a small strut that folds out at the back to support the pack on the ground. This strut enables the parent to comfortably put the pack on from a table top with the baby sitting in the pack; this device should never be used to convert the pack into a seat for the baby.

Soft packs, or sling carriers, can be worn in which the baby is carried in front, rather than on the back. These should not be used before the baby can hold up his or her head, at about four months, unless they have a built-in neck support. As the child gets heavier, however, a backpack is more practical.

The Baby's Temperature

A newborn baby is unable to control body heat as efficiently as an older child. External changes in temperature can vary a baby's body temperature considerably. Unless a baby is kept adequately warm, he or she could suffer from hypothermia. This does not mean that the parents must constantly check the baby's temperature with a thermometer, but they must be aware of potentially dangerous situations.

Cold. A baby's bedroom must be maintained at a temperature of at least 65°F (18.3°C). The room should be kept slightly warmer for babies under 8 pounds (3.6 kg). A thermostat heater is an efficient method of keeping the room warm throughout the night. During the winter, warm the baby's crib with a hot water bottle before placing him or her in it, but remember to remove the bottle first. Never use an electric blanket on a baby's bed. Also, before putting the baby to bed, cuddle him or her. A tiny baby does not move much during the night and is unlikely to warm up. A cuddle before bed warms the baby.

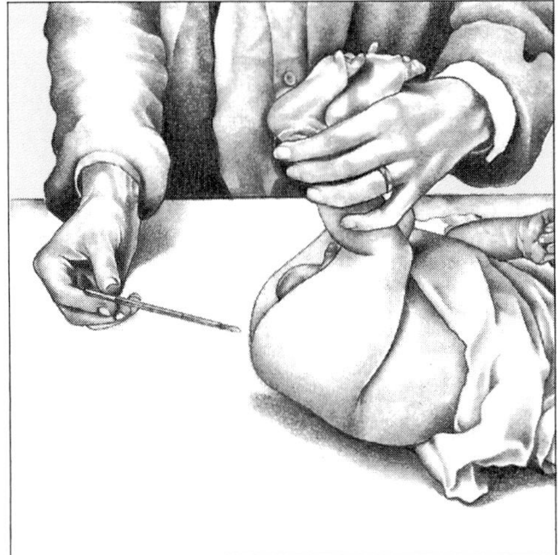

Taking a rectal temperature: Lay the baby on his or her back. Dip the end of the thermometer in petroleum jelly. With one hand, hold the baby's legs up and gently insert the bulb into the anus. Do not push if the thermometer meets an obstruction. Slide the thermometer in about 1 inch (2.5 cm).

Heat. During hot summer weather a baby should wear light, loosely fitting, cool clothing. As long as he or she is protected from direct sun, the baby can lie outside in nothing but a diaper. Overdressing, causing overheating, is one of the most common reasons for irritable babies during the summer.

Never leave a small baby or child unattended in a car. This is especially important during the summer, especially if the car is in direct sun, because the baby can become dangerously overheated. A baby under the age of three months is unable to lose excess heat.

During car journeys, check frequently to make sure that the sun is not shining directly on the baby. Also, protect the baby's head from the sun.

Illness. When a baby becomes ill, he or she may or may not have a temperature above normal. A reading from a thermometer is an inaccurate guide to a baby's state of health. Other warning signs also must be considered.

The most common noticeable signs that a baby has an infection or illness are a sudden loss of appetite; irritability or lethargy; and vomiting or diarrhea. These signs are a more accurate indication than a temperature reading.

However, during an illness the physician may ask the parent to monitor the baby's temperature. It is dangerous to place a thermometer in a baby's mouth and difficult to keep one underneath a baby's arm for a sufficient length of time. The safest way to take the baby's temperature is with a rectal thermometer. (*See page 98.*)

A rectal thermometer has a rounded, stub end. This type of thermometer can be used for taking oral temperatures as well, so when buying a thermometer, buy a rectal one.

Finally, do not keep a baby's room too hot if he or she is ill. If the baby has a high temperature, keep him or her covered with light clothes and a sheet. The physician may recommend sponging with tepid water to keep the baby's temperature down.

Rectal Temperature. Make sure that the mercury ribbon is first shaken below the thermometer's normal mark. Then take the baby's rectal temperature using the method described below.

It usually takes three to five minutes for a rectal thermometer to register the body temperature. Although the normal body temperature varies from person to person, the average is 98.6°F (37°C) for an oral temperature, and 99.6°F (37.6°C) for a rectal temperature.

Wash the thermometer carefully after use with cool water and soap. An alcohol pad, available at drugstores, is also acceptable for cleaning thermometers. Never use hot water because this will break the bulb.

Baby carriage. *See* BABY CARE.

Baby feeding. *See* BABY CARE.

Baby, premature. *See* BIRTH, PREMATURE.

Baby transport. *See* BABY CARE.

Bacillus (bə sil′əs) is a general term for any rod-shaped bacterium of class Schizomycetes and for bacteria of the genus *Bacillus.* Some bacilli are harmless and found everywhere. Others cause disease, such as *Bacillus anthracis.*

See also ANTHRAX; BACTERIA.

Back refers to the rear trunk of the body extending from the neck to the pelvis. The back is composed of various bones, or vertebrae; these are stacked in a column and form the spine, or backbone. The back also contains numerous muscles that are used to produce body movement and act as a support for the spine.

See also MUSCULAR SYSTEM.

Backache. *See* BACK PAIN.

Backbone. *See* SPINE.

Back care. The spinal region from the neck to the buttocks is very susceptible to injury or disease. Backache, which is

Proper **back care** should include sleeping on a firm mattress. To prevent backache, a mattress should follow the body contours while allowing for minimum curvature of the spine, *top.* A soft mattress that causes the spine to curve excessively, *bottom,* can cause severe backache.

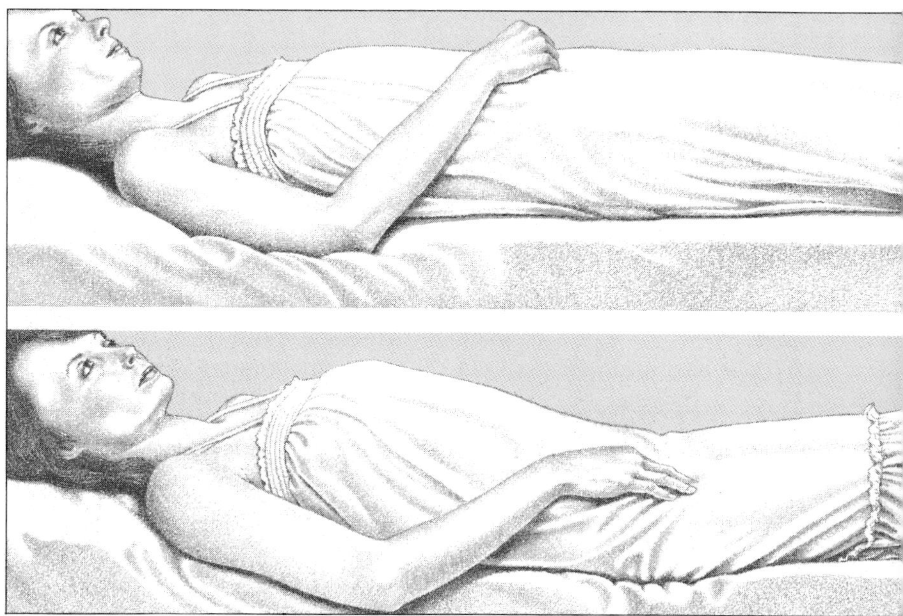

a symptom of a variety of disorders often stemming from a muscle, ligament, or bone injury, is one of the most common complaints among adults. With proper care, many disorders that produce acute or chronic backache can be avoided. Correct posture and the avoidance of too much physical stress are important ingredients for good back care. Some of the more common causes of back pain and methods of treating or avoiding those ailments are discussed in this article.

Lower Back Pain. Low back pain is one of the most common physical complaints and often affects young adults or persons in early middle age. The symptoms vary from morning back stiffness and difficulty in getting out of chairs to sudden pain in the sides and an inability to stand upright or move.

Lower back pain is usually caused by strained ligaments and muscles in the area surrounding the spine or an intervertebral disk that has partially slipped. The injury can occur while doing unaccustomed back exercise.

The treatment for lower back pain varies according to the severity of the pain or the disability. Good posture and care taken while bending and lifting can reduce the possibility of lower back pain.

Whiplash Injury of the Neck. A whiplash injury occurs when an accident jerks the head backward and forward like a whiplash. The sudden powerful force that causes the injury is often the result of an automobile accident. The ligaments in the neck are stretched or torn, internal bleeding may occur around the site of the injury, and sometimes an intervertebral disk in the neck may tear, causing pain down the shoulder and arm and tingling in the hand.

A whiplash injury is not at first apparent, but a few days after the accident the person experiences dizziness, severe headaches, and the inability to turn the head. Treatment depends on the severity of the injury. Whiplash injuries can be prevented by the use of headrest attachments on the seats.

Lordosis and Kyphosis. Lordosis refers to the forward or inward curvature of the spine. Abnormal or excessive lordosis usually affects the lumbar region of the spine and can cause backache. It is common among obese per-

Spinal column

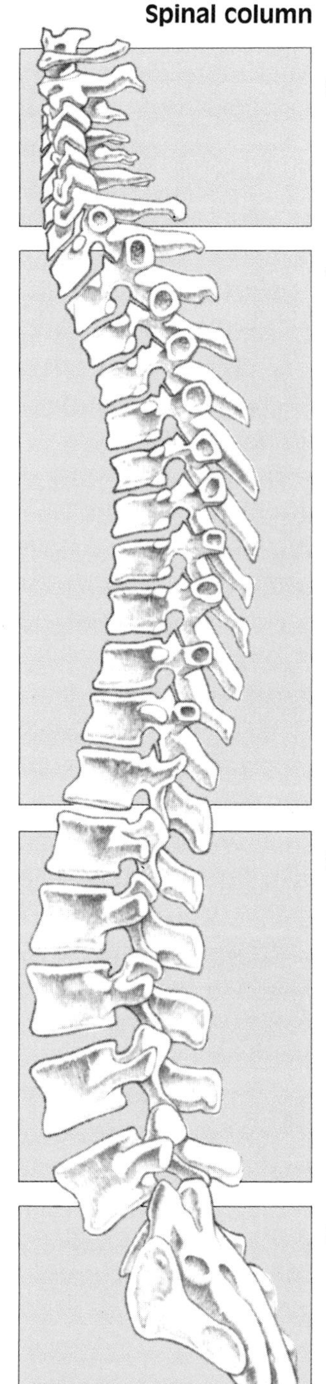

Cervical region: seven vertebrae, the first of which supports the skull

Thoracic region: twelve vertebrae, each carrying a pair of ribs.

Lumbar region: the five largest and strongest vertebrae, the area most commonly affected by back ailments.

Sacrum: triangular in shape, consisting of five fused vertebrae.

Coccyx: triangular in shape, consisting of four fused vertebrae

Proper postures

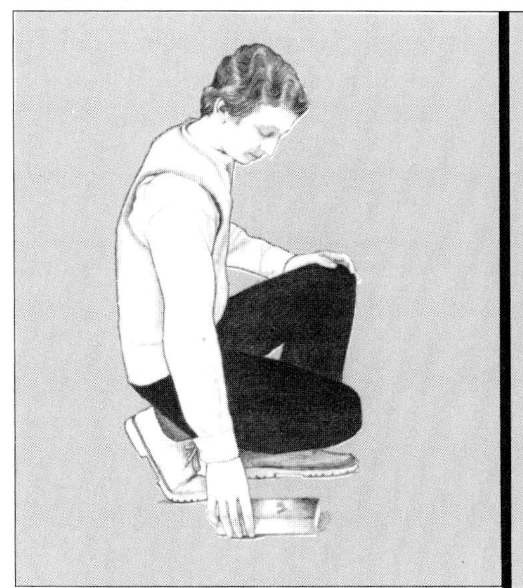

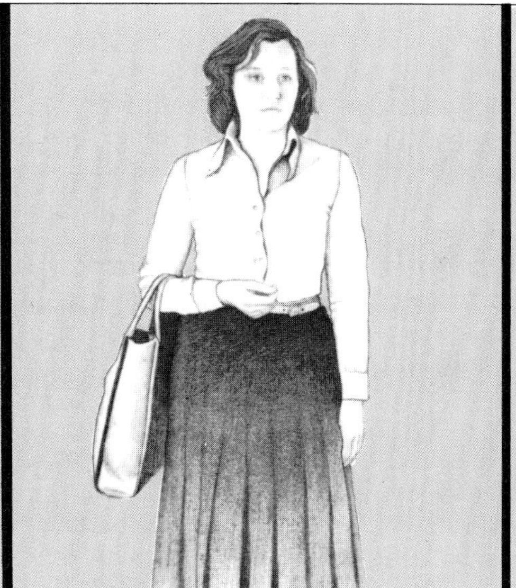

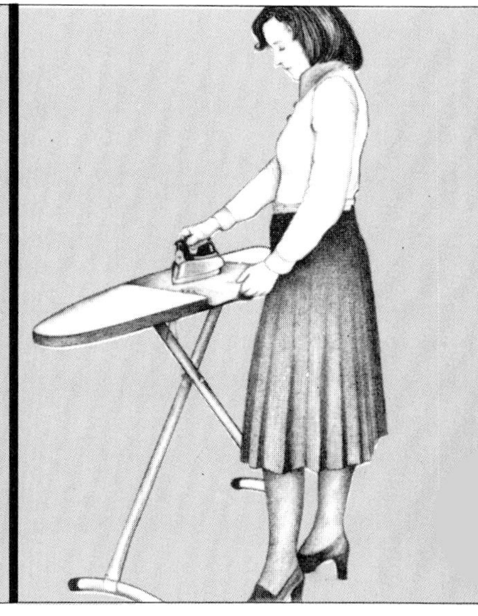

Lifting

To lift a small object from floor level, the back should be kept straight and the knees should be bent. The placement of the free hand on the raised knee will support the body. The back should be kept straight and the leg muscles should be used as a standing position is resumed.

Carrying a handbag

A handbag should be carried on one arm. This ensures that the weight of the bag is over the hip. The body is therefore balanced, with the trunk and spine upright. A heavy load should be divided into two bags and carried one in each hand with arms at the side.

Standing and working

Ideally all work surfaces should be at waist level. If a surface is too low, the body's weight should be transferred to one leg. This enables the person to keep his or her back straight. As work is done, weight should be transferred from one leg to the other.

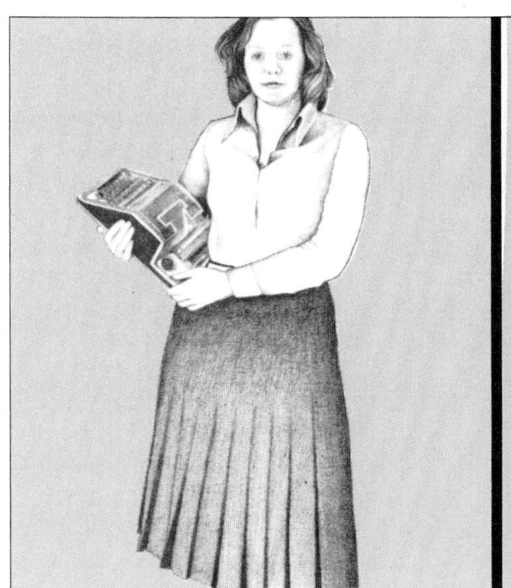

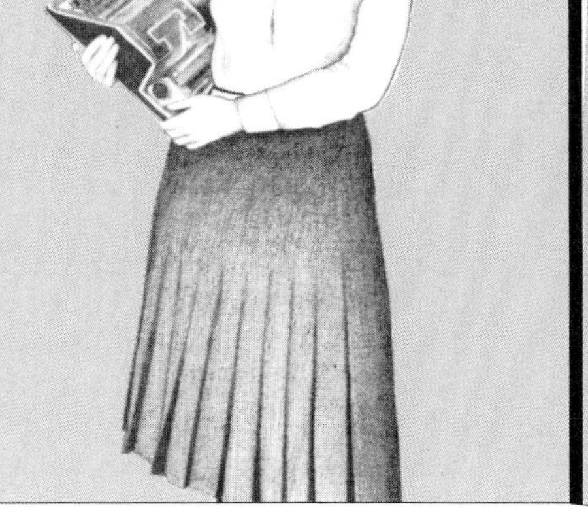

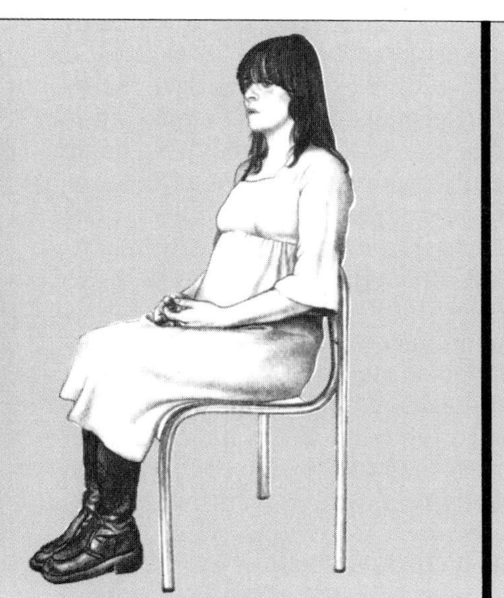

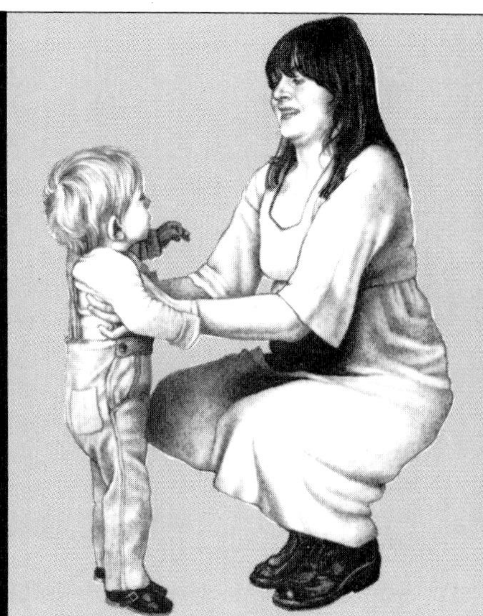

Carrying an object

Instead of carrying a heavy object in front of the body, a person should carry it on one of his or her hips. The weight is then taken through the pelvis and transmitted down each leg, and the back remains straight.

Sitting when pregnant

During pregnancy, it is essential to support the back while sitting. An upright chair with a high back is more comfortable than a low chair or sofa. To reduce pressure in the veins of the leg, both feet should be flat on the floor. Legs should not be crossed.

Lifting when pregnant

A pregnant woman with a small child can find pregnancy very tiring. When she lifts her youngster, she should bend at the knees instead of at the waist, lift the small child with both hands, and keep the back straight as she lifts.

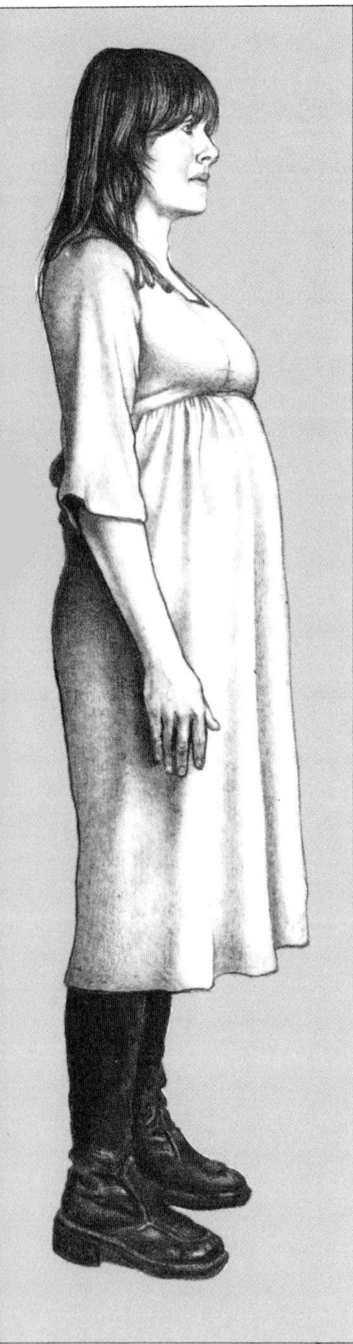

Back care: During pregnancy the small of the back supports much of the weight of the fetus. A pregnant woman should stand with her feet slightly apart, her hips swung forward, and her back straight.

sons and during pregnancy, but also may be caused by incorrect posture.

Abnormal kyphosis is an excessive curvature of the spine in the thoracic region. It can result in the condition popularly known as hunchback. It is frequently associated with scoliosis, a lateral curvature of the spine that is usually caused by incorrect posture. It also can be caused by an injury to the back, by congenital malformation, or by various disorders that affect the spine.

Herniated Disk. An intervertebral disk consists of fibrocartilage. The outer part is called the anulus fibrosus, and the soft inner core is known as the nucleus pulposus. As the spine bends, pressure is exerted on the disks. If the pressure is too great, the soft center can rupture through the outer ring and press on a nerve running from the spinal cord to another part of the body. The pain of the injury is felt in the area that the nerve supplies. The injury most commonly affects the lumbar intervertebral disks, because they take the most strain. If this occurs the pain is felt in the buttock and down the leg to the foot (sciatica).

A person can herniate a disk by lifting a heavy object, or by doing some form of vigorous exercise to which the body is not accustomed. Treatment varies according to the severity of the injury. Herniated disks are more common in young men than women and do not usually occur after the age of 50.

Coccygodynia. Coccygodynia is persistent, severe pain in the lowest area of the spine, the coccyx. The pain increases during defecation and when sitting, but is reduced, or absent, when the person stands. The condition may last for many months following an injury to the coccyx. The most common way to injure the coccyx is by falling heavily backward in a sitting position.

See also BACK PAIN; SPINE.

Back disorders. *See* BACK CARE.

Back pain is a discomfort most commonly located in the lumbar (lower) region of the spine and surrounding tissues. It is an extremely common ailment and is most often caused by injury or stress to a muscle, ligament, bone, or nerve. Low back pain can become chronic if the cause of the discomfort is not properly treated.

Q: *What are common causes of back pain?*

A: The most common causes of back pain are sudden tears or strains of the muscles, tendons, or ligaments of the back. The area of such tears is tender to the touch, and the pain is increased by moving about.

Pain also can be caused by chronic strain to the back caused by curvatures of the spine (lordosis, kyphosis, scoliosis), having one leg shorter than the other, bad posture, or repetitive lifting of heavy objects. *See also* LORDOSIS; KYPHOSIS; SCOLIOSIS.

Q: *What is a slipped disk?*

A: A "slipped," or herniated, disk occurs when one of the intervertebral disks, which serve to separate the vertebrae and act to absorb the shock of motion, slips out of place. This displacement can compress a spinal nerve and place a strain on the surrounding ligaments. This can also result in sciatica, where pressure on the sciatic nerve causes pain down one or both of the legs. *See also* DISK, HERNIATED; SCIATICA.

Q: *What other spinal disorders cause back pain?*

A: Pain can result from osteoarthritis, where the roughened surface of the bone results in local irritation. In osteoporosis, the bones become brittle due to lack of calcium; vertebrae can, therefore, collapse, resulting in pain and possible nerve compression. In young and middle-aged people, a disorder that causes the vertebrae to fuse together (ankylosing spondylitis) produces pain and gradual stiffening of the spine. Also cancer can spread to a vertebra with resulting pain. *See also* SPONDYLITIS, ANKYLOSING.

Chronic deformities of the spine (lordosis, kyphosis, scoliosis) can result in pain, as can a condition called spondylolisthesis, in which one or more vertebrae are not correctly formed. This can lead to partial dislocation of the spine. *See also* SPONDYLOLISTHESIS.

Q: *What nerve disorders cause back pain?*

A: A tumor of the spine can cause back pain. But, more commonly, back pain of neurologic origin results from inflammation of a nerve. See also NEURITIS.

Q: *Apart from causes directly associated with the spine, what other disorders can result in backache?*

A: A low ache in the back often occurs in women before the onset of menstruation or as part of a painful menstrual period (dysmenorrhea). Other gynecological disorders may also cause backache.

Pain from a kidney infection (such as pyelonephritis) often occurs in the lower or mid-back. A dull ache high in the back may be a symptom of a chest disorder.

Q: *What is the treatment for back pain?*

A: Painkilling drugs, such as acetaminophen or aspirin, can be taken to relieve pain due to a minor strain of a ligament or muscle. For more severe pains, a physician may prescribe a strong, anti-inflammatory and/or muscle relaxant drug.

Rest can be a very important aid in back pain treatment. The patient should rest in a position that will straighten out the lower back, such as on the back with the knees supported in a bent position by a pillow, or lying on the side with the head supported by a pillow. A firm mattress is essential.

Treatment by physical therapy may include exercise, massage, or local heat. The spine may be carefully stretched using traction; a patient is usually hospitalized for this treatment.

If back pain is severe, prolonged, or accompanied by serious symptoms, such as a fever or a weakness in a leg, it is important that a physician be consulted immediately.

Q: *What everyday precautions can help relieve or prevent back pain?*

A: Correct posture, a firm mattress, and strengthening of the muscles by means of careful exercise all can help to relieve some types of backache. Maintaining correct body weight (by dieting, if necessary) also helps to prevent backache. Being overweight puts extra strain on the spine. It is important to remember, when lifting objects, to bend at the knees and hips, rather than at the waist. This allows use of the more powerful leg muscles and avoids strain on the back. Also, when carrying something in the arms, it should be held close to the body, rather than with outstretched arms.

See also BACK CARE.

Bacteremia (bak tə rē'mē ə), or bacteraemia, is the medical name for bacteria in the blood.

See also BLOOD POISONING.

Bacteria (bak tir'ē ə) are a large group of microscopic, single-celled organisms, some of which can cause diseases in humans. Classified by shape, there are four different types of bacteria: spirochetes, which are either rigid, flexible, or curved coils; cocci, which are sphere-shaped; bacilli, which are rod-shaped; and vibrios, which are comma-shaped.

See also BACILLUS; COCCUS; SPIROCHETE; VIBRIO.

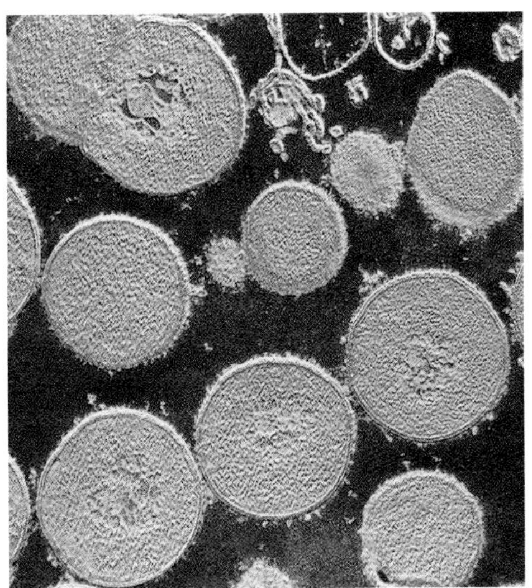

Bacteria are classified by shape, the ones pictured here being cocci, because of their spherical form. The full name is *Streptococcus pneumoniae,* a bacteria associated with pneumonia in humans.

Bacterial endocarditis. See ENDOCARDITIS, BACTERIAL.

Bad breath, or halitosis, is a condition in which an offensive odor is emitted from the mouth. Smoking and poor oral hygiene are probably the most common causes of bad breath. The condition also can be caused by the odor of acetone in untreated or poorly controlled diabetes, ammonia in liver disease, or by sinus or throat infections.

Adequate dental care should correct most cases of bad breath. If bad breath continues even after such care, a physician should be consulted.

Bagassosis (bag ə sō′sis) is an asthma-like condition caused by inhaling the spores of a fungus that infects sugar cane. The attacks occur in those who have worked with sugar cane for several months and come several hours after contact with the plant. Repeated attacks lead to fine scarring of the lungs and to the development of pneumoconiosis. Treatment of the attack is systemic; prevention of further attacks requires a change of job or environment.

See also PNEUMOCONIOSIS.

Bag of water is the common name for the protective fluid-filled sac that surrounds a fetus in the uterus and that breaks during labor. Its medical name is amniotic sac.

See also AMNION.

Balance, or body equilibrium, is controlled by the part of the brain called the cerebellum. Changes in body position are detected by the three semicircular canals of the inner ear; by the eyes; and by sensors in the body that send messages to the brain.

Q: *What can go wrong with the sense of balance?*

A: Various disorders can affect balance. Some are minor or only temporary. For example, some persons traveling by automobile, ship, or airplane experience motion sickness. Middle ear infection, known medically as otitis media, can also upset the sense of balance by affecting the semicircular canals. Dizziness, caused by an inadequate supply of blood and thus of oxygen to the brain, is the sensation that precedes fainting. Loss of balance may be due to emotional stress, or it may be a symptom of anemia, heart disease, or a circulatory disorder. Vertigo, in which balance is so severely affected that the room seems to be spinning around, may be a symptom of Ménière's disease or some other ear disorder.

Any person who suffers recurrent or persistent loss of balance should consult a physician.

See also MÉNIÈRE'S DISEASE; MOTION SICKNESS.

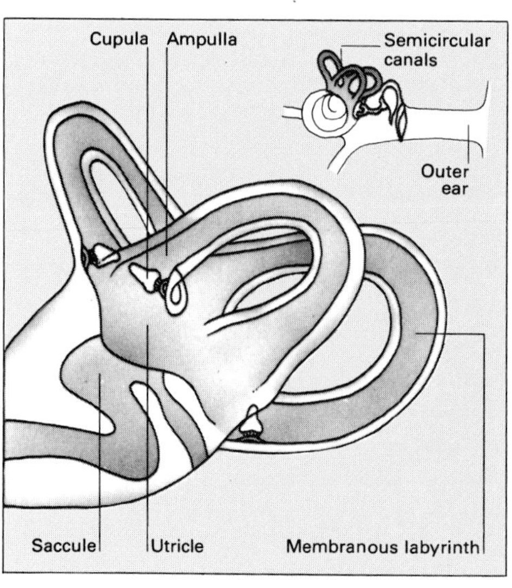

Balance is monitored by fluid within the ears' semicircular canals.

Balanitis (bal ə nī′tis) is inflammation of the end of the penis (the glans penis), accompanied by itching and a slight discharge. It is caused by a failure to keep the glans clean. Balanitis is more common in men and boys who have not been circumcised, particularly if they suffer from phimosis (the inability to pull back the foreskin). Prevention and treatment depend on keeping the area washed and clean. A physician should be consulted if the disorder does not clear up promptly.

See also PHIMOSIS.

Balanoposthitis (bal ə nō pos thi′tis) is an inflammation and ulceration of the glans penis, similar to balanitis. The cause, however, is usually a common sexually transmitted disease, and the treatment often includes an antibiotic drug.

See also BALANITIS.

Baldness is the partial or complete loss of hair. A tendency to go bald is inherited; the age at which the balding process begins and the pattern it takes are often similar in successive generations. Male pattern baldness is extremely common and entails the loss of hair at the front of the scalp or the crown of the head. No therapy has yet been successful in preventing male pattern baldness.

Temporary baldness may be caused by a skin disease, anticancer medication, endocrine disorder, or emotional stress. Normal hair growth can be restored in most of these cases.

Some women may experience partial hair loss or hair thinning as they grow older, but complete baldness in women is extremely rare.

See also ALOPECIA.

Ball joint. *See* JOINT.

Balloon angioplasty. *See* ANGIOPLASTY, BALLOON.

Bamboo spine is another name for the condition known medically as ankylosing spondylitis. The name refers to the X-ray appearance of the spine in this disease.

See also SPONDYLITIS, ANKYLOSING.

Barber's itch, known medically as sycosis barbae, is a form of folliculitis that affects a man's face. It first appears as scattered pimples that later dry out.

See also FOLLICULITIS.

Barbiturate (bär bich′ə rāt) is the name of a classification given to a group of sedative and sleep-inducing drugs derived from barbituric acid. Barbiturates act by depressing the central nervous and respiratory systems; with larger doses, blood pressure may also be depressed. Physicians use barbiturates, injected into a vein, as anesthetics. Barbiturates are used in the treatment of epilepsy and are occasionally prescribed for sleeplessness (insomnia) and to reduce anxiety.

Q: *Are barbiturates addictive?*

A: Barbiturates are mildly addictive and, after prolonged use, can alter the normal pattern of sleep. Because of the dangers of drug addiction and overdosage, physicians prefer to prescribe other kinds of sleep-inducing drugs. Barbiturates should never be taken with alcohol; the combination of the two drugs can be fatal.

See also DRUG ADDICTION.

Barium (bãr′ē əm) is a metallic chemical element. The metal and its salts, particularly barium sulfate, show up clearly on X-ray photographs. A patient undergoing certain types of X-ray examinations may be asked to swallow a mixture of barium sulfate and water, called a barium meal, which is fairly tasteless unless artificially flavored. Via X rays, a physician can watch the progress of the barium while it is swallowed, as it enters and leaves the stomach, and then as it moves through the small intestine to reach the colon (large intestine). A barium enema, a barium sulfate mixture passed into the rectum and colon, shows the outline of the colon. Barium is used to help diagnose various conditions affecting the digestive tract.

See also BARIUM ENEMA.

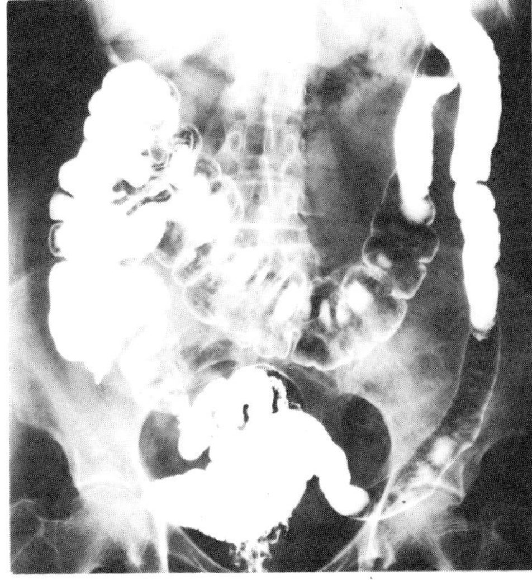

Barium is a metallic element that shows up on X rays of the digestive tract.

Barium enema (bãr′ē əm en′ə mə) is the infusion of barium sulfate into the rectum and colon, in order to facilitate fluoroscopic and X-ray examinations. In this way, tumors, obstructions, and other abnormalities in the rectum or colon can be seen in an X ray.

The patient must adhere to a strict diet prior to the examination, in order to clear the lower intestinal tract. Afterward, a cleansing enema removes the barium sulfate. Today the most common form of barium enema includes air contrast study. Air is pumped into the colon following the administration of the barium. This enhances the visualization of structures.

See also BARIUM; ENEMA.

Barotitis (bãr ō tī′tis), also known as aerotitis, is an inflammation of the middle ear caused by a sudden fluctuation in pressure in the ear, such as occurs during flying or scuba diving. Usually a condition, such as a cold, is present; the Eustachian tube is, therefore, blocked, and the middle ear is unable to adjust to pressure changes. Barotitis usually clears up once the person is on the surface. Yawning, wiggling the ears, or trying to force air through the nose while it is pinched are measures that can open up the Eustachian tube. People with acute sinusitis or otitis media should be advised not to fly or dive. Chronic barotitis should be treated to avoid complications.

Barotrauma (bar trô′mə) is damage to a part of the body caused by a change in atmospheric or water pressure. It is particularly common in the middle ear when the Eustachian tube is blocked. (The Eustachian tube connects the middle ear to the back of the throat and acts as a pressure equalizer.) The barotrauma causes pain in the ear and, in severe cases, may rupture the eardrum. A similar condition may occur in the nasal sinuses or lungs, especially among deep-sea divers.

See also BAROTITIS; EUSTACHIAN TUBE.

Bartholin's cyst (bär tō'linz sist) is a small collection of fluid at any of the four Bartholin's glands at the vaginal orifice. It is caused by a blockage of one or more of these vaginal ducts. Symptoms include a feeling of vaginal stretching and occasional discomfort, particularly during intercourse (the condition called dyspareunia). The condition may call for the surgical removal of the affected gland in order to prevent repeated infection.

See also BARTHOLIN'S GLAND.

Bartholin's gland (bär tō'linz) is one of a pair of lubricating glands at the vaginal orifice.

See also BARTHOLIN'S CYST.

Basal cell carcinoma. *See* CARCINOMA, BASAL CELL.

Basal metabolic rate, BMR, is a measure of the amount of energy used by a person while at rest. Measurement of BMR is usually used in medical research, rather than clinical practice.

Bath, giving a. *See* NURSING THE SICK.

Bathing a baby. *See* BABY CARE.

Bath, medicinal. Medicinal bathing is the use of special waters for therapeutic purposes. Bathing in hot water that ranges from 98-112°F (37-45°C) relaxes muscles, dilates blood vessels, and improves circulation. Warm baths that range from about 90-97°F (32-36°C) may relieve sleeplessness and ease tension. Cold baths of less than 75°F (24°C) can reduce swelling. Whirlpools and water massages are used to treat a variety of arthritic and muscular problems.

For many years, people have visited health resorts called "spas" for medicinal baths. Most spas are on the site of a natural spring that yields bubbling, heated, or mineral-filled water. The benefits of the baths do not come solely from being in the water; drinking the water can also have medicinal benefits. Additional benefits may result from the relaxation, favorable climate, controlled diet, and exercise that are a usual part of an overall spa program.

Battered child syndrome. *See* CHILD ABUSE.

BCG vaccine (bacille Calmette-Guérin) is a preparation of live, but markedly weakened, tuberculosis organisms that is used as a vaccine to give protection against the harmful, natural form of the disease. In countries where tuberculosis is still common, the BCG is given in infancy. (The BCG is not commonly used in the United States.) A skin test is carried out first to show if a natural immunity has been acquired. The BCG vaccine was first used by Leon Calmette and Camille Guérin.

See also TUBERCULIN TEST; TUBERCULOSIS.

Bedbug (*Cimex lectularius* or *cimex hemipterus*) is a small blood-sucking insect that can infest bedding and bite humans or other animals. The insect is red-brown, oval, flat, and wingless. Its bite is painful and causes swelling, itching, and sometimes infection. It may transmit relapsing fever. The bite can be treated with a corticosteroid cream or other anti-inflammatory preparation. The infested bedroom furniture should be disinfected.

See also RELAPSING FEVER.

Bedmaking. *See* NURSING THE SICK.

Bedpan, use of. *See* NURSING THE SICK.

Bedsore, known medically as decubitus ulcer or pressure sore, is a skin and tissue injury caused by impaired blood supply and tissue nutrition. It is caused by prolonged pressure over bony prominences due to lying too long in the same position.

Q: *Where do bedsores form and what do they look like?*

A: The parts of the body most likely to be affected are the pressure areas: the bone at the lower end of the spine (the sacrum), the buttocks, and the heels. The shoulder blades and elbows may also develop these sores. The area first becomes slightly red with cracked skin, which turns dark blue before ulcerating as dead tissues disintegrate.

Q: *Can bedsores be prevented?*

A: Yes. Patients who cannot move themselves must be moved every few hours. Patients must not sit in bed or in a chair for long periods. The patient should be lifted, not slid, when moved. The skin is to be kept clean and dry. Bedclothes must be kept clean, dry, and free from creases. Additional protection

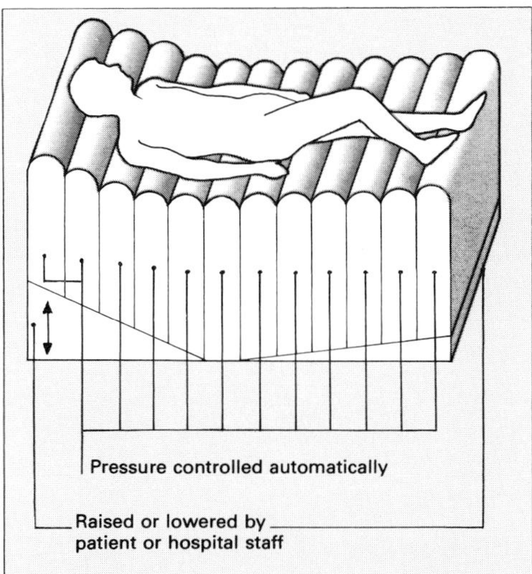

Bedsore problems can be prevented by using a variable-pressure air bed.

can be given to the pressure areas by using foam pads and real or artificial sheepskin. A variety of air mattresses and other types of beds are available to help prevent decubitus ulcers. A well-balanced diet helps to prevent bedsores.

Q: *What is the treatment if an ulcer has formed?*

A: The patient should not lie on the ulcer, although this may be awkward. The ulcer should be cleansed according to a physician's advice. Specific ointments or dressings may be prescribed. Care must be taken to turn the patient frequently to treat the bedsore and prevent new ones. The sores generally heal over a period of time if they are carefully tended. The best treatment, however, is prevention.

See also ULCER.

Bedsore prevention. *See* NURSING THE SICK.

Bed-wetting, known medically as nocturnal enuresis, is habitual urination in bed. It is a fairly common problem of childhood. A calm, reassuring approach on the part of the parents is the key factor in dealing with bed-wetting. Eventually almost all children resolve this problem.

Q: *At what age does a child usually stop wetting the bed?*

A: As the nervous system matures, the reflexes that control the bladder come under the voluntary control of the brain even while the child is asleep. This occurs at different ages in different children, but by the age of three or four most children achieve bladder control. Bed-wetting, however, can still be considered normal up to the age of six.

Q: *What causes bed-wetting in an older child?*

A: Usually the cause of such bed-wetting is emotional. In such a situation, it is wise to consult a physician because the cause needs investigation. Some authorities state that the method by which a child is taught toilet training is an important factor in bladder control at night.

In some cases there is a physical cause. There may be a urinary infection, or possibly a structural defect in the urinary tract, present from birth. Diabetes mellitus can also cause enuresis. Rarely, there may be a disorder of the nerves that serve the urinary system.

Q: *What should be done about bed-wetting?*

A: The child should never be scolded or punished. The parents should be calm, rational, and understanding in dealing with the problem. A physician may be able to help by suggesting methods that other parents have found successful.

See also BABY CARE.

Bee sting is a wound caused by the venom of bees and is usually followed by pain and swelling. Most people are not seriously allergic to bee venom and experience no serious complications from occasional bee stings. Treatment involves application of an ice pack to alleviate the pain, and then washing the wound with soap and water. If a person has been stung in the mouth, give the victim a mouthwash of sodium bicarbonate and water.

Multiple bee stings, or an extreme allergic reaction to bee venom, may be more serious. In these cases, emergency medical attention should be sought. In a hypersensitive person, a single bee sting may result in death due to anaphylactic shock. If a victim stops breathing, give artificial respiration as quickly as possible. Persons who are extremely allergic to bee stings should carry an emergency treatment kit containing epinephrine (adrenaline).

See also ARTIFICAL RESPIRATION; BITES AND STINGS: FIRST AID; EPINEPHRINE; SHOCK, ANAPHYLACTIC.

Bee sting: treatment. *See* BITES AND STINGS: FIRST AID.

Behavior modification. *See* BEHAVIOR THERAPY.

Behavior therapy, often used interchangeably with behavior modification, is a form of psychological treatment based on learning theory. Behavioral therapists believe that maladaptive behavior and thinking is learned or conditioned and, therefore, can be unlearned. New, more constructive behavior can then be taught or shaped. Little attention is paid to intrapsychic or unconscious forces. Instead, behavior therapy focuses directly on overt behavior. It has been found to be particularly effective with anxiety and fear, using techniques such as relaxation training, desensitization, and assertiveness training. To increase the probability of success, behavioral therapists also attempt to remove the reinforcing consequences of maladaptive behavior as well as to reward appropriate behavior.

Belching, sometimes called burping, is the noisy emission of gas from the stomach via the esophagus. It is common for babies to belch after a feeding, but adults also belch, especially if they have eaten too rapidly or taken carbonated drinks. Air swallowing (aerophagia) is a nervous habit that often results in belching.

See also AEROPHAGIA.

Belladonna (bel ə don′ə) is an extract of the deadly nightshade plant. It contains atropine, an alkaloid drug used in various forms to treat intestinal disorders and a variety of other medical problems. It is also used in eye examinations to dilate the pupils. Side effects include a dry mouth. An overdose may cause an excited, confused mental state and may have fatal consequences.

See also ATROPINE.

Bell's palsy is paralysis of the muscles of the face, caused by acute malfunction of, or damage to, the nerve that supplies them. An attack frequently occurs without apparent cause.

Q: *What are the symptoms of Bell's palsy?*

A: Facial features lose their symmetrical arrangement, and the mouth droops at one corner. Paralysis of the muscles results in loss of control over saliva or tears, so that the patient may dribble or appear to cry.

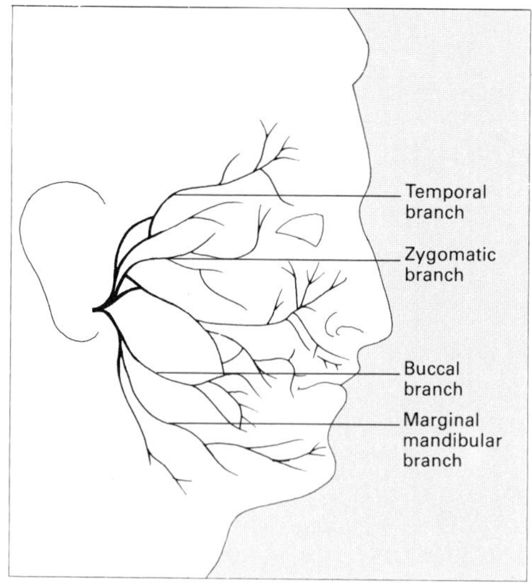

Bell's palsy is a disorder of the branches of the nerves that control the facial muscles.

Q: *What is the treatment for Bell's palsy?*

A: It is important that a physician is consulted immediately because swift treatment with corticosteroid drugs may help. Many patients recover spontaneously; about 70 percent recover completely within 4 to 6 weeks, and about 20 percent make a partial recovery. Surgery to the affected nerve may restore partial nerve function.

Benadryl® (ben′ə drəl) is the antihistamine drug diphenhydramine. It can be used to relieve the symptoms of allergies such as hay fever.

See also ANTIHISTAMINE.

Bends, also called decompression sickness or caisson disease, is a disorder caused by the formation of nitrogen bubbles in the blood and tissues after a person changes too quickly from an environment of high atmospheric pressure to one at normal pressure. Symptoms of the bends include painful joints, tightness in the chest, vomiting, giddiness, abdominal pain, and visual disturbances. Sometimes the victim suffers from convulsions and paralysis may follow. In severe cases, the condition can be fatal.

Q: *How are the bends treated?*

A: The victim must be returned immediately to a high-pressure atmosphere, either at the original work site or in a decompression chamber. The patient is then brought back very slowly to normal atmospheric pressure. This allows enough time for the dissolved nitrogen to be safely reconverted to its normal gaseous form and breathed out via the lungs.

Q: *Can the bends cause permanent damage?*

A: Damage to the joints may leave permanent arthritis. The nervous system may also be damaged, causing paralysis or signs of a stroke.

Benign (bi nīn′) describes a condition that is usually nonrecurrent and seldom causes severe problems. It is the opposite of malignant. A benign tumor is noncancerous and usually not, therefore, an immediate health threat, although treatment may be instituted at a later date for health or cosmetic purposes.

See also MALIGNANCY; TUMOR.

Benzedrine® (ben′zə drēn) is a registered trademark for an amphetamine, a drug that causes wakefulness.

See also AMPHETAMINE.

Benzocaine® (ben′zō kān) is a surface, or topical, anesthetic. It is used to make the passage of instruments more comfortable during an examination of internal organs (endoscopy). Benzocaine is also an ingredient in some lozenges used to relieve a sore throat, in sprays for soothing irritated skin, and in suppositories for relief of hemorrhoids.

See also ANESTHETIC; HEMORRHOID.

Beriberi (ber′ē ber′ē) is a disease caused by a deficiency of vitamin B_1 (thiamine) in the diet. The disease involves nerve degeneration (peripheral neuritis) and muscle disease (myopathy), particularly affecting heart muscles. Symptoms include fatigue, diarrhea, loss of weight, and heart failure. Beriberi is prevalent in eastern and southern Asia, but is relatively rare in the United States. It is sometimes associated with chronic alcoholism because many alcoholics fail to eat a properly balanced diet.

There are two types of beriberi: dry and wet. Dry beriberi results in the loss of strength and of some feeling in the limbs due to nerve degeneration. Wet beriberi is caused by accumulated fluid in the limbs (edema) and in the abdomen (ascites) because of a heart malfunction; nerve degeneration is commonly present as well.

Beriberi is treated with vitamin B_1, and this cures most cases of the disease. Care should be taken to provide the patient with a balanced diet.

Beta blocker is a drug that relieves stress on the heart by blocking the effects of adrenalin in the heart cells and blood vessels. Beta blockers have been shown to be particularly successful in reducing heart attacks among those who have already suffered them. Physicians often use beta blockers in treating heart patients, people who have hypertension, and persons suffering from angina and irregular heart beat. They are also used to treat migraine headaches, hyperthyroidism, and glaucoma. They are not prescribed for persons suffering from asthma or lung disorders, as they tend to constrict breathing passages. They should be used with caution in patients with diabetes mellitus.

See also ANGINA PECTORIS; HEART DISEASE; HYPERTENSION.

Biceps (bī′seps) is a muscle with two heads. The biceps muscle of the upper arm (biceps brachii) is Y-shaped, the single muscle branching into two strands higher up. This muscle flexes the arm at the elbow. The biceps muscle of the thigh (biceps femoris) flexes the leg.

Bicuspid (bī kus′pid), also known as a premolar, is a double-pointed tooth that tears and grinds food. Adult humans have eight bicuspids, located in pairs between the canines and the molars.

See also TOOTH.

Bicycle safety. Even though a bicycle is relatively simple to operate, a cyclist still must exercise careful planning and defensive driving in order to assure a safe journey. It is advisable to check with your local police department for city and/or state ordinances pertaining to bicyclists. These may vary from city to city and from state to state.

When bicycling, do not wear wide-bottomed pants, flapping skirts, trailing scarves, or any other loose clothing that may catch in the wheel spokes or on the gear chain. Pants bottoms should be tucked into socks or secured with bicycle clips. Shoes should have low heels. During the daytime, bright-colored or fluorescent vests or belts can be worn over normal clothing.

For cycling at night, when it is especially difficult for car drivers to see a cyclist, it is even more important to wear conspicuous clothing. Retroreflective material should be sewn onto clothing and retroreflectors should be mounted onto the bicycle. Otherwise, retroreflective vests or belts can be worn over normal clothing. A lit light at the front of the bicycle is now required by law in all states for nighttime bicycling. Some states also require a lit light at the back.

Bicyclists should always wear a helmet to provide head protection in case they fall or are knocked down. It is especially important to provide infants or small children with the same protection when riding with an adult. Head-related injuries account for 75 percent of all bike fatalities. Some states have therefore made the wearing of helmets mandatory.

A cyclist should never carry a passenger on a bicycle built for one driver, except in the case of an adult with a small child in a seat directly behind the adult. Otherwise, one seat, one cyclist.

Choosing a Bicycle

When choosing a bicycle, pick one that you will be able to drive with comfort and confidence. When you are on the seat, the toes of both feet should be able to touch the ground without tilting the bicycle. The thigh, leg, and heel of the foot on a pedal at its lowest should form a straight line as you ride along. The seat should be almost parallel to the ground. The handlebars should almost always be level with the seat.

Keep the bicycle clean and well oiled, and make sure that there are no loose parts. Pay special attention to the brakes, tires, and lights. Regularly check the tightness and alignment of the wheels, handlebars, pedals, and chain.

At all times, cyclists must give clear and positive hand signals when turning. Do not weave in and out of traffic or ride close to moving vehicles. Special care is needed at crosswalks, near parked cars, and on uneven road surfaces.

Bile (bīl), or gall, is an alkaline liquid produced by the liver. The liquid is a dark yellow-green color, and it contains cholesterol, bile salts, a reddish pigment called bilirubin, a green pigment called biliverdin, some proteins, and urea. It passes down the common bile duct to enter the duodenum (the first part of the intestine). A branch joins the bile duct to the gall bladder, in which bile can be stored until it is needed.

Q: *Why is bile needed?*

A: Bile helps to break down fats in food so that they can be absorbed, and it neutralizes the acidity of the stomach contents when they reach the duodenum. The presence of fats in the duodenum causes the release of a hormone that stimulates the contraction of the gall bladder and the production of bile.

Q: *Are there any bile disorders?*

A: The most familiar is jaundice, in which a blockage of the bile ducts causes bilirubin to circulate in the blood, giving the skin a characteristic yellow color.

See also BILE DUCT; BILIRUBIN; CHOLECYSTITIS; CHOLESTEROL; COLIC, BILIARY; GALL BLADDER; GALLSTONE; JAUNDICE.

Bile duct is the passage through which bile flows from the liver and gall bladder into the duodenum of the small intestine. Problems associated with bile ducts include stones that block the ducts, leading to pain; serious, life-threatening infections; and tumors.

See also BILE.

Bilharziasis (bil här zī′ə sis), or schistosomiasis, is a parasitic infection caused by a species of fluke of the genus *Schistosoma*. It is transmitted to humans through contaminated water, as well as through snails. Bilharziasis is fairly common in the tropics and in the Orient. Treatment is difficult; prevention is more effective. Chlorination of fresh water, and proper disposal of human feces are very effective in eliminating the disorder.

Biliary colic. *See* COLIC, BILIARY.

Bilirubin (bil ə rü′bin) is a reddish-yellow pigment formed mainly by the decomposition of hemoglobin in worn-out red blood cells. The blood carries it to the liver, where it combines with the bile and is passed on to the duodenum, eventually being excreted.

Jaundice is caused by an accumulation of bilirubin in the body. In newborns, special "bililites" help to remove excess bilirubin. Jaundice, however, often occurs in healthy, newborn babies. It may also occur if the mother and infant have incompatible blood groups.

See also JAUNDICE.

Billroth I and II are gastrectomies, that is, surgical procedures used in the treatment of stomach cancer and peptic ulcers. Billroth I involves the removal of the lower portion of the stomach. The remaining stomach is then connected directly to the duodenum, the upper part of the small intestine.

Billroth II involves the removal of both the lower portion of the stomach and the duodenum. The remaining stomach is then connected directly to the jejunum, the middle portion of the small intestine.

See also INTESTINE.

Biofeedback (bī′ō fēd bak) is a type of relaxation therapy in which the patient learns to control such bodily functions as heart rate, blood pressure, muscle tension, or brain wave activity. Continuous auditory and/or visual feedback on a particular body function is provided to assist the patient, in a trial and error process, to achieve the desired results. Biofeedback can be used to lower blood pressure, prevent headaches, and reduce chronic pain. For many problems, such as anxiety or headaches, simpler forms of relaxation training may be as effective as biofeedback.

Biomedical engineering is the use of engineering principles to solve medical problems and further medical research. It provides the tools to perform many medical tasks.

Biomedical engineers design artificial structures and control devices to replace or assist defective parts of the body. For example, a cardiac pacemaker is used to regulate the heartbeat when the natural pacemaker is defective. Other devices have been developed to replace hearts, kidneys, and other organs.

The application of various forms of energy to diagnose and treat disorders is also a feature of biomedical engineering. For example, internal body structures can be viewed or treated by energy in the form of X rays, nuclear radiation, and ultrasound. Lasers, which produce powerful beams of light, make possible bloodless surgery on small blood vessels, individual nerve fibers, and damaged retinas. Cryogenic (extremely cold) and electric probes can be used to correct disorders deep within the brain. Lifetime pacemakers powered by nuclear energy also have been developed.

Biomedical engineers also design and build measurement equipment, such as complex patient monitoring systems that take measurements in and on the body during surgery and treatment. These systems measure blood pressure; electrical activity in the brain, heart, muscles, and nerves; exchange of gases in the lungs during anesthesia; pulse and breathing rate; and body temperature. Monitoring systems also have automatic warning devices that signal when a patient's condition becomes critical.

Biopsy (bī′op sē) is the removal of a small piece of living tissue for the purpose of examining it under a microscope to see whether disease is present.

There are several ways in which a biopsy can be performed: (1) through a small cut in the skin; (2) by a tube passed through the mouth into the . testine to remove a small piece of intestinal lining; (3) through an instrument such as a sigmoidoscope or cystoscope; or (4) with a special needle to reach the liver or kidney.

Biotin (bī′ə tin), also known as vitamin H, is one of the vitamins of the vitamin B complex. It is found in many foods; particularly rich sources are liver, kidney, milk, egg yolks, and yeast. Biotin deficiency occurs only in association with a deficiency of others of the vitamin B group.

See also VITAMIN.

Bipolar disorder. *See* MANIC-DEPRESSIVE ILLNESS.

Birth control. *See* CONTRACEPTION; FAMILY PLANNING.

Birth defect. *See* CONGENITAL ANOMALY.

Birthmark, or nevus, is a blemish on the skin that is present at birth. Birthmarks do not usually cause problems, although there are some abnormal marks, such as a port-wine stain, which may require treatment.

Q: *What are the main types of birthmarks?*

A: The most common birthmark is a simple skin discoloration (nevus pigmentosus), which may be any color from light yellow to black. A mole is typical of this type of birthmark. It does not need treat-

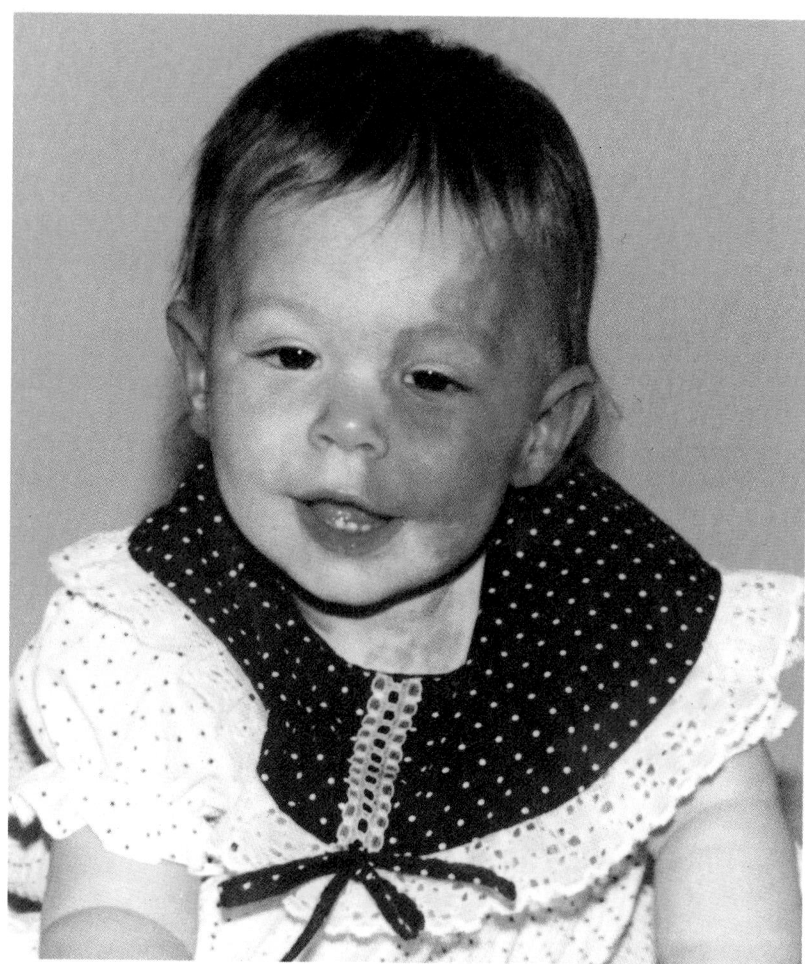

A **birthmark** is caused by expanded blood vessels below the skin.

ment, unless it is irritated by clothing or is disfiguring.

Rarer types of birthmarks are generally the result of having a cluster of blood vessels just below the surface of the skin. Typical of this type is the strawberry nevus. It is a slightly raised reddish or purplish mark that appears most often on the face, head, neck, or arms. It grows rapidly for the first year after birth and then decreases in size. In most children it disappears by the age of five.

A port-wine stain is a complex birthmark, sometimes flat, sometimes raised and bumpy. It does not disappear but grows in proportion with the rest of the body. Like a strawberry nevus, it is caused by expanded blood vessels below the surface of the skin.

Q: *Why should some birthmarks be removed?*

A: If birthmarks of the port-wine stain type are large enough or serious enough to cause danger in case of injury, they may be removed by plastic surgery. In many cases, removal of a birthmark is not medically advised, but cosmetics can be used to reduce any embarrassment that the blemish might cause.

Birth, premature. Premature birth occurs when an infant is born earlier in pregnancy than normal. There is no single measure of fetal weight or development that is used to determine premature birth, but the designation usually implies that the infant was born before the thirty-sixth week of gestation. A premature birth may occur spontaneously, or it may be medically induced.

The incidence of premature birth is higher for women who have not had proper prenatal care and whose obstetric history is abnormal. Other contributing factors include cigarette smoking and diets deficient in protein or calories.

Premature birth and low birth weight are major causes of neonatal mortality. In infants born before 34 to 36 weeks of gestation, the lungs may be immature, and the infant may thus have problems in breathing. Physicians, therefore, try to prevent premature delivery if at all possible.

Fortunately, improved neonatal care has helped many premature infants survive.

Bisexuality (bī sek shü al′ə tē) is (1) the condition of being attracted to both sexes, or (2) the combining of both male and female organs in one individual, animal, or plant.

See also HERMAPHRODITE; HOMOSEXUALITY.

Bite is a puncture or other wound of the skin caused by a living organism. The most common bites are those of dogs, cats, snakes, spiders, and various insects. Most bites are relatively harmless and require only a thorough cleansing with soap or an antiseptic. But some bites are serious (such as the bite of the black widow spider) and require specialized medical treatment.

Human bites are quite serious as they often become infected if not properly treated; proper medical attention may be necessary.

See also BITES AND STINGS: FIRST AID; RABIES; SNAKEBITE.

First aid for bites and stings

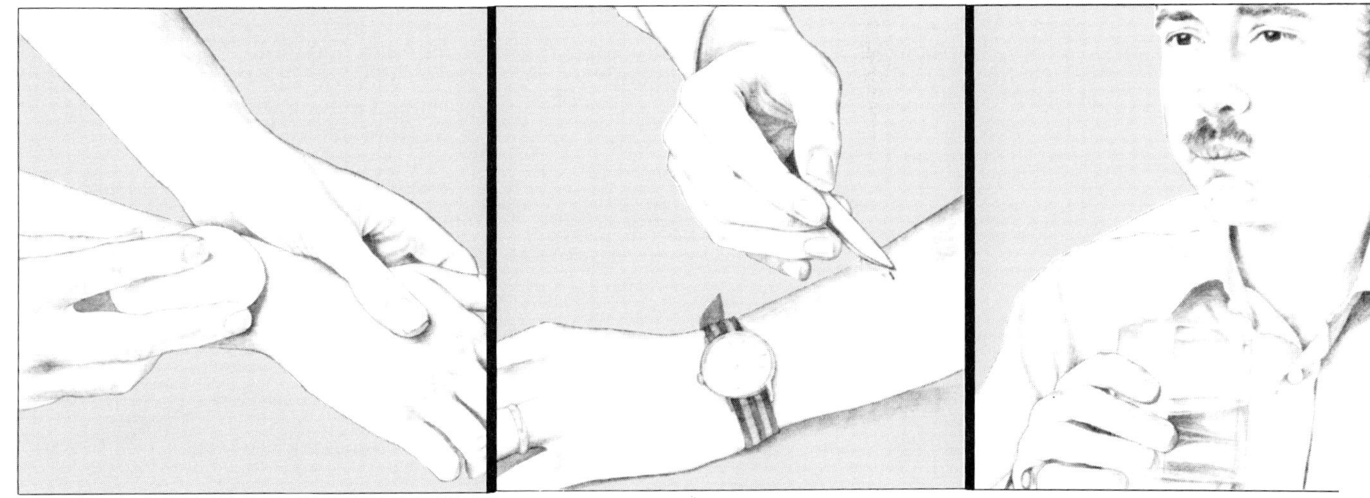

1 If the victim has been bitten or scratched by an animal, the wound must be washed with soap and water. Control any bleeding by pressing firmly on a dressing over the wound until bleeding stops. Then the wound should be dressed and bandaged. Summon immediate medical attention if the wound is severe.

2 If a stinger with its venom sac is present, carefully remove the stinger by gently scraping it from the skin. This is preferable to using a tweezer, which often results in the injection of additional venom.

3 If the victim has been stung in the mouth, he or she should be given ice to suck and mouthwashes of sodium bicarbonate solution. This can be made by dissolving one teaspoon of sodium bicarbonate in a glass of water. This solution will help to reduce the swelling. Summon immediate medical aid.

Bites and stings: first aid. Poisonous bites and stings are relatively rare but can be extremely dangerous. Poisons from different poisonous creatures require different medical treatment, so it is important to identify the creature or preferably to kill or capture it for expert identification. If you have identified the creature as being poisonous or if you only suspect it, summon emergency medical aid.

Treatment. Follow the individual instructions listed later in this article according to the type of animal bite that has occurred. Emergency treatment may be necessary if a victim experiences anaphylactic shock or stops breathing entirely. Anaphylactic shock is characterized by faintness; pallor; nausea; vomiting; difficulty in breathing; wheezing; swelling of the throat, mouth, or face; hives; weak pulse; or rapid heartbeat. If a victim is suffering from anaphylactic shock, put him or her on the ground and remain with the victim while emergency aid is summoned. If the victim stops breathing, give artificial respiration. If a victim's heart stops, give external cardiac compression.

See also ARTIFICIAL RESPIRATION; HEART ATTACK: FIRST AID; SHOCK, ANAPHYLACTIC.

Bites and Stings

Name	*Toxic substances*	*Symptoms*	*Treatment*
Ant Genus: *Pogonomyrmex; Solenopsis.*	enzyme; formic acid; vasodilator	Sharp stinging pain; whiteness at point of bite; itching; in severe cases, fever and ulceration; multiple bites may cause death.	1. Identify insect. 2. If reaction is severe, take victim to a hospital immediately. 3. Apply cold compress.

(*continued* on pages 114 and 115)

Name	*Toxic substances*	*Symptoms*	*Treatment*
Bee For example: honeybee; bumblebee. Genus: *Apis; Bombus; Xylocopa.*	enzymes; hemolytic agents; neurotoxin; vasodilator	Local pain; burning sensation; whiteness at site of sting; swelling and redness; multiple stings may cause generalized swelling, respiratory distress, and shock; rarely death.	1. Identify insect. 2. Carefully remove stinger. 3. Apply ice cubes. 4 Administer oral antihistamines and analgesics as needed. 5. Multiple stings may require immediate hospitalization.
Hornet or wasp Genus: *Polistes; Seliphron; Vespa; Vespula.*	enzymes; hemolytic agents; neurotoxin; vasodilator	Similar to the signs and symptoms of a bee sting.	Treat as a bee sting.
Mosquito Genus: *Aedes; Anopheles; Culex.*	anticoagulant in saliva; disease-causing organisms in saliva	Slight local pain; swelling; itching. Organisms in mosquito bite may cause a variety of diseases, including malaria and yellow fever.	1. Hydrocortisone cream relieves irritation. 2. Do not scratch. 3. Antimalarial drugs and insect repellents, if in malarial region.
Scorpion Genus: *Centruroides; Tityus; Leiurus.*	neurotoxin; enzymes	Acute burning pain at site of sting; restlessness; confusion; chest and abdominal pain; respiratory distress; in some cases, convulsions and death.	1. Identify scorpion. 2. Apply ice cubes. 3. Take victim to a hospital. Antivenin is available in some areas for some types of scorpions.
Tick Genus: *Dermacentor; Ixodes; Ornithodoros.*	not known	Itching; local skin irritation. Poisonous species cause pain; redness; swelling; muscle cramps. Some species carry typhus, Rocky Mountain spotted fever, and Lyme's disease.	1. Apply petroleum jelly, alcohol, or gasoline to tick, to loosen its jaws. 2. Use tweezers to carefully remove tick. Do not leave jaws embedded. 3. Wash skin carefully.
Jellyfish For example: Portuguese man-of-war. Genus: *Physalia.* Other species have less serious effect.	sea anemone toxin; vasoconstrictor	Acute stinging or burning sensation; rash; blistering; shock; rarely causes death, unless from drowning as a result of shock.	1. Remove all tentacles with gloved fingers if possible. 2. Wash area with seawater, then with vinegar. 3. Apply hydrocortisone cream. 4. Take victim to a hospital.

Name	*Toxic substances*	*Symptoms*	*Treatment*
Black widow spider Genus: *Latrodectus.*	neurotoxin	Delayed pain; cramp-like pain in chest, abdomen and legs; muscle rigidity; nausea; fever; bite is sometimes fatal.	1. Identify spider. 2. Apply ice cubes. 3. Lay the victim down; keep bitten part at or below the level of the heart. 4. Take victim to a hospital.
Brown recluse spider Genus: *Loxosceles.*	cytotoxin; enzymes; hemolytic agent	Delayed pain; whiteness at bite, surrounded by red swelling; blistering; bleeding into tissues; vomiting; fever; only rarely, heart failure and death.	1. Identify spider. 2. Lay the victim down. 3. Keep bitten part at or below the level of the heart. 4. Take victim to a hospital.
Tarantula spider Genus: *Aphonopelma; Eurypelma.*	variable, depending on species and location	Slight pain like a pinprick; poison is usually mild and may be harmless.	1. Identify spider. 2. Wash bite with warm salted water.
Gila monster Genus: *Heloderma.*	neurotoxin (heloderma venom)	Local pain; swelling; nausea; respiratory distress; heart failure; in some cases, death.	Treat as snakebite.
Copperhead Genus: *Agkistrodon.*	enzymes	Shock; local pain; swelling; vomiting; blood in stools; may be fatal.	General treatment is the same for any snakebite. 1. Lay the victim down. 2. Calm and reassure the victim. 3. Keep the bitten part still. 4. Keep bitten part at or below the level of the heart. 5. Take victim to a hospital or poison-control center for treatment with the specific antivenin. 6. If the victim cannot be moved, summon medical help at once. 7. Clean the bite, but do not apply a tourniquet, do not cut or suck the bite, do not apply ice. 8. If victim is unconscious, place in recovery position.
Coral snake Genus: *Micrurus; Micruroides.*	enzymes; neurotoxin	Shock; numbness; headache; vomiting; swollen face; sore throat; rapid heartbeat; may be fatal.	
Fer-de-lance Genus: *Bothrops.*	enzymes	Shock; local pain; bleeding from bite; blood does not clot; bleeding into tissues; respiratory distress; may be fatal.	
Rattlesnake Genus: *Crotalus.*	enzymes	Shock; local pain; swelling; bleeding into tissues; vomiting; dry mouth; problems with speech and vision; may be fatal.	
Water moccasin Genus: *Agkistrodon.*	enzymes	Shock; local pain; vomiting; blood in stools; tiny bleeding spots on skin; may be fatal.	

Black death. *See* BUBONIC PLAGUE.

Black eye is a swollen bruise of the eyelids and eye socket. It is usually caused by direct injury, or it may be the result of a fractured skull. The dark color of the skin results from the escape of blood into the eye socket and the thin tissue surrounding it. The blood tends to drain into the eyelids, making the eye difficult to open. It may also spread down the cheek. Cold packs applied with pressure as soon as possible after the injury help the damaged blood vessels to contract, and reduce the swelling. Any problems or defects in vision, or a black eye after a head injury, require immediate medical attention.

Blackhead, or comedo, is a plug of hardened secretion in the duct of an oil gland in the skin. It is dark because of the effect of oxygen on the secretion, not because of dirt or other particles.

See also ACNE.

Black lung is the common name for the lung disorder anthracosis. The normal pink color of the lungs is turned black by the inhalation of coal dust or smoke. Once a common disorder only among coal miners, anthracosis is now also found in city dwellers.

Q: *What are the symptoms of anthracosis?*

A: In the early stages the symptoms resemble those of bronchitis, with coughing and shortness of breath. If the cause is not removed, over a period of years the coughing gradually gets worse. Diagnosis is confirmed by an X-ray examination.

Q: *What is the treatment for anthracosis?*

A: The lung damage caused by the inhaled dust cannot be repaired, nor can it be treated directly. Breathing clean air halts the progress of the disease and may help reduce the severity of the symptoms. A victim should avoid further exposure to dust particles.

See also ANTHRACOSIS; PNEUMOCONIOSIS.

Blackout is a temporary loss of consciousness. It is most often caused by an inadequate supply of blood to the brain (fainting), but also may occur during an epileptic seizure or during a mild stroke.

If a victim has not regained consciousness within a few minutes, and has not completely recovered within 15 minutes, summon medical help and treat for unconsciousness. If a blackout lasts longer than several minutes, it may be caused by an underlying illness, and the victim should seek medical advice on recovery. Repeated blackouts are also an indication that further medical attention is needed.

An alcoholic blackout is a little different. Alcoholics will often suffer memory loss (amnesia) for a period during which they have been drinking heavily. Although they may not have lost consciousness at any time, this forgotten period is referred to as a blackout. A history of alcohol-induced blackouts is strongly suggestive that a person suffers from alcoholism.

See also FAINTING: FIRST AID; UNCONSCIOUSNESS: TREATMENT.

Bladder is any hollow body structure, usually referring to the bladder that collects and stores urine. It is a strong, muscular organ that receives urine from the kidneys, and then releases the urine out of the body through the urethra tube.

Q: *How much liquid does the bladder hold?*

A: In most adults, the bladder holds a little more than one pint (475ml) of urine. This quantity may be much greater as a result of certain bladder disorders. Between 700 and 2000ml (.7 to 2l) of urine are usually excreted each day.

Q: *Is the bladder in a child weaker than in an adult?*

A: No, but a child's bladder is smaller, and he or she often feels

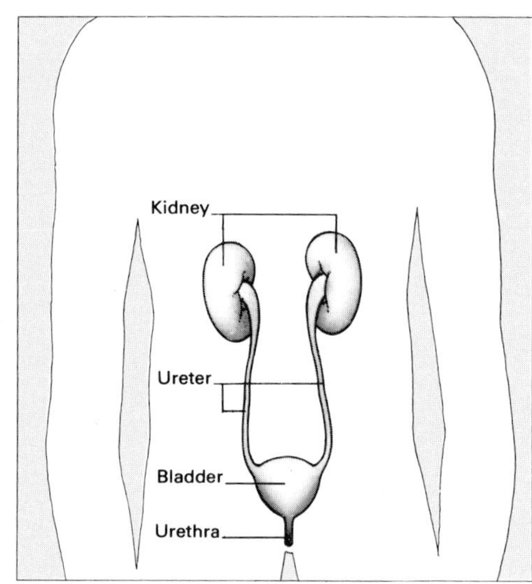

The **bladder** collects urine from the kidneys and passes it out of the body through the urethra.

nervous when the bladder is full.

See also BLADDER DISORDERS; URETHRA.

Bladder disorders. The following table lists some common disorders that affect the bladder, grouped according to their chief symptoms. The symptoms may also indicate other clinical disorders; this is not a complete list. A good medical history and physical examination by a physician are essential for adequate diagnosis. For more information, *see* the individual entry for each disorder.

Symptom	*Disorder*
Blood in the urine	Calculus (a stone in the kidney, ureter, or bladder)
	Cystitis (bladder inflammation)
	Tumor
Difficult urination	Prolapse (of uterus or vagina)
	Prostate gland (enlargement)
	Stroke (nerve damage affecting bladder control)
Frequent urination	Cystitis
	Diabetes (glucose in urine; thirst)
	Fibroid (benign tumor in the uterus)
	Incontinence
	Prostate gland (enlargement)
	Stroke
	Urethritis (inflammation of urethra)
Painful urination	Calculus
	Cancer (of the cervix)
	Cystitis
	Gonorrhea
	Peritonitis (of the pelvis)
	Prostatitis (prostate inflammation)
	Urethritis

Bladder infection occurs in the organ of the body that gathers, holds, and eventually releases urine. There are many types, causes, and symptoms of bladder infections. One of the more common bladder disorders is cystitis, a bladder inflammation that is painful, may be recurrent, and causes urine to turn cloudy. Bladder infections may also cause difficulty in urination, frequent urination, and bloody urination. Treatment for bladder infections varies, but some methods include increased liquid intake and antibiotics.

See also BLADDER; CALCULUS; CYSTITIS.

Bland diet. *See* DIET, SPECIAL; NUTRITION.

Blastomycosis (blas tō mī kō'sis) is an infection caused by a yeast-like fungus. The infection occurs in the skin and lungs, causing a slow form of pneumonia with lung inflammation. The infected person usually has a cough, shortness of breath, chills, chest pains, and a fever. The disease is most common in men living in the southeastern and central portions of the United States. Recovery is usually swift, following the administration of an antibiotic which kills the fungus.

Bleeding is the release of blood from damaged blood vessels following a cut, wound, or an internal hemorrhage. Blood in mucus that is coughed up or in stools could be a symptom of an internal disorder and should be reported to a physician.

See also BLEEDING: FIRST AID; BLOOD, SPITTING OF; BLOOD, VOMITING OF; HEMORRHAGE.

Bleeding: first aid. For slight bleeding, pressure applied by a sterile gauze bandage held firmly or bandaged over the wound usually stops the flow of blood. For more severe bleeding, it may be necessary to locate the vein or artery above the bleeding point and press it against the bone behind it. When pressure is properly applied, external bleeding should cease. With internal bleeding it is important to recognize the general signs (which apply to both external and internal bleeding): pallor; cold, clammy skin; a weak, rapid pulse; and fast, shallow breathing. The victim may also feel faint or even pass out. Internal bleeding is extremely dangerous, and medical assistance should be sought immediately. Do not give a person suspected of internal bleeding any food or drink. If the victim has been stabbed and the implement is still in the wound, do not remove it. If the victim has an open wound in the chest, cover it to prevent air entering the chest. If there is bleeding from the leg or uterus, lay the person down with

First aid for bleeding

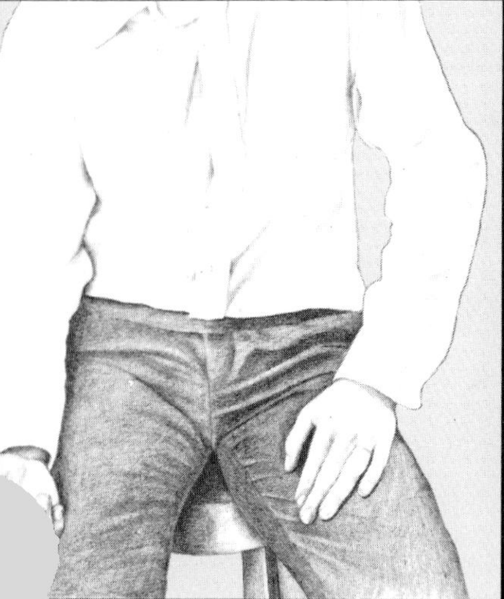

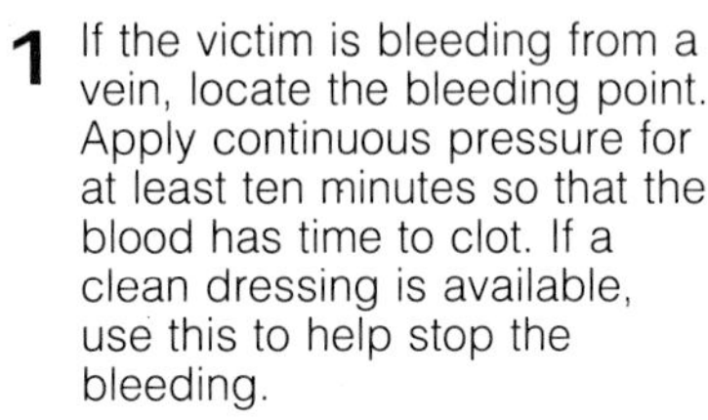

1 If the victim is bleeding from a vein, locate the bleeding point. Apply continuous pressure for at least ten minutes so that the blood has time to clot. If a clean dressing is available, use this to help stop the bleeding.

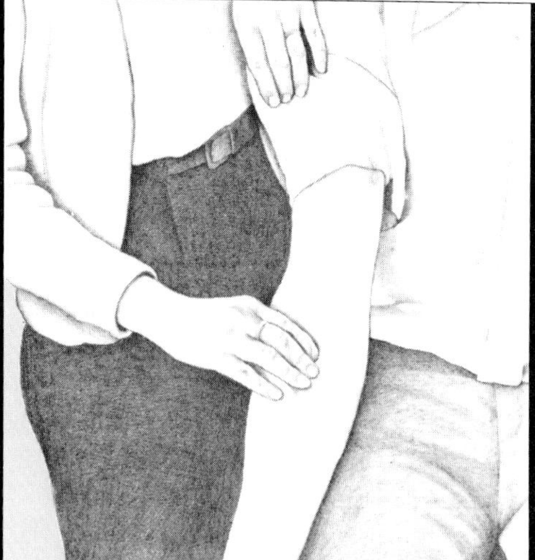

2 Continue to apply pressure over the dressing until the bleeding stops. Raise the injured part if possible while continuing to apply pressure. Lay the victim down with the legs raised. If the victim goes into shock, *see* SHOCK: TREATMENT.

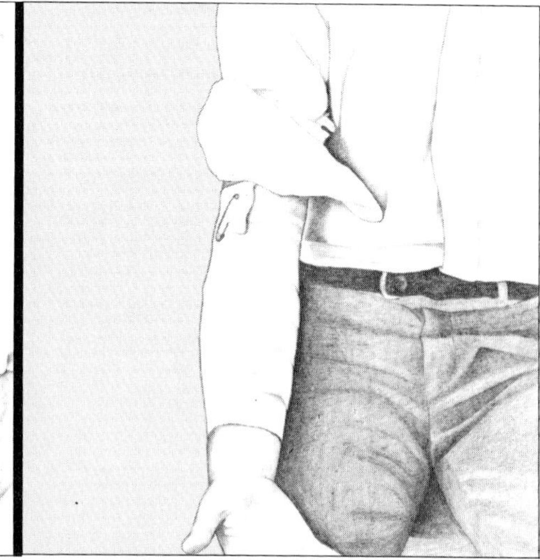

3 Wash the wound and remove any foreign body that comes out easily. If the victim has been stabbed, *do not* remove the implement. Apply a clean dressing and a firm bandage. *Do not* bandage too tightly. Keep the injured part raised and summon medical help as soon as possible.

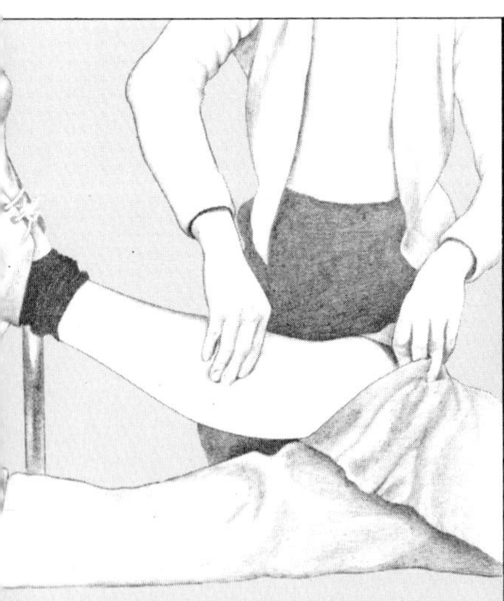

4 If the victim is bleeding from a varicose vein, raise the affected leg as high as possible. Apply pressure to the bleeding point. When the bleeding stops, cover the area with a clean dressing, bandage the whole leg, and summon medical help.

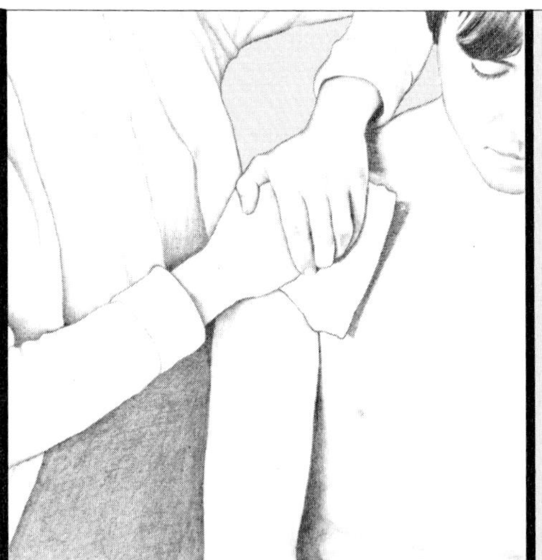

5 If the victim is bleeding from a deep wound, cover the wound with a clean dressing, such as a handkerchief. Apply firm pressure for at least ten minutes, or until the bleeding has stopped.

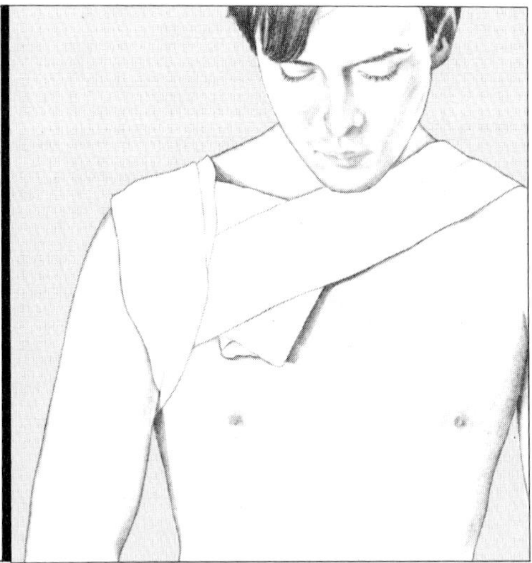

6 When the bleeding has stopped, apply a firm bandage to keep the dressing in place. *Do not* remove the dressing or the bandage as this may reopen the wound. Summon medical help as soon as possible.

legs raised. Keep the victim warm and comfortable but do not overheat.

The sudden loss of large quantities of blood may result in the condition of shock, in which the skin becomes cold and clammy and the blood pressure drops severely. Watch the victim's pulse and breathing. If the victim has stopped breathing, give artificial respiration. Bleeding from an artery can be recognized by the rhythmic pumping of the blood from the wound and its bright scarlet color. Bleeding from a vein is recognizable by the fact that the blood is much darker and flows more smoothly.

Blepharitis (blef ə rī′tis) is a disorder affecting the eyelids. Redness and inflammation of the eyelids accompany the disorder. If the lids are infected, a sty (an infected swelling of a hair follicle) may appear. The cause of blepharitis is usually an increased oil secretion from the glands on the lid margins or an infection of these glands. Sometimes it is a result of allergy.

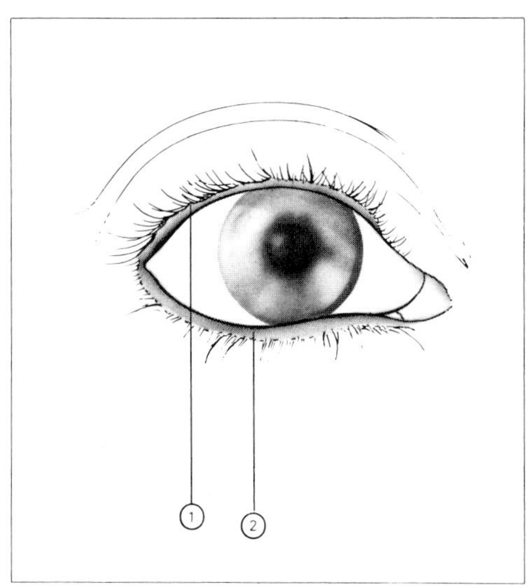

Blepharitis is an inflammation that can affect both rims (1, 2) of the eyelid.

Q: *What is the treatment for blepharitis?*

A: The eyelids should be cleansed regularly with a warm solution of salt water. A mild antiseptic may be applied to the rims. A physician may prescribe antibiotic or corticosteroid drugs, but continued treatment with these may cause a skin allergy.

See also EYELID; STY.

Blindness is the absence of vision in one or both eyes. It may be present at birth, or it may occur suddenly in one or both eyes at a later stage in life. Commonly blindness involves a gradual deterioration of vision until the stage when no sight remains. It may be caused by various disorders affecting the eye itself or may result from a disorder of the visual center of the brain. The medical term for blindness in which the eye appears to be normal is amaurosis. Temporary blindness, commonly called a blackout, can occur with some minor disorders, such as fainting.

Q: *Why are some babies born blind?*

A: Congenital blindness is sometimes caused by infection of the mother by rubella (German measles) at some time during the first three months of pregnancy. The disease causes the lenses in the baby's eyes to be opaque. Other causes of congenital blindness are defects in the formation of the eye and various metabolic disorders.

Q: *What are the causes of gradual blindness?*

A: Any of the following disorders may cause gradual blindness: pressure within the eyeball (glaucoma); the formation of opaque patches in the eye lens (cataract); a retina damaged as a result of high blood pressure (hypertension), diabetes, or degenerative disease of the retina; pressure on the optic nerve from a tumor (for example, pituitary gland adenoma); or recurrent ulcers on the cornea, which may be caused by a form of conjunctivitis (trachoma) common in hot, dry climates. Treatment of the cause usually arrests the condition and, in some cases, may restore sight.

Q: *What causes sudden blindness?*

A: The retina, the part of the eye onto which light rays are focused, may become detached from the layer enclosing it (the choroid), and blindness can result. Detached retina may be caused by an accidental blow to the eye, or it may occur spontaneously in people with the vision defect myopia (nearsightedness). Bleeding behind the retina or inflammation of the optic nerve (retrobulbar neuritis) may cause blindness in one eye. A blocked

Blindness may be caused by a cataract on the lens, preventing light penetration.

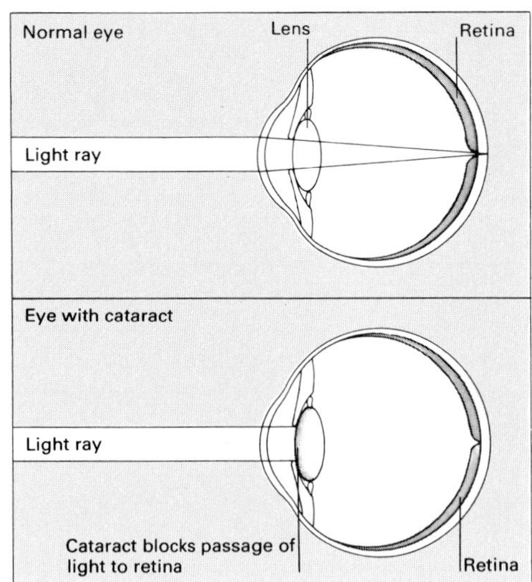

vein or artery supplying the eye can also result in sudden blindness. Sudden blindness in one eye occurs much more frequently than sudden blindness in both.

Q: *What causes temporary blindness?*

A: Temporary blindness may be caused by a spasm of the arteries during a bad migraine headache, by low blood pressure that precedes fainting, or by a small blood clot (embolus) that is passing through an artery that serves the eye.

Q: *How can a person adapt to being blind?*

A: Many schools and agencies provide education and training for people who are born blind or become blind later in life. Blind persons learn to use Braille and other techniques to help them retain their independence. Blind persons are employed in practically every profession, including computer programming, engineering, law, music, teaching, and many other fields.

See also AMAUROSIS; COLOR BLINDNESS; NIGHT BLINDNESS.

Blister (blis′tər) is a raised area on the skin that contains fluid derived from blood serum. It generally forms as a result of skin irritation, rubbing, or pinching. Excessive heat also causes blistering.

Q: *What is the best treatment for blisters?*

A: Normal blisters are most effectively treated by applying a mild antiseptic cream and by covering them with a clean, dry pad to prevent further rubbing. If a blister bursts, it should be kept as clean as possible with an antiseptic solution. A blood blister is best wrapped in a firm dressing with a little pressure, to prevent further bursting of blood vessels.

See also BLISTER, BLOOD; BLISTER: TREATMENT.

Blister, blood. A blood blister is a raised, hemispherical section of skin containing blood from broken vessels.

See also BLISTER.

Blister: treatment. Blisters may be caused by a variety of injuries, such as friction from ill-fitting shoes, burns, scalds, exposure to certain chemicals, and contact with irritant plants. Many diseases, such as chickenpox, eczema, impetigo, and herpes simplex, also produce blisters.

For blisters caused by a burn or a scald, *see* BURNS AND SCALDS: FIRST AID.

For blisters caused by contact with an irritant plant or chemical, *see* POISONING: FIRST AID.

If a disease is suspected as causing the blister, if the blister persists after treatment, or if there is increased redness and pain or other symptoms of infection after the apparent cause has been removed, a physician should be consulted.

Blocker (block′ər) is a drug or chemical that inhibits the action or secretion of a substance, the activity of a part of the body, or the transmission of stimuli along the nervous system.

See also BETA BLOCKER; HISTAMINE H_2-RECEPTOR ANTAGONIST.

Blood is the body's "transportation system," the liquid that carries oxygen and essential nutrients to all parts of the body. It also carries waste products, such as carbon dioxide, to the organs that eliminate them from the body.

Q: *What else does blood do?*

A: Heat from inner parts of the body is carried in the blood to the skin to keep the temperature of the body stable. The blood also carries defenses against infection (antibodies) to all body tissues and transports vital chemicals and hormones that are used in the control of body functions.

Q: *How much blood does the body contain?*

A: In an adult of average size there is

include a red blood cell count, a white blood cell count, a differential white cell count, a platelet count, and a blood smear, which reports any abnormalities in the red blood cells. The actual counting of cells is usually done by an electronic counter, in which a computer recognizes the patterns of each cell type. In some laboratories, parts of the CBC may still be done manually. A complete blood count is a starting point in the exploration of possible diseases or conditions. A physician may request additional blood tests at the same time, or the CBC results may suggest areas for further investigation.

Blood disorders. Disorders of the blood are generally categorized by physicians according to the nature of the complaint. There are disorders of blood production, disorders within the blood cells, infections in the blood, and disorders of the blood clotting mechanism.

The following table lists the most common disorders that are caused by blood disease or malfunction and their basic characteristics.

Disorder	*Basic characteristic*
Agranulocytosis	Reduced production of white blood cells
Anemia	Reduced production or loss of red blood cells
Blood poisoning	Infection of blood stream by bacteria
Christmas disease	Defective blood clotting
Hemophilia	Defective blood clotting
Leukemia	Uncontrolled and disorderly increase of white blood cells
Malaria	Parasitic infestation of red blood cells
Mononucleosis	Excess of large white blood cells
Myeloma	Cancer of the bone marrow
Polycythemia	Excessive production of red blood cells
Purpura	Bleeding under the skin
Sickle cell anemia	Deformity of red blood cells in which the cells take on a sickle shape
Thalassemia	Deformity of red blood cells
Thrombocytopenia	Decreased number of blood platelets

Of the conditions listed, most are serious and require immediate medical treatment. However, many characteristics cited here may also be indicative of some other clinical disorder. An accurate medical history and physical examination by a physician are essential for adequate diagnosis of a problem. Each disorder also has its own article in this encyclopedia.

Blood group or blood type. Blood is classified into groups according to the presence of particular antigens, or proteins, on the blood cells. A knowledge of a person's blood group is important when a blood transfusion is necessary in tissue and organ transplants, in cases of disputed paternity, and in preventing problems with newborn children. The two most important classification systems are the ABO system and the Rhesus (Rh) system.

Q: *What is the ABO system?*

A: The ABO system distinguishes four blood groups: A, B, AB, and O. All blood can be classified in one of these groups.

A and B represent proteins that are found on the surface of blood cells. O represents the absence of either of these proteins. Since a person receives two genes for blood groups (one from each parent), one can fall into four groups: A, representing either two A genes (AA) or one A gene and an O gene for which there is no protein produced; B, similar to A; O, if one receives O genes from both the parents; or AB. People develop antibodies that fight against the proteins they do not possess. For example, someone with type A would have antibodies against type B blood. If someone is given a transfusion of blood against which he or she has antibodies, a serious reaction can occur. Since a person with AB blood has both groups, he or she may receive A, B, O, or AB blood. Conversely, since a person with O blood has neither protein, he or she cannot receive A, B, or AB blood, but O blood can be given to people with any ABO type.

Q: *What is the Rh factor?*

A: The Rhesus system defines two blood types: blood in which the

Rh factor is present (Rhesus positive, or Rh+), and that in which it is not (Rhesus negative, or Rh−). In Western countries, about 85 percent of people are Rh+.

The Rhesus system and the ABO bear no correlation whatsoever with each other, but for the sake of clarity the ABO and Rhesus classifications are generally combined when stating a blood group (for example, A+, O−, etc.).

Q: *Is one blood group more common than the others?*

A: Yes. Recent statistics show the following world incidence of blood groups: group O, 46 percent; A, 42 percent; B, 8 percent; AB, 4 percent.

See also ANTIBODY; HEMOLYTIC DISEASE OF THE NEWBORN; RH FACTOR.

Blood, passing of. The passing of blood through the rectum can be caused by any one of several conditions or a combination thereof. Blood that has turned black and tarry may be an indication of acute gastritis or an ulcer. It may also stem from a disturbance in the beginning or the near-beginning of the gastrointestinal tract. The darker color of the blood results from being partially digested. Red blood is more often passed when the cause is farther down the gastrointestinal tract, such as a colon polyp, hemorrhoids, or colitis.

Red blood can also result from upper gastrointestinal problems in which the blood passes through the system so rapidly that its color is not affected by digestion.

Blood may also be passed in the urine, indicating a problem in the kidneys or bladder. Any passage of blood is potentially serious, and a physician should be consulted.

Blood poisoning, also called bacteremia, is the presence of bacterial infection in the bloodstream. Once infection has spread to the blood, it may be carried in the blood to other parts of the body. Frequent, intermittent, high fever, shaking chills, and red streaks leading from a wound are all symptoms. In extreme cases, abscesses may appear throughout the body, both on the skin and in internal organs such as the liver or brain. Severe blood poisoning may be fatal if hospital treatment is delayed.

See also PYEMIA; TOXEMIA.

Blood pressure is the pressure blood exerts against the walls of the arteries. The amount of pressure depends upon the strength and the rate of the heart's contraction, the volume of blood in the circulatory system, and the elasticity of the arteries. Two measurements are taken, the highest and lowest values for pressure, which correspond to the two main stages in the pumping action of the heart.

Q: *How is blood pressure measured?*

A: Blood pressure is usually measured by an instrument called a sphygmomanometer. To measure the pressure, an inflatable cuff, or wide band, is placed around the patient's upper arm and a stethoscope is applied to the artery just below the cuff. By listening for changes in the sound of the pulse, the individual measuring the blood pressure knows how much to inflate the cuff, in order to stop blood from flowing in the arteries of the arm. Air is slowly let out of the cuff until the blood begins flowing again. At this stage, the sphygmomanometer records what is called the systolic blood pressure. Additional air is let out of the cuff until the sounds become muffled. The instrument then indicates the diastolic pressure. The systolic pressure corresponds to the contraction of the heart muscle, and the diastolic pressure corresponds to a relaxation of the

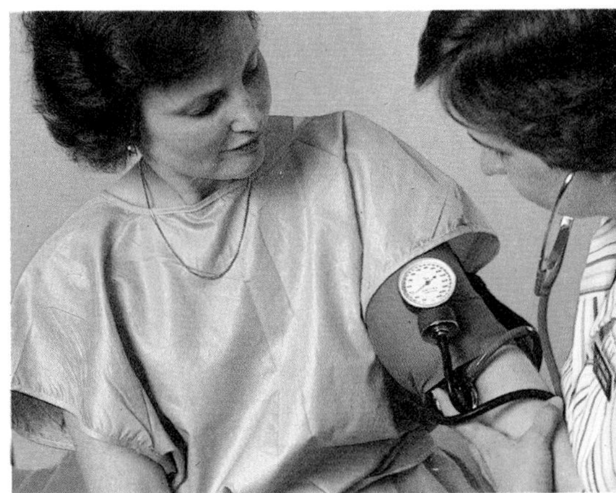

Blood pressure is measured by an instrument called a sphygmomanometer.

heart. The two pressures are expressed in the following way: systolic/diastolic—120/80. See *also* SPHYGMOMANOMETER.

Q: *What is considered a normal blood pressure reading?*

A: A healthy (normal) blood pressure reading varies with age, activity, and altitude and from person to person. Bearing in mind these qualifications, values between 100/60 and 140/90 are generally considered normal. A single blood pressure reading, unless very high or very low, should not be considered abnormal. An average of several readings taken on different days is generally used.

Q: *What does high blood pressure mean?*

A: High blood pressure, also called hypertension, is itself a major disorder that requires treatment. Untreated, this sustained rise in blood pressure can damage the heart, blood vessels, and kidneys.

Other serious disorders that cause blood pressure to rise well above the normal level include congestive heart failure and head injuries. See *also* HYPERTENSION.

Q: *What causes low blood pressure?*

A: Low blood pressure (hypotension) can result from shock and some diseases. It can cause fainting. See *also* HYPOTENSION.

Blood serum is the clear to pale-yellow liquid part of blood that separates from clotting blood. It is blood minus its fibrin and the blood cells.

See *also* SERUM.

Blood, spitting of. Spitting of blood, known medically as hemoptysis, is a symptom of bleeding somewhere in the respiratory tract. The frothy and bright red blood may come from the nose, mouth, or throat (the upper respiratory passages), the lower respiratory passages, or the lungs. The seriousness of the disorder depends on the cause.

Q: *What can cause the spitting of blood from the upper respiratory passages?*

A: The most common and least serious reason for blood in the sputum (the substance spat out) is that coughing has ruptured a small blood vessel in the nose, mouth or throat. Any infection or damage in the mouth, throat, or back of the nose may also cause bleeding.

Q: *What causes the spitting of blood from the lower respiratory passages?*

A: Bleeding from this region is caused by damage or infection in the trachea (windpipe) or the bronchi (tubes to the lungs). Serious disorders to be excluded include bronchiectasis, pulmonary embolus, pneumonia, tuberculosis, and lung cancer. Damage to a bronchus from breathing in a foreign body, such as a peanut, also causes blood in the sputum.

See *also* FLUKE; PNEUMOCONIOSIS; TUBERCULOSIS; WORM.

Blood test. See BLOOD COUNT, COMPLETE.

Blood transfusion (trans fyü'zhən) is the transference of blood from one person to another. A patient is usually given a transfusion using blood supplied by a blood bank, where the blood has been stored under refrigeration after collection from the donor. Usually in a transfusion, the blood is allowed to flow slowly by gravity into a vein in the patient's arm. A person facing elective surgery can "bank" his or her own blood in the months before surgery. This way there is no chance of incompatibility or of receiving blood that might contain infectious agents of various viruses including the hepatitis virus and the virus responsible for AIDS.

Q: *When is a transfusion necessary?*

A: A transfusion may be carried out because a patient is extremely anemic, either as a result of disease or from a loss of blood through bleeding. A transfusion may also be considered necessary in the treatment of acute shock. See *also* ANEMIA; SHOCK.

Q: *Can a person's blood be completely replaced by a transfusion?*

A: Yes. This type of transfusion (exchange transfusion) is sometimes necessary in newborn babies or persons suffering from extreme uremic poisoning. See *also* HEMOLYTIC DISEASE OF THE NEWBORN.

Q: *What precautions are taken before transfusing blood?*

A: The blood of the donor must be tested to ensure that the donor is not anemic. In addition, blood is now tested for the presence of infection by viruses. A sample of the donor's blood is mixed (cross-matched) with a sample of the recipient's blood beforehand to make sure that the blood groups are compatible.

See also BLOOD GROUP.

Blood typing. *See* BLOOD GROUP.

Blood vessel is any tube in the body through which blood circulates. This includes arteries, veins, and capillaries.

See also ARTERY; CAPILLARY; VEIN.

Blood, vomiting of. Vomiting of blood, known medically as hematemesis, is a condition that is extremely serious and must be evaluated immediately. Acid in the stomach makes the color of the blood dark, often black. For this reason, this type of vomited blood is sometimes described as "coffee grounds."

Q: *What causes vomiting of blood?*

A: A common cause of vomiting blood is acute gastritis that occurs after excessive alcohol intake, aspirin ingestion, or nonsteroidal anti-inflammatory medication intake.

Vomiting blood can also be caused by a peptic ulcer in the stomach or duodenum or by cancer of the stomach. The vomiting of blood is only rarely associated with hemophilia, leukemia, or other blood disorders. A benign form of hematemesis occurs frequently following a nosebleed.

Q: *What treatment can be given to someone who repeatedly vomits blood?*

A: The person should lie down and be covered with a blanket or coat to treat for shock. Medical assistance should be called immediately.

See also BLOOD DISORDERS; CANCER; GASTRITIS; ULCER, PEPTIC.

Blow-out fracture of orbit. *See* ORBIT, BLOW-OUT FRACTURE.

Blue baby is a baby born with a congenital, or inborn, heart defect or incompletely expanded lungs, which causes a bluish tinge to the skin. Because of the heart defect, some blood bypasses the lungs and thus misses the normal oxygenation process. This phenomenon is known as a "right to left shunt" of blood to the left side of the heart. Thus a mixing occurs of nonoxygenated blood from the right side, or pulmonary circuit, with oxygenated blood. This results in only a partial oxygenation of blood. The left side of the heart then pumps this partially mixed blood to the rest of the body. Any complication in breathing makes the bluish tinge darker. In most cases, blue babies can be treated by surgery.

See also HEART DISEASE, CONGENITAL.

Blurred vision. *See* VISION, BLURRED.

Body odor is the offensive smell caused by the breaking down of stale sweat on the skin. Sweat, especially in the armpits and groin, mixes with dead skin cells and decomposes. The odor produced varies from one person to another and also depends upon diet. Treatment of body odor includes a daily shower or bath and a change of underwear, plus the use of a deodorant or antiperspirant.

See also ANTIPERSPIRANT; DEODORANT.

Body temperature. *See* TEMPERATURE.

Boil, also called furuncle, is an infection of the hair roots or sweat glands caused by the *staphylococcus* bacteria. Boils commonly occur in the armpit, on the back of the neck, in the groin, or on the buttocks, but can also appear elsewhere. A red, painful lump forms, gradually grows bigger, and then breaks down to form pus in the center. The pus normally discharges spontaneously. If a boil does not heal within two weeks or if a series of boils develops, one should seek medical attention. It is possible that some underlying disease is allowing the boils to recur.

See also STAPHYLOCOCCUS.

Boil: treatment. Apply moist heat to encourage the boil to come to a head and drain on its own. Cutting open of the boil frequently spreads the infection. Boils on the nose or face and multiple boils should be treated with antibiotics, depending upon the culture and sensitivity results. Recurrent boils are also treated with antibiotics and may take two to three months to heal. Family and friends who may be the source of reinfection must also be treated.

Bolus (bō′ləs) is (1) a lump of chewed food ready to be swallowed; (2) an oral medicine in a large, soft mass, usually not prepackaged; or (3) an intravenous medication given rapidly over a short period of time.

Development of a boil

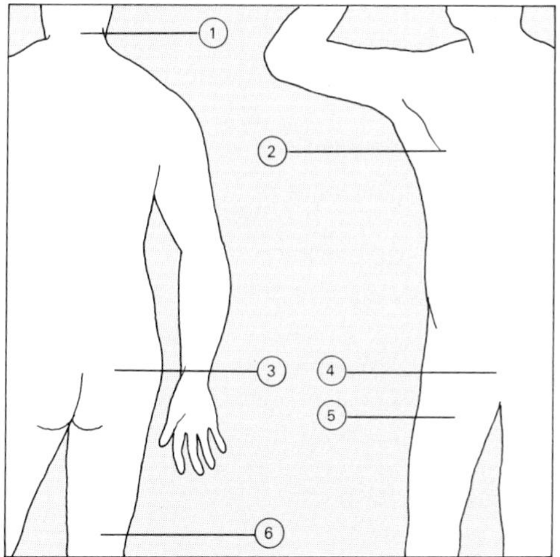

A **boil** occurs more frequently in areas where the skin is constantly rubbed: (1) at the back of the neck; (2) under the arms; (3) on the buttocks; (4) around the groin; (5) at the top of the thigh; and (6) behind the knees. Boils on or in the nose, or in the outer ear, are extremely painful as they develop because the tissues do not stretch easily, and the pressure is localized and intense.

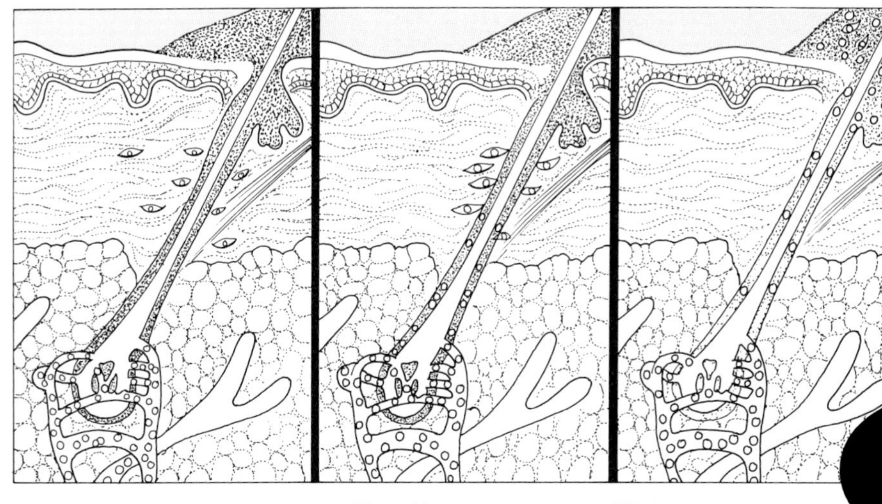

1 First a red swelling forms deep in the hair follicle. The skin around the hair itches.

2 The skin around the hair forms a tight, red lump. The developing boil is extremely painful.

3 Within three days, a yellow head forms. The boil bursts to discharge pus. The pain subsides.

Bone is the hard, rigid tissue that forms the body's skeleton. It supports the body and surrounds and protects its internal structures. Bone is made of tough fibers embedded with calcium-containing salts, which make up 67 percent of its substance. Usually hollow, bone acts as a storage place for calcium and the soft, blood-forming tissue called marrow.

See also BONE DISORDERS.

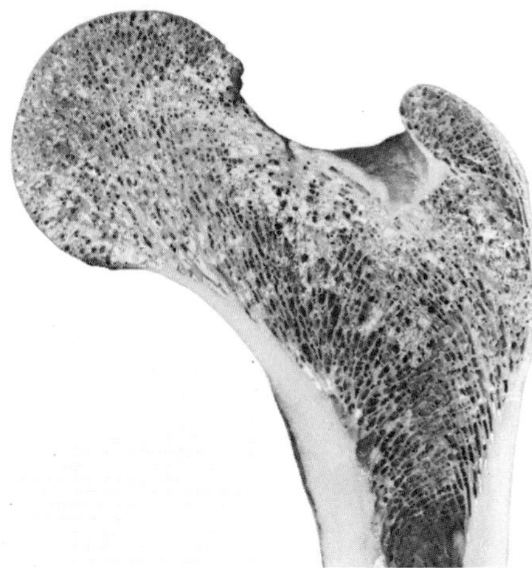

Bone is honeycombed in specific directions for maximum strength, as in the femur pictured here.

Bone disorders. The following table lists disorders that affect bones, grouped according to cause. Each has a separate article in this encyclopedia.

Cause	*Possible disorder*
Bacterial infection	Osteomyelitis (most commonly caused by staphylococcus; may follow dental abscess or trauma in some cases)
Congenital (present at birth)	Achondroplasia (dwarfism caused by lack of growth hormone) Osteogenesis imperfecta (abnormally fragile bones)
Hormone imbalance	Achondroplasia (dwarfism caused by lack of growth hormone)
Inflammation	Osteitis (inflammation of bone)
Physical damage	Fracture Paget's disease of bone (bone deformity of unknown cause)

Cause	*Possible disorder*
Tumor	Osteoma (nonmalignant tumor of bone) Osteosarcoma (malignant tumor of bone)
Vitamin deficiency	Osteomalacia (bone softening in adults due to lack of calcium caused by vitamin D deficiency) rickets (bone softening in children due to lack of calcium caused by vitamin D deficiency)

Bone marrow (mar'ō) is the soft, blood-forming tissue that fills the cavities of bones. It is either yellow, because of fat content, or red, because of developing blood cells.

Bone marrow transplant is the intravenous transfer of bone marrow from a donor to a recipient. The procedure is used on people who suffer from aplastic anemia, a deficiency in red cell production. It is also used to treat immunodeficient patients. There is a particularly high success rate in producing remission in some types of acute leukemia. Complications in bone marrow transplants occur frequently, including rejection of the transplant by the recipient, infection, and hemorrhaging.

See also BONE MARROW; IMMUNODEFICIENCY DISEASE.

Booster shot (büs'tər) is an additional injection given some time after an initial injection to maintain a person's immunity to a disease.

See also IMMUNIZATION.

Boric acid (bôr'ik) is a white crystalline powder that was once commonly used as an antiseptic solution or as an ointment. Large doses taken orally are poisonous and, therefore, use of boric acid has been limited to ophthalmic, or eye, preparations.

Bornholm disease. *See* PLEURODYNIA, EPIDEMIC.

Bottle-feeding. *See* BABY CARE.

Botulism (boch'ə liz əm) is a rare, severe form of food poisoning. It occurs when food that contains a toxin produced by the organism *Clostridium botulinum* is eaten. This organism is usually found in food that is improperly canned or preserved. The toxin attacks the central nervous system. Disturbances in vision and general weakness are the most common initial symptoms. This is followed by paralysis.

Prompt medical treatment is essential, because the disease develops rapidly and has a high mortality rate.

See also FOOD POISONING.

Bowel (bou'əl) is the popular name for intestine.

See also INTESTINE.

Bowel, impacted (bou'əl, im pak'tid). An impacted bowel is excessive accumulation of feces in the rectum. This results in an inability to defecate.

The condition is often caused by a combination of different factors: an improper diet, usually not including enough roughage; inadequate exercise; anxiety; and a habit of irregular bowel movements. Sometimes it is a side effect of pregnancy, a diagnostic procedure, or medication. Other causes might include abdominal muscle weakness, intestinal tumors, or anal lesions. Impacted bowel is common in the elderly.

The specific causes of the impacted bowel must be ascertained, in order to ensure the proper treatment. This might mean dietary changes, to include plenty of fresh fruits and vegetables and liquids; regular exercise, which might include training the abdominal muscles; an attempt to establish a consistent time of day for a bowel movement; reduction of anxiety; and specific medical therapy for the more serious problems causing bowel impaction. Bulk agents and stool softeners are often helpful.

See also CONSTIPATION; DIET.

Bowlegs, or genu varum, are legs that curve outward, so that when the feet are together there is a gap between the knees. Babies often have bowlegs when they begin to walk. The curvature corrects itself gradually, although sometimes overcompensation in the young child produces knock-knees (genu valgum), the inward curving of the legs at the knees, which peaks at three to four years of age.

By the time the child becomes a teenager, the legs are normally straight.

Q: *Can older persons develop bowlegs?*

A: Yes. Legs that become bowed later

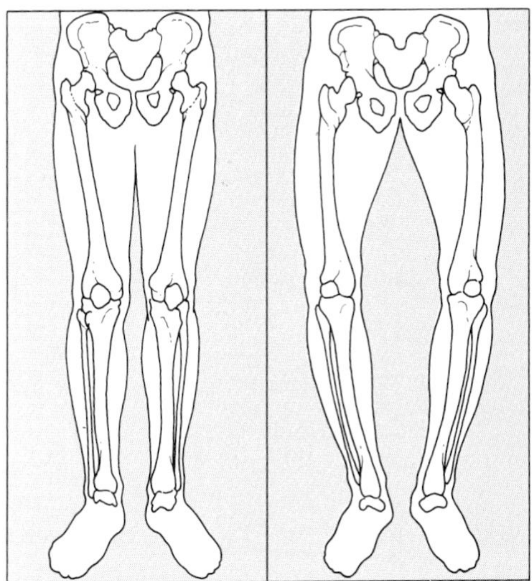

Bowlegs, *right,* curve outward, unlike normal legs, *left.*

in life may be caused by osteomalacia, a softening of the bones (rickets, in children), or by Paget's disease of bone.

See also OSTEOMALACIA; PAGET'S DISEASE OF BONE; RICKETS.

Brace is any device that supports or holds in position a part of the body. The Milwaukee brace, a large trunk brace used to correct scoliosis, is an example. Used in the plural, braces are an appliance for straightening misaligned teeth.

See also SCOLIOSIS.

Brachial plexus (brā'kē əl pleks'əs) is a network of nerves in the neck, extending under the clavicle and into the axilla (armpit). These nerves stimulate and control the muscles and skin of the chest, shoulders, and arms.

Erb's palsy, a paralysis of the brachial plexus, sometimes affects the newborn. It is caused by a sudden traction during childbirth, but is easily cured by splinting and physical therapy. Traction injuries to the brachial plexus can also occur in older persons. Other disorders of the brachial plexus include inflammation and degeneration, such as in toxin exposure or postinfectious polyneuritis.

See also NERVOUS SYSTEM.

Brachium (brā'kē əm) is the part of the upper arm from the shoulder to the elbow. The term is also used to describe arm-like anatomical structures, for example, the brachium conjunctivum, a band of fibers in the brain.

Bradycardia (brad ə kär'dē ə) is a slow pulse rate. A pulse rate below 60 is considered to be bradycardia. Any symptomatic individual with bradycardia should receive an immediate medical evaluation; an underlying heart disorder may be present. As a medical disorder, bradycardia can follow a virus illness, such as influenza or infectious hepatitis. Resting bradycardia occurs in normal healthy individuals, including those who exercise regularly. Bradycardia also occurs with the underactive thyroid disorder, myxedema, and with a heart block. Symptomatic bradycardia, that is, less than 50 beats per minute or with pauses in the beat of 2.5 seconds, often requires the insertion of a pacemaker.

See also MYXEDEMA.

Brain is the master control center of the body. It receives, processes, and stores the information that floods into it from inside and outside the body. It issues "instructions" for body action. It is the seat of human consciousness, intellect, memory, emotions, and personality.

The brain is a delicate structure weighing about 3 pounds (1,380 g) and containing from 10 to 100 billion nerve cells (neurons) and a far greater number of glia (support and disease control cells). Although making up only about 2 percent of the total body weight, the brain uses about 20 percent of the oxygen consumed by the entire body when at rest.

The brain has a triple defense network: the bones of the skull; three covering membranes called meninges; and cerebrospinal fluid (produced in the four brain cavities called ventricles), which forms a thin, cushioning layer between the soft tissues of the brain and the hard bones of the cranium.

The brain works somewhat like both a computer and a chemical factory. Brain cells produce electrical signals and send them from cell to cell along pathways called circuits. As in a computer, these electrical circuits receive, process, store, and retrieve information. Unlike a computer, however, the brain creates its electrical signals by chemical means. The proper functioning of the brain depends on many complicated chemical substances produced by brain cells.

The human brain has three main divisions: (1) the cerebrum, (2) the cerebellum, and (3) the brain stem.

The **brain** has three major divisions—the cerebrum, the cerebellum, and the brain stem. The cerebrum and the cerebellum are both divided into two hemispheres. Each hemisphere of the cerebrum contains four divisions or lobes.

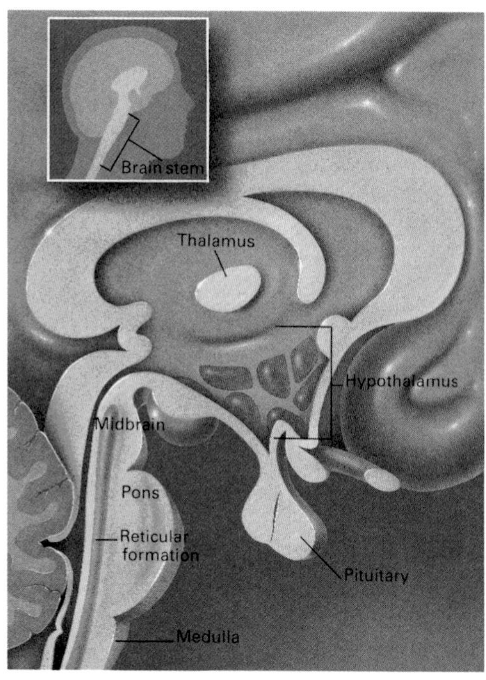

The brain stem is a stalk-like structure that connects the cerebrum with the spinal cord. Various parts of the brain stem control vital body processes such as breathing, heartbeat, eye movements, hunger, thirst, and body temperature.

Information of physical sensation passes to the brain's sensory cortex. The impulses stimulate the reticular activating system in the brainstem, which alerts the whole cortex. The motor cortex then relays information for action along motor nerves.

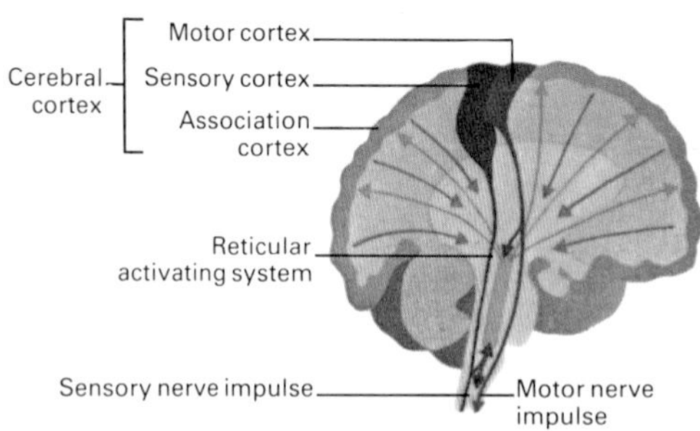

Nerve pathways cross as they pass through the brain stem. These pathways link each side of the cerebrum with the opposite side of the cerebellum. Thus, each cerebral hemisphere controls the opposite side of the body.

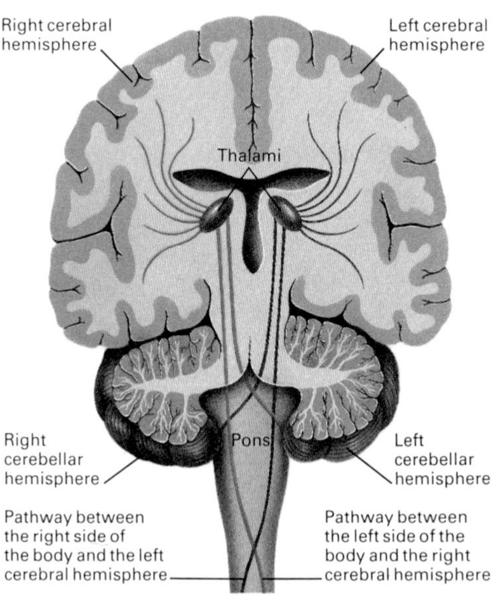

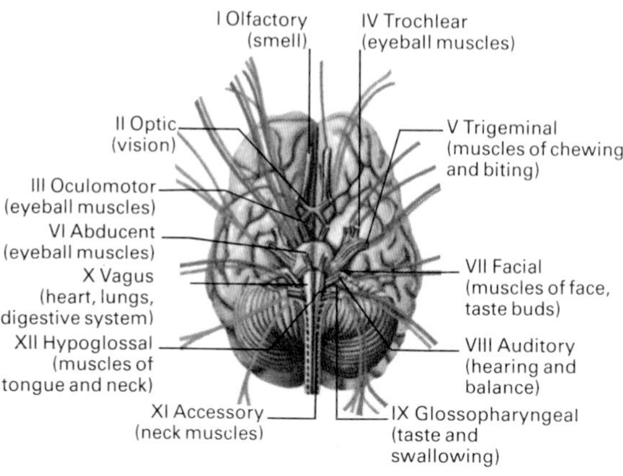

Arising from the underside of the brain are 12 pairs of cranial nerves that receive and relay information to and from many organs. Nerves carrying incoming messages are shown in green; those sending out instructions in orange.

The cerebrum, about 85 percent of the weight of the brain, is covered by a thin layer of nerve cell bodies called the cerebral cortex. This folds in upon itself and so forms a surface with many ridges and grooves, thus increasing the surface area of the cortex. Sensory messages from all over the body are received by the somesthetic cortex. Nerve impulses to control the skeletal muscles are sent out by the motor cortex. The association cortex is, however, the largest portion of the cerebral cortex. It analyzes, processes, and stores all incoming information, making possible our higher mental abilities, such as thinking, speaking, and remembering.

A fissure (large groove) divides the cerebrum into halves called the left cerebral hemisphere and the right cerebral hemisphere. The two parts are connected by bundles of nerve fibers, the largest of which is the corpus callosum. Studies suggest that the left hemisphere largely controls our ability to use language, mathematics, and logic. The right hemisphere is the main center for creative, artistic, or musical ability, the recognition of complicated visual patterns, and the expression of emotion.

Each hemisphere is divided, in turn, into four lobes (regions). The frontal lobe is at the front and regulates body movement and coordination, planning and consciousness, speech, and smell. The temporal lobe is at the lower side and controls hearing and speech. The temporal lobe, the thalamus, and the hypothalamus together form the limbic system, which plays a central role in the production of emotions. The parietal lobe is in the middle and regulates touch interpretation and body position. The occipital lobe is at the rear and governs vision, visual images, and reading. This is only a partial listing of the functions of each lobe.

The cerebellum, located below the back part of the cerebrum and also divided into hemispheres, is mostly responsible for balance, posture, and the coordination of movement. Together with the cerebral cortex, the cerebellum largely regulates voluntary movements. Nerve pathways connect the right half of the cerebellum with the left cerebral hemisphere and the right side of the body. Pathways from the left half connect with the right cerebral hemisphere and the left side of the body.

The brain stem is a stalk-like structure connecting the cerebrum with the spinal cord. Its bottom part is called the medulla oblongata, which controls breathing, heartbeat, the involuntary muscles, blood flow, and many other vital body processes. The major sensory and motor pathways between the body and the cerebrum cross over as they pass through the medulla. Each cerebral hemisphere thus controls the opposite side of the body.

Just above the medulla is the pons, nerve fibers, which connect the hemispheres of the cerebellum and link the cerebellum with the cerebrum. Above the pons the midbrain helps control movements of the eyes and the size of the pupils.

At the upper end of the brain stem are the thalamus and the hypothalamus. The right and left halves of the thalamus act as the central exchange for nerve impulses between the body and the cortex and between the parts of the brain. The hypothalamus regulates body temperature, hunger, thirst, and other internal conditions. It also controls the activity of the nearby pituitary gland, the master gland of the body, which regulates the body's rate of growth, its sexual and reproductive processes, and other functions.

Deep within the brain stem lies a network of nerve fibers called the reticular activating system, which helps regulate the brain's level of awareness. Sensory messages that pass through the brain stem stimulate the reticular activating system, which in turn stimulates activity and alertness throughout the cerebral cortex.

See also BRAIN DISORDERS; NEURON.

Brain disorders. The following table lists some disorders that affect the brain and basic characteristics of each condition. Each has a separate article in this encyclopedia.

Disorder	*Basic characteristic*
Abscess	Collection of pus in brain tissue
Alzheimer's disease	Premature aging of brain cells, appearing in middle age onward
Anoxia	Oxygen starvation to the brain during childbirth
Blood clot (extracerebral)	Subdural or epidural hematoma pressing on brain
Cerebral Hemorrhage	Rupture of blood vessel in brain
Coma	Prolonged unconsciousness
Concussion	Temporary unconsciousness following a blow to the head
Down's syndrome	Mental retardation that also produces Mongolian-like features
Encephalitis	Inflammation of the brain

Disorder	*Basic characteristic*
Epilepsy	Convulsions with or without loss of consciousness
Glioma	Malignant tumor of the brain
Hydrocephalus	Abnormal accumulation of cerebrospinal fluid within the skull, causing possible retardation
Meningioma	Tumor of the brain
Meningitis	Inflammation of the membranes that surround the brain
Multiple sclerosis	Destruction of material coating the nerves; poor muscle movement and coordination
Rubella (in pregnancy)	Possible mental retardation of the newborn
Schizophrenia	A disorder in the neurotransmitters of the brain resulting in psychosis
Spina bifida	Incomplete development of the spine protecting the spinal cord
Stroke	Rupture of blood vessel in brain or blockage of blood vessel to brain
Syphilis (final stage of infection)	Paralysis; loss of sense of position and balance
Vitamin B deficiency	Temporary degeneration

Brain stem (brān′stem) is the base of the human brain lying beneath the cerebrum and the cerebellum. It connects the spinal cord with the forebrain and controls reflex, motor, and sensory functions.

See *also* BRAIN.

Braxton Hicks contraction (brak′stən hiks), commonly known as false labor, is an irregular tightening of the uterus after the third month of pregnancy. Not experienced by all pregnant women, the contractions are painless, even though they may increase in duration and intensity throughout the pregnancy. Near childbirth they are sometimes difficult to distinguish from true labor.

See *also* LABOR PAIN, FALSE.

Breakbone fever. See DENGUE.

Breast is the front of the chest. The same term is used in the plural to describe the mammary glands in women. Breast development is one of the secondary sexual characteristics that distinguish women from men. The function of breasts is to produce milk after childbirth to feed the baby. Each breast in an adult female contains 15 to 20 milk glands or lobes, surrounded by fatty tissue, each of which contains a duct ending in a lactiferous sinus, that leads to the nipple. Breasts develop in girls at the onset of puberty in response to hormones produced by the ovaries and the pituitary gland. See *also* ADOLESCENCE.

Q: *Is it normal for one breast to be slightly larger than the other?*

A: Yes. The difference is partly caused by a variation in the size of the underlying muscles that supply the shoulder. The muscles tend to be larger on the dominant side (for example, the right side of a right-handed person).

Q: *When do the breasts produce milk?*

A: Milk production is a response to special hormones that are produced at the end of pregnancy. The start of milk production in the breasts coincides with the birth of the baby. Early milk is a thin, yellow fluid (colostrum) that differs in composition from normal breast milk that is secreted later. Production of milk not during pregnancy (galactorrhea) is sometimes caused by a tumor of the pituitary gland. Treatment consists of surgical removal of the tumor. See *also* PREGNANCY AND CHILDBIRTH.

Q: *Do males ever grow female-type breasts?*

A: Such a condition (gynecomastia) may occur in adolescent boys. A boy should be reassured that the condition will last only for 6 to 12 months. In an adult male, hormone imbalance or disease may cause female characteristics. See *also* GYNECOMASTIA.

Q: *Is it natural for the breasts at times to feel different and change in size?*

A: Such changes accompany different stages of the menstrual cycle. Before menstruation, the breasts may feel "tight" and congested; some pain may be experienced, often accompanied by a tingling sensation in the nipples. These changes settle down as soon as the menstrual period begins. However, changes in the breasts, such as thickening and lumps, may mean breast cancer and need to be reported to a physician immediately. Regular, monthly self-examination of the breast can detect cancer early.

See also BREAST EXAMINATION.

Q: ***Why do some women have bigger breasts than others?***

A: Differences in breast size and shape are largely due to inherited factors. Being overweight increases the size of the breasts with extra fatty tissue.

Q: ***In addition to breast self-examination, what other procedures can be done to detect breast cancer?***

A: Mammography of the breasts at age 35 and annually after age 40 is recommended by the American Cancer Society.

Breastbone. *See* STERNUM.

Breast disorders are disorders that can affect the female breast. It should be noted that most lumps in the breast are benign (noncancerous) and respond rapidly to treatment. Usually benign breast cysts can be aspirated, or drained, using a needle and syringe by a physician in his or her office. If a woman develops a lump, however, she should contact her physician as soon as possible. Hormonal changes caused by the menstrual cycle or the taking of birth control pills may cause breast pain or tenderness.

The following table lists some disorders and the basic characteristics of each condition. Each disorder also has a separate article in this encyclopedia.

See also CONTRACEPTION; PALPATION.

Disorder	*Basic characteristic*
Adenoma	Nonmalignant fibrous growth
Cancer (of breast)	Malignant tumor
Cyst, sebaceous	Nonmalignant growth of fatty tissue
Mastitis	Inflammation
Paget's disease of the nipple	Inflammation of areola and nipple

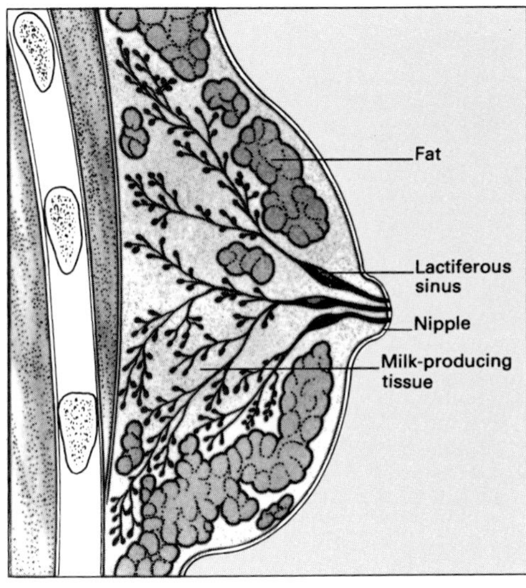

Breast disorders can affect any part of the milk-producing tissue and related breast structure.

Breast examination is self-examination of a woman's breasts, to detect any unusual lumps or other changes that might indicate cancer. The earlier the detection of cancer, the more likely a cure. For breast examination techniques, *see* illustrations on page 134.

The self-examination should be carried out each month, a few days after menstruation, when the breasts are stimulated by the least amount of estrogen. It is important to examine the breasts at the same time each month, because a woman's cycle produces natural changes in the breast tissues that may be confusing. A woman who detects a lump should see her physician immediately. It must be remembered, however, that the majority of breast lumps are not caused by cancer. There are many other reasons for breast lumps; and they all need evaluation by a physician.

See also BREAST LUMP.

Breast-feeding. *See* BABY CARE.

Breast lump is a change in the density of an area of the breast. This may be caused by an infection, a cyst, or a tissue growth. An infection can be easily treated with antibiotics. A cyst can form from stimulation of estrogen. The cyst can be drained with a needle or may clear up on its own.

One in nine American women will develop breast cancer. Women of all ages should examine their breasts monthly. Mammograms or X ray examination is also recommended for all women over 35 years of age. For lumps

Steps for breast examination

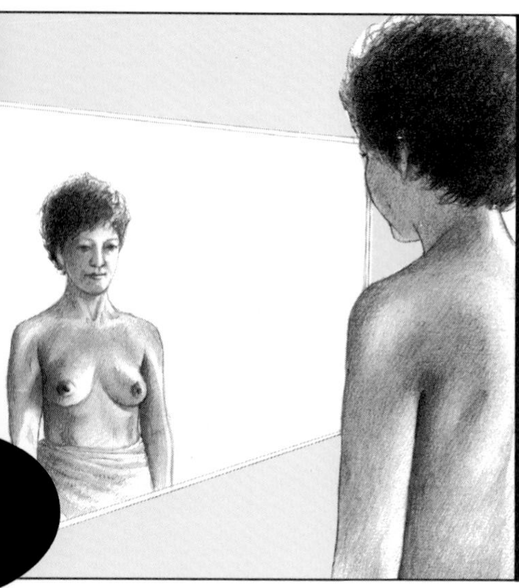
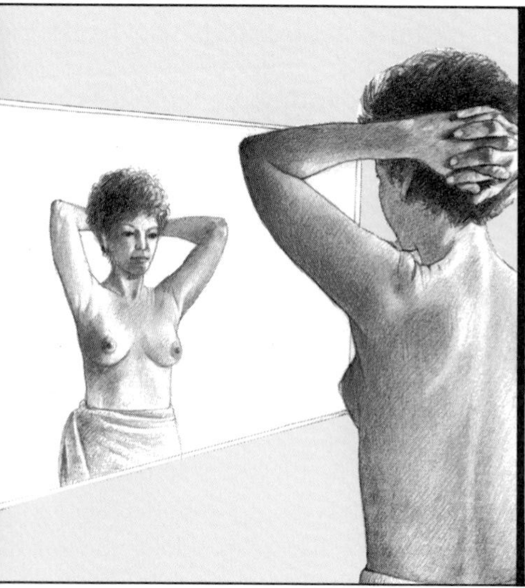
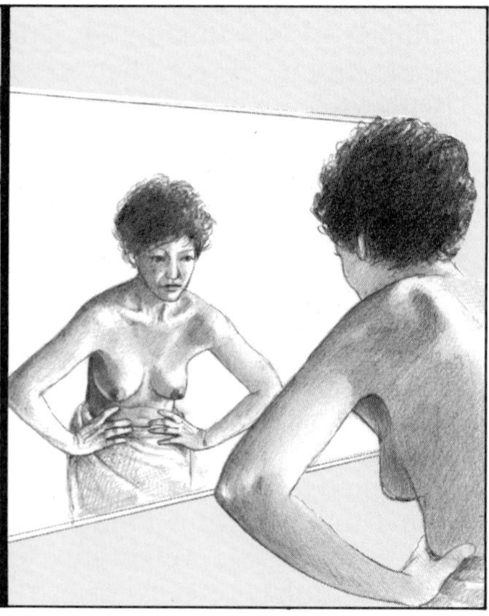

1 While standing in front of a mirror, look carefully to check your breasts for changes in appearance, including the scaling or puckering of skin or a discharge from the nipples.

2 While still in front of a mirror, place your hands behind your head and press forward. Look in the mirror to note any changes in the normal shape of your breasts.

3 Put your hands on your hips and bend toward the mirror. Pull your shoulders and elbows forward. Again, look in the mirror to note any changes in the normal shape of your breasts.

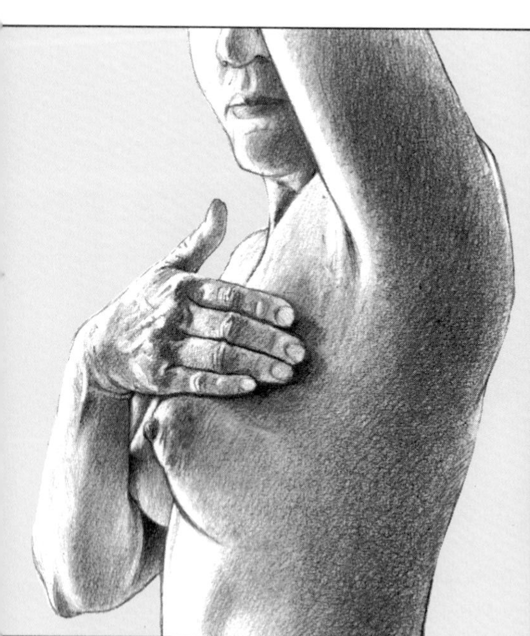
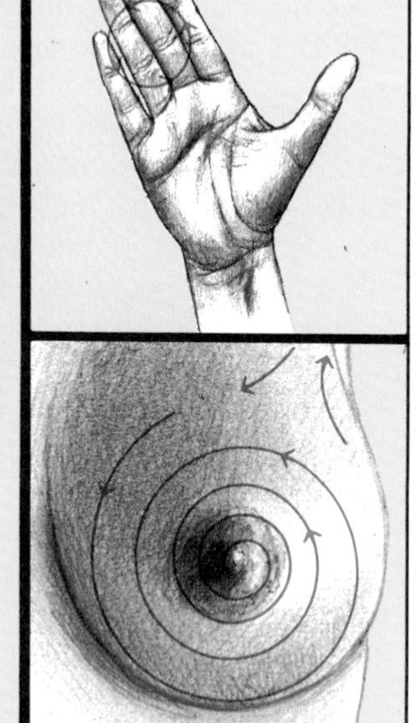
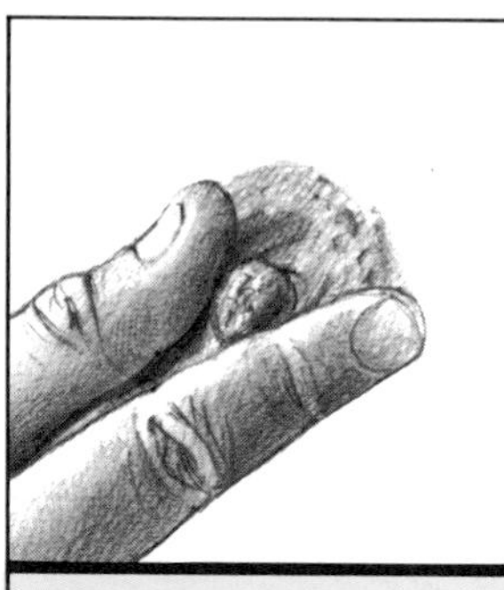

5 Squeeze your nipple gently, *left.* Note any discharge. Then repeat steps 4 and 5 on your right breast.

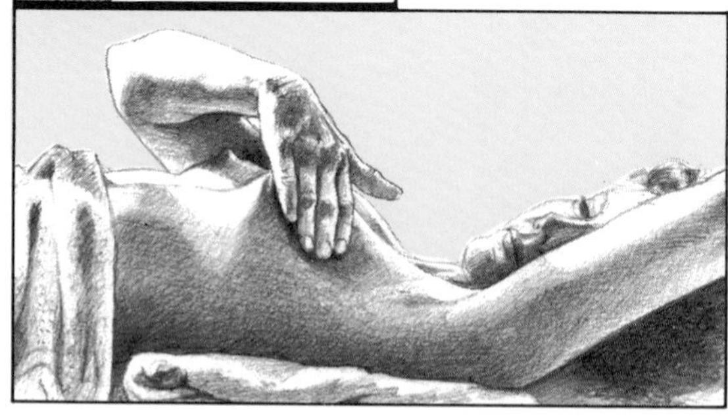

4 With your left arm raised, firmly examine your left breast using three or four fingers of your right hand. Begin at the outer edge of your breast and press the flat part of your fingers, *top right,* in small circular movements around the breast moving gradually toward the nipple, *bottom right.* Check the entire breast in this manner, paying particular attention to the area between the breast and the armpit, including the armpit itself. Note any unusual lump under the skin, especially if it was not noticed in an earlier exam.

6 Now lie on your back and raise your left arm over your head. Place a pillow or folded towel under your left shoulder. This position, with breast slightly flattened, makes examination easier. Repeat steps 4 and 5 using the circular motions described in step 4. Then repeat on your right breast.

which may be cancerous, a biopsy is recommended. Early detection of cancer improves the opportunity for cure.

See also BREAST; BREAST EXAMINATION; CANCER PREVENTION; CYST: BREAST; MAMMOGRAPHY; THERMOGRAM; ULTRASOUND.

Breast pump is a small suction device that helps draw milk from a nursing mother's breast. It may be made of plastic or glass and operated by hand or by electricity. A mother may need to use a breast pump if a distended breast causes pain or if a baby has a cleft palate or is premature and, therefore, unable to suck efficiently. A working mother may wish to use a breast pump to express and store milk while she's at work. This milk can be fed to the baby while the mother's away.

Breathalyzer (breth'ə li zər) is an apparatus that is used to analyze exhaled air. The best known breathalyzer is the one used by civil authorities to ascertain whether or not the alcohol content of a motorist's blood is within the legal maximum. One simple type of breathalyzer is a tube containing bichromate crystals that change color when alcohol-rich air is blown through them. A more complicated type analyzes exhaled air electronically.

Breath, bad. See BAD BREATH.

Breath-holding attack occurs when a child stops breathing during a period of severe crying or in anger. Such attacks occur most commonly in children between the ages of one and four years. An attack is preceded by a cry or wail, after which the breath may be held for as long as 20 to 30 seconds. The child may turn blue in the face and fall to the ground as if unconscious, making occasional convulsive movements. After recovery, the child may be confused for 10 to 15 seconds.

Q: *Is a breath-holding attack serious?*

A: Although these attacks are frightening to witness, they are not serious. However, a physician should be consulted to rule out any other cause of unconsciousness.

See also TEMPER TANTRUM.

Breathing. See RESPIRATION.

Breathing disorders. See LUNG DISORDERS.

Breathing stoppage: first aid. See ARTIFICIAL RESPIRATION.

Breathlessness, known medically as dyspnea, is a normal reaction to greater than usual exertion, such as vigorous physical exercise. The normal result of physical exercise is an increase in the amount of carbon dioxide in the blood. Breathing rate automatically increases to get rid of the carbon dioxide through the lungs.

A wide range of lung disorders can also be responsible for breathlessness, such as asthma or pneumonia.

Persons with heart disorders often have difficulty with breathing. A moderate degree of anemia also causes shortness of breath after exercise.

Breech birth (brēch) is the delivery of a baby, buttocks, knees, or feet first, rather than head first. This position can be dangerous for the baby, so a Cesarean section may have to be performed.

See also PREGNANCY AND CHILDBIRTH; CESAREAN SECTION.

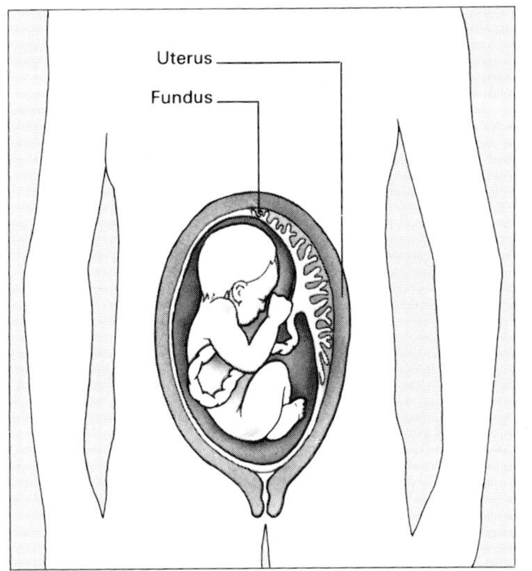

Breech birth occurs when labor begins with the baby in a position other than head first.

Bridge is (1) a band of protoplasm connecting adjacent elements of a cell in plants and animals; (2) the upper, bony part of the nose; or (3) a partial denture, which is false teeth in a mounting attached to real teeth.

Briquet's syndrome. See SOMATIZATION DISORDER.

Broken tooth: treatment. See TOOTH, BROKEN: TREATMENT.

Bromide (brō'mīd) is a compound of bromine and another element, usually potassium bromide. It calms nervousness and causes sleep by depressing the nervous system. It was once widely used as a sedative. Because bromide may produce serious mental disturbances as side effects, a condition known as "bromism," it is rarely used for that purpose anymore.

Bronchial dilator (brong'kē əl dī lā'tər), also called bronchodilator, is a drug that widens the airways to the lungs. It enlarges the bronchi and, therefore, improves the breathing of patients with bronchial asthma and other chronic chest disorders, such as emphysema and bronchitis. Depending on the specific preparation, a bronchial dilator may also increase the blood pressure and heart rate and stimulate the respiratory center in the brain. It may also cause anxiety and muscle tremors.

Bronchial pneumonia. *See* BRONCHOPNEUMONIA.

Bronchiectasis (brong kē ek'tə sis) is a chronic disorder of the bronchi and bronchioles, the tubes that carry air in and out of the lungs. The tubes become weakened and stretched and do not allow normal drainage of fluid secretions from the lungs. This inelasticity of the bronchi may result from a recurrent infection, tuberculosis, cystic fibrosis, aspiration of a foreign body (such as a peanut or a button), an obstructive tumor, collapse of the lung (atelectasis), or an abnormality present at birth.

Q: *What are the symptoms of bronchiectasis?*

A: Bronchiectasis may show few symptoms. Sometimes the patient has a cough with thick phlegm, which occasionally contains blood. There may be a slight fever and a general feeling of being unwell.

Q: *How is bronchiectasis treated?*

A: A physician may prescribe antibiotic drugs to prevent complications at the beginning of any respiratory infection for a patient with a history of bronchiectasis. It is important also to drain the secretions from the lung, and for this reason the patient is taught correct breathing and how to use postural drainage. If repeated infections still occur, the physician may rarely recommend a lobectomy, an operation to remove the diseased area.

See also BRONCHIOLE; BRONCHUS; LOBECTOMY; POSTURAL DRAINAGE.

Bronchiole (brong'kē ōl) is any of the many narrow branches of the bronchi, the tubes that carry air to and from the lungs.

See also BRONCHUS; LUNG.

Bronchiolitis (brong kē ō lī'tis) is an acute viral infection of the bronchioles, the small bronchial tubes in the lower respiratory tract. Affecting primarily infants under 18 months of age, it starts typically as the common cold and proceeds through wheezing and coughing to a high fever and very shallow respiration.

Antibiotics and other drugs are not routinely used. Rather, humidity and oxygen are administered via a Croupette® or vaporizer; fluids are provided intravenously; and the airways are regularly suctioned to remove secretions. Without complications bronchiolitis clears up in seven to ten days.

Bronchitis (brong kī'tis) is an inflammation of the bronchi, the air passages to the lungs. It may be either acute or chronic. Bronchitis often follows a common cold or any infection of the nose and throat.

Q: *What are the symptoms of acute bronchitis?*

A: There is a slight fever, 100-102°F (37.8 to 38.9°C), with an irritating, dry, painful cough that starts to produce thick, yellow sputum after two or three days. At this stage the fever often recedes, and the pain from coughing diminishes. Even after the condition improves, a slight cough commonly remains for another week or two.

Q: *What is the treatment for acute bronchitis?*

A: The patient needs bed rest in a warm, humid room, with frequent steam inhalations from a vaporizer to soften the infected mucus in the bronchi. Hot drinks should be given; they help the patient cough up and spit out phlegm, and they prevent dehydration. Any sedative cough medicine may be taken at night to help the patient sleep. A cough syrup, with an expectorant, may help during the day.

If the condition appears to worsen and the fever increases, a physician should be consulted. An antibiotic may be needed to combat the infection.

Q: *How soon after an attack of acute bronchitis may a person return to work?*

A: All crowded places should be avoided for at least 10 days to allow the mucosal lining of the bronchi to heal before taking the increased risk of encountering new infection.

Q: *What causes chronic bronchitis?*

A: Chronic bronchitis is caused by repeated attacks of acute bronchitis. It is aggravated by smoking and by harmful environmental conditions, such as air polluted by chemicals, smoke, and dust.

Q: *What are the symptoms of chronic bronchitis?*

A: The major symptom is a cough which is usually worse in the mornings, when the bronchi have not drained overnight. The patient produces clear, mucous sputum. The sputum becomes thicker and yellow if any additional infection occurs.

The constant, vigorous coughing may break the fine tissues of the lungs and produce a condition called emphysema. A patient with emphysema tires quickly and becomes breathless after exercise. Heart failure may occur. *See also* EMPHYSEMA; HEART FAILURE.

Asthma, obesity, and smoking all complicate and worsen chronic bronchitis. When these conditions are treated as well, the bronchitis usually also improves.

Q: *Can chronic bronchitis be treated?*

A: A close watch is kept on any colds or respiratory infections. The physician usually prescribes antibiotics at the first sign of a bronchitic attack to prevent the possibility of secondary bacterial infection and further damage to the bronchi and lungs. Breathing exercises, and sometimes postural drainage, can help to keep the bronchi clear. The physician will also recommend stopping smoking and, if possible, a change of working conditions.

See also POSTURAL DRAINAGE.

Bronchogram (brong'kō gram) is an X-ray picture that shows the structure of the lungs. It is taken after a dye, which is opaque to X rays, has been introduced into the lining of the windpipe (trachea), from where it spreads downward to the lungs.

See also LUNG.

Bronchopneumonia (brong kō nü mōn'yə), also called bronchial pneumonia, is a contagious infection of the lungs. This type of pneumonia is localized, mainly in the smaller branches of the bronchial tubes, called bronchioles.

Bronchopneumonia can be caused by pneumococci, certain other bacteria, or by viruses. The bronchioles become inflamed as they clog with pus and mucus, resulting in one or more of the following symptoms: coughing, chest pains, fever, blood-streaked sputum, chills, distended abdomen, and difficulty in breathing.

Treatment is with antibiotic drugs and bed rest. Hospitalization for diagnostic tests may be necessary for some patients.

See also PNEUMONIA.

Bronchoscopy (brong kos'kə pē) is an examination of the trachea (windpipe) and the lungs. The trachea is examined prior to the removal of objects that have been accidentally inhaled, such as peanuts, or before a tracheal specimen is taken for a culture or biopsy.

A bronchoscope is the instrument used in a bronchoscopy. There are two types of bronchoscopes in use today. The first type consists of a long, inflexible tube with a light at one end; the second and newer type utilizes fiberoptic technology.

See also FIBEROPTICS.

Bronchus (brong'kəs) is either of two tubes that carry air in and out of the lungs. The bronchi branch out from the lower end of the windpipe (trachea) and separate, with one going to each lung. They are kept permanently open by rings of cartilage and are lined with special hair-like cells that sweep dust and mucus upward toward the throat. The bronchi themselves divide further into narrower branches and finally into the extremely narrow bronchioles.

See also BRONCHIOLE.

Brucellosis (brü sə lō'sis) is an infectious disease, principally of cattle, goats, pigs, dogs, and occasionally of humans. It is caused by bacteria of the genus *Brucella*, which are found in the milk of infected animals. Human beings contract the disease by consuming infected milk or meat, especially from cattle, or by handling diseased animals. In humans, brucellosis is more commonly known as undulant fever or Malta fever.

See also INFECTIOUS DISEASE.

Bruise is a visible, purplish mark beneath the surface of the skin. It is caused by the escape of blood from small blood vessels. Most bruises result from a blow or from pressure, but sometimes a bruise occurs spontaneously in elderly people. The color of the bruise fades away gradually, becoming purplish-blue, brownish, and then yellow, before disappearing.

Bruises may be slightly painful, but they are not usually serious. But a bruise that appears with no apparent cause may be a sign of a disorder such as leukemia or hemophilia. A bruise near a bone that appears some days after an injury may indicate a fracture and requires immediate medical attention.

See also HEMOPHILIA; LEUKEMIA.

Bruise: treatment. Bruising is a minor form of internal bleeding. It is commonly caused by a sharp blow or knock that is painful when it happens, but can also occur after a blow that, at the time, went unnoticed. Bruising is also common around the sites of other injuries. Before treating bruising, check for other injuries such as a fracture.

Bruising that occurs apparently spontaneously can be a sign of several different conditions. Consult a physician immediately.

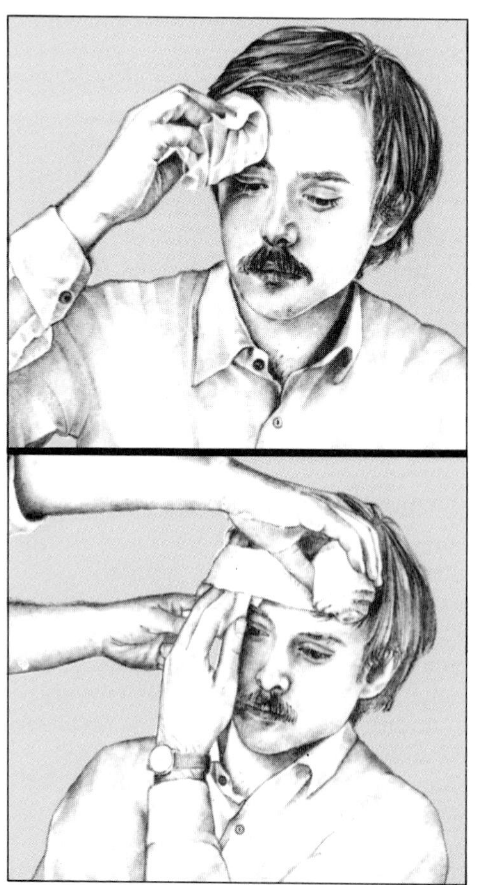

Treatment for a bruise: rest a bruise as much as possible. This may be difficult on the face or at a joint, but immobility allows the blood to clot more rapidly. This in turn prevents further bleeding beneath the skin. To discourage swelling, apply an ice pack or a cold compress to the bruised area.

When the bruised area is already swollen, a bandage should be applied to hold an ice pack or cold compress on the bruise. Replace the ice pack or cold compress as often as necessary. The cold also helps to numb the pain.

Most bruises are not at all serious; if the victim is in good health, generally, there should be no cause for alarm. The bruise should eventually disappear of its own accord. All bruises are individual; there is no set healing time, although the process of healing can be gauged, to some extent, by the coloration.

Usually, bruises are red at first before turning blue, then brown, and finally yellow, as the blood is gradually reabsorbed. But bruises may not proceed through the whole sequence; they may start half-way through, especially around the face. Blood blisters are another form of bruising. They display the same sequence of coloration, generally more vividly. *See also* BLISTER, BLOOD.

Bruising that occurs some days after an injury near a bone may indicate a fracture. A physician should be consulted if this is a possibility, because if a broken bone is left untreated, it may cause severe complications in the future. *See also* FRACTURE.

Bruising in the abdominal region may be a sign of internal injury.

A black eye is another form of a severe bruise. Usually, it is the result of a blow just above the eye or between the eyes. But a black eye following an injury to the eye itself should always be checked by a physician, because it may be a sign that there is some damage to the structure of the eye. A black eye following an apparently unrelated head injury is a possible indication of a fractured skull.

Persons with such blood disorders as hemophilia bruise easily, sometimes without apparent cause. *See also* HEMOPHILIA.

Bruising in persons taking anticoagulant drugs may be a sign that the dosage has been set too high and should be regulated lower by the prescribing physician. *See also* ANTICOAGULANT.

Bruxism (bruk'siz əm) is the habitual grinding of teeth. It probably functions as a release of tension, both during the waking hours in times of stress and, as is more usual, during sleep. In either case the habit is largely unconscious and compulsive. Wearing an occlusive dental bit at night may be helpful in many cases.

Bubo (byü'bō)is a swollen lymph node (a junction of the vessels of the lymphatic system), often containing pus. Buboes most commonly occur in the groin or armpit. They can accompany infectious disease (for example, bubonic plague) and often develop in conjunction with venereal diseases.

See also BUBONIC PLAGUE; LYMPH NODE; SEXUALLY TRANSMITTED DISEASE.

Bubonic plague (byü bon'ik) is a form of plague in which the lymph nodes become painful, tender, and swollen, forming buboes. Early symptoms are a high fever, rapid pulse, low blood pressure, restlessness, and mental confusion. These are followed by coma and death unless promptly treated.

See also BUBO; PLAGUE.

Budd-Chiari syndrome (bud'ke ar'ē) is a blockage in the veins that carry blood from the liver. It is perhaps caused by clotting disorders, thrombosis, trauma, or the presence of cancer cells. The condition greatly enlarges the liver, which becomes tender, and causes hypertension (high blood pressure) in the other veins to the liver. The condition also triggers a build-up of fluid in the abdominal cavity (ascites).

See also ASCITES.

Buerger's disease (ber'gərz), known medically as *thromboangiitis obliterans*, is a rare condition, characterized by inflammation of the arteries and veins of the arms and legs. It is more common in men especially those who smoke. The symptoms vary in intensity. Commonly the disease produces tender, swollen areas over the inflamed veins, followed by coldness of the feet and hands. Pain occurs in the calves during walking (intermittent claudication), due to arterial blockage. The poor circulation may result in gangrene.

Q: *What is the treatment for Buerger's disease?*

A: The patient, if a smoker, stops smoking; this often produces an immediate improvement. Medications and/or surgery are sometimes beneficial.

See also CLAUDICATION, INTERMITTENT; GANGRENE.

Bulbar paralysis (bul'bər pə ral'ə sis) is paralysis of the muscles of the tongue, lips, palate, and throat. The cause is generally a degeneration of the nerve nuclei in the brainstem, usually occurring over age 50 or in conjunction with amyotrophic lateral sclerosis or multiple sclerosis. The patient has difficulty swallowing and speaking and may inhale saliva and food.

See also AMYOTROPHIC LATERAL SCLEROSIS; MULTIPLE SCLEROSIS.

Bulimia (byü lim' ē ə) is an eating disorder characterized by binge eating of high calorie foods, often followed by purging with a laxative or self-induced vomiting. Binge eating is usually followed by depressive moods and self-deprecating thoughts. Bulimia may be associated with another eating disorder, anorexia nervosa, in which individuals attempt to severely restrict their food intake in order to lower their weight to dangerously low levels. The binging and purging of bulimia is, as in anorexia nervosa, a way to fulfill their occasional urge to eat and still maintain their weight. Bulimia, which is rarely seen in males, usually begins in late adolescence and is often associated with an attempt to lose weight. At first, bulimics learn that binging/purging is a useful method of maintaining weight. At some point, however, they lose control of the ability to stop binging.

Some researchers believe the disorder may develop through excessive parental pressure and standards. Bulimics tend to be perfectionists with high standards and poor self-esteem. It has been found that some bulimics display brain chemistry characteristics of certain forms of depression. *See also* ANOREXIA NERVOSA; DEPRESSION.

Bulimics often develop hernias, ulcers, a dependence on laxatives or diuretics, and damage to tooth enamel from the acid in the digestive fluids of the vomit. Repeated vomiting may result in a ruptured esophagus, and the victim may bleed to death before help arrives. The violent purging may also upset the body's electrolytes, which can cause heart failure in extreme cases.

Q: *Can bulimia be detected in its early stages?*

A: Usually not. The bulimic typically hides the overeating and purging pattern, sometimes for years.

Q: *How is bulimia treated?*

A: Bulimia is usually treated on an outpatient basis, often combining individual and family therapy. Some bulimics respond to antidepressant drug therapy. In recent years, support groups have formed to help bulimics and their families understand and cope with the disorder. *See also* ANTIDEPRESSANT.

Bulla (bůl′ə) is a medical term that may describe one of three things: a large fluid-filled vesicle, a blister, or a space within an organ, such as a lung.

See also VESICLE.

Bunion (bun′yən) is a painfully enlarged condition of the joint of the big toe, which causes a bony bump to develop on the inside edge of the foot and the toe to turn in toward the other toes (hallux valgus). This protrusion rubs the inside of the shoe and causes a callus or even bursitis in the joint. The condition is aggravated by pointed shoes and/or high heels. Therefore, it is much more common in women. It also has a tendency to run in families. Loose, comfortable shoes should be worn, but padding the joint should be avoided, because it increases the pressure on the joint. In severe cases, the malformation can be surgically corrected.

See also BURSITIS; CALLUS; HALLUX VALGUS.

Bunion: treatment. *See* CORNS AND BUNIONS: TREATMENT.

Burn is an area of tissue damage, caused by heat (including friction and electricity), by cold, by a caustic chemical, or by radiation. Burns are classified according to the depth of the tissue damage.

First-degree burns produce a redness of the skin, like a sunburn, and they heal without scarring.

Second-degree burns cause the destruction of deeper structures within the skin, resulting in blistering.

Third-degree burns destroy the full thickness of the skin, leaving an open area. The deeper tissues (fat or muscle) are also destroyed.

First- and second-degree burns tend to be more painful than third-degree burns, because the nerve endings are damaged but not completely destroyed. Extensive third-degree burns are a life-threatening emergency. Large areas of burned skin cause the loss of the body fluid of the surrounding tissues, which can lead to dehydration and the rapid onset of shock, particularly in children. For this reason, intravenous rehydration may be necessary, as well as local treatment and painkilling drugs. Third-degree burns require a skin graft to prevent disfiguring scars. Recent developments in artificial skin hold great promise for burn victims.

See also BURNS AND SCALDS: FIRST AID.

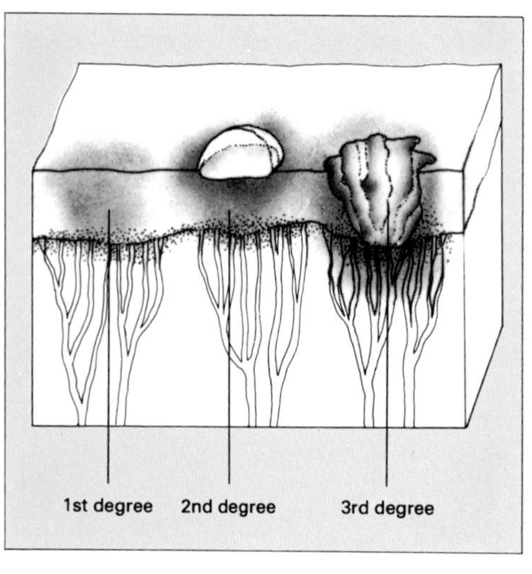

A **burn** can be of three types: 1st degree reddens the skin, *left;* 2nd degree blisters the skin, *center;* or 3rd degree destroys the skin, *right.*

Burnout is the loss of mental and physical energy following a period of prolonged job-related stress. It is sometimes characterized by physical illness and the extinction of motivation or incentive. In extreme cases there may also be suicidal tendencies.

Several factors combine to cause this condition. These factors include the following: frustration over the gap between job expectations and actual job performance; long working hours and job-related anxiety during nonworking hours; pressure from superiors; low pay; unsafe work situations; and lack of emotional support from co-workers and family.

A period of rest and psychological counseling is usually sufficient to deal with burnout. The pinpointing of the precise causes at the workplace, however, is also necessary. If their elimination is not possible, then learning to deal in a nonstressful way with the job situation becomes essential. The individual must learn to balance life priorities in order to prevent recurrences of burnout. Appropriate time and energy must be allocated to other areas of life including: (1) relationships with family, friends, and others; (2) recreation and humor; (3) physical exercise; (4) rest and relaxation; (5) intellectual and emotional growth; and (6) spiritual growth. If burnout still recurs, a job or career change should be considered as a possible alternative.

Burns and scalds: first aid. Burns are caused by contact with dry heat. Scalds result from contact with moist heat. The effects of burns and scalds are similar. See illustrations on page 142.

In first-degree burns, the damage is limited to the outer layer of the skin, resulting in redness, warmth, an occasional blister, and tenderness. Mild sunburn is an example of a first-degree burn. In second-degree burns, the injury goes through the outer layer and involves the deeper layers of skin, causing blisters. In third-degree burns, the full thickness of skin is destroyed and a charred layer of seared tissue is exposed. The seriousness of a burn depends on the amount of skin burned, the location of the burn, and the depth of the burn.

The aims of first aid are to remove the victim from any smoke or fumes; to reduce the effect of heat on the skin; to relieve pain; to prevent fluid loss; to prevent infection; to treat for shock; and to summon emergency medical aid. Correct first aid is essential for rapid recovery.

If the victim's clothing is on fire, push the victim to the ground and move him or her away from the flames immediately. When smothering the clothing, do not use highly flammable material such as nylon. If necessary, roll the victim over to smother burning clothing. If the victim's clothing has not caught on fire, but is smoldering, remove it at once and extinguish the smoldering.

Do not remove burned clothing once the flames have been extinguished. The burned clothing helps to protect against infection and prevents fluid loss. Also, the burned clothing may adhere to the wound. Its removal is painful and requires expert medical supervision.

If the victim's clothing is saturated with hot liquid, remove the clothes quickly but carefully.

For small burns, ice or cold water will stop further tissue damage and lessen pain. Oral pain medications should also be given.

For large burns, the victim will be in a state of shock. Immediate medical attention is vital for the recovery of the burn victim.

See also SHOCK.

Burping. *See* BABY CARE.

Bursa (bėr'sə) is a small, sac-like structure, found mainly in joints, that protects bones and tendons from friction (for example, in the elbows and knees). Bursae are filled with a thick, compressible fluid.

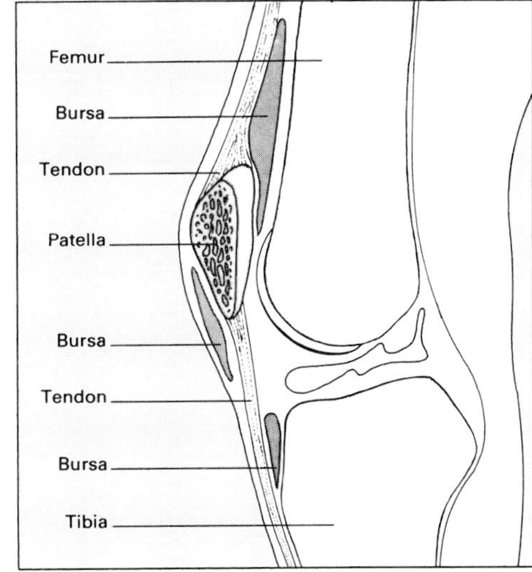

A **bursa** is a fluid-filled sac that protects bones and tendons from friction.

Bursitis (bər sī'tis) is inflammation of a bursa. In most cases the cause is unknown, but it can be caused by such factors as injury, infection, and repeated friction. It is treated by rest; use of cold, followed by heat; anti-inflammatory drugs; and sometimes an injection of a corticosteroid drug.

See also BURSA.

Bursitis, prepatellar (bər sī'tis, prē pə tel'ər). Prepatellar bursitis, commonly called housemaid's knee, is an inflammation of the bursa in front of the kneecap.

See also BURSITIS.

Buttock (but'ək). Buttocks are composed of fat and gluteal muscles, which form the two fleshy hind parts of the body where the legs join the back.

Byssinosis (bis ə nō'sis) also called cotton workers' disease, brown lung, or Monday fever, is an allergic reaction to cotton dust. The symptoms are coughing, breathlessness, and constriction in the chest. Symptoms initially occur only on the first working day of each week (hence "Monday fever"). Later, symptoms occur throughout the week, and eventually there is lung scarring and pneumoconiosis.

See also PNEUMOCONIOSIS.

First aid for burns and scalds

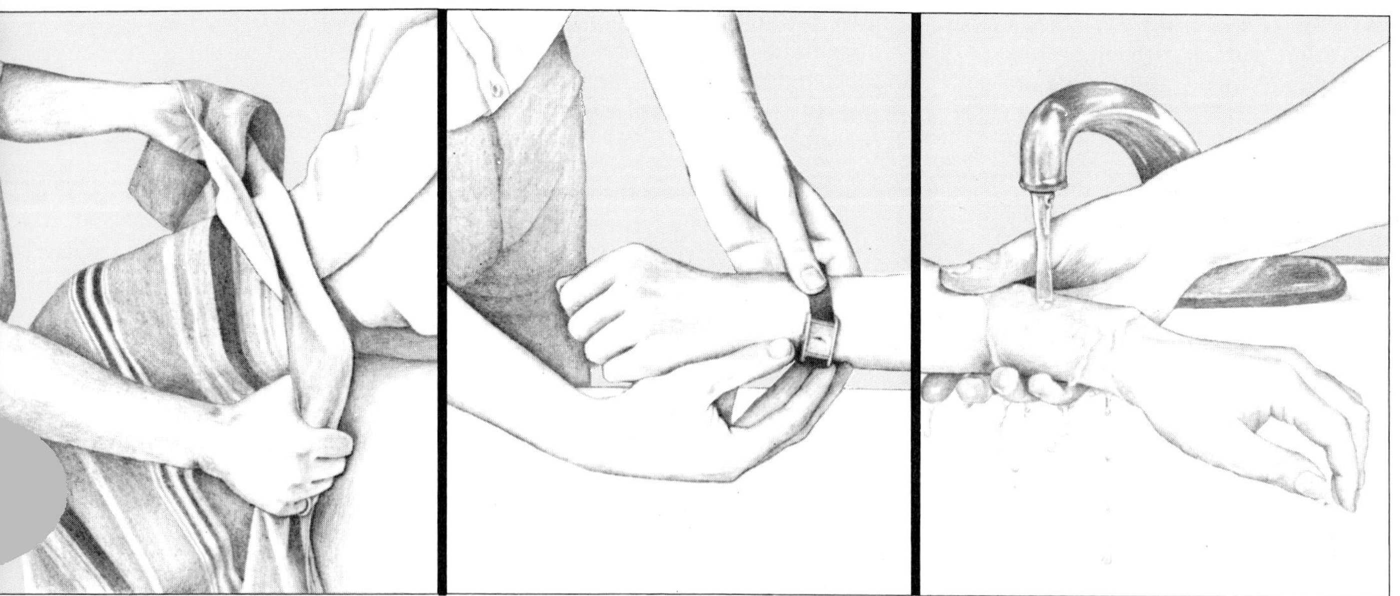

1 If the victim's clothing is on fire, push the victim to the ground. Use a large piece of nonflammable material, such as a blanket, rug, or coat, to smother the flames.

2 If possible, remove any restrictive items, such as rings, bracelets, belts, and shoes. The burned area may swell later, making it impossible to remove such items.

3 For first-degree burns, keep the burned area under running cold water for at least ten minutes or until the pain has subsided. *Do not* immerse second degree or third-degree burns in water.

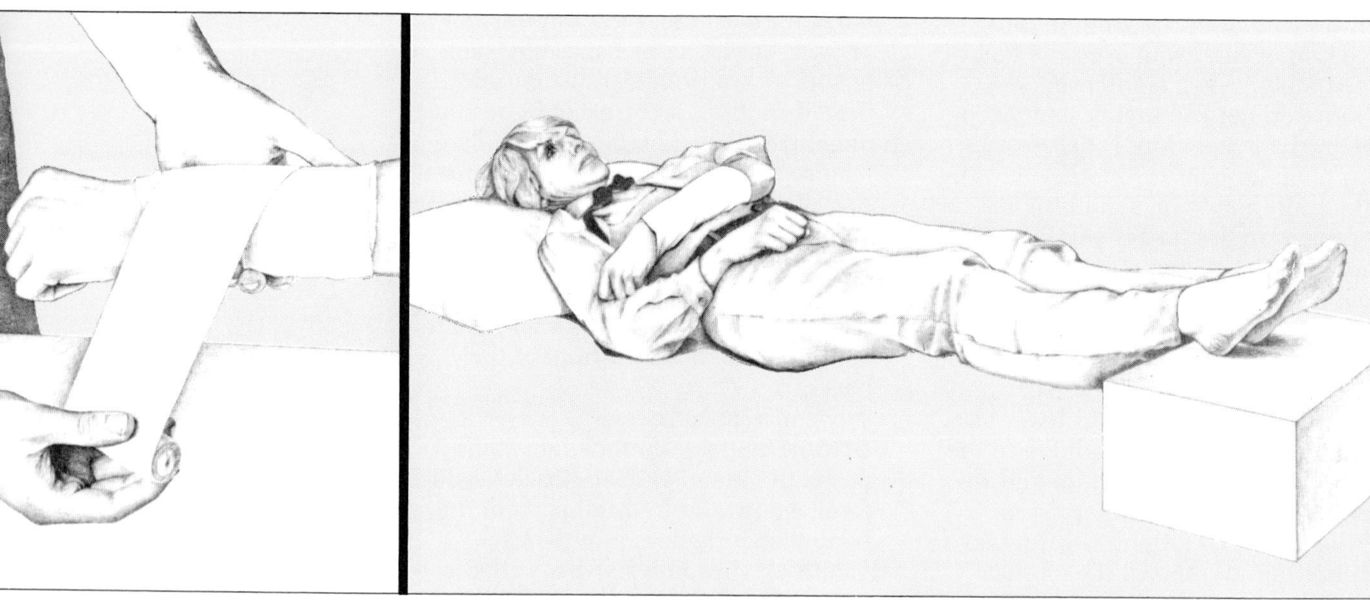

4 Cover the burned area with a sterile dressing. If none is available, use a clean dry sheet. The burned area should be touched as little as possible. *Do not* apply any lotions or ointments.

5 If the victim is conscious, administer small, cold drinks at frequent intervals. *Do not* give alcohol. If unconscious, the victim should be placed in such a position as to maintain a clear airway. If possible, raise the burned area and the victim's legs above the level of the head to reduce the effects of shock. Summon emergency medical aid.

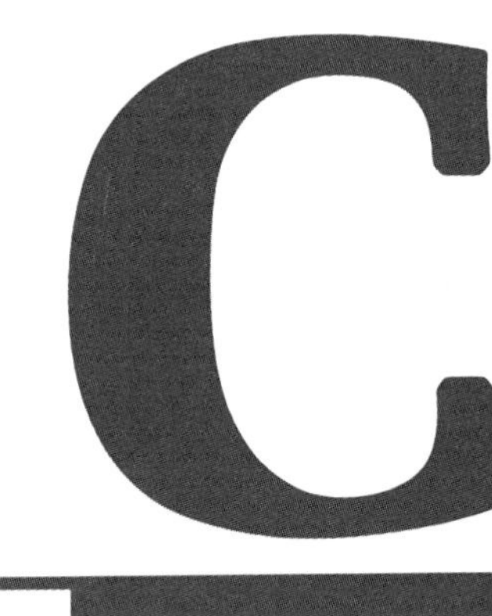

CABG. *See* CORONARY ARTERY BY-PASS SURGERY.

Cadmium (kad′mē əm) is a metallic element. Both the metal and its compounds are poisonous. They are widely used in industry, for example, in batteries, electroplating, welding, photography, and ceramics. If cadmium salts are swallowed, violent diarrhea and vomiting result. More serious poisoning results from prolonged breathing of cadmium oxide fumes, which may cause a cough, pains in the chest, and general weakness. Emphysema may result, causing further difficulty in breathing; it may be fatal if not treated swiftly.

Caesarean section. *See* CESAREAN SECTION.

Caffeine (kaf′ēn) is a stimulant alkaloid drug, present in coffee, tea, and some carbonated drinks. Caffeine stimulates the central nervous system and the production of urine from the kidneys. It also increases the pulse rate. A large cup of strong, freshly ground coffee contains about 100 milligrams of caffeine. Excessive intake of caffeine may lead to insomnia, a rapid or variable pulse rate, and a feeling of anxiety and apprehension. Following prolonged caffeine ingestion, a sharp reduction in caffeine intake may on rare occasions produce acute withdrawal symptoms, such as headache, sweating, tremor, and an inability to concentrate. Caffeine has been linked to birth defects in laboratory animals, so many physicians advise pregnant women to avoid excessive caffeine consumption.

Caisson disease. *See* BENDS.

Calamine lotion (kal′ə mīn) is a liquid preparation containing zinc oxide. It has a soothing effect when applied to inflamed or irritated skin. It is useful to counteract itching of the skin, such as that encountered with chickenpox.

Calcaneus (kal kā′nē əs) is the heel bone.

See also HEEL.

Calciferol (kal sif′ə rōl) is a fat-soluble substance from the vitamin D family, which is found in milk and fish-liver oils. It is used as a dietary supplement in the treatment of disorders associated with low calcium levels in the body, such as rickets.

See also RICKETS.

Calcification (kal sə fə kā′shən) is the accumulation of calcium salts in body tissues. The vast majority of calcium entering the body is deposited in bones and teeth; a tiny percentage remains in body fluids such as the blood. The temporary build-up of calcium-containing tissue at the site of a bone fracture (callus) helps in the healing process. An abnormal calcium build-up in the arteries, lungs, kidneys, or other tissues may interfere with the organ's function and cause serious problems.

See also CALLUS.

Calcium (kal′sē əm) is an alkaline metallic element whose compounds occur widely in the body, primarily in bones. Calcium ions are essential for good health; the body requires calcium for muscle contraction, nerve impulse transmission, blood coagulation, and other functions. Insufficient calcium in the body can lead to such bone disorders as rickets. An abnormally high build-up of calcium can lead to muscle weakness and eventually to coma.

Infants need about 0.6 grams of calcium daily; small children require about 0.8 grams; adults need between 0.8 and 1.3 grams; men require 0.8 grams; young women require 1.2 grams; and women past menopause require 1.5 grams. Pregnant women and nursing mothers should increase their daily intake by about 0.5 grams. Calcium intake is supplied through a well-balanced diet, and its absorption is controlled through vitamin D. Foods rich in calcium include milk, yogurt, cheese, and other dairy products.

Calcium channel blocker (nifedipine, diltiazem, and verapamil) belongs to a class of drugs that inhibits the entry of calcium ions into vascular and heart muscle cells. This action decreases muscular contraction strength (especially spasms of arteries), making these drugs useful in the treatment of migraine, high blood pressure, and angina due to coronary artery spasms. A similar action on heart conduction cells slows electrical conduction in the heart; therefore, they are useful in the treatment of certain cardiac arrhythmias.

See also ANGINA PECTORIS; HYPERTENSION; MIGRAINE.

Calculus (kal′kyə ləs) is a stone-like mass that may form in ducts or hollow organs of the body, especially the gall bladder, kidneys, and ureters.

Calculi are composed mainly of crystalline substances: certain salts, cholesterol, and some protein. Because of their hardness, calculi can obstruct a duct or an organ, resulting in inflammation through infection.

Q: *Why do calculi form?*

A: Calculus formation may be due to a combination of factors, rather than to any one factor. Such factors include local infection, high levels of calcium or other salts in the blood, some conditions that cause a reduction in the flow of bodily fluids, and a genetic predisposition.

Q: *What symptoms might indicate that calculi have formed?*

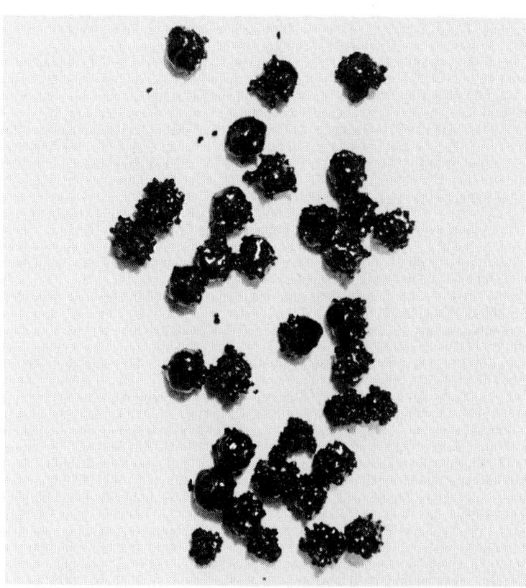

Calculus is a "stone," such as these gallstones, that forms in hollow organs of the body, often causing obstruction.

A: Symptoms depend upon the part of the body involved. For example, calculi in the gall bladder may either cause no symptoms or may cause vomiting, jaundice, and severe pain if they lodge in and obstruct the bile duct. The only way to determine if calculi have formed is to conduct tests, such as X rays or ultrasound examination, on parts of the body suspected to be involved. *See also* COLIC; CYSTOSCOPY; GALLSTONE.

Q: *How are calculi treated?*

A: Treatment depends upon the site of the calculi and on the severity of the symptoms. For many cases, surgical removal of calculi is necessary. However, a recent innovation, extracorporeal shock wave lithotripsy, offers a nonsurgical approach to the removal of kidney and gall bladder stones. With the patient seated in a large tub of water, shock waves are focused on the stone until it crumbles (usually in about 45 minutes) and can be passed out of the body. Recovery with this approach takes days, instead of the weeks required following surgery. And, since lithotripsy does not damage the kidney, it can be repeated if kidney stones recur. *See also* LITHOTOMY; LITHOTRIPSY.

Caldwell-Luc operation (kald′wel-lük′) is an operation to relieve chronic sinusitis by improving the drainage of the maxillary sinus, one of the cavities behind the nose. To improve drainage, a new opening is made through the upper jaw above one of the second molar teeth. This allows drainage of fluid from the sinus into the mouth. Once the sinus has drained, the opening is allowed to heal. The operation is named after American physician George Caldwell and French laryngologist Henry Luc.

See also SINUSITIS.

Calf (caf) is the thick, fleshy part of the back of the leg below the knee. The calf is formed by the gastrocnemius and soleus muscles.

See also MUSCLE.

Caliper (kal′ə pər) is an instrument used to measure the diameter or thickness of a solid or a convex body, such as the triceps skin fold of the arm, which is measured to evaluate obesity.

Callus (kal'əs) is an area of skin that has become thickened and coarsened as a result of constant rubbing or pressure. The term callus also describes the temporary bone-like tissue that forms between the broken ends of a bone fracture as a normal part of the healing process

See also CALCIFICATION.

Calorie (kal'ər ē) is a unit of heat energy. In dietetics and medicine, calories are a measure of the energy value of food. Different foods yield various calorie levels when eaten and digested. For example, an ounce (28 grams) of sugar will produce about 100 calories. The average calorie expenditure of a normally active 150-pound (67.5-kilogram) man is about 2,700 calories a day, but individual calorie requirements vary according to age, sex, build, level of activity, and metabolic rate. If a person takes in more calories than he or she needs, a weight gain results.

See also METABOLISM.

Canal is a tube or a duct in an animal or plant that carries liquid, air, food, or other solid matter from one part or organ to another. The alimentary canal is an example.

Canaliculus (kan ə lik'yə ləs) is a small canal or duct in the body.

See also CANAL.

Canalis (ka nā'lis) is the Latin word for canal and is still sometimes used in medical terminology. For example, the Latin medical term for alimentary canal is *canalis alimentarius.*

See also CANAL.

Cancer (kan'sər) is a disease in which certain body cells multiply without apparent control, destroying healthy tissue and organs and endangering life. The disease is a leading cause of death in many countries. In North America only diseases of the heart and blood vessels kill more people. Cancer occurs in most species of animals and in many kinds of plants as well as in human beings.

Cancer strikes people of all ages but especially middle-aged persons and the elderly. It occurs about equally among people of both sexes and can attack any part of the body. The parts most often affected are the skin, the digestive organs, the lungs, and the female breasts.

Without proper treatment, most kinds of cancer are fatal. In the past, the methods of treatment gave patients little hope for recovery, but the methods of diagnosing and treating the disease have improved greatly since the 1950's. Today, about one-third of all persons treated for cancer recover completely or live much longer than they would have lived without treatment. Much research remains to be done to find methods of preventing and curing the disease. To help further this research, many countries have anticancer programs.

There are more than 100 identifiable forms of cancer. Although lung cancer is the most deadly form (accounting for about 30 percent of total cancer deaths annually; *see* table below), cancer can attack virtually any part of the body with devastating results.

There are three main classifications of cancer: carcinoma, which is cancer of the epithelial tissue that forms the skin and the linings of the internal organs; sarcoma, which is cancer of connective tissue, such as cartilage, muscle, or bone; and fluid cancer, such as

The following statistics are listed according to types of cancer and the percentage of distribution among men and women who have cancer.

Incidence of cancer in men		*Incidence of cancer in women*		*Incidence of deaths from cancer among men*		*Incidence of deaths from cancer among women*	
lung	20%	breast	29%	lung	34%	lung	21%
prostate	20%	colorectal	15%	colorectal	11%	breast	18%
colorectal	15%	lung	11%	prostate	11%	colorectal	13%
urinary	10%	uterus	9%	leukemia & lymphomas	8%	leukemia & lymphomas	7%
leukemia & lymphomas	7%	leukemia & lymphomas	6%	urinary	5%	ovary	5%
oral	4%	ovary	4%	oral	2%	uterus	4%
all other sites	24%	all other sites	26%	all other sites	29%	all other sites	32%

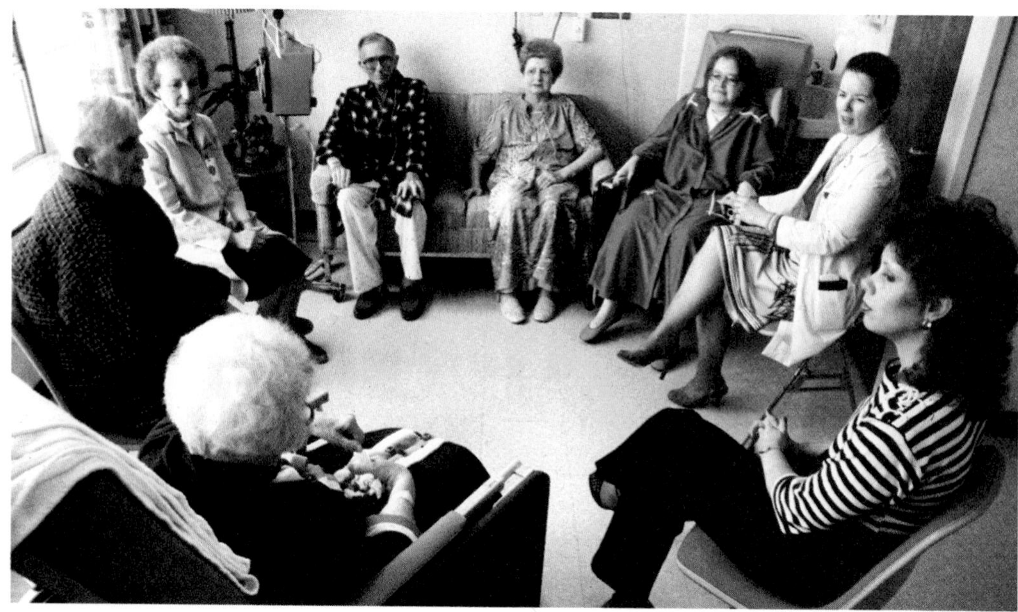

Cancer counseling sessions help individuals cope with the trauma of their disease.

leukemia or lymphoma, which affects the blood stream and the lymph system. Some experts prefer to include sarcoma in the third category, because blood and lymph are forms of connective tissue.

Some Common Types of Cancer

Bladder Cancer is the most common malignancy of the urinary tract. An early symptom may be a small amount of blood in the urine (microhematuria), although this is more often associated with conditions of the kidneys. A more common sign of bladder cancer is gross hematuria, where the urine becomes red.

About 70 percent of those who get bladder cancer are men, many of whom are between the ages of 50 and 70. If the malignancy has developed in the bladder wall itself, it spreads rapidly to underlying muscles and is very difficult to treat. However, if the cancer has not spread before treatment is initiated, the recovery rate is about 70 percent. Recurrence of bladder cancer is relatively common.

Papillary cancer of the bladder is a very common form of the disease. It does not grow into the bladder wall itself; rather, it is attached to it by a kind of stem. As such, it is easily removed by a surgical procedure.

Bone Cancer is relatively rare and usually affects persons under the age of 20. The most common symptom is pain, especially at night. Because children often experience pain due to falls and rough play, it is easy to dismiss this early symptom. Any child whose pain persists for more than a week should be taken to a doctor. Other danger signals to look for include prominent veins, unusually warm skin over the bone, and swelling. An X ray can often detect the presence of bone cancer, and a biopsy will confirm any suspicious findings.

Chemotherapy is usually used to treat bone cancer, sometimes in combination with surgery and radiation. In some cases the diseased portion of the bone can be removed surgically and replaced with a metal prosthesis. This is then followed by chemotherapy.

Unfortunately, by the time the symptoms are recognized, the cancer is usually well advanced and the fatality rate is therefore high.

Brain Cancer can strike persons of any age, but its most frequent victims tend to be younger adults. Symptoms include headaches, blurred vision, nausea, difficulty in walking, and personality changes. Loss of vision in the eye on the side of the tumor may also occur.

Because the brain is tightly confined within the skull and plays such a vital role in the management of the entire body, any tumor, even a benign one, is considered dangerous. The usual treatment is surgery, often followed by radiation or chemotherapy. If a tumor is inoperable, radiation therapy is usually applied. The development of sophisticated scanning techniques has made it possible to locate and evaluate brain tumors much more precisely than in the past. As a result, the chances of successful treatment have been greatly enhanced.

Breast Cancer is the most prevalant form of cancer among women, afflicting about 130,000 women annually in recent years. Factors that increase the risk of acquiring breast cancer include a family history of the disease, a high-fat diet, early menstruation, late menopause, and a first childbirth after the age of 40. Women who have had cystic breast disease or malignancies in other parts of the body also run a somewhat higher risk of getting the disease.

Breast cancer is most likely to strike women between the ages of 35 and 55, to about the age of 65. In rare instances, men also develop breast cancer.

As with other types of cancer, the most important factor in successful treatment is early detection. All women should examine their breasts monthly and see a doctor about every two years. Women over the age of 40 should have periodic mammograms (breast X rays) and see their physician for a breast examination annually. *See also* BREAST EXAMINATION; MAMMOGRAM.

Possible indications of breast cancer include a lump in the breast, a change in its shape or contour, swelling, thickening, pore enlargement, retraction or scaliness of the nipple, nipple discharge, pain, or tenderness.

Any suspicions of breast cancer should be confirmed by a mammogram. It will not only detect lumps, but help determine whether a lump is cancerous. For accuracy in certain diagnoses, however, a biopsy must be performed. In this procedure, the lump and some of the tissue surrounding it are removed surgically and examined for cancer. In some cases it may be possible to perform a needle biopsy, in which a hollow needle is inserted into the lump, in order to withdraw some of the fluid for analysis.

Treatment of a cancerous breast will vary according to the nature and extent of the cancer, the opinion of the doctor or doctors, and the wishes of the patient. In some cases the breast is removed completely, along with surrounding tissues and underlying muscles. This is called a radical mastectomy, and for many years it was the only treatment available. Now, in some cases in which the cancer is fairly small and localized, it is possible to remove only the lump and some of the surrounding tissue. This procedure is sometimes called a "lumpectomy." It is followed then by radiation or chemotherapy, possibly both.

Nearly 70 percent of all female breast cancer patients recover and remain free of the disease 5 years or longer after treatment.

Cervical Cancer involves the cervix, the neck-like, narrow opening at the base of the uterus. There are no symptoms in the earliest stages, but cancer can be detected by a Pap smear. This is a simple diagnostic test in which scrapings from the surface of the cervix are analyzed for cancer. Visible symptoms of the disease can include vaginal discharge, irregular bleeding, and spotting after intercourse or douching.

Factors often identified as increasing the risk of cervical cancer include obesity, early sexual activity, multiple sexual partners, and a history of viral genital infections. All women who are sexually active or over the age of 20, should have a pelvic examination once a year, especially if any of the risk factors are applicable.

If the cervical cancer has not spread, the cancerous area can be removed surgically and followed up with radiation or chemotherapy. Cancers that involve a large part of the cervix or that have spread into the uterus may require a hysterectomy.

Colorectal Cancer is cancer of the large intestine (colon). In the Western world this is one of the more common types of cancer. Its incidence rises with age, beginning around 40 and reaching a peak between 60 and 75. Men and women are affected about equally.

Adenocarcinoma affects the sigmoid colon or the rectum, sections nearest the external opening at the anus. Three-fourths of all colorectal cancers are of this variety.

Symptoms of colorectal cancer vary, depending on the site of the growth in the colon or rectum. Generally, there is a change in bowel habits, such as constipation, diarrhea, or episodes of both, and occasionally nausea or anemia. Stools may become either flattened or

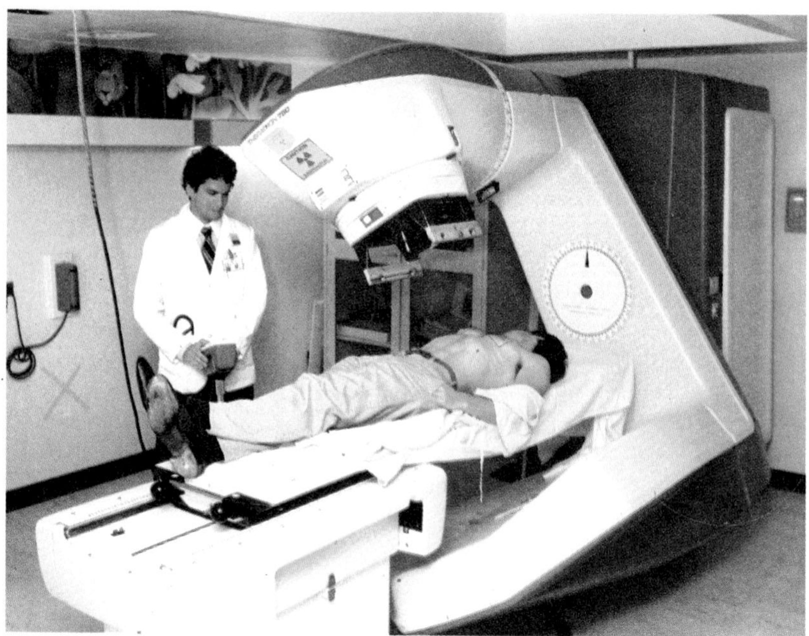

Cancer can be treated with radiation therapy using cobalt 60, which kills cancer cells.

pencil-shaped, and they may contain blood, visible or not. Because colorectal cancer is slow-growing, physical symptoms may not appear for quite some time. The best prospect for an early diagnosis lies in regular physical examinations that include stool testing for blood and a proctoscopic examination.

Like most cancers, a specific cause can not be demonstrated. However, world-wide studies have shown that populations with a high incidence of colorectal cancer eat less fiber and more animal protein, fats, and refined carbohydrates than less susceptible populations. The exact role a refined diet plays in allowing cancer to grow has not yet been established.

Treatment usually involves a wide surgical removal of the colon (colectomy) and if possible the rejoining of the cut ends. If the growth is near the end of the colon or rectum, a colostomy may be necessary. Sometimes, if there is indication that the cancer may have spread, the regional lymph nodes are also removed. Radiation, chemotherapy, or immunotherapy may be used during certain stages of cancer.

The survival rate 5 years after surgery for patients with colorectal cancer is about 50 percent, the chances increasing the earlier the detection is made.

Leukemia, sometimes called blood cancer, is a disease of the bone marrow, where blood cells are produced. It is characterized by an increase in abnormal, immature leukocytes (white blood cells), which then interfere with the production and function of normal white blood cells, needed by the body to fight infections.

Leukemia is the most prevalent type of cancer in children, though the incidence of the disease in adults is far higher, roughly 8 to 1. Males are twice as likely to get the disease. The mortality rate is about 30 percent.

Symptoms include fatigue, blood in the stool, bleeding gums, frequent infections and bruises, enlarged spleen and lymph nodes, pain in the bones or joints, and weight loss.

Leukemia may be diagnosed by examining blood smears under a microscope, but confirmation requires an examination of the bone marrow. The marrow sample is obtained by inserting a needle into the hip bone or sternum of the patient, while using a local anesthetic.

People who suffer from certain kinds of chronic leukemia are able to live for years with little or no therapy. Acute leukemia, on the other hand, requires aggressive chemotherapy. With the development of several new and highly effective anticancer drugs, the recovery rate among acute leukemia patients has greatly improved in recent years. This is particularly true of children suffering from lymphocytic leukemia, a type of blood cancer affecting primarily lymphocytes, cells vital to the functioning of the body's immune system.

Lung Cancer is the leading form of cancer among men in the United States and is on the rise among women. In 1986 there were about 150,000 new cases of the disease diagnosed in the United States and approximately 120,000 deaths attributed to it.

Those at greatest risk are smokers, and the risk increases with the number of cigarettes smoked. Among men who smoke more than two packs of cigarettes a day, the death rate from cancer of the lung is roughly 15 to 20 times higher than among men who do not smoke. Other factors influencing risk include the number of years of smoking, the age at which smoking commenced, and how deeply the smoker inhales.

One of the most common symptoms of lung cancer is a persistent cough. Other symptoms include chest pain, shortness of breath, and blood coughed up from the lungs (hemoptysis).

Surgery is the usual treatment for lung cancer, but only half the cases are operable at the time of diagnosis. This may involve the removal of a cancerous tumor or an entire lobe of the lung. Because many cases of lung cancer are not diagnosed until they are fairly well advanced, radiation and chemotherapy are also often necessary.

Prostate Gland Cancer involves the large gland surrounding the male urethra just below the bladder, affecting about 96,000 men annually. The typical patient is about 73 years of age at the time of diagnosis. However, because the disease progresses very slowly, a significant percentage of men have it without knowing it. For this reason all men over 40 should have a proctoscopic examination once a year.

Only when the disease is well advanced do symptoms occur. One of the main symptoms is difficulty in urination, resulting from an enlarged prostate, normally about the size of a chestnut, which then obstructs the flow of urine. There may be a need to urinate frequently, particularly at night. Urination may be accompanied by a painful or burning sensation. Blood may appear in the urine, and urination may be difficult to start and stop.

These symptoms occur more frequently with a benign enlargement of the prostate, called benign prostatic hypertrophy (BPH).

Advances in prostatic surgery and radiotherapy have greatly reduced the incidence of impotence in the treatment of this disease. A form of hormone therapy called LH-RH has none of the side effects of conventional estrogen therapy.

The survival rate for prostate gland cancer patients is under 70 percent.

Skin Cancer is the most common form of cancer in the United States and, fortunately, the most treatable, having less than a two percent mortality rate. About 400,000 cases are reported annually, frequently occurring in patients with other forms of cancer. For these reasons the disease is not included in tabulating new cases of cancer, which amount to over 900,000 annually.

A common cause of skin cancer is excessive exposure to the sun, the most frequent victims being people with fair skin. Many of them live in the southern and southwestern states, where the sun is strong and the skin is frequently exposed to it. Skin sensitivity to the sun may also be increased by antibiotics, certain drugs, and birth control pills.

Symptoms of skin cancer may include any change in the appearance of the skin, such as a wound that does not heal, or any sudden change in a birthmark, mole, or wart. Any mole that bleeds, enlarges, itches, shows up after age 30, or becomes tender should be examined by a doctor immediately. Special precautions with moles are extremely important because they are often starting points for malignant melanoma, a deadly form of skin cancer that can spread to other parts of the body.

Most forms of skin cancer can be cured with surgery or with topical anticancer drugs.

Stomach Cancer, on a steady decline in North America and western Europe, occurs in about 2 or 3 percent of all cancer cases, accounting for about 24,600 new cases each year. Stomach cancer is more likely to affect men than women; incidence peaks between the ages of 50 and 59.

While a direct cause has yet to be found, stomach cancer is often associated with gastric ulcers, exposure to asbestos, and various dietary factors, in-

Although **cancer** chemotherapy may produce undesirable side effects at times, these medications are often important in the treatment of cancer.

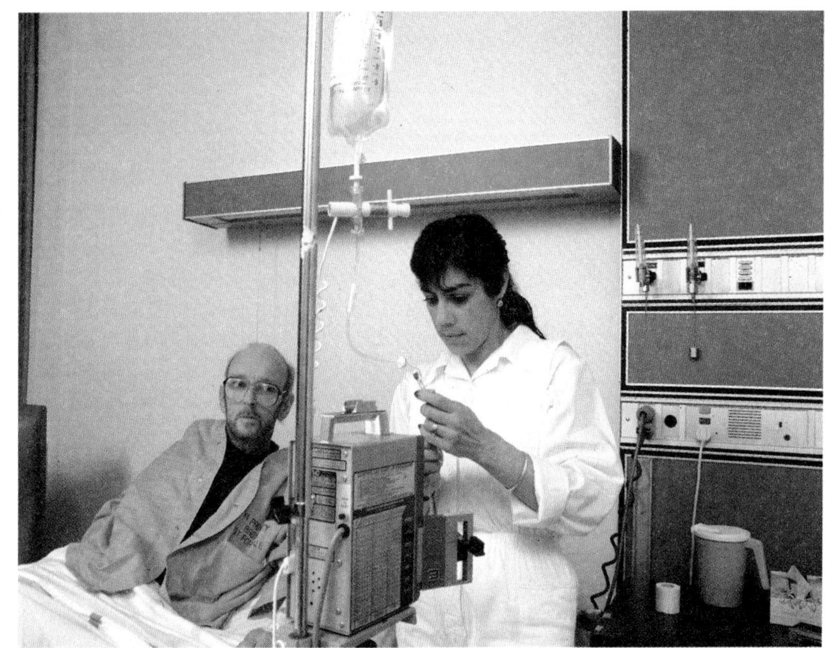

cluding the excessive consumption of nitrates and smoked or salted fish and meats.

Symptoms include vague stomach discomfort, unexplained weight loss, and anemia. Diagnosis is accomplished by means of X-ray films, biopsy, endoscopy, and gastric analysis.

Usually radiotherapy and chemotherapy are not effective. Excision of the tumor is usually recommended, with a survival rate of about 40 percent.

Testicular Cancer is cancer of the male testes, often involving an undescended testicle. Usually affecting men between the ages of 20 and 35, tumors develop more often in the right than in the left testicle. Testicular cancer accounts for less than .005 percent of all cancer cases annually.

Early symptoms are almost nonexistent, the disease revealing itself only in later stages. These later symptoms include lung problems, obstruction of the passage of urine between the kidneys and the bladder, or a lump in the abdominal area.

Accurate diagnosis includes internal examination of the scrotum by means of a light instrument and urine tests. Depending on how advanced the cancer is at the time of diagnosis, treatment may include any combination of radiotherapy, chemotherapy, and surgical excision. Prognosis is often very good.

Uterine Cancer is known medically as endometrial cancer, a disease of the membrane lining the uterus. Occurring most often in women between the ages of 40 and 60, it may be associated with ovary malfunction, a history of infertility, estrogen therapy, and a combination of hypertension, obesity, and diabetes.

The main sign of uterine cancer is abnormal bleeding from the vagina; back pain is a secondary symptom. A dilatation and curettage test usually provides the most accurate diagnosis. This involves the scraping of the inside of the uterus with an instrument in order to obtain pieces of tissue for laboratory analysis.

Because of the rapid spread of the disease, a hysterectomy is the usual treatment; 70 percent is the normal survival rate. Radiotherapy is often administered before and after the operation.

Q: *What causes cancer?*

A: There is no one cause of cancer. Most experts agree that people develop cancer mainly through repeated or prolonged contact with one or more cancer-causing agents, known as carcinogens. In addition, scientists suspect that some people may inherit a tendency toward some forms of cancer, such as breast and colon cancer.

Carcinogens increase the probability of cancer because they damage body cells, eventually causing at least one cell to become cancerous. The most common chemical carcinogen is the tar found in tobacco smoke. Industrial chemicals, such as arsenic, asbestos, and some oil and coal products, can increase the risk of cancer. Chemical carcinogens polluting air and drinking water can raise the risk of cancer for entire communities. In microscopic concentrations they are also used in some food and agricultural processes.

Some natural substances, such as the molds that grow on corn and peanut crops, are also suspected carcinogens. Diets that are high in fat may play a role in colon cancer. Overexposure to the ultraviolet rays in sunlight can cause skin cancer, particularly in people with fair, sensitive skin. Large doses of X rays are also a cancer hazard, as are radioactive substances.

Q: *How does cancer develop?*

A: Although definite causes of cancer remain hard to identify, the behavior of cancer cells is easily recognized. Unlike normal cells in the human body, cancer cells grow at an unrestrained rate. They do not grow larger than normal cells, as is commonly believed, but they last longer and divide more frequently. In the process of their uncontrolled growth, cancer cells compete with healthy cells for space and nourishment. In so doing, they may take over, replace, or kill normal cells. The rate at which this process takes place varies greatly from one form of cancer to another.

The cancer cells, dividing at an uncontrolled rate, form a cluster of cells called a tumor. Benign tumors do not spread to other parts of the body; malignant (cancerous) tumors do.

The spread of cancer (metastasis) occurs when some cancer cells break away from the tumor and travel through the lymphatic system or the bloodstream. These cancer cells may then lodge in other organs or tissues and cause new tumors to form. Cancer can also spread by invading tissues that surround the tumor. Once cancer has metastasized, it is very difficult to treat.

Q: *What are the symptoms of cancer?*

A: Cancer has no symptoms in its earliest stages, though they may appear before the cancer begins to spread. The American Cancer Society lists seven warning signals, any one of which may indicate that the disease is developing:

(1) Any changes in bowel or bladder habits. These might indicate cancer of the colon, bladder, or prostate.

(2) A sore that does not heal. This could be a warning that mouth or skin cancer is developing.

(3) Unusual bleeding or discharge. Blood in the urine may be a symptom of bladder or kidney cancer. Blood or mucus in the stool may indicate bowel cancer. Any unusual vaginal discharge or bleeding might be a sign of cancer of the female reproductive organs.

(4) A thickening or a lump in the breast or elsewhere in the body.

(5) Persistent indigestion or difficulty in swallowing. These may be signs of stomach cancer or cancer of the esophagus or throat.

(6) Obvious change in a wart or a mole. Any sudden change in their size, shape, or color could signal skin cancer.

(7) Nagging cough or chronic hoarseness. A persistent cough may be a sign of lung cancer, especially if accompanied by spitting of blood and loss of weight.

Anyone experiencing any of these symptoms for two or more weeks should promptly consult a physician. Though not definite indications of cancer, any one of these symptoms should be considered a possible warning sign of cancer. Authorities agree that early detection of cancer is the most important ingredient in successful treatment. Certain types of cancer can be detected in the early stages of development through self-examination. Breast cancer and testicular cancer are common examples.

Q: *How is cancer treated?*

A: Physicians have three main methods of treating cancer: (1) surgery, (2) radiation therapy or radiotherapy, and (3) drug therapy or chemotherapy. In many cases, treatment consists of two, or possibly all three, methods, a procedure called combination therapy.

Surgery is the main method of treating cancers of the breast, colon, rectum, lung, stomach, cervix, and uterus. Some brain tumors can also be removed surgically.

Surgery involves removal of the tumor and repair of the affected organ. In addition to the tumor itself, certain types of apparently healthy tissue may also have to be removed to help prevent the further spread of the disease. For example, a mastectomy (breast cancer operation) involves a partial or full removal of the cancerous breast and certain neighboring lymph nodes. This is done because cancer cells may have infected these glands and could spread from there to other parts of the body.

Some forms of cancer, such as those involving the skin and areas of the head and neck, can be treated with radiotherapy alone. The diseased body part is exposed to radiation from X rays or radioactive substances, such as cobalt 60. Radiation kills normal cells as well as cancerous ones, so care must be taken to administer radiation doses that do not endanger life.

Improvements are constantly being made in radiation equipment to increase the effectiveness of radiotherapy. For example, the supervoltage X-ray machine and the cobalt bomb produce radiation that has greater penetrating power and is less damaging to normal tissue than ordinary radiation. Two other modern engineering devices, the

Cancer spreads when one or more cancer cells break away from the primary tumor and travel through a blood or lymph vessel. These cells may then form new tumors at other body sites.

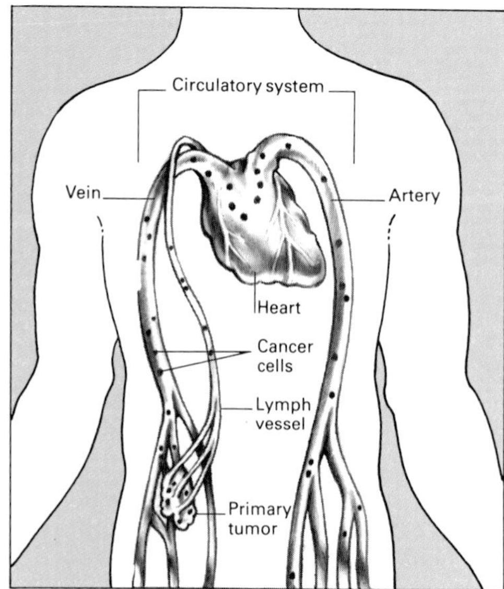

linear accelerator and the cyclotron, are even more efficient in this respect. Beams of high-energy electrons produced by linear accelerators are increasingly used to treat deep-seated tumors. High-energy neutron beams produced by cyclotrons are being used experimentally to treat advanced cancers of the head, neck, breast, esophagus, lung, and rectum.

Chemotherapy is particularly effective against leukemia and lymphoma, but is also used against other forms of cancer. These anticancer drugs function like radiation in that they kill normal cells and have side effects ranging from nausea and hair loss to high blood pressure.

The controversial drug Laetrile is used in other countries, because it is supposed to have fewer side effects than other cancer therapies. However, many experts in the United States and elsewhere feel that Laetrile is not only ineffective in treating cancer, but also dangerous. It is therefore not licensed for use in this country.

Researchers are continually looking for drugs that will be less harmful to healthy body cells. They are also investigating a natural, protective body substance called interferon that cells produce themselves to defend against invading viruses.

Q: *What are the body's natural defenses against cancer?*

A: The immune system that protects against invading bacteria and viruses also fights cancer cells. A strong immune system might be the reason why many people will never develop cancer. Some people may have a weak immune response to cancer cells, thus enabling the disease to develop.

Q: *Can cancer be prevented?*

A: Avoiding known cancer-causing agents, such as tobacco smoke and asbestos, can certainly reduce the risk. Many physicians and researchers now believe that certain foods contain substances that may help to prevent cancer. Such foods include broccoli, cauliflower, cabbage, spinach, carrots, whole-grain breads, cereals, and some seafoods. A reduced intake of fats may also help prevent some cancers from forming.

Large doses of vitamins A, C, and E have been proven effective in treating some cancers in laboratory animals. However, it is not advisable to take megadoses of these vitamins, as toxic effects may result.

Alertness to the seven warning signs mentioned above and regular medical checkups are certainly good defenses against cancer.

See also BIOPSY; BREAST EXAMINATION; CANCER PREVENTION; CHEMOTHERAPY; COLOSTOMY; FIBROCYSTIC DISEASE OF THE BREAST; HODGKIN'S DISEASE; MAMMOGRAM; MASTECTOMY; PAP SMEAR TEST; PROCTOSCOPE; PROSTATE GLAND; RADIOTHERAPY; TUMOR.

Cancer prevention takes a number of forms, most of which are related to personal habits. According to statistics compiled by the American Cancer Society, about 450,000 Americans die from cancer each year.

Of these deaths, about 135,000, or 30 percent, are caused by cigarette smoking. As a result of these statistics, the single most important means of cancer prevention in this country has become the abandonment of smoking.

The American Cancer Society has also developed a list of other recommendations, mostly dietary, that can lessen the risk of getting cancer:

- Avoid obesity. One study conducted by the Society over a period of 12 years showed a marked increase among obese people in cancers of the uterus, gall bladder, kidney, stomach, colon, and breast.

- Cut down on fat intake. Epidemiological and laboratory studies indicate that excessive fat intake increases the likelihood of developing cancers of the breast, colon, and prostate. The average American diet presently consists of 40 percent of calories in the form of fat. The National Academy of Sciences recommends a reduction to 30 percent.
- Increase the consumption of such high-fiber foods as whole-grain cereals, fruits, and vegetables.
- Include foods rich in vitamin A, such as dark green and deep yellow vegetables, and certain fruits that are rich in carotene. Studies have indicated that such foods lower the risk of cancer of the larynx, esophagus, and lung. Examples of foods rich in carotene are carrots, tomatoes, spinach, apricots, peaches, and cantaloupes. *See also* CAROTENE.
- Include food rich in vitamin C. Epidemiological studies indicate that persons whose diets are rich in ascorbic acid (vitamin C) are less likely to get cancer, particularly of the stomach and esophagus. Citrus fruits are high in vitamin C.
- Include "cruciferous" vegetables, such as cabbage, broccoli, Brussels sprouts, kohlrabi, and cauliflower. Epidemiological studies have demonstrated that consumption of these vegetables reduces risk of cancer, particularly cancers of the gastrointestinal and respiratory tracts.
- Exercise moderation in the consumption of alcoholic beverages. Heavy drinkers have been shown to be at high risk for cancers of the oral cavity, larynx, esophagus, liver, and lung.
- Exercise moderation in the intake of salted, smoked, and nitrite-cured foods. Smoked foods such as hams and sausages absorb carcinogenic tars similar to those in cigarettes.
- Avoid overexposure to the sun, particularly if one is fair-skinned. Almost all of the 400,000 cases of nonmelanoma skin cancer in the U.S. each year are diagnosed as sun-related.

Cancer screening center offers early detection programs for cancer, appropriate counseling, and follow-up services. A basic screening package would typically include laboratory tests of the blood, urine, and stool and a physical examination of possible cancer sites, such as the mouth, throat, skin, breasts in women, and testes and prostate in men.

The results of the lab tests and the examination are reviewed with the patient; if deemed necessary, further tests can be conducted. Such additional tests might include breast X rays for women and examinations of the colon.

If the patient's medical history, the family history, the physical examination, or the laboratory tests indicate an increased potential for cancer developing in the body, the screening center will provide advice and information on appropriate prevention techniques, in order to reduce the risks for cancer. These may include changing the dietary intake, adjusting the work situation, or alleviating emotional stress.

As part of the screening service patients are also instructed in self-examination techniques for the breasts and testes.

If any of the tests indicate the presence of cancer, the patient is then referred to an appropriate specialist for further diagnosis and treatment. In patients whose test results are negative, follow-up examinations are usually scheduled in 18 to 24 months.

See also CANCER; CANCER PREVENTION.

Candida (kan'də də) is a genus of a yeast-like fungus, including the species *Candida albicans.* Candida albicans is usually present in the mucous membranes of the intestinal tract, vagina, mouth, and skin. Occasionally, *candida albicans* may cause infections of the mouth, vagina, or gastrointestinal tract, and in rare situations these infections may be serious.

See also CANDIDIASIS.

Candidiasis (kan də dī'ə sis), also called moniliasis, is an infection caused by the microorganism *Candida albicans,* a fungus resembling yeast normally found in the intestine, on the skin, and in the mucous membranes of the mouth. A change in environment favorable to the fungus, combined with the weakening of the host's defenses, can allow the microorganism to increase in number and cause the infection.

Q: *What environments encourage candidiasis?*

A: Antibiotic treatment for some other condition, such as bronchitis, kills many of the bacteria normally present on the skin and in the intestine. This allows the fungus to grow, thus causing the infection. Altered hormone levels in the body, such as those that occur during pregnancy and while taking contraceptive pills, also make it easier for the fungi to grow. The infection may accompany other disorders, such as diabetes mellitus, leukemia, or conditions that require treatment with corticosteroid drugs, all of which lower the body's immunity to *Candida albicans*.

Q: *Which parts of the body are affected by candidiasis?*

A: It mostly affects areas of the body that are moist and warm. In babies, the mouth is a common area for thrush (oral candidiasis), where the infection results in small, white patches on a red, inflamed background. Similar conditions occur in the vagina, a common area for the infection in women.

There are various areas on the skin that can become infected. These are in the groin, around the anus, beneath the breasts (particularly in overweight women with pendulous breasts), in folds of skin of people who are obese, and in the armpits.

Candidiasis may occur as a form of diaper rash in babies, if the buttocks are allowed to remain moist with urine.

Q: *Can candidiasis be sexually transmitted?*

A: Yes. Inflammation of the end of the penis (balanitis) may occur in uncircumcised men after intercourse with a woman with candidiasis. Both partners must be treated.

Q: *How is candidiasis treated?*

A: Skin infections are treated with fungicidal creams or lotions, and vaginal infections may be treated with suppositories. The rare internal forms of candidiasis are, under the care of a physician, treated with potent fungicidal drugs.

See also BALANITIS; FUNGAL INFECTION.

Cane. *See* WALKING AID.

Canine. *See* TOOTH.

Canker sore (kang′kər), known medically as aphthous ulcer, is a small and painful whitish ulcer, usually in the mouth or on the lips. It is probably caused by a virus that normally lives in the body cells without causing symptoms. In the presence of a disorder, such as the common cold, or even during menstruation, ulcers may form.

Various brands of throat drops or ointment stop the pain and help mouth ulcers to heal. A physician may prescribe an antibiotic rinse to produce rapid healing.

See also ULCER.

Cannabis (kan′ə bis) is another name for marijuana.

See also MARIJUANA.

Canoeing safety. *See* WATER SPORTS SAFETY.

Capillary (kap′ə ler ē) is the smallest type of blood vessel in the vascular system. Capillaries connect the smallest arteries with the smallest veins; most are so narrow that only one blood cell can pass along them at a time. The capillary wall is the conduit for material passing from an artery to a vein. The function of capillaries is to carry oxygen-rich blood to the tissues, to pass

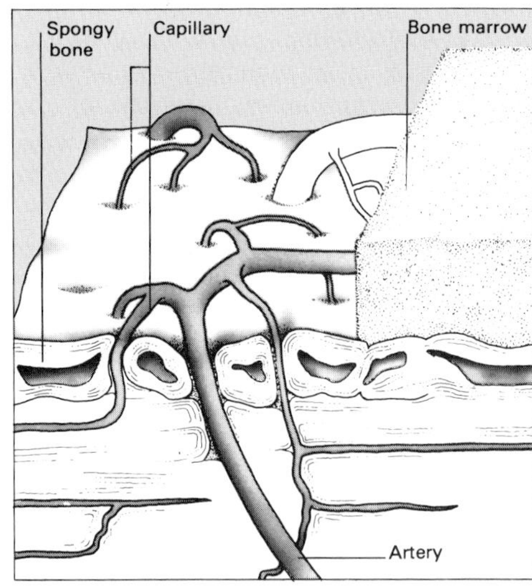

A **capillary** absorbs blood that is formed in the bone marrow and conveys it to the arteries.

food substances to tissue cells, and to carry away waste products, such as carbon dioxide.

See also VASCULAR SYSTEM.

Capsule (kap′səl) is either a small, soluble case, usually made of gelatin, containing a single dose of a drug (the covering prevents the patient from tasting the drug), or a membrane or ligament enclosing part or all of an organ.

See also TABLET.

Capsulitis (kap səl ī′tis) is inflammation of any membrane that encloses an organ or structure. There are various forms of the disorder, but the most common affects the membranes of large joints, especially the hip and shoulder. The inflammation causes stiffness and pain when the joint is moved.

An affected joint should be rested, and a physician may recommend painkilling drugs (analgesics) and anti-inflammatory drugs for the first few days. If capsulitis takes a long time to improve, the physician may prescribe corticosteroid drugs, physiotherapy, or shortwave diathermy.

See also BURSITIS.

Carbohydrate (kär bō hī′drāt) is an organic compound furnishing most of the energy needed in a healthy diet. Carbohydrates exist as "simple" sugars (sucrose, glucose, fructose, and lactose) or as glucose polymers (starch or "complex carbohydrate," glycogen, and cellulose). Simple sugars rapidly and temporarily raise blood sugar. It is preferable to eat more complex carbohydrates which are digested and absorbed more slowly.

Foods high in carbohydrate content include bananas, bread, rice, cereals, potatoes, and corn. During the digestion of such foods, the carbohydrates are broken down into the energy-producing sugar, glucose,and ultimately, into water, carbon dioxide, and energy.

If little or no carbohydrate is in the diet, the body uses the protein from muscles and enzymes to provide energy. Fat stores are also a source of energy.

See also NUTRITION.

Carbolic acid (kär bol′ik), also called phenol, is a very poisonous, corrosive substance derived from coal tar. Low concentrations of carbolic acid are used in various antiseptic formulas.

See also ANTISEPTIC.

Carbon dioxide (kär′bən dī ok′sīd) is a colorless, odorless gas that occurs in the atmosphere (0.035 percent by volume) and is produced in body tissues as a waste product of energy-generating processes. Dissolved in the blood, carbon dioxide is carried to the lungs, and from there it is exhaled as a gas. Some carbon dioxide also leaves the body in urine and in perspiration.

If the level of carbon dioxide in the blood rises above normal, the brain automatically stimulates the lungs into working faster. The increase in breathing rate is necessary to rid the body of the extra carbon dioxide, but it may be harmful in other ways. Solid carbon dioxide (dry ice) is used medically in simple cryosurgery to destroy warts.

See also ACIDOSIS; CRYOSURGERY.

Carbon monoxide (kär′bən mon ok′sīd) is a poisonous, inflammable gas that is colorless and, in its pure state, odorless. It is present in the exhaust fumes from all internal combustion engines, in the gas produced from burning coal, and in sewers. Carbon monoxide is dangerous if inhaled because it is, in preference to oxygen, easily absorbed by hemoglobin in the blood, thus preventing the blood from carrying oxygen. This results in asphyxiation, which can cause brain damage or death.

Q: ***What are the symptoms of carbon monoxide poisoning?***

A: Symptoms vary greatly, but the victim normally has a pink or blotchy face and chest and complains of dizziness, difficulty in breathing, nausea, faintness, ringing in the ears, and throbbing temples. The pupils of the eyes become dilated, and the victim may lose consciousness.

Q: ***What action should be taken for carbon monoxide poisoning?***

A: Remove the victim as quickly as possible from the source of the fumes. Fresh air and artificial respiration aid the recovery of the victim, but an oxygen mask, using 100 percent oxygen, is the best treatment.

See also ARTIFICIAL RESPIRATION; ASPHYXIA.

Carbon tetrachloride (kär′bən tet rə klôr′īd) is a clear, colorless liquid with anesthetic and sleep-inducing (narcotic) properties. In these respects carbon tetrachloride resembles chloroform, but it is too poisonous to be used as an anesthetic. The most common uses of carbon tetrachloride today are in the chemical industry.

Q: *What are the poisonous effects of carbon tetrachloride?*

A: Small doses taken orally may cause giddiness, headache, and vomiting, and symptoms of severe kidney and liver damage may occur within weeks. The toxic effects are increased if carbon tetrachloride fumes are inhaled.

Carbuncle (kär′bung kəl) is an inflamed bacterial infection of the skin, which is usually due to the bacterium *Staphylococcus aureus*. It is similar to a boil, except that a carbuncle tends to spread locally, sometimes forming clusters with several openings that discharge pus. Carbuncles occur most commonly on the back of the neck, buttocks, and thighs. The infection is usually treated with antibiotics taken under medical supervision, but sometimes a physician has to make an incision to drain a carbuncle.

See also BOIL.

Carcinogen (kär sin′ə jən) is any substance that is known to cause cancer, for example, tobacco tar or asbestos.

See also CANCER.

Carcinoma (kär sə nō′mə) is a type of cancer that forms on the epithelial tissue that covers the inside and outside of most body organs. It develops most commonly in the skin, large intestine, stomach, lungs, prostate gland, or breast. The tumor is malignant and tends to spread (metastasize) to other parts of the body. Treatment usually involves the surgical removal of the tumor and some of the normal surrounding tissue.

See also CANCER.

Carcinoma, basal cell (kar sə no′mə, ba′səl sel). Basal cell carcinoma is a common form of skin cancer. It usually appears on the face, tip of the nose, eyelids, or ears. Although it is classified as a cancer, it spreads only by local ulceration and not by metastasis

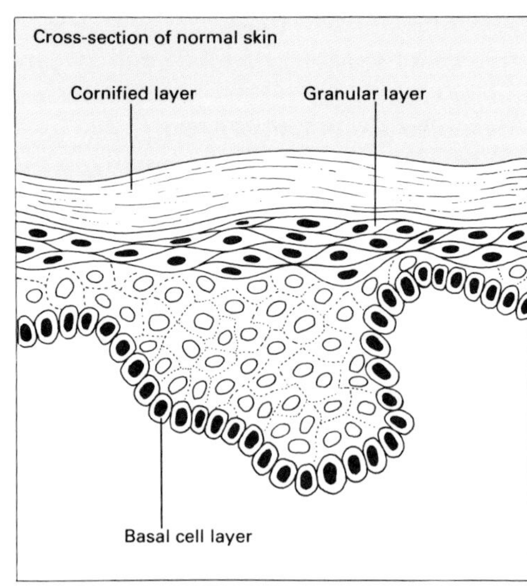

A **basal cell carcinoma** is a malignant growth that begins in the basal cells, usually on the face.

(movement of malignancy through the blood and lymph). Most patients are over the age of 50.

At first, the sore appears as a small, pear-like nodule, which slowly grows and ulcerates in the center to form a small scab. Early treatment achieves a cure rate of more than 95 percent.

Carcinoma in situ (kär sə nō′mə in si′tü) is a premalignant cell change that occurs in superficial epithelial tissue. Although the cell change has not yet spread to the membrane underlying the epithelial tissue, it shows the characteristics of a cancerous cell change that would spread. Carcinoma in situ is often seen on the uterine cervix and may also occur in the esophagus, anus, penis, prostate, and vagina. Treatment includes surgery.

See also CANCER; EPITHELIUM.

Cardiac (kär′dē ak) describes anything pertaining to the heart.

See also HEART.

Cardiac arrest (kär′dē ak ə rest′) is the sudden stoppage of the heart. Cardiopulmonary resuscitation should be started immediately following cardiac arrest in order to prevent heart, lung, kidney, or brain damage.

See also CARDIOPULMONARY RESUSCITATION; HEART STOPPAGE.

Cardiac asthma. *See* ASTHMA, CARDIAC.

Cardiac catheterization (kär′dē ak kath ə tər i zā′shən) is a technique that enables a physician to diagnose certain heart problems with a very high degree of accuracy. The catheter is a narrow, flexible tube that is inserted into the heart via a vein or artery in the arm or leg. This allows exploration of the valves, the chambers, the coronary arteries, and the other major blood vessels; measurement of blood pressure; and analysis of blood gases. Once the physician has completed these tasks, a contrast media (dye) is injected into the heart through the catheter to facilitate further diagnosis by means of an angiogram, a picture of the vessels of the heart. Using a fluoroscope, image intensifier, television system, and video recorders, the physician can determine immediately whether additional views will be necessary.

Cardiac catheterization is most often used when less invasive means of diagnosing heart problems have not provided adequate information to allow the physician to properly diagnose and/or treat the problem. The procedure very often precedes coronary by-pass surgery, an operation requiring substantial detailed information about the heart and its blood supply.

Q: *Is the patient given a general anesthetic during cardiac catheterization?*

A: No. Only a local anesthetic and mild sedative are used. The patient remains awake during the entire procedure.

Q: *How long does the procedure last?*

A: Cardiac catheterization requires two to three hours.

Q: *How does the doctor know when the catheter has reached the heart?*

A: The doctor monitors the progress of the catheter on a fluoroscope. *See also* FLUOROSCOPE.

Q: *Is this process painful?*

A: Insertion of the catheter causes some discomfort, similar to insertion of an intravenous needle. When the dye is injected, some patients experience a hot flash, burning sensation, or nausea. For many, the chief discomfort is caused by having to lie still for a long period of time, sometimes in awkward positions.

Q: *Are there any risks associated with cardiac catheterization?*

A: There are a number of risks, including stroke, heart attack, infection, damage to the vein or artery, swelling, bleeding, and allergic reaction to the contrast medium (dye).

Q: *What are the chances of a complication developing during the procedure?*

A: In facilities that perform at least 200 catheterizations in the course of a year, complications occur in less than 4 percent of cases. Most of these are minor.

See also ANGIOGRAM; CORONARY ARTERY BY-PASS SURGERY; HEART DISEASE, CORONARY.

Cardiac massage (kär′dē ak mə säzh′) is the repeated compression of the heart in order to restore and maintain the heartbeat and blood flow following cardiac arrest.

See also CARDIAC ARREST; CARDIOPULMONARY RESUSCITATION.

Cardiac murmur. *See* HEART MURMUR.

Cardiac muscle (kär′dē ak mus′əl) is the medical term for heart muscle, the involuntary muscle that forms the bulk of the heart wall.

See also HEART; MUSCLE.

Cardiac pacemaker. *See* PACEMAKER, ARTIFICIAL; PACEMAKER, NATURAL.

Cardiogram (kär′dē ə gram) is a graph that records the electrical activity of the heart muscle. The term cardiogram is often used colloquially for electrocardiogram, which is also abbreviated as EKG or ECG.

See also ELECTROCARDIOGRAM.

Cardiology (kär dē ol′ə jē) is the medical specialty that involves the study of the heart and its functions and the diagnosis and treatment of its disorders.

See also HEART; HEART DISEASE.

Cardiomyopathy (kär dē ō mī op′ə thē) is a general term for diseases of the heart muscle. Cardiomyopathy is characterized by a progressive weakness and enlargement of the heart and irregular heart rhythms. Heart failure may result.

There are various possible causes for cardiomyopathy: (1) genetic factors; (2) infection caused by rheumatic fever or viruses; (3) beriberi and other vitamin B deficiency disorders; and (4) excessive alcohol intake; (5) chronic diseases such as diabetes mellitus and generalized coronary atherosclerosis.

Cardiopulmonary resuscitation (kär dē ō pu̇l′mə ner ē ri sus ə tā′shən), also known as CPR, is an emergency life support procedure. It consists of artificial respiration and manual cardiac massage, applied to prevent irreversible brain damage or death in the case of cardiac arrest. It should be performed only by someone trained in the technique, after making sure that the victim's heart has stopped or respiration has ceased.

To see if a victim's pulse has stopped, check the pulse rate in the neck. If no pulse can be felt, assume that the victim's heart has stopped and start CPR at once if you are properly trained. Persons untrained in CPR should notify emergency medical aid as soon as possible; those performing CPR should alert someone else to notify medical assistance.

To administer CPR to an adult or a large child, the rescuer first initiates mouth-to-mouth resuscitation. For complete instructions, *see* ARTIFICIAL RESPIRATION. The rescuer then places the heel of one hand parallel to and over the lower part of the victim's sternum (breastbone), 1 to 1.5 inches (2.5 to 3.8 cm) from its tip. The rescuer puts the other hand on top of the first and brings the shoulders directly over the sternum. The rescuer's fingers should not touch the victim's chest.

Keeping the arms straight, the rescuer pushes down forcefully on the sternum. This action, called *external cardiac compression*, forces blood from the heart through the pulmonary artery to other parts of the body. The rescuer alternately applies and releases the pressure at a rate of about 60 compressions per minute. After every 15 compressions, the rescuer briefly gives the victim artificial respiration.

If the victim is a small child, the rescuer uses only one hand for the compressions. Pressure is applied at about the middle of the sternum. To treat an infant, the rescuer exerts pressure with the index and middle fingers at the middle of the sternum. In all cases, the compressions must be accompanied by artificial respiration. Treatment should continue until professional help arrives.

CPR is best performed by two persons. One administers external cardiac compression, and the other provides artificial respiration. The rescuers position themselves on opposite sides of the victim so they can switch jobs easily if either becomes fatigued.

For illustrations of CPR procedures, *see* HEART ATTACK: FIRST AID.

Cardiovascular system (kär dē ō vas′kyə lər), comprising both the heart and the blood vessels, circulates blood throughout the body. It carries essential supplies of food and fuel to every living cell and exchanges them for potentially harmful waste products. The adult circulation consists of thousands of miles of tubing containing about 10 pints (4.7l) of blood. The blood is kept flowing round the body by the pumping action of the heart.

Blood is made up of a pale yellow liquid (plasma) containing dissolved nutrients and wastes, plus blood cells, hormones, proteins and other substances. Most numerous of these cells are the disk-shaped red blood cells. Their color comes from the presence of the substance hemoglobin, which combines with oxygen. When red corpuscles charged with oxygen approach body cells, the oxygen is delivered in exchange for the waste product carbon dioxide. Other two-way transportation of materials takes place between the body cells and the plasma, and all unwanted substances are carried away in the blood for excretion by the kidneys, lungs, and liver. Plasma also contains white blood cells, which help to fight infection, and platelets, which are involved in blood clotting.

In its passage through the body, blood is carried in tubes known as arteries and veins. Most arteries transport oxygen-rich (oxygenated) blood, whereas most veins transport carbon dioxide-rich (deoxygenated) blood. The largest artery is the aorta, which stems directly from the heart. The aorta and other large arteries have thick walls lined with muscle. Blood flow is assisted by the contraction of this muscle and the impetus given by the heartbeat. The "push" from the heart can be felt as the pulse wherever large arteries run near the body surface.

As they penetrate the tissues, arteries split into narrow branches called arterioles, which in turn divide into capillaries. It is through the very thin capillary walls that the blood gives up its oxygen and nutrients and receives carbon dioxide and wastes. Deoxygenated blood in the capillaries flows into narrow veins (venules), and then into veins. The two largest veins, the venae cavae, return this blood to the heart. Veins have thin walls compared with those of arteries, and blood moves through the veins much more slowly. Blood flow in the veins is assisted by the action of muscles in surrounding tissues, and backflow is prevented by one-way valves.

The deoxygenated blood delivered to the heart along the veins is no use to body cells until it has been recharged with oxygen. To ensure reoxygenation, the circulation has a second "loop." In this part of the system, blood rich in carbon dioxide travels from the heart along the pulmonary artery to the lungs, where carbon dioxide is exchanged for oxygen breathed in. The pulmonary artery is the only artery to carry deoxygenated blood. The newly oxygenated blood is carried back to the heart along the pulmonary vein, the only vein to transport oxygenated blood.

The heart is a muscular organ about the size of a clenched fist. The structure and action of the heart are designed to serve the two loops of the circulation. Inside, the heart is divided vertically by a muscular wall. On each side of this wall is an upper chamber (atrium) and a thicker, lower chamber (ventricle). Blood moves through each side of the heart systematically. Deoxygenated blood is delivered into the right atrium. It then enters the right ventricle, from where it is pumped out into the pulmonary artery and to the lungs. Oxygenated blood returning in the pulmonary veins flows into the left atrium. This blood enters the left ventricle and is then pumped into the aorta for circulation.

The flow of blood in each side of the heart is controlled by a series of valves. The pumping action of the heart is achieved by the contraction of the cardiac muscle, of which the heart is largely composed. The rhythm of the heartbeat is regulated by bursts of electrical impulses sent out by a concentration of specialized heart tissue called the pacemaker.

Under the influence of the pacemaker, the heart of an adult at rest beats at a rate of 60 to 80 beats a minute. The pacemaker also helps to en-

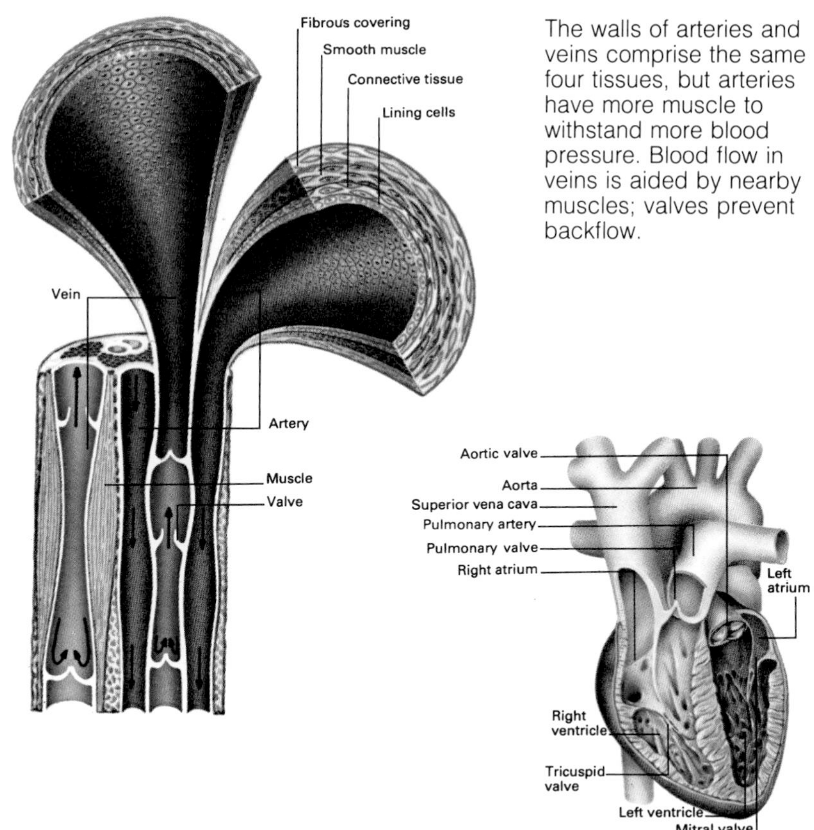

The walls of arteries and veins comprise the same four tissues, but arteries have more muscle to withstand more blood pressure. Blood flow in veins is aided by nearby muscles; valves prevent backflow.

Blood flow in the heart is controlled by valves. The tricuspid valve controls flow from right atrium to right ventricle; the mitral valve controls flow from left atrium to left ventricle. Valves also guard the entrances to the aorta and pulmonary artery in order to prevent backflow of blood after the heart contracts.

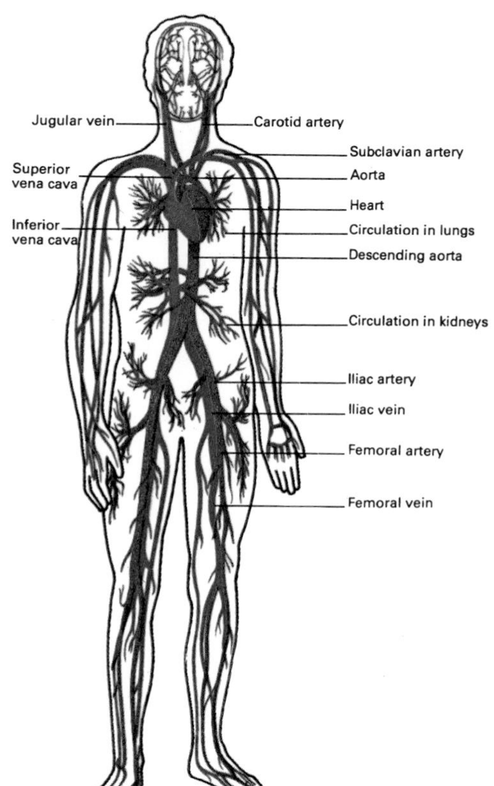

The human circulation is made up of 60,000 miles (96,500km) of tubing. Branching from the aorta are arteries taking oxygen-rich blood to all body parts. The blood returns to the heart in the veins and is then carried to the lungs to be reoxygenated.

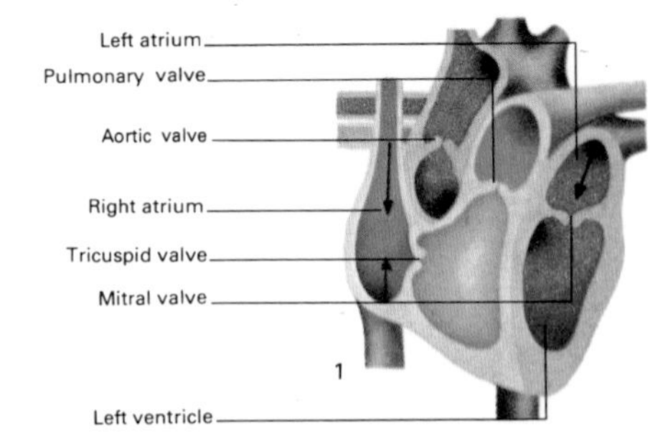

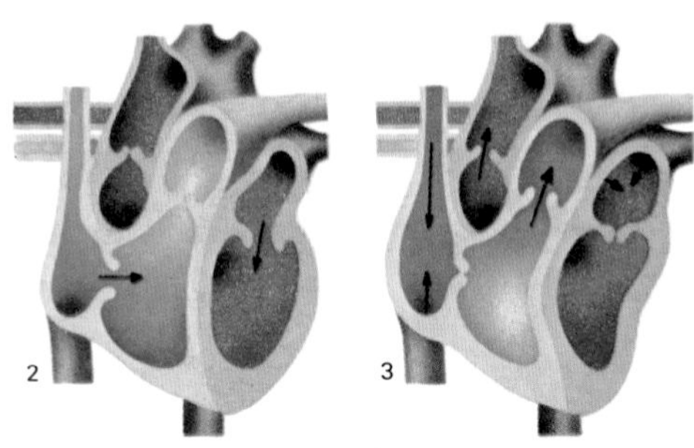

As a heartbeat begins (1) right and left atria fill with blood. The atria contract (2) forcing blood into the right and left ventricles. The ventricles then contract strongly (3) so that blood is pushed into the aorta and pulmonary artery.

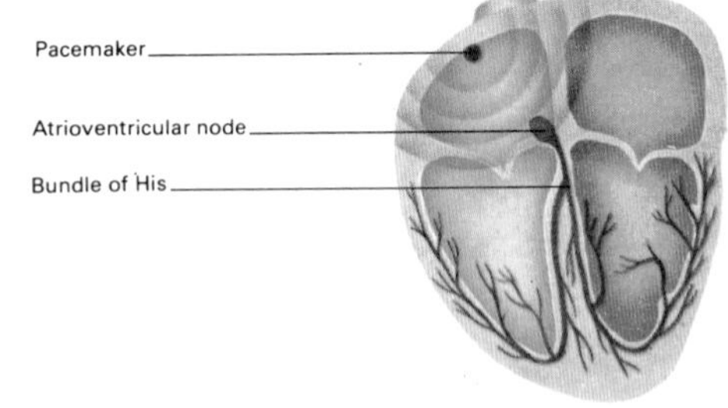

The pacemaker, *right,* sets the heart beating by sending out nerve impulses that pass to the atria, then to the ventricles via other special nerve tissues.

An electrocardiogram (EKG) records the waves of nerve impulses of each heartbeat. The P wave starts just before the atria contract; the QRS wave indicates the contraction of the ventricles; and the T wave indicates the recovery period before the next contraction.

sure the correct sequence of activities during each heartbeat; first the two atria contract, followed rapidly by the ventricles. The powerful contraction of the ventricles pushes blood into the aorta and pulmonary artery. This period of contraction (systole) is followed by a period of relaxation (diastole), during which the heart refills. The complete sequence is accompanied by electrical activity of the muscle, which can be monitored as an electrocardiogram (EKG).

See also BLOOD; BLOOD CELL, RED; BLOOD CELL, WHITE; ELECTROCARDIOGRAM; HEART (and other related entries beginning with HEART); PLATELET.

Cardioversion (kär dē ō vėr′zhən), or electroversion, is the restoration of normal rhythm to an irregular heart through the use of carefully controlled electric shock. It may be necessary when the rhythms normally controlled by the natural cardiac pacemaker have been replaced by irregularities, such as heart muscle fibrillations or other arrythmias.

See also ARRYTHMIA; FIBRILLATION; PACEMAKER, NATURAL.

Care of the chronically ill. *See* NURSING THE CHRONICALLY ILL.

Care of the dying. *See* DYING, CARE OF THE.

Care of the sick. *See* NURSING THE SICK.

Caries (kãr′ēz) is the progressive deterioration of teeth or bones. Caries is usually accompanied by inflammation of the surrounding soft tissue. The term is most often used to refer to tooth decay (dental caries).

See also TOOTH DECAY.

Carotene (kar′ə tēn) is a yellow-orange pigment present in many plant and animal tissues. When such a plant or animal is eaten as food, the carotene is digested and stored in the liver until it is converted by the liver into vitamin A. Carotene is abundant in yellow vegetables such as carrots and corn, and it can also be found in eggs.

See also VITAMIN.

Carotid artery. *See* ARTERY.

Carpal tunnel syndrome (kär′pəl tun′əl) causes a numbness or pain in the wrist or hand, especially in the fingers (except the little finger). The sensation may be particularly noticeable at night. Carpal tunnel syndrome occurs when a ligament across the front of the wrist becomes swollen and compresses the median nerve that supplies the first three fingers. The condition is more common in women and becomes worse with excessive use of the wrist, as with repetitive movements encountered in some occupations or athletic activities. It may occur during pregnancy, menopause, or before the menstrual period, when fluid may build up in the ligaments. It may also occur with mild arthritis; in rare cases, it may result from a hormone disorder.

Resting the wrist, sometimes using a splint, and use of anti-inflammatory drugs may improve the condition. If these fail, a physician may inject a corticosteroid drug into the ligament. Sometimes, a minor operation is needed to cut free the ligament to relieve the pressure on the nerve.

Carpus (kär'pəs) is the medical name for the wrist. A carpal bone is any of the eight small bones in the wrist.

See also WRIST.

Carrier (kar'ē ər) is a person who harbors or passes on germs that cause disease in others while remaining unaffected by those germs himself or herself. Carriers are responsible for the spread of such diseases as typhoid and diphtheria. An individual infected with hepatitis B virus may become a chronic carrier of that virus. A carrier may also be a person who has a recessive gene disorder, such as hemophilia, which is passed on genetically. A disease-carrying organism, such as a mosquito, is also sometimes known as a carrier, or vector.

Car safety. See AUTOMOBILE SAFETY.

Car seat, baby. See BABY CARE.

Car sickness. See MOTION SICKNESS.

Cartilage (kär'tə lij) is dense, semitransparent connective tissue that is capable of withstanding great pressure and tension. Cartilage forms part of the structure of the skeleton in some ribs and between vertebrae of the spine. It is also present in the nose and in the covering on surfaces of joints. In a developing fetus, cartilage becomes impregnated with deposits of calcium salts.

Q: *What is a torn cartilage?*

A: A torn cartilage commonly refers to a disorder of the knee. The cartilage tears away from the ligament that holds it in position. A piece of cartilage may become free to move around in the knee joint. This can cause pain, swelling, and sometimes a "locking" of the knee that holds the leg in one position. No weight can be placed on the leg.

Q: *How is a torn cartilage treated?*

A: A minor tear can be treated effectively with a firm bandage around the knee and by taking as much rest as possible. More serious tears require the removal of part or all of the cartilage in an operation (meniscectomy). Sometimes small areas of torn cartilage can be removed through an arthroscope. Osteoarthritis may affect the knee joint later in the patient's life.

See also ARTHROSCOPY.

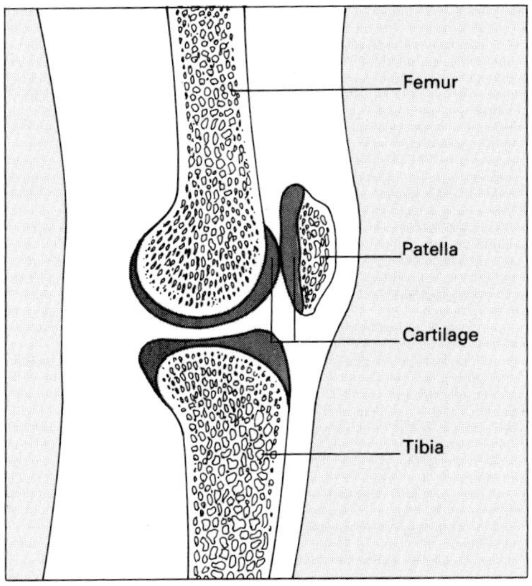

Cartilage in the knee cushions the bones against shock and prevents them from rubbing together.

Caruncle (kar'ung kəl) is any small fleshy lump, such as those occurring at the inside corner of the eye or under the tongue. An abnormal reddened caruncle sometimes appears at the opening of the urethra in women. An urethral caruncle may cause bleeding and pain on urination and may be extremely sensitive to friction. The condition is not serious in itself and can be removed surgically if it causes discomfort.

Cast is a plaster or fiberglass mold used to support a fractured or dislocated bone while it is mending. In dentistry, a cast is a mold made of a person's teeth and inner jaw area for the purpose of producing and properly fitting dentures.

See also DENTURE; FRACTURE.

Castration (kas trā'shən) is the surgical removal of the genital organs. The term is commonly taken to mean the removal of the testicles (orchidectomy), although medically it also applies to the removal of the ovaries (oophorectomy). Castration may be necessary if the growth of a cancerous tumor is stimulated by sex hormones, as happens, for example, with cancer of the prostate or cancer of the breast. The removal of one or both testicles or ovaries is sometimes necessary if they have been seriously damaged by infection. In women, the ovaries may be removed at the same time as the uterus (hysterectomy).

Q: *Does castration affect sexual desire and fulfillment?*

A: The operation in men subdues the sexual drive (libido). Intercourse is still technically possible, but unlikely. The semen does not contain sperm. Growth of body hair is reduced, but the depth of the voice remains unchanged. If a boy is castrated before puberty, secondary sexual characteristics (such as hair growth and deepening of the voice) do not develop.

Castration in women does not reduce a woman's ability to have sexual intercourse or her enjoyment of it, but the possibility of conception is permanently removed. If ovaries are removed before puberty, secondary sexual characteristics (such as breast development) fail to occur. Removal of the ovaries of a young woman will result in "sexual menopause"; the resulting sudden loss of female hormones may cause severe hot flashes and a loss of bone, leading to osteoporosis.

See also STERILIZATION.

Catabolism (kə tab′ə liz əm) is the destructive half of the metabolic process, in which complex living tissues are broken down into simpler substances or waste matter, thereby producing energy.

See ANABOLISM; METABOLISM.

Catalepsy (kat′ə lep sē) is a trance-like state in which the muscles of the body are more or less rigid. In this state, a person's arms or legs remain in any position in which they are placed. Catalepsy may occur during hypnosis and in such organic and psychological disorders as schizophrenia and epilepsy.

Catalyst (kat′ə list) is a substance that speeds up a chemical reaction, while itself remaining practically unchanged. Catalysts in cells and bodily fluids are known as enzymes.

See also ENZYME.

Cataplexy (kat′ə plek sē) is the momentary loss of muscular power and control without the loss of consciousness. These momentary attacks of paralysis usually last only a few seconds and seem to be caused by such emotional responses as surprise, fear, anger, or joy. Cataplexy may be associated with narcolepsy.

See also NARCOLEPSY.

Cataract (kat′ə rakt) is an opaque (nontransparent) area in the lens of the eye. Cataracts cause a gradual, painless deterioration of sight, beginning with an inability to see detail clearly and a distortion of sight in the presence of bright lights.

Q: *What causes cataracts?*

A: Cataracts often develop in elderly persons as a result of a degeneration of the lens tissue. Cataracts may also occur due to hereditary factors or as a result of some kind of damage to the fetus early in the pregnancy, for example, infection with rubella (German measles). Injury to the eye later in life may also cause cataracts, or they may accompany a disease, particularly diabetes. Some medications, steroids, for example, may produce a predisposition to the formation of cataracts.

Q: *How are cataracts treated?*

A: If vision is seriously impaired, the lens is removed in an operation or broken up by ultrasound and removed through a tiny slit. After an initial period of adjustment, clear vision may be restored with the assistance of strong eyeglasses or contact lenses. In some cases, an artificial lens is placed in the eye at the time the cataract is removed.

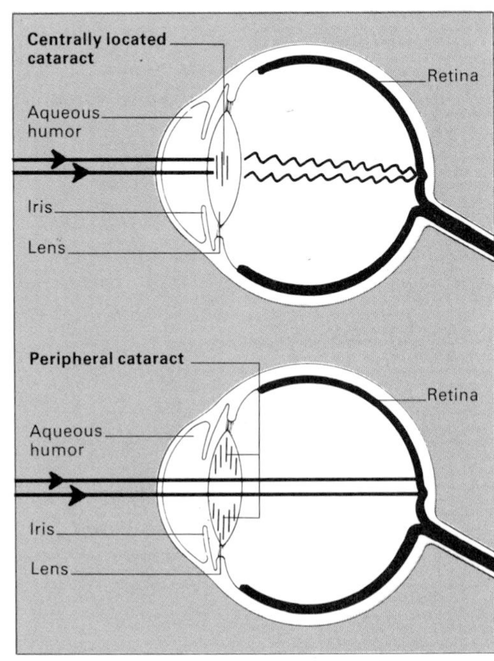

A **cataract** centrally located (1) will result in more sight loss than a peripheral cataract (2).

Catarrh (kə tär′) is an obsolete term for an inflamed condition of a mucous membrane, usually that of the nose or throat, causing a discharge of mucus. This condition is actually a symptom of various infections, such as the common cold, hay fever, laryngitis, or rhinitis.

Cathartic (kə thär′tik) is a substance, castor oil, for example, that induces one or several watery bowel movements. Cathartics may be used to cleanse the bowel prior to barium X rays or prior to a colonoscopy.

See also COLONOSCOPY.

Catheter (kath′ə tər) is a tube inserted into a body cavity to extract or inject fluids. A catheter is usually made of flexible plastic or of rubber. One type of catheter is inserted into the bladder in order to allow drainage of urine. Another type is used to administer intravenous fluids.

CAT scan. *See* COMPUTERIZED AXIAL TOMOGRAPHY SCANNER.

Cat-scratch fever is a disease caused by a bacteria, as yet unnamed, that is transmitted by the scratch or bite of a healthy cat. It develops 7 to 14 days after the scratch or bite. Inflammation of the affected area heals in a few days, but lymph nodes in the area remain slightly swollen and tender. A mild fever and general feeling of being unwell may persist from two weeks to a month.

Causalgia (kô zal′jē ə) is a severe burning pain in an area where nerves have been injured, particularly the palm of the hand or the sole of the foot. The surface skin often becomes thinner and reddish, and slight changes such as a cool breeze may aggravate the burning sensation. The pain may cause the patient to become severely emotionally disturbed. Causalgia is difficult to treat. If painkilling drugs and warm, wet compresses are not effective, a physician may try local anesthetic injections or surgery to cut the damaged nerves.

Cautery (kô′tər ē) is an artificial way of destroying tissue for medical reasons. It is done using heat, cold, corrosive chemicals, electricity, or (the most recent method) a beam of laser light. Tissue may be cauterized to treat wounds that are likely to become infected or to destroy a lumpy scar. In surgery, an electric cauterizing needle is often used to stop bleeding from small blood vessels. Other examples of cautery include the use of silver nitrate to stop recurrent nosebleeds.

Cavity (kav′ə tē) is either a hole in a tooth, caused by decay, or an enclosed space inside the body. Examples of the latter type of cavity include the abdominal cavity, which contains internal organs below the diaphragm, and the oral cavity, which is the space inside the mouth.

See also ABDOMEN; TOOTH DECAY.

CBC. *See* BLOOD COUNT, COMPLETE.

Cecostomy (sē kos′tə mē) is an artificial opening made surgically by joining the first part of the large intestine (cecum) to the wall of the abdomen. It may be a permanent or temporary measure to treat a blockage of the colon caused by a condition such as cancer.

See also COLOSTOMY; ILEOSTOMY.

Cecum (sē′kəm) is the sac-like first section of the large intestine, just beyond the point at which the lower part of the small intestine (ileum) joins the large intestine. Attached to the cecum is the vermiform appendix.

Celiac disease (sē′lē ak) is a metabolic disorder caused by a sensitivity to gluten, a protein found in some grains, for example, wheat, barley, and rye. With celiac disease, the cells lining the small intestine are damaged and prevent the normal absorption of food, particularly fats. The disorder primarily strikes young children. It is also known as nontropical sprue.

Q: *What are the symptoms of celiac disease?*

A: Babies and young children with the disease fail to gain weight normally, may develop a swollen abdomen, and excrete loose, fatty stools. They may also suffer repeated respiratory infections, dry skin, and eventually, signs of anemia, rickets, and other deficiency disorders. Adult patients may experience stool problems, as well as breathlessness and muscle cramps. The abdomen may be swollen, and the fingers may show clubbing.

Q: *What is the treatment for celiac disease?*

A: Patients should be permanently put on a gluten-free diet and treated for anemia and any other deficiency disorder that is present. The diet should also be low in fats, with a high level of protein and vitamins to ensure adequate nourishment. With proper treatment, chances for a full recovery are excellent.

See *also* CLUBBING; DIET, SPECIAL; GLUTEN; SPRUE.

Cell is the basic unit of all living matter; all plants and animals are composed of cells. An adult human body contains about 10 trillion (10,000,000,000,000) cells. Most cells only measure a few thousandths of a millimeter in diameter.

Each human being starts life as a single cell, a fertilized egg, which divides into more cells during the embryonic development. In the course of this duplication, cells begin to differentiate into muscle cells, skin cells, nerve cells, and so on. Cells continue to divide and differentiate throughout a person's life.

Q: *How do cells reproduce?*

A: Most human cells reproduce through the process called mitosis. In mitosis, a cell divides and forms into two identical daughter cells. Each daughter cell then doubles in size and becomes capable of dividing. During the period between divisions, the cell grows and carries on its normal activities, which include a duplication of its chromosomes, a process which precedes mitosis.

Q: *What makes one cell different from another?*

A: Scientists are not exactly sure how cells establish their different functions, but they think that DNA (deoxyribonucleic acid), the hereditary material carried by the chromosomes, controls differentiation partly by directing the production of certain enzymes. As these enzymes appear in a cell, their chemical reactions cause the cell to become specialized.

The variations between cells reflect the tasks of different cells. Some of the cells nearest to the "basic" design include the hexagonal liver cells, which perform many complex chemical reactions. Other simple cells are those that provide support and lining in many tissues. Often these column-shaped cells produce the sticky substance, mucus, and are edged with minute hair-like projections (cilia), which can move substances along. The fat cells found beneath

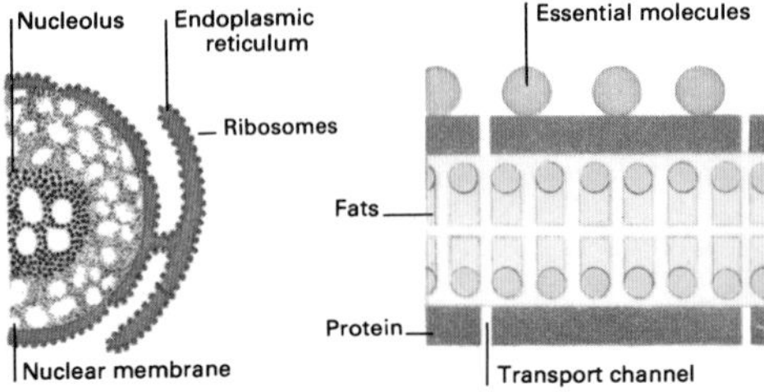

In the nucleus, information is housed in the chromosomes. The nucleolus aids protein synthesis. Substances pass in and out of pores in the membrane.

The cell membrane consists of two layers of protein enclosing a layer of fat. Special areas in the membrane allow molecules to enter and leave the cell.

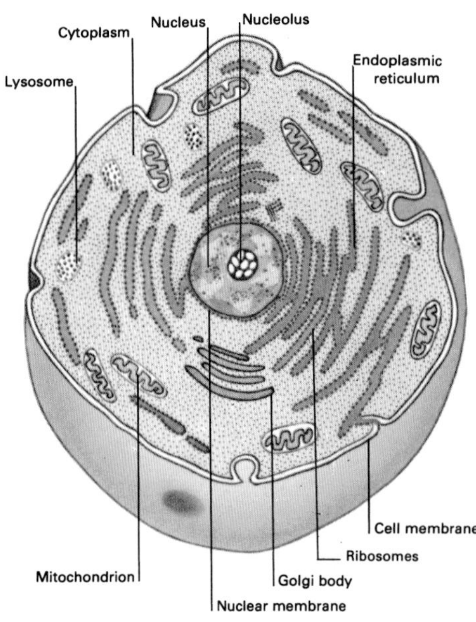

All body cells have the same basic constituents. The cell is enclosed in a membrane and comprises the cytoplasm and nucleus. The cytoplasm contains organelles vital to cell activity, such as mitochondria, for energy production; and the endoplasmic reticulum, running from the membrane to the nucleus, that bears ribosomes essential to protein building. Instructions for protein manufacture are given by the DNA of the nucleus.

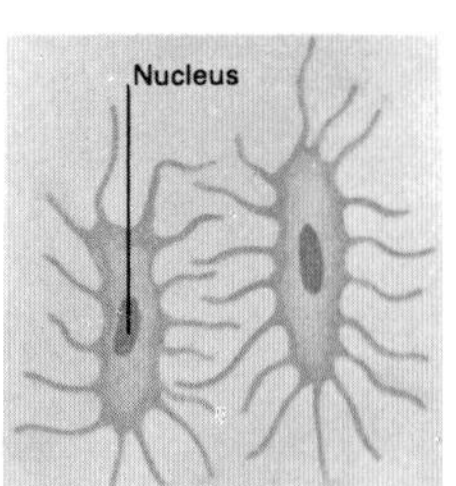

Cells called osteoblasts make the hard substances in bone. The minerals are molded by the cells' long cytoplasm-filled arms.

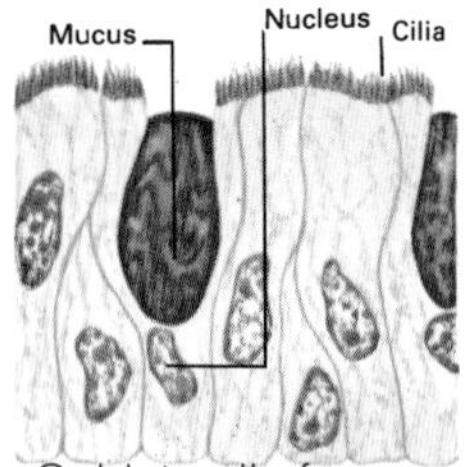

Goblet cells form part of a mucous membrane. They secrete mucin, which combines with water to form slippery mucus.

the skin and around many organs are simple cells whose cytoplasm is packed with globules of fat. The fat is used to provide insulation and energy. Red blood cells, which carry oxygen and carbon dioxide within the circulation, are unusual in having no nuclei in their mature form. In contrast, many of the white blood cells, part of the body's defense system against disease, have very large nuclei.

Three of the most specialized sorts of cells are muscle cells, nerve cells, and reproductive cells. Muscle cells are greatly elongated and have the power of contraction made possible by special proteins that can slide over one another. Because muscle contraction is energy-intensive, muscle cells have huge numbers of mitochondria.

Nerve cells are also elongated but have specialized membranes for transmitting the electrical impulses of nerve messages. Each nerve cell ends in a cell body bearing projections that lie close to similar projections on adjacent nerve cells. Messages "jump the gaps" with the aid of chemicals made in the nerve cells.

Reproductive cells (sperm from the male and eggs from the female) are unique in containing only half the usual number of chromosomes.

Q: *What are the components of a cell?*

A: A thin covering called the cell membrane or plasma membrane encloses the cell and separates it from its surroundings. The cell has two main parts: (1) the nucleus and (2) the cytoplasm.

The Nucleus is the control center that directs the activities of the cell. A *nuclear membrane* surrounds the nucleus and separates it from the cytoplasm. The nucleus contains two types of structures, *chromosomes* and *nucleoli.*

Chromosomes are long, threadlike bodies that normally are visible only when the cell is dividing. Chromosomes consist chiefly of two substances—DNA and certain proteins. Lined up along the chromosomes are the *genes,* the basic units of heredity. *Genes* control the passing on of characteristics from parents to offspring. Each gene consists of part of a DNA molecule. DNA determines a person's height, eye color, shape of hands, texture of hair, and thousands of other characteristics.

Nucleoli are round bodies that form in certain regions of specific chromosomes. Each nucleus may contain one or more nucleoli, though some cells have none at all. Nucleoli help in the formation of *ribosomes,* the cell's centers of protein production. Nucleoli are made up of proteins and *RNA* (ribonucleic acid). RNA is chemically similar to DNA and plays an important role in making proteins.

The Cytoplasm is all the cell except the nucleus. Proteins are made in the cytoplasm, and many of the cell's life activities take place there. Many tiny structures called *organelles* are located in the cytoplasm. Each has a particular job to do. These organelles are called *mitochondria, lysosomes,* the *endoplasmic reticulum, centrioles,* and *Golgi bodies.*

Mitochondria are the power producers of the cell. A cell may contain hundreds of mitochondria. These sausage-shaped structures produce almost all the energy the cell needs to live and to do its work.

Lysosomes are small, round bodies containing many different enzymes, which can break down many substances. For example, lysosomes help white blood cells break down harmful bacteria.

Endoplasmic Reticulum is a complex network of membrane-enclosed spaces in the cytoplasm. The surfaces of some of the membranes are smooth. Others are bordered by ribosomes—tiny, round bodies that contain large amounts of RNA. Ribosomes are the cell's manufacturing units. The proteins the cell needs in order to grow, repair itself, and perform hundreds of chemical operations, are made on the ribosomes.

Centrioles look like two bundles of rods. They lie near the nucleus and are important in cell reproduction.

Golgi Bodies, also called *Golgi complex* or *Golgi apparatus,* consist of a stack of flat, bag-like struc-

Types of cells

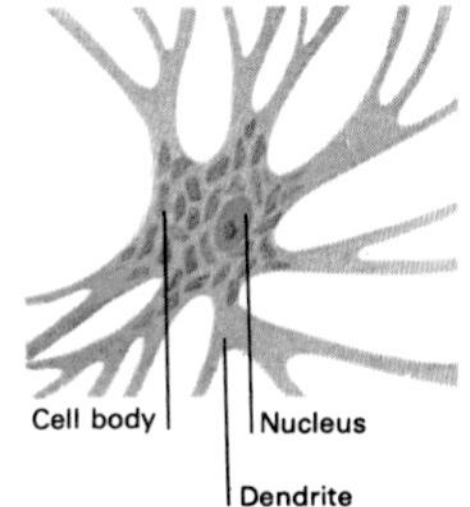

The transmission of impulses between nerve cells is achieved with the help of outgrowths (dendrites) from each cell body.

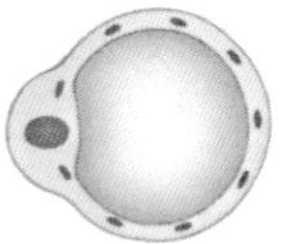

Spherical fat cells can expand to accommodate large stores of energy-rich fats. They have small nuclei.

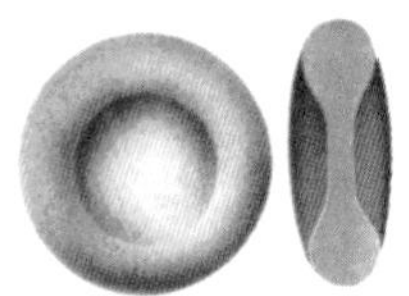

Mature red blood cells, flattened concave disks that have no nuclei, carry oxygen and carbon dioxide.

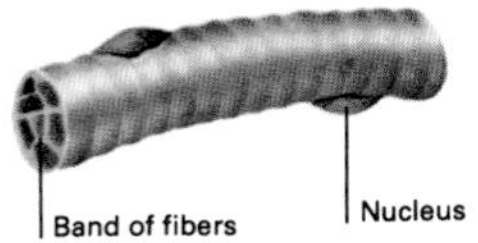

Elongated cells of skeletal muscle look striped because they contain filaments that move to make the muscle contract.

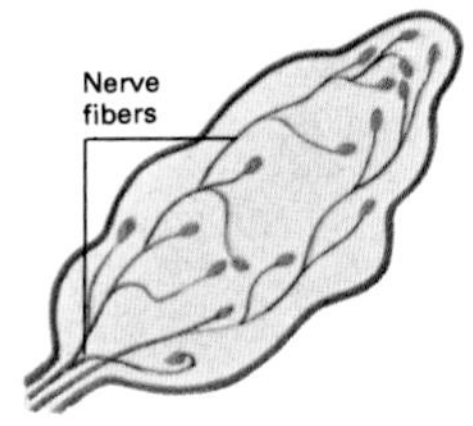

Cold is detected in the skin by end bulbs of Krause, *above,* made of nerve fibers enclosed within a thin covering membrane.

tures that store and eventually release various products from the cell.

Membranes enclose the entire cell, the nucleus, and all the organelles. The membranes hold the cell and each of its parts together. Most membranes consist of a double layer of a fatty substance called *phospholipid*. Proteins occur at various points and extend to different depths within the double layer of phospholipids. Only needed materials can enter the cell and its parts because of the structure and chemical composition of the membranes. *See also* LIPID.

Q: ***What about advances in cell research?***

A: Building on Gregor Mendel's discovery of the laws of heredity, scientists have worked on unraveling the secrets of DNA. Researchers are trying to determine the answers to many questions: What causes a cell to die? Can errors in the cell's genetic code be corrected?

If scientists discover what causes a cell to die, they may be able to slow the aging process and increase the span of human life. As scientists learn more about DNA and the genetic code, they may be able to alter the code and erase hundreds of inherited mental and physical defects. They may find a way to control cancer. If scientists learn how a cell differentiates, they may be able to alter mature nerve cells, which do not reproduce. Then these cells could be replaced if damaged or destroyed. Or perhaps scientists may be able to replace worn-out or diseased tissues or encourage the stump of an amputated leg to regrow. By manipulating hereditary processes, scientists may free farm crops and livestock of hereditary diseases. Thus, agricultural production may be greatly increased.

One of the most promising areas of future cell research is the field of genetic engineering. This field developed during the 1970's after scientists discovered techniques for removing genes from one organism and inserting them into another. This procedure is called *recombinant DNA research*. Experiments with recombinant DNA have helped scientists to learn more about the structure and function of genes. Many researchers believe that recombinant DNA research will lead to advances in agriculture, medicine, and industry. However, many people feel that such research is dangerous, and the government has placed strict guidelines on recombinant DNA research in the United States.

See also DEOXYRIBONUCLEIC ACID; GENETIC ENGINEERING.

Cellulitis (sel yə lī'tis) is a diffuse infection in the tissue under the skin, commonly associated with a small cut, abrasion, or boil. Poor blood circulation and diabetes mellitus often play a role in the development of cellulitis. The condition is characterized by skin or other tissue surrounding the infection becoming red, swollen, and tender. Treatment includes antibiotics and, sometimes, the soaking of the affected area in warm water.

Cellulose (sel'yə lōs) is a carbohydrate that does not change chemically during the human digestive process; as cellulose is indigestible, it passes through the intestinal tract unchanged. It is present in fiber-containing foods, such as green vegetables, fruits, and whole-grain wheat bread. Cellulose aids in the elimination of waste products from the intestine. For this reason, it is sometimes used in the treatment of constipation.

See also CARBOHYDRATE; NUTRITION.

Celsius. See CENTIGRADE.

Centigrade (sen'tə grād), or Celsius, is a scale of temperature measurement in which 0° centigrade (written 0°C) is the freezing point of water at sea level, and 100°C is the boiling point of water at sea level. The other common system of temperature measurement is the Fahrenheit scale. The normal average human body temperature is 37°C (equal to 98.6°F).

See also FAHRENHEIT.

Central nervous system. *See* NERVOUS SYSTEM, CENTRAL.

Cerebellum (ser ə bel'əm) is the part of the brain that controls the coordination of body movements, posture, and balance. The cerebellum, however, has no power to initiate movements. It is located just behind and above the brainstem.

See also BRAIN.

Cerebral cortex (ser′ə brəl kôr′teks) is the layered "gray matter" of the brain that forms the outer layer of each hemisphere of the cerebrum. The cerebral cortex receives and interprets nerve impulses from the sense organs and directs voluntary movement. It is also concerned with higher mental functions, such as intelligence, memory, and perception.

See also BRAIN; CEREBRUM.

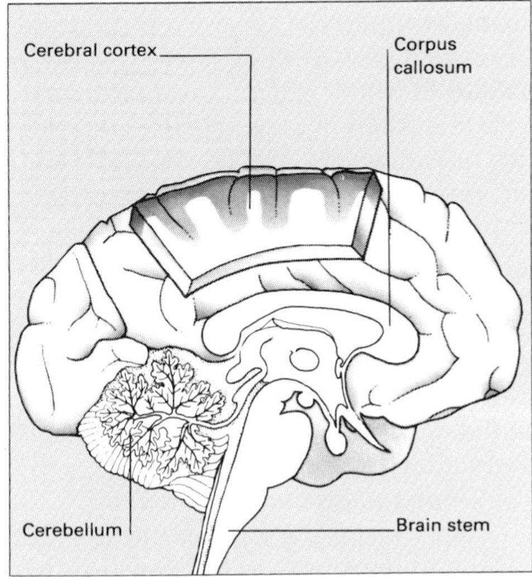

The **cerebellum** coordinates body movements; the **cerebral cortex** controls higher mental functions.

Cerebral hemorrhage. *See* HEMORRHAGE, CEREBRAL.

Cerebral palsy (ser′ə brəl pôl′zē) is a general term for various disorders resulting from brain damage that occurs before, during, or shortly after birth. It may cause severe crippling and mental retardation, or the symptoms may be so mild that they hardly interfere with the patient's activities. All cerebral palsy victims have at least some loss of voluntary muscle control.

Q: *What causes cerebral palsy?*

A: The type of brain damage that can produce cerebral palsy may result from disease, faulty growth, or injury. One or more of these causes may occur before, during, or shortly after birth. In many instances, a specific cause is never found. Cerebral palsy can not be inherited.

Before birth, brain damage may result from a disease of the mother. For example, German measles can severely harm an unborn child, even though the mother may have had only mild symptoms or none at all during pregnancy. Faulty growth of the child's brain may occur if the mother is severely malnourished during pregnancy. Brain damage occurs in some cases of premature birth.

During the birth process, brain damage may result from a difficult delivery, in which there is direct damage to the baby's head and brain. Some events during birth can lead to a lack of oxygen in the brain. Brain cells die if they do not have oxygen—even for a few minutes—and the body can never replace them. Problems during birth can also cause tearing in parts of the baby's brain.

After birth, a baby may develop cerebral palsy if disease or injury damages the brain. During the first year of life, infections and accidental dropping of the child are the most frequent causes of the condition. In some cases, child beating has caused cerebral palsy.

Q: *What are some symptoms of cerebral palsy?*

A: Some of the more common symptoms of cerebral palsy are lack of balance, clumsy walk, unclear speech, shaking, jerking movements, and convulsions. In some persons with cerebral palsy, there is also mental retardation, learning disability, and/or severe hearing and sight problems. Symptoms of cerebral palsy are sometimes apparent at birth. However, in most cases, a definitive diagnosis of cerebral palsy may not be made until the child is between one and two years old.

Q: *How is cerebral palsy treated?*

A: Since cerebral palsy is a permanent, nonprogressive brain disorder, there is no cure. Therefore, treatment for the condition is aimed at helping the victim make best use of his or her physical and mental abilities. The degree of success in the treatment of cerebral palsy is largely dependent upon the extent of brain damage involved.

In general, treatment for cerebral palsy usually includes physiotherapy, speech therapy, medications, surgery, biofeedback, and special education. Psychological support is also very important in helping people with cerebral palsy and their families.

For many people with cerebral palsy, a physician may prescribe braces and other devices that provide support and can also aid in walking.

Cerebrospinal fluid (ser ə brō spī′nəl flü′id), or CSF, is a clear, watery substance that flows around the brain and spinal cord, protecting and insulating these structures. The fluid assists the supply of nutrients to the brain, and it assists in the disposal of waste substances. A blockage in CSF flow, as may occur with a blood clot, congenital structural abnormalities, or certain infections, can result in serious complications, such as hydrocephalus.

See also HYDROCEPHALUS.

Cerebrum (ser′ə brəm), or forebrain, is the largest part of the brain, composing about 70 percent of that organ. It is situated beneath the roof of the skull and consists of two hemispheres that are separated lengthwise by a layered division. The outer layer of each hemisphere is the cerebral cortex, the section of the brain sometimes referred to as "gray matter."

Within the cerebral hemisphere is white matter consisting of three kinds of fibers that connect the hemispheres, convey impulses to and from the cortex and the spinal cord, and connect different areas of the cortex with each other. The cerebrum performs a variety of duties, including controlling the sensory and voluntary motor functions, as well as such higher processes as thought and memory.

See also BRAIN.

Cerumen (sə rü′mən) is the wax-like substance produced by cells of the external canals of the ears.

See also EARWAX.

Cervical (sėr′və kəl) refers to any cervix, or neck-like structure, for example, the upper seven bones of the spinal column (cervical vertebrae) or the neck of the uterus (cervix uteri).

Cervical cancer (sėr′və kəl) is a malignant growth in the uterine cervix.

See also CANCER.

Cervical cap (sėr′və kəl) is a contraceptive device made of flexible material and shaped like a cup. It fits over the cervix of the uterus and prevents sperm from entering the cervical canal. Initial fitting should be done by a physician or a nurse. Afterwards, the user may need to practice inserting the cap properly. To be effective, the cervical cap must be inserted perfectly.

This method of contraception is at least as effective as the diaphragm, and it is more comfortable. Some users may experience vaginal infections, particularly if the cap is not removed and cleaned properly.

See also CERVIX; DIAPHRAGM.

Cervical erosion (sėr′və kəl i rō′zhən) is an abnormal change in the tissue of the surface wall of the cervix, the neck portion of the uterus. Natural healing of the disorder involves the downward growth of tissue cells from the endocervical canal. But it is not uncommon for healing to be incomplete and for the area to become ulcerated. This may cause an abnormal discharge from the vagina and occasional bleeding, particularly after sexual intercourse.

Q: *What causes cervical erosion?*

A: Infection in the vagina, the stimulus to hormone production resulting from pregnancy, or the use of birth control pills may cause cervical erosion.

Q: *How is cervical erosion treated?*

A: A physician may introduce an antiseptic and antibiotic compound into the vagina to kill the infection and allow the cervical cells to regrow. If this fails, cautery of the damaged area is the usual treatment. This does not usually require hospitalization.

Q: *How soon after cautery can a woman resume sexual intercourse?*

A: A woman should not have sexual intercourse until a further physical examination confirms that the area has healed properly.

See also CAUTERY.

Cervical rib (sėr′və kəl) is a small extra rib with which some people are born. It is an appendage to the seventh cervical vertebra in the neck. The extra rib generally does not cause problems. If, however, it puts pressure on the adjacent nerves and blood vessels, there is pain in the arm and hand and, possibly, symptoms similar to Raynaud's phenomenon. If a cervical rib causes such symptoms, it should be removed.

See also RAYNAUD'S PHENOMENON.

Cervical smear (sėr'və kəl smir), also known as Pap smear, is a test for the early detection of cancer cells of the cervix, the neck of the uterus.

See also PAP SMEAR TEST.

Cervical spondylosis. See SPONDYLOSIS, CERVICAL.

Cervicitis (sėr və sī'təs) is the inflammation of the neck of the uterus (cervix). Cervicitis does not always have symptoms, but when they occur they may include a thick discharge from the vagina, pain during sexual intercourse, bleeding after sexual intercourse, and lower back pain. The cause of cervicitis often remains unknown, but it may be caused by cervical erosion or by vaginal infections. It may become chronic because of reexposure to the germ or due to such factors as multiple sex partners or poor nutrition.

Antibiotic medication may help cure cervicitis, but chronic infections may have to be destroyed using cautery or cryosurgery.

See also CAUTERY; CERVICAL EROSION; CRYOSURGERY.

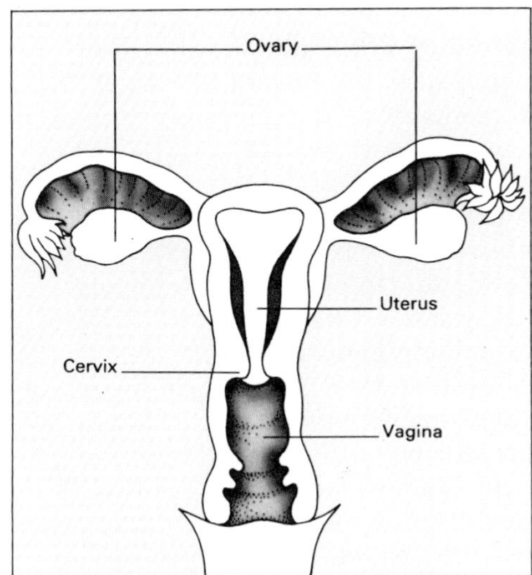

The **cervix** of the uterus is the narrow opening from the vagina to the uterus.

Cervix (sėr'viks) is the neck or any part of an organ that resembles a neck. The cervix of the uterus is the narrow opening at the base of the uterus that protrudes slightly into the vagina.

Cesarean section (si zăr'ē ən) is the delivery of a baby through a surgical opening in the abdominal and uterine walls into the uterus. This method may be preferable to natural birth through the vagina for various reasons: (1) if the mother's birth canal is too narrow for normal childbirth; (2) if a misplaced placenta blocks the exit from the womb (placenta previa); (3) when the fetus is in an unusual position (for example, head up, feet down); (4) when signs of fetal distress or potential illness occur; or (5) when the mother is ill.

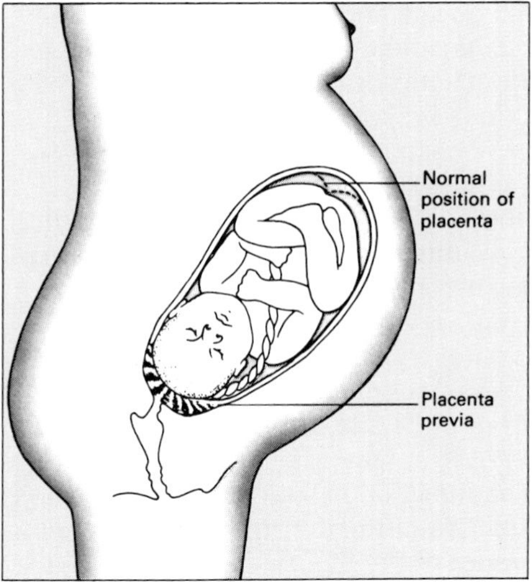

A **Cesarean section** may be necessary if the placenta obstructs the birth canal (placenta previa).

The United States has a high rate of Cesarean section operations; approximately 15 percent of births are delivered in this manner.

Q: ***Can a woman who has had a Cesarean section have a normal delivery for her next baby?***

A: Yes, unless the reason for surgical delivery was a narrow birth canal or some permanent illness in the mother.

See also PREGNANCY AND CHILDBIRTH.

Cestodiasis (ses tō dī'ə sis) is the infestation of the intestine by worms of the subclass Cestoda (phylum Platyhelminthes). The most common parasitic worms in this group are tapeworms. Symptoms of cestodiasis may include diarrhea, abdominal discomfort, or anemia.

See also TAPEWORM.

Chafing (chā'fing) is a skin irritation caused by rubbing the affected skin on another skin surface or on wet clothing. The most common areas of chafing are the groin, the anal region, and between the fingers and toes. Chafing is usually accompanied by itching and burning; an infection can occur if the superficial skin is broken. If the chafed area is kept clean and dry, the irritation usually heals itself.

Chagas' disease (chä'gəs) is a disorder transmitted by the bloodsucking bite of an insect that carries the causative agent, *Trypanosoma cruzi*. It is one form of trypanosomiasis. With acute Chagas' disease, there is a red swelling around the site of the bite, which, if on an eyelid, may cause the eye to close. The infection enters through the conjunctiva of the eye, the mucous membranes of the mouth or nose, or a skin abrasion. Symptoms of Chagas' disease may include fever, general enlargement of the lymph nodes, and a rapid heartbeat. Gastrointestinal symptoms, such as dilation of the esophagus or colon, may also occur. The parasite can also be carried through the bloodstream to the heart and cause inflammation leading to chronic heart failure.

Q: *What is the treatment for Chagas' disease?*

A: There is no effective form of treatment, and the disorder has a high death rate, particularly among children. However, the disease often runs its course without complications.

Q: *Is there a higher incidence of Chagas' disease in some countries?*

A: Yes. Chagas' disease is most common in Central and South America, and it occurs, although rarely, in the southwest United States.

Chair, tip-up. *See* NURSING THE SICK.

Chalazion (kə lā'zē ən), or meibomian or tarsal cyst, is a small, localized inflammation of the eyelid. It forms when an oil-producing gland (a tarsal gland) becomes blocked with secretion. A chalazion is not malignant or painful; but if treatment is advised, it can be removed surgically.

See also STY.

Chancre (shang'kər) is a small, painless red ulcer that is usually an early sign of the sexually transmitted disease, syphilis. It usually appears on the genitals, but may occur elsewhere depending on the site of the infection, for example, the lips or skin. Several chancres may occur simultaneously. A chancre appears within four weeks after infection and becomes an ulcerous sore that heals slowly during the next month. It may leave a small scar. It is important to consult a physician to receive early treatment for the underlying disease.

See also SYPHILIS.

Chancroid (shang'kroid), also called soft chancre or soft sore, is a highly contagious sexually transmitted disease. It is caused by bacteria (*Hemophilus ducreyi*) and is common in the tropics. About three or four days after contact with the infection, the patient develops a small, red ulcerating sore on the genitals. This becomes painful and the local lymph nodes swell and may discharge. Other symptoms may be a slight fever and a general feeling of being unwell.

Q: *How is chancroid treated?*

A: Because the red sore of chancroid resembles the sore that occurs as a sign of syphilis, the patient must also be tested for syphilis. Appropriate antibiotics should heal the chancroid. The patient's sexual partner(s) should be treated as well.

See also SEXUALLY TRANSMITTED DISEASE.

Change of life is the informal term for menopause, the time of life when a woman's menstrual periods end.

See also MENOPAUSE.

Changing a diaper. *See* BABY CARE.

Chapping (chap'ing) is a condition where skin is irritated, cracked, or inflamed due to overexposure to cold, wet weather. Chapped skin is particularly likely to occur around the lips. Preventive measures include the use of water-repellent cream on the hands and face during outdoor activities. Ointment can also be used on the lips. If possible, chapped skin should be protected by warm, dry clothing.

Charcot's joint. *See* JOINT, CHARCOT'S.

Charley horse is the common term for pain and stiffness in a muscle, usually in the leg. A charley horse may be the result of a muscle strain that occurs during strenuous activity.

See also CRAMP; CRAMPS AND SPASMS: TREATMENT.

Cheilitis (kī lī'tis) is inflammation and cracking of the lips. Frequent causes are sunburn, allergic reaction to cosmetics, dermatitis, and vitamin deficiency.

See also DERMATITIS.

Cheilosis (kī lō′sis) is a condition in which the lips redden and fissures or lesions occur at the corners of the mouth. Cheilosis is usually caused by a deficiency of the vitamin B complex, especially riboflavin. Vitamin B tablets and emollient skin cream can improve the condition.

See also FISSURE; LESION.

Chelating agent (kē′lā ting) is a substance that combines chemically with metals such as lead and mercury. Chelating agents are used to combat poisoning by such metals. There are various chelating agents, including penicillamine and EDTA, edetic acid. A physician decides which agent is best for a particular form of poisoning.

Cheloid. *See* KELOID.

Chemical dependency is a compulsive desire, both physical and psychological, to take drugs. A person can be chemically dependent on alcohol or nicotine; on street drugs, such as marijuana, cocaine, or heroin; on hallucinogenic drugs, such as LSD or mescaline; or on prescription drugs, such as amphetamines, codeine, barbiturates, or tranquilizers.

Treatment of the chemically dependent individual often involves a prolonged hospital stay in order to minimalize the physical side effects and to ease the psychological stresses brought about by withdrawal from chemical dependency.

See also ALCOHOLISM; DRUG ABUSE.

Chemical poisoning: first aid. *See* POISONING; FIRST AID.

Chemonucleolysis (kē mō nü klē ol′i sis) is the dissolving of the nucleus pulposus, usually by means of a chemolytic agent, such as chymopapain, that breaks down the protein structure. The nucleus pulposus is the pulpy cushioning substance between the vertebrae, which spills out and puts pressure on the spinal cord when the disk containing it is ruptured. Chemonucleolysis may be used in selected cases on persons with herniated disks, as an alternative to back surgery.

See also DISK, HERNIATED; NUCLEUS PULPOSUS; SPINE.

Chemosis (kē mō′sis) is excessive swelling of the mucous membranes that line the eyelids and surface of the eyes (conjunctiva). It may be caused by a physical injury, infection, or contact with an irritating substance such as chlorine. Chemosis may also appear in acute conjunctivitis. Chemosis may be a temporary reaction, but if the condition does not clear up within several hours, a physician should be consulted.

See also CONJUNCTIVITIS.

Chemotherapy (kē mō ther′ə pē) is the treatment of disease through the use of chemical agents that have a destructive (toxic) effect on an infecting organism or on malignant cells. The term usually refers to the use of cytotoxic chemicals to destroy cancer cells. Cytotoxic drugs include methotrexate and cyclophosphamide. The treatment of bacterial infections with penicillins or other antibiotics is also a form of chemotherapy. Many types of cancer chemotherapy have negative side effects; these side effects may include the possible destruction of healthy tissue.

See also CANCER.

Chest, or thorax, is the upper part of the trunk of the body. It extends from the base of the neck to the diaphragm, which separates the chest from the abdomen. The framework of the chest consists of twelve pairs of ribs, which are connected to the spine at the back, and the intercostal muscles in between them. The upper seven pairs of ribs are connected at the front to the breastbone (sternum). The lower five pairs do not connect directly to the sternum; three pairs are connected indirectly by carti-

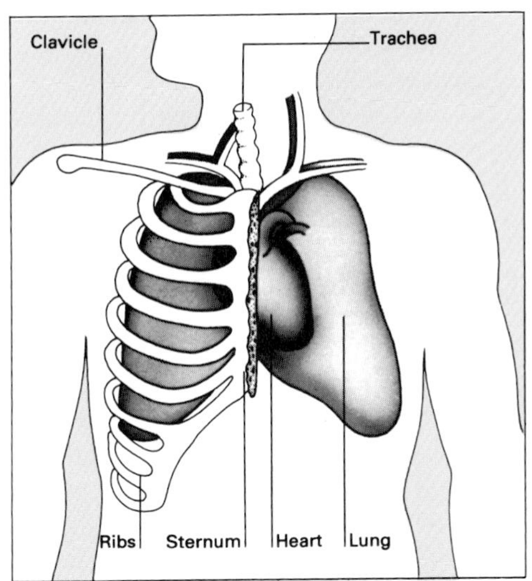

The **chest** contains the ribs, most of the respiratory organs, and the heart.

lage, and the other two pairs to the spine only.

The thoracic cavity enclosed by this frame contains the heart; the respiratory apparatus, including the two lungs in their surrounding membrane (pleura); the lower part of the trachea, and the bronchi; various glands; the esophagus (gullet); the two vagus nerves and two phrenic nerves; and the major blood vessels. Movement of the diaphragm and intercostal muscles changes the volume of the thoracic cavity during breathing.

Chest exercise. *See* EXERCISE.

Cheyne-Stokes asthma. *See* ASTHMA, CARDIAC.

Cheyne-Stokes respiration (chān-stōks′ res pə rā′shən) is an abnormal breathing pattern that is first shallow and infrequent and then increases gradually to become abnormally deep and rapid, before fading away completely for a brief period. Breathing may be stopped for about 5 to 30 seconds, before the next cycle of shallow breathing begins. Cheyne-Stokes respiration is often accompanied by changes in the level of consciousness; it most commonly occurs in seriously ill patients with brain or heart disorders. It may occur during sleep.

Q: *Is Cheyne-Stokes respiration always associated with serious disorders?*

A: No. The breathing pattern can occur in elderly people, especially when they have taken sleeping pills. Poor circulation and acidosis may also be causes of the disorder. Cheyne-Stokes respiration may also strike an otherwise healthy person due to hyperventilation.

Q: *Is there any treatment for Cheyne-Stokes breathing?*

A: If the breathing abnormality is associated with a heart or brain disorder, it improves when the cause is treated. Sometimes, a physician prescribes the drug aminophylline.

Chickenpox (chik′ən poks), or varicella, is a virus infection characterized by a rash of small red spots that first appears on the back and chest and then spreads to cover the rest of the body. The rash is usually preceded for a few days by a slight fever, sore throat, and discharge of mucus from the nose. The spots develop quickly into clear, oval blisters of various sizes. These become milky in color and within three or four days shrivel up as scabs, which may take another week to fall off. One or two more waves of rashes may occur in the next two to three days. The rash is often very itchy. During the acute stage of the disorder, which lasts for three or four days, the patient's temperature may rise as high as 102–104°F (39–40°C); a physician should be consulted. There is no vaccine against chickenpox.

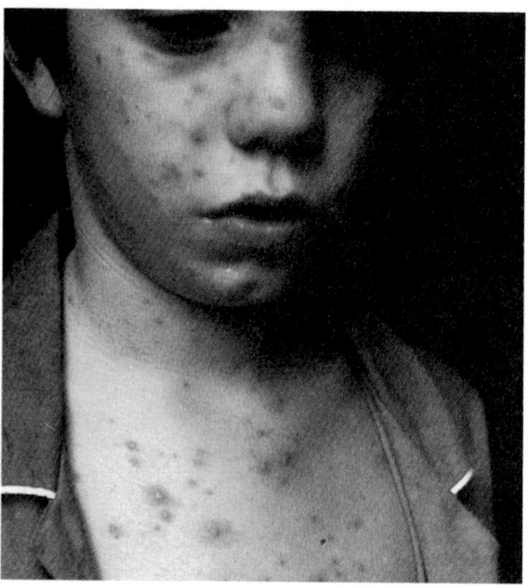

Chickenpox is a contagious viral disease that produces an itchy, blister-like rash.

Q: *Is chickenpox contagious?*

A: Yes. The first symptoms appear 12 to 17 days after contact with the disease. The contagious stage extends from about five days before the outbreak of the rash until all of the blisters have crusted. It is advisable to isolate the patient once the spots appear. The disease is spread through direct contact with the rash or tiny droplets that are exhaled by infected persons.

Q: *How long is chickenpox likely to last?*

A: The acute illness lasts for three or four days, but it is usually another seven to ten days before the spots have disappeared.

Q: *Are some people more likely than others to get chickenpox?*

A: Yes, children. Adults are less likely to catch chickenpox because, by the age of 15, about 75 percent of children have had chickenpox, and it is unusual to get the disease a second time. People in poor health and the elderly should avoid contact with a child with chickenpox, because the infection may cause the related disorder, shingles (herpes zoster), which is more common in adults. *See also* SHINGLES.

Q: *How is chickenpox treated?*

A: Calamine lotion has a soothing effect on the irritating spots, and a physician may prescribe an antihistamine drug (also useful for its sedative effect) to reduce the irritation. It is most important to keep the patient from scratching the spots, because further infection can easily result if the skin is broken. For this reason, babies and small children may sometimes have to wear gloves. A physician may prescribe acetaminophen, which is taken every four hours to reduce the fever and headache. A child must be encouraged to drink plenty of liquids. Nightwear and bedclothes should be light and preferably made of cotton, because wool and synthetic fabrics are likely to be irritating to the skin.

Q: *Where else do spots occur apart from the back and chest?*

A: Spots may spread to the rest of the trunk and face, as well as to the limbs. Spots may also appear in the mucous membranes, such as those of the mouth and vagina, or in the ears.

Q: *Can complications result from chickenpox?*

A: Complications are rare, but chest infections, such as bronchitis and pneumonia, sinusitis, and middle ear infection (otitis media), may occur. These can all be treated effectively with prescribed antibiotics. A more serious possible complication is encephalitis (brain inflammation). *See also* ENCEPHALITIS.

Q: *How long is it before a child is back to normal after chickenpox?*

A: A child may be irritable and unusually tired for about a week after the symptoms of chickenpox have disappeared, so it is important that he or she does not return to school too soon after the illness.

Chigger (chig'ər), or jigger, is the common name of a mite that is found in tall grass and weeds. The chigger attaches itself to the skin, generally on the legs, feet, around the waist, or in the armpit or groin, where it causes irritation and intense local itching. A swelling forms where the insect attaches and feeds, and this may become ulcerated and infected. This swelling is treated by opening it with a sterilized needle to remove the chigger. Antiseptic cream is then applied. Clothing that was worn should be washed immediately to help prevent further infestation. Persons walking in areas where chigger infestation is present should use insect repellents and should bathe and change clothes shortly after exposure to the chigger.

Dirt that enters the skin as the chigger becomes attached may cause tetanus if the individual has not been immunized.

See also CHIGOE.

Chigoe (chig'ō), often called jigger, is a burrowing flea found in the tropics of America and Africa. The pregnant female flea burrows into the skin, usually of the feet, causing intense inflammation. Infection can lead to loss of a toe.

Chilblain (chil'blān) is an inflammation of the skin, usually occurring on the toes, fingers, ears, or face. The inflammation is due to cold, damp weather that damages small blood vessels and nerves in the skin. People with poor blood circulation are especially prone to chilblains. Tobacco increases the risk of chilblain, as it constricts the blood vessels. A chilblain may cause aching, burning, and itching, especially when the body becomes warmer. Some children form ulcers that may leave scars after healing.

Treatment includes warm, protective clothing and gentle warming of affected areas. The affected areas should not be rubbed, and extreme heat should not be applied directly; these measures may cause further damage. Corticosteroid creams may help soothe the itching skin.

Child is a person between about 18 months and 13 years of age. Childhood is thus the stage of development between infancy and adolescence.

During childhood most boys and girls nearly double their height and quadruple their weight. They begin to develop sexually. Their behavior, thought processes, emotions, and attitudes all undergo significant changes.

The Stages of Childhood

There are four major stages in a child's development: the toddler stage, the preschool years, the early school years, and the preteen years.

The Toddler Stage lasts from about 18 months to 3 years of age. A child's physical growth is generally slower during this second 18 months of life than it was during the first 18 months.

By 18 months of age, most children can feed themselves, walk and run a short distance, stack some blocks, and say a few meaningful words. A toddler is expected to improve all these skills.

One of the first standards that all children are expected to learn is control of the bowels and bladder—a process called toilet training. However, the age when such control becomes possible varies greatly among children. Most toddlers have started to develop it by the age of two years. Patience and positive encouragement for successes are much more effective in helping the child gain control than are punishment or shaming.

The development of language skills—especially the building of sentences—is a major challenge. Most two-year-olds use one or two words for an entire thought. Parents can not always be sure what the words mean. For example, a child who says "milk" or "milk gone" may mean anything from "I want some milk" to "I just spilled my milk." By three years of age, however, most children can link several words together to form a fairly complete sentence. They can speak about 900 words—an enormous increase over the average 10 to 20 word vocabulary at 18 months of age.

Playing with toys not only tests skills, but is also a way of learning to play with children of the same age, thus developing social relationships. Until the age of about two years, the toddler seldom plays directly with other children, partly because of the lack of social skills, partly because of shyness, and also because of a feeling of possessiveness about toys and belongings. Slowly, sociability increases out of a similarity of interest and friendship. By three years of age, children start to realize that they have things in common with other children. They then begin to regard them as equals.

Toddlers form their strongest attachments to their parents or substitute parents. In most cases, the mother is especially looked to for help, comfort, and companionship. Above all, toddlers want to feel assured that they have their parents' acceptance and approval. As a result, they are sensitive to any sign of rejection or disapproval.

Anger is a frightening thing to a small child, not only parental anger toward him or her, but also the child's anger toward the parents. The parent should indicate that his or her anger expresses displeasure with what the child has done, and not a dislike for the child. After the angry emotion has passed, it is important that the parent show physical signs of affection toward the toddler. It is equally important that the child learn that losing one's temper never achieves anything, otherwise he or she may start using anger as a weapon to succeed when other methods have failed. The toddler with temper tantrums eventually learns to control them when he or she finds they are ignored and are a waste of energy and time.

The toddler needs abundant praise and attention for good behavior. "Positive reinforcement" does more to model desired behavior than does any negative punishment.

The Preschool Years extend from about three to five years of age. Preschoolers are highly active and constantly exploring the world around them. At the same time, they are beginning to learn that there are certain standards of behavior—things they should and should not do.

By about three or four years of age, the majority of children have become increasingly aware of themselves and of other people. They are not only more conscious of their own actions, but they have also begun to realize that other people have feelings like their own. Children then start to govern some of their actions according to the pleasure or displeasure that they give another person.

Many standards of behavior are taught to children of preschool age. These standards include obedience, truthfulness, respect for property, and

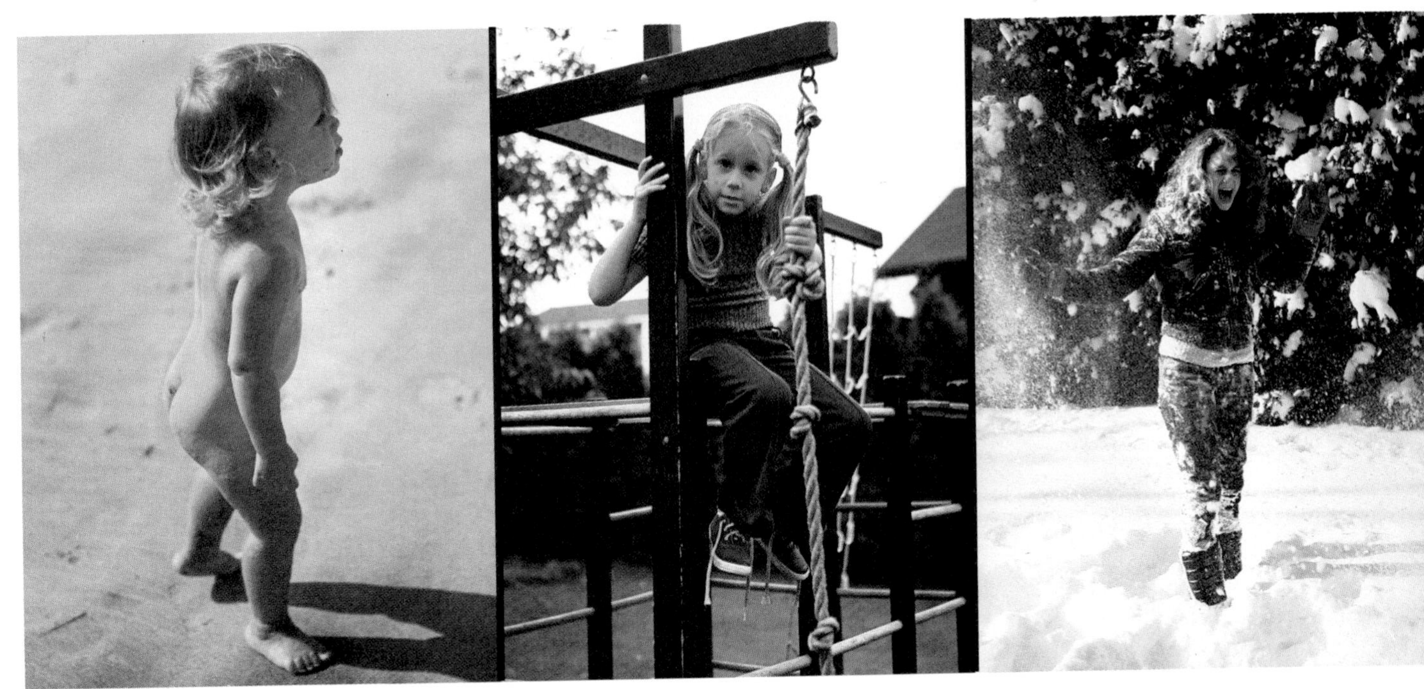

A **child** undergoes significant physical changes throughout childhood. Here are three photos of the same child at two years, *left*, six years, *center*, and twelve years, *above*.

various sex role standards—that is, the roles that people are expected to play as males or females. Today there is much less rigidity in sex role standards than in previous times.

Preschoolers also learn standards of behavior through an unconscious process called identification. The process often begins during the toddler stage, but it becomes fully developed during the preschool years. Children identify with another person if they feel that they have the same physical and psychological characteristics as that person. Most children identify with one or more members of their family, especially their parents.

Preschools. Many children begin to attend preschool at age three or four. A good preschool allows children to develop social skills and an interest in learning and discovery. There should be adequate staff to work with the children, and attention should be paid to maintaining a safe environment. Parents should observe the preschool class "in action" as part of the process of choosing a preschool.

Social Skills are also being developed as the preschooler's friendships are constantly being tested by disagreements and quarrels. Similar interests and enthusiasms, and the need for a friend with whom to play games, help to resolve most disagreements in the same way that the child has learned to cope with disagreements in the family. By sharing and enjoying experiences with other children, the preschooler begins to feel the benefit of independence from his or her parents.

The preschool child will assert his or her independence from others who try to prevent him or her from doing what he or she wishes. This rapidly leads to quarrels with brothers and sisters, who are also trying to do what they wish. The conflict is healthy and natural, even if it leads to lost tempers and tears. It is important that the parents not interfere at the onset of every quarrel. Children must learn that fairness and justice can be achieved from a balance of interest. They soon find out that the sole possession of a favorite toy may lead to the loss of a companion in some other game. Giving and taking in the home is an introduction to the outer world, where the same balance has to be achieved to maintain friendships that are built without family bonds.

Inevitably, a violent and vicious fight must be stopped, as the older or larger child usually wins. Even so, it is important that the parent not take sides. The parent is there to prevent real harm. At this point the children frequently ask, either directly or indirectly, for parental judgment on the quarrel. An explanation of the judg-

Development of drawing skills

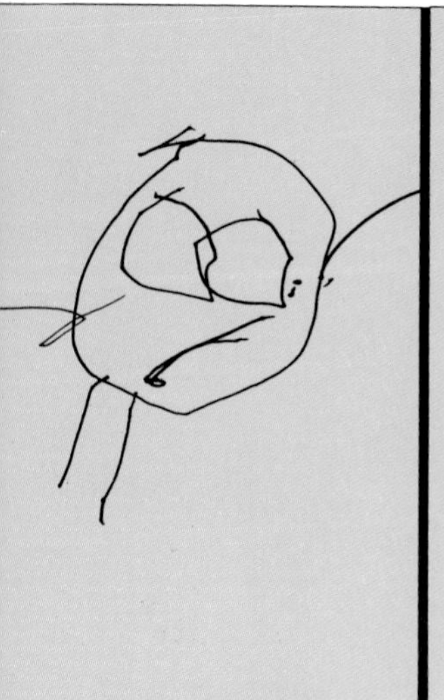

Two-year-old child
This picture shows a two-year-old child's drawing of a person. The head and facial features are the most prominent parts in the drawing. This is because, even at this age, a child learns to associate specific facial expressions with adult approval or disapproval.

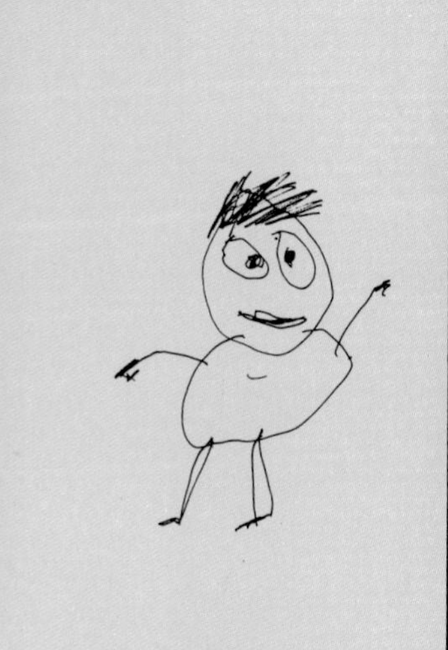

Three-year-old child
This picture shows a three-year-old child's drawing of a person. The head and face are still the major components of the drawing, but the body also appears, although in a very rudimentary form and out of proportion with the head.

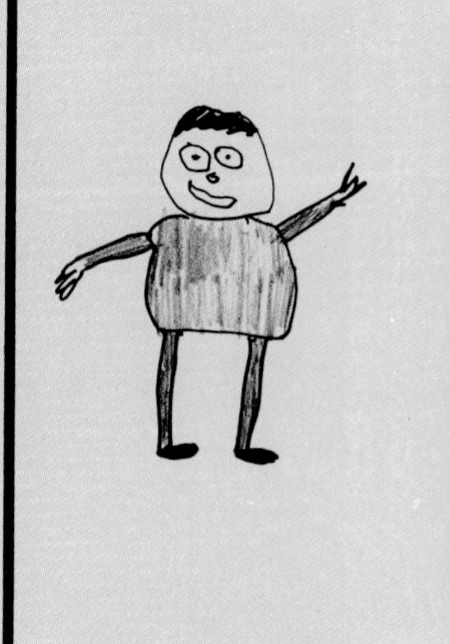

Seven-year-old child
This picture shows a seven-year-old child's drawing of a person. The child's nervous system has by now developed sufficiently to enable him or her to draw a relatively life-like picture that shows all the main features—head, body, arms and hands, and legs and feet.

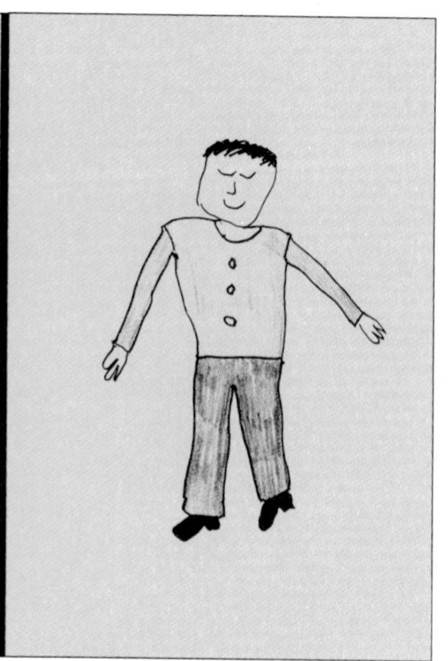

Fourteen-year-old child
This picture shows a fourteen-year-old child's drawing of a person. By this age, the nervous system has matured almost completely and the child has a high degree of coordination between hand and eye. This can be seen in the drawing in which the person's features are in life-like proportions.

ment should be given. At the same time the parent should point out that, no matter who was right in the quarrel, violence on either side is not an acceptable way of resolving a problem. It should be stressed that both children are equally at fault in this and must be aware of it.

Discipline. Most parents use rewards and punishments to teach their children standards of behavior. This is a form of discipline that the child understands readily, provided it is consistent and fair. A word of praise or a hug is usually a sufficient reward. Punishment usually consists of a strong "no," always accompanied by an explanation.

Punishment should only be an occasional weapon used in the longer process of discipline. It is important, however, not to get into a habit of threatening punishment without carrying it out. Physical punishment should generally be avoided. If it must be used, it should be immediate and directly related to the offense. A sharp smack on the hand of the naughty preschooler may be needed if the child is about to do something harmful to himself or herself or to another. A normal, affectionate relationship will not be harmed by such disciplinary action. Anger also makes a strong impression on the child. However, too much parental anger and temper soon loses its effect. Disapproval at the right moment is frequently a sufficient punishment.

Sex Education. All children ask questions, and sooner or later these include queries about sex. Simple questions need simple, direct, and honest answers, not lengthy lectures. A child may find it difficult to believe an answer and may ask the same question two or three days later. It is often easier for a child to believe that a newborn baby is bought at the shop, than it is to understand that it takes nine months to grow inside the mother's tummy after the father has implanted a seed in an egg located there. Honest, direct, understandable answers to questions are the best approach.

In helping to illustrate an answer, examples should be used. For instance, if the mother becomes pregnant again, the child can be allowed to feel the growing baby moving around inside. A description of how the cat has kittens is a help toward understanding childbirth. Watching an animal suckling its young introduces the topic of breast-feeding. Children may see dogs mating. If a child asks about it, he or she is ready to know. Parents may wish to mention the fact that it is possible to prevent fertilization by using contraception.

The whole topic should be discussed openly enough so that the child does not feel that questions about sex are different from his or her questions on any other subject. This leaves the child free to ask about sex when he or she is ready to understand.

It is always difficult to know how much a child remembers and whether he or she has linked up apparently isolated questions into a complete understanding. By the time the child goes to school, much of the initial curiosity has died down. There is often an apparent lack of sexual interest until puberty. The child has an increased understanding, but decreased interest.

Safety. A major problem for parents is to warn preschool children of the dangers of strangers, without making them frightened of an outside world that may already be causing stresses and anxieties. A child is more likely to be puzzled rather than frightened by a man who exposes himself. If a child is frightened by the experience, it should be explained that such people are in need of help and seldom do any harm. Care should be taken in the future not to let the child out alone where it may happen again.

The true molester is a far more serious problem. Children must be told never to accept rides from strangers or to believe people who say that they have been sent to collect them from school.

The Early School Years, which last from age five to eight, mark a major turning point in a child's psychological development. Children continue to improve their physical skills during this stage, but the period is distinguished mainly by important advances in a child's mental, emotional, and social development.

By the fifth year, most children have been taught basic standards of social behavior and have learned to judge whether particular actions are right or wrong. The majority of three- and four-year-olds do not know they have a choice in their actions. If something they do displeases their parents, they feel anxious, ashamed, or sorry, but they do not blame themselves for the action. By about five years of age, however, most children start to realize that they can choose one action rather than another. Children then begin to feel guilt, as well as shame, if they behave wrongly. Such children are thus ready to begin a more formal education. School-age children have to discover how to cope with a new environment and how to compromise their desire for freedom with the restrictions of school discipline. The parents can help in this adjustment by showing an interest in their children's work and play and by talking to the teachers about their progress. Such involvement is appreciated by both the teachers and the children.

A child may have anxieties and fears about the first few days at any school. This is normal, and most schools will let the parent stay for a little while until the child has met the new classmates and teachers and has had a look around the school. Most children fit into a pattern of school life and discipline in a few days.

Problems may arise for some children from bullying or from teasing. The reasons why a child becomes a bully are complicated. It may be because of problems or tensions at home that are not noticeable to outsiders. It is difficult to take a bully in hand without causing problems between families. School authorities should be notified. The child being picked on should be told that the bully may be a very unhappy child and that violence on his or her side would not make the situation better.

Teasing may be aimed at some obvious or imagined defect. A birthmark or deformity may be commented on by other children, or they may pick on some minor problem, such as blushing. Teasing always continues if the child reacts openly to it, but the teasing soon stops if the child is able to ignore it. Sometimes, a child is called a nickname by which he or she becomes known throughout school life, regardless of the initial reaction. Parental reassurance and acceptance is vital to help the child who is subject to teasing. The attitude of those the child loves gives him or her the best basis for ignoring teasing. A physical problem that may be amenable to treatment should be discussed with the child's physician if the problem is a source of unhappiness or teasing for the child.

It is very important for parents to show an active, daily interest in the child's schooling. Such support is essential. It is often surprising how, with just a little reassurance, a child is able to cope with most school problems by himself or herself.

Intellectual/Emotional Maturation. Every schoolchild is expected to learn to solve problems, a skill that improves with practice. A five-year-old may try to solve a problem by choosing the first solution that comes to mind. But a six- or seven-year-old thinks about other possible solutions and recognizes why one is better than another. Children this age also begin to see how things are alike and how they differ. Finally, children gain confidence in their mental powers and start to enjoy solving problems correctly.

By the age of seven or eight, most children begin to rationalize their beliefs—that is, to find reasons for holding them. They may thus decide that the standards of behavior they have learned are good or bad. Children this age also increasingly compare themselves with other youngsters. Such comparisons contribute to a child's opinion of himself or herself. Such a self-image formed during childhood can influence a person's behavior throughout life.

Children actually begin to form a self-image during the preschool years as they identify with their parents or other family members. A child's self-image is favorable or unfavorable, depending on the attitudes and emotions of the persons with whom the child identifies. For example, children who see mainly negative qualities in their parents will likely view themselves in a negative light. Children form a more favorable self-image if they have a better impression of their parents. When children compare themselves with other children, they reinforce or alter their basic self-image.

The Preteenage Years extend from about age 8 to 13. This stage is also known as preadolescence. During preadolescence, the rate of physical growth, which had been declining since infancy, increases sharply. The preteenager begins to grow heavier and taller and to develop the sexual characteristics of an adult. Most girls, for example, have their first menstrual period by age 12 or 13. Most boys develop hair on their body and face, and their voice deepens. The entire stage during which a person matures sexually is called puberty. Some children reach sexual maturity before age 13. But the majority do not become sexually mature until the early teenage years.

During the preteenage years, a child's circle of friends and acquaintances, the peer group, plays an increasingly important role in the child's development. Preteens begin to look chiefly to their peer group, rather than to their parents, for acceptance and approval. They judge themselves according to peer group standards, adjusting their self-image accordingly. A child's behavior may also change noticeably under peer group pressure.

During late preadolescence, children may begin to worry if a new standard of behavior conflicts with an earlier one. They often relieve such anxieties by talking them over with their friends. Nevertheless, older preadolescents feel a growing need to keep their beliefs consistent. They may therefore revise or reject a conflicting standard. Children this age also begin to reason that a "wrong" action may be permitted under some circumstances.

Individual Differences among Children

Two main forces—heredity and environment—account for the individual differences among children. Heredity is the process by which children inherit physical and mental traits from their parents. Environment consists of all the things in a child's surroundings that affect the child's development of the inherited traits.

Individual differences among children are caused by heredity and environment acting together, not separately. In general, heredity limits what the environment can do in influencing a

Toys for different ages

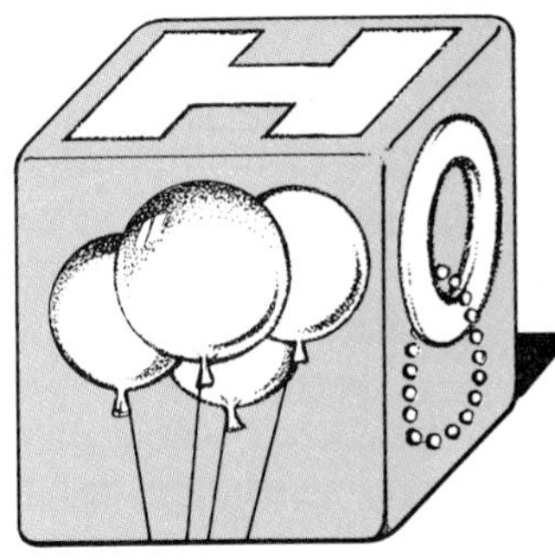

Up to six months

Balloons or streamers for the baby to watch. Toys hung across the crib or carriage within the baby's reach. Rattles that small hands can easily grasp. Teething rings, or interesting toys, too large to swallow but satisfying to bite or chew on.

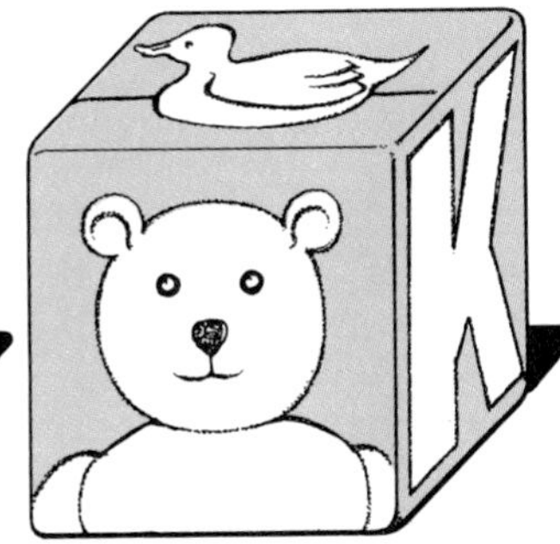

Six to eighteen months

Soft toys to hold and snuggle. Plastic bath toys. Jugs and cups for pouring. Toys on wheels to push or pull. Balls to roll and follow. Household objects, such as paper to rattle and tear. Blocks to pile up and knock down. Hammer and pegs.

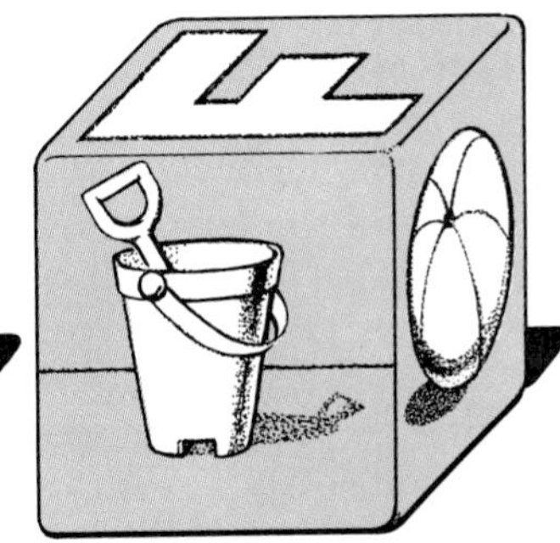

Eighteen months to three years

Bucket and spade for the sand box. Swings and slides. Simple jigsaw puzzles. Toy telephone. Thick crayons and large sheets of paper. Paints and big brushes. Blackboard and chalk. Dolls to dress and undress. Miniature cooking utensils. Dollhouse.

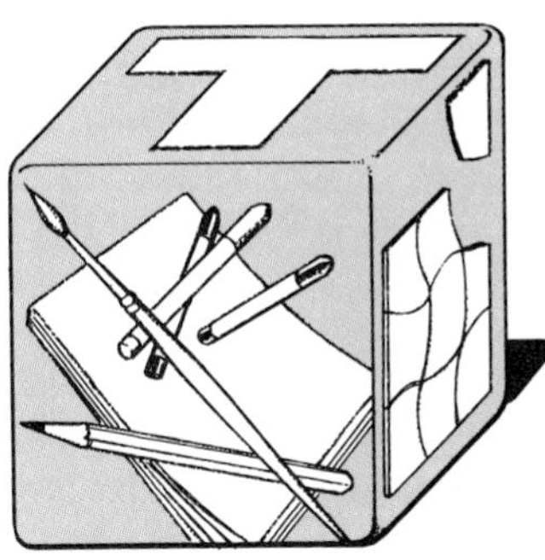

Three to five years

Ready-mixed and powder paint with plenty of paper. Pencils and crayons. Construction sets with large pieces in wood or plastic. Toys to "play house" with. Garage, fort, or farm sets. Blunt scissors and a scrap book. Dominoes. Simple card games. Tricycle.

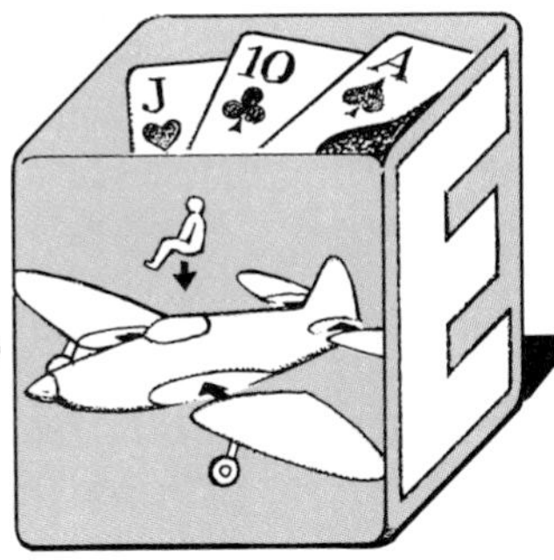

Five to eight years

Construction sets with small pieces. Modeling kits for careful painting and gluing. Carpentry tools (begin a set). Dice, board games, more complicated card games. Glove puppets; string puppets for an older child. Scooter or bicycle for outdoors.

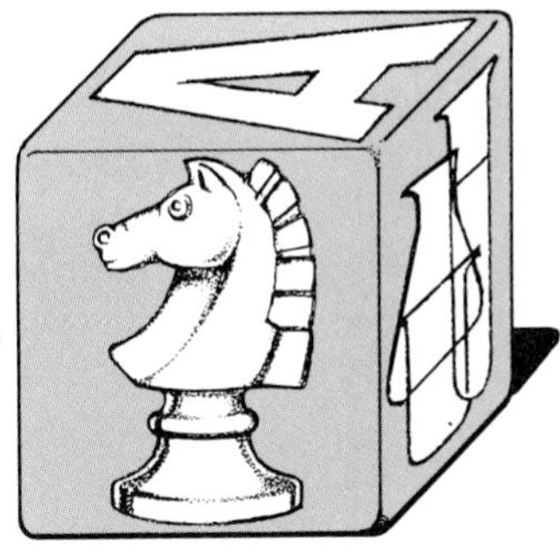

Eight years and over

Practical chemistry sets and realistic scientific equipment. Weaving, basketmaking, or other craft sets. Sewing and mending sets. Board games—checkers, chess, Monopoly®. Toy theater. Magic sets. A box with clothes and masks for dressing up.

child's development. For example, every child inherits a tendency to grow to a certain height. Not even the best environmental conditions will enable a child to grow much taller than this height. Children need the right conditions, including proper nourishment and exercise, to grow as tall as their heredity allows. Heredity and environment together thus determine the physical differences among children. The two forces together also account for individual differences in intelligence.

Physical Differences. Children differ greatly in their physical appearance and rate of growth. For example, the normal weight for 9-year-old boys ranges from 56 to 81 pounds (25 to 37kg). Their normal height may be 50 to 56 inches (130 to 140cm). The normal ranges for 9-year-old girls are slightly lower. But most girls grow rapidly at about 9 to 12 years of age. Girls are normally heavier and taller than boys during these years. At about age 12, however, most boys start to grow rapidly, and the girls' growth rate declines. By age 14, most boys are again heavier and taller than most girls their age. Some children begin this rapid growth a year or two earlier or later than the majority. Children are not necessarily abnormal if their height and weight vary somewhat from the normal ranges for their age.

Differences in Intelligence among children are usually measured by IQ (intelligence quotient) tests. These tests are designed to indicate a child's general mental ability in relation to other children of the same age. Each child's performance on the tests is rated by an IQ score. On most such tests, about two-thirds of all children score from 84 to 116. About one-sixth score below 84, and one-sixth score above 116.

The IQ scores of persons related by blood generally differ less than do the scores of unrelated persons. Some experts, therefore, conclude that general mental ability is largely inherited and is only slightly affected by environment. Other experts, however, believe that environment has a strong influence on a person's intelligence. Their view is supported by studies of culturally deprived children. Children are considered culturally deprived if their home life lacks the kinds of experiences that will help them profit from formal schooling. Many such children have an IQ score below 80. In a number of cases, culturally deprived children have dramatically improved their score after receiving educational and environmental enrichment.

Some experts question the usefulness of IQ tests on the grounds that they do not measure basic mental skills. These experts point out that intelligence involves a variety of separate powers, such as memory, logic, evaluation, and originality. A child may have little ability in some of these areas, but exceptional talent in one or more other areas. The critics, therefore, believe that children should be tested and evaluated for each mental skill separately. IQ testing is also often culturally biased, so that children from different cultures may test poorly because of unfamiliarity with objects or phrases used in the testing.

Special Problems of Childhood

Some children develop patterns of behavior that are a problem to themselves and to the people around them. Such behavior may be a symptom of a deeper psychological or physical disorder or may represent a reaction to family stress.

A child's behavior is a problem if it differs widely from normal behavior; has undesirable consequences or side effects; and distresses the child or the parents. All three conditions generally must be present before behavior becomes viewed as a problem. For example, a child who shows exceptional ability in school differs greatly from most other school children. But the child's behavior is not considered abnormal because it does not usually have undesirable consequences or cause psychological distress.

Two of the most common behavioral problems of childhood are unrealistic fears and aggressive and antisocial behavior.

Unrealistic Fears. All children are afraid on occasion, as fear is a normal emotion. Fears are unrealistic if they occur regularly in the absence of real danger. In some cases, such fears may be directly related to a frightening past experience. For example, a child who has a fear of all animals may have developed the fear after being attacked by an animal. In other cases, unrealistic fears may be only indirectly related to a past event. For instance, a child who feels extreme guilt over an action may expect severe punishment. The child may then develop an abnormal fear of death, accidents, or illness.

Aggressive and Antisocial Behavior. Psychologists define aggression as angry, hostile behavior that is intended to hurt or upset others. Such behavior in young children can result from frustration. Children may feel frustrated if their demands are not met or if their feelings of worthiness and self-respect are threatened. If a child's anger becomes intense, it may erupt into a tantrum—a common form of aggression in young children.

Children can learn to control aggression if they are taught at an early age that some of their demands will not be met. A child who develops such a frustration tolerance is less likely to have severe or frequent tantrums. Children may have great difficulty developing the necessary tolerance if their parents are overly strict or overly permissive. If parents are too strict, a child may feel increasingly frustrated in trying to meet their high goals. If they are too permissive, the child may react aggressively to any frustration. In addition, parents encourage aggression if they are frequently angry and hostile themselves.

Violent behavior on television may heighten the aggressive tendencies of a child who considers such behavior permissible. Children are less likely to be influenced by TV violence if they have learned that violent behavior is wrong. In the end, the day-to-day behavior of parents themselves has a more powerful influence on their children than do isolated events and experiences.

Most children learn to control aggression by the preteenage years. They may do so partly by channeling their energies into hobbies, sports, schoolwork, and other activities. Some children, however, do not learn to deal with aggression effectively. Instead, they may relieve feelings of frustration and hostility by antisocial behavior, such as bullying other children, stealing, or destroying property. Such behavior worsens if the peer group encourages it.

Other special problems may also be symptoms of psychological or physical disorders. These problems include hyperactivity or extreme restlessness; poor performance in school; extreme shyness; and bedwetting.

Hyperactivity. Most hyperactive children can not concentrate on anything for more than a few minutes at a time. Scientists do not know the exact cause of the disturbance. Although some physicians claim that some cases may be caused by an allergy to certain chemical additives in food, especially particular food colorings and dyes, there is little solid evidence to support this theory; it remains controversial.

Poor Performance in School is frequently caused by a child's failure to learn to read. In many cases, however, reading problems can be avoided if parents prepare their children for learning to read. Parents should, thus, make a practice of reading stories and poems to their children during the toddler and preschool years. Parents should also acquaint their children with books and other reading materials and help them build a vocabulary. Children who lack such preparation may fall behind their classmates in learning to read. Children also need a motive for learning to read. Parents help provide such a motive if they show that they value learning.

Failure in reading may be due to a physical or psychological problem, such as poor eyesight, poor hearing, or extreme shyness. The reading ability of most hyperactive or mentally retarded children is severely limited.

School avoidance may develop in the child who is performing poorly in school, who is threatened or teased by other children, or when family problems have made the child insecure about being away from home. The physician should be consulted promptly if this becomes a recurrent problem so that the child can be helped to return to school.

Extreme Shyness. In some cases, children become overly shy if they are dominated by older brothers and sisters. Shyness may also begin as an inherited tendency. However, the precise causes of extreme shyness are not well understood.

Bed-wetting. A habit of bed-wetting after about five years of age may reflect a physical problem, such as bladder infection, or may be due to psychological distress. Parents should not punish or threaten a child who has the problem. In every case, a physician should be consulted to evaluate the problem and recommend the appropriate form of treatment.

The Role of Parents

Mothers and fathers can best promote the development of their children in three major ways: understanding a child's basic needs; reinforcing appropriate behavior; and serving as models of appropriate behavior.

Understanding a Child's Basic Needs. All children have certain basic physical and psychological needs. Both sets of needs must be met if a child is to develop normally. Poor physical health may harm a child's psychological development, and psychological problems may affect a child physically.

Physical Needs. Children need regular, nourishing meals, adequate sleep, proper clothing, and a clean, comfortable home. They also require a reasonable amount of play and exercise and enough space to play in. In addition, children who learn good health habits and safety practices reduce the risk of diseases and accidents.

If a child should become sick, the parent will often realize it before the child does. No longer cheerful and enthusiastic, the little boy or girl becomes tearful and quiet at the onset of illness. A child on the verge of illness, like one who is overtired, may rebel against the idea of giving up a game or going to bed.

Young children find it difficult to explain what is the matter with them. Vomiting and diarrhea are obvious signs of illness, but a child may not mention a headache or sore throat. Symptoms can be misleading; for example, aching limbs or stomachache may be caused by tonsillitis or influenza. A child with a high fever may feel hot and seem sleepy, but yet complain of nothing. A parent usually knows all the variations of behavior in the child and can assess most accurately whether something is seriously wrong.

Improved health care has greatly increased the life expectancy of children in many countries during the 1900's. For example, such diseases as diphtheria and whooping cough formerly killed thousands of children every year. The development of immunization programs has sharply reduced the death rate from these diseases. Most children receive their first immunizations before 18 months of age. A child should be reimmunized for diphtheria, polio, tetanus, and whooping cough at about four to six years of age.

Psychological Needs. Basic psychological needs are the same for all children, although they may be modified by the skills and personality traits of a particular child.

Toddlers need to develop self-confidence, and so they must feel loved, wanted, and respected. They should also have enough verbal stimulation and variety in their routine to help them develop language skills. Preschoolers especially need close contact with adults they like and admire. Such contacts help promote normal emotional development and attachment.

Children are expected to behave more responsibly after they reach school age. They must, therefore, be able to comprehend that required standards of behavior are predictable and stable. Preteens have a strong need to feel as successful as other children their age. Success often means measuring up to the sex role valued by society. The preteen thus requires freedom to develop the appropriate masculine or feminine qualities. Overly rigid gender stereotyping is limiting and frustrating for many adolescents.

Reinforcing the Child's Behavior. Parents motivate a child when they encourage the child to adopt a certain type of behavior. Rewarding good behavior is the most effective means of motivation. Persistent misbehavior should be punished, but punishment should be just. Children will understandably be upset if they are punished for behavior that they continually see in their parents. Children should be made to feel that they were personally responsible for improvements in their behavior.

Appropriate rewards and punishments work in most cases of problem behavior. Children whose parents regularly encourage schoolwork are more likely to succeed in school than are children who lack such encouragement. A child who is taught to control aggression is less likely to become a bully than is a child who is not taught such control. Motivation is not always effective, however, because other factors also influence a child's behavior. For example, children can not be motivated to learn to read if they believe they lack the ability. Parents may also be unable to motivate a child who feels resentful or hostile toward them.

Serving as Models of Appropriate Behavior. Children model themselves largely on their parents, mainly through identification. Children identify with a parent when they believe they have the qualities and feelings that are characteristic of that parent. The things parents do and say—and the way they do and say them—therefore strongly influence a child's behavior. Parents should strive to provide a consistent role model of appropriate behavior for their children.

A parent's actions also affect the self-image that children form through identification. Children who see mainly positive qualities in their parents will likely learn to see themselves in a positive way. Children who observe chiefly negative qualities in their parents will have difficulty seeing positive qualities in themselves. Children may modify their self-image, however, as they become increasingly influenced by peer group standards during the preteenage years. This peer group influence may also be a positive or negative experience.

Loss and Grieving

Isolated events, even dramatic ones, do not necessarily have a permanent effect on a child's behavior. Children interpret such events according to their established attitudes and previous experiences. For example, children who know they are loved are better able to accept the divorce of their parents or a parent's early death. But if children feel insecure, they may interpret such events as a sign of rejection or punishment.

Death is a difficult subject for children and parents to deal with. Often, the death of a favorite pet is the first introduction to the idea of life and death. As the child is unable to think of abstract ideas before the preteenage years, death must be discussed in a matter-of-fact way; and a logical explanation of what happens after death must be given. It is just as difficult for a child to accept that his or her puppy is dead and buried in the ground, as it is to accept the death of a grandparent or parent.

Parents should not be afraid to show grief after the death of a loved one. The child must learn about emotions and how to express them. This is a way of learning how to cope with his or her own feelings. The child should realize that not only does life continue, but grief also becomes less acute with time. It is difficult for a child to deal with personal emotions if the parents seem to have none. A child may think the parents callous or may feel that feelings of grief are abnormal and wrong and should be suppressed.

Parenting is a rewarding but complex and demanding job. Often, parents are confused as to whether they are doing the "right" thing in disciplining or teaching their children. Sharing experiences and concerns with other parents and with the physician often provides support and reassurance.

Child abuse is the physical, emotional, or sexual mistreatment of a child. The child's parent or guardian is the most common abuser. Child abuse includes such acts as severely beating a child, starving a child, or having an incestuous relationship with a child. Child neglect is the failure of the parent or guardian to take care of the child's physical, educational, medical, and/or emotional needs. Child abuse or neglect may result in permanent physical or psychological damage. Abuse can sometimes be fatal, especially in younger children.

Because child abuse is usually an act of private violence (done in the home), the exact incidence is difficult to determine. Reports of child abuse have increased in the United States over the last few years, but this may be due more to an increased awareness of the problem, as well as improved methods of reporting it, rather than to an actual increase in the incidence of abuse.

Q: *What causes child abuse?*

A: Child abuse is the result of a complex set of variables that involves the parent, child, and the external environment. Often, there is a failure or breakdown in self-control on the part of the parent or guardian. Many experts cite four primary reasons for this breakdown.

(1) *Childhood Experience of the Abusive Parent.* Abusive individuals often received little warmth or affection themselves as children and consequently are unable to bestow warmth and affection on their own children. Studies have shown that over 90 percent of the parents in abusive households were abused as children. Abusive parents typically lack self-esteem and are prone to frustration and temper tantrums.

(2) *The "Different" Child.* Children who differ from accepted norms may inadvertently trigger abuse from a parent. Such children

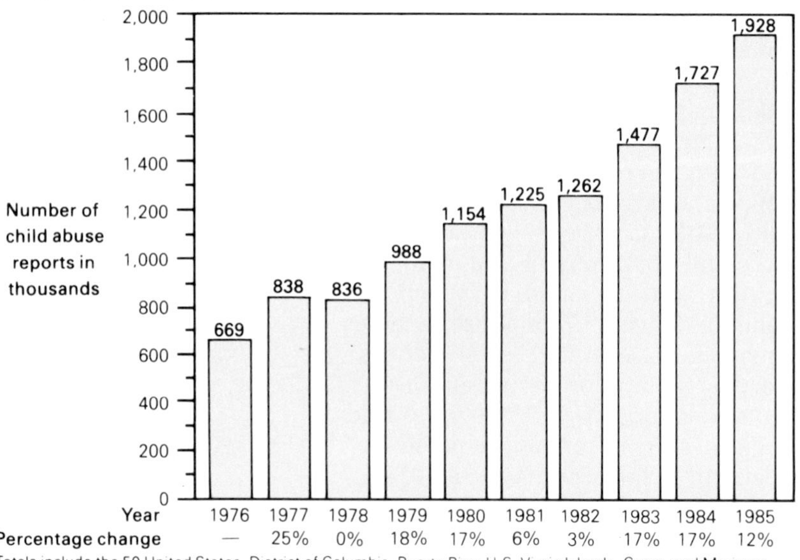

Reports of **child abuse** have increased in the United States over the last few years. This may, however, be due to an increased awareness of the problem, rather than an actual increase in the incidence of abuse.

may be hyperactive, have special physical or emotional needs, or simply cry a lot. A premature baby or a child with congenital abnormalities may also unwittingly help foster abuse by a frustrated parent who is prone to violence. In some cases an abused child may not measure up to other siblings in such areas as academics or athletics. The age of the child is also an important ingredient in abuse. Small children are more likely to be victims of abuse, because they are more demanding of parental time and attention and are less able to defend themselves.

(3) *The Isolated Parent.* A parent may lack a network of family or friends to provide support during stressful periods. Such a parent may lash out at a child when there is nowhere else to turn.

(4) *A Crisis Situation.* A crisis may precipitate abuse, particularly when support is unavailable. Abuse may occur as a result of a major crisis, such as a parent losing a job, or it may be triggered by a minor event, such as a bathtub overflowing. Alcohol, money problems, drugs, and other health problems may also contribute to child abuse.

Q: *What are some signs of child abuse?*

A: Obvious physical signs, such as burns, welts, or bruises, are common indications of child abuse, particularly when they are recurrent, and the explanations are vague or suspicious. Symptoms of emotional abuse are more difficult to spot. A child who is excessively moody or conspicuously lacking in self-esteem may be a victim of persistent criticism or ridicule on the part of a parent. Sexual abuse is also difficult to identify. Usually there are no physical symptoms, and both the child and the parent are normally reluctant to reveal the incestuous relationship.

Although reporting of possible child abuse cases is important in helping to modify a destructive environment, care must be taken not to suspect parents or guardians without cause. Not all burns and bruises, even highly unusual ones, are signs of child abuse.

Q: *How should child abuse be treated?*

A: Treatment of families affected by child abuse should be undertaken with a view toward a long-range, comprehensive resolution. Ideally, a number of professionals will be involved, including a social worker, physician, psychologist or psychiatrist, and perhaps others. It is extremely important to approach the family in a helping, rather than accusatory or punitive, manner. In some cases the abused child may be removed from the home, either temporarily or, on occasion, permanently.

Being aware of a situation that helps foster abuse may help prevent its occurrence. High-risk parents, such as those who were abused as children, should be made aware of the cyclical nature of violence. An organization called Parents Anonymous exists to help families in which a child is abused. Parental stress hotlines are available for parents who are having difficulties coping with their children.

Medical professionals are bound by law to report cases of suspected child abuse or neglect. All persons, however, have a moral responsibility to report such cases. An individual who makes a report in good faith is immune from any legal action against him or her by the alleged abusing party. Many states have a toll-free telephone number for reporting suspected cases of child abuse or neglect.

Childbirth is the process of having a baby.

See also CHILDBIRTH: EMERGENCY DELIVERY; CHILDBIRTH, NATURAL; PREGNANCY AND CHILDBIRTH.

Childbirth: emergency delivery. Labor is divided into three stages. During the first stage regular abdominal pains begin as the woman's uterine muscles start to tighten and relax in a rhythmic pattern. These pains become longer and stronger as labor progresses. There may be a low backache and a discharge of bloodstained mucus. The "breaking of waters" may also occur during this first stage when clear fluid (the amniotic fluid) is expelled. The first stage may last an average of 13 to 14 hours (each woman is a little different), but is usually shorter for women who have had previous children.

The second stage of labor is the birth of the baby. The third stage is the delivery of the afterbirth (placenta).

Action. Keep calm. There is usually ample time to prepare for the birth. Summon medical assistance. If medical help is on its way, collect the mother's belongings and be ready for the transfer to a hospital. If aid is unlikely to arrive in time, prepare to help with the birth. (See accompanying illustrations for step-by-step instructions.)

If in a public place, find somewhere that provides privacy and is quiet and warm. It is essential that everything is scrupulously clean. Nobody with a cold or any other infection should help. Scrub your hands thoroughly, preferably under running water. If they become soiled later, wash them again.

By the start of the second stage of labor, the birth canal is fully dilated and the top of the baby's head is visible. Instruct the mother to continue to push. When most of the baby's head has emerged, the mother should not bear down and should not hold her breath during the contractions. Ask the mother to pant; this allows the rest of the baby's head to emerge slowly. The head of a newborn baby may be misshapen. Do not be alarmed. The head has been temporarily deformed by its passage through the birth canal, and it eventually reverts to normal shape.

Do not interfere with the progress of the birth by attempting to pull the baby out. If a membrane is covering the baby's face, it must be carefully torn. If the baby emerges with the umbilical cord around the neck, try to ease the cord over the head. Take great care not to stretch or break the cord.

Rarely will the baby's buttocks, foot, or arm emerge first. If so, do not interfere. If any part other than the head emerges first, make arrangements for immediate careful transportation to a hospital.

The contractions begin again shortly after the delivery of the baby. This is the third stage of labor, the delivery of the afterbirth (placenta). *Do not* try to speed up this process by pulling on the umbilical cord.

If the contractions continue and a second head appears instead of the placenta being expelled, the mother is bearing identical twins. *Do not* cut the cord. Attend to the first baby, then follow the same procedures to deliver the second baby. The placenta will follow with two cords attached.

If the birth appears to be normal, but the contractions continue after the placenta has been delivered, the mother is probably bearing nonidentical twins. This is like two separate births; follow the same procedures as for a single birth.

If there is much bleeding after child-

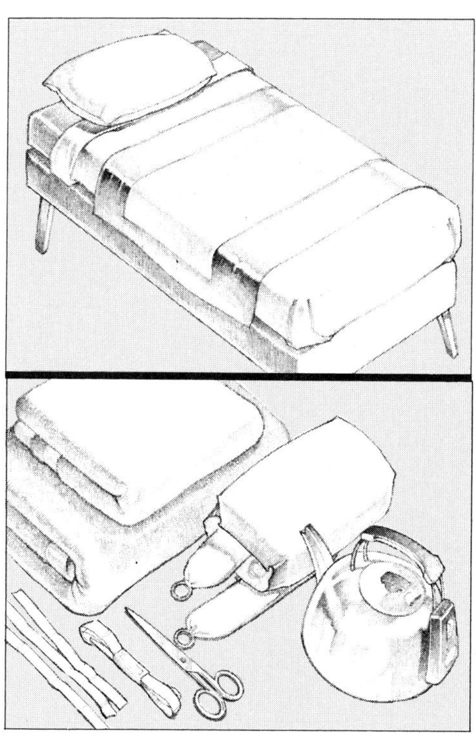

Prepare a clean surface, preferably a bed, for the mother to lie on. Protect the surface with a sheet of plastic or newspapers covered with a clean towel or sheet.

Ask the mother to empty her bladder; if it is full, labor will be impeded. Do not allow her to use the bathroom because the birth may occur suddenly.

Assist the mother to the bed.

There should now be plenty of time to gather the things you will need for the birth and after delivery:

Blankets or towels to wrap the baby in;

Swabs or clean handkerchiefs;

Sanitary napkins;

Scissors and cloth tape;

Boiling water for sterilizing the tape and scissors.

What the contractions mean

The abdominal pains during labor are caused by regular contractions of the uterus. In some mothers these contractions become more frequent as labor progresses, being two minutes or less apart when birth is imminent. But there are many exceptions, and the interval between contractions is not a reliable indication of the imminence of childbirth.

The effect of the contractions is to gradually dilate the birth canal until it is wide enough to allow the baby's head to pass through. The contractions also push the baby downward and eventually cause the baby to emerge.

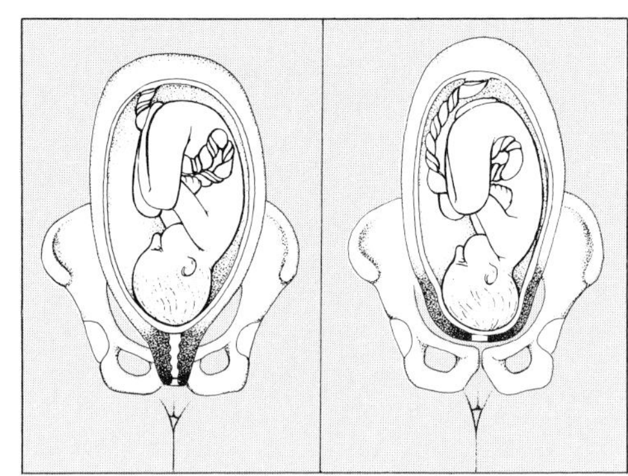

Instructions for emergency delivery

1 During the first stage of labor, the amnion (a sac surrounding the baby) may rupture, resulting in an outpouring of clear fluid. Do not be alarmed; this is quite normal.
Lay the mother on her back and remove all her clothing below the waist. Cover her with a blanket.

Ask the mother to bend her knees and let them fall part. Encourage her to relax between each contraction.

2 Contractions will now be longer and stronger; the mother will have the urge to bear down with each contraction.

Tell the mother to push with each contraction and to relax between contractions. She may have a bowel movement during a contraction. If so, wipe it away from the front backward. Do not soil the birth canal.

Remember, your hands must be clean; if they get dirty, wash them again.

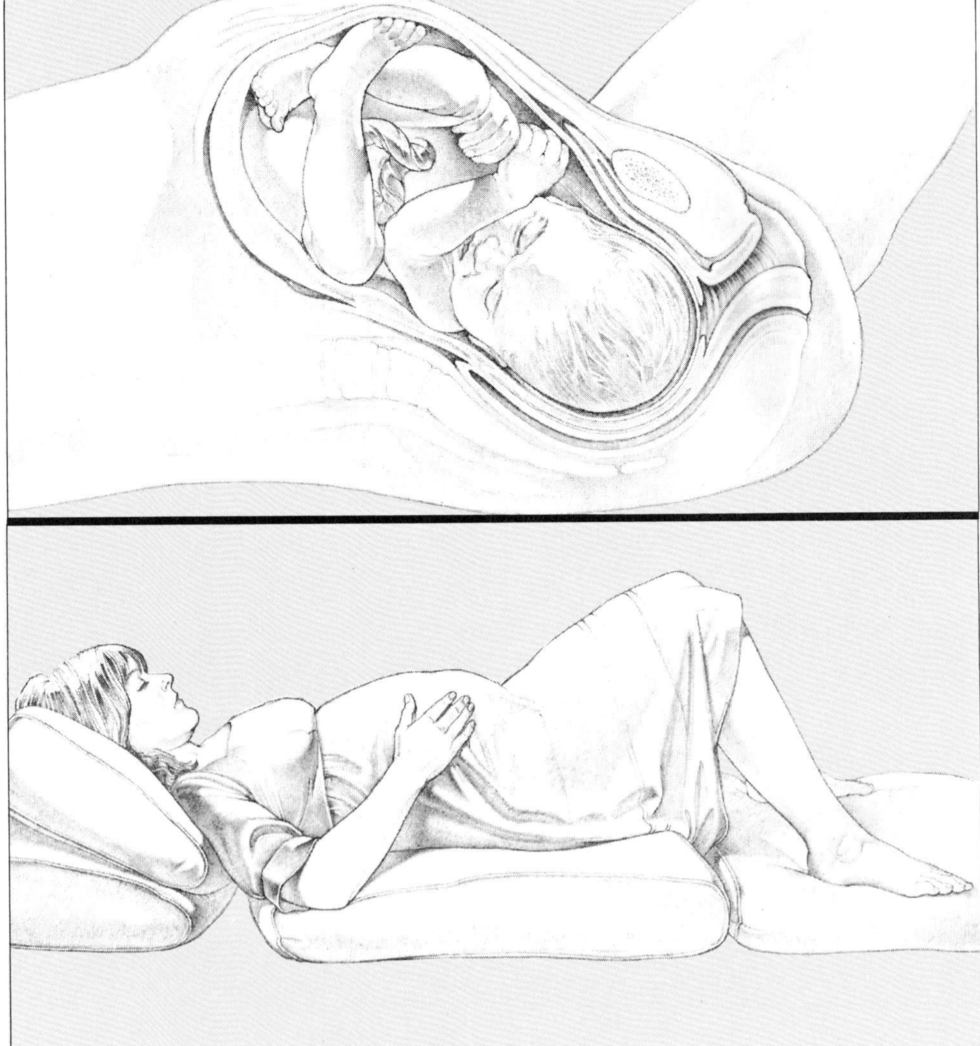

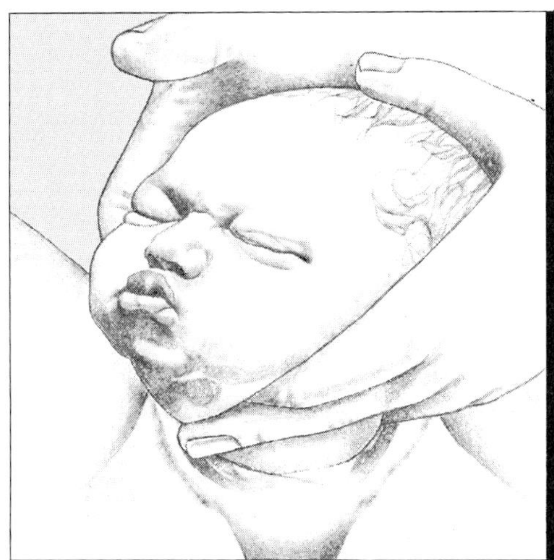

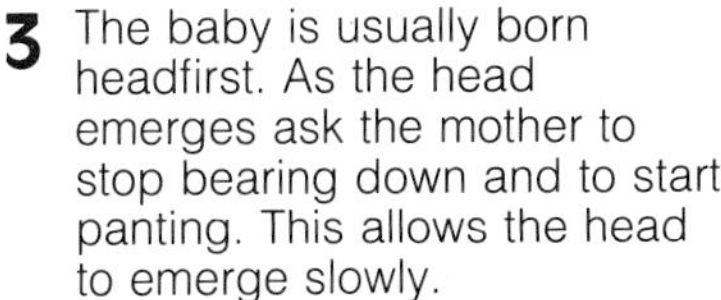

3 The baby is usually born headfirst. As the head emerges ask the mother to stop bearing down and to start panting. This allows the head to emerge slowly.

Do not interfere with the baby's head, only support it gently with cupped hands.

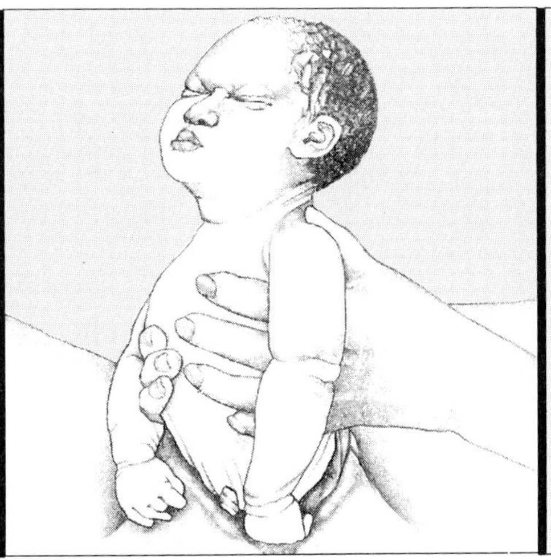

4 The shoulders and body will emerge fairly quickly. *Do not* try to pull the baby out.

Hold the baby gently under the armpits and lift toward the mother's abdomen. The baby will be slippery, so hold him or her firmly.

Do not pull or stretch the cord.

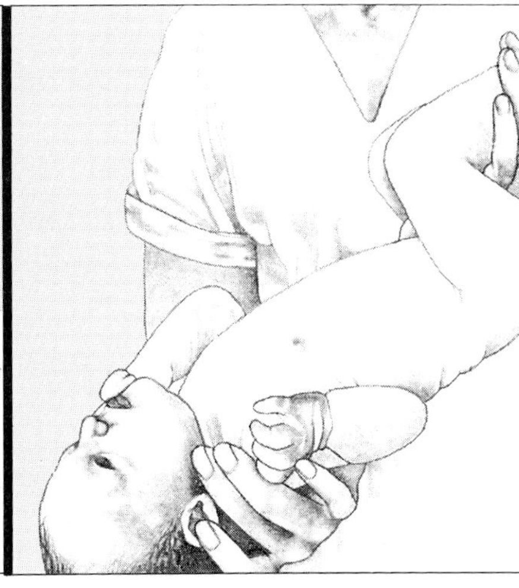

5 Cradle the baby carefully in your arms, with the head positioned low to allow any fluid to drain from the nose and mouth.

If the baby does not start to breathe immediately, wipe out the nose and mouth and begin artificial respiration. *See* ARTIFICIAL RESPIRATION.

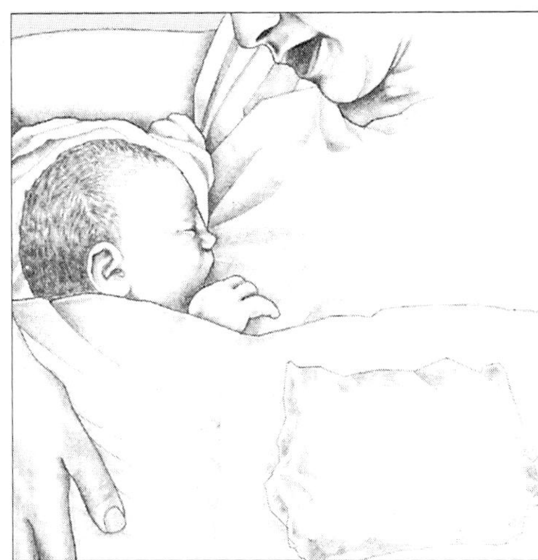

6 The baby can now be wrapped in a blanket and placed by the mother's side. Remember, the baby is still attached to the mother by the cord.

When the placenta has been delivered, wrap it and place it next to the baby. The placenta must be inspected by an obstetrician.

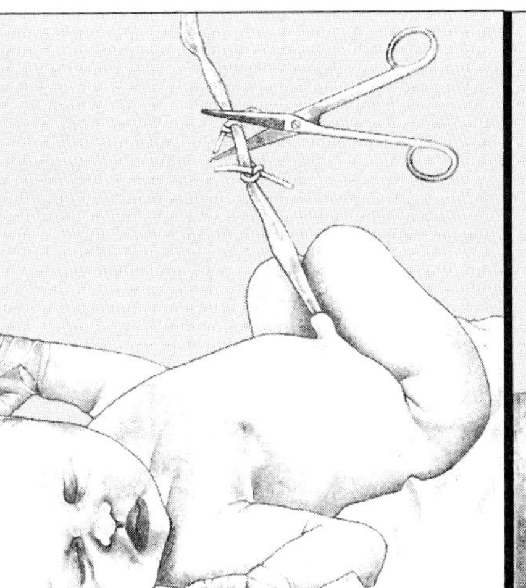

7 *Do not* cut the cord unless medical help is unavailable. Wait until the placenta has been delivered and sterilize a pair of scissors and three pieces of cloth tape.

Tie the tape very firmly round the cord six inches and eight inches from the baby's navel. Cut the cord between the two ties.

8 Tie the third piece of sterilized tape four inches from the baby's navel.

Inspect the cord regularly to ensure that no bleeding has occurred.

Wash the mother, wiping her from front to back. Fix a sanitary napkin in position.

birth, place a sanitary napkin in position, raise the mother's legs, and gently massage her abdomen just below the navel. This stimulates the uterus to contract and should stop the bleeding. If the bleeding does not stop, urgent medical assistance is required.

Childbirth, natural. Natural childbirth describes a method of having a baby without the use of drugs or without the technique known as Cesarean section. Because natural childbirth avoids the use of painkilling drugs or anesthesia, it is considered by many to make the delivery process a more natural event.

Usually, natural childbirth is discussed as part of an educational process that begins when a woman and her partner discover she is pregnant. This process, which may include prenatal classes, is meant to reduce any anxiety a woman may have about the pregnancy and thereby enable the woman to better enjoy the stages of pregnancy. After discussing the option of natural childbirth, some women decide it is the method they prefer, while other women decide against it.

Q: *What are some methods of natural childbirth?*

A: There are many different methods of natural childbirth, often named after the physician who first introduced that particular method. Examples are the Lamaze, Leboyer, and Dick Read methods. These methods are usually introduced in a prenatal class, which ideally is attended by both the mother-to-be and the father-to-be.

Prenatal classes explain what is happening at the various stages of pregnancy and exactly what happens during labor. It is explained that the hard effort that is necessary during labor is similar to that needed for any athletic event, and appropriate physical and psychological tips are given. The basis of the instruction in the classes is to teach the woman, and her partner, how she can help herself and her attendants during labor.

Whatever method is taught, it is essential for the woman to realize that everything is being done to help her and that some labors are much more difficult than others, even when perfectly normal. Some women do need painkilling drugs, but this is not a sign of failure on the part of the mother or of the method. Other problems may arise that force the obstetrician to use forceps or vacuum extraction or to perform a Cesarean section.

Q: *In what ways can a woman help during labor?*

A: Muscular tension can be lessened by special exercises, such as breathing in a manner that relaxes. In the first stage of labor, before the uterus is open, breathing during contractions should be a series of deep breaths that become rapid and more shallow as the pains increase, returning to slower, deeper breathing as the pains lessen. This difficult stage, which is often lengthy and tiring for the mother, can be made easier by applying gentle pressure to the area over the sacrum bone. Such pressure shifts the weight of the body from the spinal column to the pelvis.

In the second stage of labor, when the fetus is being expelled from the uterus and down through the pelvis, the breathing pattern is different. Rapid, short, puffing breaths are taken, and then the breath is held for a few moments while the mother pushes down with her abdominal muscles during contraction.

The obstetrician indicates when to "push," and this pattern of puffing and pushing alternates until the baby is expelled from the birth canal. During this second stage, if the father is present, he can help by supporting the mother's back with his arm and holding her legs bent.

The third stage of labor is the expulsion of the placenta. This is not a lengthy process, and the woman should be asked to give a further push or cough as the placenta is expelled.

See also PREGNANCY AND CHILDBIRTH.

Childhood disorders. See Age-by-age Chart, Appendices.

Children, care of sick. See NURSING THE SICK CHILD.

Children in hospital. See HOSPITALIZATION: CHILDREN.

Chill is the sensation of cold often caused by exposure to a frigid environment. A shivering attack often accompanies a chill. A mild fever sometimes follows a chill, and this may be the first indication of an impending infectious illness.

Shaking chills are one of the signs of bacteremia or bacterial infection in the bloodstream.

Chin is the front of the lower jaw, or mandible, below the mouth.

Chinese restaurant syndrome. *See* MONOSODIUM GLUTAMATE.

Chip is a very small piece of a bone or a tooth. Bone chips, usually cancellous (the porous or latticed parts of the inside of a bone), are sometimes used to fill in a bone fracture in order to speed healing.

Chiropractic (kī rə prak′tik) is an alternative system of therapy based on the theory that most diseases are the result of misalignments or subluxations of the spinal column, which cause disruption of the "flow of energy" through the spinal cord. In making diagnoses, chiropractors may use X rays along with standard physical and laboratory examinations. They do not prescribe drugs or perform surgery.

Some chiropractors confine their practice to the treatment of joint and muscle disorders, but others treat a wide range of illnesses. While manipulation has been found useful for certain joint and muscle disorders, it must be noted that the effectiveness of chiropractic in the treatment of medical illness has not been confirmed by scientific research.

In the United States there are nine chiropractic colleges that are recognized by the Council on Chiropractic Education. These colleges offer a four-year program that leads to the degree of Doctor of Chiropractic (D.C.).

Chlamydia (klä mid′ē ə) refers to a class of microorganisms that function as parasites and cause a number of diseases afflicting humans. Probably, the most well known form of chlamydia is the sexually transmitted variety—*chlamydia trachomatis.*

In men, *chlamydia trachomatis* causes an inflammation of the urethra, the structure serving as a channel for semen, or a swelling of the epididymis, a tube transporting sperm from the testicles to the penis. In women it can do damage to the uterus and trigger pelvic inflammatory disease (salpingitis). *Chlamydia trachomatis* can also set off conjunctivitis, a swelling in the eye. Although rare in the United States, *chlamydia trachomatis* infections of the eye are, in developing countries, the most common cause of blindness in newborns.

The other major form of chlamydia, *chlamydia psittaci,* is responsible for a pneumonia in humans.

See also CONJUNCTIVITIS; EPIDIDYMIS; SALPINGITIS; SEXUALLY TRANSMITTED DISEASE; URETHRA.

Chlamydiosis (klä mid ē ō′sis) is a generic term for all the infections caused by the bacteria, *Chlamydia.*

See also CHLAMYDIA.

Chloasma (klō az′mə) is a patchy yellowish-brown discoloration of facial skin caused by a concentration of the pigment melanin. It may occur in pregnant women and is called "the mask of pregnancy." Chloasma may also appear in Addison's disease and in some women who take birth control pills.

See also ADDISON'S DISEASE; MELASMA.

Chloramphenicol (klôr am fen′ə kōl) is a wide-spectrum antibiotic drug. It is used in the treatment of typhoid fever and some forms of meningitis and as drops or ointments for skin, eye, or ear infections. It is used with caution because it may cause serious, and even fatal damage, to the blood-forming cells in the bone marrow.

Chlorhexidine (klôr heks′i dēn) is a disinfectant that is used on its own or with antibiotics to clean wounds or to sterilize the skin.

Chloroform (klôr′ə fôrm) was one of the first general anesthetics and, like ether, was in common use in the United States until the 1950's. Since then, it has been gradually replaced by safer, less toxic drugs. It is still used in many developing countries.

See also ANESTHETIC.

Chloroquine (klôr′ə kwīn) is a drug that is taken by persons in malaria-stricken regions to prevent them from getting that disease. The standard preventive dose is 300mg per week, but larger doses are required if a person actually gets malaria. In some parts of the world, however, some malarial organisms are resistant to the drug. Prolonged, high doses may cause permanent eye damage, intestinal disturbances, headaches, and itching of the skin. Chloroquine has also been used in the treatment of amebiasis, lupus erythematosus, and rarely, rheumatoid arthritis.

See also MALARIA.

Chlorpromazine (klôr prō′mə zēn) is a neuroleptic or antipsychotic drug used to reduce hallucinations and delusions in persons with mental illness, such as schizophrenia. It is also used as a sedative in anesthesia and in treating overdoses from psychedelic and amphetamine drugs. It is manufactured under the trade name Thorazine®.

Choking is the inability to breathe following the obstruction of the larynx or windpipe (trachea) by food, mucus, or a foreign object that has been swallowed or inhaled. Choking can also be caused by external compression of the neck.

See also CHOKING AND COUGHING: FIRST AID.

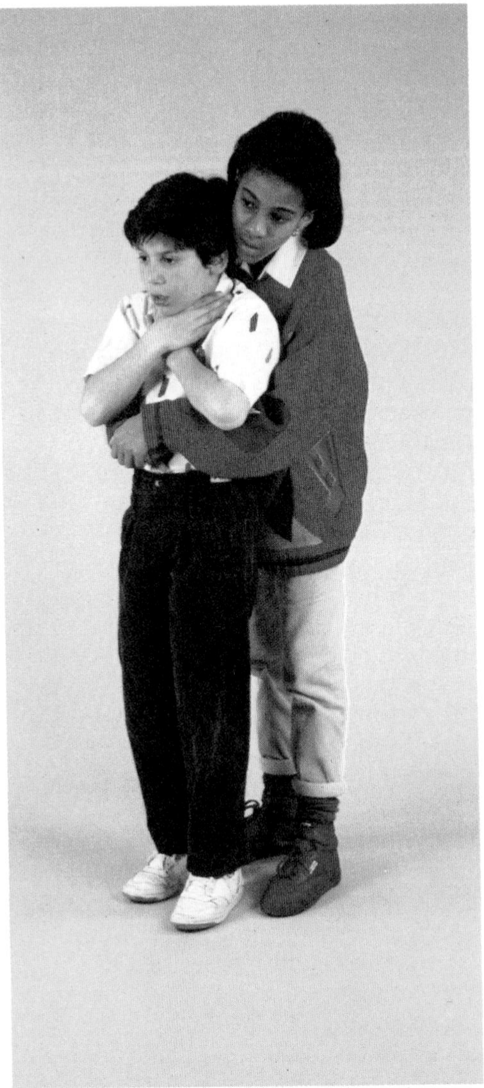

Children choking: first aid

Children should be taught to perform the Hemilich maneuver as described in steps 2 and 3 on page 191. They are often with school classmates at times of choking emergencies. They are also the right size to perform the maneuver on each other since an adult could break a child victim's ribs.

Choking and coughing: first aid. Choking is the interruption of breathing caused by an obstruction in the airway. The unmistakable sign of a choking victim is the inability to speak. The victim may also be coughing and struggling for breath. Lack of sufficient oxygen causes the victim's face to turn purple and then blue in color; after a short time, the victim collapses.

The most common cause of choking is food lodged in the windpipe. Another cause is muscle spasms that result from inhaling poisonous fumes. An acute asthmatic attack may also cause the victim to choke and cough. Choking may result in death by asphyxiation in approximately four to six minutes.

Action. The type of emergency assistance depends upon the cause of the choking attack. In the case of food or another object blocking the windpipe, the most effective method to remove the object is a technique called the Heimlich maneuver. To perform this maneuver, stand behind the victim and place your arms around the victim's waist. Make a fist and place it so that the thumb is against the victim's abdomen, slightly above the navel and below the ribcage. Grasp your fist with your other hand and then press your fist into the victim's abdomen with a quick upward thrust. This action forces air out of the victim's lungs and blows the object from the windpipe.

If the victim has collapsed or is too large for you to support or place your arms around, lay the person on his or her back. Then face the victim and kneel straddling the hips. Place one of your hands over the other, with the heel of the bottom hand on the victim's abdomen, slightly above the navel and below the ribcage. Then press your hands into the victim's abdomen with a quick upward thrust.

When applying the Heimlich maneuver, be careful not to apply pressure on the victim's ribs. Such pressure may break ribs.

Babies. To remove an obstruction from a baby, hold the baby face down and give the baby four firm blows between the shoulders, using the heel of your hand. If this does not work, flip the baby face up and give four chest thrusts as if for external cardiac compression. (For step-by-step instruc-

First aid for choking

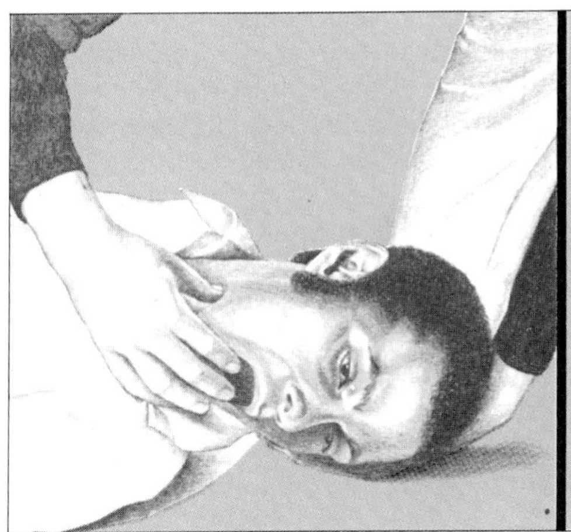

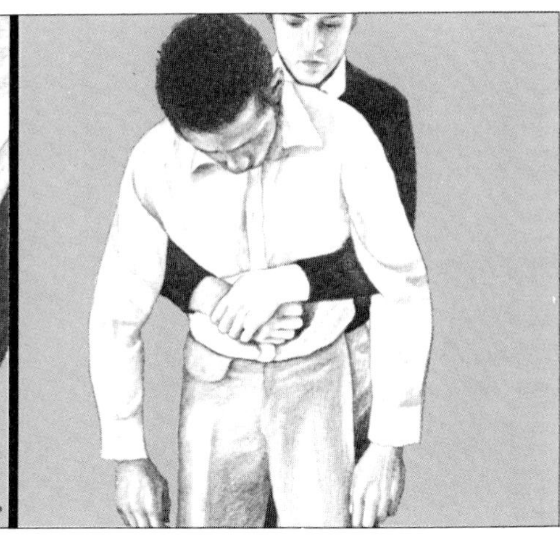

1 To clear the airway, turn the victim's head to one side. Using your fingers, remove any obvious obstructions, such as dentures or food. If an obstruction can not be removed by hand, it must be forced out.

2 Stand behind the victim with the arms firmly around the lower part of the victim's chest.

Make a fist with one hand and grasp it firmly with the other hand. Both hands should be placed centrally just below the victim's ribs.

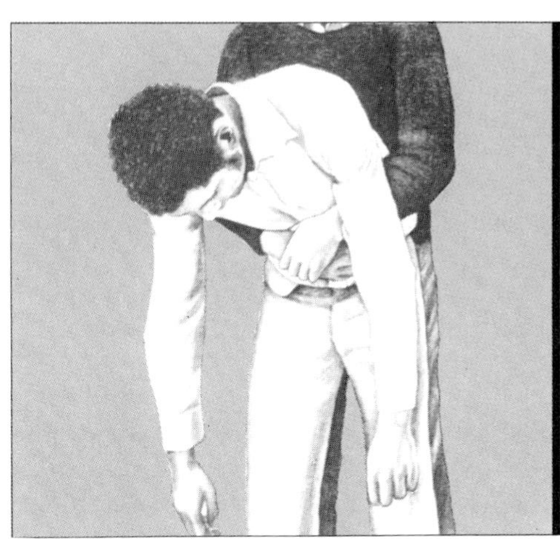

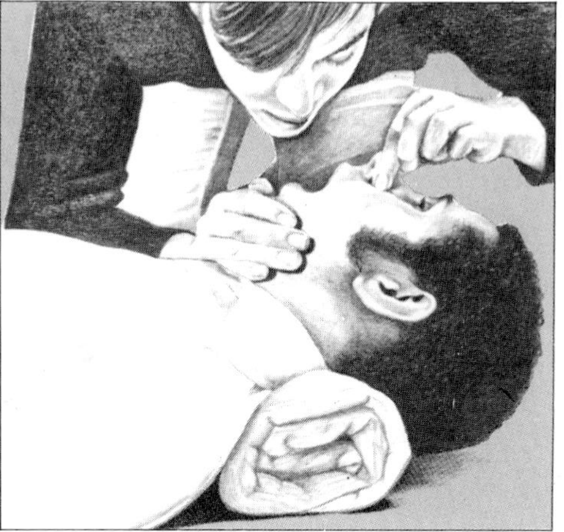

3 The victim should be leaning forward with the head and arms hanging down. Give a firm, inward and upward thrust against the victim's abdomen. It may be necessary to repeat this maneuver a few times in order to force the victim to cough up the obstruction. (Steps 2 and 3 illustrate the Heimlich maneuver.)

4 When the obstruction is out, give artificial respiration if the victim is not breathing. For instruction, *see* ARTIFICIAL RESPIRATION.

When choking has been relieved and normal breathing has been restored, lay the victim in the recovery position. For instruction, *see* FAINTING: FIRST AID. Summon emergency medical aid or take the victim to a hospital.

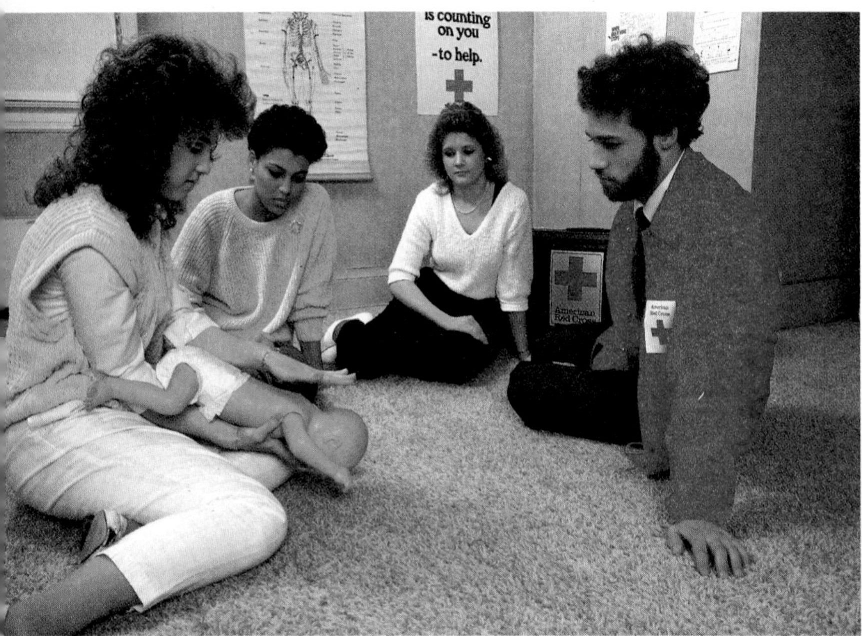

Baby choking: first aid

Hold the baby face down. Give the baby four sharp blows between the shoulders, using the heel of the hand. If unsuccessful, flip the baby face up and give four chest thrusts as if for external cardiac compression. *See* HEART ATTACK: FIRST AID. When the obstruction is out, give artificial respiration if the baby is not breathing.

tions, *see* HEART ATTACK: FIRST AID). If the victim is not breathing following the removal of the object, give artificial respiration. *See also* ARTIFICIAL RESPIRATION.

Poisonous Fumes. If choking is caused by poisonous fumes or smoke, immediately remove the victim to fresh air. If the victim is in an enclosed space, get additional help if possible. Before entering the enclosed space, breathe in and out several times, then take a deep breath and hold it. Go in and get the victim out. If the victim can not be removed at once, cut off the source of danger; open all windows and doors and get out. Do not take a breath until it is safe to do so. Return to remove the victim as soon as it is safe to do so.

Ensure that the victim's airway is clear and loosen all clothing around the victim's neck, chest, and waist. If the victim has stopped breathing, give artificial respiration. If the victim's heart has stopped, use cardiac compressions. *See also* ARTIFICIAL RESPIRATION; HEART ATTACK: FIRST AID.

Asthmatic Attack. If choking is caused by an asthmatic attack, ask the victim to intertwine his or her fingers; with the palms downward or outward, instruct him or her to brace the hands and the arms against a table or a wall so that the rib cage is expanded. Allow the victim to use an inhaler or to take any tablets that a physician has prescribed. Summon emergency medical help if the symptoms continue.

Cholangiogram (kol an′jē ə gram) is an X ray of the gall bladder and bile ducts taken after a radiopaque dye, a substance that can be seen in an X ray, is introduced into the structures. The dye may be injected into a vein (intravenous), into the hepatic ducts (transhepatic), or during surgery directly into the biliary ducts (intraoperative). The latter is done to ensure that there are no stones in the ducts following the removal of the gall bladder (cholecystectomy).

See also CHOLECYSTOGRAM, ORAL.

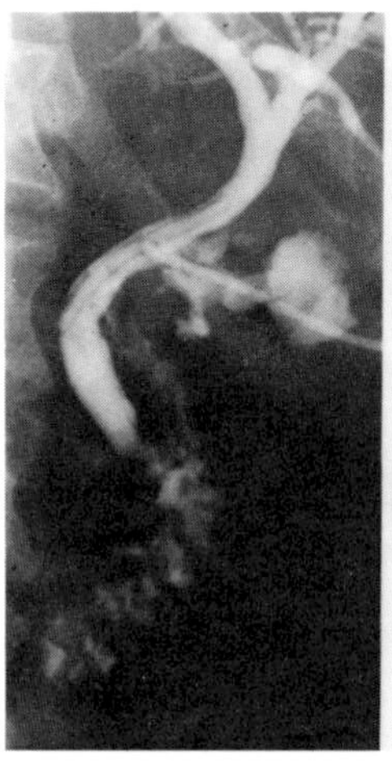
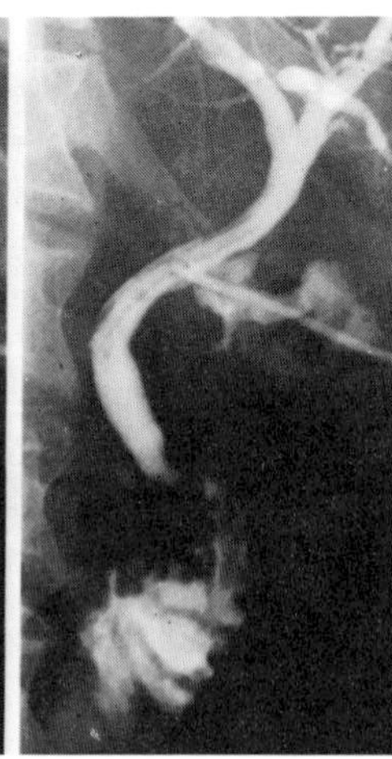

An intravenous **cholangiogram** is an X ray of the gall bladder and bile ducts taken after a radiopaque dye is injected into a vein.

Cholangitis (kol ən jī′tis) is inflammation of the bile ducts. It is usually caused by an obstruction of the bile ducts that link the liver with the gall bladder and duodenum. The obstruction may be caused by the presence of gallstones or a cancer, or it may occur following the removal of the gall bladder (cholecystectomy). Pain in the upper abdomen is accompanied by a high fever, often with vomiting, hot and cold sensations, and jaundice. Dark urine and pale feces can be other signs of the disease. A severe bile duct obstruction may require surgical removal; but less severe blockage may be treated with antibiotics.

Cholecystectomy (kol ə sis tek′tə mē) is the surgical removal of the gall bladder.

Cholecystitis (kol ə sis tī′tis) is an inflammation of the gall bladder. Acute cholecystitis is almost always caused by gallstones that are unable to pass through the cystic duct. Chronic cholecystitis may occur in middle-aged persons, especially women, who are overweight and may or may not have gallstones.

Q: *What are the symptoms of cholecystitis?*

A: In acute cholecystitis, there is usually severe, sudden, or gradual pain in the right upper abdomen, with nausea, chills, vomiting, high fever, and sometimes referred pain in the back or the right shoulder blade. The symptoms of chronic cholecystitis are less severe and include discomfort in the right upper abdomen, gas, belching, heartburn, or indigestion.

Q: *How is cholecystitis treated?*

A: Antibiotics and, if vomiting has been severe, hospitalization for intravenous fluids are preliminary treatments for acute cholecystitis. If there is no improvement, the gall bladder is removed (cholecystectomy). Sometimes it is necessary to drain the gall bladder (cholecystotomy) to allow the patient to become well enough for the gall bladder to be completely removed. For patients with chronic cholecystitis, weight loss and a low-fat diet are usually tried first.

Cholecystogram, oral (kôl ə sis′tə gram). An oral cholecystogram is an X-ray examination of the gall bladder. It is used to diagnose gallstones and chronic inflammation of the gall bladder (cholecystitis). The patient is given a fat-free meal on the evening before an examination and is then deprived of solid food. The same evening, the patient swallows a compound containing iodine. Twelve to sixteen hours later, a series of X rays are taken of the gall bladder. The iodine compound becomes concentrated in the gall bladder and makes abnormalities, such as gallstones, visible on X rays. The patient is then given a fatty meal, and more X rays are taken. Absorption of fats from the meal causes the gall bladder to contract and permits the bile ducts to become visible.

An oral cholecystogram gives a definite result in most cases. However, if the gall bladder and the bile ducts can not be seen on the X rays, an intravenous cholangiogram may be necessary. Other alternatives to an oral cholecystogram include ultrasound and special scans using radioactive dyes. Ultrasonography in particular is gradually replacing cholecystograms.

See also CHOLANGIOGRAM, INTRAVENOUS; ULTRASOUND.

Cholelithiasis (kol ə lə thī′ə sis) is the presence of gallstones in the gall bladder or bile duct. Patients with gallstones usually have too much cholesterol in their bile. When the cholesterol levels become too high and can no longer remain in solution, tiny crystals form that group together to build gallstones. Besides cholesterol-based stones, there are mixed stones (containing calcium, bilirubin, and cholesterol), bilirubin stones, and uric acid stones. Gallstones occur much more frequently in women than in men. A typical gallstone patient is female, middle-aged, and overweight. However, anyone with abnormally high levels of cholesterol has a much greater risk of developing gallstones. Other factors thought to be involved in the formation of gallstones include glandular or genetic predisposition and repeated infections of the bile duct and/or gallbladder.

Q: *What are the symptoms of cholelithiasis?*

A: Many gallstones are "silent" (dormant) and produce no symptoms.

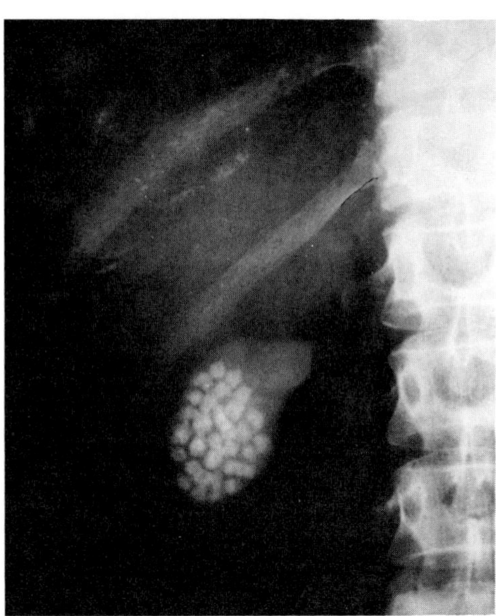

Cholelithiasis is the formation of gall stones, which are usually caused by an excess of cholesterol.

Symptoms that can occur are pain in the right upper abdomen; gas; belching; a spasm in the bile duct, causing severe pain; sweating and vomiting, when a stone moves from the gall bladder; and jaundice, if a stone blocks the common bile duct. Cholelithiasis increases the chances of damage to the pancreas and increases the chance of cancer of the gall bladder.

Q: *How is cholelithiasis treated?*

A: The usual treatment for symptomatic gallstones is the removal of the gall bladder. A new nonsurgical technique called shock wave lithotripsy is also effective in many cases. Medications are now available that will, in some cases, dissolve certain types of gallstones.

Cholera (kol′ər ə) is an acute infectious disease of the small intestine caused by bacteria *(Vibrio cholerae)*. Cholera produces an intestinal toxin that triggers an outpouring of watery fluid from the walls of the intestine. Symptoms are severe diarrhea and vomiting, with massive loss of body fluids, muscle cramps, and shock caused by dehydration. Cholera is transmitted by water, milk, or other foods, especially shellfish that have been contaminated by the feces of infected persons. Cholera is mainly an epidemic tropical disease in Asia and Africa.

Q: *How is cholera treated?*

A: The patient requires replacement of fluids by drinking or by intravenous injection to counteract the dehydration. Antibiotic drugs are also prescribed. During the recovery period, glucose and potassium tablets may be given.

Q: *How successful is the treatment of cholera?*

A: When proper treatment is available, it is usually effective and the patient recovers completely within two weeks. Even when treated, the death rate in adults is about 5 percent and in children 10 percent.

Q: *Can cholera be prevented?*

A: People in epidemic areas are advised to avoid unsterilized water, fresh fruit, and shellfish. Cholera vaccinations provide some protection for at least three months. These vaccinations consist of two injections given one to four weeks apart.

Cholesterol (kə les′tə rōl) is a fatty substance found in all animal tissues. The substance makes up an important part of the membranes of each cell in the human body. The liver uses cholesterol to manufacture bile acids, which aid in digestion. Cholesterol is also utilized in the production of certain hormones, including sex hormones.

Q: *How is cholesterol produced?*

A: The human body manufactures most of its own cholesterol. All body cells are capable of production, but most is made by liver cells. Cholesterol also enters the body in food, particularly from butter, eggs, fatty meats, shellfish, and organ meats, such as liver and brains.

Q: *How is cholesterol transported in the body?*

A: Three types of special molecules called lipoproteins—high-density lipoproteins (HDL), low-density lipoproteins (LDL), and very low-density lipoproteins (VLDL)—transport cholesterol from the liver through the bloodstream to cells throughout the body.

Q: *Is cholesterol harmful?*

A: Although the body needs cholesterol, high levels of LDL-type and VLDL-type cholesterol have been linked to certain diseases, particularly atherosclerosis (hardening of the arteries). One large study of middle-aged men with elevated cholesterol levels showed that for each one percent reduction in blood cholesterol level the chance of heart attack was reduced by two percent. Because of this, many physicians have recommended a diet low in cholesterol and saturated fats to reduce risk of heart attacks and atherosclerosis elsewhere in the body. Each person's ability to maintain a healthy level of cholesterol is determined partially by inheritance and partially by diet. Foods high in saturated fats and cholesterol should be reduced in quantity and frequency. Consultation with a physician or nutritionist will help direct effective changes toward a more healthy diet and lifestyle. Several books are also available for this purpose. Adults should have their blood cholesterol checked every five years by their physician in order to control this very important health risk factor. It should be checked more often if other cardiac risk factors are present.

Q: *What is "good cholesterol"?*

A: HDL-type cholesterol is sometimes referred to as "good cholesterol" because, unlike the other types, high levels of HDL-type cholesterol may actually provide protection against heart attack. Exercise and a diet high in fish may improve the HDL level.

See also APPENDIX IV.

Choline (kō′lēn) is a member of the B complex vitamins and is essential to the functioning of the liver. It acts as a check on the build-up of fats in the liver. A lack of choline may result in cirrhosis of the liver, which can lead to a host of other conditions, including bleeding ulcers, kidney damage, abnormally high cholesterol levels, and hardening of the arteries. Some researchers are now experimenting with choline to attempt to alleviate symptoms of Alzheimer's disease. The best sources of choline are found in liver, kidney, wheat germ, and egg yolk.

See also NUTRITION; VITAMIN.

Chondroma (kon drō′mə) is a slow-growing, usually benign tumor of cartilage that may occur wherever cartilage is present in the body. It may or may not cause pain. Depending on its location, it may also increase the likelihood of bone breakage. Chondroma occurs most commonly in adolescents and young adults.

Chondromalacia (kon drō mə lā′shē ə) is the softening of cartilage in joints, especially that behind the kneecap (patella). It most commonly occurs following a knee injury and is characterized by pain and swelling. There may be some degenerative change in the cartilage as a result of the injury.

Chondrosarcoma (kon drō sâr kō′mə) is a malignant (cancerous) tumor that forms from cartilage cells. It may develop outside or inside a bone.

See also CANCER.

Choosing a physician. See PHYSICIAN CHOICE.

Chordotomy. See CORDOTOMY.

Chorea (kô rē′ə) is a disorder of the nervous system that is characterized by spasm of the facial muscles and involuntary contortions of the limbs. The two common forms of chorea are unrelated: Sydenham's chorea (St. Vitus's dance) and Huntington's chorea. *See also* CHOREA, HUNTINGTON'S.

Q: *What is Sydenham's chorea?*

A: Sydenham's chorea is a disorder in which the small arteries of the brain become inflamed. It is an allergic reaction to streptococcal infection, such as meningitis, some forms of pneumonia, and scarlet fever. Sydenham's chorea commonly follows several months after an attack of rheumatic fever and is most likely to occur in children between the ages of 5 and 15.

The symptoms of Sydenham's chorea include facial contortions, grunts, and occasional difficulty in speaking. Sometimes only one side of the body is affected.

Q: *How is Sydenham's chorea treated?*

A: Bed rest is essential. Sedative drugs help to control the involuntary contortions, and antibiotic drugs are usually prescribed to fight infection. The disease is often treated with regular high dosages of aspirin. Recovery may be complete within 3 or 4 months, but further attacks occur in about 30 percent of cases.

Chorea, Huntington's (kô rē′ə, hun′ting tūnz). Huntington's chorea, or disease, is an inherited disorder of the central nervous system, which usually affects an equal number of males and females between the ages of 30 and 50. The symptoms of Huntington's chorea are the gradual onset of involuntary, jerky, and contorted movements of the limbs. Mental deterioration and severe personality change are associated symptoms. The patient may eventually need institutional care.

Q: *Can Huntington's chorea be treated?*

A: No effective form of treatment has been found for the disorder. There is a 50 percent chance that a child of someone with Huntington's chorea will develop it later in life. The traditional medical advice has been that a person who has a parent with the disorder should not have children. There is now in the experimental stage a blood test that can identify the defective gene responsible for Huntington's chorea long before any symptoms appear. The availability of this test may bring up difficult ethical and legal questions concerning who has the right to know the results.

See also GENETIC ABNORMALITY; GENETIC COUNSELING.

Choriocarcinoma (kôr ē ō kär sə nō'mə) is a malignant (cancerous) growth of the outer layer of the membrane (chorion) that surrounds a fetus in the womb. It is a relatively rare condition in the United States, occurring in about 1 out of every 45,000 pregnancies. Choriocarcinoma is more likely to occur in women over the age of 40. An obstetrician looks for signs of the disease in pregnant women who have had the formation of a hydatidiform mole, which leads to an unusually large uterus for that stage of pregnancy. But mole formations are not necessarily a sign of choriocarcinoma; they occur in about 1 out of every 2,000 pregnancies (especially in older women), and over 80 percent of these moles are benign. Other symptoms of choriocarcinoma may include vaginal bleeding and extreme nausea. After the removal of a hydatidiform mole, the effectiveness of treatment can be assessed by measuring human chorionic gonadotropin (HCG) levels in the blood. Normally, these levels should drop dramatically after the removal of the mole. If the levels do not drop, this is a sign of a choriocarcinoma. Repeated blood tests are made to determine the level of these hormones in the mother's bloodstream. If this level remains above normal, treatment with anticancer drugs (chemotherapy) is given to destroy the growth. The hydatidiform mole may also be suctioned from the uterus; occasionally, a hysterectomy will be performed (especially with older patients).

Choriocarcinoma may, on rare occasion, appear in the testes.

See also MOLE, HYDATIDIFORM.

Chorionic villus biopsy (kôr ē on'ik vil'əs bī'op sē), also known as CVB, is a relatively new technique employed during the first trimester of pregnancy, in which ultrasound guides the gynecologist's instrument towards the placenta in a mother's womb, in order to obtain a tissue sampling. This can be helpful in determining the possible presence of genetic defects in the fetus. More conventional methods can not be used until after 11 weeks of gestation.

However, because the accuracy and safety of this technique has yet to be clinically established, a CVB should be used only when the risk of a genetic disorder is clearly higher than the risk of using this unproven method.

See also AMNIOCENTESIS.

Choroid (kôr'oid) is the middle coat of the eyeball that contains the dark coloring matter and blood vessels. The term choroid plexus is applied to a small group of specialized blood vessels in the cavities (ventricles) of the brain, which produce cerebrospinal fluid.

Choroiditis (kôr oi dī'tis) is inflammation of the middle coat (choroid) of the eyeball. The symptoms of the disorder are a gradual blurring of vision, distorted vision, floating black spots, and sometimes pain or reddening. Untreated, choroiditis may have serious complications.

Christmas disease, or hemophilia B, is an inherited deficiency of a plasma protein active in the formation of blood clots. The condition has the same symptoms as classic hemophilia (hemophilia A), prolonged bleeding from slight injuries and internal bleeding without any known cause. Christmas disease is usually less severe than classic hemophilia; its severity is dependent on the extent of the plasma protein deficiency. Transfusion of blood plasma containing the correct clotting factor is the appropriate treatment. The condition gets its name from the patient in whom it was first discovered.

See also HEMOPHILIA.

Chromosome (krō'mə sōm) is a threadlike structure in the nucleus of a cell. It is made up of many hundreds of genes, the messengers that carry the "instructions" that determine a person's hereditary makeup. There are 46 chromosomes (arranged as 23 pairs) in each human cell except the ova (eggs) and sperm, which have only 23 chromosomes.

Q: *What happens to the chromosomes when a cell divides?*

A: The chromosomes divide at the same time as the cell, so that the 2 new cells, each with 46 chromosomes, are identical to the parent cell. Exceptions are the cells that

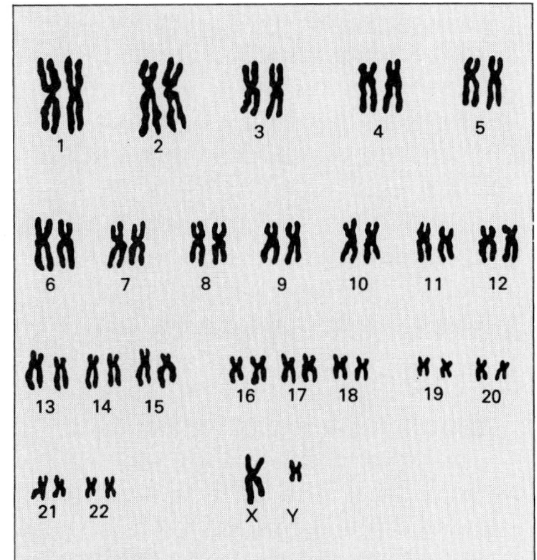

Chromosomes of a male include 22 pairs (XX), plus one odd set (XY).

form sperm and ova, which divide to produce sex cells (gametes) with only 23 chromosomes each. This means that when a sperm joins an ovum at fertilization to form a new cell of 46 chromosomes, it does so with half the genes from the mother and half from the father.

Q: *How do chromosomes decide the sex of an individual?*

A: The male chromosome is called Y. It is smaller and contains fewer genes than the female chromosome. Each sperm contains either an X or a Y chromosome; each ovum contains a single X chromosome. When a sperm and an ovum combine to form a new individual, the fertilized ovum contains either two X chromosomes (XX) and is female, or it contains an X and a Y (XY) and is male.

See also CELL; GENE.

Chronically ill, nursing of. *See* NURSING THE CHRONICALLY ILL.

Chronic obstructive pulmonary disease. *See* PULMONARY DISEASE, CHRONIC OBSTRUCTIVE.

Chrysotherapy (kris ə ther′ə pē) is the medical term for any treatment that uses gold salts or any other gold compound.

See also GOLD SALTS TREATMENT.

Chylomicron (kī lō mī′kron) is one of the minute particles of emulsified fat, usually about a micron in diameter, carried in the blood to bodily tissues for their utilization.

Chyme (kīm) is the pulpy mass of partly digested food in the stomach. Chyme passes from the stomach into the small intestine as a semiliquid acid.

See also DIGESTIVE SYSTEM.

Chymopapain injection. *See* CHEMONUCLEOLYSIS.

Cicatrix (sik′ə triks) is the medical name for a scar.

See also SCAR.

Cigarette smoking. *See* SMOKING OF TOBACCO.

Cigar smoking. *See* SMOKING OF TOBACCO.

Cilia (sil′ē ə) are the fine, hair-like projections on many cells of the body that sweep particles along. Microscopic cilia are found, for example, in the airways to the lungs (bronchi). Eyelashes are an example of large cilia.

See also CELL.

Cimetidine. *See* HISTAMINE H_2-RECEPTOR ANTAGONIST.

Circadian rhythm (sėr kā′dē ən) is the daily biological pattern in which sleep, hunger, variation in body temperature, and other physiological changes occur. Moving to a distant time zone may disturb the rhythm, and the body may take 10 days to adjust completely to the change.

Circulation (sėr kyə lā′shən) is the flow of blood from the heart, through the arteries and capillaries, and back to the heart via the veins. The term may also be applied to the circulation in the eye or to the lymphatic system.

See also BLOOD; CIRCULATORY SYSTEM; HEART.

Circulatory system (sėr′kyə lə tôr ē) is the network of tubes through which nutrients are supplied to all parts of the body. This network consists of the blood vessels, the heart, and the lymphatic system.

The circulatory system is often subdivided into various parts. The systemic circulation refers to the usual flow of oxygenated blood from the heart, through arteries to capillaries, where the oxygen is removed, and then back to the heart via the veins.

The pulmonary circulation is the passage of deoxygenated blood from the heart to the lungs and the return of oxygen-rich blood back to the heart.

There are also two portal circulation systems in which the blood flow starts and ends in the capillaries. One flows from the intestine to the liver (the he-

The **circulatory system** consists of the systemic circuit to the body and the pulmonary circuit to the lungs.

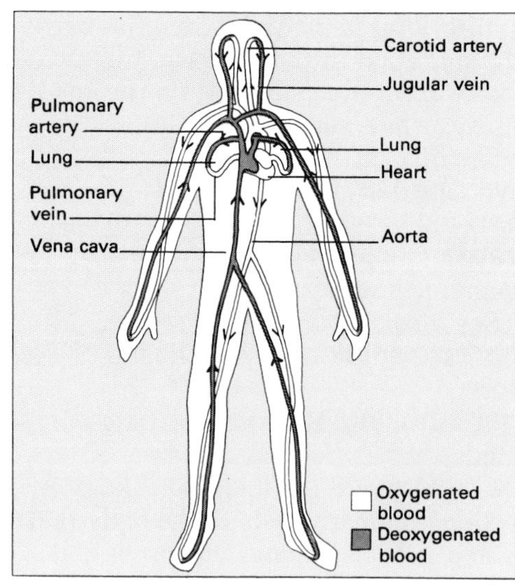

patic portal system); the other flows from the hypothalamus of the brain to the anterior lobe of the pituitary gland.

The fetal circulatory system is somewhat different. In the fetal circulation, the blood by-passes the lungs by moving from the pulmonary circulation directly into the systemic circulation, through a special duct (ductus arteriosus). The placental circulation passes blood through the placenta of the fetus in order for it to receive oxygen.

See also BLOOD VESSEL; CIRCULATION; HEART; LYMPHATIC SYSTEM.

Circumcision (sėr kəm sizh′ən) is the surgical removal of all or part of the foreskin (prepuce) of the penis. In infancy it is usually carried out for social or cultural reasons. In later life it is less common and is usually performed for medical reasons.

Q: *How is circumcision performed?*

A: There are two common methods. (1) In newborns, a special bell-shaped piece of plastic or metal is applied over the end (glans) of the penis, and the foreskin tissue is compressed in such a way as to prevent bleeding. The foreskin is then cut off, and the device is removed. (2) In adults, the foreskin is carefully cut and stitched. An anesthetic is not used for newborn babies, but it is used for a child or an adult.

Q: *Are there any risks involved in the circumcision operation?*

A: Mistakes are extremely rare but can occur. Too much or not enough skin may be removed, as may part of the glans itself. Damage may be caused to the urethra, or severe bleeding may occur.

Q: *What are the medical reasons for circumcision?*

A: In some rare instances, the foreskin is unusually long and the exit unusually narrow (phimosis); or the glans, inside the foreskin, may become infected by bacteria (balanitis) or from diaper rash. This causes the foreskin to become scarred and abnormally tight. Sometimes, the foreskin stays retracted (paraphimosis). All of these conditions can be corrected by circumcision. *See also* BALANITIS; PHIMOSIS.

Q: *What are the social reasons for circumcision?*

A: These differ from culture to culture. Often, circumcision forms part of a religious rite or an initiation into adulthood. Frequently, circumcision may seem desirable because it is in the tradition of the family or because the majority of boys in the neighborhood are circumcised. In the United States today, social and religious factors are the major reasons for circumcisions.

Q: *What possible advantages are there in not being circumcised?*

A: Ulceration of the glans is more common in those who are circumcised than in those who are not circumcised.

Q: *Does circumcision have any effect on the incidence of cancer of the penis or cancer of the cervix?*

A: Current medical evidence suggests that circumcision has no effect one way or the other on these two types of cancer. There is no medical reason for routine circumcision of newborn boys.

Cirrhosis (sə rō′sis) is a type of permanent and progressive liver damage. Any chronic liver disease, especially those caused by alcohol abuse or viral hepatitis, can lead to the formation of fibrous scars and nodules. These scars and nodules connect to involve large areas of the liver. Once present, cirrhosis is permanent, but its progress can be stopped if the cause is removed. Untreated, it can be fatal.

Q: *What are the causes of cirrhosis?*

A: In the U.S. the most common cause of cirrhosis is alcohol abuse, accounting for up to 85 percent of all cases. Other causes include infections, such as hepatitis and cholangitis; autoimmune disease; some rare inherited diseases, such as Wilson's disease and hemochromatosis; and some drugs and chemicals, such as carbon tetrachloride. In some parts of the world, virus infections or parasites, such as liver flukes, are more common causes. *See also* AUTOIMMUNE DISEASE; CARBON TETRACHLORIDE; CHOLANGITIS; HEPATITIS; WILSON'S DISEASE.

Q: *What are the symptoms of cirrhosis?*

A: Early symptoms can include weakness and a feeling of tiredness, loss of appetite, nausea and vomiting of blood, and constipation or diarrhea. Symptoms of advanced cirrhosis include jaundice, broken blood vessels, a hard liver, a swollen abdomen, and swollen ankles. Some men suffering from the disorder experience an enlargement of their breasts, loss of pubic hair, and shrinking of the testicles (causing impotence).

Q: *How is cirrhosis treated?*

A: In cirrhosis caused by drinking alcohol, the only useful treatment is to stop drinking completely.

In cirrhosis caused by autoimmune disease, steroids and immunosuppressive drugs may be prescribed. Specialized care over a long period includes a high-protein diet with extra vitamins. Antibiotic drugs may be prescribed if there is infection (cholangitis). Occasionally, the accompanying high blood pressure in the liver can be reduced by a surgical by-pass operation. *See also* IMMUNOSUPPRESSIVE DRUG; STEROID.

Q: *Can cirrhosis cause complications?*

A: Cirrhosis results in a kind of scar tissue that interferes with the flow of blood through the liver. This raises the blood pressure in the veins within the abdomen, especially at the lower end of the esophagus, which becomes dilated and congested (esophageal varices), and the rectum (hemorrhoids). If esophageal varices burst, severe internal bleeding and vomiting of blood (hematemesis) can result.

Other complications of cirrhosis include jaundice, coma, bleeding disorders, peptic ulcers, and accumulation of fluid in the abdomen (ascites). *See also* COMA; HEMORRHOID; JAUNDICE.

Claudication (klô də kā'shən) is the medical term for limping that is usually caused by pain. Intermittent claudication is pain in the legs that is a symptom of arterial disease; the pain occurs during and after exercise.

See also CLAUDICATION, INTERMITTENT.

Claudication, intermittent (klô-də kā'shən, in tər mit'ənt). Intermittent claudication is pain or cramp in the calf muscle after exercise. Relieved by rest, the pain recurs when the muscle is again exercised.

Q: *What causes this form of pain?*

A: The cramp-like pain is the result of an inadequate blood supply, and therefore inadequate amounts of oxygen, to the calf muscles; this is caused by a disorder, usually arteriosclerosis, of the blood vessels. Sometimes, the pain may follow blockage of an artery by an embolus (clot of blood or other material from elsewhere in the body) or by Buerger's disease (chronic inflammation of the blood vessels). Occasionally, intermittent claudication occurs following an injury to the leg and subsequent blood vessel damage. *See also* ARTERIOSCLEROSIS; BUERGER'S DISEASE.

The condition commonly develops in smokers and in those with diabetes mellitus. The symptoms become worse if the patient becomes anemic or develops hypothyroidism. *See also* HYPOTHYROIDISM.

Unless the onset is sudden because of embolus or thrombosis, there is a gradual deterioration in blood supply to the muscles. The symptoms tend to become worse, and finally, any form of activity causes pain.

Q: *Are there any dangers in intermittent claudication?*

A: Yes. The condition is a sign of poor blood supply to the leg. Other tissues also suffer, possibly resulting in gangrene of the toes and feet. Sudden blockage of the blood vessel may lead to an infarction (area of dead tissue) in the muscles, and the gradual deterioration may result in peripheral neuritis (inflammation of nerves). *See also* INFARCTION; NEURITIS.

Q: ***How is intermittent claudication treated?***

A: It is essential that a patient who smokes stop smoking, because this may prevent any further progress of the condition and allow him or her to lead a relatively normal life without further discomfort. A physician may prescribe a drug that makes the blood vessels widen (vasodilator) or that causes the blood cells to flow more readily. Such drugs are, however, seldom successful.

If the symptoms are severe and the patient is suffering from considerable incapacity, angioplasty or surgery is indicated. An arteriogram locates the diseased section, and arterial surgery is performed to graft in a new segment of artery or plastic tubing. This treatment often gives complete relief from symptoms. *See also* GRAFT.

Claustrophobia (klôs′trə fō′bē a) is an irrational fear of being in any confined area or enclosed space, such as a windowless elevator. Such situations may cause anxiety or even panic in some individuals.

See also PHOBIA.

Clavicle (klav′ə kəl), or collarbone, is one of two bones that connect the breast bone (sternum) with the shoulder blades (scapulas).

See also SCAPULA; STERNUM.

Clawfoot is another name for pes cavus. *See also* PES CAVUS.

Claw hand is a deformity of the hand, characterized by widely spread, curved fingers, so that the hand resembles a claw. It is usually the result of a nerve injury.

Cleft palate (kleft pal′it) is an abnormal fissure, present at birth, in the roof of the mouth. In normal development of the fetus, separate tissues fuse together to form the palate, upper lip, and upper jaw. If the tissues fail to fuse, a cleft palate is the result. Often, a cleft palate is accompanied by a similar division in the upper lip, called a harelip. These defects affect females more often than males and sometimes run in families. *See also* HARELIP; PALATE.

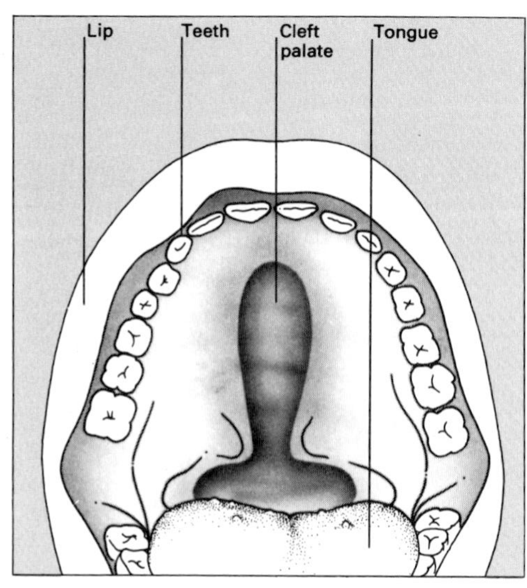

Cleft palate occurs when the roof of the mouth does not develop completely.

Q: ***Does a cleft palate cause feeding problems for a baby?***

A: Yes. A cleft palate and harelip interfere with the natural sucking ability of a newborn baby, and the child must be fed with a bulb syringe or spoon or with a special long nipple on a baby bottle.

Q: ***Can a cleft palate be corrected?***

A: Most cases of cleft palate can be repaired by a series of operations. Plastic surgery is necessary to repair a harelip. If proper treatment is not started at a reasonably early age, the child may develop speech difficulties. Speech therapy may be necessary in any case for a person with a cleft palate. *See also* PLASTIC, SURGERY.

Climacteric. *See* MENOPAUSE.

Clinic, community. Community clinics generally provide primary care for patients who are not hospitalized. Some clinics are part of a hospital. The physicians and medical workers who staff such clinics are hospital employees or volunteers. Other clinics are run by physicians in group practices or by community organizations. Group practice clinics and some community clinics operate for a profit, while other community clinics are nonprofit organizations. The physicians and medical workers who staff these clinics charge the patients a small fee or none at all. The U.S. government provides financial aid for some community clinics, which are called neighborhood health centers.

A number of clinics have both specialists and general practitioners on their staff. Some group practice clinics have specialists only. Among the concerns of specialized clinics are alcoholism, cancer detection and treatment, dental care, diabetes, infant care, mental health, drug addiction, prenatal care, and venereal disease.

Clitoris (klit'ər is) is a small, soft, sensitive area of tissue that is part of the female genitalia. It is situated below the pubic bone and is partially enclosed by the thin folds of the labia minora. The clitoris plays an important part in the sexual stimulation of the female and, like the male penis, becomes erect during sexual excitement.

See also LABIUM.

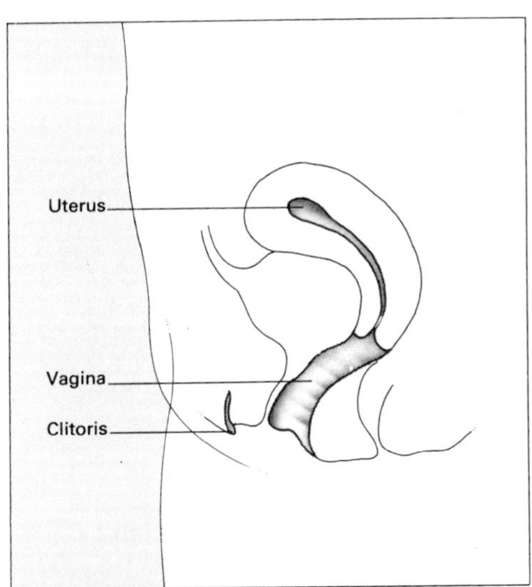

The **clitoris** is made of erectile tissue similar to that of the male penis.

Clone (klōn) is any group of individuals produced asexually from a single ancestor. In biology, a clone is an exact duplicate of a single cell that simply splits off from the parent cell. In tissue culture, a clone is a cluster of cells produced by a single parent cell.

See also CELL.

Clonic (klon'ik) refers to the alternate, rapid contraction and relaxation of muscles, such as would occur in a seizure.

Clostridium (klos trid'ē əm) is a genus of spore-bearing, rod-shaped, or spindle-shaped bacteria that are able to grow in the absence of oxygen. These bacteria are common in soil and in the intestines of animals. Some species are harmless to humans, but others produce toxins that are highly dangerous and potentially fatal. Different *Clostridium* species are responsible for tetanus (lockjaw) and botulism (food poisoning).

See also BACTERIA; BOTULISM; FOOD POISONING; TETANUS.

Clot (klot) is the jelly-like substance formed when a liquid coagulates. In medicine, the term is normally used to mean a blood clot.

See also BLOOD CLOT.

Clubbing (klub'ing) is a condition characterized by the splaying of fingers and toes and the rounding of the nails. In most cases, clubbing is a sign of a more serious underlying heart, liver, or lung disorder. It may also be a symptom of celiac disease, colitis, chronic dysentery, or other intestinal disorders. The precise mechanism of the enlargement is unknown, but if the cause is found and successfully treated, clubbing may disappear.

See also CELIAC DISEASE; COLITIS.

Clubfoot, known medically as talipes, is a deformity of the foot present at birth. In the most usual form (talipes equinovarus), the sole of the foot is turned inward and the heel upward. It is more common in boys than in girls and may affect both feet.

Treatment is most effective when started soon after birth. The foot is held in the correct position by a metal brace or a plaster of Paris cast. An orthopedist may recommend an operation to correct the condition.

Cluster headache. *See* HEADACHE, CLUSTER.

CMV. *See* CYTOMEGALOVIRUS.

CNS. *See* NERVOUS SYSTEM, CENTRAL.

Coagulation (kō ag yə lā'shən) is the formation of a clot in blood, lymph, or other liquid. It is a normal part of the healing process following an injury or surgery. Blood coagulation is a complicated process that involves many factors. If any of these factors are missing, coagulation occurs slowly or not at all. Hemophilia is an example of a disease caused by a missing coagulation factor.

See also AGGLUTINATION; BLOOD CLOT.

Coarctation (kō ärk tā'shən) is a narrowing of a tube. The term usually refers to the narrowing of the aorta, the chief artery leading from the heart. This is usually a congenital defect (present at birth). Coarctation of the aorta prevents normal blood flow, causing high blood pressure in the head and arms and low blood pressure in the rest of the body. It may be treated by surgery, in which the narrowed section of the aorta is removed.

See also AORTA; BLOOD PRESSURE.

Cobalt (kō'bôlt) is a metallic element, traces of which are found in most foods and are easily absorbed in the digestive system. Cobalt is most commonly used in medicine as cobalt 60, a radioactive isotope, which emits beta particles and gamma-ray radiation to destroy malignant tissue. The source of cobalt 60 is always well shielded in lead casings.

Cobalt treatment (kō'bəlt) is a type of radiotherapy used against cancer.

See also CANCER; RADIOTHERAPY.

Cocaine (kō kān') is an illegal, mood-altering drug. It is a fine white powder consisting of cocaine hydrochloride from the leaves of the coca shrub and other compounds. The shrub is indigenous to Peru and Bolivia, the countries from which most cocaine comes. There are an estimated five million users of cocaine in the United States. Use of the drug can lead to serious physical and/or psychological problems, sometimes resulting in death.

Surgeons used cocaine as a local anesthetic over a century ago. Today, except in certain kinds of nose and throat surgery, the use of cocaine in surgery has been replaced by synthetic, local anesthetics. The use of cocaine as an illegal stimulant of the central nervous system, however, has grown to alarming proportions in recent years, prompting drug enforcement officials to redouble their efforts in combating the growth, importation, distribution, and sale of the drug.

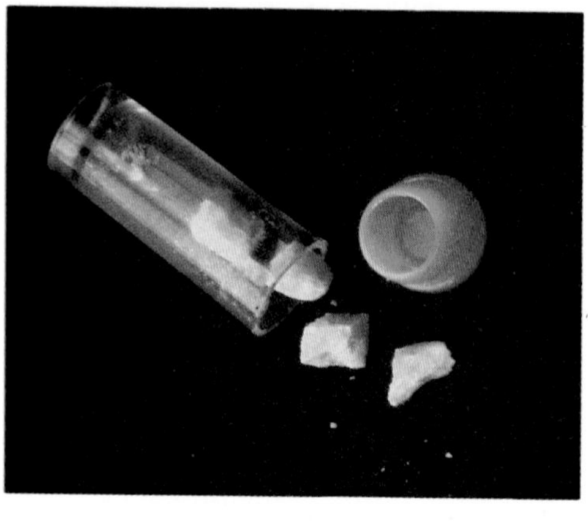

A form of **cocaine** known as "crack" is a smokeable, freebase form of the drug.

Cocaine gained widespread acceptance in the 1970's when it was viewed as a harmless "recreational" drug that produced the desired "high" without the danger of addiction or typical drug-related side effects. Many persons in the public eye—movie stars and sports heroes, for example—were users of cocaine. It quickly became fashionable in other sectors of society, especially among those who could easily afford its once high price. Before the price came down, cocaine use was directly associated with wealth and success. Those who used the drug claimed that the cocaine rush not only produced the intended euphoric "high," but also resulted in higher levels of performance in whatever activity they happened to be engaged in.

Addiction. Since the 1970's and early 1980's, scientific research and painful experience have demonstrated that cocaine, far from being a harmless recreational drug, is not only highly addictive, but also very dangerous, even potentially lethal. Further, the much-touted euphoria and elevation of performance levels have turned out to be either transitory or illusory.

According to research done by the American Council for Drug Education, cocaine affects the same part of the brain that reinforces basic instinctual drives such as hunger, thirst, and sexual desire. This is the brain's "reward center." Cocaine causes the release of a neurotransmitter called dopamine in the brain's nerve endings. When the level of dopamine increases, the reward center is falsely notified that a basic need has been satisfied; the reward center then provides the pleasure response or euphoric high. With the repeated use of cocaine, the reward center is "reprogrammed," thus encouraging the user to obtain and use more cocaine to supplant survival-oriented drives.

Once a person's brain has accepted cocaine as necessary to basic survival, that person is addicted, and the drive to obtain and use cocaine takes precedence over important areas of life, such as nutrition, sleep, sex, and career. According to the American Council for

Drug Education, cocaine addiction is characterized by four major features: cravings and compulsions to obtain and use the drug; inability to limit or control use; continued use despite adverse consequences; and denial that the problem exists.

Of the many serious problems associated with cocaine addiction, one of the more apparent ones is the "crash" that follows the "high." Though the level of dopamine initially rises when a person takes cocaine, producing the "high," it soon falls off, dropping to a level below normal and producing the "crash." With repeated use of the drug, an overall depletion of dopamine levels occurs and chronic depression sets in. The addict requires ever-increasing amounts of the drug to attain the desired high. Eventually, however, the addict's tolerance reaches a level so high that no amount of cocaine will produce euphoria.

Side effects of cocaine use can include a substantial drop in weight because of loss of appetite. Addicts who inhale cocaine often develop sensitive and ulcerated nasal membranes. This can even lead to a perforation of the nasal septum. Addicts who inject cocaine intravenously are also at greater risk for contracting infectious diseases, such as AIDS, due to the habit of sharing needles and syringes. Among the psychological effects are irritability, sleeplessness, paranoid thoughts, and possible full-blown, paranoid psychosis.

Persons with plasma pseudocholinesterase deficiency are at risk for sudden death from even small amounts of cocaine because this enzyme is essential for its metabolism. Cocaine deaths are usually caused by severe disturbances of the heart rhythm (ventricular fibrillation), heart attack (myocardial infarction), repeated convulsions, or depression of the respiratory center in the brain.

Crack. In recent years, a form of cocaine, known by its street name of "crack" or "rock," has emerged as an even greater menace than cocaine in its more familiar powdered form. Crack is freebase cocaine, a smokable form of the drug, that has been extracted ("freed") from the hydrochloride salt of cocaine and formed into pellets using baking soda and water. The name comes from the cracking sound the drug makes when heated and smoked.

Cocaine taken in this way is rapidly and efficiently absorbed into the bloodstream. It reaches the brain in 8 to 10 seconds and, in this concentrated form, produces a very rapid and intense high. The high lasts only a few minutes, however, so the user requires another dose very soon to sustain the high. Repeated doses of the highly concentrated form of the drug cause the user to become addicted very quickly.

With crack, all the medical and psychological problems produced by powdered cocaine are magnified. The extremely high levels of cocaine in the blood greatly increase the possibility of serious toxic reactions, such as high blood pressure, irregular heartbeat, fever, and potentially fatal brain seizures. Among serious respiratory problems suffered by crack smokers are wheezing, chest congestion, chronic cough, and impairment of lung function. Psychological consequences often include radical changes in personality and behavior, which can range all the way from irritability and withdrawal to paranoid reactions and suicidal behavior.

Treatment programs for cocaine addiction are available in cities throughout the country. There are several sources of information about the drug:

American Council for Drug Education, 204 Monroe, Rockville, MD 20850.

National Clearinghouse for Alcohol and Drug Information, P. O. Box 2345, Rockville, MD 20852.

National Federation of Parents for Drug-Free Youth, 8730 Georgia Avenue, Suite 200, Silver Springs, MD 20190.

PRIDE, Inc., 100 Edgewood Avenue, Suite 1002, Atlanta, GA 30303.

See also DRUG ABUSE; DRUG ADDICTION.

Coccidioidomycosis (kok sid ē oi dō mī kō′sis), also known as San Joaquin Valley fever or desert fever, is indigenous to hot, dry regions, such as the southwestern United States and northwestern Mexico. Caused by a fungus carried in dust particles, the disease occurs in two forms. The primary (pulmonary) form affects the respiratory system, causes symptoms similar to those of the common cold, and usually does not need to be treated. It clears up by itself.

The secondary (progressive) form can develop from the primary form; it affects the lungs and, occasionally, the spinal fluid. Skin lesions, arthritis, weight loss, and low-grade fever are also seen. It is potentially fatal, but medical therapy with amphotericin B is often successful.

Coccus (kok'əs) is a sphere-shaped type of bacteria, which can be the cause of many infections. Streptococcus, pneumococcus, and gonococcus are examples of this type of bacteria.

See also STREPTOCOCCUS.

Coccyx (kok'siks) is the final bone of the spine, usually formed from four small bones, fused together and joined to the sacrum. The coccyx is sometimes called the tailbone.

See also SACRUM; SPINE.

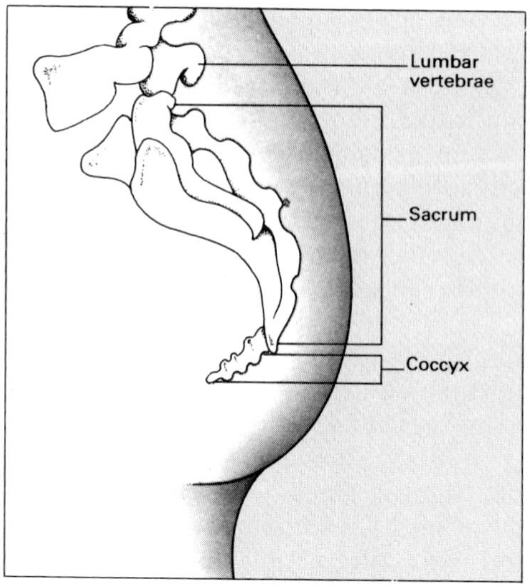

The **coccyx** is a bone at the base of the spine formed from four small bones.

Cochlea (kok'lē ə) is the spiral-shaped portion of the ear, which contains the inner ear parts. The cochlea includes the sensory cells (hair cells) and the nerve endings that transmit sound to the brain.

See also EAR.

Codeine (kō'dēn), known medically as methylmorphine, is a drug derived from opium. It is used as a painkiller, a cough suppressant, and a treatment for diarrhea. Prolonged use of large quantities may produce mild addiction. Many painkilling preparations contain a small amount of codeine in addition to acetaminophen or aspirin. In the United States codeine is available only by prescription.

Cod-liver oil (kod'-liv ər) is purified from the fresh livers of codfish. The oil contains a high concentration of vitamins A and D and was once used to supplement children's diets.

See also VITAMIN.

Coil (koil) is the common name for a type of intrauterine device (IUD) used in contraception.

See also CONTRACEPTION.

Coitus. See SEXUAL INTERCOURSE.

Colchicine (kol'chə sēn) is an alkaloid drug obtained from the roots of the autumn crocus. It is used to treat gout and biliary cirrhosis. A side effect is diarrhea.

See also DIARRHEA; GOUT.

Cold, known medically as an upper respiratory infection, is a contagious virus disease. It is a droplet infection caught by inhaling airborne water droplets from a sneeze of a patient with the disorder or by contact with hands that have touched an infected mouth or nose. Symptoms appear about 48 hours after exposure to the virus, which may be any one of, or a combination of, more than 100 different types. Colds are more frequent among the young and are more likely to occur during the winter months.

Q: *What are the typical symptoms of a cold?*

A: Early symptoms of a cold include a runny nose, watering eyes, a headache, and a sore throat. Later, there may be a stuffy nose, a slight cough, and aching muscles. The patient may also have a chill and a slight fever.

Q: *Can a cold be serious?*

A: A cold, although extremely annoying, is seldom serious. However, babies, young children, and patients with asthma, bronchitis, a heart disorder, or kidney disease, who have symptoms of a cold, may be at risk and should seek medical advice.

Q: *Can a cold be cured?*

A: There is no cure for a cold. Home treatment to relieve the symptoms includes regular doses of a mild painkiller such as acetaminophen; an antihistamine to help dry up the nasal discharge; a cough medicine; and lozenges for the sore throat. Contrary to popular belief, antibiotics do not cure a cold (or any other virus infection). The patient should drink plenty of fluids and avoid contact with others to prevent spreading the infection.

An ordinary cold should clear up in three or four days. If it does not or if additional symptoms occur, such as earache, pain in the face, higher fever, or a combination of sore throat, cough, and shortness of breath, a physician should be seen.

Cold abscess. See ABSCESS, COLD.

Cold exposure: treatment. See HYPOTHERMIA: TREATMENT.

Cold sore, or fever sore, is a small blister that appears, becomes an ulcer, and then heals with a scab. Cold sores usually occur around the lips and nose, but they are also common in the genital region and tend to recur.

Cold sores, known medically as herpes simplex, are caused by the herpes simplex virus type 1 (HSV1). This virus is present in many people and produces no symptoms when the person is in good health, but causes cold sores when another infection, such as the common cold, occurs. Sometimes, stress or exposure to wind, sunlight, certain foods, or drugs can cause cold sores. In some women, cold sores appear with the menstrual period. Acyclovir, in the form of an ointment, can be an effective drug used to treat cold sores.

See also HERPES GENITALIS.

Colectomy (kə lek'tə mē) is an operation to remove part or all of the large intestine (colon). It is usually performed to treat cancer of the colon or severe colitis. After a total colectomy or a partial colectomy, close to the anus, an artificial opening is made in the wall of the abdomen (ileostomy or colostomy). When only a part of the colon is removed, the two ends are joined, but a temporary colostomy may be done to help speed healing.

See also COLITIS; COLON; COLOSTOMY; ILEOSTOMY.

Colic (kol'ik) is an acute spasm accompanied by severe pain in the abdominal cavity. The pain is usually localized in one of the ducts or hollow organs in the abdomen, such as the colon, the ureters, or the gall bladder.

Q: *What causes colic?*

A: Colic in adults is usually severe. When its cause is an obstruction, such as a gallstone in the bile duct or a kidney stone in the ureter, the person may vomit and double up with pain. Colic may also accompany menstruation, lead poisoning, and other medical conditions.

The precise cause of infant colic has not been determined, but it seems to be the result of a combination of factors. Often, a family history of irritable bowel syndrome may be present. Some believe it is caused by immaturity in the digestive system or the nervous system, by individual differences in temperament and parental responses to them, or by a reaction to cow's milk proteins or other elements that may be in formula or breast milk. The baby's abdomen is slightly distended; the legs are drawn to the abdomen, often with passage of gas by rectum; and there are prolonged periods of crying, usually at the same time each day.

Q: *How is colic diagnosed and treated?*

A. Adult colic is usually diagnosed using special X-ray techniques; it is treated by eliminating the cause, such as removal of a gallstone.

Infant colic is usually diagnosed by observing the signs. The infant should be comforted until the pain subsides; special attention should be paid to diet and feeding methods. The infant usually thrives despite the colic. For the parent, coping with the frustration and guilt over the distress may require time away from the infant, when someone else takes care of the colicky baby.

Colic, biliary (kol'ik, bil'ē er ē). Biliary colic is an extremely severe pain in the upper right-hand part of the abdomen. The pain, which comes and goes, is often accompanied by sweating and vomiting. It is the result of a spasm of the gall bladder or of obstruction of the bile ducts, either of which is caused by one or more gallstones.

Q: *What is the treatment for biliary colic?*

A: Injections of antispasmodic drugs reduce the pain, which usually ceases altogether when the gallstone passes into the duodenum, is removed, or lodges at the side of the bile duct. An oral cholecystogram can confirm the presence of gallstones, and the gallstone (and bladder if it is diseased) can be removed by an operation.

See also ABDOMEN; GALL BLADDER.

Colic, renal (kol′ik, rē′nəl). Renal colic is an acute, severe pain in the lower back, usually caused by the passing of a kidney stone through the ureter, the tube connecting the kidney with the bladder. The pain originates over the kidney and pulses down and forward into the groin and, in the male, into the scrotum. It has been described as one of the most severe pains known.

See also CALCULUS.

Colitis (kō lī′tis) is inflammation of the colon (large intestine). There are two kinds of colitis. The more common, milder form is called irritable bowel syndrome. The other more severe form, which includes ulcerative colitis, is inflammatory bowel disease. This term is frequently misunderstood, and it is important to note that most people who believe they have some form of colitis have something entirely different.

See also COLITIS, ULCERATIVE; COLON; INFLAMMATORY BOWEL DISEASE; IRRITABLE BOWEL SYNDROME.

Colitis, mucous. *See* IRRITABLE BOWEL SYNDROME.

Colitis, pseudomembranous. *See* ENTEROCOLITIS.

Colitis, ulcerative (kō lī′tis, ul′sə rā tiv). Ulcerative colitis is a disorder of the large intestine, in which the colon becomes inflamed and ulcerated. It usually occurs in persons between 15 and 35 years old. The underlying cause of the disorder is not known.

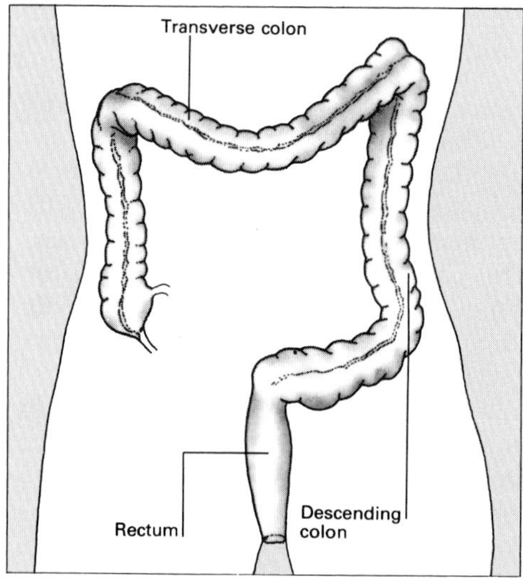

Ulcerative colitis first affects the rectum and then progresses to the colon.

Q: *What are the symptoms of ulcerative colitis?*

A: The most common symptom is a series of attacks and bloody diarrhea that vary in severity and duration from one person to another and from one attack to another. They may start suddenly or gradually and may occur as frequently as 10 or 15 times in 24 hours. The attacks are often accompanied by pain and spasms around the anus (tenesmus). Attacks may also cause fever, loss of appetite, and weight loss.

With mild attacks, the symptoms are less alarming. The patient may feel tired, but usually there are no signs of generalized illness.

The symptoms usually disappear between attacks, although some patients may suffer from mild diarrhea.

Q: *Can ulcerative colitis cause complications?*

A: Yes. The most serious complications are associated with a sudden attack of bloody diarrhea, perforation of the intestine, peritonitis, and intestinal bleeding.

Persons with ulcerative colitis may also develop anemia, arthritis, inflammation of the eyes, or tender nodules under the skin. If ulcerative colitis persists for longer than about 10 years, there is a greater than average chance of developing cancer of the colon.

Q: *How is ulcerative colitis diagnosed and treated?*

A: A positive diagnosis may require an internal examination of the colon and a barium enema X ray.

Mild attacks of ulcerative colitis are usually treated with antidiarrheal drugs, a low-fiber diet, and rest. Sulfonamide drugs may control the symptoms of a severe attack. Treatment with corticosteroids may also be necessary.

Persons who suffer an extremely severe attack may require hospital treatment. If complications develop, such as peritonitis or intestinal bleeding, emergency surgery may be necessary.

The outcome of ulcerative colitis is variable. However, most patients suffer repeated attacks over many years, and about 30 percent eventually require some form of surgery.

Patients with recurrent ulcerative colitis should have regular internal examinations of the colon to check for early signs of intestinal cancer. In some cases, it is necessary to remove part or all of the colon (colectomy) and form an opening to the skin (colostomy).

See also COLITIS.

Collapsed lung. See LUNG, COLLAPSED.

Collarbone. See CLAVICLE.

Collarbone fracture: first aid. See FRACTURE: FIRST AID.

Colles' fracture (kol'ēz frak'chər) is a fracture of the radius bone in the forearm, just above the wrist. Part of the radius shifts and causes the wrist to be unnaturally positioned upward. A regional anesthetic to numb the involved arm is normally given while an orthopedist restores the bone to its original position. The forearm is immobilized in a cast for about six weeks, after which physiotherapy is needed to restore normal movement to the wrist.

Coloboma (kol əbō'mə) is any one of a group of congenital eye defects that may appear as a white swelling or as a gap. It may also appear as a groove or cleft in the iris, the lens, or the choroid. Sometimes, the eyelid is also involved. Vision may be impaired. There is no treatment for the condition.

See also EYE.

Colon (kō'lən) is the part of the large intestine that extends from the cecum to the rectum. ("Large" refers to diameter, not to length.) Sections of the colon have different names. For example, the ileum of the small intestine joins with the cecum of the colon. Where the colon extends upward, it is called the ascending colon; where it crosses the abdomen, it is called the transverse colon; and when it moves downward toward the pelvis, it is called the descending colon. The last part is the sigmoid colon, which meets the rectum.

See also INTESTINE.

Q: *What is the function of the colon?*

A: Although most of the digestive process occurs in the small intestine, the colon absorbs excess water and salts to be taken into the blood. This function of conserving and recycling is an important one; without it, dehydration can take place. After the excess water and salts have been absorbed by the blood, the remaining contents of the colon take on the consistency of feces, which are stored in the rectum until passed through the anus.

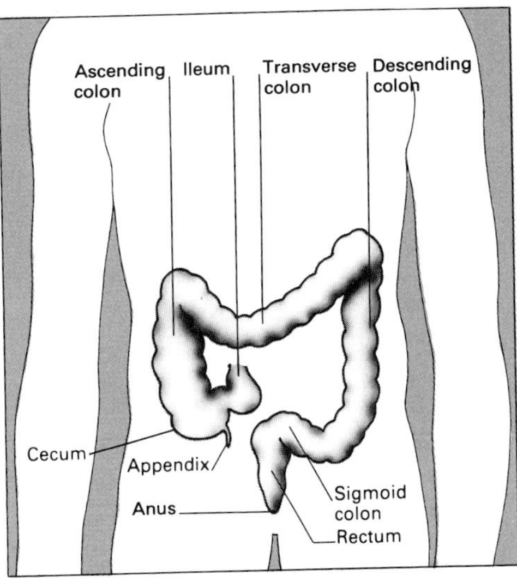

The **colon** receives indigestible fiber from the ileum and passes it along to the anus by peristalsis.

Colonic irrigation. See ENEMA.

Colonoscopy (kō lən os'ko pē) is an examination of the colon with a colonoscope, a lighted instrument, inserted through the anus, which allows the physician to see the interior of the large intestine.

See also COLON.

Color blindness is an inherited defect of vision, resulting in a person's inability to distinguish between specific colors. Partial color blindness is more common than total color blindness, in which a person sees everything as shades of gray. The most common form of partial color blindness leads to an inability to distinguish between red and green; rarely, the difficulty is between blue and yellow.

Color vision depends on the stimulation of the approximately eight million cone cells in the light-sensitive membrane at the back of the eye (retina). The three colors distinguished by the eye—red, green, and blue—cause three different pigments in the cone cells to react. Absence or defect in one or more of these pigments at birth results in defects of color vision.

Q: *How common is color blindness?*
A: The defect is genetically determined as an X-linked pattern and is passed on to about 10 percent of the male population. Only about 1 percent of all women have some form of color blindness. Total color blindness is rare.
Q: *How is color blindness diagnosed?*
A: There are several different tests that may be used. For example, Ishihara's test is composed of a series of colored cards on which numbers or lines of equal shade can be read by a person with normal color vision but not by someone with defective color vision.

Colostomy (kə los'tə mē) is an artificial connection, produced by surgery, between the large intestine (colon) and the surface of the body at the abdominal wall. A special bag over the opening in the abdominal wall is usually necessary to collect stools. *See also* COLON.
Q: *Why might a patient need a colostomy?*
A: A diseased area of colon may have to be removed (partial colectomy). Then the two ends on each side of the removed portion may be brought to the surface. This type of colostomy may be temporary, until the two ends can themselves be joined surgically. But if the whole of the lower part of the colon is diseased and has to be removed, the upper part alone may be brought to the surface. This type of colostomy is permanent. *See also* COLECTOMY.
Q: *What adjustments might a colostomy patient have to make?*
A: Once the patient has learned how to deal with it, a colostomy is usually not a major inconvenience. The diet should be regulated to avoid constipation or diarrhea. Some patients find that a morning enema via the colostomy (colostomy irrigation) clears the colon for the day, and the bag may not be required.

While still in the hospital following colostomy surgery, nurses with special knowledge and skills help the patient with the initial adjustment and teach the patient about the care of their colostomy. The patient gains confidence from the emotional support of other colostomy patients. This can come from the many colostomy societies, which offer help and mutual advice.

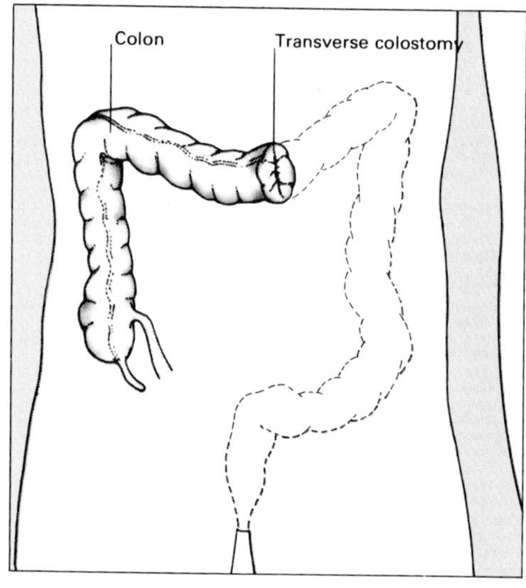

A **colostomy** performed on the transverse colon is managed post-operatively with a special bag for collecting stools.

Colostrum (kə los'trəm) is the yellow fluid secreted by a woman's breasts for a few days before and after childbirth. It contains about 20 percent protein, including the mother's antibodies to the diseases that she has had. Colostrum has a higher concentration of salts, but less fat and carbohydrates than normal breast milk.

See also ANTIBODY; PREGNANCY AND CHILDBIRTH.

Colposcopy (kol pos'ko pē) is an examination of the tissues of the cervix and the vagina with a colposcope, a special magnifying lens.

Coma (kō'mə) is a deep, and sometimes prolonged, unconscious state. It may result from a head injury, stroke, reaction to drugs or alcohol, or an epileptic seizure. It may also be caused by a disease such as diabetes, liver failure, or uremia (retention in the blood of substances usually excreted by the kidneys).

Treatment is to place the patient in the recovery position and to keep the airway open. (For instructions, *see* FAINTING: FIRST AID.) Breathing and pulse rate should be monitored. The patient should be hospitalized at once.

Comatose (kom'ə tōs) describes the condition of being in a coma, a stupor caused by illness or injury.

See also COMA.

Comb, long handled. See NURSING THE SICK.

Comedo. See BLACKHEAD.

Comminuted fracture. See FRACTURE, COMMINUTED.

Common cold. See COLD.

Communicable disease is a disease that is transmitted from one person to another, either directly, by touching the secretions of the body, or indirectly, via some inanimate object such as a drinking glass, doorknob, or contaminated water source. Communicable diseases may also be spread via animals, such as flies, mosquitoes, or ticks. The following is a list of contagious diseases, each of which has a separate entry in this encyclopedia.

Acquired immune deficiency syndrome	Paratyphoid
Bronchopneumonia	Pertussis (whooping cough)
Candidiasis	Plague
Chickenpox	Pleurodynia
Chlamydia	Pneumonia
Cholera	Poliomyelitis
Cold	Puerperal fever
Conjunctivitis	Ringworm
Diphtheria	Roseola
Gonorrhea	Rubella (German measles)
Hand-foot-and-mouth disease	Scarlet fever
Hepatitis	Sexually transmitted disease
Herpes genitalis	Smallpox
Influenza	Syphilis
Leprosy	Trachoma
Measles	Tuberculosis
Meningitis	Typhoid fever
Mononucleosis	Vaccinia
Mumps	Yaws

Complete Blood Count. See BLOOD COUNT, COMPLETE.

Complex (kom′pleks) is a psychological term, introduced by Carl Jung, for an idea or group of ideas repressed into the unconscious. It is because these ideas have a strong emotional charge that complexes may influence a person's behavior. Examples of complexes include the Electra complex, the sexual love of a daughter for her father; Oedipus complex, the sexual love of a son for his mother; and inferiority complex, a state of mind in which a person feels inferior to others.

The term complex is often loosely used to mean an obsession. Complex also refers to the lines traced by an electrocardiograph that represent the beating of the heart. A complex may also be a collection of symptoms that make up a syndrome.

Compound fracture. See FRACTURE, COMPOUND.

Compress (kom′prəs) is a pad of material used to apply heat, cold, or medication to a part of the body.

Compulsion (kəm pul′shən) is an irrational impulse to perform an action normally not indulged in. The compulsion is repetitive and, if resisted, leads to anxiety. Alcoholism, compulsive gambling, eating disorders, and other addictions are examples of compulsive behavior.

See also OBSESSION; PHOBIA.

Computerized axial tomography scanner is often abbreviated to CAT scan. It is a machine that passes X rays through a patient's body from various angles. A computer can utilize the images from the X rays to construct a cross-sectional view of the inside of the body. By layering these planes, the computer can create a three-dimensional image of internal organs and structures. Since different types of tissue absorb different amounts of X rays, a physician can distinguish various

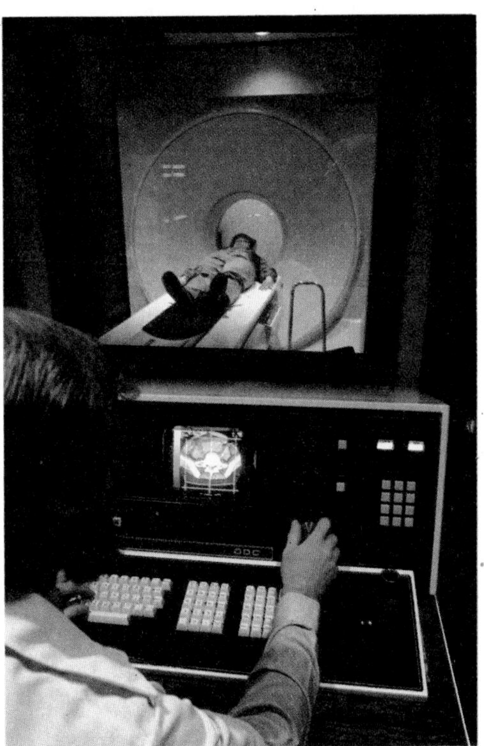

A **computerized axial tomography scanner** (CAT scan) painlessly detects tumors and other disorders. Detailed visualizations of tissues are produced.

structures within the body, differentiating a solid tumor from a fluid-filled cyst, for example, or a blood-filled hematoma in brain tissue.

See also RADIOLOGY; TOMOGRAPHY; X RAY.

Conception (kən sep′shən) is the moment in the reproduction cycle when a sperm fertilizes an ovum. This usually takes place in a woman's fallopian tube. The fertilized egg then passes into the uterus, where it becomes implanted in the wall and develops first into an embryo and then into a fetus.

See also PREGNANCY AND CHILDBIRTH.

Concussion (kən kush′ən) is an injury to a part of the body resulting from a blow or from a violent shaking. Concussion usually refers to an injury to the brain, which is commonly caused by a head injury. It may also result from a fall in which the point of impact is the lower end of the spine.

Q: *What are the symptoms of brain concussion?*

A: The symptoms of brain concussion vary according to the site and extent of the injury. Brain concussion usually, but not always, produces unconsciousness. The return to consciousness often occurs gradually. Following the initial injury, there may be headache, difficulty in concentrating, nausea, vomiting, difficulty in focusing, and a feeling of depression and irritability. Events immediately before the injury may be forgotten at first (retrograde amnesia), but the memory of them usually returns.

Q: *How is brain concussion treated?*

A: A physician should be consulted in all cases of concussion because there may be more serious brain damage. Bed rest is essential for at least a day after the injury. The physician may prescribe painkillers to relieve the headache. Alcohol, sedatives, and tranquilizers may aggravate the symptoms. The patient should avoid sports and work until he or she is completely recovered.

Q: *What should one be alert to when observing a person with a concussion?*

A: The key sign is level of consciousness. Is the person conscious? Can the person be aroused? Other signs worth observing include unequally dilated pupils, an inability to feel or move some body part, or persistent vomiting.

Conditioned reflex (kən dish′ənd rē′fleks) is either a modification of an inborn reflex or a completely new automatic response that is developed as a result of an individual's experience. Conditioned reflexes were first demonstrated by Ivan Pavlov in the 19th century. He taught a dog to salivate at the sound of a bell by first teaching the dog to associate the ringing of a bell with the appearance of food.

See also REFLEX.

Condom (kon′dəm), or prophylactic, is a soft, flexible covering for the penis, usually made of rubber, which is used during sexual intercourse to help prevent pregnancy or the spread of sexually transmitted diseases, such as gonorrhea, syphilis, herpes, and AIDS.

See also ACQUIRED IMMUNE DEFICIENCY SYNDROME; CONTRACEPTION; SEXUALLY TRANSMITTED DISEASE.

Condyloma (kon də lō′mə) is an infectious, wart-like growth on the genitals or near the anus. There are two types: (1) condyloma accuminatum, which is the result of a sexually transmitted viral infection; and (2) condyloma latum, which is a complication of syphilis and which appears flat or ulcerated.

See also SYPHILIS; WART.

Cone (kōn) is a photoreceptor cell, shaped like a cone, in the retina of the eye, which enables a person to see colors. There are three in each eye, one each for red, blue, and green. Other colors are visualized by stimulating different combinations of the three cones.

See also EYE.

Congenital (kən jen′ə təl) refers to any characteristic or condition that is present at birth.

Congenital anomaly (kən jen′ə təl ə nom′ə lē) is a mental or physical abnormality that is present at, and usually before, birth. Some anomalies may be medically insignificant and may not appear for some time. In other cases, the anomaly may pose a direct threat to life and requires immediate attention. There are, however, some anomalies that can not be treated.

Q: *What are examples of congenital anomalies?*

A: Congenital anomalies include bone disorders, cataract, cleft palate, cretinism, Down's syndrome, congeni-

A **congenital anomaly** is a defect that occurs in only a few of every 1,000 newborn children.

tal heart disease, hemophilia, joint disorders, pyloric stenosis, and spina bifida. Blindness, deafness, hydrocephalus, and jaundice are also often due to congenital anomalies, although in other cases they are the result of an event that occurred after birth. Each of the above examples is defined elsewhere in this encyclopedia.

Limbs or organs may be malformed, duplicated, or entirely absent. Organs may fail to move to the correct place, as in cryptorchidism; fail to open correctly as in imperforate anus; or fail to close at the correct time, as in patent ductus arteriosus. Congenital anomalies often occur together. For example, 33 percent of babies born with Down's syndrome also have heart disease.

Q: *What may cause the development of congenital anomalies?*

A: Congenital anomalies arise from the faulty development of a fetus, caused either by genetic disorders or other factors. Some anomalies arise from a combination of factors, and the underlying cause is far from clear in all cases.

Q: *How are genetic disorders responsible for congenital anomalies?*

A: Inherited congenital anomalies generally result from the presence of abnormal genes or chromosomes. Heredity is determined by corresponding pairs of genes, called alleles. One of these paired genes is dominant and the other recessive, and it is the dominant gene that governs the transmitted trait or characteristic. Thus, if the abnormal gene of a pair is dominant, the abnormal or anomalous trait will be conveyed to the embryo. If the abnormal gene is recessive, then both genes in the pair have to be abnormal for a congenital anomaly to occur.

Some congenital anomalies, such as hemophilia, are linked to a defect of one of the sex chromosomes. Many genetic disorders, however, are neither wholly dominant, recessive, nor sex-linked, but may be caused by more than one abnormal pair of genes. *See also* CHROMOSOME; GENE.

Approximate incidences of some congenital anomalies

Defect	Ratio M:F	Incidence per 1,000
Congenital heart disease	1:1	
Pyloric stenosis	4:1	
Clubfoot	2:1	
Down's syndrome	1:1	
Spina bifida	1:1	
Hydrocephalus	1:1	
Microcephaly	1:2	
Congenital dislocated hip	1:6	
Harelip and cleft palate	2:1	
Klinefelter's syndrome	1:0	

Q: *What other factors may cause congenital anomalies?*

A: Infection in the mother is a common cause of abnormality in a baby. For example, an attack of rubella during the first three months of pregnancy may cause her child to be born deaf or have cataracts, heart disease, jaundice, or other anomalies. Cytomegalovirus (CMV) and toxoplasmosis also cause congenital anomalies. *See also* CYTOMEGALOVIRUS; RUBELLA; SYPHILIS; TOXOPLASMOSIS.

Certain drugs taken by a woman during pregnancy are often responsible for abnormalities in the child. For example, large doses of corticosteroids can cause a variety of congenital defects, as can some anticonvulsants given to control epilepsy. Other drugs include anticancer drugs; narcotics and sedatives; tranquilizers and antidepressants; antibacterials, especially tetracycline; anticoagulants; drugs prescribed to treat cardiac conditions and hypertension; oral hypoglycemics used to treat diabetes in the mother; and, of course, heavy consumption of alcohol. Other drugs may cause gross abnormalities, such as the defects arising from thalidomide. A pregnant woman should, thus, avoid taking any medication without first consulting with her physician.

Injury to a pregnant woman or to a fetus is another cause of congenital anomalies. For example, limbs may be malformed if an intrauterine device (IUD) is not removed early in the pregnancy. Smoking during pregnancy is implicated as one factor in the incidence of abnormally low birth weight in babies, and malnutrition seems to be related to a high incidence of congenital anomalies. The age of the woman at the time she conceives can also be a factor. For example, Down's syndrome occurs more frequently when conception occurs after the age of about 35.

Congenital anomalies have also been attributed to the effects of X-ray examination made early in a pregnancy.

Q: *Is it possible to diagnose congenital anomalies in a fetus?*

A: Yes. The most reliable method of diagnosis is to examine a sample of fluid from the amniotic sac, sometime between the fifteenth and eighteenth week of pregnancy. The sample is obtained by amniocentesis. Microscopic examination of the cells in the fluid then reveals possible abnormalities in the chromosomes. Congenital anomalies that can be diagnosed in this way include Down's syndrome, spina bifida, and anencephaly. Sometimes, the diagnostic use of ultrasound can detect abnormalities of the skull or spine. *See also* AMNIOCENTESIS.

Q: *Can congenital anomalies be treated?*

A: Treatment depends entirely on the nature and severity of the condition. Many anomalies can be treated, but for some there is no treatment.

Q: *In what circumstances might abortion be considered?*

A: Abortion might be considered if serious fetal disorders are found early in a pregnancy. The decision to abort rests with the parents and is made after considering the advice of the physician and specialists on the nature of the disorder and the consequences of abortion.

Q: *Are congenital anomalies more likely to occur in first-born babies?*

A: No. Statistics disprove this commonly held belief.

Q: *Does a congenital anomaly in a baby indicate that subsequent babies will be similarly affected?*

A: Genetic counseling deals with such questions. In many cases it is possible to state risks numerically. For example, a baby with congenital heart disease is likely to be followed by a similarly affected child in 2 percent of pregnancies instead of the ordinary risk of one percent. Spina bifida occurs in about 1 child in every 1,500, but if a previous child was born with the condition, there is about a 1-in-20 to 1-in-50 chance that it will occur in a later child. *See also* GENETIC COUNSELING.

Congenital heart disease. *See* HEART DISEASE, CONGENITAL.

Congestion (kən jes'chən) is the swelling of body tissues due to the accumulation of blood or tissue fluid. It may be a reaction to infection or injury, or it may be caused by a blockage in veins returning blood to the heart.

Congestive heart failure. *See* HEART FAILURE, CONGESTIVE.

Conization (kōn i zā'shən) is the removal of tissue in the shape of a cone. This procedure is often utilized for cancer *in situ* of the cervix and may circumvent the need for a hysterectomy.

See also CANCER.

Conjunctiva (kon jungk tī'və) is the thin, mucous membrane that lines the eyelid and covers the white of the eyeball, or sclera.

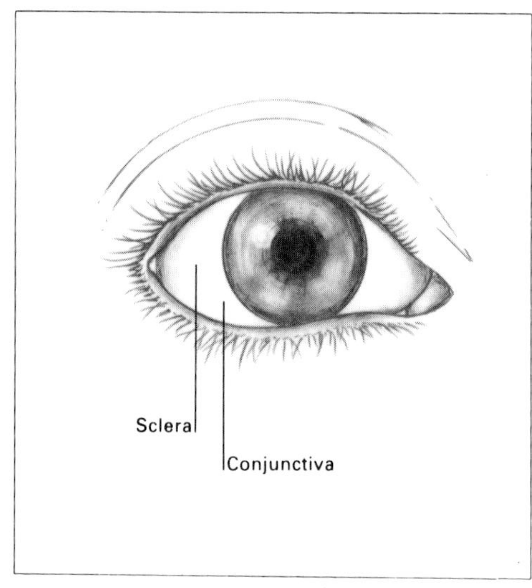

Conjunctiva lines the inside of the eyelids and covers the white portion of the eyeball.

Conjunctivitis (kən jungk tə vī'tis), also called "pink eye," is inflammation of the membrane covering the eye (the conjunctiva). Acute conjunctivitis frequently occurs with viral respiratory illnesses, such as the common cold or influenza, and may be highly contagious. More severe attacks are usually caused by bacterial infections. Conjunctivitis that is not associated with respiratory disorders may be caused by irritants, such as dust, cosmetics, or smoke, or by an allergic reaction to a specific substance, such as pollen or penicillin. Conjunctivitis may also result from the eye disorder trachoma and from a number of other rare afflictions or conditions. Suspected conjunctivitis should always be evaluated promptly by a health professional.

Q: *What are the symptoms of conjunctivitis?*

A: The eye tends to water profusely and the white of the eye is bloodshot or pink. The eye is painful when moved and may be oversensitive to bright light. Sometimes, there is a discharge of pus from the eyelids.

Q: *How is conjunctivitis treated?*

A: A physician usually prescribes an antibiotic drug and other treatments, such as eyedrops. Prolonged use of drops, however, may aggravate the inflammation. Conjunctivitis known to be caused by an allergy may be treated with corticosteroid drugs. Dark glasses give protection against bright light, but a patch over the eye may increase the inflammation. If the eye is painful, a mild painkiller such as acetaminophen gives relief. It is important not to rub the eye, because this may transmit the conjunctivitis to the other eye. For the same reason, patients with conjunctivitis must wash their hands often and use separate towels in order to prevent transmission of the disease. *See also* CORTICOSTEROID DRUG.

Connective tissue is any tissue that connects and supports other tissues or organs—for example, the fibrous tissue of ligaments. Dense connective tissue includes cartilage and bone.

See also BONE; CARTILAGE.

Consciousness (kon'shəs nis) is a state of awareness. The individual is aware of his or her own feelings and mental activity and of the immediate world and is, thus, able to respond to external stimuli. Being conscious is usually synonymous with being awake. Thus, an individual loses consciousness by falling asleep, sometimes when suffering a blow to the head, or while undergoing general anesthesia in preparation for an operation.

See also UNCONSCIOUSNESS.

Constipation (kon stə pā'shən) is the difficult or infrequent excretion of feces. The frequency of bowel movements considered to be normal depends on the individual; "normal" may range from movements three times a day to three times a week. Greater intervals of time between movements than is customary for a particular person are a sign of constipation. The condition is not an illness in itself, but it may be a symptom of one. A physician should be consulted if the condition persists.

Q: *What causes constipation?*

A: Constipation is most often caused by insufficient bulk in the diet or the habit of ignoring the desire to defecate. This gradually makes the rectum tight as the feces accumulate there, especially if a person's diet contains little vegetable fiber and a lot of highly processed food. Some effects of hormones produced during pregnancy may aggravate the problem. A marked change in diet, for example, as a weight-losing measure, may cause constipation. Painkilling drugs taken regularly are often a cause. Drugs that are used as treatment for hypertension, rheumatic disorders, or depression may also cause constipation. Sometimes an anal fissure, a small tear at the opening, causes bowel movements so painful that babies and children avoid having them, which only aggravates the constipation. Colon cancer, depression, or hypothyroidism may also, at times, be associated with constipation. Thus, persistence of the condition should always be medically evaluated.

Q: *Why are babies often constipated?*

A: Hot weather, insufficient fluid in the diet, or a fever may cause slight dehydration in babies. This means that most of the fluid in the colon is absorbed into the bloodstream, leaving the feces hard and difficult to pass. If a baby is constipated from birth, it may be a sign of a developmental failure in the intestine called Hirschsprung's disease.

Q: *Are laxatives an effective treatment for constipation?*

A: Laxatives are sometimes used for immediate relief from constipation, but they should be used sparingly and never taken if other symptoms indicate that the patient may have appendicitis. The regular use of strong laxatives that contain chemicals and vegetable irritants (for example, senna or cascara) may actually maintain constipation, instead of alleviating it. *See also* APPENDICITIS; LAXATIVE.

Q: *How else can constipation be treated?*

A: Treatment must be aimed at removing the cause, such as a drug side effect, improper diet, or depression. Nonirritant purgatives, called bulking agents, help to return the bowel to its normal rhythm; if the feces are hard, special softening laxatives may be recommended. An attempt should be made to establish some regularity in bowel movements and eating habits. A diet containing vegetable fiber, bran, cellulose, or other bulk produces large, soft feces, which are easily passed.

Q: *Does constipation affect certain groups of people more than others?*

A: Constipation occurs more frequently with advancing age. Those who spend many hours sitting down are more susceptible to constipation than those who are physically active.

Consultation (kon səl tā′shən) is the conferring of two or more physicians on the diagnosis or treatment of a patient. Sometimes a physician has a patient with a medical problem that requires specialized expertise. For example, a family-practice physician may have a patient with a severe gastrointestinal problem. The family-practice physician then requests a consultation from a gastroenterologist, who examines the patient and performs special diagnostic procedures (such as endoscopy), and then writes a consultation report, which includes a diagnosis. The primary physician makes a final diagnosis based on the consultation with the gastroenterologist. Although a consultant provides important information, the patient's medical problem is, thus, still managed by his or her own family physician. In other cases, the patient is referred for treatment to the consulting physician for the duration of the illness.

Contact lens is a glass or plastic lens that fits over the cornea of the eye to correct a vision defect. Contact lenses adhere to the cornea and move with the eyeball, providing greater peripheral vision than conventional eyeglasses. The soft, hydrophilic plastic lenses, which allow fluids to pass through, are more comfortable to wear than the older, harder types and can be worn for longer periods of time. Soft lenses, however, do require special handling and care.

Q: *What are the advantages and disadvantages of contact lenses?*

A: Apart from good general vision, contact lenses are being studied as a means of keeping medication in contact with the eyeball for persons with keratitis (inflammation of the cornea). Hard lenses may also temporarily retard the progress of myopia and conical corneas (keratoconus).

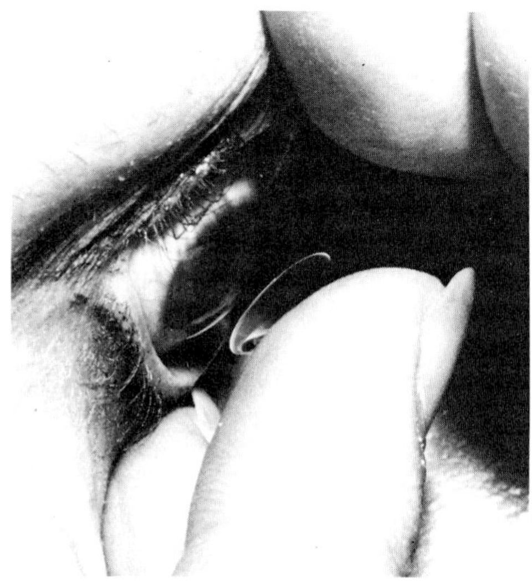

A **contact lens** is shaped to fit over the cornea of the eye. Such lenses are an alternative to conventional eyeglasses.

Contact lenses can require skillful fitting and can be expensive. In the time needed for the eye to become used to a lens, conjunctivitis may occur. Lenses must not be worn when the eye is inflamed, even with the mild conjunctivitis that occurs with a cold. The lenses must be removed and sterilized periodically. Lenses can also cause an allergic reaction.

Most people believe contact lenses are more convenient than conventional eyeglasses, after they have worn them for awhile.

Contagion (kən tā'jən) is the spreading of disease by direct or indirect contact.

See also COMMUNICABLE DISEASE.

Contagious disease. *See* COMMUNICABLE DISEASE.

Continence (kon'tə nəns) is the voluntary control of the bladder and the bowels.

See also INCONTINENCE.

Contraception (kon trə sep'shən), or birth control, is the prevention of pregnancy. There are various contraceptive methods. Some are designed to prevent the male sperm from fertilizing the female egg (ovum) and others to prevent the fertilized egg from developing. The most suitable method is a matter of personal choice and medical advice and often involves trying various methods. The failure rate of each method is expressed as the number of pregnancies per 100 that occur in women using that method each year.

Q: *What forms of contraception require no artificial aids?*

A: There are two common "natural" methods: coitus interruptus and the rhythm method. Coitus interruptus is the withdrawal of the penis from the vagina before ejaculation. Although it is a widely practiced method, it is extremely unreliable, because some sperm nearly always escape before orgasm. The technique also induces stress during intercourse, and many couples find this method frustrating. The failure rate is about 30–40 per 100.

In the rhythm method, or safe period, intercourse is avoided on the days before and following ovulation, when an egg is released from an ovary and travels along a fallopian tube to the uterus. These so-called "safe" days are calculated using the date of ovulation, with the knowledge that the egg survives for a maximum of one day and the sperm for a maximum of six days, or an average of four days. Ovulation usually occurs between 12 and 16 days before a menstrual period is due. A woman can calculate her own ovulation time using either the calendar method or the temperature method, although neither method is totally reliable.

Q: *What is the calendar method?*

A: For this method, a record of menstruation must be kept for at least six months. Counting the first day of menstruation as day 1, the first "unsafe" day is found by subtracting 18 from the shortest recorded cycle, and the last by subtracting 11 from the longest cycle. Thus, if a woman's shortest cycle was 27 days and her longest 32, she must avoid intercourse from days 8 to 22.

Q: *How does the temperature method work?*

A: Each month a woman's body temperature rises slightly at the time of ovulation. She can record this rise if she takes her temperature every morning before (and not after) getting out of bed. The "safe" period is usually from two days after ovulation until five days before the next expected rise in temperature. The failure rate is about 20-30 per 100.

Q: *What are the artificial aids to contraception?*

A: Two methods use simple physical barriers between the sperm and the egg: the condom and the diaphragm. The condom, worn by the man, is a sheath of thin rubber or plastic and often has a small teat at the end to collect the ejaculated sperm. The condom is rolled onto the erect penis just before intercourse. After orgasm the penis must be withdrawn from the vagina before it becomes flaccid, or the condom may fall off in the vagina. For added protection the woman should use a spermicide.

The condom is probably the most widely used form of artificial contraceptive and has a failure rate of about 10-20 per 100.

The diaphragm is a dome-shaped piece of rubber or plastic attached to a flexible wire ring. It is placed deep inside the vagina, covering the cervix, to prevent sperm from entering the uterus. A cervical cap or vaginal sponge works in a way similar to the diaphragm. The technique and rates are the same as for the diaphragm.

Q: *How does a woman choose the correct size of diaphragm?*

A: The first fitting must be made by a family physician or gynecologist. After an examination, a woman is given the correct size of diaphragm and taught how to fit it herself. She should fit it each night as a matter of habit, whether or not she has intercourse. For maximum effectiveness, the diaphragm should be used with a spermicide and left in place for at least six hours after intercourse. The failure rate is about 15 per 100, if the diaphragm is used by itself, and 3 per 100, if a spermicide is used.

Q: *How do spermicides work?*

A: Spermicides are chemicals available as jellies, foams, or suppositories that kill sperm in the vagina. They are inserted high into the vagina with an applicator, at least five minutes before intercourse, and must be reapplied before further intercourse. The contraceptive sponge also contains a spermicide. Spermicides should never be used alone, but always in conjunction with another method, such as a condom or diaphragm. Some spermicides may have additional benefits in reducing, but not eliminating, the risk of transmitting certain diseases, such as AIDS.

Q: *How does an IUD work?*

A: The intrauterine device (IUD) is a small, flexible piece of plastic that is inserted into the uterus through the vagina. It is usually shaped as a coil, loop, or ring and may contain copper, zinc, or progesterone, which is believed to increase the effectiveness of the plastic; exactly how an IUD works is not known.

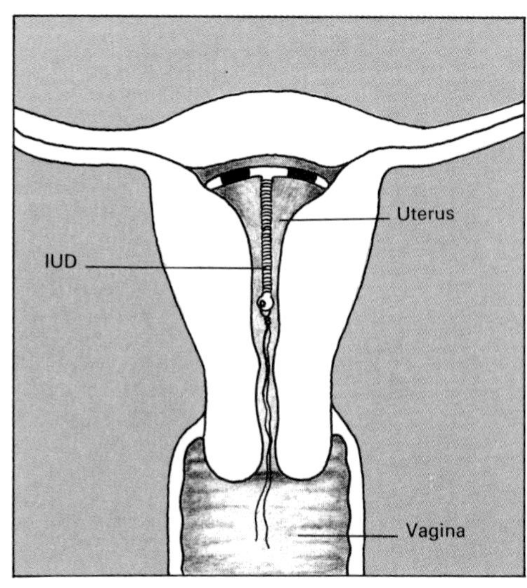

One form of **contraception,** the IUD, is thought to be effective by preventing the implantation of a fertilized egg.

Serious pelvic infections and the deaths of several IUD users has brought about the withdrawal of most IUD's from the U.S. market.

Q: *What is the birth control pill?*

A: Oral contraceptives, or the pill, were introduced in the 1950's as hormone preparations used to prevent pregnancy. The pill must be prescribed by a physician. It is by far the most reliable contraceptive, and possible side effects are its only drawback. Recently, side effects have been greatly reduced by using the lowest dosage of hormone capable of preventing pregnancy. *See also* CONTRACEPTIVE, ORAL.

Q: *How does the pill work?*

A: There are many different types of birth control pills, but they all contain synthetic preparations of one or both of the hormones, known as estrogen and progesterone. The estrogen works by preventing ovulation each month in the same way as the natural hormones do during pregnancy. As a result, there is no egg to be fertilized by the sperm. The progesterone has three functions: (1) it helps to prevent ovulation; (2) it thickens the cervical mucus, thus presenting a barrier to the sperm; and (3) it affects the lining of the uterus, making it unreceptive to a fertilized egg.

Q: *What is the combined pill?*
A: This pill has both estrogen and progesterone hormones. One pill is taken each day for three weeks in the menstrual cycle, thus allowing menstruation to occur in the fourth week, when no pills are taken. The withdrawal of hormones usually produces a lighter and shorter period. The first course of pills is started on the fifth day after menstruation starts, but additional contraceptive precautions must be taken for at least two weeks during the first course. The failure rate is about 0.025 per 100.

Q: *How does the progesterone-only pill work?*
A: This so-called "minipill" relies solely on the effects of progesterone. The dosage is continual and low, and menstruation occurs irregularly, sometimes with breakthrough bleeding between periods. It is essential that the pill be taken each day, preferably at the same time. If two consecutive pills are missed, the couple must use an additional means of contraception until the woman's next period. Even when used correctly, the minipill incurs a higher risk of pregnancy than the combined pill. The failure rate is about 10 per 100.

Q: *Who should use the progesterone-only pill?*
A: The progesterone-only pill is meant for women with conditions that might be aggravated by added estrogen, such as high blood pressure, diabetes, or a history of blood clots. In the absence of such conditions, the progesterone-only pill should not be used. The combined pill is far preferable.

Q: *What are the side effects of the pill?*
A: Common side effects of the pill are occasional nausea and weight gain, which may occur in the early weeks of use; an increase in tenderness of the breasts and in vaginal discharge; variable effect on the skin, with either an improvement in, or worsening of, acne, and occasionally a brownish discoloration of the face (chloasma); slight fatigue or weariness in muscles, loss of sexual drive, and mild depression; increase or decrease in headaches and migraine; and spotting and breakthrough bleeding. Possible spotting (slight blood loss from the uterus) may occur; however, the pill should be continued for the rest of the cycle. If mid-cycle (breakthrough) bleeding occurs beyond the first three months on the pill, the physician may select another pill with different hormone levels.

In general, if any adverse symptoms persist for more than two or three months, a gynecologist should be consulted, because a different preparation may be needed.

Q: *What are the more serious complications associated with the pill?*
A: A woman's fertility may be affected temporarily after she stops taking the pill and before the return of normal menstruation. This happens more often to women whose periods have previously been irregular. Although diabetes is not caused by the pill, mild diabetes may be made worse by it. Hypertension may occur in some women, particularly in those who have had high blood pressure in pregnancy. Recent studies have shown that thrombosis and its complications of deep vein thrombosis, stroke, and heart attack increase significantly (three to four times) in women taking a pill containing estrogen. This latter complication is almost entirely among women over age 35 and among those who smoke cigarettes. For this reason the pill should be avoided by women over age 35. Women on the pill who smoke should be encouraged to quit smoking.

Q: *Is it true that the pill can cause cancer?*
A: Research is still continuing, but there is no conclusive evidence that the pill causes cancer of the breast or the uterus. There is, in fact, some research suggesting that use of oral contraceptives may lower the incidence of some types of cancer.

Q: *Can any woman take the pill?*
A: The pill should be prescribed only after a physician has made a thorough examination and selected the type of pill most suited to the

woman. Any woman using the pill should have regular examinations of the breasts and pelvis and cervical smear (Pap) tests. See also PAP SMEAR TEST.

Q: *Is there a surgical form of contraception?*

A: Yes. Surgical sterilization may be performed on men or women to make them infertile. It is a minor operation for either, but one that is difficult to reverse. Male sterilization is achieved by means of a vasectomy, female sterilization by means of a tubal ligation or laparoscopic sterilization. See also STERILIZATION.

Q: *How should a woman and a man decide which contraceptive to use?*

A: The couple should choose the safest and most effective form of contraception for each partner. Since contraception is no longer considered only the woman's concern, it is important that the man consider the hazards associated with some methods and share the responsibility of using appropriate protection. Two sources of information for choosing contraceptive methods are the woman's family physician and/or gynecologist and Planned Parenthood.

Contraceptive, oral (kon trə sep′tiv, ôr′əl). Oral contraceptive, which is known more popularly as the birth control pill or simply as "the pill," is the most effective of the reversible (not permanent) methods of birth control. The failure rate is less than 0.2 percent a year.

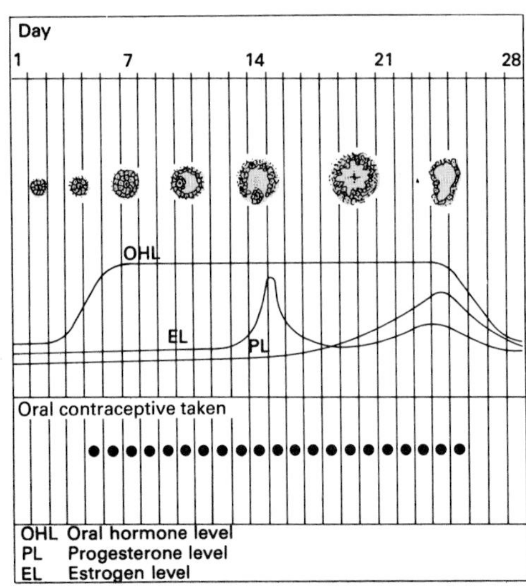

An **oral contraceptive** changes the levels of hormones in the blood and stops ovulation.

Oral contraceptives contain two synthetically produced female hormones, estrogen and progesterone. They cause the suppression of the pituitary gland that would normally stimulate the ovary to release an egg cell. Without the presence of an egg, conception can not take place. Oral contraceptives also act on the cervix, the lining of the uterus, and on the fallopian tubes, rendering them inhospitable not only to an egg or embryo, but to sperm as well.

Pills are sold in packs geared to the normal 28-day menstrual cycle. In a typical pack there will be 21 active birth control pills and 7 placebos, vitamin and iron tablets. The woman takes a birth control pill every day for 21 days, then takes a placebo pill each day for the next 7 days. During the 7 days she is not taking active birth control pills, a woman normally experiences withdrawal bleeding.

Birth control pills must be prescribed by a doctor, but not before the doctor has conducted a thorough physical examination and has taken a comprehensive medical history. The reason for these precautions is to minimize the risk of harmful side effects. The most serious of these are blood clots, stroke, and heart attack. These complications are more likely to occur in women over the age of 35 who smoke, and to a lesser degree in women between 30 and 35. For this reason, older women who smoke or have other risk factors in this age group should probably not take the pill. Therefore, women who should avoid the pill include those who smoke, those whose medical histories include any kind of heart or vascular problems, and those who have had incidence of cancer in the reproductive organs or an impaired liver function. Women who suspect they are pregnant should not take the pill, nor should women who are taking medications that might lessen the pill's effectiveness.

Side effects include dizziness or faintness, shortness of breath, chest pain, pain in the legs, severe headaches, breast lumps, muscle weakness or numbness, vision changes, loss of vision, speech irregularities, severe depression, and yellowing of the skin.

There are also some peripheral benefits from taking oral contraceptives, such as relief from the painful cramps and heavy bleeding of the normal menstrual cycle. The reduced loss of blood also makes iron deficiency and anemia less common. The pill has also been credited with lowering the incidence of ovarian cysts, uterine cancer, and pelvic infections and alleviating problems with acne.

See also CONTRACEPTION; CYST, OVARIAN; DYSMENORRHEA; MENSTRUAL PROBLEMS; MENSTRUATION; PREGNANCY AND CHILDBIRTH.

Contraceptive sponge. *See* SPONGE, CONTRACEPTIVE.

Contrecoup (kôn trə koo′) is an injury to one side of the body, as a result of a blow to the opposite side of the body. For example, a blow on the back of the head can cause the front parts of the brain to be rotated and bruised.

Contusion (kən tü′zhən) is a superficial injury in which the skin is not broken, often producing a bruise. There may be pain, swelling, and a discoloration of the skin.

See also BRUISE; BRUISE: TREATMENT.

Convalescence (kon və les′əns) is a period of recovery from the end of an acute stage of an illness or operation to the return to a normal level of health and activity. During this period, a person may be weak and in need of both physical and psychological help.

Q: ***What practical measures should be provided during convalescence?***

A: Most of the specific measures provided during convalescence are, of course, determined by the physician. There are, however, some general measures that are applicable to most people during convalescence. For example, conditions favoring rest should be provided. Meals should be small in size, but more frequent than normal to help encourage the return of a healthy appetite. Prolonged bed rest may be harmful if it results in decreased muscle strength (deconditioning), skin damage, social isolation, lethargy, or depression. Early in the convalescent period, a person should begin light exercises at bedside to use arms and legs. Later, as the person's strength returns, regular exercise, such as walking, should be encouraged to help restore normal muscle tone. The person's morale will benefit from companionship, especially during a long convalescence.

Convulsion (kən vul′shən) is a series of sudden muscular spasms, activated by the brain and involving contortions, as muscles alternately contract and relax. Loss of consciousness is also usual. A convulsion (also called a seizure) may occur as a symptom of various disorders: epilepsy; infection in the brain (for example, encephalitis or meningitis); drug withdrawal; diabetes; high fever, particularly in children; brain tumor; arteriosclerosis (in elderly people); injuries to the head (for example, after a severe automobile accident); toxemia in pregnancy; and poisoning.

Q: ***What immediate treatment should be given?***

A: Most importantly, the patient should be protected against injuring himself or herself. All hard objects or surfaces should be out of reach of the extremities. No spoons, pencils, or other hard objects should be placed in the mouth. An unconscious patient should be turned on his or her side, which will have the effect of keeping the airway open to prevent choking. A convulsion in a feverish child may be prevented by sponging with cool or tepid water, so that heat is lost by evaporation. A diabetic should be given sweets or sugar because the convulsions may be caused by excess insulin. Extra sugar is not harmful to a diabetic in such circumstances.

See also CONVULSION: FIRST AID.

Convulsion: first aid. A convulsion is a sudden, usually violent, involuntary muscle contraction. A convulsive seizure is a series of such contractions.

Convulsions may be caused by a high fever, particularly in children under the age of two; head injury; drug overdose; poisoning; low blood sugar in diabetics; alcohol withdrawal; infection; or grand mal epilepsy.

In general, with the exception of convulsions caused by head injury, convulsions from all causes are initially treated in the same way. With head injury, treat the victim as for shock, and summon emergency medical aid.

If the convulsions are caused by poisoning, drug overdose, diabetes, or a head injury, the victim may not recover

First aid for convulsions

1 At the beginning of an epileptic attack, the victim loses consciousness and falls down, sometimes with a cry as air is forced out of the lungs. The victim may then become rigid for a few seconds. This is usually followed by convulsions and noisy breathing.

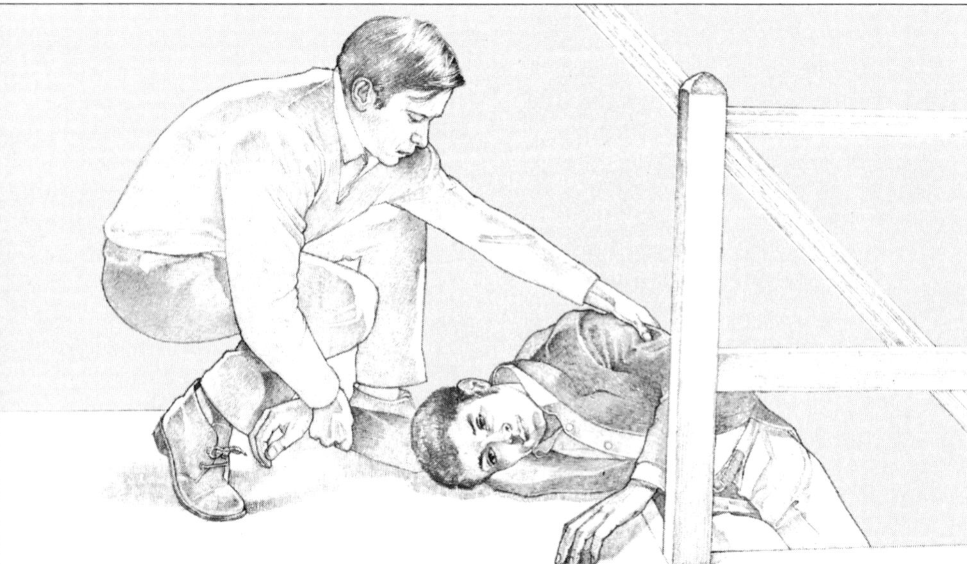

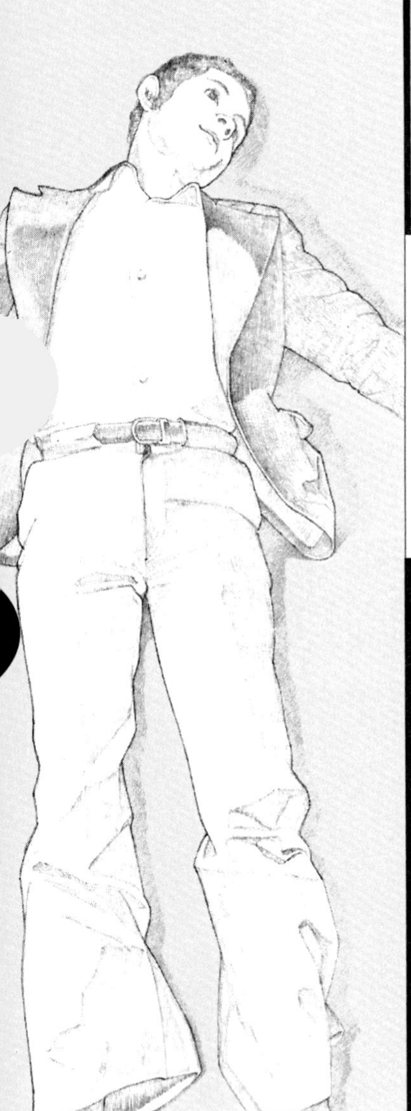

2 Lower the victim to the ground before he or she falls down. *Do not* attempt to stop the convulsions by forcibly restraining the victim because this may injure the victim.

Guide the victim away from any hazards so that he or she will not be injured. The jaw may be clenched, and bloodstained froth may appear in the mouth. *Do not* attempt to force open the victim's mouth during the convulsions.

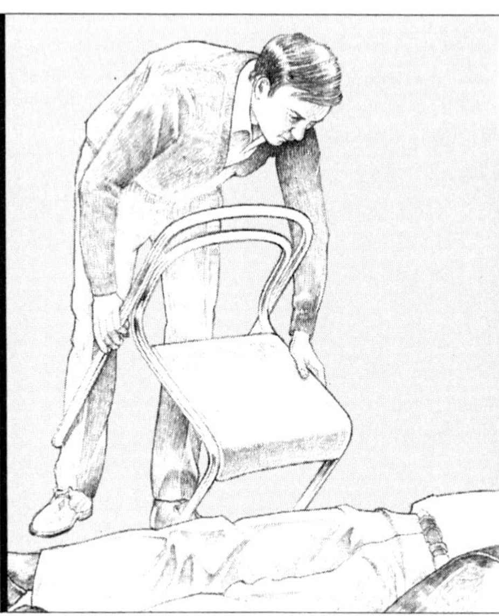

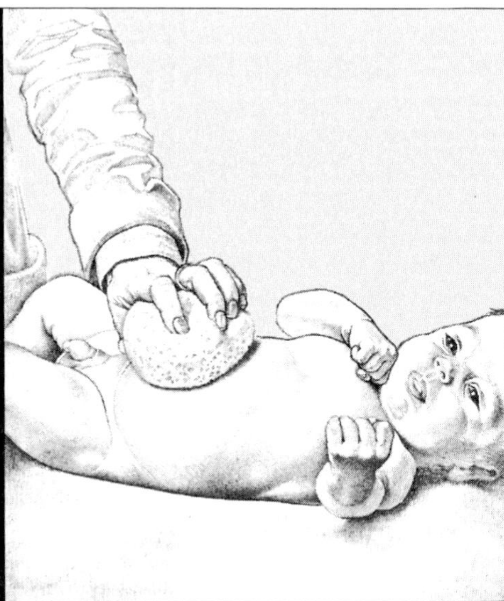

3 Remove any dangerous objects from near the victim. When the convulsions have finished, loosen the victim's clothing around the neck, chest, and waist; place the victim in the recovery position.

4 If a child's fever precipitates convulsions, follow the procedure outlined here. When the convulsions stop, sponge the child's body with tepid water. Consult a physician as soon as possible.

consciousness after the convulsion. Summon emergency medical aid immediately.

Action. Before an epileptic seizure, the victim may have a brief premonition, called an "aura," of the convulsion. If possible, help the victim to lie down before he or she collapses.

The violent muscular actions usually begin after a brief period of rigidity. Move away any furniture that the victim could hurt himself or herself on.

An epileptic seizure lasts for about a minute. Then the victim relaxes and may go into a trance-like state or fall asleep. Do not restrain the victim during the seizure. If a seizure lasts for longer than three minutes, seek emergency medical aid.

When the actions have stopped, examine the victim for any injuries that may have been sustained during the seizure. Stay with the victim, who may be distressed and confused. Ask bystanders to keep away.

Allow the victim to sleep. When the victim awakens, advise him or her to consult a physician.

If the victim is not breathing when the convulsions have stopped, check that the tongue is not blocking the airway. If the airway is clear and the victim is still not breathing, give artificial resuscitation.

See also ARTIFICIAL RESPIRATION.

Cooley's anemia. *See* THALASSEMIA.

Coombs' test (kümz) is a test for the presence of antiglobulins in red blood cells. The test is used in diagnosing certain anemias, specifically those caused by the destruction of red blood cells.

See also ANEMIA; HEMOLYSIS.

COPD. *See* PULMONARY DISEASE, CHRONIC OBSTRUCTIVE.

Cordotomy (kôr dot′ə mē) is an operation to cut some of the nerves in the spinal cord. It is a method sometimes used by surgeons for relieving chronic severe pain.

See also SPINAL CORD.

Corn (kôrn) is the thickening of the skin on or between the toes. It is usually produced by friction or pressure caused by tight or ill-fitting shoes. If present on exposed surfaces, a corn is hard; if it occurs between the toes, it is soft and may become inflamed.

See also BUNION; CORNS AND BUNIONS: TREATMENT.

Cornea (kôr′nē ə) is the clear transparent layer on the front of the eyeball. Its curvature is greater than that of the other layers of the eyeball. It acts with the lens to bend light rays and focus them onto the retina at the back of the eye.

See also EYE; RETINA.

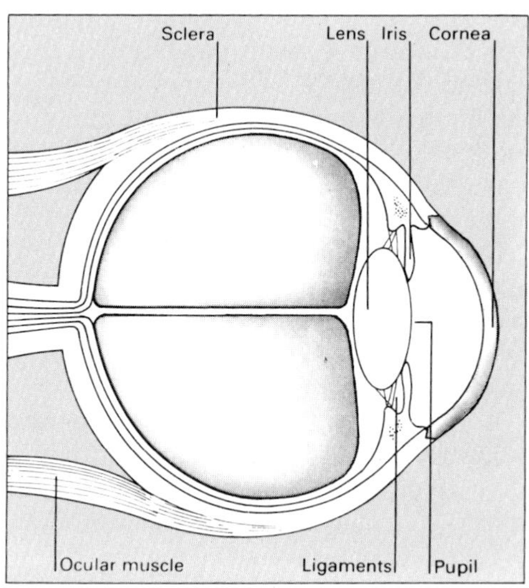

The **cornea** is the transparent front layer of the eyeball.

Corneal graft (kôr′nē əl graft), known medically as keratoplasty, is a surgical procedure in which a damaged cornea is replaced by a healthy cornea, usually taken from a deceased donor. Because the cornea has no direct blood supply and, therefore, no rejection syndrome, transplantation does not require the careful tissue matching required for other organs. A cornea, removed from the eye of a donor within four to six hours of death, can be preserved for several days in an antibiotic and nutrient medium at 4°C, before it is needed for a corneal graft.

Q: *How might the cornea be damaged?*

A: Scarring of the cornea from injury or infection, such as herpes or other diseases, often renders it useless. If the damage is severe, a graft may not be possible.

See also CORNEA.

Corns and bunions: treatment. A corn is a painful thickening of the outer layer of the skin of the toes. Corns are usually caused by the pressure of tight shoes. Inside a "hard" corn, usually a hard growth on the upper surface of a toe, is a cone-shaped core that extends downward and presses on a nerve, causing pain. "Soft" corns are usually found between two toes; they remain soft because of the heat and moisture. Hard corns can also appear on top of the foot and even on the sole—anywhere that friction with the shoe occurs.

Do not attempt to lance or pare a corn (or bunion) with a sharp blade. This is dangerous and can cause serious infection.

A bunion is a painful swelling at the base of the big toe. The large joint of the big toe becomes inflamed and thickened and bends the toe inward toward the other toes. Bunions are usually caused by ill-fitting shoes.

Do not put padding between the bunion and the shoe. This only causes extra pressure on the toes. Padding between the big toe and the second toe may, however, relieve pain.

Action. Anyone with either corns or a bunion should first ensure that thereafter he or she wears properly fitting shoes.

To treat corns, soak the feet in hot water and then rub the corn gently with an emery board or pumice stone. This should painlessly remove the superficial, hard skin and leave a softer surface that can be protected with a dressing.

A variety of corn remedies are available, many of which contain salicylic acid, which softens hard skin and may provide temporary relief. But it is also advisable to consult a podiatrist or physician, who can remove corns and give advice about preventing their recurrence.

The only complete and final cure for bunions is surgical removal of the bunion and part of any overgrown bone beneath it.

Coronary (kôr′ə ner ē) generally refers to the heart. The term "coronary" is also sometimes used to mean a heart attack, in which case it is actually an abbreviation of "coronary thrombosis."

See also HEART ATTACK; HEART DISEASE, CORONARY.

Coronary artery by-pass surgery is an open-heart operation that allows blood to flow around blockages in coronary arteries. It may be performed only

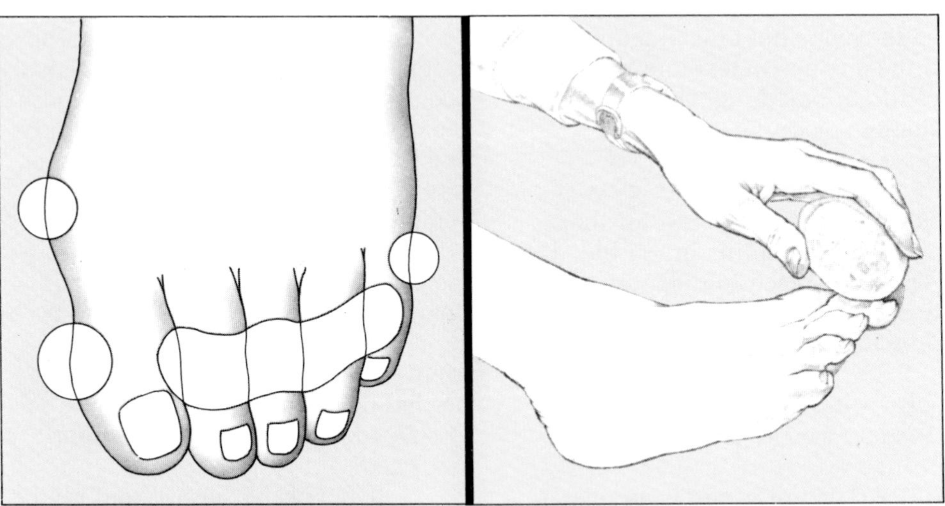

Corns are caused by friction from shoes that are too tight. A hard, painful thickening of the skin is formed where the inside of the shoe rubs the foot or toe. The most common site is the upper surface of a toe that is bent in order to fit in the shoe. When toes are pressed together by tight shoes, soft corns may form between them. The best treatment for a corn is to wear wider and longer shoes. Shoes that come to a point, or that have high heels, are common causes of corns. Soaking a corn in hot water softens the top layers of the hardened skin. An emery board or a pumice stone can then be used to gently file away the hardened skin.

if a short section of a coronary artery is blocked.

The surgeon typically first removes a short segment of vein from the patient's leg; this vein will be used to by-pass the blockage in the coronary artery. One end of this segment is then attached to the aorta. The other end is attached to the affected coronary artery at a point beyond the blockage. The surgeon may construct several by-passes, depending on the number of blocked arteries.

Artery by-pass surgery is performed on patients with coronary artery disease, the narrowing of the arteries of the heart due to the build-up of plaque and fatty deposits. The operation increases the blood supply flowing through the heart, thus increasing the heart's oxygen supply and relieving chest pains.

The hospital recuperation usually lasts 10 to 14 days, including time immediately following the operation in an intensive care unit. In one out of five cases, thrombosis (the formation of a blood clot in an artery or vein) occurs in the by-pass within one year after the surgery. The mortality rate is 1 in 100 operations.

Despite obvious successes, the operation is still somewhat controversial. Recent studies have suggested that treatment with medication only is just as effective as by-pass surgery. Medical therapy also does not involve the risks associated with a surgical procedure. In addition, a third option, a newly developed technique called balloon angioplasty, which does not require open-heart surgery, has become available. Persons with coronary artery disease should work closely with their physicians to determine which of these treatment options is appropriate in their cases.

See also ANGIOPLASTY, BALLOON; ARTERIOSCLEROSIS; HEART DISEASE, CORONARY.

Coronary heart disease. *See* HEART DISEASE, CORONARY.

Corpus albicans (kôr′pəs al′bi kanz) is a pale scar that develops over the decaying corpus luteum on the surface of an ovary.

See also CORPUS LUTEUM.

Corpuscle (kôr′pə səl) is the medical term for any small, rounded body. It is usually applied to blood cells, red blood corpuscles (erythrocytes) and white blood corpuscles (leukocytes).

See also BLOOD CELL, RED; BLOOD CELL, WHITE.

Corpus luteum (kôr′pəs lü′tē əm) is a small, yellow, hormone-producing structure that develops in an ovary at the site of a released egg (ovum). In addition to the hormone called estrogen (also produced by the ovaries and the adrenal glands), the corpus luteum produces progesterone. These hormones prepare the lining of the uterus (endometrium) for the implantation of a fertilized ovum. If conception takes place and an ovum becomes fertilized, the corpus luteum remains; if not, it degenerates and shrinks when menstruation starts.

See also CONCEPTION; HORMONE; MENSTRUATION.

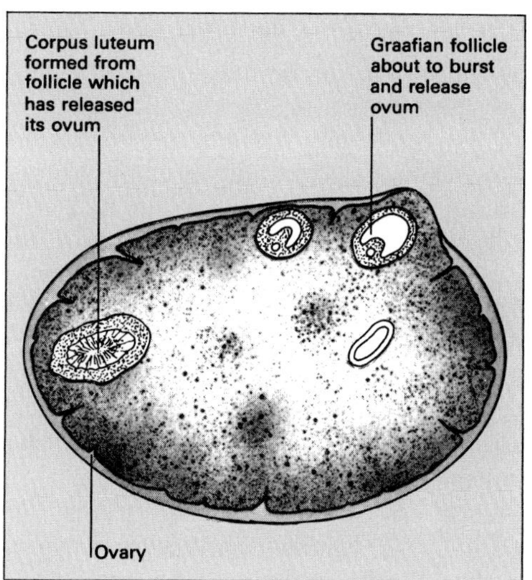

Corpus luteum is a structure that develops in an ovary and secretes progesterone.

Cortex (kôr′teks) is the outer layer of an organ, as distinct from the inner portion (medulla). For example, the cerebral cortex is the layer of nerve cells (gray matter) on the surface of the brain, and the adrenal cortex is the outer layer of an adrenal gland.

Corticosteroid (kôr tə kō ster′oid), or corticoid, is a steroid hormone produced in the outer layer (cortex) of the adrenal glands. The term is also used for a number of synthetic derivatives (corticosteroid drugs) that have properties similar to those of the natural hormones.

There are three main groups of naturally occurring corticosteroids: (1) aldosterone, which regulates the excretion of sodium and potassium salts through the kidney; (2) cortisol (hydrocortisone), which promotes the synthesis and storage of glucose and regulates fat distribution within the body; and (3) sex hormones, which have only a minor effect on the body of an adult. Aldosterone and cortisol are essential to life, and they affect many chemical processes within the body. They work together to maintain a constant internal environment, despite the fact that the body is always subjected to changes.

Corticosteroid drug (kôr tə kō ster′oid) is a synthetic derivative of the corticosteroid hormone, used to treat Addison's disease, allergies, rheumatic disorders, and inflammation. The use of corticosteroid medications requires great caution. Long-term use can lead to numerous complications, such as fluid retention, weight gain, increased blood pressure, osteoporosis, and depression. Suddenly stopping corticosteroids can also lead to potentially fatal complications because they suppress the natural production of corticosteroids by the adrenal glands. The glands cannot suddenly begin producing these substances again. As a result, low blood pressure, shock, and, in come cases, death can occur. Extremely close supervision and monitoring by a physician is required whenever these drugs are used. Nevertheless, when used with proper supervision for brief periods, they can be both extremely effective and safe.

Corticosteroids are not synonymous with "sex hormones," although these are frequently confused. The two are entirely different drugs.

See also ALDOSTERONE; CORTICOSTEROID; CORTISOL.

Corticotropin. *See* ADRENOCORTICOTROPIC HORMONE.

Cortisol (kôr′tə sōl), or hydrocortisone, is the most important naturally occurring corticosteroid. It controls the level of glucose, fats, and water in the body. Several synthetic cortisol drugs are available. They all work in preventing the body's normal reaction to disease or damage. This effect can be useful in treating such conditions as allergy or inflammation.

See also CORTICOSTEROID; HORMONE.

Cortisone (kôr′tə zōn) is one of the corticosteroid hormones. It is inactive until changed into cortisol by the liver.

See also CORTICOSTEROID; CORTISOL.

Coryza. *See* COLD.

Cosmetic surgery. *See* SURGERY, COSMETIC.

Costal chondritis. *See* TIETZE'S SYNDROME.

Cough is an action that clears an irritated area of the lungs or throat. It is a common symptom of a number of disorders, such as the common cold, influenza, or a minor respiratory illness. A cough may also accompany a serious lung disorder or heart disease.

Any cough that lasts for more than a few days should be discussed with a physician. *See also* COLD; HEART DISEASE.

Q: *Should medicine be taken to stop a cough?*

A: Coughing is a useful and protective mechanism, and treatment that completely suppresses it could do more harm than good. When a person coughs, a deep breath is taken in, the vocal cords close, and pressure builds up within the lungs. When the cords open, a violent expulsion of air takes place as the body attempts to expel any foreign material in the throat or lower respiratory tract.

Cough syrups that help the person to bring up phlegm are called expectorants, and many kinds are available without prescription from a drugstore. Other preparations containing antihistamines may help to dry up secretions. A cough suppressant, sometimes prescribed by a physician, contains a drug such as codeine or dextromethorphan. *See also* ANTIHISTAMINE; CODEINE.

Q: *Apart from infection, what else can cause a cough?*

A: Smoking can produce a cough, especially in the morning, because the lining of the air passages to the lungs (the bronchi) is damaged and the lungs fail to empty themselves naturally during the night.

Asthma, lung cancer, and other serious disorders produce symptomatic coughing.

Q: *What can be done for a dry cough?*

A: Eating something dry, a soda cracker or a cookie, may help to stop the irritating tickle. In a dry, overheated room, a vaporizer can relieve congestion of the nose and throat membranes.

Sometimes a dry cough, especially in a child, can be exhausting and debilitating, as in pertussis (whooping cough) or some of the virus illnesses that commonly occur during the winter months. In such cases, a medicine that suppresses the cough is to some extent helpful, but should be used only on medical advice. *See also* PERTUSSIS.

Coughing: first aid: *See* CHOKING AND COUGHING: FIRST AID.

Cowpox (kou'poks), or vaccinia, is an infection of cattle that can cause a mild illness in human beings. It is the virus originally used by Edward Jenner in 1796 for vaccinating human beings against smallpox. In the milk cow, the udder and teats are affected by a slight eruption. Similar, pus-filled blisters appear on the skin of human beings who have either been inoculated with cowpox vaccine or have been in contact with infected cows.

See also INOCULATION; VACCINATION.

Coxalgia (kok sal'jē ə) is the medical name for pain in the hip.

Coxa vara (kok'sə vä'rä) is a deformity of the thighbone (femur). The angle of the neck of the bone, at the part leading to the hip joint, is reduced. This makes the knee move inward. Coxa vara is much more common than the associated condition, coxa valga, in which the bone angle is increased.

There are various possible reasons for coxa vara. It may be congenital; or caused by a fracture, or a softening of the bone from rickets, osteomalacia, or parathyroid disease. The condition may also result from any injury during childhood that causes the head of the thighbone to slip or move out of position. The patient has a limp because one of the legs acts as if it were shorter than the other. There is often pain in the hip (coxalgia).

Treatment depends upon the symptoms, which should be treated by a bone specialist.

See also OSTEOMALACIA; RICKETS.

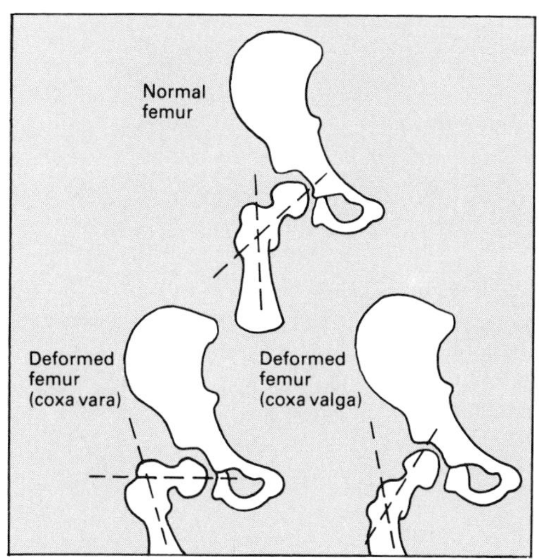

Coxa vara is a deformity of the thighbone that causes the knee to move inward. Coxa valga is less common.

Coxsackie virus (kok sak'ē vī'rəs) is one of a family of viruses that can produce a number of disorders, including a severe, influenza-like illness (epidemic pleurodynia) and a virus form of meningitis. It is named for a town in New York where it was first isolated in 1948. Diagnosis is usually made by means of blood tests after the patient has recovered, and treatment is symptomatic.

See also MENINGITIS; PLEURODYNIA, EPIDEMIC.

CPR. *See* CARDIOPULMONARY RESUSCITATION.

Crab lice. *See* LICE.

Crabs. *See* PEDICULOSIS PUBIS.

Crack. *See* COCAINE.

Cramp (kramp) is a sudden, involuntary, and often painful contraction of a muscle or a group of muscles. The affected muscles may become hard and knotted. Cramps in the abdomen are sometimes called colic, and cramps in the leg are popularly called a charley horse. Cramps may occur after prolonged exercise, such as swimming; or at night, especially in the elderly and usually affecting the leg muscles; or at the start of menstruation. The causes of cramps are not fully understood; but in some cases, cramps may be caused by salt loss from excessive sweating or diarrhea or from poor blood circulation. *See also* CHARLEY HORSE; COLIC.

Q: *How can cramps be treated?*

A: Because the causes of cramps are so little understood, there is no single treatment for all types of cramps. Stretching and warming the affected muscle may help. Drinking water to which salt has been added may relieve cramps

Treatment for cramps and spasms

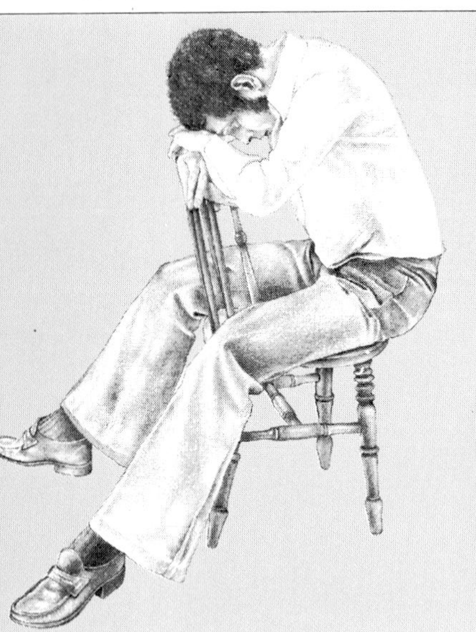

During an asthmatic attack, let the victim sit, with the arms at chest height. *Do not* lay the victim down because this makes breathing more difficult. Allow the victim to use any prescribed medication.

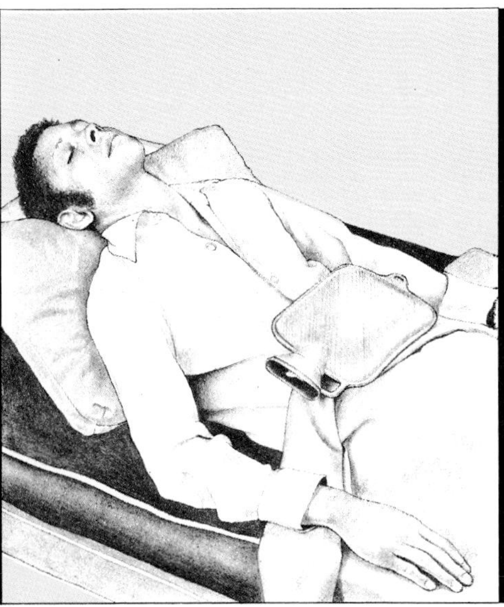

If the victim is having intestinal cramps, lay the victim down. Keep the victim warm and comfortable, possibly with a hot water bottle. If the spasms are severe or if the victim is vomiting, summon emergency medical aid.

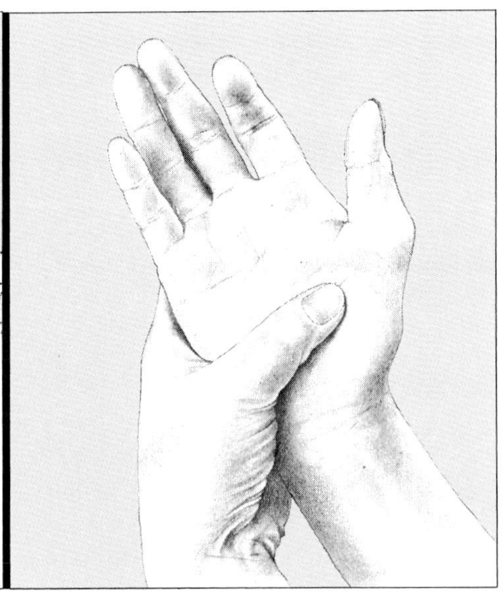

If the cramps are caused by excessive activity, such as swimming, running, or rowing, immediately stop the activity. Rest and massage the affected part.

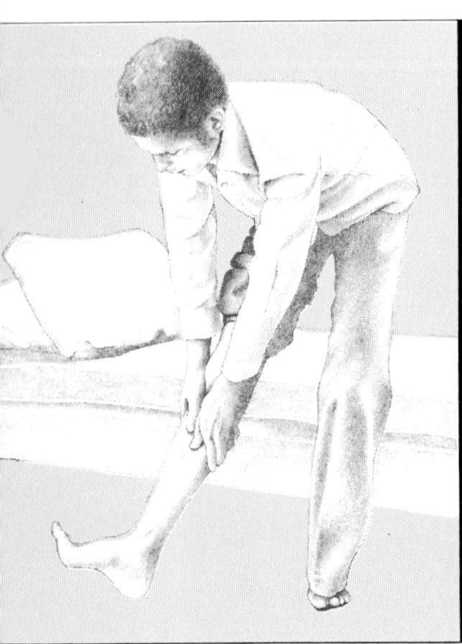

If the victim has night cramps in the legs or the feet, move the feet to stretch the affected muscles. Night cramps in the legs or feet may also be relieved by massaging the affected part.

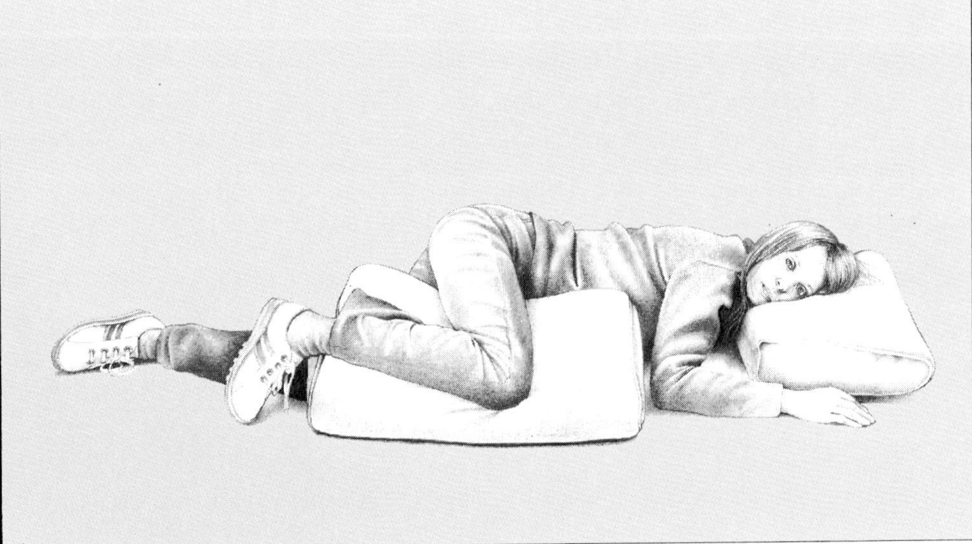

Menstrual cramps usually last for about 3 minutes, with an interval of about 15 minutes between attacks. If a woman has menstrual cramps, it may help to perform light exercise.

If exercise is ineffective, the woman should rest in bed. Gentle heat applied to the woman's abdomen or middle of the back may relieve the pain. If it does not, give the woman painkillers.

caused by salt loss. If cramps occur frequently, especially in the calf muscles after walking (intermittent claudication), a physician should be consulted because there may be a more serious underlying cause, such as a disorder of the blood circulation.

See also CLAUDICATION, INTERMITTENT; CRAMPS AND SPASMS: TREATMENT.

Cramps and spasms: treatment. A spasm is a sudden, involuntary muscular contraction, either of a single muscle or of a group of muscles. A convulsion is a general spasm that affects the whole body. Spasms may be caused by various factors, such as muscular fatigue, electrolyte inbalance, or emotional stress. Although the term muscle spasm usually refers to large, voluntary muscle groups, small muscles in the walls of arteries, the bronchial tubes, or the larynx can also contract in a spasm. Asthma is an example of a spasm in the bronchial tubes. *See also* ASTHMA; CONVULSION; CRAMP.

Strong spasms of large muscles of the chest, abdomen, arms, or legs can produce moderate to severe pain. Such painful muscle spasms are commonly known as cramps. Excessive salt loss may cause cramps. Certain chemicals and drugs, if ingested in large quantities, may also cause cramps. *See also* DRUG OVERDOSE: FIRST AID.

If cramps are caused by excessive salt loss, replace the lost salt by drinking a glass of water to which one-half teaspoon of salt has been added. Rest the affected part until the cramps stop.

Cramps may occur during vigorous exercise even in healthy persons, particularly if exercise is taken after eating or drinking. This can be dangerous if the cramps occur while swimming. Avoid exercise immediately after eating or after drinking alcohol.

If cramps or spasms persist or recur frequently, consult a physician; there may be a more serious underlying cause.

Cramps, menstrual. *See* DYSMENORRHEA.

Craniotomy (krā nē ot'ə mē) is an operation to make an opening in the skull, as a preliminary to brain surgery.

Cranium (krā'nē əm) is the anatomical name for the skull. It usually refers to

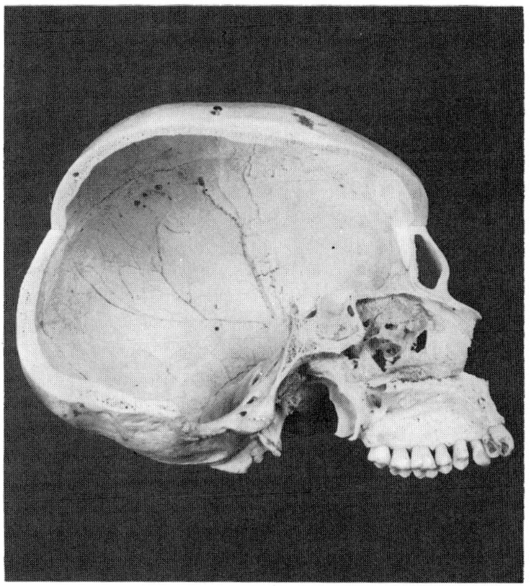

The **cranium** is that portion of the skull that encloses the brain.

the part that surrounds the brain, but excludes the bones of the face and the jaw.

Cretinism (krē'tə niz əm) is a condition of stunted body growth and impaired mental development. The symptoms, which appear during early infancy, are the gradual development of a characteristic coarse, dry skin, a slightly swollen face and tongue, umbilical hernia, and an open mouth that drools. The baby is usually listless, slow-moving, constipated, and a slow feeder. Cretinism is the result of a congenital deficiency in the secretion of the hormone thyroxine from the thyroid gland. In some cases, this is thought to be caused by an insufficient amount of iodine in the diet of the child's mother during pregnancy. Thyroid testing on newborns to detect cretinism is now a routine test in many states.

Q: *How is cretinism treated?*

A: After the condition has been diagnosed with the help of blood tests, treatment with thyroid hormone promotes normal physical and mental development. It is essential that treatment be started during the first six weeks of life or irreversible changes may take place.

See also THYROID GLAND.

Creutzfeldt-Jakob disease (kroits'felt-yä'kob) is a rare, degenerative brain disease of middle and late life, caused by a slow virus, as yet unidentified. Death usually occurs within one year of diagnosis.

Crib. *See* BABY CARE.

Crib death. *See* SUDDEN INFANT DEATH SYNDROME.

Crohn's disease (krōnz), known medically as regional ileitis or regional enteritis, is a chronic, inflammatory condition of the intestine. There is no known cause for the disease, although it may be hereditary. It is usually confined to the lower end of the small intestine (ileum), but may involve the large intestine (colon). The symptoms of Crohn's disease include intermittent attacks of diarrhea and abdominal pain, weight loss, and fever. Rarely, the intestine may become blocked or ulcerate into adjacent areas via fistulas. Treatment involves a nutritious diet, pain-killing drugs, antibiotics, and sometimes corticosteroids. If complications occur, the physician may recommend surgery to remove the diseased section of intestine, though the inflammation has a tendency to recur.

See also COLON; CORTICOSTEROID; ILEUM.

Cross-eye. *See* STRABISMUS.

Cross-infection is the infection of one patient by another. This is a serious problem in hospitals, especially if the disease-producing organism is resistant to most antibiotics.

Croup (krüp) is an acute breathing disorder, most often occurring in young children, age one through four. The mucous membrane of the larynx, trachea, and bronchial tubes becomes inflamed and swollen and produces excessive mucus. Laryngotracheobronchitis is synonymous with croup.

Q: *What causes croup?*

A: Respiratory infections caused by various kinds of virus can often result in croup. However, a more serious but less common kind of croup, called membranous croup, occurs most often as a symptom of diphtheria. *See also* DIPHTHERIA.

Q: *What are the symptoms of croup?*

A: For most cases of croup, there is loss of appetite, fever, difficulty in breathing, and a barking cough that ends with a whistle upon inhalation. Only in the most severe cases of croup do certain other symptoms occur, such as cyanosis (blue-tinged skin) due to insufficient oxygen. This condition is a medical emergency.

Q: *How are most cases of croup treated?*

A: The mildly ill child may be cared for at home. He or she should be made comfortable and be given plenty of liquids. Rest is important. A vaporizer is an extremely important aid to breathing. If a vaporizer is unavailable, creating a steamy environment in the bathroom by running a hot shower will make the baby more comfortable.

Crush syndrome, also called compression syndrome, is the failure of the kidneys and liver to function after severe injuries, especially a crushed leg. It occurs because large amounts of proteins from damaged muscles have been released into the circulation system, and the kidneys cannot cope with them; shock is another factor. Treatment of this very serious condition requires hospitalization. Kidney dialysis may be necessary until the kidneys recover.

See also KIDNEY DIALYSIS.

Crutch. *See* WALKING AID.

Cryosurgery (krī ō sėr′jər ē) is a surgical technique in which tissues are exposed to extreme cold, usually below −4°F (−20°C), using liquid nitrogen or carbon dioxide. It is used to remove cataracts, malignant tumors, and hemorrhoids. Cryosurgery is also used in brain surgery, to repair detached retinas, to treat cervical erosion and warts, and to reduce bleeding.

Cryptorchidism (krip tôr′ki diz əm), or cryptorchism, commonly known as undescended testicles, is the congenital condition in which one or both of the testicles have not descended into the scrotum. It is often accompanied by a hernia in the groin. *See also* SCROTUM.

Q: *Why does cryptorchidism occur?*

A: The reason is not known. The testicles develop in the abdomen of a fetus, and before birth they descend through the abdominal wall into the scrotum. If this fails to happen, cryptorchidism results. In many male babies the testicles appear to be absent, because the attached muscles pull them up to the abdominal wall. This is perfectly normal and should not be confused with cryptorchidism.

Q: *How is cryptorchidism treated?*

A: If the testicle can be located outside the abdomen, an operation may be performed to fix the testicle in the scrotum (orchiopexy). If the testicle is in the abdomen, major surgery is involved. It may still

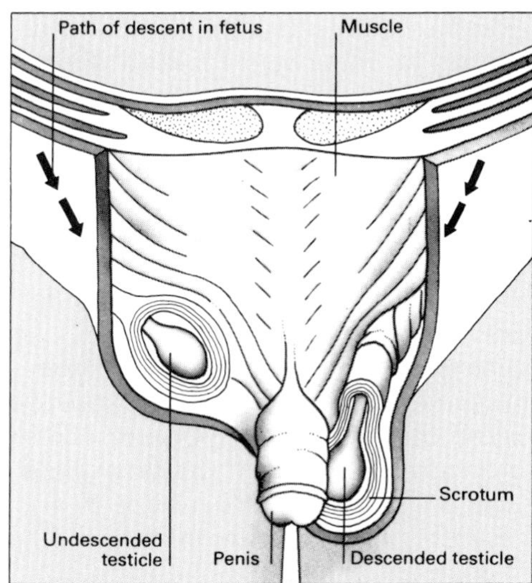

Cryptorchidism is the failure of a testicle to descend into the scrotum.

not be possible to find the testicle. An alternative, but less certain, method is the administration of human chorionic gonadotropic hormone, which may stimulate the testicle to descend. An undescended testicle seems to place one at greater risk for testicular cancer later in life. It is still not certain whether orchiopexy reduces that risk.

See also ORCHIOPEXY.

Culture (kul′chər) is the procedure for growing microorganisms in a suitable medium, usually carbohydrates, proteins, and minerals dissolved in sterile water. A tiny sample from the patient (blood, urine, mucus, etc.) is carefully put into a clean container with a medium to encourage growth of colonies of any bacteria, viruses, or fungi present in the sample. Once the type, or types, of organisms have been identified, appropriate antibiotic therapy can begin.

See also BACTERIA; VIRUS.

Curare (kyů rä′rē) is the general name for a wide variety of chemical extracts derived from several South American trees. Curare causes rapid paralysis of the muscles throughout the body and was originally used on poisonous arrows by South American Indians. A refined preparation of curare, called tubocurarine, may be used as a muscle relaxant during general anesthesia and to help diagnose myasthenia gravis.

See also MUSCLE RELAXANT DRUG; MYASTHENIA GRAVIS.

Curettage (kyů ret′ ij) is the scraping clean of the interior of a body cavity with a spoon-shaped instrument or by suction.

See also DILATATION AND CURETTAGE.

Cushing's syndrome (kush′ingz) is a rare glandular disorder. It is characterized by excessive production of cortisol and similar corticosteroids by the adrenal glands. Cushing's syndrome may occur spontaneously, or it may be caused by a tumor of the adrenal glands or a tumor of the pituitary gland; this causes an excessive amount of corticotropin (ACTH) to be produced and the adrenal glands to be overstimulated. Cushing's syndrome may also result from prolonged medication with large doses of corticosteroid drugs. See also ADRENAL GLAND; CORTICOSTEROID; CORTICOSTEROID DRUG; CORTISOL; PITUITARY GLAND.

Q: *What are the symptoms of Cushing's syndrome?*

A: The symptoms include fatty swellings on the back of the neck; a characteristic "moon face"; fatigue; weakness; obesity of the trunk, while the limbs remain thin; and skin discoloration with pink streaks. In addition, there may be diabetes mellitus and, on occasion, hypertension. There may also be excessive hair growth, reduced sex drive in men, and the cessation of menstruation in women. In cases where the cause is cancer, Cushing's syndrome may be fatal.

Q: *How can Cushing's syndrome be treated?*

A: There are drugs available that may temporarily control the symptoms, but surgical removal of either the tumor or the overproductive tissue is the most common treatment. Radiation therapy is also sometimes used. If an adrenal gland is surgically removed, there will be lack of the hormones that it normally produces. Such a lack may be compensated by taking corticosteroid drugs.

Cut is an opening in the skin, such as a wound or a gash, made by a knife or some other sharp object.

See also CUT: TREATMENT.

Cutaneous (kyü tā′nē əs) refers to the skin. For example, cutaneous nerves are sensory nerves that are situated in the skin.

Cuticle (kyü'tə kəl) is a layer covering the free surface of epithelial cells. It may be horny or calcified, as in tooth enamel. The term is also used for the thin outer layer of the skin, adjacent to a fingernail.

See also EPITHELIUM; NAIL.

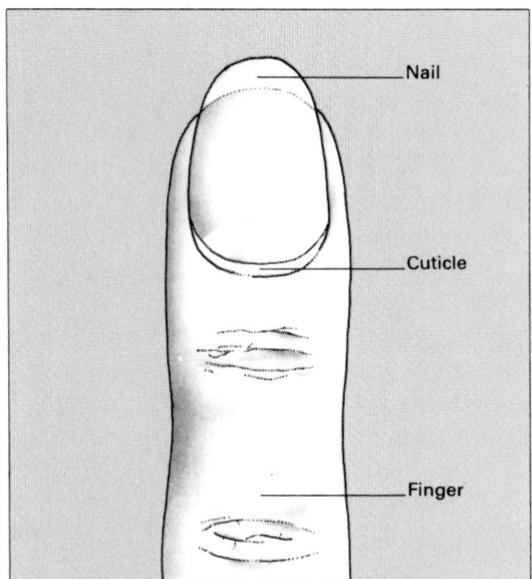

Cuticle is the hard skin around a fingernail or toenail. If it is injured, a hangnail may form.

Cut: treatment. A cut is a break in the skin that permits the escape of blood, which may lead to infection. Incised cuts, for example, made with a sharp blade, usually bleed profusely. Lacerated cuts involving torn tissues bleed less than incised cuts, but heal with more difficulty. Punctured cuts may have relatively small openings but may be deep, causing serious injury to the underlying tissues. Most cuts are minor injuries and do not require expert medical attention.

If the victim has a deep and dirty cut, a physician should be consulted, because antitetanus injections may be necessary. Any large cut should be examined by a physician, because stitches may be necessary. *See also* TETANUS.

Action. The first action is to control bleeding. If damage to internal parts of the body is suspected, emergency medical aid should be summoned. Control heavy bleeding by applying firm pressure over the wound. *Do not* attempt to remove minor debris; such action may cause more bleeding.

If the cut is deep or there is an object impaled in the wound, *do not* tamper with the wound. However, it is imperative that bleeding be controlled. Summon emergency medical aid.

If the victim has a small puncture wound, wash it with soap and water, and dry it carefully. Cover the wound with a clean, dry dressing. If a fish hook is deeply impaled or is embedded in a part of the face, *do not* attempt to remove it. If the fish hook is in any other part of the body, push the shank through the skin until the barb appears. Cut off the barb with clippers or pliers and remove the shank from the wound. Wash the wound and cover it with a clean dressing. Consult a physician immediately.

If the wound discharges pus when the dressing is changed, if it becomes inflamed and painful, or if there are other symptoms of infection, consult a physician.

See also BLEEDING: FIRST AID; INFECTION.

CVB. *See* CHORIONIC VILLUS BIOPSY.

Cyanosis (sī ə nō'sis) is a bluish discoloration of the skin, most easily seen in the lips. It is caused by a lack of oxygen in the blood, which may be caused by constriction of blood vessels to the skin in cold environments, failure of the lungs to oxygenate the blood fully, pneumonia, heart failure, asphyxiation, or overdose of certain drugs. It also occurs in children with some forms of congenital heart disease. Treatment depends on the cause.

See also BLUE BABY.

Cybernetics (sī bər net'iks) is the comparative study of the human and animal nervous system and certain mechanical systems, in order to better understand communication and control of impulses and responses in both types of systems.

Cyclosporine (sī klə spôr'in) is a metabolic by-product of a type of soil fungus. Since it has antifungal and immunosuppressive qualities, it is being utilized in organ transplant patients to prevent rejection.

See also TRANSPLANT SURGERY.

Cyst (sist) is an abnormal swelling or sac that usually contains fluid. Cysts can occur in almost any body tissue, but they are most frequently found in the skin, breasts, and ovaries, where they may grow to a large size. There are several kinds of cysts: (1) nonmalignant tumors with cells producing liq-

Treatment for cuts

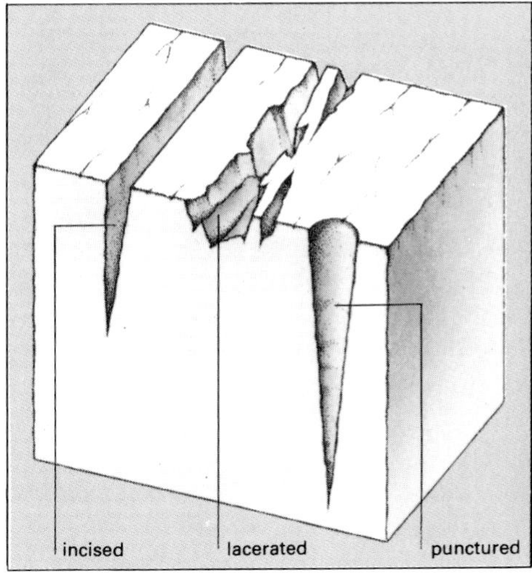

Types of cuts

An incised cut is a clean cut made with a sharp edge.

A lacerated cut has irregular, torn edges.

A punctured cut is a wound that penetrates deeply into the skin.

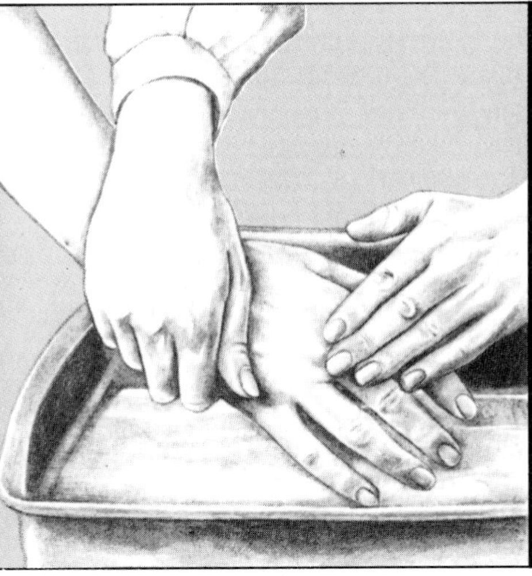

1 If the cut is small, wash the wound with soap and water, rinse it thoroughly and dry.

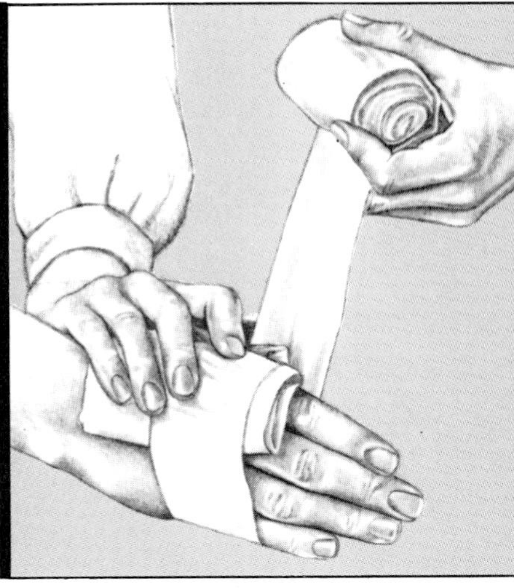

2 Apply a clean dressing over the cut. *Do not* touch the part of the dressing that will be applied to the wound. *Do not* apply any salves or ointments.

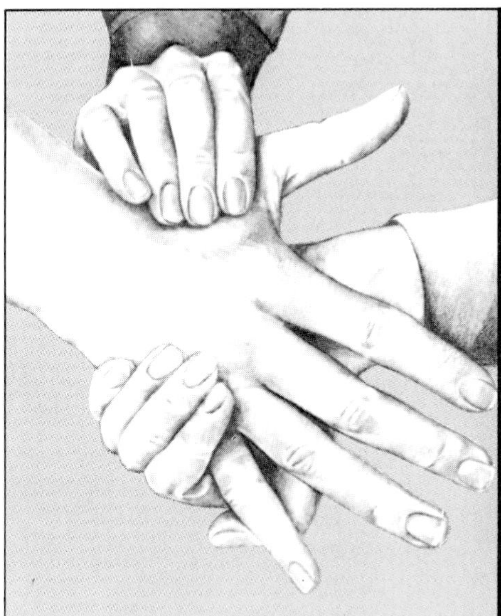

3 If the cut is deep, control any bleeding by pressing clean gauze directly over the wound with the palm of the hand. *Do not* wash or tamper with the wound.

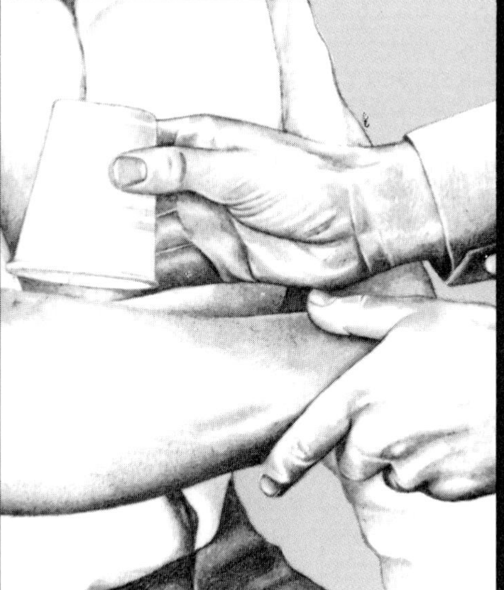

4 If the impaled object that caused the wound is still embedded in the skin, *do not* remove it. Carefully cut away any clothing from around the wound.

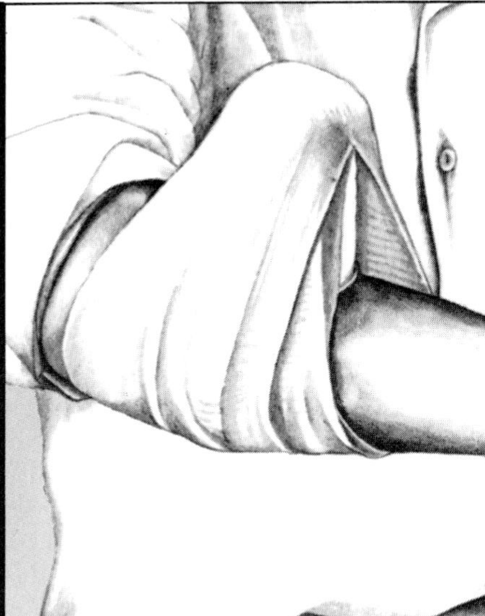

5 Cover the impaled object with anything that will prevent it from being moved, such as a cup. Bandage the protective cover in place. Summon emergency medical aid.

uids that cannot escape; (2) cysts containing cells of tissues that are normally found elsewhere in the body (for example, a dermoid cyst may contain elements of skin and hair); (3) cysts caused by parasitic infection (hydatid cyst); and (4) ordinary glands that have become blocked (sebaceous cyst). Treatment, if any, depends on the type of cyst.

See also TUMOR.

Cyst, breast (sist). Breast cysts are benign and rather common. On occasion, a woman may have several or recurrent cysts; this condition is referred to as fibrocystic breasts. Although no treatment is usually needed, large or painful cysts can be easily drained with a needle. It is especially important that women with fibrocystic breasts perform monthly self-examinations in order to detect subtle changes in their breasts.

See also FIBROCYSTIC DISEASE OF THE BREAST.

Cyst, dermoid (sist, dėr′moid). Dermoid cyst is a nonmalignant cyst formed from surface skin cells. The cyst may contain elements of skin, hair, sweat glands, and bone, which form a small, hard swelling in the body. A dermoid cyst is caused by a fault in the folding of tissues during embryonic development or by a wound that forces surface skin cells under the skin. Dermoid cysts are often found in the ovary, but may occur elsewhere, such as the lungs or the thyroid. The usual treatment is surgical removal of the cyst.

See also CYST.

Cyst, hydatid (sist, hī′də tid). Hydatid cyst is a kind of cyst that forms in body tissues, especially those of the liver. It encloses the larvae of a type of tapeworm (*Echinococcus granulosus*). This parasite can infest dogs, foxes, wolves, cattle, and sheep. It is passed on to human beings in food that has been contaminated with the eggs of the tapeworm.

Q: *What are the symptoms of hydatid cysts?*

A: Frequently, there are no symptoms, although there may be a dull ache on the right side of the abdomen and the liver may become enlarged. Blood tests and ultrasound examinations may help in the diagnosis.

Q: *How is hydatid cyst disease treated?*

A: When the condition has been confirmed, the only treatment is to remove the cyst, or cysts, through surgery.

See also CYST; TAPEWORM.

Cysticercosis (sis ta sėr kō′sis) is a disorder caused by infection with the pork tapeworm (*Taenia solium*) or beef tapeworm (*Taenia saginata*). The tapeworm larvae penetrate the intestinal wall and spread throughout the body, causing small cysts in the muscles, eyes, heart, liver, lungs, peritoneum, or tissues of the central nervous system. During the first weeks of infestation, there may be no symptoms, but later fever, headache, and aching muscles usually occur. Other symptoms, such as epilepsy, personality changes, or other neurologic problems, may take many years to appear. A physician may diagnose cysticercosis by means of X rays, blood tests, and biopsy. The usual therapy involves the removal of any cyst that causes specific problems or treatment with the drug praziquantel.

See also CYST; TAPEWORM.

Cystic fibrosis (sis′tik fī brō′sis) is a noncontagious, inherited disorder, in which mucous secretions from several parts of the body become thick and sticky and interfere with normal functioning. Commonly affected are the lungs, pancreas, and sweat glands. Mucus in the lungs can block the bronchi, making breathing difficult. Thick mucus can also block the ducts of the liver and the pancreas, causing improper digestion.

Q: *What are the symptoms of cystic fibrosis?*

A: In most cases, persons with cystic fibrosis seem to be born healthy, but begin showing signs of this disorder between infancy and adolescence. Such signs may include greasy, foul-smelling stool; chronic cough; persistent wheezing; recurrent respiratory problems; and decreased growth rate.

Q: *How is cystic fibrosis diagnosed?*

A: Along with observation of symptoms common to this disorder, special tests often help in this diagnosis. It seems that the sweat glands are also affected by this disorder. They produce excessive amounts of salt, which can be detected by testing perspiration samples.

Q: *How is cystic fibrosis treated?*
A: There is no known cure for this disorder, but treatment with many new antibiotics is allowing children with cystic fibrosis to reach adulthood. Treatment usually involves alleviating symptoms. For example, antibiotics to fight infections and special diets to combat malnutrition may be prescribed. Sometimes, digestion can be improved by adding missing digestive enzymes to the diet. Bronchial drainage is done repeatedly to loosen and remove mucus in the lungs.

Cystitis (sis tī′tis) is acute or chronic inflammation of the bladder. It causes frequent, painful, and cloudy urination, sometimes with blood. Milder symptoms may be only a slight increase in the frequency of urination, accompanied by a burning sensation. Fever and backache may occur, particularly if infection has spread to the kidneys (pyelonephritis). The pain during urination may be so severe that children refuse to pass urine. *See also* BLADDER.

Q: *What causes cystitis?*
A: Cystitis is usually caused by infection of the bladder, usually ascending from the urethra. Causes other than infection may be the aftereffects of radiotherapy for bladder tumors. *See also* URETHRA.

Q: *Can other disorders increase the chances of getting cystitis?*
A: Yes. The presence of any abnormality that affects the bladder may make cystitis more likely: an obstruction that affects the normal flow of urine (for example, an enlarged prostate gland); pouches in the bladder resulting from a birth defect; the presence in the bladder of stones (calculi) or a tumor; or, in tropical countries, schistosomiasis. A distended uterus during pregnancy may obstruct the normal flow of urine and cause cystitis. *See also* SCHISTOSOMIASIS.

Q: *How is cystitis diagnosed and treated?*
A: Cystitis is usually diagnosed by testing a urine sample for the presence of infection. The disorder can be treated effectively by simple methods. Large quantities of fluids (at least one glass of water every hour) should be drunk. Potassium citrate mixture, an old-fashioned remedy, often brings relief from the burning pain that accompanies urination. In most cases, a short course of an antibiotic drug, prescribed by a physician, is required to cure the cystitis. After an attack of cystitis, a physician may test a urine specimen again to make sure that the infection has disappeared.

Q: *Does treatment differ if another attack of cystitis occurs?*
A: No, but the disorder should be more fully investigated. This may involve blood tests, examination of the prostate gland, and X rays with intravenous pyelography (IVP) and a cystogram. Sometimes the physician examines the bladder with a special instrument (cystoscope), to make sure that stones or other abnormalities are not present. Urine specimens may have to be examined on several occasions to make sure that a low-grade infection is not present all the time and to rule out the rare possibility of tuberculosis. Recurrent (chronic) cystitis commonly affects women. In men, however, even a single episode of cystitis warrants a diagnostic evaluation. *See also* CYSTOGRAM; PYELOGRAM, INTRAVENOUS.

Q: *Why is chronic cystitis a common problem in women?*
A: In women, the urethra is short, and this makes it easy for bacteria to reach the bladder. Sexual intercourse may move more bacteria into the urethra (honeymoon cystitis).

Q: *What precautions might prevent honeymoon cystitis?*
A: Simple measures, such as emptying the bladder immediately after intercourse, may remove any bacteria that have passed up the urethra. Hygiene is also very important. The anus should be wiped from front to back to prevent intestinal bacteria from entering the vaginal area. Sometimes, however, cystoscopy is done to make certain there is no anatomical reason for the cystitis. *See also* CYSTOSCOPY.

Cyst, meibomian. *See* CHALAZION.

Cystogram (sis′tə gram) is a special X ray, taken after a radiopaque dye has been placed in the urinary bladder,

A **cystogram** is an X ray of the bladder after a radiopaque dye has been injected into it.

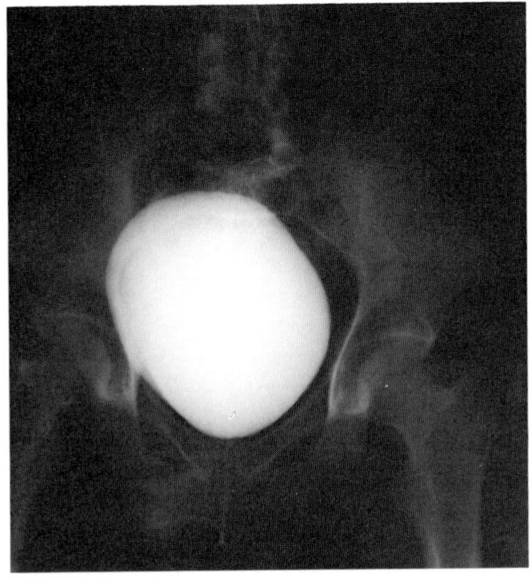

usually after the bladder has been emptied by means of a catheter. X rays can be taken before and during urination, to detect the presence of stones, tumors, or defects in the bladder.

See also CALCULUS.

Cystoscopy (sis tos'kə pē) is the examination of the inside of the bladder, using a special instrument equipped with a lens and a light (cystoscope). The cystoscope is introduced through the urethra, the tube that carries urine from the bladder to the outside of the body. Long, thin instruments can be passed into the bladder to take a biopsy of a tumor, to crush stones, or to treat the bladder tissue.

Cyst, ovarian (sist, ō vâr'ē ən). An ovarian cyst is a swelling, abnormal sac-like growth on an ovary. It can be less than an inch or as much as 10 inches (250 mm) in diameter. Some cysts are painless as well as harmless. Others may cause great pain and result in serious complications.

Cysts most commonly occur in women between the ages of 20 and 40. In about 85 percent of cases, they are benign (noncancerous).

Some cysts will disappear on their own. If they persist, enlarge, or produce symptoms, they should be removed surgically.

Cysts occurring in women over age 50 have a higher chance of being malignant. Cancerous cysts must always be removed, along with both ovaries, both fallopian tubes, the uterus, and possibly the omentum and selected lymph nodes. Ovarian cancer usually requires additional treatment of chemotherapy or radiation therapy.

See also CHEMOTHERAPY; OMENTUM.

Cyst, sebaceous (sist, si bā'shəs). Sebaceous cyst, sometimes called a wen, epidermal cyst, or pilar cyst, is a swelling in the skin, caused by a blocked sebaceous gland. The gland continues to produce waxy sebum and becomes enlarged.

Sebaceous cysts can occur anywhere on the body, but are most common on the scalp. They grow gradually and only rarely become malignant (cancerous).

See also CYST.

Cytology (sī tol'ə jē) is the study of the structure, function, and formation of cells. It is now widely used in the early diagnosis of cancer, especially cancer of the cervix. A Pap test is a well-known example of a cytologic study.

See also CERVICAL SMEAR.

Cytomegalovirus (sī tō meg ə lō vī' rəs), CMV, is a cluster of viruses causing many diseases in humans, especially in infants. Cytomegalovirus infection is characterized by swollen glands, fever, and fatigue. In adults, CMV may take the form of mononucleosis or hepatitis; in newborns, jaundice and low birth weight. In the most severe cases of infected infants, CMV may result in brain damage, deafness, blindness, and death. In patients with cancer, transplanted organs, or AIDS, CMV can cause severe disease of the lungs. There are no specific drugs available to prevent or treat CMV-related illnesses.

Cytoplasm (sī'tə plaz əm) is the living substance or protoplasm of a cell outside of the nucleus.

See also CELL.

Cytotoxic drug (sī tə tok'sik) is a drug that destroys cells or prevents their multiplication. It is mainly used in immunotherapy and in the treatment of cancer; it is occasionally used to treat other disorders, such as psoriasis and rheumatoid arthritis. The administration of cytotoxic drugs must be carefully controlled; excessive doses may cause serious blood disorders, hair loss (alopecia), and reduced resistance to infection.

See also CANCER.

D

Dacryocystitis (dak rē ō sis tī'tis) is inflammation of the tear sac, caused by a blockage of the duct or by infection from the nose. The symptoms are pain, swelling, and tenderness in the corner of the eye, with a discharge of pus and tears that can not drain normally. To treat the condition, a physician may apply hot compresses and/or antibiotic solution directly to the tear sac to prevent infection of the cornea. In addition, oral antibiotics may be prescribed, or surgical removal or intubation of the tear sac may be required.

See also EYE; INTUBATION.

Dalmane® (dal'mān) is a preparation of flurazepam hydrochloride, a drug of the benzodiazepine group. Dalmane is used primarily as a sleep-inducing agent.

See also FLURAZEPAM HYDROCHLORIDE.

D and C. *See* DILATATION AND CURETTAGE.

Dander (dan'dər) is the small, dry scales from the skin, hair, or feathers of animals that may cause an allergic reaction in individuals with a sensitivity to it.

See also ASTHMA.

Dandruff (dan'drəf) is a minor condition in which the scalp is dry and scaling, often caused by surface skin glands that do not secrete enough moisture. Dandruff tends to get worse when it occurs with seborrhea (a disorder of the sebaceous glands). To treat dandruff the hair should be washed two or three times a week with shampoo containing selenium sulfide or salicylic acid. A physician may prescribe a preparation containing corticosteroid hormones, to be applied at night.

See also SEBORRHEA.

Dangerous plants. *See* POISONING: FIRST AID.

Dapsone (dap'sōn) is a sulfone-type drug used to treat leprosy, dermatitis herpetiformis, brown recluse spider bites, and AIDS. It is considered to exert its action through an immunosuppressive effect. Side effects can include anemia, fever, nausea, and rash.

See also AIDS; BITES AND STINGS: FIRST AID; DERMATITIS; LEPROSY.

Darvon® (där'von), a preparation of the drug propoxyphene hydrochloride, is a painkiller, available in a number of forms. Its uses are similar to those of acetaminophen; it can, however, produce adverse effects, such as dizziness, sedation, nausea, vomiting, headache, skin rashes, abdominal pain, and constipation. Persons with respiratory disorders should use Darvon and its derivatives with caution and never with other depressants, antidepressants, or alcohol. Because Darvon is a narcotic, persons taking the drug for a long period can develop a tolerance to it or even some dependence on it.

DDT is an abbreviation of dichlorodiphenyl-trichloroethane, now known also as chlorophenothane. DDT was once an extremely effective odorless insecticide. Many pests, however, have now developed an immunity to it. DDT is no longer used when substitutes are available, because its use is thought to contaminate the food supply of animals and human beings. When ingested orally, DDT causes acute poisoning.

Deaf-mute. *See* HEARING IMPAIRED.

Deafness is the inability to hear. It can affect one or both ears, either totally or partially. Deafness may be present at birth (congenital deafness), or it may occur later, suddenly or gradually.

Q: *Are there any obvious signs that a person may be deaf?*

A: Yes. Deafness may be suspected if a person fails to react to sounds at various levels or speaks more loudly than is necessary. A child who is partially deaf may give the impression of being bored or uninterested and will have difficulty in learning to speak. Such a child may not progress well at school, and it is often a teacher's report that first leads a parent to suspect

Conductive **deafness** can be caused by otosclerosis, a hereditary disorder caused by the gradual build-up of extra bony tissue around one of the small bones (stapes or ossicle) in the middle ear.

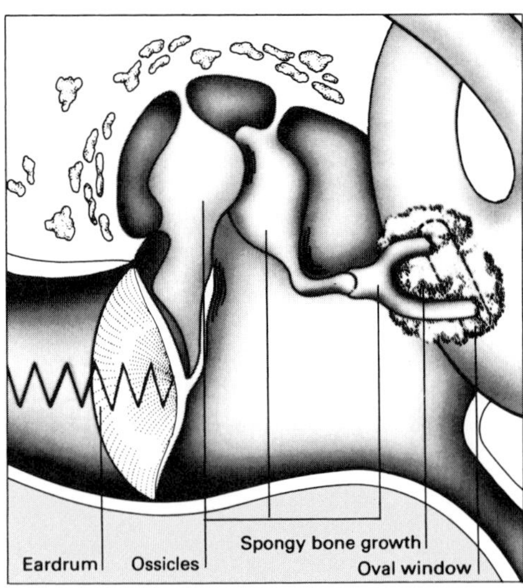

that the child may have impaired hearing. Deafness in an older person can lead to a sense of isolation, which can make the person bad-tempered. The degree of hearing loss, however, depends on the kind of deafness involved.

Q: *What different kinds of deafness are there?*

A: It is usual to categorize deafness as being either conductive deafness or sensorineural deafness. Some persons, however, suffer from a combination of the two.

Q: *What is conductive deafness?*

A: Conductive deafness is hearing loss resulting from interference with the transmission of sound waves through either the outer or the middle ear. Conductive deafness can be either a temporary or a permanent condition.

Q: *What causes conductive deafness?*

A: Conductive deafness can have many causes, perhaps the most common of which is earwax (cerumen) that obstructs the ear canal and prevents sound waves from reaching the inner ear. Another common cause of conductive deafness is infection of the middle ear (otitis media), which often arises from various childhood diseases, particularly those involving the upper respiratory tract. To prevent hearing loss, children under the age of three who are subject to recurrent otitis media should be treated with antibiotics. Infections of the upper respiratory tract often cause swelling in or around a Eustachian tube. This tube connects the middle ear with the nasopharynx and helps equalize air pressure on both sides of the eardrum. When the pressures are unequal, as often happens during upper respiratory tract infections, deafness can result. Flying in aircraft, or deep-sea diving, can also change pressure within the ear and cause conductive deafness. *See also* BAROTRAUMA.

Q: *How is conductive deafness diagnosed?*

A: In addition to direct observation of the signs, otologists and audiologists (specialists in problems of the ears and of hearing) use various tests to diagnose this kind of hearing impairment. One such test involves the use of a tuning fork. If the sound of a vibrating tuning fork is heard more clearly when the fork is placed close to the ear, the deafness is likely to be conductive. Specialists may then use an audiometer to determine the degree of deafness and X-ray photographs of the skull to pinpoint obstructions that may be causing the deafness.

Q: *How is conductive deafness treated?*

A: Treatment depends on the cause. For example, if earwax is the cause, removal of the wax often restores hearing. This removal should, however, be done only by a trained person; an untrained person may force the wax deeper into the ear or puncture the eardrum.

Other forms of treatment for conductive deafness may also include antibiotics, as in the case of otitis media; draining the fluid build-up from the middle ear; and surgery, in the case of a punctured eardrum or an immobile stapes. Surgery in cases of otosclerosis, called stapediolysis and stapedioplasty, are common and highly successful procedures.

Q: *What is sensorineural deafness?*

A: Sensorineural, or nerve, deafness arises from the inability of nerve impulses to reach the auditory center of the brain because of nerve damage either to the inner ear or to the brain. For example, nerve damage to the cochlea, which contains

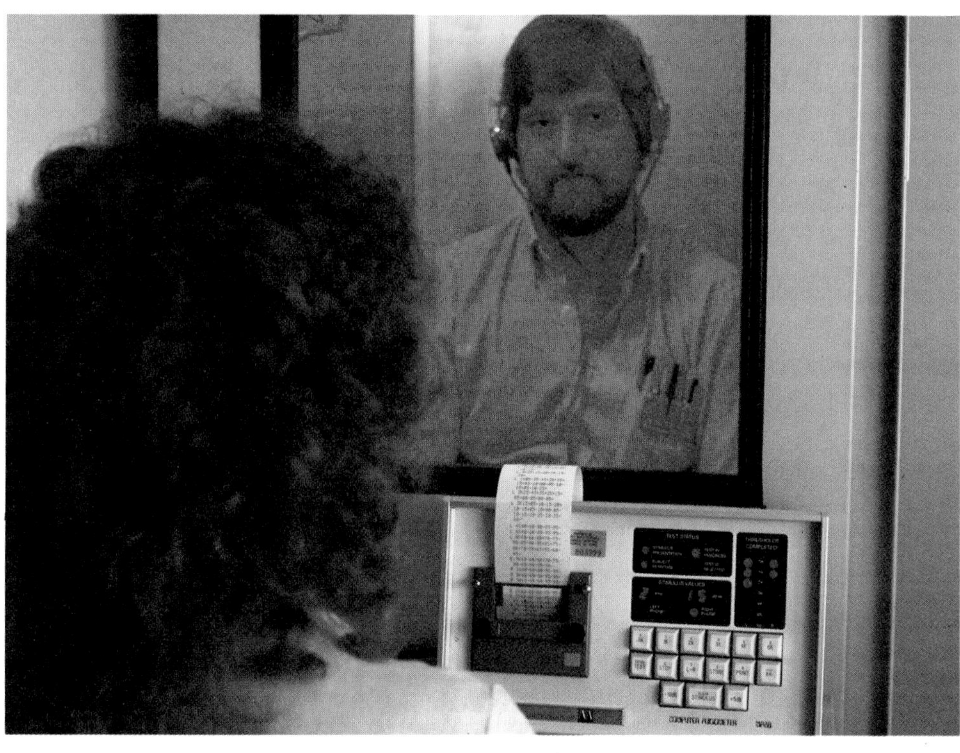

The degree of **deafness** or the kind of impairment is often tested by audiologists using special equipment.

the sense organ for hearing (the organ of Corti), damage to the ear's auditory nerve, and nerve damage to the cerebral cortex of the brain can all result in sensorineural deafness.

Q: *What causes sensorineural deafness?*

A: Diseases are a common cause of sensorineural deafness. The diseases include arteriosclerosis, chicken pox, influenza, Mèniére's disease, meningitis, mononucleosis, mumps, Rh disease, and syphilis.

Many children born with sensorineural deafness have mothers who contracted rubella (German measles) during the first three months of pregnancy.

Other causes of sensorineural deafness include tumors of the brain or the middle ear, concussion, blows to the ear, and repeated loud sounds. The toxic effects of certain drugs can also cause sensorineural deafness in some persons.

Q: *How is sensorineural deafness diagnosed and treated?*

A: Together with observation of the obvious signs of deafness, audiologists and otologists use electronic equipment to detect and diagnose sensorineural deafness. Such equipment, which includes various types of audiometers, can also help specialists to determine if tumors or other problems are involved in causing the deafness. Most cases of sensorineural deafness can not be treated. However, an operation called a cochlear implant, in which a tiny electronic device is surgically implanted, can be helpful.

Q: *Can hearing aids help all hearing-impaired persons?*

A: No. Hearing aids amplify sound, but such devices are helpful only to persons who retain some hearing.

See also AUDIOGRAM; CERUMEN; EAR.

Death occurs when all activity of the brain ceases and life is completely extinct. It may come at the end of a long illness or be sudden and unexpected as the result of an accident or a heart attack. But in every case, every individual person can spare his or her loved ones a great deal of unnecessary anguish by thinking out clearly, in advance, all the details and instructions surrounding arrangements for his or her own death. The funeral will have to be organized; the family must be comforted and cared for; and any other special circumstances, such as a part of the body left for medical research, must be taken into account.

Q: *What is the first thing to think about when death has occurred?*

A: A death certificate will be issued and signed by a physician familiar with the deceased or the physician who was in attendance at the time of death. When a person dies in a hospital, the certificate will be signed by an attending physician and is obtained from the hospital business office along with any personal effects belonging to the deceased. Receipt of these is usually acknowledged by signature. Copies of the certificate are made available from the health department. In the event of an accidental or unexplained death, the certificate will be issued by the medical examiner's or coroner's office. The coroner may not be able to state the cause of death without performing an autopsy.

Q: *Isn't an autopsy too harrowing for the relatives to bear at this time?*

A: It is as distasteful to the hospital staff as it is to the bereaved to have to face the decision to perform an autopsy at this most grievous time. But legal authorities may require a medicolegal autopsy to determine the cause of death in certain instances, such as an accident or if the deceased had not been seen by a physician within a specified time period. An autopsy for medical or educational reasons may provide the family with specific information concerning the cause of death, or it may advance medical research by adding to the data on conditions, diseases, and treatments. For this type of autopsy, the survivors must give their consent.

Q: *How are the arrangements made for the funeral?*

A: The services of a capable funeral director can considerably ease the administrative burden of death arrangements. It may be wise to speak with more than one funeral director about specifics such as what services are provided and at what cost. Then, on notification by the family, the funeral director obtains permission to remove the body to the funeral home, consults with a responsible relative on details of casket, service, burial or cremation, hours of visiting so that people can pay their respects, whether the head and shoulders are to be on view or the coffin closed, and so on. The director should also take care of press obituaries.

Q: *Who takes care of medical bequests by the deceased?*

A: If the deceased has left his or her body to a medical school, the funeral director will usually convey the body there for a small fee. In cases of sudden, accidental death in young, fit people, consideration must be given to kidney, heart, and liver donation if facilities are available. If the deceased has bequeathed his or her corneas for transplant or experimental use, the local eye bank (which works closely with the Lions Clubs) will send a technician immediately upon notification. Speed is essential, and it is important to know about such bequests ahead of time.

Q: *What is the best way to help the bereaved relatives?*

A: Somebody must take charge of affairs, and most families look to one or two members to do this. Often it will be the eldest child of the deceased, or an old and trusted friend who may be executor of the estate. It is usually better that the individual concerned be able to be fairly detached, in order to take the burden off the most grieving survivor especially in the choice of a funeral director. The telephone will be in frequent use for a time, and it is advised that the family member who is in charge use a phone nearby, leaving the home phone clear for calls of sympathy and help from other relatives and friends. The family lawyer should be told immediately, particularly if the deceased has left any special instructions. The family priest, minister, or rabbi should also be informed at the earliest opportunity.

Death is a test of a family's strength; it can bring out the best or the worst in family and friends. Perhaps the best guide to conduct is to try to act in a manner that would have been approved of by the deceased.

Q: *What is the grief process?*

A: Death in the Western world has become a private affair that is concealed as far as possible. Grief is therefore a socially difficult emotion. A bereaved family may find themselves isolated because friends and relatives feel unable to cope with another person's grief.

At first, grief takes the form of shock and numbness; then great waves of emotion sweep over the person, accompanied by uncontrollable tears; and finally the person becomes calm. This cycle of emotion can continue for some weeks, even months. The emotional, tearful phase should not be suppressed. It acts as a necessary relief from bereavement.

Grief is often accompanied by tremendous fatigue. There is a great deal for the family to organize. For the single bereaved person, the burden is even greater. He or she also has to deal with a quiet home and a loss of routine; there are usually feelings of guilt; and gone is the feeling of being wanted and needed. The person needs company and others to talk to. It is a time for other members of the family to give support and help to prevent a deepening of the depression that follows a death.

Professional persons offer a great deal of support to the bereaved. A family physician can lend moral support and make sure that good health is maintained despite the physical and mental stress of bereavement; a lawyer can handle the financial and legal future; and a member of the clergy can offer spiritual support.

Gradually the bereaved person's life returns to normal and he or she resumes social contacts. Grief remains, but with understanding and sympathy the bereaved can adjust to the loss of a loved one and get on with living his or her life.

See also DYING.

Debility. *See* WEAKNESS.

Débridement (dā brēd män′) is the cleansing of a wound by the surgical or nonsurgical removal of foreign matter and dead or damaged tissue or bone.

Decalcification (dē kal sə fə kā′shən) is the loss of calcium salts from the bones and teeth. This condition may occur in persons who are confined to bed for long periods of time and in persons who are subjected to long periods of weightlessness. Decalcification may result from various disorders: overactive parathyroid glands, causing osteitis fibrosa; rickets and osteomalacia, caused by vitamin D deficiency; and osteoporosis. Local decalcification may be caused by bone tumors (osteosarcomas), or the spread of cancer from other parts of the body. Decalcification may lead to the formation of stones in the kidneys and bladder.

See also CALCULUS.

Deciduous (di sij′ü əs) is the term used to refer to the teeth that appear in infancy and are later replaced by the permanent teeth.

See also TOOTH.

Decompression sickness. *See* BENDS.

Decongestant (dē kən jes′tənt) is a drug or other agent that reduces any congestion of mucus produced by various mucous membranes, particularly those in the nose. Decongestants should be taken according to the prescribed dosage and for no longer than two or three weeks; if the recommended dosage is not strictly followed, the chemical effects of the drugs may further irritate the mucous membranes and prolong the presence of mucus.

See also MUCOUS MEMBRANE.

Decubitus ulcer. *See* BEDSORE.

Defecate (def′ə kāt) is the medical term for having a bowel movement. It also applies to the release of feces from an artificial opening that has been made in the intestines, such as a colostomy or an ileostomy.

See also COLOSTOMY; DIGESTIVE SYSTEM; ILEOSTOMY.

Defibrillation (dē fī brə lā′shən) is the term used for stopping the trembling, or fibrillation, of the heart muscle by means of drugs or an electric shock. In certain conditions, for example, coronary heart disease, the heart may stop beating while the heart muscle continues to fibrillate. Sometimes, normal

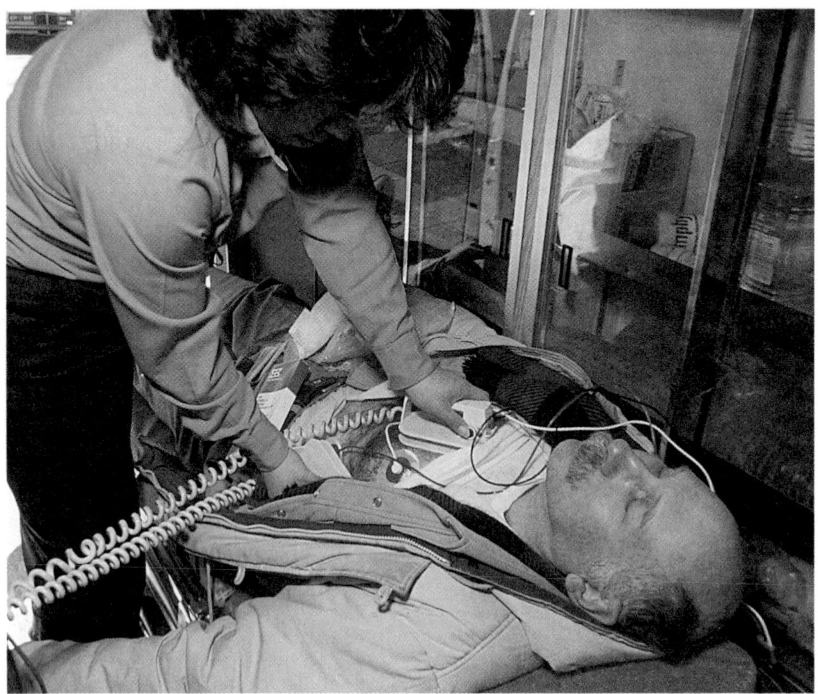

Defibrillation, the stopping of fibrillation, or trembling of the heart, can sometimes be accomplished via electric shock from a cardiac defibrillator.

heart contractions can be restored by electric shocks from a machine called a cardiac defibrillator.

Deficiency disease is a disorder that is caused by a lack or deficiency of a substance that is essential to the proper functioning of the body, such as various vitamins, minerals, and proteins. Deficiency diseases often result from an inadequate diet, but they can also be caused by metabolic disorders, such as pernicious anemia (which is caused by inadequate absorption of vitamin B_{12}); intestinal disorders; overexcretion of the substance in the urine, feces, or by vomiting; the presence of a parasite, for example, a hookworm or tapeworm; or by a prolonged illness.

Q: *What are the most common deficiency diseases?*

A: The most common deficiency diseases are those caused by a lack of vitamins or minerals. They include anemia (lack of iron); scurvy (lack of vitamin C); beriberi (lack of vitamin B_1); night blindness (lack of vitamin A); rickets and osteomalacia (lack of vitamin D); and goiter (lack of iodine).

Q: *How are deficiency diseases treated?*

A: In most cases the disorder is treated by a special diet that is rich in foods that restore the deficient substance. The diet is sometimes supplemented with vitamin tablets or specific drugs.

Q: *What are some of the symptoms of deficiency diseases?*

A: Scurvy may cause bleeding from the gums. Vitamin B deficiencies can cause cracking at the corners of the mouth and a magenta-colored tongue. Vitamin D deficiency can, when it is severe, result in rickets and body deformities involving long bones.

See also VITAMIN.

Dehydration (dē hī drā'shən) is the excessive loss of water from the body. In normal conditions an adult needs about 5 pints (2.4l) of water each day to replace that which is lost by breathing, sweating, urinating, and defecating. If this fluid loss is not replaced, dehydration results.

The major symptom of dehydration in adults is thirst; muscle cramps may occur if dehydration is combined with fatigue. Dehydration is potentially serious, especially in babies and young children. Danger signs are drowsiness, constipation, wrinkled skin, lack of elasticity in the skin, dry skin, coated tongue, lack of urination, irritability, confusion, and a depressed "soft spot" (fontanel) in a young baby's skull. The major causes of dehydration include diarrhea, vomiting, excessive water loss through sweating caused by fever or high air temperatures, illness such as diabetes, and a reaction following surgery.

Q: *How is dehydration treated?*

A: A seriously dehydrated baby should be hospitalized immediately. A lesser degree of dehydration can be treated with small and frequent drinks of water or milk and water. In adults, dehydration can usually be treated with water to which a little salt has been added. If the cause is a disorder such as cholera or diabetes, hospital treatment is required.

Delhi boil. *See* LEISHMANIASIS.

Delirium (di lir'ē əm) is a state of mental confusion and extreme excitement, commonly accompanied by hallucinations and continual but aimless physical activity. Delirium is the immediate result of a disturbance in brain function, but the disturbance itself can be caused by any, or by a combination of several, generally serious conditions.

High fever, particularly from pneumonia, can cause delirium, as can malaria, meningitis, encephalitis, liver or kidney disease, or high blood pressure (hypertension). Another cause is alcoholism, which can lead to delirium tremens, a dangerous disorder that involves both visual and auditory hallucinations, usually accompanied by other serious medical problems. Drug overdoses and some mental disorders, such as schizophrenia, can also cause delirium.

Delirium can be reduced with sedatives or tranquilizers, but hospitalization is generally necessary for treatment of the underlying serious condition.

See also DELIRIUM TREMENS.

Delirium tremens (di lir'ē əm trē'mənz) (d.t.'s) is a form of delirium that occurs with withdrawal from alcohol among alcoholics. It is a potentially fatal condition, and hospitalization is urgently necessary. Delirium tremens may be complicated by epilepsy, pneumonia, and heart and liver failure, resulting from severe alcoholism.

Q: *What are the symptoms of delirium tremens?*

A: The symptoms of delirium tremens include sweating, tremor, fever, tachycardia or increased heart rate, chest pain, gastrointestinal symptoms, sleeplessness, anxiety, and nausea. There is often an aversion to food. Persons with delirium tremens may suffer delusions and hallucinations and become extremely agitated. For example, such persons may experience strange skin sensations, see monstrous creatures, and make wild gestures with the hands. If untreated, the symptoms will progress, and the patient may have a seizure.

Q: *What is the treatment for delirium tremens?*

A: Initial treatment usually consists of bed rest, sedation, and a controlled diet. Long-term treatment aims at helping patients to overcome their addiction to alcohol.

See also ALCOHOLISM.

Delivery is the final stage of childbirth. The term also includes the expulsion of the placenta.

See also PREGNANCY AND CHILDBIRTH.

Delivery, emergency. *See* CHILDBIRTH: EMERGENCY DELIVERY.

Delusion (di lü'zhən) is a steadfast and unshakable belief that is held in the face of contrary evidence. Examples include delusions of persecution (a belief that others are plotting against one); delusions of grandeur (a belief that one is an important figure, for example, Jesus Christ); and delusions of control (a belief that one's thoughts and actions are being controlled by others). Arguing against delusions is futile as the person will wrongly interpret irrelevant or insignificant observations, occurrences, or information to support his or her delusional belief.

The presence of delusions often reflects a serious psychiatric disorder, such as manic-depressive illness, severe depression, schizophrenia, or paranoia. Physical causes, such as organic brain syndrome, should be evaluated.

Q: *How are serious delusions treated?*

A: Delusions can be resolved or be controlled if drug therapy is successful in treating the underlying psychiatric or physical disorder. Some long-standing delusions can, however, be resistant to treatment. Hospitalization may be necessary if an individual is either a danger to himself or herself or to others, or if an individual simply can not function.

See also AFFECTIVE DISORDER; MENTAL ILLNESS; SCHIZOPHRENIA.

Dementia (di men'shə) refers to an organic brain syndrome that results in a deterioration in intellectual functioning; this includes deficits in memory, particularly short-term memory; impairment in abstract thinking; impairment in the ability to learn new information; impairment in problem solving; and impairment in judgment. Changes in personality, emotional response, and impulse control often occur. In some cases, as in Alzheimer's disease, dementia is a chronic and progressive condition, which leads, eventually, to a loss of most intellectual functions and to a loss of responsiveness to one's environment.

Dementia can, however, be reversed if the underlying organic cause, for example, hydrocephalus, hypothyroidism, or brain tumor, can be successfully treated. It is, therefore, important to explore all possible explanations for dementia before resigning oneself to the progressive loss of intellect.

In the older individual, depression can mimic dementia (pseudodementia).

Support programs can help families cope with the heavy emotional demands of caring for a family member afflicted with chronic, progressive dementia.

See also ALZHEIMER'S DISEASE.

Dementia, presenile. *See* ALZHEIMER'S DISEASE.

Demerol® (dem′ə rōl) is a preparation of meperidine hydrochloride, a synthetic painkiller (narcotic analgesic) with similar effects and uses as morphine. Demerol has less sedating action than morphine and has no cough-suppressant effects; it is also less constipating than morphine. Like morphine, Demerol is addictive.

The main use of Demerol is as a painkiller. It is especially useful in the treatment of colic, caused by gallstones or kidney stones, because it has an antispasmodic effect, which is not shared by morphine. Demerol may be combined with other drugs, such as antihistamines, as a form of preanesthetic medication.

Q: *Can Demerol produce adverse side effects?*

A: Yes. Demerol can cause dizziness, drowsiness, sweating, nausea, vomiting, and a dry mouth. Occasionally, it can also cause retention of urine, palpitations, and convulsions.

See also MORPHINE.

Dendrite (den′drīt) is one of the tubelike extensions of the cell body of a neuron. Dendrites receive impulses that are conducted to the cell body.

See also CELL.

Dengue (deng′gā), also known as breakbone fever, is an acute tropical disease, caused by a virus infection transmitted by the mosquito *Aedes aegypti, A. albopictus,* or *A. polynesiensis.* The disease is rarely fatal. Symptoms include fever, skin rash, headache, and severe pains in the eyes, muscles, and joints. The symptoms often subside after the fifth or sixth day, but then return for another three or four days.

There is no specific treatment, although painkilling drugs and plenty of fluids may ease the symptoms. An attack of dengue is often followed by a period of depression and severe debility, before normal health returns.

Dental care. *See* TOOTH CARE.

Dental caries. *See* TOOTH DECAY.

Dental disorders. The following table lists some common disorders of the teeth and gums. These disorders are usually treated by a dentist, by an orthodontist, or by a periodontist.

Many entries are defined elsewhere in this encyclopedia.

See also DENTIST; ORTHODONTIST.

Symptom	*Possible disorder*
Teeth	
Decay	Plaque (saliva and food sugar containing harmful bacterial enzymes)
Sharp pain	Abscess
	Tooth decay affecting the dentin
Temperature sensitive	Tooth decay affecting the enamel and dentin
Dull, throbbing pain	Abscess
	Tooth decay affecting the tooth pulp (soft inner part of tooth containing nerves and blood vessels)
	Impacted or emerging tooth
Acute pain, loose tooth	Abscess at base of tooth
	Infected gingivitis
	Periodontitis
	Plaque (saliva and food sugar containing harmful bacterial enzymes)
	Deciduous teeth (in young children only)
Overcrowded teeth	Malocclusion
Speckled enamel	Excessive amount of fluoride
Gums	
Irritation	Gingivitis
	Plaque (saliva and food sugar containing harmful bacterial enzymes)
An open sore	Canker sore (ulceration of the mouth or lips)
	Badly fitting dentures
Pus-filled swelling	Abscess due to badly fitting dentures
	Pyorrhea

Dental floss (flôs) is a waxed or unwaxed thread used to clean between the teeth.

Dentifrice. See TOOTHPASTE.

Dentin (den'tin) is the hard substance that makes up a tooth. It surrounds the central pulp and is itself covered by harder external enamel.

See also TOOTH.

Dentist (den'tist) is a person whose profession is the care of teeth. A dentist fills cavities in teeth, cleans, straightens, or extracts them, supplies artificial teeth, and treats diseases of the mouth and gums.

Denture (den'chər) is a set of artificial teeth. The term may refer to any number of teeth attached to a plastic or metal appliance (plate), which is fitted to the upper or lower jaw. The appliance may be removable or permanently fixed. Dentures should be cleaned at least once a day.

Deodorant (dē ō'dər ənt) is an agent used to destroy or disguise odors of the body or the breath. Most body odors arise from the decomposition of bacteria in a mixture of dead skin cells and sweat, usually because a person does not wash often enough. Most commercial skin deodorants contain an antiperspirant, such as aluminum chloride, which reduces sweating by forming a hydroxide gel in the sweat ducts; usually perfumes are also added. However, care should be taken in the use of deodorants because some can cause skin reactions in those people who are allergic to them. *See also* BODY ODOR.

Bad breath is often caused by food decomposing between the teeth. Commercial mouthwashes and deodorants disguise the smell of bad breath but do not treat the cause.

Deoxyribonucleic acid (dē ok sə rī bō nü klē'ik) is commonly known as DNA. It is a complex protein that makes up the substance of genes. It is found mainly in the nucleus of a cell, controlling its life—and the lives of organisms made up of cells—in two ways.

First, it passes on all hereditary information from one generation of cells to the next. Second, DNA determines the form and function of the cell by regulating the kinds of proteins it produces. Thus, DNA is the master plan of all life.

DNA molecules lie tightly coiled in the chromosomes of a cell. Each chromosome probably contains one extremely long DNA molecule. On the average, a single human chromosome consists of a DNA molecule that is about 16 inches (41cm) long. But the DNA molecule is a thread so thin that its details can not be seen even when magnified by a powerful electron microscope. Scientists have figured out its structure on the basis of its chemical composition. They also have bounced X rays off the atoms in a DNA molecule and studied the patterns the scattered X rays made on photographic plates.

The patterns show that the molecule is a double helix—that is, a double thread, held together by crosspieces and coiled like a spring. In other words, DNA looks like a twisted rope ladder. All DNA molecules have this shape, whether they come from the cells of a cactus, a turtle, or a human being.

The DNA ladder consists of six pieces. The long threads that make up the sides of the ladder contain alternating units of phosphate and a sugar called deoxyribose. The rungs of the ladder are made up of four compounds called bases. The bases are adenine, cytosine, guanine, and thymine (abbreviated A, C, G, and T). They are attached to the sugar units of the ladder's side pieces. Each rung consists of two bases: A-T, T-A, C-G, or G-C. No other combination is possible, because only the A-T and C-G pairs are chemically attracted to each other. In addition, only these pairs make rungs of the proper length

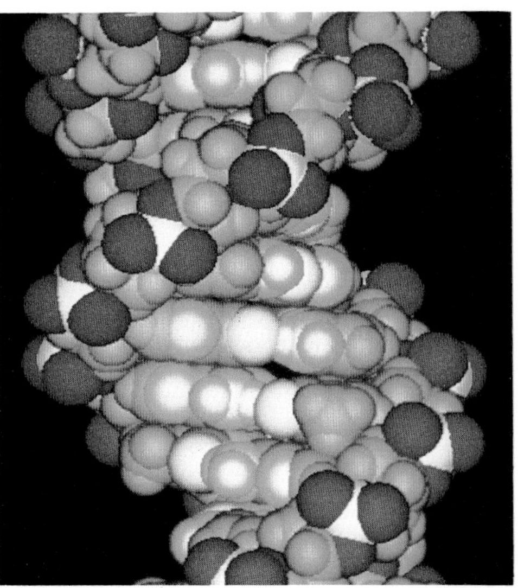

Deoxyribonucleic acid (DNA) molecules, which lie coiled in the chromosomes of a cell, control cellular life as well as the lives of organisms made up of cells.

to fit between the ladder's side pieces. Any other combination is too big or too small. The order of the bases in one strand (half) of the ladder determines the order of the bases in the other strand. For example, if the bases in one strand are ATCGAT, the bases in the opposite strand would be TAGCTA. Before a cell divides, the DNA duplicates. The ladder splits lengthwise, separating the bases of each strand. Then, with the help of special enzymes, each half ladder picks up free bases with their attached sugars and phosphates. But the bases in each half ladder can pick up only their matching mates. The A's attach to T's, the T's to A's, the G's to C's, and the C's to G's. In this way, each new ladder becomes a duplicate of the original ladder. When the cell divides, each of the new daughter cells receives identical DNA molecules.

The duplication and passing on of DNA thus ensures two results. First, the daughter cell is an exact duplicate of the parent cell. Second, the daughter cell has the blueprint (DNA) for the development of its descendants.

The second way DNA controls life is by regulating the kinds of proteins a cell produces, determining its form and function. Inside the nucleus, DNA contains the blueprint for every protein made in the cell. Acting rather like a factory foreman, DNA instructs its chemical cousin, ribonucleic acid (RNA), to manufacture new proteins in the cytoplasm of the cell, according to the DNA structure of the cell's genes.

The way RNA carries out its instructions is discussed under its own heading. The finished protein either becomes a part of the structure or function of the cell or is sent out into the body to fulfill its function as an enzyme, a hormone, an antibody, etc.

See also CELL; PROTEIN; RIBONUCLEIC ACID.

Depersonalization (dē pėr sə nə lə zā′ shən) refers to feelings of unreality or strangeness. In depersonalization, one experiences oneself, one's body, or one's thinking as strange or unfamiliar. Occasionally, there is the feeling of being outside of one's body, observing oneself as if one were another person. The same sense of unreality and unfamiliarity can also be applied to the external world in addition to the self. Isolated incidents of depersonalization are normal; however, if it continues for long periods of time or recurs frequently, it may be a symptom of depression, schizophrenia, or panic disorder. Treatment is directed toward the underlying conditions.

See also MENTAL ILLNESS.

Depilatory (di pil′ə tôr ē) is a substance or device that removes hair. Chemical depilatories remove the hair painlessly without damaging the root. Electrolysis is a method of removing hair permanently. It destroys each hair root by an electric current. Electrolysis is particularly useful on sensitive areas of the body, but it is impractical for areas of dense hair growth and may cause inflammation and pain.

See also ELECTROLYSIS.

Depression (di presh′ən) is a mental state characterized by prolonged feelings of despair and/or a pervasive loss of interest or pleasure. A person experiencing a depressive episode may describe the feeling as sad, hopeless, down, or discouraged. Other symptoms may include sleep disturbance, appetite or weight change, loss of energy, agitation, irritability, withdrawal from others, poor concentration, indecisiveness, loss of libido, feelings of worthlessness or guilt, and thoughts of death or suicide. Some depressed individuals experience an increase in physical symptoms such as headaches, chest pains, or fatigue, sometimes not being aware of the underlying depression. The abuse of alcohol or other drugs may also indicate serious depression. It is important to assess for these symptoms as not all depressed persons can label their mood as depressed. *See also* DRUG ABUSE.

Q: *Can depression be normal?*

A: Yes, to some degree. Almost everyone suffers from periods of sadness, grief, loneliness, or discouragement under certain circumstances. It is normal for a person to be depressed by the terminal illness or death of a relative or friend, for example. But this type of depression is generally temporary and does not usually cause the person to cease functioning for any significant period of time. When the depressive mood persists and is associated with other symptoms, a depressive or affective illness may be suspected.

Q: *What causes depression?*

A: The precise underlying causes are not known. Almost anybody can become depressed if subjected to enough emotional stress, but some persons seem to become depressed more easily than others. A personal trauma or stressful event may trigger a depressive episode. Such psychological stress accounts for about half of all cases of severe depression. Other causes include side effects of a surgical operation or medication, alcohol or drug abuse, or withdrawal from drugs. Some types of depression, such as premenstrual syndrome or menopausal depression, are apparently related to a person's metabolism and age. Depression can also result from an underlying physical problem, such as thyroid disease.

Many behavioral scientists believe that some types of depression may have roots in the experiences of a person's childhood. Studies undertaken by researchers indicate that some types of depression may run in families. There is growing evidence that vulnerability to depression may be genetically transmitted. This means that severe depression may result from biochemical imbalances in brain function. Thus, depression may be caused by a combination of several factors: early psychological losses, poor upbringing, genetic predisposition, or biochemical imbalance.

Hereditary origins of depression may be suspected in persons who persistently become depressed for no apparent reason. Such persons display many of the common signs of depression for weeks or even months at a time. They then appear to make a gradual and complete recovery, but their depression usually recurs. Manic-depressive illness, characterized by alternating periods of elation (the manic phase) and periods of severe depression, is the best example of a hereditary mental illness. *See also* MANIC-DEPRESSIVE ILLNESS.

Q: *What are the dangers of depression?*

A: In all types of depression, the main danger is that of suicide. The risk of suicide is always present and can not be judged by the apparent depth of the depression. It is important to talk to the depressed person about suicidal thoughts in a direct manner. Bringing up the issue of suicide will not put the thought into a person's mind. If the depressed individual has thought of a concrete plan for suicide or has made past suicide attempts, a referral to a mental health professional should be made immediately. *See also* SUICIDE.

Q: *How is depression treated?*

A: Treatment for depression depends on the type and the severity. For example, the so-called normal depression that stems from the death of a relative or from a divorce usually needs no medical treatment, particularly if the individual has good support from caring family and friends.

Individuals with persistent depressive symptoms or a severe depression will probably need treatment. This may include individual counseling, family therapy, drug therapy (such as antidepressants), or hospital confinement. Hospitalization may be necessary for suicidal patients and for those persons who can no longer function in their daily lives. *See also* FAMILY THERAPY.

Electroconvulsive therapy may be necessary if the depressed person does not respond to psychotherapy or drug therapy; when the person's medical condition does not allow for the use of antidepressants; or if a quick recovery from the depressive symptoms is necessary. *See also* ELECTROCONVULSIVE THERAPY.

Dermatitis (dėr mə tī′tis) is inflammation of the skin. There are many different causes, and treatment depends on the diagnosis by a dermatologist. Most forms of dermatitis respond to skin preparations containing corticosteroid drugs. If infections are present, the physician may also prescribe antibiotics and, sometimes, antifungal agents.

See also ECZEMA.

Dermatographia (dėr mə tə graf'ē ə) is a form of urticaria (hives). It is a sensitive condition of the skin, in which scratching or rubbing produces raised red areas. The term literally means "skin writing," and gentle drawing of a blunt point over the skin causes visible lines to appear and remain for a time. Usually, dermatographia is not a serious condition and does not require medical treatment.

Dermatology (dėr mə tol'ə jē) is the branch of medical science concerned with diseases of the skin and the treatment of skin disorders.

Dermoid cyst. *See* CYST, DERMOID.

DES. *See* DIETHYLSTILBESTROL.

Desensitization (dē sen sə tə zā'shən) is a method of treating an allergy. Tests on the patient identify the substance causing an allergy. Sensitivity is reduced by regular injections of the specific allergen in solutions of increasing strength.

Desensitization is also a procedure used in behavior therapy of phobias. The patient is gradually exposed to distressing stimuli until a toleration point is reached.

See also ALLERGY.

Detached retina. *See* RETINA, DETACHED.

Deviated nasal septum. *See* SEPTUM, DEVIATED.

Devil's grip. *See* PLEURODYNIA, EPIDEMIC.

Dexedrine® (dex'ə drēn) is a preparation of dextroamphetamine sulfate, a central nervous stimulant chemically closely related to amphetamine. It is used to treat narcolepsy and attention deficit disorder in children.

Like most other amphetamines, Dexedrine increases blood pressure, dilates the pupils of the eyes, increases respiration rate, and suppresses appetite. Because it suppresses the appetite, Dexedrine was once widely prescribed as a weight reducing drug. However, it is inadvisable to use Dexedrine as an appetite suppressant primarily because it is addictive. The drug has been widely abused, so physicians tend to be cautious about prescribing it.

See also ATTENTION DEFICIT DISORDER; NARCOLEPSY.

Dextrocardia (deks trə kär'dē ə) is a congenital abnormality in which the heart is located in the right side of the chest instead of the left. Dextrocardia is often associated with reverse positioning of all the organs, known as *situs inversus*. In the absence of other associated abnormalities, this condition produces no real problems, although it may cause some confusion in diagnosis of other conditions.

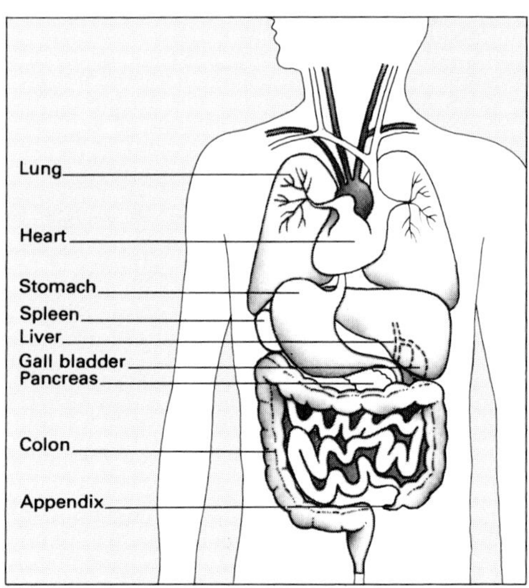

Dextrocardia is an abnormality in which the position of the heart, as well as other internal organs, is reversed.

Diabetes (dī ə bē'tis) is the name of two metabolic disorders that are generally serious. The term by itself is commonly used as an abbreviation of diabetes mellitus, which is one of the two major forms; the other is diabetes insipidus.

See also DIABETES INSIPIDUS; DIABETES MELLITUS.

Diabetes insipidus (dī ə bē'tis in sip' ə dəs) is a disorder that arises from a hormonal imbalance that makes the kidneys overactive or renders them unable to reabsorb the water passed to them from the blood. A person who has the disorder urinates excessively (polyuria) and has a raging thirst (polydipsia) and an increased appetite. These are symptoms also of diabetes mellitus, but the two disorders are otherwise unrelated. *See also* DIABETES MELLITUS.

Q: *What are the causes of diabetes insipidus?*

A: Diabetes insipidus generally occurs because of a lack of vasopressin, an antidiuretic hormone (ADH) that controls the body's urine output. The hormone is produced in the hypothalamus (a part of the brain) and is stored in and secreted by the pituitary gland. The normal secretion of vasopressin can be disturbed by any disease or injury to either the pituitary gland or the hypothalamus. Other causes of diabetes insipidus include diseases such as encephalitis, meningitis, and syphilis. In extremely rare cases, the cause may be the impaired ability of the kidneys themselves to hold water.

Q: *How is diabetes insipidus treated?*

A: Following diagnosis by skull X rays and special tests, a physician may advise an injection of ADH to correct the hormone deficiency. Recent treatment involves synthetic ADH used as a nasal spray. If the cause of the disease is a kidney disorder, treatment with a diuretic is sometimes effective. Diabetes insipidus can not be cured, but treatment greatly improves a patient's condition.

Diabetes mellitus (dī ə bē′tis mel′ə təs), or sugar diabetes, is a disorder in which the body can not make use of sugars and starches in a normal way. A key element in the proper use of sugar and starches is the hormone insulin, which is secreted by special cells (beta cells) within the pancreas; these cells are known as the islets of Langerhans. Diabetes results from either a lack of insulin or an inability of the body to use the insulin properly, but the cause of diabetes is not known. Persons may inherit a tendency toward diabetes. Obesity may also be a factor in the onset of diabetes. *See also* INSULIN; ISLETS OF LANGERHANS.

There are two major forms of diabetes mellitus: Type I, sometimes called insulin-dependent, or juvenile-type, diabetes; and Type II, sometimes called noninsulin-dependent, maturity onset, or adult-type, diabetes. One is usually found in persons under age 25; the other, in persons over age 40.

Diabetes is a serious, sometimes fatal, disorder. There are about seven million known diabetics in the United States and an estimated five million unknown diabetics. According to the U.S. National Commission on Diabetes, the disorder and its complications cause more than 300,000 deaths a year in the United States, making it a leading cause of death.

Q: *What causes the imbalance in blood-sugar levels?*

A: Normally, food digested in the body releases glucose, a form of sugar, into the blood. This increase in blood sugar level causes beta cells in the pancreas to release insulin, which aids in transporting glucose from the blood to storage in such tissues as the liver and muscle.

In persons with Type I diabetes, the pancreas is unable to produce insulin. In Type II diabetes, the pancreas produces some insulin, but the tissues do not respond to it properly. As a result, in both cases, high concentrations of sugar build up in the blood after eating (hyperglycemia). A vicious circle then begins. *See also* HYPERGLYCEMIA.

The fatty acids released from tissue throughout the body are converted by the liver into biochemicals called ketone bodies. These also pour into the bloodstream causing a condition in which the blood becomes dangerously acidic (ketoacidosis). This can lead to diabetic coma and, if untreated, to death.

Q: *What are the symptoms of diabetes?*

A: The general symptoms of diabetes include increased frequency of urination and persistent thirst. In Type I diabetes these symptoms are often accompanied by weakness and increased appetite.

A physician can diagnose diabetes by testing for sugar in the urine and blood. A glucose tolerance test determines how well the body uses and stores sugar. *See also* GLUCOSE TOLERANCE TEST.

Q: *What is the treatment for diabetes mellitus?*

A: Any diabetic who has lapsed into a coma requires immediate emergency medical attention and must be hospitalized.

Type I diabetics need daily injections of insulin. A physician determines the correct dosage, and patients are taught how to prepare and administer the insulin themselves. The technique is simple, even for children. Some diabetics use a portable pump that delivers insulin directly to the body through an artificial opening. Recently, home serum glucose monitoring systems have gained widespread use, rendering urine testing much less useful.

A strict diet is important in controlling diabetes to keep the levels of insulin and sugar in the blood from fluctuating too widely. Careful regulation of activity, food intake, and insulin is also necessary to prevent insulin shock (hypoglycemia), in which the insulin level rises too high and blood sugar drops too low. *See also* HYPOGLYCEMIA.

The first signs of insulin shock are mild hunger, dizziness, sweating, and heart palpitations; then follows mental confusion and coma. Diabetics can stop insulin shock by consuming some substance high in sugar and should always carry sugar or candy. It is advisable for diabetics to have an identification card, tag, or bracelet so that they will receive emergency care.

Type II diabetes is much easier to control. Some cases are treated with diet alone, others with diet plus oral antidiabetic drugs. Some cases are treated with insulin.

Most Type II diabetes can be controlled with diet alone, at least at the onset of the illness, if the patient maintains proper body weight. Approximately 90 percent of all adult-type diabetics are overweight at the time of diagnosis.

Q: ***What complications arise from diabetes mellitus?***

A: Diabetics have increased fatty acids in their blood. This predisposes diabetics to atherosclerosis, a type of arteriosclerosis, which may lead to heart disorder and damage to small and large blood vessels. Nerve tissue degeneration resulting in loss of sensation is another complication of diabetes. Diabetics often have blurred vision or diabetic retinopathy leading to other eye problems, and reduced resistance to infections of all types. Generally, the longer the diabetic condition exists, the more prone the patient is to complications, such as retinopathy and kidney disease. *See also* ARTERIOSCLEROSIS.

Q: ***Is it safe for a diabetic woman to have a baby?***

A: There is some risk involved, particularly in longstanding or complicated diabetes. Despite every precaution, approximately 4 percent of all babies carried by women with diabetes die before or shortly after birth. And maternal deaths of diabetic women are approximately double the expected rate. However, most diabetic women who have not suffered from the disease for a long period of time have perfectly healthy children. There is, however, definitely a need for special care during pregnancy and childbirth and just after. During pregnancy, a diabetic woman's blood sugar level may vary widely, which means that if she needs insulin, her insulin requirement will vary also. Usually, the physician takes regular blood-sugar tests and instructs the woman about testing her urine to be sure she has proper insulin dosage.

The fetus carried by a diabetic woman is usually larger than normal. The newborn infant of a diabetic mother may be particularly prone to hyaline membrane disease, a respiratory disorder; hypoglycemia; and severe congenital anomalies (malformations). After the first week, however, the progress of those babies that survive should be the same as that of other children. *See also* HYALINE MEMBRANE DISEASE.

Most medical experts recommend that diabetic women have no more than two pregnancies, because pregnancy tends to aggravate the disorder.

Q: ***Can diabetes be prevented?***

A: Maintaining proper body weight is the best precaution for an individual with a family history of diabetes, especially if a glucose tolerance test reveals that the person's sugar-processing mechanism is not normal.

Diacetylmorphine (dī as ə təl môr′ fēn) is the medical term for heroin. It is highly addictive, and its importation and medical use in the United States are illegal.

See also HEROIN.

Diagnosis (dī əg nō′sis) is the process by which a physician identifies a disease or disorder from its symptoms, signs, and history. In order to get information for making a diagnosis, the physician may ask the patient to undergo an X-ray examination or various medical tests.

Dialysis. *See* KIDNEY DIALYSIS.

Diaper changing. *See* BABY CARE.

Diaper rash is inflammation of a baby's skin in the area covered by the diaper. The red inflamed area around the buttocks and genitalia may ooze and crust. Diaper rash is usually caused by bacteria in the feces reacting with the urine to produce ammonia. The longer a baby lies in a wet, dirty diaper, the stronger the ammonia becomes. The rash may be aggravated by the diaper's moisture, and the chemical effect of any detergents or soaps left in a diaper that has not been properly rinsed after washing.

Q: *What is the treatment for diaper rash?*

A: Frequent changing of the diaper is essential. Exposure to the air without any covering is the surest way to heal the skin. The urine in the diaper must be able to evaporate, so plastic pants should not be worn until the rash has disappeared. Various soothing applications, such as calamine lotion, zinc compound cream, or petroleum jelly, are effective and should be applied frequently after careful washing of the inflamed area. If the area becomes infected, a physician may prescribe antibiotic or antifungal creams.

See also BABY CARE.

Diaphoretic (dī ə fə ret′ik) is a substance that increases sweating, for example, camphor, opium, and, though rarely used, pilocarpine.

See also PERSPIRATION.

Diaphragm (dī′ə fram) is any thin tissue that separates one structure from another. The term is most commonly applied to the large sheet of muscle between the abdominal cavity and the chest cavity.

See also DIAPHRAGM, CONTRACEPTIVE.

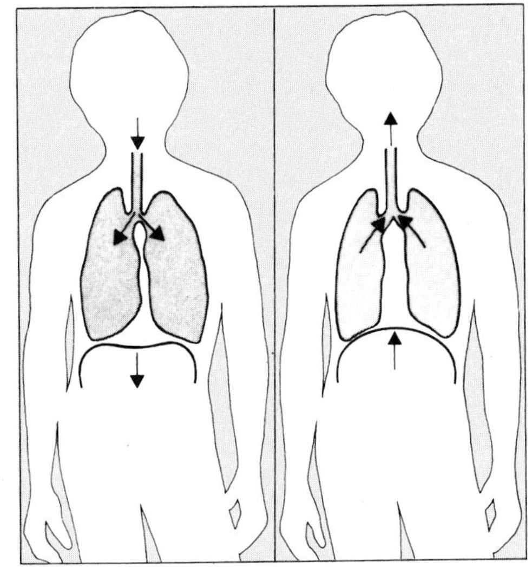

The **diaphragm** contracts and flattens during inhalation, then expands and relaxes during exhalation.

Diaphragm, contraceptive (dī′ə fram, kon tra sep′tiv) is a device, often made of molded rubber, which is inserted into the vagina so that it covers the opening of the uterus and prevents entry of spermatozoa. A spermicide—a drug that kills sperm—is usually applied to the diaphragm before insertion. The diaphragm thus physically and chemically blocks the entrance of the sperm. A woman is usually fitted for a diaphragm in a physician's office. The diaphragm is selected according to several factors specific to the woman. These factors include the size of the vagina; the strength of the muscles surrounding the vagina; and the position of the uterus. A diaphragm must be refitted following childbirth or following a significant change in weight.

See also CONTRACEPTION.

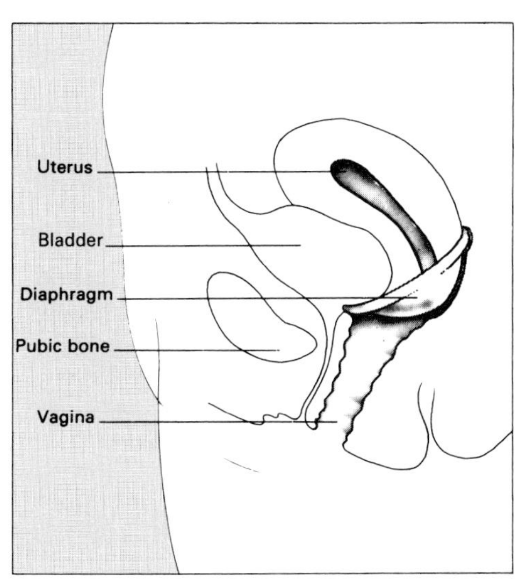

A **contraceptive diaphragm,** which is usually made of molded rubber, blocks spermatozoa from entering the uterus during sexual intercourse. Used in conjunction with a spermicide, the diaphragm is a safe and fairly effective method of contraception.

Diarrhea (dī ə rē′ə) is a condition characterized by frequent bowel movements and feces that are soft or watery, and that may contain blood, pus, or mucus. The condition can prevent the body from absorbing necessary water and salts into the bloodstream, which may lead to dehydration. Diarrhea can be acute or chronic. *See also* DEHYDRATION.

Q: *What can cause acute diarrhea?*

A: Attacks of mild acute diarrhea can often be traced to a simple dietary cause, such as eating rich food, or to an emotional upset. But serious acute diarrhea may be caused by cholera, dysentery, food poisoning, otitis media, viral infection, salmonella, shigella, Campylobacter, or Yersinia. Among other causes of serious acute diarrhea are chemical poisoning and certain respiratory infections. *See also* CHOLERA; DYSENTERY; FOOD POISONING; OTITIS.

Q: *How is acute diarrhea treated?*

A: All persons with acute diarrhea should drink plenty of fluids to prevent dehydration. Most persons with mild acute diarrhea benefit from a diet of bland foods, such as boiled or poached eggs, crackers, custards, gelatins, and rice. In some cases physicians may prescribe antidiarrheal or antispasmodic preparations to help ease the symptoms.

Persons with serious acute diarrhea usually need immediate medical help because of the high risk of dehydration. Signs that dehydration is taking place include a decrease in urine output, dark or light brown urine, sunken eyeballs, rapid pulse rate, vomiting, constant thirst, and drowsiness or even unconsciousness. Dehydration is a serious condition that may prove fatal, especially to infants and young children.

Q: *What can cause chronic diarrhea?*

A: Chronic diarrhea may be a symptom of various serious disorders. Among such disorders are infections of the colon, intestinal cancer, sprue, and infestation of the intestines with worms.

Q: *How is chronic diarrhea treated?*

A: All persons with chronic diarrhea should drink plenty of fluids, to avoid dehydration. Treatment for chronic diarrhea depends partly on the cause, which may be determined by diagnosis of the symptoms and by the results of certain tests. These tests may include sigmoidoscopy, barium enema, and stool-sample examination.

Diarrhea, traveler's (dī a rē′ə). Traveler's diarrhea is an intestinal disorder that can be caused by several factors: a change in diet, which disturbs the microorganisms in the intestine; excessive intake of fruit; large quantities of alcohol; or true intestinal infections. Usually in true traveler's diarrhea, or "turista," a toxin affects the small intestine from the bacterial organism *E. Coli*. The symptoms include severe stomach cramps, vomiting, and frequently watery diarrhea.

Plenty of fluids should be drunk to prevent dehydration. A bland diet and antidiarrheal drugs usually control the symptoms until there is a natural improvement. A physician should be consulted if the symptoms persist for more than 12 hours, if the diarrhea is bloodstained, or if there is a high fever. Traveler's diarrhea may be prevented by taking Septra® before and during a trip to regions known for "turista."

See also DIARRHEA.

Diastole (dī as′tə lē) is the normal period of relaxation of the heart muscle; it alternates with the period of contraction (systole). During the diastole, the heart cavities fill with blood; the diastole of the atria (upper chambers) occurs momentarily before that of the ventricles. The diastolic blood pressure is the point of least pressure in the arteries, because blood is not being pumped by the heart during this phase.

See also HEART; SYSTOLE.

Diathermy (dī′ə thėr mē) is the painless production of heat within the body tissues by means of a high-frequency electric current. Physiotherapists use shortwave diathermy to relieve the symptoms of stiff, painful joints and muscles. Surgical diathermy, or electrocoagulation, is a method of sealing blood vessels using an electrically heated probe.

Diathermy is also used in experimental processes to assist in treatment of various forms of cancer.

See also CAUTERY; HYPOTHERMIA.

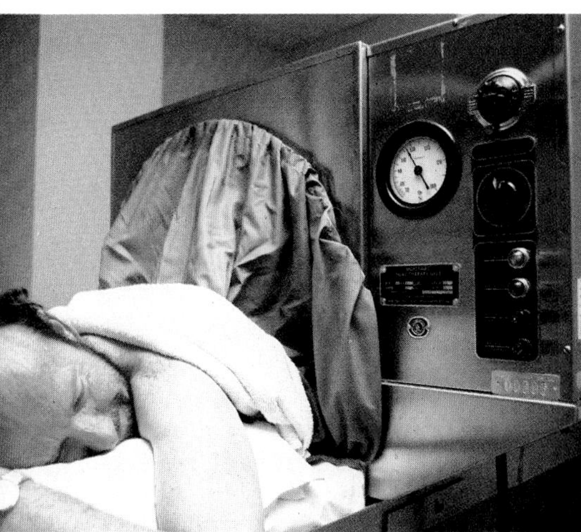

Diathermy is the painless production of heat in body tissues using a high frequency electric current.

Diathesis (dī ath′ə sis) is a constitutional or hereditary tendency to develop a particular disease or disorder. With some disorders that apparently run in families, it is the diathesis that is inherited, not the actual disorder. It may be possible to avoid developing such a disorder by taking appropriate preventive measures.

Diazepam (dī az′ə pam) is the generic name for the tranquilizing drug commonly known as Valium®.

See also VALIUM.

Diet refers to the types of food a person eats regularly. Diet also refers to a set of practices to control the types and amounts of food eaten in an effort to promote health.

A healthy diet should provide the body with all of the substances necessary to maintain growth, to keep in good health, and to repair damaged tissues. These substances should come from food that contains proteins, fats, carbohydrates, vitamins, minerals, and water. A healthy diet should also contain the exact amount of food to satisfy the body's energy needs and no more. In children, and in pregnant women, sufficient calories and protein must be consumed to allow for proper growth. When a body takes in more food than it can use for energy, the excess may be stored as fat. *See also* WEIGHT PROBLEM.

Q: *How is the energy content of foods measured?*

A: Foods are measured for their heat energy value in metric units called calories. One calorie is the energy needed to raise the temperature of one gram of water one degree centigrade. Nutritionists use the kilocalorie (1,000 calories), properly written Calorie (with a capital C), to express the energy content of foods. By convention, in this context, the kilocalorie is written calorie. Protein and carbohydrates have about four calories per gram. Fat has about nine calories per gram.

The daily number of calories needed depends on a person's age, size, physiological state, and level of physical exercise. Generally, men need more calories than women, and youngsters need more than older persons.

Ideally, carbohydrates should make up 58 percent of the diet; fat should make up around 30 percent (10 percent as saturated fats), and only 12 percent of the diet should come from protein.

Q: *What foods make up a balanced diet?*

A: Nutritionists classify foods for a balanced diet in various categories. One such system, the Basic Four, places foods into four groups: a milk group, a meat group, a bread and cereal group, and a fruit and vegetable group.

A healthy diet is based on three things: moderation (not too much of one thing and not too little); variety (within the food groups as well as between the different food groups); and balance (a match between intake of calories and the body's energy needs). Meat, poultry, fish, eggs, beans, peas, and nuts make up the meat group. They are rich sources of protein, vitamin B, iron, niacin, phosphorus, and some carbohydrates. A balanced diet requires one or two servings of these foods per day.

Leafy, green, and yellow vegetables provide folic acid, vitamin A, the B vitamins, vitamin C, calcium, iron, and nonnutritive fiber. A person should have at least one serving from this group each day.

Citrus fruits, green vegetables, and tomatoes supply vitamins A and C, calcium, and iron. At least one daily serving is recommended.

Potatoes, other vegetables, and

noncitrus fruits provide carbohydrates, minerals, and small amounts of most vitamins. One potato and another food from this group is recommended in the daily diet.

Whole-grain bread, breakfast cereal, and enriched flour are rich sources of carbohydrates, vitamins, and minerals. Some, such as bran, also supply fiber. Nutritionists recommend at least four daily servings.

Butter and fortified margarine supply vitamin A and fats.

Milk and such milk products as cottage cheese, yogurt, and cheese provide vitamin A, vitamin B_2, calcium, protein, and fats.

See also NUTRITION.

Diethylstilbestrol (dī eth əl stil bes′ trōl), commonly abbreviated DES, is a synthetic female hormone (estrogen) used primarily to treat menopausal symptoms, as well as estrogen-sensitive carcinoma of the breast or prostate.

DES should *not* be used during pregnancy; it causes vaginal cancer in female offspring.

Diet, special. Special diets are sometimes prescribed by physicians for patients suffering from or recovering from various disorders, or for healthy children or adults who have special nutritional requirements. It must be emphasized that no person, healthy or unhealthy, should make any radical or long-term change in his or her diet without first consulting a physician or nutritionist. *See also* NUTRITION.

High-calcium Diet. A diet rich in calcium is usually advised for pregnant and nursing women. For the duration of a woman's pregnancy, and also while she is nursing her baby, her food has to supply both her own needs and those of her baby. Her food should be rich in proteins, calcium, iron, and vitamins. In particular, she needs over twice the usual amount of calcium required by a normal healthy adult.

Milk, in quantities of up to two pints (.94 liters) a day, is especially recommended. Other foods rich in calcium include cheese, all kinds of fish, and the vegetables broccoli and spinach. This high-calcium diet should be followed from the beginning of preg-

Current diet

Fat
42% of kcalories

Protein 12%

Complex carbohydrate
22%

Sugar
24%

Recommended diet

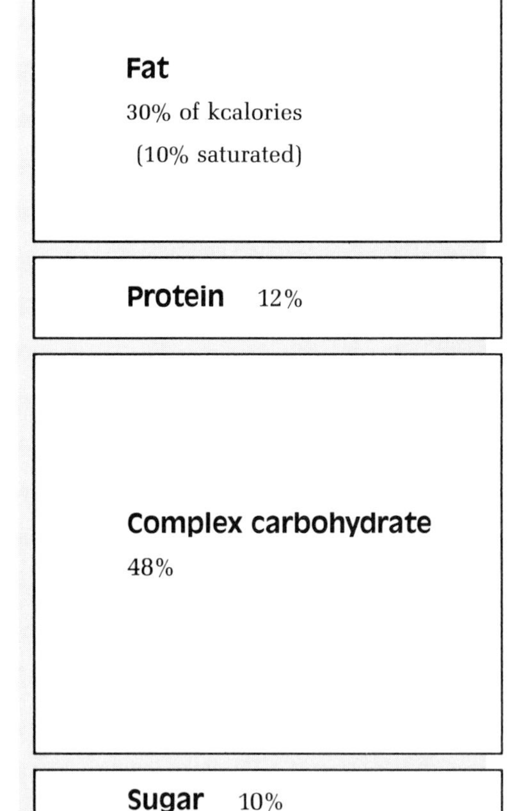

The *Dietary Goals for the United States,* prepared by a Senate committee, suggest that Americans need to make changes to their current **diet.** The recommended diet has a lower percentage of calories coming from fat and sugar and a higher percentage of calories coming from complex carbohydrates.

nancy. Symptoms of nausea and vomiting are often an indication that the amount of fat in the diet is too high, and constipation is usually an indication that the fluid intake is inadequate. A pregnant woman should be guided by her physician in her choice of foods and in the methods of preparing them. If there are signs that she is gaining too much weight, her diet will be adjusted so that the calories are restricted while the protective factors (protein, calcium, iron, and vitamins) remain adequate.

A high-calcium diet with plenty of milk is also suitable for adolescents, who require more than the normal amount of calcium to sustain the rapid physical development that takes place between the ages of 12 and 15. Because of social pressures, adolescents are often careless about their eating habits, and it is the responsibility of parents to make sure that their adolescent children eat regular and nutritious meals.

Low-fat Diet. This diet is considered suitable for patients suffering from gall bladder disease. It can also help to prevent the onset of atherosclerosis and coronary heart disease.

All foods with a high fat content should be excluded from the diet. Fats to be omitted include butter, margarine, lard, and cooking fats. Foods with a high fat content include whole milk, milk products such as cheese and cream, egg yolks, pastry, nuts, chocolate, peanut butter, creamy sauces, and preserves. Meats and fish to be omitted include duck, ham, pork, sausage, salmon, herring, and all fish that is canned in oil.

A low-fat diet should consist of foods that have high carbohydrate and protein contents and that are easily digestible. Such foods include skimmed milk, cottage cheese, white fish, and certain meats such as liver and veal. All excess fat should be trimmed from meat before cooking, and all food should be cooked by some other means than frying.

Low-sodium Diet. This diet is usually prescribed for patients suffering from disorders associated with the retention of body fluid. Such disorders include kidney and liver diseases, high

Nutritional values of common foods

Food	Portion	Calories	Protein (gm)	Calcium (mg)	Iron (mg)	Vitamins A (I.U.)	C (mg)	D (I.U.)	Thiamine (mcg)	Riboflavin (mcg)	Niacin (mg)
Apple, raw	1 large	117	0.6	12	0.6	180	9	0	80	60	0.4
Banana, raw	1 large	176	2.4	16	1.2	860	20	0	80	100	1.4
Beans, green, cooked	1 cup	27	1.8	45	0.9	830	18	0	90	120	0.6
Beef, round, cooked	1 serving	214	24.7	10	3.1	0	0	0	74	202	5.1
Bread, white, enriched	1 slice	63	2.0	18	0.4	0	0	0	60	40	0.5
Broccoli, cooked	⅔ cup	29	3.3	130	1.3	3,400	74	0	70	150	0.8
Butter	1 tablespoon	100	0.1	33	0.0	460	0	5	tr.	tr.	tr.
Cabbage, cooked	½ cup	20	1.2	39	0.4	75	27	0	40	40	0.3
Carrots, raw	1 cup, shredded	42	1.2	39	0.8	12,000	6	0	60	60	0.5
Cheese, cheddar, American	1 slice	113	7.1	206	0.3	400	0	0	10	120	tr.
Chicken, fried	½ breast	232	26.8	19	1.3	460	0	0	67	101	10.2
Egg, boiled	1 medium	77	6.1	26	1.3	550	0	27	40	130	tr.
Liver, beef, fried	1 slice	86	8.8	4	2.9	18,658	10	19	90	1,283	5.1
Margarine, fortified	1 tablespoon	101	0.1	3	0.0	460	0	0	0	0	0.0
Milk, whole, cow's	1 glass	124	6.4	216	0.2	293	2	4	73	311	0.2
Oatmeal, cooked	1 cup	148	5.4	21	1.7	0	0	0	220	50	0.4
Orange, whole	1 medium	68	1.4	50	0.6	285	74	0	120	45	0.3
Pork, shoulder, roasted	2 slices	320	19.2	9	2.0	0	0	0	592	144	3.2
Tomatoes, raw	1 large	40	2.0	22	1.2	2,200	46	0	120	80	1.0
Potatoes, white, baked	1 medium	98	2.4	13	0.8	20	17	0	110	50	1.4
Rice, white, cooked	1 cup	201	4.2	13	0.5	0	0	0	20	10	0.7
Sugar, white, granulated	1 tablespoon	48	0.0	0	0.0	0	0	0	0	0	0.0

gm = grams; mg = milligrams; mcg = micrograms; I.U. = International Units; tr. = trace.

blood pressure, and congestive heart failure. During the acute stage of illness a low-protein diet is combined with the low-sodium diet, and such foods as sugar, cornstarch, and puddings are recommended. When the patient begins to recover, the low-protein diet is replaced by a high-protein diet, with plenty of eggs, curd or cream cheese, and fresh meat and fish. A combined low-sodium/high-protein diet may be advised as a long-term measure.

The main dietary source of sodium is salt, so all foods with a high salt content should be avoided. These foods include bacon, ham, sausage, ice cream, chocolates, cheese (except unsalted curd and cream cheeses), canned meats and fish, cakes and cookies. Avoid also salted sauces, dressings, ketchup, and gravies.

Permissible meats and fish with a low salt content include lean mutton, rabbit, and turbot. Most vegetables, including potatoes, are permitted, but should be cooked without salt. Rice and spaghetti, sugar and preserves, and unsalted nuts and butter are all permissible. It is also possible to buy bread, cereals, and other products that have been specially prepared for low-sodium diets.

Low-residue Diet. This diet is usually recommended for patients suffering from inflammation of the intestinal tract and various other digestive disorders.

The patient should take small amounts of easily digested food at regular and frequent intervals. Recommended foods include eggs, milk, cottage or cream cheese, creamed soup, cooked vegetables, stewed fruit, plain cakes, and jello. Meats that are recommended include lean beef and chicken. Avoid pork, veal, raw fruit and vegetables, cereals with whole wheat, nuts, pastry, and all food that is fried, spiced, or seasoned.

All food should be chewed thoroughly. The patient should have plenty to drink, but should avoid alcohol and should not smoke.

High-residue Diet. This diet, which is also known as a high-fiber diet, is recommended for patients suffering from constipation. The patient should eat plenty of bulky foods with a high cellulose content. The patient's normal diet should be supplemented with whole-grain bread and cereals, raw and stewed fruits and vegetables, salads, and buttermilk, as well as plenty of water.

Low-purine Diet. This diet is usually recommended to patients suffering from gout and includes foods with a high carbohydrate content and a low fat content. Recommended foods include skimmed milk, fruit, vegetables, and enriched bread and cereals. Avoid liver, kidney, sweetbreads, anchovies, sardines, and herrings. Beans, lentils, spinach, and soups are also not advised. Fruit juices are recommended, but coffee, tea, chocolate, cocoa, and alcohol should all be avoided.

Gluten-free Diet. This diet is prescribed for patients suffering from celiac disease or nontropical sprue, which are caused by sensitivity to the protein gluten. Gluten is found in wheat, barley, and rye. All traces of these cereals must, therefore, be eliminated from the diet.

Avoid all bread and cakes that are made with wheat, barley, rye, or oat flour, and all drinks that contain malt. Also avoid pasta, sausages, and ice cream, and take care that desserts, sauces, gravies, and sweets do not contain wheat, barley, or rye products.

Permissible foods include fruit, vegetables, most meats and fish, and carbohydrate foods such as rice and sago, which are not associated with the forbidden cereals. It is possible to buy gluten-free flour for baking at home, and many other gluten-free foods.

Diabetic Diet. A strictly controlled diet is an important part of the treatment of patients suffering from diabetes mellitus. Their food must be free of all sugar, but must contain adequate calories and nutrients. The amount of calories and the proportions of carbohydrate, protein, and fat should remain constant for every meal and for every day. Most physicians prohibit alcohol and advise diabetics to eat small amounts at frequent and regular intervals. A patient will receive an individual dietary program from his or her physician.

The American Diabetes Association and the American Dietetic Association have developed a system of food exchanges that enable individual diabetic patients to choose a varied diet while remaining within the necessary restrictions. The foods permissible for the diabetic patient are divided into six lists: milk and milk products, vegetables, fruits, bread and cereals, meat and other high-protein foods, and fats. Each list gives the amounts of different foods having the same nutritional value in carbohydrate, protein, and fat. The patient is able to choose different foods, while keeping the amount of calories and the nutritional value constant.

Slimming Diets. If you weigh more than is considered normal for your height and sex, then you should try to lose the excess weight to improve your physical fitness.

If you are overweight or obese, this is because the food you eat contains more calories than you use in physical activity. The aim of all slimming diets is, therefore, to reduce the amount of calories you take in, while retaining the necessary amounts of proteins, minerals, and other nutrients. There is no easy or simple way of doing this, and you should be cautious of diets you hear of or read about that claim to have a "magic formula" for losing weight. Beware especially of diets that allow you to eat as much as you want of certain categories of foods, and also of diets that claim that grapefruit, lemon, or other citrus fruits can speed up the conversion of fat to energy. There is no scientific evidence to support this claim.

Claims made by manufacturers of commercial diet aids may be misleading. Many of the pills that claim to reduce appetite are ineffective, and even those that are prescribed by physicians can sometimes have disturbing side effects, notably restlessness and emotional tension. Artificial sweeteners that may be used instead of sugar in drinks and in cooking do indeed contain less calories than sugar, but they also may have side effects. It is far more sensible to adjust your eating habits and accustom yourself to unsweetened drinks and foods. Substitute foods and low-calorie drinks and foods that are specially prepared for dieters are expensive, and often have less satisfactory taste than the natural products they claim to replace. Foods with bulking agents that swell inside your stomach can make you feel so full that you actually eat less food, but these also can have dangerous side effects.

The slimming diets that are most effective are of two types: the low-carbohydrate diet and the calorie-controlled diet. Both of these diets may be followed with complete safety, and they require no artificial aids. However, they do require a certain degree of commitment and self-discipline. They are most effective, especially if you wish to improve your physical fitness, when combined with a program of physical exercises.

Whichever type of diet you choose, remember that if you make yourself eat slowly, you will probably eat small total amounts. Also, several small meals a day are less fattening than two or three set meals containing the same amount of food.

Low-carbohydrate Diet. With this diet, you simply eat only the most nutritious foods and reduce or eliminate altogether from your diet the foods that have the highest fat and sugar contents. This should result in a reduction in the amount of calories in your diet without any reduction in essential nutrients.

The following lists of foods are intended as a guide to what you should and should not eat. The first category includes foods with high sugar or fat content; you may eliminate these from your diet completely without losing any essential nutrients. The second category includes foods that contain some fat or sugar, but also contain essential nutrients; you should eat these foods only occasionally, and only in small amounts. The third category includes foods that contain high amounts of essential nutrients, low amounts of fat and sugar, and relatively low amounts of calories; these foods should form the main part of your diet.

Foods to avoid:	sugar, sweets, chocolate; cream, butter, margarine, oils and fats; cakes, pies, pastries, cookies, puddings; honey, syrup, jam, marmalade; fruit canned or bottled in syrup, dried fruit; fried potatoes, chips, nuts; salad dressing, or mayonnaise; spirits and liqueurs; most commercial soft drinks.

Foods to eat in restricted amounts only:	fatty meats, such as salami, paté, sausages, and bacon; milk, eggs, cheese (except cottage cheese); bread and cereals (wholemeal varieties are preferable); potatoes, rice, pasta; oily fish, such as sardines and herrings; thick creamy soups; prepacked and canned foods; wine, beer, cider.
Foods that may be eaten in unrestricted amounts:	liver, kidney, heart, brain; poultry (except duck), game; white fish, seafood; green and root vegetables; salads; fresh fruit; skimmed milk; cottage cheese, natural yogurt; clear soups, herbs, spices; water, low-calorie soft drinks; tea and coffee without milk.

If you follow this diet with reasonable self-discipline, you should lose weight at a rate of roughly one or two pounds a week.

Calorie-controlled Diet. The average adult male uses roughly 2,500 calories a day; the figure for females is slightly lower. A person who is on a calorie-controlled diet sets a target figure and plans his or her meals so that the food taken in during the day does not exceed this amount of calories. This target figure will vary according to personal needs, and your physician should be able to advise a suitable figure with which to start the diet. The lower your target figure, the more weight you will lose; but a target figure of below 1,000 calories a day can be dangerous.

To calculate the amount of calories your food contains you will need a detailed calorie chart, giving the number of calories in stated amounts of specific foods. An abridged version of such a chart is on p. 252. You can obtain a more comprehensive chart from your physician. A calorie-controlled diet will probably consist mainly of the foods recommended in the low-carbohydrate diet. The number of calories varies according to the method of cooking, and you should therefore avoid all kinds of fried foods.

If your daily food intake contains 1,000 calories less than the amount you use in physical activity, your average weight loss should be about two pounds a week.

Vegetarian Diet. Most people who follow a vegetarian diet in Western countries do so for moral reasons, not because of economic necessity. A vegetarian diet may be more healthy than a conventional diet, and research has shown that a vegetarian diet can significantly reduce the chances of heart disease.

A vegetarian diet can be as rich, varied, and nutritious as any diet that includes meat. The main vegetarian protein sources are soya, legumes such as kidney beans and broad beans, nuts, cheese, and eggs. Fats are provided by nuts, oil in salads, and vegetable fats used in cooking. Vitamins and minerals are provided by vegetables, which should be steamed or cooked in minimal amounts of water in order to retain these nutrients. Roughage is provided by whole foods eaten raw, and by brown rice and wheat germ cereals, which should be preferred to polished rice and products made from white flour. Dried skimmed milk mixed with water has a higher proportion of protein and calcium than fresh milk.

Vegetarians who exclude from their diets all animal products including eggs, cheese, and honey may need to supplement their diet with yeast extract or vitamin tablets to avoid vitamin B deficiency.

Digestion (də jes′chən) is the process of breaking down food into smaller particles so that it can be absorbed into the body's bloodstream for nourishment.

See also DIGESTIVE SYSTEM.

Digestive system (də jes′tiv) is the series of organs that process and convert food into simpler substances that the body uses for nourishment. Starch and complex sugars are digested to simple sugars; fats to fatty acids and glycerine; and proteins to amino acids. These simpler substances consist of small molecules that can then pass through the intestinal wall and into the bloodstream for distribution to all parts of the body. The digestive system consists of the alimentary canal—mouth, pharynx, esophagus, stomach, and small and large intestines—aided by secretions from the liver and pancreas.

Action of the digestive system			
Site	Secretion	Food content	Action
Mouth	Saliva, alkaline	Starch	Water to aid lubrication of food, which converts starch to maltose
Stomach	Gastric juice, acid	Proteins	Provides acid medium for pepsin and kills most bacteria Absorbs only alcohol
Duodenum	Pancreatic juice, bile, intestinal juice, alkaline	Fats Starch Proteins	Bile emulsifies fat for absorption
Ileum	Succus entericus	Fats Starch Proteins	Most absorption of food occurs here
Colon			Absorption of water

The **digestive system** breaks down food into elements that can be absorbed by the body.

The digestive system

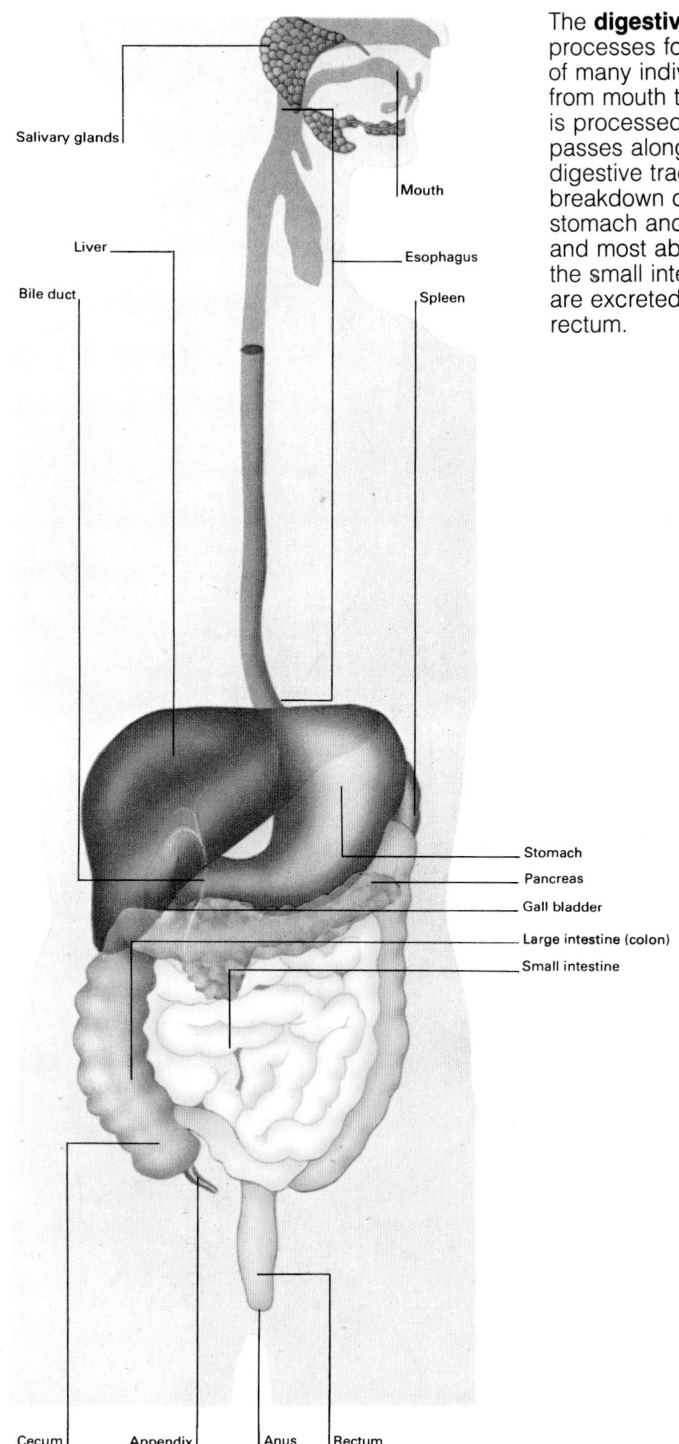

The **digestive system** processes food by means of many individual organs, from mouth to anus. Food is processed for use as it passes along the digestive tract. Most food breakdown occurs in the stomach and duodenum, and most absorption in the small intestine. Wastes are excreted through the rectum.

Q: *What happens to food in the mouth?*

A: The teeth break up food by chopping and grinding it into fine particles. Glands in the mouth lubricate and moisten food with saliva, which also contains a digestive enzyme. The tongue conveys food to the throat, and the pharynx muscles push it down the esophagus (gullet), a muscular tube about 10 inches (25cm) long that leads to the stomach.

Q: *What happens to food in the stomach?*

A: The stomach both stores and helps to digest food. The stomach of an average adult can hold about one quart (0.9l). The muscular stomach churns food around and mixes it with gastric juice, which includes hydrochloric acid to provide the acid medium needed for the enzyme pepsin to break down protein. The partly digested food (chyme) passes from the stomach to the small intestine, usually after two to five hours.

Q: *How does the small intestine function?*

A: The digestive process is completed in the small intestine, a narrow muscular tube about 20 feet (6m) long. Enzymes from the pancreas mix with enzymes from the duodenum. Bile, made by the liver and stored in the gall bladder, also enters the small intestine. Bile helps in the digestion of fats.

The digested food particles are then absorbed by lymph or blood vessels in the intestinal wall. Tiny finger-like projections (villi) on the

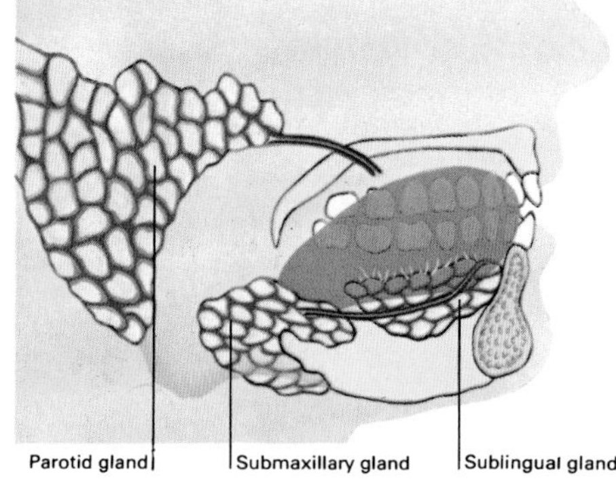

Three large pairs of salivary glands and many smaller ones pour out some 2.5 pints (1.2l) of saliva a day. Saliva contains an enzyme that starts the digestion of carbohydrates.

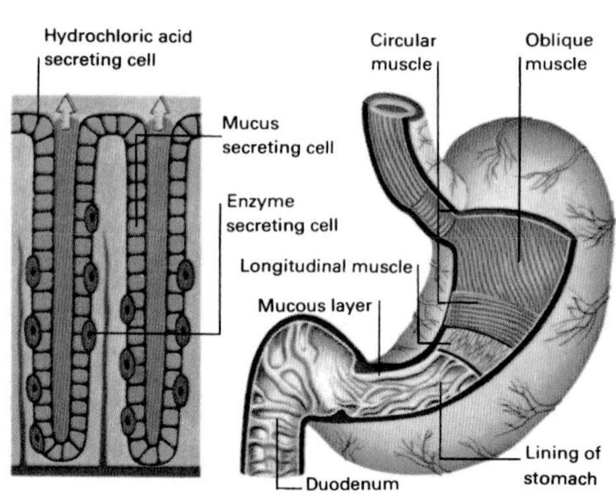

The muscles of the stomach churn food and push it into the duodenum. Glands on the stomach wall secrete mucus, enzymes, and hydrochloric acid, which aid digestion.

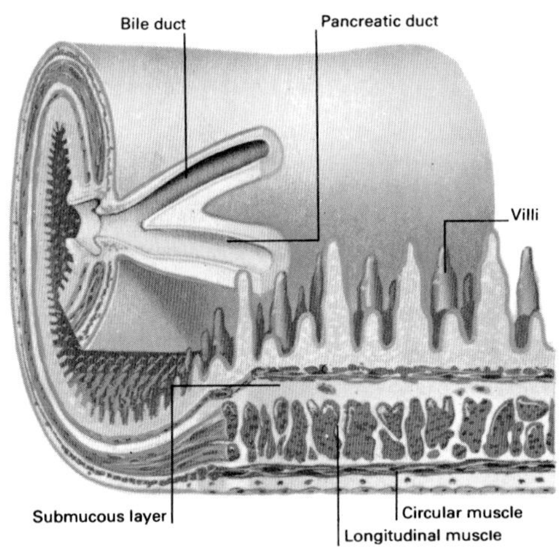

In the duodenum, glands on the inner wall secrete digestive juices. These mix with juices from the gall bladder and pancreas. Digested food is absorbed by the villi and carried by the bloodstream to the liver.

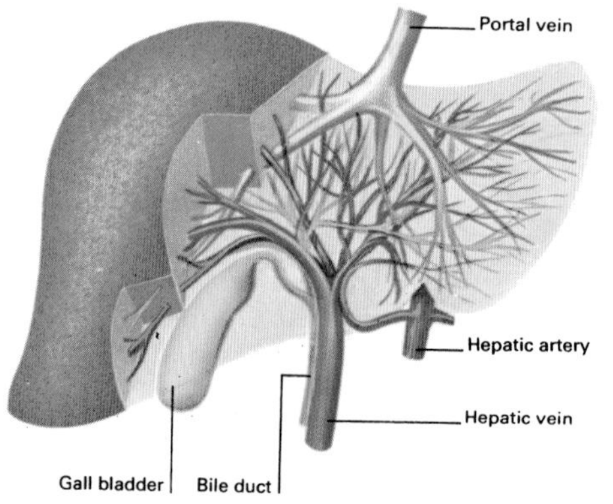

When digested food reaches the liver, essential substances (sugars, vitamins, minerals) are extracted for storage; spent blood leaves via the hepatic vein. Bile formed in the liver is stored in the gall bladder until needed for digestion.

walls of the small intestine increase the surface area that can absorb the food. The digested particles are then carried by the bloodstream to the liver, which converts them into substances needed by the body.

Q: *What is the role of the large intestine?*

A: Eaten material that can not be digested as food, such as plant fiber, passes into the large intestine, which is about 5 feet (1.5m) long. There, water is removed from the liquid waste, and bacteria convert it to its final form, feces. The waste material is excreted from the body through the end of the large intestine (rectum).

Q: *How does food move through the digestive system?*

A: Food is propelled along by wavelike contractions of muscles in the stomach and intestines. This is called peristalsis. The food moves in one direction only. Sphincters, circular muscles that close tightly, prevent the food from moving backward. There are sphincters at the lower end of the esophagus, at the exit from the stomach, at the lower end of the small intestine, and at the exit from the rectum.

Q: *What are common diseases or disorders of the digestive system?*

A: One fairly common disorder is ulcers of the stomach or duodenum, the first part of the small intestine. If bile stagnates in the gall bladder because of a blocked bile duct, gallstones can form and must be removed surgically. Disorders of the intestinal tract include colitis, diverticulitis, diverticulosis, and enteritis.

Digital subtraction angiography. *See* ANGIOGRAPHY, DIGITAL SUBTRACTION.

Dilantin® (dī lan′tin) is an anticonvulsant drug; the generic name is phenytoin sodium. It is principally used to treat epilepsy. It can take several months of dosage modification and combination with other anticonvulsant drugs to control the epileptic attacks, and it must be taken strictly as directed by a physician to minimize side effects, toxicity, and drug interactions with other anticonvulsants.

See also EPILEPSY.

Dilatation and curettage (dil ə tā'shən and kyů ret'ij), commonly abbreviated to D and C, refers to dilatation (stretching) of the cervix, the neck of the uterus, and curettage (scraping with an instrument called a curette) of the inside of the uterus. D and C is a surgical procedure, performed while the patient is under light, general anesthetic. Because pieces of tissue removed by D and C can be microscopically examined in a laboratory, the technique is valuable for the diagnosis of gynecological disorders.

It is also used to clean the inside of the uterus; to remove polyps; to remove any placental tissue remaining after a spontaneous abortion; after childbirth; or as a method to produce an abortion.

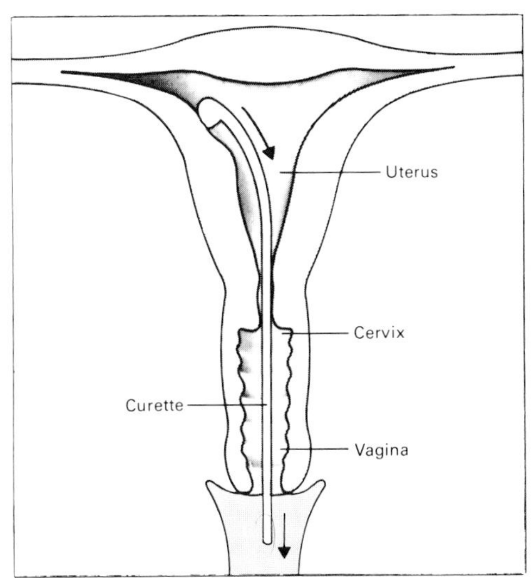

Dilatation and curettage, or D and C, is done under a general anesthetic. A curette is used to scrape the uterus lining.

Diopter (dī op'tər) is the unit of measurement of the focusing power of a lens.

Dioxin (dī ok'sən) is any of 75 related chemicals (principally isomers), all of which consist of carbon, chlorine, hydrogen, and oxygen. In common usage, however, the term refers only to the most toxic and widely known of the group, the compound 2,3,7,8-tetrachlorodibenzo-p-dioxin (TCDD). Dioxin is a contaminant of a herbicide that was used throughout the world on both grasslands and on woody shrubs and trees. Because of its toxicity, dioxin is no longer manufactured in the United States. Soil and water in parts of the United States (and other parts of the world) have, however, become contaminated with dioxin due to improper disposal of industrial waste products. Dioxin was a contaminant in Agent Orange, a defoliant used by the United States during the Vietnam War. Exposure to dioxin can cause headaches and a painful skin rash known as chloracne; dioxin is purported to cause birth defects and cancer, but this has not been proved scientifically.

See also AGENT ORANGE.

Diphtheria (dif thir'ē ə) is an acute infectious disease caused by the bacillus *Corynebacterium diphtheriae.* This bacterium usually grows on the membranes of the nose and throat, but can affect other mucous membranes and occasionally infects the skin. Diphtheria is now a rare disease because of widespread vaccination against it. It occurs most often in children under the age of 10.

Q: *How is diphtheria spread?*

A: The disease is usually spread by minute airborne droplets that are breathed out by an infected person. As a result, it can spread extremely rapidly. The diphtheria bacillus can be transmitted by a carrier, a person who is immune to the disease, who does not exhibit any symptoms, and who may be unaware of the infection.

Q: *What are the symptoms of diphtheria?*

A: Before any symptoms become apparent, there is an incubation period of up to five days; this period varies and symptoms may appear after only one day. There is a sudden onset of a sore throat and fever, accompanied by rapidly increasing feelings of ill health and weakness. A typical symptom is a thick, white, crust-like membrane at the back of the throat. The inflamed tissues are painful, and the lymph nodes in the neck often become swollen, but the infection rarely spreads any further.

Q: *Are there any complications associated with diphtheria?*

A: Yes. The crust-like membrane may obstruct breathing. In severe cases, this complication may need urgent treatment to prevent suffocation. Another complication is that the toxin produced by the infection

Diphtheria most commonly affects the mucous membranes of the nose and throat. Following an incubation period of up to five days, there is a sudden onset of sore throat and fever. A typical, secondary symptom is a thick, white crust-like membrane at the back of the throat. In severe cases, this membrane can obstruct breathing.

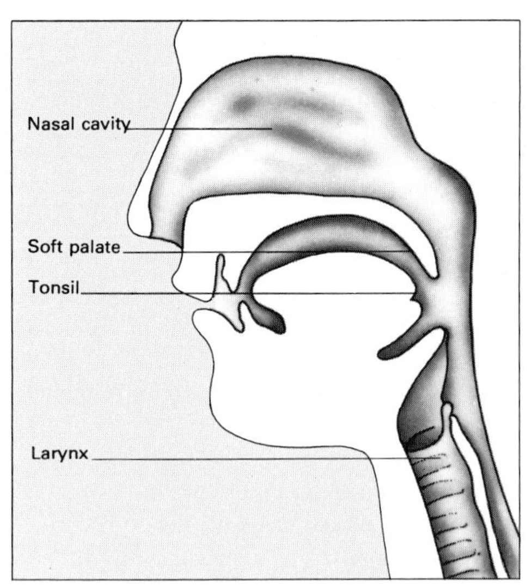

may cause nerve damage (neuritis), heart muscle damage (myocarditis), and kidney damage. There may also be localized paralysis resembling poliomyelitis.

Q: *How may diphtheria be treated?*

A: A patient with diphtheria requires hospital treatment in isolation. This usually involves the administration of diphtheria antitoxin and antibiotics. The antitoxin counteracts the effects of the toxin, and the antibiotics kill the bacteria. Complete bed rest is essential during the acute stage of the disease, with a gradual return to normal activity afterward.

Q: *Can diphtheria be prevented?*

A: Yes. Diphtheria immunization is usually carried out in the first year of life. It is usually combined with pertussis and tetanus immunization as a DPT shot.

Diphyllobothrium latum (dī fil ō both'rē əm lā'təm) is the largest of the parasitic tapeworms that infest human beings. The adult worm lives in the intestine and may grow to about 30 feet (9m) long. Most cases of infestation arise from eating raw or undercooked fish. The first sign of infestation is often worm segments in the feces. Treatment is usually with drugs that kill the worm.

Diplegia (dī plē'jē ə) is paralysis of like parts on both sides of the body, for example, both arms or both legs.

See also PARALYSIS.

Diplopia. *See* VISION, DOUBLE.

Dipsomania. *See* ALCOHOLISM.

Disarticulation (dis är tik yə lā'shən) is an amputation through a joint.

See also AMPUTATION.

Discharge (dis chärj') is the loss of a substance through a body opening. It may be the result of a normal body process, such as urination. The term is more commonly used, however, to refer to an abnormal expression of fluid; for example, the discharge of bloody mucus from the ear.

Discipline of children. *See* CHILD.

Disease (də zēz') is a disorder in the structure or function of any organ or system of the body. The disorder is often recognizable by a known set of signs and symptoms, the cause of which may or may not be known.

Disinfectant (dis in fek'tənt) is a substance that destroys infection-causing organisms. The term is generally applied to chemicals used for treating such things as surgical instruments and sickroom floors.

See also ANTISEPTIC.

Disk (disk) is any flat, round, plate-like structure. In medicine, the term commonly has two meanings. The optic disk is the point at which the optic nerve enters the back of the eye. An intervertebral disk is a fibroelastic ring with a soft, gelatinous center, which lies between each pair of vertebrae of the backbone. The intervertebral disks act as shock absorbers and enable the backbone to flex. Occasionally an intervertebral disk ruptures, causing the condition known as slipped disk, or herniated disk.

See also DISK, HERNIATED.

Disk, herniated (disk her'nē āted). A herniated disk, also known as a prolapsed intervertebral disk, is a disorder of the spine. The disks between the bones of the spine (vertebrae) are composed of gristle-like fibrous tissue with a soft center. A disk can rupture as a result of strain, allowing its soft center to pass through the ruptured outer fiber. The soft tissue protrudes into and compresses the spinal canal, which contains the spinal cord. Pressure on the spinal nerves produces pain, felt either locally (backache) or as referred pain in another part of the body, as in sciatica. Muscle weakness, paralysis of muscle function, and loss of sensation is possible in severe cases.

In childhood and adolescence, the disks are flexible and pliable, and so strain at this stage is unlikely. The disks harden in later life, and the soft centers gradually solidify. By the age of 45 or 50, the center is of the same tough composition as the outer edge.

The disks of the neck (cervical region) and those of the lower spine (lumbar region) are the most likely to rupture because they are the most mobile. A herniated disk in the thoracic spine, behind the chest, can occur in rare cases. *See also* BACK PAIN; NECK, STIFF; SCIATICA.

Q: ***What are the symptoms of a herniated disk?***

A: In the neck, it is usually the result of a twisting injury that develops into a stiff neck. The pain is intense when the patient tries to move or cough. Gradually the pain spreads as the disk presses on the nerves that affect one shoulder and arm. Loss of sensation in the skin and muscle weakness may develop because of nerve damage. If the disk protrudes deeply into the spinal cord, there is loss of sensation lower down the body. It may cause disruption in the nerves controlling walking, or it may cause difficulty in urinating.

The symptoms in the lower spine are usually caused by a herniated disk either between the fourth and fifth lumbar vertebrae or between the fifth lumbar and first sacral vertebrae. There is severe pain in the back, making it difficult to move. The pain gradually improves over a matter of days.

The back pain may be followed by sciatica, with shooting pain going down one buttock, the thigh, leg, and foot. A tingling sensation is common and is aggravated by coughing, sneezing, or bending. The patient walks with a limp because of spasms in the back muscles, and he or she is unable to raise the affected leg at right angles to the body.

A herniated disk higher in the lumbar region causes pain in the groin and in the front of the thigh.

Q: ***How is a herniated disk treated?***

A: Painkilling drugs may be prescribed in mild cases. A herniated disk in the neck usually involves immobilizing the neck with a stiff collar. This helps the patient sleep or drive a car without too much pain. In addition, anti-inflammatory drugs, physiotherapy in the form of short-wave diathermy and massage, and in severe cases, hospitalization and continuous traction may be recommended. If conservative measures fail, surgical removal of the herniated disk may be necessary. *See also* DIATHERMY; TRACTION.

A herniated disk in the lumbar region is treated with rest, painkillers, and anti-inflammatory drugs. Strict bed rest remains extremely important since even standing up dramatically increases the pressure upon the disks. Traction and/or a surgical corset that immobilizes the spine are commonly used in severe cases.

Manipulative treatment, such as osteopathy, can also help in the treatment of a herniated disk by temporarily reducing pressure on the disk. *See also* OSTEOPATHY.

Q: ***Are there any other disorders that have symptoms similar to those of a herniated disk?***

A: Osteoarthritis, tumors of the spinal cord, and secondary tumors of the vertebrae produce similar symptoms. Cervical rib trouble may produce disk-like pains down an arm. Spondylolisthesis, in which one vertebra slips forward on another, and ankylosing spondylitis cause similar back pains.

See also SPONDYLITIS, ANKYLOSING; SPONDYLOLISTHESIS.

Disk, slipped. See DISK, HERNIATED.

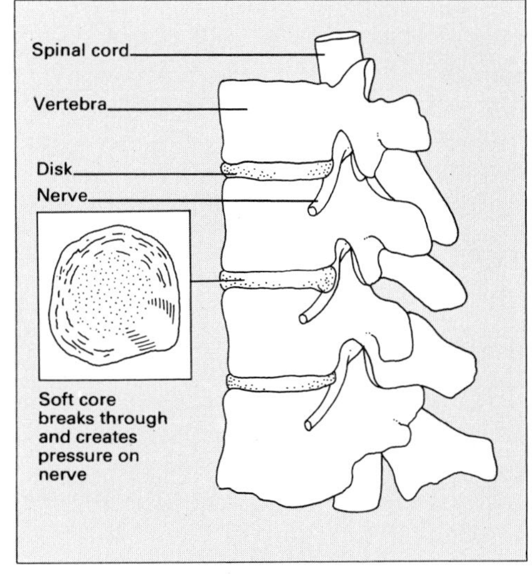

Due to a sprain, a disk, the gristle-like fibrous tissue between vertebrae, can rupture. The rupture allows the disk's soft center to pass through the ruptured outer fiber and protrude against the spinal canal. The **herniated disk** puts pressure on the spinal nerves, causing intense pain.

Dislocation (dis lō kā'shən), or luxation, is the displacement of a structure from its normal position in the body. In most joints, dislocations of bones are rare, except as a complication of a fracture or as a result of weakened joint ligaments. Dislocations most commonly occur in the shoulder, where there may be a congenital weakness of the surrounding ligaments. A dislocation always involves torn ligaments, and it may take several weeks for the tears to heal. Various surgical operations have been devised to strengthen or replace weak ligaments and, so, overcome the problem. Occasionally, one or both hips may be dislocated from birth (congenital hip dislocation), and early diagnosis and treatment are required to prevent permanent disability.

See also HIP DYSPLASIA.

Dismemberment (dis mem'bər mənt) is the amputation of a limb or a portion of a limb of the body.

Disorientation (dis ôr ē en tā'shən) is a loss of normal awareness of place, time, or identity. Such mental confusion may occur in serious physical illnesses, with fever, as a result of certain drug treatments, or as a symptom of a mental illness.

Distal (dis'təl) is a term used in medicine to refer to an object away from the center or point of origin. For example, fingernails are at the distal ends of the fingers.

See also PROXIMAL.

Diuresis (dī yu̇ rē'sis) is an increase in urine output. It occurs in such conditions as diabetes mellitus. Coffee, tea, alcohol, and some medications (diuretics) cause diuresis.

See also DIURETIC.

Diuretic (dī yu̇ ret'ik) is one of a group of agents that act on the kidneys to increase urine output. This increase in the urine output is accompanied by a loss of sodium and, sometimes, potassium salts. Alcohol, tea, and coffee are mild, but nonmedical, diuretics.

Q: *Which disorders may diuretics be used to treat?*

A: Diuretics are used to treat virtually any disorder in which there is an excessive build-up of fluid in the body (edema). These include disorders of the heart, liver, and kidneys. Some weak diuretics are used to decrease excessive fluid pressure within the eyeball (glaucoma). Diuretics are used to treat certain lung disorders in which fluid accumulates in the lung tissue (pulmonary edema). They may also be used to decrease high blood pressure (hypertension) and to treat overdosage of certain drugs.

Q: *Can diuretics produce any adverse effects?*

A: Yes. The adverse effects of diuretics vary according to the specific drug used. The commonly prescribed diuretics may cause nausea, weakness, skin rashes, and allergic reactions. All diuretics should be used with care by diabetics and by those with impaired liver or kidney function. Dehydration and shock can occur in some cases, especially among the elderly.

Q: *Why is it necessary to take a potassium supplement along with some diuretics?*

A: Some diuretics cause increased urinary excretion of potassium. If the level of potassium falls too low in the blood, this can result in an irregular heartbeat, especially among persons who are also taking digitalis. Diet alone, through the eating of foods rich in potassium (for example, oranges, bananas, and peanuts), may in some cases correct this.

Diverticulitis (dī vər tik yə lī'tis) is a common disease of the bowel, the main part of the large intestine. Diverticulitis develops from diverticulosis, which involves the formation of pouches (diverticula) on the outside of the colon. Diverticulitis results if one of these diverticula becomes inflamed. Bacteria may subsequently infect the outside of the colon if an inflamed diverticula bursts open. If the infection spreads to the lining of the abdominal cavity, (peritoneum), this can cause a potentially fatal illness (peritonitis). Sometimes inflamed diverticula can cause narrowing of the bowel, leading to an obstruction. Also, the affected part of the colon could adhere to the bladder or other organ in the pelvic area. Diverticulitis most often affects middle-aged and elderly persons.

Q: *What are the symptoms of diverticulitis?*

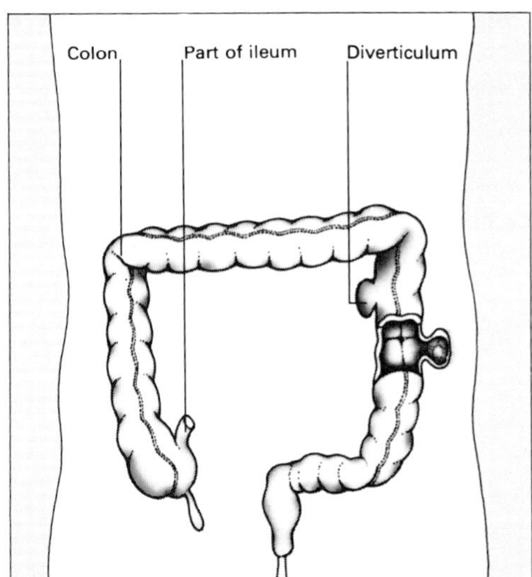

Diverticulitis occurs when a small pocket in the bowel, a diverticula, becomes inflamed.

A: The symptoms of diverticulitis include localized abdominal pain and tenderness, loose bowel movements or constipation, and fever. A blood test shows an increased number of white blood cells.

Q: *What is the treatment for diverticulitis?*

A: An acute attack of diverticulitis is usually treated with antibiotics. When the infection has been controlled, patients suffering from such an attack are also placed on a high-fiber diet. However, recurring acute attacks or complications, such as peritonitis, require surgical treatment.

See also DIVERTICULOSIS; PERITONITIS.

Diverticulosis (dī vər tik yə lō'sis) is a disorder of the bowel, mostly of the colon, that generally affects people over 50 years of age. Diverticulosis involves the formation of pouches (diverticula) on the outside of the colon. The inflammation of these pouches can result in diverticulitis.

Diverticulosis may be the result of a diet low in roughage (fruit and vegetable fibers). Symptoms are few except for occasional abdominal pain and rectal bleeding. A barium enema X ray examination, sigmoidoscopy, or colonoscopy is used to reveal the presence of diverticula.

Treatment for diverticulosis includes a high-fiber diet, which aids in passing waste through the colon and, thus, reduces intestinal pressure. This could help to prevent diverticulitis from developing. However, in cases of severe bleeding, surgery is necessary.

See also COLON; DIVERTICULITIS.

Diverticulum (dī vər tik'yə ləm) is a small finger-like pouch, most often found in the intestinal wall, but also occurring in other parts of the body. Diverticula may occur normally, or they may result from a rupture of intestinal mucous membrane.

There are true diverticula consisting of all layers of bowel wall, and false diverticula, which are due to herniation of mucosa through the muscular coat of bowel wall. False diverticula are much more common.

See also DIVERTICULITIS; DIVERTICULOSIS.

Diverticulum, Meckel's (dī vər tik' yə ləm, mek'elz). This is a 0.4–4.8 inch (1–12cm) long pouch that protrudes from the wall of the ileum. It is present at birth and represents the yolk stalk of the embryo. In most persons, the stalk structure disappears at birth. It is not unusual, however, for Meckel's diverticulum to persist; it does not usually require treatment unless it becomes inflamed or bleeds. Often the problem is discovered incidentally during unrelated surgery.

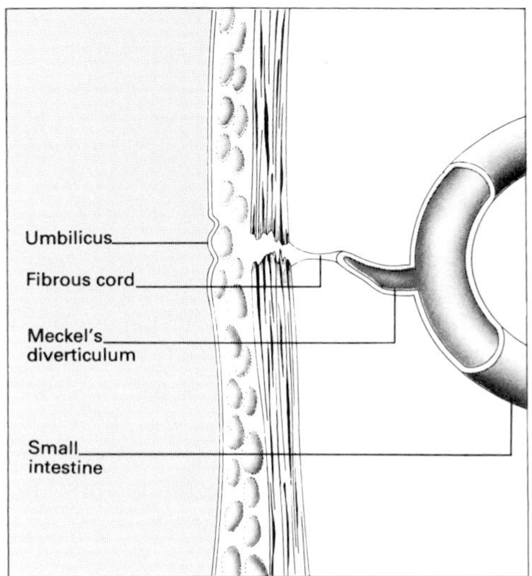

Meckel's diverticulum is a pouch that protrudes from the wall of the illeum.

Diving safety. See WATER SPORTS SAFETY.

Dizziness is a sensation of unsteadiness or lightheadedness. Dizziness should not be confused with vertigo, which is a feeling of movement, either of the external world rotating about the person, or of the person spinning.

See also BALANCE; VERTIGO.

DNA. *See* DEOXYRIBONUCLEIC ACID.

Doctor/patient relationship. *See* PATIENT/PHYSICIAN RELATIONSHIP.

Dominant (dom′ə nənt) is a term used in the study of heredity to describe a gene that affects the physical characteristics (phenotype) of an individual in preference to another gene of the same type. For example, the gene for brown eyes is dominant over the gene for blue eyes (which is said to be recessive). Therefore, in the case of a person who has received a gene for brown eyes from one parent and a gene for blue eyes from the other parent, the person would have brown eyes because that is dominant for that gene pair.

The term dominant is also used by psychiatrists to describe persons with strong, overpowering personalities.

See also HEREDITY; RECESSIVE.

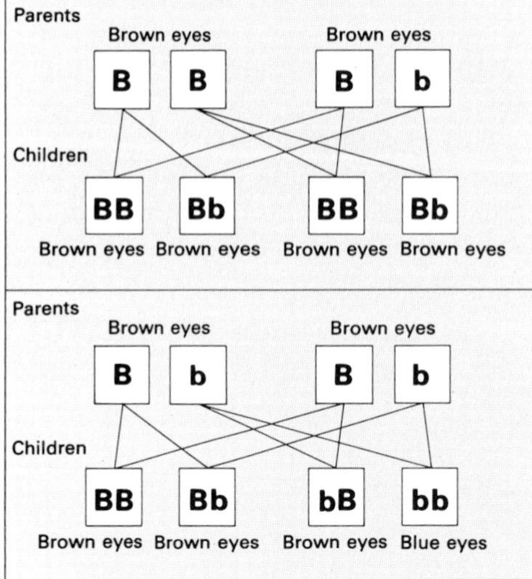

The **dominant** gene for brown eyes (B) prevails unless two recessive genes (bb) coincide.

Dopamine (dō′pə mēn) is a compound produced by the body. It is found in large quantities in the basal ganglia of the central nervous system and acts as a neurotransmitter in many areas of the nervous system. Chemically synthesized, dopamine is used in the treatment of such disorders as shock, acute heart failure, renal failure, and Parkinson's disease. The signs and symptoms of Parkinson's disease are caused by a deficiency of dopamine in the substantia nigra (a layer of pigmented gray substance) of the basal ganglia (masses of gray matter in the cerebral hemisphere) of the brain.

See also BRAIN; LEVODOPA; PARKINSON'S DISEASE.

Dorsal (dôr′səl) refers to a region of the back (dorsum) or the dorsum (back) of any organ or structure. The opposite of dorsal is ventral.

Double vision. *See* VISION, DOUBLE.

Douche (düsh) is a stream of vapor, water, or antiseptic fluid directed against a part of the body. It may be used either for personal hygiene or to treat a local disorder. The term is usually used to describe the washing of the vagina. The vagina cleanses itself naturally and is also cleansed in the normal bathing process, so there is little reason for a healthy woman to use a vaginal douche. Occasionally a physician may prescribe a medicated douche for some kinds of vaginal infections. However, some studies have shown that douching may force contaminated water into the uterus and fallopian tubes. Therefore, directions concerning water pressure should be carefully followed. Despite popular belief, there is no evidence that a vaginal douche following sexual intercourse is an effective method of contraception.

Down's syndrome (dounz), or trisomy 21, is a congenital defect that causes mental and physical abnormalities. It usually is caused by an extra chromosome. There are 47 chromosomes instead of the normal 46. The defect is usually caused by an extra number 21 chromosome. The syndrome is associated with increasing age of the mother and not with the number of pregnancies. A mother between the ages of 35 and 39 has a 1.5 percent chance of having a child with Down's syndrome; a woman over the age of 40 has a 5 percent chance of having a child with Down's syndrome. The physical characteristics include a flat, round head, which is also smaller than normal; small, low-set ears; a flattened nose; skin folds over the inner corner of the eyes; a large tongue that protrudes from a small mouth; and a typical pattern of creases on the palm. However, the most important feature is delay in gross motor development. An affected child may have an intelligence quotient (IQ) of 50 to 60, although this can vary.

Q: *Are there any other abnormalities associated with Down's syndrome?*

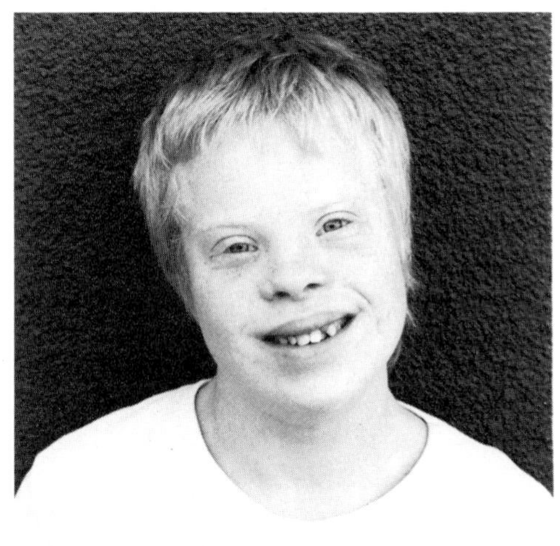

Down's syndrome is a congenital anomaly that results in mental and physical abnormalities. It is usually caused by an extra chromosome.

A: Yes. Down's syndrome is often associated with other congenital disorders, such as heart defects, intestinal defects, chronic respiratory and ear infections, visual problems, and an increased susceptibility to acute leukemia.

Q: *What can be done to help children with Down's syndrome?*

A: There is no medical treatment that can cure Down's syndrome. However, with specialized education, most affected children can learn to look after themselves and to lead useful lives. Parents of a child with Down's syndrome should discuss education with their physician and a pediatrician who has a special interest in the disorder.

Q: *After the birth of one affected child, what is the likelihood of subsequent children having Down's syndrome?*

A: Because Down's syndrome is rarely inherited, there is an extremely good chance that any subsequent children will be normal, unless the mother is over the age of 40. Although it is very rare, Down's syndrome can be inherited. It is, therefore, advisable to seek genetic counseling before embarking on another pregnancy. *See also* GENETIC COUNSELING.

Q: *Can Down's syndrome be detected during pregnancy?*

A: Yes. By testing a sample of the fluid from around the fetus in the womb (amniocentesis), a geneticist can, while there is still time to consider an abortion, predict whether a baby will be born with Down's syndrome. A new test, chorionic villus sampling, may be able to provide the same information as amniocentesis much earlier in the course of the pregnancy. *See also* AMNIOCENTESIS; CHORIONIC VILLUS BIOPSY.

DPT vaccine (vak′sēn) is a combination of diphtheria, pertussis (whooping cough), and tetanus vaccines, used in immunizing infants. Some studies have reported serious side effects following routine immunization of infants and small children with DPT vaccine. These effects have been linked to the pertussis portion in the vaccine. If an allergic reaction, high fever, shock-like state, severe crying episode, convulsion, or unconsciousness follow a DPT immunization, the pertussis portion of the vaccine can be left out for the remainder of the series. If an infant or small child has some neurological disorder, or has had any type of seizure, the matter should be discussed with a physician and thoroughly studied before DPT immunization is carried out.

Dracunculiasis (drah küng kū lī′ə sis) is an infection, often called guinea worm disease, caused by the infestation by the nematode worm *Dracunculus medinensis*. Dracunculiasis is characterized by sores on the legs and feet through which larvae are discharged by the female. Intense itching and burning may develop. It is caused by ingesting contaminated water or shellfish and is common in highly populated tropical and subtropical areas.

Drawsheet. *See* NURSING THE SICK.

Dream is a series of thoughts, emotions, and experiences that occur during sleep. Any of the senses may contribute to a dream, but most dreams are visual and are accompanied by rapid eye movements (REM). Everybody dreams, although not everybody can remember dreaming.

The purpose of dreams is not known. But persons who are deliberately deprived of dream sleep become irritable and restless. Dream deprivation may also cause emotional problems. Many psychiatrists believe that the events

First aid for drowning

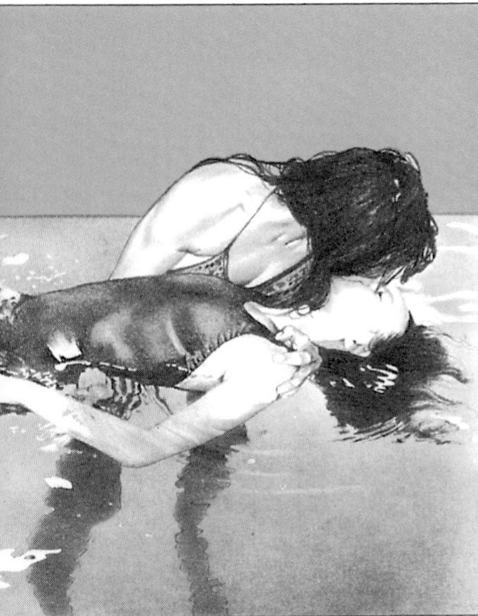

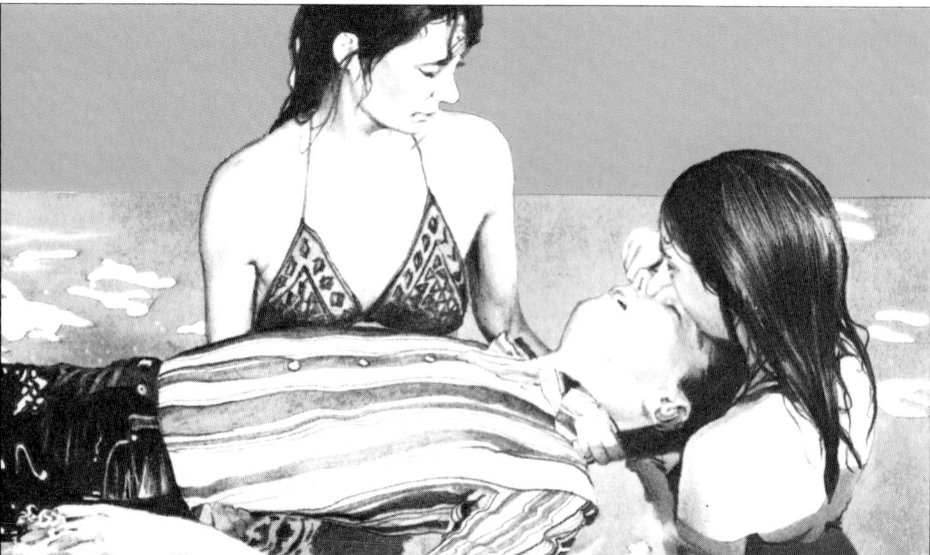

1 If you are alone, it is best to begin artificial respiration once you get the victim ashore. However it may be necessary to begin while still in the water (*see* ARTIFICIAL RESPIRATION). Continue to resuscitate the victim while wading ashore.

2 If other people are available, give artificial respiration once you are in shallow water. One person should support the victim's head and body while another gives artificial respiration.

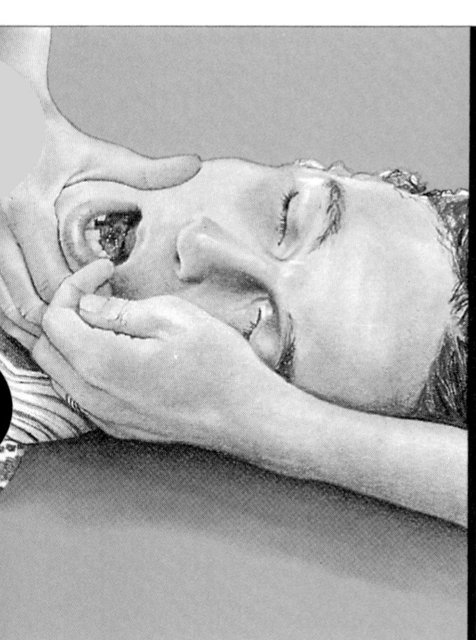

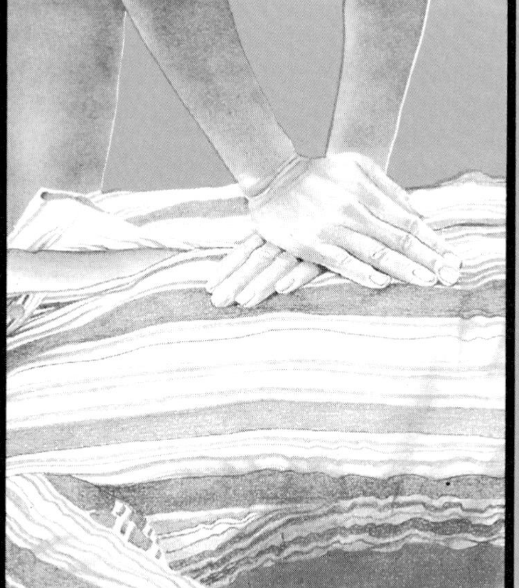

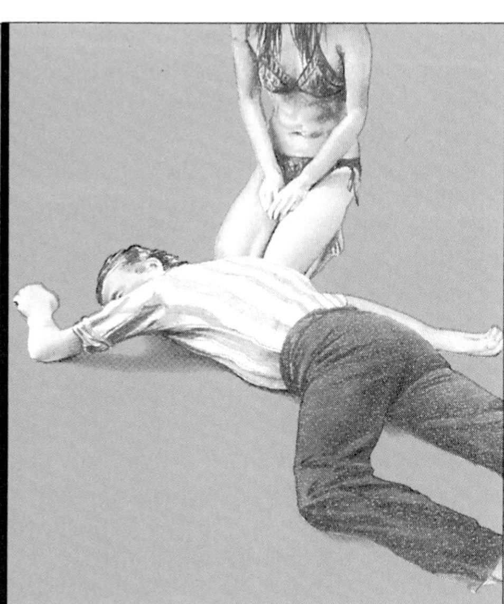

3 When ashore, clear the victim's airway of any obvious obstruction, using two fingers. Lift the victim's neck and tilt the head back so that the tongue does not block the throat.

4 If the victim's heart has stopped, give external cardiac compression. With palms down, press on the victim's chest over the heart area, just to their left of center. Press firmly at a rate of about 60 compressions per minute (*see* HEART ATTACK: FIRST AID).

5 When the victim's heartbeat and breathing have been restored but are still weak, place him or her in the recovery position, face down, head to one side. *Do not* leave the victim alone; the breathing may stop again.

within dreams relate to the dreamer's life and that by studying a patient's dreams they can find clues to the underlying causes of the dreamer's condition.

See also NIGHTMARE; SLEEP.

Drop foot. *See* FOOT DROP.

Drop wrist. *See* WRIST DROP.

Drowning: first aid. Drowning is suffocation in water or some other liquid. It occurs when liquid prevents oxygen from reaching the lungs and nourishing the blood.

Many deaths are caused every year by drowning. It can happen in a swimming pool or bath tub as easily as in the ocean. *Never leave young children unattended near any body of water.* And *do not* go swimming alone. Even expert swimmers can get into difficulty while swimming.

Signs. A drowning person may be blue around the lips and cheeks. There may be froth coming out of the mouth and nose. The victim may be gasping for breath or may have stopped breathing completely.

Action. A drowning person may be in a state of panic. His or her erratic movements and flailing may endanger the rescuer's life. Do not attempt to rescue a drowning person if you are alone, unless you are trained in water rescue and lifesaving techniques.

Call for a lifeguard or send someone while you keep the victim's position pinpointed. If a lifeguard is not available, throw a line or extend a pole or branch toward the victim. If the water is of standing depth and there are other people in the vicinity, summon their help to make a human chain out to the victim.

Begin artificial respiration as soon as possible, first making certain the victim's air passage is clear. Enlist the help of others if possible. If the victim's heart has stopped, give external cardiac compression. *See also* ARTIFICIAL RESPIRATION; CHOKING AND COUGHING: FIRST AID; HEART ATTACK: FIRST AID.

Do not attempt to drain water out of the victim's lungs. Determine whether the victim is suffering from shock and treat accordingly. *See also* SHOCK: FIRST AID.

Keep the victim warm with blankets or clothing. Do not give the victim alcohol to drink. Expert medical attention is necessary, even if the victim seems to have made a complete recovery, because near-drowning may lead to serious complications, such as pneumonia and heart problems.

Drug is a chemical substance used to treat or prevent diseases. Drugs can, however, also cause harm if used improperly. *See also* DRUG ABUSE.

Classified according to their effect on the body, drugs can be placed in about a dozen categories. Categories of particular importance include the following: (1) drugs that kill or impede the growth of bacteria and thus cure or prevent infectious diseases; (2) drugs that affect the heart and blood vessels; (3) drugs that affect the nervous system.

Drugs used for infectious diseases include antibiotics, such as penicillin and sulfonamides (sulfa drugs). Physicians often prescribe these drugs to treat pneumonia, meningitis, or cystitis.

Drugs that prevent infectious diseases include vaccines and antiserums and immunoglobulins. Vaccines stimulate the body's immune system to make antibodies to specific diseases, such as cholera, diphtheria, measles, smallpox, and polio. These antibodies will combine with specific antigens of the bacteria or virus to render the organism harmless. Antiserums and immunoglobulins are similar to vaccines, except that they already contain the antibodies necessary to neutralize the antigens of such infectious diseases as diphtheria, tetanus, hepatitis, and rabies.

Drugs that affect the heart and blood vessels are referred to as cardiovascular drugs. These include antiarrhythmics to normalize an irregular heartbeat, cardiotonics to strengthen the pumping capacity of the heart, vasodilators to enlarge small blood vessels, and antihypertensives to treat high blood pressure.

Drugs that affect the nervous system include analgesics, anesthetics, hallucinogens, stimulants, and depressants. Analgesics relieve pain and can be either narcotics (analgesia plus sedation or drowsiness) or non-narcotics. Examples of narcotics include codeine, heroin, and morphine. One of the most widely used non-narcotic analgesics is aspirin.

General anesthetics eliminate sensation by producing a state of unconsciousness and are often used during surgical operations. Halothane and thiopental are examples.

Hallucinogens, often called psychedelic drugs, cause a person to hallucinate or experience something that exists only in the mind. Hallucinogens include LSD (lysergic acid diethylamide), marijuana, and mescaline.

Stimulants increase the activity of the nervous system, thus diminishing the perception of fatigue or tiredness. They include caffeine, cocaine, and amphetamines. Stimulants are seldom prescribed by doctors because they can cause drug dependency. *See also* DRUG ADDICTION.

Depressants depress the nervous system and diminish tension and worry. Tranquilizers (antianxiety agents), sedatives, hypnotics, and alcohol are all depressants. Benzodiazepines are the most commonly used antianxiety agents. Barbiturates are also used as sedatives and include phenobarbital, pentobarbital, and secobarbital. Other nonbarbiturate sedatives include chloral hydrate and paraldehyde. Like stimulants, depressants can become addictive.

Other drugs besides those discussed above include diuretics, which increase the formation of urine; hormones, which control certain body functions; vitamins, which are necessary for maintaining health; antitumor (antineoplastic) drugs, which destroy cancer cells; and immunosuppressive drugs, which help prevent the body from rejecting a transplanted organ.

Drug abuse is the harmful use of mind-altering drugs. Although the term usually refers to problems with illegal drugs, it can also include harmful use of legal, prescription drugs.

The abuse of drugs is an increasingly serious problem, among both teenagers and adults. The incidence of drug use is increasing among even younger children of 9 or 10 years of age, which should be a matter of concern for all parents. Drug abuse occurs throughout society, and parents must not be complacent because they have provided a good home for their children.

Smoking and drinking alcohol are also serious problems among adolescents. Although these drugs are generally more socially acceptable, they are potentially more harmful than some of the less acceptable drugs.

Reasons for Drug Abuse. The reasons behind drug abuse are complex. Some persons take drugs out of curiosity or because of social pressures from their friends. Others may turn to drugs as a form of escape, or to rebel against their parents or against what they consider to be an unfair society. Some children may smoke, drink alcohol, or take drugs because they think it is grown-up to do so. Once a young person has been introduced to the subculture of drug users and suppliers, it is often difficult for him or her to break out.

Effects of Drug Abuse. Amphetamines, cocaine, nicotine, LSD and other hallucinogens, and certain chemicals used in glue and some solvents are habit-forming. A person who takes such substances regularly can become psychologically dependent on them. The user of a habit-forming drug feels compelled to continue taking the drug in order to maintain the state of well-being produced by it, but the drug is not essential for the physical needs of the body. When deprived of the drug, a habituated person becomes restless, irritable, and anxious.

Heroin and barbiturates are physiologically addictive. These drugs alter the body chemistry so that the drug becomes necessary for the normal physical functioning of the body. Such physical dependence takes about six weeks of regular drug use to develop. Because of this effect on the body chemistry, an addict develops painful, physical withdrawal symptoms if the drug is discontinued suddenly. In addition to developing physical dependence, an addict also develops tolerance to the drug, so that larger doses are necessary to produce the desired effects. *See* DRUG ADDICTION.

Sudden withdrawal from addictive drugs produces a painful physical illness. Several hours after the last dose of heroin, an addict may develop stomach cramps, chills, nausea, diarrhea, uncontrollable shaking, and profuse sweating. Sudden withdrawal from barbiturates is extremely dangerous and may even be fatal. For this reason, barbiturate withdrawal should be done gradually, preferably under expert medical supervision.

Drug abuse

Drug	*Medical use*	*Short-term effects*	*Long-term effects*
Alcohol	Rarely used.	Relaxation; euphoria; drowsiness; lack of coordination; loss of emotional control.	Habituation; liver and brain damage; obesity with excessive use; addiction with prolonged use.
Amphetamines (Benzedrine®; Methedrine®; Dexedrine®)	Relief of depression; reduction of fatigue; occasionally, for treatment of obesity.	Increased alertness; loss of appetite; insomnia; euphoria; large doses can produce hallucinations.	Habituation; irritability; restlessness; weight loss; mental disturbances.
Antidepressants (dibenzodiazepines; MAO inhibitors)	Treatment of depression.	Mental stimulation; elevation of mood; occasionally, trembling, insomnia, confusion, and hallucinations. MAO inhibitors may interact adversely with some foods and other drugs.	Dry mouth; blurred vision; fatigue; skin rashes; palpitations; occasionally, jaundice.
Barbiturates (Amytal®; Nembutal®; Seconal®; phenobarbital)	Treatment of insomnia and relief of nervous tension.	Intoxication; relaxation; drowsiness; lack of coordination; loss of emotional control; relief of anxiety; occasionally, euphoria. An overdose or in combination with alcohol can be fatal.	Habituation; irritability; weight loss; addiction. Severe withdrawal symptoms if the drug is suddenly discontinued.
Cocaine	Anesthesia of the eyes, ears, or nose.	Increased alertness; reduction of fatigue; reduction of appetite; insomnia; euphoria. Large doses may cause hallucinations, convulsions, and death.	If sniffed, ulceration of the nose. Other long-term effects similar to those of amphetamines.
Hallucinogens (LSD; psilocybin; STP; DMT; mescaline; phencyclidine)	Rarely used.	Hallucinations; lack of coordination; nausea; dilated pupils; irregular breathing; sometimes anxiety, paranoia, confusion, and depression.	May precipitate mental disturbance and chronic personality changes in susceptible individuals. Occasionally, recurrence of original hallucinatory experience without taking more of the drug. May cause chromosome damage.

Drug	*Medical use*	*Short-term effects*	*Long-term effects*
Marijuana	Rarely used.	Relaxation; euphoria; alteration of time perception; lack of coordination. Large doses may produce hallucinations.	Long-term effects have not been definitely established. Prolonged, heavy use may lead to insomnia and depression on sudden withdrawal.
Narcotics (Opium; heroin; codeine; Demerol®; methadone)	Treatment of severe pain.	Sedation; euphoria; relief of pain; lack of coordination; impaired mental functioning.	Constipation; loss of appetite; weight loss; temporary sterility; addiction, producing painful withdrawal symptoms on stopping use of the drug. The use of unsterilized hypodermic needles may cause severe infections.
Nicotine	None.	Mental stimulation; relaxation; relief of tension.	Cancer, particularly of the lungs; heart and blood vessel disease; bronchitis.
Tranquilizers (Librium®; phenothiazines)	Treatment of anxiety and other mental disorders.	Relaxation; relief of anxiety; general depression of mental functioning.	Drowsiness; dry mouth; blurred vision; skin rashes; tremors; occasionally, jaundice.
Miscellaneous (Amyl nitrite; antihistamines; toluene and other solvents – "glue sniffing")	None, except for antihistamines for allergies and amyl nitrite for angina.	Euphoria, lack of coordination; impaired mental functioning.	Variable. Some of these substances can cause liver and kidney damage.

Experimentation with drugs does not always lead to addiction. For example, most people who smoke or drink alcohol do not become physically dependent on these drugs. But psychological dependence can develop relatively rapidly. The regular use of "soft" drugs, such as marijuana, does not necessarily result in addiction to "hard" drugs. However, experimentation with drugs must not be ignored; parents should explain to their children the dangers of even casual drug use.

Preventive Measures. Parents should establish codes of behavior to guide their children and should be prepared to use discipline to enforce these rules. But the parents should explain the reasons for the rules so that their children can see that they are not just arbitrary restrictions. Parents should learn how the various drugs affect the mind and body and should explain these effects to their children. Parents should also abstain from smoking and drinking.

Drug use is less common in families where a good relationship exists between parents and children. Parents should take an active interest in their children. They should help the children with their homework and help to fill their leisure time creatively.

If parents suspect that a child is using drugs, they should try to act calmly but decisively. The sooner the parents act, the greater the likelihood of their preventing addiction. It may be difficult to determine whether or not a child is taking drugs, but there may be several indications. For example, alteration in the child's behavior, such as apathy, furtiveness, or unusual aggressiveness; indifference to personal appearance; change in school habits, such as being late or missing school; change in work habits, such as poor homework; refusal to wear short-sleeved clothes in an effort to hide needle marks in the arms; stealing or borrowing money to pay for drugs; and being seen in the company of known drug users. Parents should be on the alert for these signs, but should also take care not to appear too authoritarian.

At the first suspicion of drug use, the parents should consult the family physician. If the physician is unable to deal with the problem, he or she can refer the parents to a specialist in drug problems.

Drug addiction, or drug dependence, is the uncontrollable craving for a drug. Such craving may occur periodically or continuously and is usually accompanied by an overwhelming compulsion to obtain the drug. The addict becomes preoccupied with thoughts about the anticipated effects of the drug.

The uncontrollable craving for a drug may be of physical origin, psychological origin, or both, and with some drugs the craving may develop in as short a time as 24 hours. In a person who is physically addicted to a drug, the body's chemical processes are altered so that the drug becomes essential for some of the normal metabolic functions. Psychological dependence on a drug does not involve a modification of the body's chemistry, but the addicted person believes that the drug is necessary in order to function normally.

Q: *Why do people take drugs for nonmedical reasons?*

A: There are many reasons for the nonmedical use of drugs. For example, some people with difficult problems, such as unemployment or large debts, become anxious, frustrated, and depressed. They feel trapped by problems that seem to have no solution and seek a release from reality in the effects of drugs.

Other people may take drugs out of boredom or curiosity, and some because their friends do and they feel the need to conform. This need to conform with friends is, perhaps, strongest among teenagers.

Q: *Are some people more likely than others to become dependent on drugs?*

A: Yes. In general, the likelihood of a person becoming dependent on a drug involves three interrelated factors: an individual's personality; the social environment; and the type of drug involved.

Some people are more sensitive than others to the effects of drugs and may feel euphoric states more intensely. This may result in a relatively rapid attraction to and dependence on drugs. In others, feelings of tension or depression may be more acute, and the relief provided by drugs correspondingly greater, and so the dependence more probable.

A person's environment affects the likelihood of drug dependence in many ways. For example, poor housing and unemployment are known to cause depression and anxiety, two states that are common causes of drug addiction. It is also likely that dependence on a drug will be greater in a person who has to steal to get money for the drug than it will in a person who does not. There is for some people a special attraction in doing something illegal or merely antisocial, and this attraction may put people in danger of becoming drug dependent.

In some cases, the nature of the drug taken affects the likelihood of

Drug addiction accounts for thousands of hospital emergency room admissions each year.

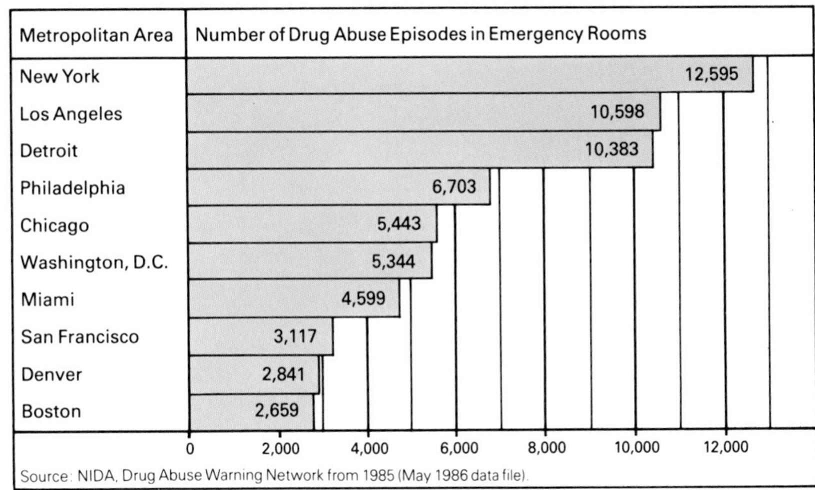

dependency. For example, a person taking heroin is more likely to become drug dependent than a person taking barbiturates.

Q: *Which drugs may cause dependency?*

A: There are many drugs on which people can become dependent. These drugs can be categorized as those that depress the central nervous system; those that stimulate the central nervous system; and those that produce hallucinations and also affect the central nervous system. The main group of drugs that depress the central nervous system are the narcotics, such as codeine, heroin, meperidine, methadone, morphine, and paregoric. Other drugs in this category include alcohol, barbiturates, nicotine, tranquilizers, and some sleeping pills.

Drugs that stimulate the central nervous system include cocaine and the amphetamines, such as Benzedrine, Dexedrine, and Methedrine.

Drugs that produce hallucinations are known as hallucinogens, or psychedelics. Some of the more common hallucinogens are LSD, psilocybin, mescaline, and THC.

Marijuana is classified as a mild hallucinogen, but it is much less powerful than other drugs in this category.

Q: *What effects do depressants produce?*

A: Depressants slow down the activities of the central nervous system. If this system slows down too much, the body's vital functions may stop, which could be fatal. Dependence on depressants usually takes the form of both physical and psychological dependence. The narcotic depressants can cause dependence much more quickly than other depressants.

The short-term effects of depressants include euphoria, relief of pain, and prevention of withdrawal symptoms. The long-term effects include depression, malnutrition, and constipation. The addict may also become infected with AIDS, hepatitis, or tetanus by using unsterile needles. If the drug is stopped, the addict will suffer withdrawal symptoms.

Q: *What symptoms may be caused by withdrawal from a depressant?*

A: The symptoms of depressant withdrawal vary according to the drug involved, but are often extremely severe and may be fatal. For example, within about 18 hours of the sudden withdrawal of alcohol from an alcoholic there may be convulsions and delirium (delirium tremens). Delirium tremens (d.t.'s) may also occur when an addict stops taking sleeping pills.

Other symptoms of depressant withdrawal include weakness; high blood pressure and pulse rate; profuse sweating; gooseflesh; diarrhea; vomiting; severe abdominal cramps; and sometimes, cardiovascular collapse. The diarrhea and vomiting may cause dehydration.

Q: *What effects do stimulants produce?*

A: The short-term effects of stimulants include excitation, sleeplessness, hyperactivity, and euphoria. In the long term, some heavy users of stimulants may also experience hallucinations, delusions, and toxic psychosis.

Dependence on stimulants is both psychological and physical. Amphetamines are perhaps the most dangerous of the stimulant drugs, and many amphetamine addicts develop a high tolerance as part of their dependence on the drug. Tolerance usually occurs rapidly, and the addict has to take large dosages to achieve the desired effects. The larger amounts may cause the stimulant addict to stay awake for several days, during which the addict may hallucinate, become disoriented, and suffer from paranoia. Following this ordeal the stimulant addict may sleep for a day or more. On waking, the addict usually feels severely depressed and often takes another dose of the drug to relieve the depression, which begins the cycle all over again.

Q: *What symptoms may be caused by withdrawal from a stimulant?*

A: The symptoms of stimulant withdrawal include severe depression, muscle pains, apathy, and a strong desire to take more stimulants. These symptoms are felt most keenly by amphetamine addicts. Generally, however, the symptoms of stimulant withdrawal are milder because stimulants are less physically addictive than depressants.

Q: *What effects do hallucinogens produce?*

A: The effects of hallucinogens vary widely, both between individuals and even in the same individual on different occasions. The main effects include exhilaration, sensory distortion, and illusions. But in some cases there may be feelings of paranoia and panic. Occasionally, "flashbacks" may occur. These are brief recurrences of a previous hallucinatory state that may occur weeks or months later without the person having taken a hallucinogen.

Hallucinogens do not seem to produce physical dependence, but may produce psychological dependence. The long-term effects are not known. But scientists are trying to determine whether long-term usage of hallucinogens can cause chromosome damage or genetic aberration.

Q: *Are babies of drug-dependent women born drug dependent?*

A: Yes, although the symptoms of drug dependence in babies vary according to the drug involved. For example, the newborn child of a heroin-addicted mother may be of small size and generally poor health. The baby may display withdrawal symptoms in the form of irritability, high-pitched crying, trembling, sweating, vomiting, and diarrhea. The withdrawal symptoms usually occur within about three days of birth, but withdrawal from barbiturate dependence usually takes longer. Methadone-dependent babies may exhibit breathing distress, convulsions, and fever. Cocaine-addicted babies are usually small at birth, irritable, and may have physical defects. They do not readily bond with their mothers and may have learning disabilities. *See also* FETAL COCAINE SYNDROME.

Q: *What is the clinical treatment for drug dependence?*

A: The first stage of treatment is withdrawal of the drug (detoxification). In cases of physical dependence this usually involves a gradual reduction of the addict's intake over a period of about 10 days. Sometimes a less harmful substitute with similar effects is administered, for example, methadone instead of heroin. The treatment of alcoholism may also include vitamin supplements and the administration of a deterrent drug, such as Antabuse. This drug produces nausea whenever alcohol is drunk. Withdrawal may be delayed if the person is in poor health. *See also* ANTABUSE; METHADONE.

In addition to withdrawal, treatment may also include a program of mental and social rehabilitation, which may involve psychiatric counseling. The treatment of drug dependence is often not completely successful, although the success rate varies from drug to drug.

The rehabilitation programs, such as therapeutic communities and Alcoholics Anonymous, greatly increase the chances of success.

See also ALCOHOLISM; DRUG ABUSE; DRUG OVERDOSE: FIRST AID.

Drug overdose: first aid. The symptoms of drug overdose vary with the type of drug taken. Many drugs cause severe drowsiness or even unconsciousness if too much is taken at one time. An overdose may also result from taking small doses too frequently.

Signs. In many cases, the initial signs of a drug overdose are vomiting, restlessness, and lack of coordination. These symptoms are often followed by unconsciousness.

If a single large dose has been taken at one time, the symptoms usually appear rapidly. If an overdose has been caused by taking small doses too frequently, the symptoms are likely to appear gradually over a longer period and may be more difficult to recognize.

Action. The first aid treatment of a drug overdose is the same for all drugs. First, act quickly. If time is wasted, more of the drug will be absorbed.

Do not leave the victim alone. Ask somebody else to summon emergency medical aid. If the victim is conscious,

First aid for drug overdose

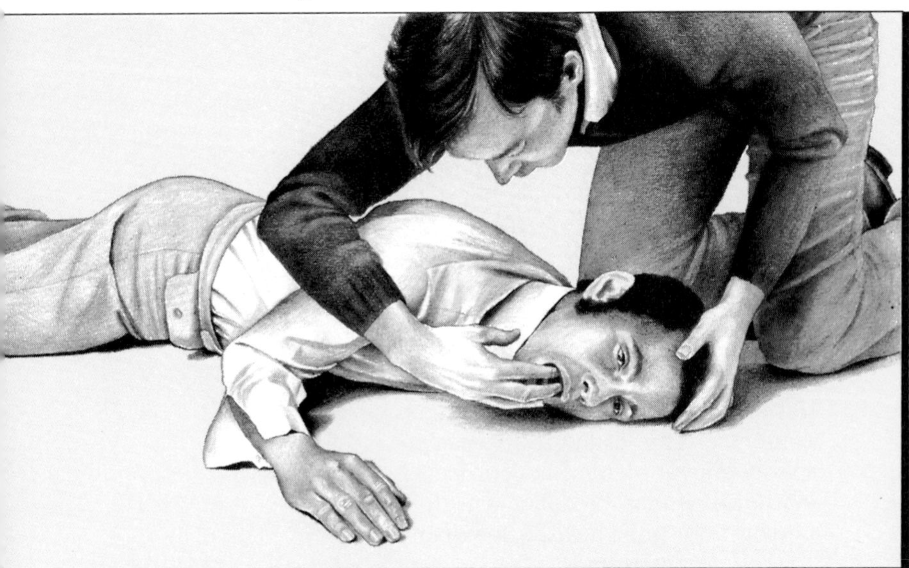

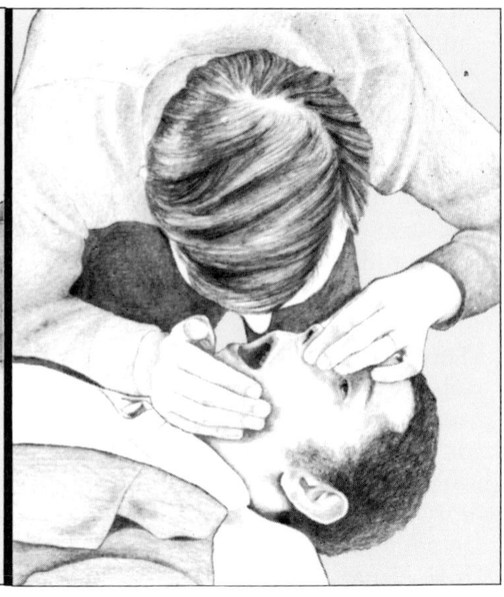

1 If the victim is conscious, induce vomiting by putting your fingers down the victim's throat or giving syrup of ipecac. *Do not* give salt water to drink. This may be harmful. *Do not* attempt to induce vomiting if the victim is unconscious or if the victim has taken a drug overdose by either injection or inhalation. If the victim is unconscious, place him or her in the recovery position, face down, head to one side.

2 Keep a close check on the victim's breathing and pulse at all times. If the victim stops breathing, give artificial respiration (*see* ARTIFICIAL RESPIRATION).

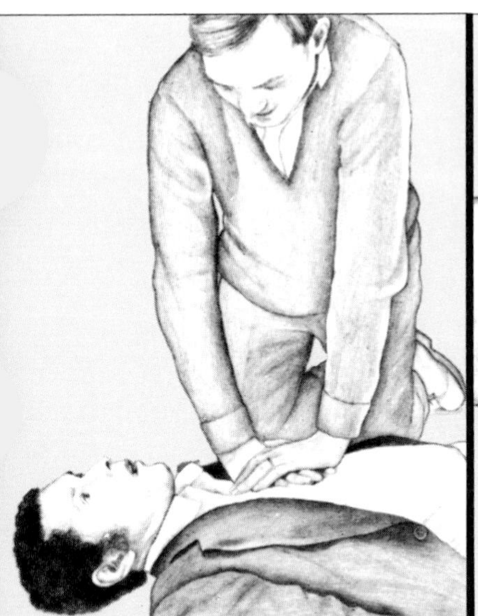

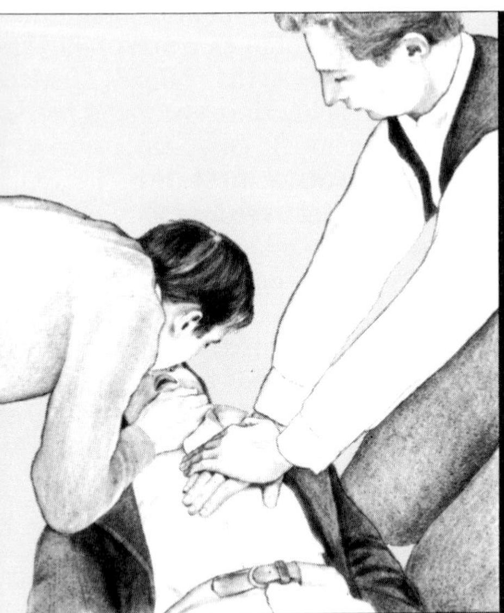

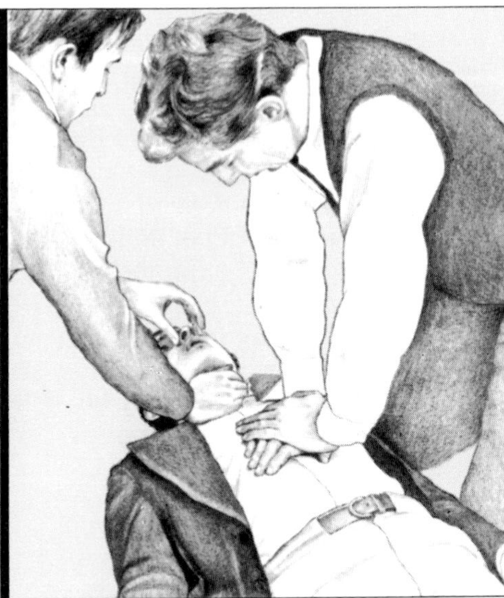

3 If the victim's heart stops, give external cardiac compression (*see* HEART ATTACK: FIRST AID). If the victim has also stopped breathing and help is unavailable, you will have to alternate between external cardiac compression and respiration.

4 If the victim's heart and breathing have both stopped and help is available, one person should kneel at the victim's shoulder and give cardiac compression; another person should kneel at the victim's other side and give artificial respiration.

5 The person giving external cardiac compression should press the victim's chest at a rate of 15 times in 11 seconds. Only a trained person should use this method. The person giving artificial respiration should ventilate twice within 15 seconds.

Drug overdose: first aid

Name	*Examples*	*Signs and symptoms of overdosage*
Acetaminophen	Tylenol®; Parafon forte®.	Nausea; vomiting; pallor; sweating; kidney failure; jaundice; difficulty breathing; delirium; and unconsciousness.
Alcohol	Beers; wines; spirits.	Changes of mood; lack of coordination; slurred speech; sweating; rapid pulse; vomiting; drowsiness; and unconsciousness.
Amphetamines	Benzedrine®; Dexedrine®; Methedrine®.	Excitement; dilated pupils; talkativeness; insomnia; tremors; exaggerated reflexes; bad breath; vomiting; diarrhea; fever; irregular, rapid heart rate; hallucinations; delirium; convulsions; and unconsciousness.
Anticoagulants	Dicumarol®; Coumadin®; Panwarfarin®:	Nosebleeds; pallor; bleeding gums; bruising; blood in the urine and feces; shock; and coma.
Antidepressants	(1) tricyclic compounds—Tofranil®; Elavil®. (2) MAO inhibitors—Nardil®; Parnate®.	(1) Dry mouth; dilated pupils; vomiting; irregular heart rate; retention of urine; hallucinations; lack of coordination; exaggerated reflexes; agitation; convulsions; unconsciousness; and hypertension. (2) Agitation; hallucinations; exaggerated reflexes; irregular heart rate; sweating; retention of urine; convulsions; and muscular rigidity.
Antihistamines	Tripelennamine; diphenhydramine; chlorpheniramine, promethazine.	Excitement or depression; drowsiness; headache; irregular heart rate; nervousness; disorientation; lack of coordination; high fever; hallucinations; fixed, dilated pupils; delirium; convulsions; and coma.
Atropine	Hyoscyamine; scopolamine; stramamine.	Dry mouth; hot, dry skin; flushing; high fever; dilated pupils; irregular heart rate; excitement; confusion; convulsions; delirium; and unconsciousness.
Barbiturates	Amytal®; Nembutal®; Seconal®; phenobarbital.	Drowsiness; headache; confusion; lack of coordination; slurred speech; lack of reflexes; slow breathing rate; and coma.
Benzodiazepines	Librium®; Valium®; Mogadon®; Xanax®.	Drowsiness; dizziness; lack of coordination; and, in rare cases, coma.
Caffeine	Coffee; tea; Nō-Dōz®; APC.	Restlessness; excitement; frequent urination; rapid pulse; nausea; vomiting; fever; tremors; delirium; convulsions; and coma.
Cannabis	Hashish; marijuana.	Overdose usually causes only sleepiness.
Chloral hydrate	Noctec®; Somnos®.	An overdose of chloral hydrate produces symptoms similar to a barbiturate overdose, but chloral hydrate may also cause vomiting.

Name	*Examples*	*Signs and symptoms of overdosage*
Cocaine	Cocaine; crack.	Stimulation followed by depression; nausea; vomiting; anxiety; hallucinations; sweating; difficulty breathing; convulsions; cardiovascular collapse; severe hypertension.
Contraceptive pill		Overdose may cause nausea and vomiting. It does not usually require emergency medical aid, but it is advisable to consult a physician.
Digitalis	Lanoxin®; Crystodigin®; Purodigin®.	Vomiting; excessive salivation; diarrhea; drowsiness; confusion; irregular heart rate; delirium; hallucinations; and unconsciousness.
Diuretics	Hygroton®; Lasix®; Dyazide®.	Massive urine output and irregular heart rate. Rarely there may also be skin rashes and abnormal sensitivity to light.
Glutethimide	Doriden®.	Drowsiness; lack of reflexes; pupil dilation; slow breathing rate; and coma.
Hallucinogens	LSD; psilocybin; mescaline; phencyclidine (PCP).	The symptoms of an overdose are not always readily distinguishable from the normal effects of these drugs, which vary betweeen individuals. The effects include hallucinations; nausea; confusion; and lack of coordination. In some cases, especially with PCP, there may be paranoia; delusions; extreme anxiety; aggressive and violent behavior; depression; seizures; coma; cerebral hemmorrhage; and even death.
Ipecacuanha	Ipecac syrup.	Nausea; vomiting, sometimes bloodstained; diarrhea; abdominal cramps; irregular heart rate; and cardiac arrest.
Iron	Iron supplement tablets and syrup.	Nausea; vomiting, sometimes bloodstained; abdominal pain; pallor; headache; confusion; convulsions; and unconsciousness.
Narcotics	Opium; heroin; morphine; Methadone®; codeine.	Pinpoint pupils; drowsiness; shallow breathing; muscular relaxation; coma; slow pulse and respiratory arrest.
Phenothiazines	Chlorpromazine; prochlorperazine; trifluoperazine.	Sleepiness; dry mouth; lack of coordination; muscular rigidity; tremors; uncontrollable facial grimacing; low body temperature; irregular heart rate; convulsions; and coma.
Quinine	Antimalarial drugs.	Vomiting; deafness; blurred vision; dilated pupils; headache; dizziness; rapid breathing; irregular heart rate; and unconsciousness.
Rauwolfia alkaloids	Reserpine.	Flushing; dry mouth; abdominal cramps; diarrhea; irregular heart rate; tremors; muscular rigidity; and unconsciousness.
Salicylates	Aspirin and many aspirin-containing painkillers.	Abdominal pain; nausea; vomiting; restlessness; noises in the ears; deafness; deep, rapid breathing; fever; sweating; irritability; confusion; delirium; convulsions; and coma.

ask what happened. Try to keep the victim conscious. The victim should be given syrup of ipecac to induce vomiting. Watch that the victim does not choke from inhaling the vomit.

If the victim is unconscious, place in the recovery position, face down, head to one side. *See also* FAINTING: FIRST AID.

If the victim vomits while unconscious, check to see that the victim's air passage is clear. Use your fingers to remove any obvious obstructions. *See also* CHOKING AND COUGHING: FIRST AID.

Closely watch the victim's breathing and pulse. Immediately give artificial respiration if breathing stops, or external cardiac compression if the heart stops, *See also* ARTIFICIAL RESPIRATION; HEART ATTACK: FIRST AID.

An overdose of some drugs may cause convulsions. Do not restrain the victim, but guide him or her away from hazards to prevent injury. *See also* CONVULSION: FIRST AID.

Look for evidence to determine whether the victim has taken a drug. There may be pills in the victim's mouth, or empty pill containers nearby. Drug addicts may have a hypodermic syringe; they may also have needle marks on their skin, usually on the inside of the forearm.

Keep pill containers, pills, and specimens of the victim's vomit. These will help to determine which drug has been taken.

Poison control centers, located nearly worldwide, can provide information on effects of poisoning, as well as reference to treatment locations.

Drunkenness. *See* ALCOHOLISM; INTOXICATION.

D.t.'s. *See* DELIRIUM TREMENS.

Duchenne type muscular dystrophy. *See* MUSCULAR DYSTROPHY.

Duct (dukt) is any narrow tube in the body that carries secretions or fluids from one part of the body to another.

Ductless gland (dukt'lis) is another name for endocrine gland. It secretes substances directly into the bloodstream.

See also ENDOCRINE GLAND.

Ductus arteriosus (duk'təs är tir ē ō'səs) is a blood vessel that joins the main artery leading to the lungs (the pulmonary artery) with the main artery that leads from the heart (the aorta). This link is present in a fetus so that the blood supply by-passes the lungs,

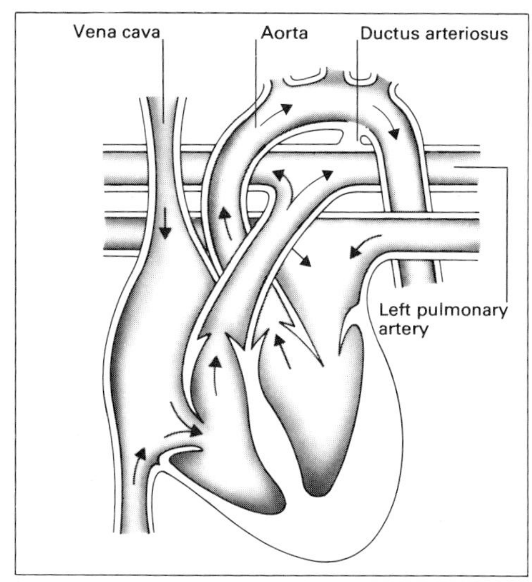

Ductus arteriosus is the blood vessel that by-passes the fetal lung; it normally closes after birth. If this fails to occur, either drug treatment or surgery may be necessary.

which do not function until after birth. The ductus arteriosus closes off soon after birth. Failure to close is a common type of congenital heart disorder, especially in a premature infant. The disorder is treated with the drug indomethacin; if not responsive to indomethacin, the condition may be corrected by tying off the vessel in a surgical operation.

See also BLOOD VESSEL.

Dumb. *See* MUTE.

Dumping syndrome (dum'ping) is a digestion disorder that occurs in a patient who has had an operation for removing a large part of the stomach. Symptoms of sweating, dizziness, nausea, abdominal cramps, belching, vomiting, shortness of breath, and weakness may sometimes be accompanied by pain, headache, or diarrhea. The cause of dumping syndrome is not fully understood, but what happens is that the stomach "dumps" its contents too quickly into the small intestine. The symptoms can be largely avoided by eating several small meals instead of one or two large ones. The meals should be high in fat and protein and low in carbohydrates.

Duodenal ulcer. *See* ULCER, PEPTIC.

Duodenum (dü ə dē'nəm) is the first part of the small intestine, surrounding the head of the pancreas. It is about 10 inches (25cm) long and receives partially digested food from the stomach. The digestive process is continued in the duodenum by the enzyme-containing fluids from the pancreas and the glands lining the duodenal wall and by the action of bile from the liver and gall bladder. When the digestive processes have been completed in the duodenum, the food passes into the jejunum.

See also DIGESTIVE SYSTEM.

Dupuytren's contracture (dyü pwē trônz′ kən trak′chər) is the inability to straighten the fingers, due to a thickening of the fibrous tissue lining the palm. Occasionally Dupuytren's contracture can involve the soles of the feet as well. The cause is not known, but it may be inherited.

Dupuytren's contracture is more common in men over the age of 40, and incidence is higher in alcoholics and epileptics. Treatment may involve a surgical operation to remove the thickened fibrous tissue and release the ligaments.

Durable power of attorney. *See* LIVING WILL.

Dura mater (dür′ə mā′tər) is the tough, fibrous, outermost membrane surrounding the brain and spinal cord.

See also BRAIN; MENINGES.

Dutch cap (duch kap) is a slang term for the diaphragm contraceptive device.

See also CONTRACEPTION; DIAPHRAGM, CONTRACEPTIVE.

Dwarfism (dwôr′fiz əm) is the physical condition of being abnormally undersized. A dwarf may have normal body formations that are proportionally smaller throughout (commonly called a midget), or the condition may involve disproportionate stunting (achondroplasia). Dwarfism may be caused by abnormal fetal development (congenital), malnutrition and other environmental factors, or hormone deficiency. Treatment of dwarfism depends on the cause. *See also* ACHONDROPLASIA.

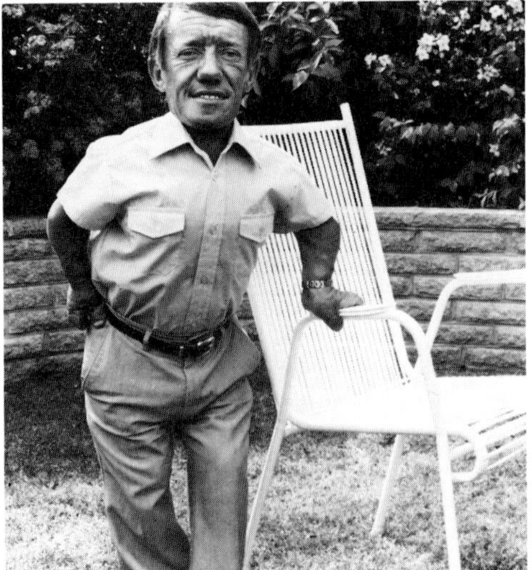

Dwarfism of the achondroplastic variety retards the growth of the long bones.

Q: *Which types of dwarfism are congenital?*

A: The most common congenital disorder is achondroplasia, the form of dwarfism in which growth of the long bones is retarded. An achondroplastic dwarf has a normal sized head and trunk, but proportionally short arms and legs. If one parent has the condition, there is a 50 percent chance with each pregnancy that the child will be affected. There are other rare congenital disorders associated with dwarfism.

Q: *What environmental factors can result in dwarfism?*

A: Malnutrition deprives the body of food and vitamins essential to normal, healthy growth. Stunted body growth in malnourished children can, if treatment is started early enough, be offset by a normal diet. Chronic illness may retard or arrest growth during the childhood years. It has also been shown that the normal rate of growth may be affected by emotional deprivation, especially if the warm supportive environment that children need is lacking and instead replaced with hate and violence. Malnutrition, brought about by child abuse, can also contribute to producing dwarfism. *See also* CHILD ABUSE.

Q: *How do hormonal deficiencies cause dwarfism?*

A: Growth hormone is produced by the pituitary gland at the base of the brain. If for any reason the pituitary gland of a child is underactive, dwarfism results. The body of a child with this deficiency remains small, but is correctly proportioned. There is no mental impairment.

In cases where hormonal deficiencies are the cause of dwarfism, the treatment is to replace the hormones of the malfunctioning glands, whether pituitary, thyroid, adrenal, or pancreatic.

See also CRETINISM.

Dyazide® (dī ə zīd′) is a drug compounded of triamterene and hydrochlorothiazide. Dyazide is a diuretic (which increases the quantity of urine) and an antihypertensive (which is used to lower mild forms of high blood pressure). The drug's main use is in the control of edema (retention of fluids) that occurs with heart failure, cirrhosis of the liver, and nephrotic syndrome of the kidney.

See also DIURETIC; EDEMA.

Dying is a natural process involving the progressive degeneration of those body functions essential to maintain life. To be dying of old age is the best example of this: the body's organs are worn out and eventually cease to function. Drug treatment and other applications of medical knowledge have made it possible to postpone the dying process.

Q: *Should a dying person be made aware of the situation?*

A: Many patients prefer to know if they are to die from their illness and press the physician for a frank opinion. If direct questions are asked, it is generally because the patient wants honest answers. Close associates of the patient sometimes prefer that their friend or relative be spared the anguish of knowing, but the wishes of the patient must be the primary consideration. In other cases, the patient suspects the prognosis but prefers not to have it confirmed. It is unlikely that a physician will offer the information unless directly requested.

Q: *How strong does fear seem to be in people who are dying?*

A: It seems that most people dread that time in the future when they will know that death is imminent. However, people who are dying and know it usually manage to come to terms with the fact. It seems clear from experienced witnesses, such as physicians and nurses, that the dying process is not frightening in itself: as death draws near, the patient tends to become peaceful and accepting of a death that may well be desired by the final stages.

Q: *What is it about a drawn-out death that people think will be frightening?*

A: The fear of pain and suffering is probably the most common fear for those who contemplate their dying. This is why people often say that they would prefer to die instantaneously (for example, from accident or injury). Another fear is that approaching death will bring remorse or terrifying revelations.

Q: *What type of requests might a dying person make?*

A: It is natural for the patient to wish to be with close friends; such companions are of most comfort during this time, and their understanding and concern may reduce the loneliness of the ordeal. The patient may feel the need to speak in confidence with certain people who are trusted, sympathetic, or admired. During such intimacies, it is likely that death will be discussed freely, and this can be a type of therapy. If other people can allay his or her alarm and fear, the dying person may more readily embrace what is natural and inevitable. Some patients cope with the thought of death by making sure that affairs consequent upon their death will cause as little inconvenience as possible to those who must attend to them. Matters of the will may be settled, funeral arrangements decided, and the patient may wish to participate in discussions about what everyday adjustments may have to be made, both short-term and long-term.

Q: *Might a person be conscious immediately before death?*

A: Yes. Sometimes a patient remains weak but alert until the moment of death. The presence of the family at this time must surely be of comfort. Often when a patient appears to be unconscious, the sense of hearing still remains; this should be considered at all times when discussing the illness in the presence of the patient.

Q: *Is it always obvious when a patient dies?*

A: No. Although a pallor and stillness typically occur with death, the exact moment of death is difficult to define even for physicians and nurses. Breathing prior to death may follow a cycle of being alternately shallow and deep for any length of time before death finally occurs during a shallow period. See also CHEYNE-STOKES RESPIRATION. Within a few minutes of the event, the eyes become staring and the muscles of the face sag.

Q: *What is a hospice?*

A: A hospice is a specialized center for the care of dying patients. Services provide a comprehensive team approach to the problems of the patients and their families in order to maximize their physical and psychological comfort. Hospices specifically do not provide the aggresive diagnostic and therapeutic care provided in hospitals. Hospice programs may be housed in a section of a hospital, exist as a free-standing facility, or provide terminal care to people in their own homes.

See also DEATH.

Dying, care of the. The sadness and inevitability of death brings problems and difficulties that few persons have the knowledge or experience to cope with alone. Most persons would like to die at home close to family and familiar possessions. Every help must be given to the patient who wishes to die at home and not in a hospital. The expense of prolonged hospitalization is often prohibitive, and this is an additional psychological as well as financial burden for the patient and family.

Some persons have more experience of helping with the dying than others. The physician knows about the patient's physical needs and has the skill to prevent or relieve pain. He or she becomes a leader and supports the family during the weeks ahead. A member of the clergy can give a spiritual support that may not have been needed by the patient or the family for many years.

At the onset of a terminal illness, the physician and family are faced with the decision of what to tell the patient. If the course of the illness is rapid, the decision may not have to be made. The problem usually arises when an inoperable cancer is present; when there is an incurable muscular disorder; or when a cardiac condition begins to rapidly deteriorate. Often the patient's mental state remains unaffected and alert.

Every physician must be free to tell the patient what he or she feels is necessary and appropriate. The problem is discussed with the patient's family. The physician does not like to lie to the patient, because the patient will lose confidence in the physician if he or she were ever to discover the truth. Often the dying patient never asks a direct question about his or her condition. This does not mean that the patient is not aware of what is happening, but that he or she prefers to help the family, the physician, and himself or herself by maintaining the pretense that all will be well. The patient may not want to know how many months or years he or she has got to live. It is enough for the patient to know that he or she is not going to suffer.

Sometimes, however, the patient wants to know exactly what is the matter, what can be done about it, the likelihood of successful treatment, and eventually, the length of time the physician expects him or her to live. Most physicians give truthful answers to direct questions such as these. This honesty may in itself help the patient through moments of mental anguish. It also gives the patient a chance to put his or her affairs in order. The patient may not want the family to know that he or she understands the predicament. This makes it easier for them all to maintain a facade of cheerfulness. Recent surveys suggest that patients increasingly want to know about their disease and its exact prognosis, rather than being "protected" from bad news.

Sudden Death. The violence of a car crash or the swift death caused by a heart attack gives the individual no time to know what is happening. Even death that occurs a day or two after an accident, operation, or acute illness is too entangled with the treatment of the condition for the patient to realize that he or she is dying. There is little time for the physician to discuss the matter with the family, other than to warn them of the possibility. The patient rarely suffers, but the family is left unprepared and appalled by the disaster.

The family needs expert help from the physician, the nurses, and the clergy. Medical help can soften the initial grief. The children and relatives can help each other. The very fact that they are being constructive produces an unexpected strength to cope with funeral arrangements, lawyers, and the hospital. Friends and neighbors can help the bereaved family in a practical way by helping with the shopping and other domestic chores.

Adjusting to life after the sudden death of a loved one is difficult. The surviving relative needs a chance to talk over the death. The bereaved person may suffer from a feeling of guilt and needs encouragement and support. Grief sometimes takes the form of anger directed at the outside causes of death. The bereaved person is looking for someone to blame for the disaster. This feeling passes as the bereaved person's normal perspective on life returns, but it can be alarming to the family and friends who are trying to help.

Acute and despairing grief is understandable and common after a sudden death. As grief lessens, the support and care of the family and friends can gradually be softened. The relative or friend can come to terms with the situation as he or she would have been able to do had the death been gradual and anticipated.

Gradual Death. The period of normal life must be maintained for as long as possible. At first, it is difficult for someone to accept that a relative has a fatal illness. One day the relative is complaining of a variety of symptoms, some of which might be severe, and the next day the physician gives the family the information that they fear most of all. They might be told after the relative has had an operation or after some minor investigation.

Usually, there is some form of treatment that produces a temporary improvement in the patient's health. Although this gives a false hope to relatives, it helps the patient's morale. If the physician recommends a short vacation for the patient, it is wise to accept the advice.

It is sensible to discuss the practicalities of the situation with the physician. The family needs to know how the disease will progress and how to make the patient comfortable and happy. Although patients and families frequently want to know exactly how long the patient can expect to live, this is the hardest question for a physician to answer; there is usually no way for the physician to predict this with any accuracy. The physician can advise them on the possibilities of caring for the patient at home in the later stages of the illness, and whether special arrangements need to be made.

The normal routine of life should be continued for as long as possible. It is important for the patient's morale, as well as for his or her financial situation, to work for as long as possible.

Weekends should be set aside for the patient's recuperation. He or she may suffer from a loss of stamina and endurance, so additional rest is advisable. The physician may suggest a mild sedative at night to ensure a good sleep for the patient and to reduce any worry or anxiety.

Effects of Gradual Weakening. Increasing weakness and onset of symptoms means that sooner or later the patient's period of normal life comes to an end. The patient often suffers from a gradual loss of vitality, and an increasing fatigue makes a full day's work impossible. A relatively minor illness, such as a feverish cold, can develop into bronchitis and rapidly reduce the patient's strength. Other symptoms become worse, or new symptoms develop. The patient may suffer from weight loss, weakness, and a loss of appetite. Other problems that frequently occur with the terminally ill are nausea at the sight of food; vomiting after a meal; and constipation. The patient's weakness and lethargy lead to a feeling of profound depression and misery. The patient's awareness of the developing situation is magnified by worry. He or she is fearful of becoming a burden to the family.

The physician can help in a positive manner. He or she can prescribe antidepressant drugs to help the patient's mood; a change of treatment to improve the patient physically; and support for the patient's family.

Although the patient is weaker, he or she can remain independent and continue getting up and going to bed, going to the bathroom, and getting dressed and undressed unaided. He or she can still enjoy short walks or drives and visits to friends and neighbors. Such trips should be planned carefully to coincide with the patient's strongest time of day. Although the trips may be exhausting, the patient will enjoy them.

The family routine begins to change. Make household rearrangements small and gradual. The patient needs a chair that is easy to get into and out of. Organize a downstairs room with a day bed. The patient will then be able to be with the family for most of the day without having to use the stairs. Encourage friends and colleagues from work to visit the patient. Work out a sensible daily routine and encourage the patient to relax.

If the patient is not in pain at this stage, his or her anxiety is increased by the onset of vague discomforts and aches. He or she needs reassurance from the physician, who may prescribe mild painkillers, antidepressant drugs, or a sedative to be taken at night to ensure a good sleep for the patient.

If the patient talks about the future, do not ignore his or her comments. He or she needs reassurance about what will happen to the family. It is important to remain both hopeful and realistic about the future, whether or not the patient knows the truth.

The Role of Friends. The role of the friend is a very important one. Friends want to help the patient and the family. The friend may not know the details of the illness, but has probably guessed the outcome. He or she can give the family and patient both moral and practical support. Visits from the friend ought to be brief, but they offer the patient an opportunity to talk about cheerful subjects, such as family, work, or old times. It is wise to avoid talking at length about the illness at the early stage, unless the patient shows signs of wanting to.

The friend can show appreciation of the work being done by the family and offer to stay with the patient if the family needs a little time away from home.

If the patient shows signs of wanting to talk about his or her illness and future, the friend can listen quietly. The patient can discuss practical problems with the friend that may be difficult to say to the family, for example, who will care for and guide the family in the future. Do not ignore the questions by convincing the patient that he or she is going to pull through in the end, when the patient obviously needs practical reassurance.

During the later stages of the patient's illness, the friend can help the family with chores, such as shopping. Sometimes, the patient's courage and strength prevent him or her from showing real emotions to the family, but such emotions may be revealed to a friend. The patient may feel that the physician does not have the time to listen, and the friend can be a sympathetic listener to whom the patient can pour out his or her worries and fears. Often, a sudden release of emotion can be of enormous value to the patient.

Physical Care of the Patient. The bedridden patient accentuates the practical problems of dealing with a terminally ill patient. The routine of caring for a chronically sick person is by now well established. The family must realize that deterioration is going to continue. Although the patient's loss of weight makes some aspects of nursing easier, the skin is more likely to be damaged without the protection of fat and muscle. It may take two adults to move the patient on and off the bedpan. A visiting nurse can help with bedbathing and can show the family how to carry out the more complicated procedures. The physician may advise the family on the use of drugs and how to insert suppositories to treat constipation or other symptoms.

Pain may become a permanent part of the patient's life. The physician prescribes painkilling drugs in adequate amounts and explains how to use them. Do not wait until the patient complains of pain before giving the drugs. It is easier and more effective to administer them at regular intervals.

Nausea and vomiting are often more distressing symptoms for the family and patient to deal with than pain. The symptoms may be combined with hiccupping, which exhausts the patient. The physician can prescribe drugs to control this. These drugs can also have a sedative effect if taken with painkillers. Although they can produce confusion and drowsiness, the drowsiness often benefits the patient. The drugs may prevent the patient from feeling thirsty, so it is important to encourage him or her to drink. Assist the patient by offering frequent drinks of cool, sweetened fluid, such as fruit juice, iced water, or herbal teas that freshen the mouth but do not have strong flavors.

If the patient is suffering from a heart or lung disease, coughing may be one of the symptoms. This distresses and exhausts the patient. The family also finds it disturbing. It is most important to control the coughing at night and so allow the patient and family a peaceful sleep. Try changing the patient's position in bed. A steam inhalation at bedtime reduces irritation and helps to prevent sleep-disturbing cough. Broken sleep is exhausting for the family and the patient. If sleeplessness continues, it is sensible to arrange alternative care every other night if possible.

Another symptom of heart or lung disease is shortness of breath. Coughing, or the smallest physical activity, can make the patient gasp for breath. This causes great distress. The physician may prescribe oxygen that can be used effectively after a bad bout of coughing or rapid physical movement.

The patient's strength and personality may cope with pain in a surprising manner. However, incontinence of urine and feces is a humiliation few can tolerate. The situation requires immense care and tact, as well as tolerance, from those nursing the patient because they must cope with the physical and psychological misery that incontinence produces. It is important that, despite the unpleasantness, the family should not let the patient feel that he or she is an intolerable burden. Incontinence must be accepted with sympathy and understanding.

As the patient becomes physically weaker, the physician administers more drugs. The mental state of the patient changes from an alert, realistic individual, to one who is often confused about time and place. This confusion varies, and periods of normal discussion fluctuate with moments of drowsiness and loss of reality. Often the patient is aware that he or she has been confused and is apologetic for the trouble caused.

Visitors should come for only a short time. It is best if they know the patient well and can remain peaceful and silent. If necessary, they can just hold the patient's hand. This physical contact is a form of communication that can produce peace and contentment.

During the patient's deterioration, the appetite is usually lost. Offer the patient small amounts of his or her favorite foods, jellies, or soups. Serve small portions of food frequently.

If at any time the family feels that they can not cope with the situation any longer, discuss the problem with the physician. It may be that the time has come for the patient to be hospitalized and it is wise to accept the physician's advice on this.

The Moment of Death. The time of death is sometimes difficult for the physician to estimate beforehand. The patient may become unconscious some hours, even days, before death or may remain alert and conscious to the end. Painkilling drugs sometimes produce a state of semicoma that can be misinterpreted by the family as a forerunner to death. The patient may develop an alarming breathing pattern called Cheyne-Stokes respiration, in which breaths increase in rapidity and volume until they reach a climax, then gradually subside and stop altogether. This period can last from five seconds through a minute before the process begins again. The syndrome is common in sick or elderly persons. Although it can be a forerunner to death, it is just as likely to last for several months or even to disappear altogether.

Do not be alarmed if the patient's breathing makes a groaning or croaking sound. It does not mean that he or she is in pain. When a dying patient slips into a coma, the position of the neck and body produces the noise, which can be reduced by gently turning the patient's shoulders or body.

Another alarming noise the dying patient may make is known as the "death rattle." This happens because the unconscious patient is unable to cough up the secretions that accumulate in the back of the throat.

The attitude of the family and the patient alters at this stage. As the patient suffers from increased weakness, lethargy, discomfort, and pain, he or she begins to come to terms with dying. Death is no longer frightening. Often a person's last days are spent more happily in the knowledge that he or she is dying, than in a state of uncertainty and doubt. It is easier for the family and patient to talk about death in a way that may not have been possible earlier in the illness. It brings comfort to everyone, and often a closeness not experienced before.

The patient or family may need additional comfort from a member of the clergy or from a physician. The length of life remaining to the patient no longer matters. The important thing is the quality of the patient's last days or hours. The physician is aware that the application of medical skill can sometimes prolong the patient's suffering and bring no real benefit. Although the physician may prescribe large doses of painkilling drugs if necessary, he or she is unlikely to start the patient on new treatment.

The actual moment of death is difficult to define, and for the family, difficult to accept. Even when the patient has stopped breathing, and a pulse can not be felt, the heart gives feeble contractions for another minute or two. Even a physician may find it difficult to give an exact time of death, but must leave it to the expert to make the diagnosis.

If the family is present at the moment of death, it is comforting for everyone to stay quietly at the bedside with his or her own thoughts. Each member of the family needs a chance to touch or to kiss the dead relative, and such physical contact helps to bring home the reality of death.

Often no one is present when the patient dies, for he or she may have been left alone to sleep. Although death is expected, it is still a shock for the member of the family who first enters the room. It is sensible to tidy the bedclothes and comb the patient's hair before telling the rest of the family. When they come in to see the body, it has an appearance of calm and peacefulness.

The Reaction of Children. A child's reaction to death depends on many factors. A child's first experience with death is often the death of a pet. A child under the age of eight can not understand that death is irreversible and may expect the mother or father to bring the pet back to life. After the age of eight or nine, the child's understanding is usually as rational as an adult's understanding.

However, it may still be difficult for the child to understand that someone in the family is dying; neither is it important that the child should understand. What is important is that the child sees that the family is united and involved in caring for the sick relative. The child can then become part of the team and help in caring for the patient.

If the patient slips into a coma, or is confused by drugs or illness, it is wise to keep the child out of the sickroom. The child may be frightened to see the familiar and loved person in this state, and the child's presence does not help the patient.

When the patient is about to die, the family may decide to send the child away to a neighbor or relative. Although this sending away is well intentioned, the experience can be frightening for the child, who may feel that death is going to involve another member of the family while he or she is away. The parents need to give the child a careful explanation about everything that will happen during his or her absence. Often, however, the child can stay at home and continue to feel part of the family.

The parents may decide to let the child see the dead relative. If the child does want to, someone should take him or her into the room and only stay long enough for the child to see how peaceful the person looks in death. If the child does not want to see the body, the family must respect that decision.

The parent may explain carefully and simply to the child what happens between the death of the relative and the funeral. A young child can not understand a funeral or cremation service, so it is probably wise to leave the child with a close friend during the service. An older child may want to take part in this important family occasion.

Parents may be confused by the child's reaction to bereavement. The child may seem indifferent or aggressive or may seem grief-stricken or guilty. The parents must encourage the child to discuss his or her feelings. The child must be reassured that these feelings are not unusual, but that they become unreasonable if taken to extremes.

The child soon learns that the sadness is made easier by sharing the emotion with the family. As time passes, the grief becomes less acute, and the child gains a better understanding of the concept of death.

Death of a Baby. The intrauterine death of an embryo ends in a miscarriage (spontaneous abortion). Ten percent of pregnancies end in this way, commonly between the sixth and tenth weeks, and usually because of an abnormality in the embryo. With care, subsequent pregnancies are usually successful.

Stillbirth is the term used to describe a fetal death occurring after the twenty-eighth week of pregnancy. The mother may become aware that the baby's movements have stopped, and an obstetrician can check for fetal movement.

If the fetus is dead, the mother and father must be told. Labor is induced with drugs if it has not begun within a few days. The mother is usually kept under sedation until the baby is born. It is important that the baby's father is with the mother for the delivery to give comfort. The parents find it easier to cope with the reality of the death if they are able to see the baby immediately after the birth.

The parents need to know the chances of subsequent pregnancies ending in this way. They also need time to mourn the loss of the dead baby before embarking on another pregnancy.

Perinatal death refers to death occurring between the moment of birth and a week after birth. Because the majority of babies are now born in a hospital, the number of perinatal deaths has dropped. However, if death does occur, the parents need the same help and support that parents of a stillborn child need.

Sudden infant death syndrome (SIDS) is commonly referred to as "crib death." Sometimes a perfectly healthy baby between the ages of three weeks and seven months is found dead in the crib. There is never an adequate explanation. The parents are left shocked and grief-stricken. They feel desperately guilty and in some way responsible. All that is definitely known about crib death is that it is not caused by choking, smothering, strangulation, or any of the other popular myths. Neither does it run in families. *See also* SUDDEN INFANT DEATH SYNDROME.

Before the parents can recover from the shock, they need careful counseling. A psychiatrist, family social agency, guidance clinic, or member of the clergy may help.

Death of an Older Child or an Adolescent. From the age of three years onward, a child begins to understand the concept of death and dying. The dying child feels protective toward his or her parents. Although the child desperately needs to talk about what is going to happen, he or she may never get close to the subject. The child may attach himself or herself to a nurse or physician while still relying on the parents. By doing this, the child is sharing the emotional responsibility. The parents may find this difficult to accept, but must realize that someone else can perhaps give more help by listening dispassionately to the child's fears and anxieties.

The child who seems to have no idea about what is happening is better left in ignorance, but the child who asks "Am I going to die?" may be happier knowing the truth. He or she can then talk more openly about the worries and uncertainties and bring comfort to himself or herself as well as to the parents. The child may be comforted by knowing the religious beliefs that surround death. Often it is the moment of death that the child fears. He or she needs to know that dying is usually calm and peaceful.

An adolescent in the same situation has reached a more logical and dispassionate view of life. He or she may reject the comfort that religious beliefs can bring. An adolescent rightly feels that life is unjust and unfair. He or she has been striving to find independence only to discover that he or she is totally dependent on the family once again. It takes a wise physician or friend to help the isolated adolescent.

Parents who lose a child at any age need help and sympathy after the death. The physician's job is to help the bereaved parents. This help must also be extended to brothers and sisters also, whose grief may go unnoticed by the overburdened parents.

Dysarthria (dis är′thrē ə) is the inability to speak clearly. The causes of the disorder include paralysis and lack of coordination of the tongue and muscles of the face and of those supplying the voice box. Disease of the muscles or nerve disorders may also be causative factors.

Dysentery (dis′ən ter ē) is an inflammatory disease characterized by severe diarrhea, with blood and mucus in the stools. It is accompanied by pain in the abdomen and, sometimes, contracting spasms of the anus with a persistent desire to empty the bowels (tenesmus).

Dysentery may have several causes, such as parasites (worms), chemical irritants, bacteria, and protozoa (amebae). But there are two main infectious forms that affect humans: Sonne dysentery, caused by bacteria *(Shigella sonnei)*; and amebic dysentery, caused by an ameba *(Entamoeba histolytica)*. Both forms are transmitted by contaminated water or food. Dysentery is particularly common in tropical countries where standards of hygiene are poor.

Q: *What precautions can a person take to prevent catching dysentery?*

A: Because dysentery is more common in tropical countries, it is important in such localities to avoid eating uncooked foods and to ensure that all foods are prepared in the most hygienic way. It is essential not to drink unboiled water, because this may carry the infection. All foods must be kept covered to prevent flies from contaminating them with the disease.

See also DYSENTERY, AMEBIC; DYSENTERY, SONNE.

Dysentery, amebic (dis'ən ter ē, ə mē'bik). Amebic dysentery is an intestinal disorder caused by the parasite *Entamoeba histolytica*.

Q: *What are the symptoms of amebic dysentery?*

A: Amebic dysentery may take some time to appear. Often some other minor intestinal disorder causes it to flare up, resulting in recurring attacks. The attacks are accompanied by colicky abdominal pain and, sometimes, fever. Intermittent attacks may already have gone on for several months, causing the patient to feel vaguely unwell, before a major attack necessitates consulting a physician.

Q: *How is amebic dysentery diagnosed?*

A: A physician diagnoses amebic dysentery by examining the feces for the infective organism, and by examining the inside of the colon with a lighted tube (sigmoidoscope). The physician can often see small ulcers in the colon; specimens from these ulcers contain the infection.

Q: *How is amebic dysentery treated?*

A: It can be treated with a variety of drugs. The drug metronidazole is usually effective in uncomplicated cases.

Q: *What are the complications of amebic dysentery?*

A: The infection may form a palpable mass inside the intestine to infect the liver, forming a liver abscess. It may also extend into the lung to produce a lung abcess. Both are serious conditions and require specialized treatment.

Dysentery, Sonne (dis'ən ter ē, sun'ē). Sonne dysentery is an intestinal disorder caused by the bacterium *Shigella sonnei*.

Q: *What are the symptoms of Sonne dysentery?*

A: There are several forms of *Shigella* infection, which cause dysentery of varying severity. The symptoms start after about 48 hours with the acute onset of vomiting, diarrhea, and abdominal pains. A high fever may occur, and diarrhea continues for several days with blood and mucus in the stools. In babies and young children, life-threatening dehydration may occur rapidly. *See also* DEHYDRATION.

Q: *What is the treatment for Sonne dysentery?*

A: It is most important to ensure that the patient drinks plenty of fluids. A physician may prescribe antispasmodic and antidiarrheal drugs to control the worst of the symptoms until the condition improves naturally. This may take up to 10 days, longer in severe cases, although the patient is often better within 48 hours. Babies and children may have to be admitted to a

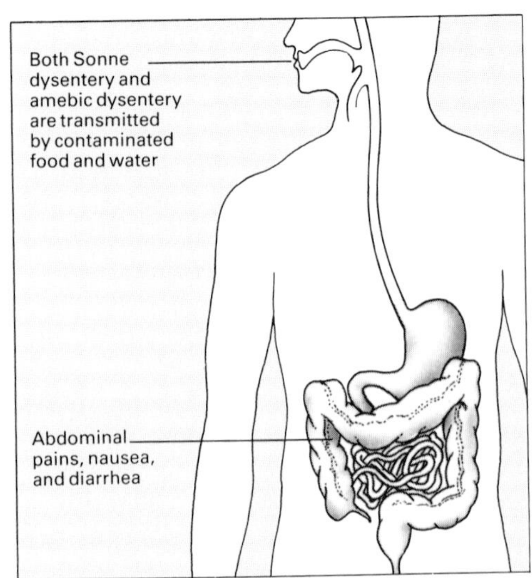
Both Sonne dysentery and amebic dysentery are transmitted by contaminated food and water
Abdominal pains, nausea, and diarrhea

Dysentery is an intestinal disorder that can be caused by bacteria or the ingestion of amebae.

hospital for intravenous infusion, if serious dehydration occurs. Antibiotics are used only in the severest cases.

Q: *What are the complications of Sonne dysentery?*

A: Sometimes a patient develops an eye inflammation, such as conjunctivitis or iritis. Because the stools may remain infectious for some weeks, it is necessary for the patient to take great care with personal hygiene, washing the hands thoroughly after each bowel movement. The physician may culture the patient's feces on several occasions to check whether the infective organism has disappeared.

Dysgeusia (dis gü'zē ə) is the condition of having an impaired sense of taste.

Dysesthesia (dis es thē'zē ə) is a condition characterized by abnormal sensation, such as the sensation of being pricked by pins and needles or the sensation of insects crawling on the skin.

Dyskinesia, tardive (dis kin ē'zē ə, tär'div). Tardive dyskinesia is the impairment of the ability to voluntarily move the muscles of the face, mouth, and neck. This results in fragmentary, repetitive movements. It predominantly affects the elderly; it results often after long-term administration of antipsychotic drugs. If a patient develops any symptoms of tardive dyskinesia, antipsychotic drugs must be stopped immediately. Unfortunately, the condition is usually irreversible. No treatment has been found to be consistently successful.

Dyslexia (dis lek'sē ə) is an imprecise term used to describe a variety of reading and writing disorders. It may be a disturbed understanding of what is read, ranging from a minor disability to a complete and permanent inability to read that is inconsistent with the individual's intelligence. It is often accompanied by an inability to spell correctly. The specific causes of dyslexia are disputed, but it may be due to congenital or acquired brain damage, probably affecting the speech centers. Reading disorders tend to run in families; many more boys are affected than girls. Dyslexia is not a sign of low intelligence, and some affected individuals may benefit from special teaching.

See also LEARNING DISABILITY.

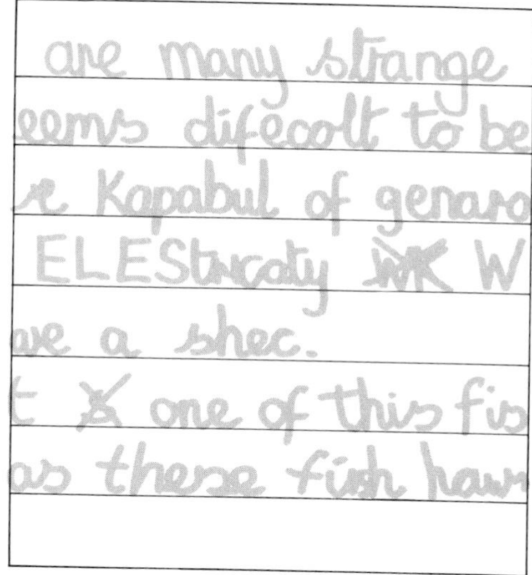

Dyslexia may be a cause of poor spelling but does not indicate a lack of intelligence.

Dysmenorrhea (dis men ə re'ə) is pain associated with menstruation. Primary dysmenorrhea occurs for no apparent cause. Secondary dysmenorrhea, usually happening later in life, has an underlying cause.

Q: *What are the symptoms of primary dysmenorrhea?*

A: The pain begins just before or at the onset of menstruation and is centered in the lower abdomen. It may be cramp-like, and it lasts for the first day or two of the menstrual period. The abdominal pain is often accompanied by backache, nausea, vomiting, headache, frequent urination or bowel movements, and occasionally by dizziness and fainting. The pain is thought to be a result of uterine contractions.

Q: *How is primary dysmenorrhea treated?*

A: Prostaglandin-inhibiting drugs may be prescribed. They should be started one or two days before menstruation and continued for the first two or three days of the period. The drugs should be taken regularly, not just when pain reappears. Painkilling or antispasmodic drugs may be helpful. If these measures fail to control the symptoms, certain hormonal drugs, such as birth control pills, will prevent ovulation and stop the pain. Finally, the gynecologist may recommend a D and C. *See also* DILATATION AND CURETTAGE.

Q: *Are the symptoms of secondary dysmenorrhea different from those of primary dysmenorrhea?*

A: Yes. The pain usually starts earlier in the cycle and lasts longer after causing a dull ache deep in the pelvis.

Q: *What are causes of secondary dysmenorrhea?*

A: Secondary dysmenorrhea is usually caused by some gynecological disorder, such as inflammation of the uterus (endometritis) or of the fallopian tubes (salpingitis), or by the spread of intestinal imflammation. In some cases the cause may be degenerating fibroid tumors, having an intrauterine device (IUD) in place, or endometriosis, in which tissue resembling womb lining occurs in other parts of the pelvic cavity. *See also* ENDOMETRITIS; INTRAUTERINE DEVICE; SALPINGITIS.

Q: *How can secondary dysmenorrhea be treated?*

A: The treatment must be directed at the cause. If there is infection, prolonged treatment with antibiotics may be necessary. Occasionally a cause such as an ovarian cyst has to be dealt with surgically.

Q: *Are there any other reasons for a woman to experience dysmenorrhea?*

A: Yes. It is common for menstruation to be accompanied by mild abdominal discomfort, a feeling of pressure in the pelvis, headache, and slight nausea. These symptoms can be much worse if the woman is overtired or has been under emotional stress. Dysmenorrhea is not a behavioral or psychological disorder.

See also MENSTRUATION

Dyspareunia (dis pə rü′nē ə) is painful sexual intercourse. There are two forms of the condition, primary dyspareunia and secondary dyspareunia.

Q: *What causes primary dyspareunia?*

A: Primary dyspareunia occurs during initial attempts at sexual intercourse. One cause can be vaginismus, the involuntary contraction of the muscle around the vagina, which makes intercourse difficult or even impossible. Vaginismus is usually the result of a woman's psychological reaction to her fears and anxieties about sexual intercourse. These fears and anxieties are often associated with a history of sexual abuse or attempted rape. Dyspareunia can also have physical causes such as inadequate lubrication; hymenal tears; a bruised urethral opening; cysts, boils, inflammations, or infections (for example, infection of the Bartholin's glands); or an allergic reaction to some contraceptive foams or jellies. And finally, there may be some congenital abnormality of the reproductive tract, such as a rigid hymen or a septum in the vagina.

Q: *What causes secondary dyspareunia?*

A: Secondary dyspareunia usually develops years after first-time sexual intercourse. Dryness and thinning of the lining of the vagina after menopause can cause pain, as can major displacements of the uterus, ovaries, or bladder. Scars from episiotomy repair can cause painful intercourse. Vaginal infections, herpes genitalis, pelvic inflammatory disease, endometriosis, and various tumors can all cause dyspareunia.

Q: *How is dyspareunia treated?*

A: In both primary and secondary dyspareunia, the pain can be expected to disappear after the underlying cause has been treated.

See also BARTHOLIN'S GLAND; EPISIOTOMY; SEXUAL INTERCOURSE; VAGINISMUS.

Dyspepsia. *See* INDIGESTION.

Dysphagia (dis fā′jē ə) is difficulty in swallowing.

Dysphasia (dis fā′zē ə) is the lack of coordination of speech and failure to arrange words in a comprehensible way. It is a less severe form of aphasia. Dysphasia commonly follows brain damage caused by a stroke or injury involving the side of the brain that controls speech. There is a tendency for the condition to improve naturally, and careful speech therapy can teach the patient how to talk, even though this may take many months.

See also APHASIA; SPEECH.

Dysphonia (dis fō′nē ə) is any voice impairment or difficulty in speaking.

Dysplasia (dis plā′zhə) means any abnormal development. It is most often used as a combining form, for example,

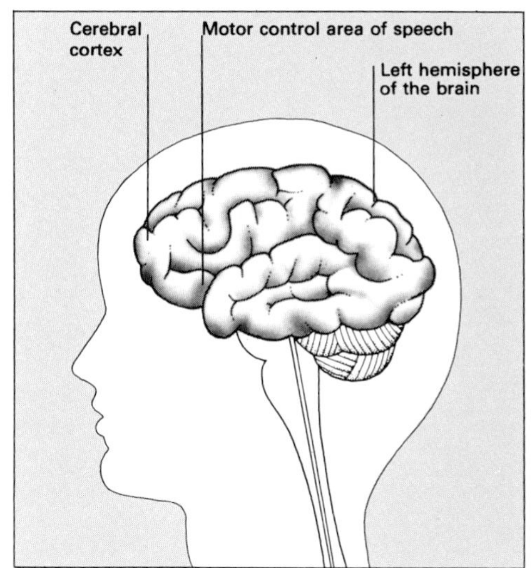

Dysphasia is a speech defect caused by damage to the left side of the brain.

chondrodysplasia or epidermodysplasia.

Dysplasia also refers to abnormally developing precancerous cells, for example, cervical dysplasia represents changes in the cells of the opening to the uterus that can become cancerous over a several-year span.

Dyspnea (disp nē′ə) is the medical term for breathlessness. The essential characteristic of dyspnea is that shortness of breath can occur without undue physical exertion. This is often a symptom of a disorder.

See also BREATHLESSNESS.

Dystrophy (dis′trə fē) refers to a wasting condition caused by improper nutrition. The word dystrophy is, however, used in some medical terms, for example, muscular dystrophy, in which the wasting condition is not due to nutritional problems.

Dysuria (dis yu̇r′ē ə) is painful or difficult urination. It is a symptom of various disorders, including cystitis, prostatitis, urethritis, stones in the bladder, or gonorrhea or other sexually transmitted diseases. Rarely, it is caused by cancer of the cervix in women or pelvic peritonitis. Any person with dysuria should consult a physician, so that the precise cause can be diagnosed and treated.

See also BLADDER DISORDERS.

E

Ear is the organ of hearing and balance. It consists of a series of sensitive structures that detect sounds and create impulses in the auditory nerve leading to the hearing center in the brain. The ear is divided into three sections: (1) the outer ear; (2) the middle ear; and (3) the inner ear.

Q: *What is the function of the outer ear?*

A: The outer ear has two main parts: the visible, curved flap on the outside of the head, called the auricle or pinna, and the auditory canal. The funnel-shaped auricle picks up sound waves and passes them along the auditory canal to the middle ear. In the outer third of its length, the auditory canal has a lining of fine hairs and a number of glands that secrete wax (cerumen). The hairs and the cerumen protect the ear's delicate structures by collecting much of the foreign matter that routinely enters the canal.

Q: *How does the middle ear function?*

A: The middle ear is separated from the outer ear by the eardrum, or tympanic membrane. As sound waves vibrate the eardrum, they set up vibrations in three tiny bones (ossicles) in the middle ear; the bones are called the hammer (malleus), anvil (incus), and stirrup (stapes). The auditory ossicles intensify and pass on the vibrations

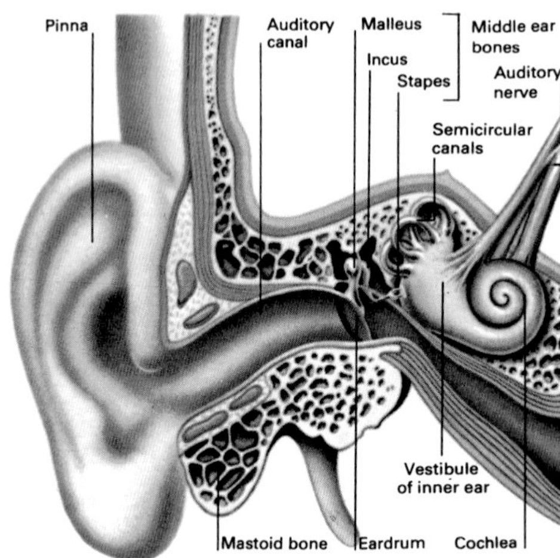

Sounds received by the ear's pinna pass along the auditory canal to the eardrum. Vibrations are carried by three bones to the cochlea, from which nerve impulses are sent to the brain.

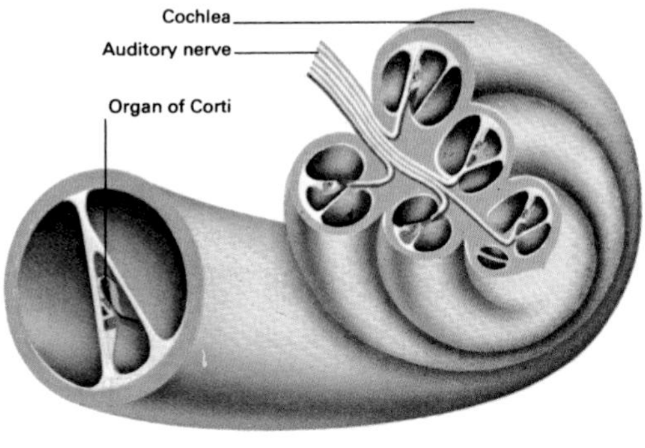

The spiral cochlea is divided internally into three compartments. In the central section is the organ of Corti, with hairs that vibrate in response to sounds. This creates nerve impulses that travel to the brain for analysis.

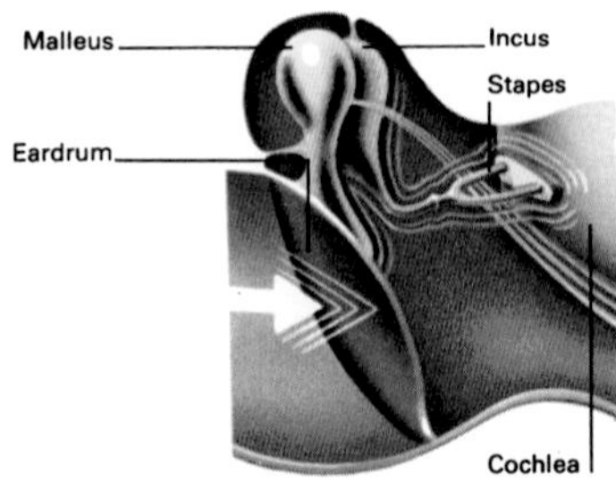

The malleus, incus, and stapes bones of the middle ear amplify sound waves and carry them to the cochlea.

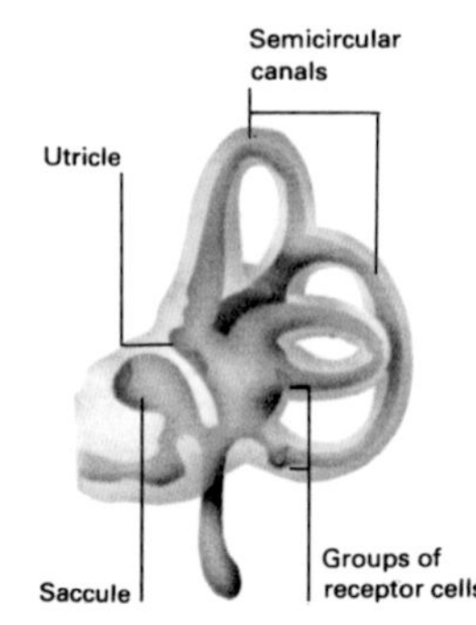

The semicircular canals detect body movement in three planes as the fluid they contain stimulates receptor cells. Utricle and saccule register the position of the head.

to a membrane of the inner ear called the oval window.

Pressure in the middle ear is kept equal to outside atmospheric pressure, allowing the eardrum to vibrate, by means of the Eustachian tube, which connects the middle ear with the back of the throat (pharynx). Two small muscles join the ossicles to the surrounding bone. These muscles contract in reaction to loud noises and protect the inner ear by limiting its vibration.

Q: *How does the inner ear function as an organ of hearing?*

A: The inner ear, or cochlea, is a tube that is coiled like a snail's shell and is filled with fluid. It contains the organ of Corti. Vibrations of the oval window activate the nerve endings within the organ of Corti causing impulses to pass along the auditory nerve to the hearing center in the brain, where sound is registered and interpreted.

Earache (ir'āk) is a variable and often intense throbbing pain deep inside the ear. Normally, atmospheric air pressure inside the middle ear is maintained by a channel (Eustachian tube) that connects with the back of the throat. If this tube becomes blocked during a respiratory infection, a build-up of pressure in the middle ear affects the sensitive eardrum and causes pain. Sudden changes in atmospheric pressure (for example, when flying or diving) can cause a similar condition—barotrauma—in the middle ear.

Inflammation in the outer ear (for example, a boil) also causes pain because the lining adheres tightly to the underlying bone.

Pain may be referred to the ear from disorders elsewhere in the body, for example, the neck, the pharynx, or the sinuses.

Q: *Can infection spread to the ear from other parts of the body and cause earache?*

A: Yes. Infection can spread from the throat along the Eustachian tube to the middle ear. The eardrum becomes inflamed from the inside, and pus forms. The pressure of the pus may be enough to burst the eardrum, in which case there is a discharge from the outer ear. The infection can also spread to the mastoid portion of the ear (temporal) bone just behind the outer ear or, in the most serious cases, through the bone to the brain. Infection of the middle ear is referred to as otitis media.

Q: *What conditions affecting the outer ear can cause earache?*

A: Accumulated wax that becomes hardened and is manipulated against the skin of the ear canal can irritate the auditory canal and cause earache. The most common reason for accumulation of ear wax is compression of wax into the ear by the use of cotton swabs. Cotton swabs should be used to clean the outer surface of the ear; they should never be pushed into the ear canal. If particles lodge in the outer ear, interference with the auditory canal may cause pain. Skin infections, such as boils, and inflammations resulting from swimming, cuts, or bruises can also sometimes cause earache.

Q: *How is earache treated?*

A: Because of potential damage to the ear, if an earache persists, a physician should be consulted. Until the cause is determined, little can be done other than to take pain-killing drugs. Middle ear disorders are treated with antibiotics, decongestant nasal drops, or antihistamines. Occasionally, surgical opening of the ear drum is necessary. Infections in the outer ear are treated with antibiotic eardrops. Any foreign object or lump of hardened wax in the outer ear should be removed by a physician.

See also BAROTRAUMA; EAR CARE; EAR DROPS: ADMINISTRATION; OTITIS.

Ear care. Part of your daily cleanliness routine should be careful cleaning of the outer part of the ear (pinna) to remove wax secreted by glands in the ear canal. Wipe a clean, damp washcloth around the outside contours of the ear as well as behind it. Never try to reach the wax in the invisible, deeper part of the ear with a cotton swab or a finger; you could push the wax deeper into the ear canal. Once this has happened, the wax, which usually moves along the canal to the outside and flakes off, hardens to a dark orange lump that irritates the wall of the ear canal and

Proper **ear care** includes protection against loud noises. Permanent deafness can occur from exposure to noise at levels of over 125 decibels (dB). Temporary deafness is likely at levels over 85 decibels.

Jet taking off 30 yards (27m)	140dB
Permanent deafness likely	125dB
Pneumatic jackhammer 2 yards (1.8m)	100dB
Inside subway train	90dB
Temporary deafness likely	85dB
Busy restaurant	65dB
Rustling leaves	20dB

causes the skin to peel. The build-up can completely cover the eardrum and cause temporary deafness. The plug then has to be removed by a physician.

Wax also tends to trap water in the canal after swimming or washing the hair. This may cause temporary deafness. Tip your head to one side and gently pull the external ear forward. The water can then flow out of the ear.

Protection from Injury. The eardrum is vulnerable to many kinds of injury that can result in partial or even total deafness. Never strike an adult or child across the ear; this can force air down the canal and burst the drum.

The ear can also be injured by high levels of noise. Loudness is measured in decibels. Exposure to noise at a level of more than 85 decibels causes temporary impairment of hearing. Continued exposure causes increasing, irreversible deafness. The first symptom of noise damage is a buzzing or ringing in the ears when the noise stops. The buzzing may take days to subside. This can happen in discothèques, if you are part of a band, or if you work in noisy surroundings.

Because of these dangers, if you work around high-level noise—for example, jet engine maintenance—you must protect your hearing with plugs or ear guards.

If you have a perforated eardrum, do not allow water or other foreign materials to enter the ear canal. Use airtight earplugs for bathing. Do *not* use eardrops unless prescribed by a physician.

Ear Infections. Ear infections need prompt medical treatment. Whenever you have an acute earache, consult your physician.

Infection can enter the ear when you are swimming or diving, particularly in hot climates. It is a sensible precaution to wear earplugs when swimming. A boil in the ear canal is extremely painful because the surrounding tissues are tight. Never squeeze the boil, but see a physician immediately.

Foreign Bodies. It is not uncommon for a child to push a bead or any other small toy into the ear. It is most important that parents never try to remove the foreign body. This must be done by an expert. Similarly, should an insect get lodged in the ear, see a physician.

Nose Blowing. An infection of either the nose or the throat can easily reach the ear and cause a painful infection of the middle ear (otitis media). The chance of the infection spreading can be reduced by carefully blowing the nose. If the nose is blown violently, mucus can move up the Eustachian tube to the middle ear. Blow your nose gently, and make sure the nostrils are open before you begin to blow.

The Eustachian Tube. The purpose of the Eustachian tube is to maintain an equal pressure on each side of the eardrum. Sometimes, an upper respiratory tract infection can block the Eustachian tube and cause temporary deafness.

A blocked Eustachian tube can usually be cleared by swallowing and gritting the back teeth at the same time. If the block lasts for more than a few hours, medical attention should be sought. The situation is potentially dangerous because any sudden change in pressure can rupture the eardrum.

Q: *How does the ear act as an organ of balance?*

A: The inner ear also contains three fluid-filled loops, called semicircular canals, set at right angles to one another. Any movement of the head affects the fluid in one or more of them. The ends of the canals contain receptor cells that register movements of the fluid and pass the information to the brain.

The whole system of canals and cavities in the inner ear is called the labyrinth. Disease or injury that causes malfunction of the labyrinth will cause vertigo, a sensation that the individual or the environment is spinning.

Another area of the inner ear, the saccule and utricle, contains sensitive cells with fine hairs that include small "stones" (otoliths) of calcium carbonate. When the head is held upright, the otoliths press on certain receptors. If the head is moved, the otoliths press on other receptors. In this way, receptors register any position of the head and pass this information to the brain. The sense of balance comes from a combination of movement and position of the head.

See also BALANCE; EAR CARE; EAR DISORDERS; VERTIGO.

Ear disorders. The following table lists some of the disorders that affect the ear and the basic characteristics of each disorder. Each disorder has a separate article in this encyclopedia.

Disorder	*Basic characteristics*
Boil (inside and outside the ear)	Abscesses, causing pain and diminished hearing
Deafness	Near or total loss of hearing
Earwax	Impaired hearing, tinnitus, pain
Labyrinthitis	Inflammation of inner ear, resulting in balance disturbances and sometimes hearing loss
Mastoiditis	Inflammation of the mastoid process
Ménière's disease	Severe episodes of vertigo, hearing loss, and ringing in the ear (tinnitus)
Otitis (externa, media, or interna)	Inflammation of outer, middle, or inner ear
Otomycosis	Fungus infection of auricle and/or auditory canal
Otorrhea	Discharge from the ear
Otosclerosis	Hereditary condition characterized by bone changes in inner ear, resulting in hearing loss
Tumor (in auditory canal, middle ear, or acoustic nerve)	Impaired hearing, deafness, balance disturbances and ear noises (tinnitus)
Vertigo	Spinning sensation

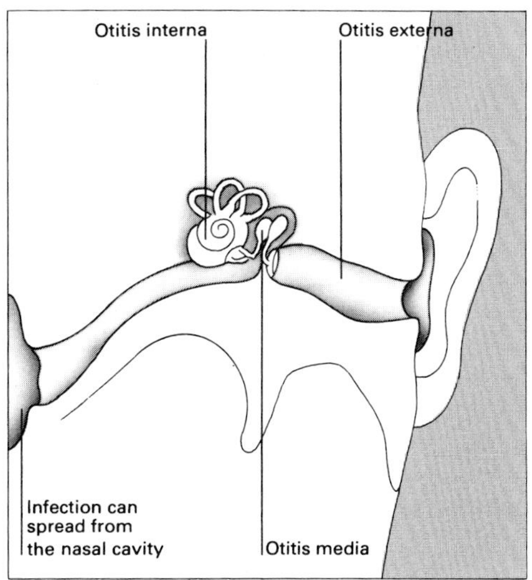

Ear disorders that cause inflammation (otitis) are classified according to the part of the ear affected. Otitis of the outer ear is called otitis externa; otitis of the middle ear is called otitis media; and otitis of the inner ear is called otitis interna.

The following table lists some general health disorders, that may cause ear problems, grouped according to symptom. The symptoms listed may also indicate other clinical disorders. A good medical history and physical examination by a physician are essential for adequate diagnosis of a problem.

Symptom	*Associated Disorders*
Auditory hallucinations	Drug addiction
	Narcolepsy
	Schizophrenia (and other mental disturbances)
Earache	Cold
	Ear, foreign body in
	Ear, water trapped in
	Gumboil
	Influenza
	Otitis (externa or media)
	Pharyngitis (sore throat)
	Pimple
	Sinusitis
	Teething in small children
	Tonsillitis
Impaired hearing/deafness	Tumor
	Congenital causes: rubella, certain drugs taken during

	pregnancy, and several hereditary syndromes
	Fluid behind eardrum due to otitis media
	Hemorrhage into inner ear caused by trauma
	Meningitis
	Syphilis
	Viruses causing influenza, mumps, measles, chickenpox, and mononucleosis
	Wax impaction
Outer ear skin problems	Carcinoma, basal cell
	Cyst, sebaceous
	Dermatitis
	Eczema
	Impetigo (aural)

See *also* EAR CARE.

Ear drops: administration. Unless the instructions on the ear-drop container state otherwise, warm the ear drops by placing the container in a bowl of warm water. Drops containing an antibiotic should not be heated. The patient should lie on his or her side with the head flat and the affected ear uppermost. Take hold of the earlobe and carefully pull it back to create as large an opening as possible. Draw up the medicine into the dropper. Rest the end of the dropper over the ear opening and allow the prescribed number of drops to trickle gently into the ear. Allow a few moments before placing a small plug of cotton in the outer ear to prevent the liquid from leaking out. The patient should continue to lie in this position for about five minutes.

If the eardrum is perforated or if a child has infection-preventing tubes in his or her ears, ear drops should not be used unless prescribed by a physician.

Eardrum, known medically as the tympanic membrane, is a layer of fibrous tissue and mucous membrane at the end of the auditory canal that separates the outer ear from the middle ear. It transmits sound vibrations to the inner ear through the auditory ossicles.

See *also* EAR; EAR DISORDERS.

Ear, foreign body in: treatment. Do not attempt to remove any foreign object from the ear, as this could cause serious damage. Lay the victim down with the affected ear facing up, and calm the victim. Obtain medical attention as soon as possible.

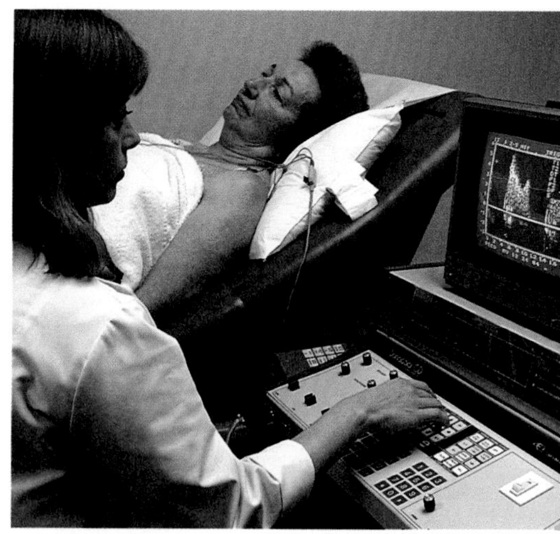

Echocardiogram, used in the diagnosis of heart disease, is a graphic recording of the echo produced when ultrtasonic sound waves are reflected from the heart.

Ear, ringing. See TINNITUS.

Earwax, or cerumen, is the fatty substance produced by special glands in the auditory canal to help protect the ear from potentially harmful organisms and other foreign matter that routinely enter the canal. Some people may experience some degree of hardened wax build-up in the ear. Hardened wax should be removed by a physician, but it can be softened through the administration of a warm solution of olive oil, bicarbonate of soda, or an over-the-counter solution for softening earwax. See EAR DROPS: ADMINISTRATION for proper administering technique.

ECG. See ELECTROCARDIOGRAM.

Echocardiogram (ek ō kär′dē ō gram) is a record of the echo produced when ultrasonic sound waves are reflected from the heart. Analysis of the echo pattern can aid diagnosis of heart disorders, such as fluid around the heart or abnormalities of the heart valves.

See *also* ULTRASOUND.

Echogram (ek′ō gram) is a record of the echo produced when ultrasonic sound waves are reflected from various body tissues. It is used to assess fetal conditions and to help diagnose problems such as tumors or gallstones.

See *also* ULTRASOUND.

Echolalia (ek ə lā′lē ə) is the meaningless repetition of words. In young children it may occur to some degree during the normal process of speech development. When it occurs in adults, it is usually a symptom of schizophrenia. It is most common in childhood schizophrenia and autism.

See *also* AUTISM; SCHIZOPHRENIA.

Eclampsia (ek lamp'sē ə) is a serious disease that occurs in women during the final four months of pregnancy or, much less commonly, after the delivery of the baby. Preeclampsia, the early stage of this disease, is relatively common, characterized by elevated blood pressure and protein in the urine. Rarely does preeclampsia develop into eclampsia, which is characterized by convulsions, hypertension (high blood pressure), and finally a coma, which may be fatal. The cause of eclampsia is not known. See *also* PREECLAMPSIA.

Preventive prenatal care, which includes a proper diet for the pregnant woman, is thought to decrease the likelihood of preeclampsia and, therefore, eclampsia.

Q: *What is the treatment for eclampsia?*

A: Immediate hospitalization is essential. Treatment varies, but drugs are commonly used to prevent further convulsions and to reduce blood pressure. If treatment appears to be failing, labor is induced immediately or a Cesarean section is performed.

See *also* TOXEMIA.

ECT. See ELECTROCONVULSIVE THERAPY.

Ecthyma (ek thī'mə) is an ulcerative adult form of the skin infection impetigo. Ecthyma frequently occurs on the legs and may result in scarring after the ulcers heal.

See *also* IMPETIGO.

Ectoderm (ek'tə dėrm) is the outer layer of cells of an embryo. Skin, hair, nails, teeth, the nervous system, and the sense organs all grow from the ectoderm.

See *also* ENDODERM; MESODERM.

Ectomorph (ek'tə môrf) is a person characterized by a body structure that is derived mostly from the ectoderm. Such a person is inclined to be relatively thin. It was once believed that an ectomorph is predisposed by heredity to be fragile and nervous.

The ectomorph is one of three hypothetical body types, first proposed around the turn of the century, to explain certain aspects of personality. The other two types are called endomorph and mesomorph. If the terms are used at all anymore, they are limited to describing a person's physical build without regard to that person's personality.

See *also* ECTODERM; ENDOMORPH; MESOMORPH.

-ectomy (ek'tə mē) is a combining form designating a surgical operation for removing a part of the body, for example, thyroidectomy, tonsillectomy, etc.

Ectopic beat (ek top'ik) is an abnormal heartbeat or an artificial stimulation of the heart. In the former, the heart begins a beat in a spot other than in the sinoatrial node in the right auricle, the heart's natural pacemaker near the point where the major veins enter the heart.

In the latter, the heart is electrically stimulated to start beating, also in a spot other than the sinoatrial node. This generally occurs with the use of an artificial pacemaker.

See *also* HEART.

Ectopic pregnancy. See PREGNANCY, ECTOPIC.

Ectropion (ek trō'pē ən) is the turning outward of an edge, most commonly the eversion of an eyelid so that it does not lie close to the surface of the eyeball. It may be caused by the atrophy of the lid muscles or, rarely, by damage to the facial nerve. The condition may also result from an infection of the eyelid. Ectropion is fairly common among elderly persons.

Q: *Can an ectropion be treated?*

A: Yes, in most cases the condition can be corrected through minor surgery.

Q: *Can ectropions affect any other parts of the body?*

A: Yes. If the uterine cervix is, for example, damaged during childbirth, the edges of the cervix may turn inside out.

See *also* ENTROPION.

Eczema (ek'sə mə) is a red, itchy, noncontagious inflammation of the skin. Eczema may be acute or chronic, with red skin patches, pimples, crusts, or scabs occurring either alone or in combination. The skin may be dry, or it may discharge a watery fluid, resulting in an itching or burning sensation. The affected skin may then become infected.

The various causes of eczema are classified as either external (irritations, allergic reactions, exposure to certain microorganisms, or chemicals) or constitutional (an inherited predisposition).

Q: *How is eczema treated?*

A: The treatment depends on the cause. For example, if eczema is an allergic reaction, the allergen must be identified and removed. Symptomatic treatment may include the use of ointments containing corticosteroids or lotions that dry up the discharging of fluids from the skin.

Edema (i dē'mə) is a localized or general swelling caused by the build-up of fluid within body tissues. Excess fluid may be a result of poor circulation of the blood; a failure of the lymphatic system to disperse the fluid; various diseases and disorders; or a combination of factors.

Other causes of edema include fluid retention caused by disease of the heart or kidneys or a reduction in the amount of protein in the blood, which may occur as a result of cirrhosis, chronic nephritis, malnutrition, or toxemia of pregnancy (preeclampsia). Localized edema may result from injury or infection.

Q: *How is edema treated?*

A: The treatment depends on the underlying cause of the edema. Diuretic drugs, which make the kidneys eliminate excess salt and water, often produce an immediate improvement. Edema caused by varicose veins or pregnancy can be prevented by wearing elastic stockings. Edema of the ankles may be helped by lying down with the feet raised.

EEG. *See* ELECTROENCEPHALOGRAM.

Effusion (i fyü'zhən) is the escape of fluid from blood or lymph vessels, so that it accumulates in closed body spaces. Effusion may be a symptom of a circulatory or kidney disorder. It is frequently a precursor of congestive heart disease. Effusions can occur around the lungs (pleural effusion), around the heart (pericardial effusion), or within a joint such as the knee.

See also EDEMA.

Egg is the common name for the female reproductive cell, the ovum.

See also OVUM.

Ego (ē'gō) is one of the three parts of the psyche (the self). It functions as a kind of mediator between the unconscious and instinctual part of the self (the id) and the moral and conscience-motivated part of the self (the superego). The ego acts as an agent of reason and consciousness, helping a person to process thoughts and feelings, to maintain a level of reality, and to cope with the demands of life.

Ejaculation (i jak yə lā'shən) is the discharge of semen at the height of orgasm from the male urethra, the tube connecting the sperm duct with the end of the penis.

See also PENIS.

Ejaculation, premature (i jak yə lā'shən, prē mə chůr'). Premature ejaculation is defined most commonly as an ejaculation, during sexual intercourse, that occurs before one or both partners want it to. Premature ejaculation is common when the sex act is a new experience. It is not considered a problem unless it persists beyond that stage.

Ejaculation may be effectively delayed by using either the "stop and start" method or the "squeeze" method. Using the stop and start method, the couple simply ceases any form of stimulation for approximately 30 seconds.

With the squeeze method, the female partner squeezes the coronal ridge of the penis for about 10 seconds. This causes a 10 to 25 percent loss of erection and decreases the male partner's sense of arousal.

If the problem persists, sex therapy, focusing on stimulation of other body areas, is usually successful in the treatment of premature ejaculation.

See also SEXUAL PROBLEMS.

Ejaculation, retrograde (i jak yə lā'shən, ret'rə grād). Retrograde ejaculation is the discharge of semen into the bladder rather than into the urethra and on to the outside. This condition usually occurs after prostatectomy, the removal of all or part of the prostate, the gland that secretes a lubricating substance used to transport sperm cells.

See also EJACULATION.

EKG. *See* ELECTROCARDIOGRAM.

Elation (i lā'shən) is a psychological term referring to an ecstatic, optimistic, excited, and self-satisfied state of mind—all out of accord with reality. Such a state of mind can be a prelude to the onset of mania or a manic-depressive illness. It may also reflect an already existing mania or manic-depressive illness.

Elation, when inappropriate to an individual's circumstances, may be a form of denial of psychological or physical problems. Depression often follows in such cases.

See also AFFECTIVE DISORDER; DEPRESSION; MANIC-DEPRESSIVE ILLNESS.

Elavil® (el'ə vil) is a preparation of amitriptyline hydrochloride, a tricyclic antidepressant. It is especially effective in treating depressed patients with sleep disorders. It is also being used in treating individuals with chronic pain or nerve injuries. For unknown reasons, Elavil appears far more effective in reducing discomfort in these patients than even narcotic analgesics.

See also ANTIDEPRESSANT, TRICYCLIC.

Elbow is a hinge joint between the lower end of the upper arm bone (humerus) and the upper end of the two bones of the lower arm (radius and ulna). Two muscles in the upper arm, the biceps and the triceps, control the action of the elbow. When the biceps contracts, the arm bends; when the triceps contracts, the arm straightens.

See also ELBOW INJURIES; FUNNY BONE.

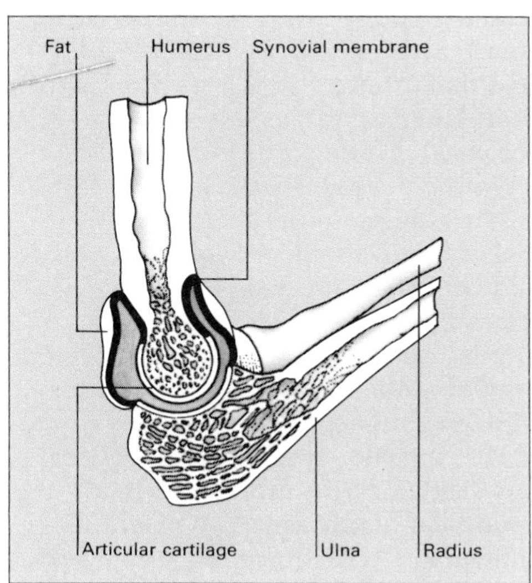

Elbow is the hinge joint that allows the upper and lower arms to move in relation to each other.

Elbow fracture: first aid. See FRACTURE: FIRST AID.

Elbow injuries are disorders that affect the elbow as a result of trauma. Common elbow injuries include fractures, which may be caused by the severe trauma resulting from a collision, and dislocations, which may be caused by falling on an outstretched hand. Like other joints, the elbow is also vulnerable to sprains, twists, and torn ligaments. *See also* ELBOW, TENNIS.

Q: *What complications might result from a fracture?*

A: The chief risk with an elbow fracture is that the main artery supplying the forearm and hand may become blocked by pressure from the broken bone. This blockage may stop the blood flow and thereby destroy the muscles that the artery supplies. For this reason the pulse should always be checked at the wrist immediately after the accident. If the pulse is absent, urgent hospital attention is needed. Temporary paralysis may result if there is pressure on nerves.

If a fracture sets badly, friction of the ulnar nerve on the back of the bones of the elbow may cause tingling in the forearm and in the fourth (ring) and fifth (little) fingers of the hand. Muscles in the hand may also become weak. If the symptoms are severe, surgical repositioning of the nerve to the front of the elbow may be necessary.

Q: *What is ankylosis, or "locked elbow"?*

A: The bones of the elbow or surrounding muscle fibers join together, resulting in a stiffening of the joint. "Locked elbow" may occur after infection or inflammation of the tissues surrounding the elbow joint. It is a difficult condition to treat. Mobility in the joint is often restored by heat therapy, exercise, and manipulation.

Q: *Why does an elbow become inflamed?*

A: Inflammation of the elbow can be a form of bursitis, in which the fluid-filled sac (bursa) surrounding the joint becomes swollen. This may be the result of injury, or it may be a symptom of such conditions as gout or rheumatoid arthritis. "Students' elbow" (olecranon bursitis) is inflammation of the bursa at the elbow, caused by constant rubbing on a flat surface, such as a desk or table. If the bursa becomes infected, a physician may prescribe antibiotic drugs.

Elbow, tennis. Tennis elbow is a strain in the ligaments of the forearm near the elbow, caused by repeated stress, particularly stress produced by sudden twisting movements. It is called tennis elbow because it often results from playing tennis, though it can also be caused by other types of activity.

Q: *What are the symptoms of tennis elbow?*

A: Pain and tenderness on the outer, bony part of the elbow, often accompanied by aching in the muscles of the outer side of the forearm, are the usual symptoms.

Q: *How is tennis elbow treated?*

A: Treatment may not be needed in mild cases. Temporary reduction of the aggravating activity is often sufficient to alleviate the problem. If pain persists or becomes worse, anti-inflammatory medications and application of a heating pad may help. If these fail, injections of corticosteroid drugs may be effective.

Electra complex (i lek'trə), according to Freudian theory, refers to a young girl's possessive love for her father. Due to the fear of punishment, the entire conflict is repressed into the unconscious during the phallic stage of psychosexual development. This dilemma is then successfully resolved through identification with the mother, from whom the young girl learns much of her value system. Through this learning of moral values, the superego is developed. The analogous male version is the Oedipus complex.

See also OEDIPUS COMPLEX; SUPEREGO.

Electric shock: first aid. Electric shock is a traumatic state caused by the passage of electric current through the body. The kind and amount of damage depends on the intensity, type, and duration of the current; the point where the electricity first touched the body; and the path it took through the body. Burns may be superficial or very deep with widespread tissue death. Severe shock may cause muscle contractions, respiratory paralysis, unconsciousness, and cardiac arrest. A high-voltage electric shock may cause a sudden muscle spasm that may throw the victim away from the power source with extreme force, resulting in further injuries, such as a fracture. Lightning causes injuries similar to those sustained from a high-voltage electric shock.

Action. Do not attempt to rescue the victim if he or she is still in contact with, or is close to, a high-voltage electric current, such as a live wire lying near or on the victim. Insulating material, such as rubber or dry wood, will not protect you against such high voltages. Summon the police and emergency medical aid. Remain at least 60 feet (18m) from the victim, and wait until being officially informed that it is safe before giving any first aid.

If the victim is in contact with a low-voltage current, such as most domestic power supplies, then it is generally safe to attempt to rescue the victim provided the correct precautions are taken. Summon emergency medical aid even if you decide to attempt a rescue. Examine the victim for injuries and give appropriate first-aid treatment.

If the victim is unconscious, *see* FAINTING: FIRST AID. If there is any serious bleeding, *see* BLEEDING: FIRST AID. To treat any burns, *see* BURNS AND SCALDS: FIRST AID.

Electric shock therapy. *See* ELECTROCONVULSIVE THERAPY.

Electrocardiogram (i lek trō kär'dē ə gram), EKG or ECG, is a record of the electric currents that the heart uses to stimulate its muscles during every heartbeat. These currents normally progress in a regular and orderly fashion, beginning in the natural pacemaker found in the right auricle; this is known as the sinoatrial node. The EKG traces the current as it passes down through the atria, through the atrio-ventricular node, and then through a specialized conduction system (the bundle of His) into the muscles of the ventricles. The electric currents are monitored by a highly sensitive machine known as an electrocardiograph. (See page 454 for a sample EKG.)

Q: *How is an electrocardiogram obtained?*

A: Electrodes (small metal plates) are placed against the patient's skin at both wrists and ankles. Six or more electrodes are placed in a specific pattern on the patient's chest over the heart. A combination of different impulses picked up by the electrodes produces the electrocardiogram. These elec-

First aid for electric shock

1 *Do not* touch a victim who is still in contact with a high-voltage electric current. Summon the police and emergency medical aid. If the victim is in contact with a low-voltage current (household power supply), cut off the current. If this is impossible, stand on some dry insulating material (wood or newspaper). Break the electrical contact using dry wood, rubber or plastic, or newspaper.

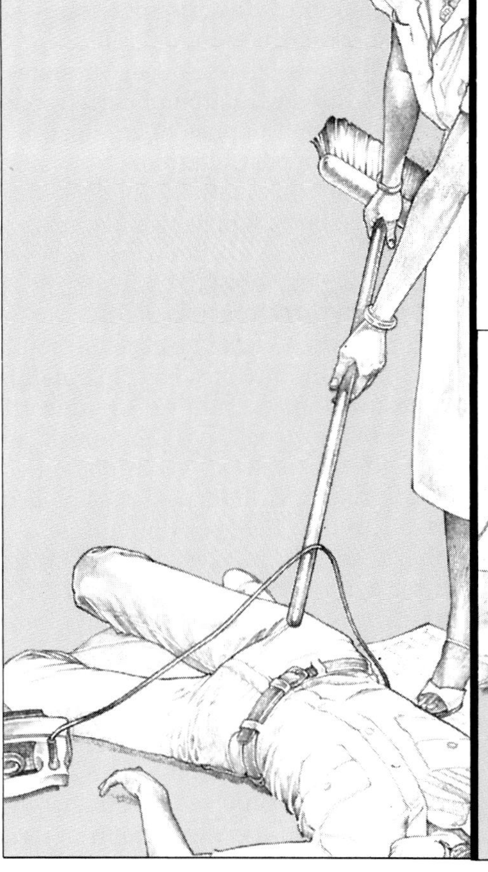

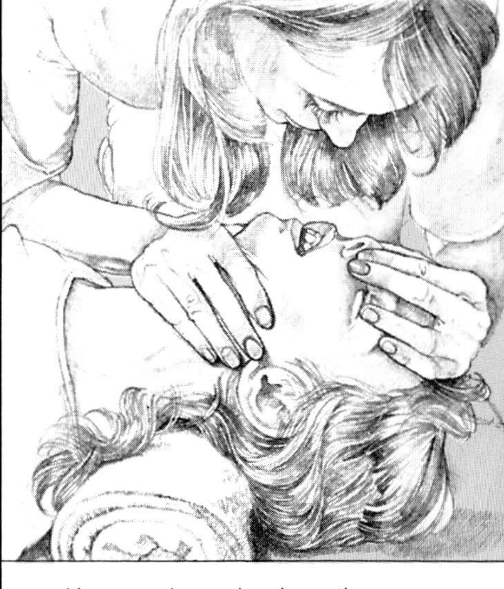

2 Keep a close check on the victim's breathing and heartbeat. If he or she is not breathing, give artificial respiration. *See* ARTIFICIAL RESPIRATION.

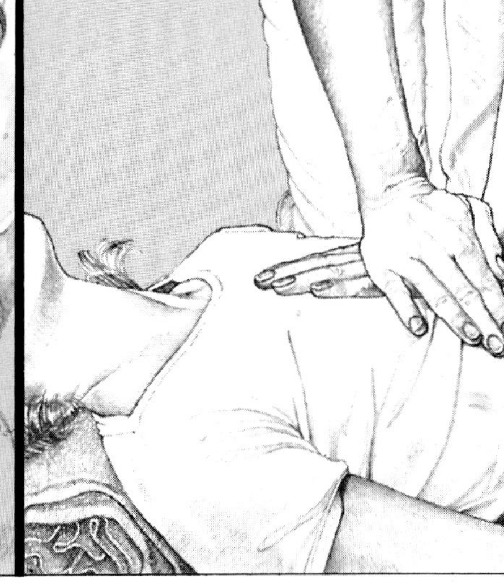

3 If the victim's heart has stoppe(give external cardiac massage. *See* HEART ATTACK: FIRST AID. If tł victim has also stopped breathing and help is unavailable, alternate between external cardiac massage and mouth-to-mouth resuscitation.

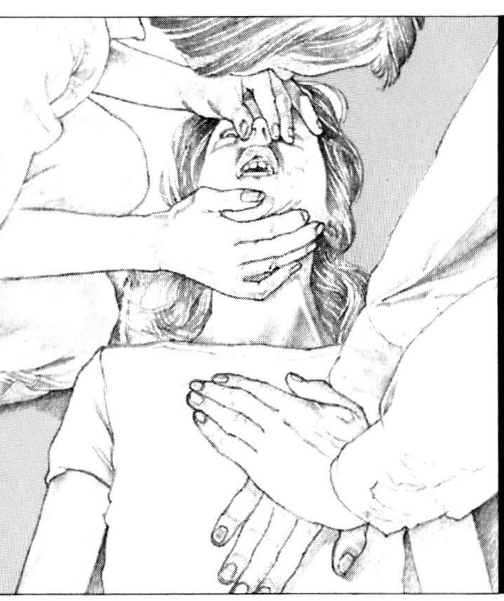

4 If the victim's heart and breathing have both stopped and help is available, one person should kneel at the victim's left shoulder, giving cardiac massage, while another kneels at the right side, giving mouth-to-mouth resuscitation.

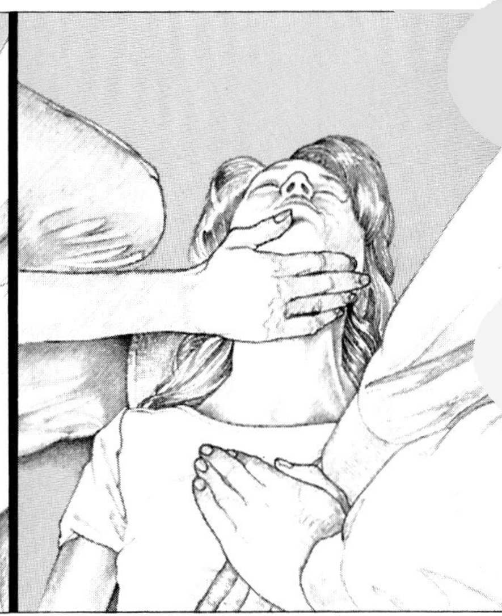

5 The person giving cardiac massage should press the victim's chest over the area of the heart at a rate slightly fasteı than once a second. The perso giving artificial resuscitation should ventilate the victim's lungs once every five seconds.

trodes allow the physician to evaluate the flow of electric current in several different directions.

Q: *What is the purpose of an electrocardiogram?*

A: A study of the recording assists a physician in the diagnosis of certain heart disorders. The EKG of a healthy person makes a certain pattern. Heart damage or disease changes this pattern in identifiable ways. Changes are usually due to lack of oxygen supply to certain areas of the heart; past heart attack; or irregular rhythms.

See *also* ARRHYTHMIA; HEART ATTACK; HEART DISEASE.

Electroconvulsive therapy (i lek trō kən vul′siv), or ECT, is the passage of an electric current through the brain to induce alterations in the brain's electrical activity. It is sometimes called either shock or electroshock therapy. ECT is sometimes used to treat major acute or chronic depression, but it is increasingly being replaced by drug therapy. When an ECT is applied, muscle-relaxant drugs are used to prevent injury to the patient during the convulsion that follows the electroshock; a general anesthetic is also normally applied so that the patient does not perceive the seizure. Recent advances in ECT, including the use of lower voltages and the application of the shock to only one side of the brain, have made ECT both safer and more effective.

See *also* DEPRESSION.

Electrocution (i lek trə kyü′shən) is the execution or accidental death of an individual caused by the passage of a high-voltage of electric current through the body.

Electrode (i lek′trōd) is either of the two terminals of a battery or any other source of electricity. It may also be a conductor by which a current is brought into a liquid or a gas.

Electroencephalogram (i lek trō en sef′ə lə gram), or EEG, is a record of the electrical activity in the brain. It takes the form of irregular lines traced on a moving strip of paper. The instrument that monitors the brain's electrical activity is known as an electroencephalograph.

Q: *How is an electroencephalogram obtained?*

A: Electrodes are attached to the patient's scalp, and the difference in electrical potential between two sites on the skull is monitored. Changes in the usual brain rhythms are recorded during rest, sleep, and during mental concentration. It is a safe and painless procedure.

Q: *What is the purpose of an electroencephalogram?*

A: The test assists physicians in the diagnosis of epilepsy and in the identification of sites of tumors or lesions in the brain. An EEG is also used in the definition of clinical death when a patient has been kept alive by artificial means. When no electrical activity is recorded for a legally determined amount of time, brain death is said to have occurred.

Electrolysis (i lek trol′ə sis), in medicine, is the destruction of certain body tissue through the use of an electric current. It is possible to destroy hair follicles by this method. In electrolysis, excessive body hair is usually removed through the use of an electric needle.

See *also* HIRSUTISM.

Electromyogram (i lek trō mī′ə gram) is a recording of the electrical impulses produced by the muscles. One method of measuring an impulse is by inserting a needle electrode into the muscle and monitoring electrical variations on an oscilloscope. A loudspeaker may also be utilized to listen to the muscle. A physician uses an electromyogram in the diagnosis of muscle disorders and to identify the specific location of any nerve problems or damage.

Electron microscope (i lek′tron mī′krə skōp) is a microscope that uses a beam of electrons instead of light rays to magnify objects. With a light microscope one can only see specimens that are larger than the wavelength of light, which is about 5,000 angstroms. (One angstrom is one ten-millionth of a millimeter.) With an electron microscope a beam of electrons is passed through the specimen under study, and a two-dimensional image is recorded on a fluorescent screen, a photographic plate, or a television screen.

Since electrons have wavelengths a fraction of an angstrom long, images of bacteria, viruses, and even atoms are made visible for diagnosis.

Electron microscopy (i lek'tron mī kros'kə pē) is a technique utilizing the electron microscope to produce images of specimens 1,000 times greater than those produced with light microscopy.

See also ELECTRON MICROSCOPE.

Electronystagmogram (i lek trō nī stag'mə gram) is a measurement of the electric activity of extraocular muscles, those which move the eyeball. The purpose is to evaluate and record eye movements, such as those movements that occur with vertigo.

See also EYE; VERTIGO.

Elephantiasis (el ə fan tī'ə sis) is a chronic condition characterized by gross swelling of the skin and underlying tissues. The legs and external genitalia are most commonly affected. The first symptoms are periodic attacks of painful skin inflammation (dermatitis) accompanied by fever; the skin surface may become ulcerated and discolored.

Q: *What causes elephantiasis?*

A: Elephantiasis, which occurs most commonly in tropic and subtropic countries, is caused by an infestation of the lymph channels by the filarial worm *Wuchereria bancrofti* or *Brugia malayi*. The worm enters the body through the bite of an infected mosquito. If the infestation is not successfully treated, the lymph vessels that normally drain fluid away from the tissues become obstructed after many years, and elephantiasis results.

Q: *Is there any treatment for elephantiasis?*

A: Drugs poisonous to the filarial worm are available. Treatment for swelling of the lymph vessels (lymphedema) depends on severity. Mild cases of elephantiasis in the legs may require only rest with the legs raised, an elastic stocking, and scrupulous foot care to prevent further infections. Elephantiasis of other parts of the body may require surgery.

See also DERMATITIS; FILARIASIS.

Ellipsoid joint. See JOINT.

Embolism (em'bə liz əm) is an obstruction of an artery, or less commonly, a vein, by material that has been carried there in the bloodstream. This material is called an embolus and may be a blood clot (thrombus), a clump of cancer cells, fat globules from the site of a broken bone (fat embolus), infected tissue from an abscess, or an air bubble (air embolus). *See also* THROMBUS.

Q: *What are the symptoms of an embolism?*

A: If the embolus is small, there may be no immediate symptoms. A large embolus can totally obstruct a blood vessel, and the area of tissue supplied by it dies. If this occurs in the heart, the patient suffers myocardial infarction. An obstructed vessel in the brain causes a stroke. If an embolus blocks the femoral artery, the patient experiences acute cramp-like pain in the leg, which quickly becomes white and cold. An embolus in the lung (pulmonary embolism) produces symptoms similar to those of coronary thrombosis: severe pain, shock, collapse, and the coughing of bloodstained mucus. An embolus in the kidney causes hematuria (bloody urine). *See also* HEART DISEASE, CORONARY; HEMATURIA; INFARCTION; STROKE.

Q: *How can an embolism be treated?*

A: Treatment depends on the size, nature, and location of the embolus. Severe obstructions, such as those occurring with pulmonary embolism, require emergency hospital treatment. The patient is treated for shock and given oxygen and anticoagulant drugs. Sometimes, surgery (embolectomy) is performed, particularly if the embolus is in an artery of the arm or leg.

Embryo (em'brē ō) is the developing organism from implantation of the fertilized egg (ovum) about two weeks after conception until the end of the second month of pregnancy.

See also FETUS; PREGNANCY AND CHILDBIRTH; REPRODUCTION, HUMAN.

Emergency delivery. See CHILDBIRTH: EMERGENCY DELIVERY.

Emergency room. See HOSPITAL.

Emergency treatment. See FIRST-AID FUNDAMENTALS.

Emetic (i met'ik) is a substance that induces vomiting. There are two kinds of emetics: one works by irritating the stomach, for example, common salt or syrup of ipecac; the other type stimulates a reflex center in the brain when injected intravenously, for example, the drug apomorphine.

Emetics are used in the emergency treatment of certain types of poisoning and drug overdoses; emetics can cause complications if they are not vomited. A poison control center should always be contacted prior to administering an emetic, as vomiting of some poisons can be dangerous.

See also POISONING: FIRST AID.

EMG. *See* ELECTROMYOGRAM.

Emphysema (em fə sē'mə) is the pathological stretching of body tissue due to the accumulation of gas or air in the tissue or organ. Pulmonary emphysema is a chronic lung disease in which the air sacs (alveoli) of the lung degenerate until the elastic fibers in them are destroyed. This leads to a decrease in lung elasticity, resulting in the accumulation of some carbon dioxide in the lungs after each exhalation. The victim must, therefore, breathe harder to expel carbon dioxide from the lungs and to pull oxygen into the lungs.

More than two million Americans suffer from emphysema; most are white males over the age of 40. When emphysema occurs early in life, it is usually associated with a rare genetic deficiency that limits lung elasticity; cigarette smoking is, however, by far the most common cause of the condition. Emphysema and other chronic obstructive pulmonary diseases are major causes of death in the United States.

Q: *What are the symptoms of pulmonary emphysema?*

A: There is gradually increasing breathlessness during exercise, and the chest moves less easily than normal, producing a constricted feeling. There may also be frequent bouts of coughing and production of sputum. The patient feels generally unwell.

Q: *What causes pulmonary emphysema?*

A: Emphysema is often seen in an advanced stage of chronic bronchitis, a lung disorder often caused by cigarette smoking. Emphysema may also follow asthma or tuberculosis, two conditions that also damage alveolar walls. Heavily polluted air and prolonged exposure to certain dusts, for example, coal dust, aggravate respiratory disorders and can lead to emphysema.

Q: *How is pulmonary emphysema treated?*

A: There is no cure for emphysema. The only effective method of dealing with the condition is to avoid smoking and to treat any diseases that precede the illness. Once emphysema develops, treatment is directed toward preventing further lung damage. Affected persons should stop smoking, make sure that all respiratory infections receive immediate medical attention, and perform breathing exercises to clear any mucus from the lungs. The patient should stay as active as possible but avoid overexertion. Persons with severe emphysema may require oxygen equipment and a respirator at home.

See also BLACK LUNG; SMOKING OF TOBACCO.

Empirin with codeine® (em'per in with kō'dēn) is a prescription preparation of aspirin and codeine. It is primarily used as a pain reliever, but because it contains aspirin, the preparation also has fever-reducing and anti-inflammatory properties.

Q: *Does Empirin with codeine produce any adverse effects?*

A: Yes. It can cause nausea, vomiting, pain, and bleeding from the stomach. For this reason, Empirin with codeine should not be taken by those with any stomach disorder. It can produce an allergic reaction, such as a skin rash, in those sensitive to either aspirin or codeine. Empirin with codeine may increase blood clotting time, so it should not be used by hemophiliacs or by those taking anticoagulant drugs. It can also cause sweating, dizziness, swelling of the throat, and hives. Large doses can produce ringing in the ears (tinnitus) and mental confusion. Prolonged use can cause kidney and liver damage, anemia, and drug dependence. Empirin with codeine should not be used by those with impaired kidney or liver functioning, those with respiratory disorders, such as bronchitis, or those suffering from anemia. Some persons prefer to use an alternative preparation that combines codeine and acetaminophen.

See also ACETAMINOPHEN; TINNITUS.

Empyema (em pē ē′mə) is the accumulation of pus in a body cavity, usually the pleural cavity between the lung and the chest wall. It generally occurs because of a secondary bacterial infection that accompanies a lung disorder, for example, pneumonia or pleurisy. Infection may also come from the outside, for example, as the result of a stab wound. The symptoms of empyema include fever and sweating, other serious illness, chest pain, and cough.

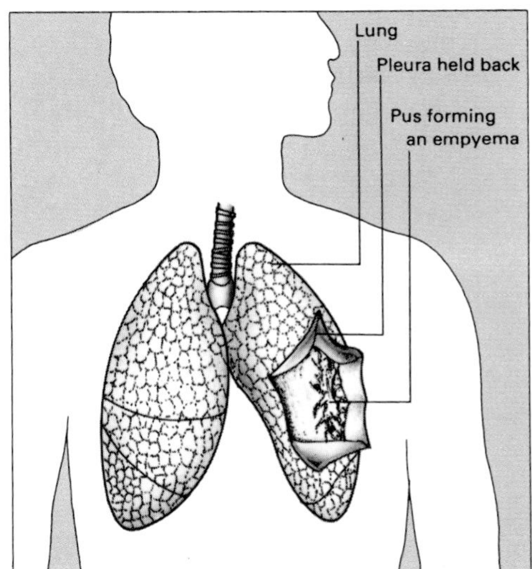

Empyema is a collection of pus in a body cavity, usually between the pleura and the lung tissue.

Q: *How is empyema treated?*

A: The pus must be removed. This can be done either by sucking it out through a hollow needle (aspiration) or by a surgical operation to remove part of a rib and drain the pus away through a tube. Antibiotic drugs are prescribed to combat the infection, and the underlying cause is treated at the same time.

Enamel. See TOOTH.

Encephalitis (en sef ə lī′tis) is an inflammation of the brain, usually caused by a viral infection, but also occasionally caused by other organisms. Encephalitis viruses are often transmitted by various carriers, such as ticks and mosquitoes; this form of the disease is more common in tropical climates. Encephalitis can also occur as a complication of virus infections, for example, mumps, measles, herpes simplex, chickenpox, rabies, and some of the *Coxsackie* viruses. Lead poisoning and allergic reactions may also lead to encephalitis. *See also* COXSACKIE.

Q: *What are the symptoms of encephalitis?*

A: Headaches, high fever, and vomiting are early symptoms. The patient's mental state varies from irritability and lethargy to confusion, delirium, convulsions, and, in severe cases, coma. The severity of the symptoms depends on the age of the victim and the type of virus infection. Diagnosis of encephalitis is made by blood tests, electroencephalogram, lumbar puncture (spinal tap), and (on occasion) brain biopsy.

Q: *How is encephalitis treated?*

A: If the encephalitis is traced to a bacterial infection, antibiotic drugs are effective. The number of deaths and neurologic aftereffects from herpes simplex encephalitis have been reduced by early intravenous treatment with vidarabine. However, encephalitis caused by most viruses has no specific treatment. Particular attention is paid to supportive care: a respirator may be used if the patient has difficulty breathing due to coma; fluids are given intravenously if the patient is unable to drink. If encephalitis is the result of a tumor or abscess in the brain, surgery is necessary to treat it. Despite the lack of specific treatments for encephalitis, many severely ill patients recover completely.

Encephalocele (en sef′ə lə sēl) is a hernia of the brain, a protrusion of a portion of the brain through the cranium. This may occur in newborn infants.

See also BRAIN DISORDERS.

Encephalomyelitis (en sef ə lō mī ə lī′təs) is a disease closely related to encephalitis, which is an acute inflammatory disease of the brain. Encephalomyelitis is the same acute inflammatory disease, but it affects both the brain and the spinal cord. Damage is chiefly to the white matter of the brain and spinal cord. Causes, symptoms, treatment, and prognosis are the same as for encephalitis.

See also ENCEPHALITIS.

Encephalopathy (en sef ə lop′ə thē) is the general name for any dysfunction of the brain tissues.

See also BRAIN DISORDERS.

Encopresis (en kō prē′sis) is the involuntary passage of fecal matter. The term is used only in reference to older children and adults. It does not refer to defecation in the infant or small child who is not yet toilet trained.

See also DIARRHEA; ENURESIS.

Endemic (en dem′ik) refers to a disease or microorganism that is indigenous to a region or population.

See also EPIDEMIC; PANDEMIC.

Endocarditis (en dō kär dī′tis) is inflammation of the endocardium, the inner lining of the heart. The area most commonly affected is the lining of the heart valves; the membrane lining the heart's chambers is also sometimes affected. Bacteria are the usual cause of the inflammation and reach a deformed heart valve from the blood stream. Therefore, the risk of bacterial endocarditis is greatly increased if there is a congenital heart deformity or if the valves have been damaged by rheumatic fever. Severe inflammation or rapid onset of the disease is called acute bacterial endocarditis. Subacute bacterial endocarditis, which has a slower onset of the disorder, is far more common. If untreated, all types of endocarditis are fatal. However, with proper treatment, about 75 percent of all patients survive.

Q: *How does the infection enter the bloodstream?*

A: The bacteria may enter the bloodstream following either surgery or the extraction of an infected tooth. Bacteria may also be released into the bloodstream following a tonsillectomy or via the uterus of a woman shortly after the delivery of a baby. Endocarditis may also result following an infection caused by blood poisoning, such as can occur from intravenous drug use.

Persons with a history of rheumatic or congenital heart disease should take antibiotic drugs just prior to visiting a dentist or before any surgical procedure. The dentist or surgeon should be informed. A course of antibiotics may be prescribed after the surgery.

Q: *What are the symptoms of endocarditis?*

A: Symptoms begin gradually with fatigue, chills, aching joints, and intermittent fever. If the condition is not diagnosed at this stage, increasing pallor due to progressive anemia and loss of appetite follow. Small blood spots may appear on the skin and under the nails, caused by infected clots (emboli) that have broken away from the site of the heart infection. *See also* EMBOLISM.

Q: *How is endocarditis treated?*

A: If endocarditis is suspected, hospitalization is necessary, and treatment with large doses of antibiotics is continued for at least six weeks. Penicillin is the antibiotic most commonly used, until a more specific one is selected after tests. Bed rest is an essential part of treatment. The patient may be given a blood transfusion if anemia is severe. Medical care should continue for several years.

Endocarditis, bacterial. *See* ENDOCARDITIS.

Endocarditis, subacute bacterial. *See* ENDOCARDITIS.

Endocardium (en dō kär′dē əm) is the smooth membrane that lines the cavities of the heart.

See also ENDOCARDITIS; HEART.

Endocrine gland (en′dō krin) is a ductless body organ that produces hormones that affect and help control various other organs. There are seven such glands that make up the endocrine system: thyroid, parathyroids, ovaries and testes, adrenals, pineal, pituitary, and pancreas islet cells.

See also ENDOCRINE SYSTEM; HORMONE.

Endocrine system (en′dō krin) is a network of ductless glands of internal secretion. The endocrine glands produce and/or store various hormones, which are secreted directly into the bloodstream.

The chief endocrine gland is the pituitary, situated beneath the brain and divided into two lobes. The front (anterior) lobe produces a group of stimulating (tropic) hormones that are carried to other endocrine glands—the thyroid, adrenals, and sex glands—to trigger hormone production. Other anterior pituitary hormones exert their influence directly. They include prolactin, which maintains milk production from the breasts, and growth hormone. The back (posterior) lobe of the pituitary stores two hormones: ADH (vasopressin), which is carried to the kidneys to help control body water content; and oxytocin, which assists the contraction of the uterus during labor and encourages the flow of milk from the breasts after the birth of a baby.

The pineal gland secretes melatonin. The function is uncertain in humans but may help regulate sexual development and menstruation.

Each of the adrenal glands, situated over the kidneys, is divided into an outer (cortex) and inner (medulla) region. The medulla makes the hormones adrenaline (epinephrine) and noradrenaline (norepinephrine), which help to prepare the body for "fight or flight" in response to danger. The hormones of the cortex include steroids involved in the metabolizing of sugars and proteins and in balancing body water content.

The thyroid gland lies below the voicebox or upper part of the windpipe. It secretes hormones that control the rate at which cells use nutrients. Attached to the back of the thyroid are the four small parathyroid glands whose hormones regulate the amounts of calcium and phosphate in the blood, an activity vital to bone building.

The amount of glucose in the blood is governed by cells in the pancreas, situated beside the duodenum. The endocrine cells of the gland are clustered in small masses and make two hormones: glucagon, which raises blood glucose levels, and insulin, which decreases them.

The sex glands—ovaries in a female and testes in a male—produce hormones that control the production of mature sex cells and help to determine a person's total sexual development.

Endocrinology (en dō kri nol′ə jē) is the study of the endocrine glands and the treatment of diseases affecting these glands.

See also ENDOCRINE SYSTEM.

Endoderm (en′dō dėrm) is the inner layer of cells formed during develop-

Endocrine System

The endocrine glands produce hormones, long-acting chemicals that travel in the blood and influence body activities.

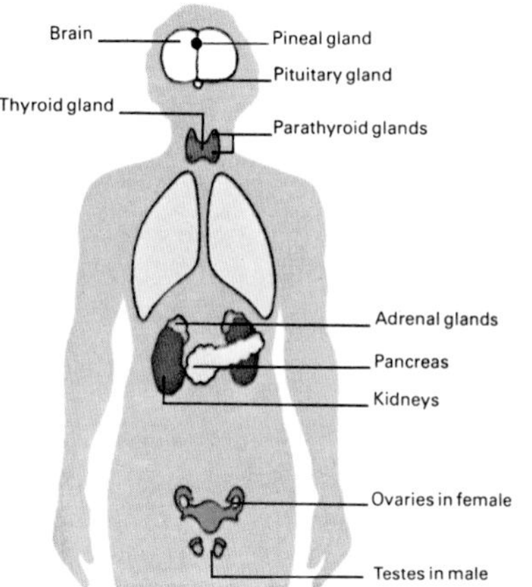

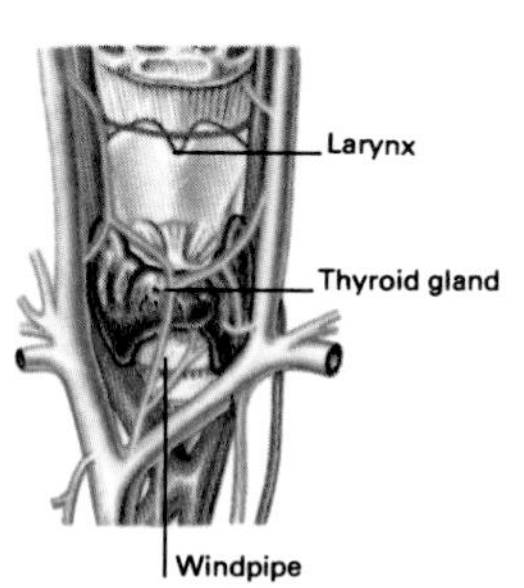

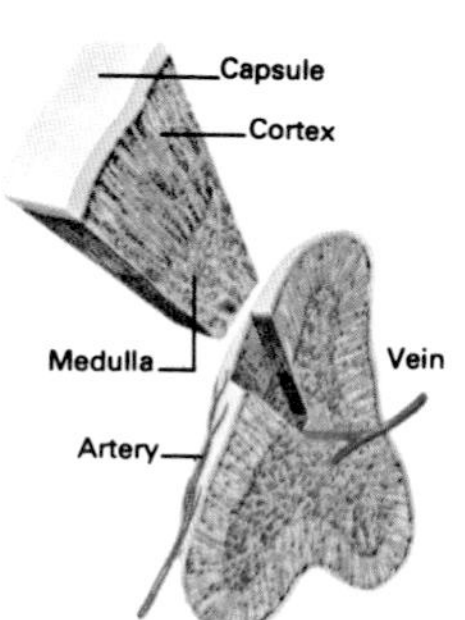

The adrenal gland's cortex makes steroid hormones. The medulla's hormones prepare the body for "fight or flight."

Hormones of the thyroid gland contain the mineral iodine and help control the rate at which the body burns and stores sugars.

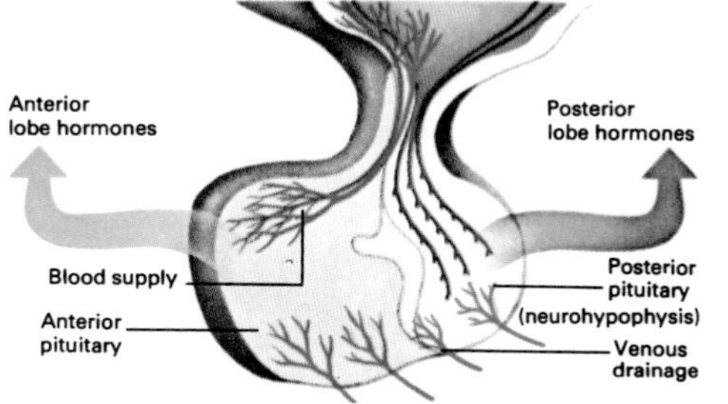

The pituitary, governed by the hypothalamus of the brain, is the chief endocrine gland, controlling the activities of the other glands.

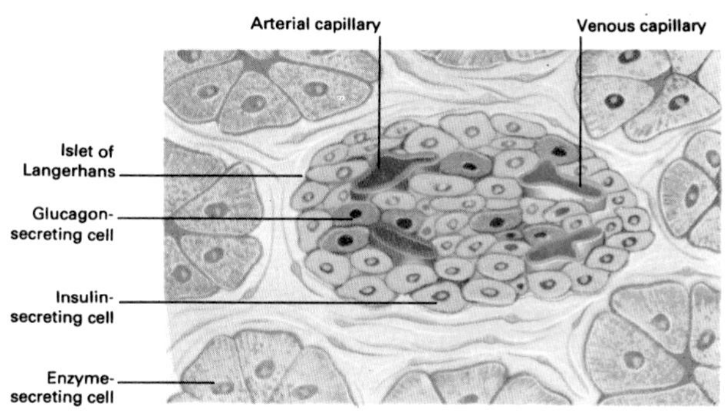

Cells in the islets of Langerhans in the pancreas produce insulin, which decreases the amount of blood sugar, and glucagon, which increases it. The gland also secretes digestive enzymes.

ment of an embryo. The lining of the organs of the digestive system develops from the endoderm.

See also ECTODERM; MESODERM.

Endodontia (en dō don′shə) is a branch of dentistry dealing with diseases of the dental pulp, the soft, inner part of a tooth containing blood vessels and nerves.

See also TOOTH DECAY.

Endometriosis (en dō mē trē ō′sis) is a condition in which fragments of the lining of the uterus (endometrium) spread to other tissues, such as the wall of the uterus, the ovaries, the peritoneum, or the bowel. The causes of the disease are unknown, but its incidence is higher in white women and in women who defer pregnancy. The fragments are benign, but may cause complications if they lodge in a critical location, leading to an organ dysfunction.

Q: *What are the symptoms of endometriosis?*

A: Often, there are no definite symptoms, and the condition is found only during a surgical operation for some other disorder. When present, symptoms include heavy periods, often more frequent than usual, accompanied by pain (dysmenorrhea); pain during sexual intercourse (dyspareunia); sometimes infertility; and sometimes pain on defecation during a period.

The abnormally placed fragments of endometrium pass through the same monthly cycle as does the normal endometrium; they swell before a period and then bleed. Because there is no outlet for the blood, cysts form. These occasionally rupture, causing severe abdominal pain. The symptoms usually disappear during pregnancy, which may cure the condition, and after menopause.

Q: *How is endometriosis treated?*

A: In mild cases, painkilling drugs may lessen the symptoms. Rarely, the fragments of endometrium can be found and removed surgically. All of the symptoms are relieved by artificially inducing menopause by irradiation or surgical removal of the ovaries, so that the uterus and the abnormal tissue cease to be stimulated by ovarian hormones. The hormone pills used for contraception may also help, and these work without sterilizing the patient. A woman with the symptoms should consult a gynecologist.

See also ENDOMETRIUM.

Endometritis (en dō mĕ trī′tis) is inflammation of the endometrium, the tissue that lines the inner surface of the uterus. The inflammation is caused by bacterial infection, which may spread to the rest of the uterus and to other tissues. The infection may follow gonorrhea, infection of the cervix, or any gynecological procedure, such as childbirth, abortion, or the insertion of an intrauterine contraceptive device (IUD).

Q: *What are the symptoms of endometritis?*

A: The symptoms include fever, low backache, abdominal pain, foul-smelling vaginal discharge, and painful periods.

Q: *How is endometritis treated?*

A: The usual treatment is with antibiotic drugs to combat the infection.

See also ENDOMETRIUM.

Endometrium (en dō mē′trē əm) is the tissue that lines the inner surface of the uterus. The endometrium is under hormonal influence and undergoes various changes during the menstrual cycle. During the cycle, the endometrium becomes thicker and develops a copious blood supply. If an egg is fertilized, it implants in the endometrium, and the placenta forms. If fertilization does not occur, the endometrium is shed each month, causing the menstrual flow.

See also MENSTRUATION.

Endomorph (en′dō môrf) is a person characterized by a predominance of structures developed from the endodermal layer of the embryo. Such a person is inclined to be soft-skinned and fat; some also ascribe to endomorphs the characteristics of being easy-going and good-natured.

The endomorph is one of three hypothetical body types first proposed around the turn of the century to explain certain aspects of personality, the other two being called ectomorph and mesomorph. If the terms are used at all today, they are in the context of describing a person's physical build without regard to that person's personality.

See also ECTOMORPH; ENDODERM; MESOMORPH.

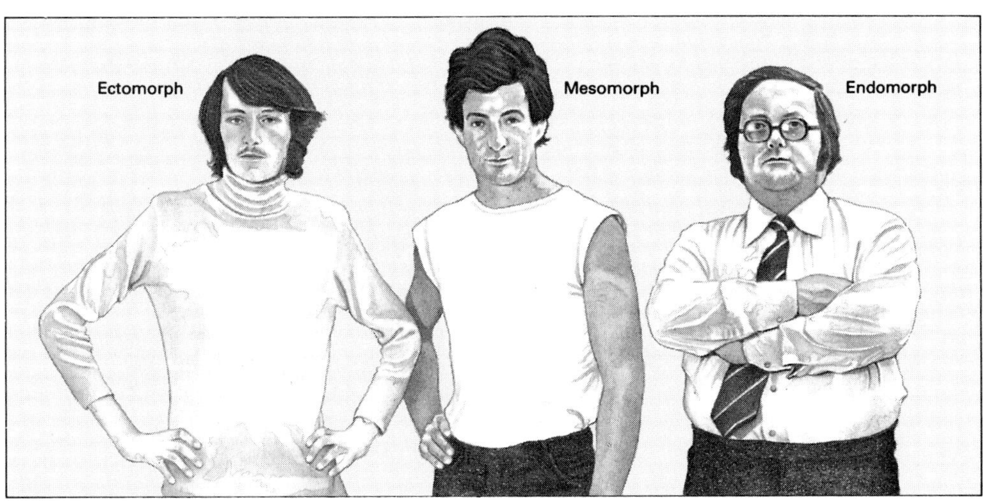

During the 1940's, W.H. Sheldon, an American psychologist, established a system of categorization for different body types: endomorph, mesomorph, and ectomorph. The **endomorph's** body is characterized by a round head, a round and large abdomen, large internal organs, rather short arms and legs with slender wrists and ankles, and a large proportion of body fat.

The **mesomorph** has the body of a classical athlete: a square head, a large heart, broad and muscular chest and shoulders, arms and legs with powerful muscles, and little body fat.

The **ectomorph's** body is essentially linear in shape: a thin face with a high forehead, a narrow chest and abdomen, long and thin arms and legs, little muscle, and a minimal amount of body fat.

These three shapes rarely occur in their classical forms. Most people can be described as a combination of two of the three types.

Endoplasmic reticulum (en dō plaz′mik ri tik′yə ləm) is a network of microcanals in a cell's cytoplasm. Ribosomes are sometimes attached to the microcanals' surface. Together with the ribosomes, the network functions in the production and transport of proteins and fats within the cell.

See also CELL; RIBONUCLEIC ACID; RIBOSOME.

Endorphin (en dôr′fin) is a chemical substance made of proteins and produced in the pituitary gland of the brain. It acts on the central and the peripheral nervous systems in suppressing pain.

Enkephalin is a type of endorphin and also a natural pain killer, working to inhibit the transmission of pain in the pathway for pain perception. This lessens the emotional and the physical impact of pain.

Research is revealing how these two natural opiates might also serve other roles. Enkephalin might be involved in the development of psycho-pathological behavior in some people. Endorphin might also exert profound effects on moods, higher production being associated with a person's sense of well-being. Increased levels of these chemical substances might also prevent an immune system from being weakened by such psychological states as depression or bereavement. People prone to depression, alcoholism, or drug addiction are often deficient in endorphin levels.

Q: *What can people do to increase or enhance endorphin levels?*

A: Regular aerobic exercise is believed to elevate endorphin levels. This is the so-called "runner's high." Meditation, prayer, and relaxation response training also elevate endorphin levels.

Endoscopy (en dos′kə pē) is an examination of the interior organs and body cavities using a light and pliable tube (endoscope). Endoscopes make use of fiber optics, fine glass tubes that conduct light even when bent or twisted. Endoscopy can be done either via a natural body opening or a surgical incision. The colon, stomach, and lungs are commonly examined by endoscopy.

Endothelium (en dō thē′lē əm) is a very thin tissue that lines lymphatic and blood vessels, the heart, and various other body cavities.

See also EPITHELIUM.

Endotracheal tube (en dō trā′kē əl) is a hollow cylinder that is inserted through the mouth or nose and passed down the throat into the windpipe (trachea). It is used to deliver oxygen or general anesthetic gases under pressure and to prevent the inhalation of foreign material during a surgical procedure.

Enema (en′ə mə) is the introduction of a liquid into the rectum and colon through the anus, either to clear the rectum or to administer medications. For example, soap and water is used to flush out constipated feces, and oil is used to lubricate the large intestine. A barium enema (a suspension of barium sulfate in water) is used in X-ray examinations to diagnose disorders of the large intestine, such as diverticulitis, ulcerative colitis, and cancer.

Q: *Are there any dangers from the regular use of enemas?*

A: Constant home use of enemas as a treatment for chronic constipation is very dangerous, because the bowels' natural ability to expel feces is weakened. There is also a possibility that an underlying disorder of the intestine may be masked. Enemas should be given only under medical guidance.

Enkephalin. *See* ENDORPHIN.

ENT is an abbreviation for ear, nose, and throat, the medical specialty called otorhinolaryngology.

See also OTORHINOLARYNGOLOGY.

Entamoeba histolytica (en tə mē'bə his tə lī'ti kə) is a species of ameba that infects the intestines of human beings. It is the primary cause of amebic dysentery and amebic abscess.

See also DYSENTERY, AMEBIC.

Enteric fever (en ter'ik) is an infection of the typhoid and paratyphoid group. Although it primarily affects the intestinal tract, the major symptoms are due to bacteria in the blood stream.

See also PARATYPHOID; TYPHOID FEVER.

Enteritis (en tə rī'tis) is inflammation of the intestine, particularly the small intestine. If the stomach is also inflamed, the condition is known as gastroenteritis; if the colon is involved, it is called enterocolitis.

Enteritis can be due to infection by a virus or bacteria, food poisoning, or chemical irritation. Symptoms of the condition are diarrhea, abdominal pain, and vomiting. Treatment is directed at the cause and at preventing dehydration. Frequently, simply limiting the diet to clear liquids (such as apple juice or broth) for several days will resolve the enteritis.

See also CROHN'S DISEASE; ENTEROCOLITIS; GASTROENTERITIS.

Enterobiasis (en tər ō bī'ə sis) is infestation of the intestines by the parasitic worm *Enterobius vermicularis.* It is commonly known as pinworn or threadworm.

See also WORM.

Enterocolitis (en tər ō kə lī'tis) is an inflammation of both the colon and the small intestine. It may be caused by a variety of microorganisms, both viral and bacterial. Another cause of the inflammation is an upsetting of the normal balance of bacteria and other microorganisms in the intestines. This can occur after the administration of a broad-spectrum antibiotic for another infection. Severe diarrhea can result. A third possibility is a decrease of the blood supply to the intestinal walls, resulting in gangrene.

Mild cases of infectious enterocolitis resolve without treatment. Sometimes, antibiotic treatment is necessary, although with some causes, for example salmonella, antibiotics can actually make the condition worse. An operation may be needed if gangrene has occurred.

See also OPPORTUNISTIC INFECTION; SALMONELLA.

Enterostomy (en tə ros'tə mē) is a surgical opening in the abdominal wall, which forms an artificial anus. The term is also used to describe an artificial opening between two parts of the intestine.

See also COLOSTOMY; ILEOSTOMY.

Entropion (en trō'pē on) is the turning inward of an edge or margin. It occurs most commonly on the edge of the lower eyelid, following infection, or as a condition of old age. An entropion can be corrected with minor surgery under local anesthetic.

See also ECTROPION.

Enuresis (en yu̇ rē'sis) is involuntary urination. Nocturnal enuresis, or bed-wetting, is common in children. Involuntary urination is not considered a medical problem in children until they have reached at least the age of four.

See also BED-WETTING.

Enuresis, nocturnal. *See* BED-WETTING.

Environment and health. The quality of the environment has a great impact on the quality of health. When the air, water, and other parts of our environmental life-support system are relatively clean, then good health is easier to maintain. However, when our life-support system is poisoned with large amounts of pollutants, toxic conditions can represent a health hazard. Environmental contaminants are not only a national health concern, they are a worldwide problem with grave implications for human survival. Among the issues threatening the environment today are air, water, and soil pollution; chemical and solid waste disposal; destruction of natural habitat; and accidents involving radioactive material.

Technology has proven to be a double-edged sword in its impact on the environment: just as technological advances in industry have improved the standard of living and our health—the by-products of many of those advances have provided the fodder for polluting agents to flourish.

Chemical Waste Disposal. Chemical waste disposal represents a major threat to public health. According to governmental estimates, there are at least 10,000 hazardous waste dumps across the United States that should be cleaned up as soon as possible. In addition, there are over 250,000 other sites that will probably need cleaning up in the next several years. Many of these sites are composed of buried steel drums filled with chemical by-products, or refuse, from industrial products. These drums often leak, spilling poisons into the earth; these poisons pollute not only the soil surrounding the sites, but also they often contaminate the groundwater used to supply neighboring communities.

Scientists are still unsure of the full health impact of these chemical waste sites; it may be decades before the full ramifications of these sites are known. Already, severely impacted communities, such as Love Canal in New York, have been rendered largely uninhabitable because of the toxicity of the soil and water. The prime danger seems to be from the heavy metals, such as mercury, arsenic, lead, cadmium, and zinc. For example, the breathing of cadmium oxide fumes has been linked to emphysema. (Cadmium and its compounds are widely used in such industries as electroplating and welding.)

The United States government, through the Environmental Protection Agency (EPA), has undertaken a program to clean up some of the worst chemical dump sites. Some critics say the program has been ineffective and underfunded. A major stumbling block appears to be how the cleanups should be funded: should the government undertake the major financial responsibility or should the companies responsible for the dump sites pay part of the cleanup costs?

Air Pollution. Most air pollution results from combustion (burning) processes. The burning of gasoline to power automobiles and the burning of

Environment and health are both adversely affected by smog, one of the most common causes of air pollution.

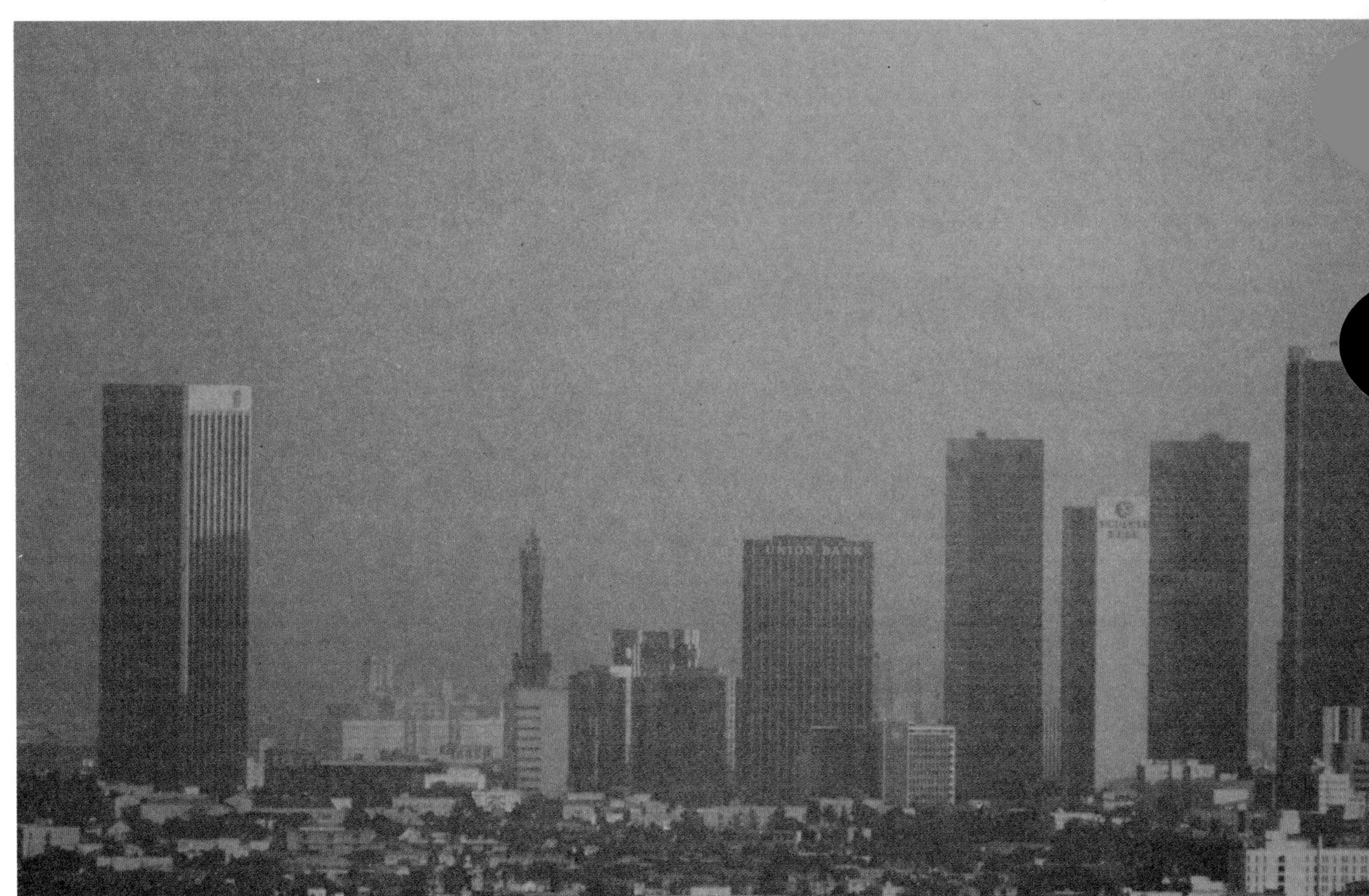

coal to help manufacture industrial products are examples of such processes. Each time a fuel is burned in a combustion process, some type of pollutant is released into the air. The pollutants range from small amounts of colorless poison gas to clouds of thick black smoke. One of the most common forms of air pollution is smog.

Air pollution can have serious consequences to human health. Particulates can settle in the lungs and worsen such respiratory conditions as asthma and bronchitis. Some experts believe that particulates can even help cause such diseases as cancer, emphysema, and pneumonia. Pollutants like aldehydes, that come from the thermal decomposition of fats and oil, irritate nasal and respiratory tracts, while ammonias from chemical processes such as dye-making inflame the upper respiratory passage. Carbon monoxide and other pollutants from automobile fumes reduce the oxygen-carrying capacity of the blood and in this way inhibit the normal growth of body tissue. Poison gases in the air can also restrict the growth of, and eventually kill, nearly all kinds of plants. Sulfur wastes in the air can result in acid rain, which destroys trees and other plant life.

Technological advances have helped reduce some causes of air pollution. For example, several types of devices, including scrubbers, have been developed to prevent particulates from leaving industrial smokestacks. And, since the early 1970's, some of the more serious poisoning by automobile fumes has been lessened by reducing the lead content of many gasolines, as well as adding catalytic converters to cars.

Water Pollution. The pollutants that affect water come mainly from industries, farms, and sewerage systems. Industries dump huge amounts of waste products into bodies of water each year. These wastes include chemicals, wastes from animal and plant matter, and hundreds of other substances. Waste from farms includes fertilizers, pesticides, and animal wastes. Most of these materials drain off farm fields and into nearby bodies of water. Sewerage systems carry wastes from homes, offices, and industries into the water. Nearly all cities have waste treatment plants that remove some of the most harmful wastes from sewage. However, most of the treated sewage still contains some pollutants.

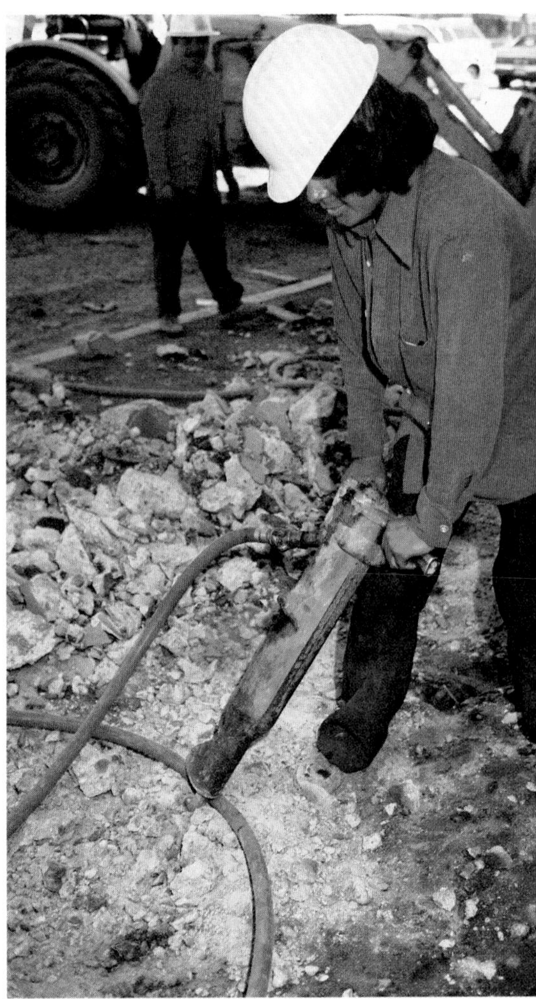

Noise pollution, here caused by the drilling of a jackhammer, also damages **environment and health.**

Purifying agents that are added to the water supply of most cities in an attempt to eliminate the danger of infection and bacteria have also raised health concerns. For instance, chlorine has been widely used to neutralize sewage contamination, but there is now some concern that large amounts of chlorine may cause some genetic damage. So too, there is the controversy about the addition of fluoride to drinking water to decrease dental decay. While fluoride has been given widespread medical approval, some physicians still believe that it has damaging health effects not yet apparent.

Some experts contend that the natural variations in the chemical content of the water (that is, the amount of calcium, making the water "hard" or "soft") may have an effect on the incidence of arteriosclerosis and coronary heart disease. Increasingly, public health officials are investigating the correlation between geographical location and the incidence of various ailments.

In the meantime, years of dumping industrial waste into lakes, rivers, and oceans has killed a significant portion of life in and around the water and has poisoned many of the species that have survived. The effects of oil spills, such as on the Alaskan coastline in 1989 by the tanker *Valdez*, are obvious and graphic. More silent but serious forms of pollution are also present. Dangerous levels of mercury have been absorbed by fish in water polluted by the dumping of industrial wastes high in mercury content. These fish often end up on our dinner tables. In this way, human pollution is returned by nature to humans.

As with air pollution, technological advances, such as the pretreatment of industrial wastewater, have improved some aspects of water cleanup. But more still needs to be done.

Radioactive Waste. The burying or dumping of radioactive waste from nuclear power plants is another environmental concern. Such waste takes years to decay and remains radioactive for decades. There is also considerable anxiety about the dangers of accidents in nuclear power stations, such as those that occurred in Harrisburg, Pennsylvania, in 1979, and much more ominously at Chernobyl in the Soviet Union, in 1986. One result of the Chernobyl disaster, which spilled radioactive waste over a very large area, is an expected rise in cancer cases in many parts of Western Europe. This reinforces the reality that environmental accidents in one part of the world have a direct impact on many other geographical areas.

Solid Waste. People throw away billions of tons of solid material each year, and much of this waste ends up littering roadsides, floating in lakes and streams, and collecting in wilderness areas. Examples of solid wastes include scraps of metal and paper; cans and other packaging material; and junked automobiles, tires, and stoves.

Solid wastes present a serious environmental problem because most of the methods used to dispose of them result in damage to the environment. Solid waste dumps provide homes for such disease-carrying animals as rats. Burning solid wastes produces smoke that causes air pollution. When wastes are dumped in water, they contribute to various forms of water pollution.

The production of solid wastes is increasing rapidly. In addition, more and more wastes that are difficult to dispose of are being produced. Tin and steel cans that rust and can be absorbed by the soil are being replaced by aluminum cans that stay in their original state for many years. Paper and cardboard packaging that decays and burns easily is being replaced by plastics that will not decay and that give off harmful gases when burned. Solid medical waste disposal, especially with the AIDS virus, will be a challenge in the next decade.

Other Kinds of Pollution. Acid rain has become an increasingly serious environmental problem. This pollutant forms when moisture in the air combines with nitrogen oxide and sulfur dioxide released by factories, automobiles, and power plants that burn coal or oil. The reaction between the moisture and the chemical compounds produces nitric and sulfuric acids that fall to the earth with rain or snow. The acids pollute lakes and streams, resulting in the death of fish and the contamination of drinking water. Acid rain can

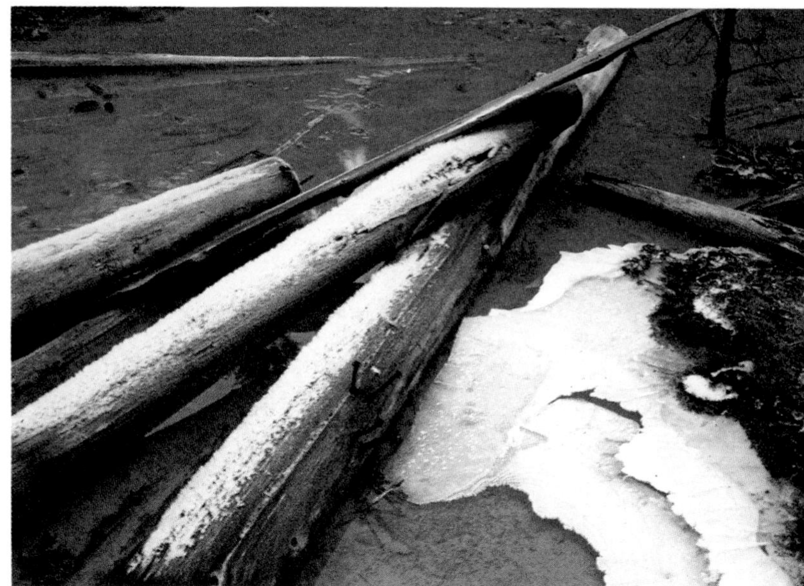

The dumping of industrial chemicals into a creek produces water pollution, which harms **environment and health.**

also harm crops and reduce the fertility of soil. It is another example of a pollutant that is created in one area and adversely impacts on another area.

Noise is also recognized as an environmental pollutant. People in and near cities are exposed to loud noise much of the time. The noise comes from such things as airplanes, automobiles, construction projects, and industry. The noise causes discomfort to many people; in extreme cases, loud noise can damage hearing or even cause deafness.

The depletion of forests and other natural habitats is another environmental concern. These natural habitat regions are the source of much plant and animal life, and their commercial development has led to the elimination of many plant and animal species. This lack of diversity may have serious ecological consequences in the future.

The Future. An increased awareness that health and environment are intricately linked has led many people to search for ways that allow for continued economic development without continuing environmental deterioration. Recycling of natural and synthetic materials is one way of reducing pollution. Other conservation efforts and new technological developments also hold out exciting possibilities for improvement in our environment. Many environmental groups have been formed to call public attention to the problems of pollution. These groups feel it is necessary to inform others of the threats to our environment in order to create a climate in which effective steps can be taken to eliminate the worst, if not all, environmental hazards.

Enzyme (en′zīm) is a chemical substance, produced by living cells, that acts as a catalyst and speeds up the rates of chemical changes in other substances. All enzymes are complicated proteins.

Q: *What kinds of enzymes are there?*

A: Enzymes that bring about the breakdown of complex substances into simpler compounds are found particularly in the digestive juices. Invertase (sucrase) is one of the enzymes responsible for the digestion of carbohydrates. Ordinary table sugar, sucrose, is broken down into smaller compounds (fructose and glucose), which the body can digest. Other digestive enzymes break down proteins into amino acids and break down fats into fatty acids.

Q: *Can deficiency of an enzyme cause disease?*

A: Yes. The absence of a particular enzyme is often inherited. The disorder known as phenylketonuria is caused by the absence of an enzyme called phenylalanine hydroxylase, which normally prevents the build-up of the amino acid phenylalanine by converting it to tyrosine. The conditions of lactose intolerance and cystic fibrosis are also associated with deficiencies of one or more digestive enzymes.

See also DIGESTIVE SYSTEM.

Epidemic (ep ə dem′ik) is an outbreak of an infectious disease or condition that afflicts many persons at the same time and in the same geographical area.

See also ENDEMIC; IMMUNIZATION; PANDEMIC; QUARANTINE.

Epidemic pleurodynia. *See* PLEURODYNIA, EPIDEMIC.

Epidemiology (ep ə dē mē ol′ə jē) is that branch of medicine dealing with the causes, distribution, and control of diseases, especially infectious diseases. *See also* INFECTIOUS DISEASE.

Epidermis. *See* SKIN.

Epidermolysis (ep ə dėr mol′ə sis) is a loosened state of the epidermis, the outermost layer of skin.

Epididymis (ep ə did′ə mis) is an ob-

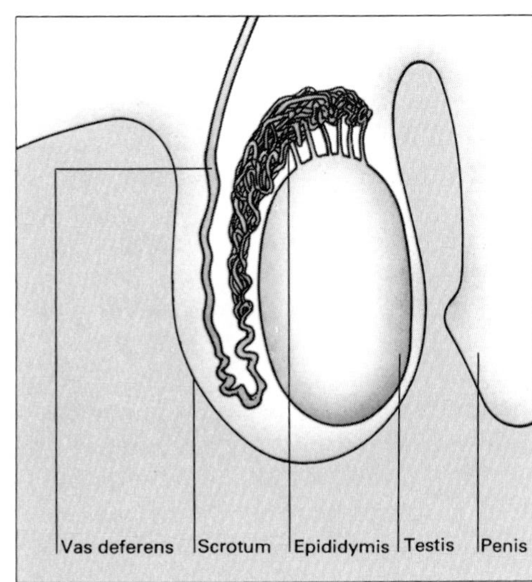

Epididymis is a twisted tube about 20 feet long leading from the testis to the vas deferens.

long structure at the side of the testicle (testis), consisting of a tightly coiled tube 18 to 20 feet (5.5-6m) long. Connected with the epididymis are about 20 small tubes through which the sperm flow from the testis. The sperm gradually mature in the epididymis, before traveling along the spermatic cord during ejaculation.

See also SPERM; TESTIS.

Epididymitis (ep ə did ə mī'tis) is inflammation of the epididymis. The inflammation causes the epididymis to become swollen and painful. The man may need to urinate more frequently, and urination may be painful. In some cases fever may occur.

The condition may be caused by the spread of a bladder infection, such as cystitis, or it may be a complication of gonorrhea, prostate disorders, a permanent catheter, or tuberculosis. Epididymitis can be effectively treated with antibiotic drugs and bed rest with support for the scrotum. Painkilling drugs may be prescribed until the pain subsides.

See also EPIDIDYMIS.

Epidural (ep ə dùr'əl) refers to anything that is situated upon or outside of the dura mater, which is the outermost membrane that surrounds the brain and spinal cord. Epidural anesthesia, for example, refers to an anesthetic that is injected into the epidural space of the spinal column.

See also DURA MATER.

Epidural anesthetic. *See* ANESTHETIC, EPIDURAL.

Epiglottis (ep ə glot'is) is a leaf-shaped structure in the throat that lies just behind the base of the tongue and over the opening of the larynx and windpipe (trachea). The epiglottis prevents food and liquids from passing into the trachea during swallowing.

See also LARYNX; TRACHEA.

Epiglottitis (ep ə glə tī'tis) is the swelling of the epiglottis, the lid-like structure that prevents food and drink from entering the windpipe (trachea) during swallowing. Symptoms associated with epiglottitis include spasmodic coughing, drooling, sore throat, high fever, and difficult or raspy breathing. The more severe cases of epiglottitis usually strike children; respiratory arrest can occur. Intubation or tracheotomy may be necessary to aid in breathing until the epiglottic swelling subsides. Intravenous antibiotics are necessary for treatment.

A bacterium, *Haemophilus influenzae*, is the most common cause of epiglottitis. Epiglottitis, caused by this organism, can now in most cases be prevented because of the vaccine against *Haemophilus influenzae* that has been developed. This vaccine is recommended for children between the ages of two and five or six.

See also EPIGLOTTIS.

Epilepsy (ep'ə lep sē) is a symptom of brain dysfunction characterized by periodic, recurrent seizures. Seizures occur in various forms, ranging from brief periods of impaired awareness to severe convulsions with loss of consciousness. Some persons with epilepsy experience an aura, a physical sensation such as a smell, at the beginning of a seizure.

Seizures used to be described as grand mal, petit mal, psychomotor, and focal. But the International Seizure Classification groups and describes seizures according to the area of the brain involved. The two major classes are partial seizures, which involve only a portion of the brain, and generalized seizures, which involve all of the brain.

See also CONVULSION: FIRST AID.

Q: ***What are partial seizures?***

A: Partial seizures involve only a part of the brain. Therefore only a specific area of the body or a particular level of consciousness is affected. Partial seizures with simple symptoms (traditionally called focal seizures) produce brief twitching movements of specific muscle groups, such as those controlling an arm or leg. If the area of the brain affected controls sight, hearing, or another of the senses, brief visual, auditory, or other hallucinations are experienced. The person retains consciousness in addition to the localized symptoms described above. Partial seizures with complex symptoms (traditionally called psychomotor seizures) involve impairment of consciousness and involuntary complicated acts. During a typical complex partial seizure, the person appears to be conscious but is unresponsive, or inappropriately responsive, to his or her surroundings. He or she may perform purposeless activities, such as lip-smacking, picking at his or her clothing, or aimless wandering. This type of seizure may be brief, last for several hours, or progress to a generalized seizure.

Q: *What are generalized seizures?*

A: Generalized seizures affect all of the brain. The two most common forms are absence seizures (traditionally called petit mal) and tonic-clonic seizures (traditionally called grand mal). Absence seizures consist of brief lapses of consciousness lasting usually 5 to 30 seconds. The person may stare blankly and appear to be daydreaming or experience slight movements of the facial muscles, head, or arms. When the seizure ends, the person resumes his or her previous activity and has no awareness of the seizure. Absence seizures commonly begin in childhood and may be as frequent as 50 to 100 a day or may occur only a few times a month. This type of seizure activity often resolves after puberty.

Generalized tonic-clonic seizures are what most people think of as epilepsy. The seizure begins with a sudden loss of consciousness. The person falls and the muscles become rigid (the tonic phase). The person may also give a sharp cry, which is caused by the sudden contraction of the abdominal muscles forcing air from the lungs through the larynx. Because there is a brief cessation of breathing, the skin may turn blue. The clonic phase then follows, consisting of jerking contractual movements of the major muscle groups. Breathing resumes, but is heavy and irregular, causing frothing of saliva. The person may bite his or her tongue or lose bladder or bowel control. Following the seizure, the person may have a headache, be confused, and want to sleep. Generalized tonic-clonic seizures usually last from three to five minutes.

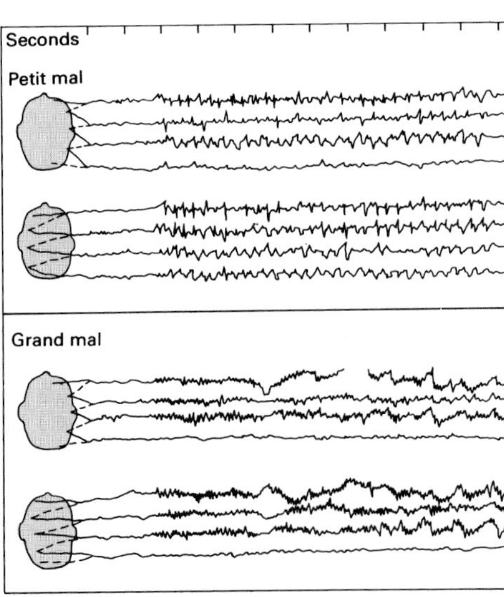

Epilepsy produces changes in the brain's electrical activity. These irregularities can be monitored by electrodes that are attached to the head. An electroencephalograph records the electrical activity for medical evaluation. The wave forms shown here indicate differences in voltage from different parts of the brain. *See also* ELECTROENCEPHALOGRAPH.

Q: *What are some of the rarer forms of epilepsy?*

A: Rare forms of epilepsy include Jacksonian seizures in which motor activity begins in the distal portion of a limb, such as a toe or thumb, and "marches" or progresses up the limb to involve major portions of the whole body. Autonomic seizures are partial seizures involving the part of the brain that controls the autonomic nervous system. Seizure activity includes headaches, stomachaches, nausea, vomiting, fever, or similar symptoms that recur without apparent cause. In atonic seizures, the person experiences a loss of muscle tone and falls with no convulsive activity. In myoclonic seizures, the individual experiences brief muscle jerks, sometimes violent enough to throw him or her to the ground. In unilateral seizures, only one hemisphere, or half, of the brain is involved and consequently seizure activity is limited to one side of the body.

Q: *What are the causes of epilepsy?*

A: Seizures are caused by the uncontrolled discharge of electrical energy by brain cells. An electroencephalograph (EEG) is used to record the electrical activity of the brain to help in the diagnosis of epilepsy. In about two-thirds of epilepsy patients, no cause can be found for the uncontrolled electrical activity, and in these persons, epilepsy is termed idiopathic. For the remaining one-third, an underlying cause can be identified, and the epilepsy is called symptomatic.

Any severe injury to the brain or central nervous system can result in epilepsy. Some of the more common causes are prenatal damage, injury during birth, brain tumors, head injury, metabolic disorders, poisoning, cerebrovascular disease, and serious infections during childhood.

Q: *Can epilepsy be an inherited condition?*

A: A number of genetic disorders, usually rare, include recurrent seizures as a symptom. In such cases, it is the genetic disorder and not a predilection toward seizures that is inherited.

The risk of epilepsy in relatives of those with idiopathic epilepsy is several times higher than that of the general population; but even with these people, the risk is low, less than 3 percent.

Q: *Does epilepsy develop only in childhood?*

A: No. Epilepsy may develop at any age, but because most cases are diagnosed in patients 18 or younger, epilepsy is often mistakenly regarded as a childhood condition. Seizures that develop after childhood are more likely to have an underlying cause, for example, a tumor or stroke. Because epilepsy is not cured, but controlled by currently available treatment, it is usually a lifelong disorder.

Q: *Are there other disorders with symptoms similar to epilepsy?*

A: Yes. Breath-holding spells in children may resemble convulsive seizures. Fainting in adults may be mistaken for epilepsy. Heart disease causing rapid changes in the pulse rate may cause symptoms similar to those of epilepsy.

High fever in young children can cause convulsions called febrile seizures. In otherwise normal children, febrile seizures do not usually have any serious consequences, but a physician should be consulted. In children with a family history of epilepsy or other neurological disorders, an increased chance of developing epilepsy may be present and preventive treatment may be prescribed.

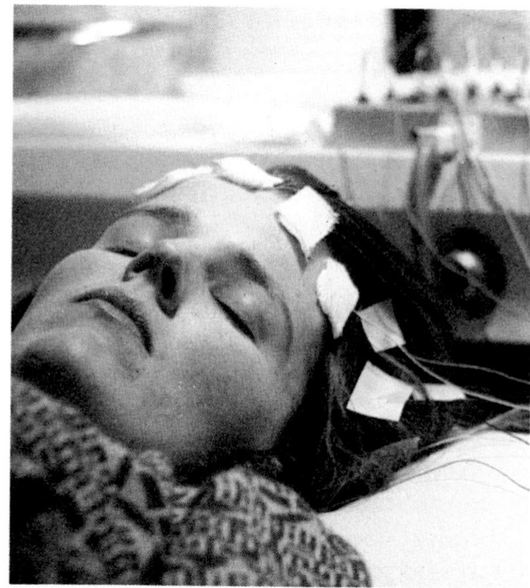

Epilepsy may be diagnosed with the help of an electroencephalograph.

Q: *How is epilepsy treated?*

A: There are many anticonvulsant or antiepileptic drugs approved for use in the United States. Not all are effective for every type of seizure. A physician will begin by prescribing a single drug and increase the dosage until seizures are controlled. If side effects appear, the dosage will be reduced until a balance between a minimum of side effects and a maximum of satisfactory control is achieved. If a single drug is not satisfactory, a second drug is usually added.

A large percentage of patients experience several different types of seizures. Sometimes the type of seizure experienced by a person may change as he or she grows older. Patients should be checked regularly by their physician.

Because the individual's body chemistry causes him or her to absorb anticonvulsant drugs in an individual way, the physician periodically takes blood samples to determine the level of drug present in the patient's system. Blood level monitoring allows the physician to accurately tailor the drug dosage to each individual to achieve maximum seizure control with a minimum of drug side effects. Some of the most commonly used anticonvulsants are phenobarbital and phenytoin for generalized tonic-clonic seizures; trimethadione, valproic acid, or ethosuximide for absence seizures; and primidone or carbamazepine for complex partial seizures.

Surgery may be used infrequently to treat epilepsy when the condition does not respond to medication or when its cause can be traced to such things as a scar on the brain or a tumor. But surgery will only be used if it can be determined that the scar or tumor is located where it can be safely removed.

Q: *What complications can result from seizures?*

A: Sometimes one seizure will immediately follow another and result in continuous seizure activity. This condition (called status epilepticus) can be life-threatening in the case of generalized tonic-clonic seizures and requires emergency medical treatment to prevent cardiac arrest or respiratory failure.

In generalized tonic-clonic, myoclonic, and atonic seizures, the person may injure himself or herself by falling against hard or sharp objects. In other seizure forms, such as absence or complex partial seizures, status epilepticus results in prolonged periods of impaired consciousness that prevent the person from behaving normally.

Untreated seizures prevent the patient from carrying out a normal life. With current treatment, more than 50 percent of persons with epilepsy can achieve complete seizure control and lead a normal life. Another 30 percent can achieve partial control over their seizures and engage in most activities.

Q: *Is epilepsy a permanent condition?*

A: In most cases, epilepsy is permanent. However, with consistent treatment, seizures may decrease in frequency after a number of years, and drugs can be gradually reduced or withdrawn. Physicians will usually begin reduction if a patient remains seizure-free for several years, but seizures often recur following drug reduction. A patient should never reduce medication without the advice of a physician. Abrupt withdrawal of anticonvulsants may result in an increase in the number and severity of seizures. Such withdrawal has also been known to trigger incidents of status epilepticus.

Q: *What precautions should a person with epilepsy take?*

A: Persons with epilepsy, whose seizures are controlled, can lead normal lives. However, they should be aware that excessive use of alcohol, poor eating habits, and lack of rest may precipitate seizures. All states permit a person with epilepsy to drive if he or she has been seizure-free for a specific period. The person whose seizures are less well controlled, or are triggered by a specific stimulus, should limit activities accordingly so as not to endanger himself or herself. The patient should always take his or her medication exactly as prescribed and report any changes in seizure activity or drug side effects to a physician so that dosage can be adjusted.

Q: *Should a woman with epilepsy consider bearing a child?*

A: A woman with epilepsy should consult a physician before becoming pregnant. Pregnancy has been known to increase both the number and severity of seizures. Further, some anticonvulsants have been shown to be associated with an increase in the incidence of certain birth defects, primarily cleft palate.

Q: *What should a person do if someone has a seizure?*

A: It should be kept in mind that most seizures are of short duration and that there is nothing a nonphysician can do to stop the seizure. Consequently, activity should focus on preventing a person with a seizure from hurting himself or herself.

A person with a seizure should be helped to lie down if he or she is not already down. The area around the epileptic should be kept clear of people and objects that could cause injury. Under no circumstances should anything be forced between the victim's teeth nor should anyone try to hold the victim's tongue to "prevent it from being swallowed." This kind of action could result in injury to the victim as well as to the rescuer. If the victim appears to be choking, he or she should be turned onto his or her side with the face down to prevent obstruction of the airway. Medical assistance should be requested.

Epilepsy, temporal lobe (ep'ə lep sē tem'pər əl lōb). Temporal lobe epilepsy is a form of epilepsy in which the seizure originates in the temporal lobe of the brain. Also called psychomotor seizure, it is characterized by the absence of convulsions, acts that are abnormal, and behaviors that are automatic. Loss of consciousness or memory, hallucinations, both auditory and visual, asocial behavior, and the automatic continuance of routine activities may be present in temporal lobe epilepsy.

See also EPILEPSY.

Epinephrine (ep ə nef'rin), also known as adrenalin, is a hormone secreted by the inner part of the adrenal gland; epinephrine enables the body to meet conditions of physical stress.

Epinephrine can be used for a variety of purposes: checking local hemorrhaging; relieving allergic reactions, such as asthma, hives, and anaphylaxis; prolonging local anesthetic action; and stimulating the heart.

See also ADRENAL GLANDS; ASTHMA; HIVES; ENDOCRINE SYSTEM; SHOCK, ANAPHYLACTIC.

Episiotomy (i piz ē ot'ə mē) is an incision in the edge of the birth canal. It is commonly made near the end of the second stage of labor, to prevent tearing of the birth canal or to facilitate the delivery of the baby.

See also PREGNANCY AND CHILDBIRTH.

Epispadias (ep ə spā'dē əs) is a congenital defect of the male penis. The urethra, the duct connecting the bladder to the tip of the penis, opens at some point in back of the head of the penis, often resulting in incontinence and sexual dysfunction. Epispadias can usually be corrected by reconstructive surgery.

Epithelium (ep ə thē'lē əm) is a thin layer of cells forming a tissue that covers surfaces of the body and lines hollow organs. It is compactly arranged with little intercellular substance, can regenerate itself very quickly, and performs protective, secretive, and other functions.

See also SKIN.

Epsom salts. *See* MAGNESIUM SULFATE.

Epstein-Barr virus (ep'stīn-bär), EBV, is a virus that causes infectious mononucleosis and has also been suspected of causing certain types of cancer. It is also believed to cause a prolonged syndrome characterized by chronic fatigue.

See also MONONUCLEOSIS.

Equilibrium (ē kwə lib'rē əm) is a state of balance: for example, the state of a chemical system, when no further change occurs in it, or the state of mental or emotional balance.

Erb's palsy. *See* BRACHIAL PLEXUS.

Erection (i rek'shən) is a state of the penis, clitoris, or other bodily organ or part, in which the erectile tissue has become distended and rigid by the accumulation of blood.

In some cases, such as nipple erection or erection of the fine hairs on the skin, the process involves muscle contraction rather than the concentration of blood.

See also SEXUAL INTERCOURSE.

Ergosterol (ėr gos'tə rōl) is a steroid substance that is now obtained mainly from yeast, but was originally obtained from ergot. Ergosterol is exposed to ultraviolet rays to yield vitamin D_2, which is sometimes used in the treatment of rickets.

See also ERGOT; RICKETS.

Ergot (ėr'gət) is a fungus, *Claviceps purpurea*, that grows as a parasite on rye. It is extremely poisonous, but its alkaloid chemicals are the source of many drugs.

Ergot poisoning can occur by eating rye bread made from contaminated grain or by taking an overdose of an ergot drug. The poison causes blood vessels to contract. This gives rise to symptoms such as extreme thirst, vomiting, diarrhea, tingling in the limbs, and, occasionally, convulsions. The victim needs immediate emergency medical attention. If the patient survives, cataracts and gangrene may develop as secondary complications.

Two of the many drugs derived from ergot are ergonovine and ergotamine. Ergonovine causes the womb to contract and may be prescribed after childbirth to stop bleeding. Ergotamine acts on the blood vessels in the head and is used to treat migraine.

See also ERGOSTEROL.

Erosion (i rō'zhən) is the breaking down of body tissues.

See also CERVICAL EROSION.

Eruption (i rup′shən) is the rapid breaking out of a skin rash or skin lesions, which accompanies certain diseases (for example, mumps or scarlet fever), drug reactions, or allergic reactions.

See *also* ALLERGY.

Erysipelas (er ə sip′ə ləs) is an acute, serious streptococcal skin infection. It tends to spread rapidly, causing inflammation, blisters, fever, nausea, and vomiting. Occasionally, the skin infection extends as a red line up a limb. Erysipelas is treated with penicillin and erythromycin. A physician should be consulted if erysipelas is suspected.

See *also* STREPTOCOCCUS.

Erysipeloid (er ə sip′ə loid) is an unusual bacterial skin infection, resembling erysipelas. Erysipeloid produces red swellings on the skin, with tingling and itching. It is usually confined to the hands and seldom makes the patient ill. The symptoms last for several days before spontaneous recovery occurs. Erysipeloid is generally acquired by handling contaminated fish or meat products, and it is more common in the summer. Although no treatment is necessary, antibiotics can shorten the time taken for recovery.

See *also* ERYSIPELAS.

Erythema (er ə thē′mə) is a severe redness of the skin or mucous membrane associated with some local inflammation. Minor examples include blushing and mild sunburn. More severe forms of erythema include erythema multiforme and erythema nodosum.

See *also* ERYTHEMA MULTIFORME; ERYTHEMA NODOSUM.

Erythema infectiosum. See FIFTH DISEASE.

Erythema multiforme (er ə thē′mə mul tə fōr′mā) is characterized by spots, pimples, vesicles, or lesions that commonly appear on the legs. It can have different causes, including pregnancy, drug sensitivity, or allergic reactions. Treatment depends upon pinpointing the exact cause; a physician should be consulted because of the potentially serious nature of the disease.

Erythema nodosum (er ə thē′mə, nü dō′səm) is a condition in which red, oval nodules appear on the skin. Over a period of several weeks, the nodules change from a red to a brown color. Erythema nodosum often occurs on the shins and may be accompanied by fever, aches, and fatigue. It usually follows a streptococcal throat infection. In children, the condition can be associated with rheumatic fever. In adults, it may occur with sarcoidosis, tuberculosis, or ulcerative colitis. Certain drugs, such as the sulfonamides, may also produce erythema nodosum. The treatment consists of bed rest and aspirin until the condition improves; corticosteroids may relieve the symptoms. If the cause of the condition is a streptococcal infection, penicillin should be taken for at least one year.

Erythredema. See PINK DISEASE.

Erythroblastosis fetalis. See HEMOLYTIC DISEASE OF THE NEWBORN.

Erythrocyte. See BLOOD CELL, RED.

Erythromycin (i rith rō mī′sin) is an antibiotic drug from the mold *Streptomyces erythreus.* Erythromycin is a medium-range antibiotic and is widely used clinically. It produces few side effects; there may be some abdominal pain with nausea, vomiting, and diarrhea, but these usually clear up within a few days. It is usually only given to patients with infections immune to penicillin: for example, pneumonia caused by *Mycoplasma pneumoniae* or *Legionella pneumophila,* as well as infections caused by *chlamydial* organisms. Erythromycin is routinely employed as an alternative to penicillin G in patients who can not tolerate penicillins, usually due to allergic reaction. Erythromycin is one of the safest antimicrobial agents and seldom causes serious adverse reactions. Rarely, it causes hepatitis; therefore, erythromycin should be prescribed with care to those with impaired liver function.

See *also* ANTIBIOTIC; HEPATITIS.

Escape from sinking car. See AUTOMOBILE SAFETY.

Esophageal speech. See SPEECH, ESOPHAGEAL.

Esophagus (ē sof′ə gəs), also known as the gullet, is a muscular tube about 10 inches (25cm) long that extends from the pharynx at the back of the throat to the stomach. In the neck, the esophagus lies behind the trachea and continues behind the aorta and heart to join the top of the stomach.

The esophagus conveys food and drink from the pharynx to the stomach. This is achieved partly by gravity and partly by peristalsis (rhythmical waves of muscular contractions). When a person breathes in, air is directed to the

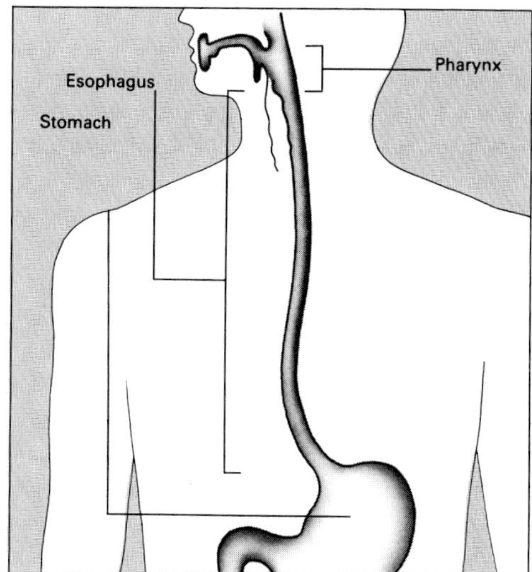

The **esophagus** is a muscular tube that conveys food and drink from the pharynx to the stomach.

larynx and the trachea. At the same time, however, saliva is able to run down the esophagus. At the point where the esophagus and the stomach join, there is a ring of muscle (the cardiac sphincter) that prevents the stomach contents from passing back up the esophagus.

See also ACHALASIA; DYSPHAGIA; HEARTBURN; HIATUS HERNIA.

Estrogen (es′trə jən) is any of a group of chemically similar hormones that cause female sexual development; estrogen is produced mainly by the ovaries, but also by the adrenal glands.

At the onset of puberty, estrogens stimulate the development of pubic hair and of secondary female sex characteristics, such as rounded hips and breasts. Estrogens also play an essential part in the hormonal control of menstruation, being partly responsible (with progesterone) for the cyclical changes in the lining of the womb. As a woman grows older, her ovaries secrete smaller amounts of estrogen. After the level of estrogens in the blood becomes too low to stimulate the uterine lining (endometrium), menstruation ceases and the woman is said to be in menopause. Men also produce estrogens, but their function is as yet unclear.

Estrogens have a number of medical uses. For example, synthetic estrogens are a component of most types of contraceptive pills and are also used in the treatment of menstrual disorders and in estrogen replacement therapy (ERT) at menopause. In men, synthetic estrogens are used in the treatment of cancer of the prostate gland.

Prolonged use of estrogens may be harmful to some patients. For example, the use of birth control pills has been associated in some women with blood clots, high blood pressure, and diabetes. Some studies have also linked the use of large amounts of estrogen drugs during menopause with higher rates of cancer of the uterus. However, this risk can be minimized if estrogens are used in conjunction with progesterone during menopause.

See also HORMONE; PROGESTERONE.

Estrogen Replacement Therapy (es′trə jən), ERT, is used to maintain a steady estrogen level after menopause.

Usually given now in combination with progesterone (in order to reduce the risk of uterine cancer), ERT relieves postmenopausal symptoms, for example, dryness of the vagina, inability to sleep, and hot flashes. It also inhibits the onset of osteoporosis, a bone-thinning disease affecting more than 15 million American women—characteristically, thin, Caucasian females who also smoke and have a family history of the disease. ERT may also lessen the chance of heart disease and breast cancer.

Side effects of ERT include cyclic vaginal bleeding, similar to menstruation, tenderness of the breasts, and a possible increase of blood pressure. Long-term effects are still being studied.

Women who take estrogen alone and continuously are at an increased risk of uterine cancer and should be screened regularly by their physician.

See also ESTROGEN; MENOPAUSE; OSTEOPOROSIS; PROGESTERONE.

Ether (ē′thər) is the general name for a class of organic chemical compounds derived from alcohols. Ether is used as a cleansing agent and was once widely used as an anesthetic.

See also ANESTHETIC.

Eustachian tube (yü stā′kē ən) is the narrow tube about 1.5 inches (4cm) long that connects the back of the nasal passages with the cavity of the middle ear. The Eustachian tube allows the pressure on each side of the eardrum to equalize. During swallowing, the lower end of the Eustachian tube opens mo-

The **Eustachian tube** connects the nasal cavity with the middle ear and equalizes pressure on both sides of the ear drum.

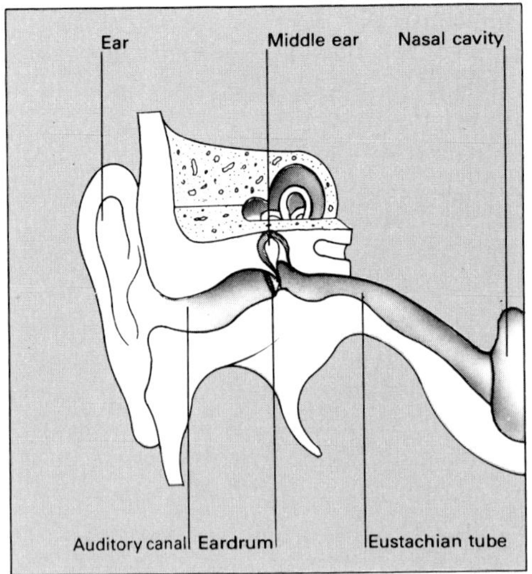

mentarily. A blockage of the Eustachian tube with swollen tissue, due to infection (otitis media), can lead to temporary deafness. If the tube is blocked and pressure suddenly changes, as may happen during flying or diving, the eardrum may rupture.

See also BAROTRAUMA; EAR; EARACHE; OTITIS.

Exanthem. *See* RASH.

Exercise is the performance of certain physical activities to tone and condition the body and to improve the state of health. There are many benefits, both physical and psychological, to regular exercise.

Exercise enables a person to stay physically fit. However, it is important to remember that physical fitness and good health are not the same, although one influences the other. Healthy people may be physically unfit because they do not exercise regularly. Physically fit people perform their usual tasks easily without tiring and still have energy for other interests.

Better physical performance, however, is only one benefit of exercise. Regular vigorous exercise also increases the efficiency and capacity of the heart and lungs. Fit people also have greater resistance to disease and tend to recover faster if they do become ill. In addition, exercise helps people to maintain proper weight; individuals who exercise regularly tend to be more slender and look better than those who are unfit. Physically fit people are also able to resist the effects of aging better than the unfit.

With regard to the psychological effects of exercise, there is some evidence that people who get regular exercise may be happier, more alert, and more relaxed than those who lead sedentary lives. Exercise can improve a person's ability to cope with both the physical and mental stress that accompanies everyday life. If you come home after a working day feeling stale and tired, a few physical exercises can immediately improve your general outlook and restore your energy.

Physical Fitness is a combination of qualities that enable a person to perform well in vigorous physical activities. These qualities include agility, endurance, flexibility, and strength. A person's level of physical fitness depends largely on how frequently and intensely he or she exercises. Most health experts agree that an individual should exercise at least three times a week to maintain physical fitness. The President's Council on Physical Fitness and Sports recommends a 30-minute workout of continuous exercise; the exercise need not be difficult or strenuous. However, as a person's condition improves, he or she should increase the number of times each activity is performed. Every workout should include three basic types of exercises: (1) flexibility exercises, (2) endurance exercises, and (3) strength exercises.

Flexibility exercises, such as bending, turning, and twisting movements, stretch the connective tissues and move the joints through a wide range of motions. These exercises cut the risk of injury from strenuous exercise and reduce muscle soreness; they should be performed before and after each workout. *See* Sports and Exercise Table, pages 321–322

Endurance exercises include cycling, running, and swimming. These activities, also called *aerobic exercises,* raise the rate of heartbeat and breathing and strengthen the circulatory and respiratory systems. *See* Sports and Exercise Table, pages 321–322

Strength exercises include pullups, pushups, situps, and exercises with weights. These exercises strengthen the arms and shoulders and other muscular parts of the body.

Physical Fitness Programs are part of most school curriculums and are also offered in many communities.

School physical education programs help children develop good physical fitness habits for life. The President's

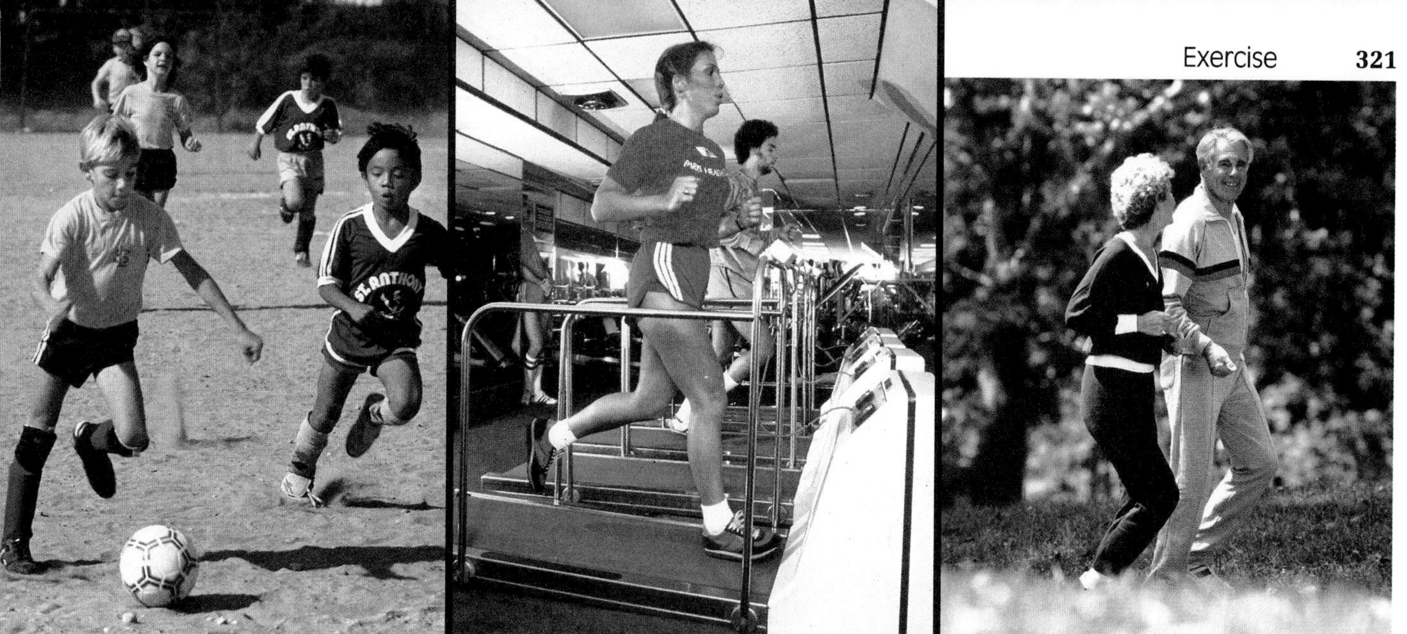

Sport	Special Exercises	Complementary Exercises
Archery	grip exercise: squeeze a rubber ball hard in each hand; one arm dumbbell rowing; shoulder turns with bar.	bench press; pushups.
Badminton	wrist exercise: hold a dumbbell rod in each hand, with the forearms horizontal, and rotate the wrists; holding a dumbbell rod like a racket, move as during a game; skipping.	exercise the other arm; chinning; one arm dumbbell rowing.
Baseball	sprinting exercise: run hard for 30 yards (27.4 meters), lie down, do 2 pushups, sprint 30 yards; grip exercise.	exercise the other arm.
Basketball	squat jumps: squat down with the hands on the floor, then jump up, stretching the arms as high as possible over the head; squat; press with dumbbells.	basketball exercises all muscle groups.
Canoeing	situps; shoulder turns with bar; bench press; press with dumbbells; flying exercise; chinning.	leg exercises; skipping; facedown, legs raise.
Cycling	squat; deep kneebends with dumbbells; legs curl; situps; setups; leg exercises.	chinning; hanging, reverse arch; shoulder turn.
Football	pushing exercises against an immobile object; all advanced exercises; weight training with professional supervision; sprinting exercises (*see baseball*).	football exercises all muscle groups.
Golf	knee exercise: stand with feet slightly apart, and turn the hips and knees in one direction, then the other, simulating golfing movements; grip exercise.	golf uses most muscle groups to a slight extent; a more vigorous, aerobic exercise is also recommended.
Handball	wrist exercises (*see badminton*); leg exercises.	handball exercises all muscle groups.
Hiking	thigh and hip exercise; while standing, balance a weight, such as a sandbag, on the foot, and lift the leg as high as possible, bending the knee; leg exercises; seesaw movement.	hiking exercises all muscle groups.
Horseback riding	thigh grip exercise; squeeze a large medicine ball hard between the knees; wide kneebends; squat; leg parting; one arm dumbbell; rowing.	abdominal exercises; back and chest exercises.

The choice of various types of exercise depends upon personal preference and need. Various sports offer a wide range and variety of exercise. The table at *left* and on page 322 outlines a selection of sports, the parts of the body each sport builds, as well as the type of exercises one should execute in relation to that sport.

Sport	*Special Exercises*	*Complementary Exercises*
Rock climbing	grip exercise (*see archery*); bench press; shoulder turns with bar; hanging, reverse arch; situps; chinning; leg side raise.	rock climbing exercises all muscle groups.
Rowing	squat jumps (*see basketball*); chinning; situps; pushups; skipping; running.	shoulder raise; facedown, legs raise; leg back raise.
Running (Jogging)	leg exercises; legs raise, on angled board; shoulder turns, with bar.	running exercises all muscle groups.
Skating	ankle exercise; stand with feet slightly apart, and rock the ankles from side to side; deep kneebends with dumbbells.	back and chest exercises; press with dumbbells.
Skiing	thigh strength exercise: lean the back flat against a smooth wall with the feet together about 2 ft. (0.6m) away, then bend the legs so that the back slides down as low as possible, and push up again; adapt ankle exercise (*see skating*) and knee exercise (*golf*) to the movements of skiing; leg exercises; seesaw movement.	skiing exercises all muscle groups.
Soccer	ankle exercise (*see skating*); knee exercise (*see golf*); leg exercises; legs curl; neck exercises; shoulder turns, with bar.	soccer exercises all muscle groups.
Squash and Racquetball	wrist exercises (*see badminton*); leg exercises; skipping; situps.	exercise the other arm.
Swimming	straight arm pull-over; shoulder turns, with bar; situps; shoulder raise; alternate legs raise.	chinning.
Tennis	wrist exercises (*see badminton*); leg exercises; skipping; straight arm pull-over; hanging, reverse arch; seesaw movement.	exercise the other arm.
Volleyball	squat jumps (*see basketball*); press with dumbbells; hanging, reverse arch; straight arm pull-over.	one arm dumbbell rowing; chinning.
Waterskiing	squat; deep kneebends with dumbbells; one arm dumbbell rowing; chinning.	hanging, reverse arch; shoulder raise.

Council recommends that all elementary and high schools provide a daily exercise period of at least 20 minutes. This program should include vigorous activities designed to develop agility, endurance, flexibility, and strength. There should also be performance tests to measure students' progress, as well as instruction in running, throwing, and other skills. Special physical fitness programs should also be provided for handicapped and mentally retarded students. All of these programs should teach simple exercises in the lower grades and progress to more complicated ones as the children mature. Older pupils can participate in such activities as gymnastics, swimming, dual and team sports, and intramural sports, which involve competition among students of the same school, as well as interscholastic sports, in which schools compete against one another.

Community programs contribute to the physical fitness of the people by increasing the opportunities for regular exercise. In many communities, schools become recreation and fitness centers during evenings and weekends and on days when the regular classes are not in session. Schools can offer sports and exercise equipment and such facilities as gyms, playing fields, and swimming pools. Some communities also have trails for cycling and jogging.

Many businesses, labor and service organizations, churches, private clubs, and park and recreation agencies provide facilities and instructors for community fitness and exercise programs.

Exhaustion (eg zôs'chən) is a state of extreme fatigue, often accompanied by a reduced ability to respond to external stimuli.

See also FATIGUE; HEATSTROKE.

Exocrine gland (ek'sə krin) is a type of gland that opens onto a skin surface or epithelium through a duct or tube. Examples are sweat glands, parotid glands, or lacrimal glands.

See also GLAND.

Exophthalmos (ek sof thal'məs) is abnormal protrusion of the eyeballs. It is usually a symptom of hyperthyroidism, but may have other causes, such as a tumor behind the eye. A physician should be consulted so that the underlying cause can be treated; otherwise, permanent eye damage may result.

See also HYPERTHYROIDISM; THYROTOXICOSIS.

Expectorant (ek spek'tər ənt) is a substance that aids the loosening and the discharge of phlegm.

Exploratory surgery. See SURGERY, EXPLORATORY.

Exposure (ek spō'zhər) is a debilitated body state that results from being subjected to extremes of hot, cold, or windy weather without adequate protection. Lack of treatment can lead to loss of consciousness and further complications. Prolonged exposure may lead to death.

Exposure: treatment. See HYPOTHERMIA: TREATMENT.

Extradural hematoma. See HEMATOMA, EXTRADURAL.

Extrasystole (eks trə sis'tə lē) is a disturbance of the natural rhythm of the heart. An extra heartbeat occurs as a premature and weak beat. When the next heartbeat is due, the heart muscles are still recovering from the extrasystole and do not respond; the heart misses a beat.

The sensation of a missed beat is usually felt in the chest or throat. It may cause anxiety, but in an otherwise normal heart, extrasystoles are no cause for alarm. They are common in many healthy persons while resting, especially in those who smoke or drink a lot of coffee. However, if extrasystoles continue after exercise or occur with some regularity, a physician should be consulted.

Extrauterine pregnancy. See PREGNANCY, ECTOPIC.

Extravasation (ek strav ə sā'shən) is the escape of a body fluid from its normal containing vessel into the surrounding tissue.

See also BLEEDING.

Extrovert (eks'trə vert) is a psychological term that describes a person whose interests center on external objects and actions, rather than on self-concerns (introvert). As such, extroverts tend to feel more comfortable interacting with others than do introverts. A balance between extroversion and introversion probably represents optimal psychological health rather than an extreme on either end of the continuum.

See also INTROVERT.

Exudate (eks'yů dāt) is a fluid that penetrates the walls of cells and blood vessels and seeps into adjoining tissues. The process is a body defense mechanism associated with inflammation caused by infection. Blood vessels dilate and become more permeable, allowing a fluid rich in serum protein and containing antibodies and white blood cells to escape. Pus and nasal mucus are also termed exudates.

Eye is one of a pair of organs of sight. It is an almost perfect sphere about one inch (2.5cm) in diameter.

Each eye is protected at its back and sides by the bones of the skull and at the front by two lashed eyelids. The outer covering of the eye, the sclera or "white," is both protective and structural. Light penetrates the sclera only at the front of the eye, where the outer surface bulges into the transparent cornea, a delicate structure overlaid with a thin defensive membrane, the conjunctiva. Under each upper eyelid is a tear-secreting lacrimal gland whose constant activity keeps the conjuctiva moist and free from germs.

Light entering the eye passes through the cornea and then through a watery fluid, the aqueous humor, in the front of the eye. Behind the fluid is the iris, a ring of muscle with a central hole, the pupil. The cornea focuses light rays so that they pass through the pupil. The iris determines how much light enters the eye. In dim light its muscles relax to let in more light; in bright light

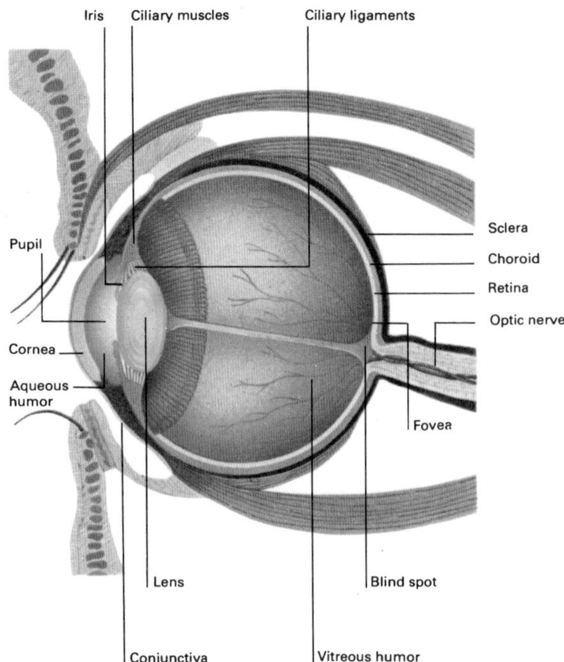

The **eye** is protected by the sclera, the outer covering or "white" of the eye and by the conjunctiva, a thin membrane covering the cornea. Light is focused by the cornea and lens onto the retina, which is nourished by blood vessels in the choroid. Impulses created on the retina leave the eye and are transmitted to the brain along the optic nerve.

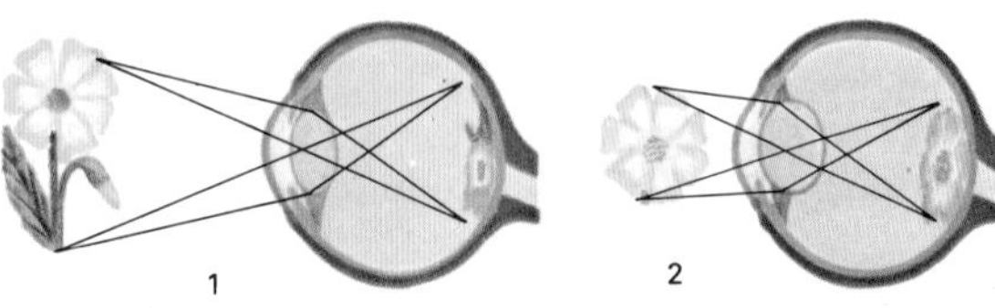

To focus on distant objects (1) muscles relax, making the lens long and thin. To focus on near objects (2) muscles contract, making the lens short and fat.

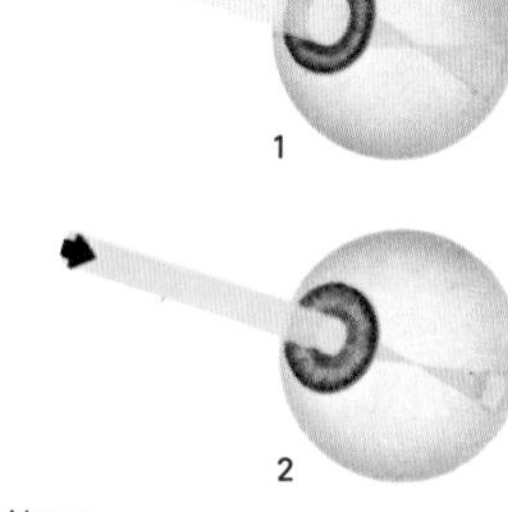

The pupil, a hole in the center of the iris, adjusts by reflex to control the amount of light entering the eye. The pupil becomes wider in dim light (1) and smaller in bright light (2).

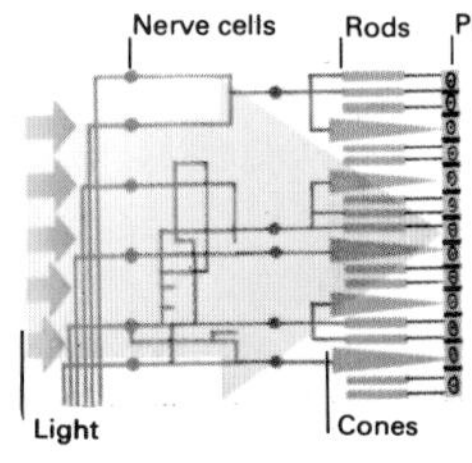

Two types of receptor cells in the retina interpret light. The cones detect color; the rods, shades of black and white. Both generate nerve impulses to the brain.

its muscles contract to reduce pupil size and restrict light entry.

The fine focusing of light is achieved by the lens, a soft, transparent structure lying behind the iris. The lens is held in place by ligaments attached to internal eye muscles. The actions of these muscles bring about changes in the shape of the lens so that close and distant objects can be focused upon. For viewing near objects, the muscles make the lens shorter and fatter; for viewing distant objects, the lens becomes longer and thinner. This process is known as accommodation.

From the lens, light passes through the thick jelly (vitreous humor) that fills the center of the eye. The light is projected onto the retina, a light-sensitive layer inside the sclera from which it is separated by the choroid, a dark layer of tissue rich in blood vessels. The retina contains two sorts of light-receptor cells: rods, which detect shades of black and white; and cones, which are sensitive to color. In response to light, the rods and cones generate nerve impulses that pass along the optic nerve to the brain to be interpreted as vision. The concentration of cones is densest at a single spot called the fovea. The fovea is the region that gives the greatest visual sharpness. Visual sharpness (acuity) depends on the number and density of the rods and cones, since each cell can record only the presence of light and, in cones, its color. There are about 10 million cones and 100 million rods in each eye. Where the optic nerve leaves the back of the eye, there are no rods or cones; this is called the blind spot.

Eye care. The eyes are highly sensitive organs and, although they have a defense system of their own, their delicate structure makes them susceptible to injury and disease.

The eyes must be protected from accidents. Blindness can result from injuries inflicted with sharp sticks, fireworks, toy guns, and other objects that children may use as missiles during play. Parents must be firm with their children and explain the possible consequences of careless play. Eyeglass lenses should be made of an unbreakable substance, particularly for children.

Eye cosmetics can produce a violent

allergic reaction, particularly the kind containing particles of "glitter." A contact dermatitis may develop after years of use, producing swelling (edema) and itching around the eyelids, sometimes involving the whole face. It is a sensible precaution to use hypoallergenic cosmetics that are now on the market.

Clean all traces of makeup off the eyes each night. Use a mild soap and water or a mild cleansing oil. If particles of makeup are left on overnight, there is a higher risk of irritation. Mascara tends to make the eyelashes brittle, and they can be damaged on the sheets at night.

A cosmetic that should never be used regularly, if at all, is false eyelash glue. If misapplied it can block the natural flow of tears from the lacrimal glands.

Eyestrain can be avoided by using common sense to develop good habits for reading and close work.

Always read in good light, but ensure that the light does not reflect directly off the page. Too much glare makes reading uncomfortable. When reading, hold the book at least a foot away from the eyes and relax the muscles that control the lens by looking at a distant object about once an hour.

Adults should have their eyes tested every few years. Children should have their eyes tested once a year. Poor vision can harm a child's social and educational development and may be mistaken for low intelligence. Early detection of any vision defect enables correction that will permit the child to make maximum use of remaining vision.

Every adult over the age of 40 should have an eye examination every 2 years, in order to identify and treat any disorders before vision is irreparably damaged.

Eyeglasses are prescribed to correct farsightedness (hypermetropia) and nearsightedness (myopia), and some other visual disorders. The lenses must be prescribed by an ophthalmologist. Farsightedness may develop with increasing age (presbyopia) because the lens of the eye becomes less elastic. Any disturbance of clear vision strains the eyes and needs swift correction. Otherwise the patient may suffer from recurring headaches.

See also FARSIGHTEDNESS; MYOPIA; OPHTHALMOLOGY; PRESBYOPIA.

Eye disorders. The following table lists some of the disorders that affect the eye and the basic characteristics of each condition. Sometimes, an eye disorder is symptomatic of some other disorder (for example, diabetes, nephritis, or stroke). Each disorder has a separate article in the encyclopedia. *See also* BLINDNESS.

Disorder	*Basic characteristics*
Adenoma (of pituitary gland)	Loss of vision due to pressure on optic nerve by a tumor
Amaurosis	Progressive loss of sight, leading to blindness
Amblyopia	Decreased vision without structural defects in the eye
Aphakia	Absence of the lens of the eye, causing blurred vision
Astigmatism	Distorted and blurred vision
Blepharitis	Inflammation of the eyelid
Cataract	Blurred vision and loss of sight
Chalazion	Lump on the eyelid
Coloboma	Cleft in the iris, the choroid, or other part of the eye
Color blindness	Inability to identify one or more primary colors
Dacryocystitis	Inflammation of tear sac
Detached retina	Flashes of light, followed later by sensation of curtain drawn over the eye
Diabetes	Dimness of vision, loss of sight
Ectropion	Inside of eyelid is turned outward
Entropion	Edge of eyelid is turned inward toward the eyeball
Exophthalmos	Bulging eye or eyes
Farsightedness	Hyperopia, diminished ability to see things at close range
Glaucoma	Increased pressure within eye, resulting in gradual loss of vision
Glioma (optic)	Tumor of optic nerve, with loss of vision

Disorder	Basic characteristics
Hemianopia	Defective vision or blindness in half the visual field
Hypertension	Damage to retina due to effect of high blood pressure on blood vessels
Iritis	Inflammation of iris with sensitivity to light
Keratitis	Blurred vision due to inflammation of cornea
Migraine	Blurred vision and flashes of light associated with intense headache
Myopia	Nearsightedness, objects can be seen distinctly only when close to eyes
Nephritis (chronic)	Deterioration of retina as result of kidney disease
Night blindness	Defective or complete loss of vision in the dark
Ophthalmia (and sympathetic ophthalmia)	Inflammation of the eye or the conjunctiva
Panophthalmitis	Infection of the whole of the eye
Papilledema	Swelling of the optic nerve and sudden blindness
Presbyopia	Diminished ability to see things at close range, due to aging
Retinitis	Inflammation of retina
Retinitis pigmentosa	Degeneration of retina, leading eventually to blindness
Retrobulbar neuritis	Inflammation of optic nerve and sudden blindness
Sarcoma	Tumor, causing pain and blurred vision
Scotoma	A blind or partly blind area in the visual field, surrounded by area of normal vision
Stroke	Temporary or permanent loss of vision or blind spots due to interruption of blood supply to brain
Sty	Infection of one or more of the small glands of the eyelid
Tay-Sachs disease	Impairment of sight, resulting in blindness

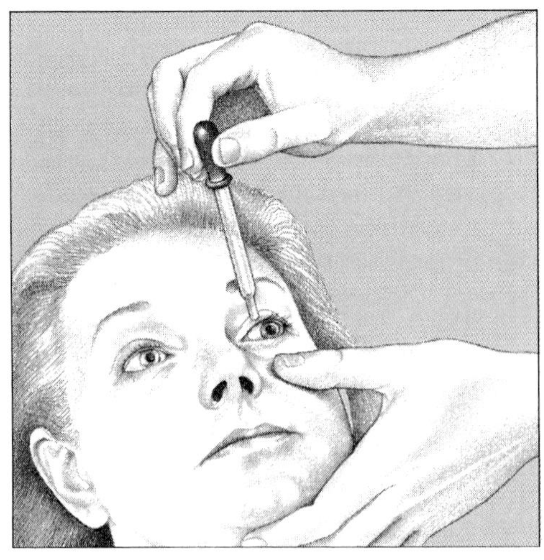

Eye drops should be applied to the inner corner of the eye while the patient looks upward.

Eye drops: administration. Ask the patient to look upward, with the head resting on a pillow. Gently ease down the lower lid with one hand. Apply the eye drops with the other. Try to place the drops toward the inner corner of the eye. Ask the patient to shut the eye for a few seconds immediately after; this ensures that the liquid is distributed evenly. Gently swab away excess liquid with a piece of cotton.

Eye, foreign body in: treatment. A foreign body can become lodged in the eye. If a soft object, such as an eyelash, becomes lodged between the lid and the eyeball, instruct the victim to close the eye. Lead the victim to a good light source, and gently open the eye. If the foreign body is not visible, instruct the victim to look up, down, then to either side as you gently deflect the eyelid in the opposite direction. When the particle is located, lift it from the eye with the dampened corner of a clean handkerchief.

Never try to remove a particle that is stuck to the white of the eye or lying over the center of the eye. Also never attempt to remove a hard foreign body from the eye unless watering has moved the particle to the inner corner. In both cases, the eye should be covered with a raised eye pad that does not touch the lid or the eyeball; the victim should then be taken to a physician.

Eyeglasses are prescribed to correct certain visual defects. Recently, contact lenses have become an alternative to eyeglasses for many visual defects.

Q: *What visual defects can eyeglasses help correct?*

A: Eyeglasses are commonly used to correct astigmatism (distortion of the cornea); hyperopia (farsightedness); myopia (nearsightedness); and presbyopia (defective vision due to hardening of the lens with age). As well as these disorders, eyeglasses may be required by young children to correct a congenital disorder. *See also* ASTIGMATISM; HYPEROPIA; MYOPIA; PRESBYOPIA.

Q: *Are there special eyeglasses for particular conditions?*

A: Yes. With increasing age many people need eyeglasses with divided lenses for each eye, called bifocals. These correct vision for both near and far objects. Trifocals correct vision for the middle distance as well as for near and far vision. Eyeglasses may have permanently tinted lenses, or they may be of variable darkness according to the light intensity. Dark lenses are used by albinos; those with certain chronic eye disorders, such as iritis and photophobia; and in conditions of extremely bright light to prevent blindness. Eyeglasses may be made with plastic or unbreakable glass lenses to prevent injury to the eyes.

Eyeglasses do not make the eyes lazy nor worsen a person's eyesight. But, because some vision defects worsen with age, this may seem to be the case. It is advisable to have an eye examination every few years, even if there is no eye problem. After age 40, it is best to have the eye exam at least every two years. *See also* IRITIS; PHOTOPHOBIA.

Q: *Is there any difference between eyeglasses and contact lenses?*

A: The choice between contact lenses and conventional eyeglasses is, in most cases, a matter of personal preference. An ophthalmologist may advise against the use of contact lenses in severe forms of astigmatism or myopia.

Eye infection: treatment. Blepharitis is an inflammation of the edges of the eyelids. The condition can give rise to infected eyelash follicles. If the membrane covering the eye becomes infected, the patient develops "pink eye" (conjunctivitis). The condition may be accompanied by a pain, discharge of pus, and sensitivity to bright light. If the infection is confined to one eye, it can be easily spread to the other eye during the early stages when the patient is unaware of the infection. For this reason, always clean the eyes separately by wiping with a cotton ball from the inner to the outer corner. Discard the ball immediately and use a fresh one for the other eye.

See also BLEPHARITIS; CONJUNCTIVITIS.

Eye injury. See EYE DISORDERS.

Eyelid is one of two movable folds of skin that protect the front of each eyeball. When closed, the eyelids cover the visible area of the eye. The upper lid is larger and capable of more movement than is the lower one. It contains a fibrous plate of tissue that gives additional protection to the eyeball. Each eyelid has on its undersurface a mucous membrane, called the conjunctiva. The conjunctiva is lubricated by tears produced by the lacrimal apparatus.

Q: *Which disorders affect the eyelids?*

A: Eyelid disorders include black eye, blepharitis, chalazion, conjunctivitis, ectropion, entropion, ptosis, and sty. The eyelids are also susceptible to general skin disorders such as eczema and rodent ulcer.

See also BLACK EYE; BLEPHARITIS; CHALAZION; CONJUNCTIVITIS; ECTROPION; ECZEMA; ENTROPION; EYE; PTOSIS; STY.

Eye, watering. A watering eye is caused by a variety of conditions, including blockage of the lacrimal apparatus, inflammation of the eyes, allergies, or foreign bodies.

See also EYE DISORDERS; LACRIMAL GLAND.

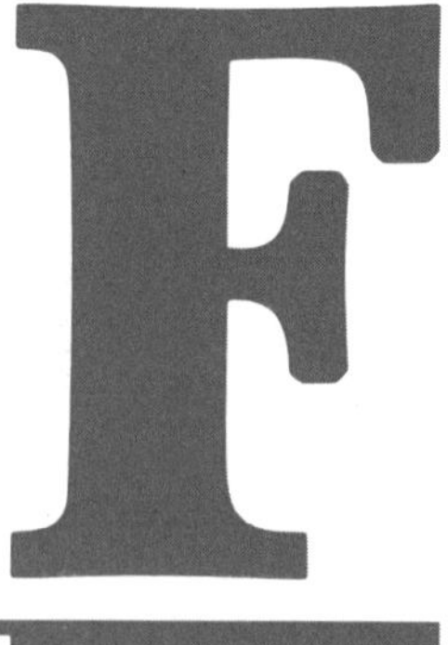

Fabry's disease (fā'brēz) is a hereditary disease attacking the heart, kidneys, and central nervous system. It is caused by an enzyme deficiency genetically linked to the female chromosome and passed on by women to their male offspring. The victims usually die in their early 20's.

See also NERVOUS SYSTEM, CENTRAL.

Face-lift. *See* SURGERY, COSMETIC .

Face presentation. *See* PREGNANCY AND CHILDBIRTH.

Facial injury: first aid. *See* HEAD INJURY: FIRST AID.

Facial paralysis (fā'shel pə ral'ə sis) is weakness of the muscles of the face, caused by damage to the nerve that supplies them (the facial nerve).

See also BELL'S PALSY.

Fahrenheit (far'ən hīt) is a temperature scale on which the freezing point of water is 32° and the boiling point of water is 212°. The normal human body temperature is 98.6°F.

See also CENTIGRADE.

Fainting (fānt'ing), or syncope, is a temporary loss of consciousness. It is usually caused by a temporary deficiency in the blood supply to the brain, often following a sudden drop in blood pressure.

See also FAINTING: FIRST AID.

Fainting: first aid. Fainting is a temporary loss of consciousness that occurs when there is an inadequate supply of blood to the brain. A faint may begin with a feeling of giddiness or dizziness, or it may occur as a sudden collapse.

There are many causes of fainting. Although most of them are relatively minor, fainting may be a symptom of an underlying illness. If the victim has not regained consciousness within a few minutes and completely recovered within 15 minutes, summon medical help and treat for unconsciousness. *See also* UNCONSCIOUSNESS: TREATMENT.

If a faint lasts longer than 10 minutes, its cause may be an underlying illness. The victim should seek medical advice on recovery.

Action. The aim of first aid is to restore an adequate supply of blood to the brain. If the person is conscious, ask whether he or she is a diabetic. If so, give the person sugar or any sugar-containing substance; artificial sweeteners will not be of any help.

There may be some warning before a faint. The person may feel unsteady and giddy; the face becomes pale with beads of perspiration appearing; the skin becomes cold and clammy; the pulse feels weak and erratic; and there may be attacks of nausea. If fainting is imminent, place the person in a lying position in a current of fresh air. Loosen any clothing around the person's neck and waist.

If lying is impossible, place the victim in a sitting position and instruct the person to lower the head between the knees and to take slow, deep breaths. If the person is unconscious, check for breathing and pulse. If absent, give artificial respiration. If breathing is present, lay him or her down in a current of fresh air and loosen any clothing around the neck and waist. Treat any injury that may have been sustained during the faint. If there has been no injury, place the victim in the recovery position. *See also* ARTIFICIAL RESPIRATION.

When consciousness has been regained, do not allow the victim to stand up immediately. Gradually raise the victim to a sitting position and give sips of water.

Fallopian tube (fə lō'pē ən), or oviduct, is a muscular tube that extends from the uterus to an ovary. It is about 4 inches (10cm) long. There are two fallopian tubes, one for each ovary.

After ovulation, the egg (ovum) passes from an ovary along the fallopian tube to the uterus. Finger-like tissue at the end of the tube nearest the

Fainting: first aid

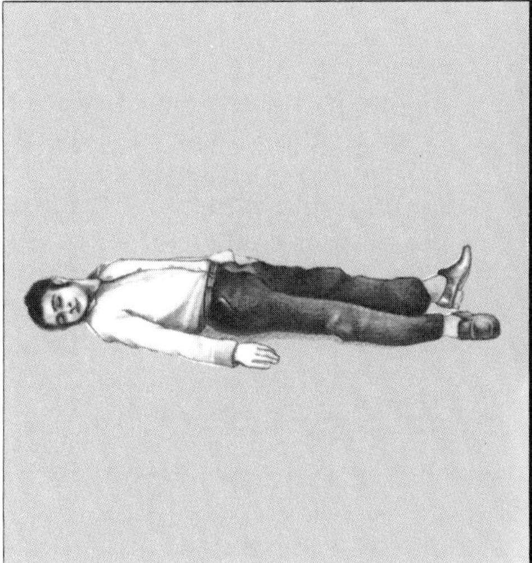

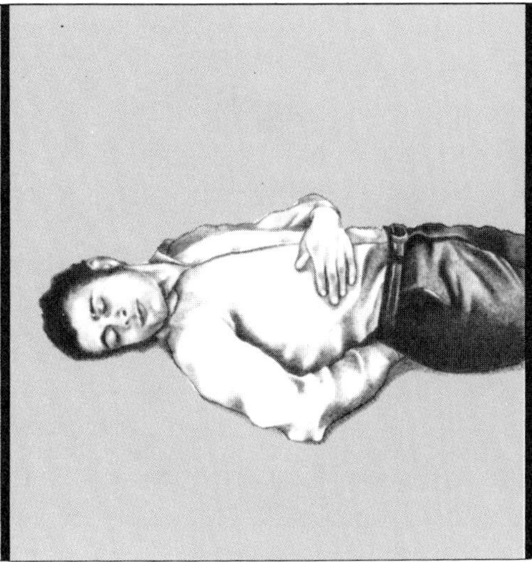

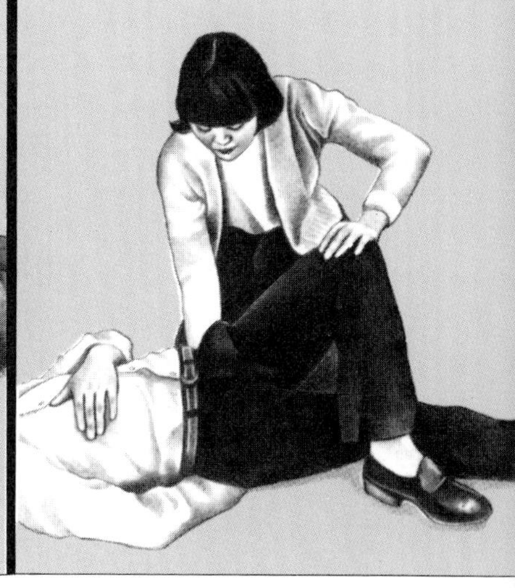

1 To turn the victim into the recovery position, first lay the victim face-up on the ground. If the victim is breathing, loosen the clothing, especially around the neck and waist. If the victim is not breathing, use artificial respiration. *See* ARTIFICIAL RESPIRATION. Place the victim's arms beside the body. Turn the victim's head toward the right side. Treat any injury suffered during the faint.

2 Tuck the right arm under the victim's buttock. Place the victim's left arm across the chest.

3 Bend the victim's left leg at the knee and cross the left leg over the right leg so that the thigh makes a right angle with the body. Gently pull the victim's right arm under the body.

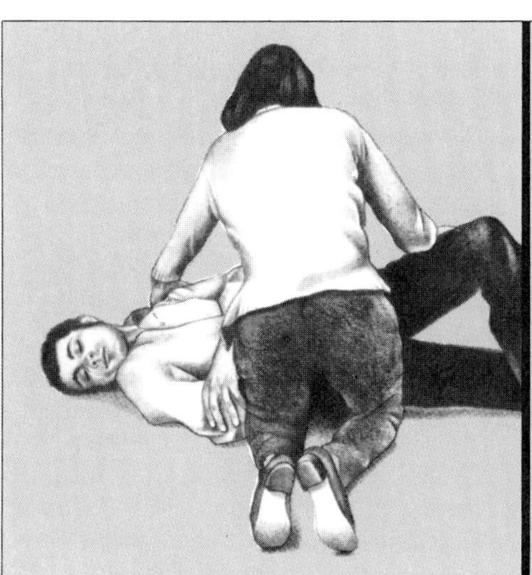

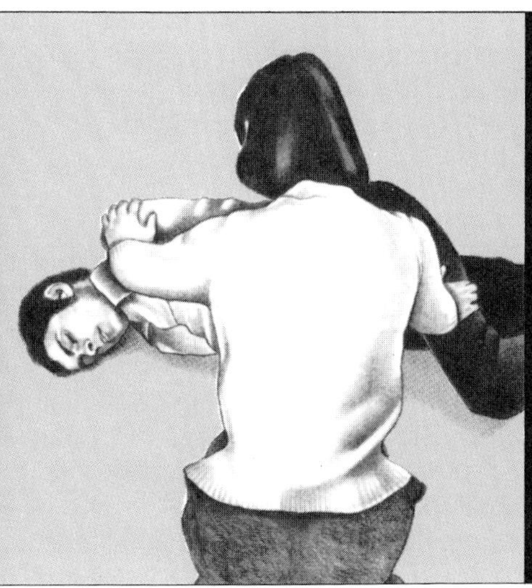

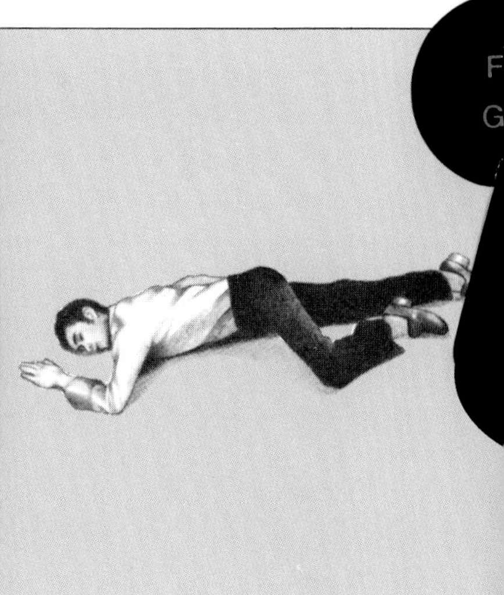

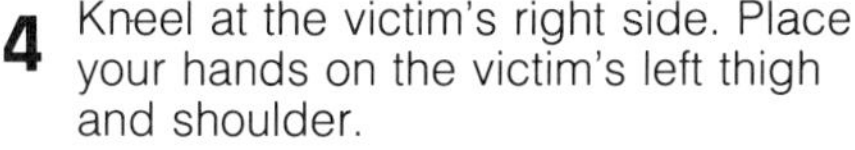

4 Kneel at the victim's right side. Place your hands on the victim's left thigh and shoulder.

5 Gently pull the victim toward you. Ensure that the victim's air passage remains unobstructed throughout the procedure.

6 To complete placing the victim into the recovery position, place the victim's left arm on the ground, palm downward with the arm bent at the elbow. Gently lift the victim's head upward and backward. With the victim's head turned to one side, the air passage should remain clear even if the victim vomits.

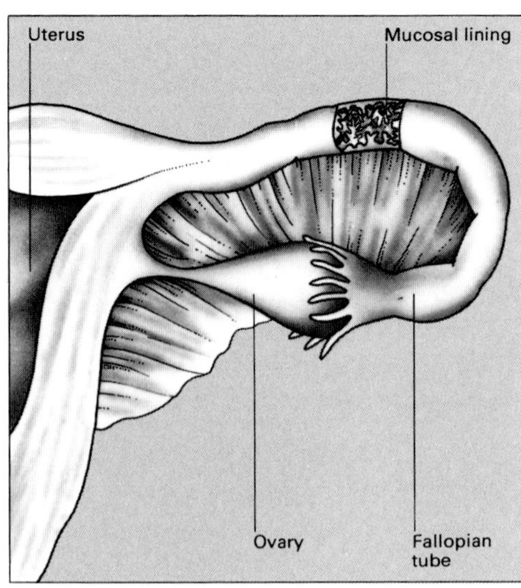

The **fallopian tube** extends from the ovary to the uterus and is lined with mucous membrane.

ovary helps to direct the egg into the tube, and hair-like cells inside the tube propel the egg along it. Sperm swim up the tube from the uterus and meet the egg. If the egg becomes fertilized, fertilization usually takes place while the egg is in the fallopian tube. If for any reason the movement of the fertilized egg is prevented, it may implant in the fallopian tube instead of in the lining of the uterus, resulting in an ectopic pregnancy.

Q: *Can a disorder of the fallopian tubes cause sterility?*

A: Yes. After inflammation (salpingitis), any scar that remains may block the tube, damage the finger-like tissue at its opening, or damage the hair-like cells. If the inflammation and scarring occur in both tubes, the woman is in danger of being unable to conceive.

Q: *Does sterilization of a woman involve the fallopian tubes?*

A: Yes. The surgical cutting and tying of both fallopian tubes is the usual method of sterilization of women.

See also PREGNANCY AND CHILDBIRTH; PREGNANCY, ECTOPIC; SALPINGITIS; STERILIZATION.

Fallot's tetralogy (fa lōz′ te tral′ə jē) is a congenital heart malformation that comprises four separate problems: (1) a hole in the wall between the left and right ventricles; (2) narrowing of the artery that leads to the lungs (pulmonary artery); (3) misplacement of the aorta; and (4) an increase in the thickness of the muscle of the right ventricle.

Q: *What are the symptoms of Fallot's tetralogy?*

A: The main symptom is a bluish tinge to the skin (cyanosis), caused by the presence in the arteries of blood that has not been properly oxygenated. Fainting sometimes occurs, and a child with the disorder is often breathless.

Q: *How is the condition treated?*

A: Cardiac surgery during childhood may correct the condition.

See also CYANOSIS.

False labor pains. *See* LABOR PAINS, FALSE.

False pregnancy. *See* PREGNANCY, FALSE.

False teeth. *See* DENTURE.

Family physician is the primary health care provider of the individual and the family. He or she provides diagnosis and treatment of the majority of an individual's health problems for all age groups.

When complicated problems warrant referral to specialists, the family physician remains the team leader, coordinating the patient's health care. This approach avoids complications that might arise from the uncoordinated ordering of tests and medications by a variety of specialists. The family physician is also responsible for caring for a family's psychological as well as physical needs, especially during times of severe illness. Appropriate specialists can be called upon when the care of a certain patient may need specialized procedures or when the particular expertise of a specialist will contribute to the patient's care.

See also FAMILY PRACTICE.

Family planning is the regulation or limitation of the size of a family by practicing birth control, therefore, deciding when and how many children will be born.

See also CONTRACEPTION.

Family practice is that specialty of medicine dealing with the total health care of the individual and the family. It is not limited to persons of a particular age or sex, nor is it concerned with a specific organ or disease. It integrates all the fields of medicine—clinical, biological, behavioral, and preventive—in order to give the individual or the family primary medical attention.

Family therapy is a form of psychological counseling that focuses on the entire family. This form of therapy assumes that an individual's emotional problems can be best understood when examined in the context of how the family interacts or behaves together. It is, thus, important for the therapist to observe how family members actually communicate and interact with each other. Through observing and modifying these family patterns of behavior, which are often subconscious, the therapist can help family members work out their mutual problems. Family therapy can be particularly effective in treating childhood behavioral problems, which are often a reflection of family or marital conflict. In some cases, understanding family dynamics can make the treatment of an individual's health problems more effective.

Family therapists can be psychologists, psychiatrists, or social workers who have received specialized training in family therapy.

Famine fever. See FEVER, RELAPSING.

Farsightedness, hyperopia or hypermetropia, is a disorder of vision. Distant objects are seen clearly, but close objects appear blurred. This occurs because light rays from nearby objects are not focused normally on the back of the eye (retina). This may be because the refractive power of the eye lens is too strong, or (more commonly) because the eyeball is not long enough from front to back. Farsightedness may be inherited, or it may develop after the age of 40 as the lens of the eye becomes less elastic (presbyopia). Corrective eyeglasses or contact lenses are prescribed to restore normal vision.

See also EYEGLASSES; MYOPIA.

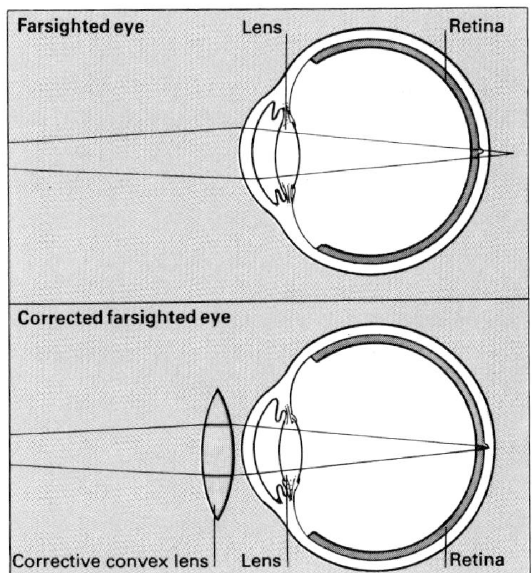

Farsightedness occurs when rays of light entering the eye are brought into focus behind the retina. It commonly occurs after the age of 40 as the lens of the eye becomes less elastic.

Fascia (fash'ē ə) is a sheet of tough fibrous tissue that covers, supports, and separates muscles. *See also* MUSCLE.

Fasting is deliberate abstinence from food over a period of time. It is a medical requirement for some gastrointestinal examinations (for example, fluoroscopy and X-ray studies), blood tests (for example, a glucose tolerance test), and before a general anesthetic. The fast required is generally 8 to 12 hours.

Fasting is a requirement in some religious rites; it is also used as a means of political or social protest. Some people fast as a means of losing weight rapidly, but this method is not recommended.

Q: *What happens to the body's metabolism during fasting?*

A: In the absence of food, the body's energy requirements are supplied first by the body's sugar, then by reserves of fat. The "burning up" of fat is incomplete, resulting in mild ketosis, due to the production of by-products of fat metabolism.

Pangs of hunger occur during the first few days of a fast, but then become less noticeable.

Q: *What precautions should be taken by a person who is fasting?*

A: A person who intends to fast for more than two days should seek the advice of a physician. Vitamin supplements are recommended. When a fast is broken, a normal diet should be resumed gradually, beginning with light, easily digested foods.

See also KETONE; WEIGHT PROBLEM.

Fat is one of the three kinds of energy-giving foods in the diet. Fats are an extremely rich source of energy, with a calorie content of about 255 calories per ounce (9 calories per gram). This is twice as much as provided by the other foods (proteins and carbohydrates). The most common fat-containing foods are butter, cream, eggs, fatty meats, margarine, oily fish, and vegetable oils.

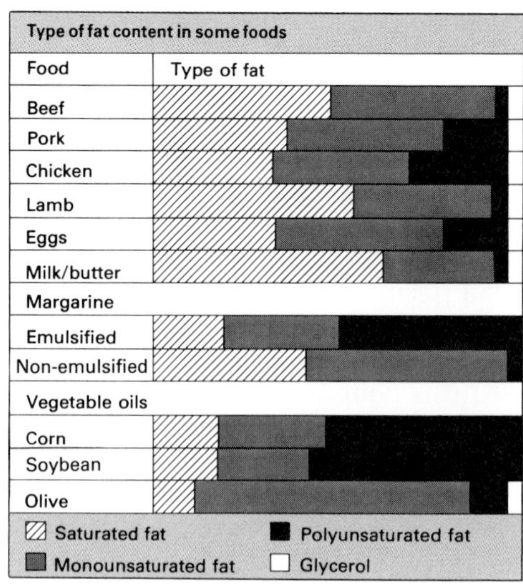

Animal meats are usually high in saturated **fats** and have been linked with atherosclerosis (vascular disease).

Q: *What are the functions of fats in the body's metabolism?*

A: Most fats are burned up (oxidized) to produce energy (in addition to carbon dioxide and water). Other fats become an essential part of cells. Fats that are not required immediately as a source of energy are stored in layers of fatty (adipose) tissue under the skin. They are available as fuel for energy at any time. The stored fats surround and protect internal organs, such as the kidneys, and act as insulation that prevents heat loss. Certain "essential" fatty acids are required for normal metabolism and health. Fats also provide an environment in which vitamins A, D, E, and K can dissolve. Some fat is stored in the liver.

Q: *What is the difference between saturated and unsaturated fats?*

A: Saturated and unsaturated fats differ chemically in the way their carbon and hydrogen atoms are arranged. Basically, unsaturated fats can absorb hydrogen, whereas saturated fats can not. Most animal fats are saturated fats; saturated vegetable fats include coconut oil and palm oil. Unsaturated fats include cottonseed oil, safflower oil, corn oil (all polyunsaturated fats that may be constituents of margarine), and olive oil. Fish oil may lower blood levels of certain harmful fats.

Q: *What is the significance of this distinction?*

A: Research suggests that large amounts of saturated fats in the diet may be associated with increased plasma cholesterol and atherosclerosis. Surveys have shown that countries with high living standards, such as the United States, have a high incidence of atherosclerosis. But whether or not this is directly caused by a staple of "rich man's food," such as meat, eggs, cream, and so on (foods high in the saturated fats), is still under investigation.

Q: *Should fats be reduced in the diet?*

A: Yes. Currently, Americans consume 42 percent of their calories as fat. Dieticians advise reducing this to 30 percent.

See also NUTRITION; APPENDIX IV.

Fat embolus (em′bə ləs) is a globule of oil, fat, or bone marrow that obstructs an artery or vein. Such an obstruction can occur after the fracture of a large bone or after some forms of orthopedic surgery.

See also EMBOLISM.

Fatigue (fə tēg′) is a feeling of tiredness or weariness and is usually a signal for rest and relaxation. It lessens concentration, slows down the reflexes, and breaks down the ability to cope with stress.

The changes in the body that produce fatigue are not fully understood. The external causes that may trigger its onset include a particularly stressful day, heavy physical exercise, inadequate sleep, mental strain, boredom, a long period of dieting, or even poor posture. Chronic (persistent) fatigue often occurs as a symptom of infection, deficient diet, depression, or an underlying disorder, such as anemia, diabetes, tuberculosis, or cancer. Persistent or severe fatigue should be brought to the attention of a physician.

See also SLEEP; STRESS.

Fatty acid is any one of a group of carbon chains that make up "fat." Essential fatty acids are required for membrane formation and synthesis of important compounds. Humans need only 15 to 25 grams of fat in a day, yet, many American diets provide over 100 grams of fat.

See also FAT; NUTRITION; APPENDIX IV.

Fatty degeneration (di jen ə rā′shən) is a disorder involving the accumulation of fat in cells, especially those of the liver and the heart. It occurs because the cells are deprived of certain chemicals that make the disposal of fat possible. Metabolic disorders, anemia, or poisoning by alcohol, drugs, or industrial chemicals, such as dry-cleaning fluids, may cause fatty degeneration.

Favism (fā′viz əm) is a form of acute hemolytic anemia caused by inhaling or swallowing fava pollen or the fava bean. It is caused by an inherited metabolic sensitivity of the red blood cells. The symptoms are headache, fever, vomiting, diarrhea, and sometimes coma. Treatment includes blood transfusions. The offending bean should then be avoided. Favism occurs primarily among peoples of the eastern Mediterranean region.

Favus (fā′vəs) is a form of ringworm affecting the scalp. It is caused by the fungus *Trichophyton schoenleini*, which is rare in North America.

See also RINGWORM.

Febrile convulsion (fē′brəl kən vul′shən) is a seizure brought about by a rapidly rising or very high fever. The convulsion usually affects only about 4 percent of children between the ages of 6 months and 8 years. Sometimes, a family history of febrile convulsions is present. As the fever goes down, the risk of convulsions also diminishes.

See also CHILD; FEVER.

Fecal analysis (fē′kəl) is the medical examination of a patient's feces to aid in the diagnosis of various disorders.

See also FECES.

Feces (fē′sēz) are the waste or end products of digestion that accumulate in the bowel (large intestine) and are expelled through the anus during defecation. The expelled product is commonly called a stool or a bowel movement. Feces are composed of undigested or indigestible food, especially vegetable fiber such as cellulose; water; mucus and other secretions from the glands that supply the intestinal tract; bacteria; enzymes that have assisted digestion; inorganic salts; and, occasionally, foreign substances.

Q: *What is the normal appearance of feces?*

A: Feces are normally brown or dark brown in color, soft, and formed. Bile pigments give feces their characteristic color. The typical odor is caused by nitrogen compounds that are produced by the action of bacteria. Medical examination of the feces for abnormalities is important in the diagnosis of certain disorders of the intestinal tract.

Q: *What disorders affect the color of feces?*

A: Black feces may result from taking drugs, such as bismuth or iron tablets, or from drinking red wine. The presence of blood in the feces may make them either black or bright red in color. This can occur because of infection, ulceration of the intestine or stomach, diverticular disease, malignant or nonmalignant tumors, abrasive foreign bodies, fissures, or hemorrhoids. Pale yellow or white feces suggest a disorder of bile production, usually an obstruction of the bile ducts. In children, greenish feces indicate that food has passed quickly through the digestive tract.

Q: *What disorders affect the consistency of feces?*

A: Hard, nodular feces are associated with constipation, which may be a symptom of some other disorder. Diarrhea produces excessively watery feces. Feces that are flat and ribbon-like may be caused by an obstruction in the rectum. With jaundice, the feces may be pale and greasy. *See also* CONSTIPATION; DIARRHEA.

Q: *What disorders can be revealed by an analysis of feces?*

A: Worms and amebic dysentery are detected by inspecting the patient's feces. Chemical and microscopic analysis of a stool may show up abnormal amounts of fats, proteins, or sugars or small amounts of blood, which may indicate a disorder of digestion or malabsorption of food.

Feet. See FOOT.

Felon (fel′ən) is an infection of the fingertip.

See also PARONYCHIA.

Femur (fē′mər) is the thighbone, the

bone that extends from the hip to the knee. It is the longest and strongest bone in the body, with some of the most powerful muscles attached to it.

Fenestration (fen ə strā'shən) is the surgical creation of an opening in an organ or bone.

Fertility (fėr til'ə tē) is the capability to produce offspring. In a woman, fertility is the capability of an egg (ovum) to be fertilized and the resulting fetus to be carried. In a man, it is the capability of sperm to fertilize an ovum.

See also FERTILIZATION.

Fertilization (fėr tə lə zā'shən) is the union of an egg (ovum) and a sperm to produce a single cell (zygote) that then develops into an embryo. Fertilization usually takes place in a fallopian tube.

See also PREGNANCY AND CHILDBIRTH.

Fetal alcohol syndrome (fē'təl) refers to the pattern of birth defects among infants born to mothers who consumed alcohol during their pregnancies. Such children may suffer from physical abnormalities, such as growth retardation or facial malformation, and/or mental disabilities, such as hyperactivity. It is not known exactly how much alcohol needs to be consumed to increase the likelihood of giving birth to a handicapped child. Most physicians urge pregnant women to abstain from alcohol.

See also ALCOHOL ABUSE.

Fetal cocaine syndrome (fe' təl) refers to the problems of infants born to mothers who used cocaine during their pregnancies. The use of cocaine only once during pregnancy may result in a disastrous outcome.

Women who use cocaine during pregnancy are at an increased risk for spontaneous abortion, premature labor, and premature separation of the placenta from the uterus. The fetus may develop overall growth disturbances and be smaller than expected. Abnormalities of the fingers and toes, the gastrointestinal tract, or the genitourinary tract may also occur. Prior to delivery, the fetus may develop an irregular heartbeat (arrhythmia) or have a heart attack or stroke.

Many fetal cocaine syndrome babies are born without apparent physical defects, however they have other special needs. Some tend to be more irritable and may be tremulous. They are at an increased risk for seizures and sudden infant death syndrome. They also tend to be poor feeders.

The long-term effects of cocaine on children remains to be seen. Questions have been raised regarding more subtle forms of brain dysfunction, learning disabilities, or hyperactivity.

See also DRUG ABUSE.

Fetal monitor, electronic (fē'təl). Electronic fetal monitor, or EFM, is an apparatus for observing and recording the heart rate of a fetus and for keeping track of the frequency, length, and strength of the mother's uterine contractions.

Fetus (fē'təs) is an unborn baby from two months after conception to the time of birth.

See also PREGNANCY AND CHILDBIRTH.

Fever is abnormally high body temperature. In adults, the normal temperature, taken orally, is 98.6°F (37°C). When taken under the armpit, it is about 1°F (0.56°C) lower than the oral temperature. The rectal temperature is about 1°F (0.56°C) higher. Children have a greater range of body temperature than adults, so a moderate temperature increase in children is of less significance than the same increase in an adult. For practical purposes, fever may be defined as a temperature that is at least 0.5°F above normal on two recordings taken at least two hours apart.

Q: *What are the symptoms that commonly accompany a fever?*

A: The accompanying symptoms depend on the underlying cause of the fever. Often, an individual complains of fatigue and headache. Small children become irritable and may cry easily. A rapidly rising fever may cause shaking chills.

Q: *What causes a fever?*

A: Fever is usually caused by infection. The infecting microbes produce toxins that disturb the normal functioning of the hypothalamus, the heat-regulating center in the brain. Poisoning, drug overdose, and certain illnesses also have this effect, as does damage to the hypothalamus. Fever may also occur with certain blood disorders, breathing problems, and psychological or emotional disorders.

Q: *When is a fever considered to be serious?*

A: Any fever that is accompanied by mental confusion or disorientation

Fever: treatment

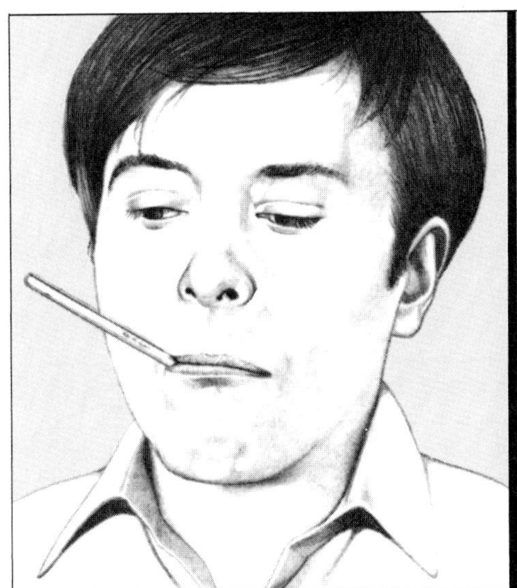

Before taking an oral temperature, make sure that the mercury has been shaken down. Place the bulb of the thermometer beneath the tongue. After about three minutes, remove the thermometer and note the mercury level.

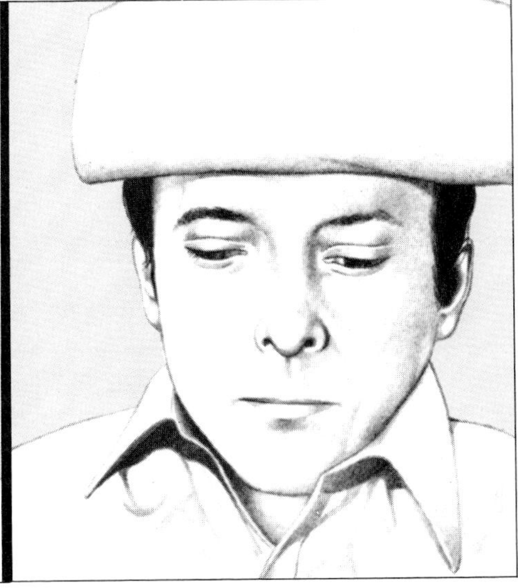

If the patient is uncomfortable, put some crushed ice in a sealed plastic bag and wrap the bag in a dry cloth. Place the bag on the patient's forehead.

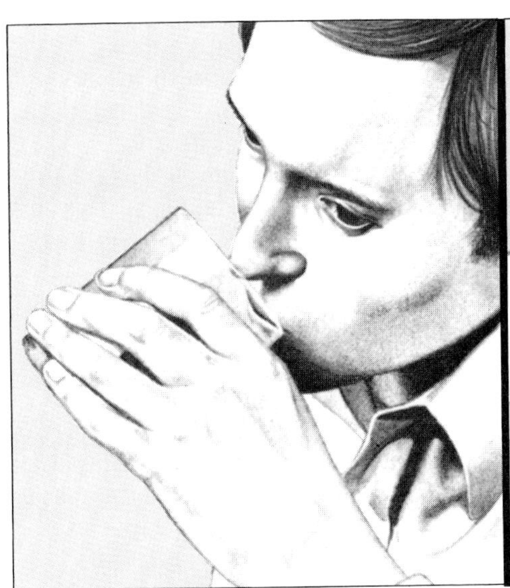

Give the patient plenty of fluids to drink, especially fruit juices or water.

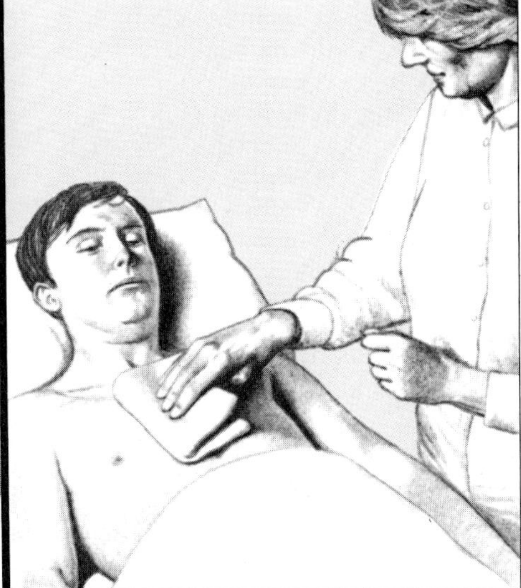

If the fever is over 102°F (38.8°C), place the patient on a waterproof sheet (or in an empty bath) and sponge the body down with lukewarm, not cold, water. Check the patient's temperature every two to four hours until it has decreased. A physician should be consulted.

Fever patterns are an important diagnostic aid. Some diseases reflect the life cycle of the invading organism. For example, malarial protozoa break out from the red blood cells every 72 hours, causing a rapid rise in body temperature.

It is thought that fever helps the body in its fight against disease. One possible reason for a fever may be that some microorganisms can not live in temperatures over 1°F (0.5°C) above normal body temperature.

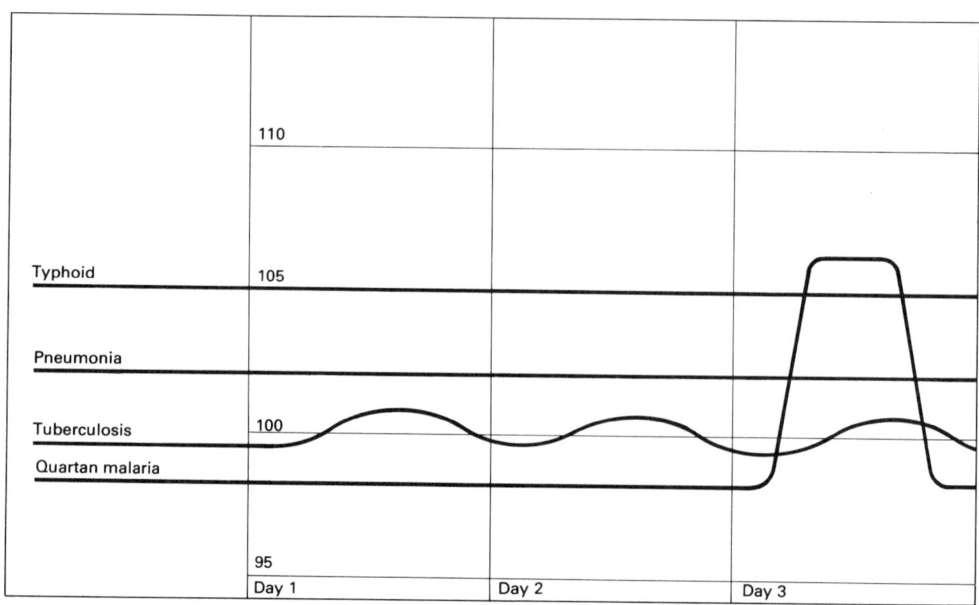

is serious and requires expert medical attention. If the temperature rises above 102°F (38.9°C) or 101°F (38.3°C) in an infant, if a continued fever has no obvious cause, or if a fever is accompanied by vomiting or diarrhea, consult a physician. Any fever in an infant under two months may be serious. Medical attention should be sought.

See also FEVER: TREATMENT.

Fever, relapsing. Relapsing fever is any one of several infectious diseases characterized by recurrent episodes of chills, fever, nausea, and neuromuscular pain. It is caused by *Borrelia* spirochetes transmitted by lice or ticks.

Treatment usually includes the administering of an antibiotic. Bed rest and acetaminophen can help reduce the symptoms.

See also FEVER: TREATMENT.

Feversore, or fever blister, is a sore that occurs on the lips, often during a fever.

See also COLD SORE.

Fever: treatment. Fever is an increase in body temperature and a symptom of a wide variety of illnesses, such as viral or bacterial infection, neurologic disease, malignancy, poisoning, congestive heart failure, and severe trauma. Fever can also be brought about in otherwise healthy people through exercise, dehydration, or anxiety. Childhood immunizations often cause fever.

Although there are individual differences, the accepted normal body temperature, measured orally, is 98.6°F (37°C). The underarm temperature is usually 1°F (0.56°C) lower than the mouth temperature. The rectal temperature is about 1°F (0.56°C) higher than the mouth temperature.

Young children often have a temperature slightly above 98.6°F (37°C). In the elderly, the temperature tends to be slightly lower. A temperature of 104°F (40°C) is more common in infants and children than in adults and carries a different medical significance.

Fever may be accompanied by shivering, sweating, headache, restlessness, loss of appetite, weakness, confusion, and delusions.

Action. Take the patient's temperature. If it is less than 102°F (38.8°C), take the following steps. (*See* illustrations on page 335.)

Put the patient to bed in a cool, quiet room. Do not be alarmed if the patient has no appetite. Encourage the patient to drink plenty of fluids, especially fruit juices. *Do not* give alcohol.

Acetaminophen may be given to help reduce the temperature. The maximum adult dosage is 2 tablets every 4 to 6 hours, not to exceed 8 tablets in 24 hours. Children's acetaminophen preparations should be used for children in the appropriate dosages.

If the fever has not gone within 24 hours or rises above 102°F (38.8°C), consult a physician.

See also TEMPERATURE, TAKING OF.

Fiber, dietary. *See* NUTRITION.

Fiberoptics (fī bər op′tiks) is a technique, employing a fiberscope, used for conducting or transmitting light and images around bends and corners. A fiberscope is a bundle of very thin glass or plastic fibers enclosed in a tube, the "tail" of which contains a light source and the "head" a lens. The bundle may be bent or twisted without distorting the image, transmitted by the fibers to a screen for viewing by the physician performing the examination.

This technique is useful in viewing internal organs or cavities, such as the lungs or the colon, without cutting the body open.

See also ENDOSCOPY.

Fiberscope. *See* FIBEROPTICS.

Fibrillation (fī brə lā'shən) is rapid, irregular twitching of muscle fibers. Any muscle can fibrillate, and the fibrillation sometimes accompanies degenerative disorders, such as motor neuron disease. It may also occur in skeletal muscle that has recently been deprived of its nerve supply. The most serious site of fibrillation is the heart, in which the condition affects either of the two pairs of chambers: the atria or the ventricles.

Q: *What is atrial fibrillation?*

A: Atrial fibrillation is extremely rapid twitching of the muscle of the upper chambers of the heart (atria). The atria no longer contract rhythmically, causing inefficient pumping of the blood. The pulse at the wrist is irregular because the main chambers (ventricles) of the heart are not receiving a regular stimulus from the atria.

Atrial fibrillation may be caused by many kinds of heart disease, such as coronary artery disease due to atherosclerosis or heart valve disease due to rheumatic fever. It may also be caused by hyperactivity of the thyroid gland (thyrotoxicosis) or by alcohol abuse. In some cases, however, the cause can not be identified.

Q: *What is ventricular fibrillation?*

A: This condition resembles atrial fibrillation in its action but affects the lower chambers of the heart (ventricles). The disorder is rapidly fatal, because the weak, rapid heartbeats pump little or no blood into the circulation. Ventricular fibrillation may be caused by coronary thrombosis, drugs such as digitalis, excess diuretic use, or electric shock.

Q: *How is fibrillation in the heart treated?*

A: Atrial fibrillation is effectively treated either with digitalis or with other drugs used to bring the rhythm of the heart under control. All such drugs are used under medical supervision. If fibrillation is associated with a thyroid disorder, thyroid treatment is necessary. Ventricular fibrillation is an emergency treated as a cardiac arrest. Regular heart rhythm is restored using a special machine that causes defibrillation.

See also TACHYCARDIA.

Fibrillation, atrial. *See* FIBRILLATION.

Fibrillation, ventricular. *See* FIBRILLATION.

Fibrin (fī'brən) is an insoluble web of protein that forms the framework of a blood clot. Synthetic fibrin, made from gelatin (fibrin foam), is sometimes used as a surgical dressing to stop a hemorrhage.

See also FIBRINOGEN.

Fibrinogen (fī brin'ə jən) is a soluble protein in the blood plasma. It is essential for the clotting of blood. Through the action of the enzyme thrombin, fibrinogen is converted into the insoluble protein fibrin.

See also FIBRIN.

Fibroadenoma (fī brō ad ə nō'mə) is a benign tumor formed from epithelial and fibroblastic tissue. Epithelial tissue lines hollow organs and covers the surface of the body. Fibroblastic tissue is the connective and supporting membrane between body parts.

Most fibroadenomas are surgically removed to confirm they are benign and because they can continue to grow. In most cases they can be removed under local anesthesia.

Fibrocystic disease of the breast (fī brō sis'tik), also known as chronic cystic mastitis, is the presence of one or more cysts in the breast tissue, making the breasts lumpy. This condition affects primarily women before the time of menopause. While the cysts themselves are not serious, they may pose a threat by obscuring or delaying identification of causes of other lumps in the breast, including cancer.

Q: *What are the symptoms of fibrocystic disease of the breast?*
A: The first sign may be some premenstrual pain or tenderness in the breasts, but more often the lumps are discovered by routine self-examination. If the cysts happen to be near the surface, they may also be moved around within the breast. Usually both breasts are affected with one or more lumps of various sizes. These benign cysts are quite common, occurring in one out of five women before menopause. Nodules that appear after menopause almost always have other causes.
Q: *How is fibrocystic breast disease treated?*
A: A physician must examine any lump to rule out other causes, such as infection, fibroadenosis, benign tumor, or cancer. Testing may include mammogram, thermogram, and biopsy. Once the diagnosis is made, no further treatment is necessary. Avoidance of caffeine reduces breast tenderness in some women with fibrocystic disease. However, patients with fibrocystic disease should be scheduled for examinations every six months, because they are almost three times more likely to develop breast cancer later in life than unaffected women. All women are encouraged to examine their own breasts each month. Regular mammograms are recommended after the age of 40.

See also BREAST EXAMINATION; CANCER; MAMMOGRAM; PALPATION.

Fibrocystic disease of the pancreas. *See* CYSTIC FIBROSIS.

Fibroid (fī′broid), known medically as leiomyoma uteri, is a benign tumor that consists mainly of muscular and fibrous tissue, forming in the muscle of the uterus. One or several fibroids may be present. They are of various shapes and are firm and slow-growing. They may range in size from less than 1 inch (2.5cm) to more than 1 foot (30cm) across.

Q: *What are the symptoms of a fibroid?*
A: Often a fibroid produces no symptoms and is discovered only in a gynecological examination. Possible symptoms may include heavy menstrual bleeding (menorrhagia), occasionally with pain (dysmenorrhea). If a fibroid causes pressure on the bladder, urination is more frequent. A large fibroid can sometimes be felt through the abdominal wall.
Q: *What causes a fibroid?*
A: Each month the uterus increases in size in response to the sex hormones and then decreases at the time of menstruation. It is likely that an area of muscle in the uterus fails to shrink with the rest of the uterus. Each month, the area grows slightly larger under the stimulus of hormones and, as the bulk increases, a fibroid is formed. After menopause, fibroids decrease in size as the uterus becomes smaller.
Q: *Can fibroids affect fertility?*
A: Sometimes fibroids cause sterility. They may also be a factor in producing a miscarriage.
Q: *How are fibroids treated?*
A: Fibroids need treatment only if they produce symptoms. In women who wish to become pregnant, symptomatic fibroids may be removed while preserving the uterus. A hysterectomy (surgical removal of the uterus) may be needed for intolerable symptoms of pain or bleeding in women who do not desire future pregnancies. Very rarely does a fibroid degenerate into a malignant cancer.
Q: *Are fibroids a common condition?*
A: Yes. It is estimated that 20 percent of women have fibroids by the time menopause begins.

Fibroma (fī brō′mə) is a benign (noncancerous) tumor of connective tissue. It may occur anywhere in the body, for example, in the fibrous covering of bone (periosteum) or nerve. It has a firm consistency, is irregular in shape, and grows slowly. A fibroma is not painful unless it causes pressure.

Fibromyalgia (fī brō mī al′jē ah) is a condition characterized by generalized aching and specific points that "trigger" pain. Often the patient experiences a disturbed sleep pattern with morning fatigue. It usually develops in tense, middle-aged persons, who develop symptoms that include stiffness in the neck, shoulders, and trunk, sometimes aggravated even by movement. No specific laboratory study confirms the problem, and there is disagreement among experts as to its cause. Fibromyalgia is also known as fibrositis and trigger point syndrome.

The muscular aches and pains of fibromyalgia are best treated by rest, gentle massage, stretching exercises, and locally applied heat or ice. Aspirin or other anti-inflammatory drugs are also used to treat the pain and stiffness. Small doses of tricyclic antidepressants are sometimes useful. Injection of trigger points with local anesthetic will temporarily relieve pain and allow initiation of a stretching program.

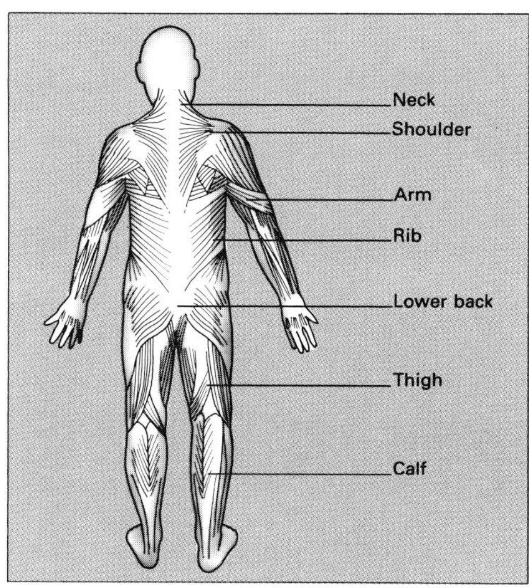

Fibromyalgia primarily affects the sites shown above.

Fibrosarcoma (fī brō sär kō'mə) is a rare, malignant tumor formed from fibroblasts, the cells of connective fibrous tissue. A fibrosarcoma is treated by surgical removal.

See also CANCER; TUMOR.

Fibrosis (fī brō'sis) is the formation of fibrous scar tissue. It is a normal reaction to infection or injury and may occur in the lungs, following pneumonia, or form adhesions in the peritoneum, following peritonitis.

See also PERITONITIS; SCAR.

Fibrous tissue (fī'brəs) is tissue containing or composed of fibers that hold organs and other structures in place.

Fibula (fib'yə lə) is the long, slender bone on the outside of the lower leg, extending from just below the knee to the ankle. Its lower end forms the outer side of the ankle joint. Unlike the shinbone (tibia), the fibula does not bear

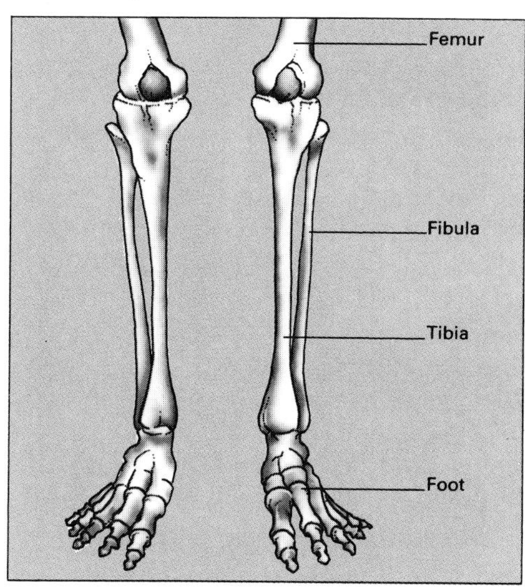

The **fibula** is a long, thin bone extending from the knee downward to the ankle.

weight but serves as an attachment for some of the leg muscles.

Fifth disease, more commonly known as erythema infectiosum, is an infection, probably caused by a virus, which mostly affects children. It is characterized by a reddish rash, usually lasting no more than 10 days. The rash first appears on the cheeks with a chapped or "slapped" appearance. Later, a rash develops over the trunk. Fever is rare. No treatment is necessary, as fifth disease clears up by itself. The child need not stay home from school.

Filariasis (fil ə rī'ə sis) is a general term for infection by any of several tropical worms of the superfamily *Filarioidea.*

See also ELEPHANTIASIS; ONCHOCERCIASIS; WORM.

Filling, in dentistry, is the process of repairing a tooth cavity. It may also refer to the material placed in the cavity.

See also TOOTH DECAY.

Finger is any of the digits of the hand. A finger consists of three bones (phalanges), except for the thumb, which has only two. The phalanges are connected by hinge joints. Tendons along the upper and lower surfaces of the fingers move the joints. These are controlled by muscles in the forearm. Other muscles in the hand help with fine finger movements.

See also DUPUYTREN'S CONTRACTURE; FROSTBITE; HEBERDEN'S NODE; RAYNAUD'S PHENOMENON; SKELETON.

Finger amputation: treatment. Summon emergency medical aid immediately. Try to stop the bleeding by raising the person's arm and applying pressure over the end of the finger stump. The severed finger or part of a finger should be saved and placed in a clean plastic bag which should then be immersed in ice water. In some cases, a severed finger or part of a finger can be rejoined to the hand with a good chance for survival, as long as prompt attention and immediate medical care are given.

Finger fracture: first aid. See FRACTURE: FIRST AID.

Fingernail. See NAIL.

Finger, ring stuck on: treatment. Place the finger in ice, then cover it with oil or grease and try to slip the ring off. If this method is ineffective and the blood circulation is constricted, urgently seek medical attention.

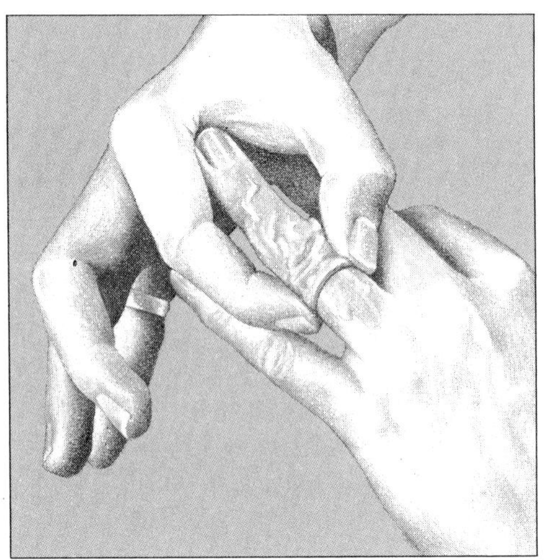

After covering the finger with oil or grease, gently try to slip the ring off. If this does not work, do not panic and do not use force to remove the ring. This will cause more swelling and further block the supply of blood to the finger. Seek medical attention.

Firearm safety. Firearms are probably the most potentially lethal pieces of equipment that are kept in the private home. About 2 percent of all accidental deaths in the United States are caused by gunshot wounds; the majority of accidental deaths are caused by handguns. In 1983, approximately 1,700 persons died as a result of accidents involving firearms, and thousands more suffered serious wounds.

Firearms are now manufactured to a high standard of safety and precision; almost all accidents involving firearms are caused by human, not mechanical, failure. Therefore, it is important that all families that possess firearms take rigorous safety precautions. Children should never be allowed to handle a gun, even in play.

Cleaning. Guns that are allowed to become dirty are unreliable and extremely dangerous, so all guns should be cleaned regularly. Simple and inexpensive gun-cleaning kits can be bought from any gun shop, but it is possible to clean the barrel with normal mineral oil and a soft rag secured firmly to the end of a straight stick. Follow the manufacturer's instructions for cleaning. Oil with gun oil before reassembling. Check that everything is in working order after you have reassembled the gun.

If you drop the gun at any time, inspect all the parts and clean them thoroughly before using the gun again. This is especially important when outdoors, as a small object or a piece of dirt in the barrel can cause the gun to explode when fired.

Storage. Lock all firearms in a cabinet or rack. Deactivate the gun by removing the firing pin. Never leave a gun on open display, where it will be a temptation to children and intruders. Store the ammunition separately. If you keep two different types of shotgun, it is essential to keep the ammunition for each gun in a separate place. A cartridge that is too large for the gun can lodge halfway down the barrel, and at the next firing both cartridges may explode simultaneously and kill or injure the user.

Trigger Locks. It is sensible to install trigger locks on all guns in the home. This is an essential precaution if there are children in the house. Simple versions are inexpensive; the more complicated devices are expensive and highly sophisticated. One popular idea for the handgun is a magnetically released trigger lock. The owner of the gun wears a magnetic safety ring on the middle finger of the trigger hand, and the trigger lock can not be released by anyone not wearing this ring. Another modification is the puzzle safety handgun. This handgun does not fire unless the user makes the extra directional movement that is built into the thumbpiece. This means that a person who is not familiar with the gun is unable to seize it and fire it.

Loading and Unloading. Always assume that a gun is loaded until you have checked that it is not. The only safe way to check whether a gun is

Number of deaths in accidents involving firearms

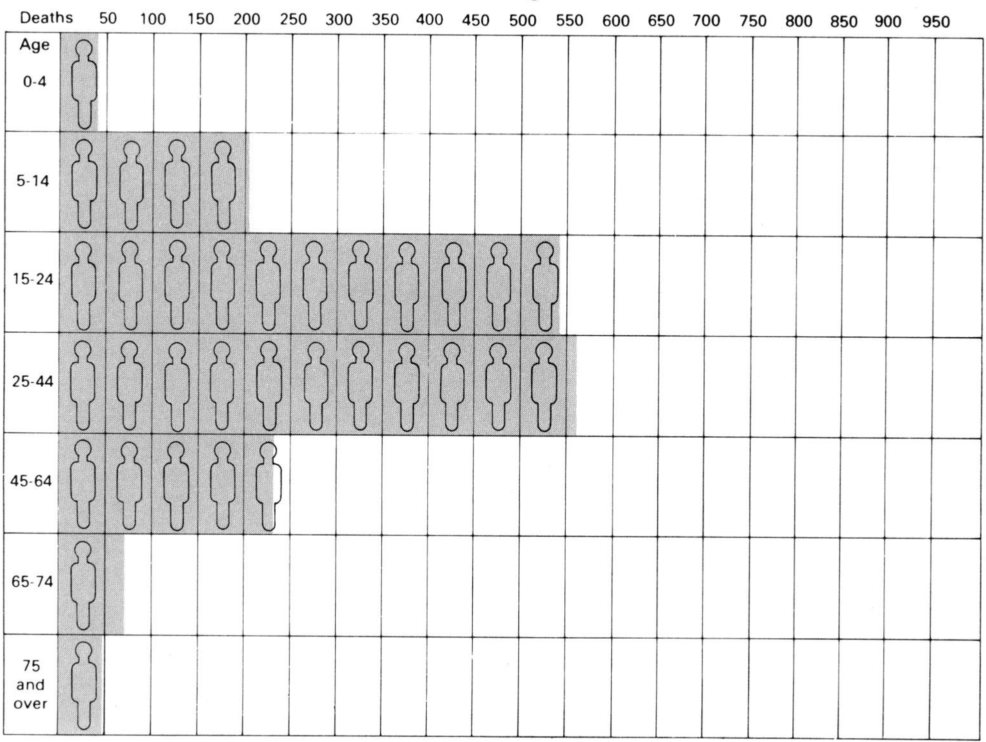

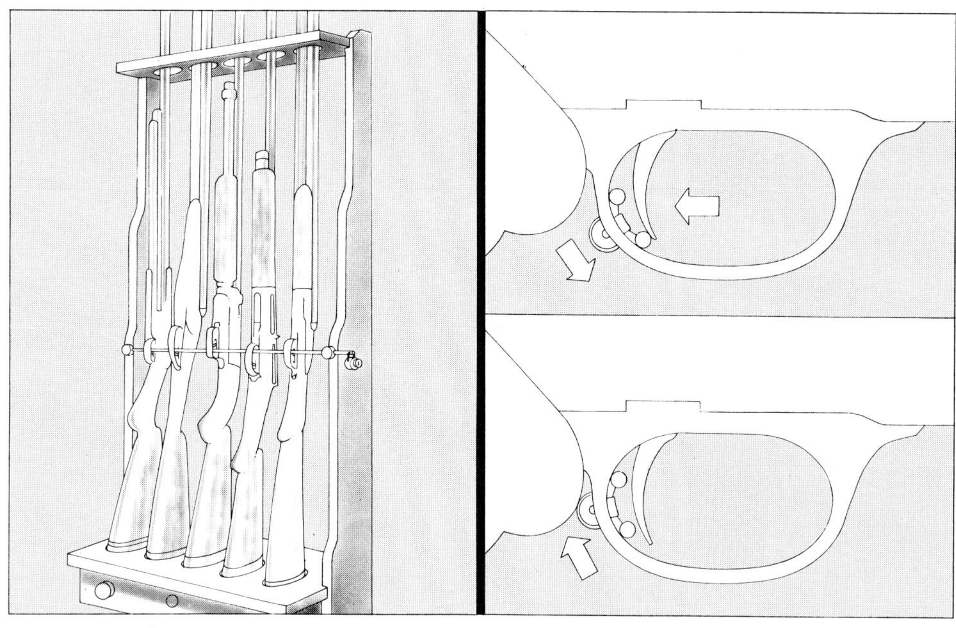

It is safer to store all firearms out of sight. However, if you must have them on display, secure them in a locking wall cabinet. Make sure that all firearms are stored unloaded.

A trigger lock lessens the likelihood of a person picking up a gun in anger and firing without thinking. It is also an invaluable precaution if there are children in the house.

loaded is to open the action and check the chamber and the magazine whenever you pick up a gun. Never look down the barrel from the front of the gun to see if it is loaded, and never pull the trigger indoors to check it. If there is a bullet in the gun, it could ricochet round the room and kill someone.

Ideally, always unload the gun when leaving the range or field, when you do not intend to fire it immediately, and also when placing it in a rack, a case, or a vehicle. In some situations, however, it may be wiser to keep the gun loaded; many shotgun accidents occur when a gun is fired unintentionally while it is being loaded or unloaded, so a user may actually increase the risk of an accident by loading or unloading a gun when it is not strictly necessary. You should learn how to carry a loaded gun in a safe, vertical position when crossing rough ground and obstacles, and when bending down to retrieve game. It is particularly important to keep the gun upright and off the ground if you trip and fall.

Hunting. You should hunt in small groups of only two or three people, and always know where your companions are positioned. You should fire a gun only when you can see your chosen target clearly; never fire at random into bushes or trees where you have seen signs of movement. For your own protection, always wear some item of brightly colored clothing, such as a cap or sweater, which makes you clearly visible to your companions.

Firearm safety should be based on a proper respect for guns and an awareness of their lethal potential. This respect should be instilled in children from the moment they first come into contact with guns. Teach them never to point a gun at anyone, even in jest. Both children and adults should have considerable experience in firing with blank cartridges before being allowed to shoot with live ammunition.

Fire prevention and control. The home is such a familiar place that fire hazards may all too easily go unnoticed. There are a variety of precautions that should be taken to minimize the possibility of a fire breaking out in the home. All homes should be equipped with smoke detectors, which should be tested regularly and whose batteries should be promptly replaced when they wear out.

Multilevel homes should have at least one smoke detector per floor. A good location for a smoke detector is directly outside a bedroom and at the top of every flight of stairs, especially those leading to a basement. Avoid placing one in the kitchen itself, since heat and fumes from cooking may set off a false alarm.

The installation of smoke detectors in a home or commercial property may lower its household insurance rates.

Local or Area Heating. Space heaters and unguarded coal or wood fires in open fireplaces are a common source of fires in the home. An open fireplace should be protected with a fire screen whenever a fire is burning in it. The screen should cover the entire opening of the fireplace.

With coal or wood fires, there is a danger of the chimney catching fire. The flue should be cleaned regularly to remove flammable tars that may have accumulated. The fire should not be allowed to become too hot or to roar up into the chimney. If wood is used as fuel, hardwoods from trees that shed their leaves should be chosen; they produce less flammable tars than softwoods.

Gas and oil space heaters should never be used in bedrooms. Elsewhere in the home, this type of heater should be vented to the outside and anchored to the floor. The floor beneath the heater should be protected with a layer of sheet metal or masonry tiles. The fuel lines should be protected against damage and placed out of the general path of travel. Portable gas or oil space heaters should not be used in homes where children are present.

Electric heaters are also a fire hazard. It is essential to keep them in good repair and to replace wires that are worn. If an electric heater is fitted with a fan, this should be kept operable at all times to prevent the heating coils from overheating. A protective grill should be fitted over the heating coils.

All types of heaters should be approved by a nationally recognized testing agency. They should be installed and operated strictly in accordance with the manufacturer's instructions.

Cigarettes. If people in the household smoke, there should be enough ash-

Fire prevention and control

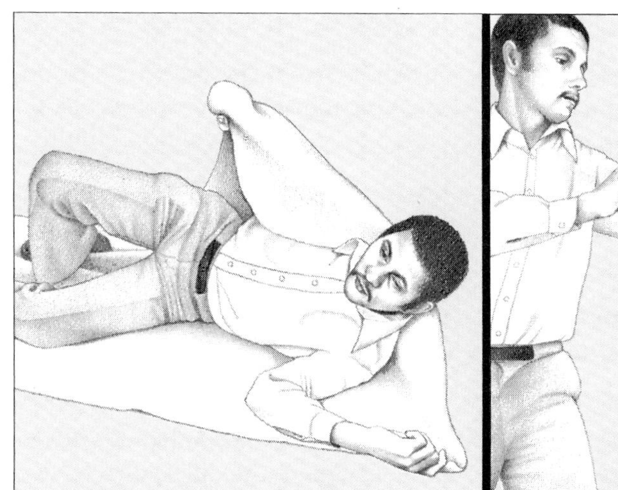

If your clothing catches on fire, lie on the ground immediately. This slows the flames from spreading up the body. Once on the ground, roll around to smother the flames. If there is a rug or blanket close at hand, wrap yourself in it.

If a pan of grease catches on fire, immediately turn off the heat. Put the fire out with a fire extinguisher or quickly slide a rigid cover, such as a lid, over the pan. *Never use water on a grease fire.* Extinguishers that are suitable for fighting grease fires should be marked either "All-class" or "Class B."

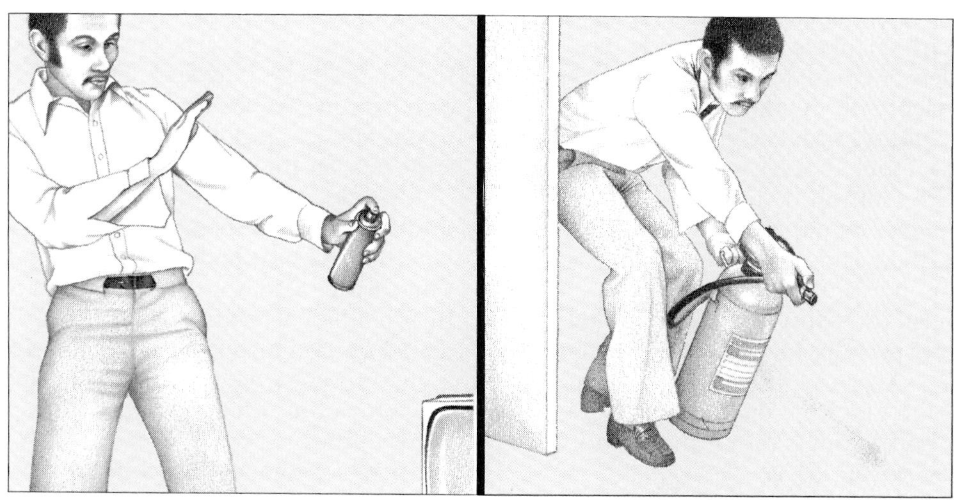

An electrical fire should *never* be fought with water unless the electrical equipment has first been unplugged. Extinguishers that are suitable for fighting electrical fires should be marked either "All-class" or "Class C."

Keep a fire extinguisher near potential fire hazards. In the event of a fire, position yourself a safe distance from the blaze. Direct the extinguisher's spray at the base of the fire and sweep the spray left and right. The best general extinguisher for all fires contains carbon dioxide.

trays available to prevent them from using wastebaskets or other flammable receptacles for ashes and butts. All ashtrays should be emptied into a metal container at night. Never smoke in bed or when drowsy.

Children. Keep matches and lighters out of the reach of children at all times. Children should wear flame-resistant clothing. Never put toys on the mantel or hang a mirror over a flame or heat source. A child may be tempted to stand too near to the fire in order to reach for something.

Small children should never be left alone in the house. If it is necessary to leave the children, ask a friend, neighbor, or relative to look after them while you are out.

Electrical Appliances. All electrical appliances should be kept in good repair. They should be grounded and fitted with appropriate fuses. Electric sockets should have childproof covers. Electrical equipment should always be unplugged when not in use.

Electric blankets are a common fire hazard. Never sleep on top of an overblanket nor beneath an underblanket. Electric blankets should never be folded or creased. They should never be used to dry damp bedding or be put on a child's or elderly person's bed if bed-wetting is likely.

Fire Control. If you discover a fire, get everyone out of the house. To this end, there should already be an escape route, previously planned and rehearsed. It is very important to have one, especially in case of fires on upper floors. After everyone is safely outside, call the Fire Department. If you are the last person out, shut all doors and windows as you leave.

If the fire is small and in its early stages and you are certain that you can tackle it without danger to yourself, make sure that everyone is safe before you begin. You should also make sure that the fire extinguisher is suitable for the type of fire. Most extinguishers are labeled as to the types of fires they best control. "All-class" extinguishers are suitable for any type of fire. When using an extinguisher, be careful not to scatter burning material with the jet.

Every room should have a second exit in the event that the usual one is blocked by fire or smoke. Usually the second exit is a window. On second and third floors, this should lead to a roof or balcony where you can wait for help to arrive. If there is no such structure, you should use a rope, a chain ladder, or some other aid to climb down.

If you are trapped in a room by a fire somewhere else in the building, you should shut the door and block any cracks with material, such as bedding, to prevent smoke from filling the room. Then go to a window and shout for help. If smoke fills the room, lean out of the window. If this is impossible because of flames from below, lie on the floor where the air is clearer. If you have to escape before help arrives, throw bedding, clothes, or even cardboard boxes onto the ground to break your fall. Lower yourself or a child to full arm's length before dropping. If you are in a room above the second floor, drop only as a last resort.

First-aid fundamentals. First aid is the immediate care given to a victim of an accident, sudden illness, or other medical emergency. Proper first aid can save a victim's life, especially if the victim is bleeding heavily, has stopped breathing, or has been poisoned. First aid can also prevent the development of additional medical problems that might result from an injury or illness.

Emergency treatment should be administered by the person on the scene who has the best knowledge of first aid. The treatment should be continued until professional medical help is available. First aid also involves reassuring a victim, relieving the pain, and moving the victim, if necessary, to a hospital or clinic.

Persons interested in taking a first aid training course should contact their local chapter of the American Red Cross.

General Rules for First Aid

Analyze the situation quickly and decide whether you can help the victim. If you decide to treat the victim, begin at once. If you are confused or unsure of yourself, do not attempt to give treatment. In many cases, the wrong treatment causes more damage than no treatment at all. For professional help in giving first aid, call a hospital, the fire department, or the police.

The general steps to take in any situation requiring first aid include the following: provide urgent care for life-threatening emergencies; examine the victim for injuries; treat the victim for shock; and call a physician.

Provide Urgent Care. Certain medical emergencies require immediate care to save the victim's life. If the victim is bleeding severely, has been poisoned, or has stopped breathing, treatment must begin at once. A delay of even a few minutes can be fatal in these cases. *See also* ARTIFICIAL RESPIRATION; BLEEDING: FIRST AID; POISONING: FIRST AID.

Do not move a victim who may have a broken bone, internal injuries, or damage to the neck or spine, unless absolutely necessary to prevent further injury. If the victim is lying down, keep the person in that position. Do not allow the victim to get up and walk about. Never give food or liquid to a person who may require surgery.

If the victim is unconscious, turn the head to one side to help prevent the person from choking on blood, saliva, or vomit. Do not move the head of a person who may have a broken neck or a spinal injury. Never pour liquid into the mouth of an unconscious person. *See also* UNCONSCIOUSNESS: TREATMENT.

Make certain that the victim has an open airway. The airway consists of the nose, mouth, and upper throat. These passages must remain open in order for the victim to breathe. *See also* ARTIFICIAL RESPIRATION.

Examine the Victim for Individual Injuries only after treating the person for any life-threatening emergencies. The victim may suffer from diabetes, heart trouble, or some other disease that can cause sudden illness. Many persons with such medical problems carry a medical tag or card. The tag or card lists instructions for care that should be followed exactly. If you must examine the victim's purse or wallet to look for a medical card, you should do so in the presence of a witness, if possible.

Make the victim comfortable, but handle the person as little as possible. If necessary, shade the victim from the sun or cover the victim to prevent chilling. Loosen the person's clothing, but do not pull on the victim's belt, because this pressure could further damage an injured spine.

Remain calm and reassure the victim. Explain what has happened and what is being done. Ask any spectators to stand back.

Treat for Shock. Shock results from the body's failure to circulate blood properly. Any serious injury or illness can cause a victim to suffer from shock. When a person is in shock, the blood fails to supply enough oxygen and food to the brain and other organs. The most serious form of shock may result in death.

A victim in shock may appear fearful, light-headed, weak, and extremely thirsty. In some cases, the victim may feel nauseated. The skin appears pale and feels cold and damp; the pulse is rapid and faint; and breathing is quick and shallow, or deep and irregular. It is best to treat a seriously injured person for shock even if these signs are not present. The treatment will help prevent a person from going into shock.

To treat shock, place the victim on his or her back, with the legs raised slightly. If the victim has trouble breathing in this position, place the person in a half-sitting, half-lying position. Warm the victim by placing blankets over and under the body.

Call for a Physician. Send someone else to call for a doctor, an ambulance, or other help while you care for the victim. If you are alone with the victim, you must decide when you can safely leave to call for assistance. Always treat the victim for any life-threatening conditions before leaving to summon aid.

When telephoning for help, be ready to describe the nature of the victim's illness or injury, the first-aid measures you have taken, and the exact location of the victim. Also be prepared to write down any instructions a physician may give you. Repeat the instructions and ask questions to clarify instructions you do not understand.

If you decide to take the victim to a hospital emergency room, it may help to first telephone the hospital to say you are coming. The hospital staff will then be better prepared to treat the victim's particular problems. Transportation by ambulance is preferable, as trained paramedical personnel will then be available to attend to the victim.

First-aid supplies include a variety of materials.

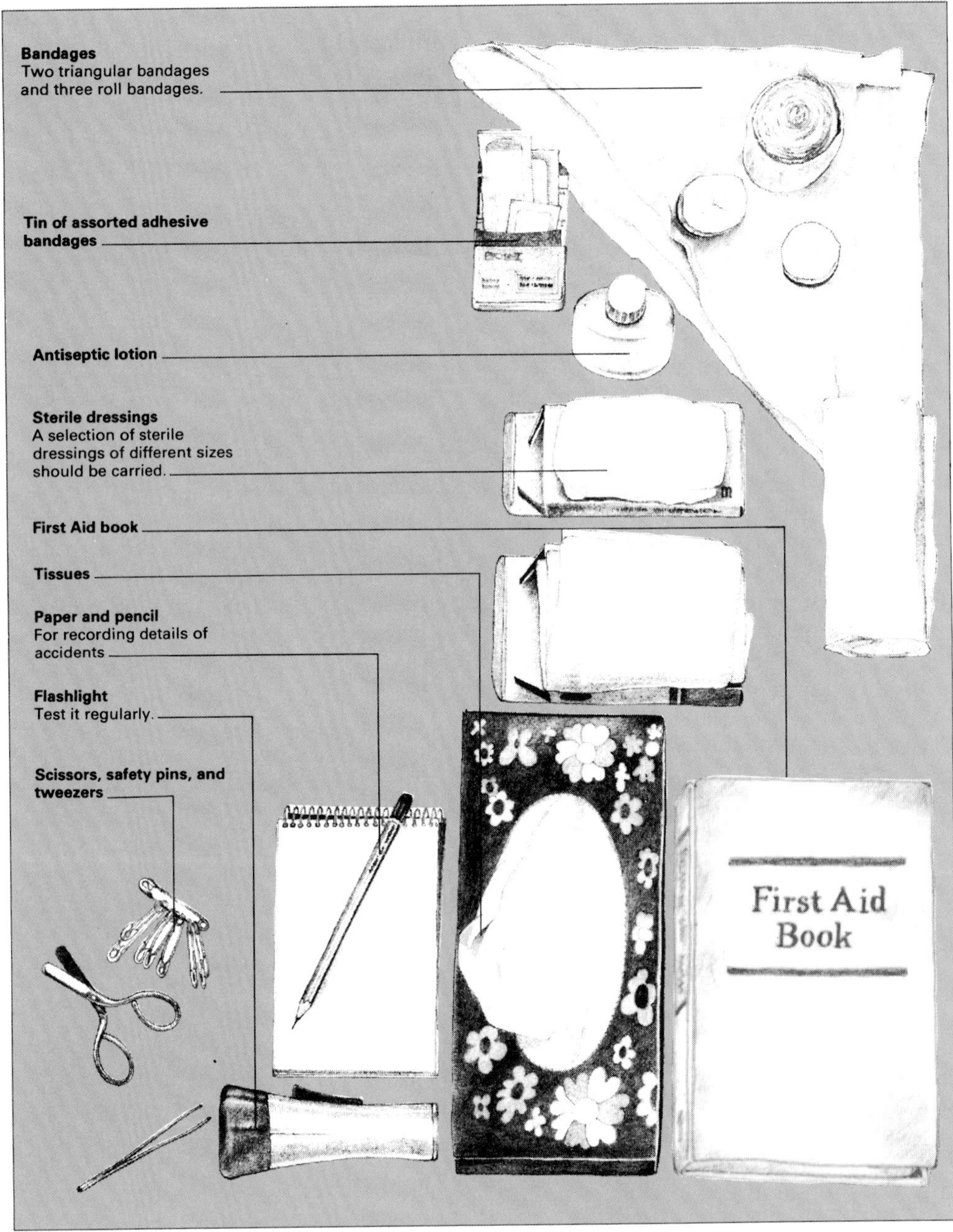

Every home should have a list of emergency phone numbers posted on or near the telephone. However, if such numbers are not available, the operator can assist you in contacting the proper person or emergency unit. Every home, as well as each car that members of the family drive, should also have a first-aid kit.

Emergency First-aid Kit

The home first-aid kit should be located in the kitchen, the most common site of home accidents, or in some other easily accessible place. The kit should also be convenient to the backyard, another common accident site, particularly among families with active children. Too often, families store the first-aid kit in an upstairs bathroom, and precious time is wasted retrieving the kit in the event of an emergency.

Wherever you choose to locate the first-aid kit, it should be well out of the reach of small children. Many medicines still do not come in so-called childproof containers and, therefore, can pose a danger to children. Also, the home medicine chest undoubtedly contains such potentially dangerous items as scissors, safety pins, and prescription medicines.

The first-aid kit you carry in your car is as important as the one you keep at home, if not more so. In an automobile accident, there is a greater likelihood that more than one person will be injured. Necessary supplies will be very difficult, if not impossible, to borrow, as you might at home. Remember, too, that the kit could be vitally important in the treatment of accident victims in other cars, whether or not your own vehicle is involved.

The emergency kit for the car should be placed in some easily accessible and visible location within the passenger compartment of the car. Mark it with a red cross, so that a nonfamily member could find it if necessary. Do not put the emergency kit in the trunk of the car. This location would not only delay access but might even make access impossible in certain kinds of accidents. If your car were struck from the rear, for example, you might not be able to get the trunk open.

In addition to the items you would have in a home first-aid kit (*see* accompanying illustration), items for the car should include a CB radio (for summoning emergency services), a battery-operated, flashing emergency light, and a blanket. You can buy a good quality first-aid kit that has everything you need or assemble your own from components you purchase separately. If you have family members who are prone to car sickness, you may want to include motion sickness remedies and perhaps a few plastic bags just in case.

It is extremely important to keep any medicines well stocked and up-to-date and to replace the equipment as it is used. Items of ordinary household use, such as scissors and flashlight, should never be borrowed from either kit. Bandages, once used by children for games, should never be rewound and put back in the medical kits. They should be replaced by new bandages.

Transporting an Injured Person

Do not move the victim if medical help is available. If the victim's life is endangered by hazards, such as fire or traffic, the priority is to move the victim away. Remember that transportation may aggravate the victim's condition.

The priorities of action are emergency rescue, if necessary, followed by treatment of breathing difficulties, bleeding, poisoning, and unconsciousness. Any injured limb should be supported and, if the extent of injury is in doubt, treated as a fracture and splinted before moving the victim. *See* FRACTURE: FIRST AID.

The victim should be made comfortable and the most practical method of transportation ascertained. Be sure to ask for assistance when faced with an emergency. Remember, time is all-important. Other persons can phone or go for assistance, locate emergency supplies and equipment, and assist you at the scene of the emergency. In the case of auto accidents, for example, it is extremely important to warn oncoming traffic in order to prevent additional accidents.

The method of transportation chosen depends upon the nature and severity of the injury, the number of people available, the distance to be traveled, and the terrain to be traversed. During the journey, keep a careful watch on the victim's condition, ensuring that the air passage is clear at all times, that there is no further bleeding, that the victim does not become unconscious, and that fractures remain immobilized. The journey itself should be as smooth and as safe as possible.

Transportation on a stretcher is the least tiring method and should be used wherever possible. Always transport an unconscious victim on a stretcher. In many instances, however, no stretcher will be available and you will have to move the victim by other means.

If conditions require unassisted and immediate removal, you may have to drag the victim. Though haste may be essential to a successful rescue, you must nevertheless make sure to drag the victim in a way that will minimize the risk of further injury. To do this, grasp the victim by the shoulders and pull in the direction of the long axis of the body. To protect the spinal cord against possible additional injury, be very careful not to bend or twist the victim's neck or trunk. Never attempt to drag an injured person sideways. If you should find it impossible or extremely difficult to drag the victim by the shoulders, drag the victim by the ankles instead, observing the same precautionary measures as with the shoulder drag.

Transporting an injured person

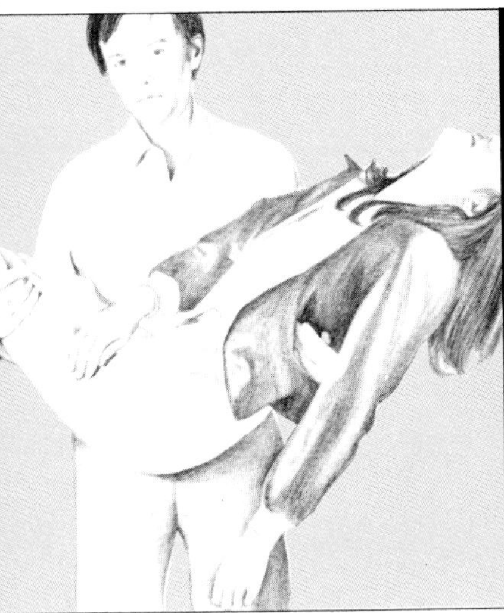

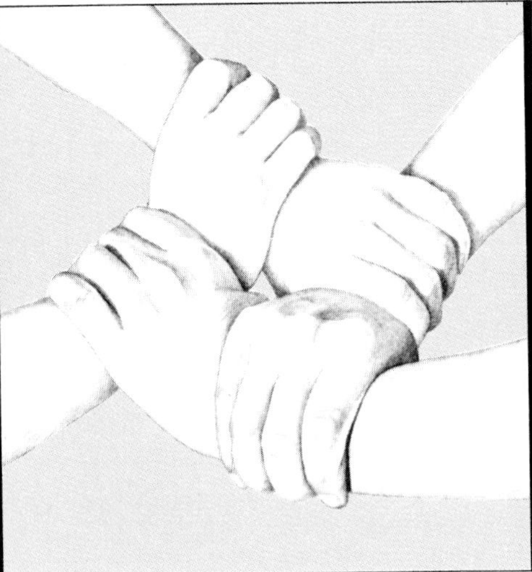

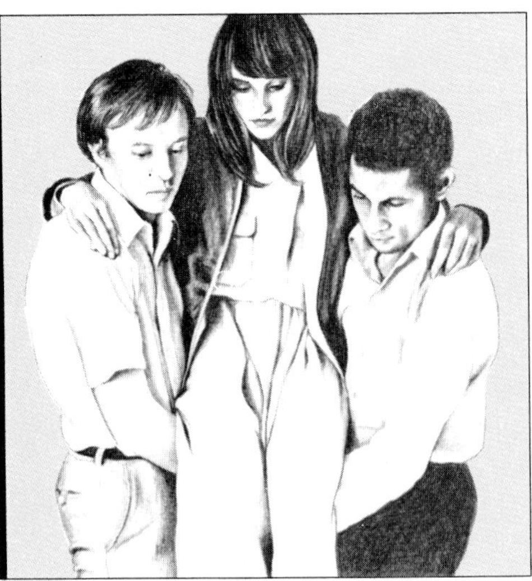

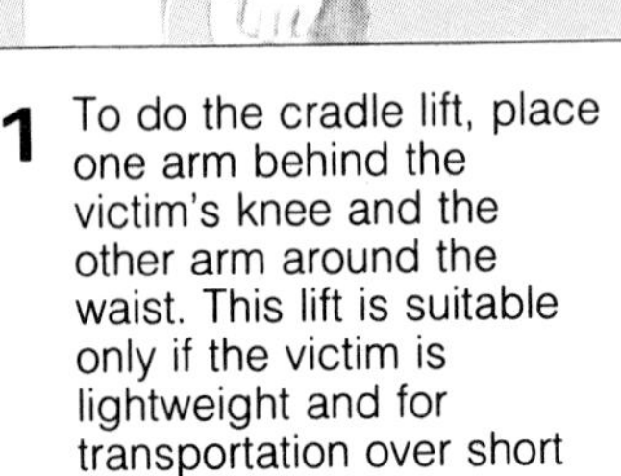

1 To do the cradle lift, place one arm behind the victim's knee and the other arm around the waist. This lift is suitable only if the victim is lightweight and for transportation over short distances.

2 For the four-handed lift, two first aiders stand facing each other behind the victim. Each grasps the top of his or her own left wrist with the right hand. Each first aider then grasps the other's right wrist with his or her own left hand.

3 To continue the four-handed lift, the victim places an arm around the neck of each first aider and sits on their interlocked hands. This lift is tiring, and so is suitable only for short distances.

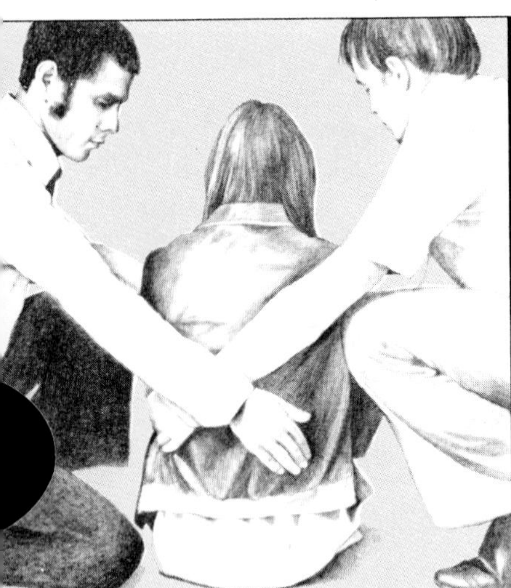

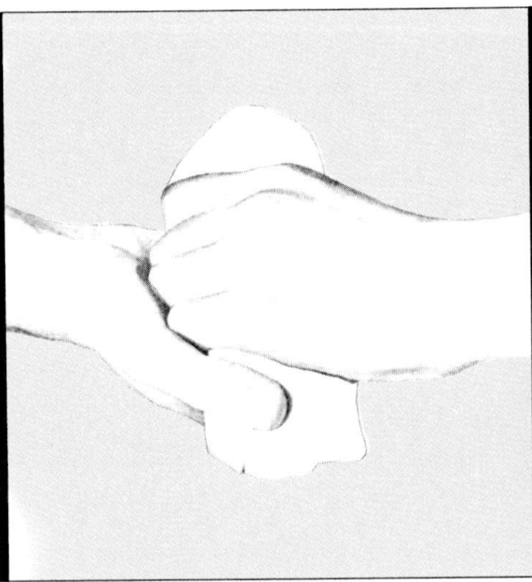

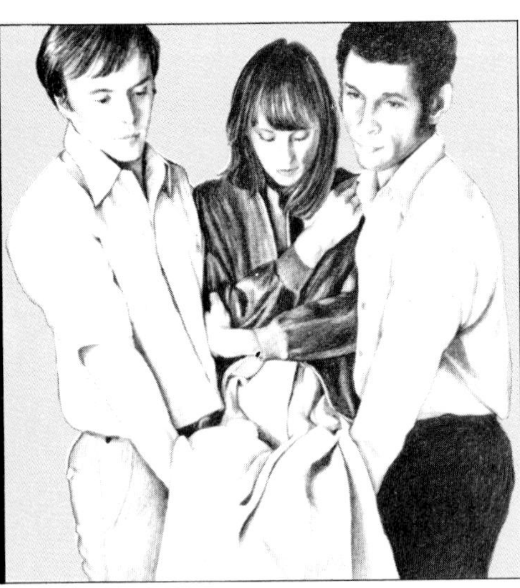

4 The two-handed lift is useful when the victim's arms are disabled. Two first aiders stand facing each other and bend down, one on each side of the victim. Each first aider places an arm behind the victim's back, just below the shoulders. They then raise the victim into a sitting position.

5 The two-handed lift continues with the first aiders passing their other arms underneath the victim's thighs and clasping their hands in a hook grip. The first aider on the victim's left side has the palm upward and holds a handkerchief to prevent being hurt by the other's fingernails.

6 The first aiders rise at the same time and step off with their outside feet. The first aiders should walk forward with a crossover step, not with sideways paces.

Transporting an injured person

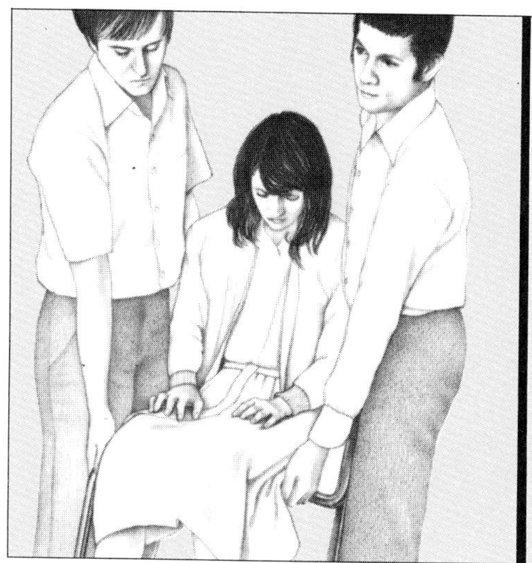

1 Sit the victim on a straight-back chair. Two first aiders stand, one on each side of the chair, each holding one front chair leg and one rear chair leg. The chair is then tilted slightly backward and lifted. This method should be used only if the victim is conscious and not seriously injured.

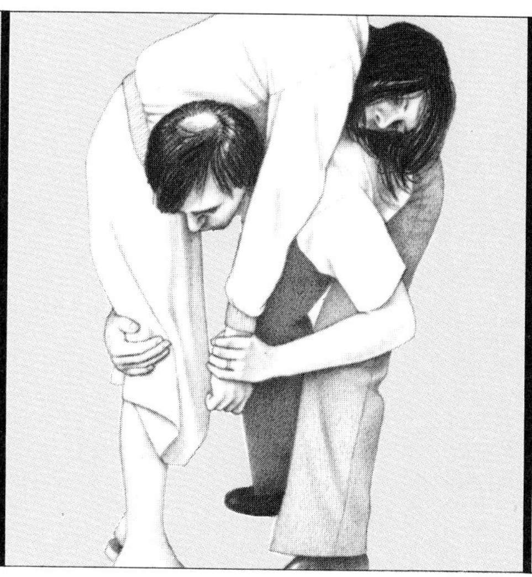

2 The victim should be helped to an upright position. The first aider should grasp the victim's right wrist with his or her left hand. The first aider then bends down with his or her head under the victim's extended right arm. The first aider places his or her right arm around the victim's legs and takes the victim's weight on his or her right shoulder.

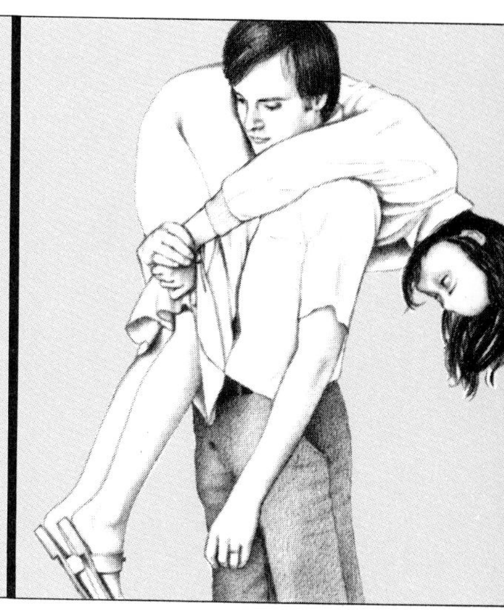

3 The first aider then rises to an upright position. He or she pulls the victim across both shoulders and transfers the victim's right wrist to his or her right hand. This lift should not be used unless it is necessary to carry the victim only a short distance as the first aider may suffer a back strain from lifting the victim.

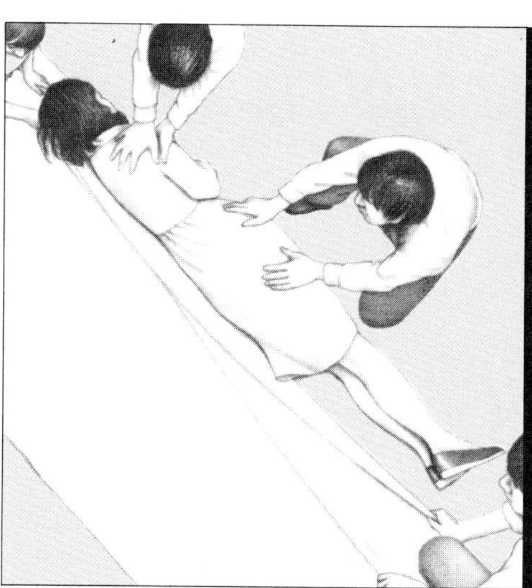

4 A blanket should be rolled lengthways for half of its width. One first aider supports the victim's head and neck, another the victim's feet. Two other first aiders roll the victim gently toward them. The rolled edge of the blanket is then placed alongside the victim's back.

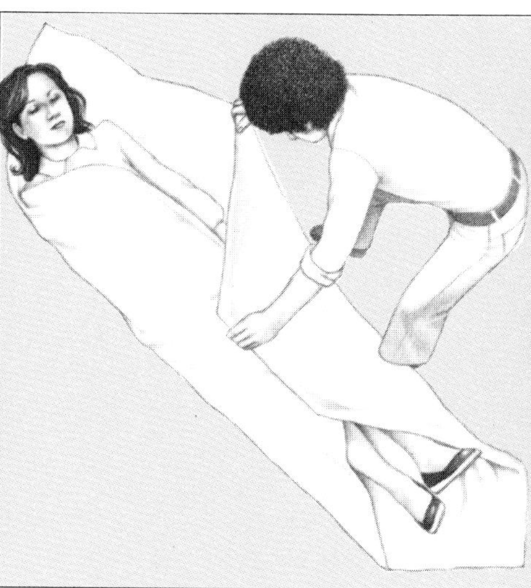

5 The victim should be turned onto the back over the roll of the blanket and then onto his or her other side. The first aider unrolls the blanket and turns the victim onto the back. Finally, the first aider rolls the edges of the blanket to form hand grips.

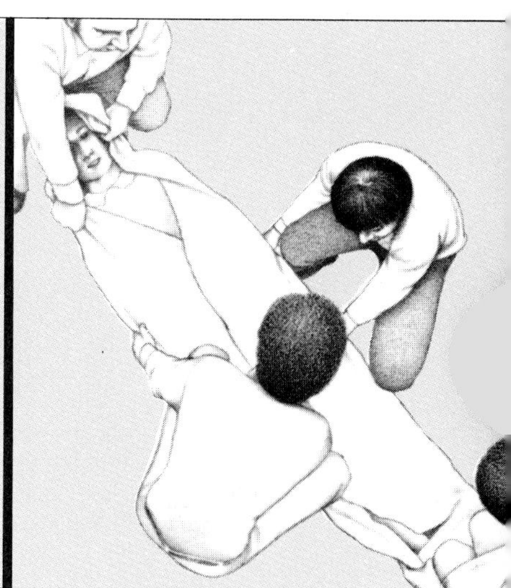

6 One first aider grasps the blanket by the side of the victim's neck, another grasps the blanket around the victim's feet. Two other first aiders stand on each side of the victim and grasp the rolls of blanket to support the victim's back and thighs. The first aiders then rise together and lift the victim onto a stretcher.

Improvising a stretcher

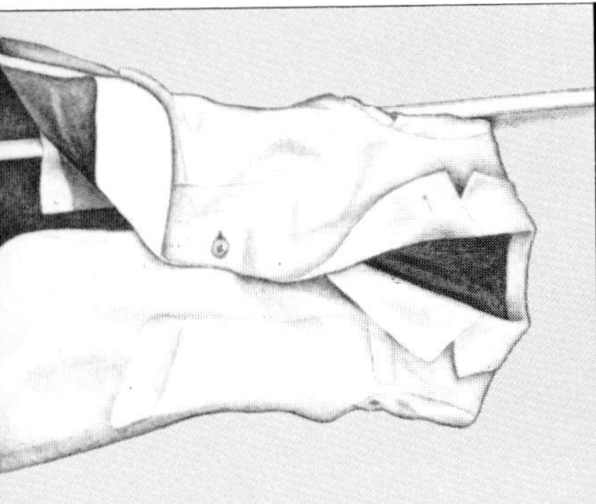

1 A stretcher can be improvised by using anything that provides a firm, flat surface and is large enough to accommodate the victim. For example, a door, a broad plank, or an ironing board can be used. A layer of padding should be placed on the surface and covered with a blanket. One form of stretcher can be made using two jackets and two strong poles. Turn the jacket sleeves inside out. Lay the jackets down with the bottom hems touching and button the jackets. Thread the poles through the sleeves.

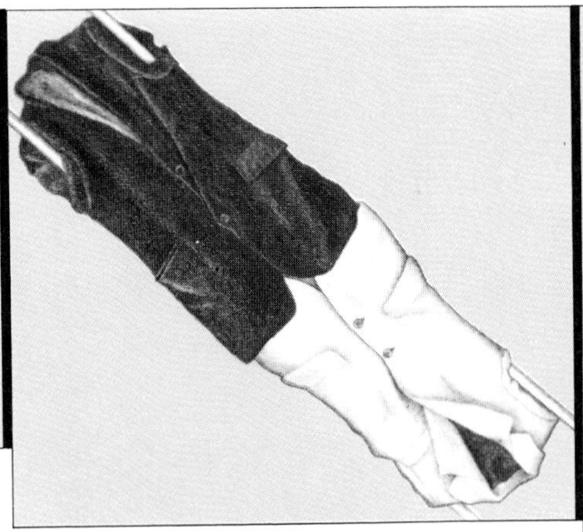

2 Lash a strip of wood perpendicularly between the poles at each end to ensure that the poles stay apart and that the stretcher stays taut. Always test an improvised stretcher before using it to transport the victim.

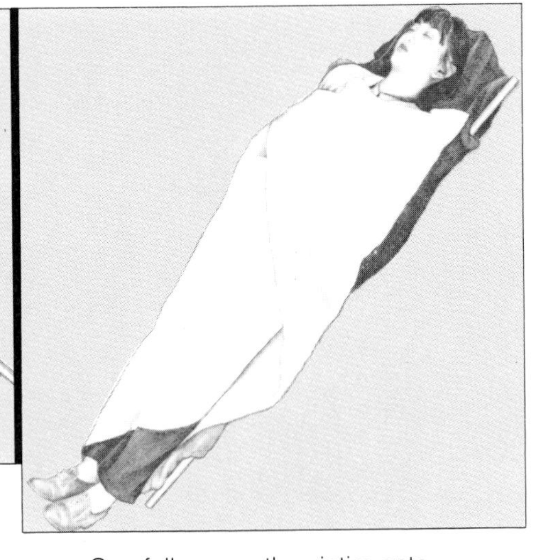

3 Carefully move the victim onto the stretcher using the blanket lift illustrated earlier in this article. During the journey, the victim should be kept warm and comfortable, but not overheated; one blanket should be sufficient for most conditions.

Head and Facial Injuries. If conscious, the victim should be moved into a sitting position with the head tilted forward. With a single first aider and a lightweight victim, the cradle lift may be used. If the victim can walk, the human crutch method may be used. Standing at the victim's side, place one arm around the victim's waist and the victim's arm around your neck. If another assistant is available, the four-handed lift or the chair lift may be used. If unconscious, the victim should be transported face-upward on a stretcher.

Chest Injuries. Chest injuries can be serious and may be accompanied by other injuries. If the victim is unconscious or there are signs of internal injury (impaired breathing or an open chest wound), transport the victim in a semi-reclining position on a stretcher.

If the victim is conscious and there are no obvious signs of internal injury, transport as a walking or sitting case. When there is only one first aider, a victim who can walk may be assisted using the human crutch method. When other assistance is at hand, either the chair lift or the two-handed lift may be used.

Arm Injuries. Arm injuries may be associated with chest injuries. In case of such an injury, the victim should be transported using one of the methods for chest injuries.

When there is only one first aider and the victim has injured only one arm, the human crutch may be used, the support being given on the uninjured side. If the victim has injured both arms, the cradle lift may be used. If help is available, either the two-handed lift or the chair lift may be used.

Hip, Pelvic, and Abdominal Injuries. These injuries often involve damage to internal organs. The victim should be transported face-upward on a stretcher.

Leg Injuries. Where possible, all persons with leg injuries should be transported on a stretcher; this is essential for serious leg injuries.

When there is only one first aider and the victim has a minor leg injury, the piggyback method may be used. The first aider bends down, back to the victim, whose arms are then placed around the first aider's neck. On bending further, the first aider lifts the victim and grasps behind the victim's knees. If other assistance is at hand, the chair lift or the four-handed lift may be used.

Neck and Spinal Injuries. *Do not* move the victim unless it is vital to do so; incorrect handling may cause paralysis. If it is essential to transport the victim, a stretcher must be used and the victim moved in a face-up position.

Before moving the victim, stiffen the stretcher by placing boards across it; a door would be suitable. Use extreme care when moving the victim onto the stretcher. The victim's body should be moved as a rigid whole. This requires six people, one supporting the head and neck, another supporting the feet, and two on each side of the victim supporting the body and legs. The journey itself should be as smooth as possible.

Multiple and Internal Injuries. *Do not* transport the victim unless it is essential to do so. If it is necessary to move the victim, a stretcher must be used. *Do not* give the victim food or drink during the journey.

See also MEDICINE CHEST.

First-aid kit. *See* FIRST-AID FUNDAMENTALS.

Fishhook removal: first aid. A fishhook is one of the more likely objects to penetrate the skin. If only the tip of the hook enters the skin, it is usually safe to pull the hook out as it entered the skin. If, however, the hook is more deeply embedded and the portion of the hook could tear the skin upon removal, it is best to have a physician remove it. If no medical help is near, the hook should be pushed through, until the barb of the hook appears. A wire cutter should then be used to cut off the barbed end.

It is very important to thoroughly clean the wound and cover it with a compress. A physician should be seen promptly, due to the likelihood of infection and to determine whether tetanus booster shots are needed.

See also INFECTION; TETANUS.

Fish oil contains "omega-3 fatty acids," which differ structurally from "omega-6 fatty acids," which are found in most domestic meats.

Evidence is accumulating that omega-3 fatty acids may reduce the chances of getting atherosclerosis, rheumatoid arthritis, migraine headaches, and other heart and inflammatory diseases, whereas omega-6 fatty acids appear to increase those same chances.

A further benefit of fish oil consumption is in the production of eicosanoid compounds, which regulate communication between cells. The type of eicosanoid produced from omega-3 fatty acids, as opposed to omega-6 fatty acids, seems to better regulate immunological responses, such as the body tissue's response to injury or disease.

Research is still being conducted, though many researchers already agree that fish consumption should be increased from the national level of one fish meal a week to as many as four fish meals a week.

Fissure (fish′ər) is the medical term for a crack or groove. It can be a natural division in a structure such as the brain, liver, or spinal cord; or it can refer to a crack-like sore. An anal fissure, the most common example, is a tear in the skin of the anus. It is usually caused by passing hard, constipated feces. Pain from the fissure is sharp, and there may be bleeding during defecation. In small children, the pain may prevent defecation, thus worsening the constipation.

Q: *How is an anal fissure treated?*

A: Anal fissures often heal on their own after several days or when the constipation ceases. Warm sitz baths are soothing; a stool softener will help constipation. An anesthetic ointment may be applied to the area to relieve pain. If the condition does not improve, the fissure may have to be removed surgically. Any scars can be removed as well.

See also CONSTIPATION.

Fistula (fis′chủ lə) is an abnormal channel from a hollow body cavity to the surface (for example, from the rectum to the skin) or from one cavity to another (for example, from the vagina to the bladder). A fistula may be congenital (bladder to navel), the result of a penetrating wound (skin to lung), or formed from an ulcer or an abscess (appendix abscess to vagina, or tooth socket to sinus).

The repeated filling of an abscess or a wound by the fluid contents of some body cavity prevents healing and encourages the formation of a fistula. An anal fistula, for example, begins with inflammation of the mucous lining of the rectum, perhaps triggered by tuberculosis or Crohn's disease. The area becomes an abscess as it is constantly reinfected by feces; eventually a fistula breaks through to the skin near the anus.

Q: *How is a fistula treated?*

A: The usual treatment is an operation to remove the fistula channel completely and drain any abscess so it does not recur.

See also COLOSTOMY; ILEOSTOMY.

Fit. *See* CONVULSION.

Flatfoot is a common disorder in which the arches of the foot are inadequately supported, causing a downward collapse of the bony structure of the foot. Normally, the bones of the foot form three arches to raise the sole. Support is provided by strong ligaments in the sole and by the muscles, especially those of the big toe. Flatfoot occurs when the larger, inner arch of the bone collapses. The sole of the foot may then contact the floor along its entire width.

All children have flat feet for a short time after they start walking. A slight outward twist of the foot (called a valgus deformity) can cause flatfoot to become a permanent condition, because it forces the inner arch of the foot downward. If the arch appears when a person with flatfoot stands on tiptoe, it is an indication that the foot is still supple enough to form a normal arch with corrective treatment. Flatfoot may produce no symptoms, or it may cause pain or a susceptibility to fatigue in the feet.

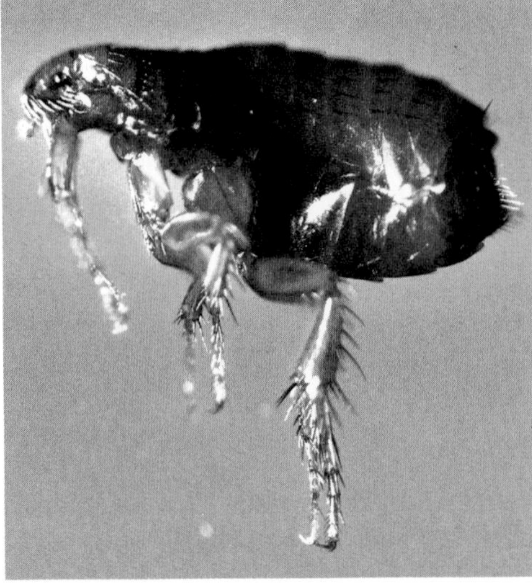

The **flea** is a parasitic insect that afflicts a variety of animals, including humans.

Q: *Are there any other causes of flatfoot?*

A: Occasionally, flatfoot may be associated with muscular disorders or paralysis. It also occurs sometimes in children who have been treated for congenital clubfoot.

Q: *What is the treatment for flatfoot?*

A: For a child, a podiatrist may suggest wedging the heels of the shoes on the inner side of the foot and doing remedial exercises. For an adult, there is no medical need to correct flat feet unless they disturb the patient. If there is pain, orthotic arch supports may be placed in the shoes.

Flatulence (flach'ə ləns) results from excessive gas in the stomach and intestines. A person may belch and pass "gas" (flatus) from the rectum. Although some gas is normally produced from fermentation in the large intestine, most intestinal gas is swallowed air. Flatulence often accompanies indigestion; it may also result from the swallowing of air (aerophagia), caused by nervous habit, eating too rapidly, or poorly fitted dentures. Commercial products for the relief of indigestion help to reduce flatulence. When the condition is caused by aerophagia, it may be best treated after evaluation by a physician.

See also AEROPHAGIA.

Flatus (flā'təs) is gas in the intestines. Excess flatus causes flatulence.

See also FLATULENCE.

Flea (flē) is a wingless, jumping, bloodsucking insect that belongs to the order *Siphonaptera*. Most fleas are parasitic on one specific species of animal, including human beings. *Pulex irritans* injects its saliva into the skin of human beings as an irritating bite.

Q: *Can animal fleas afflict people as well?*

A: Yes. Fleas from cats and dogs (*Ctenocephalides felis* and *C. canis*) may bite human beings, but they do not stay long on human skin. One of the rat fleas, *Xenopsylla cheopis*, carries bubonic plague if the rat it lived on was infected. This flea can pass on the disease in its bite. The same rat flea may carry a form of typhus.

See also LICE; MITE.

Flexible sigmoidoscopy. *See* SIGMOIDOSCOPY, FLEXIBLE.

Flu. *See* INFLUENZA.

Flu, intestinal. *See* GASTROENTERITIS.

Fluke (flük) is a flatworm of the class *Trematoda*, which can cause various parasitic infections in human beings. The life cycle of a fluke is complex. A small organism (miracidium) hatches from an egg, invades a snail, and develops there. When it changes into a small cyst-like structure (cercaria), it is excreted by the snail and finds its home in plants, crabs, or fish. If human beings or animals consume water, fish, or shellfish containing the cysts, flukes that evolve from the cysts invade the human tissues, producing clinical symptoms. Flukes mate in the intestines of their hosts, and eggs excreted in the feces or droppings begin the life cycle again.

See also WORM; SCHISTOSOMIASIS.

Fluorescein (flü ə res′ē in) is a dye that is used intravenously in tests to study blood flow in the eye and to diagnose certain disorders of the retina. It may also be applied to the surface of the eye, in order to diagnose corneal injuries or ulcers.

Fluoridation (flůr ə dā′shən) is the addition of fluoride to the water supply to reduce tooth decay. Some water supplies naturally contain an adequate amount of fluoride; the addition of more is potentially harmful to teeth.

See also FLUORIDE.

Fluoride (flü′ə rīd) is a chemical compound of fluorine. Fluoride, in the form of calcium fluoride, occurs naturally in the soil and in the water supply in some regions. Many municipalities add fluoride to the water supply. It helps in the formation of bones and teeth and in the prevention of tooth decay. It may also be helpful in preventing osteoporosis. A prolonged, excessively high intake of fluoride may cause discoloration of the teeth and weakening of the tooth enamel in children whose teeth are still developing. Rarely, bone disorders, such as osteosclerosis, may occur.

See also OSTEOPOROSIS.

Fluoroscope (flůr′ə skōp) is a machine that aids in diagnosis. It projects onto a screen continuous X-ray pictures of what is happening inside a person's body. The screen, which looks like a television screen, is activated when X rays strike it. By using a fluoroscope, a physician can study the movements of internal organs and the passage of contrast materials through those organs. Although fluoroscopy is still sometimes used (for example, in orthopedic surgery), it has been largely replaced by ultrasound examination, which imparts no radiation.

See also ULTRASOUND.

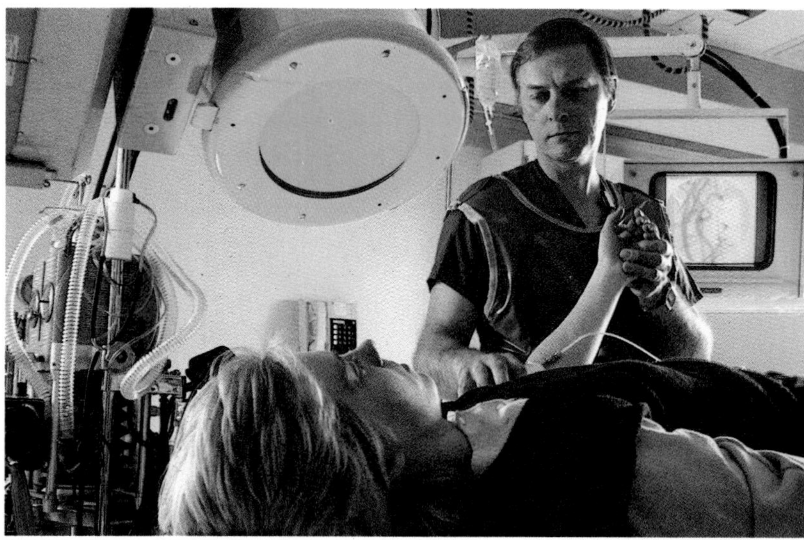

A **fluoroscope** is a type of X-ray device that projects a moving image onto a screen.

Flurazepam hydrochloride (floor az′ə pam hī drə klôr′īd) is a prescription sedative used for insomnia. Because the drug may produce a physical and psychological dependence, it should be used with caution and only for brief periods under a physician's care.

See also DALMANE.

Flush (flush) is sudden redness of the skin, particularly of the face and neck. The cheeks may be flushed with a fever, or flushing may be part of such illnesses as chronic pulmonary tuberculosis. A hot flush, or flash, is accompanied by a sudden feeling of heat caused by an oversensitivity of the surface blood vessels to minor changes of temperature or emotion. This often occurs in women at time of menopause, due to decreased estrogen levels in the body.

See also MENOPAUSE.

Flutter (flut′ər) is a state of extremely rapid, regular vibrations or pulsations.

Atrial flutter occurs in the upper chambers (atria) of the heart, where the number of contractions can rise to between 200 and 400 per minute. The lower chambers (ventricles) cannot contract at such a rapid speed. They go into ventricular flutter, contracting on every third or fourth atrial beat, causing a rapid or sometimes weak pulse.

Flutter of the heart may be caused by many kinds of heart disease, particularly rheumatic valve disease, or by stimulation from an overactive thyroid gland, called thyrotoxicosis. Sometimes, no cause can be found.

Diaphragmatic flutter is rapid pulsations of the diaphragm, occurring sporadically or lasting for an extended period. The cause is unknown.

See also FIBRILLATION.

Fly is a winged insect that belongs to the order *Diptera*. The housefly, like other flies, feeds on decomposing organic matter and can pick up disease germs on its feet and legs. A fly that settles on food contaminates it by shedding germs from its feet, in its droppings, and through its mouth while it is feeding. Illnesses that may be spread by flies include bacillary dysentery and other intestinal disorders, cholera, conjunctivitis, poliomyelitis, sandfly fever, and typhoid.

Foley catheter (fō′lē kath′ə tər) is a rubber tube with a balloon tip. After insertion into the bladder, the tip is filled by means of a syringe with a sterilized liquid or with air, in order to keep the catheter in place. This type of catheter allows for continuous draining of the bladder, primarily during and shortly after surgery.

Folic acid (fō lik) is a vitamin of the B group.

See also VITAMIN.

Folk medicine is any nonorthodox, but traditional way of treating illnesses and injuries. It may use herbal mixtures, physical manipulations, religious rituals, or a combination of these. It differs from orthodox medicine in that the treatments are not the products of scientific medical research. Folk medicine was the starting point from which the science of medicine developed. It is not, however, a simple alternative. Some old remedies have now been incorporated into standard medical practice because their effectiveness has been scientifically proven.

Many folk remedies that do not work are useless rather than harmful. Harm might occur indirectly if a person uses such remedies instead of consulting a physician.

Follicle (fol′ə kəl) is a small, roughly spherical cavity or a small secretory gland. An example of a follicle is the skin socket out of which a body hair grows.

Follicle-stimulating hormone (fol′ ə kəl-stim′yə lāt ing), or FSH, is a hormone that stimulates the growth of an ovarian follicle in the first half of each menstrual cycle. It also affects sperm formation in men. The hormone is produced by the frontal lobe of the pituitary gland. When the ovarian follicle has matured, the membrane surrounding it bursts, and a single egg cell (ovum) is released.

See also OVULATION.

Folliculitis (fə lik yə lī′tis) is an inflammation of the hair follicles on the skin. It first appears as scattered pimples that later dry out and form crusts around the follicles. The affected area is itchy, and nearby lymph nodes may become swollen. In most cases, folliculitis is caused by streptococcus or staphylococcus bacteria. Sycosis barbae on the face and neck of males is a form of folliculitis, caused by shaving.

Q: *How is folliculitis treated?*

A: The application of antiseptic creams or lotions to the infected area reduces the infection. Warm soaks or compresses aid healing. A physician may prescribe antibiotic drugs.

Fontanel (fon tə nel′), or fontanelle, is a gap between the bones of the skull of a newborn baby. At birth, there are six fontanels in a baby's skull. The two main ones lie along the centerline of the scalp, one toward the front of the skull just above the forehead and the other toward the back of the skull. The bones of a baby's skull are still unjoined at birth. The fontanels allow the bones to overlap and the skull to change shape during birth to fit through the birth canal.

Q: *Is it possible to see any of the fontanels on a baby's head?*

A: Yes. The fontanel at the front of the skull, sometimes known as the "soft spot," can usually be seen and felt. It bulges when the baby cries and may form a hollow if the baby has become dehydrated.

Q: *Is it possible to harm the fontanel?*

A: No, not through normal handling. A tough membrane covers the gap

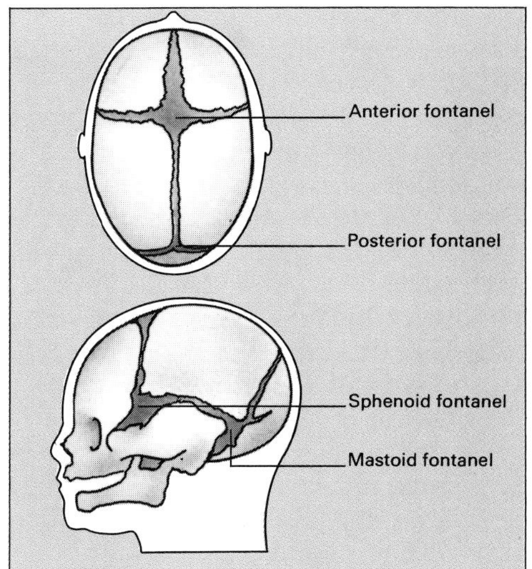

A **fontanel** is a space between the unjoined bones of the baby's skull.

and protects the brain. The area can be touched and washed without harming the baby.

Q: *When do the fontanels disappear?*

A: They are usually closed by the time the child is two years old.

Food poisoning is an acute illness caused by eating contaminated or poisonous food. The usual symptoms are vomiting, diarrhea, and sharp abdominal pain. Cramps, headache, and sweating may be additional symptoms. The patient may collapse with weakness and exhaustion. Food poisoning is rarely fatal (except botulism), and recovery usually takes place after about 6 to 24 hours.

Q: *What are the causes of food poisoning?*

A: There are several possible causes of food poisoning, the most common of which involve bacteria.

(1) Bacteria in contaminated food may grow in the food and produce their own toxin. The germs usually enter the food from a staphylococcal infection (such as a boil, abscess, or other skin infection) in a person who has handled the food during processing. Although cooking kills the germs, it does not destroy the toxin that has been produced. Poisoning from the toxin takes place one to eight hours after eating contaminated food. Toxins produced in foods from other kinds of bacteria are rare, botulism (from the bacteria *Clostridium botulinum*) being one example. Botulism causes severe weakness and difficulty in breathing. It can be fatal if not treated.

(2) Another type of poisoning occurs when bacteria contained in food develop in the intestines of the patient (for example, salmonella or shigella bacteria). Salmonella bacteria are found in many animals, and the foods most likely to contain them are meats (especially chicken and processed frozen meat) and duck's eggs. The bacteria need time to grow in the intestines, and so symptoms may not appear for one or two days. Proper cooking and food handling greatly decreases the risk of such infection.

(3) Water and foods such as unwashed fruit and vegetables may be contaminated by chemicals such as pesticides or by lead from automobile emissions.

(4) Many plants and some animals are naturally poisonous to human beings. These include some types of fungi and some shellfish. Food poisoning results with varying severity if these substances are eaten.

(5) Certain foods may cause severe allergic reactions in some individuals.

Q: *What is ptomaine poisoning?*

A: Ptomaines are foul-smelling products of bacteria present in putrefying food. They were once believed to cause food poisoning. It is now known that so-called ptomaine poisoning is bacterial infection of the intestines.

Q: *How is food poisoning treated?*

A: The physician may treat any water and salt deficiency, a consequence of the vomiting and diarrhea. More severe vomiting may require use of antinauseant medication. Some infections require antibiotic therapy.

Q: *What measures can be taken to avoid food poisoning?*

A: Persons involved in the processing or preparation of food should be checked for skin infections. All fresh fruit and raw vegetables should be washed thoroughly before being eaten. Cooked food should be covered, cooled quickly, and stored in a refrigerator to prevent the growth of bacteria. Food that is reheated should be eaten at once and not kept warm, because this encourages the growth of bacteria.

Food poisoning: treatment. *See* POISONING: FIRST AID.

Foot is joined at the ankle to the lower end of the leg. The calcaneus, which is the largest bone in the foot, forms the heel. Above the calcaneus, and resting on the front part of it, is the talus bone, from which extend three long, narrow bones (metatarsals) that connect to the first three toes. The cuboid bone is also in front of the calcaneus, and from it the fourth and fifth metatarsal bones connect with the fourth and fifth toes. The arch of the foot is raised higher on the instep because the talus projects farther forward than does the cuboid bone. The weight of the body is taken by the calcaneus and transmitted to the heads of the metatarsal bones.

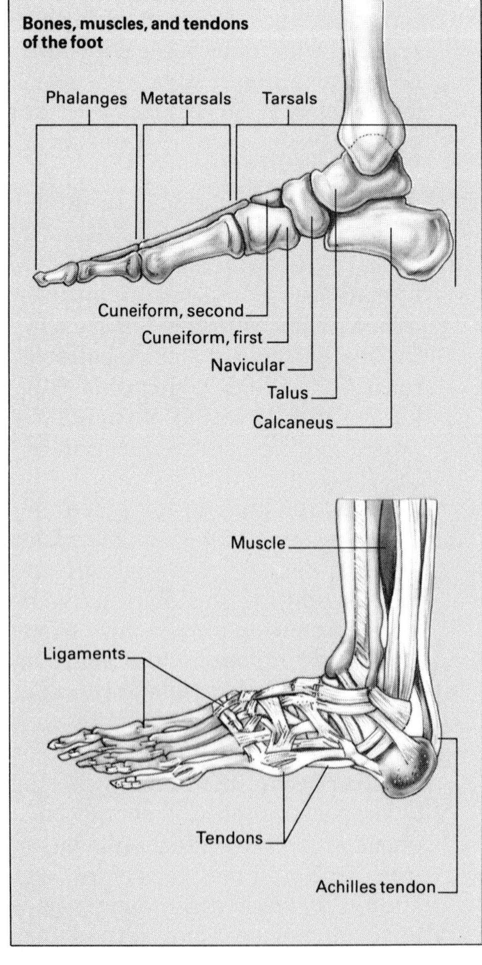

The **foot** is formed from 26 bones and a complex set of muscles and ligaments.

See also FLATFOOT; FOOT CARE; FOOT DISORDERS; HEEL; TOE.

Foot care. Good foot care can prevent many foot problems from developing. A person can avoid or moderate such problems as a sprain or an infection by taking several precautions. (1) Avoid walking or running barefoot on cement or other hard surfaces. (2) Do not wear platform or high-heeled shoes for long periods of time. (3) Use foot powders or lotions to avoid recurrence of athlete's foot or other types of foot infections. Diabetics and other persons with poor circulation are especially prone to foot problems, such as infections and ulcers. They should obtain their physicians' advice on the extra care their feet require.

Routine Foot Care. You should wash your feet at least once a day and dry thoroughly between the toes. You should change stockings or socks daily. It is also advisable to change the type of shoes worn at least once a day. Toenails should be kept trimmed straight across, in order to minimize the occurrence of ingrown nails.

Badly fitting footwear is the major cause of foot problems in modern society. It is important to choose footwear carefully, particularly when buying shoes for children.

Good shoes give support under the instep and heel and give enough room for the toes to spread inside the shoe. When trying on shoes, wear your normal socks or stockings. Try on both shoes and walk around in them. If there is any discomfort, do not buy them.

Children's feet should be measured regularly since their feet grow quickly and also change shape. The soft bones can be easily deformed by badly fitting shoes. Shoes should be discarded when they become too small. Shoes mold themselves to the first wearer's feet and should preferably not be handed down from one child to another.

The choice of materials for footwear is important. Shoes should be made of a natural material, such as leather, suede, canvas, or rope. Socks should be made of wool or cotton. Synthetic materials do not absorb sweat nor allow it to evaporate. A damp foot is vulnerable to infection.

See also FOOT DISORDERS.

Foot disorders. The following table lists some of the disorders that affect the feet and the basic characteristics of each condition. Each disorder is discussed elsewhere in this encyclopedia.

Disorder	*Basic characteristics*
Athlete's foot	Skin eruptions, usually between the toes
Blister	Collection of fluid under the skin causing top layer to puff out
Bunion	Thickening of the skin over the joint at the base of the big toe and extension of metatarsal bone
Bursitis	Inflammation of sac around joint
Callus	Hard, thickened areas of skin on the foot
Cellulitis	Inflammation of skin and underlying tissue
Chilblain	Itching, swelling, and painful reddening of skin
Clubfoot (talipes)	Forepart of the foot is twisted out of direction
Corn	Hard, cone-shaped, thickened areas of the skin on the toes
Flatfoot (pes planus)	Lack of support of the arches of the foot
Foot drop	Difficulty in lifting front part of foot
Frostbite	Reddened or whitened skin with swelling, blistering, and numbness
Ganglion	Cystic tumor on a tendon
Gangrene	Dead tissue
Gout	Inflammation of joint of big toe usually, but also of instep or heel
Hallux valgus	Inclining of big toe toward other toes
Hammertoe (claw toe)	Toe is bent at its two joints, with corns over the bends
Immersion foot	Blueness of skin
Ingrown toenail	Edges of nail overgrown with tissue, causing pain and possible infection
Maduromycosis	Swollen feet with ulcers
Metatarsalgia	Pain in the metatarsal region
Osteoarthritis	Inflammation and degeneration of bone and cartilage that form joints
Pes cavus	Abnormally high arch
Plantar wart	Viral skin infection on the sole of foot
Polydactylism	Extra toes
Rheumatoid arthritis	Inflammation and degeneration of joints

Foot drop is a condition in which the toes drag and the foot hangs, caused by weakness or paralysis of the muscles on the side of the shinbone. It may occur as a result of damage or inflammation of the nerves supplying the muscles. A muscle disorder, such as myasthenia gravis or one of the muscular dystrophies, can also cause foot drop.

The treatment of foot drop depends on the underlying cause. If foot drop remains after the treatment, the patient may wear a special splint or a spring on the shoe to prevent stumbling. Occasionally, a physician recommends an operation called an arthrodesis, which stops ankle movement, so that the ankle is fixed with the foot at right angles to the leg. Alternatively, the base of a tendon may be transplanted from one side of the foot to the other, to strengthen the movement of the foot.

Foot fracture: first aid. *See* FRACTURE: FIRST AID.

Foot, immersion (i mer′zhən). Immersion foot is a condition resembling frostbite, in which the blood vessels contract and the foot becomes blue. Ulcerations may form. If neglected, it can lead to gangrene, particularly in a person suffering from arteriosclerosis, diabetes mellitus, or hypothyroidism. Immersion foot is caused by exposure to wet, damp conditions, such as icy water, for a prolonged period of time.

Forceps (fôr′seps) are pincers that are used in surgery for holding, seizing, or extracting. A different type of forceps is used in obstetrics for some deliveries, in order to help guide the infant's head out of the birth canal.

Foreign body is a particle or small object from outside the body that has lodged itself into the skin, onto surface organs (for example, the eyes, ears, or nose), or inside the body.

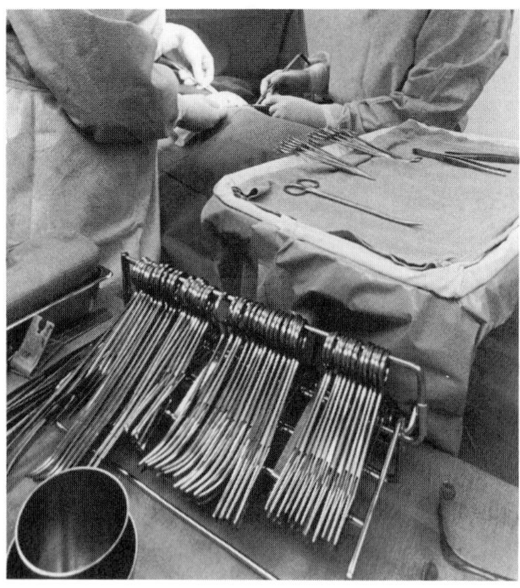

Forceps are pinchers sometimes used during surgery to expose tissue or a body organ.

Foreign body in ear: treatment. *See* EAR, FOREIGN BODY IN: TREATMENT.

Foreign body in nose: treatment. *See* NOSE, FOREIGN BODY IN: TREATMENT.

Foreign objects in stomach: treatment. *See* STOMACH, FOREIGN OBJECTS IN: TREATMENT.

Forensic medicine (fə ren′sik) is the branch of medical science that is related to the law and legal processes. It applies medical knowledge to legal (especially criminal) problems.

Foreskin (fôr′skin), or prepuce, is the fold of skin that covers the end of the penis (glans penis). Before a boy reaches the age of about three, the foreskin is held down by fine strands of tissue; after this age, it can be pulled back. Because the foreskin is subject to irritation and inflammation (balanitis), it should be pulled back and the penis washed regularly as a standard part of male hygiene.

See also BALANITIS; CIRCUMCISION.

Formaldehyde (fôr mal′də hīd) is a pungent, poisonous gas. It is a component of formalin, a solution used in medicine as a disinfectant and preservative.

See also FORMALIN.

Formalin (fôr′mə lin) is a watery solution of the organic chemical formaldehyde, with some added methanol (methyl alcohol). It is used in medicine as a disinfectant and preservative. As a disinfectant, formalin is a component of soaps produced for hospital use. Clothing, towels, and samples of feces and sputum may be sterilized in formalin. Body tissues soaked in formalin become hard, and the solution is therefore used to preserve surgical specimens for examination by a pathologist.

Formic acid (fôr′mik) is an organic chemical found in nettle plants and some insects, including ants. It is a clear, pungent liquid that is chemically related to formaldehyde and methanol (methyl alcohol).

Formication (fôr mə kā′shən) is the sensation of insects crawling over the skin. It is a form of paresthesia (an abnormal sensation without cause). Formication is sometimes a symptom of delirium tremens, and it is a common side effect of alcohol and cocaine withdrawal.

See also DELIRIUM TREMENS.

Formula. *See* BABY CARE.

Fovea (fō′vē ə) is any small cup-shaped depression that occurs naturally on many structures in the body; an example is the pit in the head of the thigh bone (femur). The term most commonly refers to the fovea centralis retinae, the depression on the retina of the eye onto which light is naturally focused and which contains only cones and no blood vessels. It is the area of greatest visual acuity.

See also EYE.

Fracture (frak′chər) is a broken bone. Any bone in the body can accidentally be broken (fractured), but some bones, because of their awkward shapes or vulnerable positions (for example, the long bones of the arms and legs), tend to fracture more often than others. Chunky bones such as the carpals in the wrist and the tarsals in the ankle are less liable to fracture.

Q: *What can cause a bone fracture?*

A: Most fractures occur as the result of injury or accident. Sometimes, a bone breaks following repeated minor strains. Some bones have a tendency to fracture easily because they are weak from disease or osteoporosis. *See also* OSTEOPOROSIS.

Q: *Do bones always fracture in the same way?*

A: No. Physicians recognize six main kinds of fractures: (1) A transverse fracture is a straight break in a bone from side to side; (2) an oblique fracture is an angled break in a bone (for example, diagonally); (3) a spiral fracture is one in which the bone breaks as a result of a twisting action; (4) a comminuted fracture is one in which the bone is broken and splintered into more than two pieces at the fracture site; (5) a greenstick fracture is one in which a break occurs on one side of a bone and the other side bends but, like a green twig, remains intact. It usually occurs in children because the bones are pliable; (6) a depressed fracture is when a piece of bone is driven inwards, as in a skull fracture.

Q: *Can fractures damage tissues other than bone?*

A: Yes. A medical description usually classifies a fracture in terms of the effect that it has on surrounding tissues. A simple (or closed) fracture does not pierce the surface of the skin. A compound (open) fracture is accompanied by a surface wound, caused either by the original impact or by a broken bone piercing the skin. A complicated fracture is one that damages a nearby structure, such as a blood vessel, nerve, or body organ. An impacted fracture is a type of fracture in which one end of the broken bone becomes wedged or compressed into another bone.

Q: *What is the standard treatment for fractures?*

A: The basis of treatment for all fractures is to relocate the bone in its normal anatomical position and to hold it there until new bone has had time to heal the break. A plaster of paris or fiberglass cast is often used for this purpose.

Q: *How are unstable fractures treated?*

A: Unstable fractures may be held together with screws, metal plates, thick pins (for the hip), or wires.

Q: *How is a complicated fracture treated?*

A: A complicated fracture is treated in the same way as other fractures except that repair of the internal damage is given priority. Open fractures often require antibiotic therapy.

Q: *Is a fractured bone always displaced?*

A: No. With some fractures, particularly those of the hand, foot, or skull, the bone breaks but does not change position.

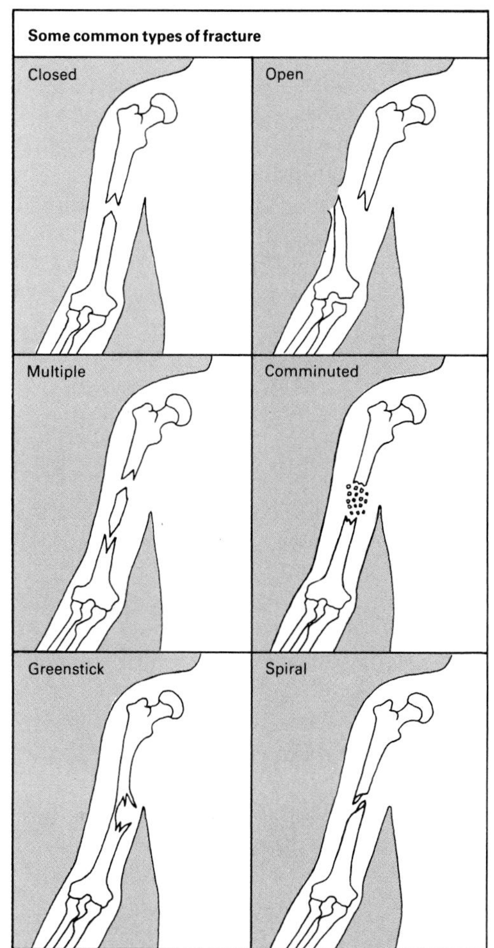

In a **closed fracture,** the broken bone does not pierce the skin. In an **open fracture,** both the bone and skin break. In a **multiple fracture,** the bone is broken in more than one place. A **comminuted fracture** is one in which the bone has splintered at the site of the fracture. A **greenstick fracture** is one in which the bone does not break completely. A **spiral fracture** is one in which the bone is broken by a twisting motion.

Q: *How long does a fracture take to heal?*

A: It depends on the type of fracture and what kind of bone is involved. The healing process takes anywhere from three weeks to three or more months.

Q: *Are there complications that can prolong the healing time?*

A: Fractures in elderly persons often take a long time to heal (called delayed union), especially when there is an underlying bone disease. With some bone diseases, the bone fails to repair itself at all (called nonunion). In that case, a bone graft from a healthier portion of bone may be inserted at the site of the fracture. Sometimes not enough blood reaches the site of the fracture; this is common in fractures of the neck of the femur (thighbone) in old people. Hip joint replacement is sometimes needed for severe hip fractures.

Q: *Are there any other possible complications of fractures?*

A: Yes. If the bone has not been set in its correct position, shortening of the limb may result. A poor joining of the fractured bone (called malunion) results if one end is allowed to rotate slightly so that the contour of its break does not lock smoothly with the other piece of bone. This problem is most common with multiple fractures, in which it is not always possible to set all the bone fragments in their exact, original positions. Infection may occur, especially with an open fracture or as a post-operative complication following a simple fracture.

Q: *Can nearby muscles be exercised while the bone is healing?*

A: Yes. It is essential that the patient exercise the muscles while a limb is in a cast. Physiotherapists teach muscle contraction exercises that can be done while the limb is immobile (isometric exercises). After the cast or splint has been removed, the nearby joint is usually stiff, and therapy is necessary to restore the full range of movement. Swimming is an excellent means of restoring muscle power. A high protein diet with additional vitamins is another measure that speeds the return of normal use to a fractured bone.

Fracture, comminuted (frak′ cher kom′ə nü tid). A comminuted fracture occurs when the bone is broken and splintered into more than two pieces at the site of the fracture.

Fracture, compound. A compound fracture is a bone fracture in which the broken bone causes a surface wound. The bone itself may or may not pierce the skin surface. A compound fracture is more serious than a simple fracture (one that does not cause a surface wound), because the compound fracture is more susceptible to infection.

Fracture: first aid. Fractures often occur as a result of a fall or a collision. The bones of the arms and legs are particularly vulnerable to breakage, but any bone in the body can be fractured. The type of first aid administered depends upon the kind of fracture and its location in the body. All first aid procedures include the following steps: (1) if there is bleeding at the fracture site, treat for bleeding before treating the fracture; (2) if excessive blood loss has led to shock, lay the victim down and treat for shock; (3) do not attempt to straighten an injured limb if it is deformed; (4) move the injured limb as little as possible; (5) if the victim has an open fracture (with a wound on the skin surface), do not bandage tightly over the injury site. Apply a clean dressing gently over any wound; (6) contact medical personnel as soon as possible.

A dislocation, which is the displacement of the bone at a joint, has many of the same symptoms as a fracture. These symptoms include possible deformity of the limb and pain and numbness immediately surrounding the injured area. If there is uncertainty as to whether the injury is a fracture or a dislocation, always treat for a fracture.

See also BLEEDING: FIRST AID; SHOCK: TREATMENT.

The Arm or Elbow. When the lower end of the forearm is fractured, there is often little or no deformity. It is a fairly common fracture and is often mistaken for a sprained wrist. If the fracture is closed, an ice bag and limb elevation may be used to prevent further swelling. *Do not* let ice come into direct contact with the skin. Use ice for only 10 minutes at a time to avoid tissue damage. In the case of a severe break, do not give the victim food or drink, in the event a general anesthetic is needed later.

The Hand or Finger. Fractures of the hand and fingers may be complicated by bleeding into tissues, which causes swelling. Remove jewelry, such as rings, only if doing so does not aggravate the injury. If the fracture is closed, an ice bag and limb elevation may be used to prevent the swelling. *Do not* let ice come into direct contact with the skin. Use ice for only 10 minutes at a time to avoid tissue damage.

The Hip, Thigh, or Knee. Fractures of the hip may be complicated by injury to the organs of the pelvis. *Do not* move the victim, because there may also be injuries to the spine. *Do not* try to straighten the fractured bone or raise the victim's legs. *Do not* give the victim food or drink, in case a general anesthetic is needed later. Keep the victim

Fracture: the arm or elbow

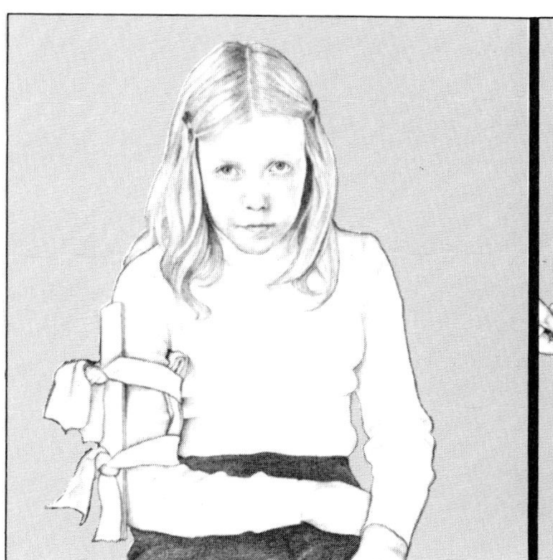

1 Immobilize the fracture by tying a splint on the outside of the victim's injured arm. Use two bandages; one above the fracture and one below it. The splint should be long enough to extend from above the fracture to well below it. Tie the bandages over the splint on the outside of the victim's arm. Place padding between the arm and the chest.

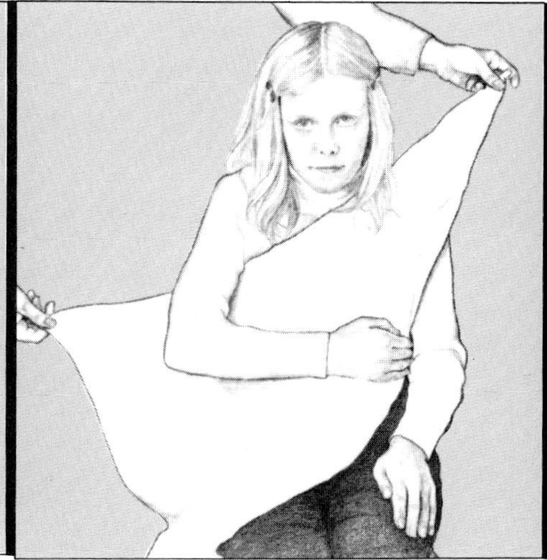

2 If the arm is found in the bent position or if the elbow can be bent, use a triangular bandage or scarf to make a sling. Place the bandage with the apex at the victim's elbow, one tip over the opposite shoulder with the longest edge along the length of the body. Carefully fold the injured arm across the chest.

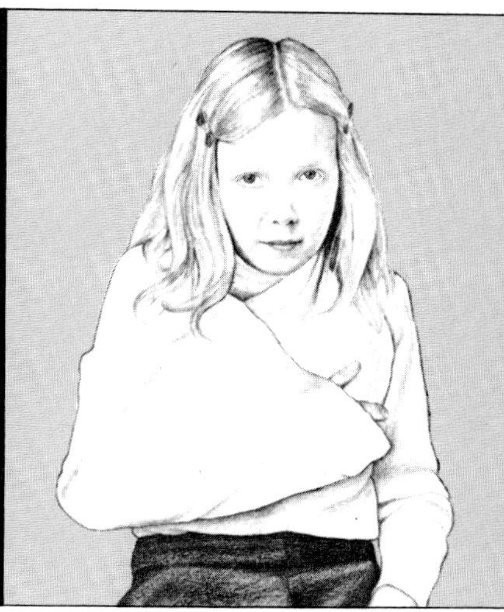

3 Bring the lowest corner up to the neck and tie the ends on the injured side. Pin the corner at the elbow edge to give more support to the arm. If the victim has an open fracture, follow the same procedure but apply a clean dressing over any open wound.

lying down and observe the pulse and breathing. If breathing stops, give mouth-to-mouth resuscitation. Summon medical aid as soon as possible. *See also* ARTIFICIAL RESPIRATION.

The Foot, Ankle, or Toe. Fractures of the foot, ankle, and toe are common injuries, often caused by a fall. They are also usually relatively minor, so before treating them, make a check for and treat any more serious injuries. It is often impossible to distinguish between fractures, dislocations, and bad sprains, the obvious sign in all three being pain and swelling. If in doubt, always treat the injury as a fracture. *Do not* allow the victim to attempt standing on an injured limb. Lay the victim down and summon medical assistance. If it is necessary to transport the victim, a stretcher should be used. For methods of transportation, *see* FIRST-AID FUNDAMENTALS.

The Shoulder or Collarbone. A fracture of the collarbone is usually caused by a fall on an outstretched hand or a fall on the point of a shoulder. The injury is relatively easy to recognize; the arm on the injured side is partially limp, and a swelling or deformity can be felt or seen over the fracture site. *Do not* give the victim food or drink, in case a general anesthetic is needed later. Incline the victim's head toward the injured side to relieve pain. Move the arm on the fractured side as little as possible.

The Spine or Ribs. A fractured spine is an extremely serious injury. If the victim is incorrectly handled, the spinal cord may be permanently damaged, resulting in paralysis. Symptoms of a fractured spine include severe pain in the back, loss of limb sensation, and loss of limb control. *Do not* move the victim. Rib fractures can also be very serious. If the ribs have punctured the lungs, the victim will have pain and difficulty breathing and may cough up blood or be in shock. If the ribs have penetrated the skin surface, there may be an open, "sucking" wound. Treat bleeding only if it is severe enough to endanger life. Treat any "sucking" chest wounds immediately with an airtight dressing. If the victim stops breathing, give artificial resuscitation. For instruction, *see* ARTIFICIAL RESPIRATION. Summon medical aid as soon as possible.

Fracture: the hand or finger

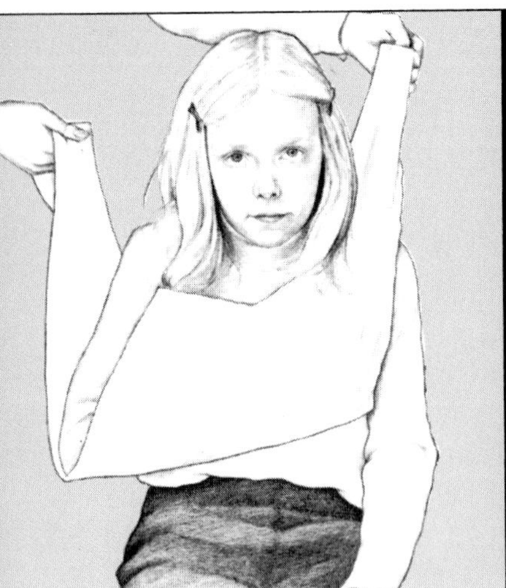

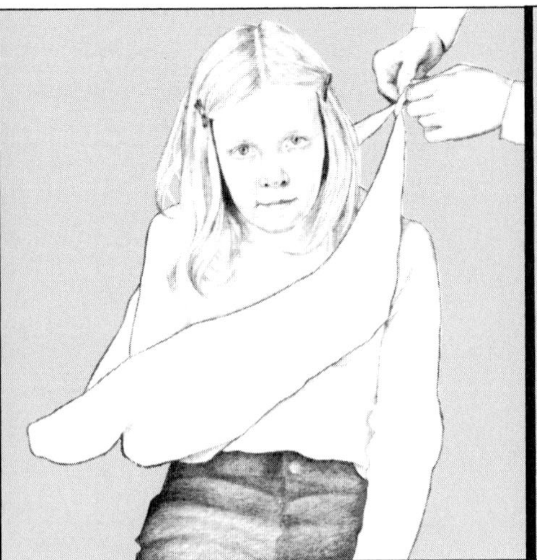

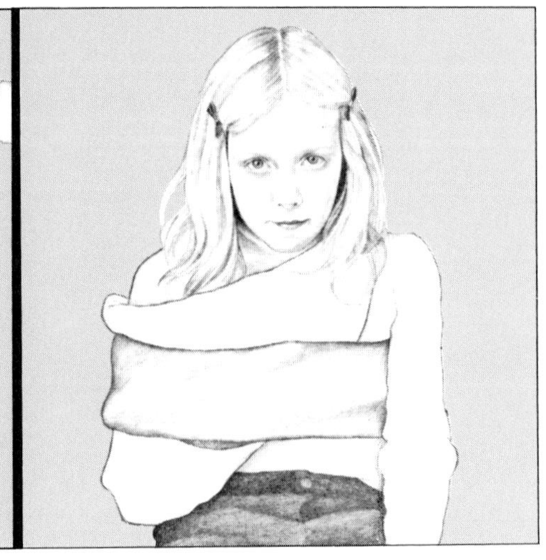

1 Fold the injured arm across the chest. Place a triangular bandage over the arm with the apex at the elbow or mid-forearm and the longest side down the length of the body. While supporting the arm, turn the lower portion of the bandage under the hand, arm, and elbow. Protect the hand by gently placing it in a fold of soft padding.

2 Take the lower corner of the bandage behind the back and over the shoulder. Pin the corner at the elbow edge to give more support to the arm. Tie the two ends at the shoulder.

3 Provide further support for the injured arm by using a broad bandage. Place the bandage over the sling, around the chest and injured arm, and under the other armpit. Tie the bandage at the back.

Fracture: the hip, thigh, or knee

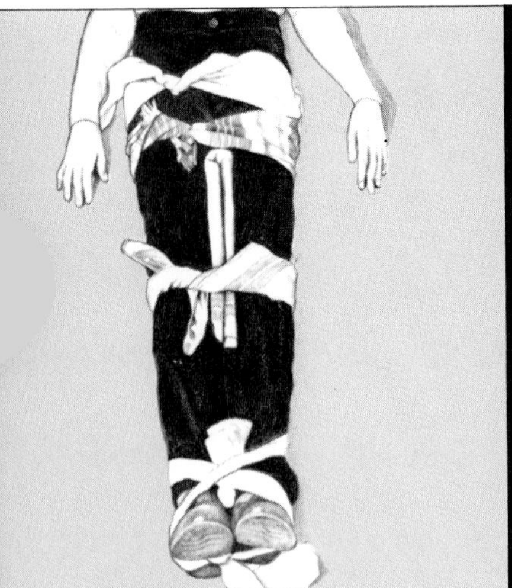

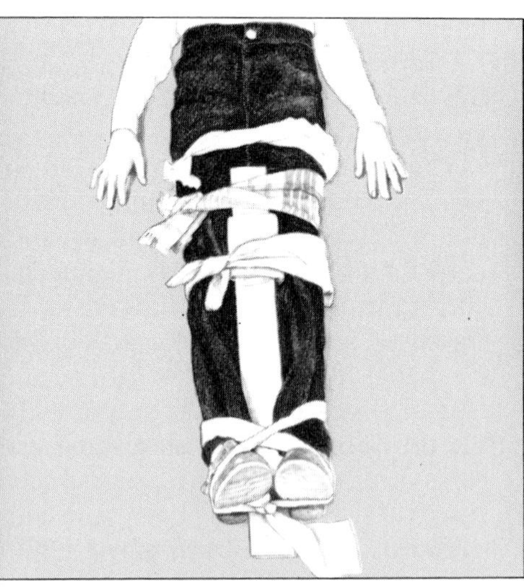

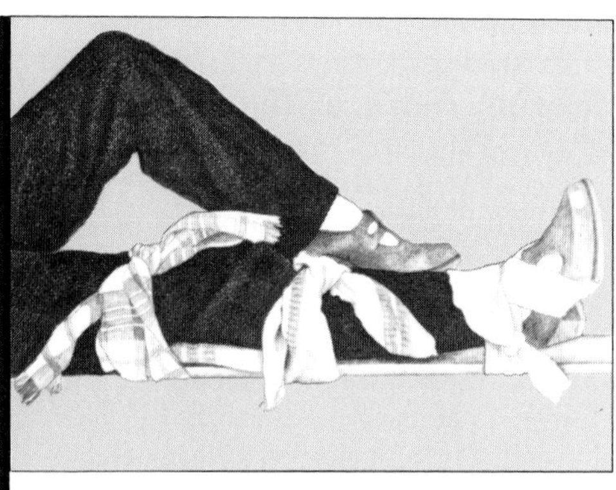

1 With a suspected hip fracture, gently put the victim's legs together with padding between the thighs, knees, and ankles. Put two broad bandages around the hips, overlapping on the injured side, and one broad bandage around the knees. Wind a narrow bandage around the feet.

2 With a suspected fracture of the thigh, use the method described in step one. If a splint is available, pad it and put it between the legs.

3 With a suspected knee fracture, place a long, padded splint behind the knee. The splint must be rigid; a length of wood or metal is ideal. Place further padding between the knee and the splint, and between the ankle and the splint.

To secure the splint, use a broad bandage around the thigh, a broad bandage below the knee, and a narrow bandage around the foot and ankle.

Fracture: the foot, ankle, or toe

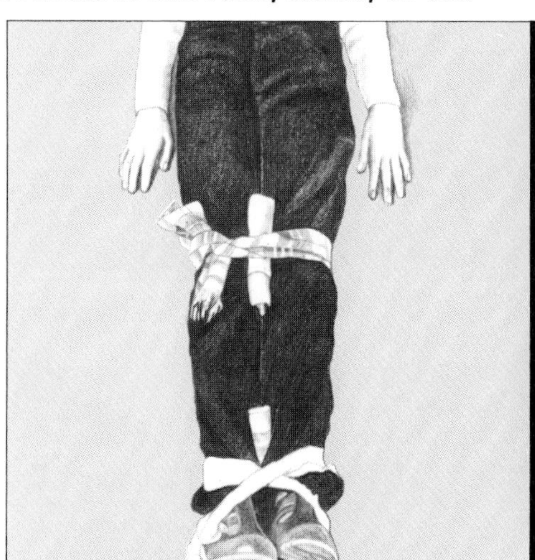

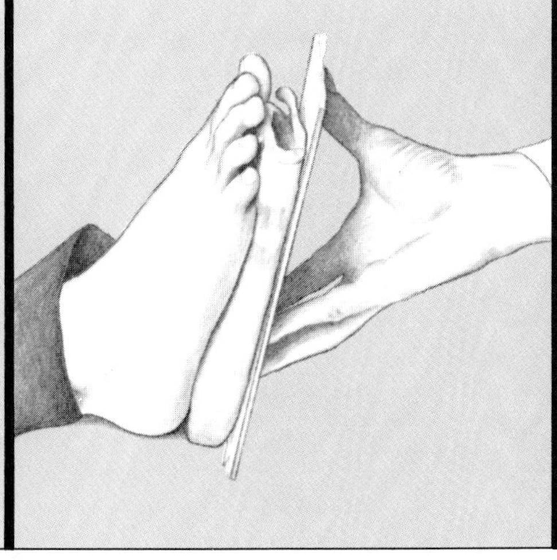

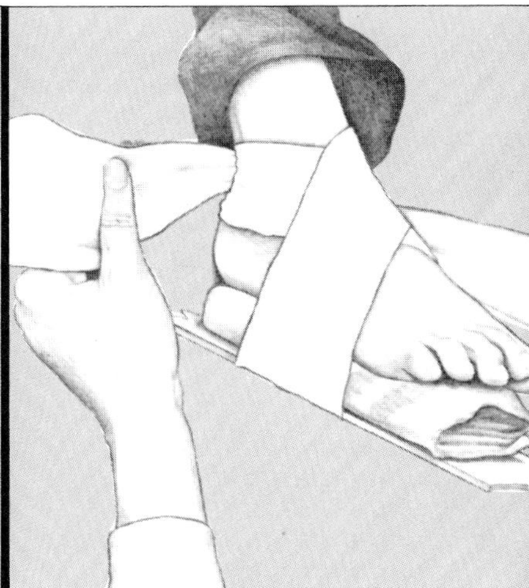

1 With a fracture of the leg, lay the victim down, with both legs straight, and the uninjured leg beside the injured leg. Place padding between the thighs, knees, and ankles; tie a broad bandage at the knees. Tie a narrow bandage around the feet.

2 With a fracture of the foot or toe, carefully remove the victim's footwear. Raise the injured foot. Place a broad padded splint against the sole of the foot. (A pillow could be used or a folded newspaper with a scarf as the padding.)

3 Tie a narrow bandage around the foot in a figure-of-eight, to secure the splint. If only one or two toes are fractured, an alternative is to use an uninjured toe as a splint. Place padding between the toes and tie a narrow bandage around the injured and uninjured toes.

Fracture: the shoulder or collarbone

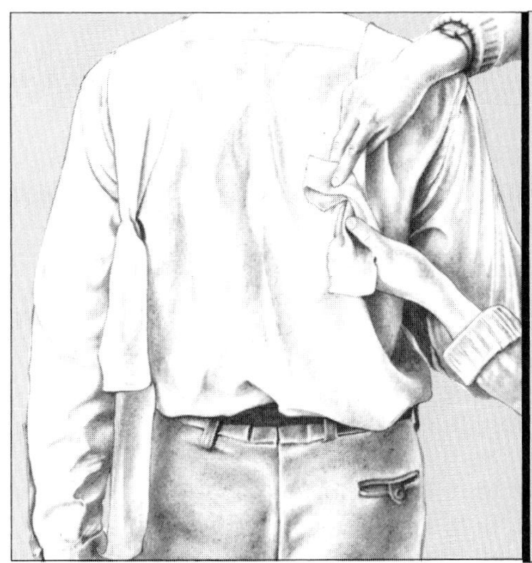

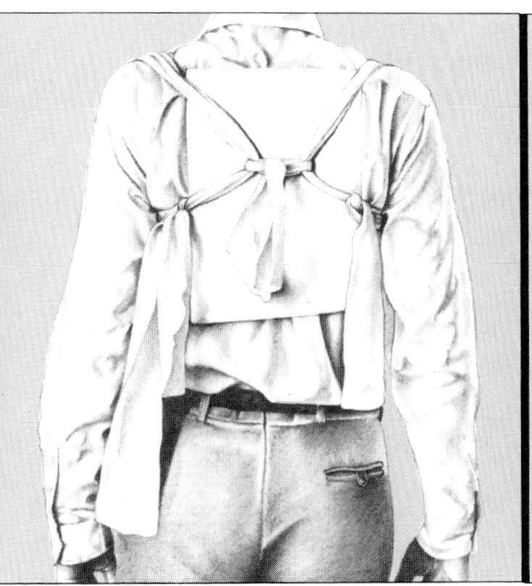

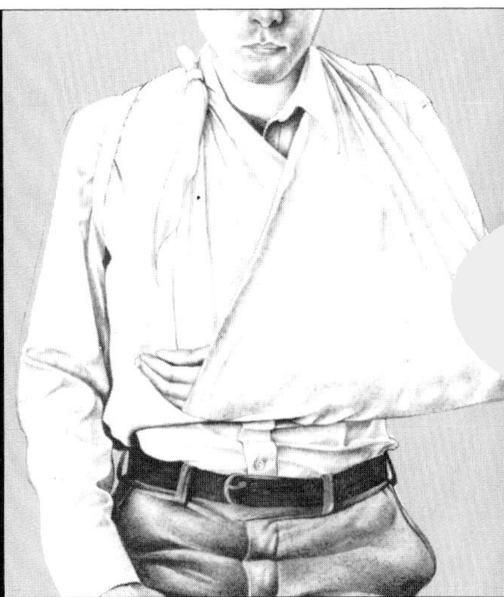

1 Sit the victim down. Fold the two triangular bandages into narrow bandages. Pass each bandage under the armpit and around the shoulder, and tie the bandages just below the shoulder blade.

2 Put padding between the shoulder blades. Use a third bandage to hold together the two bandages encircling each shoulder. The third bandage must be tight, as it is necessary that the shoulders are braced well back and kept in this position.

3 Fold the arm on the injured side across the chest. Place a triangular bandage with the apex at the victim's elbow and one tip over the shoulder on the injured side. Fold the bandage under the arm, bring the tip up to the shoulder on the uninjured side, and tie the two ends. Pin the corner to provide support for the elbow.

Fracture: the spine or ribs

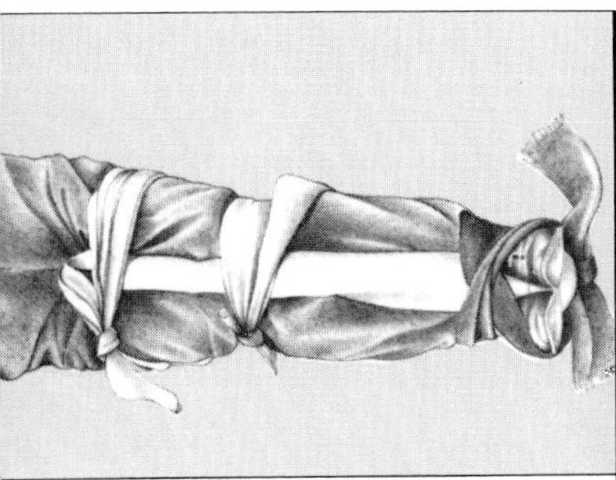

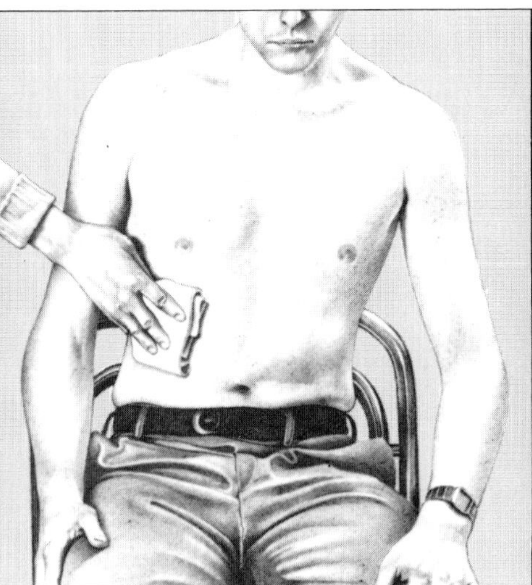

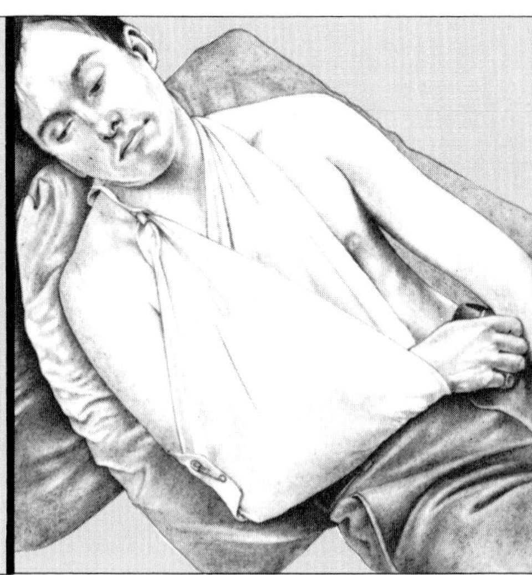

1 If medical assistance is available, *do not* move a victim with spinal fractures. If medical assistance is not available, prepare the victim for transportation. Using the utmost care, slide a wide board (a door will do) under the victim. Place padding between the thighs, knees, and ankles. Tie broad bandages around the thighs and knees, and a narrow bandage around the feet. If the victim is unconscious, *do not* use the recovery position because this may cause further damage. For specifics on the recovery position, *see* FAINTING: FIRST AID.

2 If the victim has rib fractures and there is no open chest wound or lung damage, place the victim in a lying position and put bandages round the chest. If the ribs have penetrated the skin, put an airtight dressing over the wound immediately.

3 Keep the airtight dressing in place and support the arm on the injured side in a triangular sling. Lay the victim down on the injured side. If the ribs have punctured the lungs, keep the victim's head and shoulders raised. *Do not* bandage the ribs.

Fracture, greenstick. A greenstick fracture is a fracture where the bone breaks on one side of the bone and the other side bends but, like a green twig, remains intact. A greenstick fracture usually occurs in children because their bones are more pliable.

Fracture, open. An open fracture is a fracture in which there is an open wound at the site of the broken bone. It is a type of compound fracture.

See *also* FRACTURE, COMPOUND.

Fragilitas ossium. See OSTEOGENESIS IMPERFECTA.

Fraternal twins. See TWINS.

Freckles (frek′əlz) are small, brown or yellowish-brown patches of pigment on the skin. They usually appear in response to sunlight, as the body's cells produce more of the dark pigment melanin as a protection against further harmful action by the sun's ultraviolet rays. Freckles tend to fade in the absence of sunlight. People who freckle easily should protect themselves from too much sun exposure because overexposure can lead to skin damage.

Friedreich's ataxia (frēd′riks ə tak′sē ə) is a serious, rare, inherited disorder of the central nervous system. It is caused by the imperfect development of some nerve fibers in the spinal cord. The first symptom of Friedreich's ataxia is poor coordination of muscles in the legs, usually beginning in childhood or early adolescence. The feet later become de-

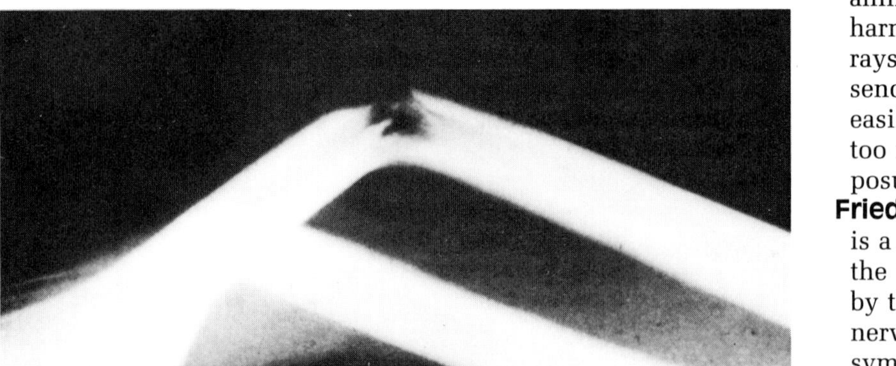

A **greenstick fracture** is an incomplete fracture in which the bone is bent and only partially broken.

formed (claw feet), the gait becomes unsteady, and poor muscle coordination spreads throughout the body. Commonly, the spine curves to one side, and the patient becomes increasingly hunched. The patient usually develops a sputtering, hesitating speech pattern.

Q: *What are the complications of Friedreich's ataxia?*

A: Friedreich's ataxia is a cause of paraplegia in children and young persons. If the heart becomes involved, heart failure may result. Diabetes is a frequent complication, and the patient is also more liable to get pneumonia.

Q: *How is Friedreich's ataxia treated?*

A: Although no effective treatment is known, attempts can be made with physiotherapy to slow the tightening process of the muscles. Death usually occurs within 10 to 20 years and is usually the result of a secondary infection.

Frigidity (fri jid'ə tē) is an abnormal aversion to sexual intercourse and the subsequent inability to reach orgasm. The term is usually applied to this condition in women. The cause of frigidity is often psychological; for example, it may be caused by a fear of becoming pregnant. Emotional problems may prevent vaginal secretions during sexual arousal, resulting in a dry genital area and a lack of sexual desire. A physician or other health professional can often determine the reasons for a woman's frigidity once her sexual history is known; appropriate treatment can then begin. Sympathetic and careful counseling is a necessity.

Frigidity can sometimes be caused by a physical abnormality, such as a vaginal infection or a tight hymen.

See also DYSPAREUNIA; IMPOTENCE.

Fröhlich's syndrome (frā'liks) is a rare glandular disorder of childhood, more common in boys than in girls. It is caused by a disturbance in the hypothalamus, the part of the brain that acts as a link between the nervous system and the endocrine hormone-secreting system. In Fröhlich's syndrome, essential pituitary hormones are not produced, so that the sex organs remain underdeveloped. Excess fatty tissue is distributed in areas normal for the female build: thighs, hips, and breasts. If the condition begins in early childhood the patient may be a dwarf; if it occurs just before puberty, the child is usually fat and sluggish. Fröhlich's syndrome in a girl causes extreme obesity.

Q: *What is the treatment for Fröhlich's syndrome?*

A: Provided treatment is started early enough, Fröhlich's syndrome can be most effectively treated with modern hormone therapy, such as the administration of pituitary hormones. This reduces the excess weight and restores development to the sex organs. If a brain tumor is the cause, the tumor is removed as part of the treatment.

Frontal lobe syndrome (frun'tal lōb) is a condition characterized by a change in personality and behavior. It may result from a tumor in the frontal lobe region of the brain or trauma to that region. In frontal lobe syndrome, the patient may exhibit outbursts of violence, show irritability or boastfulness or both, or may become severely depressed and neglectful of personal appearance.

Before the general use of antipsychotic drugs, partial frontal lobotomies were often performed to control the outbursts. These are no longer performed.

See also LOBOTOMY.

Frostbite (frôst'bīt) tissue is an acute reaction to extreme cold. Particularly vulnerable areas of the body include the toes, fingers, ears, and the tip of the nose. Superficial frostbite may only damage the skin, but severe frostbite affects the deep tissues and may result in gangrene.

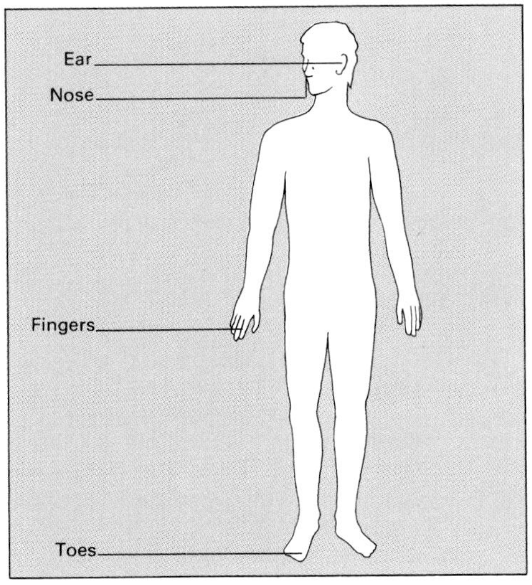

Frostbite is most likely to affect a person's fingers, toes, nose, and ears.

Q: *What are the symptoms of frostbite?*

A: The affected area turns unnaturally white. The victim is unaware of the condition because there is no sensation of pain at this stage. Within a few hours blood seeps back into the tissues turning them purple or black. The area becomes red, swollen, and painful. The skin may blister, and the blisters break down into ulcers. In severe cases, the circulation does not return on warming, and the damage leads to gangrene.

Q: *What causes frostbite?*

A: In extreme weather conditions of cold and wind, the blood and tissue moisture in the affected area freezes. In severe cases, the blood vessels supplying the area shut down, preventing normal circulation even when gently warmed.

Q: *How is frostbite treated?*

A: The affected area must be warmed gradually, preferably at the same time as the rest of the body or by immersing the area in warm water. Rubbing must be avoided, as it increases the damage to the already injured tissues. If the area remains white after warming, a physician must be consulted immediately. If gangrene sets in, amputation may be necessary.

Q: *How can a person avoid frostbite?*

A: During extremely cold weather, clothing must be well-fitting, warm, and wind-resistant. Tight shoes, socks, or gloves cut down the circulation and endanger the specific area. People with diabetes or any form of circulatory disorder are more likely to develop frostbite.

Frostbite: first aid. Frostbite occurs when areas of tissue freeze in cold weather conditions. It is more likely to occur if the conditions are damp or windy. The underlying tissues, as well as the skin, may be affected. Frostbite may result in blistering and ulceration of the affected part. In severe frostbite, gangrene may follow.

The areas most commonly affected are the nose, ears, cheeks, fingers, and toes. Frostbite usually occurs without pain. The frostbitten part becomes numb and stiff and appears white. Because of the numbness, the symptoms may not be noticed. There may be an area of red, inflamed skin between the yellowish-white, frostbitten part and the normal tissues. Stiff fingers or toes

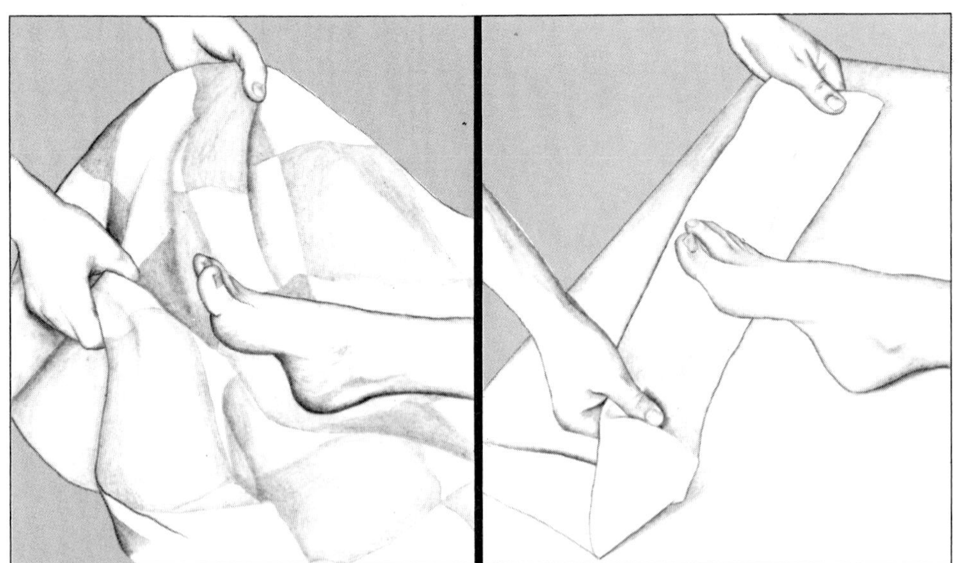

1 Gently warm the affected part. If the toes are frostbitten, wrap them in a dry blanket, but do not rub them. Do not apply direct heat to the frostbitten area. Seek medical attention as soon as possible.

2 The injury caused by frostbite resembles a burn and is vulnerable to infection. Cover the frostbitten area with a sterile dressing. Take the victim to a hospital as soon as possible.

may be an indication that frostbite is occurring or has occurred.

Treatment. It is important to promptly recognize the signs of frostbite so that first aid can be given at the earliest opportunity. First of all, try to rewarm the affected part, but be careful about the way this is done. Warm parts of the face by covering them with warm hands that are not frostbitten. Warm frostbitten hands by placing them in the armpits, next to the skin. Warm frostbitten feet by wrapping them in a blanket or by warming them against the abdomen of another person.

A person who has frostbite may also be suffering from hypothermia, so protect the victim from further cold. *Do not* apply direct heat to the frostbitten part. For example, do not warm the feet or hands in front of a fire. *Do not* rub a frostbitten area, either directly with the hands or with snow. *Do not* exercise the frostbitten part, and do not try to walk on frostbitten feet.

When safely out of the cold, the frostbitten part may be rewarmed by immersion in warm water measuring 100-105°F(37-40°C). Do not use water hotter than 105°F (40°C), since this may cause additional tissue damage.

Aspirin, acetaminophen, or other painkilling drugs may be required to relieve the pain that occurs as frostbitten tissues gradually become warm again.

See also HYPOTHERMIA; HYPOTHERMIA: TREATMENT.

Frozen section is a technique in which an area of tissue (from a biopsy) is frozen. A thin slice is then cut off for examination under a microscope. The technique is useful for immediate preliminary diagnosis of any disease process affecting the biopsied tissue. This technique also allows the surgeon to decide if sufficient tissue has been removed to successfully treat the disease.

Frozen shoulder. *See* SHOULDER, FROZEN.

Fructose (fruk'tōs) is a natural sugar found in honey and many fruits. It is used as a food sweetener and as a nutritive substance in some intravenous solutions.

FSH. *See* FOLLICLE-STIMULATING HORMONE.

Fugue (fyüg) is a rare, temporary disturbance of consciousness in which a person in some ways behaves as though conscious. On "waking" from a state of fugue, a person suddenly realizes that he or she cannot account for, nor remember in any way, the time during which the fugue lasted. The condition is thought to represent a hysterical state of repressed emotions concerning some unfaceable crisis. A fugue may also be associated with epilepsy or concussion caused by a head injury.

A fugue differs from amnesia, in which state a person acts consciously but without memory of previous events.

See also AMNESIA: HYSTERIA.

Fulguration (ful gyə rā'shən) is the destruction of living tissue, using electric current. It is sometimes used to treat skin tumors.

See also DIATHERMY.

Fumigation (fyü mə gā'shən) is a method of disinfecting an area using poisonous fumes.

Fungal infection (fung'gəl) may be caused by microscopic fungi or their spores. Many of these disorders are difficult to treat because the fungi resist most antimicrobial agents. The following table lists some of the common fungal disorders and the basic characteristics of each condition. Each disorder has a separate entry elsewhere in this encyclopedia.

Disorder	*Basic characteristics*
Actinomycosis	Fibrous masses about the mouth or tongue, that burst and become sinuses or ulcers; also abscesses in the lungs
Aspergillosis	Lumps in the skin, ears, sinuses, and especially, the lungs
Athlete's foot	Skin eruptions on the foot, usually between the toes
Blastomycosis	Lesions all over the body but, especially, infection of the lungs
Candidiasis	White patches inside the mouth, that later become shallow ulcers; may also occur in the vagina
Histoplasmosis	Infection of the lungs, ulcers in the gastrointestinal tract, and possible skin lesions
Ringworm	Raised, round sores of the skin, scalp, or nails

Funny bone is at the inner, lower end of the humerus (upper arm bone). The ulnar nerve lies over this section of the humerus, close to the surface of the skin at the back of the elbow. A blow on the ulnar nerve is painful and often accompanied by tingling or numbness in the fingers of the affected hand.

See also ELBOW; HUMERUS.

Furosemide (fyůr ə sem′īd) is one of the powerful diuretics. It is available in tablet and injection form. Furosemide, whose trade name is Lasix®, is used to treat edema, a retention of fluid that accompanies disorders such as heart failure, kidney disease, and cirrhosis of the liver. It may also be prescribed in the treatment of high blood pressure and is sometimes used in the treatment of overdoses of certain drugs, such as barbiturates, because it increases the flow of urine.

Q: *Can furosemide produce any adverse side effects?*

A: Yes. Furosemide may cause nausea and diarrhea, and it may, in rare cases, result in deafness. The use of furosemide may also cause a decrease in the levels of sodium, calcium, and potassium in the blood. For this reason, potassium supplements should be prescribed when furosemide is taken for a long period of time.

See also DIURETIC.

Furred tongue. *See* TONGUE, HAIRY.

Furuncle. *See* BOIL.

Fused joint. *See* JOINT.

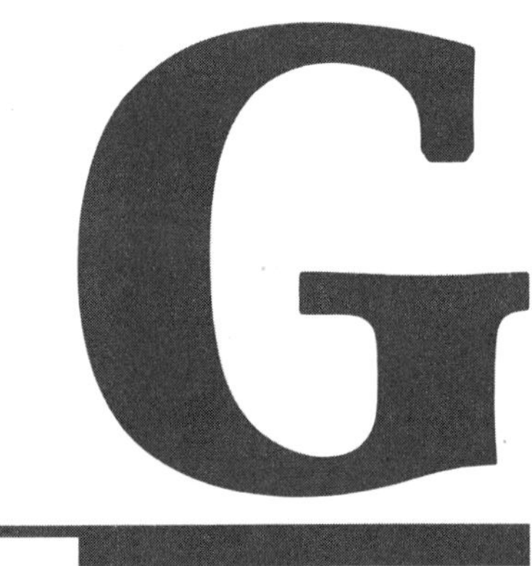

Gait (gāt) is the method, tempo, and quickness of the walking step.

Galactorrhea (gə lak tə rē'ə) is an excessive or spontaneous flow of milky fluid from the breasts, not related to pregnancy or nursing. The condition should always be evaluated by a physician, as it can be a symptom of particular diseases or a side effect of certain drugs.

Gall (gôl) is another name for bile.
See also BILE.

Gall bladder (gôl blad'ər) is a pear-shaped organ beneath the right side of the liver. It is approximately 3 to 4 inches (7.6–10.2cm) long and about 1 inch (2.5cm) wide. The function of the gall bladder is to store bile, a digestive liquid continually secreted by the liver. The bile emulsifies fats and neutralizes acids in partly digested food. A muscular valve in the common bile duct opens, and the bile flows from the gall bladder into the cystic duct, along the common bile duct, and into the duodenum (part of the small intestine).
See also BILE; CHOLANGITIS; JAUNDICE.

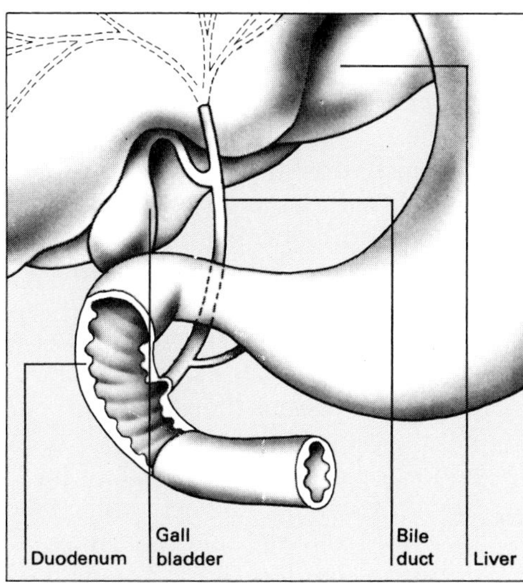

The **gall bladder,** situated underneath the right lobe of the liver, secretes bile into the duodenum.

Gallstone (gôl'stōn), a type of calculus, is usually a mixture of cholesterol, bilirubin (a bile pigment), and protein. Resembling a stone, the calculus forms in the gall bladder or sometimes in the common bile duct or hepatic ducts. The size of a gallstone can vary from a tiny crystal to a lump the size of a small egg. Usually, more than one gallstone is formed. The incidence of formation increases with age, especially among women.
See also CALCULUS; CHOLELITHIASIS.

Gamma globulin (gam'ə glob'yə lin) is a plasma protein, a component of blood serum that contains antibodies. It can be extracted from the blood of a person who is immune to a certain infection and injected into another person who has been exposed to the disease (hyperimmune globulin). These extracts can provide temporary immunity to infectious hepatitis, rubeola (measles), poliomyelitis, tetanus, yellow fever, or smallpox. Gamma globulin injections do not seem to be of much benefit against mumps or rubella (German measles). *See also* ANTIBODY; IMMUNIZATION.

Q: ***Are gamma globulin extracts used to give immunity to any other conditions?***

A: Yes. A special preparation of gamma globulin, Rh_o (D) immune globulin, is given to a mother who has Rh- (Rh negative) blood after she has given birth. *See also* HEMOLYTIC DISEASE OF THE NEWBORN.

Q: ***How important is an adequate amount of gamma globulin in the blood?***

A: There is a serious risk of infection if a person has a low level of gamma globulin. For example, in a rare, inherited disorder called agammaglobulinemia, there is almost no gamma globulin in the blood. Infections of all kinds occur more often and are more serious. Decreased gamma globulin levels sometimes result from the treatment of leukemia or cancer by chemotherapy. The only treatment in such circumstances is regular doses of gamma globulin.

Ganglion (gang'glē ən) is an anatomical term for a bundle of nerves within the nervous system that acts as a relay station outside the brain and spinal cord. A basal ganglion, however, is located within the brain and spinal cord. Ganglions are present throughout the autonomic nervous system.

As a surgical term, a ganglion is a cyst-like, benign tumor that appears in the sheath of a tendon, particularly in the wrist.

See also CYST.

Gangrene (gang'grēn) is the decay and death of tissue caused by a lack of blood supply to an area. It is a complication of external or internal injury or of damage to an artery. External causes include infected bedsores or other skin ulcers; crushing injuries; deep burns; frostbite; boils; and chemical damage of the skin. Internal causes include blood clotting (thrombosis) in a diseased artery; an embolus; severe arteriosclerosis; diabetes; a strangulated hernia; torsion of the testes; Buerger's disease (a rare disorder of the leg arteries); and Raynaud's phenomenon (spasm-like contraction of the arteries in the arms and legs).

Medically, gangrene is considered either "dry" or "moist."

Q: *What is dry gangrene?*

A: Dry gangrene is the withering and drying out of tissue without infection by bacteria. This process may continue unnoticed for weeks or months, especially in elderly persons. Dry gangrene is most often a complication of advanced diabetes or arteriosclerosis.

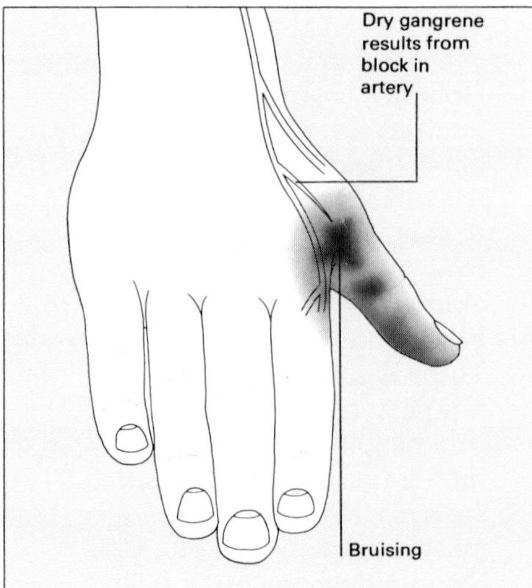
Dry gangrene results from block in artery
Bruising

Dry **gangrene** is frequently associated with advanced diabetes or arteriosclerosis (hardening of the arteries).

Q: *What is moist gangrene?*

A: Moist gangrene occurs usually in the toes, feet, or legs after a crushing injury or some other factor that causes a sudden stoppage of blood. The gangrene spreads rapidly as invading bacteria thrive and multiply unchecked by the defenses normally carried in the blood. *See also* GAS GANGRENE.

Q: *What are the symptoms of gangrene?*

A: Areas of both dry and moist gangrene are conspicuous by a red line on the skin that marks the border of the gangrenous tissue. Dry gangrene causes some pain in the early stages. The area becomes cold, and the skin changes in color to brown, then black. Moist gangrene begins with swollen skin that may be blistered, red, and hot. The area then becomes cold as the tissues die, and the skin appears bruised. The putrefactive bacteria produce an offensive odor.

Q: *Which parts of the body are susceptible to gangrene?*

A: The limbs, especially the ends of the toes and fingers, are most commonly affected. The intestine may become gangrenous if an artery supplying it is twisted (volvulus), obstructed by a hernia, or diseased by arteriosclerosis. Bone gangrene is also possible.

Q: *What is the treatment for gangrene?*

A: The only treatment is surgical removal, with large doses of the proper antibiotics.

Q: *Can any measures be taken to guard against gangrene?*

A: Patients who have severe arteriosclerosis or diabetes should take particular care of their feet and hands, especially the nails; these conditions increase the risk of infection from even a very minor injury, for example, one caused by cutting a nail too short. This is because the narrowed blood vessels in their fingers and toes can not conduct sufficient blood to combat infection. People with diabetes are at especially high risk, because they may have a loss of sensation in their hands and feet and therefore may not perceive the warning signal of pain in an affected extremity. Any abrasion should be treated immediately.

Gardnerella vaginalis (gard ner el′ah vaj i nal′əs) is a form of vaginitis caused by *gardnerella*, a slow-growing bacteria. It can be, but is not always sexually transmitted. It usually shows no symptoms, but may appear as a thin, white, malodorous discharge. Antibiotics may be prescribed, but metronidazole (Flagyl®) is the treatment of choice. Treating the male partner is recommended.

See also SEXUALLY TRANSMITTED DISEASE; VAGINITIS.

Gas. *See* FLATULENCE.

Gas gangrene (gang′grēn) is a type of moist gangrene that is usually a complication of a crushing injury. The infection is caused by the bacterium *Clostridium welchii,* which thrives without oxygen and releases a foul-smelling gas as well as a poisonous toxin. The bacteria breed in the damaged tissue and spread rapidly to healthy tissue. Symptoms include a high fever, putrid-smelling pus, and the formation of gas bubbles under skin. Urgent hospitalization is necessary. Death occurs within about two days if the condition is not treated.

See also CLOSTRIDIUM.

Gas poisoning. Many poisonous gases are released when solids and liquids, such as mineral acids, ammonia, cyanides, and mercury, are heated. Others are specially manufactured as war gases. Poisonous gases affect the body in various ways, and many are potentially fatal.

Q: *What are some examples of the effects of poisonous gases?*

A: Carbon monoxide, and mixtures that contain it, prevent the blood from carrying oxygen to tissues; hydrogen sulfide causes respiratory paralysis; carbon tetrachloride damages the liver and kidneys; carbon disulfide produces nerve damage and ultimately causes paralysis and psychoses; tear gases, such as xylyl bromide, severely irritate the eyes, nose, and throat; the various nerve gases prevent the proper functioning of nerve impulses; lung irritant gases, such as chlorine and phosgene, attack the eyes, nose, throat, and lungs; vesicant gases, such as mustard gas and lewisite gas (containing arsenic), cause blisters and ulcers on the skin; nauseant gases, such as chloropicrin, induce vomiting; nose irritant gases, such as diphenylchlorarsine, cause pain, sneezing, depression, and sometimes vomiting.

Q: *How can people come in contact with such gases?*

A: Carbon monoxide is the most poisonous gas likely to be present in domestic surroundings. For example, when an automobile engine has been left running in an enclosed space, such as a garage, carbon monoxide can accumulate to toxic levels. Carbon tetrachloride is used in dry cleaning. Hydrogen sulfide is a poisonous gas produced in some chemical processes. Tear gases are used by police and military personnel. Carbon disulfide is used in the rubber industry and in making rayon.

See also POISONING: FIRST AID.

Gastrectomy (gas trek′tə mē) is the surgical removal of part or all of the stomach. The operation is performed to remove a perforated or bleeding stomach ulcer (partial gastrectomy), to remove scarred tissue that obstructs the passage of food, or to remove a cancerous growth.

Q: *How is the digestive process affected after a gastrectomy?*

A: The small intestine is capable of maintaining the preliminary breakdown of proteins that normally takes place in the stomach. After the total removal of the stomach, however, a patient may have to make some dietary adjustments.

Q: *What dietary adjustments may have to be made?*

A: Supplements of vitamins and iron may be necessary. The absorption of vitamin B_{12} depends on the presence of gastric (stomach) juices; after a total gastrectomy, injections of this vitamin must be given. Iron supplements reduce the risk of anemia if a gastrectomy interferes with the amount of iron normally absorbed during digestion. After a partial gastrectomy, the patient has to adopt a routine of eating smaller amounts of food, more often.

See also DUMPING SYNDROME; VITAMIN.

Gastric ulcer. *See* ULCER, GASTRIC.

Gastritis (gas trī'tis) is an inflammation of the stomach lining. The inflammation may be caused by viral infection, alcohol, smoking, certain drugs, poisoned food, or stress. Gastritis may be acute or chronic.

Q: *What are the symptoms of gastritis?*

A: Acute gastritis causes vomiting, hairy tongue, thirst, severe stomach pain, and mild fever. Dehydration may occur. Chronic gastritis usually produces few symptoms, although in some cases a person may experience one or more of the following discomforts: mild indigestion; slight nausea; a bloated feeling after a small meal; a bad taste in the mouth; and vague stomach pain.

Q: *How is gastritis treated?*

A: Acute gastritis improves of its own accord if the precipitating factor or factors are eliminated. Antacid preparations and/or histamine blockers and antinauseant drugs are often prescribed. Chronic gastritis can be treated only by eliminating the causative factor, for example, alcohol, smoking, or highly spiced or other foods that are difficult to digest. Antacid drugs are recommended for the treatment of chronic gastritis.

See also TONGUE, HAIRY.

Gastroenteritis (gas trō en tə rī'tis) is any inflammation of the lining of the stomach and intestinal tract. The inflammation is usually caused by a bacterial infection. If it occurs in infants, there is severe liquid loss, and the patient may require hospitalization to prevent or treat dehydration. But gastroenteritis can also be caused by alcohol, certain drugs, food allergies, contaminated food, and certain bacterial infections. The symptoms of gastroenteritis are vomiting, abdominal cramps, diarrhea, and in severe cases, dehydration.

Q: *How is gastroenteritis treated?*

A: In most cases, the symptoms are treated, not the cause. The patient must stop drinking alcohol and must replace essential nutrients, especially liquids, that are lost through vomiting or diarrhea. Care must be taken to prevent dehydration. Once vomiting or diarrhea has stopped, normal diet must be resumed very slowly over a period of several days. Most relapses of gastroenteritis occur when a person prematurely returns to his or her normal diet.

Drug treatment of symptoms is rarely needed, and antinauseant drugs and antispasmodics are best avoided. Similarly, most cases of gastroenteritis do not require treatment with antibiotics.

See also DEHYDRATION; DIARRHEA; STOMACH.

Gastroenterology (gas trō en tə rol'ə jē) is the branch of medicine that deals with the gastrointestinal tract, that is, the organs from the mouth to the anus.

See also BILE DUCT; GALL BLADDER; INTESTINE; STOMACH.

Gastroenterostomy (gas trō en tə ros'tə mē) is an artificial opening that is made between the stomach and the small intestine. The operation (gastroenterotomy) is necessary if the muscle that surrounds the stomach opening is scarred and unable to pass food normally from the stomach. When removing part of the stomach (partial gastrectomy), a surgeon may perform a gastroenterotomy to connect the remaining part of the stomach to the small intestine. The lower opening is made into the jejunum (the part of the small intestine just beyond the duodenum).

See also DUMPING SYNDROME; ULCER, PEPTIC.

Gastrointestinal series (gas trō in test'tə nəl), or GI series, is an investigation of the gastrointestinal tract in which a series of X-ray photographs are taken. This is made possible when the patient swallows a tasteless solution of barium. X rays are taken as the radiopaque barium passes through the esophagus, stomach, and intestines. The barium solution shows the outline of these hollow organs. The barium is usually given to the patient early in the morning when the stomach is empty.

A lower GI series, or barium enema, is used to visualize the large intestine, or colon. In this case, however, the barium solution is given as an enema, rather than being swallowed.

See also BARIUM.

Gastrointestinal tract (gas trō in test′ tə nəl) is that series of organs from the mouth to the anus, specifically the esophagus, stomach, and intestines.

Gastroscopy (gas tros′kə pē) is the examination of the internal surface of the stomach through a special instrument (gastroscope) that is passed through the mouth and down the esophagus. The gastroscope may be either a straight tube or flexible fiberscope. Gastroscopy is a type of endoscopy.

See also ENDOSCOPY; FIBERSCOPE.

Gastrostomy (gas tros′tə mē) is an opening that is made from the outside surface of the abdomen into the stomach. The operation (called a gastrotomy) may be performed if there is some obstruction in, or damage to, the lower end of the esophagus that prevents foods from passing on down (for example, cancer, or severe scarring following acid poisoning). A gastrostomy allows the patient to be fed through the opening directly into the stomach. Gastrotomies are often performed as a temporary measure after major gastrointestinal surgery to allow stomach and abdominal tissue to heal completely.

Gaucher's disease (gō shāz′) is a rare inherited disorder caused by the absence of an enzyme that is necessary for the processing by the body of a particular group of fatty acids. The age of onset varies greatly. There is no treatment for this disease. Children generally die of the disease within one to two years after its onset, but death in adults usually results from a complication, such as pneumonia.

Gene (jēn) is the basic unit of heredity that carries "instructions" for a particular characteristic. Within the nucleus of nearly all human cells there are 23 pairs of chromosomes. Each cell contains thousands of genes. Exceptions are sex cells (eggs and sperm), which contain only 23 single chromosomes each. When an egg and a sperm fuse at fertilization, the resulting embryo carries genes from each parent cell.

See also HEREDITY.

Generic (jə ner′ik) refers to an officially accepted drug name that does not belong exclusively to one manufacturer. The generic name often gives a clue as to the chemical properties or pharmacological classification of the drug. Usually a generic drug product costs less than the comparable brand-name product.

Genetic abnormality (jə net′ik) is a disorder caused by an abnormality of a gene or by an incorrect number of genes. (The table on pages 374 and 375 lists genetic abnormalities. Each entry is defined elsewhere in this encyclopedia.)

Q: *What genetic abnormalities commonly occur?*

A: Conditions such as achondroplasia, hemolytic disease of the newborn, sickle cell anemia, Down's syndrome, and cleft palate are among the most common genetic abnormalities. There are more than 2,000 genetic disorders, some of which are extremely rare, such as phenylketonuria, an inherited metabolic disorder. *See also* PHENYLKETONURIA.

Q: *Are all genetic abnormalities immediately apparent?*

A: No. Some genetic abnormalities, such as Tay-Sachs disease, affect the metabolism in subtle ways and may not become apparent until several months after birth. Others, such as Huntington's chorea, may not appear until the individual reaches middle age.

Q: *Can normal parents have children with genetic abnormalities?*

A: Yes. The effects of an abnormal gene may be masked by a normal gene in either one or both of the parents. In such a case, the parents will appear to be completely normal, but their children may be affected. Hemophilia is an example of a condition in which this situation could occur. Genetic abnormalities in children with normal parents may also occur if there is a spontaneous mutation, or change,

Genetic Abnormalities

Abnormality	*Characteristics/Symptoms*	*Treatment*
Achondroplasia (fetal rickets)	Large head, small face; bulky forehead; short, thick limbs; normal trunk	None
Agammaglobulinemia (Bruton's disease)	Susceptibility to infection	Injections of gamma globulin
Albino	No pigment in eyes, hair, and skin; extreme sensitivity to sunlight	None; protection of skin and eyes from sunlight
Ankylosis	Stiffening of a joint	Physical therapy
Celiac disease (celiac sprue)	Swollen abdomen; pale, foul-smelling stool; vomiting; diarrhea	Gluten-free diet; possible elimination from diet of all milk products
Chorea, Huntington's	Facial muscle spasms; involuntary movements of the limbs; mental deterioration	None
Christmas disease (hemophilia B)	Prolonged bleeding from injuries	Transfusion of blood with correct clotting factor
Cleft palate	Fissure in the palate of the mouth	Plastic surgery
Cystic fibrosis (fibrocystic disease of the pancreas)	Chronic cough; persistent wheezing; respiratory problems	No effective cure; special diets, antibiotics, and bronchial drainage help alleviate symptoms
Down's syndrome (mongolism)	Sloping forehead; small ears; skin folds over the inner corner of the eyes; mental retardation	None; specialized education to help the child adjust to society
Dwarfism	Abnormal underdevelopment of the body	If the pituitary gland is underproducing, injections of growth hormone; with other causes, no effective treatment
Epilepsy	Periodic, recurrent seizures; abnormal behavior; possible loss of consciousness	No effective cure; anticonvulsant drugs to control the seizures
Farsightedness (hyperopia)	Distant objects seen clearly; close objects blurred	eyeglasses; contacts
Friedreich's ataxia	Muscular weakness and uncoordination; hunching of the back; clawed feet	None
Gaucher's disease	Enlarged spleen; darker skin pigmentation; abnormal bone growth	None
Hemolytic disease of the newborn (erythroblastosis fetalis)	Anemia; jaundice; enlargement of liver and spleen	blood transfusions
Hemophilia	Spontaneous internal bleeding	Injections of missing clotting factor

Abnormality	*Characteristics/Symptoms*	*Treatment*
Hirschsprung's disease (megacolon)	In children: vomiting & retarding of growth; in adults: severe, continuous constipation; distended abdomen	Surgical removal of abnormal section of intestine
Klinefelter's syndrome	Postpuberty, male breasts increase in size; testes remain small; mental retardation	No specific treatment
Myopia (nearsightedness)	Distant objects appear out of focus; close objects seen sharply	Corrective lenses
Myotonia congenita (Thomsen's disease)	Muscles do not relax readily after contracting.	No cure, but drug treatment can control disorder
Osteogenesis imperfecta (Fragilitas ossium)	Brittle bones, deformities; blue discoloration of the whites of the eyes; progressive deafness	No effective treatment
Phenylketonuria (PKU)	mental deterioration; irritability; vomiting; convulsions	A PKU-free diet during childhood
Polycystic kidney	Blisters; red teeth; purple or pink urine	Avoidance of sunlight
Retinitis pigmentosa	Rod cell degeneration; night blindness; daytime vision deterioration; telescopic vision	No definitive treatment
Sickle cell anemia	Abnormal, sickle-shaped red blood cells; severe anemia	No specific treatment; therapy directed toward alleviating symptoms as they arise
Tay-Sachs disease (gangliosidosis)	Brain cells degenerate; spasticity; convulsions; blindness; progressive loss of mental & physical abilities	No known treatment
Thalassemia (hemolytic anemia)	Breathlessness; pallor; fatigue; jaundice; leg ulcers	No effective treatment
Turner's syndrome (gonadal dysgenesis)	Female anomaly; short stature; webbing of the neck; multiple birthmarks; underdeveloped secondary sexual characteristics	No effective treatment
Von Recklinghausen's disease (neurofibromatosis)	Nodules at birth; skin spots; scoliosis	Treatment of severe symptoms
Wilson's disease (Hepatolenticular degeneration)	Cirrhosis of the liver; anemia; and chorea	Penicillamine

of the parental genes or if there is a fault in the process of egg or sperm production.

Q: *Can genetic abnormalities be treated?*

A: Although most genetic abnormalities are untreatable, there are a few that can be treated. Those suffering from phenylketonuria can be given a phenylalanine-free diet during the first few years of life while the nervous sytem is developing, after which they can lead a normal life. Those with celiac disease can prevent the occurrence of any symptoms by having a gluten-free diet throughout their lives. Cleft palate and spina bifida may be treated surgically, although with spina bifida, the success of the treatment depends upon the initial severity of the condition.

See also CONGENITAL ANOMALY; GENE; GENETIC COUNSELING; HEMOPHILIA; HEREDITY; MUTATION.

Genetic counseling (jə net′ik) is a branch of medicine that provides and interprets information about human genetics. The main objective of genetic counseling is to prevent the occurrence of congenital anomalies, abnormalities present at birth. *See also* CONGENITAL ANOMALY.

Q: *What types of congenital anomalies may be caused by a genetic disorder?*

A: Although genetic disorders causing birth defects are comparatively rare, the range of such disorders is wide. For example, some genetic disorders, such as cleft palate, are apparent at birth; others, such as Huntington's chorea, do not appear for a number of years. For a more detailed account of genetic disorders, *see* GENETIC ABNORMALITY.

Q: *What information will a genetic counselor require?*

A: A counselor will need to know the ages of the couple; whether either of the couple, or any of their close relatives, has a congenital abnormality; and whether either has had children with an inherited disorder. A counselor will need as complete a family health history as possible, perhaps going back for several generations. A counselor may also perform certain tests to determine whether either of the couple has an inherited disorder of which they may be unaware.

Q: *Are there any disorders that do not affect the parents but which may occur in their children?*

A: Yes. If both parents have one recessive gene for the same disorder, neither will exhibit any abnormality. However, if a child inherits both recessive genes, one from each parent, then the disorder will manifest itself. In such a case, there is a 25 percent chance that the child will inherit both genes and so manifest the disorder.

Q: *What information does a genetic counselor give?*

A: A counselor explains about dominant and recessive genes; the kinds of chromosomal abnormalities that may occur; and why certain conditions occur. If the couple has a child with a genetic disorder, a counselor explains the chances of a second child suffering from the same disorder. Similarly, if one or both parents has an inherited disorder, a counselor tells them about the chances of a child inheriting the same disorder.

A genetic counselor's task is to provide as much information as possible. The genetic counselor does not advise whether or not to have a baby; that decision rests with the couple. But many couples have found the decision easier to make when they know the facts.

Q: *Can anything be done to warn a pregnant woman of an abnormal fetus?*

A: Yes. In the fourth month of pregnancy, amniocentesis, the sampling of fluid from the bag around the fetus, may be performed. This fluid can be tested for abnormal substances and for chromosomal abnormalities that may indicate an inherited disorder. For example, an abnormally high level of the substance alpha fetoprotein (AFP) is produced by fetuses with either anencephaly or spina bifida. Amniocentesis may be combined with ultrasound techniques to give further information about the fetus. These techniques can detect many but not all abnormalities. If an abnormality is detected, the pregnancy may be terminated if the parents wish it. A new technique, chorionic villus biopsy, can allow a genetic study of the fetus to be performed much earlier than amniocentesis. Chorionic villus biopsy can be done in the second month of pregnancy. Test results are usually available within one week.

See *also* AMNIOCENTESIS; CHORIONIC VILLUS BIOPSY.

Q: *How can genetic counseling be obtained?*

A: If a couple wants genetic counseling, they should consult their family physician or an obstetrician, who will refer them to a genetic counselor.

Genetic engineering (jə net′ik) is the intervention into, and manipulation of, the material containing hereditary traits (genes), which is passed from parents to offspring. Genetic engineering has been used by scientists to discover ways of creating new forms of life, as well as to gain greater insight into the causes of human birth defects and hereditary diseases. Genetic engineering has come under attack by those who feel that science has gone too far in search of a perfect human species.

See *also* GENE.

Genitourinary system (jen ə tō yůr′ə ner ē) is the reproductive and urinary system of women and men, sometimes referred to as the GU system. This includes the kidneys, ureters, bladder, and urethra in both sexes. In women, the ovaries, fallopian tubes, uterus, vagina, labia, and clitoris are also part of the GU system. In men, the testes, prostate gland, vas deferens, and penis are included in the GU system.

See *also* UROGENITAL SYSTEM.

Genu valgum. See KNOCK-KNEE.

Genu varum. See BOWLEGS.

Geriatric medicine (jer ē at′rik) is the branch of medicine dealing with aging and the conditions and diseases that affect the elderly.

Germ (jėrm) is any microorganism, especially one that causes disease, such as a specific bacterium, virus, fungus, or protozoan. The term also describes embryonic living matter that has the capacity to develop into an organ, part, or organism (for example, the dental germ from which a tooth develops). Germ cell is another name for a single egg (ovum) or sperm.

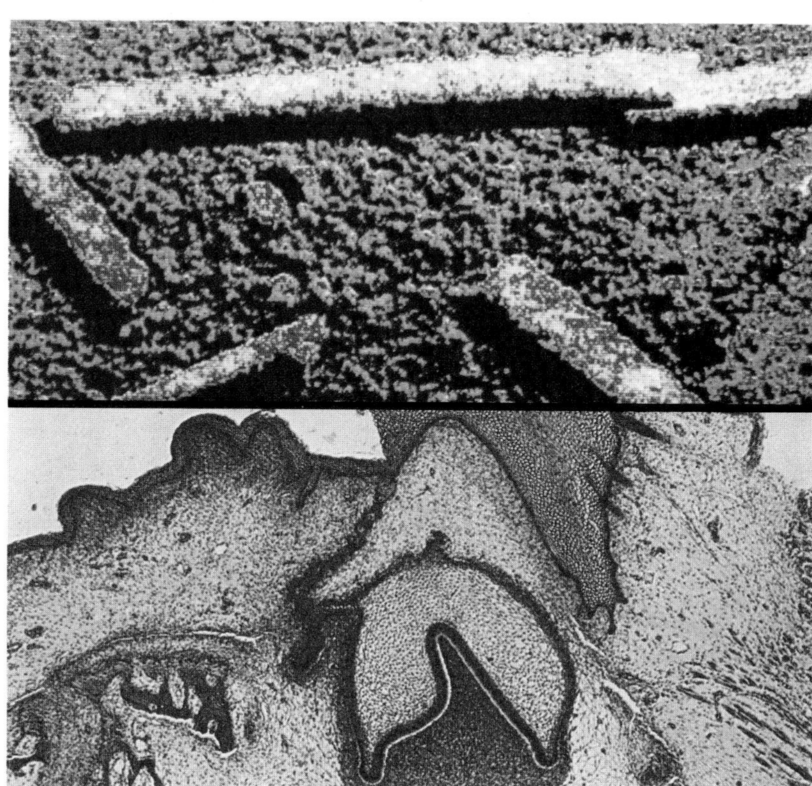

A **germ** is a microscopic animal, especially one that causes disease. The tobacco mosaic virus, *top,* is a germ that causes tobacco mosaic, a disease that attacks the leaves of tobacco plants.

The word germ also refers to the earliest form of a living thing. The tooth germ, *bottom,* is a bud-like thickening in the connective tissue of the jaw that will develop into a tooth.

German measles. See RUBELLA.

Gestation (jes tā′shən) is the time from conception to birth. In humans this usually lasts 266 days.

See *also* PREGNANCY AND CHILDBIRTH.

GI. See GASTROINTESTINAL TRACT.

Giardiasis (jē är dī′ə sis) is an infection caused by the protozoan *Giardia lamblia,* which lives in the small intestine. *Giardia* usually enters the body when a person drinks contaminated water. However, it can also spread between people who are in very close contact, for example, in households or day-care centers. The protozoan sometimes interferes with fat absorption, causing a swelling of the abdomen, burping, vomiting, nausea, diarrhea, weakness, and weight loss. The infection commonly lasts two to three months. All patients with giardiasis, even those showing no symptoms, should be treated with drugs to eradicate the organism.

Gigantism (jī gan′tiz əm) is a condition of abnormal growth that occurs before puberty and results in excessive size and stature. An overproduction of growth hormone is the cause.

GI, lower. See GASTROINTESTINAL SERIES.

Gingivitis (jin jə vī′təs) is inflammation of the gums accompanied by any combination of pain, swelling, and a tendency to bleed. If the inflammation is left untreated the teeth may become loose or fall out. The most common cause of gingivitis is the accumulation of dental plaque as a result of poor dental hygiene. Gingivitis may also be caused by ill-fitting dentures, vitamin C deficiency disease, known as scurvy, or generalized inflammation of the mouth (stomatitis). It may also result as a complication of diabetes, leukemia, or pregnancy. While most cases of gingivitis are responsive to improved oral hygiene, cases in which the gums become tough and fibrotic may require removal (gingivectomy) of the inflamed tissue.

See also DENTAL DISORDERS.

GI series. *See* GASTROINTESTINAL SERIES.

Gland is a body organ that is made up of specialized tissue that secretes a fluid. There are two types of glands: an exocrine gland, which secretes fluid into a duct or tube; and an endocrine gland, which secretes directly into the bloodstream.

See also ENDOCRINE GLAND; EXOCRINE GLAND.

The human body contains two types of **glands:** exocrine glands, which secrete fluids into a duct or tube; and endocrine glands, which secrete fluids directly into the bloodstream. Some body organs contain both exocrine and endodrine glands.

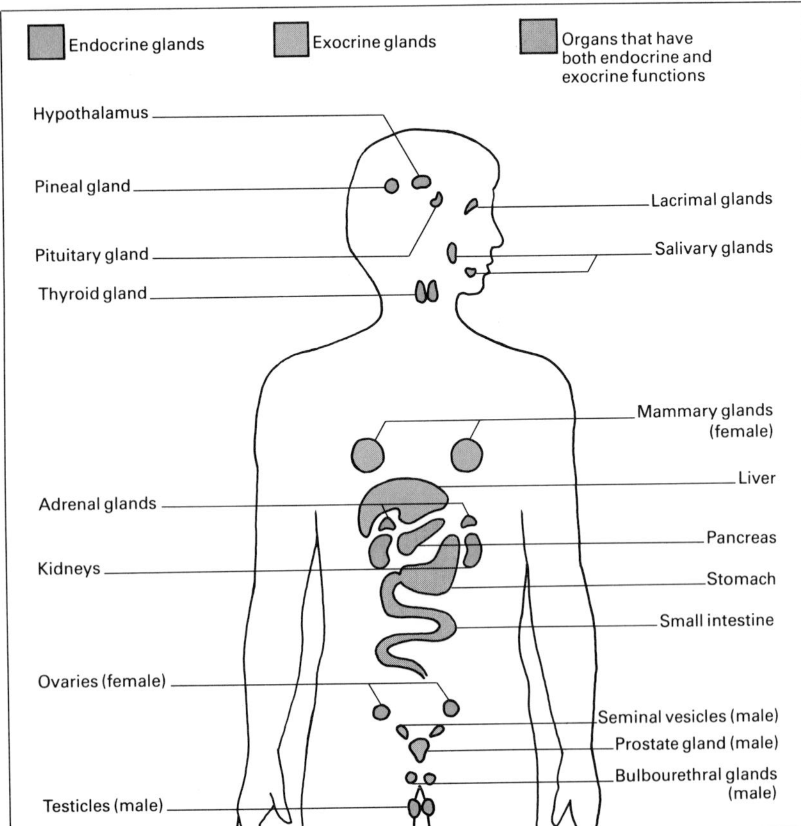

Glandular fever (glan′jə lər) is an archaic name for infectious mononucleosis.

See also MONONUCLEOSIS.

Glaucoma (glô kō′mə) is a group of eye diseases characterized by the build-up of fluid pressure within the eyeball. The pressure severely affects the eye lens and optic nerve, resulting eventually in blindness unless the condition is detected and treated before damage becomes permanent.

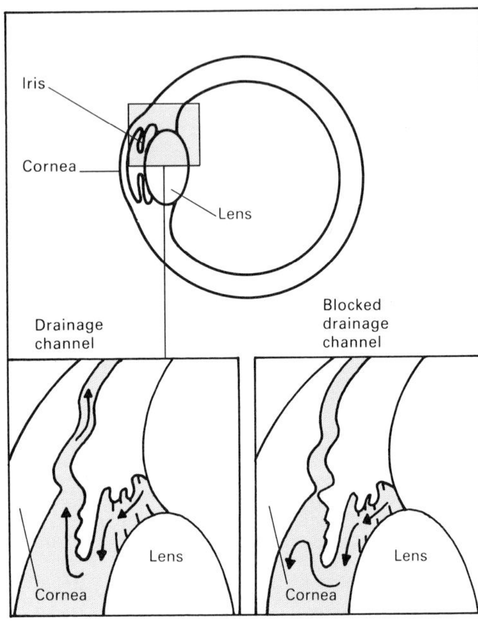

Glaucoma is a disease in which the aqueous humor, the fluid that nourishes the cornea and the lens, does not drain properly. Pressure on the eye increases and, if untreated, destroys the optic nerve.

Primary glaucoma usually occurs without known cause. A high incidence of glaucoma in certain families suggests that it may be an inherited tendency. It is more common in farsighted persons.

Secondary glaucoma is a complication of other eye disorders, such as inflammation of the iris (iritis). Diabetics seem more likely to develop this condition than nondiabetics.

Q: *What are the symptoms of glaucoma?*

A: Acute glaucoma usually occurs suddenly with pain and a dramatic blurring of vision. The patient begins to notice rainbow-colored halos around lights and bright objects and a loss of vision at the sides of the field of view (tunnel vision). Eyesight deteriorates, and blindness results if treatment is not obtained promptly.

Chronic glaucoma occurs slowly and without pain, so that an individual is usually unaware of the disorder until it is well advanced.

Q: *How does glaucoma cause loss of vision?*

A: The pressure of the fluid (aqueous humor) in the front of the lens increases the pressure in the fluid (vitreous humor) behind the lens. The resulting pressure on the retina at the back of the eye reduces the flow of blood and damages the light-sensitive rods and cones. If untreated, the pressure destroys the optic nerve. Peripheral, or side vision, is lost first, followed by total loss of vision. *See also* EYE.

Q: *How is chronic glaucoma detected before eyesight deteriorates?*

A: A physician measures the pressure in the eye with a special instrument called a tonometer, which is placed over the eyeball. This simple test is painless, fast, and accurate. Everyone over the age of 40 should have a glaucoma check once a year.

Q: *How is glaucoma treated?*

A: If the condition is detected early, drug treatment prevents later damage to sight. Various eye drops can be used at regular intervals to reduce pressure within the eyeball. An ophthalmologist may prescribe pilocarpine, which increases the size of the opening through which the aqueous humor drains. Other eye drugs may also be used. Diuretic drugs, such as acetazolamide, help to decrease the amount of aqueous humor produced.

If drug treatment fails, surgery is necessary. An ophthalmic surgeon makes a small hole near the rim of the iris to create a new outflow channel for the fluid.

See also IRIDECTOMY.

Glioma (glī ō′mə) is a tumor in the weblike tissue that supports nerves and the brain. A glioma may develop slowly or grow rapidly. In many instances gliomas are malignant (cancerous). Gliomas may be treated either by surgical removal or with radiotherapy.

See also RADIOTHERAPY.

Globulin (glob′yə lin) is one of two simple proteins in the blood plasma, the other being albumin. Globulins can be divided into alpha, beta, and gamma subgroups. The blood clotting agents fibrinogen and prothrombin are both globulins.

See also ALBUMIN; BLOOD.

Globus hystericus (glō′bus his ter′ə kus) is the common "lump in the throat," which often occurs when one is crying. It can be associated with anxiety, depression, or some other emotional conflict. Although the "lump" is actually not physically present, the sensation of it can be very real, and it may interfere with eating.

An individual experiencing globus hystericus should consult a physician in case there is a physical reason for the symptom. If not, it is important to identify the psychological and emotional issues as soon as possible. The condition can then be alleviated by counseling, medication, or a combination of both.

Glomangioma (glō man jē ō′mə), also know medically as a glomus tumor or angioneuroma, is the painful, benign (noncancerous) enlargement of the glomus, a collection of tiny arteries with nerve endings. Glomera are found in the nailbeds and the pads of the fingers, toes, ears, hands, and feet. Usually located beneath a fingernail, a glomangioma causes purplish-red discoloration with slight swelling, extreme tenderness, and sometimes shooting pain. The only treatment is surgical removal.

Glomerulonephritis (glə mer ə lō ni frī′tis) is a form of nephritis that involves the glomeruli, clusters of tiny blood vessels that filter the blood to extract urine in the kidneys. Glomerulonephritis may be either acute or chronic.

Q: *What are the symptoms of acute glomerulonephritis?*

A: Acute glomerulonephritis sometimes follows a sore throat caused by a streptococcal infection. It is more common in children than in adults. A few weeks after the onset of infection, the patient may suddenly suffer from headaches and abdominal pain. The face swells, and the patient passes blood-stained, "smoky," or brown urine. These symptoms last for several

Glomerulonephritis occurs when the glomeruli within the kidney are damaged due to a reaction to streptococcal bacteria. The damage leads to blood in the urine and the retention of salt, water, and waste substances in the bloodstream.

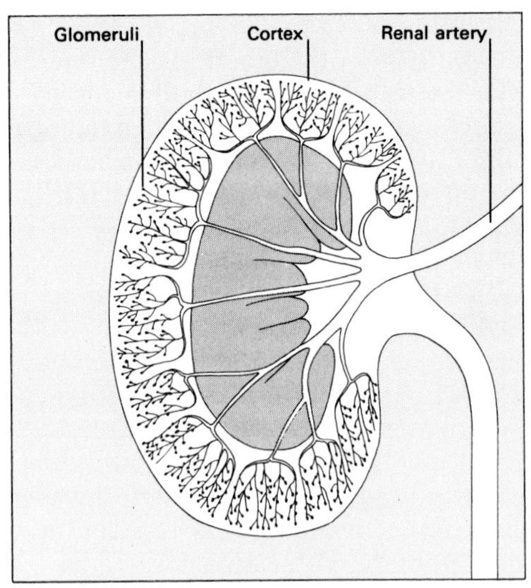

days, and the condition gradually improves within a few weeks.

Q: *What causes acute glomerulonephritis?*

A: In most cases, it results from a reaction to one of the types of streptococcal bacteria that cause sore throats or skin infections. The reaction damages the glomeruli and leads to hematuria (blood in the urine) and the retention of salt, water, and nitrogenous waste substances in the bloodstream. In some cases, the cause of glomerulonephritis is not known.

Q: *How is acute glomerulonephritis treated?*

A: In most cases, the disease is mild enough to be treated by a restriction of salt and fluid intake, with total bed rest. If a bacterial infection is present, a physician usually prescribes antibiotic drugs. If there is high blood pressure, other drugs may be prescribed to reduce it. Occasionally, glomerulonephritis in adults causes severe kidney damage that necessitates kidney dialysis until the kidneys recover.

Q: *What are the symptoms of chronic glomerulonephritis?*

A: The symptoms develop slowly over a period of several months, and the condition may not be detected until it is in its final stages. The symptoms are those of kidney failure: poor appetite, fatigue, and anemia. There is also high blood pressure and the risk of heart failure. Usually, chronic glomerulonephritis is detected during a routine examination, when protein and small amounts of blood are found in the urine.

Q: *How is chronic glomerulonephritis treated?*

A: Treatment involves a strict diet with restriction of salt and protein intake and drugs to reduce high blood pressure. In severe cases, kidney dialysis and, eventually, kidney transplantation may be necessary.

See also NEPHRITIS.

Glomerulus (glə mer′ů ləs) is a cluster of capillaries within the kidney that are involved in filtering the waste products from the blood.

See also KIDNEY.

Glossitis (glo sī′tis) is inflammation of the tongue. Acute glossitis is often associated with other mouth disorders, such as gingivitis or generalized stomatitis. Symptoms of acute glossitis include a painful, sometimes ulcerated tongue, thick and sticky saliva, and difficulty in swallowing. The patient may also complain of unpleasant taste and odor.

Chronic glossitis is associated with chronic ill health, anemias, and tooth infections. Other causes include gastritis, smoking, alcohol consumption, and sometimes the use of antibiotic drugs.

Q: *How is glossitis treated?*

A: Acute glossitis is treated with antiseptic mouthwashes and an anesthetic solution to reduce pain. Chronic glossitis is treated by improving the general health of the patient.

Glucagon (glü′kə gon) is a hormone, produced by the islets of Langerhans in the pancreas, that raises the body's blood sugar level by stimulating the breakdown of glycogen to glucose. Glucagon preparations are sometimes used in the emergency treatment of insulin shock, when a diabetic's blood sugar level falls too low.

See also ISLETS OF LANGERHANS.

Glucose (glü′kōs) is a monosaccharide, a simple sugar that is essential to body cells for energy. Because it does not have to be broken down in the lower digestive system, it passes directly into the bloodstream from the small intestine and is stored as glycogen in the liver. Glucose is classified as a carbohydrate and is found in most sugars and starches.

The amount of glucose in the blood is called the blood sugar content, which is carefully regulated by the pancreatic hormone insulin and, to a lesser extent, by other hormones. Insufficient insulin produces high blood sugar, as in diabetes mellitus. Glucose preparations are used in the treatment of dehydration and other disorders. *See also* DIABETES MELLITUS; GLYCOGEN; INSULIN.

Q: ***What other disorders are associated with abnormal blood sugar levels?***

A: High blood sugar, hyperglycemia, is associated with acromegaly, hemochromatosis, hyperthyroidism, and hyperadrenalism. Low blood sugar, hypoglycemia, is associated with Addison's disease, insulin shock, hypopituitarism, and myxedema, a severe form of hypothyroidism. *See also* GLUCOSE TOLERANCE TEST; HYPERGLYCEMIA; HYPERTHYROIDISM; HYPOGLYCEMIA; HYPOTHYROIDISM.

Glucose monitoring device (glü'kōs) is a small electronic unit, used by many persons with diabetes, to help maintain control of blood sugars. The devices are about the size of a small portable radio, lightweight, and relatively inexpensive. They can measure glucose levels in a single drop of blood. Because they are easy to use and portable, they are useful in helping many diabetics take better care of themselves.

See also DIABETES; DIABETES MELLITUS; GLUCOSE.

Glucose-6-phosphate dehydrogenase deficiency (glü'kōs fos'fāt dē hī drə' jə nās) is an inherited condition in which the red blood cells are completely or partially lacking in glucose-6-phosphate dehydrogenase, an enzyme in the liver and kidneys that helps metabolize glycerol to glucose. Because it is transmitted by a gene on the X chromosome, this disorder is seen almost entirely in men. In addition, certain ethnic groups are more susceptible to the deficiency. About 10 percent of American black males have the disorder. Italians, Greeks, and other people from the Mediterranean basin are also more prone to the disease. In persons affected with the disorder, an exposure to certain drugs, including aspirin, can lead to hemolysis, the breakdown of red blood cells. Hemolysis may also be caused by conditions of acute stress in persons with the deficiency. Treatment entails the elimination of the cause.

See also HEMOLYSIS.

Glucose tolerance test (glü'kōs tol'ər əns) is a procedure that a physician carries out to determine whether a patient is able to use and store glucose normally. The test is most commonly carried out to diagnose diabetes mellitus in patients with symptoms suggestive of diabetes. In some persons, however, an abnormally elevated fasting blood sugar level on two occasions may be sufficient to diagnose diabetes. The glucose tolerance test may also be used during pregnancy to test for gestational diabetes.

After a period of fasting, the patient's blood and urine are tested for glucose. Then, a measured quantity of glucose is administered as a drink or by injections. Further blood and urine samples are taken at regular intervals for two to four hours. A normal result shows a maximum level of glucose in the blood about an hour after the dose, followed by gradual return to the normal level during the second hour. An abnormal result reveals an unusually high rise in the blood sugar level, an extremely slow return to normal, and sugar in the urine (glycosuria).

See also DIABETES MELLITUS; GLUCOSE.

Gluten (glü'tən) is a protein found in wheat and other grains. Persons with nontropical sprue and celiac disease are believed to be allergic to gluten.

See also CELIAC DISEASE; DIET, SPECIAL; SPRUE.

Glycerol (glis'ə rōl) is a colorless, sweet, syrupy liquid, which is soluble in water and alcohol. It is obtained from animal and vegetable oils and fats. Glycerol preparations are called glycerin and are used in chapped-skin ointments and some drug preparations.

Glycogen (gli'kə jən) is a starch-like carbohydrate that is stored in the liver and muscles in small amounts. It acts as an energy reserve for the body, because glycogen can be quickly metabolized into glucose when needed. The balance between glycogen and glucose is maintained by various hormones. Insulin, for example, causes the conversion of glucose into glycogen. Glucagon, on the other hand, is responsible for glycogen breakdown.

See also GLUCAGON; GLUCOSE; INSULIN.

Glycosuria (glī kə sŭr′ē ə) is the medical term for glucose in the urine.

See also GLUCOSE TOLERANCE TEST.

Goiter (goi′tər) is an enlargement of the thyroid gland. The resulting bulge on the neck may become extremely large, but most simple goiters are brought under control before this happens. Occasionally a simple goiter may cause some difficulty in breathing and swallowing.

Q: *What causes a goiter?*

A: Iodine is the principal component of thyroxine, the thyroid gland's hormone. If there is not enough iodine in the diet, there is insufficient thyroxine, and the pituitary gland responds by releasing more thyroid-stimulating hormone. This causes enlargement of the thyroid gland.

However, a goiter may also be caused by overactivity of the pituitary gland or by overactivity of the thyroid gland itself (hyperthyroidism). Other causes include reduced activity of the thyroid gland because of inflammation (thyroiditis), so that the gland swells in order to produce more thyroxine. Some types of drugs can produce a goiter. During adolescence or pregnancy, a goiter may appear as the thyroid gland copes with the body's need for more thyroxine. Sometimes a goiter is caused by a tumor on the thyroid gland.

Q: *How is a simple goiter treated?*

A: Iodized salt added to the diet is an effective treatment, as well as a preventative measure. The best drug for treating goiter caused by hypothyroidism (underactivity of the thyroid gland) is thyroxine. Such treatment prevents the pituitary gland from secreting too much thyroid-stimulating hormone. Lumps or nodules on the thyroid gland are removed surgically in case they are cancerous. Inflammation (thyroiditis) may be part of a general illness, and the goiter improves when the patient recovers. Goiters resulting from the hormone requirements of adolescence or pregnancy disappear when the demand for thyroxine is reduced naturally.

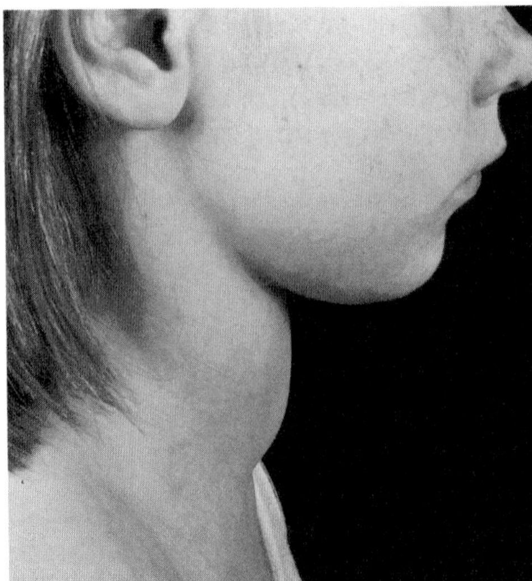

A **goiter** is an enlargement of the thyroid gland caused by an insufficient amount of iodine in the diet. The pituitary gland responds to this insufficiency by producng additional thyroid-stimulating hormone, which triggers the enlargement of the thyroid.

Gold salts treatment refers to the use of gold salts, usually in combination with other drugs, in the treatment of severe rheumatoid arthritis. Because gold salts can cause extremely dangerous, even fatal, toxic reactions, treatment must be carefully supervised by a physician.

See also ARTHRITIS, RHEUMATOID.

Gonad (gon′ad) is a sex gland in which reproductive cells develop. Ovaries and testes are gonads.

See also REPRODUCTION, HUMAN.

Gonorrhea (gon ə rē′ə) is a highly contagious venereal (sexually transmitted) disease. It is common throughout the world and is widespread in the United States, where authorities estimate there are three million cases annually. If left untreated, it can lead to sterility and can be the cause of congenital blindness.

If reported to a physician promptly, gonorrhea can be treated successfully with antibiotics, although no immunity is given against reinfection. Any person who has an urethral or vaginal discharge should report it to a physician at once. This consultation is important; it not only increases the chances of successful treatment, it also allows the early detection of other sexually transmitted diseases that may also be present.

Q: *What are the symptoms of gonorrhea?*

A: In a male, a thick, yellow-green discharge from the penis occurs within 2 to 14 days after infection. Inflammation and pain in the urethra (the tube through which urine is passed) are common, and urination becomes slow and difficult. A small number of males may develop no symptoms at all, although they are still capable of spreading the infection to a sexual partner.

In a female, the infection may produce no symptoms; so a woman is often unaware that she may be infecting the person, or persons, with whom she comes into sexual contact. Occasionally, however, symptoms do develop slowly. These include vaginal discharge, painful or frequent urination, or pain in the lower abdomen. Gonorrhea in the rectum or throat is usually asymptomatic.

Q: *What causes gonorrhea?*

A: Gonorrhea is caused by the gonococcus bacterium, *Neisseria gonorrhoeae*. In most cases, the bacteria cause inflammation of the mucous membranes of the urogenital tract, but they may also affect the membranes of the throat, the conjunctiva, or the rectum.

Q: *How is gonorrhea diagnosed?*

A: For a male, a test (Gram's stain) of the urethral discharge produces a reliable diagnosis. In a female, this diagnosis is less reliable; it is sometimes difficult to detect the difference between the gonorrhea organism and others that resemble it but occur normally. Positive diagnosis can, however, be made from a culture.

Q: *How is gonorrhea treated?*

A: All cases of gonorrhea, even if only suspected, must be treated by a physician. The patient's partner must also see the physician. There is no home cure for the disease, nor will it disappear if left alone. Antibiotic treatment with penicillin is usually successful. Some strains of the bacteria are resistant to penicillin, however, and these must be treated with other antibiotics.

Q: *What are the possible complications of gonorrhea?*

A: Neglected cases of gonorrhea become chronic. In a male, infection spreads from the mucous membranes into deep tissues, such as the bladder, prostate gland, and epididymis. Sometimes the urethra becomes scarred, which makes urination slow and difficult; and in some cases, sterility may result.

In a female, the chronic infection may spread to the uterus, fallopian tubes, and ovaries and cause sterility. A pregnant woman with untreated gonorrhea may infect her baby's eyes as the baby passes through the birth canal.

An infection that spreads via the bloodstream throughout the body is more common in women than in men. There is fever and infection with swelling of the joints, skin, tendons, and liver. The heart and brain are rarely affected.

Q: *How can a person avoid catching gonorrhea?*

A: A person can avoid catching gonorrhea by using a condom (sheath), which provides some protection against the disease.

See also SEXUALLY TRANSMITTED DISEASE.

Gout (gout) is a hereditary, metabolic disorder characterized by inflammation and pain in affected joints. Gout occurs more frequently in men than in women. It is caused by an excess of uric acid in the blood and tissues. Crystals of the acid form under the skin and in the joints, causing local pain. In normal circumstances, uric acid above a certain low concentration is excreted in the urine. Gout occurs either when too little uric acid is excreted or when there is too much of the acid for the kidneys to excrete. Alcohol intake may increase the incidence of attacks of gout.

Q: *What are the symptoms of gout?*

A: An attack begins suddenly with severe pain and swelling in a joint. The overlying skin becomes red and shiny. A severe attack may cause fever and nausea. Untreated, an attack of gout lasts between three and seven days. Even when the symptoms disappear, further attacks are likely. An infection in a joint can appear very similar. A physician should be consulted.

Q: *What brings on an attack of gout?*

A: In general, the causes of acute attacks of gout are not known, but minor injuries and some drugs, for example, diuretics, can bring on an attack.

Q: *How is gout diagnosed?*

A: A physician has to make sure that the inflamed joint is not the result

Gout is caused by the formation of uric acid crystals under the skin and in joints, causing pain and swelling.

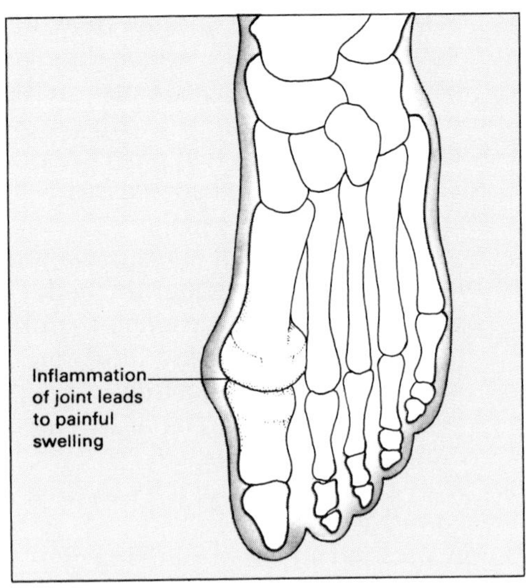
Inflammation of joint leads to painful swelling

of infection, osteoarthritis, or acute rheumatoid arthritis. A diagnosis of gout is made after the fluid from an inflamed joint is examined for crystals. A blood test to check the uric acid level is often performed.

Q: *How is gout treated?*

A: During an acute attack, the joint is rested until the pain subsides. The drug colchicine can bring relief within a few hours, but possible side effects make it unsuitable for the elderly and for patients with heart, liver, or kidney disorders. Other drugs prescribed for an acute attack include phenylbutazone, ibuprofen, naproxen, and indomethacin.

After an attack, treatment is aimed at reducing the blood level of uric acid, by means of drugs and an increased intake of fluids. Colchicine can be taken regularly, as can probenecid, sulfinpyrazone, or allopurinol. Aspirin negates the effect of the drugs and should be avoided; acetaminophen is an acceptable substitute.

Q: *Does gout have any complications?*

A: Yes. If gout is not treated in its early stages, the condition may become chronic. Chronic gout results in deposits of uric acid (tophi) in the joints. These deposits may cause permanent arthritis. The most serious danger from the metabolic disorder which causes gout is that uric acid crystals may be deposited in the kidneys.

Graafian follicle (grä′fē ən fol′ə kəl) is the mature cavity within an ovary that contains the egg (ovum) before ovulation. When the follicle ruptures under the influence of luteinizing hormone (LH), the ovum is released. The corpus luteum develops within the ruptured follicle.

See also CORPUS LUTEUM.

Graft is the surgical procedure in which healthy tissue is transferred from one part of the body to another or to a second body, in order to repair structural damage. Skin is the tissue most commonly grafted, although cartilage, bone, tendon, blood vessel, nerve, muscle, cornea, and whole organs, such as the heart, kidney, or liver, can be grafted. Synthetic grafts are often used to replace diseased blood vessels.

The technique of skin grafting is invaluable in the treatment of deep burns and similar injuries. Healing time is reduced, and the grafted skin is stronger and less disfigured than the scarred tissue that would otherwise have formed.

See also TRANSPLANT SURGERY.

Grand mal. *See* EPILEPSY.

Granulocytopenia. *See* AGRANULOCYTOSIS.

Granuloma (gran yü lō′mə) is a tumorlike mass or nodule of tissue that is produced by chronic inflammation, due either to infectious disease or to the presence of a foreign body. Granulomas may disappear by themselves or last until the infection goes away. They may become gangrenous (dead tissue) or spread. Many granulomas can be effectively treated with antibiotic drugs.

Some of the diseases producing granulomas are leprosy, yaws, syphilis, granuloma inguinale, and tuberculosis. Some of the nonliving, foreign causes are splinters or gravel under the skin, sutures, or talc.

See also GRANULOMA INGUINALE.

Granuloma inguinale (gran yü lō′mə ing wə nä′ lē), or Donovanosis, is a venereal (sexually transmitted) disease caused by the bacterium *Calymmatobacterium granulomatis.* The first symptom is a small, painless lump in the genital area. If neglected, this rapidly breaks down and forms a deep ulcer that spreads slowly. New ulcers may develop and cover the entire genital area, buttocks, and abdomen. Effective treatment can be given with antibiotic drugs. All persons with granuloma inguinale should be tested for syphilis, because the two diseases often occur together.

See also SEXUALLY TRANSMITTED DISEASE.

Graves' disease. *See* THYROTOXICOSIS.

Greenstick fracture. *See* FRACTURE, GREENSTICK.

Grief is a normal emotion of intense sorrow experienced in response to a significant loss, such as the death of a friend or relative. Signs of normal grief include lack of strength, sleep disturbance, tightness in the throat or chest, a preoccupation with the deceased, and withdrawal from social contact.

Q: *How may someone be helped during the initial stages of grief?*

A: There are many ways to help a grieving person; for example, giving practical help with the domestic chores or providing emotional support by listening to the grieving person as he or she talks about the loss. The person may also be helped by talking to a clergyman. Encourage the person to take a rest during the day in order to maintain physical strength. A physician may prescribe sedatives to aid in sleeping or tranquilizers for times of acute stress, such as a funeral. The use of such drugs should be limited to a brief period of time—no more than a few days.

Q: *How may a grieving person be helped after the initial stages?*

A: The grieving person should be continually invited to participate in family and social events, even if the invitations are refused. Expert advice on any legal or financial problems may help to relieve the person's anxiety.

Despite the good will and efforts of family and friends, some people seem to cling morbidly to grief. This prolonged grief is sometimes a sign of underlying guilt, remorse, or anger, and the person may require counseling.

To resolve the grief process, an individual must accept the reality of the loss, experience the pain of grief, adjust to a life style without the deceased, and reinvest emotional energy elsewhere. Occasionally an individual will show little emotional reaction to the loss; then weeks, months, or even years later, someone or something will trigger a delayed grief reaction.

Grippe (grip) is another term for the contagious disease influenza.

See also INFLUENZA.

Gristle. *See* CARTILAGE.

Group therapy is a therapeutic technique based on discussions and interactions among a group of people who have similar problems. Group therapy has proven effective in the treatment of various problems, such as alcoholism and drug abuse.

For some individuals, group therapy can offer a more positive approach than individual counseling, as group members can provide both constructive feedback and a good support network for each other. Group therapy is usually less expensive than individual counseling.

Growth is normal development as a result of a variety of biological and social factors. Physical development, which is most pronounced during childhood and adolescence, can be disrupted by a variety of disorders. *See also* ADOLESCENCE; CHILD.

Sometimes a tumor is also referred to as a growth. *See also* TUMOR.

Guillain-Barré syndrome (gē yän′-bä rā′) is an inflammation of the nerves. Symptoms usually begin with symmetric weakness in the legs, progressing to paralysis of the muscles of the legs, arms, trunk, and occasionally, the face. The cause is unknown, but many patients have reported respiratory infections preceding the onset of Guillain-Barré syndrome. Treatment consists primarily of skilled nursing care in the early stages because of the potential risk of paralysis of the muscles for breathing. In some cases, patients require a respirator or other mechanical device to aid with breathing. Gradual return to health generally occurs after a few weeks or, in some cases, months.

Gullet (gul′it) is a common term for the esophagus.

See also ESOPHAGUS.

Gum, in medicine, is the dense, fibrous tissue that surrounds the necks of the teeth. The gums are covered by a mucous membrane. It is important to keep the gums healthy by massaging them when cleaning the teeth, and by keep-

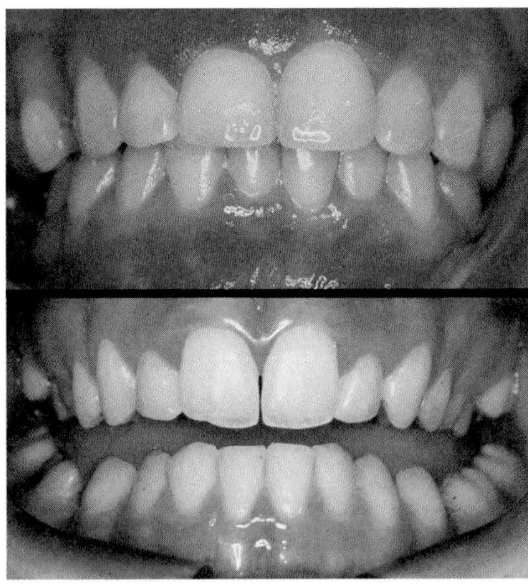

Red, swollen **gums,** *top,* are often a sign of gingivitis. Healthy gums, *bottom,* have a more pinkish color.

ing the teeth free of plaque, tartar, and food particles.

Fairly common gum disorders include canker sore, gingivitis, gumboil, periodontitis, and Vincent's infection. Spongy, ulcerated gums may be a symptom of diabetes mellitus, leukemia, tuberculosis, stomatitis, and digestive disorders. Gums that bleed easily usually indicate gingivitis, but such a condition may also be caused by scurvy or inflammatory illnesses, such as pyorrhea.

The color of the gums can be a useful diagnostic aid; a red line around the edge usually indicates gingivitis, pyorrhea, or scurvy.

See also TOOTH CARE.

Gumboil (gum′boil), known medically as a parulis, is a swelling of the gum. It is a type of abscess, usually caused by local infection at the root of a tooth. Other causes include irritation or injury to the gum, either from dentures or a toothbrush. The affected area of gum is typically red, swollen, extremely tender, and painful.

Q: ***How is a gumboil treated?***

A: Painkilling drugs and hot mouthwashes relieve some of the symptoms. A dentist may prescribe an antibiotic drug such as penicillin. The gumboil may burst of its own accord or it may have to be cut open.

See also TOOTHACHE: TREATMENT.

Gumboil: treatment. See TOOTHACHE: TREATMENT.

Gumma (gum′ə) is a soft tumor of the tissues, usually seen in the third stage of syphilis. A gumma may also occur as a reaction to yaws. Gummata occur alone or in groups and usually affect the liver. Sometimes the heart, brain, testes, bone, and skin are affected. On the skin, gummata may ulcerate. These ulcers are painless but heal slowly and may leave the skin badly scarred. Treatment with penicillin is usually effective.

See also SYPHILIS; YAWS.

Gun safety. *See* FIREARM SAFETY.

Gut is a popular term for the intestine.

See also INTESTINE.

Gymnasium. *See* EXERCISE.

Gynecological disorders. (gī nə kō läj′ i kəl). The following table lists, by the chief symptom, some of the disorders that affect the reproductive organs of women. It is important to remember that some of the symptoms are not necessarily abnormal; for example, vaginal discharge is heavier than normal at certain times during the menstrual cycle and before intercourse. Not all of the disorders listed below require medical attention, but if there is any doubt, a physician should be consulted.

See also BREAST DISORDERS; MENSTRUAL PROBLEMS; PREGNANCY AND CHILDBIRTH; SEXUAL PROBLEMS.

Symptom	*Related disorder*
Absence of, or missed period (Amenorrhea)	Adrenal glands or thyroid gland disorders
	Anemia
	Anorexia nervosa (psychological avoidance of eating)
	Cancer
	Cyst in an ovary
	Ectopic pregnancy (development of a fetus outside the uterus)
	Malnutrition
	Menopause (cessation of periods)
	Pregnancy and childbirth
	Tuberculosis
Aches and pains in abdomen or back	Cervical erosion (bacterial destruction of the wall of the cervix)
	Chronic cervicitis (inflammation of the cervix)
	Cyst (in an ovary)
	Endometritis (inflammation of the lining of the uterus)

Symptom	*Related disorder*
	Fibroid (benign muscle tumor in the uterus)
	Gonorrhea (early stages)
	Menstruation (normal)
	Miscarriage, threatened
	Ovulation (normal)
	Premenstrual syndrome
	Prolapse (displacement of the uterus)
	Sālpingitis (inflammation of a fallopian tube)
Bleeding after intercourse	Cervical erosion
	Chronic cervicitis (inflammation of the cervix)
Difficult or painful intercourse (Dyspareunia)	Bartholin's cyst (cyst in a gland in the vagina)
	Endometriosis (displacement of tissue from the lining of the uterus)
	Fissure, anal
	Frigidity (psychological aversion to sexual intercourse)
	Hemorrhoid (piles)
	Hymen, thick or tough (membrane across the vagina)
	Obesity, extreme
	Prolapse (displacement of the uterus)
	Rectocele (hernia of the rectum)
	Salpingitis (inflammation of a fallopian tube)
	Vaginismus (spasm in the muscles of the vagina)
	Vaginitis, atrophic
	Vulvitis (inflammation of the vulva)
	Vulvovaginitis (inflammation of the vulva and the vagina)
Enlarged uterus	Cancer
	Fibroid (benign muscle tumor in the uterus)
	Pregnancy and childbirth
Genital itching or soreness	Allergy
	Anxiety
	Diabetes mellitus
	Leukoplakia (itchy white patches on the vulva)
	Lichen planus (itchy inflammation)
	Scabies (itchy skin disease caused by mites)
	Stress
	Vaginitis (inflammation of the vagina)
Headache, dizziness, moody spells	Menopause (cessation of menstruation)
	Premenstrual syndrome
Heavy or irregular bleeding	Cervical erosion
	Ectopic pregnancy (development of a fetus outside the uterus)
	Endometriosis (displacement of tissue from the lining of the uterus)
	Endometritis (inflammation of the lining of the uterus)
	Fibroid (benign muscle tumor in the uterus)
	Hepatitis (inflammation of the liver)
	Menopause
	Menorrhagia (heavy periods)
	Metrorrhagia (irregular periods)
	Pneumonia (inflammation of the lungs)
	Polyp (in the uterus)
	Salpingitis (inflammation of a fallopian tube)
	Tumor (in the uterus or ovary)
Hot flashes	Menopause (cessation of menstrual periods)
Infertility	Endometriosis (displacement of tissue from the lining of the uterus)
	Fibroid (benign muscle tumor in the uterus)
	Frigidity (psychological aversion to sexual intercourse)
	Gonorrhea (advanced)
	Hyperplasia, endometrial (abnormal overgrowth of endometrium of the uterus.)
	Salpingitis (inflammation of a fallopian tube)

Symptom	*Related disorder*
Ovarian problems	Amenorrhea (absence of periods)
	Cyst (in an ovary)
	Oophoritis (inflammation of an ovary)
	Tumor (in an ovary)
	Turner's syndrome (sex chromosome abnormality)
Painful period (Dysmenorrhea)	Endometriosis (displacement of tissue from the lining of the womb)
Postmenopausal bleeding	Cancer (of the uterus)
	Endometritis (inflammation of the lining of the uterus)
	Estrogen (drug therapy)
	Vaginitis (inflammation of the vagina)
Urinary problems (related)	Cystitis
	Urethritis, nonspecific (inflammation of the urethra)
	Stress incontinence (involuntary urination)
Vaginal discharge	Cervical erosion (bacterial destruction of the wall of the cervix)
	Cervicitis (inflammation of the cervix)
	Gonorrhea
	Polyp (in the cervix)
	Salpingitis (inflammation of a fallopian tube)
Vaginal discharge, with inflamed vulva	Endometritis (inflammation of the lining of the uterus)
	Tumor
	Vaginitis, including Trichomonas vaginalis infection and vaginal mycosis
	Vulvitis

Gynecology (gī nə käl'ə jē) is the branch of medicine that specializes in diseases of women, particularly of the reproductive organs.

Gynecomastia (gī nə kä mas'ti ə) is the appearance of an enlarged breast or breasts in a boy or man. In men of 50 years or older, only one breast is generally affected; in children and young men, both breasts are affected. At puberty, sensitivity to female hormones produces gynecomastia in about 30 percent of boys. These hormones are produced normally by the adrenal glands before the major development of the testes. Apart from the embarrassment that the condition may cause, there is no medical need to worry and no need for treatment in younger males. Gynecomastia at this age generally disappears naturally after 6 to 12 months when the proper hormonal balance is established.

In older men, gynecomastia may have a number of causes. Treatment with estrogens or steroids can cause the symptoms, as can an estrogen imbalance brought on by cirrhosis of the liver. Rarely, it may be due to a tumor of the pituitary gland or the testis or a hormone-secreting tumor in another organ. A biopsy may be taken by a physician to rule out breast cancer.

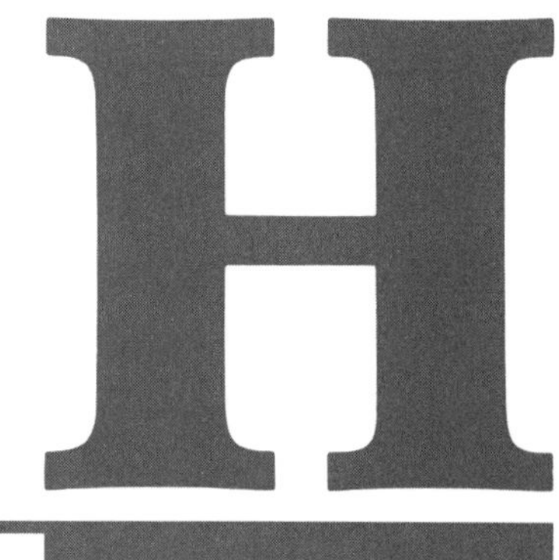

Habit spasm. *See* TIC.

Hair is a fine, thread-like structure that grows from the skin. It consists of cells of a tough protein called keratin, which grows in the hair follicle, a small pit in the outer layer of the skin (epidermis). A hair follicle produces and nourishes a hair. The root of the hair (hair bulb) is embedded at the base of the follicle, and it is here that growth takes place. The greasy secretions of a sebaceous gland at the side of the follicle drain into the follicle and lubricate the hair shaft, which can be raised by muscle attached to the follicle. Each hair has a definite period of growth, after which it is shed, and the follicle begins pushing up a new hair. The lifespan of a hair varies according to where on the body it is situated. For example, eyebrow hairs last from three to five months, and hairs on the head last from two to five years.

There are three concentric layers of cells in a hair, and color is formed in the middle layer. Hair color is produced at the base of the follicle by special cells, which inject colored pigments into each cell. Color is a hereditary factor. Dark hair color usually dominates over light hair color. For example, if a child has one parent with black or brown hair and one parent with red or blonde hair, the child's hair is likely to be dark-colored.

Q: *What is the function of hair?*

A: Among humans, hair has both a cosmetic and protective function. Hair around the eyes, ears, and nose serves to prevent dust, insects, and other matter from entering these organs. In addition, the eyebrows decrease the amount of light reflected into the eyes.

Q: *Why does hair fall out?*

A: All body hair falls out gradually and is replaced by new hair. The follicle does not die when a hair falls out; it goes into a resting period before producing a new hair. Baldness results when hair replacement fails to keep up with hair loss. Abnormal hair loss may be caused by folliculitis or some other disorder. *See also* FOLLICULITIS.

Q: *What factors affect the growth and condition of hair?*

A: Hair growth is dependent on hormones, particularly the sex hormones. A woman's hair, for example, has a tendency to become greasier just before menstruation, because hormones then stimulate more sebaceous gland secretions. Hormonal changes during pregnancy delay the resting phase of hair growth. A decreased thyroid gland or pituitary gland function makes hair become thin, dry, and brittle.

See also ALOPECIA; BALDNESS; HAIR CARE.

Hair care. Healthy hair results from regular brushing and shampooing and a well-balanced diet. Brushing removes dirt, dust, and tangles and spreads the natural oil of the scalp through the hair. Normal hair should be shampooed about once or twice a week, but oily hair may need to be washed more often.

Routine Hair Care. You should brush the hair daily to remove dirt and dead hair follicles. Do not brush too vigorously, because you may uproot hairs and leave small ridges on the scalp that are vulnerable to infection. The best type of brush to use is made from natural bristle. The best type of comb is one that is saw-cut. Clean the brush and comb every time you wash your hair.

Hair can be washed twice a week without disturbing the natural balance of the oils. Greasy hair may need more frequent washing. After shampooing, a vigorous massage of the scalp stimu-

Hair care

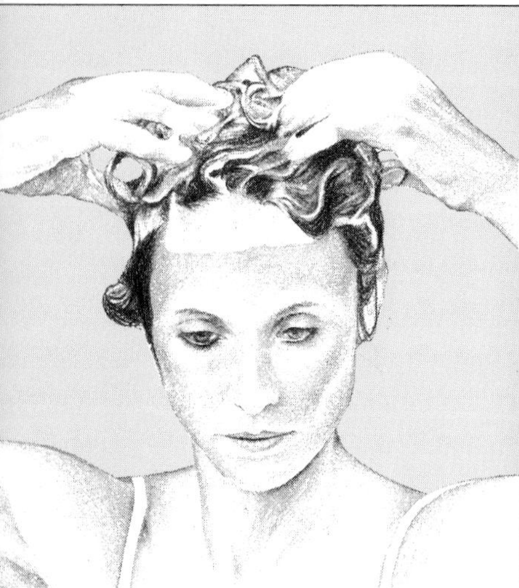

1 Massage shampoo into the hair and scalp with your fingertips. Use one or two applications of shampoo and carefully rinse the hair with clear water after each application to make sure that all of the lather is removed.

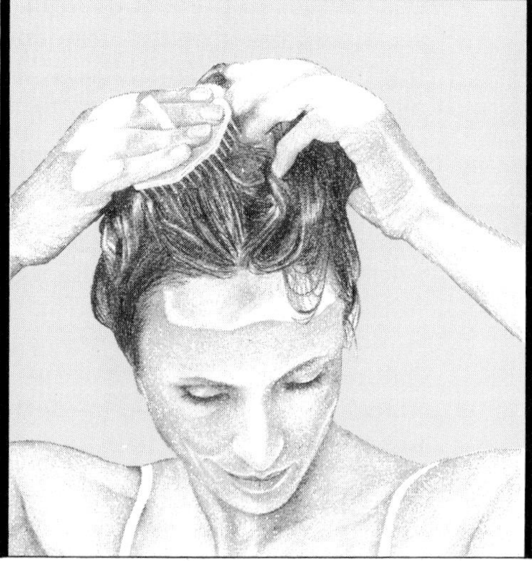

2 Washing removes not only grease and dirt from the hair but also the natural oils. A special, soft plastic massager may be used to massage hair that is naturally dry. Conditioners, which coat the hair with a layer of wax, can be used after shampooing to counteract dryness.

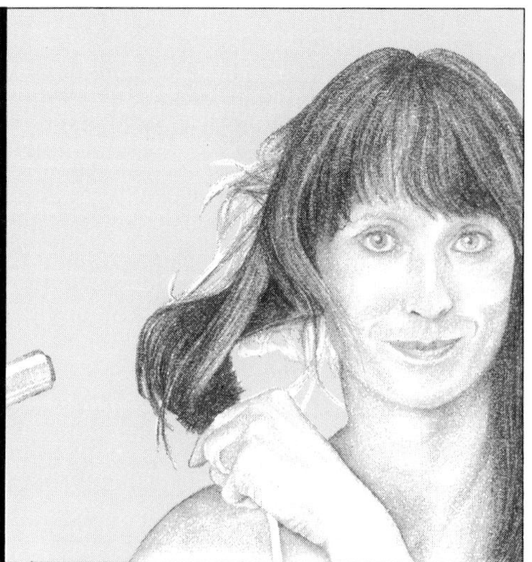

3 Dry your hair by gently rubbing it with a soft towel. Hard rubbing with a rough towel may split the ends of the hairs. Drying can also be done with an electric hair dryer. Do not hold the dryer too close to the head because you may burn the hair or even the skin of the scalp.

lates the local circulation and frees small particles that may be adhering to the skin. The hair should be rinsed thoroughly in clean water and should be brushed gently as it dries.

The basis of all shampoos is a soluble grease-removing agent. Other constituents include scents, colorants, and chemicals to make the shampoo thicker. These additional components may irritate the scalp. Commercial shampoos that claim to cure dandruff or seborrhea are unlikely to be better than standard varieties. However, shampoos that contain selenium compounds may help these conditions. But prolonged use of such shampoos may be unhealthy.

Cosmetic Hair Preparations. Many commercial hair treatments, particularly hair dyes, can produce an acute allergy or contact dermatitis. For this reason, hair dyeing should be carried out only by a trained beautician. A person who is susceptible to allergy should ask for a patch test before any new dye is used on the scalp.

You should not attempt bleaching with hydrogen peroxide, dye stripping, or permanent waving at home. These methods can seriously damage the hair. Continual dyeing and bleaching tends to make the hair brittle. Regular use of other preparations, such as hair oils and hair sprays, may encourage dandruff. *See also* DANDRUFF.

Hair Disorders. Alopecia (baldness), caused by changes in a person's hormones, occurs naturally in some people and, thus, can not be prevented. The condition is more common in men, and the pattern of hair loss tends to be inherited. Partial hair loss may affect women after menopause. Sometimes, hair loss occurs after a severe emotional shock, a severe illness, or childbirth. Occasionally, the body reacts against the hair substance. Sudden alopecia may occur for no apparent reason. *See also* ALOPECIA; BALDNESS.

In some cases, a hair transplant may disguise baldness. Nonproductive hair follicles are replaced with productive follicles from another area of the scalp. This procedure is expensive and the results vary. It does not arrest hair loss, which may continue behind the patch of transplanted hair.

Barber's rash is a chronic infection of the hair follicles by staphylococcus bacteria. Small, recurrent boils appear around each hair on the shaved area. It is most common in men, but women who shave axillary hair can also suffer from the condition. A person with barber's rash can either stop shaving or sterilize all shaving equipment after use. A mild antiseptic applied to the area after shaving may also help.

Hirsutism is an abnormal growth of hair. It is more common in women than men and among some ethnic groups more than others. It is usually caused by an inherited predisposition or by hormonal changes in the body. Sudden abnormal hair growth might be a sign of a gland disorder and therefore should receive medical attention. *See also* HIRSUTISM.

Surrounding Skin Disorders. Ringworm (tinea capitis) is a fungal infection of the scalp. It produces bald patches on the head that are covered with scaling skin and stumps of hair. Ringworm must be treated swiftly by a physician, because it is highly infectious. Anyone contracting ringworm must use a separate brush and comb, which should be sterilized daily.

Seborrhea is overactivity of the sebaceous glands of the skin. If this occurs on the scalp, the hair becomes greasy soon after it has been washed. The activity of the glands can not be altered. The hair should be washed daily. Selenium-based shampoos may also help.

A person with suspected head lice must see a physician. Towels, brushes, and combs must be sterilized after use and must not be used by others.

The crab louse infests the pubic hair, eyelashes, and eyebrows. It may be transmitted during sexual intercourse or picked up from bedclothes or towels.

Both varieties of lice should be treated swiftly, because lice can transmit relapsing fever and typhus or cause crusting, oozing skin similar to impetigo.

See also LICE; PEDICULOSIS PUBIS; RINGWORM; SEBORRHEA.

Hair, excess. See HIRSUTISM.

Hair loss. See ALOPECIA.

Hair pulling, or trichotillomania, is the abnormal desire to pull out one's own hair. The condition is usually associated with the mentally retarded or with young children.

Hair pulling may be caused by a variety of conditions, including anxiety, depression, and family stress. The child often receives much attention for hair pulling, which, in turn, strengthens the urge to engage in the act. In some children, hair pulling can become a very strong, compulsive habit. Therapy can include behavior modification and family or individual counseling. Recently, the use of clomipramine, a medication prescribed for obsessive compulsive disorders, has been found useful for trichotillomania. Until the underlying causes for the condition are cleared up, the only solution is to keep the hair too short for pulling.

Hairwashing. See HAIR CARE; NURSING THE SICK.

Halitosis. See BAD BREATH.

Hallucination (hə lü sə nā'shən) is a false or imagined sensory phenomenon that is not caused by external stimuli. In an hallucination, a person may see, hear, feel, taste, or smell something that is not there.

Q: *What causes hallucinations?*

A: Hallucinations may occur as a result of fatigue, particularly if it is accompanied by dehydration and illness that produces a high fever, especially in children. Many drugs produce hallucinations, including sedatives used after a surgical operation. In drug addiction and alcoholism, the hallucinations may be aggravated by a lack of vitamin B; they are also quite common during physical withdrawal from alcohol. In some severe forms of mental illness, such as schizophrenia, hallucinations become an integral part of the condition.

See also HALLUCINOGEN.

Hallucinogen (hə lü'sə nə jen), or hallucinogenic drug, is one of several substances that distort a person's perception of self and surroundings. These drugs temporarily change the functioning of the brain. They affect the senses, emotions, reasoning, and the brain's control of muscles and certain body functions.

Hallucinogenic drugs are sometimes called psychedelic (mind expanding) drugs. The most powerful of these is LSD. This drug and two others, STP and DMT, are chemically synthesized.

Other hallucinogenic drugs come from plants, for example, peyote and mescaline. In the United States, laws prohibit the manufacture, distribution, and possession of these drugs, except for government-approved research.

The effects of hallucinogenic drugs are sometimes called "trips." The users may hallucinate during a trip and see objects, distorted in size and shape, which change constantly. The person may step out of a window not realizing the danger of being hurt or even killed. Some hallucinogen users can have a vivid recall of past events, experience overwhelming fear, success, sadness, or horror, or feel intense love or joy. Some drug users claim that, during a trip, they have gained a new understanding of God, the universe, and themselves.

A common adverse reaction to these drugs consists of an acute panic or paranoid reaction, sometimes referred to as a "bad trip." This occurs when, due to the effects of the drug and the drug-induced hallucinations, the user feels threatened by his surroundings. When this happens, it is advisable to isolate the user in a darkened, quiet room while someone talks to him or her in a calm, reassuring manner. This process is commonly referred to as "talking someone down." Medical care should be sought for the user while this is being done.

The effects of hallucinogens may last from one hour to several days. It is believed that these effects may reappear several months later as flashbacks, but there is no conclusive evidence to prove this. The experience and its effects vary greatly from user to user and from one experience to another, and are influenced by the amount and type of drug taken, the circumstances in which the drug is used, and the user's personality and mood at time of use. Hallucinogens are not addictive, but some scientists believe they cause birth defects.

See also LYSERGIC ACID DIETHYLAMIDE; MESCALINE.

Hallux rigidus (hal'əks rij'i dəs) is stiffness and pain in the first joint of the big toe. The condition is usually caused by arthritis of the first joint and may, in turn, cause deformity in the gait, the step, or the toe itself. Occasionally, it may be caused by repeated injury to the joint.

See also HALLUX VALGUS.

Hallux valgus (hal'əks val'gəs) is a deformity of the big toe, usually caused by tight-fitting shoes. The toe is angled toward the other toes, with the toe joint becoming inflamed, forming a bunion. Osteoarthritis may also develop, causing hallux rigidus. The usual treatment is to have the big toe straightened, with the arthritic bone and bunion surgically removed.

See also HALLUX RIGIDUS.

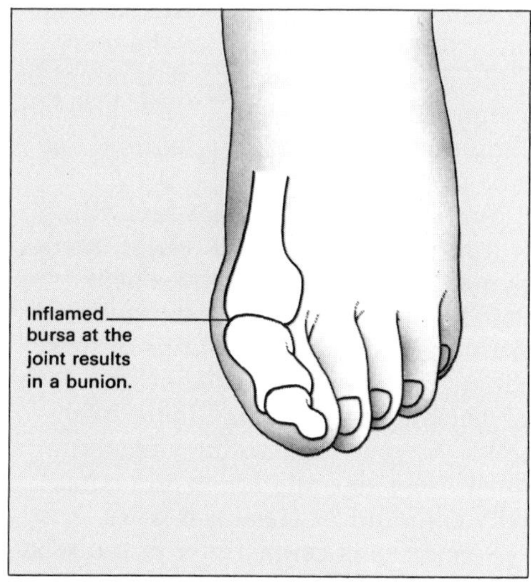
Inflamed bursa at the joint results in a bunion.

Hallux valgus is a misshapen big toe that is often caused by poorly-fitting shoes. This distorts the position of the toes.

Hammer. *See* MALLEUS.

Hammertoe (ham'ər tō) is a toe deformity in which the first and second joints of the toe are bent downward at a right angle, creating a claw-like appearance. Hammertoe occurs most frequently in the second toe and is most often caused by wearing shoes that are too small and narrow.

When the problem is mild, this condition is treated by having the patient wear pads around or underneath the toe. In more severe cases, surgery is the preferred treatment.

Hamstring (ham'string) is one of several tendons that connect the muscles at the back of the thigh to the lower leg. The term also refers to the muscles at the back of the thigh.

Hand is the end part of the arm; the hand's function is to grasp objects. Five long metacarpal bones form the palm of the hand. These bones connect the wrist (carpus) with the fingers and the thumb. The long bones are jointed to smaller bones at the base of each finger and the thumb. There are three separate bones (phalanges) in each of the four fingers and two in the thumb. The fingertips are extremely sensitive to pain, temperature, and touch and are protected by the nails. *See also* NAIL.

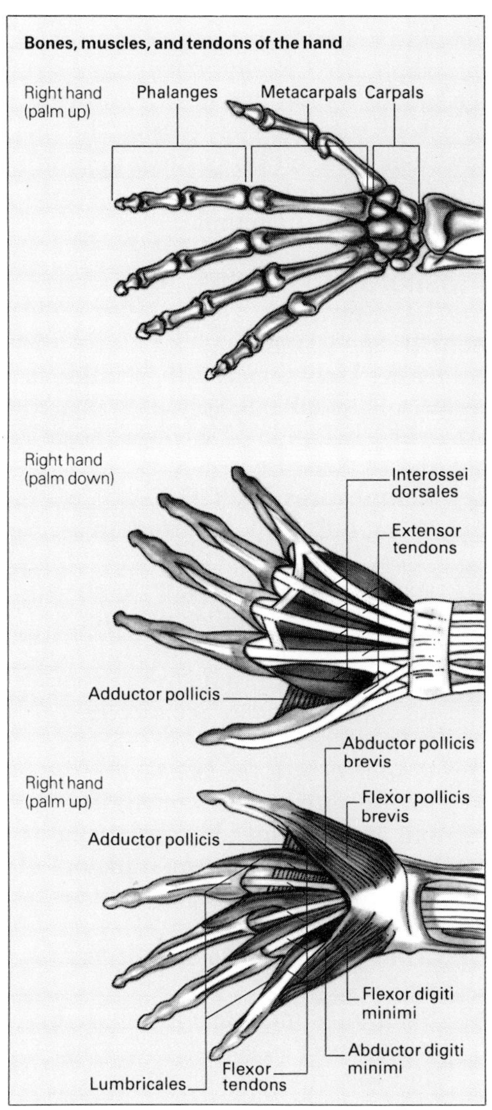

The **hand** consists of 27 bones (including those in the carpus, or wrist) and a complex network of tendons and muscles.

Q: *How does the hand move?*

A: The main muscles that control hand movements are in the forearm, connected to the fingers by long, strong tendons. When the muscles on the back of the forearm contract, the fingers open. To prevent friction, the tendons are enclosed in synovial (lubricated) sheaths. Twenty muscles within the hand allow the hand and fingers to make a variety of precise movements.

Hand care. The hand is a mechanically complex and highly sensitive structure containing 27 bones and a network of tendons and muscles. Misuse can easily damage the hand.

Injury. Injury accounts for the majority of hand problems. But many forms of damage can be avoided, and adequate care can lessen the possibility or effect of injury.

A form of inflammation of the tendon sheath (de Quervain's disease) is caused by continual overuse of the thumb in occupations that involve a pincer movement of the hand, for example, haircutting. The person experiences pain in the thumb. Minor surgery is usually necessary to relieve the condition, but it may be avoided if a person heeds the warning signs of discomfort and stiffness in the thumb and wrist after a day's work. The thumb should be rested for several days, and work resumed slowly during the following months.

The thick skin that covers the palm helps to prevent minor cuts and abrasions and usually heals quickly and cleanly. However, a puncture wound may introduce infection into the deeper tissues of the hand. Any deep puncture wound of the hand should be seen by a physician.

General Care. A routine for washing the hands is of extreme importance, not merely as a matter of normal cleanliness or social acceptability, but also as a protective measure. Failure to keep the hands clean can lead to impairment of the sense of touch. A surface coating of dirt or of chemicals, not properly washed from the hands, can have serious consequences.

Most parents teach their children to wash their hands before meals and after using the bathroom. Few parents, however, are equally careful to teach exactly how the hands should be properly washed.

To rinse, soap, and rinse again is not enough. Attention should be paid also to cleaning the finger tips, between the fingers, the backs of the hands, and the top of the wrist. Dirt under the nails must be removed with an instrument designed for the purpose, as soon as may be convenient, and certainly before the next meal. *See also* NAIL CARE.

Rings should be removed for any manual work, including housework. If the ring catches on a projection, it can strip the flesh off the finger or, in very severe cases, amputate the finger.

During the last three months of pregnancy, the hands swell slightly, and a ring can become too tight. A tight ring constricts the blood flow out of, but not into the finger, resulting in sudden swelling. Once this occurs, the finger needs emergency medical attention, and the ring must be cut off. *See also* FINGER, RING STUCK ON: TREATMENT.

Tenosynovitis is inflammation of the sheath surrounding a tendon. Normally, each tendon moves easily within the tendon sheath. Overuse can inflame the tendon and cause grating and pain. The condition can become so serious that the patient can hear the tendon grating. This is known as tenosynovitis crepitans. A physician should be consulted at the first sign of pain.

Trigger finger is another type of mechanical disorder of a tendon. A lump develops on the tendon of a finger through overuse. The patient wakes with a flexed and painful finger, which straightens with an audible and visible snap. Surgery is the primary treatment for the condition.

Hand-foot-and-mouth disease is a virus infection that occurs in young children, sometimes as a minor epidemic. Small blisters or a rash appear on the palms of the hands, the soles of the feet, and on the gums. It is a mild condition that lasts for about three or four days before recovery occurs naturally. It is totally unrelated to hoof-and-mouth disease seen in animals.

Hand fracture: first aid. *See* FRACTURE: FIRST AID.

Hangnail is a partly detached piece of dry skin at the base of a fingernail. Treatment involves clipping the hangnail as close to the skin as possible.

Hangover is the informal name for a collection of symptoms caused by drinking an excessive amount of alcohol. Since alcohol is a diuretic, the person suffering from a hangover is somewhat dehydrated. This causes the symptoms of headache, muscle cramps, thirst, dizziness, and fatigue. Withdrawal from alcohol causes the symptoms of nausea, vomiting, and nervousness. The effects of alcohol on the stomach lining can also cause nausea, vomiting, and abdominal pain.

See also ALCOHOL ABUSE.

Hansen's disease. *See* LEPROSY.

Hardening of the arteries. *See* ARTERIOSCLEROSIS.

Harelip (hăr′lip), or cleft lip, is a congenital split in the front of the upper lip. The cleft may vary in size from a notch to a fissure that extends across the whole lip. Usually, it extends from the mouth up into the nostril and may be associated with cleft palate. The treatment for cleft lip is surgery, usually when the infant is about 10 weeks old or weighs 10 pounds.

See also CLEFT PALATE.

Hashimoto's thyroiditis. *See* THYROIDITIS, HASHIMOTO'S.

Hashish. *See* MARIJUANA.

Hay fever, known medically as allergic rhinitis, is an allergic condition characterized by irritation of the eyes, nose, and throat. *See also* ALLERGY.

Q: *What causes hay fever?*

A: When dust or pollen from trees, grass, flowers, weeds, mushroom spores, and animal hair is inhaled, some people's bodies produce an excessive amount of histamine, a chemical that produces the symptoms of hay fever. *See also* HISTAMINE.

Q: *Who is at risk for hay fever?*

A: Hay fever is most common in people with a family history of similar complaints or a personal history of eczema, hives (urticaria) and/or asthma.

Q: *What are the symptoms of hay fever?*

A: Symptoms include a runny, itchy, stuffy nose; sneezing; and itchy and watery eyes. Patients may complain of ear fullness, sinus congestion, and a cough due to postnasal drip.

Q: *How is hay fever treated?*

A: The ideal treatment is avoidance of the allergen. However, since this is not always possible, a variety of antihistamines, decongestants, and intranasal steroids may be prescribed. Topical decongestants are effective, but should not be used for longer than three days to avoid rebound swelling and rhinitis. Immunologic therapy, or hyposensitization, is useful in individuals who do not respond to the above treatments. They are given small, gradually increasing inoculations of extracts of the allergen to which they are sensitive. These injections are given weekly, usually for one year with maintenance therapy injections every 2 to 4 weeks for 3 to 5 years. About 80 percent of patients benefit from hyposensitization.

Head has three medically related definitions: the top part of the body, including the face and scalp, which contains the brain and the organs for seeing, hearing, tasting, and smelling; the end of a bone at the point of attachment or origin; the larger extremity of a body or organ.

See also BRAIN.

Headache (hed'āk) is a pain or ache across the forehead or within the head itself. It is not a disorder but a symptom. Possible causes of headaches include conditions associated with emotional disturbances or muscular tension; disorders of the blood vessels of the brain; neuralgia, caused by disorders of nerves in the head; conditions, especially infections, affecting the ears, sinuses, mouth, or the membrane that surrounds the brain; head injuries; conditions that affect the skull; and increased pressure within the brain.

Q: ***What are the most common causes of headache?***

A: One of the chief causes of a headache is tension in the muscles of the neck and jaw.

Another common cause is migraine, in which the headache often occurs in only one-half of the head (hemicrania) and may be accompanied by nausea and vomiting. *See also* MIGRAINE.

Any generalized infection, such as influenza, may affect the blood vessels and cause a headache. Blood vessels of the brain may also be affected by external factors, such as drinking too much alcohol, smoking excessively, or inhaling or swallowing various chemicals or drugs.

Ear disorders involving inflammation, such as otitis and mastoiditis, may cause moderately severe headaches on the side of the head that is affected. Eye disorders, such as iritis, glaucoma, and eye strain, may produce frontal headaches, as well as pain around the eye. Sinusitis, particularly of the frontal sinuses above the eyes, may cause a severe ache at the front of the head, usually associated with a respiratory disorder, such as a cold or hay fever. A toothache may cause headaches as well as local pain.

A head injury often causes concussion and a generalized headache of variable intensity that seems to get worse during periods of fatigue or emotional stress. It may be accompanied by dizziness, difficulty in sleeping, and loss of concentration. The injured area may also be painful and tender.

Any head injury is potentially serious, especially if there is a history of concussion. A physician should be consulted so that the skull can be X-rayed and other tests performed.

Q: ***How may the common forms of headache be treated?***

A: Aspirin or preparations containing aspirin and acetaminophen are usually effective in removing the pain of a normal headache. If a headache persists more than a day, is extremely severe, or is associated with any neurological changes, such as localized weakness, loss of sensation, or altered vision, a doctor should be consulted immediately.

See also HEADACHE, CLUSTER.

Headache, cluster (hed'āk, klus'tər). A cluster headache is a recurrent headache associated with an increase of histamine in the body. Some of the symptoms include tearing, runny nose, dilation of the carotid arteries, which carry blood through the neck to the brain, and sudden, acute pain on one side of the head from the neck to the temple. Antihistamines provide effective relief.

Head injury is damage to the scalp, skull, or brain. It is one of the most potentially serious types of injury, be-

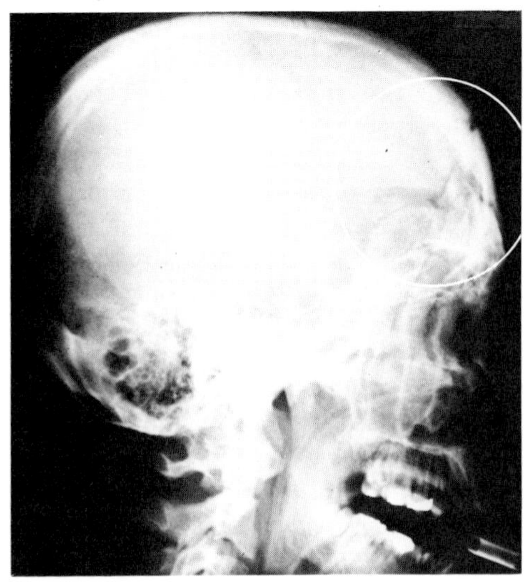

A **head injury,** such as a depressed fracture of the skull, can impair the functioning of the brain.

cause it threatens the highly complex structure and functioning of the brain.

Q: *What are the various types of skull fractures?*

A: The least serious type is a hairline fracture, in which the skull cracks, but the bone does not change position. If a fracture causes the bone to move, the displaced bone may press onto the tissue of the brain. This type of fracture, called a depressed fracture, often causes brain damage.

Q: *What is a brain concussion?*

A: Concussion is a severe jolting of the brain that causes microscopic damage to brain cells and a temporary neurological disorder. The most common disorder is a loss of consciousness. Other temporary disorders may include problems involving memory, vision, balance, muscular weakness, or paralysis. Recovery is generally complete. Companion symptoms may include headache, difficulty in concentrating, and irritability or depression.

Q: *What is a brain contusion?*

A: Contusion of the brain is bruising that damages the nerve centers in the brain.

Q: *How are head injuries treated?*

A: Although there is little that can be done to repair brain tissue already damaged, there is much that can be done to prevent further harm. Hairline fractures usually heal without complications, and an operation is seldom necessary. A depressed fracture or any type of brain hemorrhage often requires an emergency operation. Blood clots are normally removed as soon as possible, bringing about a rapid improvement.

For all head injuries that do not require surgery, rest is the best treatment. It may take weeks or months before the last symptoms of concussion disappear.

Q: *Are there any long-term aftereffects of head injuries?*

A: Yes, the brain may become infected as a result of a skull fracture. Meningitis is the most serious form of infection, but it can be treated successfully with antibiotics.

A late complication of a head injury may be a blood clot that increases in size and is discovered only several weeks after the initial injury. Brain functions tend to deteriorate until the blood clot is removed. Epilepsy can also occur as an aftereffect of a head injury, even as long as two years after the injury. In a few patients, brain damage is so severe following a head injury that they do not regain consciousness. In many of these cases, life-support systems are used to keep a patient alive, although recovery is rare. *See also* HEMATOMA, SUBDURAL.

Permanent brain damage can cause a variety of irreversible physical or mental disorders, such as weakness of the limbs (paresis), deafness, blindness, double vision, and speech-related disorders, such as aphasia. Possible mental aftereffects include personality changes and mental impairment. Repeated minor injuries to the head can cause symptoms of disturbed coordination, memory, and concentration and may also affect vision and hearing.

See also HEAD INJURY: FIRST AID.

Head injury: first aid. Head injuries are potentially dangerous because brain damage may result. Indications of brain damage include unconsciousness, headache, convulsions, drowsiness, vomiting for no apparent reason, and loss of memory of the injury. There may be unequal pupil size and paralysis.

Head injury: first aid

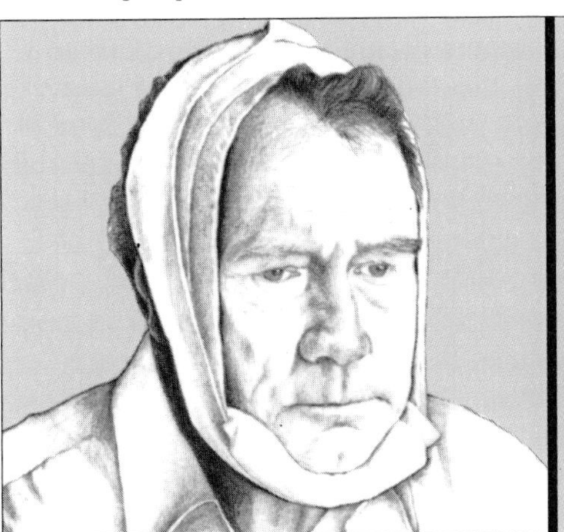

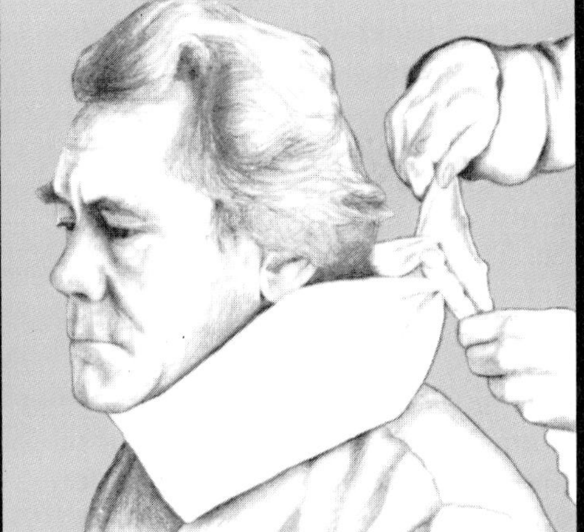

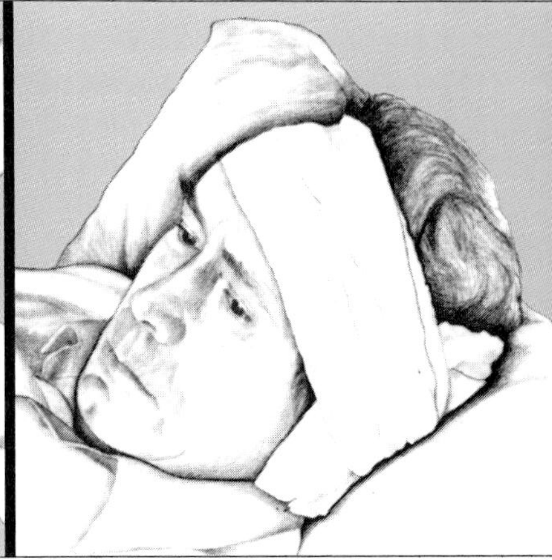

1 Jaw fracture: If unconscious, place the victim in the recovery position and ensure there is a clear air passage. For instructions, *see* FAINTING: FIRST AID. Remove any dentures and carefully support the jaw using a pad secured with a bandage. If conscious, place the victim in a sitting position with the head well forward. Remove any dentures and maintain a clear airway. Support the jaw as described above.

2 Neck injury: *Do not* move a victim with a suspected neck fracture. Proper treatment is discussed under FRACTURE: FIRST AID. If it is certain that the neck is not fractured, the neck should be supported with a collar. A collar can be made from a folded towel or newspaper. Cover this with a bandage, place it around the victim's neck, and tie the ends.

3 Ear injury: *Do not* put anything into the ear canal. Treat bleeding from a wound by pressure over the wound. Place a clean dressing over the ear and secure it with a broad bandage. Lay the victim down on his or her back with head and shoulders raised and the head inclined toward the injured side.

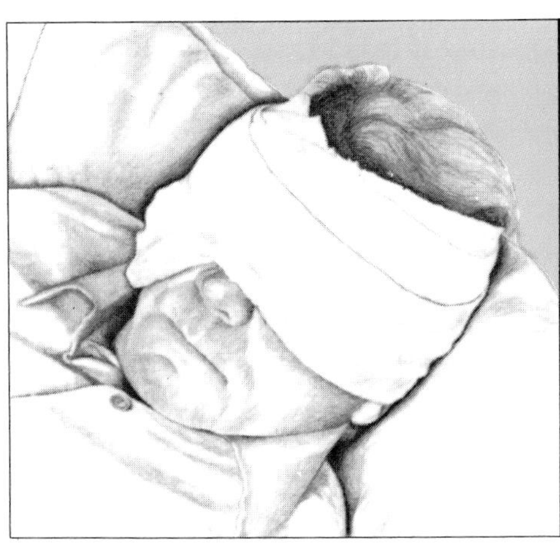

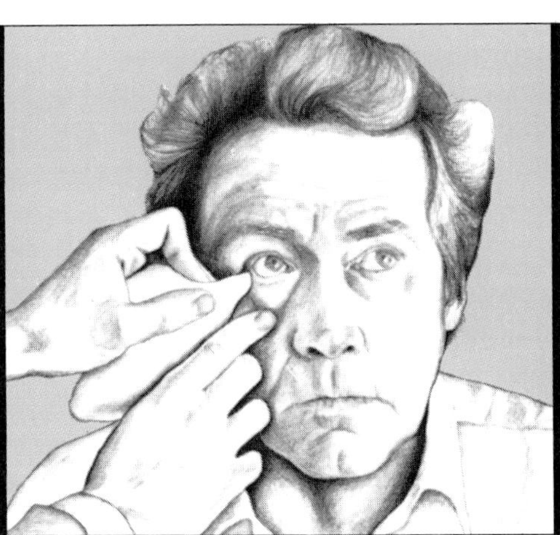

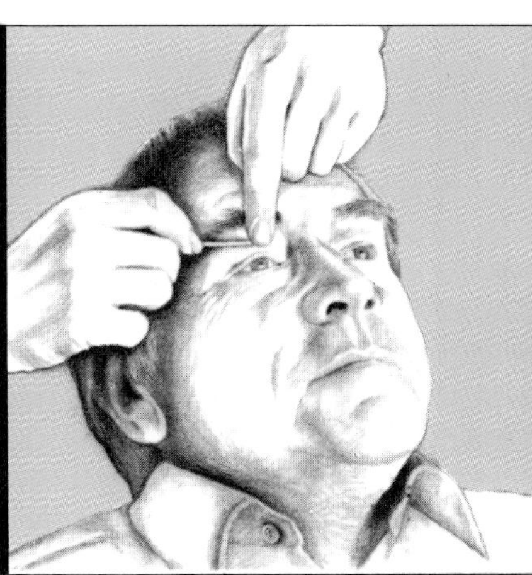

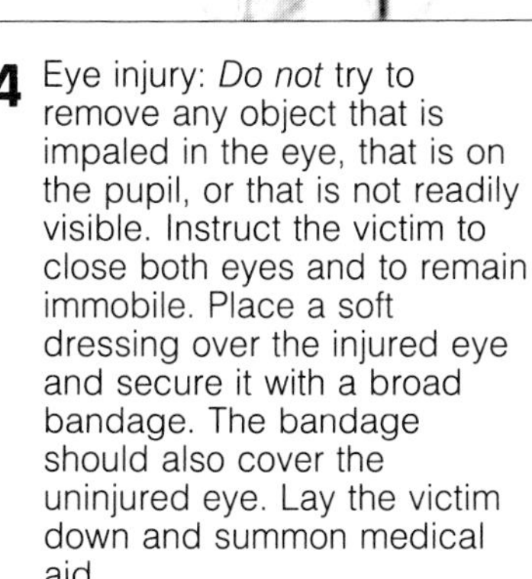

4 Eye injury: *Do not* try to remove any object that is impaled in the eye, that is on the pupil, or that is not readily visible. Instruct the victim to close both eyes and to remain immobile. Place a soft dressing over the injured eye and secure it with a broad bandage. The bandage should also cover the uninjured eye. Lay the victim down and summon medical aid.

5 If there are loose fragments in the eye, they should be removed. If the fragments are visible, place the victim in a sitting position facing a light. Pull down the bottom eyelid with a forefinger. Instruct the victim to look upward and remove the fragments with the corner of a clean handkerchief.

6 If there is a fragment under the upper lid, instruct the victim to tilt the head back. Stand behind the victim; steady your hand. Place a matchstick at the base of the upper lid and press gently backwards. Grasp the lashes and turn the lid over the matchstick. Remove the fragment with a clean handkerchief.

Bleeding from the ear without any obvious cause may indicate a fractured skull. Blood trickling from the nose together with other head injuries may indicate a fractured skull and should be treated as such. If the victim has a fractured or dislocated jaw, there will be difficulty in talking and increased salivation. The teeth may seem to be out of alignment. *Do not* try and set a dislocated jaw. Even if you attempt first-aid steps, summon emergency medical assistance as soon as possible.

Action. If the victim has stopped breathing, give artificial respiration to restore breathing. For instructions, *see* ARTIFICIAL RESPIRATION. If facial injuries are severe, utilize the mouth-to-nose method. If there is a suspected fracture of the neck or spine, *do not* move the victim. Proper treatment is discussed under FRACTURE: FIRST AID. If the victim is unconscious, place in the recovery position, as described in FAINTING: FIRST AID. The position may have to be modified, so that the wound is not in contact with the ground. Further first-aid instruction is listed under UNCONSCIOUSNESS: TREATMENT.

Treat any serious bleeding with ice, elevation, and direct pressure. Do not press too heavily if the bleeding is over a fracture site. For instruction, *see* BLEEDING: FIRST AID. Do not give the victim food or drink, in case a general anesthetic is needed later. *Do not* remove impaled objects from a wound; stabilize the objects and protect them from further movement. *Do not* try to remove objects from the ear. A broken nose will be swollen and painful. Tell the victim to breathe through the mouth and apply ice. *See also* NOSEBLEED: TREATMENT.

Health and environment. *See* ENVIRONMENT AND HEALTH.

Health insurance. *See* MEDICAL EXPENSES AND INSURANCE.

Health Maintenance Organization, or HMO, is a medical group that provides prepaid medical services. Members are charged a yearly fee and receive a full range of medical services, from checkups to hospitalization, at little or no additional expense.

There are two main types of HMO's. The most common type, a prepaid group practice, employs a group of physicians, including such specialists as internists, pediatricians, obstetricians, and gynecologists. In most of these groups, the physicians have offices in the same medical center and do not have separate private practices. Such groups as consumer organizations, insurance companies, and medical groups may organize this type of HMO. The other main type of HMO is organized by physicians who prefer to maintain their own private office and individual practice. Many of these HMO's are sponsored by county medical societies.

Although the first HMO's were set up during the 1930's, they grew slowly until the 1970's, when the United States government, insurance companies, and other organizations provided financial assistance to encourage their growth. Today, more than 400 HMO's serve almost 20 million people in the United States.

Health tests, routine. A person's main need for a physician occurs when symptoms of some disorder become apparent. Many disorders, however, do not produce obvious symptoms until the disease is well advanced. This type of disease can usually be effectively treated if it is identified at an early stage. Routine health screening tests are now a recognized and important part of preventive medicine. Many health tests can be carried out annually by your physician, but some can be carried out daily, weekly, or on a regular basis by you.

A general awareness of the normal working of your body is essential in order to recognize when it is not functioning well. A change in appetite or bowel or urinary habits, irregular menstruation, or sudden loss or gain of weight may indicate the beginning of some disorder. There are many things that you can do yourself to assess any change that may be occurring. You are more likely to notice minor alterations in bodily function than your physician, who may not see you regularly.

Physical Checkups. Many individuals decide to have a regular physical checkup by their own physician or to have one as part of the health program

Recommended weights for adults

Men

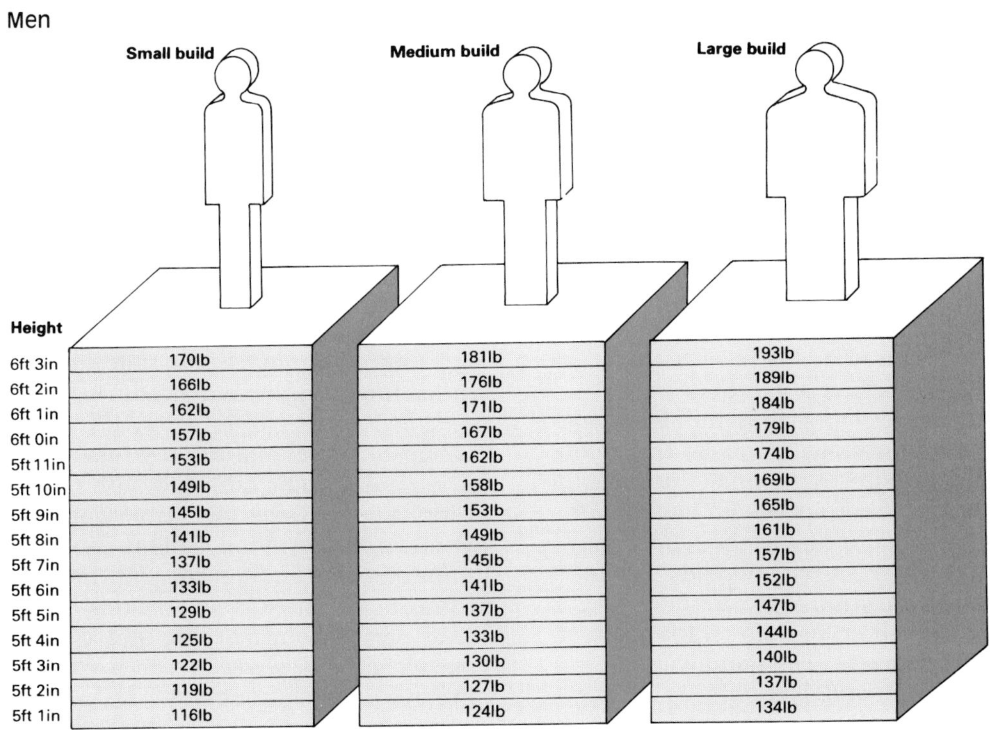

Small build
Medium build
Large build
Height
6ft 3in
6ft 2in
6ft 1in
6ft 0in
5ft 11in
5ft 10in
5ft 9in
5ft 8in
5ft 7in
5ft 6in
5ft 5in
5ft 4in
5ft 3in
5ft 2in
5ft 1in
170lb
166lb
162lb
157lb
153lb
149lb
145lb
141lb
137lb
133lb
129lb
125lb
122lb
119lb
116lb
181lb
176lb
171lb
167lb
162lb
158lb
153lb
149lb
145lb
141lb
137lb
133lb
130lb
127lb
124lb
193lb
189lb
184lb
179lb
174lb
169lb
165lb
161lb
157lb
152lb
147lb
144lb
140lb
137lb
134lb

Women

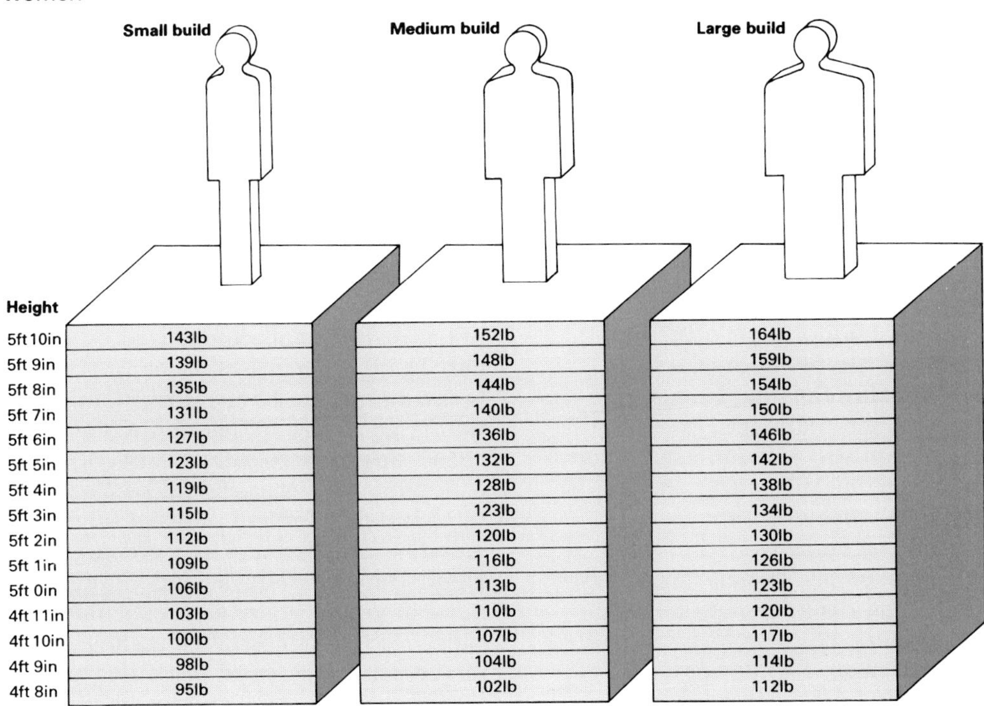

recommended by the employer. The tests are often carried out at health centers containing all the facilities and equipment needed for such assessments.

Although health care is important, it should not become a preoccupation and cause anxiety, when there is a slight disturbance in the body's normal function. This can lead to hypochondriasis, which in itself can be disabling.

One of the major problems with regular checkups is that a person may save up his or her complaints until the annual checkup. This is not recommended, because a month or two of some minor change may indicate something more serious. To avoid this, some companies now randomize the checkup so that their employees no longer look on it as a routine procedure. This may be done through the company's computer, to ensure that the randomizing does not call an individual too often or too infrequently. The employee receives a letter advising him or her to make an appointment within a short period of time.

Patients who have a particular problem, such as hypertension (high blood pressure), diabetes mellitus, or glaucoma, should have regular examinations to ensure that the condition is under control. Patients with hypertension can also be taught how to take their own blood pressure. Obesity is another problem that needs the regular attention of a physician.

Although diabetics were taught in the past to monitor their urine for sugar, today simple home devices, which measure the blood sugar directly, are more popular. However, diabetics should still learn to check their urine for ketone substances, such as acetone. *See also* KETONE.

Routine testing helps to ensure a healthy pregnancy, because many potentially fatal disorders, such as preeclampsia, can be identified and treated at an early stage. The development of the fetus can be monitored, and possible problems that may arise during labor can be detected, such as a breech birth. The obstetrician's examination includes blood pressure recording, urinalysis, and weight assessment during prenatal examinations. Usually, a pregnant woman is advised to see her obstetrician every six weeks during the first six months, each month for the next two months, and every two weeks during the final month.

Personal Health Tests. It is important to establish a daily routine of health care, including general cleanliness and care of the nails and teeth. In addition, check the margins of the gums every morning to make sure that they are pink and rise to points between each tooth. If they are rounded or slightly puffy (a possible early sign of gingivitis), you should improve your oral hygiene. Check your eyes in the mirror each morning to make sure that the whites look healthy and are not colored.

Monitor bowel and urinary habits, but do not become obsessed with regularity, because this differs from person to person. If bowel movements cause minor discomfort, increase your intake of roughage. For example, make a bran cereal part of your morning diet. Check your weight every week, even if you do not have a weight problem.

Each month a woman should examine her breasts for any unusual lumps or other changes. The examination should be carried out a few days after menstruation when the breasts are at their smallest. It is important to examine the breasts at the same time each month, because a woman's cycle produces natural changes in the breast tissue that may be confusing. A woman who detects a lump should see her physician immediately. It must be remembered, however, that the majority of breast lumps are not caused by cancer. There are many other reasons for breast lumps, and a medical examination is necessary to determine the cause. *See also* BREAST EXAMINATION.

In men, the testes should be examined monthly for any unusual lumps or growths. This is especially recommended for adolescents and young men, in whom the rate of testicular cancer is the highest. Although, as with the breast lumps, most testicular lumps will prove to be benign, they should still be brought to the attention of a physician.

Semiannual Tests. Every six months you should visit the dentist and the dental hygienist. The dentist checks the teeth and fillings and may also X-ray your teeth to detect signs of decay and to see if any uncut wisdom teeth are likely to cause problems when they erupt.

The dental hygienist clears away any tartar that may have built up around the gum margin. He or she also checks that you are cleaning your teeth correctly and not habitually missing an area at the back of the teeth. Some hygienists like to bathe the teeth in a fluoride solution for about 10 minutes. The hygienist also polishes any new fillings.

A visit to a podiatrist (foot specialist) may also be necessary periodically, especially for people susceptible to foot problems, such as diabetics. The podiatrist checks that your feet are free from infection, such as athlete's foot or plantar warts, and checks that the heels and toes are not being rubbed by badly fitting shoes. If there is a corn that is causing discomfort, the podiatrist may shave this away. It is important that you then change your footwear to prevent the corn from recurring.

Annual Tests. A yearly visit to the ophthalmologist enables him or her to test your eyes for early signs of vision deterioration. The ophthalmologist also tests the intraocular pressure of the eye with a tonometer. This detects early signs of glaucoma, a treatable disease that can cause permanent blindness if neglected. This test is particularly important after the age of 40.

During an annual checkup with your physician, he or she runs a full physical examination, including inspection of eyes, ears, nose, skin, glands, and reproductive organs. If appropriate, the physician also arranges for chest X rays and an electrocardiogram with or without exercise. The physician takes your weight, your blood pressure, and a sample of urine for analysis. The physician may also advise you to take a blood screening test and a hearing test. The physician may review and, if necessary, update your immunization program. Booster immunizations for tetanus and diphtheria should be given every 10 years.

It is now common for doctors to give their patients materials to screen their stool for the presence of blood. This is done to test for colon cancer, which is easily treatable, if found in its early stages. These test materials are also marketed directly to the public. Anyone over the age of 40 should take this test each year. Your physician may also conduct a proctoscopy, an examination of the colon, in order to detect possible colon cancer. Male patients over the age of 40 should have a rectal and prostate examination.

Female patients should have a breast and pelvic examination and a Pap smear test. Women past the age of 40 should also have a rectal examination. All women should have a baseline mammogram sometime between the ages of 35 and 40. These should be done yearly after the age of 50, earlier for women who have had breast lumps and are therefore at greater risk for developing breast cancer.

Routine Health Tests. Infancy and early childhood are times of rapid growth and development. Regular testing and examination during these periods are important. The tests can be carried out either by your family physician or by a pediatrician. Some physicians like to see the baby once a month for the first two months, every two months for the next four months, and every three months for the next eighteen months. During these consultations, the physician weighs and measures the baby and checks that he or she is developing normally. Certain tests, such as hearing tests, are carried out at specific ages. Parents are able to discuss any worries with the physician during the consultations. The physician also follows a careful immunization schedule and inspects the baby's emerging teeth. The baby will not have to visit the dentist until after the age of two-and-one-half to three years.

During later childhood and adolescence, children should have their growth and development checked regularly. Semiannual visits to the dentist are imperative during these years, because orthodontic treatment may be necessary to correct malocclusion.

See also MALOCCLUSION.

Hearing is the perception of sound. The ear is the organ that makes hearing possible.

See also DEAFNESS; EAR; EAR DISORDERS.

Hearing aid is a small, battery-powered, electronic device that amplifies sound. It is used by people who can not hear well.

Hearing disorders. *See* DEAFNESS; EAR DISORDERS; HEARING IMPAIRED.

Hearing impaired. A person who is hearing impaired has a decreased ability to detect or distinguish sounds. It has been estimated that in the United States there are as many as 18 million people who are hearing impaired. Although most of these people are not truly deaf, one-third of this group has significant hearing loss, leading to a marked reduction in the ability to understand speech.

Hearing impairment may be either congenital, meaning that the person was born with the hearing problem, or acquired. Congenital causes of hearing loss include genetic diseases and exposure of the fetus to infections (such as rubella) or drugs. Among children, the most common cause of acquired hearing loss is untreated or recurrent ear infection (otitis media). Among adults, the causes of hearing loss include otosclerosis (a disorder of the middle ear), physical trauma, sound trauma (especially in noisy work environments), or presbycusis (progressive hearing loss associated with aging).

Hearing impairment can lead to significant problems and disability, although hearing impairment as the underlying cause of the problem may not be suspected. For example, undetected hearing impairment in children can cause developmental delays and poor school performance. In adults, hearing loss can lead to irritability, confusion, or social isolation. Among the elderly, these symptoms can be mistaken for a form of dementia, if the hearing is not carefully checked.

The treatment of hearing impairment depends upon the underlying cause. Surgery, hearing aids, and other devices to amplify sound may all be helpful in some cases.

See also DEAFNESS; EAR DISORDERS; OTITIS; OTOSCLEROSIS; RUBELLA.

Heart is a strong, muscular organ, the size of a clenched fist, that pumps blood throughout the body. It is situated behind and slightly to the left of the breastbone (sternum), between the lungs. The heart is completely enclosed by a thin sac (pericardium) made of tough tissue. This sac protects the heart from rubbing against the lungs or the wall of the chest.

Q: *How does the heart work?*

A: The structure and action of the heart are designed to serve the two loops of circulation. Inside, the heart is divided vertically by a muscular wall (septum). On each side of this wall is an upper chamber (atrium) and a thicker, lower chamber (ventricle). Blood moves through each side of the heart systematically. Venous blood, which is lower in oxygen content, is delivered into the right atrium. It then enters the right ventricle, from where it is pumped out into the pulmonary artery and to the lungs. Oxygenated blood returning in the pulmonary vein flows into the left atrium. This blood enters the left ventricle and is then pumped into the aorta for circulation.

The flow of blood in each side of the heart is controlled by a series of valves. The pumping action of the heart is achieved by the contraction of the cardiac muscle of which the heart is largely composed. The rhythm of the heartbeat is regulated by bursts of electrical impulses sent out by a concentration of specialized heart tissue called the pacemaker.

Under the influence of the pacemaker, the heart of an adult at rest beats at a rate of 60 to 100 beats a minute. The pacemaker also helps to ensure the correct sequence of activities during each heartbeat. First the two atria contract, followed rapidly by the ventricles. The powerful contraction of the ventricles pushes blood into the aorta and pulmonary artery. This period of contraction (systole) is followed by a period of relaxation (diastole), during which the heart refills. The complete sequence is accompanied by electrical activity of the muscle, which can be monitored as an electrocardiogram (EKG).

See also CARDIOVASCULAR SYSTEM; CIRCULATION.

Heart, artificial. An artificial heart is a mechanical substitute for the human heart, which can be implanted in a patient to replace a damaged heart. The first mechanical heart, operating in a human for any length of time, was the Jarvik-7, which was implanted in Barney Clark in 1982 at the University of Utah. Due to medical complications, Clark survived the implantation for only a few weeks. The Jarvik-7, however, was found to have functioned well as a pump.

Many problems remain before this artificial heart can be widely used. A better power source is needed. The Jarvik-7 used compressed gas with complex equipment outside the body. A solution is also needed to the serious problem of the interaction of blood with the device, which can cause clots and other complications.

The Jarvik-7 is a totally artificial heart. Another type of artificial heart, the left ventricular assist device (LVAD), can be used without the removal of the patient's own heart. This device assists the natural heart in its pumping action, until the natural heart has healed sufficiently to take over on its own.

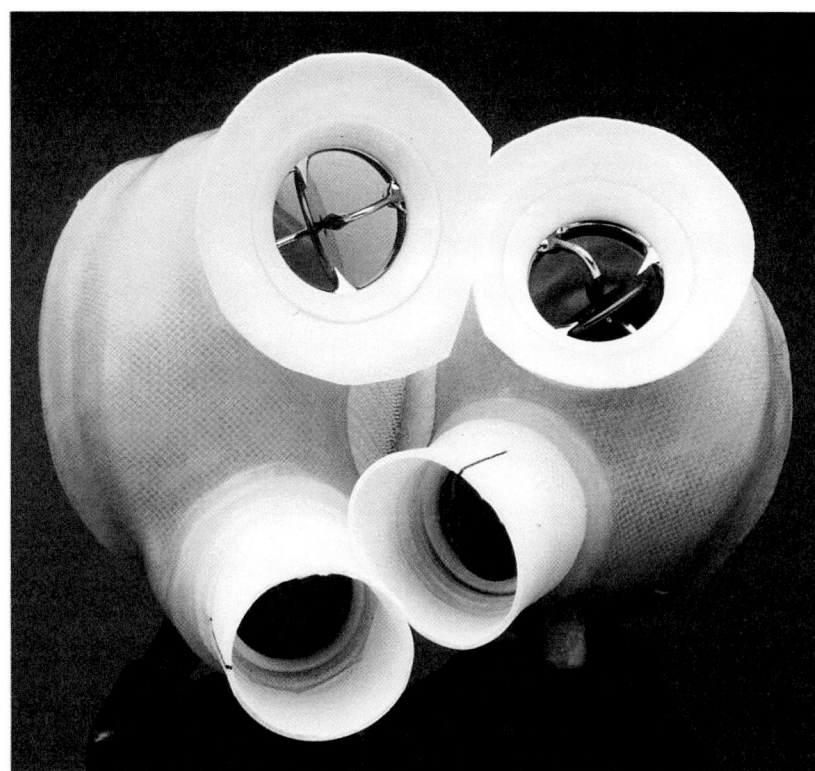

The first **artificial heart,** operating in a human for any length of time, was the Jarvik-7.

Heart attack, or myocardial infarction, begins when a section of heart muscle suddenly loses its blood supply, due to a partial or complete obstruction of the coronary arteries. Such obstruction is usually the result of coronary arteriosclerosis. If the obstruction persists longer than a few minutes, that section of heart muscle will die. This is known as a heart attack. If, however, the obstruction lasts only a short time (a few minutes), the patient will experience chest pain, angina pectoris; but there is no permanent damage. Medication is now used to dissolve blood clots early in a myocardial infarction (within 4 to 6 hours). In this fashion, the amount of heart muscle that might die can be decreased.

Heart attacks can be complicated by weakness of the pumping activity of the heart (congestive heart failure) or irregular heartbeat (arrythmia). Heart attacks are extremely serious and can result in death, if a large part of the heart muscle dies or if complications are not treated.

See also ANGINA PECTORIS; HEART ATTACK: FIRST AID; INFARCTION.

Heart attack: first aid. There are two degrees of coronary insufficiency. The milder form, called angina pectoris, is caused by a partial obstruction of the coronary artery. Because it is only temporary, no permanent damage occurs to the heart muscle. The more severe, sometimes fatal, form is caused by a complete blockage of the coronary artery, which results in death of a section of heart muscle.

Angina Pectoris. With angina pectoris, the victim feels a severe pain in the chest. It starts in the middle of the chest and may spread to the shoulders and upper arms (particularly the victim's left arm), to the abdomen, and to the neck or jaw. This pain may be accompanied by nausea, sweating, or shortness of breath.

The victim should rest immediately, using a position that is most comfortable. A sitting position is often best, because it makes breathing easier and allows the best flow of blood to the heart. Loosen any tight clothing. Call medical assistance immediately and allow the victim to rest until help arrives.

Action. Observe the victim's pulse and breathing. Feel the victim's wrist pulse. Time the number of beats per minute. There should be 60 to 100. If no pulse is felt and the victim is unconscious, see instructions for treating a severe heart attack later in this article. If the victim stops breathing, initiate mouth-to-mouth resuscitation. For instructions, *see* ARTIFICIAL RESPIRATION.

Heart attack: first aid (angina pectoris)

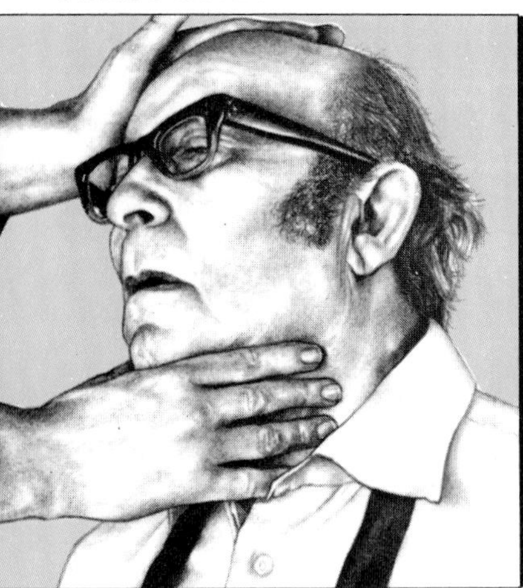

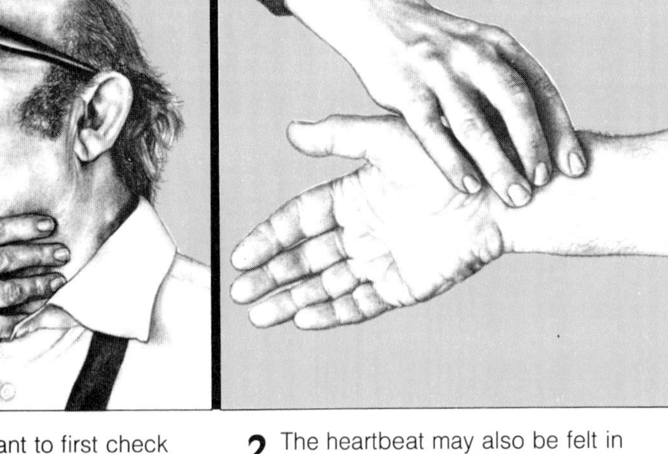

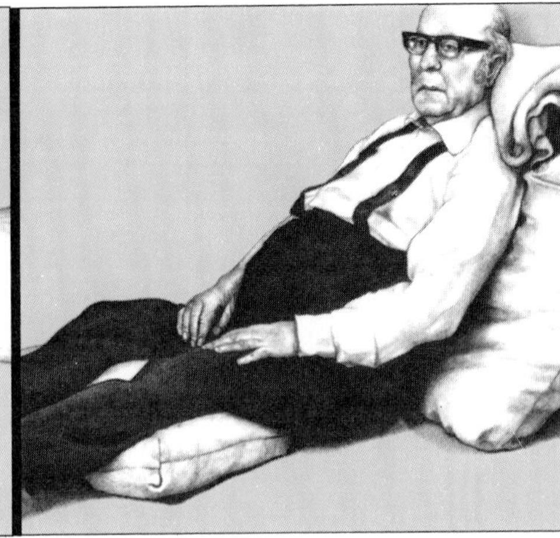

1 It is important to first check the victim's pulse rate. The strongest pulse is felt in the neck (the carotid pulse). To feel the carotid pulse, carefully place your fingers alongside the windpipe near to the angle of the jaw. Do not press too hard. If there is no pulse, refer to the instructions concerning a more severe heart attack on page 405.

2 The heartbeat may also be felt in the wrist (the radial pulse) as the blood is pumped down the arm to the hand. Place your fingers in a line along the inside of the victim's arm, on the same side as the thumb, just above the wrist. The radial pulse may be hard to detect if the heart is failing or the artery is small. If there is no pulse, refer to the instructions concerning a more severe heart attack on page 405. If there is a pulse, continue with step 3.

3 A victim with angina pectoris should rest in the most comfortable position possible until medical help arrives. Usually, the victim is most comfortable when sitting, with the back well supported. The knees may also be supported; care must be taken to ensure this support does not interfere with blood circulation in the legs. All tight clothing should be loosened.

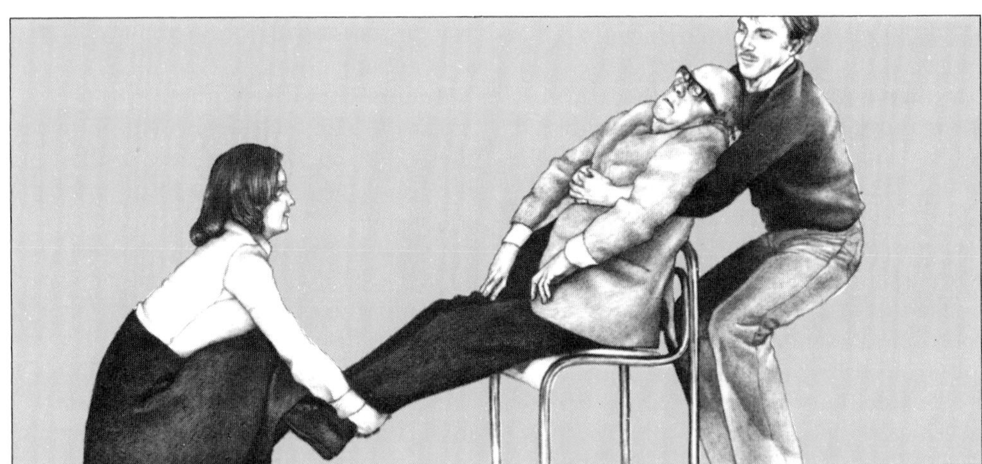

4 It may be necessary to move a victim of angina pectoris into a comfortable resting position. To do this, one person should hold the victim's legs while another person holds the victim's shoulders. You should try to move the victim as swiftly and as gently as possible. If the heart has stopped, it is important to move the victim onto the floor as quickly as possible, lifting the person as illustrated. Although this illustrated method is the most efficient, almost any other method will suffice. The victim must lie faceup, so that external cardiac compression can be started immediately. For instructions on external cardiac compression, see the severe heart attack section of this article.

Severe heart attack: first aid

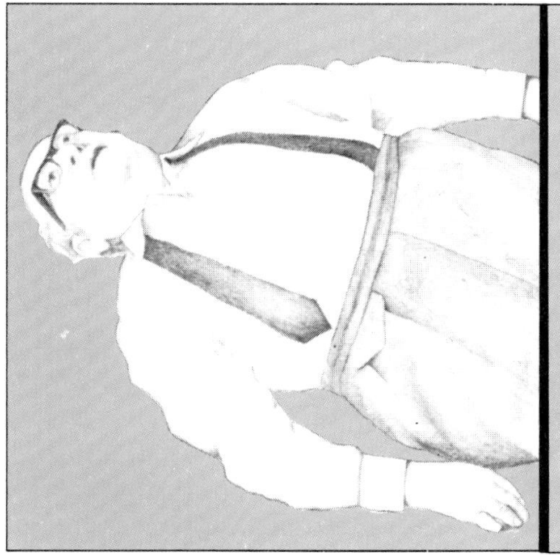

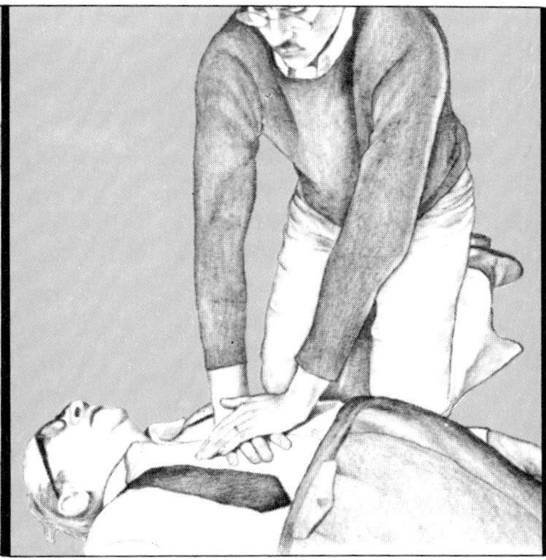

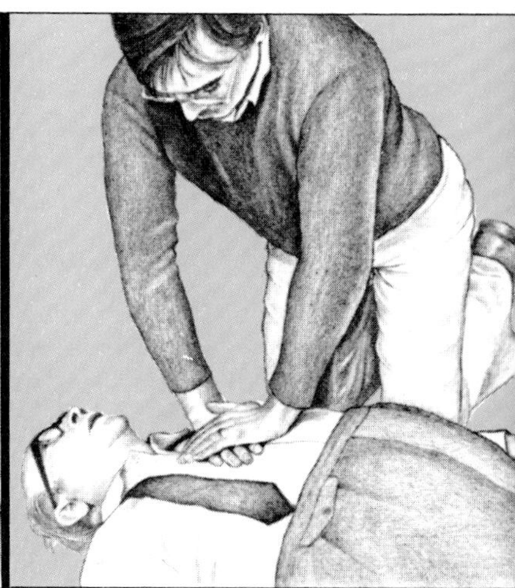

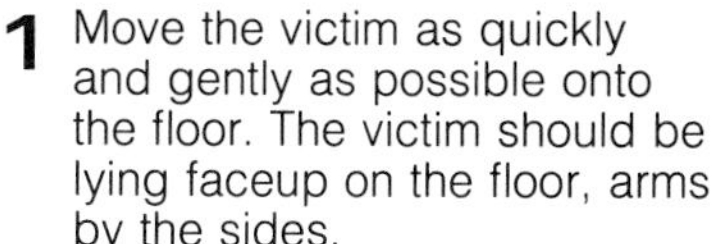

1 Move the victim as quickly and gently as possible onto the floor. The victim should be lying faceup on the floor, arms by the sides.

2 Kneel at the victim's left shoulder and place your hands, palms down, with the stronger hand under the other, over the victim's heart. The heel of your bottom hand should be over the lower half of the victim's sternum (breastbone).

3 Lean forward with the arms straight and the shoulders directly over the sternum. Push the victim's sternum down 1.5 to 2 inches (3.75 to 5 cm). Press at a rate of about 15 compressions every 11 seconds. Press firmly, but do not damage the ribcage. After every 15 compressions, briefly give the victim artificial respiration.

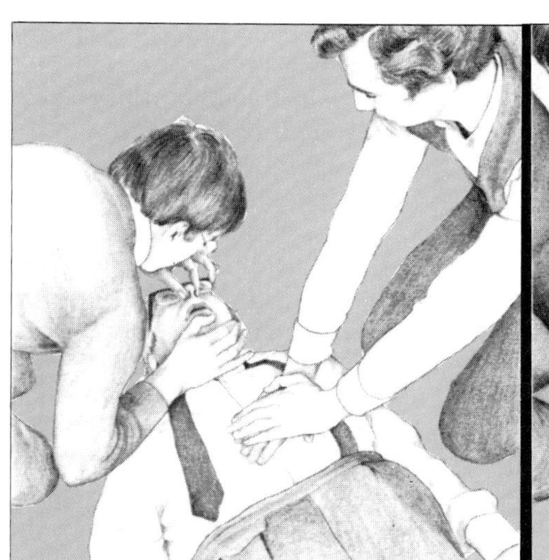

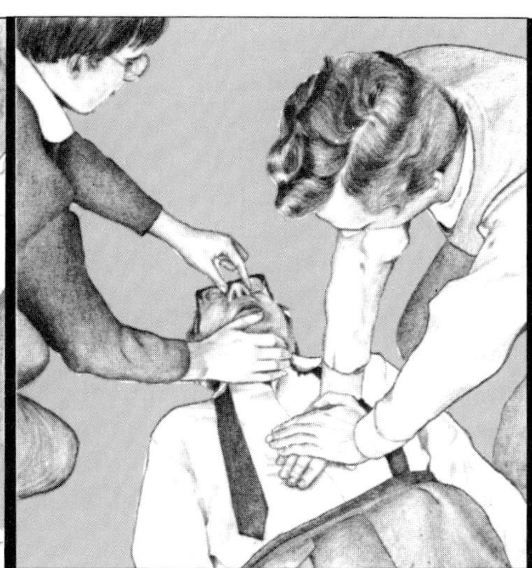

4 With two people, the one compressing the heart should kneel at the victim's left shoulder. The other person, on the victim's other side, tilts the victim's head back, holds the victim's nose, and breathes into the lungs.

5 This dual technique occupies a 15 second cycle. The person applying cardiac compression presses 20 times during this period. At the same time, the person giving resuscitation ventilates the victim's lungs twice. It is necessary for both people applying aid to establish a steady working rhythm.

If the victim has suffered angina pectoris before, tablets prescribed by a physician may be in the victim's pocket or close at hand. Before giving any tablets to the victim, ask if they are the right ones. *Do not* give an unconscious person any medication.

Severe Heart Attack. The symptoms of a severe heart attack include acute and sudden chest pains, gray facial color, sweating, rapid and feeble pulse, shallow and fast breathing, and a loss of consciousness. The heartbeat and breathing may even stop.

In case of heart stoppage, it is imperative to either restart the heart as quickly as possible or to manually circulate the blood until the heart can take over on its own. The best way to do this is by external chest compressions, which consist of manually pressing the chest wall over the heart. This should be attempted only by those trained in CPR procedures. In this way, the pumping action of the heart is artificially maintained. See illustrations on page 405 for external chest compression procedures. *See also* CARDIOPULMONARY RESUSCITATION.

Action. Call for medical help immediately. If the victim is not breathing, breathe air into the victim's lungs twice, so as to inflate them. *See also* ARTIFICIAL RESPIRATION.

Check the victim's carotid pulse on the left side of the neck, below the ear. If the pulse can be felt, do not apply external compressions. Refer to the instructions for treating angina pectoris earlier in this article.

If no pulse can be felt, start external chest compressions at once, if you are trained in CPR procedures. The heel of one hand should be placed on the lower half of the sternum (breastbone), the second hand being put directly over the first. With the elbows locked, arms straight and shoulders directly over the hands, push the victim's sternum down 1.5 to 2 inches (3.75 to 5 cm). Give 15 compressions every 11 seconds, adding up to a rate of 80 to 100 per minute.

If no other help is available, combine external cardiac compression with mouth-to-mouth resuscitation. Alternate between 15 external chest compressions and 2 artificial respirations. Keep calm, so that your own breathing is regular and so that you do not get tired.

Heartblock is a disorder in the transmission of nerve impulses between the upper chambers (atria) and the lower chambers (ventricles) of the heart. A disturbance of this mechanism causes the heartbeat to falter or become irregular (arrhythmia).

Q: *What are the symptoms of heartblock?*

A: A partial heartblock may cause no symptoms, although the irregularity of the heartbeat can be detected with a stethoscope. With a total heartblock, the contractions of the ventricles may not be fast enough to maintain an efficient blood supply. The patient may have bouts of unconsciousness. At other times, dizziness, faintness, and breathlessness may occur. *See also* STOKES-ADAMS SYNDROME.

Q: *What are the causes of heartblock?*

A: Heartblock may be associated with congenital heart disease. It can be caused by coronary heart disease, toxic effects of drugs, infection of the heart muscle (myocarditis), or damage to heart muscle from rheumatic fever.

Q: *How is heartblock treated?*

A: Patients who have temporary heartblock recover spontaneously when the acute stage of the causative illness has passed. Permanent, complete heartblock may be treated with drugs, but the treatment is not curative. The most effective treatment is the addition of an artificial heart pacemaker. *See also* PACEMAKER, ARTIFICIAL.

Heartburn, also known as pyrosis, is a burning sensation in the esophagus (gullet) caused by acid rising from the stomach. It is most frequently associated with indigestion.

See also INDIGESTION.

Heart disease is the ordinary term used to describe a variety of heart disorders. All the disorders mentioned below are the subjects of individual articles in which symptoms and treatment are discussed.

The sac surrounding the heart, the pericardium, may become inflamed (pericarditis) as a local disease or as part of a general heart inflammation, such as rheumatic fever. The heart muscle itself may become inflamed (myocarditis) or degenerate (cardiomyopathy) from a variety of causes.

Atherosclerosis (the buildup of fatty deposits in the arteries) can cause coronary heart disease, which in turn may lead to coronary thrombosis. The aortic valve is frequently involved. Affected by valvular disease, it narrows, becomes deformed, and sometimes causes a back flow of blood. The distortion of the normal blood flow from valvular disease causes heart murmurs. *See also* ARTERIOSCLEROSIS; HEART DISEASE, CORONARY; THROMBOSIS, CORONARY.

Hypertension (high blood pressure) produces hypertrophy (increase in the size of the heart muscle) and, like other forms of heart disease, may eventually cause heart failure.

Disorders of the normal electrical impulses in the heart may produce fibrillation, flutter, or heartblock. Such disorders can also occur with valvular disease, rheumatic fever, or coronary heart disease.

Other conditions that may affect the heart include angina pectoris; blue baby; dextrocardia; embolism; and bacterial endocarditis.

Electrical disorders of the heart include bradycardia, extrasystole, Stokes-Adams syndrome, tachycardia, paroxysmal atrial tachycardia, and vasovagal syncope.

Q: *How may a physician investigate the causes of heart disease?*

A: A history of previous illness, such as rheumatic fever, may help the physician to interpret any abnormal heart sounds or murmurs. But no specific cause is generally found.

There are many tests that a physician can use to assess the condition of the heart. (Many of the tests discussed have individual articles elsewhere in this encyclopedia.) Blood tests can detect anemia, hormone disorders such as thyrotoxicosis or hypothyroidism, and the levels of cholesterol and triglyceride fats. An electrocardiogram (EKG) can provide extremely useful information. A portable EKG can be worn for one or more days by a patient, going about his or her daily activities. This can supplement information gained on a single EKG, which lasts less than two minutes. EKG information may be further supplemented by coronary catheterization, angiography, ultrasound studies (echocardiography), exercise tolerance tests (treadmill tests), chest X rays, and phonocardiography, all of which help determine the movement of the heart and its sounds.

Heart disease, congenital (kən jen′ə təl). Congenital heart disease is any heart disorder that is present at birth, although the condition may not be diagnosed until later in life. The most common problems are a hole between the two ventricles; a narrowing of the aorta, the main artery from the heart; the wrong positioning of the aorta or the artery that leads to the lungs; and constriction of the valves in the left side of the heart, with weakness of the heart muscle.

Q: *What are the symptoms of congenital heart disease?*

A: The symptoms, if present at all, depend on the nature of the disorder. Many types of defects produce murmurs. A baby may have difficulty in sucking, eating, or breathing. There may also be a bluish color to the skin. An infant with congenital heart disease is likely to have frequent respiratory infections. *See also* BLUE BABY; FALLOT'S TETRALOGY.

Q: *What are the causes of congenital heart disease?*

A: Often, the cause is unknown, although genetic factors are thought to be important. Some forms of congenital heart disease may be caused by a virus infection in the mother during the first three

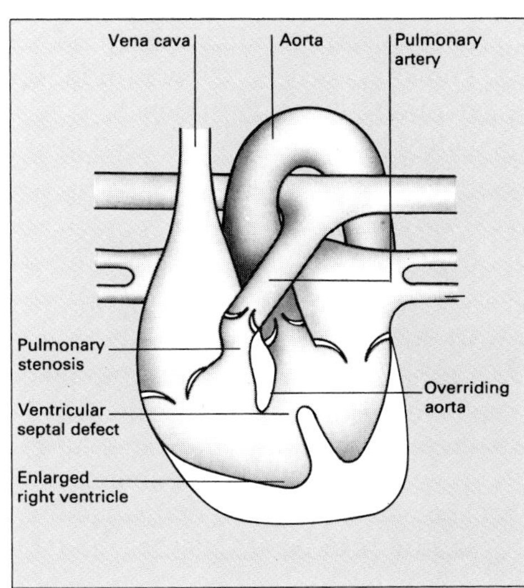

A **congenital heart disease** that affects four sites in the heart is known as Fallot's tetralogy.

months of pregnancy, such as rubella. *See also* RUBELLA.

Q: *How is congenital heart disease treated?*

A: Successful treatment depends on a speedy diagnosis. If possible, the appropriate type of heart surgery is then undertaken.

Q: *Are some babies more susceptible to congenital heart disease than others?*

A: Yes. Although about 1 percent of first-born babies have a congenital heart disease, the likelihood of it occurring in a subsequent baby is increased to 1 in 25. There is also a 1 in 25 chance that a baby born to parents, one of whom has a congenital heart disorder, will also have a heart problem.

Heart disease, coronary (kôr′ə ner ē). Coronary heart disease is any damage to the heart muscle resulting from reduced blood supply from the two coronary arteries. Normal blood supply is reduced by the narrowing of any section of an artery. The type of arteriosclerosis known as atherosclerosis, a build-up of fatty deposits in the arterial walls, is the most common cause. The artery usually affected is the first descending branch of the left coronary artery.

Q: *What are the symptoms of coronary artery disorders?*

A: Sometimes, a pain in the center of the chest (angina pectoris) occurs during exercise. Such pain usually vanishes when the exercise ceases. Often, there are no symptoms at all until thrombosis (blood clotting) shuts off the blood supply completely. This causes death of part of the heart muscle, a condition known medically as myocardial infarction. In popular usage it is called a "coronary" or "heart attack." *See also* HEART ATTACK; HEART DISEASE.

Q: *What are the symptoms of a heart attack?*

A: The patient usually complains of severe, tight, constricting pain in the chest. This may extend to the shoulders, arms, and hands, into the neck and jaw, and sometimes down into the upper abdomen. The pain may be accompanied by shortness of breath, nausea, and sweating. A patient with these symptoms should be hospitalized as soon as possible. It is also possible to have a "silent" heart attack, with no symptoms, which may only be discovered much later in an electrocardiogram (EKG). This most often occurs in elderly patients.

Q: *How long does the pain last?*

A: The pain may last from a few minutes to several hours, after which the patient is exhausted.

Q: *Does the heart stop beating?*

A: If the condition is severe, it is possible for the heart to stop beating. If the heartbeat is not restored immediately, death occurs.

Q: *How is a heart attack diagnosed?*

A: The diagnosis of a heart attack is made by studying the patient's history of pain, by observing characteristic changes in the electrocardiogram, and by detecting the presence of various enzymes in the blood.

Q: *What is the treatment for a heart attack?*

A: The first hours of treatment are the most critical. The patient may be admitted to a coronary care unit, where electrocardiographic monitoring is done to detect any irregularities in the pulse. Such irregularities may indicate that the heart may be about to stop. Pulse irregularities can be treated with drugs. Injections of painkilling drugs can be given if needed. If a blood clot was the cause of the heart attack, drugs should be administered to dissolve the thrombosis. Other drugs (for example, heparin or warfarin) can be given to prevent thrombosis. After two to three days, the most dangerous period is over, and the patient is usually permitted to get out of bed. This reduces the chance of deep vein thrombosis in the legs.

Q: *For how long may a coronary heart disease patient be hospitalized?*

A: It depends on the severity of the obstruction to the blood supply and on any complications. A patient may be hospitalized for about 10 days to 3 weeks.

Q: *What advice can be given about convalescence?*
A: The patient should live a quiet and relaxed life, without stress, and gradually take a little exercise. Anticoagulant drugs may be taken at home for several weeks. Sexual intercourse may be resumed after the first month. Heavy lifting and strains should be avoided for two months following the attack. After six weeks, the dead muscle in the heart will have been replaced by scar tissue. To strengthen the heart, the physician may recommend increasing amounts of exercise.
Q: *Does a heart attack alter the life-style of a patient?*
A: There are a number of precautions that a patient must observe for life. Most physicians advise physical exercise for 10 to 15 minutes a day. Initially, exercises may be taught at a coronary rehabilitation center, where monitoring equipment shows up any signs of heart strain in the patient.

A person who has had a heart attack must never smoke. Alcohol, too, should be avoided as it may interfere with weight reduction and control of blood pressure. Excessive use of alcohol causes direct toxicity on the heart. If the patient suffers from hypertension (high blood pressure), this must be treated and kept well under control.
Q: *What are the complications of coronary heart disease?*
A: Damage to the electrical conducting mechanism of the heart may cause atrial fibrillation, with the symptom of an irregular, rapid pulse. Congestive heart failure (due to inadequate pumping by the heart) may occur if a large amount of the heart muscle has been damaged. *See also* FIBRILLATION.
Q: *Are certain groups more prone to coronary heart disease?*
A: Four times as many men as women have coronary heart disease. It also tends to affect more men earlier in life than women. Coronary heart disease is more common in women after menopause. There is a high incidence of the disorder in the following groups: smokers; those with hypertension; those who are overweight; those with high blood cholesterol levels; those with physically inactive jobs; and those with anxious or aggressive dispositions. The possibility of a heart attack is greatly increased in those who have had one already, those who have a family history of them, and those who are diabetic.

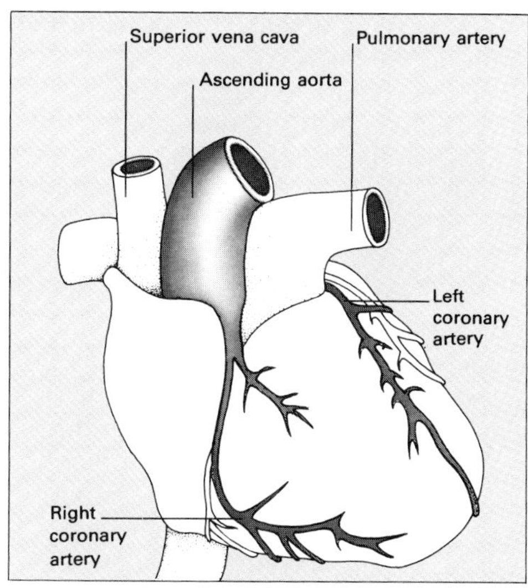

Q: *Is it possible to prevent coronary heart disease?*
A: Patients who are overweight, who are hypertensive, who smoke, or who are inactive with a high cholesterol level can reduce the chances of heart attacks by changing their habits appropriately.

Heart failure occurs when the heart's pumping ability is impaired. The heart continues to beat, but not strongly enough to maintain adequate circulation. This results in a retention of blood in the organs and tissues throughout the body. The reduction of heart function may be due to a variety of conditions: hypertension (high blood pressure); valvular heart disease; or coronary heart disease. For symptoms and treatment of chronic heart failure, *see* HEART FAILURE, CONGESTIVE.

Acute heart failure may follow a pulmonary embolus (a blood clot blocking an artery in a lung) or coronary thrombosis (a blood clot blocking an artery in the heart). The patient experiences shortness of breath and coughs up blood-stained sputum. Acute congestive heart failure may come on at night because excess fluid moves from the legs into the circulation mainstream when the

Coronary heart disease is damage to the heart muscle that is caused by a reduced blood supply from the two coronary arteries.

patient is lying down. This puts further strain on the heart.

See also HEART ATTACK: FIRST AID.

Heart failure, congestive (kən jes′tiv). Congestive heart failure is a condition in which the heart is unable to maintain the normal circulation of the blood. Heart failure does not mean that the heart stops suddenly (cardiac arrest), rather that it gradually becomes inefficient as the blood in the veins increases in volume and the veins become dilated. The lungs, liver, and intestines become congested with blood. There are many causes of congestive heart failure: weakness of the heart muscle; hypertension (high blood pressure); heart attack; a chronic lung disease (such as emphysema); disease of the heart valves; hyperthyroidism (overactivity of the thyroid gland); a viral illness; arrhythmia (irregular heartbeat); severe anemia; or pulmonary embolism. Untreated, the condition can be fatal.

Q: *What are the symptoms of congestive heart failure?*

A: The symptoms include breathlessness (as fluid backs up in the lungs), swollen ankles (a form of edema), and weakness.

Q: *How is congestive heart failure treated?*

A: A physician may prescribe a diuretic drug, which helps to relieve any swelling (edema) in the body tissues and reduces some strain on the heart. A salt-free diet is sometimes recommended to help prevent any further retention of fluids. In addition, digitalis may be used to improve the strength of the heartbeat. In some cases, drugs may also be given that dilate the arteries, thus making it easier for the heart to pump blood. Bed rest with hospitalization, if necessary, is advised for acute congestive heart failure. Oxygen may be required, and a source of oxygen should be kept available.

Heart-lung machine is an apparatus that permits the heart to be operated on safely. This machine, which utilizes an oxygenator and a pump, allows the surgeon to operate on a bloodless, unbeating heart. The heart-lung machine not only temporarily takes over the pumping activities of the heart, but also oxygenates the blood and removes carbon dioxide from it. Thus, the rest of the body is supplied with vital blood circulation during heart surgery. With this machine, many types of heart surgery that were previously impossible or extremely dangerous can now be done with comparative safety. These include heart transplants, coronary by-passes, removal and replacement of damaged valves, and repair of other structural defects.

Heart massage. *See* CARDIAC MASSAGE.

Heart murmur (mėr′mər) describes an abnormal noise produced by the blood flowing through the chambers and valves of the heart.

With any murmur, a physician must be consulted. Many heart murmurs require no treatment, although a few may require some form of heart surgery. Before undergoing surgery or dental work, a person with a heart murmur should inform his or her physician or dentist of the condition. Antibiotics may be needed before the procedure, in order to prevent bacterial endocarditis.

See also ENDOCARDITIS.

Heart pacemaker. *See* PACEMAKER, ARTIFICIAL; PACEMAKER, NATURAL.

Heart stoppage, or cardiac arrest, is a temporary or permanent failure of normal heart muscle contractions. When the heart stops, blood ceases to be pumped around the body. Various tissues, particularly those of the brain, then become adversely affected by the lack of oxygen.

Heart stoppage may be caused by a severe electric shock; a coronary thrombosis (blood clot); or heart disease, particularly when it affects the heart muscle, as in cardiomyopathy and myocarditis. Heart stoppage may also result from an irregular heart rhythm (arrhythmia) or Stokes-Adams syndrome. During heart surgery it is sometimes necessary to stop the heart deliberately. The heart is restarted by electrical stimulation (cardioversion).

See also ARRHYTHMIA; HEART ATTACK; HEART DISEASE; STOKES-ADAMS SYNDROME.

Heart surgery is any surgical operation on the heart. There are two main forms of heart surgery, open and closed. The general procedure in an open technique is to cut open the chest cavity and fully expose the heart. The patient's blood supply is then connected to a heart-lung machine, and the heartbeat is stopped. This enables the surgeon to repair the heart while the heart is empty of blood and not pumping.

In a closed technique, a small incision is made into the chest cavity, and the heart is repaired through this opening.

See also HEART-LUNG MACHINE.

Heart transplant is the replacement of an irreparably diseased heart with a healthy one.

See also TRANSPLANT SURGERY.

Heat exhaustion. *See* HEAT RELATED INJURY.

Heating pad is an electrical device used to warm a portion of the body. A heating pad is often used to relieve the pain of rheumatic disorders or to ease stiffness after muscular damage.

Heat rash. *See* MILIARIA.

Heat related injury includes heat exhaustion, heat cramps, and heat syncope.

Heat exhaustion is caused by excessive exposure to heat and the depletion of body fluids. Victims sweat profusely and may shiver and have goose bumps. Weakness, nausea, dizziness, headache, poor judgment, rapid pulse, and a normal or slightly elevated body temperature are present. Heat cramps occur in healthy individuals during or following strenuous physical activity. Muscles, oftentimes those in the calf, cramp and produce severe pain. Fainting from the heat is referred to as heat syncope.

Treatment for heat related injuries includes rest in a cool, shaded environment, along with fluid replacement. Cramped muscles should be stretched or massaged.

See also, CRAMP; FAINTING: FIRST AID.

Heatstroke, or sunstroke, is a potentially fatal reaction to heat and humidity exposure. It is an acute medical emergency. Heatstroke is caused by the body's inability to regulate its own temperature. Its onset may be gradual or sudden, with the symptoms of heat exhaustion (headache, weakness, and nausea) occurring in the initial stages. Two symptoms separate heat exhaustion from heatstroke: (1) mental confusion is mild or absent in heat exhaustion, but in heatstroke it is profound; (2) body temperature in heatstroke is markedly elevated 104-115° F. (40-46° C). In addition, some people with heatstroke stop sweating and their skin becomes hot and dry. Shock, convulsions,

Heatstroke: first aid

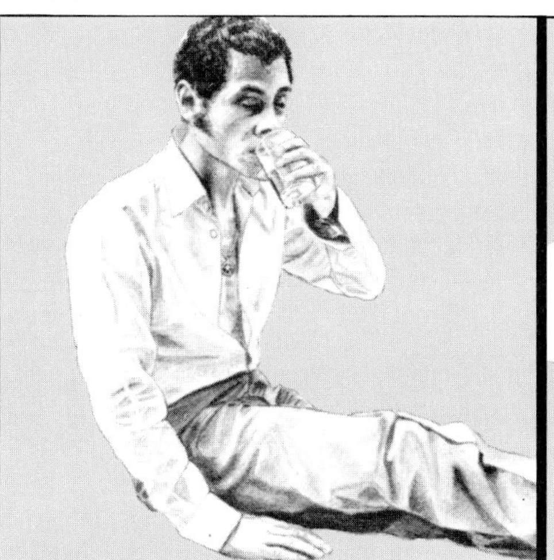

1 If the victim is suffering from heat exhaustion, place him or her in a cool, shady environment. Give the victim one-half of a glass of cold water. Untreated heat exhaustion may lead to heatstroke.

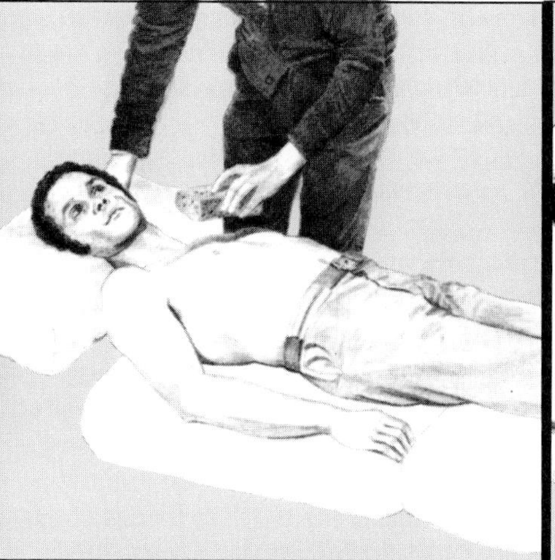

2 If the victim is suffering from heatstroke, summon emergency medical assistance immediately. While waiting, the body temperature must be reduced as quickly as possible. Place the victim in a cool, shady environment. Treat for shock (*see* SHOCK: FIRST AID). If the victim is unconscious, place him or her in the recovery position (*see* FAINTING: FIRST AID).

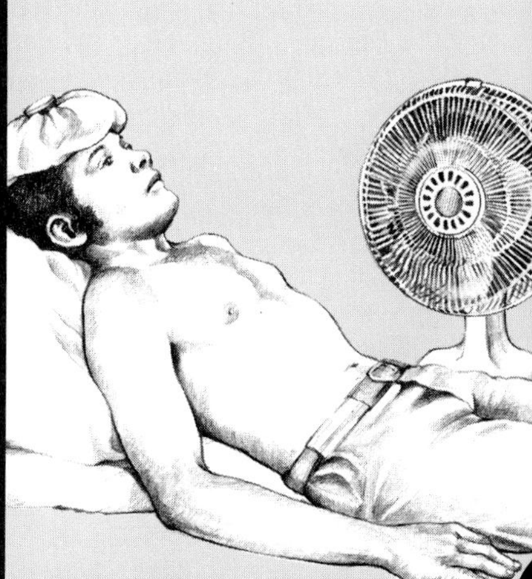

3 Remove most of the victim's clothing. Spray or sponge cool water over the victim's skin and fan vigorously (or use an electric fan). Place ice packs on the forehead and over the pulses of the neck, armpits, and groin. Wait for emergency medical assistance.

coma, and even death may occur with heatstroke.

See also HEATSTROKE: FIRST AID.

Heatstroke: first aid. This medical emergency requires prompt action. Emergency medical assistance should be summoned immediately. An attempt to lower the body temperature should be made as quickly as possible.

Action: Place the victim in a cool, shaded place and elevate slightly his or her feet. Remove most of the victim's clothing and then spray cool to tepid water onto the bare skin. Fan vigorously (preferable with a powerful electric fan). Ice packs to the head, neck, armpits, and groin also reduce the victim's temperature. The temperature must be brought down below 102° F. (39° C) as soon as possible. If this is not done immediately, the victim could suffer irreparable brain damage or die.

See illustrations on page 411.

Heat syncope. *See* HEAT RELATED INJURY.

Heberden's nodes (heb'ər denz) are small, hard lumps that sometimes form next to the joints of the fingers in persons with osteoarthritis; they occur much more often in women. There is no cure, but the discomfort of tender nodes may be lessened by wax baths and gentle heat. Disfiguring nodes can be removed surgically.

Heel is the rear part of the foot, under the ankle and behind the instep. The heel is composed of the heel bone (calcaneus), which bears the full weight of the body when standing, and a thick, firm pad of tissue beneath the calcaneus, which acts as a shock absorber.

Heimlich maneuver (hīm'lik mə nü' vər) is a first-aid procedure used to rescue a victim of choking due to an obstruction, such as food, in the windpipe. Choking is a potentially fatal condition that requires immediate action. The Heimlich maneuver consists of an abdominal thrust that forces the lodged material out of the windpipe. For a discussion and illustrations of this emergency maneuver, *see* CHOKING AND COUGHING: FIRST AID.

Heliotherapy (hē lē o ther'ə pē) is the use of direct sunlight in the treatment of disorders such as psoriasis and acne.

See also ACNE; PSORIASIS.

Hemangioma (hi man jē ō'mə) is a tumor composed of blood vessels. It is usually benign (noncancerous) and generally affects the skin, but may involve other parts of the body, such as the intestine or the nervous system. The most common hemangiomas are types of birthmarks.

See also BIRTHMARK.

Hemangioma, capillary (hi man jē ō' mə, kap'ə ler ē). A capillary hemangioma, or port-wine stain, is a birthmark or benign tumor filled with small, tightly packed blood vessels; it often appears in infants. Usually, a capillary hemangioma disappears as the infant grows into early childhood. If there is frequent bleeding or some other complication, surgical removal may be necessary.

See also BIRTHMARK; HEMANGIOMA.

Hematemesis. *See* BLOOD, VOMITING OF.

Hematocele (hem'ə tō sēl) is a cyst or a tumor filled with blood.

Hematocolpos (hem ə to kol'pos) is a rare condition in which menstrual blood is retained because the hymen completely closes the entrance to the vagina. Treatment involves making a small opening in the hymen to allow the blood to escape.

See also HYMEN.

Hematology (hem ə tol'ə jē) is the study of blood and blood-forming tissues.

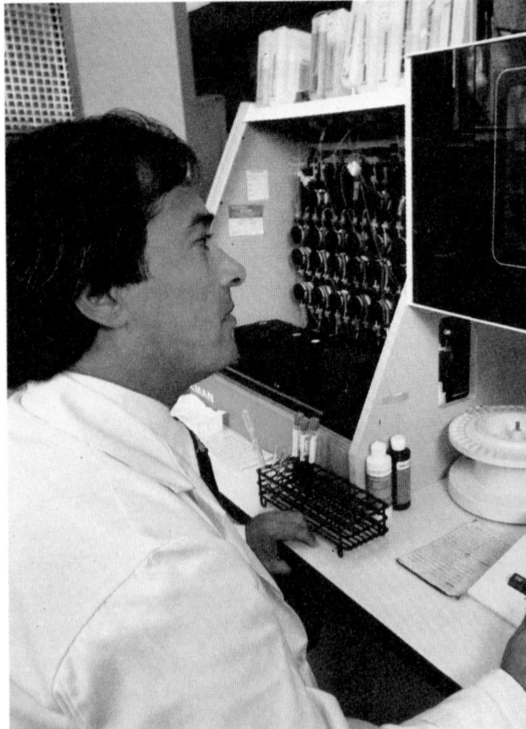

Hematology is the study of functions and diseases of the blood. Sophisticated machinery enables accurate blood analysis.

Hematoma (hē mə tō′mə) is trapped blood, often clotted, in an organ or within body tissues. A hematoma forms as a result of an accident or surgery. The blood is usually reabsorbed into the body tissues, and the clot disappears. The common name for a hematoma of the skin is bruise.

Hematoma, extradural (hē mə tō′mə, eks trə dủr′əl). Extradural hematoma is an accumulation of blood between the dura mater (the tough fibrous membrane that covers the brain) and the skull. The blood comes from a ruptured artery that supplies the internal surface of the skull. Extradural hematoma usually follows a head injury involving a skull fracture.

Q: *What are the symptoms of an extradural hematoma?*

A: The first sign may be a temporary loss of consciousness, followed by a period of apparently normal behavior. Other symptoms may begin hours or sometimes days after the injury. The patient's speech becomes slurred, and he or she walks unsteadily. The patient may suffer a headache, followed by unconsciousness, caused by the pressure of the clotted blood on the brain.

Q: *How is an extradural hematoma treated?*

A: The patient needs urgent hospitalization. X rays are taken to diagnose the condition. A surgeon then performs an operation to remove the clot. If treated promptly, the patient generally recovers fully.

Hematoma, subdural (hē mə tō′mə, sub dủr′əl). Subdural hematoma is an accumulation of blood in the subdural space, which is located between the duramater and arachnoid, two of the membranes of the brain. Usually caused by severe head injury or trauma, a subdural hematoma may take up to several weeks to develop. It is characterized by progressive neurologic deterioration and/or possible coma or amnesia.

Hematuria (hē mə tủr′ē ə) is the presence of blood in the urine. It is always a symptom of a disorder, and a person with hematuria should consult a physician immediately.

Small amounts of blood give urine a smoky or cloudy appearance. Larger amounts make the urine dark red or dark brown. But such discoloration is not always a sign of hematuria. Urine that has been standing for a while may naturally become cloudy. Reddish urine may be caused by pigments in certain foods, such as beets.

See also HEMOGLOBINURIA.

Hemianesthesia (hem ē an əs thē′zhə) is the loss of sensation down one side of the body.

Hemianopia (hem ē ä nō′pē ə) is the loss of half the normal field of vision in one or both eyes. The many types of hemianopia are classified according to which half of the vision is lost and in which eye. The most common types are homonymous hemianopia, in which the left (or right) half of each eye is blinded, and bitemporal hemianopia, in which the outer halves of both eyes are blinded.

Hemiparesis (hem ē pə rē′sis) is muscular weakness on one side of the body only. It is commonly accompanied by loss of sensation (hemianesthesia) on the same side.

Hemiplegia (hem ē plē′jē ə) is total paralysis on one side of the body only. It is commonly accompanied by a loss of sensation (hemianesthesia) on the same side. Hemiplegia is generally caused by a stroke.

See also PARALYSIS; STROKE.

Hemochromatosis (hē mə krō mə tō′sis) is a relatively rare genetic disease of iron metabolism in which iron gradually accumulates in various tissues and organs. Bronze pigmentation of the skin, cirrhosis, diabetes mellitus, heart failure, and joint changes may also occur. Such changes appear between the ages of 40 and 60 years, primarily in males.

See also CIRRHOSIS; DIABETES MELLITUS; SIDEROSIS; THALASSEMIA.

Hemodialysis. *See* KIDNEY DIALYSIS.

Hemoglobin. (hē′mə glō bən) is an iron-containing protein that occurs in red blood cells. It consists of an iron-containing pigment, called heme, and a simple protein, globin. Hemoglobin carries oxygen in the blood from the lungs to the body tissues and also carries carbon dioxide from the tissues to the lungs.

Q: *Are there different forms of hemoglobin?*

A: Yes. More than 100 types of abnormal hemoglobin have been produced by rare genetic mutations. Sickle cell anemia and thalassemia, for example, are caused by different, abnormal forms of hemoglobin.

See also SICKLE CELL ANEMIA; THALASSEMIA.

Hemoglobinuria (hē mə glō bə nůr′ē ə) is the presence of the red blood pigment hemoglobin in the urine. It is caused by the destruction of red blood cells at a rate greater than the liver's ability to remove the hemoglobin from the blood.

See also HEMATURIA; HEMOGLOBIN.

Hemolysis (hi mol′ə sis) is the breakdown of red blood cells causing the release of hemoglobin into the blood plasma. It is a normal process at the end of the life-span of each red blood cell. Hemolysis is usually slow enough for the red blood cells to be removed by the liver, spleen, and bone marrow. A reduction in the number of red blood cells in the circulation, called anemia, is caused by excessive hemolysis. If hemolysis occurs rapidly, it may produce shivering, fever, jaundice, abdominal pains, and an enlarged spleen.

See also HEMOGLOBIN.

Hemolytic disease of the newborn (hē mə lit′ik), also known medically as erythroblastosis fetalis or Rh factor incompatibility, is a serious condition affecting a baby before, during, or after birth. It is caused by an incompatibility between the blood of the baby and the blood of the mother. The condition is much more likely to occur in second or subsequent pregnancies.

Q: *What are the symptoms of hemolytic disease of the newborn?*

A: The symptoms depend on the severity of the condition. The baby may be anemic because of the destruction of fetal blood, or it may have jaundice because the yellow pigment bilirubin is released when the red blood cells break down. If too much bilirubin is released, brain damage may result. The most severe cases also include an abnormal accumulation of fluid in the body (edema), an enlarged spleen and liver, and possibly respiratory distress syndrome and congestive heart failure. *See also* RESPIRATORY DISTRESS SYNDROME OF THE NEWBORN.

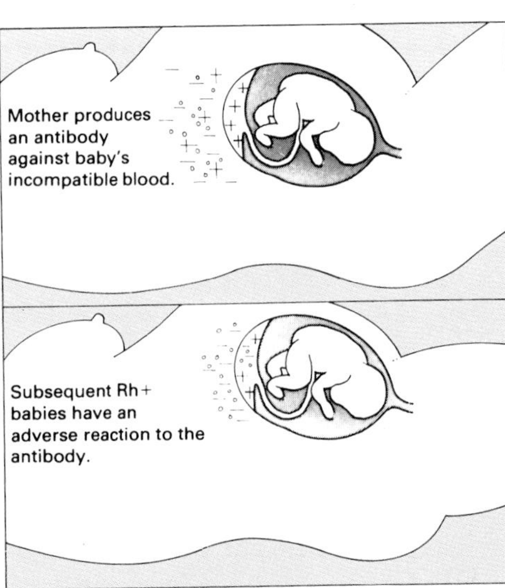

Mother produces an antibody against baby's incompatible blood.
Subsequent Rh+ babies have an adverse reaction to the antibody.

Hemolytic disease of the newborn is caused by an incompatibility between the blood of the baby and the blood of the mother. This incompatibility triggers the development of antibodies in the mother. Subsequent Rh+ babies react adversely to the antibody. Injections of anti-Rh− gamma globulin can prevent this.

Q: *How is hemolytic disease of the newborn treated?*

A: Babies born with the disease are given exchange transfusions of blood in which all the body's Rh+ blood is replaced with Rh− blood. The transfusions are usually given immediately after birth or as needed during the baby's first several weeks. If necessary, after tests on both mother and child, the baby can be given a transfusion while still in the uterus.

Q: *What can be done to prevent hemolytic disease of the newborn?*

A: Every woman should have a blood test as soon as she knows she is pregnant. If she is Rh−, the father should also be tested. If the father is Rh+, there is a possibility that the baby will develop hemolytic disease if the mother already has borne an Rh+ baby.

An injection of an anti-Rh− gamma globulin (RhoGAM®) should be given to the mother after approximately 28 weeks of gestation, as well as within the first 72 hours after delivery of an Rh+ baby. The injection blocks any fetal blood from entering the mother's blood circulation during the birth. This prevents antibodies from developing in most mothers and reduces the chances of hemolytic disease in future pregnancies. In order to be effective, this same treatment should be given after each pregnancy, whether it ends in delivery, miscarriage, or abortion, and after any amniocentesis, a procedure for testing amniotic fluid during pregnancy.

See also RH FACTOR.

Hemophilia (hē mō fil′ē ə) is a hereditary disease in which the blood does not clot properly. It is caused by a deficiency in one of the substances (clotting factors) needed for normal blood clotting. This deficiency is due to a sex-linked recessive genetic defect. Because the gene is sex-linked, hemophilia occurs in men; women merely carry the abnormal gene without developing the disease. *See also* GENE; GENETIC COUNSELING; HEREDITY.

Q: *What are the symptoms of hemophilia?*

A: Hemophilia is characterized by repeated episodes of spontaneous internal bleeding and prolonged external bleeding following even minor injuries.

Q: *How is hemophilia treated?*

A: Injections of the missing clotting factor stop any bleeding. For minor injuries, firm pressure over the affected area may stop the bleeding if the pressure is maintained long enough, often for an hour or more.

Q: *What precautions should a hemophiliac take?*

A: A hemophiliac should avoid contact sports and any activity in which minor injuries are likely. Any medical operation, either surgical or dental, requires an injection of the missing clotting factor at least a week prior to the operation. Hemophiliacs should wear an identity tag or carry a card stating that they suffer from hemophilia.

Hemoptysis. *See* BLOOD, SPITTING OF.

Hemorrhage (hem′ə rij) is internal or external bleeding as a result of a damaged blood vessel. A nosebleed is a mild hemorrhage. Rapid, heavy bleeding may cause shock; slow continuous bleeding may cause anemia.

See also BLEEDING: FIRST AID.

Hemorrhage, cerebral (hem′ə rij, ser′ə brəl). Cerebral hemorrhage is internal bleeding caused by the bursting of a blood vessel within the brain. This causes bleeding into the brain matter and damage to the surrounding tissue. A cerebral hemorrhage is a life-threatening disorder and may cause either partial or complete paralysis. Most such hemorrhages result from either the rupture of a hardened artery, as may be associated with hypertension, or from trauma to the cranial region.

See also STROKE.

Hemorrhage: first aid. *See* BLEEDING: FIRST AID.

Hemorrhage, postpartum (hem′ə rij, pōst par′təm). Postpartum hemorrhage is vaginal bleeding after childbirth, usually involving the loss of more than 17 fluid ounces (500ml) of blood during or after the third stage of labor. It is second only to infection as a cause of maternal mortality. The greatest chance for hemorrhaging is during the first hour after childbirth. The bleeding may be caused by prolonged labor, relaxant anesthesia, multiple births, or extreme distention (stretching) of the uterus. Uterine atonia (poor muscle contraction of the uterus) is a common cause of extensive bleeding following childbirth. This occurs more frequently in mothers who have borne several infants. With proper care before, during, and after delivery, postpartum hemorrhaging is usually preventable.

Hemorrhage, subarachnoid (hem′ə rij, sub ə rak′noid). Subarachnoid hemorrhage is bleeding into the space between the membranes that surround the brain. Cerebrospinal fluid circulates through this space. It most commonly occurs in people between the ages of 25 and 50 and is frequently caused by the spontaneous bursting of a blood vessel that was abnormally weak at birth or ruptured due to trauma. In the older age group, subarachnoid hemorrhage may occur when arteriosclerosis causes damage to an artery, or it may be associated with a bleeding disorder.

Q: *What are the symptoms of a subarachnoid hemorrhage?*

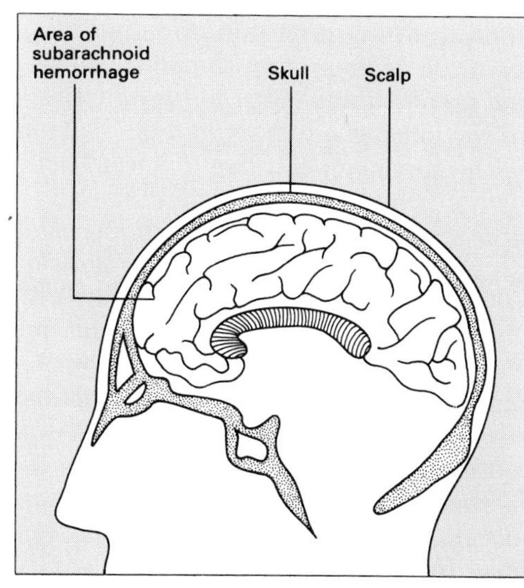

A subarachnoid hemorrhage is bleeding into the space between the membranes that surround the brain. This is usually caused by the spontaneous bursting of a blood vessel that was abnormally weak or ruptured due to trauma.

A: Most patients have a sudden and severe headache. There may also be a temporary or prolonged loss of consciousness. After the patient recovers consciousness, he or she is confused and may vomit or have convulsions. Temporary weakness of the muscles may follow or complete paralysis of one side of the body. Generally, the neck becomes stiff within a few hours.

Q: ***How is subarachnoid hemorrhage treated?***

A: About one-third of all patients die from the initial hemorrhage, and a further 15 to 20 percent die within the next month. It is therefore necessary to locate the area of bleeding as quickly as possible. Neurosurgery may repair the damage.

Hemorrhage, subconjunctival (hem'ə rij, sub kon jùnk tī'vəl). Subconjunctival hemorrhage is bleeding between the conjunctiva (the thin, transparent membrane that covers the outside of the eye) and the sclera (the fibrous tissue that forms the white of the eye). It causes the white of the eye to become red. It most commonly occurs as the result of trauma to the eye or occasionally because of hypertension. Although a subconjunctival hemorrhage usually causes no significant problems, a physician should be consulted, because the bleeding may be the result of some significant underlying disorder or be accompanied by other more serious eye problems.

See also RED EYE.

Hemorrhoid (hem'ə roid), or piles, is a painful mass of distended (swollen) veins in the lining of the anus and rectum, resulting from the formation of varicose veins around the anus. Internal hemorrhoids occur at the junction of the anus and rectum and are covered with mucous membrane. External hemorrhoids occur just outside the anus and are covered with skin. On occasion an internal hemorrhoid may prolapse, or protrude, to the outside, cutting off the blood supply. A number of treatments are available for internal hemmoroids. External hemorroids must be surgically removed. *See also,* HEMORRHOID: TREATMENT.

Hemorrhoids can occur at any age, often without apparent cause. Causes may include constipation, pregnancy,

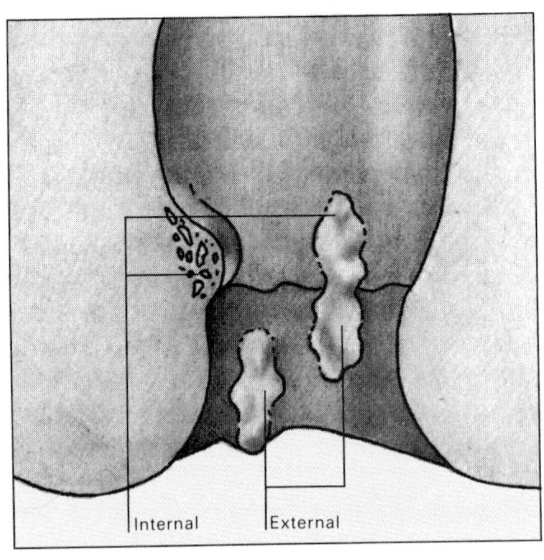

Hemorrhoids occur in the lining of the rectum and the anus. Internal hemorrhoids are covered by mucous membrane. External hemorrhoids are covered by anal skin.

liver disorders, rectal tumors, and the repeated use of laxatives. Hemorrhoids can cause itching and burning and may bleed during a bowel movement.

Hemorrhoids do not cause cancer nor do they become cancerous. But any rectal bleeding may be a sign of cancer of the colon or rectum and should be checked by a physician.

Hemorrhoidal preparations (hem ə roi'dəl prep ə rā'shenz) are substances, generally ointments and creams, that have a soothing or cleansing action on hemorrhoids (piles). Hemorrhoidal preparations act to shrink the hemorrhoids, thereby easing the irritation.

See also HEMMORRHOID: TREATMENT.

Hemorrhoid: treatment. Temporary relief from hemorrhoids may be obtained by applying a cold compress directly to the affected area until the pain subsides. This is most easily done if the patient lies face-down and another person applies the compress. Tepid water baths may also help. A person should eat a high-roughage diet to ensure regular defecation of large, soft stools. Ointments, creams, and suppositories containing corticosteroids may also ease the symptoms.

All cases of rectal bleeding should be examined by a physician to rule out cancer of the colon and rectum. If the diagnosis is hemorrhoids, the remedies mentioned above may solve the problem. However, persistent hemorrhoids may need to be removed, using one of several methods. The hemorrhoid may be frozen off during cryosurgery; hardened, using a sclerosing agent; tied off, using a rubber band at the base of the hemorrhoid; or removed surgically (hemorrhoidectomy).

Hemothorax (hē mə thôr'aks) is the accumulation of blood in the pleural cavity, the space between the lungs and the chest wall. The blood may be removed with a special syringe and needle, or a surgical operation (thoracotomy) may be necessary.

See also PARACENTESIS; PLEURA.

Heparin (hep'ər rin) is an anticoagulant substance found in the liver, lungs, and other tissues. A heparin preparation produced from animal tissues may be injected into a patient during surgery in order to prevent thrombosis (blood clotting). Bleeding, which is the most common adverse reaction, does not usually occur with the amount of dosage effective in preventing thrombosis.

See also ANTICOAGULANT.

Hepatic (hi pat'ik) is the medical term for anything concerning the liver.

See also LIVER.

Hepatitis (hep ə tī'tis) is inflammation of the liver, either acute or chronic. The most common cause of hepatitis in the United States is one of the four hepatitis viruses: the A virus, B virus, non-A non-B virus, or the D virus. Other common causes include alcohol abuse, use of certain chemicals and drugs, and autoimmune disorders. Such infections as amebic dysentery and malaria may also inflame the liver.

Q: *What are the symptoms of acute hepatitis?*

A: Initially, the person experiences a low fever, nausea, abdominal pain, and a loss of appetite. Many causes of hepatitis are accompanied by jaundice. The skin and whites of the eyes turn yellow, and the urine is dark-colored. The person often feels somewhat better once the jaundice appears, but may still feel weak and tired. The jaundice may last from one to four weeks.

The symptoms of all forms of viral hepatitis are similar. However, the symptoms of hepatitis caused by virus B take longer to develop, generally last longer, and are more severe. Viral hepatitis can be fatal. All types, except that caused by virus A, can become chronic.

Q: *How is acute hepatitis transmitted?*

A: The viruses are transmitted in different ways. Virus A is contracted by drinking water or eating food contaminated by the feces of an infected person. Virus B, virus non-A non-B, and virus D are usually spread by blood products or by contaminated hypodermic needles shared by drug users. These viruses are also spread by sexual contact.

Q: *How is acute hepatitis treated?*

A: In the initial stages, treatment involves bed rest. After the acute state has passed, the patient can gradually resume normal activities. The patient need not be totally isolated. The specific precautions to be taken depend on the type of hepatitis. For hepatitis A, it is essential that feces and urine are carefully disposed of. For type B, type non-A non-B, and type D, it is necessary to avoid contamination by blood or other body fluids. For persons who have been in close and prolonged contact with a patient with hepatitis A, injections of gamma globulin may be given. *See also* GAMMA GLOBULIN.

A vaccine to immunize against hepatitis B is now available and recommended for those persons at high risk for the disease, including homosexual men, people who need frequent blood transfusions, and some health care workers. A hepatitis A vaccine is being developed.

Q: *What are the symptoms of chronic hepatitis?*

A: Chronic hepatitis (liver inflammation lasting six months or longer) is accompanied by persistent nausea, fatigue, and jaundice. The condition may be mild or lead to cirrhosis and cancer of the liver.

Q: *How does alcohol cause hepatitis?*

A: Because of the toxic effects of alcohol on the liver, frequent use of large quantities of alcohol can result in inflammation of the liver. If left untreated, alcoholic hepatitis may lead to cirrhosis and eventually to liver failure, which has a high mortality rate.

Heredity (hə red'ə tē) is the transmission of mental and physical characteristics from parents to their children, and also the total genetic constitution of any individual. The basic unit of heredity is a gene, which occupies a specific location on strands called chromosomes in the nuclei of every cell in the body. The billions of different genes in the body (perhaps 500 per chromosome) each carry the instructions for one specific characteristic, such as the formation of hemoglobin in the red blood cells. Sometimes, the effects of several genes together determine a single characteristic. It is thought, for example, that three or four genes contribute to the determination of eye color.

Q: *What is a chromosome?*

A: A chromosome is a collection of genes in which each gene occupies a specific position on the strand. Every chromosome consists of a double strand of deoxyribonucleic acid (DNA), arranged in a helical shape. The nucleus of every body cell contains 46 chromosomes arranged in 23 pairs. In a cell that divides to form the sex cells (ovum and sperm), the number of chromosomes is halved, so that each sex cell contains only 23 chromosomes.

At fertilization the sex cells fuse. The 23 chromosomes from the egg unite with the 23 chromosomes from the sperm to form the embryo with 23 pairs of chromosomes. Hereditary characteristics are those contributed by the mother and by the father. One pair of chromosomes are the sex chromosomes, determining the sex of the new embroyo. In males one of these chromosomes is a shorter strand than the other. This short chromosome is called a Y chromosome and contains fewer genes; the longer chromosome is called an X chromosome. Males have XY sex chromosomes, and females have XX sex chromosomes.

Q: *What is sex-linked inheritance?*

A: Sex-linked inheritance is the transmission of a characteristic by genes on the sex chromosomes. Because the X chromosome is longer than the Y chromosome, not all of the genes in the sex chromosome are paired. Unpaired genes on the X chromosome exert their influence, even if they are recessive, because there is no corresponding gene to modify their effects. For example, the gene for hemophilia is recessive and is carried on the X chromosome. Therefore, hemophilia occurs almost always in men because there is no corresponding gene on the Y chromosome. There are only a very few sex-linked characteristics that are carried in the Y chromosome.

Q: *Are genes always inherited in an unaltered form?*

A: No. There may be a fault in the replication of the sex cells within the parents so that one or more genes in them differ from the genes in the rest of the body. This may result in a child who has characteristics that neither parent possessed.

Q: *Can inherited disorders be predicted before birth?*

A: Prediction of some inherited disorders is possible. Through genetic counseling, parents may be advised on the probability of a recurrent, inherited disorder if one has occurred in a previous child or in either of the parent's families. If a pregnancy has started, sampling of the amniotic fluid (amniocentesis) and testing the blood for alphafetoprotein may reveal any of a number of disorders.

See also AMNIOCENTESIS; GENETIC COUNSELING.

Hermaphrodite (hėr maf′rə dīt) is a person with both male and female organs. A true hermaphrodite often has sex chromosomes that are male in the testicular part of the sex glands and female in the ovarian part. This condition is rare in human beings; pseudohermaphroditism is more common. For example, a male may have the breasts of a female and a tiny penis, or a female may develop male characteristics. Such a condition is also termed intersex.

Q: *What may make a male appear female?*

A: This rare condition may be caused by a malfunction of the adrenal glands, triggering the production of excessive amounts of certain female sex hormones. Males with this condition may appear female with breasts, vagina, and vulva,

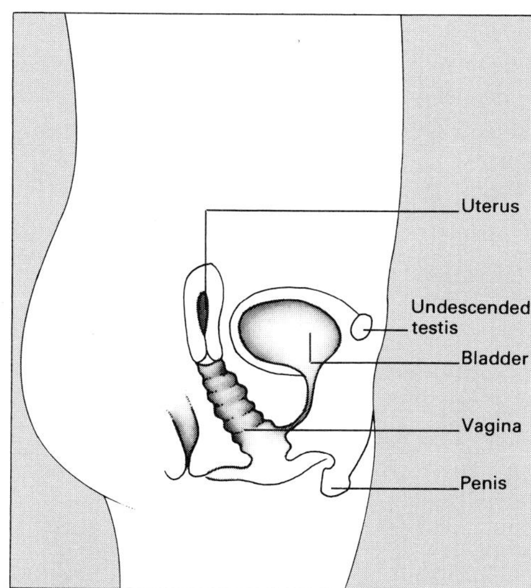

A **hermaphrodite** is a person with both female and male reproductive organs. The condition is very rare.

but no uterus. A male may also appear female because of an inherited disorder that makes the body fail to respond to the male sex hormone testosterone.

Q: *What condition may make a female appear male?*

A: In some girls, an adrenal gland malfunction may cause the development of male secondary sex characteristics (virilism), with hair growth in unusual places (hirsutism) and voice changes. It is more usual for females to develop male characteristics than for males to develop female ones.

Q: *If there is doubt about a baby's sex, what should be done?*

A: Sex must be determined as early as possible. The sex of a baby can be determined by examination of the chromosomes, usually in cells from inside the mouth and from blood lymphocytes, as well as by measurement of hormone levels in the urine and special tests to examine the vagina.

Hernia (hėr′nē ə), or rupture, is a protrusion of some tissue or organ of the body from its normal position through a wall of the cavity that contains it. It is usually caused by straining the abdominal muscles and often occurs when lifting a heavy object or exercising strenuously. A hernia may occur internally, as in a hiatus hernia, in which the stomach protrudes through the diaphragm muscle into the chest. More commonly, a hernia may manifest externally, such as when the intestine protrudes through a weakness in the abdominal muscles, causing a local swelling.

Q: *Is a hernia dangerous?*

A: Some hernias can be pushed back into the abdomen by a physician and present little danger. If a hernia can not be pushed back, it is termed irreducible. Abdominal pain, pain over the hernia, and vomiting indicate a condition called strangulation. The blood supply within the strangulated hernia is cut off, and the herniated tissue dies unless an emergency operation is performed within a few hours. A femoral hernia on the inside of the upper thigh is most likely to become strangulated because the hole is small and the ligament above the femoral artery is strong and tight.

Q: *What is the treatment for a hernia?*

A: Treatment depends on the site of the hernia. In a baby, an umbilical hernia usually disappears by the age of about four; if it does not, an operation is usually then performed. In older people, an umbilical, inguinal (groin), or femoral hernia, or one occurring in a surgical scar, is best treated with an operation called a hernia repair, which closes the weakness in the abdominal wall. Hernias in the midline of the abdomen seldom need treatment.

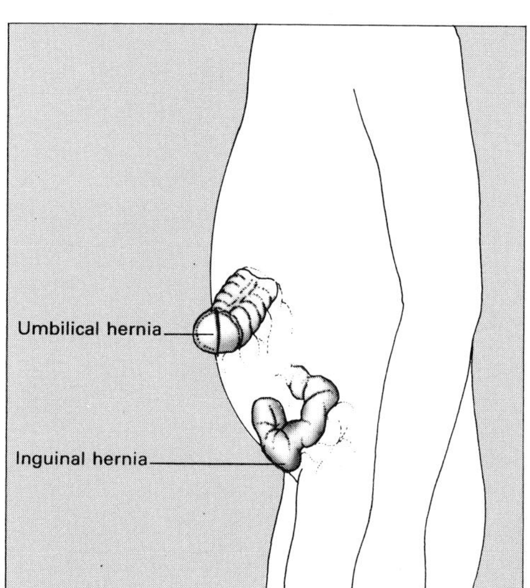

A **hernia** is a protrusion of some organ or tissue through a wall of the cavity that normally contains it. An umbilical hernia is the protrusion of intestine through the umbilicus, or navel. An inguinal hernia is the protrusion of intestine into the inguinal canal. In a male, this type of hernia sometimes fills the scrotal sac.

If the patient is too old or not well enough for an operation, a device called a truss can be worn to keep an inguinal hernia in a reduced position.

See also HERNIA, STRANGULATED: FIRST AID; HIATUS HERNIA.

Hernia, strangulated: first aid. A strangulated (tightly compressed) hernia is a potentially life-threatening disorder in which the protruding part of the intestine becomes twisted or trapped by the abdominal muscles. It is an extremely serious condition because the blood supply to the strangulated tissue is cut off, and the intestine is obstructed.

If the condition goes untreated, the interruption of the blood supply to the strangulated tissue may result in gangrene. A strangulated hernia usually requires an emergency surgical operation to restore an adequate blood supply and to repair the hernia.

In the event of a strangulated hernia, *do not* try to reduce the swelling. Summon emergency medical assistance. While waiting for medical assistance, lay the victim down and elevate the head, shoulders, and knees. If the victim vomits, turn him or her to the recovery position, as described in FAINTING: FIRST AID, in which the victim's head is turned to one side and the air passage is kept clear.

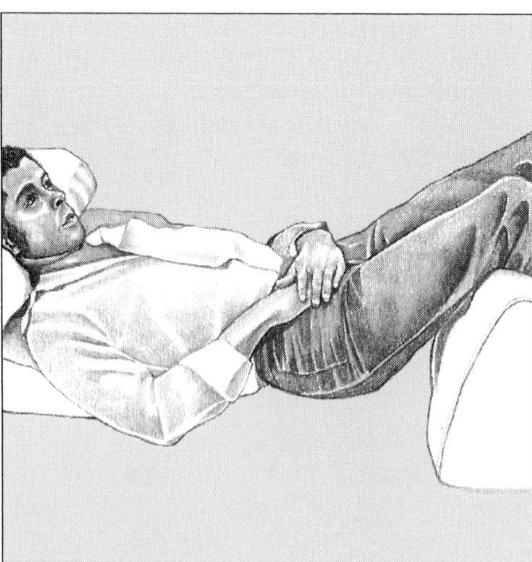

To aid a person suffering from a **strangulated hernia,** lay the victim down and elevate the head, shoulders, and knees. Summon medical aid immediately.

Herniated disk. See DISK, HERNIATED.

Heroin (her'ō in), also called diacetylmorphine, is a highly addictive drug derived from the opium poppy. Heroin is illegal in the United States, but in some countries it is used medically to stop pain in the terminal stages of cancer.

See also DRUG ABUSE.

Herpes genitalis (hėr'pēz jen ə ta'lis) is a viral infection that causes skin lesions on and around the sex organs, mucous membranes, and/or the lips of the mouth. Genital herpes (herpes simplex virus, type II) is related to cold sores (herpes simplex virus, type I) and displays similar characteristics, small blisters that eventually rupture into superficial, rounded, red ulcers. Although painful, the ulcers crust over and heal in a few days, leaving scars. At this point the virus retreats to clusters of nerve cells near the spinal cord and enters a latent stage. This latent stage can last forever or for as short a span as two weeks. When a latent period is over, the virus reinfects the original site, setting off a new round of lesions. *See also* COLD SORE.

Q: *Is genital herpes contagious?*

A: Yes. During an active period when lesions are in evidence, genital herpes is moderately contagious, as well as immediately before lesions appear when there are localized sensations of itching or tingling. It is usually contracted during intimate physical contact.

Q: *How long does it take for symptoms to appear after exposure?*

A: The incubation period is approximately four to seven days. The early symptoms include itching and soreness on or near the penis, vulva, thighs, buttocks, or mouth.

Q: *How is genital herpes diagnosed?*

A: A physician can usually diagnose herpes by examining the blisters or lesions. Diagnosis can be confirmed by taking serum from ulcerated lesions and growing tissue cultures.

Q: *Can genital herpes be cured?*

A: There is no known cure, but the antiviral drug acyclovir seems to shorten the periodic outbreaks without preventing their recurrence. While the connection is not clear, there is a definite increase in the risk of cervical cancer in women who have had genital herpes. Herpes victims should be careful to avoid infecting other individuals. Expectant mothers should inform their physicians of the condition. Newborns, for whom the infection can be fatal, may be exposed to herpes during the passage down the birth canal. Therefore, the physician may recommend a Cesarean section delivery to protect the infant from the herpes virus.

Herpes simplex. *See* COLD SORE.

Herpes zoster. *See* SHINGLES.

Heterograft (het′ər ə graft), or xenograft, is the transplant of tissues from one species to another. This is done usually when there is insufficient tissue available from the patient or other human donors. Performed as a temporary measure, the procedure often results in quick rejection.

See also TRANSPLANT SURGERY.

Hiatus hernia (hī ā′təs hėr′nē ə) is a hernia that occurs when a part of the stomach protrudes upward through the sheet of muscle (diaphragm) that separates the chest cavity from the abdomen. If the hiatus hernia is small, there may be no symptoms. Sometimes, however, the condition can become serious enough to require a major operation.

Q: *What are the symptoms of a hiatus hernia?*

A: A baby with a hiatus hernia frequently regurgitates food, which may be bloodstained. The baby may also have difficulty in breathing and swallowing.

In an adult, a typical symptom is heartburn, especially when bending forward or lying down. The pain may spread to the jaw and down the arms, similar to an attack of angina pectoris. Other symptoms include hiccups, a dry cough, regurgitation, and more forceful heartbeat.

Q: *How is a hiatus hernia treated?*

A: If the hernia is present at birth, the defect usually corrects itself. Until this occurs, the baby should sleep in a crib with the head raised and be given feedings that are thicker than usual.

An overweight adult patient must lose weight and sleep propped up on a pillow. Antacid preparations can help to relieve heartburn. The patient is generally encouraged to eat a main meal at lunchtime and have a light supper, with no food being consumed after supper.

If these measures fail to bring adequate relief or if the symptoms worsen, drugs may be used to decrease the amount of acid in the stomach or to prevent the acid from moving upward into the esophagus. Rarely, corrective surgery may be necessary.

See also HERNIA; HISTAMINE H_2-RECEPTOR ANTAGONISTS.

H.i.B. vaccine (vak′sēn) is a childhood vaccine introduced in the United States in 1986. H.i.B. stands for the bacteria *Hemophilus influenzae,* type B. Non-type B *Hemophilus* species are found in the upper airways of most children and are frequent causes of ear infections and pneumonia in infants and young children. Unfortunately, the vaccine does not protect against most of these species.

H.i.B. vaccine is, however, effective against the type of *Hemophilus* that is a common cause of severe childhood meningitis, as well as epiglottitis. Thus, all children should be given the vaccine in a single dosage at the age of two years. If a child attends day-care, where spread of these diseases is more common, the vaccine should be given at the age of 18 months. There are rarely any side effects.

See also EPIGLOTTITIS; MENINGITIS; VACCINE.

Hiccups (hik′upz) are an abrupt, involuntary intake of air caused by a spasm of the diaphragm. This spasm pulls air into the lungs through the larynx (voice box). The larynx is flanked by the vocal cords and topped by the epiglottis, a movable cap that keeps food from getting into the air passages. The epiglottis closes over the larynx when the diaphragm suddenly contracts. When the spasm of the diaphragm pulls air into the larynx, the air forcibly strikes the closed epiglottis and causes a movement of the vocal cords. These actions result in the *hic* sound that is made.

Hiccups may occur several times in a minute or even two or three times each second. They normally last for several minutes. Hiccups are rarely serious. They may be caused by overeating, minor stomach disorders, excessive drinking, or emotional stress.

Hiccups that persist for hours or days may be a symptom of a more serious disorder, such as a brain lesion, a tumor in the chest cavity, various intestinal diseases, kidney or liver disease, or uremia. These causes are all comparatively rare and in such cases there are usually other symptoms. However, if the hiccups last for many days, there is a risk of death from exhaustion.

If hiccups are persistent or occur frequently, a physician should be consulted. The physician may prescribe tranquilizers or, in extremely rare cases, recommend a surgical operation on the nerve that serves the diaphragm.

See also DIAPHRAGM (RESPIRATION); HICCUPS: TREATMENT.

Hiccups: treatment. Most of the remedies for occasional bouts of hiccups are based on the principle of altering the flow of air passing through the larynx. People can often stop ordinary hiccups by breathing deeply or by holding their breath for a short period of time. Some people prefer to stop hiccups by breathing rapidly into a paper bag. *Do not* use a plastic bag. Hiccups may also disappear spontaneously.

High blood pressure. *See* HYPERTENSION.

Hiking safety. Never set out on a hike alone. On day trips, travel with at least one companion. If the planned hike takes the party more than five hours away from habitation on any part of the route, travel with three companions. Plan the route carefully from maps and guidebooks. A person not going on the hike should be given a copy of the intended route and the estimated time the party expects to arrive at a given point. Do not stray from the plan, and let the same person know when the party is back safely. Make a note of mountain rescue posts, ranger stations, and telephone boxes that are accessible should an emergency arise. The itinerary should be within the capabilities of the slowest and least experienced of the party. Do not plan anything that puts an inexperienced walker at risk. Check the weather forecast before leaving. On the route, check weather forecasts for individual mountains. Weather conditions at the top of a mountain are often displayed on notice boards at the beginning of well-used routes. Make sure that the walk can be completed within daylight hours. Be prepared to turn back if the weather worsens.

Equipment. Make sure that the backpacks for the hike are completely waterproof. Check that the frame sits easily on the back of the person carrying it and is properly adjusted. Pack essentials, such as enough spare, dry clothing, before packing luxuries. A survival kit must be carried by each member of the hiking party. It should be lightweight and compact, and each item should satisfy one of the basic needs of first aid, shelter, signals, or fire. The kit should contain a map and compass; a signalling device (a whistle or metal mirror); matches or other fire-starting materials; a nylon rope; and a waterproof first-aid kit. The first-aid kit should include at least one elastic bandage; sterile cotton; small scissors; tweezers; a triangular bandage; gauze bandage pads in individually sealed envelopes; safety pins; antiseptic and anti-infective ointment; soap; a snakebite kit; an adequate supply of antidiarrhea medicine; lip salve; aspirin or acetaminophen; commercial antihistamine tablets; and water-sterilizing tablets. Each member of the party should carry adhesive bandages to deal with minor cuts and blisters. Each person must carry enough water for the trip. There should be at least one flashlight, a spare battery, and a spare bulb carried by the hiking party. Emergency food should include chocolate, dried fruit, glucose (dextrose), and salt. A bag of nuts, raisins, and small candies can provide nourishing snacks during the hike.

During the Hike. The pace of the hike should match the walking rate of the slowest member of the party. If one member begins to lag behind, let that person at once take the lead. Rather than one large meal halfway through the day, it is advisable to take a few small meals and to drink small amounts frequently. An overfull stomach slows down walking. Walk rhythmically to conserve energy. If one member of the party has to stop for any reason, do not walk on, expecting that person to catch up, because he or she may get into difficulty and need help.

General Accident Procedure. If a member of a party of four or more is involved in an accident that prevents further travel, two people should go in search of help. One person must stay

Hiking Equipment

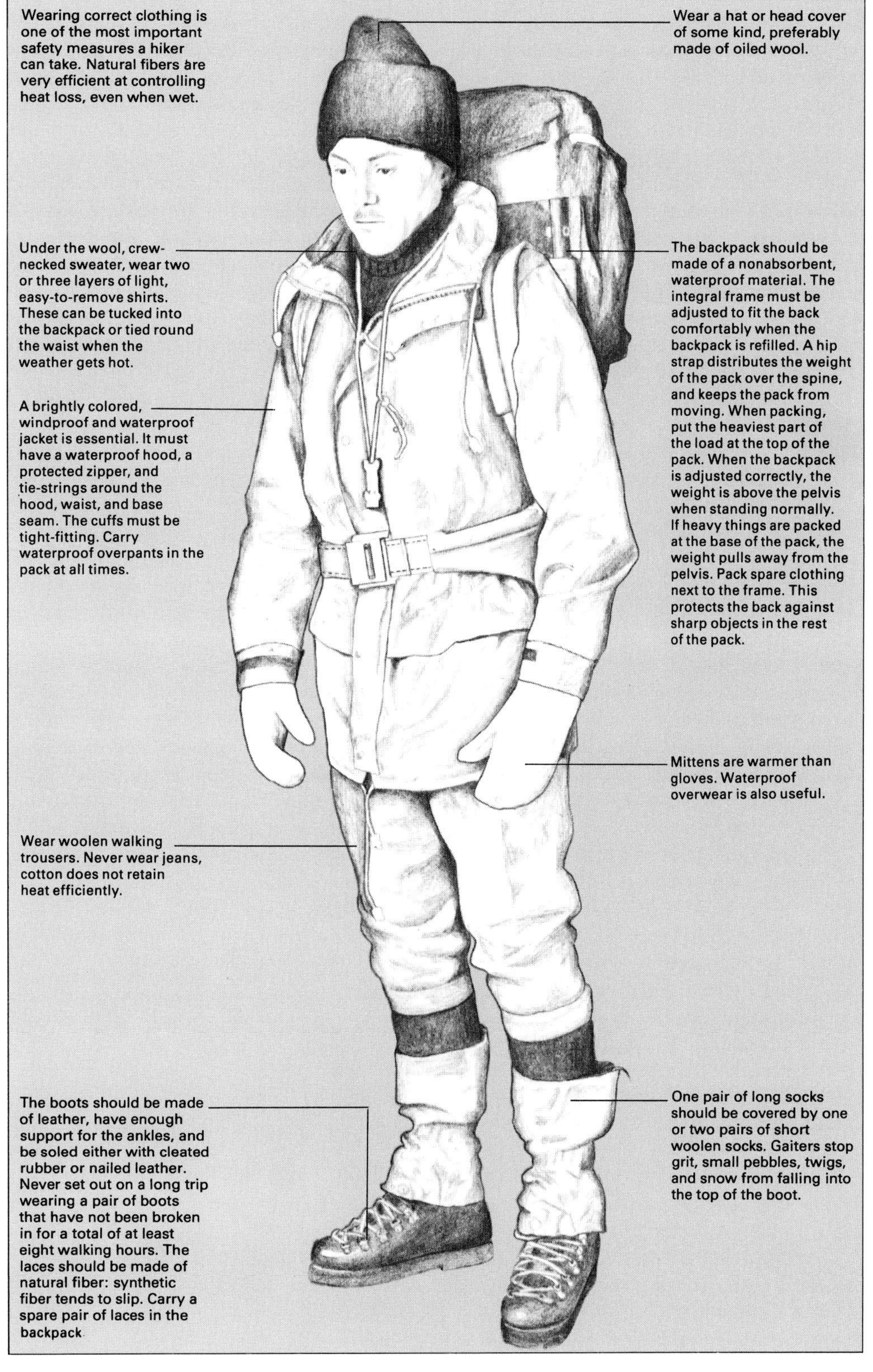
Wearing correct clothing is one of the most important safety measures a hiker can take. Natural fibers are very efficient at controlling heat loss, even when wet.
Wear a hat or head cover of some kind, preferably made of oiled wool.
Under the wool, crew-necked sweater, wear two or three layers of light, easy-to-remove shirts. These can be tucked into the backpack or tied round the waist when the weather gets hot.
The backpack should be made of a nonabsorbent, waterproof material. The integral frame must be adjusted to fit the back comfortably when the backpack is refilled. A hip strap distributes the weight of the pack over the spine, and keeps the pack from moving. When packing, put the heaviest part of the load at the top of the pack. When the backpack is adjusted correctly, the weight is above the pelvis when standing normally. If heavy things are packed at the base of the pack, the weight pulls away from the pelvis. Pack spare clothing next to the frame. This protects the back against sharp objects in the rest of the pack.
A brightly colored, windproof and waterproof jacket is essential. It must have a waterproof hood, a protected zipper, and tie-strings around the hood, waist, and base seam. The cuffs must be tight-fitting. Carry waterproof overpants in the pack at all times.
Mittens are warmer than gloves. Waterproof overwear is also useful.
Wear woolen walking trousers. Never wear jeans, cotton does not retain heat efficiently.
The boots should be made of leather, have enough support for the ankles, and be soled either with cleated rubber or nailed leather. Never set out on a long trip wearing a pair of boots that have not been broken in for a total of at least eight walking hours. The laces should be made of natural fiber: synthetic fiber tends to slip. Carry a spare pair of laces in the backpack
One pair of long socks should be covered by one or two pairs of short woolen socks. Gaiters stop grit, small pebbles, twigs, and snow from falling into the top of the boot.

with the injured person, marking the site of the accident carefully. If possible, the injured person should be moved to a sheltered spot. If this is not possible, erect a temporary shelter around him or her. This can be made from branches, a pile of backpacks, or a bank of snow. Place plastic, waterproof clothing under the injured person for protection from the damp ground. Try to keep his or her morale high until help arrives.

Hypothermia. This is a condition in which core body temperature falls suddenly below its normal level of 98.6°F (37°C). It is the most dangerous condition a hiker is likely to face and can occur under the most unexpected circumstances, even on "warm" days (60-70°F), if there is a strong wind and the hiker's clothing is wet. Hypothermia is caused by a combination of conditions: cold, wind, precipitation, hunger, and fatigue.

The most dangerous aspect of the condition is that the victim may not be aware of the danger, and nobody else may realize a person is affected until the symptoms become obvious. These symptoms include uncontrollable shivering, slurred speech, stumbling, and drowsiness. If left untreated, hypothermia may lead to death.

The treatment for hypothermia is to try to gradually rewarm the victim's whole body. Carefully remove wet, frozen, or restrictive clothing, and wrap the victim in layers of dry, warm clothing. Administer a warm, nonalcoholic, noncaffeinated drink. In acute cases, where hospitalization may be necessary, a healthy member of the hiking party should seek medical aid. Unless necessary for safety, avoid moving the victim.

To help prevent hypothermia, wear windproof, woollen clothing; wool provides better insulation than other fabrics. Wear loose garments that do not restrict blood circulation. Several layers of light clothing are better than one, heavy layer. If clothes get wet, change into dry clothing. Keep hands, head, and feet covered because they are most susceptible to heat loss.

See also HYPOTHERMIA: TREATMENT.

Hinge joint. *See* JOINT.

Hip is the part of the body at the widest portion of the pelvis, where the legs join the torso. The hip joint at the top of the leg is capable of movement in many directions. It is a ball-and-socket joint in which the ball at the end of the thighbone (femur) fits into a socket in the pelvis. The hip joint is supported by strong ligaments and is extremely secure.

Q: *What disorders can affect the hip?*

A: Congenital dislocation of the hip joint occurs spontaneously at, or soon after, birth. It may be caused by an inherited weakness, a breech birth, or a weakening of the ligaments about the joint. If diagnosed at birth, the dislocation can be treated with a splint.

Fractures of the neck of the femur occur commonly in the elderly. Surgical procedures either pin the bones together or replace the head of the femur with a metal head that fits into the hip joint.

The hip may also be involved in rheumatoid arthritis or osteoarthritis, or it may become infected, causing pyogenic arthritis.

Q: *How is arthritis of the hip treated?*

A: If treatment with drugs is not successful, various surgical operations can be performed. The most successful is total replacement of the joint with an artificial one made of metal or plastic and metal.

See also ARTHRITIS, RHEUMATOID; OSTEOARTHRITIS.

Hipbone, known medically as the innominate bone, is either of two, wide

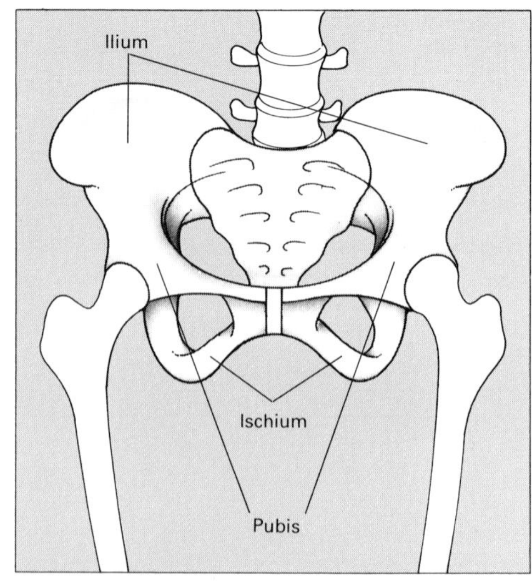

Each half of the **hipbone** consists of three bones fused together, the ilium, the ischium, and the pubis.

irregular bones, each consisting of three consolidated bones, the ilium, ischium, and pubis. The hipbone and the lower backbone together form the pelvis.

See also ILIUM; ISCHIUM; PELVIS; PUBIS.

Hip dysplasia (dis plā'zhə) is dislocation of the hip joint. It occurs when the head of the femur (thighbone) does not properly fit into or pops out of the acetabulum, the cup-shaped socket at the base of the hipbone.

Hip dysplasia can be either congenital or caused by an accident. In the former, the acetabulum is too shallow to hold the head of the femur. Physical therapy can usually deepen the cavity. An accidental hip dislocation is often accompanied by a hip fracture. A splint, traction, and physical therapy are usually effective treatment. A surgical procedure may sometimes be necessary, especially if the patient is an older person.

See also FRACTURE: FIRST AID.

Hip fracture: first aid. *See* FRACTURE: FIRST AID.

Hirschsprung's disease (hirsh' sprəngz), or megacolon, is a congenital defect of the large intestine in which there is an absence of the nerve fibers within certain segments of the intestinal muscles. As a result, the muscles in the affected area do not work, and there is no peristalsis (the rhythmic movement by which the intestine moves its contents along) in the affected section. This acts as an obstruction.

Q: *What are the symptoms of Hirschsprung's disease?*

A: There is usually severe, continuous constipation, and the abdomen becomes increasingly distended (swollen) as the intestine fills with feces. The affected child may vomit, and growth may be retarded.

Q: *How is Hirschsprung's disease treated?*

A: Most cases require a surgical operation in which the abnormal section of the intestine is removed, and the two normal ends joined together.

Hirsutism (hər'süt izm) is the excessive growth of hair or the presence of hair in areas that are not usually hairy. Medical conditions that cause excessive hair growth are usually caused by hormonal disturbances and are much more common in females than in males. An increase in hair may occur after menopause or in patients taking corticosteroid drugs.

See also ELECTROLYSIS.

Histamine (his'tə min) is a chemical that is normally present in tissue mast cells and certain white blood cells (basophils) circulating in the body. Large amounts of histamine are released in response to an injury or in conjunction with an antigen-antibody reaction, such as an allergic reaction.

Histamine causes contraction of pulmonary smooth muscle (bronchoconstriction) that results in an asthma-like disorder. Histamine also dilates small blood vessels and increases their permeability. These actions are responsible for histamine headache and the typical wheal-and-flare allergic skin reaction. Histamine is a potent stimulant of acid secretion in the stomach.

Epinephrine and H_1-receptor blocking antihistamines reverse the actions of histamine on smooth muscles; H_2-receptor blocking antihistamines, such as cimetidine or ranitidine, reverse the gastric acid stimulant action of histamine.

Q: *How can the adverse effects of histamine be treated or prevented?*

A: The most rapidly effective treatment is epinephrine (adrenaline), which is usually given by injection. Antihistamines are better at preventing reactions than treating them and are useful if an allergic reaction, such as hay fever, is expected.

See also ANTIHISTAMINE; EPINEPHRINE.

Histamine headache. *See* HEADACHE, CLUSTER.

Histamine H_2-receptor antagonists (his' tə min) inhibit the production and secretion of stomach acid. There are now a number of H_2-receptor antagonists available including cimetidine (Tagamet®), ranitidine (Zantac®), and nizatidine (Axid®). They are used in the treatment of duodenal and gastric ulcers, pancreatitis, and various other disorders in which too much stomach acid is produced. Possible side effects include dizziness, diarrhea, skin rashes, and muscular pain.

See also PANCREATITIS; ULCER.

Histology (his tol′ə jē) is the study of the microscopic structure of tissues. Pathological histology is the study of diseased tissues.

Histoplasmosis (his tō plaz mō′sis) is an infection caused by the fungus *Histoplasma capsulatum,* which grows in soil enriched with droppings from birds or bats. It is most common in the Mississippi, Missouri, and Ohio river areas. Histoplasmosis originates in the lungs when spores of the fungus are inhaled and may spread in the bloodstream to other parts of the body. Histoplasmosis may be mild or acute or, rarely, progressive and eventually fatal, if untreated. Mild histoplasmosis has no obvious symptoms. The only sign of infection is the presence of calcified spots on the lungs, which can be detected on a chest X ray. The primary acute form of severe histoplasmosis is characterized by a cough, breathlessness, hoarseness, coughing up of blood, and fever. There may also be chills, muscle pains, weight loss, and fatigue. Occasionally, the disease spreads to other parts of the body; this is called progressive disseminated histoplasmosis.

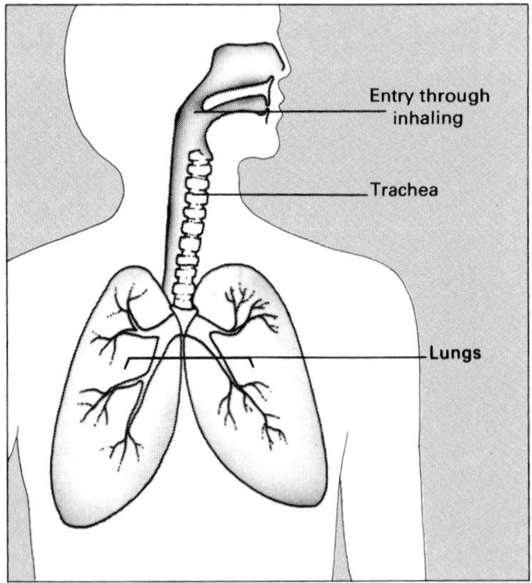

Histoplasmosis is an infection that originates in the lungs after the inhalation of spores from a fungus that grows in soil enriched with bat or bird droppings.

Hives (hīvz) or urticaria, is a condition characterized by red, slightly swollen eruptions or itchy lumps on the skin. The lumps are called angioedema when they occur with excessive swelling of soft tissues.

Q: *What causes hives?*

A: Hives is usually caused by an allergic reaction to an insect bite or sting, a drug, or certain foods, such as shellfish or eggs. Virus and streptococcus bacterial infection also cause hives in some persons; others may inherit a tendency to develop hives.

Q: *What are the symptoms of hives and how is the condition treated?*

A: Itching is usually the first symptom, followed rapidly by the formation of lumps of various sizes, which may appear anywhere on the skin. Hives in the mouth or throat may cause respiratory obstructions and are particularly dangerous.

The individual with hives should be taken immediately to a hospital emergency room. If the throat is involved, injection of epinephrine is urgently required, followed by antihistamine drugs. In most cases, hives lasts for only a few days.

See also ANTIHISTAMINE; EPINEPHRINE.

HMO. *See* HEALTH MAINTENANCE ORGANIZATION.

Hodgkin's disease (häj′kins) is a malignant (cancerous) condition involving the body's lymph nodes. The condition may spread throughout the body to the spleen, liver, and other organs.

As the disease progresses, the patient experiences weight loss, tiredness, and a general feeling of ill health.

Q: *How is Hodgkin's disease treated?*

A: Radiotherapy may be combined with cytotoxic drugs, which may have to be taken for many months. The earlier the diagnosis is made, the more successful is the treatment.

See also CYTOTOXIC DRUG; RADIOTHERAPY.

Holistic medicine (hō lis′tik) is a system of comprehensive patient care that addresses itself to all of the physical, emotional, social, spiritual, and economic needs of the individual. In this system, all factors that may affect an individual's health are taken into account by the holistic practitioner. These include heredity, nutrition, physical activity, stress, family relationships, medical care, spiritual health, and living and working conditions.

Many physicians, nutritionists, and other health care professionals practice holistic medicine, stressing the responsibility of the patient in achieving and maintaining the best possible health.

They help patients establish good eating and exercise habits and may also teach patients various methods of medical self-care. For example, a patient might learn to control a normally involuntary body process, such as the rate of the heartbeat, by means of relaxation techniques or meditation.

The idea of a holistic approach to health is as old as medicine itself. Good medical practice has always included elements of holistic medicine. Its popularity is growing because many people are beginning to realize that the most common noninfectious diseases, including cancer and heart disease, are related to specific life styles and such personal habits as smoking and diet.

The holistic health care field has attracted both legitimate health professionals and those with questionable qualifications. As a result, the consumer, who encounters a holistic program, needs to find out exactly what the program entails and what the qualifications of the director and practitioners are. The consumer should be alert, as always, to potential problems.

Homeopathy (hō mē op′ə thē) is a controversial form of medical treatment, in which disorders are treated by giving the patient minute doses of substances that produce the same symptoms as does the disorder. Most of the substances used in homeopathy are derived from herbs that have been repeatedly diluted in a mixture of alcohol and water, sometimes with a little sugar added. The dilution of the mixture is so great that very little of the original substance remains in the final preparation.

Although this form of treatment was widely used in the nineteenth and early twentieth centuries, it is widely acknowledged today to have no real effect in the treatment of disorders.

Home safety. About one-third of all accidental injuries occur in the home. Household mishaps rank second only to highway accidents as a cause of accidental deaths in the United States.

With planning, the home can be a safe and comfortable environment. Nearly all accidents that occur in and around the home can be prevented by following basic safety rules in the kitchen, bathroom, utility areas, living room, nursery and bedroom, garage, and yard.

The Kitchen. The kitchen is one of the busiest rooms in the house—and can be one of the most dangerous. Climbing and reaching cause many accidents in the kitchen. Never use a chair, table, or a pile of boxes as a ladder. Use a ladder or a stepstool, and if possible, have someone hold it for you. Careful storage reduces awkward climbing and reaching. Keep heavy objects, such as food mixers and roasting pans, on low shelves and lighter items higher up. Keep a fire extinguisher in an accessible place. Make sure mature family members know how to use it. Install childproof locks on the freezer. Keep the kitchen well ventilated.

Make sure the kitchen range is well maintained and is working correctly. Turn it off when not in use. Turn pan handles away from the front of the range, so that they are out of the reach of children, but not over another burner. Use dry hot pads to take hot pans and dishes from the oven; a dishcloth is both ineffective and dangerous. If you spill something on the floor,

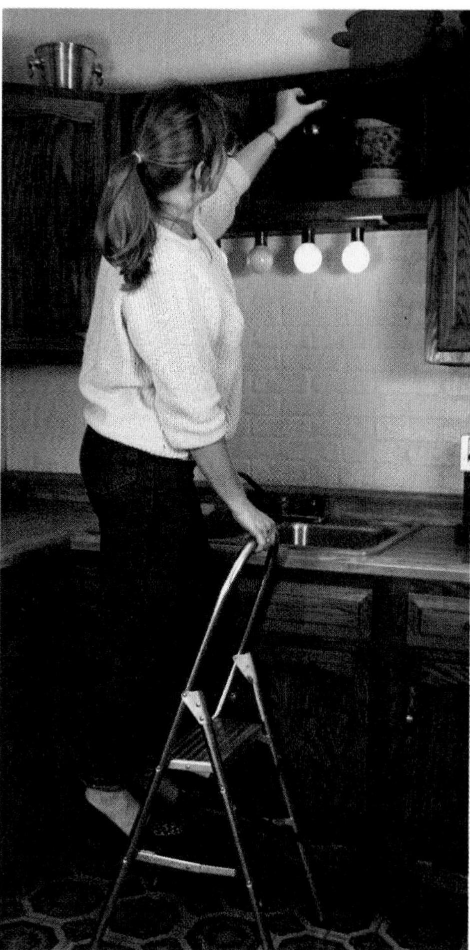

When reaching for an object in the kitchen, use a stable ladder or stepstool.

wipe it up immediately to prevent the floor from becoming slippery. If you use floorwax, buff the wax surface thoroughly, or use a nonskid product to make the floor less slippery.

Keep knives and sharp cooking utensils in a secure drawer. Wrap dangerous refuse, like razor blades, in thick newspaper before throwing away.

Keep bleaches, disinfectants, and scouring powders in a high cupboard. Never store them next to fruit drink bottles, in which case even an adult could mistakenly drink them. Store china, glass, and plastic bags in a high cabinet or cupboard. Keep pots and pans and other unbreakables in the lower cupboards. If the highest shelves are difficult for an adult to reach, keep a sturdy kitchen stepstool on hand.

With small children in the house, it is essential to keep a play area physically separate from the kitchen, but within view. This eliminates the risk of tripping over a small child or a litter of toys, while you are carrying a hot pan.

Keep potentially harmful materials in a locked cabinet, out of the reach of children.

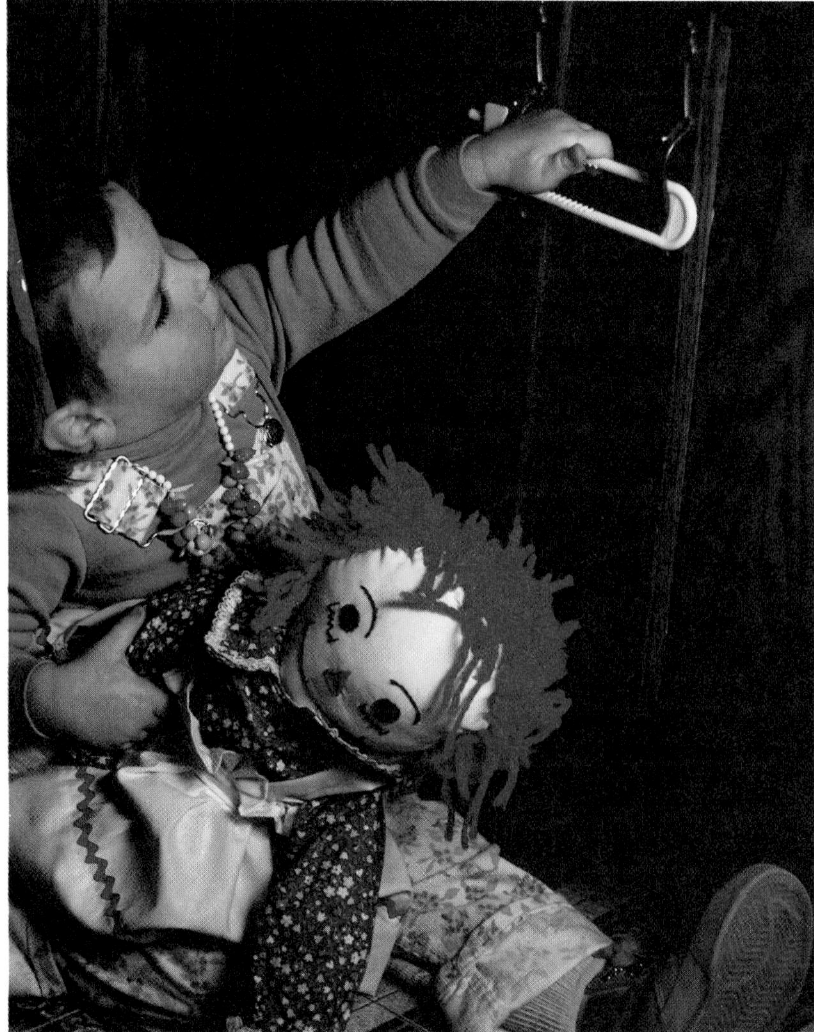

The Bathroom. Falls are one of the worst accidents in the bathroom. To prevent them, use a rubber mat or adhesive-backed plastic strips, called *appliqués,* in the bathtub or shower stall. Also, install a sturdy handrail on the wall over the tub. Keep soap in a holder to reach it easily and to prevent it from falling underfoot. Use only nonskid bathroom rugs, and wipe up spilled lotions, other liquids, and powders to prevent slipping.

Use a medicine cabinet with a lock so that aspirin and other drugs can be kept away from youngsters. Never tell children that medicine tastes like candy. Whenever you take medication, read the label carefully to be certain of the instructions. Never take drugs in the dark or take medicine prescribed for someone else. Throw out old medicines, but not where children might find them. In addition, such cleaning products as bleaches and drain cleaners should be stored in a locked cabinet to keep them away from children.

Dry your hands thoroughly before using a hairdrier or any other electric appliance. Water is a conductor of electricity, and you could be electrocuted by touching anything electrical while your hands or feet are wet. If you listen to a radio while taking a bath, use a battery-powered model and keep it well away from the water. A plugged-in radio could eletrocute you, if the radio fell into the water or if you touched it with wet hands.

Keep the bathroom well ventilated. If the room needs extra heat, have a heater installed by a professional. It should be high on the wall or ceiling, away from the bathtub or sink, and have a wall-mounted switch. Never bring a portable heater into a bathroom. Heated towel rails must be cool enough not to burn the skin if touched accidentally.

At bathtime, run cold water into the bath first. This way, if a child steps into the tub without the temperature having been first checked by hand, he or she will not be scalded.

Never leave a small child in the bath alone; a child can drown in two or three inches of water. If the doorbell or telephone rings, take the child with you, or ignore the call. Avoid leaving a small child in the bath with an older child in the bathroom. The older child could accidentally turn on the hot water and scald the younger.

Utility Areas. Safety in the utility areas depends largely on the careful use of such dangerous items as power tools, appliances, and poisonous chemicals. The chemicals, which include cleaning products, paint thinner, and insecticides, should be kept in containers that have a childproof lid or cap. Store all hazardous items in a locked cabinet so that children can not get at them.

Do-it-yourself projects can be dangerous. Select your tools carefully, handle them with caution, and clean up thoroughly after you finish working. Dress properly when you work with power tools. For example, wear shoes instead of sandals. Tuck in your shirttails, and remove any ring, watch, or other jewelry that might get caught in the tool. Use safety glasses and a dust mask when sanding or grinding. Do not use power tools if you are tired or upset. Never leave a tool plugged in if children are present.

Dispose of an old freezer or refrigerator if it is not being used—or at least remove the door. A child might use the appliance as a hiding place, become trapped inside, and suffocate.

The Living Room. All fireplaces must be protected by a firescreen that covers the entire opening. People should be discouraged from reaching over the opening or standing too close to it. Do not place combustible furnishings near the fireplace opening.

Make sure the bottom shelf of a set of shelves is high enough to prevent a small child from using it as a ladder. Keep sewing and knitting materials out of the reach of children. Cigarettes must also be kept out of a child's reach; a small child can be poisoned by eating one cigarette. Remove tablecloths and mats from the table; a child may pull the contents of the table on top of himself or herself.

Inspect all toys carefully for small detachable parts and for sharp edges. Be careful that a younger child does not get hold of a toy designed for an older child; for example, a marble or a small piece of a toy construction set. Some television sets get very hot and are potential fire hazards. They must stand on a firm base to prevent them from being knocked over. Always turn the set off before leaving the room. Make sure the set is clear of drapes and other furnishings.

The Nursery and Bedroom. The crib in the nursery must have high sides and be stable. Make sure that between the sides and the mattress there is no gap in which a child could get trapped. A child under the age of one does not need a pillow. It is dangerous to provide one for an infant because he or she may roll over onto the pillow and accidentally suffocate. You may warm the baby's crib with a hot water bottle, but remove it before putting the baby to bed. Use a hot water bottle with a thick cover and a button-down flap over the metal stopper.

If older children sleep in bunk beds, the top bed must have a guard rail. Pajamas are safer for children than nightdresses. They are less likely to catch in a heater. Make sure that all night clothes are made of flame-resistant fabric.

Central heating in the bedroom and nursery should be set at a temperature low enough to prevent a burn if the radiator is accidentally touched. Do not hang clothes to dry over a portable heater or place it near curtains.

If you decide to leave some light on at night, never dim a lamp by covering it with anything. Instead, use a low-wattage bulb, or use a low-voltage or battery-operated night light. Cover all plugs with safety covers when not in use. If a child remains fascinated by a

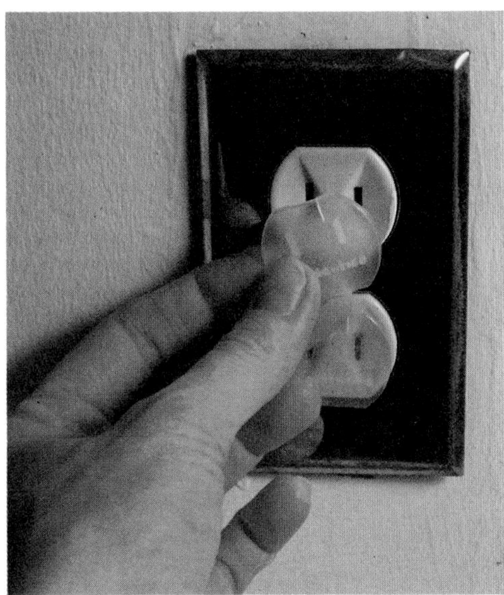

Electrical outlets, especially those within reach of children, should be covered by safety covers when not in use.

plug, move a heavy piece of furniture in front of it.

Never smoke in bed. Falling asleep with a lit cigarette is one of the most frequent causes of bedroom fires. If you use an electric blanket, make sure it is serviced regularly and discard it when electrical parts become worn or broken.

Keep all cosmetics, aerosol containers, and medicines, which must be kept in the bedroom, in a locked drawer or on a high shelf out of the reach of children.

Make sure that carpets or other floor coverings are in good repair. A loose or worn carpet or rug may cause a dangerous fall. Loose rugs on top of a polished floor are particularly hazardous.

The Garage. Keep the garage well ventilated. Never run a car engine inside the garage; poisonous gases may build up. To inspect the underside of a vehicle, it is safer to put it on a ramp than to use a jack. If you use a jack, make sure the handbrake is set and place wedges behind the wheels that are not being raised. Always clean up after each job; wood shavings and oily rags are a fire hazard. Never smoke in the garage. A fire extinguisher should be kept within easy reach, and every member of the family old enough should be taught to use it. Whenever you leave the garage, always lock the doors.

The garage should have its own electric outlet; extension cords should not be strung from the house to the garage. Special care should be taken in a garage to ensure that the electrical system is isolated from any place where water, gasoline, or any other liquid is stored or used. The electric outlet should have its own circuit breaker and be of sufficient voltage to power an electric light plus other garage appliances.

Lock the car door whenever you leave it. A small child could climb in and release the handbrake, start the engine, or get a hand trapped in the door. Take extreme care when backing out of the garage. A small child may be standing behind the car below the level of visibility from the rear-view mirror.

Inside the garage, there should be shelves and hooks on which to store potentially dangerous items out of the reach of children. All bottles and cans of chemicals must be carefully labeled and have tightly fitting lids. Only small quantities of gasoline should be kept and then only in "safety cans" bearing a UL or FM label. Ladders and sharp tools should be secured to prevent them from falling.

The Yard. If you burn waste or have a barbecue in the yard, make sure that the fire or barbecue is situated away from combustible materials. Keep children and pets at a safe distance. Keep a bucket of water or a connected garden hose nearby. Never leave the fire unattended. When you have finished, make sure the fire is extinguished by dousing

How people died in home accidents

Type of accident	*Age in years* 0–4	5–14	15–24	25–44	45–64	65–74	75 and over
All home	1,900	800	1,400	3,500	3,200	2,400	7,300
Falls	130	20	50	300	750	950	3,900
Fires and burns	600	400	300	700	750	450	800
Poisoning by solids and liquids	60	40	400	1,500	600	200	300
Poisoning by gases and vapors	30	30	140	170	140	80	110
Suffocation (ingested object)	300	40	70	140	350	300	800
Suffocation (mechanical)	190	60	40	110	40	40	20
Firearms	40	130	200	250	110	50	20
Drowning	250	30	100	80	60	30	150
All other home	300	50	100	250	400	300	1,200

Statistics are for the year 1985.

it with water. Do not leave a fire to burn itself out.

Keep ornamental paths in good repair, and sweep them regularly. Remove any uneven stepping stones, and relevel the underlying sand before replacing them. Outside steps must be kept clean. They must also be adequately lit and repaired when broken or cracked.

Check fences regularly for holes and gaps, so that young children can not get out, especially if the home is situated near a busy street. Fences should be high enough to prevent small children from climbing over. All gates should have childproof locks and be kept closed. Place swings and other recreational items on the grass. If the grass beneath wears down to dirt, move the position of the equipment.

When using a lawn mower, keep your feet away from the machine and never pull it toward yourself. The mower could run over your foot and gash it. Before mowing, remove stones, pieces of wire, and other small objects from the lawn. The blades of a power mower can hurl such objects like bullets. Never clean the grass chute while the motor of a power mower is running.

Keep your lawn and garden tools in a locked garage or shed. Never leave them lying around where someone might step on them and be hurt. Insecticides and other poisons should be locked in a cabinet or at least placed on a high shelf in the shed or the garage.

If you have a swimming pool, guard it with a fence and a locked gate. Make sure the pool is supervised whenever anyone uses it. People who use the pool should know such safety techniques as how to dive properly and how to use lifesaving equipment. Keep the pool drained or covered during periods when it is not in use.

Safety From Fire. Installing one or more smoke detectors in your home is an important step in preventing injury in the case of a fire. These smoke detectors sound an alarm at the first sign of smoke. It is especially important to have a smoke detector situated so it can be heard from all of the bedrooms. Plan an escape route from each room and hold a home fire drill periodically. All exits must be kept clear at all times. Keep at least one fire extinguisher in the house.

See also FIRE PREVENTION AND CONTROL.

Preventive measures against accidents in the home

Falls

1. Provide adequate lighting for all areas of the house.
2. Install handrails on stairways and in the bathroom.
3. Secure firmly all loose carpets and rugs.
4. Do not leave toys or other small objects lying around on the floor.
5. If there are children in the house, install safety bars at the top and bottom of stairways.
6. Do not allow young children to remain alone near open windows.

Fires and burns

1. Place firescreens around all open fires.
2. Check regularly that all electrical appliances, sockets, plugs, and leads are in good repair.
3. Switch off all electrical appliances when they are not being used.
4. Keep all flammable liquids out of the reach of children.
5. Do not hang clothes or towels to dry over cookers or heaters.
6. Buy children's clothes, especially night clothes, made of flame-resistant fabric.

Poisoning

1. Keep all medicines and other potentially dangerous substances and liquids in locked cabinets.
2. Keep all medicines and tablets in their original containers, clearly labeled.
3. Check the correct dosage for all medicines and tablets before taking them.
4. Destroy or return to the pharmacy all unused medicines and tablets.
5. Check regularly that all gas appliances are in good repair, and make sure that there is good ventilation when using them.

Suffocation

1. Keep all plastic bags inaccessible to children.
2. Check that all blankets in a baby's crib are secure and can not be pulled over the baby's face. Do not allow a young baby to sleep on a soft pillow.
3. Watch over a baby when he or she is feeding, and take appropriate action in case of choking.

Homosexuality (hō mə sek shů al′ə tē) is sexual attraction between persons of the same sex. Gay is the accepted term for homosexual. A gay female is also called a lesbian. Scientists estimate that 10 percent of the adult males in the United States are sexually attracted primarily to members of their own sex. About 5 percent of the adult females are believed to prefer their own sex.

Some people are not entirely homosexual or entirely heterosexual. A person who is sexually attracted to both men and women is called a bisexual.

Q: *Is homosexuality considered a disorder?*

A: In 1973, the American Psychiatric Association removed homosexuality from the list of psychological disorders.

Q: *What causes a person to be homosexual?*

A: Causes of homosexuality are not fully understood. Basic gender and sex-role identities are strongly developed by the time a child is three years old. Whether this development includes sexual orientation is still a matter to be determined.

Q: *Is it possible or desirable to treat homosexuality?*

A: Many homosexual people are happy as they are and would not wish to change even if it were possible. Individuals who feel guilty or embarrassed about being gay can sometimes benefit from discussions with a sex counselor or a psychiatrist.

Q: *How should parents react if they realize that their child is homosexual?*

A: Ideally, parents should be nonjudgmental. Trying to persuade a child to change sexual orientation often produces problems instead of solutions. Denying the child's gayness also creates problems. Feelings must be dealt with, not suppressed. If necessary, some form of individual or family counseling can be helpful.

Hookworm. *See* ANKYLOSTOMIASIS.

Hormone (hôr′mōn) is a powerful chemical substance produced by cells in a particular organ. Hormones then act on other organs to regulate their activity. Several organs produce hormones. For example, the endocrine glands, such as the thyroid gland, produce hormones that are carried in the bloodstream to affect activities in other parts of the body. Other hormones are produced by the gastrointestinal tract and have a more local effect, stimulating the production of digestive juices from adjacent areas of the small intestine.

See also ADRENAL GLANDS; CORPUS LUTEUM; ENDOCRINE GLAND; ENDOCRINE SYSTEM; EXOCRINE GLAND; GRAAFIAN FOLLICLE; OVARY; PARATHYROID GLAND; TESTIS; THYROID GLAND.

Hormone replacement therapy. *See* ESTROGEN REPLACEMENT THERAPY.

Horner's syndrome (hôr′nərz) is a condition that affects one side of the face. The pupil of the eye constricts (myosis); the upper eyelid droops (ptosis); and the eyeball is set deeper into its socket than usual. The skin may be red and lose the ability to sweat on the affected side of the face. Horner's syndrome is caused by paralysis of the sympathetic nervous system in the neck. This condition may result from various rare nervous disorders, occasionally from shingles, or sometimes from nerve compression caused by a tumor in the upper chest.

See also SHINGLES.

Hospice (hos′pis) is a facility and/or a system of health care devoted to the social, physical, emotional, and spiritual support of terminally-ill patients and their families.

Relying on a group approach to ease the physical and psychological pain of the patient's illness, the hospice team includes the patient and his or her family, as well as physicians, nurses, social workers, members of the clergy, and volunteers. The modern system of hospice care began with the founding of St. Christopher's Hospice in London in 1967 by Cicely Saunders, an English physician.

The hospice concept emphasizes home care. Family members are encouraged to participate in caring for the patient. The hospice staff works with the family and with the community agencies to help the patient remain at home. Staff members visit the family regularly and are available at all times for emergencies, trying to provide what the patient and the family need. Such services may include nursing care and pain control, meal preparation, laundry, or shopping. Hospice staff members are also available to sit with the patient while family members rest. After the patient's death, emotional support is provided for the family.

Hospice care is also available to inpatients—that is, patients who can not remain at home. This care may be provided in a separate hospice medical center or in a hospice unit of a hospital. In some cases, a hospice team cares for patients throughout the wards of a general hospital.

Patients are admitted to a hospice program on the basis of health needs, not according to their ability to pay. In the United States, Medicare—a government health insurance program—pays part of the cost of hospice care for elderly patients.

See also DYING, CARE OF THE.

Hospital is an institution that provides medical services. Hospitals can vary greatly in size, from fewer than 100 beds to over 1,000 beds. Every year, approximately 3.6 million patients are cared for in the 7,000 hospitals in the United States. In order to receive a state license for practicing medicine, giving patient care, and conducting education and research, all hospitals must adhere to certain laws and be subject to inspection by state officials. In addition, most hospitals are accredited by the Joint Commission on Accreditation of Hospitals.

If a physician recommends hospitalization, it is better to go to the hospital that he or she recommends, rather than requesting one that is reputed to have better facilities, but where the physician may not be as well-known.

Organization of a Typical Hospital

The basic organization of all hospitals is similar. Within a hospital there are a number of hierarchical divisions of personnel. There are four main divisions: the hospital board; the medical staff; the nursing staff; and the nonmedical staff. The better the cooperation between these groups, the better the care received by the patients.

Hospital Board. The hospital board makes major decisions about the general running of the hospital, such as policy decisions, expansion programs, and fund-raising. The link between the board and the rest of the hospital is usually the chief administrator.

Medical Staff. The medical staff is headed by a chief of staff, who always holds a medical degree, but whose position is administrative. Immediately below the chief of staff are the chiefs of various subdivisions, such as medicine, surgery, and gynecology. Should there be a complaint about a member of the medical staff, it is the responsibility of the department head and finally the chief of staff to take action. *See also* MEDICAL SPECIALISTS.

The resident staff are the most junior members of the hierarchy and are in training in the various medical specialties. They deal with the patient's immediate needs at all times. If a patient needs emergency attention, it is usually a resident who gives the initial treatment. Residents are not in sole charge of a patient but are responsible to more senior and experienced physicians. *See also* RESIDENCY.

Nursing Staff. The nurses are headed by the director of nursing, immediately below whom is the assistant director. Nursing supervisors are responsible for several floors or sections. Head nurses are responsible for individual units and organize the nurses' work on that unit.

Nurses are rated according to the length and quality of their training. An RN is a registered nurse, a rating which is at least equivalent to a college degree; an LPN is a licensed practical nurse, a slightly lower qualification than an RN; and a nursing aide is restricted to performing less skilled procedures. *See also* NURSE, LICENSED PRACTICAL; NURSE, REGISTERED.

Some of the nursing staff are responsible for training nurses and the revision of nursing care. This benefits both the medical staff and patients.

Nonmedical Staff. The nonmedical staff supply the essential auxiliary services, such as cleaning, laundry, food, and the maintenance of complicated medical equipment. The person who is responsible for the day-to-day running of all these services is the chief administrator or executive director. There are also assistant directors and directors of various departments, who are all responsible to the chief administrator.

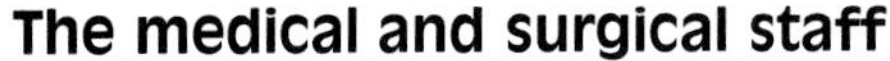

The medical and surgical staff

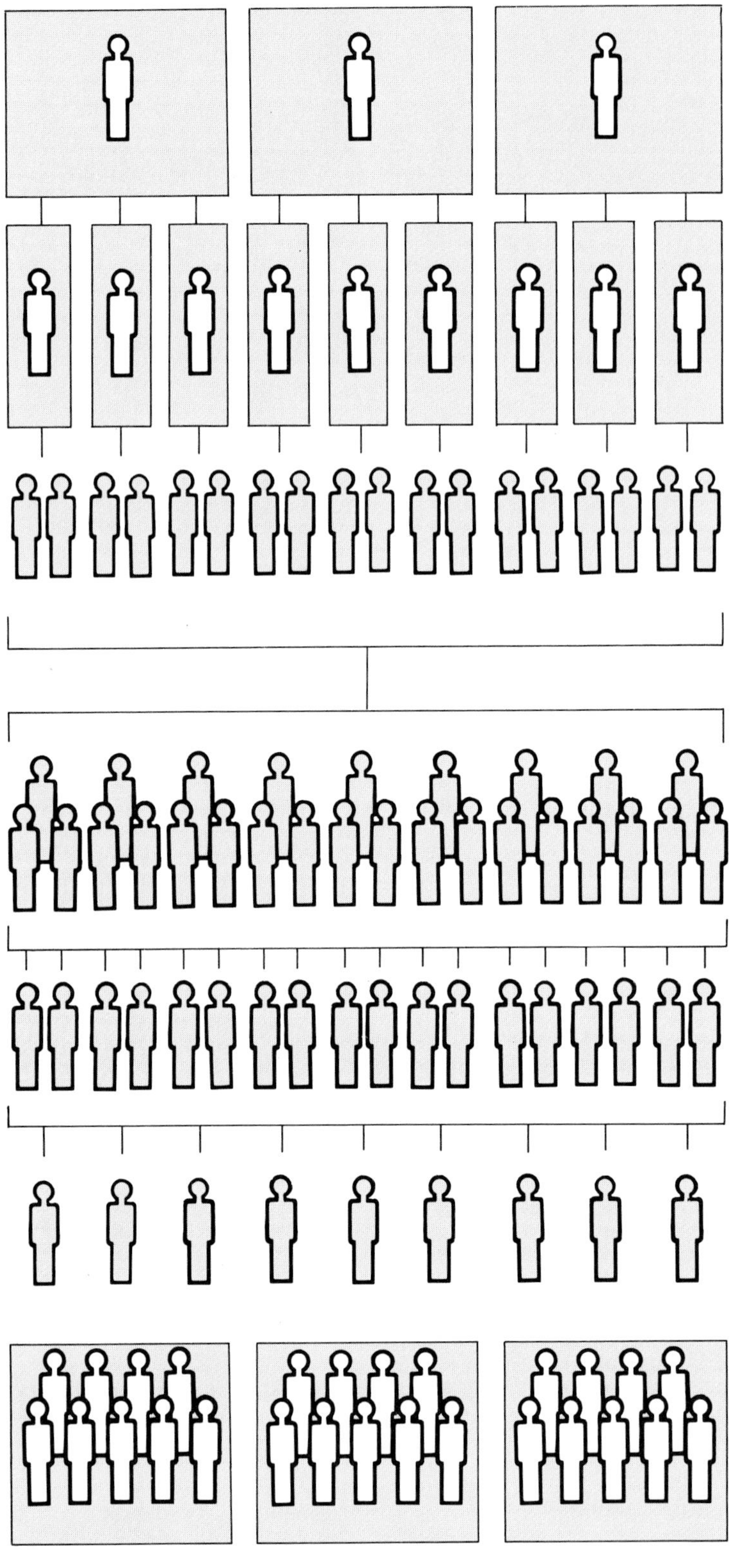

Each department of a general hospital is under the jurisdiction of a chief.

A varying number of attending physicians and surgeons have privileges at many hospitals.

A team of senior residents cares for the patients in the hospital. The team is divided into medical and surgical senior residents.

By the time a physician has reached resident stage, he or she has not yet specialized in a medical or surgical specialty.

First-year residents work long hours at the hospital to gain valuable practical experience.

Each unit has a variable number of medical aides on the team.

Support units such as pharmacy, radiography, and therapy have a structure of their own similar to the general structure, and are comprised mainly of technicians.

The nursing staff

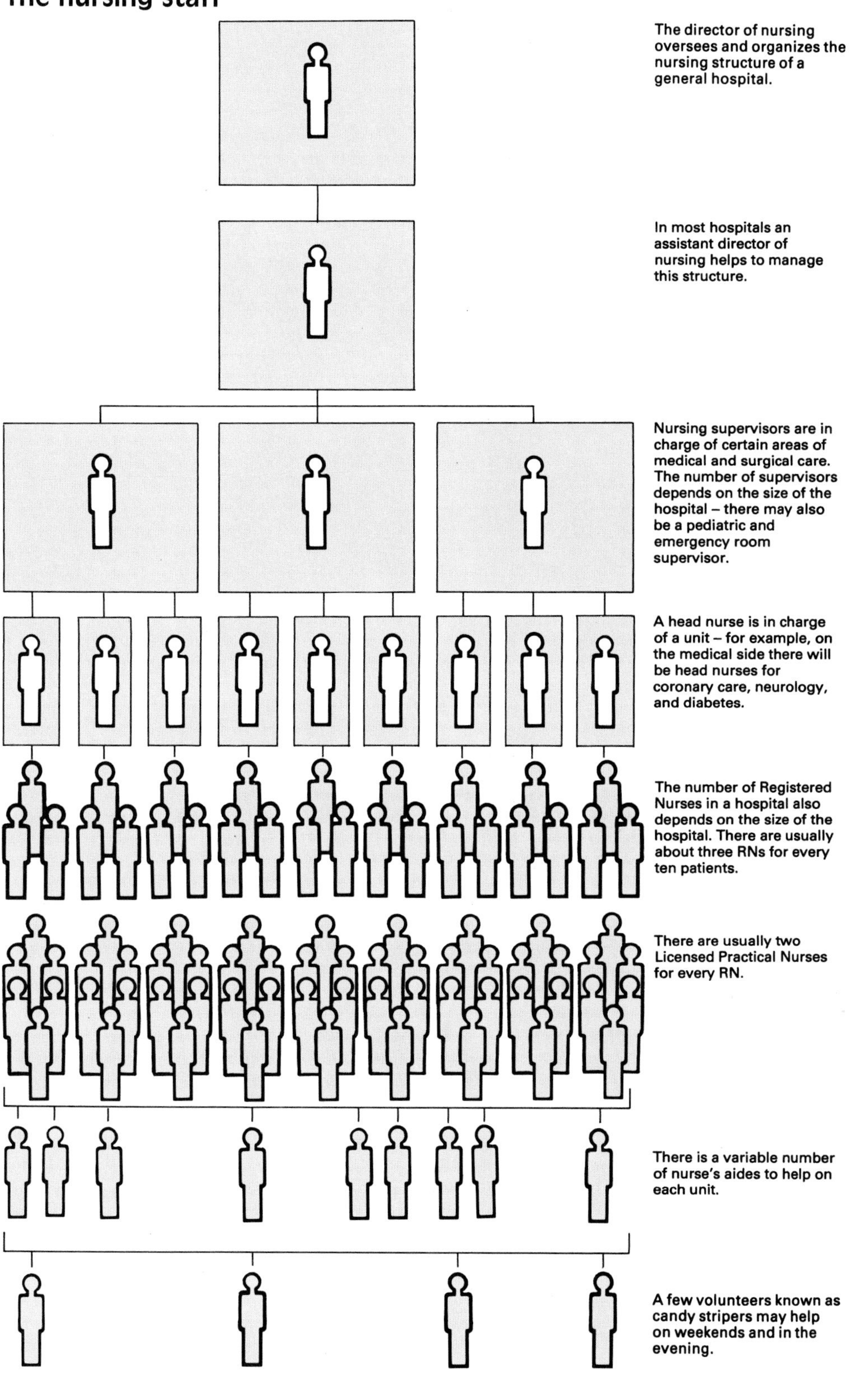

The director of nursing oversees and organizes the nursing structure of a general hospital.

In most hospitals an assistant director of nursing helps to manage this structure.

Nursing supervisors are in charge of certain areas of medical and surgical care. The number of supervisors depends on the size of the hospital – there may also be a pediatric and emergency room supervisor.

A head nurse is in charge of a unit – for example, on the medical side there will be head nurses for coronary care, neurology, and diabetes.

The number of Registered Nurses in a hospital also depends on the size of the hospital. There are usually about three RNs for every ten patients.

There are usually two Licensed Practical Nurses for every RN.

There is a variable number of nurse's aides to help on each unit.

A few volunteers known as candy stripers may help on weekends and in the evening.

Layout of a Typical Hospital

The layout of a modern hospital is dictated by the services it provides. Large hospitals have at least three functions: care of the sick inside the hospital; treating emergency and accident cases; and giving highly technical medical care to outpatients who do not require constant hospital care.

Large hospitals are complex institutions containing many specialized departments and facilities. These may include an intensive care unit; a bank of organs for use in transplant surgery; a department of renal dialysis, containing equipment for separating waste matter from blood; a department for X-ray diagnosis and treatment; and a maternity division, which usually includes a nursery and a delivery room.

Going to the hospital for the first time, either as a patient or even as a visitor, can be a stressful experience. Checking-in is less of a strain when you know how to find your way around the often large, sometimes overwhelming, medical complex.

The first floor, or street level, usually has at least two entrances, one leading into a central, hotel-like lobby, and the other into the emergency and outpatient departments.

In the lobby, near the main entrance, is the information desk and the telephone switchboard. Not far away is the admission office for patients. The cashier is in the same area. The clerk at the information desk can locate the various units and departments and direct the visitor to them, give a patient's room number, and provide the name of the doctor in charge. Information about a patient's condition, however, is best obtained from the nurse in charge of the unit in which treatment is being given.

Most of the other administrative departments, such as housekeeping, maintenance, insurance, and security, are also located near the central lobby.

For the convenience of visitors and patients, there is often a gift shop that stocks toiletries, magazines, and sometimes candy and flowers. There may also be a small cafeteria for the public, and there is usually a chapel.

The lobby has comfortable seating and cheerful furnishings. One of the marks of a good hospital (and reassuring to the new patient) is the attention and concern that all of its employees show to the public.

In the Emergency Room. The emergency room, or ER, also on the street level with its own entrance and ramp for ambulances, is often called "the trenches," or some similar nickname, by the hard-working medical team who staff it. Their combined skill and speed can make the difference between life and death for the injuried patients brought there. The units within the ER are organized so that the staff can treat as many patients as possible, as quickly as possible.

There is at least one clerk on duty in the reception area who records information, such as name, address, age, insurance details, and the patient's main complaint. These clerks are specially trained to call for assistance when a patient's symptoms suggest an urgent problem.

In many hospital emergency rooms, a registered nurse is present in the waiting area or visits it at frequent intervals for purposes of triage. This is the term used to describe the difficult, but essential, task of deciding which patients need immediate treatment.

For example, a middle-aged man suffering with chest pain, shortness of breath, and sweating, who therefore may have had a heart attack, will have priority over someone with a sprained ankle.

Patients who are severely injured or acutely ill will be given immediate emergency treatment. This may include cardiac resuscitation, blood transfusion, and tracheostomy. Patients whose injuries or disorders are not immediately life-threatening may have to wait until a physician is available before they are treated.

The job of triage is a difficult one because every patient in distress regards his or her case as urgent. An understanding attitude by the public of the problems of the ER can help the staff work more smoothly.

In the ER there is a central area used by doctors and nurses to consult with the patient's personal physician or with a specialist, to write notes, telephone for laboratory results or X-ray reports, and make arrangements for admission to the hospital. This area commands a view of the treatment area, which may be a large room divided into sections by curtains or a series of individual rooms. The X-ray department, or a branch of it, is nearby. Many ER's also have an adjacent operating room that can be used if immediate surgery is required. There may also be a small ward in which patients may be kept for overnight observation to decide whether admission to the hospital is necessary.

There is a waiting room here, too, where the patient, or one of his or her relatives, waits for the doctor to explain the results of various tests.

The Outpatient Clinic. This hospital service relies on the same support facilities as the ER and so occupies an area close to it.

Outpatient clinics have been expanding in many community hospitals to treat those patients whose illnesses do not require constant hospital supervision. *See also* OUTPATIENT.

The Surgical Unit. The surgical unit usually occupies one of the upper floors of the hospital and is composed of the operating, anesthesia, recovery, changing, and scrub rooms.

Patients are usually brought to surgery on a narrow stretcher with wheels. Patients may be brought a few minutes before they are scheduled for anesthesia; this allows a final check of their physical condition to be made, and ensures that there is a smooth transition from the anesthesia room to the operating room. The patient may be surrounded at this stage by busy nurses, orderlies, and physicians, most of whom will be wearing the special caps and masks that must be worn in the operating room itself. At this time the patient may meet the anesthesiologist and surgeon who will be responsible for his or her operation.

The anesthetic is administered in a special room near the main operating room, although in special cases the anesthetic may be administered in the operating room itself.

The operating room is lit by large mobile lights and contains several tables on which the sterile instruments to be used in the operation are placed. The operating table is in the center of the room.

Next to the operating room is the scrub room, where the surgical personnel wash up before putting on their sterile gowns and gloves.

After surgery, patients are wheeled into the recovery room where nurses can keep close watch on them until the effects of the anesthetic have worn off. At each bed station there are wall outlets for oxygen, suction, and electrical appliances. There may be as many as 20 beds in the recovery room. One nurse is usually responsible for one or two patients.

The recovery room contains machines for monitoring the patient's heartbeat and instruments for measuring blood pressure and for assisting breathing until the patient has fully recovered from the anesthetic. Other specialized equipment for patients with particular needs is also available in the recovery room, and the patient's progress in recovering from his or her operation is constantly monitored. *See also* SURGERY.

The Intensive Care Unit. The critically ill, or those whose condition suddenly might become worse, are kept under observation in the intensive care unit, or ICU. This is usually located on the same floor as surgery.

The fact that a patient is being treated in an intensive care unit should not be cause for alarm. The physician's reason may be a precautionary one.

Intensive care units are busier than the normal nursing units. The ratio of nurses to patients is higher in intensive care because there is more to do for each patient.

The concentrated attention makes it necessary to limit visiting time. A special waiting room is attached to the unit, however, so that relatives and friends can remain within easy reach of the patient.

Many patients in ICU have respiratory problems and so require respirators. In addition, most of the patients are connected to cardiac monitors to record their heartbeat. Some patients also require dialysis, and the unit may contain a hemodialyzer. This machine acts as an artificial kidney, separating waste matter from the blood.

All the nurses in ICU have had special training in the emergencies that may arise and are well-equipped to deal with them.

The Typical Nursing Floor. Most of the inpatients are cared for on a regular nursing floor. The patient's rooms are grouped near a central nursing station. Alongside the nursing station there is a room for keeping drugs and medical supplies, a conference room for doctors, a supervisor's office, and dictating equipment.

Often, there is also a general conference room for the daily discussion of patient management and for education sessions, an essential part of modern medical care. The layout of a regular nursing unit is identical on each floor, making it easy to identify and locate a room.

Staff in a Typical Hospital

When you go into a hospital many people are responsible for your health and welfare, but the role each person plays in your care is not always obvious. Your stay will be more relaxing if you know what to expect from each person, and who to talk to about a particular problem. Fortunately, most members of the staff are immediately identifiable by the identification badge they wear.

Nursing Staff. The uniform worn by nurses varies from country to country, and in the United States it has for many years been all white. However, some hospitals are replacing the white uniforms of the female nurses with pastel-colored uniforms, which give the staff a less institutional look. The male nurses usually still wear white jackets and pants.

Many nurses wear a small hat or cap that usually indicates they are graduate or registed nurses (RN). The cap may also show the badge of the nursing school. *See also* NURSE, REGISTERED.

A nursing unit has a well-structured hierarchy, and each type of nurse can be identified by his or her uniform. The director of nursing and assistant director are not often seen around the ward because their job is mostly administrative, but the nursing surpervisor is usually dressed differently from the other nurses on the unit. In some hospitals, the supervisors wear white coats over their uniforms, so the only reliable method of identifying them is via the badge they wear.

Each unit has a head nurse to organize the work, and most problems are referred to her or him. The other nurses are usually called staff nurses, and their identity badge shows the nurse's name, position, and type of qualification. For example, RN after the name stands for registered nurse and indicates that the wearer has had at least four years of training before graduation.

There are a number of specialist nurses throughout the hospital. IV team nurses, for example, are responsible for starting, maintaining, and removing all intravenous infusions, IV's. If the hospital is attached to a nursing school you may also be administered to by a student nurse whose badge states the stage he or she has reached in training. *See also* NURSE PRACTITIONER.

The letters LPN after a nurse's name stand for licenced practical nurse. This means that he or she has had a good deal of experience and practical training, but lacks the academic training of an RN. An LPN has had more training than a nurse's aide and carries more responsibilty. *See also* NURSE, LICENSED PRACTICAL.

On every ward there is at least one clerk or secretary, often dressed in a smock or short coat, who answers questions, makes phone calls to all parts of the hospital, and acts as the clerical support for the medical and nursing staff.

Medical and Surgical Staff. When you go into the hospital you will have already met the physician who is caring for you. If you see other physicians in the hospital wearing regular street clothes, they are probably also attending physicians who have private practices and are granted the privilege of admitting patients to one or more hospitals.

A staff physician sometimes wears a long white coat. In addition to the coat, the staff physician usually wears a plastic badge on the left upper part of the coat showing his or her name, degree, and department. The badge may also show a photograph of the physician. Other hospital employees, such as laboratory technicians or pharmacists, can also be identified by their badge.

The full-time medical team includes physicians at various stages of training. A first-year resident is usually a physician who graduated less than a year ago, and a resident is a physician who graduated one or more years ago. In general, first-year residents and resident physicians wear badges that indicate their level of training. *See also* RESIDENCY.

In a teaching hospital, medical students usually wear a badge displaying their status. It is a good idea to get into the habit of looking carefully at the identity badges. The badges help to introduce the wearer and make direct contact more personal.

You may also see doctors in the hospital wearing green, blue, or white overalls, possibly under their white coats. These are scrub suits or "scrubs" worn by the surgical teams in the operating room.

Other Staff. Much of the work in a hospital takes place behind the scenes. No modern hospital could function without its building engineers, laboratory technicians, maintenance and housekeeping staffs, and other support personnel. The people who bring the meals are easily recognized, and their badges bear words like Dietary Dept., Diet Aide, or Nutrition. If you are on a special diet or have a problem with food, the dietitian will develop an appropriate menu.

If your physician recommends breathing exercises or inhalation therapy, the respiratory therapist will visit you. He or she sometimes wears the job initials RT on his or her identification badge.

Inevitably, you will at some time during your hospital stay have a blood sample taken. It is usually a relatively painless procedure. The blood is drawn by a member of the laboratory staff, and the identification badge usually states laboratory, laboratory technician, or in some hospitals a new title, phlebotomist. (The word is derived from the Greek and means "one who opens veins.")

The so-called "candy stripers" are young volunteers who may be planning to be nurses. They usually help the nursing unit on the weekend, or in the afternoon, and sometimes wear a striped uniform.

Another visitor to your room may be the patient representative. This is a person who tries to visit each patient to see that all of the patient's needs are being met, and if they are not, to find out why. Not every hospital employs a patient representative, but they are becoming more common because they provide a useful link between the patient and the hospital administration. The representatives act as an official voice for the patient and may also help to uncover faults or inefficiencies that might not otherwise come to the attention of those in authority. They make the patient's stay in the hospital more comfortable because they look after the nonmedical needs of the patient and may also help investigate complaints.

There are a number of other people you may see during your stay, depending on the circumstances. These include social service workers, if you need special aftercare at home, or building engineers, if the air conditioning does not work.

During your stay you will almost certainly be taken by an orderly to a number of departments for treatment or tests. You will go there on a stretcher trolley or in a wheelchair. This is for your own safety, and even if you feel well, do not insist on walking to the department if an orderly has brought you a wheelchair. Many people, especially the elderly, get dizzy on standing after they have been inactive for a few days. It is often difficult to assess accurately how far you can walk when you have walked very little for a number of days.

When you reach the specified department, the orderly leaves you with the staff there. In a radiology department, the technicians often wear long white coats and have a dosimeter pinned on the lower front of the coat. The dosimeter is a device that records the level of radiation to which each of these technicians has been exposed over a given period of time.

The technicians are not allowed to tell you the results of any of the tests because this is the job of the attending physician. You can ask about the various procedures and why they are being done, and the technicians should explain what the procedure entails. If you do not know what a test is for, you should ask; it is a standing rule that all procedures are explained to the patient.

Specialized Staff. Some patients have to be isolated either because they have a contagious illness or because they themselves are especially vulnerable to infection. The staff in charge of the patients in the isolation unit wear masks and surgical caps.

There are several types of isolation rooms, and specialist staff care for the patients in them. For example, there may be a respiratory isolation room or an enteric (intestinal) isolation room. The staff usually have to instruct visitors about the precautions they must take before entering the rooms, for example, washing the hands, disposing of tissues, or wearing a mask. If a visitor is uncertain what to do before visiting the patient, he or she must ask because an error could be dangerous.

The staff in the intensive care unit usually wear pajama-type clothes similar to a surgeon's scrub suit. The nursing station on the unit is in the center of the floor, and glass partitions allow the staff to see patients at all times.

Most patients have a number of wires connected to the chest to monitor breathing and heartbeat, and all the patients in the unit have an intravenous line attached to the arm. The staff on the unit are highly trained in the management of the machinery on the unit. Some patients may need a respirator that is attached to them through the mouth. A large mobile cabinet beside the bed carefully monitors the volume and rate at which the air is delivered to the patient.

The staff have to restrict visiting hours, but there is usually a waiting room near the unit so that relatives can remain close to the patient.

Typical Hospital Rooms

Obviously, rooms differ from hospital to hospital. The general pattern tends to be similar, however, and the following section should help to familiarize you with a hospital room and identify most of the items to be found in it.

Except for units with a special function, such as the intensive care unit or the surgical recovery room, it is rare to see more than two beds in any room. A single room does not necessarily indicate that it is a private room paid for at private rates.

The beds in a two-bedroom are usually placed with the heads of the beds square with the wall. This means that the patients do not have to stare at each other, but have a feeling of companionship. The rooms are equipped with a dividing screen that can be drawn across to separate the beds if privacy is required.

The Bed. The modern hospital bed is operated electrically so that the patient or the nurse can adjust the height of

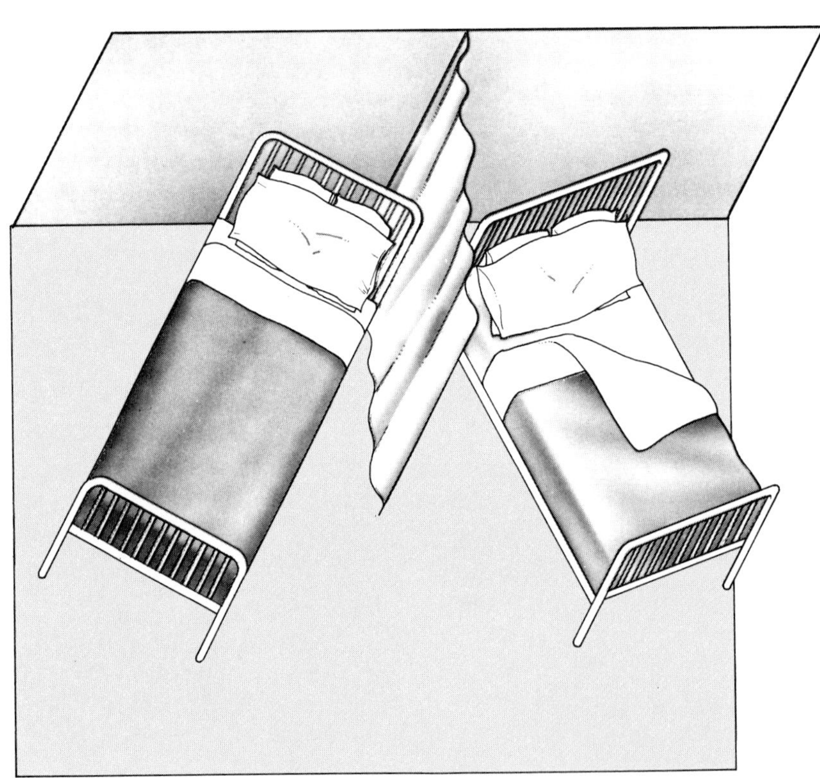

In most hospitals, a partition is placed in rooms with more than one bed. This provides a sense of privacy. Beds in shared rooms may also be turned to face away from each other to provide privacy.

the bed and the angle of either the foot or the head of the bed.

Usually, the bed should be low enough to enable the patient to sit on the edge and touch the floor with the flat of the feet. It is then safe for the patient to assume a standing position. Sometimes, however, the nurse may prefer to raise the height of the bed for bathing the patient, changing dressings, or making the bed when the patient is sitting on his or her chair. The bed height is operated by a button either on a console above the bed or on a hand-held control.

The same console has a control to raise and lower the head of the bed. This makes it easier for the patient to watch television, read, or talk to a visitor. For patients with certain disorders, it is important to be able to raise the foot of the bed to an angle of 45 degrees. For instance, if a leg is fractured or swollen, it is more comfortable for the patient if his or her legs are raised. If a cushion or pillow is used for this purpose, an uneven pressure is exerted on the leg which may impede the circulation and cause other problems. Also, the pillow may slip out of position.

Hospital mattresses are, for several reasons, firmer than mattresses sold commercially. A soft mattress allows the hip and abdomen to sink downward, causing an appreciable curvature of the spine. A firm mattress not only alleviates backache, but makes routine examination easier for the physician.

Bedsores are difficult to avoid when nursing a patient who can not move because of pain, paralysis, or a coma. A soft mattress encourages bedsores because the part of the body that sinks downward sweats more and receives less air. The skin can quickly become damp and soft, making it more susceptible to ulceration.

For patients with debilitating diseases, a variable pressure airbed that can prevent bedsores can be placed over the regular mattress. The airbed consists of a number of inflatable compartments, within which the air pressure can be varied so that different parts of the bed press on the patient's body.

On both sides of the bed are rails that can be raised or lowered. When they are down they are below the level of the mattress; they can be raised and locked into position at night. There are two good reasons for raising the bed-rails: to prevent the patient from falling out of bed when he or she is asleep and to stop the patient from getting out of bed at night unaided. The latter is important because a sick patient can become confused at night, forget where he or she is, and instead of taking a walk to the bathroom, find that he or she has walked to the top of a flight of stairs. When a patient is asleep, the muscles relax and the blood pressure drops. A patient may get out of bed too quickly, feel dizzy, and faint before a nurse arrives to help.

The console above the bed provides headphones and a radio and television tuner to enable the patient to listen to the radio or watch television. On the console, there is also a push-button bell that is used to summon assistance. When the patient presses the button, a signal is sent either to the nursing station or the nurse call station. The nurse call station can speak by microphone to the patient, then pass on the message to the nursing station.

Next to the bed is a bedside table with drawers and compartments for personal possessions. The table is usually on rollers to make bedmaking easier for the nursing staff, so the patient should not use the table as a support when getting out of bed. The patient is also often provided with a table for writing letters, reading, and eating meals.

It must be emphasized that patients should not keep anything of value in the room. Although hospitals employ full-time security personnel, it is impossible to prevent petty pilfering and, unfortunately, it does occur. If you have valuables when you come into the hospital, either give them to a relative or ask the nursing staff to lock them away for you.

Above the bed is a variable-angle wall lamp for reading, but after 10 o'clock in the evening, the lights are dimmed to a night light. The night lights allow the nursing staff to give necessary medications during the night.

Toilet Facilities. Some hospitals provide a small sink and faucets next to the bed to allow the patient to sit on the edge of the bed to wash, brush his or her teeth, or shave. The hospital

The console

The console above the hospital bed provides headphones and a radio and television tuner to enable the patient to listen to the radio or watch television. On the console, there is also a push-button bell that is used to summon assistance. When the patient presses the button, a signal is sent either to the nursing station or the nurse call station.

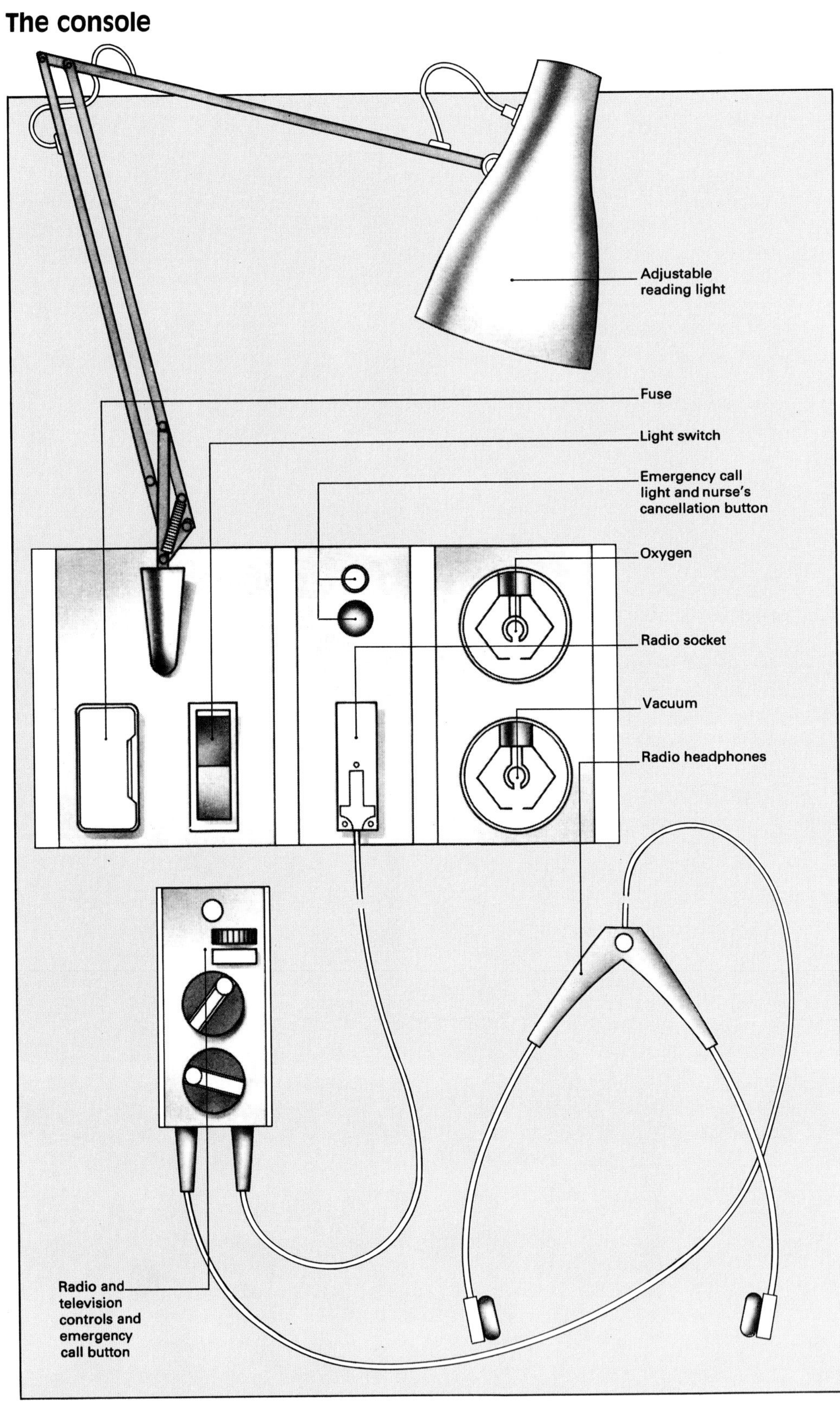

may also provide a shop to enable the patient to buy small toilet articles, such as toothpaste and soap.

The bathroom is usually near the beds and comes equipped with safety handles placed in strategic positions to help the patient use the toilet, shower, or sink. There are no locks on the doors of the bathrooms, and patients must use the "occupied" notice for privacy. The reason for this is that if a patient faints or falls in the washroom, the nursing staff will have access to the room. Sometimes, the washroom partitions do not reach to the full height of the ceiling. Again, this is to enable a member of the staff to get over the partition if a patient falls across the door on the inside. If a patient is not well enough to use the bathroom, the nursing staff may bathe the patient in bed. Similarly, the patient can use a urine bottle or a bedpan if he or she can not get to the bathroom.

The Room. Each patient is provided with a good sized chair because modern medical practice is to get the patient out of bed as soon as possible. This speeds up recovery and minimizes the possibility of complications, such as bedsores and blood clotting. Some hospitals provide a support band on the chair that is placed around the patient's chest so that there is less danger of the patient slipping off the chair onto the floor.

The windows are always kept closed, and the temperature and fresh air is controlled by central heating or air conditioning. There are two reasons for this. The hospital must be kept warm because sick patients can suffer from hypothermia very quickly, and the rooms must be warm so that the staff can bathe a patient on the bed without chilling him or her. The other reason is to stop a suicidal patient from jumping out of a window. Even if a patient vigorously protests that he or she has no intention of doing such a thing, the nursing staff can not risk the possibility.

When a patient arrives at the hospital he or she is given a small kit containing toiletry articles, such as tissues and a mouthwash. The hospital also provides a small booklet that describes the hospital and its facilities. The booklet may also contain a detachable sheet for the patient to record complaints or compliments about the hospital service.

On one side of the door to the room, there is a panel that carries information for the nursing staff. For instance, it may say "nothing by mouth" indicating that the patient is going for surgery or having some test that requires the stomach to be empty. The sign means literally nothing by mouth, not even a drink of water, and if a patient is accidently offered a drink or cookie, he or she must refuse it. Visitors must never override the instructions and smuggle food in for the patient. If a visitor is not sure what the hospital allows, particularly regarding alcohol, he or she should ask the nurse in charge. Although hospital diets can not compare with home cooking, they are adequate and the nutritional content is measured with great care. It is detrimental to the patient's health for a visitor to supply him or her with extra food.

Smoking in a hospital is now increasingly discouraged, and a patient may have to go to another room if he or she needs a cigarette. Any room that uses oxygen has signs forbidding smoking.

The Telephone. A bedside telephone is available for the patient and provides a link with home and friends. However, too many incoming calls are a nuisance, and if necessary, the calls may be intercepted by the hospital switchboard if requested by the attending physician.

Restraints. The use of restraints in the hospital often shocks and angers relatives and friends of the patient, but there is a reason for the use of restraints. If a patient is confused for any reason, particularly during the night, he or she may be restrained in bed with a device other than the bedrail. This is because the risk of the patient injuring himself or herself is high if he or she is able to wander around the floor. If the patient is very confused and is being given intravenous fluids, he or she may pull the lines out or displace them. Sometimes, it is necessary to secure the wrist to the side of the bed with a padded but snug band. The band is checked frequently by the hospital staff to make sure that it is not causing any discomfort. The restrained patient should never feel like a prisoner, and because restraints are used only under certain circumstances, the patient is often not aware that they are being used at all.

However, if relatives or friends are concerned about a restraint, they must talk to the attending physician. The physician can then explain why restraint is needed, when restraints are used, and for how long they will be necessary. Restraints are used only for the patient's own protection.

Layout of a Hospital Floor. The nerve center of the floor is the nursing station placed in the middle. It is surrounded by a counter about waist high, with a spacious desk area in the middle. The ward secretary usually sits in the middle to receive phone calls, make appointments, see that laboratory and X-ray results are placed on the appropriate charts, and deal with any other inquiries. The patient's charts are kept at the station, and physicians and nurses use the desk area to make notes. The area also contains a data processing terminal and dictating equipment. Some units have monitor screens fed by equipment in the patients' rooms and also a screen which either lights up or buzzes when the patient presses his or her call button. The nursing station receives and processes all the information for the smooth and efficient running of the floor.

Other Rooms. There are a number of other rooms on the floor containing housekeeping materials, a small kitchen where hot or cold drinks can be made and, possibly, a microwave-oven to heat food from the main kitchen. There may also be a conference room for physicians and nurses and an office for the nursing supervisor. The supply rooms contain all the instruments, syringes, fluids, dressings and drugs needed in the hospital.

Hospital admission tests. *See* HOSPITALIZATION: ADULTS.

Hospitalization: Adults. The procedures you follow on admission to a hospital vary from one hospital to another, but basically the process is the same in most institutions in the United States.

Admission Procedures

You will most probably be admitted into a short-term hospital, which is a hospital that seldom has patients for longer than a month, and usually for 3 to 10 days. Long-term hospitals treat patients with psychiatric problems or long-lasting physical illnesses.

The hospital will probably be a general hospital, that is, one that deals with a complete range of treatment. However, some patients require care in a special hospital, for example, a pediatric hospital, if the patient is a child, or a maternity hospital, if a woman is having a baby. Your physician will recommend the most appropriate kind of hospital for your particular condition.

Elective Admission is admission to a hospital after at least one day of planning before the actual date of entry. Many such admissions are for surgery. Others are for tests that can not be performed on an outpatient basis. Medical conditions that require an elective admission are less common, but if a hospital is full and the condition is not an emergency, a patient may remain at home for a day or two until a bed becomes available. *See also* OUTPATIENT; SURGERY.

The admissions office is usually located in the main lobby near the information desk. When you arrive at the desk, there are a number of questions that the admissions office clerk will ask. Your name, address, and date of birth are required, and you will probably be asked to give your employer's telephone number as well as your home number. The clerk will also need to know the name and address of your next of kin or another responsible party in case an emergency develops during your stay in the hospital. Many hospitals want to know your religion because some religious groups place restrictions on what procedures may be done, and it is important that the hospital knows this in advance. For example, some sects do not allow the use of blood transfusions, and the hospital would be liable if one were given without the patient's consent.

The clerk must know the details of your insurance coverage, and you should take any necessary identifying information with you. Your Social Security number will be required. *See also* MEDICAL EXPENSES AND INSURANCE.

During the interview, the clerk may or may not ask for your family physician's name. If you are being admitted under his or her care, the question is unnecessary because your physician

An admissions form

ACCT NO: 000-000-01 | PATIENT NAME (LAST, FIRST, MI): SMITH JOHN RICHARD | MAIDEN: | ADM DATE: 10 10 94 | TIME: 12NOON | ROOM: 107 | BED: B | ACC | SERV

ADM OR NO: 14 | FC | INS | IF PRIVATE ROOM—REASON | ADDRESS: 1313 SOUTH ST. JOHNSONVILLE | STATE: OR | ZIP: 97163 | HOME PHONE: 222-7777 | U S CITIZEN: YES

PLACE OF BIRTH (CITY & STATE OR COUNTY): INDIANAPOLIS IND | DATE OF BIRTH: 12/20/36 | AGE: 57 | SEX: M | MAR: YES | REL: PROT | RACE: W | PATIENT OCCUPATION: SALESMAN | SPOUSE/GUARANTOR OCCUPATION: EDITOR

MEDICARE ID NO | SOCIAL SECURITY NO: 672-09-1057 | TYPE OF ADMISSION: URGENT | ATTENDING PHYSICIAN: JACKSON | PHY NO: 072 | PREV TREAT THIS HOSP: NONE

FATHERS NAME: SMITH ALFRED RALPH | MOTHERS NAME (MAIDEN): PIGNATELLI | HOW BROUGHT TO HOSPITAL: AMBULANCE

SOURCE OF THIS INFORMATION: PATIENT | RELATIONSHIP | ADDRESS | STATE | ZIP | HOME PHONE: 222-7777

SPOUSE OR NEAREST RELATIVE: FREDA RACHEL SMITH | RELATIONSHIP: WIFE | ADDRESS: SAME AS PATIENT | STATE | ZIP | HOME PHONE

WHOM TO NOTIFY IN EMERGENCY: WIFE | ADDRESS | STATE | ZIP | HOME PHONE

INSURANCE | NAME OF PLAN | CITY, STATE | EFFECT DATE | EXPIR DATE | SERV CODE | I D NO
PRIMARY— BLUE-CROSS
SECOND— | COMPREHENSIVE | | 1/1/90 | 12/31/98 | | 76543

HISTORY: G.I. BLEEDING | WHEN: THIS AM | WHERE: HOME | HOW: VOMITED BLOOD

PROVISIONAL DIAGNOSIS: PEPTIC ULCER | DIAG CD: 679 | ALLERGY(S): PENICILLIN

PATIENT EMPLOYER: RT JACOBS | ADDRESS: 2742 MAIN ST JOHNSONVILLE | STATE: OR | ZIP: 97163 | HOW LONG: 10 yrs | PHONE: 222-0414

SPOUSE EMPLOYER: SELF EMPLOYED | ADDRESS | STATE | ZIP | HOW LONG | PHONE

GUARANTOR EMPLOYER: RT JACOBS | ADDRESS: AS ABOVE | STATE | ZIP | HOW LONG | PHONE

GUARANTOR NAME | ADDRESS | STATE | ZIP | HOME PHONE

BANK (NAME & ADDRESS): JOHNSONVILLE LOAN CO | TYPE OF ACCT(S): CHECKING | AMOUNT: $1000

LANDLORD OR MORTGAGE HOLDER (NAME & ADDRESS): JOHNSONVILLE SAVINGS & LOAN CO | OWN: ✓ | RENT | PAYMENTS: $100/MO

CREDIT REFERENCE (NAME & ADDRESS): MASON'S DEPARTMENT STORE | OPEN BALANCE: $250 | MONTHLY PAY: $25

NO IN FAMILY: 2 ADULT(S) 3 CHILDREN | NO EMPLOYED: 2 | GROSS FAMILY INCOME: $70,000 | PATIENT: 45,000 | HUSBAND | WIFE: 25,000

LIABILITY INSURANCE: DOES NOT APPLY | PLACE ACCIDENT OCCURRED: DNA | HOW ACCIDENT OCCURRED

PERSONS INVOLVED IN ACCIDENT | ADDRESS

PERSONS INVOLVED IN ACCIDENT | ADDRESS

CAR OR PROPERTY OWNER | ADDRESS

INSURANCE COMPANY & AGENT (NAMES) | ADDRESS

ATTORNEY'S NAME | ADDRESS

PATIENT PLATE | VALUABLES CHECKED: $100 CASH, GOLD WATCH | ENVELOPE NO: 210

I/we hereby certify that the above statements are true and I/we guarantee payment of all by the patient from admission untill discharge.

[signature] PATIENTS SIGNATURE (SEAL) | [signature] PERSON RESPONSIBLE (SEAL)

[signature] ADMITTING OFFICER (SEAL)

ADMISSION PATIENT ACCOUNTS

will have already been identified when the admissions office was notified of your arrival. If, however, your physician has referred you to another physician or surgeon for inpatient care, then make sure that your physician's name is also on your chart.

Once the clerical part of the work is complete, you will have some tests done. In some hospitals, a technician waits close to the admissions office, and in others you are escorted to the laboratory for the tests. If you have been admitted for surgery, the operation will usually be done the following day. It is important that preoperative test results be available as soon as possible, because they may affect the decision to operate. If you are found to be anemic, you may need a transfusion before surgery. Your blood group must be identified before any operation, so that blood can be standing by for transfusion if any is needed during surgery. Your blood is cross-matched to make sure that it reacts favorably with blood of the same group, and its clotting ability is also tested. Most surgeons like the patient to have a routine electrocardiogram and chest X ray done before surgery, and these are also carried out before you reach your hospital room. *See also* ANEMIA; BLOOD GROUP; ELECTROCARDIOGRAM; X RAY.

You are usually escorted to your room by a hospital patient escort, often a volunteer. Before leaving the main lobby, you may be asked to hand over

Date 10/11/94

AUTHORIZATION FOR PERFORMANCE OF OPERATIONS AND OTHER PROCEDURES, INCLUDING ADMINISTRATION OF ANESTHESIA

1 I hereby consent to and authorize the performance upon JOHN RICHARD SMITH (myself or name of patient) of the following procedures PARTIAL GASTRECTOMY & VAGOTOMY of which I have been advised, to be performed under the direction of my physician(s), DR. JACKSON (name of physician(s))

2. I further consent to and authorize:

(a) the administration of such anesthesia, and
(b) the performance of such additional operations and procedures (whether or not arising from presently unforseen conditions) considered necessary or desirable in the judgement of my doctor or of those of the Hospital's medical staff who serve me.

3. I further consent to and authorize either the photographing or televising of such operations and procedures, including appropriate portions of my body, for medical, scientific or educational purposes, providing my identity is not revealed by the picture or by descriptive texts accompanying them.

4. I hereby waive and transfer to the Hospital for study or any other purpose all rights to any organ, limb or any part of my body removed during such operations or procedures.

5. The nature and purpose of the operations, or other procedures have been explained to me. I acknowledge that no guarantee has been made as to the results that may be obtained.

(CROSS OUT PARAGRAPHS WHICH ARE NOT APPROPRIATE)

John Smith
(Signature of patient or person authorized to consent for patient)

(Relationship to Patient)

WITNESS:

Signature

Address

DATE OF SURGERY 10/13/94
SIGNATURE [signature]
CLASSIFICATION MAJOR

(TO BE COMPLETED AFTER THE SURGICAL PROCEDURE HAS BEEN PERFORMED)

FORM 7804

any valuables or money you brought in with you for storage in the hospital safe. It is advisable to have only a few dollars in your room.

Shortly after your arrival in your room, a member of the nursing staff greets you, explains the facilities, and shows you how to use the nurse call system. You are then asked to change out of your street clothes into pajamas or a nightgown, or the hospital may provide a hospital gown.

If you still have valuables and money in your possession, you can hand them to the nurse, who will place them in an envelope and give them to a security guard for storage in the hospital safe. A receipt for the valuables will be attached to your chart.

Once you are in bed, a nurse will take your temperature, check your pulse and blood pressure, and record your weight. The wristband will be checked to make sure that the name is correct. It is fixed with a permanent clasp, and you must not cut the band off until you leave the hospital. *See also* BLOOD PRESSURE; PULSE, TAKING OF; TEMPERATURE, TAKING OF.

The ward clerk will check your signature on the admitting forms and see what tests and treatments have been ordered by looking at your chart. The clerk will give you the hospital information booklet and personal toilet kit. If you have any questions, do ask.

A nurse will then ask you a number of questions about your health and the reasons for coming into the hospital. He or she will want to know general health points, such as how regular your bowel movements are. He or she will also need to know if you are taking any other kind of medicines. If you have these with you, the nurse will take them and place them in a locked closet to make sure that all the medicines you take during your stay in the hospital come from one source and are carefully recorded.

If you have been taking contraceptive pills, you may need to stop dosage before surgery. The contraceptive pill can increase the chance of postoperative blood clotting in the veins of the legs, but many women do not regard the pills as drugs, possibly because they are not treating an illness. If you are taking contraceptive pills, always inform your doctor and the hospital staff. You may be advised that for your condition the birth control pills are not contraindicated, and you may then continue to take them while in the hospital. *See also* CONTRACEPTIVE, ORAL.

You must also tell the nurse if you are allergic to any sort of medication or adhesive dressing. If you are, it should be recorded not only on the nursing notes, but also on the front of your chart and on your treatment card. The medications for all the patients on the floor are kept on a medicine cart with treatment cards for each patient. The nurse will take the cart around the floor regularly and record each medication and dosage. *See also* ALLERGY.

The process of elective admission is now complete. On a busy day it may take several hours from the time you arrive at the hospital door to the time when you are finally settled down in your hospital bed.

Emergency Admission. Although the majority of hospital admissions are elective, you may be admitted to a hospital following an accident or for some other serious emergency. When you arrive at the emergency room, the clerk on duty needs information similar to that of the admissions clerk. He or she must know your name, address, insurance details, and major injury or complaint. The clerk is trained to recognize potentially dangerous symptoms.

Once the clerk has seen you, a registered nurse (RN) examines you to see if you need urgent treatment. If the nature of your injury is not life-threatening, you may have to wait for some time in an emergency room because the staff is dealing with other patients. However distressing the wait may be, a patient's health is in far less danger if he or she is in the emergency room. Should something life-threatening happen, such as a cardiac arrest, then the patient is only seconds away from a team of experienced physicians and nurses and specialized equipment. *See also* NURSE, REGISTERED.

If you are brought to the emergency room following an accident and are subsequently admitted to the hospital, remember to ask a friend or relative to bring in a clean set of clothing before you are discharged. You must remember that the hospital cannot clean the clothes you wore on admission.

Informed Consent. Before surgery of even the most minor kind can be performed, you must give your consent in writing. If a patient is unable to do this because of age, mental confusion, or coma, the consent must be given by the nearest possible relative. The legal term for this is "informed consent," and the consent must be based on all available evidence. *See also* INFORMED CONSENT; LIVING WILL.

Major surgery, for example, open-heart surgery or the removal of a malignant tumor, carries some risk of death during or shortly after the operation, so the decision to consent is not usually granted as quickly as in an emergency. There is no immediate urgency in terms of hours, but the likely outcome without surgery in terms of life or quality of life is again so poor that the necessity to consent is obvious.

The decision to consent to elective surgery is often the most difficult to make. Although surgery in these conditions offers relief of symptoms, the disorder itself is unlikely to shorten life. A good example of this type of surgery is a total hip replacement for arthritis of the hip. Walking may be severely limited by pain and activity generally reduced, but the patient must personally decide whether the risk carried by any form of surgery is worth taking.

If elective surgery has been recommended, you must discuss the problem with your family physician, who can give you all of the facts clearly and explain any possible aftereffects before you sign the consent form.

Another point worth remembering is that if you are undergoing exploratory surgery, for example, to discover whether a lump in the breast is cancer, the consent form may include the operation that the surgeon will have to perform if the result is malignant. The surgeon waits until the pathologist's report is returned and makes the decision either to close up the incision or to remove possibly affected tissue. It would not be practical to wake up the patient, tell him or her the result, and then reopen the wound when the second consent has been signed. But if you feel that all the consequences of the operation have not been fully explained, do not consent to a further operation, until you have discussed the matter with your physician.

Postadmission Physical

One of the duties of the nursing staff, which receives a new patient on a unit, is to notify a member of the resident medical staff that the patient has arrived so that the resident or intern can take the history of the patient's illness and previous illnesses, examine the patient, and write up initial orders. The interview is likely to be lengthy, and many of the questions will be reviewed by other members of the staff. The patient must cooperate to the best of his or her ability and should never insist that, because the family physician has already taken all of the details, repetition is unnecessary. Often, the patient forgets to tell his or her own physician about something, and this comes to light only during the interview at the hospital. This medical history is the most important single factor in helping the physician to make a diagnosis. It is more important than the physical examination, the tests, or the X rays, even with the sophisticated equipment available in today's hospitals.

An intern usually comes to see you after you have settled into your room. He or she writes down all the details of your illness. *See also* INTERNSHIP.

Giving a History. The resident physician begins the interview by introducing himself or herself and explaining who he or she is. Residents vary in interview technique, but commonly the resident begins by discussing the patient's main symptoms, because obviously this is causing the patient the most concern. When the resident asks you what is wrong, you should explain the most prominent symptom or symptoms, such as shortness of breath or abdominal pain. The resident does not want your estimated diagnosis. *See also* DIAGNOSIS; SYMPTOM.

The questions that follow relate to the presenting symptom. For example, if you are complaining of abdominal pain, the resident will ask questions such as: has the pain changed position at all; has the pain become localized (concentrated in one area) or has it spread to other areas of the abdomen; and what type of pain is it (sharp, burning, spasmodic, or a dull ache).

The resident will ask questions relating to the intensity of the pain. A question commonly asked of mothers is whether the pain is as intense as labor pains. The resident will also want to know if anything makes the pain worse, such as moving a limb, or whether anything eases the pain, such as sitting up or lying down. The resident will ask if you notice any other symptoms at the same time as the pain, for instance, gas or flatus.

After the questions concerning the main complaint, the resident will probably ask about your past medical history. The questions will cover areas such as: have you had any major illnesses (do not forget to mention any childhood illnesses you have had); have you had any operations (you should mention even the most minor ones, such as having a mole removed); and have you ever been treated for a disorder (remember to mention minor disorders such as indigestion). The resident will ask a female patient about her menstrual and obstetrical history; how many children she has had; whether all the pregnancies and labors were normal; and if there were any postnatal complications. A female patient must remember to mention any blood pressure problems during pregnancy or complications, such as forceps delivery or induced labor. If you have ever been hospitalized, you will be asked the year and your home address at the time, the name of the previous hospital, and the physician whose care you were under. *See also* IMMUNIZATION; MENSTRUAL PROBLEMS.

The resident will ask you what job you do and whether it exposes you to any particular hazards or emotional tension. A patient's social history plays an important part in the diagnosis.

The physician will ask if your mother and father are still alive. If they are not, he or she will want to know of what they died. If your grandparents lived into their eighties and both parents are alive and well at the age of seventy, there is a likelihood that you will live to the same age. If you are an adopted child, you should mention it. The resident may also ask direct questions about conditions and illnesses in the family: is there any incidence of tuberculosis or has any member of the family suffered from a stroke or heart attack. *See also* HEART ATTACK; STROKE; TUBERCULOSIS.

The resident will want to know about your drinking and smoking habits. This is not an opportunity for the resident to criticize or pry into your habits, but it is essential that you answer the questions accurately. The resident has no wish to censure you, but he or she must have accurate information in order to reach a correct diagnosis. *See also* ALCOHOL; SMOKING OF TOBACCO.

The resident will then probably move on to questions related to drugs and medications. A patient often denies taking drugs regularly, only to admit, after closer questioning, that he or she has been taking antacids for indigestion for the past forty years or a laxative every morning for the past month. It is most important that you think carefully before giving your answer. The accuracy of the diagnosis could depend on it. A good example of this is the contraceptive pill. Many women do not regard this as regular medication, but during major surgery it can encourage the formation of blood clots that could prove fatal. The resident will also want to know about any allergies, such as one to adhesive tape. *See also* ALLERGY; CONTRACEPTIVE, ORAL; DRUG.

Many residents make a habit of running through all of the body's systems at the end of the interview, asking direct questions about each. This is a sort of screening that gives the patient a last chance to remember anything that may be important. The questions about the chest may include: how much do you smoke; do you ever have pain in the chest; are you ever out of breath after walking up the stairs; and do you ever cough up mucus. Questions about the bowels may include: how often do you have a bowel movement; have you ever noticed blood in the stool; or do you feel bowel discomfort at any time. Questions about the bladder may include: how often do you urinate; do you ever feel pain or burning on urinating; have you ever noticed any blood or cloudiness in the urine; have you ever suffered from stress incontinence or frequency; and have you ever had trouble urinating. A female patient will be asked questions about her menstrual cycle: is it regular; is the bleeding heavy or light; does she suffer from painful menstruation; or does she ever bleed in midcycle. *See also* ANGINA PECTORIS; BLADDER DISORDERS; BOWEL, IMPACTED; INCONTINENCE.

The Examination. After the interview, the resident will give you a thorough examination. Again, the order in which the resident examines you may vary. He or she may begin by examining the physical signs of the actual condition or by examining the head and neck, and then continue with the rest of the body. The illustrations show the main examinations and explain what the resident is looking for in each system. If the disorder is associated with a limb, the physician always begins by examining the healthy limb. This is so he or she knows what the limb usually feels like before examining the condition. A pelvic or rectal examination may also be included.

At the conclusion of the examination, the resident usually makes some comment about the impression he or she has formed. You must remember, however, that the first physician you see is usually less experienced than the consultant and will not have any results of tests or X rays, so it is unlikely that he or she will be able to make an accurate diagnosis at this point. If the first physician was an intern, you may have to go through the questions and examination again, this time by a more senior house staff member, an assistant resident, or a chief resident. Finally, you will see the physician in charge. If you ask all three for their opinion, you may get three slightly different answers, and many people get worried in this situation, because they feel that there is some uncertainty about the case. A patient may worry because one physician orders a stomach X ray, whereas another suggests a gall bladder X ray first. Both have a good reason for their opinion. The final diagnosis will be achieved either way, but techniques do differ. Another cause of worry is confusion about the terms that a physician uses. A patient may be told by one physician that he or she has a peptic ulcer, whereas another may say the patient is suffering from a duodenal ulcer. This is because a duodenal ulcer is a type of peptic ulcer, not because the diagnosis is different. The safest policy to adopt is to always talk to the physician in charge of your case. He or she can give an opinion based on the information from the other physicians and explain any confusions or misunderstandings. *See also* ULCER.

Preparation. You can prepare information in advance for the medical history. It is often difficult to recall on short notice the exact year that you had a certain operation done, for example, an appendectomy at the age of six or a tonsillectomy at the age of ten. You can find out the dates before you are admitted to the hospital. In fact, many patients forget about major operations in childhood, and the physician discovers that such operations have been performed only when he or she sees the surgical scars. If you are uncertain about the cause of death, or the age at death, of a parent or grandparent, try to get the facts from another family member. If you are taking regular medication, look carefully at the bottles and write down the name of the drug and the dosage. *See also* APPENDECTOMY; TONSILLECTOMY.

Although the outcome of your hospital stay depends on the skill and concern of those who look after you, your own participation should not be entirely passive. A patient's history is vitally important, and you should do everything in your power to ensure that the history and facts that you provide are accurate and concise. Foresight and preparation may, at least, shorten the time spent answering questions and, at most, might save your life, if the information concerns something as serious as an allergy to some drug. The first day in the hospital with all the admission procedures and repeated questions and examinations can be tiring, especially if you are not feeling well. The thoroughness with which everything is done is essential, so it is best to be tolerant.

Hospital Testing Procedures

The world of medicine is under constant reappraisal and alteration as a result of research. For instance, just a few years ago it was customary for a patient who had just undergone major surgery to rest in bed for seven to ten days because it was believed to assist recovery. Nowadays, the patient is encouraged to be out of bed and moving as soon as possible. Many studies have confirmed

Post-admission physical

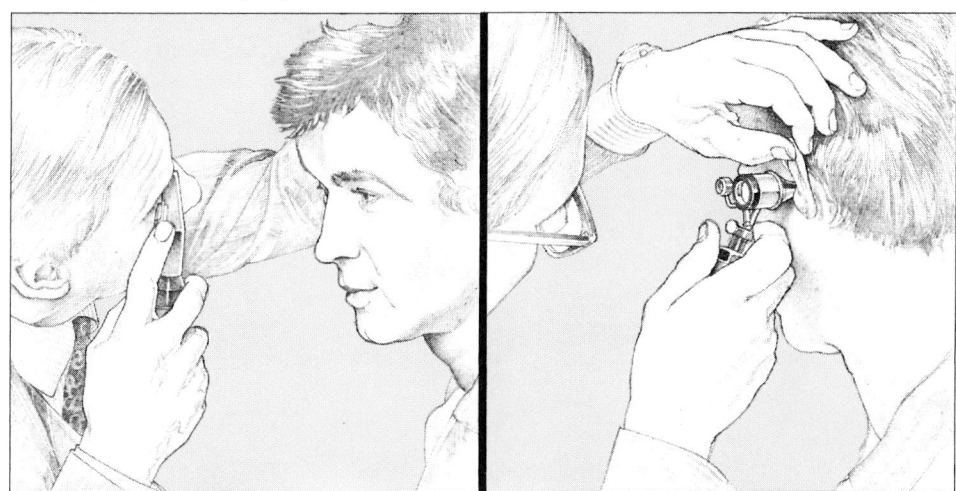

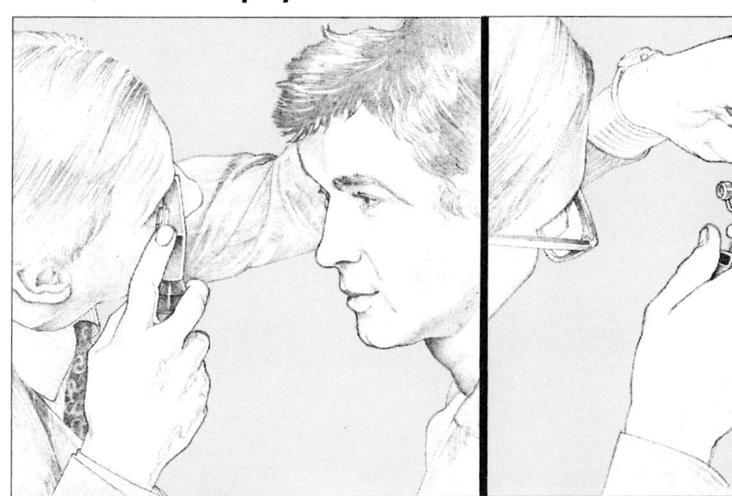

Eye examination: The physician will ask you to move your eyes in all directions to test the function of several nerves. After shining a light into each eye to test the reaction of the iris, the physician will use the ophthalmoscope to study the retina of the eye. The retina reflects the state of the small blood vessels in the body. Sometimes, the physician may also check the pressure within the eyeball.

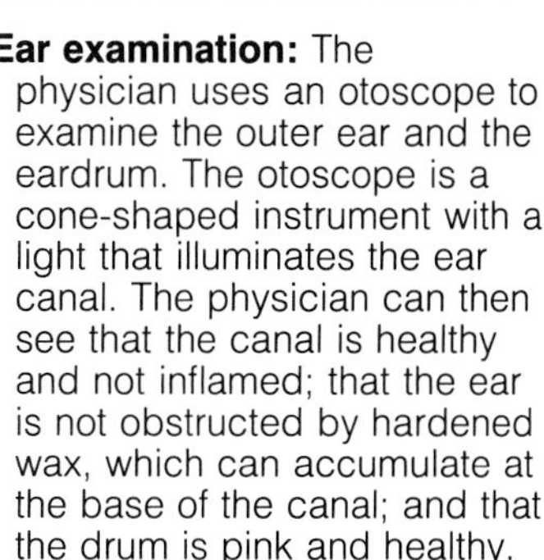

Ear examination: The physician uses an otoscope to examine the outer ear and the eardrum. The otoscope is a cone-shaped instrument with a light that illuminates the ear canal. The physician can then see that the canal is healthy and not inflamed; that the ear is not obstructed by hardened wax, which can accumulate at the base of the canal; and that the drum is pink and healthy.

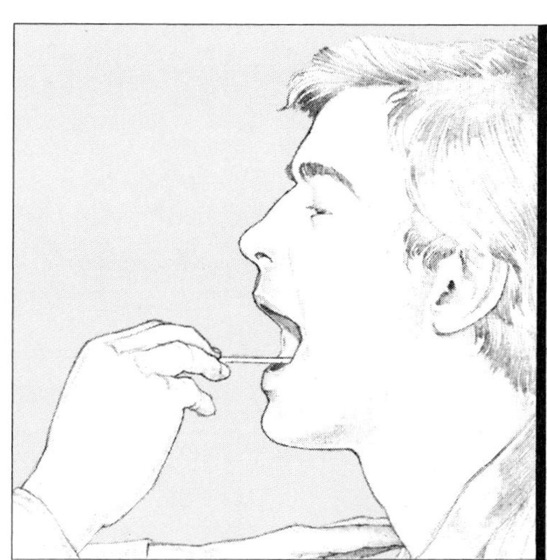

Mouth and throat examination: The physician will ask you to open your mouth wide so that he or she can see inside the mouth and throat. The physician will also press your tongue down with a wooden spatula and ask you to say "Aaah." This moves the tongue out of the way and moves organs in the back of the throat, such as the tonsils, into view. The physician can then see that there is no throat inflammation.

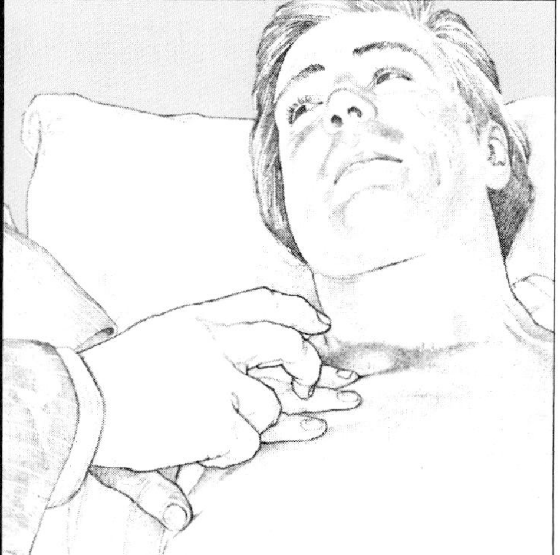

Chest examination: First, the physician will ask you to take a few deep breaths to see that both sides of the chest move normally. He or she will then tap on the chest with the fingers. A normal chest has a faint, hollow sound when examined in this way (percussed), and the presence of fluid or inflammation changes the sound. The physician is also able to tell whether or not the diaphragm is moving normally.

Post-admission physical, *continued*

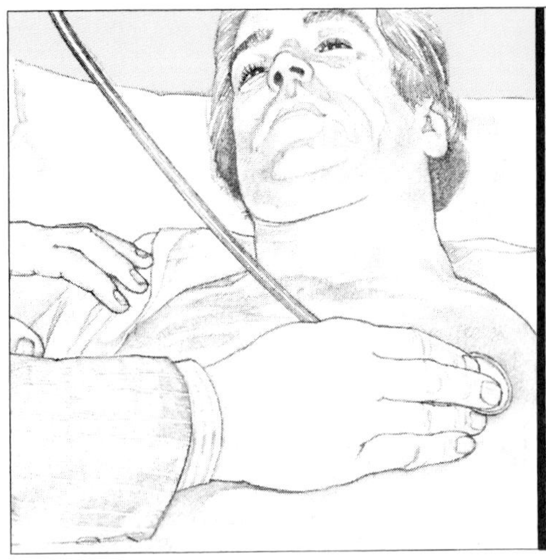

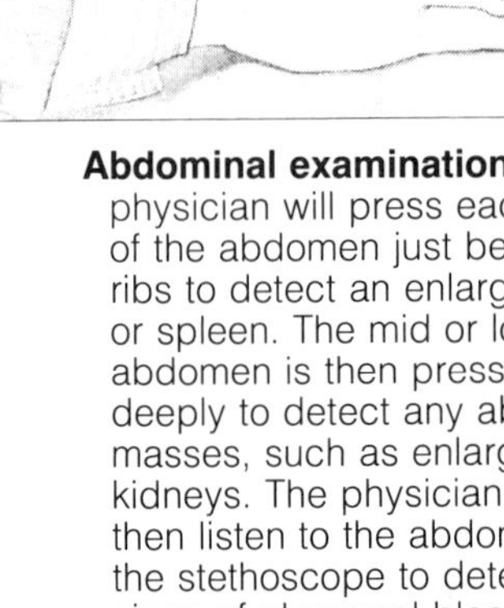

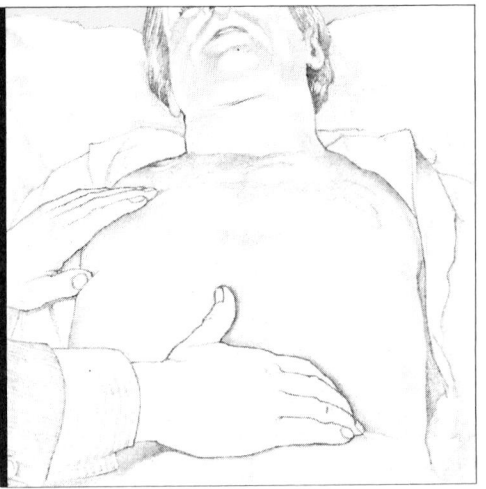

Heart examination: Initially, the physician assesses the size and position of the heart by percussion and by placing the hand on the chest wall to feel for the point of the strongest heartbeat. He or she then listens to the heart with a stethoscope to detect any abnormal heart murmurs that may indicate valve disease, abnormal heartbeat, or the presence of fluid in the sac around the heart (pericardium).

Abdominal examination: The physician will press each side of the abdomen just below the ribs to detect an enlarged liver or spleen. The mid or lower abdomen is then pressed deeply to detect any abnormal masses, such as enlarged kidneys. The physician may then listen to the abdomen with the stethoscope to detect any signs of abnormal blood flow within the abdominal cavity and internal organs.

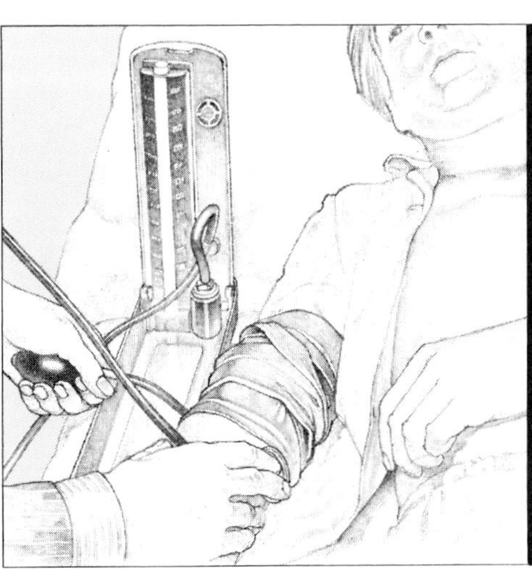

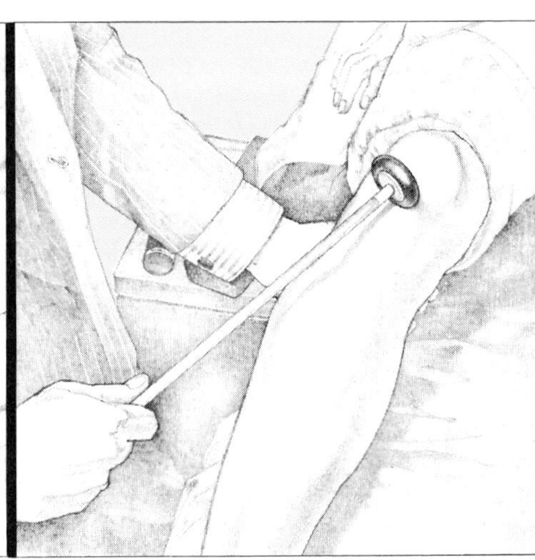

Blood pressure: The physician measures blood pressure with a sphygmomanometer. A cuff is wrapped around the upper arm and inflated to stop the blood flow. The physician places the stethoscope over the front of the elbow and listens while the pressure in the cuff is gradually released. The physician can tell at what cuff pressure the blood begins to flow again because he or she can hear it.

Reflex examination: The physician will test the reflexes of the knee and foot as part of the examination of the nervous system. The physician raises the knee with one hand and taps it with a patella hammer just below the knee cap. If reflexes are normal the foot involuntarily jerks upward. The physician will check reflexes in the foot by stroking the side or the sole of the foot with a wooden stick.

that this speeds recovery and reduces the number of postoperative complications. Some of the tests described in this section are under review at the moment, and the emphasis in many hospitals is increasingly on reducing the cost of medical care. This means that physicians are being encouraged to reduce the number of routine tests to a minimum or have the tests performed before the patient comes to the hospital if that is possible. A necessary test is never omitted, but the physician must be sure that the test is justified before ordering it.

Each nursing station has a thick book listing all of the tests which can be done, and the size of the book increases every year. This section is unable to discuss all of the possible tests a patient can have done; but by explaining the significance of the most common tests in a diagnosis, it is hoped that a patient will submit to the tests with interest, not impatience. A test is less alarming if the patient knows beforehand what to expect.

Blood Samples. You can be certain that during a stay in a hospital you will receive visits from the laboratory technician who will take a sample of blood. You will notice that the technician who draws your blood will collect it in glass tubes with rubber stoppers of different colors. For a complete blood count (CBC), the stopper is usually a mauve color because there is a chemical in the tube which stops the blood from clotting. For many other tests, the stopper is red and the tube is plain glass. The blood is allowed to clot and the clear yellowish fluid known as serum is used for testing. With modern needles and experienced personnel, the discomfort of having your blood taken is minimal. *See also* BLOOD COUNT, COMPLETE.

Complete Blood Count. When a CBC is done, the technicians calculate the number of red blood cells per cubic milliliter of blood. They also look at the size and shape of the cells, the proportion of red cells to the total amount of blood (the hematocrit), and the amount of hemoglobin (protein in the red cells that carries oxygen to the tissues) in the sample. A low red blood cell count is called anemia. If you are anemic, your body cells may not receive an adequate supply of oxygen. Common causes of anemia are loss of blood or lack of iron in the diet, but it may also be caused by a malfunction of the bone marrow that produces the cells or an increased rate of destruction of the red cells. These normally survive for about four months before being broken down. *See also* ANEMIA; BLOOD CELL, RED.

The technicians also look at the white cells. Although there is only one variety of red blood cell, there are several different types of white blood cell. They are one of the main body defenses against infection and disease. An increase in the number of normal white cells is often seen if the body is fighting an infection such as appendicitis or pneumonia. Although a normal white blood count (WBC) would not exclude the condition, it would make it less likely. An excessive number of abnormal white cells may indicate leukemia. *See also* BLOOD CELL, WHITE; LEUKEMIA.

The technicians also investigate the blood's ability to clot. If there is a break in a blood vessel wall, it is plugged by small components in the blood known as platelets, which release a chemical and start the process of clotting. A platelet count is part of the automated CBC now used universally. *See also* PLATELET.

Continuous Flow Analysis. Another test that requires a blood sample is run on a machine called a continuous flow analyzer. With barely half an ounce of blood, the technicians can run 12 to 20 different tests at appreciably less cost than if the various chemical tests were ordered individually. Several body functions are screened, and if a result is abnormal, it may provide a useful clue to some disorder or condition. Sometimes, the routine screening picks up an elevation of blood sugar long before any symptoms of diabetes have developed. Although no treatment is needed, the patient can be advised to alter his or her diet. *See also* DIABETES; GLUCOSE.

Blood Clotting Tests. In addition to the many blood tests used to help in diagnosis, there are other tests which are used to gauge the severity of a disease or the effectiveness of treatment. For instance, the victim of a heart attack has daily blood tests run to measure the level of chemicals released

Electrocardiogram (EKG)

As the breakdown of the EKG chart shows, each impulse of the heart is recorded through the sensitive electrodes placed on the patient's body. The physician is able to study the strength and the quality of each phase of the heartbeat and identify disorders such as atrial fibrillation. On this trace, the physician can see that the atrial impulse is weak and irregular, thus impeding adequate systolic impulses. Similarly, the trace of a patient who has had an infarct recently, or a patient who has suffered an infarct some time before, is easily identified by the unusual EKG trace.

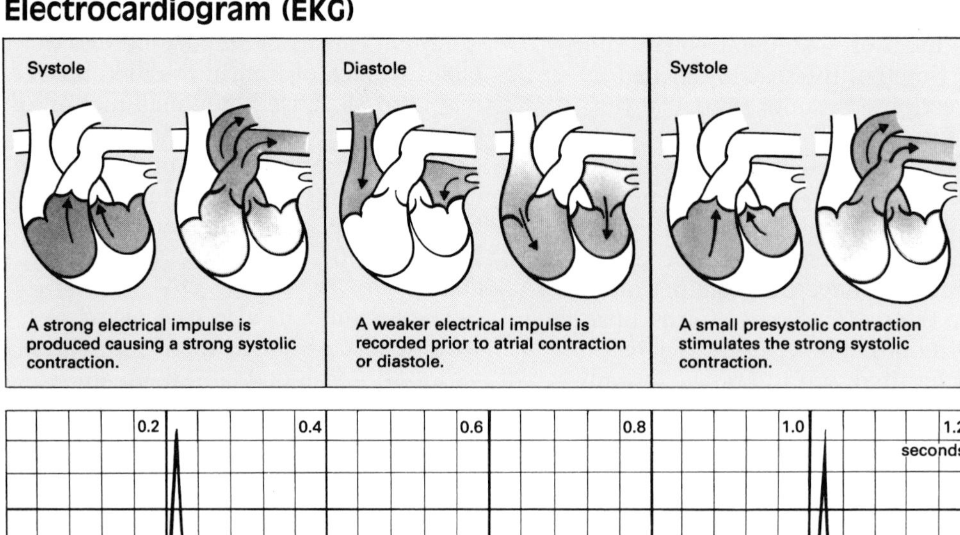
Systole
Diastole
Systole
A strong electrical impulse is produced causing a strong systolic contraction.
A weaker electrical impulse is recorded prior to atrial contraction or diastole.
A small presystolic contraction stimulates the strong systolic contraction.

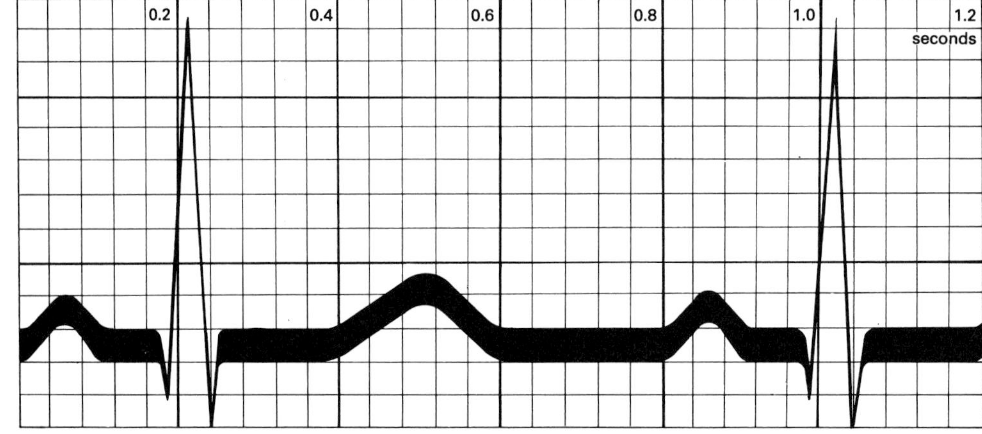
0.2
0.4
0.6
0.8
1.0
1.2
seconds

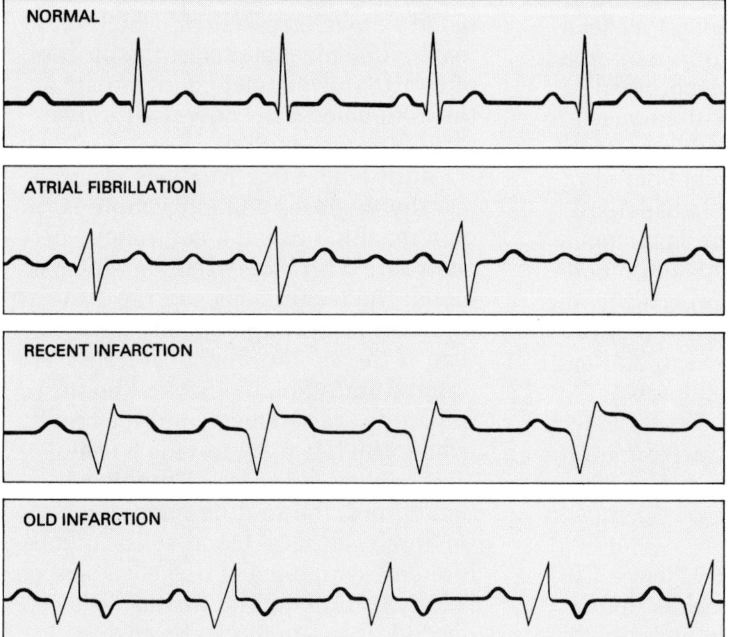
NORMAL
ATRIAL FIBRILLATION
RECENT INFARCTION
OLD INFARCTION

from damaged or dead heart cells. The more extensive the damage, the higher the proportion of chemicals in the bloodstream.

Some conditions, for instance thrombophlebitis, are treated with agents to slow down the rate of clotting. Tests are run daily while medication is given to ensure that the interference with the clotting is not too great. *See also* BLOOD CLOT.

Frequent drawing of blood can be tedious for the patient. But it makes everything more interesting if you ask the technician what the tests are for. The technician may welcome the chance to explain. Remember, he or she cannot tell you why a test has been ordered or talk about the result. This is the job of your physician.

Electrocardiograph. An electrocardiograph (EKG) records the electrical activity of the heartbeat. The test is safe and painless because the electrical impulses flow from the patient to the machine, not the other way around. Electrodes are placed on the patient's wrists, ankles, and chest, and effective contact is achieved by moistening the skin with jelly before applying the electrodes. The resulting graph is useful even if it is a normal trace, because it is changes in the EKG that are important. When a physician is faced with an EKG tracing with questionable changes, it is a great help if there are previous normal tracings for comparison. It should be emphasized that repeated EKG tests do not imply that there is something seriously wrong with your heart. *See also* ELECTROCARDIOGRAM.

X-ray Photographs. A chest X ray used to be routine for any patient in the hospital. Today, there is evidence that routine chest X rays performed on people under the age of thirty with no respiratory or cardiac symptoms are no longer justified. The amount of radiation received during a chest X ray is negligible, but any unnecessary exposure to radiation is now avoided. *See also* X RAY.

X-ray photographs of the stomach, the bowel, the gall bladder, and the kidneys demand special techniques, and the patient has to be prepared beforehand. The stomach and intestine must be completely empty, because any food that is retained reduces the quality and clarity of the X ray. The patient must fast for at least half a day before the X ray. He or she is also given laxatives followed by an enema to clear the large intestine.

For a stomach and bowel X ray, the patient has to drink a thick, chalky liquid known as a barium meal. It is completely flavorless. The patient lies down for the X ray and may have to wait long intervals between films to allow the barium to move through the system before another organ is outlined. *See also* BARIUM.

For a kidney X ray, known as an IVP (intravenous pyelogram), the patient is given a small injection. A similar procedure may be used before X-raying the gall bladder. *See also* PYELOGRAM.

Nuclear Scanning. Nuclear scanning is a simple and safe procedure. A chemical is injected into the bloodstream. It is called a radioactive tracer, and it is taken up by various organs in the body. The concentration of radioactive material in the various organs is measured with a Geiger-Müller counter, giving an impression of their size and ability to function. The test is often used as a safe screening procedure to determine whether there is an abnormality that might require further, more complicated tests. *See also* NUCLEAR MEDICINE.

Ultrasound and Echo Studies. These studies are used mainly for examinations of the heart and abdomen. The procedures are painless and completely safe. They work on the same principle as sonar, in that the sound waves or ultrasound waves reflect off different tissues at different rates, enabling an image to be formed. *See also* ULTRASOUND.

Computerized Axial Tomography. One of the more dramatic advances in recent years is the CAT scan. Information that formerly could only be obtained by exploratory surgery can now often be gathered with accuracy and safety. For instance, the investigation of certain brain diseases sometimes required a procedure called air encephalography that was painful for the patient, required the services of a neurologist, a radiologist, and a technician, and carried some danger. The CAT scan has made this procedure rarely necessary. From the patient's point of view, the scan is no more troublesome than having one's photograph

X-ray photographs

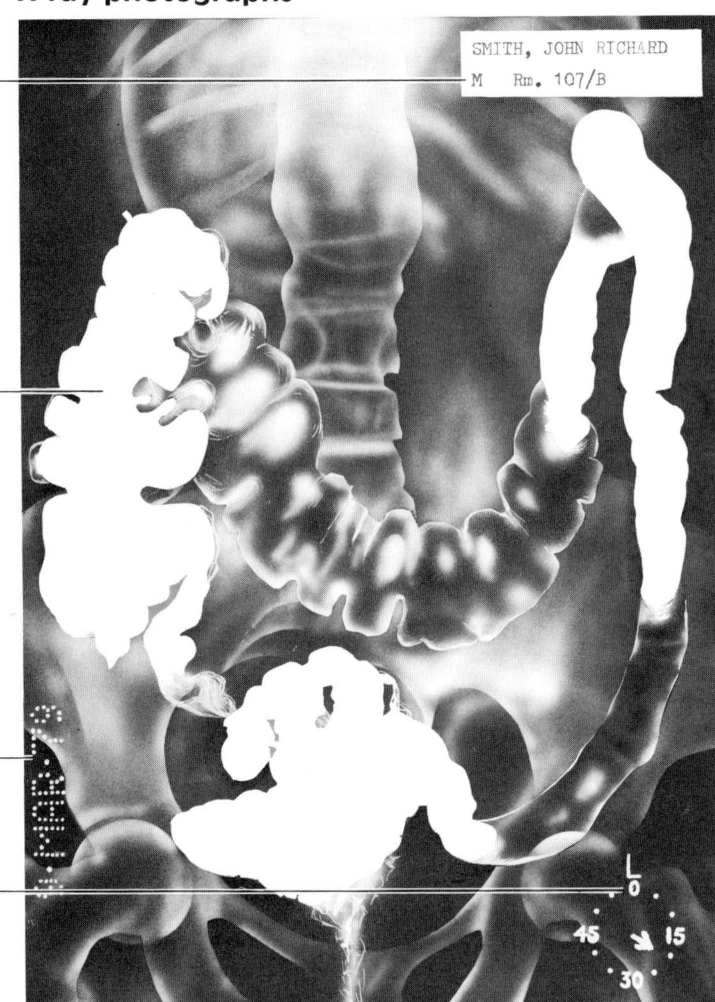

Identification
The patient's full name is clearly marked, followed by the sex and hospital room number.

Artificial dye
A dye, such as a barium salt, when swallowed or injected, is radiopaque and shows up clearly on an X ray. On this artwork representation, the large intestine from cecum to rectum is being examined; certain areas have been highlighted for clarity.

Date
The date is important for monitoring the patient's progress over several days, and perhaps several years.

Time
It is also important to know how long after the initial swallowing or injection the X ray is being taken. Above the "clock", the "L" indicates that this is the patient's *left* side.

A common use of X rays is to check whether or how a bone has been fractured. There are a number of different kinds of fracture and it is essential to know exactly what the break is like before treatment begins. It is vital to be able to see, for example, that the young child (*left X ray*) actually has a clean break in the radius at the wrist, and not the greenstick fracture more common at her age. X rays can also be used to see that any metal pin or bolt inserted to reinforce a damaged bone is fulfilling its purpose. A prosthesis, such as an artificial hip joint (*right X ray*) made of metal or plastic, can be seen to be in place and functioning properly.

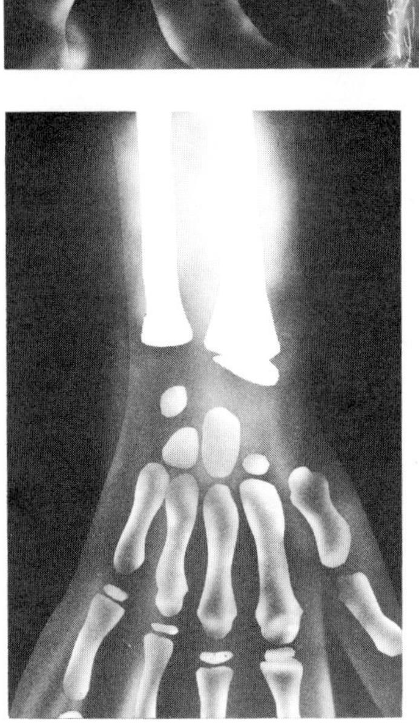

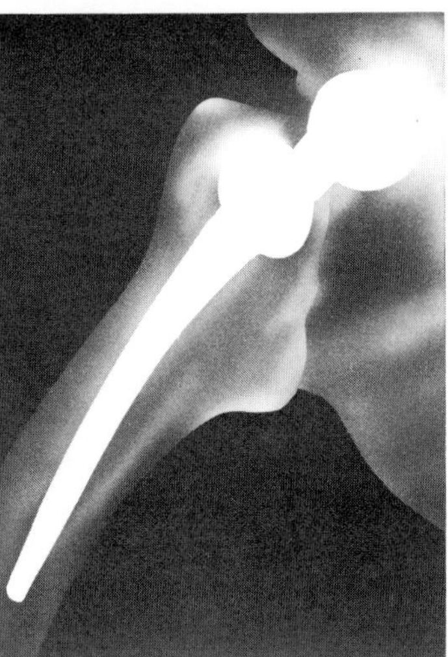

taken. *See also* COMPUTERIZED AXIAL TOMOGRAPHY SCANNER.

Stress Test. A common test of cardiac efficiency is the stress test, which is usually done as a "screen" for coronary artery disease before any disease is obvious. Although it is more commonly an outpatient procedure, it is usually done in a hospital cardiac department. Electrodes are attached to the patient, who walks slowly on a revolving rubber treadmill. The speed is gradually increased, and the heart rate is kept under constant observation for any signs of stress. *See also* STRESS TEST.

Respiratory Laboratory. This is where the efficiency of a patient's lung function is tested. The test normally involves little more than breathing in and out of a series of machines, but may also include some blood sampling. It is quite safe and, apart from the discomfort of taking a blood sample, quite painless. *See also* LUNG FUNCTION TEST.

Typical Hospital Routine

The hospital day usually begins around 6:00 a.m. The reason everything happens earlier in a hospital than at home is that with the many tests available for an accurate diagnosis, the sooner the results are obtained the better. The physician in charge can then make his or her decision as a result of the tests.

The night staff has to make a note of vital signs first thing in the morning. This includes taking your temperature and your pulse, monitoring your respiration, and possibly taking your blood pressure. This monitoring of vital signs will be repeated usually four times during the day.

Shortly after you wake up, you may be visited by a laboratory technician for a blood sample. The laboratories prefer to have the bulk of the blood specimens ready when the day staff arrives at 8:00 a.m. This enables the laboratory staff to complete its work by 5:00 p.m.

Before breakfast you are expected to wash. If you are convalescing, your physician may have indicated on the order sheet that you can have bathroom privileges. This means you can take care of your personal toilet at the start of the day, go to the bathroom, wash, or take a shower when you feel like it, depending to some extent on the availability of a bathroom.

If you are confined to bed, then toilet facilities are brought to you and assistance given if it is needed. This may be done at any time in the morning depending on how busy the floor is, how many sick patients require a lot of personal attention, or how many patients have to be prepared for early surgery or X rays.

Breakfast is usually served between 7:00 and 7:30 a.m. Patients often find that, because there is little in their day to occupy them, they look forward to mealtimes with interest because meals break up the day.

Meals. Obviously, a very sick and confused patient will be in no condition to choose his or her menu. The patient may in fact be on an intravenous drip feed. Everybody else, however, receives a daily checklist from which to choose meals for the following day. The choice you are offered depends on any special restrictions placed on your diet by your physician, and these will be written on your order sheet. The food is brought to you by a member of the dietary department. A nursing aide usually checks to see if you need any help cutting up the food or with eating and drinking.

The food should be hot, and nowadays, great efforts are made to provide food that is appetizing as well as nutritious. Apart from regular meals, there is usually some provision made for snacks at regular intervals, and these are also specified on the order sheet.

Ask the dietician what sort of diet you are supposed to be on before accepting any food or drink brought in by friends and relatives. For anything but a "regular diet," you should have nothing extra without your physician's approval.

Special Diets. Special diets are used in the treatment and management of certain disorders. For instance, if a patient is suffering from an acute liver or kidney disorder, a low-protein diet may be prescribed. Low-residue diets are prescribed for inflammation of the gastrointestinal tract, and high-residue diets for diverticular disease. Patients suffering from gout are occasionally advised to follow a low-purine diet. Purines are broken down into uric acid, and an excess of uric acid production can aggravate gout. Diabetics are kept

Medical charts, such as temperature charts, are a day-to-day record of the patient's condition.

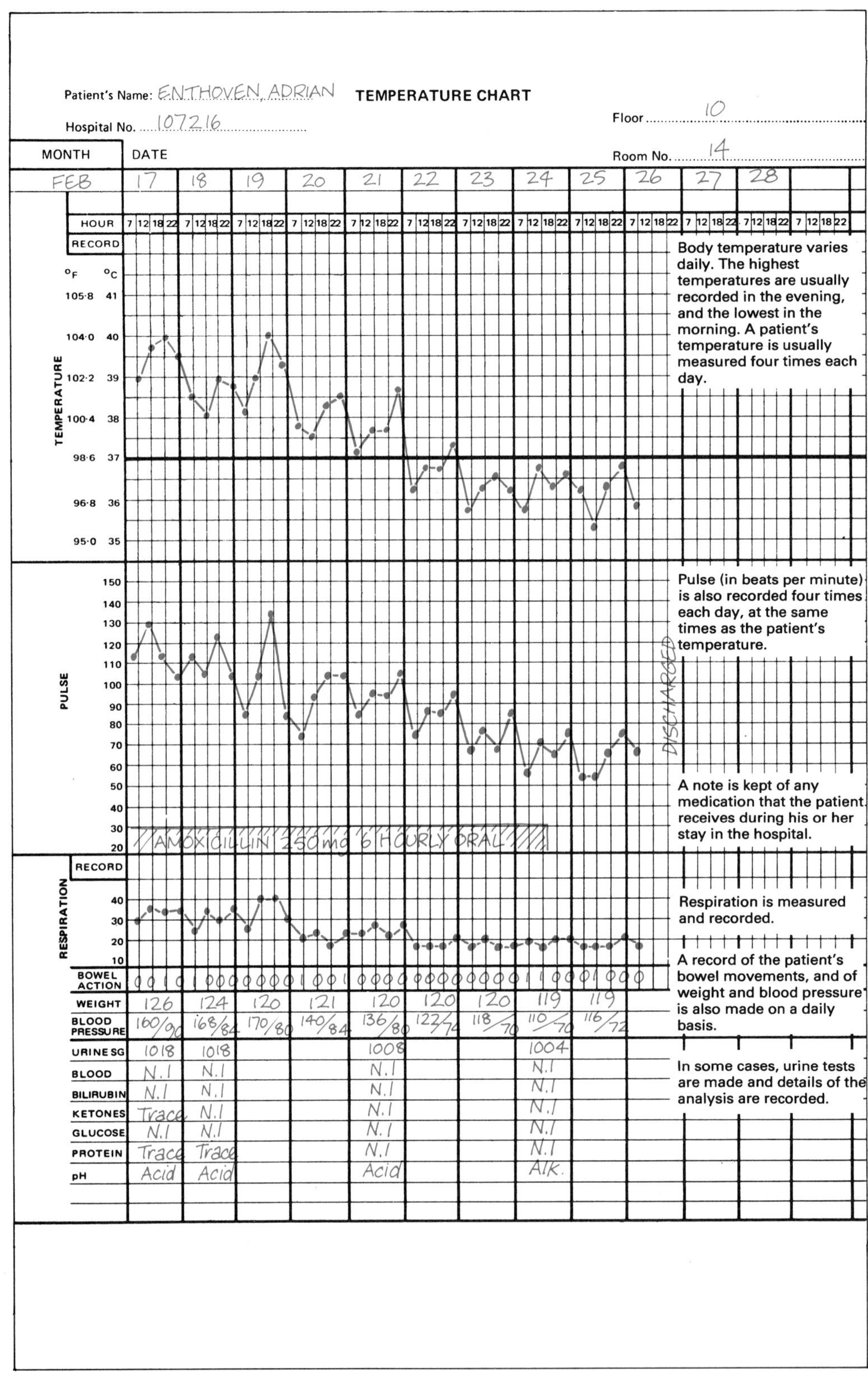

Patient's Name: ENTHOVEN, ADRIAN
TEMPERATURE CHART
Hospital No. 107216
Floor 10
MONTH
DATE
Room No. 14
FEB
17 18 19 20 21 22 23 24 25 26 27 28
HOUR
7 12 18 22
RECORD
°F °C
105·8 41
104·0 40
102·2 39
100·4 38
98·6 37
96·8 36
95·0 35
TEMPERATURE
PULSE
150 140 130 120 110 100 90 80 70 60 50 40 30 20
AMOXCILLIN 250mg 6 HOURLY ORAL
DISCHARGED
RESPIRATION
40 30 20 10
BOWEL ACTION
WEIGHT 126 124 120 121 120 120 120 119 119
BLOOD PRESSURE 160/90 168/84 170/80 140/84 136/80 122/74 118/70 110/70 116/72
URINE SG 1018 1018 1008 1004
BLOOD N.I N.I N.I N.I
BILIRUBIN N.I N.I N.I N.I
KETONES Trace N.I N.I N.I
GLUCOSE N.I N.I N.I N.I
PROTEIN Trace Trace N.I N.I
pH Acid Acid Acid Alk.
Body temperature varies daily. The highest temperatures are usually recorded in the evening, and the lowest in the morning. A patient's temperature is usually measured four times each day.
Pulse (in beats per minute) is also recorded four times each day, at the same times as the patient's temperature.
A note is kept of any medication that the patient receives during his or her stay in the hospital.
Respiration is measured and recorded.
A record of the patient's bowel movements, and of weight and blood pressure is also made on a daily basis.
In some cases, urine tests are made and details of the analysis are recorded.

on a carefully controlled diet. The catering department of each hospital produces these varied diets for the patients under care. *See also* DIET, SPECIAL.

The Order Sheet. The staff on the unit gets all of the information about your daily routine and care from the order sheet. The physician writes his or her instructions on the sheet, and the nurses consult it whenever they need information.

Instructions about your activity around the ward are written on the order sheet. "Up ad lib" or "unrestricted" means that you are free to get up and walk around the room, go to the dayroom, and use the corridor. You should not leave the unit without permission because, if you were suddenly taken ill, there would be a delay in getting help to you. "Up ad lib in room" means you may walk about the room, but not leave it. "Bathroom privileges," as previously mentioned, means that you may use the bathroom when you want to. If you do not understand the reason for a certain restriction, ask the resident physician to explain it to you.

Rounds. Throughout the day, various people go round the unit to check on the progress of the patients. The head nurse or the deputy head nurse usually make a round early in the morning (between 7:30 a.m. and 8:30 a.m.). The head nurse's comments are important to the physician in charge, and it is the nurse's responsibility to pass on all the information to the physician or the resident.

The head nurse also draws up a list of problems on which to base the plan for the day and assigns jobs to various members of the team in the nursing unit.

During the morning, one or more of the resident physicians will visit you to see how you are, correlate your progress with the information collected by the nursing staff, and discuss any changes in your condition. The resident is also there to answer any questions you may have, although you should remember that the ultimate authority rests with the physician in charge of your case.

The physicians are not encouraged to discuss the case in front of the patient. For somebody with no medical background, it is alarming to hear a group of physicians discussing possibilities, because, even if the patient does not understand the terms the physicians use, some of the words may sound threatening. If, however, you are worried by a remark made between physicians, you should promptly ask for clarification.

The physician in charge of your case may make his or her own visit at any time of the day depending on his or her schedule. It is a good idea to ask for an estimate of when the visit might be, so that you do not become unnecessarily anxious. Your physician's visit is the most important one for you because

Sample diets	*Bland diet*	*Low-fat diet*	*High-fiber diet*
Breakfast	Fruit juice Cereal, milk, and sugar Eggs (boiled or poached, not fried) Toast and butter	Fruit juice Cereal, milk, and sugar Egg (boiled or poached, not fried) Tea with skimmed milk	Fresh fruit Whole-grain cereal or bran, milk, and sugar Whole-grain bread Weak tea
Lunch	Cream soup Whitefish Creamed potatoes Cooked vegetables Stewed fruit and custard Milk or weak tea	Liver or veal or whitefish Boiled potatoes Cooked vegetables Fruit Skimmed milk	Lean meat Potatoes Vegetables, such as spinach or cabbage Stewed fruit Buttermilk
Supper	Chicken or lean meat Cooked vegetables Sponge cake or gelatin Milk or weak tea	Cottage cheese Salad (without oil or dressing) Fruit or cake Skimmed milk	Cheese or lean meat Salad Whole-grain bread Fresh fruit Weak tea

A large number of special diets are prescribed as part of the treatment of certain disorders. This chart gives sample meals for three diets commonly prescribed in hospitals. The bland diet is often prescribed for patients who have fever or who are convalescing. The low-fat diet is suitable for patients suffering from gall bladder disease. The high-fiber diet is for patients suffering from constipation.

all of the important decisions are made by him or her. Try to organize your questions beforehand so that the time may be used with maximum efficiency.

The nurse assigned to each patient has the job of dispensing all the medications. It is also the nurse's job to provide all the primary care necessary for the patient assigned to him or her. When the medication is ordered by your physician, the information is transferred to a card which is kept on the medication chart. This means that the nurse has a record about which drug he or she should administer to the patient, how often it should be given, and in what circumstances it should be given. Each dose administered will be noted on the chart by the nurse. The nursing staff carries out numerous safety checks to make sure that there are no mistakes. You can participate by learning what each tablet or capsule is, so that if you are given a new pill you can ask when it was ordered.

Dispensing medication is a very responsible job, and the nurse must concentrate on what he or she is doing.

At some time during the morning a member of the housekeeping department cleans your room thoroughly. This may be done while you are out of your room having tests or X-ray photographs. During the morning your bed is changed and tidied. You can ask for this to be done again if a restless day has made the bed untidy by the evening.

Entertainment. Television is not included automatically in the facilities provided by the hospital and must be paid for separately, although the rates are reasonable. Most hospitals provide a radio which can be listened to with headphones in order not to disturb other patients. The radio has only a limited selection of stations.

Some hospitals offer library facilities, and these are usually run by a volunteer who makes a round with a library cart each day. The volunteer department also has a cart that sells magazines, toilet articles, such as toothpaste or shampoo, and other small items. The daily newspapers are provided by regular employees, who make daily rounds, a newspaper vending machine in the lobby, or a hospital gift shop. It is therefore a good idea to keep a small amount of money with you to buy a newspaper or magazine. You can also ask a friend to bring in reading literature if the hospital does not have a library.

Visiting Hours. Few hospitals permit visiting by family and friends much before two o'clock in the afternoon, and regular visiting usually finishes at eight or nine in the evening. This leaves the morning free for the staff to carry out the bulk of the work. By the afternoon, there is unlikely to be any major activity to occupy the patient's time. This is when a visit from friends can be a welcome break in the daily routine.

There may be a limit on the number of visitors allowed in a room at any one time, which may not always be strictly enforced, unless, as occasionally happens, the system is abused and patients in nearby beds are disturbed or distressed by a crowd of noisy visitors. Relatives can always ask the head nurse on the unit if they are worried about the number of visitors allowed. Visitors should also remember that the patient is a captive audience, and a few short visits are less tiring and break the day up better than one visit that lasts an hour. If you find that you are getting unduly tired by visitors or that there are people you do not want to see, you can let your physician know. There are many ways of protecting a patient from unwanted visitors without causing personal embarrassment.

Visiting time is a good opportunity for you to take a short walk, with assistance if necessary, provided your physician has given consent. Visiting time also provides an opportunity for the family to participate in the care of the patient, encouraging the patient to drink plenty of fluids or helping the patient to brush his or her hair. Such activity is very supportive for the patient.

Visiting time and routines are very different on a children's ward, as explained in the section HOSPITALIZATION: CHILDREN.

The Night Time. Many patients find sleeping difficult at night for various reasons. The lights on the unit are turned out early, at about 9:30 in the evening, and you may have slept during the day. There are constant disturbances on the unit because patients need medication throughout the night. You may be sharing a room with a very sick patient who needs constant nursing, or you may feel feverish and unwell yourself. However, there are several nonhabit-forming drugs available to overcome sleeping problems, and these are often offered to you to be used as required.

If you are kept awake by disturbances in the unit, you must accept that other patients have needs that must be fulfilled. If the disturbance is made by the night staff and you think that the noise is unnecessary, you should talk the matter over with the hospital representative. If the noise is unavoidable (for instance, moving an emergency admission into the ward after an operation), this can be explained to you. If not, the hospital representative can take up the legitimate complaint. Patients are sometimes afraid to make a complaint about hospital employees, because their temporary dependency makes them fear a reprisal. Complaints are always handled confidentially. There are a variety of ways in which the validity of a complaint can be verified without involving the patient who made the allegation.

While the patients sleep, the night staff is working. One of their duties is to make regular rounds of all the rooms to verify that the patients are in fact asleep, that the breathing is regular, and the pulse is steady. The night rounds are important, because falls can occur during the night when a patient leaves his or her bed in order to visit the bathroom, possibly imagining himself or herself at home. You should not usually be aware of night rounds.

Checking Out of the Hospital

The day of discharge is the most important day in the patient's hospital stay. Although it may appear straightforward to the patient, there are many procedures that have to be completed before the patient can leave.

The day of discharge is usually decided 24 hours before, and the decision is made by the physician in charge of your case. He or she is the only person authorized to discharge you. All your questions should have been answered, and you should be fully aware of the outcome of your hospital stay and the type and degree of activity in which you can involve yourself.

Some hospitals have printed sheets of instructions for patients convalescing from common disorders or operations. The physician usually discusses all of these subjects with you the day before you are discharged from the hospital. After this discussion, the physician has to go to the nursing station to review your hospital record. The physician does this every day in order to see any new test results or to read the nursing reports or medicine orders.

On the day before discharge, there are additional items that require his or her attention. The order for discharge and the date of discharge have to be written on the record. The physician will have to check that a careful record has been made of the medication which the patient needs to continue taking at home and that a prescription for these drugs has been written. The physician must also add a final diagnosis or diagnoses on the face sheet of the record, and dictate a summary of all that has happened during the hospital stay. This latter piece of information may be compiled by the resident physician and may be done a few days after you have left the hospital. It is an important part of the procedure, particularly if another physician is taking over your care during convalescence at home.

The summary reviews your complete case, records the results of all the tests, describes any surgical or diagnostic procedures, states what medication you were given or may still be taking, and what treatment you were given while in the hospital. If any tissues have been removed from the body, they are sent for microscopic examination by a pathologist, and the summary includes the pathologist's report. If you received a blood transfusion during your stay, this is also recorded on the summary, a copy of which is sent to your family physician to become part of your personal medical record.

Until the discharge order is written and signed, no patient can legally leave the hospital or be released by another member of the staff. Once it is signed, other people on the unit continue the discharge procedure.

The ward clerk will notify the cashier's office, and in many hospitals the information is passed through a computer so that all areas of the hospital know which patients are being dis-

Most hospitals have a fairly standard procedure for discharging patients.

Procedure for checking out of the hospital

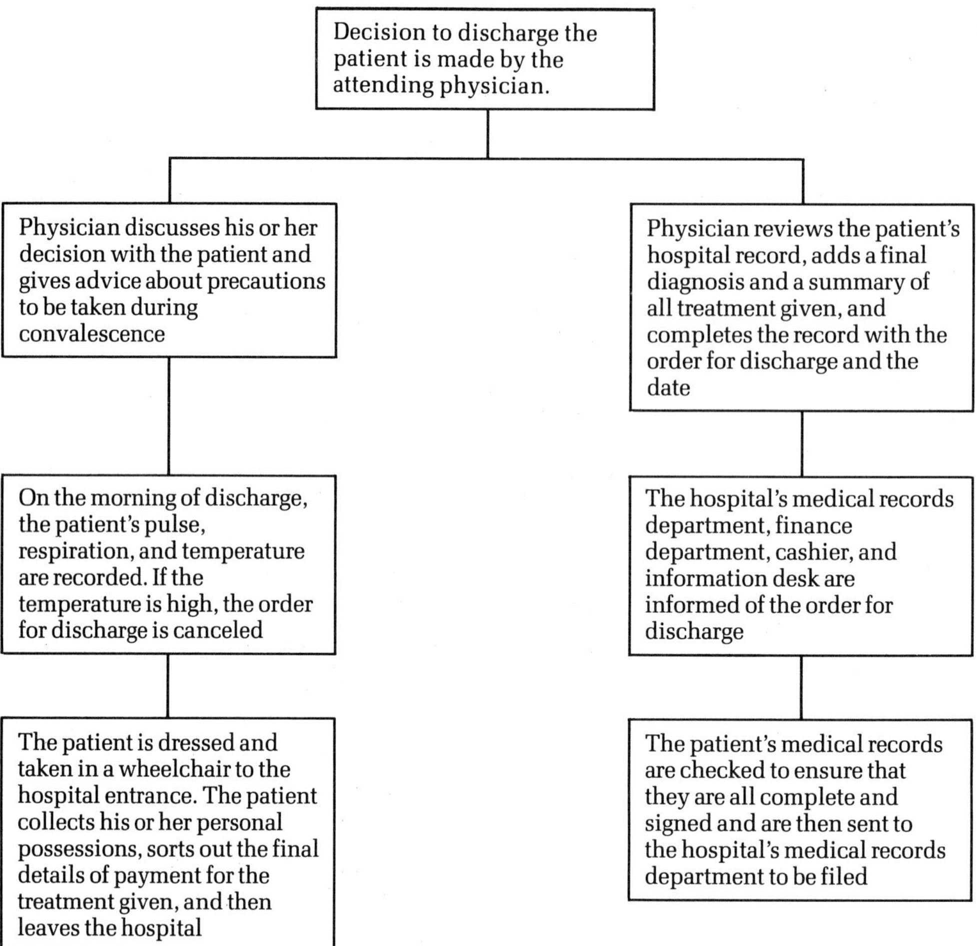

Decision to discharge the patient is made by the attending physician.
Physician discusses his or her decision with the patient and gives advice about precautions to be taken during convalescence
Physician reviews the patient's hospital record, adds a final diagnosis and a summary of all treatment given, and completes the record with the order for discharge and the date
On the morning of discharge, the patient's pulse, respiration, and temperature are recorded. If the temperature is high, the order for discharge is canceled
The hospital's medical records department, finance department, cashier, and information desk are informed of the order for discharge
The patient is dressed and taken in a wheelchair to the hospital entrance. The patient collects his or her personal possessions, sorts out the final details of payment for the treatment given, and then leaves the hospital
The patient's medical records are checked to ensure that they are all complete and signed and are then sent to the hospital's medical records department to be filed

Checklist of documents and personal possessions

Before leaving the hospital, the patient should check that he or she has collected all the following items:

- Clothes
- Money and valuables
- Other personal possessions such as toilet articles, books, letters, and writing equipment
- Medications
- Medical prescriptions
- Physician's checklist of instructions for convalescence
- Receipts for all bills paid
- Insurance forms and certificates, signed where necessary

charged. This includes the information desk, finance department, and the medical records department.

On the day of discharge all of the materials involved in your medical care are assembled by a nurse who checks that the records are complete before sending them down to the medical records department after your release.

The ward clerk usually asks you what time you will be leaving and also informs you of the hospital policy for the time of departure.

On the morning of discharge, pulse, respiration, and temperature are recorded as usual, as an additional safeguard. If a patient has even a slight temperature, he or she may not be discharged. This precaution is necessary to prevent complications after the patient has gone home.

A member of the nursing staff makes sure you have a prescription for medication, which you can collect from the hospital's pharmacy. Once at home, you should make use of a local pharmacy for refills. The nurse will check that the prescription is correctly dated and signed. The physician may have left instructions for the administration of medication before you leave the hospital. Any drugs left on the medicine cart in your name are returned to the pharmacy.

A nurse on the unit will help you to dress if you can not manage on your own. You will then be asked to wait in your room until someone comes to help you down to the hospital entrance. Even if you are feeling healthy and fit, you will be asked to sit in a wheelchair for the journey. Many hospitals have a risk management expert who is employed full-time to transport patients. This is a wise precaution for many reasons. Even if your hospital stay was short and the condition or operation minor, you will certainly have spent more time in bed than usual. Because of this, your muscles will be temporarily weaker. You may find that after a walk to the elevator and a standing wait, you feel weak and dizzy. You may even faint.

You are taken in the wheelchair to the main lobby where you can collect your valuables from the cashier's office and sort out details of payment. For weak patients, a member of the security department will deliver valuables to the room.

Discharge Against Medical Advice. Occasionally, a patient discharges himself or herself against the advice of the physicians. In such an event, the patient must sign a form confirming that the action being taken is against medical advice (known as A.M.A.) and that the hospital and medical staff concerned can not, therefore, be responsible for anything that happens afterwards. A.M.A. is obviously a dangerous practice. The reason is often dissatisfaction about the care you are receiving. If this is the case, it is safer to ask for another physician to take over your case than to leave the hospital against advice.

Hospitalization: Children. Fortunately for young patients, there have been enormous advances in the technical and professional aspects of pediatric care, as well as in the understanding of the emotional needs of hospitalized children. Twenty or thirty years ago, there was a general feeling that small patients were easier to handle if their parents did not visit them too often. Now it is recognized that, although a stay in the hospital is a worrying period for any child, the experience can be less frightening and traumatic if the parents are actively involved in the child's care and recovery.

Pediatric facilities vary from hospital to hospital. The following article is based on a modern children's hospital. A parent should not be concerned if facilities are not the same as those described, as long as there is ample evidence that the team caring for the child understands his or her needs, as well as the needs of the parents. The more involved a parent can be with the treatment, the better. Few parents would choose to stand by and watch when they could be taking an active part in their child's recovery. *See also* PEDIATRICS.

Preparing a Child for a Hospital Stay. The hospitalization of a child should be something that is openly discussed throughout a child's early life. If a friend is in the hospital, take the chance of visiting with your child so that he or she becomes accustomed to hospitals when healthy. Similarly, if a brother or sister has to go into the hospital, make sure that all the family have a chance to visit.

A child's impressions about hospitals are molded by the parents' opinions. Never let your child hear you talking about horrific medical or surgical experiences or discussing relatives who have died in the hospital, in case the child imagines hospitals are for dying in.

A child's reaction to hospitalization also depends on age. A child between the ages of 6 months and 4 years is more likely to be upset by the experience. This is why many operations are postponed until after this age. Obviously in an emergency there is no choice, but it is important that the parents are there when the child regains consciousness after an injury or anesthetic.

The adolescent from 12 years of age through the teens presents a different set of problems and needs. The upper limit of pediatric age varies from 16 to 21, depending on how large a hospital's facilities are and the availability of beds. Some hospitals are fortunate enough to have sufficient room to separate the various pediatric age groups, so that the different units can care in a more specific manner for their patients. For instance, a teenager would find little to interest him or her in a playroom, and a four-year-old would not want to play pool or table tennis. A certain amount of overlapping is a good idea, however, because the older children often enjoy helping the younger ones.

Many pediatric centers have a well established preadmission program to help prepare the patients. This may include a film or a puppet show. In the home, parents should encourage "doctor and nurse" games and intervene only if the game becomes dangerously inaccurate, for instance, if you notice the children enacting painful or violent scenes. You should explain carefully that this is not the sort of thing that happens in a real hospital.

Before Admission. It is probably kinder to delay telling a child under the age of six that he or she is going into the hospital until a few days before the event. This spares the child weeks of worry. However, an older child, particularly one of late school age, may find it easier to know in advance, so that he or she can organize schoolwork with the teacher.

Before any child goes into the hospital for elective surgery, make sure that he or she understands which part of the body is going to be operated on and how the surgeon is going to do the operation. You must be receptive to any questions the child wants to ask, because often what seems like a thorough explanation to an adult summons up horrific ideas in the mind of a child. For instance, a child may be convinced that the only way a surgeon can reach the adenoids is by taking off the nose. The child will want to know if the operation is going to hurt. You can explain that an anesthetic is given before

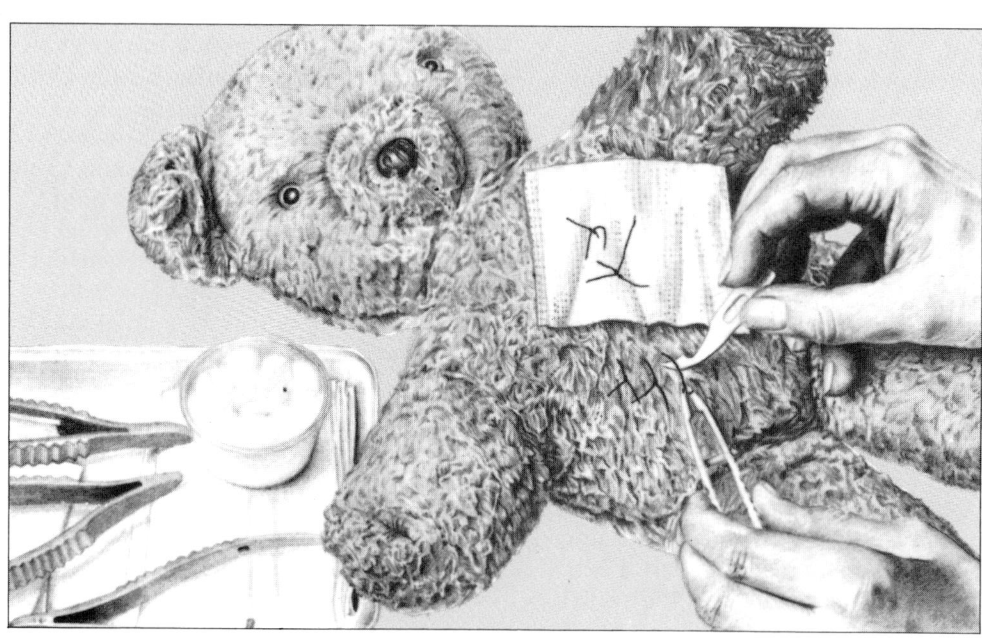

Removing stitches after an operation can be easily explained to a child by using his or her teddy bear as an example. A nurse can stitch the teddy bear up and show the child how stitches are lifted with the tweezers and gently cut with the stitch cutter. The child can also be encouraged to remove some of the stitches.

the operation, which makes him or her go to sleep. Explain that if the child is sore after waking up, the physician or nurse will give something to ease the soreness. In fact, children recuperate very quickly from surgery and are often up and about the following day with little or no apparent pain. *See also* ANESTHETIC; SURGERY.

Children always want to know about shots and needles. There is no point in trying to pretend that the child won't have a shot while in the hospital or that it won't hurt. You can explain that very small needles are used and that a shot doesn't hurt much.

Older children require detailed answers to questions and may even want to read about the condition and operation themselves. If your child asks a question which you can not answer with confidence, call your physician and get the facts right. An adolescent may not express concern or may be cross if you suggest that he or she might be worried about going into the hospital. An adolescent is of course just as worried as a younger child, because this is a time of life when the body goes through many changes. An adolescent is often more concerned with the body and any threat to it than a younger child. It may be better for an older child to discuss the operation with the physician or a nurse. You should give him or her this opportunity if it seems appropriate.

If a physician decides to admit your child to the hospital after seeing him or her as an outpatient, it is important that the child comes home with you to pack his or her things, if possible. If the child is admitted directly into the hospital while you collect the things, there is the possibility the child will think that every visit to an outpatient department will result in confinement. *See also* OUTPATIENT.

Admission. Take the child's immunization record with you. If your child is adopted or you are a legal guardian, the hospital may require you to show the necessary papers. Some hospitals send preadmission papers to you ahead of time so that you can prepare. *See also* IMMUNIZATION.

The preadmission testing may be done before you and your child are taken to the hospital room. With a small child, the blood sample can be obtained by pricking the heel or finger, which is less painful and frightening than the application of a tourniquet and a needle. *See also* BLOOD COUNT, COMPLETE.

Modern hospitals try to make the surroundings attractive and reassuring, and this is particularly evident in pediatric units. The rooms are bright and the colors cheerful. There are pictures on the walls, a playroom for convalescent children, and, sometimes, a recreation room for older children. Many nurses on children's wards wear colored smocks.

The child should not be deprived of any comforters or favorite toys during his or her stay. The nursing staff is aware of this need, so make sure that the child has his or her comforter, even if it is an old piece of cloth.

The hospital may like the child to get undressed and settled into bed. If so, you should undress the child and not leave it up to the staff. This makes the settling-in process easier for the child. Often, a child feels safer if the clothes are left in sight.

Many modern hospitals provide facilities that allow the parents to stay with the child throughout hospitalization and may provide a bed in the child's room. Obviously, not everyone is able to take advantage of the facilities because there may be other members of the family who need care at home. Make sure that the staff knows how much you would like to be involved in the care of your child and when during the day you are likely to be with him or her.

A child under the age of six is more likely to be frightened by separation from his or her parents than by the actual experience of a stay in the hospital. A child who has been left by the parents before, for instance, with a baby sitter or grandparent, is less likely to be upset because he or she knows that the parents always return. Your child is bound to be upset when you leave, and there will be tears, but never make the mistake of either saying you will only be gone for a few minutes or slipping away when the child's attention is elsewhere. The child will never trust your word again. Even when you are separated for a few minutes (such as going for an X ray), the child will think you will not be coming back.

The Day of Surgery. You will probably be allowed to see your child on the day of the operation and should be there when he or she awakes from the anesthetic. This is important because some children think that, if they wake up in another bed, their parents will not be able to find them again.

In some modern hospitals, the child is kept occupied in a playroom next to the operating suite while he or she is waiting for surgery. The child then comes in for the anesthetic in a relaxed frame of mind. Often, no preanesthetic medication is needed. The anesthesiologist may use gas right from the beginning of the anesthetic because it is easy for the child to breathe. Parents are encouraged to tell the nurse any nickname the child may have and to have a favorite toy on hand when the child wakes up. *See also* ANESTHETIC.

Visiting Hours for parents in nearly all hospitals are now unlimited. If you want to stay overnight with your child, the hospital should be able to arrange this. Visits by other people are more subject to general hospital rules, but ask the nurse in charge of the unit if you would like to bring other children in to see the young patient.

When you are at the hospital you may be encouraged to help with the care of the child, by bathing him or her and helping to give medicines. If you have any questions to ask, talk to the head nurse on the unit or the pediatrician during one of the rounds.

Convalescence. A child is well enough to be out of bed when he or she feels like it. Children's units are very different from adult units. Play is actively encouraged, and the children spend most of their time out of bed. They sometimes eat their meals at a communal table, and the children, who are too unwell to be up, can be wheeled into the main play area so that they can watch the other children.

Many hospitals employ a child-life expert as a member of the pediatric team. This worker relates to the child and is often able to aid in the adjustment to hospitalization. The child is also encouraged to learn about his or her experience of being in a hospital. Again, games of "doctors and nurses" should be encouraged, and the child may be allowed to play with instruments such as a stethoscope. As a parent you should involve yourself in these play sessions and make sure that the child-life worker and the nursing staff are familiar with any unusual words your child uses which they may not recognize.

Some hospitals employ a teacher who can help older children to keep up with their educational program. This is very important for a child coming up to exam time, because this could be an additional worry. The hospital teacher can contact the child's regular teacher to see what kind of instruction would be the most helpful, and the parents can bring in the child's schoolbooks.

Discharge from the Hospital. Despite the efforts to make a child's experience of hospitalization as free from fear and pain as possible, the child is bound to be affected in some way. Children under the age of four may refuse to let the parent out of sight for a moment when they are home again and cling as if afraid of losing the parent again. Some children revert to bed-wetting or may have sleeping and eating problems. All these problems should be temporary, but need to be handled with sympathy. If the child keeps coming downstairs in the evening, indulge the whim for a few days. *See also* BED-WETTING; SLEEP DISORDERS.

The final opportunity for the child to learn, as a result of the experience, is when it is all over, but not forgotten. At this point, not only can your child be rewarded with recognition that he or she dealt well with the experience, but it can also be pointed out that many of the child's fears were unfounded.

Outpatient Visits. During an outpatient visit, a parent's participation is important, particularly with a child under the age of three, who may be frightened by a routine examination. When the physician wants to examine the child's eyes, nose, or mouth, the parent should hold the child firmly (but not roughly). Place one hand on the child's forehead and the other around the arm. The child's legs can be firmly held between your legs. If the physician wants to look at the child's ear, the child can be held facing to one side, with the head held firmly against your chest. Talk to the child during the examination and never grip him or her tightly if struggling begins. The physician will gain the child's confidence during the examination by being completely honest, when something is going to hurt. The parent must not try to distract the child's attention or tell him or her to look the other way, if something uncomfortable is about to take place, because the child will not trust the physician during the rest of the examination. The physician usually decides whether or not to discuss the child's case in front of him or her. But, if you feel strongly against it, you can arrange to discuss the case in private.

Hot flash, or flush, is a sensation of warmth accompanied by reddening of the skin of the face. It is a common symptom of menopause.

See also MENOPAUSE.

Housemaid's knee. *See* BURSITIS, PREPATELLAR.

Human immunodeficiency virus. *See* VIRUS, HUMAN IMMUNODEFICIENCY.

Humerus (hyü'mər əs) is the bone of the upper arm, between the shoulder and the elbow. The ulnar nerve lies behind the lower, outer end of the humerus, an area known as the funny bone.

See also FUNNY BONE.

Humor (hyü'mər) is a fluid or semifluid substance in the eyeball. There are two humors, the aqueous humor and the vitreous humor, both of which help to maintain the shape of the eyeball. The aqueous humor is a transparent liquid that fills the region between the cornea at the front of the eye and the lens. The vitreous humor is a transparent, jelly-like substance that occupies the region between the lens and the retina at the back of the eye.

Q: *How is the aqueous humor produced?*

A: The aqueous humor is constantly secreted by the ciliary body around the lens, so there is a continuous flow of the humor from the lens area to the eye's front chamber. The aqueous humor is kept at constant pressure by a compensating leakage in the angle between the outer rim of the iris and the back of the cornea.

Q: *What is the function of the aqueous humor?*

A: The aqueous humor carries nutrients and facilitates the exchange of gases (oxygen and carbon dioxide) in the cornea and other tissues of the eyeball that have no blood supply.

Q: *What disorders may affect the aqueous humor?*

A: Disturbances of the drainage mechanism that maintains a constant fluid pressure in the aqueous humor may cause an increase in the pressure, a condition called glaucoma.

Q: *How is the vitreous humor produced?*

A: The vitreous humor is present from birth and remains virtually unchanged throughout an individual's life.

Q: *What disorders may affect the vitreous humor?*

A: Specks may occur in the vitreous humor caused by the degeneration of its cells with age. This is a normal occurrence. The presence of specks does not noticeably impair vision. Occasionally, a hemorrhage into the vitreous humor may occur, usually caused by an injury. A hemorrhage may also occur in diabetes mellitus, arteriosclerosis, or retinitis. A hemorrhage may be serious and a physician should be consulted.

See also GLAUCOMA.

Huntington's chorea. *See* CHOREA, HUNTINGTON'S.

Hutchinson's teeth. *See* TEETH, HUTCHINSON'S.

Hyaline membrane disease. *See* RESPIRATORY DISTRESS SYNDROME OF THE NEWBORN.

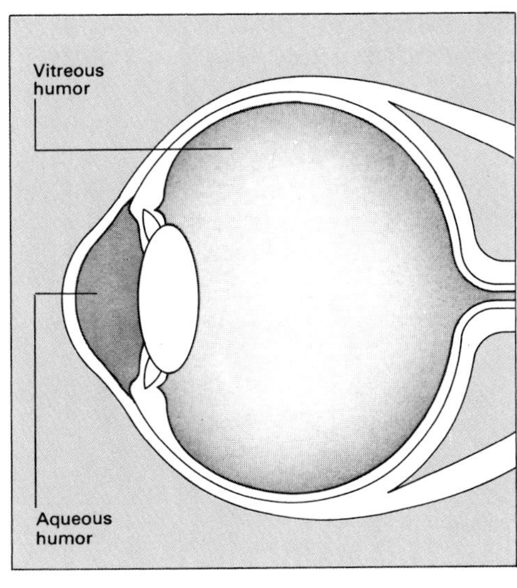

Humor, a fluid or semifluid substance, helps to maintain the shape of the eyeball. Vitreous humor occupies the region between the lens and the retina. Aqueous humor fills the region between the cornea at the front of the eye and the lens.

Hydatid cyst. See CYST, HYDATID.

Hydatidiform, mole. See MOLE, HYDATIDIFORM.

Hydrocele (hī'drō sēl) is an accumulation of fluid in any of the body's sac-like cavities. The term is most often used to describe an excess of fluid in the scrotum, the protective bag of skin that surrounds the testes.

Hydrocele is a collection of fluid in any of the body's sac-like cavities. The term, however, usually refers to an excess of fluid in the scrotum.

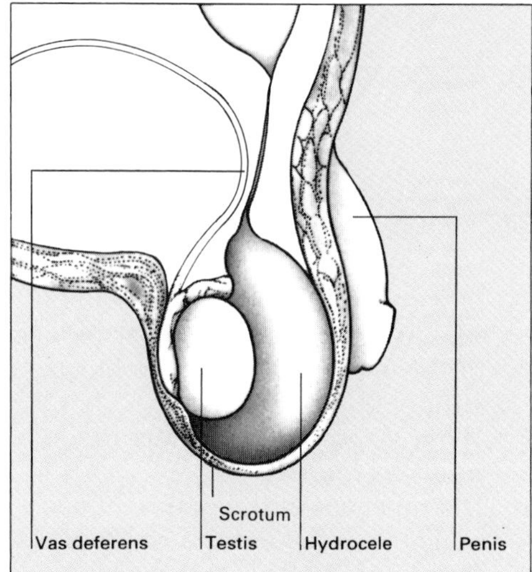

Q: *What causes a hydrocele?*

A: The male embryo has a canal that links the abdominal cavity with the scrotum. This canal usually closes before birth, but it occasionally remains open. Fluid can pass through the open canal and accumulate in the scrotum before birth.

A less common cause of hydrocele is inflammation of a testicle or the epididymis around it. An obstruction in the veins or the lymphatic drainage system from the testes may also cause a hydrocele. This condition is more common in older men. A direct blow to the genitals may also cause a hydrocele.

Q: *How is a hydrocele treated?*

A: Congenital hydrocele usually disappears on its own and does not require treatment. If it persists for more than a year, a physician may advise surgery to tighten or remove the sheath around each testis, where the fluid accumulates.

Hydrocephalus (hī drō sef'ə ləs) is an accumulation of cerebrospinal fluid within the brain, especially in infancy, often causing great enlargement of the head. Brain damage may result from the excessive accumulation of the fluid. Hydrocephalus may be associated with spina bifida.

Q: *What conditions may cause hydrocephalus?*

A: In most cases, there is a congenital blockage of the normal circulation and absorption of cerebrospinal fluid in the brain. Hydrocephalus may also be caused by a brain tumor that interferes with the usual circulation of the cerebrospinal fluid. This can occur following meningitis because of scarring of the membrane covering the brain.

Q: *What symptoms appear with hydrocephalus?*

A: The chief symptom is an abnormally large head. In severe cases, the forehead bulges and the eyes appear to have receded into their sockets. The soft spots or spaces between the cranial bones of the skull (fontanels) may seem unusually tight or tense to touch. There may be irritability, lethargy, vomiting, and neurologic and reflex deficiencies. Diagnosis is made using X rays, CAT scan, and cerebrospinal fluid examination.

Q: *How is hydrocephalus treated?*

A: In about one-third of babies born with hydrocephalus, the condition does not get worse. There are various forms of brain surgery to bypass the blockage to the flow of cerebrospinal fluid. Usually, a tube is run through a tunnel created under the skin to the abdominal cavity where the excess fluid is reabsorbed into the circulatory system.

See also MENINGITIS; SPINA BIFIDA.

Hydrochloric acid (hī drō klô'rik) is a compound of hydrogen and chlorine. Secreted in the stomach, it is an important ingredient in gastric juices.

See also DIGESTIVE SYSTEM.

Hydrocortisone. See CORTISOL.

Hydrogen peroxide (hī'drə jən pə räk'sīd) is a colorless, relatively nontoxic liquid used in a dilute solution in water as an antiseptic to clean wounds, ulcers, abscesses, septic tooth sockets, or inflamed mucous membranes. It may also be used to treat a sore throat, to soften hard wax in the ears, and to bleach hair.

Hydronephrosis (hī drō nef rō′sis) is the swelling of a kidney caused by complete or partial obstruction of urine flow. The obstruction may be caused by a calculus, tumor, enlarged prostate, urinary tract infection, or defect of the ureter. Hydronephrosis causes a gradual destruction of kidney tissues from the increased pressure. Often, there are no symptoms, but occasionally urinary tract infection will call attention to this disorder. There may also be abdominal pain or intermittent pain in the flank. If both kidneys are affected, kidney failure may result.

Q: *How is hydronephrosis diagnosed and treated?*

A: An ultrasound is the diagnostic tool of choice. The image obtained will reveal the dilation of the ureter or ureters and of the kidney collecting system. Treatment is aimed at the underlying cause of hydronephrosis. *See also* ULTRASOUND.

Hydrophobia. *See* RABIES.

Hydrotherapy (hī drō ther′ə pē) is the treatment of a disorder with water, either drinking it or bathing in it.

Hygiene (hī′jēn). Children should be taught a routine of cleanliness from the earliest practicable age. When continued, such a routine develops into a personal habit which enhances an individual's appearance and his or her health.

Personal Hygiene. Because cleanliness is a personal matter, routines differ from person to person. But careful washing of the whole body, preferably once a day, is essential. It is particularly necessary to wash the hands after using the toilet and before touching food. The activities of the day may also necessitate careful washing. A bath or shower that includes washing the hair, for example, is advisable after most sports. In addition, children should be taught not to put their fingers into their ears, nose, or any other orifice, especially if they are natural finger suckers. Although children may need encouragement to use soap and get dirt off properly, most children enjoy baths, and it should not be difficult to accustom them to a washing routine. *See also* HAIR CARE; HAND CARE.

Proper hygiene includes the careful cleaning of the ears, nose, and other areas that might get overlooked during a bath or shower. The wearing of clean clothes, especially undergarments, is also important. A clean pair of underwear should be worn daily.

A proper cleanliness routine helps moderate many skin problems, such as acne and athlete's foot. Another common condition that is moderated by good hygiene is that of body odor. Body odor is largely produced by bacteria on the skin surface that break down glandular secretions (perspiration). The areas that produce the odor, generally the feet, groin, and armpits, should be washed daily with mild soap and water; a deodorant or antiperspirant can then be applied. A deodorant serves to mask body odor, while an antiperspirant primarily works by reducing the amount of perspiration that the body generates. *See also* ACNE; ATHLETE'S FOOT; BODY ODOR.

The more perspiration the body exudes, the more odor there is likely to be; active jobs and pastimes normally increase the body's production of perspiration. But overactive sweat glands in a nonactive person may be the medical condition known as hyperhidrosis.

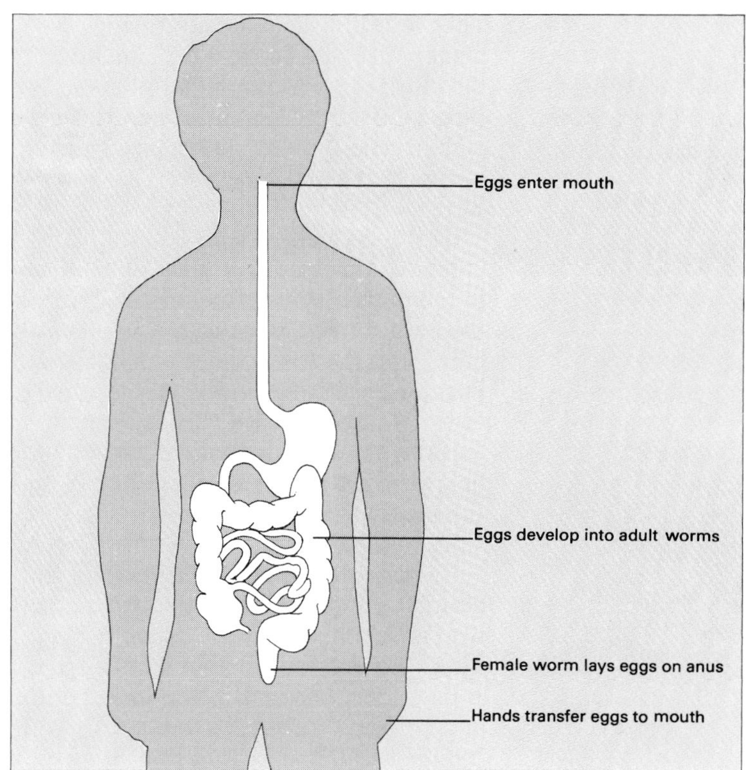
Eggs enter mouth
Eggs develop into adult worms
Female worm lays eggs on anus
Hands transfer eggs to mouth

One of the most common results of improper **hygiene**, especially in children, is infestation by pinworms (also called threadworms). The eggs of the pinworm are swallowed in contaminated water and travel to the small intestine where they develop into adult worms. The female worms move down the intestine and lay eggs in the skin around the anus at night, causing anal itching. The eggs become embedded under the nails during scratching and are transported back to the mouth via contact with the hands to restart the cycle. The eggs can also stick to the lavatory seat or be transferred to towels, bed linen, curtains, books, and clothing. As a precaution, children must be taught never to scratch around the anus and to carefully wash their hands each morning, after using the lavatory and before handling food. Many physicians treat all members of a family when one member is found to have pinworms.

This condition may occur during menopause or as a result of anxiety. If the affected areas are not kept clean, fungal infections (such as moniliasis) may invade the damp skin and cause further problems. *See also* PERSPIRATION.

Dental Hygiene. Teeth should be brushed and flossed at least twice a day to remove food or other particles from the mouth. Nutritious eating habits also help keep the teeth and gums healthy. Regular dental check-ups (about once every six months) are part of proper tooth hygiene. A dentist can treat and help prevent tooth decay and other diseases of the mouth. *See also* TOOTH CARE.

Hygiene in the Work Place. Personal cleanliness is particularly important in work situations where hygiene has a direct bearing on the health of others. A person who works in the preparation or serving of food, for example, should be checked for infection, even if only suffering a mild stomach upset. If a food handler develops an infection such as a boil or a nail infection, he or she should carefully cover the infection or stop handling food until the infection clears. Cuts on the hands and fingers may also harbor harmful bacteria, although these cuts may not appear to be visibly infected. As a general precaution, extra cleanliness is also necessary following a bout of diarrhea or vomiting. A person in food service should also wear a hair net or other hair covering to help prevent the spread of dirt or other small particles.

Taking Care of Others. Sometimes, a physical or mental disability may limit a person's ability to practice proper hygiene. This is especially true of chronically-ill, bedridden patients. In such cases, it is important that someone help the sick person maintain both a clean body and clean surroundings. A sick person may have to be bathed, with particular attention given to the genitals and other areas that may produce moisture. Changing bedclothes and linen is also important. *See also* NURSING THE SICK.

Improper Hygiene. There are a number of disorders that are primarily caused by the failure to practice proper hygiene and are therefore usually avoidable, if there is a thorough cleanliness routine.

Many of these disorders concern either the transmittal of bacteria by the hands, particularly the nails, or irritation and inflammation of the vulva, the penis, or the anus. The nails, for example, are usually implicated in infestations of pinworm and incidents of food poisoning. *See also* NAIL CARE.

Irritation and inflammation of the vulva and the vagina may be caused by various factors. But if the area is not kept sufficiently clean, the build-up of natural secretions may irritate the skin and cause intense itching. However, similar itching can be caused by too much cleaning of the vagina. Douching is seldom, if ever, necessary; the vagina's natural secretions keep it clean. Frequent douching can cause vaginal irritation.

Inflammation of the glans penis is known as balanitis. Many factors may be responsible for the condition, but a lack of personal cleanliness, particularly in uncircumcised men, can cause irritation. The penis should be washed daily with mild soap and water—including the foreskin, which should be rolled back gently for the purpose. Note that in baby boys, the foreskin is attached to the tip of the penis. If the foreskin is rolled back before the age of about three years, the tissue may tear.

Insufficient cleaning of the anal area after defecation can be a major cause of irritation and infection, especially in combination with infrequent washing. Although the chief remedy is improved hygiene and a regular washing routine, there are also forms of medical treatment that may help clear up any problems. If anal itching continues for more than two weeks, medical advice should be sought.

Hymen (hī'mən) is a thin fold of mucous membrane at the entrance to the vagina. The hymen may initially cover the vaginal opening.

Although the hymen may be ruptured through sexual intercourse, rupture or absence of the hymen is not proof of sexual activity. The hymen is often ruptured by exercise. In some cases, females do not have a hymen. When the hymen takes the form of an unperforated membrane, menstrual blood can not escape (hematocolpos).

Hyoid bone (hī'oid) is a semicircular bone that lies at the base of the tongue, just above the thyroid cartilage (Adam's

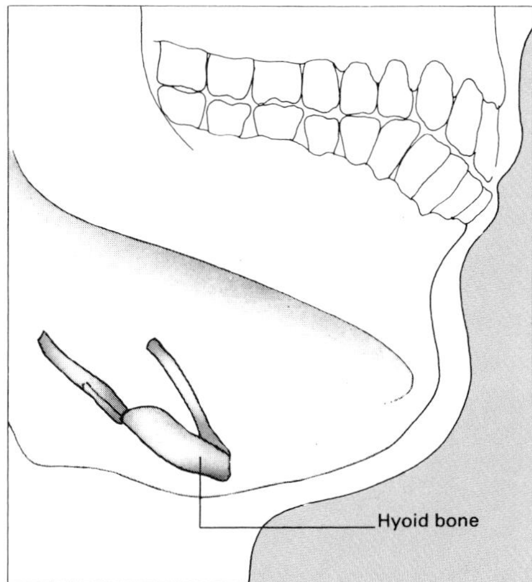

The **hyoid bone** is a tiny bone that is suspended within the jaw at the base of the tongue.

apple) and partly encircles the epiglottis.

See also EPIGLOTTIS.

Hyperactivity (hī pər ak tiv′ə tē) is either increased activity of a particular organ (for example, hyperactivity of the heart or a specific gland) or, more commonly, excessive physical activity by a person, usually a child. Hyperactivity may also be called hyperkinesis, attention deficit disorder, or minimal brain dysfunction.

The hyperactive child is usually a boy who is overactive in the classroom or in other inappropriate situations. Most hyperactive children are easily distracted and have short attention spans; therefore, they can only concentrate on a game or work assignment for a few minutes, and so they seldom carry out instructions. As a result, they tend to fall behind at school, even though most of them have normal or above-average intelligence. Other children and adults may regard hyperactive children as disobedient, stubborn, or simply "bad." Hyperactive children tend to be impulsive and lack self-control. Because of their problems with school, peers, and authority figures, hyperactive children often develop a poor self-image.

Hyperactivity affects from 1 to 5 percent of elementary schoolchildren in the United States. It may result from a physical disorder, such as a problem in the functioning of the brain, from social problems at home or in the school, or from a combination thereof. Some evidence indicates that dyes and other additives in food may aggravate hyperactive behavior in a small number of children. However, in the vast majority of cases, specific causes remain unidentifiable.

Although certain drugs, particularly amphetamines, may be used to treat hyperactivity, little is known about their long-term effects. The safest therapy combines special teaching methods, behavior modification, and family counseling. Drug treatment is generally reserved for those children whose behavior is significantly interfering with schoolwork or who do not respond to the other therapy techniques.

The prognosis for hyperactive children is uncertain. In some children, all of the symptoms are resolved by adolescence, while in others all of the symptoms persist into adulthood. Sometimes, the overactivity is curtailed in children, but the attention difficulties remain.

See also ATTENTION DEFICIT DISORDER.

Hyperacusis (hī pər ə kyü′sis) is an abnormal sensitivity to sound. To a person with hyperacusis, even ordinary levels of sound seem very loud.

Hyperbilirubinemia (hī pər bil ə rü bi nē′mē ə) is an over-accumulation of bilirubin in the blood, often associated with liver disease, anemia, or bile excretion problems.

See also BILIRUBIN.

Hyperchlorhydria (hī pər klôr hī′drē ə), also called hyperacidity, is an excessive amount of hydrochloric acid in the stomach. The excessive acidity may lead to a peptic ulcer.

See also ULCER, PEPTIC.

Hyperemesis (hī pər em′ə sis) is the medical term for excessive vomiting. It may be a symptom of conditions such as gastric flu or intestinal obstruction. When it occurs in pregnancy, it is known as hyperemesis gravidarum.

Q: *What causes hyperemesis gravidarum and how is it treated?*

A: Excessive vomiting during pregnancy is a serious form of the normal, early morning sickness that affects 50 percent of pregnant women. Hyperemesis gravidarum probably develops because of an oversensitivity of the vomiting center in the brain to the hormones produced during pregnancy, but it may also be of psychological origin. The vomiting causes dehydration and should be treated in a hospital with intravenous infusions of glucose, antinauseant drugs, and sedation.

See also VOMITING.

Hyperesthesia (hī pər es thē'zhə) is an increased sensitivity of a sensory organ, most commonly the skin.

Hyperglycemia (hī pər gli sē'mē ə) is a condition in which there is an excessive amount of glucose in the bloodstream. It results from diabetes mellitus.

See also DIABETES MELLITUS.

Hyperhidrosis (hī pər hi drō'sis) is excessive perspiration.

See also PERSPIRATION.

Hyperkinesis. *See* HYPERACTIVITY.

Hypermetropia. *See* FARSIGHTEDNESS.

Hypernephroma (hī pər ni frō mə), or Grawitz's tumor, is a malignant (cancerous) tumor of the kidney. It is the most common form of kidney cancer and is twice as common in men as it is in women. It usually occurs after the age of 40.

See also CANCER; KIDNEY.

Hyperopia. *See* FARSIGHTEDNESS.

Hyperpigmentation (hī pər pig mən tā'shən) is a darkening of the skin due to increased pigmentation. It may be caused by heredity, excessive sunlight, or insufficient corticosteroid hormones. It may also be a side effect of drugs.

See also ADDISON'S DISEASE.

Hyperplasia (hī pər plā'zhə) is an overgrowth of cells that results in an increase in the size of an organ.

See also HYPERTROPHY.

Hyperplasia, endometrial (hī pər plā'zhə, en dō mē'trē əl). Endometrial hyperplasia is the abnormal overgrowth of the endometrium of the uterus. The condition is caused by an unremitting stimulation of the endometrium by estrogen, which normally acts as a growth hormone for the endometrium. In this case, the estrogen is not counterbalanced by progesterone stimulation, and the endometrium consequently becomes unusually thickened. Abnormal uterine bleeding often occurs; a biopsy may be recommended to check for malignancy. The condition usually responds well to progesterone therapy.

See also ENDOMETRIUM.

Hypersensitivity (hī pər sen sə tiv'ə tē) is a condition in which the body or part of the body overreacts to outside stimuli. The term hypersensitivity is commonly used to refer to allergic reactions, such as those occurring with hay fever or asthma.

See also ALLERGY; ASTHMA; SHOCK, ANAPHYLACTIC.

Hypertension (hī pər ten'shən), or high blood pressure, is a condition in which a person's blood pressure is persistently above normal. Although blood pressure varies from person to person and from time to time, 140/90 or above is considered abnormal when measured while the person is at rest. Normal blood pressure is about 120/80. *See also* BLOOD PRESSURE.

Incidence of hypertension is higher in blacks than in whites and increases with age in all groups. It plays an important role as a risk factor in disease. High blood pressure is associated with a significantly elevated risk of heart attack, stroke, and kidney failure; with extremely high blood pressure, retinal damage and encephalopathy (brain tissue dysfunction) can occur.

Q: *What are the symptoms of high blood pressure?*

A: Symptoms are rare. High blood pressure is usually discovered during a routine examination. However, a very high blood pressure causes headache, heart failure, and vision disturbances.

Q: *What causes hypertension?*

A: In more than 90 percent of patients, the cause of high blood pressure remains unknown. Such patients are said to be suffering from essential hypertension. Among the known causes of high blood pressure, however, are kidney disease, diseases of the arteries, and tumors, such as those of the adrenal gland. While not technically causes of high blood pressure, the following factors have been linked to the condition: hereditary predisposition, obesity, smoking, high level of salt in the diet, a high level of stress, and excessive use of alcohol.

Q: *How is high blood pressure treated?*

A: Treatments for high blood pressure vary. Drug therapy includes the use of diuretics to rid the body of excess salt. Sometimes, the cause of high blood pressure can itself be treated.

Q: *What is the danger if blood pressure rises during pregnancy?*

A: High blood pressure in pregnancy can indicate preeclampsia. Other symptoms are fluid retention and albuminuria (protein in the urine). If the blood pressure is not rapidly reduced to normal, there is an increased chance of the mother developing eclampsia. *See also* ECLAMPSIA; PREECLAMPSIA.

Hyperthyroidism (hī pər thī′roi diz əm), also known as thyrotoxicosis, is overactivity of the thyroid gland and excessive production of thyroid hormones.

See also THYROTOXICOSIS.

Hypertrophy (hi pər′trə fē) is an increase in the size of a body tissue or organ. It may occur in the heart muscle or in the remaining kidney after one has been removed. Hypertrophy can also occur as the result of changes that take place with age, such as an enlarged prostate gland.

Hyperventilation (hī pər ven tə lā′shən) is excessive or forced respiration, which disrupts the normal balance of carbon dioxide and oxygen in the bloodstream. Hyperventilation is often caused by anxiety or emotional tension. Other causes include disorders of the central nervous system; increased metabolism from exercise, fever, infections, or hyperthyroidism; and high concentrations of certain drugs in the body.

Symptoms include faintness, dizziness, impaired consciousness, and feelings of anxiety and panic. Immediate treatment includes having the person breathe into a paper bag (not a plastic one) or, more simply, breathe slowly. Antidepressants or tranquilizers may be initially useful for some individuals who suffer from recurrent episodes of hyperventilation. Further treatment often involves teaching relaxation methods and stress management skills.

See also PANIC ATTACK.

Hypesthesia (hip es thē′zhə), or hypoesthesia, is a reduction in the normal sensation from the skin or other sense organs. It may result from nerve damage (polyneuritis) or occur with hemianesthesia following a stroke.

See also HEMIANESTHESIA.

Hypnosis (hip nō′sis), or hypnotic trance, is a change in a person's conscious awareness, induced by another person, in which a variety of phenomena may appear spontaneously or in response to verbal or other stimuli. These phenomena may include alterations in consciousness and memory; increased susceptibility to suggestion; and the production in the subject of responses and ideas that would normally be unusual. Additionally, some phenomena, such as anesthesia, paralysis, rigidity of muscles, and vasomotor changes (such as sweating and blushing) can be produced and removed in the hypnotic state.

Only a small percentage of people can not be hypnotized at all, but very few can be put into a deep hypnotic trance. Persons in a light hypnotic trance are aware of their actions and have a distinct memory of what happens. Persons in a deep trance can not remember details of what occurs. Also, contrary to popular belief, hypnosis can not be used to control the subject or make the subject do anything against his or her will.

The most common technique used to hypnotize another person is by direct command, repeated continuously in a low, monotonous tone of voice. Occasionally drugs, such as sodium pentathol, alcohol, or certain barbiturates, are used to facilitate the process.

There are various degrees of hypnosis. In light hypnosis, the subject becomes sleepy and follows simple directions easily. Under deep hypnosis, complete anesthesia, or loss of sensation, may be produced.

Hypnosis is used in research, medicine, surgery, dentistry, and psychotherapy. Physicians sometimes use hypnosis to treat patients who are nervous or irritable. Physicians may also use it to relieve pain or uncomfortable symptoms. Surgeons and dentists may use hypnosis as a form of anesthesia so that a patient undergoing a surgical or dental operation will feel no pain. Hypnotism is also used by some obstetricians as an aid during childbirth. Hypnosis can also be useful in helping patients give up habits, such as smoking, and overcome phobias, such as the fear of flying.

In treating psychiatric disorders, mental health professionals may use hypnosis to calm patients. They also may hypnotize a person to try to discover the underlying cause of his or her illness. Under hypnosis, these patients sometimes remember incidents that they had forgotten or repressed.

Usually, it is not difficult to bring a subject out of a hypnotic trance by means of a special signal. Occasionally, a hypnotist has a difficult time bringing a person out of a trance. Therefore, hypnosis should be practiced only by a qualified person, preferably someone with adequate training in a valid medical or mental health discipline, such as psychiatry or psychology. Only such persons can understand what happens to patients under hypnosis and will not overestimate the apparent cures they achieve. Many people have the ability to hypnotize others, but this ability should not become a substitute for adequate psychiatric training, nor should hypnosis be considered as anything but one of many possible therapeutic strategies.

In the late 18th century, Franz Mesmer and his followers, called *mesmerists,* were among the early users of hypnosis in Western civilization. A century later, Jean Martin Charcot set up dramatic experiments involving the use of hypnosis at his clinic, La Salpêtrière, in Paris. Among his students was Sigmund Freud, who was to conduct his first studies of the unconscious on hypnotized people.

Hypnotics (hip not′iks) are a group of drugs often used to ease anxiety or to produce sleep.

See also SEDATIVE.

Hypocalcemia (hī pə kal sē′mē ə) is a condition in which there is a lower than normal level of calcium in the blood. It may occur as a result of underactivity of the parathyroid glands, or it may be a consequence of vitamin D deficiency.

The condition is extremely serious in newborn babies, in whom hypocalcemia causes listlessness, twitching, breathing problems, and seizures. In adults, there are often no symptoms, and diagnosis is made only after a routine blood test. In severe hypocalcemia, the patient may suffer a seizure or tetany, with muscular spasms of the hands, feet, and jaw.

See also OSTEOMALACIA; PARATHYROID GLAND; RICKETS.

Hypochondria. *See* HYPOCHONDRIASIS.

Hypochondriasis (hī pə kon drī′ə sis) is a psychiatric condition in which a person has a persistent preoccupation with his or her physical health and well-being. Such individuals may fear specific diseases, such as cancer or heart problems, and overinterpret body sensations or symptoms in order to reinforce their fears. Hypochondriacal complaints may mask depression or anxiety, which should be carefully evaluated and treated.

Past medical illness in the individual or his or her family members and psychosocial stresses may contribute to the start of this disorder. Individuals with this disorder may "doctor shop" and endure multiple diagnostic and therapeutic procedures, including surgery and medications.

See also SOMATIZATION DISORDER.

Hypodermic (hī pə der′mik) describes anything applied or administered beneath the skin, as in a hypodermic injection.

Hypoglycemia (hī pō gli sē′mē ə) is a condition that occurs when the level of glucose (sugar) in the blood is abnormally low. Glucose supplies the body's cells with energy, and a low level of glucose seriously affects the brain cells. This condition most often occurs in persons with diabetes mellitus. *See also* DIABETES MELLITUS.

Q: *What are the symptoms and signs of hypoglycemia?*

A: The patient may suffer from headaches, weakness, sweating, shakiness, hunger, visual disturbances, hypothermia, mental confusion, or personality changes. In severe cases, he or she may go into a coma.

Hypokalemia (hī pō kə lē′mē ə) is a deficiency of potassium in the blood and body tissues, which may result in muscular weakness or an irregular heart rhythm. Hypokalemia is most common in persons taking diuretics. People on diuretics should have the blood potassium level closely watched, especially if they are concurrently taking the heart-stimulant drug, digoxin.

See also DIURETIC.

Hyponatremia (hī pō na trē′mē ə) is a lower than average concentration of sodium in the blood.

Hypophysis. *See* PITUITARY GLAND.

Hypopituitarism (hī pō pə tü′ə tə riz əm) is decreased function of the pituitary gland that results in an insufficient production of hormones. The pituitary gland is the chief endocrine gland of the body. Its hormones trigger hormone production in the other endocrine glands. If the pituitary gland malfunctions, the hormonal production of the entire endocrine system is affected.

Q: *What are the symptoms of hypopituitarism?*

A: The symptoms of hypopituitarism are actually symptoms of various disorders caused by the lack of pituitary hormones. These symptoms include loss of weight, tiredness, lack of sex drive (libido), low blood pressure, and a feeling of faintness. Children with the condition fail to grow normally and remain small, though properly proportioned. In men and women, the normal hair growth becomes sparse. In women, there is a failure to lactate, and menstruation ceases. If the cause of the pituitary malfunction is a tumor, headaches and vision problems also occur.

Q: *What is the treatment for hypopituitarism?*

A: If the cause of the condition is a tumor, treatment is the destruction of the tumor, using surgery or radiotherapy. If there is no tumor causing the pituitary insufficiency or if there is no improvement after surgery, a physician may prescribe drugs as substitutes for the hormones normally produced by the other endocrine glands.

See also ENDOCRINE SYSTEM; PITUITARY GLAND.

Hypoplasia (hī pə plā′zhə) is the defective or incomplete development of an organ or tissue.

Hypostasis (hī pos′tə sis) is poor circulation in a part of the body, usually the legs.

Hypotension (hī pə ten′shən), or low blood pressure, is a condition in which the blood pressure is reduced or below normal. Most physicians in the English-speaking world consider hypotension to be a symptom of some other disorder. But, in many parts of the world, hypotension is itself considered to be a disorder that can cause various symptoms, including depression, lethargy, and fatigue. This different attitude is probably the result of different methods of medical training.

Q: *What conditions may be accompanied by hypotension?*

A: Like hypertension (high blood pressure), slightly low blood pressure may be a particular person's normal pressure. Provided there are no other symptoms and the individual feels well, the low blood pressure can be considered a chance variation from average, probably associated with a prolonged life expectancy. But if low blood pressure occurs in an individual whose blood pressure is normally higher, it may be caused by some recent illness. In this case, it should be only temporary and should improve spontaneously. Some kinds of drugs, particularly antidepressants, may cause low blood pressure.

A more serious possible cause of low blood pressure is peripheral neuritis, in which the autonomic nervous system is affected so that blood accumulates in the legs because of the absence of the normal nervous response that causes the veins to contract. Disorders such as diabetes mellitus, tabes dorsalis, and Parkinson's disease may result in low blood pressure. Patients who have had a coronary thrombosis or who are in a state of shock also have low blood pressure. *See also* DIABETES MELLITUS; PARKINSON'S DISEASE; TABES DORSALIS; THROMBOSIS, CORONARY.

Q: *What are the symptoms of hypotension?*

A: Frequently, there are no symptoms and the condition is found at a routine physical examination. The person may feel dizzy, and a sudden change in position, such as standing up quickly, may cause fainting. Serious low blood pressure may bring on the symptoms of shock, pallor, and a feeling of coldness. *See also* SHOCK.

Q: *How is hypotension treated?*

A: There is a spontaneous improvement in most individuals, although treatment of the cause helps the return to normal. Drug treatment that may cause the low blood pressure should, if possible, be discontinued. Patients with peripheral neuritis are more difficult to treat. An improvement may be made by an increase in blood volume, achieved by additional salt in the diet and, sometimes, with corticosteroid drugs. *See also* NERVOUS SYSTEM, PERIPHERAL; NEURITIS.

Hypothalamus (hī pə thal′ə məs) is a part of the brain containing nerve centers that control appetite, thirst, body weight, fluid balance, body temperature, and sex drive (libido). It is located below the thalamus and above the pituitary gland and acts as a link between the nervous system and endocrine hormone-secreting system.

See also ENDOCRINE SYSTEM; PITUITARY GLAND; THALAMUS.

Hypothermia (hi pə thėr′mē ə) is a condition in which the body temperature falls below the normal level of 98.6°F (37°C). The term usually applies to a dangerously low body temperature of below 95°F (35°C), even as low as 80°F (27°C) rectally. During hypothermia, the activity of the organs slows down and their need for oxygen decreases.

Hypothermia is usually the result of accidental exposure to extreme cold temperatures. It can also occur when people have a reduced ability to produce heat by shivering, as may happen in infants and in the very elderly. The victim may be mentally confused, semi-conscious or unconscious, and may have slow or arrested respiration and heartbeat.

People who are hungry or tired, the elderly, people who are ill, children, and people who drink alcohol are particularly likely to suffer from hypothermia in cold conditions.

Hypothermia develops gradually. The greatest danger to a person in the early stages of the condition is that the confusion it causes may make a person careless. At the first sign of such carelessness, the person must find food, warmth, and shelter.

Physicians may deliberately induce hypothermia using cooling mattresses or ice as a preparation for some surgical procedures, such as on the heart or on organs being preserved for transplantation, or to counteract high, prolonged fever caused by an infectious or neurological disease.

See also HYPOTHERMIA: TREATMENT.

Hypothermia: treatment

It is important to prevent further exposure to wind and cold by protecting the victim. Replace wet clothing with dry clothes or wrap the victim in a dry, warm blanket. Give him or her food and warm, sweet liquids.

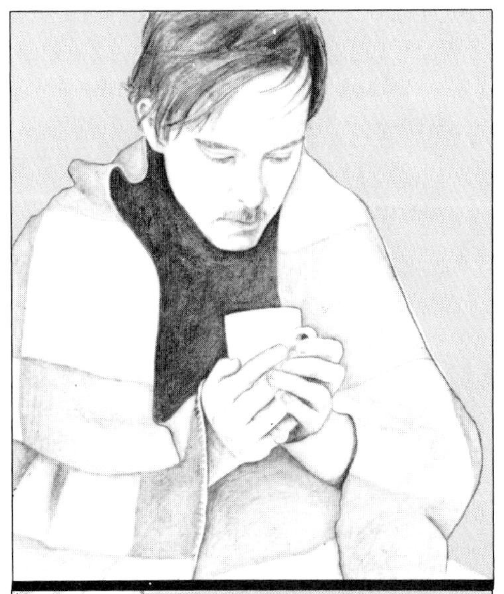

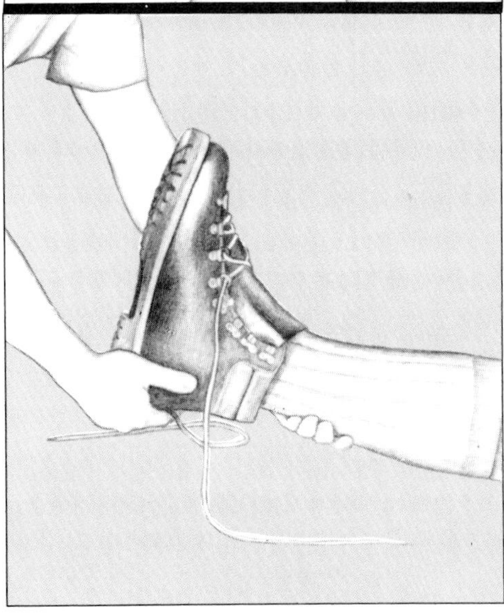

Remove wet boots or gloves that may constrict the circulation of blood. Keep the victim conscious.

Hypothermia: treatment. When a person is inadequately dressed in cold weather conditions that are also windy or wet, there is a danger that the body temperature will drop. Such a drop in body temperature affects the central nervous system and causes the symptoms of slurred speech, loss of coordination, and confusion. In severe cases, hypothermia can lead to unconsciousness, coma, and death.

It is extremely important to recognize the symptoms of hypothermia so that the correct treatment can be given as quickly as possible. The initial symptoms of hypothermia include sluggish physical and mental responses, slurred speech, muscle cramps, persistent shivering and the tendency to miscalculate one's abilities, particularly with regard to strength or endurance.

Action. First, raise the temperature of the body as a whole, and keep a constant check on the temperature to prevent any further drop. This is done by moving the victim to a warm, sheltered environment. Remove all wet, cold clothing and re-dress in dry, warm clothes or bundle in dry, warm blankets. A sleeping bag with a warm person inside may also help rewarm the victim.

Give the victim warm, sweet liquids to drink. *Do not* give alcohol to a hypothermic person. In severe cases of hypothermia, take the victim to a hospital as soon as possible. However, as the heart of a person suffering from hypothermia is extremely vulnerable to ventricular fibrillation, any sudden movement and too rapid rewarming should be avoided. There is debate as to the optimal method of in-hospital rewarming with the controversy centering on the method of whole-body emersion in hot water. Massive IV doses of corticosteroids help counteract the effects of severe, sudden shock.

See also HYPOTHERMIA.

Hypothyroidism (hī pə thī'roi diz əm) is a condition that results from an inadequate supply of hormones from the thyroid gland in the neck. When hypothyroidism develops before birth, the infant is retarded both mentally and physically. *See also* CRETINISM.

Q: *What are the symptoms of hypothyroidism?*

A: The symptoms of hypothyroidism include tiredness, weight gain, and a sensitivity to cold. The patient's skin becomes dry and puffy, especially on the face, and the hair of the scalp and the eyebrows becomes dry and brittle. The voice may become hoarse, and anemia may develop. Sometimes, there is numbness and tingling in the hands and feet. Constipation is common. In women there are menstrual disorders, such as heavy bleeding (menorrhagia) and irregular periods.

These symptoms develop gradually. Over a period of time, if the condition is untreated, the individual's personality can also change. There may be a slowing down of the thought processes, sometimes mild confusion and dementia, and occasionally symptoms that suggest paranoia. This severe form of hypothyroidism is called myxedema.

Q: *What is the treatment for hypothyroidism?*

A: A physician usually begins treatment of hypothyroidism with a small dose of one of the thyroid hormones and then gradually increases the dose. The increase generally takes several weeks, because a sudden change may cause cardiac problems, especially in an elderly patient.

Patients who receive appropriate treatment for hypothyroidism recover completely and can expect to lead a normal life. They will, however, require treatment for the rest of their lives, with occasional blood tests to ensure that the correct amounts of hormones are being given.

See also THYROID GLAND.

Hypoxia (hī pok'sē ə) is a condition in which there is a lack of, or low content of, oxygen in the body tissues, usually because of a reduction in the oxygen level in the blood, called hypoxemia.

Hysterectomy (his tə rek'tə mē) is an operation to remove the uterus. In a total hysterectomy, the cervix, or neck of the uterus, is also removed.

Q: *Why may a physician recommend a hysterectomy?*

A: A hysterectomy is performed if there is cancer of the uterus or cervix; if heavy bleeding from the uterus causes anemia; or if large fibroids cause troublesome symptoms. *See also* FIBROID.

Q: *What is the effect of a hysterectomy?*

A: Menstruation ceases, and conception is not possible.

Q: *Are the ovaries removed at the same time as the uterus?*

A: In women under the age of about 45, the ovaries are usually left in place if they appear healthy at the time of the operation. This procedure is known as a *total hysterectomy*. In older women, the ovaries are usually removed because they either will soon have no function or are already nonfunctional, and they may cause problems later in life. The ovaries, the oviducts, lymph nodes, and lymph channels are removed along with the uterus

A **hysterectomy** is an operation to remove the uterus. It is usually performed due to cancer of the uterus or cervix or due to fibroids. In a total hysterectomy, the ovaries are left in place. In a radical hysterectomy, the ovaries, oviducts, lymph nodes and channels, the uterus, and cervix are removed.

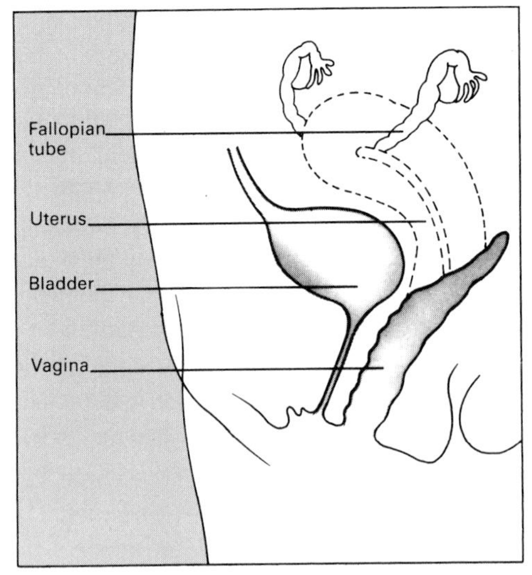

and cervix in a procedure called a *radical hysterectomy.*

Q: *How is a hysterectomy performed?*

A: The operation is usually done through the abdominal wall. An alternative method is via the vagina, leaving no external incision. Which technique is used depends on the indications for the surgery. The uterus is removed, and the top of the vagina closed to form a blind tube.

The patient usually remains in the hospital about one week and is encouraged to get out of bed as soon as possible after the surgery to prevent the risk of venous thrombosis in the legs. If the patient has varicose veins or a previous history of venous thrombosis, she may be given small doses of an anticoagulant drug for a day or two after the operation.

Q: *Does a hysterectomy affect a woman's sexual interest?*

A: There should be no effect on the woman's sexual interest. On the contrary, some women experience increased libido when the possibility of conception is no longer present. If the ovaries are removed before menopause, the physician may prescribe a course of hormones, by implant, injection, or mouth. This treatment prevents the sudden onset of the symptoms that are normally associated with menopause.

It is advisable not to resume sexual intercourse until the patient has had a postoperative check by her gynecologist about six weeks after the operation. Initially, there may be some discomfort because the top of the vagina is not as elastic as previously. Medically, there is no reason why a woman should not resume normal sexual activity subsequent to a hysterectomy.

See also GYNECOLOGICAL DISORDERS.

Hysteria (his tir′ē ə), although not part of current psychiatric terminology, refers to a condition in which the individual exhibits any one of a number of often dramatic symptoms. These include paralysis, blindness, seizures, abdominal pain, and alterations in consciousness, such as amnesia or fugue. None of these symptoms have any organic basis. Such individuals may go from doctor to doctor in an attempt to find a solution. They often undergo many diagnostic and therapeutic procedures, including surgery, and take multiple medications. However, the basis of hysteric symptoms is typically believed to be repressed psychological conflict.

A thorough physical and psychological evaluation is needed. Hysteria is usually treated with some type of psychotherapy designed to help the patient understand his or her unconscious conflicts. Treatment with drugs and hypnosis may also supplement the psychotherapy.

The psychiatric term, hysteria, is very different from the emotional outburst most people associate with the word "hysteria."

See also HYPOCHONDRIASIS.

I

Iatrogenic disorder (ī at rō jen′ik) is any disorder brought about as a result of medical treatment.

Ibuprofen (ī byü′prə fin) is an anti-inflammatory agent used in the treatment of disorders such as headache, muscular aches, and arthritis. Side effects may include gastrointestinal difficulties and skin rash. Although ibuprofen contains no aspirin, patients sensitive to aspirin may experience an allergic reaction with ibuprofen medication. Common brand names include Motrin®, Advil®, and Mediprine®.

Ice fishing safety. See WINTER SPORTS SAFETY.

Ice skating safety. See WINTER SPORTS SAFETY.

Ichthyosis (ik thē ō′sis) is a disorder, usually hereditary, in which the skin, lacking natural oils, becomes dry and scaly like that of a fish. The lifelong condition generally develops before the age of four years. There is no cure; a physician, however, may prescribe skin ointments to alleviate the symptoms.

Icterus. See JAUNDICE.

Icterus gravis neonatorum. See HEMOLYTIC DISEASE OF THE NEWBORN.

Id (id) is a term used in psychoanalysis to describe the unconscious part of the psyche (the self) that is the source of instinctual drives, such as sex and aggression. The id has a strong urge toward self-preservation.

See also EGO; SUPEREGO.

Identical twins. See TWINS.

Idioglossia (id ē ō glos′ē ə) is a speech defect characterized by unintelligible pronunciation. The condition may be caused by severe deafness in infancy, or it may occur after a stroke.

See also DEAFNESS; STROKE.

Idiopathic (id ē ō path′ik) describes a disorder or condition that occurs for no known reason. For example, while some types of hypertension (high blood pressure) have a specific cause, the most common type has no known cause and is termed idiopathic hypertension. Idiopathic disorders are frequently treatable, even though the exact cause is not known.

Idiosyncrasy (id ē o sing′ krə sē) is an unusual and possibly eccentric pattern of behavior in an individual. Medically, the term idiosyncratic is used to describe an unusual and unanticipated reaction to a drug, such as hypersensitivity, that is not related to the dose taken. It may also refer to an individual's failure to respond to a drug, even when a high dosage is administered. These unusual reactions reflect a characteristic of the individual, rather than the characteristic effects of the drug as exhibited by many people.

Ileitis (il ē ī′tis) is an inflammation of the ileum (the third portion of the small intestine), often also involving the colon. It may result from infection, previous bowel surgery, or, most commonly, an immunologic factor. The condition usually causes acute abdominal pain, similar to appendicitis. Other symptoms include diarrhea (sometimes alternating with constipation), fever, anorexia, weight loss, and a distention of the abdomen.

Q: *Who is susceptible to ileitis?*

A: The disease affects males and females equally, usually under the age of 40.

Q: *What is the treatment for ileitis?*

A: No specific treatment has been discovered. Sometimes a complete recovery will follow an initial isolated attack of acute ileitis. More commonly, the disease is chronic, in which case various drugs can help reduce the symptoms. A bypass operation or the removal of the affected bowel can also diminish the symptoms, though surgery will not eliminate the condition.

Ileostomy (il ē os′tə mē) is an opening into the small intestine that is created surgically by bringing a part of the

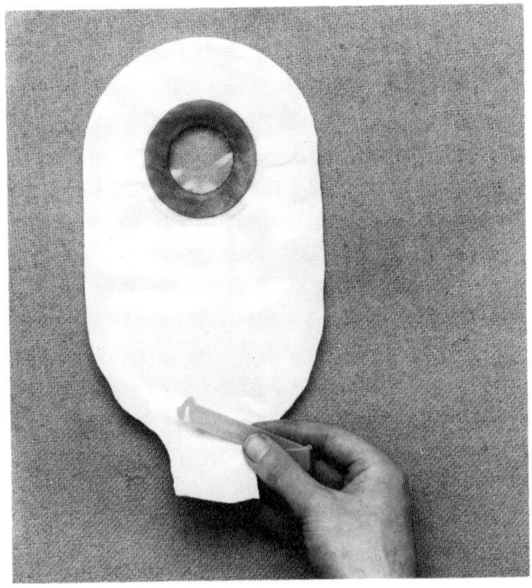

Ileostomy drainage bags fit securely over the stoma and collect the contents of the ileum.

small intestine (ileum) to the outside surface of the body at the abdomen. An ileostomy may be required as a temporary measure to by-pass the intestine during the treatment of intestinal obstruction. A permanent ileostomy is necessary following removal of the large intestine.

Q: *How are the contents of the ileum collected?*

A: The patient must wear a special kind of bag over the ileostomy to collect the liquid that drains from the ileum.

Q: *What problems might an ileostomy patient have to deal with?*

A: The three main problems are skin irritation, odor, and leakage. The skin becomes irritated if it comes in contact with the feces or if the patient develops an allergy to the materials of the drainage bag. Special pastes and ointments can be applied to protect the skin, but the most effective way to prevent irritation is to ensure that the bag fits well over the ileostomy. A secure fit also eliminates any unpleasant odor.

One of the functions of the large intestine is to absorb water from the feces as they pass along the intestine. An ileostomy patient is unable to reabsorb this fluid and may become dehydrated. Supplements of salt in the diet and extra fluids are therefore necessary.

Q: *Can an ileostomy patient lead a normal life?*

A: Yes. Once patients with ileostomies become adjusted to the social inconvenience of an ileostomy, they can lead normal lives. The various ileostomy associations can give sound, practical advice to new patients.

See *also* COLOSTOMY.

Ileum (il'ē əm) is the section of the small intestine that extends from the jejunum portion of the small intestine to the beginning of the large intestine (colon). It is about 12 feet (3.6m) long.

Disorders of the ileum, such as chronic ileitis, produce malnutrition if they continue for a long time. Tumors of the ileum are rare, but a Meckel's diverticulum may occur as a congenital anomaly of the ileum.

See *also* DIVERTICULUM, MECKEL'S.

Ileus (il'ē əs) is any obstruction of the intestine that is caused by either a mechanical blockage, such as a hernia, adhesions, or volvulus; by a functional problem, such as muscle paralysis or spasms; or by external pressure from an adjacent organ, such as a pregnant uterus. Symptoms of ileus include sudden, colicky pain, which then becomes continuous; constipation; vomiting of fecal matter; and a swollen abdomen. If not treated promptly, a person suffering from ileus can go into shock.

A physician can diagnose an ileus condition by the symptoms as well as by the absence of bowel sounds, which normally are audible through a stethoscope placed on the abdomen. An X ray of the abdomen may reveal dilated loops of intestine with large pockets of gas. The patient with ileus must take nothing by mouth and will usually have a nasogastric tube installed to empty the stomach. Treatment ultimately depends on the specific cause of the disorder.

See *also* VOLVULUS.

Ilium (il'ē əm) is the broad upper portion of each hipbone and the largest of the three bones that fuse together to form each hipbone, the other two bones being the ischium and the pubis. A number of strong muscles of the upper leg and the buttocks are attached to the ilium.

See *also* HIPBONE; ISCHIUM; PELVIS; PUBIS.

Immersion foot. See FOOT, IMMERSION.

Immunity (i myü'nə tē) is the body's ability to protect itself from disease. Immunity is either acquired or natural.

Acquired immunity is either active or passive: active acquired immunity results from having had the disease or from being vaccinated against that disease; passive acquired immunity results from fetal acquisition from the mother or from injection of antibodies.

Natural immunity is genetically determined. It is also influenced by such factors as temperature, metabolism, and diet.

Local immunity is limited to a particular area or tissue of the body.

See also ACQUIRED IMMUNE DEFICIENCY SYNDROME; ANTIBODY; BLOOD CELL, WHITE; IMMUNIZATION.

Immunization (im yü ni zā′shən) is the process of providing immunity to various infectious diseases. Such immunization is also known as inoculation or vaccination. The immunity gained by immunization may be divided into two types: passive immunity and active immunity.

Q: *What is passive immunity?*

A: Passive immunity is only temporary, helping the body to fight a disease already contracted. Such immunity to a specific disease is usually provided by injecting gamma globulin (also called immune serum globulin) containing antibodies from an immunized person or animal. Serum sickness may occur as a reaction to gamma globulin, particularly from animal sources.

Q: *What is active immunity?*

A: Active immunity is a condition in which the body's own natural immunity system is stimulated to prevent the contracting of a particular disease. This immunity is long-lasting and may even be permanent.

Active immunity is usually provided in one of three ways: (1) by injecting a dead virus, bacterium, or toxoid of the disease (as against diphtheria, influenza, tetanus, and whooping cough); (2) by injecting a weakened live organism of the disease (as against measles or mumps); or (3) by introducing a weakened, live virus through a scratch in the skin as with smallpox. Some vaccines, such as that against poliomyelitis, are taken by mouth.

See also VACCINATION.

Q: *Does active immunity give total protection?*

A: Unfortunately, not always. However, if the disease is contracted after active immunity, the effects are generally much milder than they would otherwise be.

Q: *Are there any risks in immunization for active immunity?*

A: Statistically, the risks are few. Some people may have allergies to specific vaccines. Rarely, the

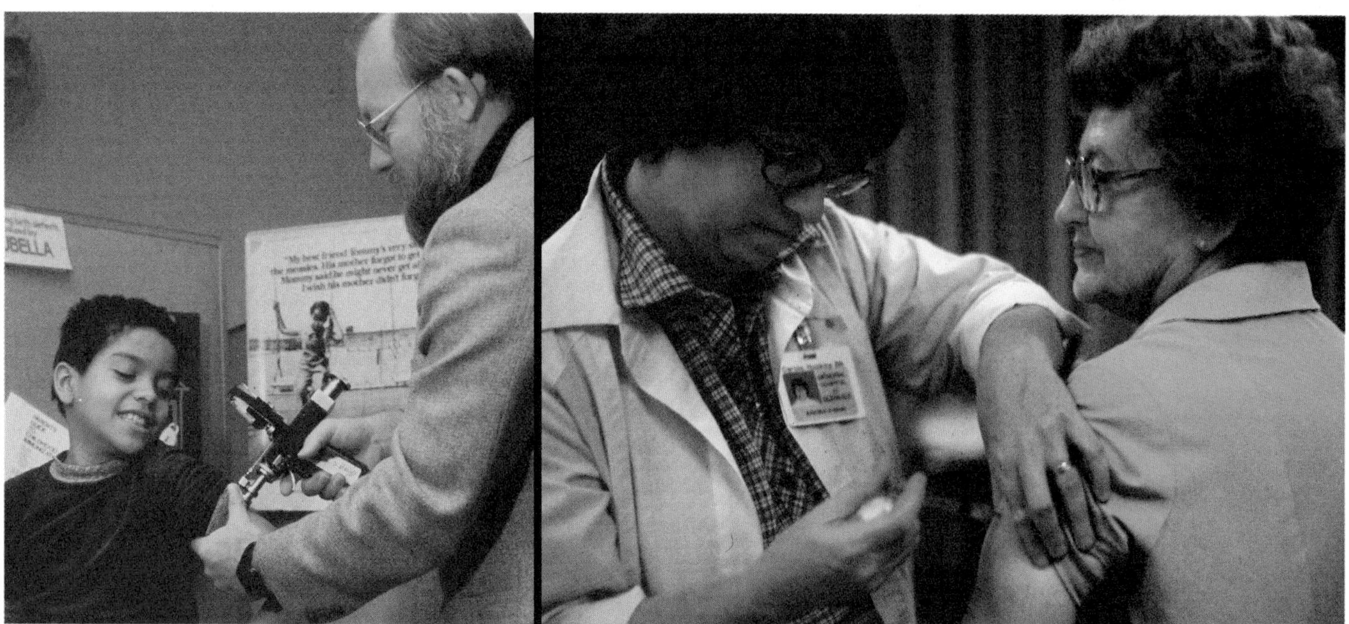

Immunization against illness is quick, relatively painless, and can be administered to people of all ages.

Routine childhood immunizations

Name and dose	*Reactions*	*Notes*
Diphtheria (from 2 months) 3 injections at bimonthly intervals. Booster in second year, at school age, and at 10-year intervals throughout life.	Sometimes local soreness. Fever normally within 1 to 2 days.	Usually given with tetanus and pertussis as Triple Antigen. Small dose used for older children and adults.
Tetanus (from 2 months) 3 injections at bimonthly intervals. Booster in second year, at school age, and at 10-year intervals throughout life.	Same as above. May include itchy skin, lasting several days. Lump at injection site may last months, but will disappear.	Usually given with diphtheria and pertussis as Triple Antigen. Further boosters following cuts or animal bites. Antitetanus serum available for injuries in unvaccinated persons.
Whooping cough, *or* pertussis, (from 2 months) 3 injections at bimonthly intervals. Booster in second year and at school age.	Same as above, but may include severe fever, loss of consciousness, and, rarely, convulsions and brain damage.	Usually given with tetanus and diphtheria in Triple Antigen. Not advised if there is a history of allergy, seizures, or prior severe reaction after receiving the vaccine.
Poliomyelitis (from 2 months) 2 doses by mouth at bimonthly intervals. Booster in second year, and at school age.	Rare. Paralysis has been reported.	Usually given orally. Not advised during bout of diarrhea; when taking corticosteroid drugs; or in first 3 months of pregnancy.
Measles (after 1 year) 1 injection at 10 to 15 months. Booster at 10 to 12 years of age.	Sometimes fever; rash within 8-10 days, for 3-4 days.	May be combined with mumps and/or rubella immunization. Not given to persons taking corticosteroid drugs; suffering from leukemia or tuberculosis; or during pregnancy. Advised for unimmunized adults.
Mumps (after 1 year) 1 injection. Booster at 10 to 12 years of age.	None.	May be combined with measles and/or rubella immunization. Not given to persons with serious illness; or during pregnancy. Advised for unimmunized adults who have not had the disease.
Rubella *or* German measles, (after 1 year) 1 injection in second year. Booster at 10 to 12 years of age.	Infrequently, slight fever; rash; aching joints.	May be combined with mumps and/or measles immunization. Not given to persons taking corticosteroid drugs; suffering from leukemia or tuberculosis; or during pregnancy. Advised for unimmunized adults, especially women.
Hemophilus influenza B (after 18 months) 1 injection in second year.	Sometimes local soreness. Rarely, fever occurs 24 hours after immunization.	Immunization may be given with DPT vaccine. If possible, give 2 months before child enters day-care to ensure protection.

whooping cough vaccine leads to brain damage. The diseases themselves, however, are much more likely to cause injury and death than are the vaccines.

Q: *Why are babies immunized?*

A: Diseases such as whooping cough and measles can lead to pneumonia, severe brain damage, permanent disability, or even death. Immunization programs begin soon after birth, but the older a child is, the more complete is the protection.

Immunodeficiency diseases (i myü nō di fish′ən sē) are a wide group of conditions in which the body's ability to defend itself against foreign substances (bacteria, viruses, etc.) is lost. In a healthy defense system the body produces a variety of white blood cells to combat various infections. Immunodeficiency diseases either suppress the production of these cells or attack them directly, thus leaving the body vulnerable to other diseases, which can become acute and chronic. Immunodeficiency also exists in fetuses and the newly born because their immune systems are not yet fully developed. Research has shown that many disorders in the immune system are congenital, waiting for a chance exposure to a specific infection to reveal themselves; other disorders, such as AIDS, are acquired.

See also ACQUIRED IMMUNE DEFICIENCY SYNDROME; BLOOD CELL, WHITE.

Immunology (im yů nol′ə jē) is the study of the body's infectious disease system and the various interrelating cells, antibodies, and chemicals that provide immunity from disease.

Immunosuppressive drug (i myü nō sə pres′iv) is a substance that suppresses the immune mechanism of the body. Immunosuppressive drugs are used to treat autoimmune disease or, after organ transplant surgery, to prevent the body from rejecting the foreign tissue of the transplanted organ.

See also AUTOIMMUNE DISEASE; TRANSPLANT SURGERY.

Immunotherapy (i myü nō ther′ə pē) is a means of fighting disease by altering the body's immune response. Often used in the treatment of allergies, immunotherapy calls for administering increasingly larger doses of offending allergens in order to gradually build up the body's ability to tolerate exposure to the offending substance. Experimentally, immunotherapy is also being used in the treatment of cancer.

If showing signs of success, immunotherapy can last from two to five years.

Impaction (im pak′shən) is a condition in which a substance is so tightly wedged that it is immovable. For example, cerumen (earwax) can be impacted in the ear canal and feces can be impacted in the bowels.

Imperforate (im pėr′fər it) describes any structure in which a natural opening is abnormally closed.

Impetigo (im pə tī′gō) is an infectious skin disease that is usually caused by staphylococcus or streptococcus bacteria. It is common among children and may appear as a complication of an existing skin condition, such as eczema or ichthyosis. Chronic impetigo in older persons is known as ecthyma.

Q: *Why is impetigo more common among children?*

A: The body's immunity is less developed in children. Frequent colds with a runny nose transmit staphylococci from the nose onto the face, especially around the mouth, where it may be reingested. Noseblowing and scratching beneath and around the nose produce minor abrasions on the skin, which allow the bacteria to enter. Other areas, such as the hands and legs, may also become infected.

Q: *What are the symptoms of impetigo?*

A: Small blisters appear on the skin. These rapidly break down to form golden-colored, crusty, oozing areas that spread. The condition may be complicated by further infection from streptococcal bacteria.

Q: *How is impetigo treated?*

A: Medical advice should be sought promptly because the infection can spread rapidly to other persons. Physicians usually prescribe an antibiotic to be taken orally. In some cases, topical applications of antibiotic ointments may be prescribed. These are usually applied after the affected areas are gently washed to remove the crusts and ooze. Because impetigo is spread by personal contact, its spread can be minimized by washing hands and using separate washcloths.

Personal hygiene is especially important during the acute and convalescent periods.

Q: *Are there any complications of impetigo?*

A: Yes. If additional streptococcal infection breaks out on the area affected by impetigo, it can cause the kidney disorder glomerulonephritis. *See also* GLOMERULONEPHRITIS.

Impotence (im′pə təns) is a man's inability to produce or maintain a penile erection. The condition interferes with sexual intercourse. Impotence may be short-lived or may last for a long time. Brief bouts of impotence may follow depression and illnesses, such as influenza, or after taking drugs or alcohol. In these cases the man can expect a swift return to former potency.

Q: *What causes impotence?*

A: Impotence often has a psychological origin, such as depression, marital conflict, or performance anxiety. There may be, however, a physical cause, such as a stroke, chronic diabetes mellitus, or alcoholism. Impotence may also occur as an aftereffect of certain surgical procedures or a side effect of certain medications. Impotence should be evaluated for both physical and psychological causes; it may result from a combination of factors.

Q: *How is impotence treated?*

A: When the impotence has a psychological basis, a physician may arrange for the problem to be discussed with a sex therapist or marriage counselor. The patient's sexual partner should be involved in such discussions and any consequent treatment because the partner's reassurance and encouragement are essential.

When impotence is the result of a physical disorder, the underlying cause must be treated first. If the physical problem can not be corrected, a surgical penile implant procedure can be done for many men to give them the mechanical ability to attain an erection.

See also INFERTILITY; STERILITY.

Incisor (in sī′zər) is a tooth having a chisel-like edge for cutting. There are eight incisors in the human mouth, with four at the front of each jaw.

See also TOOTH.

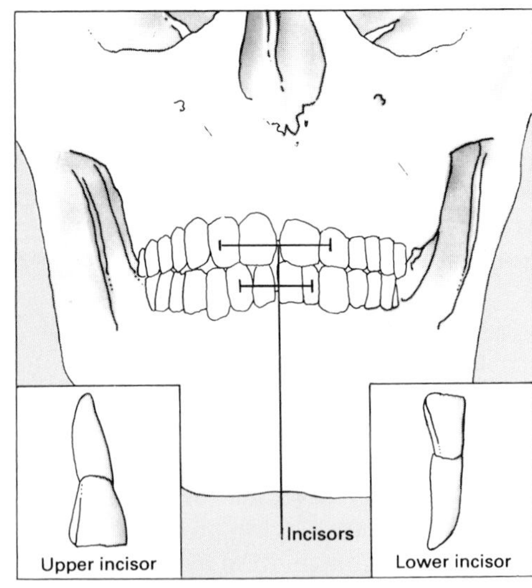

Incisors are the four front teeth in both the upper and lower jaw that are used for cutting.

Incontinence (in kon′tə nəns) is the lack of voluntary control of the bladder or bowels, particularly in an adult. Voluntary control of the bladder during the daytime is not achieved until about the age of two years, and at night may not occur until some years later.

Q: *What can cause incontinence of the bladder?*

A: Any neurological disorder that interferes with normal sensations from the bladder can prevent control of the sphincter muscle that normally closes it. Such disorders include spina bifida; damage to the spinal cord; multiple sclerosis; and nerve degeneration that occurs with conditions like diabetes mellitus, stroke, or Alzheimer's disease. Incontinence is also seen following certain attacks of epilepsy.

Incontinence may also result from partial obstruction caused by enlargement of the prostate gland (prostatomegaly) and from disorders of the muscle that controls the outflow of urine; such a muscle disorder may follow surgery or cancer. Some women develop stress incontinence because of prolapse (a displacement) of the uterus, which presses on the bladder and changes its structure so that urine escapes when the woman coughs or laughs. Incontinence may also result from an injury to the spinal cord that prevents impulses between the brain and the bladder.

Q: *What can cause incontinence of the bowels?*

A: In young children, lack of bowel control may simply be resistance to toilet training. But in older children it may occur because of stress or a psychological disorder.

Fecal incontinence is common in the senile, as is constipation. Failure to control the bowels may also be associated with neurological disorders, such as a stroke, multiple sclerosis, or the polyneuritis associated with diabetes mellitus. The condition may follow damage to the sphincter muscle that closes the anus following childbirth or an operation for anal fistula or fissure. Another factor can be cancer of the rectum or simply severe diarrhea.

Q: *How is incontinence treated?*

A: The treatment of any form of incontinence must be directed toward the cause. Special bags may be used for urinary incontinence, but fecal incontinence is more difficult to control. Special waterproof undergarments with absorbent pads may be worn to prevent leakage of stool or urine.

A new treatment involves electrical stimulation of the muscles that close the exits from the bladder and the rectum.

See also BED-WETTING; STRESS INCONTINENCE.

Incrustation (in krus tā′shən) is the formation of crusts or scabs on the skin.

See also SCAB.

Incubation period (in kyə bā′shən) is the time between exposure to an infectious illness and the appearance of the first symptoms. It is not the same as quarantine, which is a period of isolation from public contact after exposure to an infectious disease so that the infection does not spread.

See also INFECTIOUS DISEASE.

Incubator (in kyə bā′tər) is a life-support system used in hospitals for sustaining premature or seriously ill newborn babies. It is a ventilated, box-like apparatus in which the environment can be kept sterile and at constant temperature, humidity, and oxygen levels.

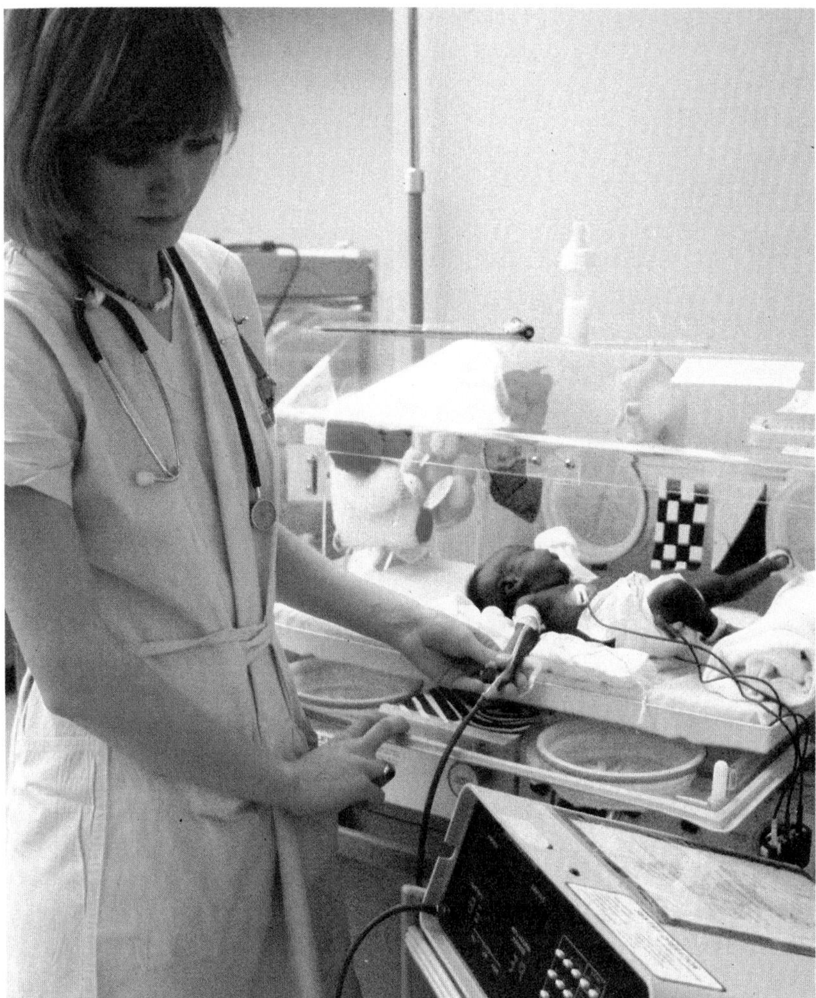

An **incubator** is a ventilated, box-like apparatus in which the environment can be kept sterile and at constant temperature, humidity, and oxygen levels. It is used as a life-support system for premature and seriously ill, newborn babies.

An incubator is also any device used to promote the growth of organisms placed inside it.

Incus (ing′kəs), commonly known as the anvil, is the second of three tiny bones in the middle ear.

See also EAR.

Inderal® (in′der ôl), or *propranolol hydrochloride*, is a beta-adrenergic blocking substance that is prescribed to treat hypertension, angina pectoris, and irregular heart rhythms (arrhythmia) and to prevent heart attacks (myocardial infarction). Principal side effects include mental depression, bradycardia (slow heart rate), and heart failure; therefore, dosages of Inderal should be carefully monitored and adjusted by a physician during the first several weeks of treatment. The dosages of Inderal should be gradually reduced before the treatment is discontinued; if treatment is stopped suddenly, a heart attack, or even sudden death, may result.

Indian hemp is another name for cannabis or marijuana.

See also MARIJUANA.

Indigestion (in də jes′chən) is incomplete or imperfect digestion. The condition is loosely defined, and it can vary according to situation and person. Acute indigestion is unpleasant, and the chronic form is debilitating. Chronic indigestion is sometimes a symptom of a more serious disorder, such as chronic pancreatitis, cardiac pain, or a peptic ulcer. Indigestion is also common during the later stages of pregnancy.

Q: *What are the symptoms of indigestion?*

A: Usually the person experiences vague abdominal discomfort and feels generally bloated. Burping may bring temporary relief. The symptoms may be severe enough to produce ill-defined pain that may or may not vary in intensity. Sometimes the feeling of discomfort increases; the patient feels nauseous and vomits. The symptoms usually last for only about two hours, although a bout of indigestion can last many weeks.

In addition to these symptoms, there may be heartburn. This produces a burning sensation beneath the breastbone that is sometimes accompanied by a bitter taste of fluid rising up into the mouth. *See also* HEARTBURN.

Q: *What causes indigestion?*

A: Indigestion is usually caused by gastritis (inflammation of the lining of the stomach), often brought on by overeating, ingestion of aspirin or ibuprofen (an anti-inflammatory substance), or an excess of alcohol. Smoking aggravates the condition. A person who has irregular meals, drinks too much strong coffee, and is anxious or depressed often develops mild gastritis. The bloated feeling may encourage aerophagia, the habit of swallowing air, which increases the indigestion symptoms. Obesity also aggravates the condition. Chronic indigestion can also be a warning sign of cancer. *See also* AEROPHAGIA; GASTRITIS.

Q: *When should someone who has indigestion consult a physician?*

A: If the symptoms are severe enough to interfere with normal life or to disturb sleep, a physician should be consulted as soon as possible.

Q: *How is indigestion treated?*

A: Treatment depends on the cause of the indigestion. Many patients find that the symptoms improve after a light, easily digestible meal or a glass of milk. Others find that an antacid medicine brings relief, particularly from heartburn.

In cases of excessive acid production, the physician may prescribe a histamine blocking agent that prevents acid from being produced. If anxiety, depression, and tension seem to be the main reasons for the indigestion, these factors should be addressed.

Indocin® (in dō′sən) is a tradename for indomethacin, an anti-inflammatory drug, available in capsule form. It is used to provide symptomatic relief of pain, swelling, and disability associated with a wide variety of inflammation of the joints. These include rheumatoid arthritis, osteoarthritis of large joints, bursitis, and gout.

Induction (in duk′shən) means causing or producing. The term has several medical applications. In one meaning, induction is the artificial initiation of childbirth. Labor is induced either by surgically rupturing the membrane around the fetus or by injecting the mother with medication. *See also* PREGNANCY AND CHILDBIRTH.

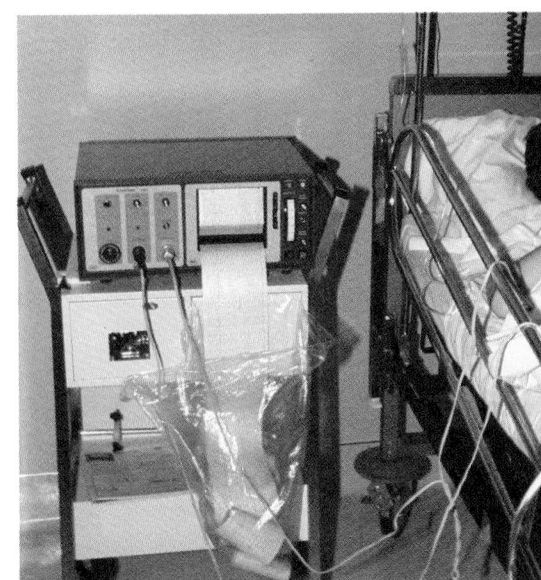

Induction of labor during childbirth can be monitored by sophisticated medical instruments.

Induction is also used to describe the beginning of anesthesia. It may refer to the intravenous injection of a short-acting barbiturate or the initial inhalation of an anesthetic gas.

In psychology, induction is a logical process of learning. The term also describes feelings reflected in another person; for example, grief in one person can induce sympathy in another.

Induration (in dů rā′shən) is an area of unusual hardness or firmness in a body tissue. The term may refer to bruising, scarring around a wound, or the hardened tissue surrounding an abscess.

Industrial diseases are disorders caused by exposure to industrial hazards, including toxic substances, temperature extremes, mechanical hazards, and biological hazards, such as microorganisms that are used in industrial processes.

See also OCCUPATIONAL HAZARD.

Infantile paralysis. See POLIOMYELITIS.

Infarction (in färk′shən) is the death of body tissue caused by a blockage of the blood supply to that tissue. The seriousness of the condition depends on the location of the infarction.

Q: *What causes an infarction?*

A: An infarction is caused by an arterial thrombosis (blood clot). The blood clot may be the result of arteriosclerosis, damage to the blood vessel, or an embolism (a blood clot from another part of the body that becomes trapped in the artery).

Q: *What are the symptoms of an infarction?*

A: The symptoms depend on which part of the body is affected. If the infarction is in the heart muscle (myocardial infarction), the patient's symptoms may range from a feeling of mild indigestion to severe pain that radiates from the left side of the chest to the left arm, neck, shoulders, back, and jaw. These symptoms are usually a sign of angina pectoris and are often the first warning of an impending heart attack.

If the infarction is in the brain, the patient suffers a stroke. In both the brain and myocardial infarctions, there are no alternative blood supplies, and the tissues die. If the infarction is in the leg, the patient experiences acute cramplike pain, and the leg becomes white and cold. If the patient does not receive immediate surgery, gangrene (death of tissue) rapidly sets in. An infarction in the kidney produces blood in the urine (hematuria).

Q: *Can an infarction be treated?*

A: No. Once the tissue has died, it can not be replaced. It can gradually heal and form scar tissue. Treatment is aimed at preventing another embolism or thrombosis from developing and causing a further infarction. Emergency surgery can replace part of the femoral artery with a graft or plastic tubing, but if the tissues have already died, amputation is the only treatment.

See also GANGRENE; HEART DISEASE, CORONARY; STROKE.

Infection (in fek′shən) is the invasion of the body by disease-producing organisms. There are six main types of infective organisms: viruses, bacteria, fungi, protozoa, worms, and rickettsia. An infection may enter the body through air that is breathed, in food or liquid that is ingested, directly through the skin, or from another part of the body.

See also BACTERIA; COMMUNICABLE DISEASE; FUNGAL INFECTION; INFECTIOUS DISEASE; PROTOZOA; RICKETTSIA; VIRUS.

Infectious disease is an illness caused by the growth of disease-producing microorganisms in the body; the infectious disease may be contagious.

The table on page 488 lists many common infectious diseases, each of which also has a separate entry in this encyclopedia. Other infectious diseases include amebic dysentery; brucellosis; cholera; epidemic pleurodynia; encephalitis; hand-foot-and-mouth disease; hepatitis; rabies; sexually transmitted diseases; smallpox; toxoplasmosis; tuberculosis; typhoid fever; typhus; yaws; and yellow fever. Each of these diseases also has a separate entry in this encyclopedia.

Infectious mononucleosis. See MONONUCLEOSIS.

Inferiority complex is a repressed state of mind in which a person believes himself or herself to be inferior to others.

See also COMPLEX.

Infectious diseases

Disease	Incubation (days)	Infectivity (days)	Duration (days)	Precautions/comments
Chickenpox	14-21	1 day before symptoms appear until 6 days after	6-8	Children should be excluded from school for 1 week after rash appears or until all sores have formed scabs. Strict precautions are needed in hospitals, or when immune-deficient persons may be exposed.
Diphtheria	2-5	14-28	Until clear	Strict isolation for persons with diphtheria infection of the throat until cultures are negative for the organism. Patients must not be allowed to work with food until the cultures are negative.
Dysentery (bacillary)	2-7	7-21	3-5	Careful hand-washing, especially after using the washroom. Patients must not be allowed to work with small children or with food until cultures are negative.
German measles (rubella)	14-21	7 days before the rash appears until 5 days after	5	Patients should remain home from work or school for 7 days after onset of rash. Contact with pregnant women must be avoided.
Influenza	1-3	When symptoms appear until 7 days after	3-5	During outbreaks in community or nursing home environment, quarantine may prevent spread.
Measles	10-14	4 days before rash appears until 7 days after	6-8	Children should be kept out of school for 4 days after onset of rash.
Meningitis, meningococcal	2-10	Up to several days after onset of infection	Varies	Contacts in home or day-care center should receive antibiotics as a precaution.
Mononucleosis	28-42	Not known; may persist for a year after infection	7-21	Spread is via saliva. Hand-washing and washing of articles soiled by oral or nasal secretions is important. Kissing is a common route of transmission among young adults.
Mumps	14-21	7 days before symptoms appear until 9 days after	10-14	Patients should remain home from work or school for 9 days after onset of swelling.
Poliomyelitis	4-13	Last part of incubation period and first week of acute illness	10-15	Because spread of disease is greatest before the onset of symptoms, there is little value in quarantine.

Disease	Incubation (days)	Infectivity (days)	Duration (days)	Precautions/comments
Roseola	2-5	Varies	5-7	There is no specific treatment.
Scarlet fever	2-5	Beginning of incubation period until 14-21 days after symptoms appear	7-10	No handling of food products until symptoms and rash disappear. Must complete at least 24 hours of antibiotic treatment before returning to work or school.
Whooping cough (pertussis)	7-21	21	42	Usually contagious before coughing begins. Patients should be isolated from infants and young children until the patient has received antibiotics for at least 5 days.

Infertility (in fėr til′ə tē) is the inability to produce offspring. It is not the same as sterility because an infertile person may have no physical disorder of the reproductive system. *See also* STERILITY.

Many couples are temporarily infertile. The likelihood of becoming pregnant on any one occasion is only about 1 percent.

With regular intercourse, 50 percent of women under the age of 30 can become pregnant within 6 months. Nearly 90 percent may be pregnant within 1 year, the remainder within 2 years. Older women usually take longer.

Q: *What should a couple do if they believe they are infertile?*

A: Taking into consideration the above statistics, it is advisable for a couple to delay any kind of investigations for at least a year. During this time they can work out the exact ovulation day of the woman. To do this, the woman takes her temperature the first thing in the morning, before having anything to eat or drink. Fourteen days before the onset of menstruation, the temperature rises by about 1°F (0.5°C). The rise in temperature occurs 24 hours after ovulation. If a temperature chart is kept for 3 to 4 months, a woman can estimate the day of ovulation. In addition, there are urine testing kits, which allow a woman to predict her day of ovulation. These kits are available without a prescription at most pharmacies.

The ovum is ready for fertilization for 24 hours. It is not known for certain how long a sperm can survive in the uterus, but it is thought to be up to 3 days. *See also* FERTILIZATION; OVULATION.

Q: *Why are some couples infertile?*

A: A sexual problem, such as complete ignorance about the mechanics of intercourse, is a more common factor than is realized. Other mechanical factors during intercourse that may prevent conception include the use of lubricants, position during intercourse, douching after intercourse, and too frequent ejaculation.

Sometimes a woman who ovulates only occasionally has a partner with a low sperm count. This means the chance of fertilization is greatly reduced.

In 50 percent of infertile couples, both partners are affected because of some physical reason. In the remaining 50 percent, half the men and half the women are physically incapacitated. Therefore, a true infertility evaluation requires examination of both the man and the woman. *See also* SEXUAL PROBLEMS.

Q: *What conditions can make a man infertile?*

A: Apart from sexual problems, infertility results if a condition or disorder affects either the total number of sperm produced during ejaculation or the number of viable, or normal, sperm produced. Such dis-

Infertility in men may be the result of inflammations, such as prostatitis and epididymitis, or a blocked vas deferens.

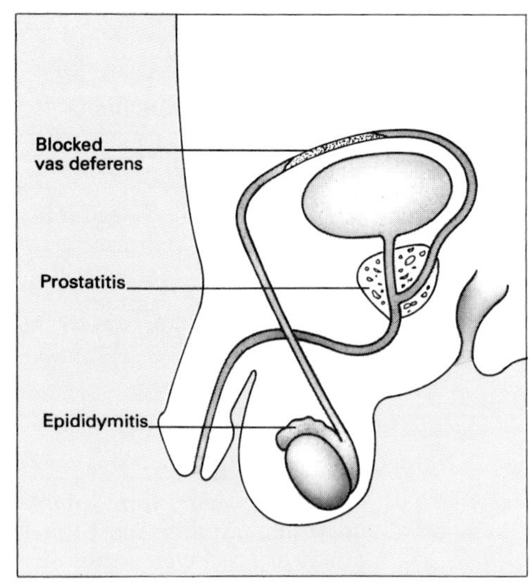

orders include any infection of the sexual organs, for example, epididymitis, venereal disease, prostatitis, mumps, blockage of the vas deferens (sperm duct), and alcoholism.

The temperature of the testicles affects the production of sperm. Undescended testicles are too warm to produce healthy sperm. In the same way, some men become temporarily infertile in hot environments or from wearing tight undershorts that hold the testicles too close to the body. More rarely, varicose veins of the spermatic cord, known as varicoceles, may cause lowered sperm counts. Other causes of infertility include certain chromosome abnormalities, Klinefelter's syndrome, cystic fibrosis, certain drugs, and irradiation of the testicles. *See also* CYSTIC FIBROSIS; EPIDIDYMITIS; IRRADIATION; KLINEFELTER'S SYNDROME; PROSTATITIS; SEXUALLY TRANSMITTED DISEASE.

Q: *How is a man's fertility assessed?*

A: A physician examines the man's testicles and then the prostate gland during a rectal examination. A sample of semen is collected and examined within two hours using a microscope to determine the sperm count. If any abnormality is noticed, the test is repeated two or three times to ensure an accurate diagnosis.

Q: *How is infertility in a man treated?*

A: General attention to health is essential. If the man is overweight, he must diet to lose weight. He should not smoke and should moderate his drinking, if necessary. Loose undershorts often help to increase the number of sperm produced, and sometimes the physician recommends bathing the testicles in cold water twice a day. If the sperm count is low, abstinence from sexual intercourse three to four days before the expected day of ovulation should increase the number of sperm ejaculated.

Infections of the reproductive organs must be treated. A varicocele can be removed by a minor operation. If no sperm are being produced or if there is a blockage in the vas deferens, it is seldom possible to cure the condition, although sometimes an operation can unblock the sperm duct. Undescended or retractile testicles have to be treated during childhood.

Sexual problems, such as impotence or premature ejaculation, require sympathetic discussion with a sex therapist or physician.

Q: *What conditions make a woman infertile?*

A: Infertility in women results if a condition or disorder affects ovulation, the movement of the ovum along the fallopian tube, the ability of the fertilized ovum to implant in the wall of the womb, or normal sexual intercourse.

Ovulation may be disrupted by anxiety or one of various hormone disorders. A hormone imbalance may occur for a few months following a course of contraceptive pills. Illness, such as tuberculosis, anorexia nervosa, or diabetes mellitus, affects ovulation. It is also thought that obesity, smoking, and alcohol affects it. An ovarian cyst also disrupts ovulation. In some cases a woman may have multiple cysts in the ovaries, a condition known as polycystic ovaries, which is also associated with infertility.

The movement of the ovum is restricted by any infection of the fallopian tube, including salpingitis, venereal disease, or an abscess. The lining of the tube becomes scarred, and even if an egg is successfully fertilized, an ectopic pregnancy is likely.

Disorders that affect the uterus include endometriosis, endometritis, polyps, and fibroids. In some women, a congenital anomaly results in a deformed uterus.

The presence of an intact hymen or vaginismus may indicate problems with techniques of sexual intercourse. Dyspareunia (painful intercourse) may indicate a gynecological infection.

Sometimes cervical secretions kill the sperm even when intercourse is successful. *See also* ENDOMETRIOSIS; ENDOMETRITIS; FIBROID; HYMEN; POLYP; PREGNANCY, ECTOPIC; SALPINGITIS; VAGINISMUS.

Q: *How is infertility in a woman assessed?*

A: Some tests can be carried out at home, for example, the temperature test for the day of ovulation described previously. A gynecological examination is necessary to see if there is any local infection in the vagina, cervix, or fallopian tubes. It is usual for a physician to check general health with a chest X ray, blood test, and urine sample. A cervical smear is taken to eliminate the possibility of local infection due to cervicitis or cancer.

A postcoital test may have to be done. Vaginal secretions are examined two to three hours after intercourse to make sure that the sperm are still moving vigorously and are not being killed by the secretions.

If the results of these tests are normal, a dilatation and curettage operation is usually performed to examine the lining of the womb. This may be followed by a salpingogram to show the shape of the womb and the condition of the fallopian tubes. *See also* DILATATION AND CURETTAGE.

Q: *How is infertility in a woman treated?*

A: Medical investigation is necessary to discover the cause of infertility. If there is an infection, it is promptly treated. However, repair operations on already scarred fallopian tubes are rarely successful. Adjustment of a womb abnormality

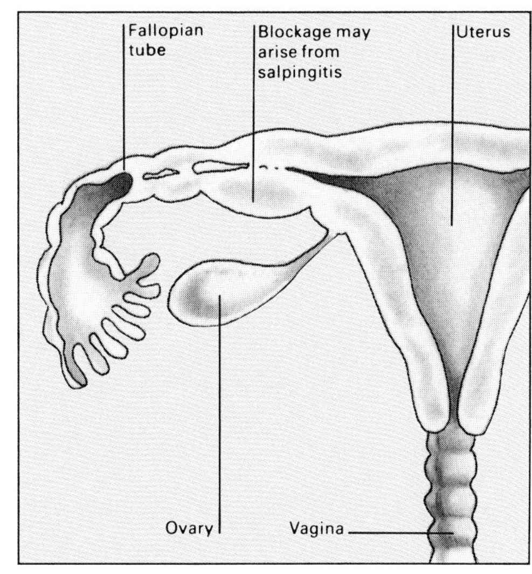

Infertility in women may be caused by a blockage in the fallopian tube.

is also difficult; it is, however, sometimes successful.

Hormone disorders are easier to treat. Ovulation can be stimulated with a drug called clomiphene combined with a small dose of estrogen. Care is taken to prevent multiple pregnancy.

In a technique known as *in vitro* fertilization, introduced in Britain during the late 1970's, infertile women become pregnant after having a fertilized ovum implanted in the uterus. The ovum is taken from the woman at ovulation, fertilized in a laboratory by sperm taken from the husband, and then replaced in the woman's womb. This technique is currently being carried out in a number of centers in the United States. The success rate, however, is only about 11 to 26 percent. *See also* *IN VITRO* FERTILIZATION.

Q: *How successful are treatments for infertility?*

A: Of those couples who seek treatment, 20 percent of the women conceive before treatment is started. A further 50 percent become pregnant within 2 years of treatment. It is important, however, that each partner follows the physician's advice. Conception may occur after years of infertility. This may also happen after the adoption of a child. There is no scientific explanation for this.

Infestation (in fes tā′shən) is the harboring of parasites, such as ticks, mites, and fleas, on the skin or in the hair. Another type of infestation is caused by worms in the body tissues or organs.

Inflammation (in flə mā′shən) is a localized reaction of body tissue to injury or disease. Inflammation may result from physical damage, infection, or surgery; or from exposure to electricity, chemicals, heat, cold, or radiation. It may also accompany autoimmune disease, cancer, or various joint disorders, such as rheumatoid arthritis or gout. *See also* AUTOIMMUNE DISEASE.

Q: *What are the symptoms of inflammation?*

A: The affected area becomes swollen and painful, and the skin becomes red and warm. If the inflamed area is large, there may also be a slight rise in body temperature, headache, and a loss of appetite. As the body repair processes start to heal and replace injured tissue, the inflammation gradually disappears. However, a collection of pus may remain. This usually discharges through the skin with the final disappearance of all the symptoms. If the pus is not discharged, it acts as a barrier to healing. In this case, a tough capsule may form around the pus, causing an abscess.

Occasionally, chronic inflammation may occur. Some infections, such as tuberculosis, act slowly, and the process of healing keeps pace with the damage. If this happens, fibrous tissue may form around the center of infection and cut off the blood supply, so that the central area of affected tissue dies. If this occurs internally, a chronic abscess is formed. If it involves the body surface, an ulcer or festering sore results. *See also* ABSCESS; ULCER.

Q: *How does the body respond to inflammation?*

A: After the initial injury or infection, damaged tissue releases chemicals, including a histamine, that causes the blood vessels in the area to expand and leak. This increased blood flow causes redness and warmth. The escape of fluid from the blood vessels causes the swelling. Pain is partly caused by compression of the nerve endings that accompanies the swelling and partly by irritation of the nerve endings by substances causing or resulting from the inflammation.

The inflow of blood carries additional white blood cells and antibodies. These remove damaged tissue and attempt to destroy any invading microorganisms by engulfing them. However, in engulfing the microorganisms, the white blood cells themselves may be destroyed. Pus is composed of dead white blood cells and dead microorganisms. *See also* ANTIBODY; BLOOD CELL, WHITE.

Q: *How is inflammation treated?*

A: Because inflammation is a natural healing process, it is advisable to interfere as little as possible. The injured area should be washed and a mild antiseptic applied. Any foreign bodies or chemicals should be carefully removed or washed away. The inflamed part should be rested. A physician should be consulted if the area of inflammation is extensive, if it becomes extremely painful, if it persists for a long time, or if an abscess or a festering sore forms.

Inflammatory bowel disease (in flam′ə tôr ē bou′əl) is a term used to describe a group of diseases, which include Crohn's disease, ileitis, and especially ulcerative colitis.

See also COLITIS, ULCERATIVE; CROHN'S DISEASE; ILEITIS.

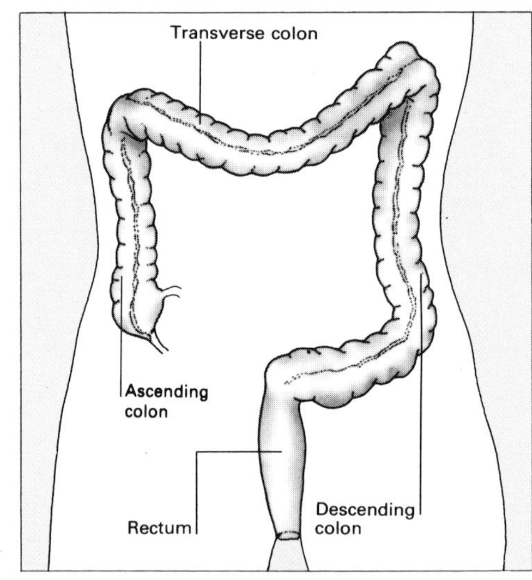

An **inflammatory bowel disease,** such as ulcerative colitis, affects both the colon and the rectum.

Influenza is a viral infection that may lead to infection of the lungs.

Influenza (in flü en′zə) is an acute, highly contagious respiratory infection caused by any of several closely related viruses. There are three major groups of these viruses, designated A, B, and C. Major influenza epidemics are usually caused by a strain of the influenza A virus.

Q: *What are the symptoms of influenza?*

A: After an incubation period of about two days, there is a sudden onset of shivering, called a chill; headache; weakness and fatigue; aching in the muscles and joints; a sore throat; a dry, painful cough; and general malaise. At the beginning of the illness there may also be vomiting and an aversion to light and noise. Initially, the body temperature may rise to about 104°F (40°C), dropping to between 102°F (38°C) and 103°F (39°C) for two or three days, then settling at between 100°F (37.5°C) and 102°F (38°C).

As the illness progresses, the cough may become less dry and painful because of the production of sputum. If no complications develop, the fever generally lasts for about five days. Recovery is usually rapid and without relapse, although it may be accompanied by some weakness and depression.

Q: *Can influenza have any complications?*

A: Yes. Influenza lowers the body's resistance to infection. This makes the patient vulnerable to invasion by other organisms that may cause secondary infections, especially of the lungs and bronchial tubes, sinuses, and ears, causing such conditions as pneumonia, bronchitis, sinusitis, and otitis media. Bronchitis can cause a chronic cough, but pneumonia is by far the most serious complication, since it is often fatal in elderly people and in patients with heart and lung diseases or malignancies. Influenza and secondary pneumonia are the major causes of sudden increases in the death rates of economically developed countries.

Q: *How is influenza treated?*

A: Influenza should be treated as any other fever. The patient should go to bed as soon as symptoms appear and should remain there until a complete recovery has been made. The patient should drink plenty of fluids, especially while there is a fever. Acetaminophen may help to relieve muscle and joint pains and to reduce fever. Aspirin should not be taken by children or young adults suffering from influenza, since it can cause a fatal reaction called Reye's syndrome. The patient should be isolated, both to prevent the spread of infection and to reduce the risk of secondary infections. If any complications develop, a physician should be consulted. Antibiotics are often prescribed to treat secondary complications. Amantadine hydrochloride is effective and recommended for patients, both children and adults, with severe infections caused by type A virus. *See also* REYE'S SYNDROME.

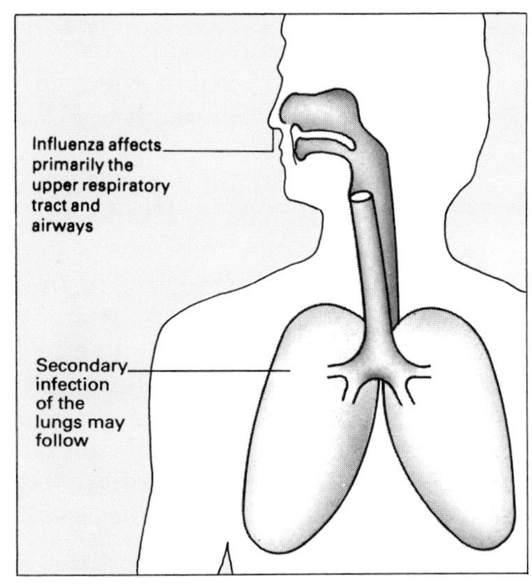
Influenza affects primarily the upper respiratory tract and airways
Secondary infection of the lungs may follow

Q: *Can influenza be prevented?*

A: Injections of dead influenza virus may confer immunity to that particular strain of influenza. The vaccination is neither immediately nor totally effective; it confers immunity about 7 days after injection and protects about 70 percent of those immunized. But the influenza virus tends to change and produce new strains, which are usually named according to their geographic origin; vaccination with one strain, therefore, does not give immunity to all of them. For this reason, vaccinations must be given each year as new strains develop.

Experiments have been performed using a modified live virus, but these have not proved as effective as vaccinations with the dead virus.

The drug amantadine hydrochloride, which is marketed under the trade name Symmetrel®, has proved useful in preventing respiratory infections due to A_2 strain of influenza virus. Amantadine hydrochloride should not, however, be used by pregnant women; it causes severe temporary dizziness.

Q: *How does influenza spread?*

A: Influenza is a contagious disease. It is spread by inhaling infected droplets in the air, which are produced by coughing and sneezing. It is also spread when nasal secretions are spread hand-to-hand, and then the injected hand touches mucosal or conjunctival surfaces. Influenza may occur at any time of the year, but is most common during winter.

Informed consent is written permission from a patient that allows a specific operation or an invasive (entering the body) procedure to be performed. This consent is also necessary in order to admit a patient to a research study. The document must be clearly written, so that the patient understands fully the risks involved; the benefits to be expected; the consequences of not having the operation or procedure (usually a test); and any alternative choices of treatment he or she may have. Informed consent is always voluntary and should be obtained from the patient only when he or she is fully competent.

Infrared radiation (in frə red′ rā dē ā′shən) is electromagnetic radiation with wave lengths from the invisible part of the spectrum. These rays' wave lengths are longer than those of the red part of the visible spectrum and are shorter than microwaves. Infrared rays occur in sunlight and in incandescent lamps. Infrared radiation is felt as heat on the body.

See also INFRARED TREATMENT.

Infrared treatment (in frə red′) is the use of infrared radiation to stimulate local and general blood circulation in order to treat various disorders and to relieve pain. It may be used by physiotherapists for muscle disorders and rheumatic diseases or in the relief of pain caused by minor muscle damage, such as sprains and strains.

A device called an infrared thermograph, which detects and photographs infrared rays, is used in the diagnosis of some disorders, particularly breast cancer. Thermography, however, is of limited use in the diagnosis of many diseases.

See also INFRARED RADIATION; THERMOGRAM.

Infusion (in fyü′zhən) is the introduction of a sterile fluid into a vein. Drugs may be administered by this method. It may also be used to maintain the balance of salts within the body.

Infusion is also a method of extracting chemicals by soaking a substance, usually an herbal plant, in water.

Ingrown toenail. See TOENAIL, INGROWN.

Inguinal (ing′gwə nəl) describes anything pertaining to the groin. For example, the inguinal nodes are lymph nodes situated in the groin.

Inhalation therapy (in hə lā′shən) is the breathing in of water, vapor, gases, or drugs into the lungs. Inhalation therapy is used to treat various respiratory disorders.

In the hospital, inhalation therapy is frequently administered to patients with pneumonia or bronchitis to loosen mucus and secretions. In patients with asthma, a bronchodilator, or medication to open up the air passages, may be used.

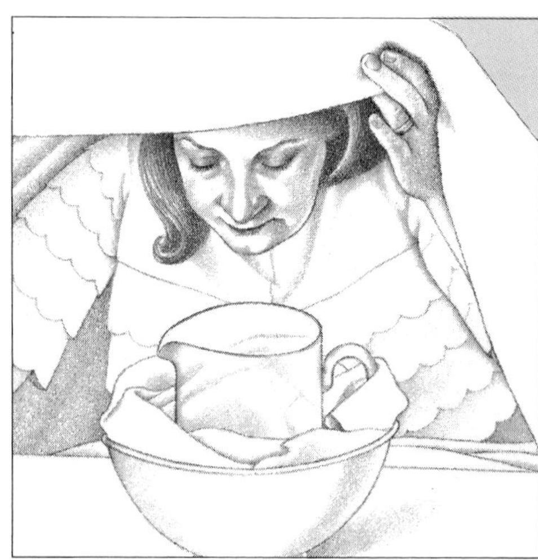

Inhalation therapy can be self-administered by placing a towel over one's head and deeply breathing in steam from a bowl of boiling water.

At home, a simple vaporizer with water may make the patient with a cold or sinusitis more comfortable. The patient with significant congestion should place a towel over his or her head and bend over a bowl of boiling water. The towel should cover the entire bowl, and the patient should breathe deeply in and out through his or her nose for ten minutes. The patient should stay in a warm environment for at least one-half hour after inhalation. Although the addition of menthol-containing fluids to the water may make the patient more comfortable, they have no medical importance.

In infants with congestion, especially those with croup, turning on a hot shower in the bathroom with the door closed will create an environment for inhalation therapy and will help the infant to breathe more easily.

Inherited disorder is an abnormality that is passed on from parents to children.

See also CONGENITAL ANOMALY; HEREDITY.

Inhibition (in ə bish'ən) is the prevention or restraint of some bodily activity by another bodily process. For example, fear may inhibit gastric secretions. The body often uses inhibition to prevent the oversecretion of a hormone. For example, if the thyroid increases its hormone production, the body will inhibit the release of thyroid-stimulating hormone.

In psychology, inhibition refers to the restraint of a particular behavior, instinctual drive, or unconscious urge. For example, in adults, anger at another person seldom leads to violence, as it more commonly does in children. This is because most adults are inhibited against violence. In this sense, inhibition is different from repression in that it may be conscious or unconscious. Repression, however, is always unconscious and automatic.

See also NERVOUS SYSTEM, AUTONOMIC; REPRESSION.

Injection (in jek'shən) is a method of forcing a fluid into the body. It is usually performed using a needle and a syringe, but may also be done using compressed air by means of a special device. An injection may be intradermal, in which fluid is injected into the superficial skin layers; subcutaneous, injected between the skin and underlying muscle; intramuscular, into a muscle; intravenous, into a vein; intra-arterial, into an artery; epidural, around the nerves of the spinal cord; intrathecal, under the meninges (membranes) of the brain; or intra-articular, into a joint.

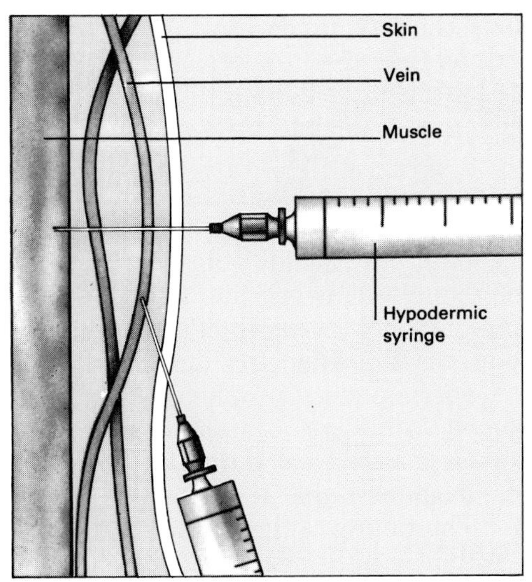

Injections can be given in many ways, including intramuscularly and intravenously.

Injured person, transportation of. *See* FIRST AID FUNDAMENTALS.

Inner ear. *See* EAR.

Innominate bone. *See* HIPBONE.

Inoculation (i nok yə lā'shən) is a method of immunization in which an inactive microorganism or toxin is injected into the body in order to stimulate the body's immune system to produce immunity.

See also IMMUNITY; IMMUNIZATION.

Insanity (in san'ə tē) is a legal term for any mental disorder, such as psychosis, that results in a person being unaware of his or her actions for which he or she is held responsible. Various legal procedures may be necessary before a person can be certified as legally insane and before medical treatment can be started. The finding of insanity by a court does not result in a person relinquishing all legal rights.

See also MENTAL ILLNESS.

Insect bites: first aid. *See* BITES AND STINGS: FIRST AID.

Insecticide (in sek'tə sīd) is any substance that kills insects. Many insecticides are also poisonous to animals and human beings. Some of the newer insecticides lose their potency and their toxicity more quickly, so that long-term hazards are less likely. In some cases, however, hazards to human beings may come from the inert ingredients used to place the insecticide in solution, as well as from the insecticide itself.

Insemination, artificial (in sem ə nā'shən). Artificial insemination is a technique in which sperm is introduced into the neck of the womb (cervix) for the purpose of fertilizing the egg (ovum) by means other than sexual intercourse. This is done with a syringe. Artificial insemination is used in some cases of infertility that are due to low sperm counts, problems in cervical mucus, or in cases of impotence.

Q: *How important is the timing of the insemination?*

A: The timing of the introduction of the sperm is critical; it should take place during ovulation (when an ovary releases an egg). The timing is estimated by following the woman's morning temperature charts, which show a sudden, slight increase in temperature on the day of ovulation, or by modern techniques, such as ultrasound examinations and hormonal tests.

Q: *Who supplies the sperm for the insemination?*

A: It is most common for the woman's husband to supply the sperm. This is known as AIH (artificial insemination by husband). The husband, although fertile, may not be able to have sexual intercourse. Or the quantity of sperm produced may be so small that the chances of conception are slight.

Artificial insemination by donor (AID) is the provision of sperm by an unknown male. This is used when the husband is infertile and both partners agree to the procedure. The physician chooses a man with qualities that are compatible with those of the future parents in vital respects, such as race and physical characteristics, absence of congenital abnormalities, and the correct blood group. The practice of artificial insemination is controversial in many countries on legal, religious, and moral grounds.

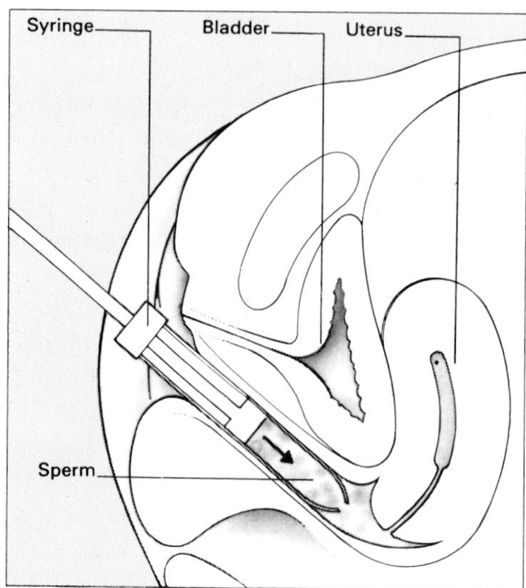

Artificial insemination is the introduction of healthy sperm into the uterus via syringe.

Insidious (in sid'ē əs) describes any condition that comes on so gradually that the affected person is unaware of its onset. Cancer is often insidious, whereas the onset of influenza is sudden or acute.

Insomnia (in som'ne ə) is the inability to fall asleep or remain asleep, resulting in long periods of wakefulness. An inability to sleep continuously through the night is not an illness in itself, nor is it necessarily the symptom of a disorder. Because of great individual differences in sleep patterns, what one person considers to be insomnia may be regarded as normal by another individual. Some people simply require less sleep. Older people, for instance, tend to sleep less, more lightly, and with more interruptions than do younger people.

Q: *How is insomnia prevented?*

A: Peace of mind is essential to falling asleep, and it is important to have a warm, comfortable bed in a quiet bedroom. The last several hours before going to bed should be as relaxed as possible. Physical exercise of some kind during the day and a walk in the fresh air after dinner are also beneficial for a good night's sleep. It also helps not to nap during the day. Stimulants, such as caffeine (in tea and many soft drinks, as well as in coffee) or those found in diet pills or cold remedies, must be avoided. Alcohol also interferes with normal sleep patterns and should be avoided.

Q: *What causes insomnia?*

A: Insomnia may be a symptom of almost any disease or disorder. Physical causes of insomnia include overeating, hunger, cold, heat, noise, excessive tea or coffee consumption before going to bed, or an uncomfortable bed. Pain is a common cause of insomnia. A cough, particularly when combined with a fever, often causes trouble in sleeping. Persistent insomnia is often caused by anxiety and depression.

Q: *How is insomnia treated?*

A: Do not stay in bed longer than 20 minutes after waking up. An insomniac should perform some kind of mental or physical activity until tired or drowsy, for example, reading, light housework, etc. A hot bath, a warm drink (such as milk), or a light snack may also help. Pain should be treated with painkillers, such as acetaminophen.

If sleeplessness is caused by anxiety or depression, it may help to discuss the problem with a physician who may then prescribe medication for a short period during the initial treatment. Psychiatric counseling may be advisable.

A further word is necessary about sleep-inducing drugs, commonly called sleeping pills. The ideal drug would permit normal sleep with regular dreaming patterns. It would be nonhabit-forming, free of aftereffects, such as lethargy or depression, and free of toxic side effects.

No drug or class of drugs meets all of these requirements; barbiturates are habit-forming, and chloral derivatives have side effects.

Additionally, any sleeping pill taken daily will lose its effectiveness within just two to three weeks, although the person taking it may already have become physically dependent on it. Therefore, sleeping drugs should never be taken without first consulting a physician.

See also SLEEP.

Insufflation (in suf la′shən) is the blowing of a fluid, gas, or powder into a body cavity. Insufflation may be used by a physician as a method of unblocking the Eustachian tube in the treatment of middle ear diseases.

Insulin (in′sə lin) is a hormone produced in the pancreas, a gland situated behind the stomach. The clustered, insulin-producing cells are called the islets of Langerhans.

Insulin controls the use of glucose, fats, and lipids by the body. An excess of insulin, sometimes caused by a pancreatic tumor, causes hypoglycemia (a low level of sugar in the blood); and a lack of insulin produces hyperglycemia (an abnormally high level of sugar in the blood), which is a symptom of diabetes mellitus. Since severe deficiency of insulin can be life-threatening, the natural insulin level in diabetic patients is augmented by insulin injections.

Insulin is obtained from the pancreases of cattle or pigs; a new insulin, identical to naturally-occurring human insulin, has recently been introduced. This new insulin is produced synthetically, using recombinant DNA (deoxyribonucleic acid), and does not stimulate the formation of antibodies against insulin, or sensitization, as the animal insulin may do.

Insulin is prepared in various ways to make it act quickly (soluble insulin), or slowly, in combination with zinc and other substances, so that only one or two injections a day are necessary. The strength of insulin is expressed in units of activity; the dosage is measured in syringes marked off in units.

See also DIABETES MELLITUS; HYPERGLYCEMIA; HYPOGLYCEMIA; ISLETS OF LANGERHANS; PANCREAS.

Insurance, health. *See* MEDICAL EXPENSES AND INSURANCE.

Insurance, malpractice. Malpractice insurance is insurance purchased by health-care professionals to cover claims of negligence, ineptitude, and improper treatment brought against them by patients. In recent years, malpractice has become a controversial topic. As lawsuits against physicians have become commonplace, the cost of such insurance has risen dramatically. Many doctors, as a result, have felt compelled to raise their medical fees to compensate for the steadily increasing insurance rates.

Integument. *See* SKIN.

Intelligence quotient (IQ) is an index of a person's intelligence, relative to the statistical average of his or her age group. The IQ is based on a variety of tests in verbal, mathematical, and writing abilities and on physical performance at set tasks. Standard intelligence tests include the Wechsler Intelligence Scale for Children (WISC) and for Adults (WAIS), as well as the Stanford-Binet Intelligence Scale.

The test score of a person is compared with those of other persons in the same age group. For example, a score between 90 and 109 is the statistical average. Such a score would then denote a normal intelligence. Any score 110 or above indicates superior intelligence to near genius or genius; a score below 90 ranges from dull normal to profoundly mentally retarded. Tests for adults are different from those for children.

Q: *Are IQ tests always accurate?*

A: No. There are many reasons why such tests may be inaccurate. Much depends on the way a child has been educated and on his or her social and cultural background. Intelligence tests may be supplemented by other performance tests and observations to provide the most accurate assessment of an individual.

Intensive care. See HOSPITAL.

Intercostal (in tər kos′təl) means situated between the ribs.

See also RIB; RIBCAGE.

Intercourse. See SEXUAL INTERCOURSE.

Interferon (in tər fir′on) is a protein substance produced by body cells in response to viral infections or certain chemicals. Noninfected cells exposed to interferon are then resistant to the virus. Research is now underway into methods of stimulating interferon production by the body. Efforts are also being made to isolate and synthesize it, so that it can be administered at the onset of a virus infection. Interferon has proven effective in treating some chronic viral infections and useful in the treatment of leukemia and other cancers. It is also being tested as treatment for immune deficiency diseases, such as AIDS.

Intermittent claudication. See CLAUDICATION, INTERMITTENT.

Intermittent porphyria. See PORPHYRIA.

Internal medicine is the area of medicine dealing with the diagnosis and nonsurgical treatment of diseases in adults. Specialists are called internists. Some internists limit their practices to specific areas of internal medicine, such as allergies, diseases of the heart and blood vessels, disorders of the digestive tract, etc.

Internship is the first year of in-hospital training following graduation from medical school.

Intersex (in′tər seks) is an individual with both male and female characteristics.

See also HERMAPHRODITE.

Intertrigo (in tər trī′gō) is the soreness and inflammation that occurs between the layers of skin that rub together. Intertrigo is a form of dermatitis. The skin becomes soft and peels off to expose reddened, sore areas that are vulnerable to infection. Intertrigo usually occurs in the creases of the neck, beneath large breasts, and in the groin. In obese people, intertrigo may also occur in the abdominal creases.

Treatment involves dieting and exercise to lose weight and keeping the skin clean and dry, with frequent washing and powdering.

See also CHAFING; DERMATITIS.

Intestinal flu. See GASTROENTERITIS.

Intestinal obstruction (in tes′tə nəl əb struk′shən) is a complete or partial blockage of the intestine. It may occur at any time and for a variety of reasons. An intestinal obstruction interferes with the normal passage of the products of digestion through the digestive system.

Q: *What are the symptoms of an intestinal obstruction?*

A: The first symptom is usually abdominal pain, followed by swelling (distention) of the abdomen. The swelling is more marked if the obstruction occurs in the lower parts of the intestine. There may also be constipation and failure to

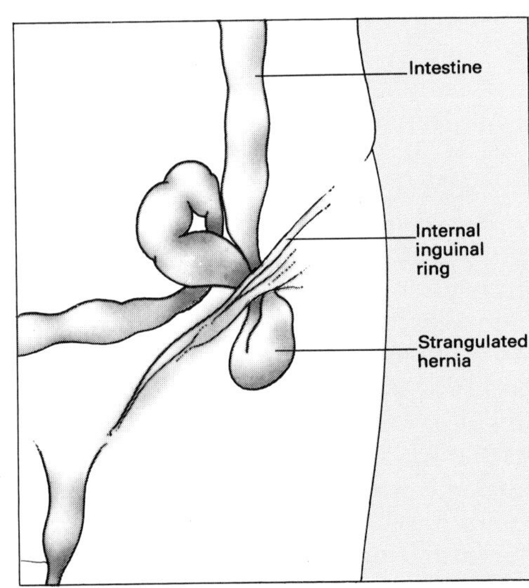

An **intestinal obstruction** may be caused by a strangulated hernia. If the symptoms are severe, the condition requires immediate surgery.

pass internal gas. Vomiting may occur, although not for some hours after the initial symptoms, unless the obstruction is in the small intestine.

Q: *What causes an intestinal obstruction?*

A: There are various conditions that may cause an intestinal obstruction. Some are comparatively simple to treat, such as an accumulation of hard feces or infestation with parasitic worms. Others are more serious, such as tumors, a strangulated hernia, or intestinal adhesions.

Q: *How is an intestinal obstruction treated?*

A: The treatment depends on the cause of the obstruction. If the large intestine is obstructed and the symptoms are not severe, there may be time for various tests, such as sigmoidoscopy and X-ray examination following a barium enema. If the symptoms are acute, an urgent surgical operation is required.

Surgery is not always necessary, but other treatments are given only if the cause is comparatively simple to treat or if the intestine can overcome the obstruction without the need for surgery. For example, if the obstruction is caused by the twisting of the intestine around an adhesion or a scar, it may untwist on its own without treatment. In all such cases the stomach is kept empty by sucking fluid up a gastric tube, and intravenous fluids are continued until it is certain that either the obstruction has disappeared or that surgery is necessary.

See also ADHESION; CROHN'S DISEASE; DIVERTICULITIS; DIVERTICULOSIS; DIVERTICULUM, MECKEL'S; HERNIA; HIRSCHSPRUNG'S DISEASE; INTUSSUSCEPTION; SIGMOIDOSCOPY, FLEXIBLE; VOLVULUS.

Intestine (in tes'tən) is the part of the digestive tract that extends from the outlet of the stomach to the anus. It is commonly called the bowel.

The intestine has two parts: the small intestine and the large intestine (the terms refer to their diameters, not to their lengths). The small intestine is the longer of the two, made up of the short duodenum and the jejunum, which together make up about two-fifths of the small intestine, and the ileum, which makes up three-fifths.

The large intestine is made up of the cecum, with the appendix, and the colon, which ends at the rectum.

The contents of the intestine are moved by a series of muscular contractions and relaxations known as peristalsis. In the small intestine, food is digested and absorbed, and the excess waste products and water pass into the large intestine. In the large intestine, excess fluid is reabsorbed, and bacterial action on the feces produces some of the essential vitamins B and K for the body.

The intestine is covered by the peritoneum which, in many places, combines to form a membrane (the mesentery). The mesentery allows the ileum and parts of the colon freedom of movement and position, while, at the same time, holding the intestine in the correct position. Blood vessels and nerves, as well as many lymphatic vessels and lymph nodes, are present in the mesentery. The veins in the mesentery join the hepatic portal vein that carries blood to the liver.

See also CECUM; COLON; DIGESTIVE SYSTEM; DUODENUM; ILEUM; JEJUNUM; MESENTERY; RECTUM.

Intestine, large (in tes'tən). The large intestine is the tubular section of the bowel, partially encircling the small intestine. It is approximately 5 feet (1.5m) long and made up of the cecum, the ascending, transverse, descending, and sigmoid portions of the colon, and the rectum. The purpose of the large intestine is to further absorb water from the digested food and to store the remaining waste until it can be eliminated from the body.

See also CECUM; COLON; INTESTINE; RECTUM.

Intestine, small (in tes'tən). The small intestine is the first, coiled, tubular section of the bowel, which carries on most of the digestive processes. It consists of the duodenum, the jejunum, and the ileum. The small intestine is 22 feet (7m) long and empties into the cecum, the first portion of the large intestine.

See also DUODENUM; ILEUM; INTESTINE; JEJUNUM.

Intoxication (in tok sə kā'shən) is a state of being poisoned. The term is commonly applied to the condition produced by an excess of alcohol. It can also refer to poisoning by drugs and the confusion and delirium caused by fever.

See also ALCOHOL ABUSE; ALCOHOLISM.

Intradermal (in trə dėr′məl) means within the skin layer. For example, rashes that occur within the substance of the skin are termed intradermal rashes.

See also SKIN.

Intramuscular (in trə mus′kyə lər) means within a muscle. For example, an intramuscular injection is one in which a solution is injected directly into a muscle.

Intrauterine device. *See* CONTRACEPTION.

Intravenous (in trə vē′nəs) means within a vein. For example, an intravenous injection is made directly into a vein. Since infusions of fluids and medicines are generally made directly into a vein, these are often referred to as "IV's (Intra-Venous).

Intravenous cholangiogram. *See* CHOLANGIOGRAM, INTRAVENOUS.

Intravenous pyelogram. *See* PYELOGRAM, INTRAVENOUS.

Introvert (in′trə vėrt) is a personality type characterized by an introspective attitude and a withdrawn, retiring demeanor, as opposed to an extrovert, who has an outgoing and sociable personality.

See also EXTROVERT.

Intubation (in tü bā′shən) is the insertion of a tube into a body opening. The term usually refers to the passage of a rubber breathing tube through the mouth or nose into the windpipe (trachea) for the administration of oxygen or anesthetic gas.

Intussusception (in təs sə sep′shən) is a form of intestinal obstruction in which one section of the intestine telescopes into the next section, akin to the finger of a glove being turned inside-out. The telescoped section of the intestine is drawn in further by the action of the intestinal muscles. Most intussusceptions occur in children.

Q: *What causes intussusception?*

A: In most cases, the cause is not known. It has been suggested that intussusception occurs most often in children who have had a recent infection that causes a swelling of lymphoid tissue in the intestinal wall. The body treats the swelling as part of the intestinal contents and pulls it along by the action of the intestinal muscles. Occasionally, a polyp, tumor, or Meckel's diverticulum may cause intussusception in adults. *See also* DIVERTICULUM, MECKEL'S.

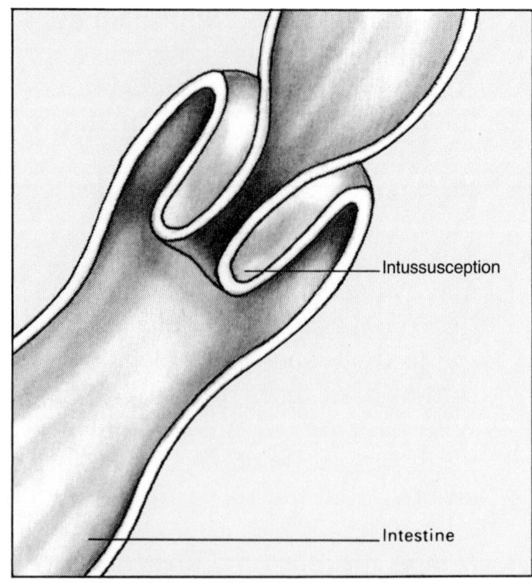

Intussusception is an intestinal obstruction in which one section of the intestine telescopes into the next section.

Q: *What are the symptoms of intussusception?*

A: In children, intussusception usually occurs suddenly, with severe pain, vomiting, and pallor. The affected child may draw up the knees and scream with the pain. As the attacks become more severe, the straining to expel feces may cause blood and mucus to be passed from the rectum. Between attacks, the child may be calm and relaxed and may appear to have recovered.

Q: *What is the treatment for intussusception?*

A: Immediate hospitalization is vital. The patient is first given a barium enema to confirm the diagnosis. The pressure of the enema sometimes restores the affected parts of the intestine to their normal positions. If this does not happen, a surgical operation is necessary.

In utero (in yü′tə rō) means within the uterus, as a fetus before birth.

In vitro (in vī′trō) is a term applied to reactions that occur outside a living body in an artificial environment. For example, drugs are often tested *in vitro* ("in glass") before being tested on a living body.

See also IN VIVO.

In vitro fertilization (in vī′trō fėr tə lə zā′shən) is a relatively new technique, in which an egg is removed from a woman's ovary and placed in a test tube or special sterile dish containing her husband's sperm. After the fertilization, the egg is placed in the woman's uterus where normal pregnancy continues.

In vitro fertilization is usually employed when the woman's fallopian tubes are blocked and can not be opened surgically. With the development of *in vitro* fertilization and its successful application, women once thought to have been infertile have successfully conceived and borne children. These children are sometimes referred to as "test-tube babies."

In vivo (in vī′vō) is a term applied to reactions that occur within a living organism.

See also IN VITRO.

Iodine (ī′ə dīn) is a nonmetallic element, which is essential in the human diet for the correct functioning of the thyroid gland. Lack of iodine in the diet leads to the formation of a goiter and hypothyroidism. *See also* GOITER; HYPOTHYROIDISM; THYROID GLAND.

Q: *Is iodine used in medical treatment?*

A: Yes. Iodine salts may sometimes be given in the early treatment of hyperthyroidism, excessive activity of the thyroid gland. Iodine dissolved in an alcoholic solution or combined with povidone (povidone-iodine) is used as an antiseptic skin preparation before surgical operations or to clean wounds. Iodine preparations are also used as diagnostic aids in special X rays, such as cholecystogram (of the gall bladder), intravenous pyelogram (of the kidney), and arteriogram (of an artery).

Radioactive iodine is used in the diagnosis of thyroid gland disease, as well as in investigations of liver, lung, and kidney disorders. The preparation loses half its radioactivity within eight days. In larger doses, it may also be used in the treatment of hyperthyroidism and cancer of the thyroid gland.

See also THYROTOXICOSIS.

Ionizing radiation. *See* RADIATION, IONIZING.

Ipecac (ip′ə kak) is a substance that is used to promote vomiting. It is usually prescribed to stimulate vomiting (emesis) in cases of poisoning or drug overdose. Ipecac can cause adverse effects if it is not vomited; therefore, it should not be given to unconscious victims. Unconscious victims may also inhale the vomit.

It is generally recommended that any households with toddler-age children keep ipecac on hand at all times as a routine safety precaution.

See also DRUG OVERDOSE: FIRST AID; POISONING: FIRST AID.

IQ. *See* INTELLIGENCE QUOTIENT.

Iridectomy (ir ə dek′tə mē) is an operation to remove part of the iris in the eye. It is most commonly performed as a treatment for glaucoma to reduce the build-up of fluid pressure in the eyeball. An iridectomy may also be done to create an artificial pupil

See also EYE; GLAUCOMA.

Iris (ī′ris) is the colored ring that surrounds the pupil of the eye. The iris is positioned in front of the lens and behind the cornea. Within the iris are muscle groups that, by contracting or relaxing, regulate how much light passes through the pupil. In bright light, some muscles of the iris relax and the pupil becomes smaller. In dim light, these muscles contract and the pupil becomes larger to admit as much light as possible. *See also* EYE.

Q: *What determines the color of the iris?*

A: Eye color, produced by pigment cells in the iris, is an inherited characteristic.

Q: *What disorders can affect the iris?*

A: The iris can become inflamed (iritis, choroiditis, or uveitis). A cleft iris is a congenital anomaly known as coloboma. An albino has no pigmentation in the iris, and so the eyes look pink because the small blood vessels are visible. *See also* CHOROIDITIS; COLOBOMA; IRITIS; UVEITIS.

Iritis (ī rī′tis) is inflammation of the iris of the eye. The iris appears muddy in color and the pupils smaller than usual. The cornea may become fogged, and vision tends to be blurred. The eye also waters continually. Pain in and above the eye, sensitivity to light (photophobia), redness, and soreness are among the other symptoms that accompany iritis.

See also IRIS; PHOTOPHOBIA.

Iron (ī'ərn) is a metallic chemical element essential to the human body. It occurs in hemoglobin, the component in red blood cells that carries oxygen. Iron is also present in enzymes (substances that produce chemical change), associated with respiration, and in myoglobin, an important protein in muscle. The body gets its iron from foods. Those rich in iron include liver, eggs, and lean meat. Pregnant women need more iron than do other adults. Growing children also need additional iron to help build new body tissue. *See also* HEMOGLOBIN.

Q: *What happens if there is insufficient iron in the body?*

A: Iron deficiency anemia occurs. The condition may be caused by a gradual loss of iron from the body because of a bleeding peptic ulcer, menstrual problems, or bleeding caused by cancer. Iron deficiency may also be caused by a sudden and severe hemorrhage. *See also* ANEMIA.

Q: *How is iron deficiency treated?*

A: The body is able to absorb iron in almost any form when taken orally. If iron deficiency does not improve after iron has been taken orally, as may happen in conditions in which there is an absence of acid in the stomach, then iron may be given by intravenous or intramuscular injection. Adverse side effects from taking a normal dose of iron are rare, but occasionally, a patient has constipation or diarrhea with mild symptoms of indigestion.

Q: *What happens if there is too much iron in the body?*

A: If taken in large doses for long periods of time, toxic deposits of iron can occur in the body. This is referred to as hemochromatosis.

Q: *How much iron does an adult require daily?*

A: The average adult needs from .5 to 1 milligram of iron a day. A female between puberty and menopause needs about twice that amount. Since the body metabolizes only a small part of the iron contained in food, a daily adult intake of 18 milligrams of iron is recommended. During pregnancy and lactation, a woman's iron intake should be between 15 and 30 milligrams a day.

Irradiation (i rā dē ā'shən) is the application of any form of radiation to a tissue or substance. In medical treatment, irradiation may be in the form of X rays, radioactive particles, heat, or ultraviolet light. Irradiation is currently used most often in the treatment of certain types of cancer.

See also RADIATION.

Irrigation (ir ə gā'shən) is the washing out of a body cavity or a wound with water or an antiseptic fluid.

See also ENEMA.

Irritable bowel syndrome (bou'əl), also called spastic colon and mucous colitis, is a recurrent intestinal disorder in which in an apparently healthy person there are bouts of abdominal pain with diarrhea or constipation. There is an abnormality of the muscular action that passes food along the colon, and this causes the constipation or diarrhea.

Q: *What causes irritable bowel syndrome?*

A: The syndrome may develop during emotional stress, such as studying for examinations, or anxieties associated with work or domestic problems. There is a tendency for it to occur in individuals who are obsessional, but it may also appear for no apparent reason. Sometimes a food allergy may be involved.

Q: *What are the symptoms of irritable bowel syndrome?*

A: The disorder first appears in young adults and is variable, with long periods in which there are no symptoms. Abdominal pain may occur as a dull ache over one area of the colon, or occasionally, there may be intermittent colic that is relieved by a bowel movement. Sometimes there is constipation or a form of diarrhea in which frequent small amounts of feces with a thin, tape-like appearance are passed. The feces may be covered with mucus. Diarrhea is often the principal symptom, usually occurring first thing in the morning or immediately after a meal. The rest of the day may be free from pain or diarrhea. The person may feel tired and mildly depressed. Weight loss is unusual.

Q: *How is irritable bowel syndrome diagnosed and treated?*

A: A physician makes a diagnosis after excluding other possibilities, such as gastroenteritis, ulcerative colitis, amebic dysentery, or other intestinal disorders that cause abdominal pain and diarrhea. If necessary, the physician may arrange for fecal analysis and a barium enema followed by fluoroscopic or X-ray examination to make sure there is no underlying disease of the intestine.

Once the physician has made the diagnosis, he or she can reassure the patient that there is no serious disorder. A diet containing additional bulk (such as bran or methyl cellulose) and the use of antispasmodic drugs usually produces an immediate improvement.

Ischemia (is kē′mē ə) is a decreased blood supply to a particular part of the body. It is caused by a spasm or a disease in the blood vessels.

The condition most commonly develops in arteriosclerosis. This may result in leg cramps, angina pectoris, if it affects the heart, or transient ischemia (TIA), if it affects the brain. Transient ischemia often, but not always, is a precursor of a stroke. Victims of TIA, however, recover completely.

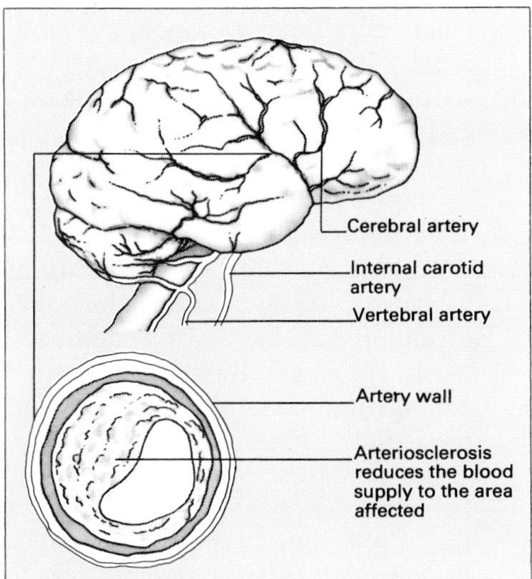

Ischemia is a reduced blood supply. When it occurs in the brain, it may precede a stroke.

Ischemia may also result from acute blockage of an artery, following an injury or a blood clot. Some tissues die much more quickly than others when they become ischemic. The brain survives for only about five minutes, whereas the kidneys can continue to function for one to two hours. The death of any tissue is known as an infarction.

See also ANGINA PECTORIS; ARTERIOSCLEROSIS; CLAUDICATION, INTERMITTENT; INFARCTION.

Ischiorectal abscess. *See* ABSCESS, ISCHIORECTAL.

Ischium (is′kē əm) is one of the three bones that form each hipbone. It joins the ilium near the hip joint and the pubis at the front. The ischium is a strong bone with a protuberant lower part, which is covered by a fluid-filled cavity (bursa) that counters pressure. This is the area that supports the body when sitting.

See also HIPBONE; ILIUM; PELVIS; PUBIS.

Ishihara's test (ish ə hä′rəs) is a method of detecting color blindness.

See also COLOR BLINDNESS.

Islets of Langerhans (läng′ər häns) are groups of cells scattered throughout the pancreas that regulate sugar metabolism.

Q: *How do the islets of Langerhans function?*

A: They secrete the hormones insulin, glucagon, and gastrin. The most important is insulin, which reduces the level of glucose in the bloodstream, by helping to convert glucose to glycogen. Glucagon has the opposite function of increasing the level of glucose in the blood. Gastrin mainly stimulates the secretion of gastric acid and pepsin, which are used in the digestion of food. *See also* INSULIN.

Q: *What happens if the islets of Langerhans fail to function properly?*

A: The production of the pancreatic hormones is upset, resulting in various disorders. The most common and well-known disorder is diabetes mellitus. In the juvenile form of diabetes, the islet cells fail to produce adequate insulin. Rarely, a tumor of the pancreas may cause overproduction of insulin, causing hypoglycemia; excess

Islets of Langerhans are clusters of hormone-producing cells scattered throughout the pancreas. They secrete insulin, glucagon, and gastrin.

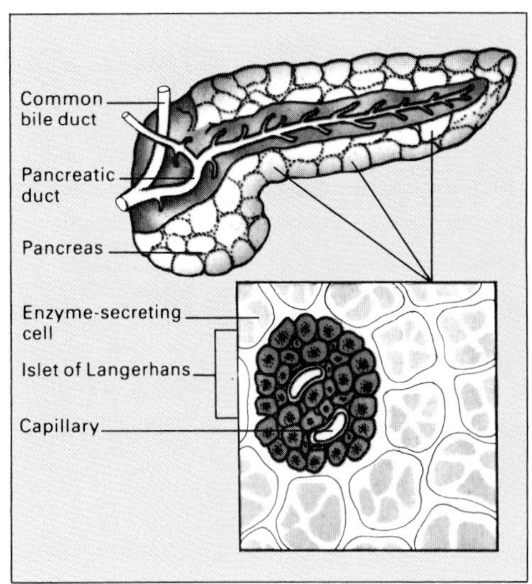

glucagon, producing hyperglycemia; or rarely, excess gastrin, causing hyperchlorhydria and a severe peptic ulcer.

See also DIABETES MELLITUS; HYPERCHLORHYDRIA; HYPERGLYCEMIA; HYPOGLYCEMIA; ULCER, PEPTIC.

Isolation (ī sə lā′shən) has various medical meanings. The most common use of the term describes the situation of a patient who is kept apart from other people to prevent the spread of an infectious disease, such as tuberculosis. A patient may also be kept in isolation during the treatment of various diseases, such as leukemia, in which the treatment itself reduces the patient's resistance to infection. In such cases, the patient is protected from being infected by visitors, rather than the other way around.

Isolation also describes the extraction and identification of bacteria or viruses that cause a particular disease.

In psychiatry, isolation is a defense mechanism in which the behavior is separated, unconsciously, from the original motive.

See also INFECTIOUS DISEASE.

Isotonic (ī sə ton′ik) describes anything, particularly muscles, that have equal tone or tension. An isotonic solution is a solution of salts in water that closely resembles the body's normal fluids in strength.

Isotope (ī′sə tōp) is any one of two or more forms of a chemical element that have the same atomic number, but different atomic weights. All isotopes of a single element have similar chemical properties. Their physical properties, however, may vary. For example, some isotopes are radioactive. Radioactive isotopes are used in the investigation and diagnosis of many disorders. They are also used in treatment, for example, to destroy cancerous tumors.

See also RADIOLOGY.

Itching, known medically as pruritus, is a symptom that is produced by a disturbance of the nerve endings just under the skin. The reasons for itching are not fully understood. Some people feel itching sensations much more easily than others, and an itching skin condition, such as measles, can cause much more distress in one patient than in another.

Q: *What conditions may cause itching?*

A: Itching may be a symptom of dry skin following sunburn or ichthyosis. There are many other skin disorders that may be accompanied by itching, including eczema, urticaria, scabies, and lichen planus. Generalized itching, which is often worse when the person is tired or warm in bed, may occur for no obvious reason. Various investigations may be carried out to discover if the cause is uremia or a liver disorder, such as jaundice or cirrhosis. Sometimes, continued itching or itching that stops and starts again is a symptom of underlying anxiety or depression. Occasionally, a malignant disease, such as Hodgkin's disease, produces itching for some years before the disease itself appears. Rarely, itching occurs during pregnancy, when it may be accompanied by urticaria. *See also* CIRRHOSIS; ECZEMA; HODGKIN'S DISEASE; ICHTHYOSIS; JAUNDICE; LICHEN PLANUS; SCABIES; UREMIA; URTICARIA.

Q: *Why do areas of itching occur?*

A: Itching in one spot may be caused by sensitivity to chemicals or materials. Examples include perfume behind the ears, nickel on jewelry, or clothing made either of wool or an artificial fiber.

Local itching around the anus (pruritus ani) may be caused by the slight, moist discharge from a hemorrhoid (piles), diarrhea, or quite commonly, an allergic reaction to anesthetic ointments used in the treatment of hemorrhoids. In children, anal itching, particularly at night, may be a sign of threadworm. *See also* HEMORRHOID; THREADWORM.

Itching of the vulva (pruritus vulvae) may occur with any form of local infection, such as vulvitis or vaginitis. It may be associated with skin infections, such as candidiasis (thrush). Genital itching is a common symptom of diabetes mellitus and may occur with leukoplakia, a condition that develops before cancerous changes in the vulva. *See also* CANDIDIASIS; DIABETES MELLITUS; LEUKOPLAKIA; VAGINITIS; VULVITIS.

Q: *How is itching treated?*

A: Areas of irritation that occur after sunburn or dry skin from any cause may be helped with soothing creams and lotions, such as calamine. If the itching persists, a physician may carry out investigations to discover the cause and prescribe the appropriate treatment.

Antihistamine and antipruritic drugs and creams may aid in controlling the symptoms. Sometimes, the physician may prescribe corticosteroid creams or ointments to be used for a short time. *See also* CORTICOSTEROID.

IUD. *See* CONTRACEPTION.

IV. *See* INTRAVENOUS.

IVP. *See* PYELOGRAM, INTRAVENOUS.

Jaundice (jôn′dis), known medically also as icterus, is a condition characterized by a yellowing of the skin and the whites of the eyes. It is a symptom, not a disease in itself. The yellow coloration is caused by an excess in the body of the bile pigment bilirubin. Normally, bilirubin is formed by the breakdown of hemoglobin during the destruction of worn-out red blood cells. It is then excreted by the liver into the bile via the bile ducts.

Q: *What causes an excess of bilirubin in the body?*

A: An excess can be caused by (1) overproduction of bilirubin; (2) the failure of the liver to metabolize bilirubin or to excrete it; or (3) a blockage of the bile ducts.

Overproduction of bilirubin may be caused by the destruction of an excessive number of red blood cells (hemolytic anemia). The liver can not, then, excrete bilirubin fast enough. This occurs in malaria, thalassemia, and hemolytic disease of the newborn.

Mild jaundice occurs as a common and normal condition in newborn babies because at birth there is both a deficiency in the enzyme that helps to excrete bilirubin and also an increased breakdown of red blood cells. In babies, the condition generally disappears within a few days as the enzyme is formed. Rarely, this enzyme deficiency can also cause jaundice in adults.

Jaundice may also result from various diseases that can affect the liver, such as hepatitis, cirrhosis, or cancer.

If the bile ducts become blocked, bile can not be excreted, and jaundice occurs. The ducts may be blocked by inflammation and infection (cholangitis); a gallstone (cholelithiasis); or cancer of the pancreas or the common bile duct. Occasionally a drug such as chlorpromazine may inhibit bilirubin excretion by the liver.

Q: *What other symptoms can occur with jaundice?*

A: Other symptoms depend on the specific cause of the jaundice. In many forms of the condition, bilirubin is excreted in the urine, which becomes dark brown in color. If the excretion of bile is obstructed, stools are almost white and the digestion of fat is impaired. If the condition has been present for some time, intense localized itching may occur due to blockage of the bile ducts.

Q: *How are the causes of jaundice diagnosed?*

A: Diagnosis requires special blood tests, in which a physician determines whether the liver is diseased; whether the bilirubin is being correctly metabolized by the liver cells; and whether there is any abnormal breakdown of the

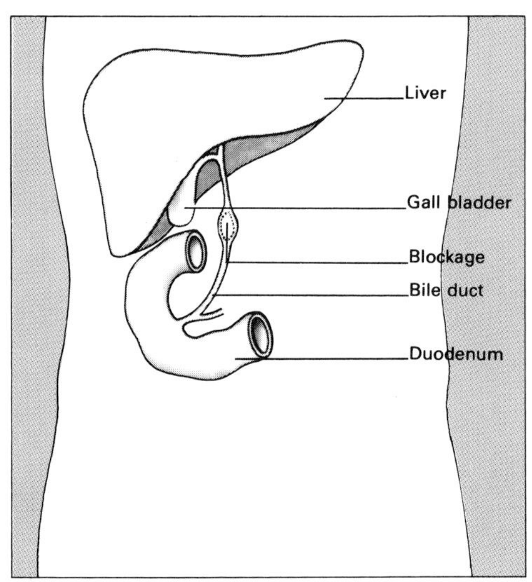

Jaundice may be caused by the failure of the liver to metabolize bilirubin or by a blockage of a bile duct.

red blood cells. The urine is examined for bilirubin, and the feces for pale coloration (which would indicate an obstruction to bile excretion). It is sometimes necessary to perform a liver biopsy to examine cells under a microscope or to examine the liver, gallbladder, and bile ducts with ultrasound to locate gallstones.

See also BILE; BILIRUBIN; CHOLANGITIS; CHOLELITHIASIS; CIRRHOSIS; HEMOLYTIC DISEASE OF THE NEWBORN; HEPATITIS; LIVER; MALARIA; THALASSEMIA.

Jaw is the name of each of the two large bones in which the teeth are embedded. Each jaw represents two bones that fuse before birth: the mandibles join in the front to form the chin; and the maxillae form most of the roof of the mouth and contain the two sinuses that open into the nose.

The upper jaw is stationary, and the lower jaw is hinged from it at small hinge joints situated in front of the ears. Powerful cheek muscles pull the lower jaw up to the upper jaw for biting. For chewing, the muscles move the lower jaw backward and forward or from side to side.

Q: *What medical problems can occur with the jaw?*

A: Because the hinge joints are small, the most common jaw problem is dislocation, resulting in the inability to close the mouth. A sudden blow is the usual cause, but dislocation may occur from yawning while leaning with the chin on one hand. Careful manipulation by a physician repositions a dislocated jaw.

Minor arthritis in a jaw joint (temporomandibular joint dysfunction) causes a clicking sensation and sometimes pain when the jaw is moved up and down.

Infection of the jaw may follow dental disorders and may cause inflammation of the nasal sinuses (sinusitis) or, rarely, inflammation of the bone (osteomyelitis).

See also JAW, BROKEN; OSTEOMYELITIS; TEMPOROMANDIBULAR JOINT DYSFUNCTION.

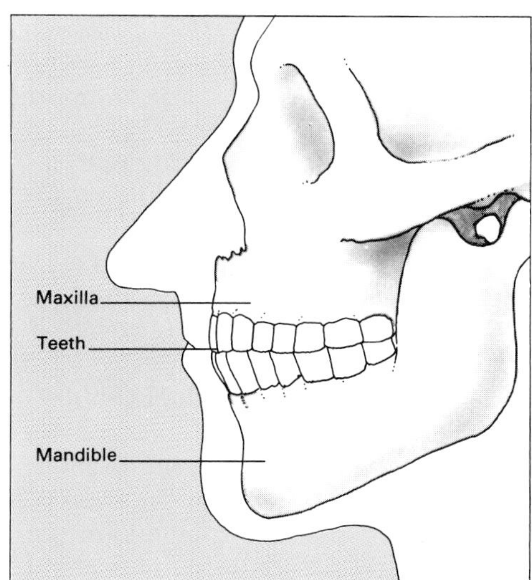

Jaw, the framework of the mouth, is formed by the maxilla and mandibular bones.

Jaw, broken. A broken jaw is a serious fracture that may require dental and maxillofacial surgery to reposition either jaw in the correct biting position. Because the upper jaw extends upward as far as the floors of the eye sockets, fractures of the maxilla may also cause a change in the position of the eye, resulting in visual problems.

Q: *How can a person eat with a fractured jaw?*

A: A person with a fractured jaw can not eat solid food. It is impossible to bite. The broken jaw is usually wired to the other jaw to reestablish the correct biting position. All food has to be sucked through a straw. Great care must be taken to ensure that choking and vomiting do not occur because a person whose jaws are wired together can not expel the vomit and may choke to death. A physician may advise the patient to carry wire cutters to use in such an emergency.

Jaw, lumpy. Lumpy jaw is a form of actinomycosis, a chronic fungus infection of the mouth, jaw, face, and neck.

See also ACTINOMYCOSIS.

Jejunum (ji jü'nəm) is part of the small intestine. It is about 4 feet (1.2m) long and connects the duodenum and the ileum. Enzymes in the small intestine continue the breakdown of food (from the stomach), which can then be absorbed through its wall into the lymphatic vessels and the hepatic portal vein. Celiac disease is a disorder of the mucous lining of the jejunum.

See also CELIAC DISEASE; INTESTINE.

Jet lag is the disorientation in the normal biological circadian rhythm, which is experienced by a person traveling from one time zone to another with more than four hours difference. The greater the time difference, the greater the degree of disorientation.

Q: *What are the symptoms of jet lag?*

A: During the time the traveler needs for his or her body to adjust to new eating and sleeping patterns, he or she may feel disoriented, tired, and "out of sync" with the new schedule, that is, sleepy during the day, awake at night, and hungry at inconvenient hours. The body temperature may also no longer be synchronized with day and night requirements.

Q: *Is it possible to prevent jet lag?*

A: The symptoms of jet lag are often made worse by overeating and by a high consumption of alcohol during the flight, which is known to cause dehydration. It is, therefore, advisable to drink plenty of nonalcoholic fluids during a long flight.

Some people believe that jet lag may be completely avoided by abstaining totally from alcohol and eating as lightly as possible during the flight, preferably on the schedule of mealtimes in the destination time zone. Additionally, a diet developed by researchers at the Argonne Research Laboratory in Illinois is thought by some travelers to help adjust the circadian rhythms prior to flying by altering the intake of food and caffeine for several days before travel. There is no medical evidence to support this; people are advised to check with their physician before following the diet, since it could have detrimental effects on certain health conditions, such as diabetes.

Q: *What is the best way to deal with jet lag?*

A: The body may take a long time to adjust to a new circadian rhythm, possibly as long as 10 days. If the stay in the new time zone is to be brief, it is often advisable not to try to adapt, but rather to retain the familiar rhythm, even at the expense of unusual hours. On a business trip this generally means that at least some working hours fall within commercial times.

A longer stay in the new time zone requires adaptation. A mild sedative, prescribed by a physician, may help to ensure proper sleep for a few nights after arrival. The body will adjust its eating habits to conform with the new sleeping pattern. *See also* CIRCADIAN RHYTHM.

Jigger. *See* CHIGGER.

Jock itch, known medically as tinea cruris, is a fungal infection of the groin, found mostly among males. The fungus flares up when the groin is kept hot, sweaty, and unaerated for a prolonged period of time. It is therefore more common during the summer months. Obesity and constrictive clothing, such as athletic supporters and tight underwear, also tend to favor the growth of the fungus.

Treatment by topical creams is usually effective. Recurrence can be minimized by wearing looser fitting clothing and by keeping the groin area dry and clean.

Joint is medically defined as an area in the body at which two bones are in contact. At a joint, the bones may be freely mobile under the control of muscles, ligaments, and tendons; they may be only slightly mobile; or they may be fixed so as to be immobile.

Q: *What are mobile joints?*

A: At a typical mobile joint, the ends of the bones are covered with tough cartilage and lined with a membrane (the synovial membrane) containing a small amount of lubricating fluid. The joint has stabilizing ligaments that limit the directions and the extent to which the bones can be moved.

Q: *Are there different kinds of mobile joints?*

A: Yes, there are several different kinds. A hinge joint acts like a hinge; examples include the elbow and the knee. A ball-and-socket joint, in which the rounded end of one bone fits inside a concave socket of the other, allows good rotation; examples are the shoulder and the hip. A saddle joint allows sliding movement in two directions; the base joint of the thumb is a saddle joint. A plane joint permits only slight sliding movement, as in the wrist bones. An ellipsoid joint allows circular and bending movements but no rotation, as in the wrist bones. A pivot joint, al-

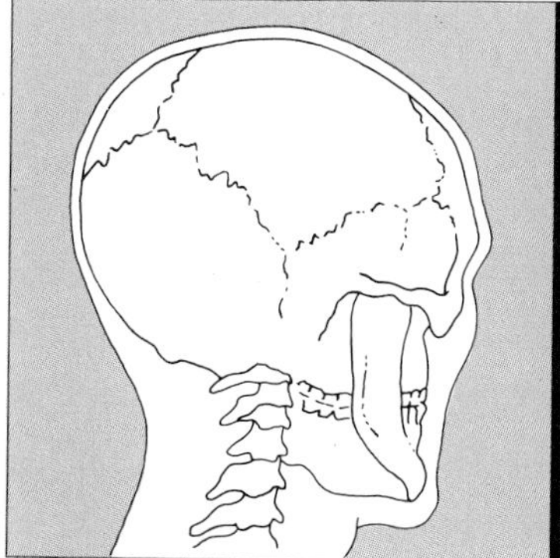
Fixed joints, such as those between the bones of the skull, permit no movement.

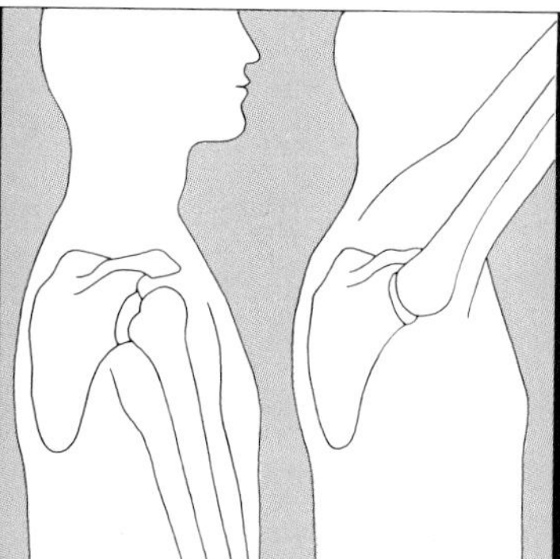
Ball-and-socket joints, like the shoulder, provide swinging and rotating movements.

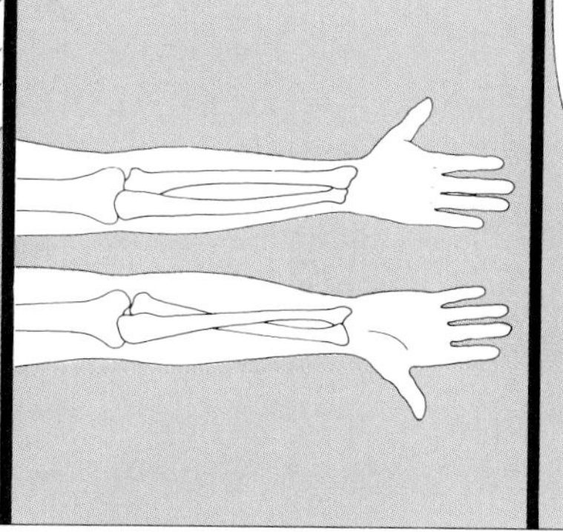
Pivot joints, such as those found in the elbow, permit a rotating kind of movement.

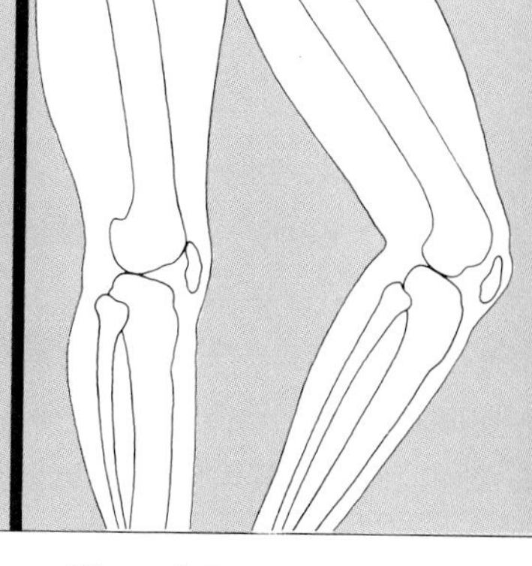
Hinge joints, such as the knee, allow backward and forward movements.

lowing rotation, is found between the two top vertebrae of the neck. A mobile joint may be capable of two types of joint movement. For instance, the elbow is both a hinge joint and a pivot joint.

Q: *What are slightly mobile joints?*

A: At a typical slightly mobile joint, the bones have a layer of cartilage between them and are held firmly together by strong ligaments. Such joints are found between the pubic bones (symphysis pubis) and the disks between the vertebrae of the spine.

Q: *What are immobile joints?*

A: Immobile joints occur where two bones are fused or fixed together before or shortly after birth. Examples are the ilium, pubis, and ischium, which together form the hipbone, and the many flat bones that combine to make up the skull.

Joint, Charcot's (shar′koz). Charcot's joint, also known as neuropathic joint disease, is an illness of one or more joints, caused by underlying neurological disorders. It is characterized by gradual degeneration of the affected joint, resulting in instability of the joint, swelling, internal bleeding, and bone atrophy.

Early diagnosis of the disease and protection of the affected joint may help prevent or reduce further damage; surgical reconstruction is of limited help, and complete recovery is rare. Amputation of the affected joint may become necessary.

The disease is named after Jean Martin Charcot, the French neurologist, a pioneer in the field in the late 19th century.

Joint disorders. There are many conditions that may involve joints: degenerative conditions, such as osteoarthritis; inflammatory conditions, such as rheumatoid arthritis; conditions involving the membranes surrounding the joints, such as synovitis; generalized disorders involving the joints, such as gout; damage to the joint involving dislocation or complicated fracture; and congenital disorders, including congenital dislocation of the hip and clubfoot.

Each of the following joint disorders has a separate article in this encyclopedia:

ankylosis	osteoarthritis
arthritis	osteochondritis
arthritis, rheumatoid	Perthes' disease
	polyarthritis
arthrodesis	rheumatic fever
bursitis	shoulder, frozen
capsulitis	spondylitis
clubfoot	spondylitis, ankylosing
disk, herniated	spondylolisthesis
dislocation	spondylosis
gout	spondylosis, cervical
hammertoe	subluxation
osteoarthropathy	synovitis

Jugular vein is any one of the four large veins in the head and neck that return blood to the heart.

See also VEIN.

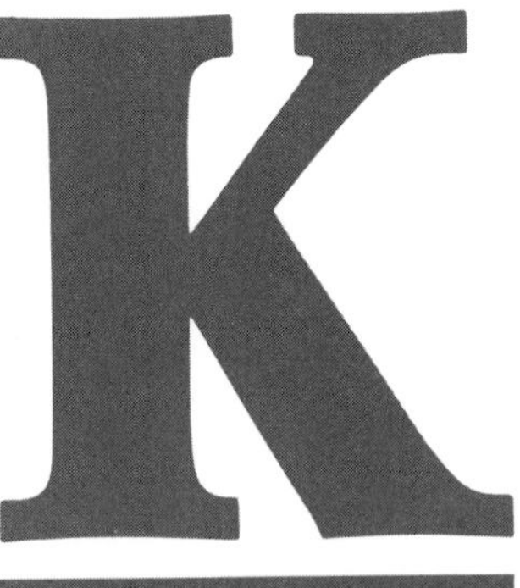

Kala-azar (kä lä ä zär′), also known as dumdum fever and Assam fever, is an infection of the liver and spleen. Occurring in tropical and subtropical regions, it is caused by a protozoan transmitted by the bite of the sand fly. Medical attention is imperative, as the condition can be fatal if left untreated.

Kaolin (kā′ə lin), or china clay, is a naturally occurring form of aluminum silicate, used medically in many antidiarrheal remedies. It has absorbent properties.

Kaposi's sarcoma (kap′ō sēz sär kō′mə) is a malignant tumor, which usually begins as soft, purplish, raised lesions on the feet and spreads through the lymphatic system. Before 1980, this tumor was seen only in elderly Italian or Jewish men or in younger people from equatorial Africa. It was a relatively rare disease. Now, however, a specific, more severe form of Kaposi's sarcoma (KS), associated with Acquired Immune Deficiency Syndrome (AIDS), has reached epidemic proportions in the United States and several other countries.

The treatment for the milder form of KS is electron beam radiotherapy, while deeper lesions are treated using X-ray therapy.

The more severe type of KS is sometimes treated with antimicrobial drugs and other forms of treatment to help restore the immune system within the cells.

See also ACQUIRED IMMUNE DEFICIENCY SYNDROME.

Keloid (kē′loid) is a mass of excessive fibrous tissue that develops at the site of a scar. Black people are more likely to form keloids than are people of other races.

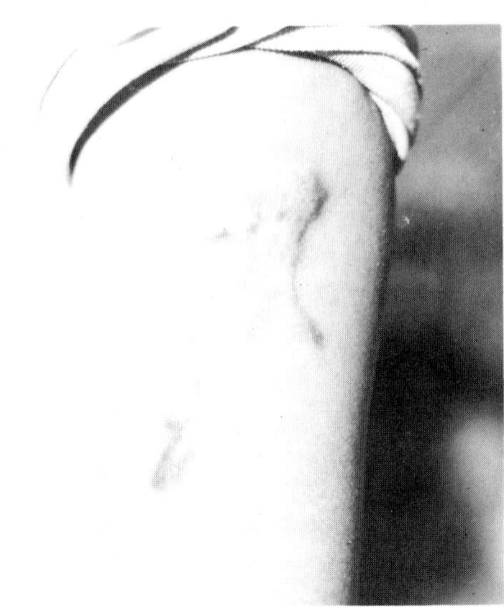

A **keloid** scar may develop when the body's healing process overresponds to an injury.

Keratin (ker′ə tin) is the tough, insoluble protein found in the outer layer of the epidermis (skin). It is the element that makes skin almost completely waterproof. In places where the skin is exposed to continuous rubbing and pressure, for example, on the hands and feet, the number of keratin cells increases and a callus results. It is also the primary component of nails, hair, and tooth enamel.

See also SKIN.

Keratitis (ker ə ti′tis) is an inflammation of the cornea, the transparent membrane that forms the front of the eye. If the condition occurs suddenly, it causes pain, sensitivity to light (photophobia), and watering of the eye. If keratitis develops gradually, only minor discomfort may result. Opaque patches in the cornea can cause the patient's vision to blur.

Q: *What causes keratitis?*

A: Keratitis is often a symptom of a more general disorder. Virus infections, such as trachoma (chronic conjunctivitis) or herpes simplex, may infect the cornea. Bacterial infection may follow any eye wound.

Keratitis is also a consequence of congenital syphilis or, rarely, tuberculosis. It most often occurs in children between the ages of 5 and 15. A deficiency of vitamin A causes dryness of the cornea, which makes it more susceptible to infection.

Q: *How is keratitis treated?*

A: Further damage to the cornea can be prevented with eye drops, containing the drug atropine, to dilate the pupil. Corticosteroid drugs reduce the inflammation. It is essential for the eyes to be examined by an ophthalmologist.

See also COLD SORE; TRACHOMA.

Keratosis. *See* SUNBURN.

Kernicterus (ker nik′ter əs) is a serious form of jaundice in the newborn, in which brain damage is caused by deposits of bilirubin in the brain. The most common cause of such severe jaundice is hemolytic disease of the newborn.

See also HEMOLYTIC DISEASE OF THE NEWBORN.

Kernig's sign (ker′nigz) may be seen as a result of a neurological test in which the patient lies flat on the back with one knee drawn up. The physician then tries to straighten the leg. If the patient unconsciously resists, it may indicate irritation of a nerve where it passes out of the spine, as may occur with meningitis.

See also MENINGITIS.

Ketoacidosis, diabetic (ke to ä si do′sis). Diabetic ketoacidosis is an acute diabetic condition characterized by electrolyte imbalance, extremely high blood sugar levels, low blood volume circulation, acidosis, and frequently coma.

See also ACIDOSIS; DIABETES MELLITUS.

Ketone (kē′ton) is a substance formed by the body during the breakdown of fats and fatty acids into carbon dioxide and water. Acetone is an example of a ketone.

Excessive amounts of ketones are formed when fat is used, instead of sugar, for providing energy. This condition, called ketosis, occurs during starvation and, sometimes, during high fevers when large amounts of heat energy are generated. It may also happen in diabetes mellitus, when the body has difficulty using sugar normally.

Ketosis. *See* KETONE.

Kidney is one of a pair of organs located at the back of the abdomen, against the strong muscles next to the spine, and behind the intestines and other organs. The adrenal glands lie on top of the kidneys.

Each kidney weighs about 5 ounces (140g) and is about 4 inches (10cm) long in the average adult. Its inner structure, which is called the renal pelvis, collects urine as it is formed and passes it out of the kidney to the bladder via the ureter. The renal pelvis also is connected to the artery and vein that carry blood to and from the kidney.

Q: *What is the function of the kidneys?*

A: The kidneys filter out water and also unwanted substances in the blood. These substances are produced by the normal working of the body. They are excreted by the kidneys in the form of urine. The kidneys also keep the salts and water of the body in correct balance.

Q: *How do the kidneys work?*

A: Blood passes through each kidney under high pressure. The blood is filtered by the glomeruli, special structures in the kidney containing clusters of capillaries that collect water, salts, and unwanted substances. The filtrate passes along a fine tube, the nephron (of which there are approximately one million in each kidney), which reabsorbs any of the water, glucose, and salts that the body still requires and allows the rest to pass into the pelvis of the kidney as urine. *See also* GLOMERULUS; NEPHRON.

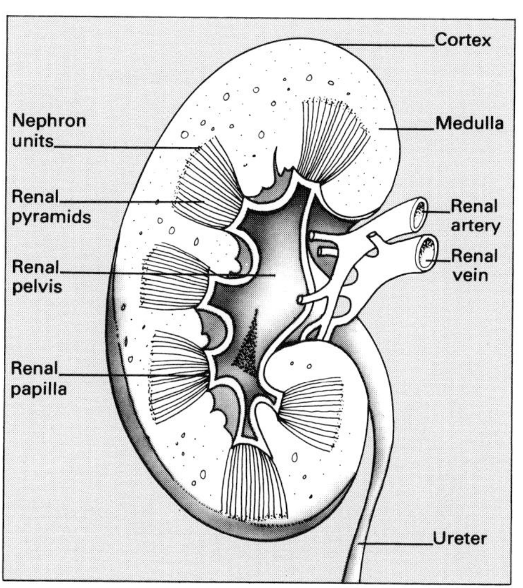

The **kidney** filters body fluids within the nephron units and expels wastes via the ureter.

Kidney, artificial. Artificial kidney is a machine that takes over the function of the natural kidneys when they are damaged by disease and can not clean the blood of toxic substances. The poisonous substances produce uremia, a serious condition that, if left untreated, leads to death.

See also KIDNEY DIALYSIS; UREMIA.

Kidney dialysis (dī al′ə sis), known medically as hemodialysis, is a method of filtering unwanted substances from the blood using a machine that acts as an artificial kidney. It is used for patients whose own kidneys are damaged or malfunctioning.

Q: *How does a kidney dialysis machine work?*

A: Blood from an artery passes into the dialysis machine and over a thin sheet of membrane that acts as a filter for unwanted substances. The purified blood is then fed back into one of the patient's veins.

A variety of machines are available, some of which are small and safe enough to be used by the patient at home. The most modern machine is portable.

Q: *Are there any problems in using such a machine?*

A: Yes. Many of the problems are associated with maintaining sterility, but most of these have been overcome by the use of machines with disposable parts. It can be difficult to find suitable veins and arteries in the patient, but it is now possible to implant a small plastic tube (called a shunt) in the blood vessels, which can then be connected to the machine.

Q: *How often should dialysis be performed?*

A: It usually is necessary to perform dialysis three times a week, for periods of four to six hours, either in a hospital, at a special dialysis center set up for the purpose, or at the patient's home.

Q: *When may dialysis be used?*

A: Dialysis is used to treat acute or chronic kidney failure. In acute renal failure, dialysis continues until the kidneys recover their normal function. In chronic renal failure, dialysis continues either for the rest of the patient's life or until a kidney transplant is performed.

See also KIDNEY; KIDNEY DISEASE; TRANSPLANT SURGERY.

Q: *Can dialysis be carried out without the use of a machine?*

A: Yes. Peritoneal dialysis does not require a machine. It is performed by inserting a sterile plastic catheter into the abdominal cavity and irrigating the peritoneum. Metabolic substances are drawn out of the capillaries of the peritoneum and irrigated out of the cavity.

Kidney disease. The body depends on the kidneys to excrete many waste products and to maintain the correct balance of water and salts. Any kidney disorder interferes with these important functions.

Q: *What are the symptoms of kidney disease?*

A: The symptoms of kidney disease depend on the underlying cause. They are often mild and vague until a late stage in the disease. Kidney disease may cause an increased amount of urine to be formed, leading to abnormally high urine output (polyuria). The formation of urine may also be diminished, leading to abnormally low urine output (oliguria).

Some kidney diseases, such as acute nephritis, may cause blood in the urine (hematuria). Other symptoms of kidney disease include acute abdominal pain (colic) and generalized edema, which is swelling due to the accumulation of water in the body tissues.

If both kidneys stop working completely, waste products accumulate in the body and poison the patient. This can be fatal and requires urgent medical attention.

Q: *What causes kidney disease?*

A: Kidney disease may be caused by many factors, such as injury, infection, cancer, or disorders in other parts of the body. In some cases, kidney disease may occur without apparent cause.

The kidney may be damaged in a serious accident, causing a rupture of its surrounding capsule and leading to severe hemorrhage. The damaged kidney may have to be surgically removed (nephrectomy). Rarely, the kidney may be damaged by radiotherapy treatment carried out for cancer. This may eventually result in high blood pressure and kidney failure.

Stones may form in the kidneys (nephrolithiasis) and cause kidney damage. This may occur without apparent cause, or it may be due to an underlying metabolic disorder. Occasionally, microscopic crystals form in the kidney tissue itself (nephrocalcinosis). These may occur for the same reasons as do stones. Rarely, babies who are given excessive amounts of vitamin D develop nephrocalcinosis.

The kidney may become infected and inflamed. This may result in various kidney diseases, such as nephritis, glomerulonephritis, or pyelonephritis. Infection of the kidneys often results from the spread of infection from the bladder.

Cancer of the kidney may occur in the renal pelvis, the collecting area for urine, or in the body of the kidney itself (hypernephroma). The latter is most common in adults, but a nephroblastoma (Wilms' tumor) may occur in young children.

Many disorders in other parts of the body have an effect on the kidney. High blood pressure gradually damages the kidneys. Because of such damage, high blood pressure often continues to be a problem after the original cause has been found and treated. Various hormone disorders, such as parathyroid gland hyperactivity, Cushing's syndrome, and hyperthyroidism, affect kidney function. Diabetes mellitus not only causes sugar in the urine (glycosuria) but may eventually cause damage to the glomeruli or to the blood supply to the kidney. A stone in the ureter may cause urinary obstruction. This may result in reverse pressure of the urine into the kidney, producing distention and progressive loss of function (hydronephrosis).

Q: *What tests are carried out to diagnose kidney disease?*

A: Suspected kidney disease can be investigated in various ways. Chemical testing of the urine detects the presence of any abnormal substances, such as protein (proteinuria), sugar (glycosuria), or hemoglobin (hemoglobinuria). The concentration of salts and urea also can be determined. Examination of urine through a microscope may detect blood (hematuria) or white blood cells resulting from infection. Tests that measure the amount of urea and creatinine (two waste products that should be excreted by the kidney) in the blood help detect kidney disease.

The kidneys may also be tested using either an intravenous pyelogram (IVP), a form of X ray, or a retrograde pyelogram. Both procedures outline the urine-collecting system and help to detect abnormalities of kidney size and shape.

An arteriogram shows the blood supply to the kidney; and occasionally a renogram, using radioactive iodine, is carried out.

Finally, if the diagnosis is still in doubt, a renal biopsy may be performed, using a long needle to obtain a small sample of kidney tissue for examination with a microscope. *See also* ARTERIOGRAM; PYELOGRAM, INTRAVENOUS.

Q: *How are kidney diseases treated?*

A: The treatment of kidney diseases depends on their cause and may involve the skilled care of a nephrologist, a specialist in kidney diseases.

See also CALCULUS; CUSHING'S SYNDROME; DIABETES MELLITUS; GLOMERULONEPHRITIS; GLYCOSURIA; HEMATURIA; HEMOGLOBINURIA; HYDRONEPHROSIS; NEPHRITIS; NEPHROLITHIASIS; NEPHROTIC

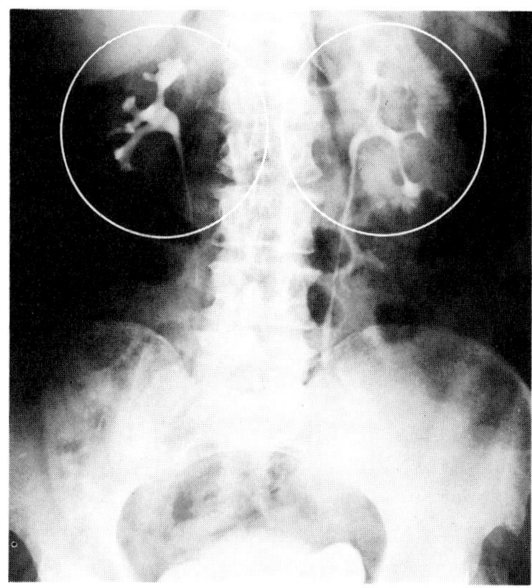

Kidney disease may be detected with an intravenous pyelogram, a form of X ray.

SYNDROME; NOCTURIA; OLIGURIA; POLYURIA; PROTEINURIA; PYELONEPHRITIS; UREMIA.

Kidney stone. *See* CALCULUS.

Kleptomania (klep tə mā'nē ə) is a compulsive and uncontrollable desire to steal. The stolen objects are not used for their monetary value as there is no criminal intent when they are taken; in fact, they often have little intrinsic value.

This psychiatric disorder is characterized by a build-up of tension as the impulse to steal strengthens, followed by feelings of release of tension and gratification after the act of stealing is completed. Stealing is not preplanned, and little thought is given to the legal consequences of being apprehended. Often, the stealing continues in an obvious manner until the patient is caught in the act. This may reflect an unconscious desire to be caught and to receive appropriate treatment.

This disorder typically starts in childhood or adolescence and can become chronic in nature. Depression and anxiety may be associated features of the disorder.

Klinefelter's syndrome (klīn'fel tərz) is a genetic disease seen in males, caused by the presence of one or more extra X (female sex) chromosomes. It is not true hermaphroditism. It is not usually diagnosed until after puberty, at which time the male breasts may become enlarged and the testicles remain unusually small. Varying degrees of mental retardation may also be present. There is no specific treatment.

See also HERMAPHRODITE; INTERSEX.

Knee is the hinge joint between the lower end of the thigh bone (femur) and the upper end of the shin bone (tibia). The front of the knee is covered by the lower tendon of the quadriceps femoris, a massive group of muscles that extend to the top of the thigh. The broad tendon that attaches this muscle to the front of the tibia contains the patella (kneecap). The patella forms a protective shield in front of the knee joint, behind which pass the main artery, vein, and nerve of the leg.

There are strong ligaments on each side of the knee that prevent its dislocation outward or inward. Inside the joint are two ligaments (cruciate ligaments) that protect the joint from dislocation forward or backward. There are also two semilunar cartilages attached to the outer edges of the internal surface of the joint, on top of the tibia.

When the leg is extended to straighten it at the knee, the bones work together so that they lock into a rigid structure.

See also KNEE DISORDERS.

Kneecap. *See* PATELLA.

Knee disorders. The knee is a complex joint capable of a large range of movements, and it has to support the full weight of the body. For this reason, it is particularly vulnerable to injury, degenerative changes, and joint disorders. With increasing age, degeneration of the knee joint through osteoarthritis becomes more likely. It occurs particularly in those who are overweight or who have a previous history of knee injury. Water on the knee (housemaid's knee) occurs particularly in persons who have to kneel frequently or continually while working.

Damage to the semilunar cartilage within the knee joint is a common occurrence that often results from excessive rotation when "locking" the leg straight. Sometimes the cartilage lining the knee degenerates (osteochondritis), and a fragment breaks off inside the joint. This causes pain, further damage, and a tendency for the knee to lock in the wrong position when not fully extended.

Occasionally, the quadriceps muscle (which passes over the knee) ruptures and causes an unstable knee joint. This condition is usually associated with a sudden strain, but sometimes there is little obvious reason. This is particularly likely to happen in the elderly.

See also BOWLEGS; BURSITIS; JOINT DISORDERS; KNEE; KNOCK-KNEE; MENISCUS; OSTEOCHONDRITIS; PATELLA.

Knee fracture: first aid. *See* FRACTURE: FIRST AID.

Knee jerk may be seen as the result of a neurological test in which the tendon of the large muscle in front of the thigh (quadriceps femoris) is tapped with a small hammer just below the kneecap (patella). This produces an involuntary kicking movement of the leg. The manner and speed with which the reaction takes place help a physician to diagnose certain neurological disorders.

See also REFLEX.

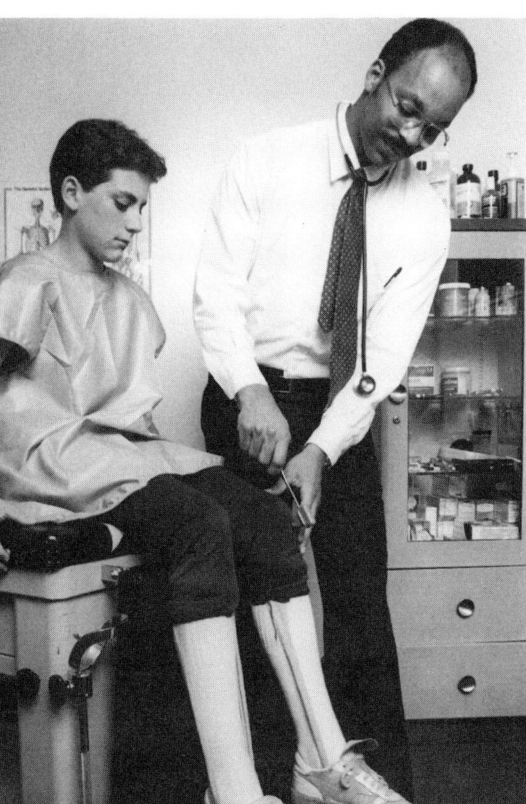

Knee jerk is a reflex reaction that is triggered by tapping the kneecap (patella) with a small hammer.

Knee, water on. Water on the knee is a form of bursitis.

See also BURSITIS.

Knock-knee, known medically as genu valgum, is a disorder in which the lower legs are curved outward so that the knees touch each other and the ankles are apart. This condition commonly occurs in childhood as a normal stage of development between the ages of about two-and-one-half and four years. As the child continues to grow, the legs gradually straighten.

Koilonychia (koi lō nik'ē ə) is a deformity of the nails. The nail becomes thin, and the normal curve of the outer surface is reversed, giving the nail a spoon-shaped appearance. This uncommon condition may occur in patients with iron-deficiency anemia.

See also ANEMIA.

Koplik's spots (kop'liks) are tiny red spots with white centers that appear on the palate, inside the cheeks, and on the tongue; they may also occur on the internal surface of the eyelids. They are the precursor of measles.

See also MEASLES.

Korsakoff's syndrome (kôr sak'ofs) is a form of mental illness. It is commonly found in brain-damaged patients suffering from alcoholism, but it may also accompany other forms of brain damage, for example, cerebral tumors, head injuries, and minor strokes.

Q: *What are the symptoms of Korsakoff's syndrome?*

A: The patient is unable to remember recent events and tends to invent plausible accounts of what he or she has been doing during the past few days or weeks. This is called "confabulation" and is a typical symptom of this syndrome. The patient will pretend to remember, and be oriented to, present situations; he or she will sometimes present elaborate responses that may sound detailed and reasonable, but which are entirely made up. Frequently, the patient may not know the day, date, season of the year, or his or her place of residence.

Q: *What is the treatment of Korsakoff's syndrome?*

A: The treatment depends on the cause. Alcoholism should be treated appropriately. Large amounts of B vitamins often produce a slow improvement.

See also ALCOHOLISM.

Küntscher nail (kint'shər) is a tubular metal nail that is inserted into the center of a bone in the treatment of a fracture. This technique is used most frequently in treatment of a broken femur or hipbone.

Kuru (kůr'ü) is a rare, slow virus of the central nervous system, affecting New Guinea natives. It produces a rapidly progressive destruction of neurologic function and is usually fatal. It is transmitted by cannibalism, specifically by eating the brains of affected corpses.

See also VIRUS, SLOW.

Kwashiorkor (kwä'shē ôr kôr) is a form of severe malnutrition in children. There is a characteristic loss of pigmentation of the hair, giving it a reddish-brown appearance. The children have dry, scaling, pale skin, as well as a protuberant abdomen, and they fail to grow normally. There is often also swelling (edema) of the feet and legs. Severe cases may lead to extreme emaciation.

Kwell® (kwel) is the trade-name for lindane of gamma benzene hexachloride, which is used to treat infestation by the itch mite (scabies) and lice. It is used topically as a shampoo, cream, or lotion.

Kyphosis (kī fō′sis) is either an excessive curvature of the spine, such as that of a "hunchback," or a more gradual, but still abnormal, curvature. It commonly affects the spine behind the chest, but may affect the lower or upper spine, if there is an excessive amount of bending forward.

It is frequently associated with scoliosis (sideways curvature of the spine) and with bone disorders that affect the vertebrae—osteoporosis in the elderly, ankylosing spondylitis, and a form of osteochondritis that affects the bones of the spine.

See also LORDOSIS; OSTEOPOROSIS; SCOLIOSIS.

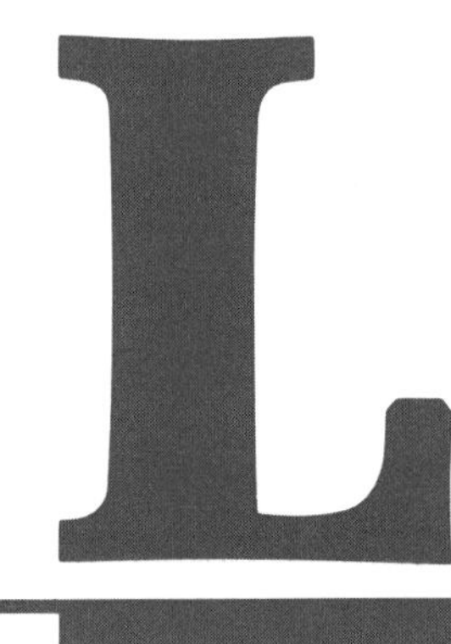

Labial (lā'bē əl) describes anything pertaining to the lips, either of the mouth or vulva.

See also LABIA MAJORA; LABIA MINORA.

Labia majora (lā'bē ə mə jôr'ə) are the two long outer folds of skin, one on each side of the vaginal opening.

See also LABIA MINORA.

Labia minora (lā'bē ə mi nor'ə) are the two inner folds of skin at the vaginal opening. They extend between the clitoris and the labia majora, the folds of skin that rim the vaginal opening.

See also LABIA MAJORA.

Labium (lā'bē əm) is the fleshy border or edge of a body structure. The term is used to describe the thick edge of a bone, the cervix (neck) of the uterus, one of the lips of the mouth, or the folds of skin surrounding the vaginal opening.

See also VULVA.

Labor is the process of childbirth by which the baby and placenta (afterbirth) are delivered. During labor, the woman's uterus contracts regularly, dilating the cervix and moving the fetus and placenta along the birth canal toward the vaginal opening.

See also PREGNANCY AND CHILDBIRTH.

Labor pain, false. False labor pains are abdominal pains that make a pregnant woman think that labor is beginning when in fact it is not. A woman's uterus normally contracts at irregular intervals throughout pregnancy. These contractions, which are termed Braxton Hicks contractions, gradually increase in frequency, intensity, and duration throughout pregnancy. Near the completion of the pregnancy, these Braxton Hicks contractions are frequently mistaken for true labor contractions.

See also PREGNANCY AND CHILDBIRTH.

Labyrinth (lab'ə rinth) is the network of fluid-filled passages in the inner ear. This network consists of three semicircular canals at right angles to each other. The labyrinth system transmits information about the position of the head to the brain. This information assists the brain in maintaining balance and equilibrium.

See also EAR.

Labyrinthitis (lab ə rin thī' tis) is an infection of the labyrinthine canals in the inner ear. It is accompanied by extreme dizziness and vomiting and often causes total hearing loss.

A bacterial infection may spread to the inner ear from a middle ear infection (otitis media); may occur with meningitis; or may follow an ear operation. The disorder requires immediate medical treatment.

See also LABYRINTH.

Laceration (las ə rā'shən) is a tear in any tissue in the body; it may be external or internal. A lacerated wound is often caused by a cut from a sharp object, such as a knife.

See also BLEEDING: FIRST AID.

Lacrimal apparatus (lak'rə məl ap ə rā'təs) is the anatomical name for the structures in each eye that produce and drain tears. The lacrimal gland lies in a notch in the upper, outer corner of the bony eye socket. The tears it secretes are carried in 12 small ducts to the sur-

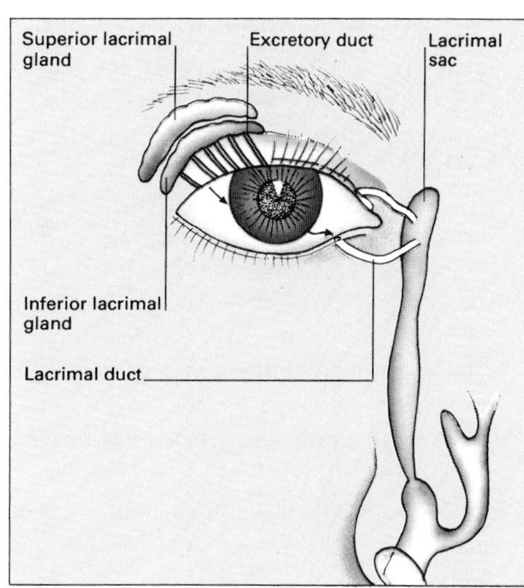

The **lacrimal apparatus** are the structures around the eyes from which tears are secreted.

face of the eyeball. They are washed across the eye by the action of blinking. Two ducts at the inner corner of the eye drain the tears into the lacrimal sac and then to the back of the nose.

See also EYE.

Lacrimal gland (lak′rə məl) is either of the two glands, one above each eye, that produce tears.

Lacrimation (lak rə mā′shən) is the medical term for the production of tears by the lacrimal gland of the eye.

See also LACRIMAL APPARATUS.

Lactation (lak tā′shən) is the process of secretion of milk from the female breast, which is used to nourish an infant. Lactation begins with the birth of the child and is controlled by a complex interaction between various hormones in the mother's bloodstream. The period of lactation is the length of time for which nursing of the child continues.

Q: *What makes the breasts start producing milk at the end of pregnancy?*

A: Throughout pregnancy, the breasts develop and increase in size in response to increased levels of the hormones estrogen, progesterone, and chorionic gonadotrophin (the chorion is the membrane that encloses the fetus). These hormones are produced by the placenta, the organ of chemical interchange between mother and fetus. The increase in breast size is caused partly by the larger number of ducts that form in the breast and partly by an increase in the amount of fatty tissue.

Milk is not formed until after the baby is born. Milk production is stimulated by the hormone prolactin produced by the pituitary gland at the base of the brain, which in turn is stimulated by changes that take place at the onset of labor.

Colostrum, a fluid rich in fat and proteins, is secreted near the end of pregnancy and for the first few days of the infant's life. It contains antibodies from the mother that help to protect the baby against disease. As soon as the baby is born, the mother's hormone levels drop rapidly, prolactin secretion starts, and milk is produced.

See also COLOSTRUM; PROLACTIN.

Q: *Why does milk secretion sometimes occur before the baby starts sucking?*

A: The contraction of the breast tissue to expel milk is partly a "let down" reflex to the baby's sucking and partly a response to the presence of the hormone oxytocin (also secreted by the pituitary gland). This hormone may be produced in response to the mother's emotional reaction when she hears the baby crying. Oxytocin also causes contraction of the uterus, and this accounts for an increase in vaginal flow when breast-feeding takes place.

Q: *How may lactation be stopped?*

A: If the woman does not want to breast-feed, fluid intake may be restricted and a tight brassiere worn to decrease milk production. Occasionally, hormones are administered to suppress lactation.

Sudden cessation of lactation may result in considerable breast engorgement and tenderness for the mother. When the infant is to be weaned, a gradual process of discontinuing breast-feeding is easier for both the infant and the mother.

Q: *Are there any dangers in using estrogens to stop lactation?*

A: Yes. An increased intake of estrogens may lead to a type of blood clot called venous thrombosis. Gastrointestinal problems may also result from the use of estrogens. Risks are greater in women over the age of 35, those who smoke, or those who have had an operation, such as a Cesarean section. *See also* THROMBOSIS, VENOUS.

Q: *Can anything be done if lactation does not begin?*

A: Frequent nursing of the infant, adequate food and fluid intake, adequate rest for the mother, and emotional support from other family members are all very helpful in successful lactation. Occasionally, medication may be needed to help the mother "let down" the milk.

Q: *Are there any problems that may occur during lactation?*

A: Yes. Lactation may gradually fail due to a combination of the mother's fatigue and an improper diet. To counter this, the mother needs additional calcium in her diet to offset the calcium secreted in the milk. The mother should also have an adequate intake of fluids and sufficient rest.

Other problems include sore nipples, engorgement of the breasts, failure to produce sufficient milk, or mastitis (inflammation of the breasts). Infection of the breast ducts usually results from a cracked nipple. With a breast infection, part of the breast becomes tender, swollen, and inflamed, and a sudden fever occurs, often starting with a shivering attack. A physician may prescribe antibiotics and painkilling drugs. If possible, breast-feeding should continue because this empties the affected area.

Lactic acid (lak′tic) is a colorless substance produced by the fermenting action of bacteria on milk or milk sugar (lactose). It occurs in sour milk and certain other foods. It is also produced during the metabolism of glucose and fat in the human body. Lactic acid levels may increase in severe liver disease and other disorders, leading to a serious condition known as lactic acidosis.

See also ACIDOSIS.

Lactose (lak′tōs) is a sugar found in milk. In the human digestive system, it is broken down into simpler substances by an enzyme (lactase) in the small intestine. Some people have an intolerance to lactose and are unable to digest it. They may experience bloating, abdominal discomfort, or diarrhea. These people must restrict, or eliminate, their intake of milk and other dairy products that contain lactose.

Lactase enzyme solutions may be added to milk to predigest the lactose. The treated milk may then be consumed by lactose-intolerant individuals.

Lameness is a condition in which a person is unable to properly use an arm or leg due to an injury or disease. The term usually refers to a permanent disability.

See also CLAUDICATION.

Laminectomy (lam ə nek′tə mē) is an operation in which a plate of bone (lamina) is surgically removed from the back of one or more vertebrae to expose the spinal cord. It is performed during any operation on the spinal cord. A laminectomy is often used to relieve pressure on a herniated vertebral disk.

Lance is a double-edged surgical knife. The term is also used to describe a minor surgical operation in which a lance is used to open and drain an abscess or boil.

Langerhans' islands. See ISLETS OF LANGERHANS.

Lanolin (lan′ə lin) is a pale, yellow, fatty substance obtained from the grease of sheep's wool. It is used in various skin preparations because it mixes with oils and with water to produce ointments that penetrate the skin. Some individuals are allergic to skin preparations containing lanolin.

Lanugo (lə nü′gō) is the fine, downy hair that covers a fetus. It begins to form in the fifth month of pregnancy and is usually shed by the ninth month. Lanugo may be visible on some premature babies.

Laparoscopic sterilization. See STERILIZATION, LAPAROSCOPIC.

Laparoscopy (lap ə ros′kə pē) is an examination of the interior of the abdomen with a lighted tube called a laparoscope. Laparoscopy is also known as peritoneoscopy.

Q: *How and why is laparoscopy performed?*

A: The examination can be carried out under local or general anesthesia. A small incision is made, usually next to the navel; the laparoscope is then passed through the peritoneum, the membranous sac

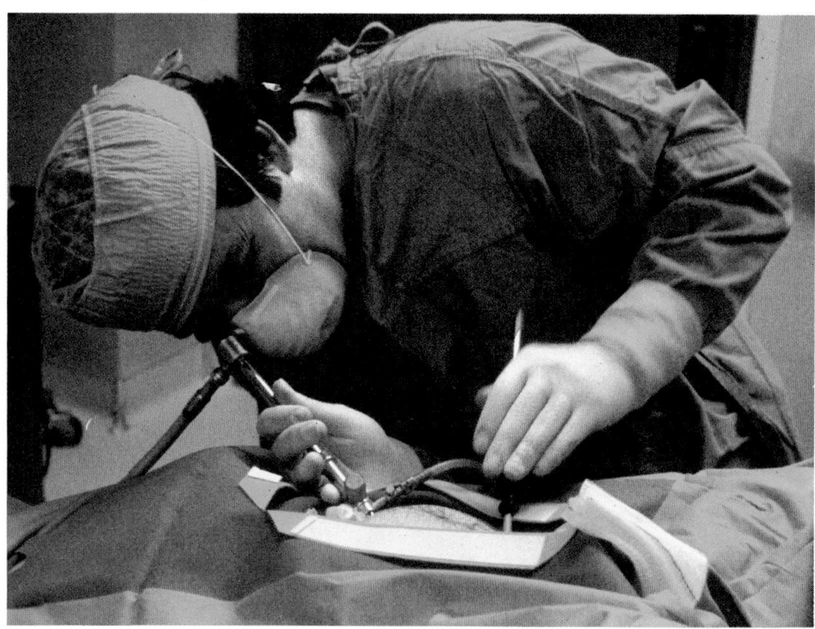

Laparoscopy is a surgical technique in which a lighted tube (laparoscope) is used to illuminate and explore the abdomen interior.

that lines the abdominal cavity. Carbon dioxide or nitrous oxide gas is passed into the peritoneal cavity through a needle to swell the abdomen and make it possible to examine the organs, such as the liver, intestine, bladder, uterus, or ovaries.

Certain kinds of cancer and cysts of the ovary can be diagnosed using this technique.

Q: *Can any surgical operations be performed with a laparoscope?*

A: Yes. A surgeon can take a small piece of tissue for microscopic examination (biopsy) or perform a sterilization operation in a woman.

See *also* STERILIZATION, LAPAROSCOPIC.

Laparotomy (lap ə rot′ə mē) is a surgical incision into the abdominal wall. The operation may be performed to explore the internal organs (exploratory laparotomy) or as a procedure preliminary to further surgery.

Large intestine. See INTESTINE, LARGE; COLON.

Laryngectomy (lar ən jek′tə mē) is an operation to remove the voice box (larynx), usually performed in the treatment of cancer. An opening is made in the windpipe (tracheotomy) so that the patient can breathe. Many of the nearby lymph glands are removed at the same time as the larynx if they are malignant.

Q: *Can a patient with a laryngectomy talk?*

A: Not immediately, and never normally as before. A patient with no larynx can, however, learn esophageal speech, in which sounds are produced from the esophagus, or learn to use an artificial larynx.

See *also* LARYNX; SPEECH, ESOPHAGEAL.

Laryngitis (lar ən jī′tis) is an inflammation of the tissues of the larynx (voice box and vocal cords). It may be acute or chronic.

Q: *What causes acute laryngitis?*

A: Any viral respiratory infection, such as the common cold or influenza, or an infection of the back of the throat, such as tonsillitis or pharyngitis, can cause acute laryngitis. Diphtheria used to be a common cause of laryngitis, but is now extremely rare in Western countries because of childhood immunization.

Overuse of the voice, heavy smoking, and alcoholism all tend to produce a hoarse voice made rapidly worse by any minor infection.

Q: *What are the symptoms of acute laryngitis?*

A: The voice is husky and sometimes disappears completely (aphonia). Talking may cause pain in the throat.

Q: *What is the treatment for acute laryngitis?*

A: It is essential to attempt to stop talking for at least 48 hours. Steam inhalations may help, and treatment of the causative condition, such as tonsillitis, may be necessary.

Q: *Are there any complications of acute laryngitis?*

A: Yes. In babies and young children, the infection may occasionally spread to the windpipe (tracheitis) and bronchi (bronchitis), causing a syndrome called laryngotracheobronchitis, or croup. This is a potentially serious disorder characterized by a fever and a barking cough. It may require hospitalization. Epiglottitis is a serious bacterial infection of the airway that also requires intensive hospital therapy.

Laryngitis in adults is seldom serious. It usually interferes with normal speech for about one week.

Q: *What are the symptoms and causes of chronic laryngitis?*

A: The chief symptom is continued hoarseness, accompanied by a slight cough and a tendency of the voice to become weaker with use. Drinking alcohol, smoking, and overusing the voice are all factors that can produce these symptoms.

Q: *How is chronic laryngitis diagnosed and treated?*

A: The diagnosis is made by a physician, who examines the vocal cords to make sure that there is no other cause for the hoarseness, such as a polyp or a tumor of the vocal cord.

See *also* LARYNGOSCOPY.

Laryngocele (lə ring′gə sēl) is an abnormal air sac near the cavity of the larynx (voice box). The air sac may appear as a tumor-like growth on the outside of the neck. The growth enlarges with increased pressure, as occurs with a cough.

Laryngoscopy (lar ing gos′kə pē) is the examination of the interior of the voice box (larynx) using an instrument called a laryngoscope.

In the technique known as indirect laryngoscopy, the laryngoscope consists of a rod with a small mirror at one end. It is passed to the back of the throat to give a reflected view of the larynx.

In direct laryngoscopy, performed under a general anesthetic, the laryngoscope is a rigid, illuminated tube which is passed down the throat to give a direct view of the larynx.

Larynx (lar′ingks) is the structure in the front of the neck that is commonly known as the voice box. It extends from the root of the tongue to the entrance of the windpipe (trachea). Until puberty, the larynx of a male differs little in size from that of a female. At puberty, it enlarges considerably in males but only slightly in females.

The "box" that makes up the larynx consists of nine cartilages that are connected by ligaments and membranes and are moved by several muscles. The largest of the cartilages, the thyroid cartilage, protrudes at the front of the neck to form the Adam's apple.

Q: *What are the functions of the larynx?*

A: The larynx forms part of the airway to the lungs. One of the nine cartilages, the epiglottis, closes the larynx during swallowing to prevent food from entering the windpipe. *See also* EPIGLOTTIS.

The other main function of the larynx is the production of speech. Inside the larynx are two vocal cords; the opening between them is called the glottis. At rest, the vocal cords are open and allow breathing to occur. During speech, the vocal cords come together, leaving only a narrow space between them. When air exhaled from the lungs passes through the cords, they vibrate and produce the sounds of speech.

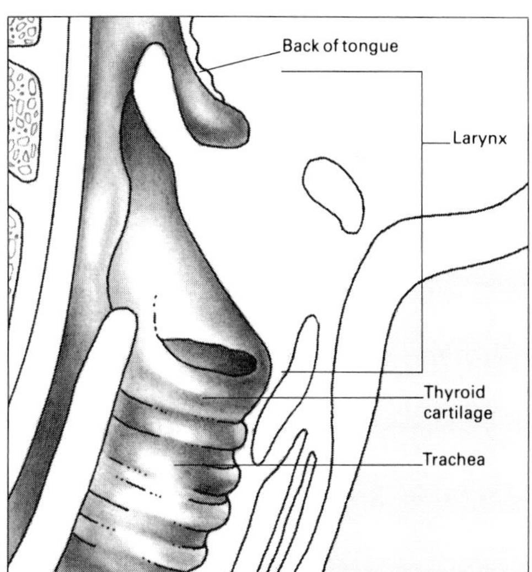

The **larynx,** or voice box, extends from the base of the tongue to the top of the trachea. It is composed of cartilage joined by ligaments and membranes.

Q: *What disorders can affect the larynx?*

A: An infection may cause laryngitis (inflammation of the larynx). Diphtheria is particularly dangerous if it involves the larynx, because the airway can become blocked by a membrane produced by the infection. Other infections elsewhere in the airway, such as a common cold or bronchitis, may spread and also affect the larynx.

The vocal cords may be damaged by overuse. This may cause small swellings on the vocal cords, often resulting in hoarseness or even a temporary loss of the voice. Cancer and other tumors of the vocal cords and larynx may also occur. In such cases, surgical removal of the larynx (laryngectomy) may be necessary. Cigarette smoking is very often associated with cancer of the larynx.

Laser (lā′zer) is an acronym for Light Amplification by Stimulated Emission of Radiation. A laser apparatus transforms and amplifies light of various frequencies into a very small and intense beam of monochromatic radiation (all one frequency) that produces very high heat and power.

See also LASER SURGERY.

Laser surgery (lā′zer) is often used to operate on the eye, as well as other places where precision is required or access may be difficult.

Common eye conditions that require laser surgery are eye tumors, retinal detachment, diabetic retinopathy (a disorder of the retina caused by diabetes), glaucoma (excessive pressure within the eyeball), macular degeneration (de-

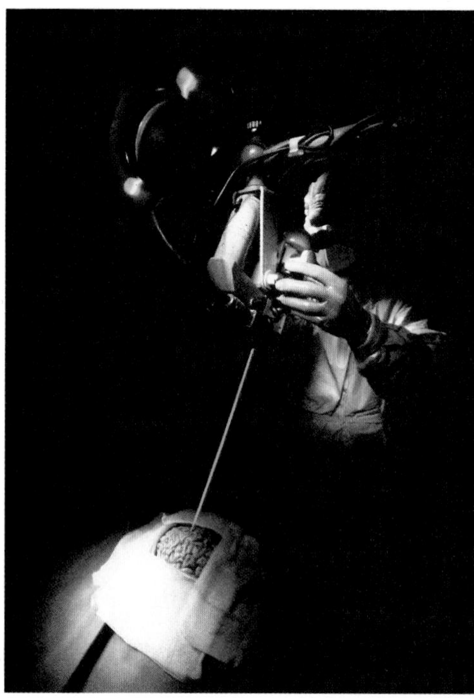

Laser equipment can be used to perform highly accurate and specialized surgical procedures.

terioration of the central vision portion of the retina), and retinoblastoma (childhood tumor of retinal tissue). Laser surgery is also often used in the treatment of venereal warts, cervical cancer, and cervical dysplasia (abnormal development of tissue at the uterine cervix).

See also ANGIOPLASTY; LASER.

Lassa fever (las′ə) is a highly contagious, often fatal disease, characterized by a high fever, chills, and malaise. In the later stages of the illness, acute abdominal pain and vomiting are common. Most cases result from the ingestion of food contaminated with a virus present in the urine of a small rat (*Mastomys natalensis*). The disease was recognized in Lassa, Nigeria, and most cases have been confined to Africa. Treatment may include a transfusion using blood or plasma from a person who has recovered from the disease.

Laughing gas is the common name for the anesthetic gas nitrous oxide.

See also NITROUS OXIDE.

Lavage (lav′ij) is the washing out of the bladder, stomach, or other body organ, usually for therapeutic purposes.

Laxative (lak′sə tiv) is any substance that speeds the emptying of the bowels (intestines). Laxatives are often used in the treatment or prevention of constipation (infrequent bowel movements).

Q: *What substances are used as laxatives?*

A: There are three main groups of laxatives, which differ in the way they affect the intestine. The group most commonly used acts by irritating the bowel wall or by direct nerve (neuronal) stimulation, causing a contraction and expulsion of the feces. Senna and cascara are examples of this type and are found in many commercial preparations. A second group of laxatives acts by attracting water from the body into the intestine, increasing the volume of feces. Milk of magnesia, Epsom salts (magnesium sulfate), and Glauber's salts (sodium sulfate) are common examples. The third group, referred to as bulk laxatives, acts as a stimulant to defecation by swelling the contents of the intestine. Bran, vegetable fiber, and general roughage are all bulk laxatives. The diet of many people in Western countries is deficient in these bulk substances; this deficiency may lead to constipation as well as other disorders, such as colorectal cancer.

Q: *What are the dangers of using laxatives?*

A: Laxatives should not be taken continually over long periods of time because the bowels may become lazy and fail to function on their own. (This is especially true of laxatives that irritate the bowel wall.) Permanent damage to the colon can occur with laxative abuse. Laxatives may also cause side effects in other parts of the body, including chemical and nutritional disturbances.

Q: *Should laxatives be used to treat all forms of constipation?*

A: No. Laxatives should never be used if constipation suddenly occurs or if it is accompanied by abdominal pain or fever. In such a case, there may be an intestinal obstruction or appendicitis, and laxatives are likely to make the condition worse. A physician should be consulted. *See also* APPENDICITIS; INTESTINAL OBSTRUCTION.

Layette. *See* BABY CARE.

Lazy eye. *See* STRABISMUS.

L-dopa (el′dō′pə) is another name for the drug levodopa.

See also LEVODOPA.

Lead poisoning is a toxic condition caused by excess lead or lead compounds in the body. Lead poisoning may result from swallowing objects that contain lead or from inhaling lead dust or fumes. Some forms of lead can be absorbed through the skin.

Lead poisoning afflicts many children who eat paint chips with a high lead content. Such paint is found in many older homes. Poisoning can also occur through drinking water that comes from lead pipes. Inhalation of lead fumes is common in smelting, battery manufacturing, and other industries that use lead. Such industries may pollute the environment with lead dust and fumes, which may cause poisoning in people who live near the plants. Another source of lead is the exhaust from automobiles that use leaded gasoline.

Lead is excreted very slowly and so tends to accumulate in the body tissues, especially in the nervous system, bones, liver, pancreas, teeth, and gums. A small amount of lead can circulate in the body without causing ill effects, but when larger amounts are ingested, the production of red blood cells is impaired, and normal body functions are disturbed. This occurs slowly and cumulatively if the lead poisoning is chronic, or rapidly and sometimes fatally if the poisoning is acute.

Q: *What are the symptoms of lead poisoning?*

A: The symptoms of chronic lead poisoning appear gradually and include fatigue, headache, irritability, dizziness, and breathlessness, caused by anemia. If the intestine becomes involved, there may also be constipation, nausea, and severe abdominal pain. Nerve damage and permanent brain damage may also result.

Acute lead poisoning causes vomiting, black or bloody diarrhea, acute abdominal pain, convulsions, delirium, and coma. The first sign is a metallic taste in the mouth, then signs of burns in the throat and esophagus (gullet). The diagnosis of lead poisoning is confirmed by the presence of anemia

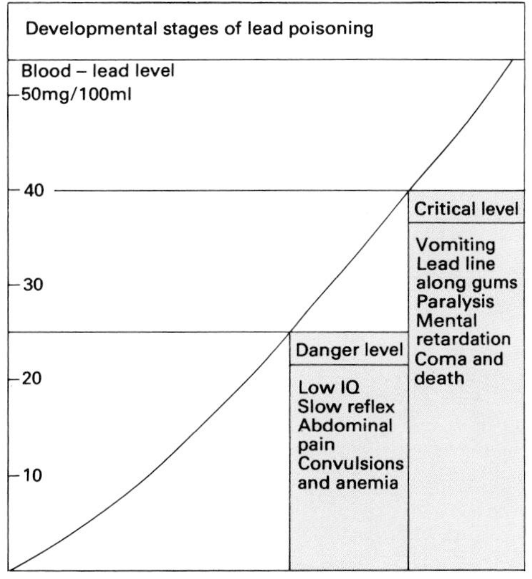

with excessive amounts of lead in the blood and urine.

Q: *How is lead poisoning treated?*

A: Acute lead poisoning requires emergency medical treatment. Initially, the stomach is often washed out. Special drugs, called chelating agents, help to remove lead from the tissues. This lead is then excreted in the urine. If lead poisoning has caused anemia, a special diet with supplementary iron may be prescribed.

Q: *Can lead poisoning be prevented?*

A: Yes, especially if precautions are strictly followed in industries that use lead. The United States government restricts the lead content of paint and certain other products and regulates industrial uses of lead. The government also sets air quality standards that limit the amount of lead that can be released into the air.

When working around the house, use only lead-free paint on indoor surfaces or any other surfaces accessible to children.

See also POISONING: FIRST AID.

Learning disability is any of a group of disorders that interfere with a child's ability to learn. They may cause a child to do poorly in school.

There are many types of learning disabilities. A learning-disabled child may, for example, have difficulty concentrating, memorizing, or coordinating certain kinds of physical movements. A learning disability may also interfere with a child's ability to speak, spell,

Lead poisoning is at a critical level when there is about 40mg lead content per 100ml of blood.

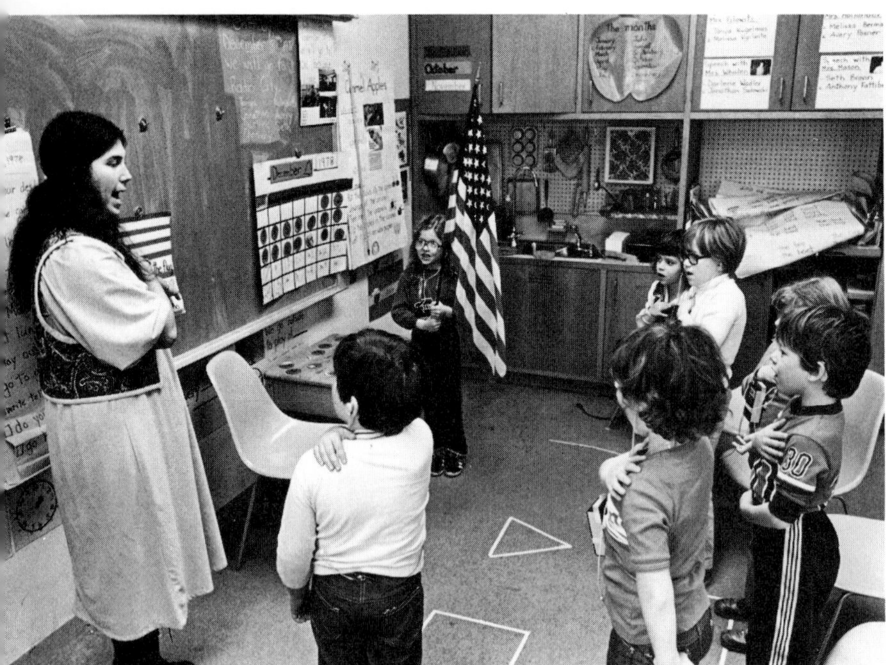

Learning-disabled children are sometimes taught in special classes. Treatment begun as early as possible offers the greatest chance for success.

understand spoken language, read, or solve mathematical problems. In the United States, from 5 to 10 percent of all children between the ages of 5 and 17 have one or more learning disabilities.

Q: *What are some of the causes of learning disabilities?*

A: It is important to remember that learning-disabled children are of normal or above-average intelligence. The major signs of learning disabilities are slow development of language skills and hyperactive behavior. Vision or hearing impairment may interfere with learning, as may a lack of adequate early learning experiences. Children with fetal alcohol syndrome also frequently have learning difficulties. *See also* FETAL ALCOHOL SYNDROME.

Q: *What are the symptoms of a learning disability?*

A: The symptoms depend on the type of disorder involved. The symptoms of one type of learning disability, dysphasia, are a child's difficulty in speaking or in understanding spoken language. Dyslexia, on the other hand, is revealed as a difficulty in reading. Dysgraphia, a third type of learning disability, produces difficulty in writing.

Still other types of learning disabilities interfere with a child's power to concentrate or to behave in a socially acceptable manner. Such a child suffers from hyperactivity, or attention deficit disorder. Hyperactive children—who are more often boys than girls—tend to speak and act impulsively and boisterously. These children are also usually impatient. Their conduct, whether at home or at school, is generally looked upon by peers and adults to be disruptive and uncontrolled. This disruptive behavior interferes both with learning in the school environment and with establishing social relationships.

Other learning disabilities display themselves as a lack of distinguishing left from right or a lack of distinguishing between letters of the alphabet that have some similarities in form, such as *b* and *d*.

Q: *How are learning disabilities diagnosed?*

A: The parent is usually the first person to suspect that a child has a learning disability. The parent usually alerts the family physician or pediatrician. Teachers also often identify children with learning disabilities. Upon examination, the physician or pediatrician may refer the child to a pediatric developmental team for further testing and evaluation. The team may include a neurologist, a psychologist, a child psychiatrist, an eye specialist, an ear specialist, an occupational therapist, and a speech therapist.

It is important to try to determine if some factor in the home environment is contributing to, or even causing, the child's learning disability. Some schools provide for the diagnosis and treatment of children with learning disabilities. Early diagnosis and treatment are important because specialized teaching techniques can help many students overcome their disabilities and succeed in school. Unless a child receives appropriate treatment, learning problems may continue into adulthood.

It is important to note that not all learning and behavioral problems are caused by learning disabilities.

Q: *How are learning disabilities treated?*

A: The method of treatment depends on the type and extent of the disability. Some learning-disabled children learn best in special classes, while many disabled children can improve their skills in regular classes with the use of supplemental learning activities. In some situations, children with hyperactivity may require medication to allow them to work effectively in school. Treatment begun as early as possible offers the greatest chance of success.

See also ATTENTION DEFICIT DISORDER; HYPERACTIVITY.

Left-handedness is a natural tendency to use the left hand, in preference to the right, in performing such tasks as writing and throwing. In most persons, the left side of the brain is "dominant," and because it controls the right side of the body, they are right-handed. In left-handed people, the right side of the brain is dominant. Left-handedness is apparently inherited.

See also RIGHT-HANDEDNESS.

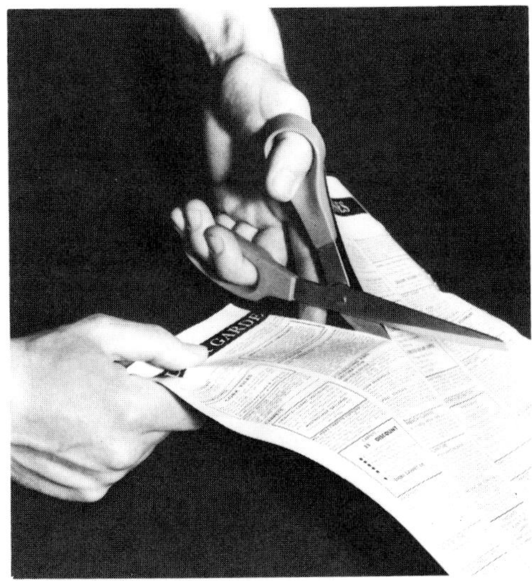

Left-handedness can be accommodated through the use of specially adapted utensils.

Leg is one of the limbs on which people stand or walk. Technically, it is only the section of the lower limb between the ankle and the knee. The part of the limb between the knee and the hip is the thigh.

See also ANKLE; KNEE; THIGH.

Legionnaire's disease (lē jə nārz′) is a potentially fatal bacterial disorder named for an outbreak at the 1976 American Legion conference in Philadelphia where 182 people were afflicted, 29 of whom died. It is caused by a previously unknown bacterium, *Legionella pneumophilia*, which is extremely difficult to culture in a laboratory. It is not known exactly how the disease is spread. In the United States, one breeding place for the bacteria was found to be in the stagnant water associated with large air-conditioning systems.

Early symptoms are similar to those of influenza—a generalized feeling of ill health accompanied by fever, muscle aches, headache, and diarrhea. Pneumonia may later develop. Definitive diagnosis can be made only by finding the bacterium in the patient's body or by finding antibodies to it in the bloodstream. Treatment is usually by the antibiotic erythromycin.

Leiomyoma (lī ō mī ō′mə) is a benign (noncancerous) tumor of smooth muscle, commonly called a fibroid when it occurs in the uterus. Leiomyomas may also occur in the gastrointestinal tract where they generally produce no symptoms, although rarely they may cause an intestinal obstruction or hemorrhage.

See also FIBROID.

Leishmaniasis (lesh mə nī′ə sis) is a group of infectious diseases of the skin and internal organs caused by various protozoan parasites of the genus *Leishmania*. Leishmaniasis is usually transmitted by sand flies.

There are two main types of leishmaniasis: visceral leishmaniasis, also called kala-azar, which attacks the internal organs, such as the stomach; and cutaneous leishmaniasis, also called Delhi boil or oriental sore, which attacks the skin. Various forms of leishmaniasis are common in tropical and subtropical regions throughout the world.

In American leishmaniasis, one of the two variants of cutaneous leishmaniasis, the ulcers form in a similar way to those of oriental sore. The ulcers usually form in the nose and throat. The ulcers also have a tendency to become infected. This can cause serious complications and may even be fatal. American leishmaniasis may last for several years, with the patient becoming increasingly incapacitated.

Q: *How is cutaneous leishmaniasis treated?*

A: Many cases of oriental sore and some of American leishmaniasis heal spontaneously and do not require treatment. When spontaneous recovery does not occur, treatment includes administering antimony drugs (compounds of metallic elements) or amphotericin B, an antifungal medication. Antimicrobial drugs are used to treat secondary infection. Visceral leishmaniasis is treated in a similar fashion.

Lens is a curved piece of transparent material that causes light rays passing through it to converge or diverge. The lens in the eye is a transparent, colorless, biconvex disk that helps to focus light onto the retina. Glass or plastic lenses are used in contact lenses, eyeglasses, and various medical instruments.

See also EYE.

Lens implant is performed on persons with cataracts, a condition in which the lens of the eye becomes clouded and vision is impaired. With a lens implant, the affected lens is removed surgically and replaced with a lightweight plastic lens.

An implanted lens is relatively free from distortion. Because it occupies the same position as the natural lens, it allows more normal vision to be achieved than eyeglasses or contact lenses, both of which are alternate methods of treatment.

Lens implants are normally not recommended for persons suffering from detached retina, glaucoma, or eye disorders caused by diabetes.

See also CATARACT.

Leprosy (lep′rə sē), or Hansen's disease, is a slowly progressive infection caused by the bacterium *Mycobacterium leprae*. The disorder is prevalent in Central and South America, in the Far East, and in the tropical countries of Asia and Africa. There are about 4,000 cases in the United States, but the vast majority of these patients were born in other countries where they may have contracted the disease.

Leprosy is contagious through the respiratory tract, but the danger of catching it from another person is very slight. Relatively few persons exposed to the disease develop it. To contract leprosy, a person must have low resistance and live in contact with a person whose body contains large numbers of the germs. Children are more likely to become infected than are adults. There are two main forms of leprosy, tuberculoid leprosy and lepromatous leprosy.

Q: *What are the symptoms of tuberculoid leprosy?*

A: Tuberculoid leprosy appears as an infection around nerve endings, causing gradual loss of feeling and the appearance of pale areas on the skin where sensation is reduced. The nerves may be felt as thickened, tender, rope-like structures. This may lead to partial paralysis, producing wrist drop or foot drop and sometimes local areas of ulceration.

Q: *What are the symptoms of lepromatous leprosy?*

A: The normal pigmentation in some areas on the skin is lost, and the skin becomes slightly reddened. There are usually many such areas scattered symmetrically across the body. The edges merge into the normal skin so that they may not be obvious in a pale-skinned person. Occasionally, there is thickening of the skin of the face, often involving the ears, to produce the "lion face" (leontiasis).

As the disease progresses, the membranes of the nose, mouth, and throat may ulcerate, producing distorted lips and loss of cartilage in the nose.

Q: *How does leprosy progress?*

A: The progress is extremely variable and depends on the level of immunity in the patient. Patients with tuberculoid leprosy often overcome the infection without much damage. But lepromatous leprosy progresses slowly, with increasing episodes of fever, enlargement in the size of affected skin areas, eye infection (iritis), lymph node enlargement, and sometimes, involvement of the testes (orchitis). Leprosy can be fatal, and it causes massive suffering throughout the world.

Q: *How is leprosy diagnosed and treated?*

A: Diagnosis can be confirmed through a biopsy of the edge of an affected skin area or nerve. Early treatment of leprosy is important in preventing deformities and other physical handicaps. Bone and tendon surgery often helps to restore the use of disabled hands and feet. Massage of affected body parts may prevent deformities. Drugs, such as dapsone, rifampin, and clofazimine, are usually successful in treating leprosy and are used in combination to prevent drug resistance. Treatment is usually continued for several years after the disease becomes inactive.

Leptospirosis (lep tō spī rō'sis) is an infectious disease caused by the spirochete bacteria of the genus *Leptospira*. It is often transmitted to humans via liquids contaminated by the urine of infected wild or domestic animals, primarily dogs, cattle, and rats. Leptospirosis is relatively rare in the United States, with only about 100 cases reported annually. Infections occur in sanitation workers, veterinarians, and farmers, but anyone can catch the disease by swimming in contaminated water.

Q: *What are the symptoms of leptospirosis?*

A: After an incubation period of one to three weeks, there is sudden onset of severe headache, muscular aching (myalgia) with shivering attacks (rigor), and fever that may last about a week. The whites of the eyes often become red and inflamed.

In severe forms of the illness (Weil's syndrome), jaundice occurs, mental confusion is common, and urinary excretion is greatly reduced resulting in uremia (a toxic condition caused by failure of the kidneys). Death may occur, especially in older victims.

Q: *How is leptospirosis treated?*

A: A patient is usually hospitalized in order to ensure careful monitoring of vital signs. Treatment with antibiotics, such as penicillin, may be effective but only if administered in the early stages of the disease.

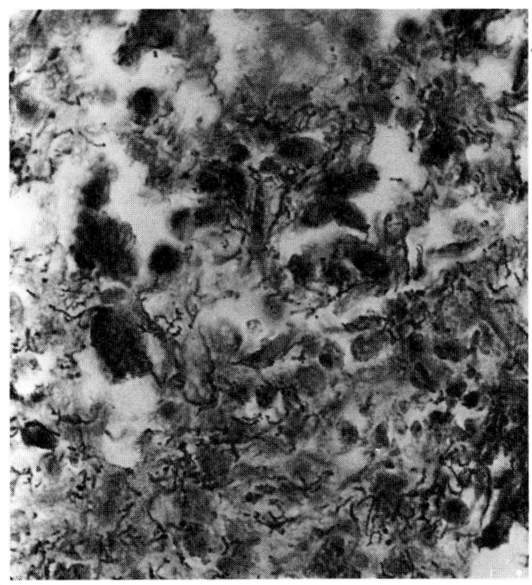

The spirochete bacteria of the genus *Leptospira* is the cause of **leptospirosis,** an infectious disease characterized by headache, muscular aching, shivering, and fever. Leptospirosis can be fatal.

Care should be taken when disposing of the patient's urine in order to prevent the spread of the bacteria.

Lesbian (lez'bē ən) is a woman who has a sexual preference for other women. Lesbianism is the female form of homosexuality.

See also HOMOSEXUALITY.

Lesion (lē'zhən) is any damaged or abnormal area of tissue, such as a wound, an injury, or an area altered by infection or tumor.

Lethargy (leth'ər jē) is a feeling of fatigue and listlessness, both physical and mental. It may occur for no particular reason, or it may follow an illness or operation. Continued lethargy, for no apparent reason, is abnormal, and a physician should be consulted.

Leukemia (lü kē'mē ə) is a malignant disease of the white blood cells (leukocytes), which play a key part in the body's defense mechanism against infection. It is a type of cancer that affects the bone marrow and other blood-forming tissues throughout the body. The cause of leukemia is not known, but seems to be associated with a failure of the developing leukocytes to mature.

Normal, mature leukocytes can not reproduce and are replaced at the ends of their lives. Leukemic cells, however, have the ability to reproduce but do not develop sufficiently to act as a defense against infection. As leukemia progresses, the leukemic cells displace normal leukocytes, leaving the patient extremely vulnerable to infection.

There are several forms of leukemia, both acute and chronic, which are classified according to the type of leukocyte affected. The major types of leukocytes involved in leukemia include lymphocytes and polymorphonuclear leukocytes.

Q: *What forms of acute leukemia are there?*

A: There are two main forms of acute leukemia, acute lymphoblastic leukemia (ALL) and acute myeloblastic leukemia (AML). ALL affects lymphocytes and occurs more often in children. AML affects the cells that form polymorphonuclear leukocytes and is more common in adults, although it can occur at any age.

Q: *What are the symptoms of the acute leukemias?*

A: The symptoms of both forms of acute leukemia are similar. The patient usually has a sudden high fever and a severe throat infection. There may also be nosebleeds, bruising under the skin, fatigue, and pain in the joints. In some patients, the onset of symptoms is slower, with lethargy, anemia, and increasing weakness.

Q: *What forms of chronic leukemia are there?*

A: There are two main forms of chronic leukemia, chronic myeloid leukemia (CML), and chronic lymphocytic leukemia (CLL). CML affects immature polymorphonuclear leukocytes and usually occurs after 35 years of age. CLL affects lymphoid tissue and lymphatic cells and usually occurs in men over the age of 50.

Q: *What are the symptoms of the chronic leukemias?*

A: The symptoms of both forms of chronic leukemia are similar. The onset is usually slow, with increasing fatigue, lethargy, and weakness. The patient may also lose weight and suffer from loss of appetite. The course of the illness is slow and may last for several years without causing major problems. However, there may be various complications, such as anemia; bleeding under the skin; recurrent fever; and the formation of nodules and ulcers under the skin.

Q: *How is leukemia diagnosed?*

A: The specific diagnosis of leukemia requires a blood count and a bone marrow biopsy. Leukemia is confirmed by the presence of large numbers of abnormal leukocytes in the blood and the typical leukemic cells in the bone marrow. With the chronic leukemias, the patient may be unaware of the disease, and a diagnosis is often made only when the patient is examined for another reason, such as during a routine checkup or before surgery.

Q: *How is leukemia treated?*

A: The treatment of acute and chronic leukemia is often similar, but it is dependent on varying factors involved in each case. The aim of treatment is to suppress the reproduction of leukemic cells. Cytotoxic drugs, which prevent cell multiplication, are used for this purpose. The rapidly-dividing leukemic cells are more susceptible to these drugs than are normal leukocytes.

The treatment of the acute leukemias usually involves the use of several cytotoxic drugs together. Once the number of leukemic cells has been reduced, corticosteroids and only one or two cytotoxic drugs need be used to maintain the improvement. With the chronic leukemias, cytotoxic drugs and corticosteroids may also be used. In some cases, a blood transfusion may be necessary.

Research into leukemia is very active. Several new drugs are being tested, and many of the latest techniques are available only in leukemia research centers. For this reason, a patient with any form of leukemia should obtain advice and treatment from an expert in this field.

Q: *Can leukemia be cured?*

A: Some children with ALL respond well to treatment. A large number treated for ALL have survived for five years without any further symptoms, and most of them (about 80 percent) can resume normal life for some time before a relapse occurs. The problem is to ensure that every leukemic cell has been destroyed. There is a tendency for recurrences in the brain and around nerves. A bone marrow transplant may help some patients who fail to respond to chemotherapy.

AML is generally fatal, but the symptoms can be controlled and the patient's life extended, especially the period of useful life. The prognosis for those with the chronic leukemias is largely dependent upon the age at which the disease occurs; as with AML, the symptoms can be controlled and life extended. Patients with CML are more likely to die as a result of leukemia than are those with CLL, because CML usually starts at an earlier age.

See also BLOOD CELL, WHITE; CANCER.

Leukemoid reaction (lü kē′moid) is a condition characterized by clinical findings resembling true leukemia, with an elevated white blood cell count. It may occur in response to infections, such as whooping cough and infectious mononucleosis, allergies, poisoning, or other disorders that cause severe physical stress. Careful clinical study is often needed to differentiate a leukemoid reaction from true leukemia.

Leukocyte. *See* BLOOD CELL, WHITE.

Leukocytosis (lü kə si tō′sis) is an increase in the number of white blood cells (leukocytes) in the blood. It is a normal response to infection and also to bodily damage, such as that caused by surgery or by an injury. An increase in abnormal leukocytes may occur in such conditions as infectious mononucleosis, leukemia, and some forms of anemia.

See also BLOOD CELL, WHITE.

Leukoderma (lü kə der′mə) is the loss of the normal skin pigmentation, resulting in the appearance of pale patches. This condition may occur temporarily following the treatment of any skin inflammation. Leukoderma may also be caused by handling chemicals that remove the pigment from the skin. Very rarely, it may be caused by leprosy. Vitiligo is a form of leukoderma for which the cause is unknown.

See also VITILIGO.

Leukopenia (lü kə pe′nē ə) is an abnormal reduction in the number of white blood cells (leukocytes) in the blood. It may occur in any acute virus infection or in forms of chemical poisoning. Leukopenia may also occur with the use of many cancer chemotherapy drugs and through alcohol abuse.

See also AGRANULOCYTOSIS.

Leukoplakia (lü kə plā′kē ə) is a condition in which thickened white patches develop on the tongue and inside the cheeks or other mucous membranes, such as those of the vulva or penis. It is a disorder of the cells of the mucous membrane that may be a prelude to cancer.

Q: *What causes leukoplakia of the mouth and how is it treated?*

A: Smoking, drinking alcohol, and chronic irritation from damaged teeth or badly fitting dentures are thought to be some of the causes. The causative agent should be eliminated or treated, and the small lesions removed by surgery.

Q: *How is leukoplakia of the vulva treated?*

A: Irritation of the vulva may be the symptom that makes a woman consult a physician. An examination may reveal the white patches of leukoplakia. The area should be examined regularly to see if there are any malignant changes. In the rare cases in which cancer is thought to be developing, parts of the vulva may be surgically removed.

Leukorrhea (lü kə rē′ə) is a whitish, somewhat thick discharge from the vagina. Normally, vaginal discharge occurs intermittently throughout the menstrual cycle, with a somewhat greater than usual amount during pregnancy. Constant leukorrhea, a change in its consistency, or a greater discharge than usual may be signs of a vaginal or uterine infection, a tumor, or various other gynecological disorders. A woman who is experiencing any abnormal vaginal discharge should consult her physician. Laboratory tests may be needed to help determine the cause of the abnormal discharge. Abnormal leukorrhea is a fairly common female disorder; in most cases, it is caused by a benign and easily treated problem.

Leukotomy (lü kot′ə mē) is the cutting of the nerve fibers that lead from the middle to the front part of the brain. This procedure is usually known as a lobotomy.

See also LOBOTOMY.

Levodopa (lē vō dō′pə) is a drug used in the treatment of Parkinson's disease. In selected areas of the brain, it increases the amount of dopamine, a chemical necessary for the normal working of brain tissue. Patients suffering from Parkinson's disease have decreased concentrations of dopamine in their brains. Treatment consists of administering initial small doses of levodopa, which are usually increased to larger doses, often producing toxic symptoms. These include loss of appetite and nausea with, occasionally, abdominal pain, constipation, and diarrhea. Lowered blood pressure may cause a feeling of faintness and dizziness, often accompanied by excessive sweating and palpitations. The patient may also develop abnormal movement disorders, such as involuntary chewing and twisting movements of the limbs.

Psychiatric problems, such as drowsiness, depression, and (sometimes) paranoia and hallucinations, may also arise. Rarely, there are problems with passing urine. In men, there may be sexual problems.

Q: *How are the toxic effects of levodopa treated?*

A: The toxic effects of levodopa are seldom a major problem if the dosage of the drug is increased slowly. A temporary reduction in dosage usually causes the symptoms to disappear.

Q: *Are there any conditions in which levodopa should not be used?*

A: Yes. The drug should be avoided, if possible, in patients who have certain pyschiatric disorders, such as schizophrenia, or the eye disorder, glaucoma, or who are taking certain other drugs, such as MAO inhibitors for depression. Persons with disease of the heart, liver, or kidneys are more likely to develop toxic effects. Additionally, levodopa should not be taken by pregnant women. Levodopa is also known as L-dopa.

See also PARKINSON'S DISEASE.

LGV is an abbreviation of lymphogranuloma venereum, a sexually transmitted disease.

See also LYMPHOGRANULOMA VENEREUM.

Libido (lə bē′do) is the psychological term for the physical and emotional energy associated with instinctual drives, primarily those actions and emotions associated with the sexual drive. The form and force of the sexual drive depends, in part, on cultural conditioning and psychological education. It also depends on biological effects produced by the sex hormones.

Libido may be increased by visual and sensory impulses; or it may be reduced by fear, anxiety, or depression. Sexual drive and desire can be altered by hormonal changes that occur during the menstrual cycle and by hormonal disorders, such as hypopituitarism. Psychiatric disorders can increase or decrease one's libido. Changes in an individual's libido should be carefully evaluated by a physician for its psychological and physical causes.

Librium® (lib′rē əm), or chlordiazepoxide hydrochloride, is a tranquilizing agent. It is usually prescribed to relieve anxiety and tension or to treat the withdrawal symptoms of persons with acute alcoholism. Side effects include possible drowsiness, mental confusion, and diminished muscular coordination (ataxia). Rarely, Librium may lead to jaundice and liver disorders. Prolonged use of Librium may lead to a dependence on the drug.

Librium should not be taken before driving an automobile or before participating in other possibly dangerous activities requiring mental alertness. It also should not be taken by pregnant women.

Lice are a group of parasitic insects that live on various animals, including humans. There are three main types of lice that infest human beings: the two varieties of *Pediculus humanus*, which live in the hair or on the body, and the crab louse, *Phthirus pubis*, which lives in the pubic hair. The head louse belongs to the same species as the body louse, but it confines itself to the scalp. Lice may cause such diseases as typhus or relapsing fever.

Q: *What symptoms do head lice cause?*

A: Often, there are no symptoms, although in severe cases there is itching of the scalp, which can cause secondary infection through scratching the infected area. Crusting and oozing then occur, similar to that of impetigo.

Head lice are most common among schoolchildren because of

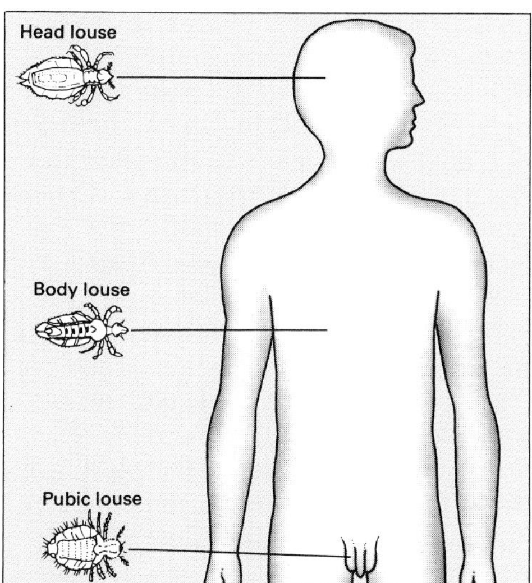

Three varieties of **lice,** parasitic animals that live on various animals, infest human beings: *Phthirus pubis* lives in pubic hair; *Pediculus humanus* lives in body hair; and a second variety of *Pediculus humanus* lives in head hair.

the frequency with which they put their heads together during work projects and games. If one child is infected, than all the other children are likely to be infected.

Q: *How is the condition diagnosed and treated?*

A: In severe cases, the lice can be seen. In most children, the diagnosis is made after finding small, shiny, pearl-colored eggs (nits) attached to the hairs.

Treatment involves careful washing of the hair with a medicated shampoo. After washing, the hair should be meticulously combed using a fine-toothed comb to remove any nits, and then inspected. A second combing may be necessary. The procedure should be repeated a week later and, on each occasion, the shampoo should be left to dry on the hair before it is washed off the next morning.

Q: *What symptoms indicate the presence of crab lice?*

A: There is intense itching in the pubic area and possible secondary infection in scratch marks. In severe infestations, the hair in the armpits, eyebrows, and eyelashes may also be involved.

Q: *What is the treatment for body lice?*

A: The diagnosis is made in the same way as for head lice by finding nits on the hairs or lice on the body. Treatment involves washing the body from the neck downward with a special solution (prescribed by a physician) and leaving it to dry. This should be done each day for three days. Treatment should not be prolonged in case it causes dermatitis.

Licensed practical nurse. See NURSE, LICENSED PRACTICAL.

Lichenification (lī kən ə fə kā'shən) is a thickening and hardening of an area of skin, usually as a result of the continual scratching of an itchy (pruritic) lesion.

Lichen planus (lī'kən plān'əs) is a recurrent skin inflammation characterized by small, itchy lesions. It usually starts at the wrists or on the legs and may spread to the trunk of the body. The condition may last for many weeks or months. Onset may be sudden or gradual; the cause is unknown.

Q: *What are the symptoms of lichen planus?*

A: The skin lesions are small, slightly raised purple or red areas that glisten. They occur on the front surfaces of the forearms, trunk, and shins. In severe cases, the lesions may occur anywhere on the body. The lesions itch and are often surrounded by scratch marks. Lesions may even occur in the mouth or on the vulva or penis. Occasionally, the nails may be involved, resulting in ridging and splitting.

Sometimes, the symptoms subside within three months; the patches lose their shiny color and become brown and scaly, before disappearing. In some patients, the condition lasts for many years.

Q: *What is the treatment for lichen planus?*

A: There is no specific treatment, although the lesions can usually be kept under control with creams or lotions containing corticosteroid drugs.

Lichen simplex chronicus (lī'kən sim'pleks kron'i kəs) is a chronic skin disorder characterized by a group of small, slightly raised skin lesions. It causes an intense desire to scratch, resulting in inflammation and possible infection. Continued scratching may lead to local thickening of the skin (lichenification). Lichen simplex chronicus is a form of neurodermatitis.

Q: *What causes lichen simplex chronicus?*

A: An allergy, eczema, or congenital dry and scaly skin may be contributory factors, but anxiety, mental tension, and emotional disturbances are probably the main causes. The condition is more common in women than in men, and it is more common in families with a history of allergies. Before diagnosing the disorder, a physician makes sure that there are no other skin conditions, such as scabies, lichen planus, or local vaginal or anal infections that may produce skin irritations.

Q: *How is lichen simplex chronicus treated?*

A: Corticosteroid creams usually give relief, and an antipruritic drug may be prescribed to combat itching.

Life expectancy is the length of time for which, according to statistical measure, an individual may expect to live. Life expectancy varies from country to country because of differences in public health and standards of living. In general, the industrialized nations have the highest life expectancy, and the developing countries, especially those in Africa, have the lowest. In the United States in the 1980's, the life expectancy of a newborn male is 72 years and that of a newborn female is 78 years. In general, females have a higher life expectancy than males. Other demographic conditions, such as a person's race, also play a factor in determining life expectancy.

Lifting a patient. *See* NURSING THE SICK.

Ligament (lig′a mənt) is a supporting band of fibrous tissue that holds a joint or body organ in place. Ligaments give support and at the same time allow movement.

Ligament, torn: treatment. *See* SPRAINS AND STRAINS: TREATMENT.

Ligation (lī gā′shən) is the tying off of a blood vessel or body tube with a suture or wire ligature. It is usually performed during surgery to stop or prevent bleeding.

See also LIGATURE; TUBAL LIGATION.

Ligation, tubal. *See* TUBAL LIGATION.

Ligature (lig′ə chůr) is a thread made of catgut, silk, nylon, or steel that is used

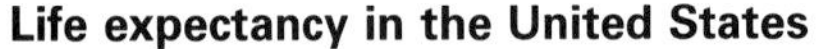

Life expectancy in the United States

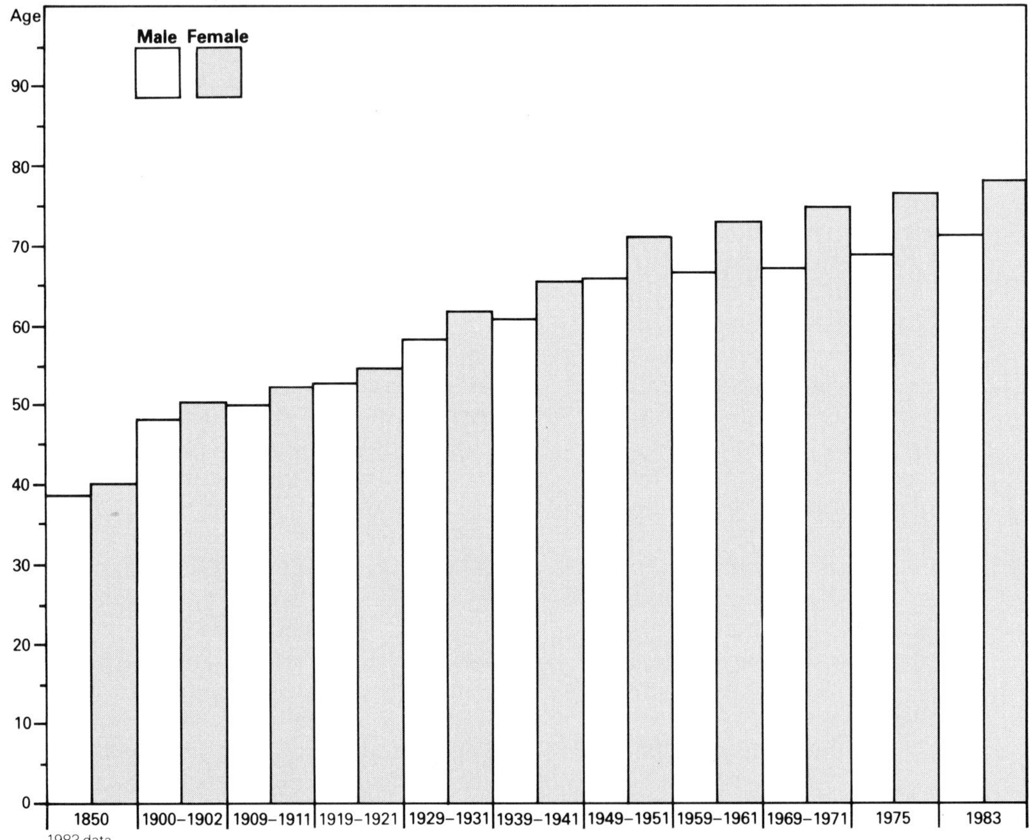

1983 data

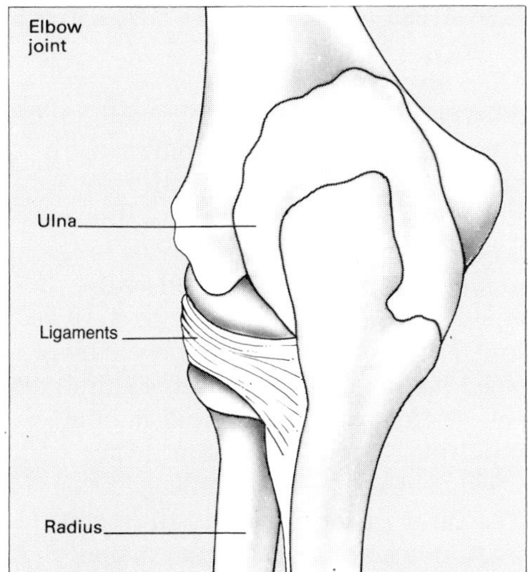

Ligaments, such as those that join the humerus, ulna, and radius bones, help bind together bones at a joint.

to tie round and close a blood vessel or any body tube.

See *also* SUTURE.

Lightening is the sensation that occurs in women late in pregnancy as the fetus descends towards the birth canal, leaving more space in the upper abdomen. If lightening does not occur during the final two to four weeks of pregnancy, a physician may conduct tests to discover if the fetus is in the proper position. Lightening may be accompanied by uterine contractions, which may be mistaken for the onset of labor.

See *also* PREGNANCY AND CHILDBIRTH.

Limbic system (lim′bik) is a group of brain structures associated with the autonomic (self-regulating) functions of the body and with certain emotions, such as anger, fear, happiness, and sexual stimulation. The limbic system is located in the rhinencephalon portion of the brain and includes such structures as the isthmus, the cingulate gyrus, and the hippocampus.

See *also* BRAIN.

Limping is a condition characterized by an awkward or abnormal gait. There are many causes of abnormal gait, including diseases of the nervous system, bones, or joints.

See *also* CLAUDICATION.

Lip is any fleshy structure bordering a body opening, usually used to refer to either of the two fleshy structures surrounding the mouth.

See *also* LABIUM.

Lipemia (li pē′mē ə) is the presence in the bloodstream of abnormally large amounts of the fatty substances called lipids (which include cholesterol). There is strong evidence that an extremely high level of such substances, the condition called hyperlipemia or hyperlipidemia, is a factor in the cause of atherosclerosis and, therefore, of coronary heart disease, strokes, and disorders of peripheral arteries. *See also* ARTERIOSCLEROSIS.

Q: *What causes an increase of the fatty substances in the blood?*

A: There is a normal increase in the lipids (particularly triglycerides) after any meal. For this reason, in a medical test the level of lipids is measured after a patient has been fasting for at least eight hours.

Hyperlipemia detected in this way may be caused by such disorders as hypothyroidism, diabetes mellitus, and a rare condition present at birth called xanthelasma, in which the body is unable to metabolize cholesterol normally.

More commonly, hyperlipemia is associated with a combination of factors, such as a mild inherited tendency, cigarette smoking, a diet containing excessive amounts of animal fats, lack of physical exercise, and obesity.

Q: *What is the treatment for high lipid levels?*

A: Treatment of any specific cause found may reduce the level of lipids. Treatment is also directed at the individual's life style. A physician may recommend a low-fat diet, regular exercise, and elimination of smoking. If life style changes are not successful, lipid-lowering drugs may be prescribed.

See *also* DIABETES MELLITUS; HYPOTHYROIDISM; LIPID; XANTHELASMA.

Lipid (lip′id) is any one of a group of fats or fat-like substances that occur in the body. Lipids include triglycerides, cholesterol, and lipoproteins, as well as fatty substances that are combined with sugars and phosphates.

Lipids are easily stored in the body, where they are an important part of cell structure and a source of reserve energy. Elevated levels of lipids in the bloodstream may lead to various disorders, including atherosclerosis.

See also ARTERIOSCLEROSIS; CHOLESTEROL; LIPEMIA; LIPOPROTEIN; TRIGLYCERIDE.

Lipoma (li pō′mə) is a benign (noncancerous) tumor that is made up of fat cells. Lipomas commonly occur under the skin and may be felt as diffuse, soft swellings, particularly over the shoulders and trunk. They seldom cause problems and are easily removed surgically. Lipomas of the breast are fairly common; they may be mistaken for malignant growths, especially if they are firmer than normal.

See also TUMOR.

Lipoprotein (lip ə prō′tēn) is a compound found in the body that consists of such lipids as triglycerides and cholesterol, combined with protein molecules. Basically, there are two kinds of lipoproteins: high-density lipoproteins (HDL) and low-density lipoproteins (LDL). Recent research in heart disease has found that a ratio of high HDL to low LDL in the body seems to offer protection against developing heart disease. Furthermore, it has been found that those who exercise regularly are more apt to have the beneficial ratio and, that those who undertake an exercise program, can improve a ratio that was formerly unfavorable.

See also CHOLESTEROL; TRIGLYCERIDE.

Liposuction (lip ō suk′shen), also known as suction lipectomy or lipolysis, is a surgical method of removing localized fat deposits using a suction apparatus. This potentially dangerous procedure should be performed only by a qualified surgeon.

See also WEIGHT PROBLEM.

Lisp is a speech defect.

See also SPEECH DEFECT.

Listeriosis (lis tir ē ō′sis) is an infectious disease caused by a nonsporulating genus of bacteria *Listeria monocytogenes*. The disease is transmitted to humans through contact with infected animals, such as shellfish or spiders, or through contact with soil or sewage contaminated by the animals. Symptoms include shock, a red rash over the lower portion of the body, and circulatory collapse. Infants and the elderly are particularly susceptible to the infection. The disease is potentially fatal; treatment with antibiotics, such as penicillin, may precede positive identification of the bacteria.

Listlessness is a condition similar to lethargy.

See also LETHARGY

Lithiasis. *See* CALCULUS.

Lithium (lith′ē əm) is an element with metallic properties used medically as lithium carbonate or lithium citrate in the treatment of manic-depressive illness or mania not associated with depression. Side effects can be very serious and may include kidney damage, excessive urination, excessive thirst, as well as tremor. Physical and mental impairment is also possible.

See also MANIC-DEPRESSIVE ILLNESS.

Lithotomy (li thot′ə mē) is an operation to remove a stone (calculus), usually from the kidney, bladder, or salivary glands, through a surgical incision.

See also CALCULUS; LITHOTRIPSY.

Lithotripsy (lith ə trip′sē) is an operation to destroy a stone (calculus) that is obstructing the bladder, gallbladder, ureter, or kidney. The stone is approached by inserting an instrument, called a lithotrite, through the urethra and either crushing the stone or shattering it with an electrical spark. In a more recently developed method, called extracorporeal or ultrasonic lithotripsy, the stone may be shattered by the use of high frequency sound waves without inserting any instruments into the body. The crushed fragments of the stone can then be passed out of the body without difficulty.

See also LITHOTOMY.

Little's disease (lit′əlz) is a form of cerebral palsy in which the legs are particularly affected. It is often accompanied by epilepsy, writhing movements of the limbs (athetosis), and mental retardation. The condition is named after the English physician, William Little.

See also CEREBRAL PALSY.

Liver is the largest and one of the most complex organs in the body. The liver gland lies in the right upper side of the abdomen under the diaphragm and ribs, and it extends across to the left side of the body, overlying the upper part of the stomach. The gall bladder and its ducts lie beneath the right side of the liver.

The liver consists of four sections, or lobes. There are two main lobes: the right lobe, which is by far the larger, and the left lobe. Two smaller lobes lie behind the right lobe. Each lobe is composed of multisided units called lobules. Most livers have between 50,000 and 100,000 lobules. Each lobule consists of a central vein surrounded by tiny liver cells grouped together. These cells perform the work of the liver.

In an average adult male, the liver weighs about 4 pounds (1.8k); it is somewhat smaller in women (1.3k). The liver is reddish-brown and has a soft, solid texture. It is covered by a tough, fibrous peritoneum. Between 2 and 3 pints of blood (about 25 percent of the total blood supply of the body) pass through the liver on the way to the heart each minute.

Q: *What are the functions of the liver?*

A: The liver probably performs more separate functions that any other organ in the body. Its primary functions are to help purify the blood of wastes and poisons and to help the body digest and store nutrients. For example, the cells of the liver process digested food, converting much of it into substances the body requires and storing the rest for future use. In this way, the sugar glucose is converted into glycogen and stored in the liver until the body needs extra energy.

The liver stores vitamins (except vitamin C) until they are required, and its reserves can last for many months. Iron and several other minerals are also stored in the liver. Liver cells also manufacture proteins and lipids.

Liver cells not only deal with food that has been digested but also recycle various substances, such as hemoglobin, that are needed by the body. In addition, the liver destroys many poisonous substances that may be absorbed into the body and acts as an organ of excretion. For example, alcohol, barbiturates, and other drugs are broken down in the liver. Bile salts and bilirubin are formed and pass into the bile ducts, to be excreted into the duodenum or stored in the gall bladder. Unwanted proteins are destroyed and changed into urea, which is carried in the bloodstream to the kidneys and excreted in the urine. Additionally, the liver also manufactures proteins that are required for clotting of the blood.

All these metabolic processes produce a considerable amount of heat that helps to maintain the body's normal temperature.

See also BILE; BILIRUBIN; DIGESTIVE SYSTEM; LIVER DISORDERS.

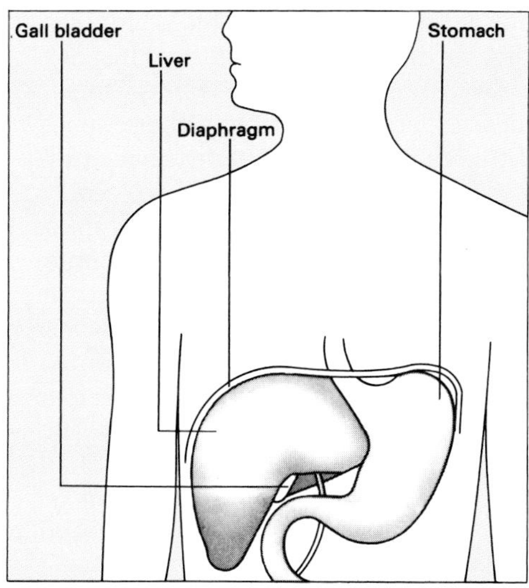

The **liver,** partially protected by the ribcage, lies just below the diaphragm.

Liver disorders are injuries or illnesses that affect the liver, the organ in the body most responsible for purifying the blood and aiding in the digestion and processing of food. Because the liver is one of the most complex organs in the body, it is susceptible to a wide variety of disorders including alcoholism, infection, poisoning, cancer, metabolic abnormalities, and obstructions. Many disorders do not produce any symptoms unless they have reached an advanced stage because the liver has a remarkable ability to regenerate itself following injury, and it has large nutrient reserves that can be used if it is damaged.

Usually, pain does not occur with liver disorders. Instead, the first symptom of many disorders is jaundice, which occurs when the bile pigment, bilirubin, accumulates in the blood. This may be caused by an inability of the liver to metabolize bilirubin or by an obstruction of the flow of bile from the liver to the intestines.

Abdominal swelling, resulting from fluid in the peritoneum (ascites), may be caused by obstruction of the hepatic portal vein. Such obstruction may also cause varicose veins to form at the lower end of the esophagus and burst, causing blood to be vomited (hematemesis) and blood in the feces (melena). The sudden blood loss and influx of protein into the intestines may cause hepatic encephalopathy. Other causes of this disorder include cirrhosis and acute viral hepatitis, caused by viral infection or poisoning. The symptoms include confusion; flapping movements of the hands; and lack of coordination (ataxia). Infection of the liver may also cause the organ to become swollen and may produce a dull ache in the upper right portion of the abdomen. Liver infections, such as those caused by acute viral hepatitis, can be quite serious, with a patient lapsing into a potentially fatal coma.

Cancerous liver tumors are usually the result of a spread of cancer from other parts of the body (metastasis). Occasionally, a primary tumor, called a hepatoma, may occur in the liver. Hepatomas are usually associated with cirrhosis, caused either by alcoholism or a nutritional deficiency.

See also BUDD-CHIARI SYNDROME; CHOLANGITIS; CIRRHOSIS; CYST, HYDATID; HEPATITIS; LIVER.

Liver fluke. *See* FLUKE.

Living will is a written statement drawn up in advance of severe illness by a healthy adult. The document states that, in case he or she were to become terminally ill, the individual does not wish certain heroic medical procedures to be instigated to prolong his or her life, if there is no possibility of full recovery. The living will concept has been espoused by many people who perceive many life-support techniques as not only frequently painful and humiliating, but also as a means to artificially prolong the dying process, rather than to extend life. A phrase commonly used by supporters of this concept is "the right to die with dignity."

Many states now have "living will laws," the overall purpose of which is to establish clear guidelines to protect both the patient's wishes and rights and physicians from legal liability. Since mental competence may be questionable when the patient is seriously ill and under the influence of drugs, the living will document, which has been signed in advance, clearly sets out the patient's wishes.

Loa loa (lo'ä lo'ä), or loiasis, is a form of filariasis, a condition in which there are microparasites in the blood and tissues. It is transmitted by the bites of flies of the genus *Chrysops*, which occur in central and western Africa. Loa loa causes temporary swellings, known as Calabar swellings, as the adult parasites move in the tissues under the skin.

See also FILARIASIS.

Lobectomy (lō bek'tə mē) is the surgical removal of a lobe from any organ, usually of the lung. A lung lobectomy is sometimes performed in order to remove a malignant (cancerous) tumor.

Lobotomy (lō bot'ə mē) is a surgical incision into the rounded, projecting part (lobe) of an organ. The term usually refers to a psychosurgical operation known in full as a prefrontal lobotomy, in which nerve fibers leading to the frontal lobes of the brain are severed. The operation may be performed in the treatment of severe forms of mental illness, such as schizophrenia and obsessive or compulsive neuroses. But it is done only for the most disabling disorders and only after all other forms of treatment have failed.

Prefrontal lobotomy may cause adverse and irreversible side effects, such as a personality change and a blunting of the emotions. With the development of modern psychotherapeutic drugs, the operation is now extremely rare and is illegal in many parts of the United States.

Lochia (lō'kē ə) is the vaginal discharge that occurs for several weeks following childbirth. During the first few days the discharge is mainly bright, red blood that gradually becomes reddish-brown in color, and then brownish-yellow. After the third week, the discharge becomes greyish-white, and the amount of lochia decreases sharply; it ceases completely soon after.

Lockjaw. *See* TETANUS.

Locomotor ataxia (lō kə mō'tər ə tak'sē ə), or tabes dorsalis, is a degenerative disease of the spinal cord that is characterized by a loss of control over walking and certain other voluntary movements and by severe pains in the legs or abdomen. It is most commonly associated with advanced syphilis.

See also SYPHILIS; TABES DORSALIS.

Logorrhea (lȯg ə rē'ə), or logomania, is an extremely rapid, often unintelligible, speech pattern over which the speaker seems to have little or no control. In a mild form, logorrhea may occur with anxiety. But in a more serious form, obsessive talkativeness is a symptom of mania and, occasionally, schizophrenia.

See also MANIA; SCHIZOPHRENIA.

Lorazepam (lor a′zē pam) is a minor tranquilizer that is prescribed to treat acute anxiety or insomnia. Side effects include drowsiness and loss of muscular coordination (ataxia). These side effects tend to increase with the age of the patient. Lorazepam should not be taken by pregnant or nursing women or children under the age of 12. It is normally not recommended for patients suffering from certain types of glaucoma. Prolonged use, especially by elderly patients, should be avoided. If absolutely necessary, such use must be closely monitored by a physician.

Lordosis (lôr dō′sis) is the curvature of the lumbar and cervical spine. The term is also used to refer to any condition characterized by an excessive curvature of the spine, with the bend towards the front (hollow back, saddle back, and sway back). Lordosis affects the lumbar region (between the ribs and the pelvis) and is the opposite of kyphosis, or hunchback.

Q: *What causes lordosis?*

A: Lordosis commonly occurs in obese people with weak back muscles and heavy abdomens. It may also develop in pregnant women.

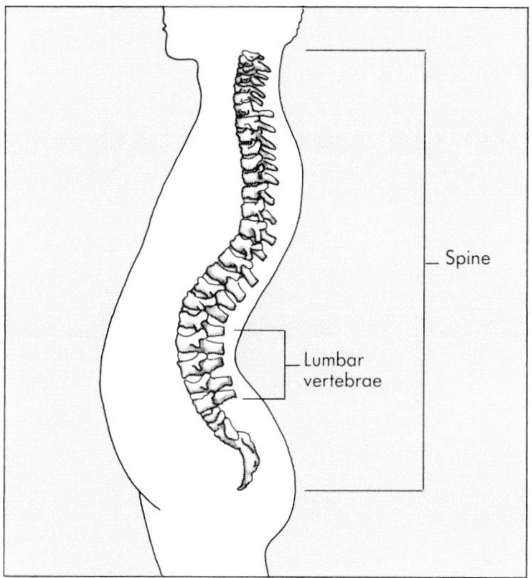

Lordosis is an excessive curvature of the spine in the lumbar region, the area between the ribs and the pelvis.

The deformity can occur when a person with kyphosis, an abnormal condition of the spinal column at the back of the chest, excessively straightens his or her spine. Any hip deformity, such as that caused by osteoarthritis, tends to make the body lean forward, which may also produce lordosis.

Q: *How is lordosis treated?*

A: Treatment must be directed toward the cause. This is the only way to encourage the spine to return to its normal shape.

See also KYPHOSIS; SCOLIOSIS; SPINAL CURVATURE; SPINE.

Loss of appetite. *See* APPETITE.

Loss of hair. *See* ALOPECIA; BALDNESS.

Loss of hearing. *See* DEAFNESS; EAR DISORDERS.

Loss of memory. *See* AMNESIA; MEMORY DISORDERS.

Loss of sensation. *See* NUMBNESS.

Loss of sight. *See* BLINDNESS.

Loss of weight. *See* DIET, SPECIAL; WEIGHT LOSS.

Lou Gehrig's disease. *See* AMYOTROPHIC LATERAL SCLEROSIS.

Low blood pressure. *See* HYPOTENSION.

Low blood sugar. *See* HYPOGLYCEMIA.

LPN. *See* NURSE, LICENSED PRACTICAL.

LSD. *See* LYSERGIC ACID DIETHYLAMIDE.

Lues. *See* SYPHILIS.

Lumbago. *See* BACK PAIN.

Lump is any abnormal swelling. Most lumps are benign (noncancerous), but some are malignant (cancerous). For this reason, anyone with a persistent, unexplained lump should consult a physician without delay.

See also CYST; FIBROMA; GANGLION; HERNIA; LIPOMA; NEUROMA; OSTEOMA; TUMOR; VON RECKLINGHAUSEN'S DISEASE.

Lumpectomy (lum pek′tə mē) is the surgical removal of a tumor or lump, with minimal disturbance to the surrounding tissue. A lumpectomy is one of the surgical procedures used in the treatment of certain breast cancers. In this procedure, only the tumor or lump located on the breast is removed, leaving the surrounding tissue undisturbed.

See also LUMP.

Lumpy jaw. *See* JAW, LUMPY.

Lung is the organ concerned with respiration. There are two lungs sited within the thorax (chest cavity), a protective cage formed by the ribs and breastbone in front and the ribs and spine at the back. Between the lungs lie the heart,

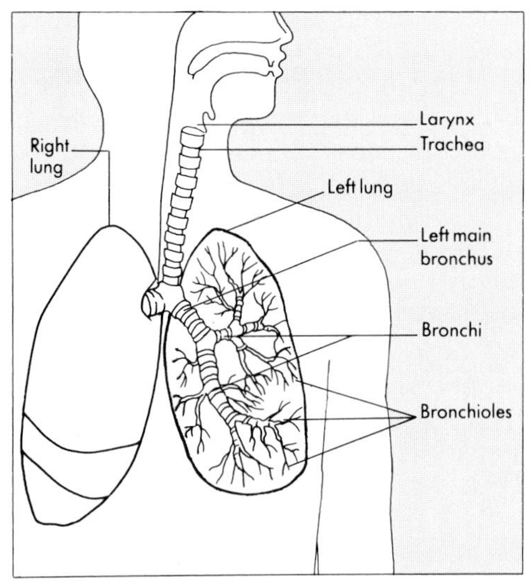

Each **lung** is filled with many bronchi and bronchioles, through which oxygen passes on its way to the bloodstream and carbon dioxide passes to be exhaled.

major blood vessels, and the esophagus.

Air enters the body through the nose and mouth and passes into the throat. From there it enters the larynx and then into the trachea (windpipe), which divides into two main bronchi, each of which leads to a lung.

Inside the lungs, oxygen from freshly breathed air enters the bloodstream. At the same time, carbon dioxide leaves the blood and enters the lungs to be breathed out.

Q: *What is the internal structure of the lungs?*

A: The right lung, consisting of three lobes, is slightly larger than the left lung, which has only two lobes. Each lobe is further divided into segments.

As the two main bronchi enter the lungs, they divide into five narrower bronchi, one for each lobe. These bronchi then divide and subdivide into narrower and narrower tubes, called bronchioles. The bronchioles terminate in tiny and extremely thin-walled air sacs called alveoli. The oxygen-carbon dioxide exchange takes place here through the moist walls of the alveoli. Oxygen passes from the alveoli into the surrounding fine blood vessels, called capillaries. Carbon dioxide passes from these capillaries back into the alveoli and is breathed out.

The lungs and the inner surface of the thorax are covered by a thin membrane called the pleura. A small amount of lubricating fluid on the pleura permits the lungs and ribcage to move against each other without friction.

The bronchi and bronchioles are lined with cells that keep them moist. These cells have small hair-like projections that sweep mucus and debris up toward the trachea and eventually to the throat.

See also LUNG DISORDERS; RESPIRATION; RESPIRATORY SYSTEM.

Lung cancer. *See* CANCER.

Lung, collapsed. Collapsed lung is a condition in which a section of lung contains no air. It may occur if there is an obstruction by a tumor or foreign body in a bronchus or if air enters the pleural cavity that surrounds the lung and compresses the lung.

See also ATELECTASIS; PNEUMOTHORAX.

Lung disorders are also called pulmonary disorders. The lungs have great reserves of capacity for air. Disorders of slow onset may therefore not cause symptoms until they have progressed for some time and caused considerable damage.

Disorders of the lung include those affecting the trachea and the bronchi, which are tubes that carry air in and out of the lungs; the bronchioles, which are the narrower tubes within the lungs; the alveoli, where the exchange of oxygen and carbon dioxide takes place; the interstitial tissue, which is the connective tissue surrounding the alveoli; the surrounding pleura and ribcage (thorax); and the blood vessels. Each of the following disorders has a separate article in this encyclopedia.

Area affected	*Possible disorder*
Trachea and bronchi	BRONCHIECTASIS (dilation of bronchi)
	BRONCHITIS
	CANCER (of the bronchus)
	CROUP (inflammation of the windpipe and bronchial tubes)
	TRACHEITIS (inflammation of the windpipe)
Bronchioles	ASTHMA
	BRONCHIOLITIS (viral lung infection of infants)
	CYSTIC FIBROSIS (formation of abnormally sticky mucus)

Area affected	*Possible disorder*
Alveoli	ACTINOMYCOSIS (fungal infection of the lung)
	ATELECTASIS (collapsed lung)
	CANCER (of the lung)
	EMPHYSEMA (destruction and enlargement of lung's air sacs)
Interstitial tissue	FUNGAL INFECTION
	PNEUMOCONIOSIS (inflammation of the lung caused by inhaling dust)
	PNEUMONIA
	SARCOIDOSIS
	TUBERCULOSIS
Pleura and thorax	CANCER (of the lung)
	EMPYEMA (pus in the pleural fluid)
	HEMOTHORAX (blood in the pleural fluid)
	PLEURISY (infection of the pleura)
	PLEURODYNIA, EPIDEMIC (Bornholm disease, a virus disorder)
	PNEUMOTHORAX (air in the pleural cavity)
	TIETZE'S SYNDROME (inflammation of the cartilage)
	TUBERCULOSIS
Blood vessels	EMBOLISM (blockage of a pulmonary artery)

Lung function test. Pulmonary function tests assess the condition and functioning of the lungs. There are a number of such tests used to investigate respiratory disorders. The various tests help a physician to diagnose a condition and determine its severity. They may also establish whether a particular treatment is effective. Some lung function tests can be performed using simple equipment, such as a spirometer, which measures the volume of air breathed in and out, or a peak flow meter. Other tests, such as the analysis of gases in exhaled air and the measurement of oxygen and carbon dioxide levels in the blood, require sophisticated equipment and a detailed analysis of the results.

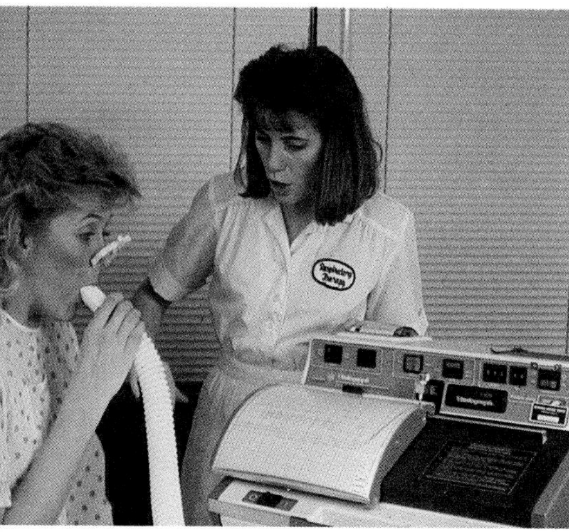

A **lung function test** can be given using a spirometer, which measures the volume of air breathed in and out.

Lung machine. *See* HEART-LUNG MACHINE.

Lupus erythematosus (lü′pəs er ə them ə tō′sis), one of a group of disorders known as the collagen diseases, takes two distinct but unrelated forms: discoid lupus erythematosus (DLE) and systemic lupus erythematosus (SLE). Both conditions affect the skin. SLE, also known as disseminated lupus erythematosus, involves other tissues and organs as well. It is purportedly an autoimmune disease. *See also* AUTOIMMUNE DISEASE.

Collagen is a fibrous, insoluble protein in connective tissue. Both DLE and SLE affect the connective tissue, but are of unknown cause or causes. It is often difficult to distinguish between the two conditions. Much confusion has arisen because the skin lesions are the same in both diseases. Other features, though, are completely distinctive.

Q: *What are the symptoms of DLE?*

A: DLE is a chronic skin disorder that occurs most commonly in middle-aged women. It produces thickened, slightly scaly, reddened patches on the face, cheeks, and forehead. The characteristic is known as "butterfly rash." The patches sometimes spread to the scalp and cause hair loss. Sunlight makes the condition worse, so in some patients it virtually disappears during the winter months. Nearly all patients with DLE remain in good health apart from the skin disorder. It is exceptionally rare for patients with DLE to develop SLE.

Q: *How is chronic DLE treated?*
A: Patients with DLE should wear hats and sunlight barrier creams to protect their skins. Also, corticosteroid skin creams may be helpful, but should be used only under medical supervision. Ultimately, some of the lesions heal on their own.

In severe cases, chloroquine (a drug used to treat malaria) may be beneficial. But, because chloroquine sometimes has an effect on the eyes, it should be used with great caution.

Q: *What are the symptoms of SLE?*
A: The patient may have the same kind of butterfly rash as in DLE. There may also be fever, arthritis, and signs of problems with lung, kidney, and heart function.

Unlike DLE, SLE is a generalized condition that may affect not only the face, but also many other tissues of the body, especially the kidneys.

Q: *How is SLE diagnosed and treated?*
A: A knowledge of the patient's history combined with discovery of abnormalities in blood tests will help diagnosis. Treatment with corticosteroids may help.

Lyme disease (lim) is a bacterial infection caused by the bacterium *Borrelia burgdorferi*. It is transmitted by the bite of certain ticks that are carried on the bodies of animals, especially white-tailed deer and white-footed field mice and other small rodents. The disease causes serious problems involving the skin, joints, nervous system, heart, and eyes. It is most common in the Northeast and upper Great Lakes.

Lyme disease progresses through three stages. In the earliest stage, within several weeks after a person is bitten, a red rash (erythema migrans) appears. The rash is circular, resembling a bull's-eye. Also at this stage, several lesions may develop on the body, often accompanied by headache, chills, fever, body aches, joint pains, and fatigue. In weeks to years, the later stages can produce many other problems, including Bell's palsy (facial paralysis), encephalitis, heart problems, and disabling arthritis attacks. *See also* BELL'S PALSY; TICK.

Q: *Is Lyme disease difficult to diagnose?*
A: Yes. There are several reasons why this is so: (1) many victims don't remember being bitten by a tick; (2) 20 to 40 percent of the victims don't get the erythema migrans rash; (3) the disease resembles many other different problems; (4) although blood tests for diagnosing Lyme disease have improved, these tests still aren't foolproof.

Q: *What is the treatment for Lyme disease?*
Q: Lyme disease can be effectively treated by several types of antibiotics, such as penicillin, tetracycline, and ceftraxone. However, there is still controversy over the question of which drug, how it should be taken (orally or intravenously), and how long the treatment should last.

Lymph (limf) is the clear fluid that is drained from around the body's cells into the lymphatic system. It carries away bacteria and waste products.

See also LYMPHATIC SYSTEM.

Lymphadenitis (lim fad ə nī′tis) is inflammation of a lymph node, which causes it to swell. It is a normal reaction to any nearby infection. For example, an infection of the upper respiratory tract is accompanied by swelling of the tonsillar glands and other glands in the neck.

See also LYMPH NODE.

Lymphadenoma (lim fad ə nō′mə) is a malignant (cancerous) tumor that affects the lymph nodes.

See also HODGKIN'S DISEASE; LYMPH NODE.

Lymphangiectasia, intestinal (lim fan jē ek tā′zhə). Intestinal lymphangiectasia is a disorder in which the body does not absorb protein or fat normally. It is characterized by diarrhea, vomiting, and pain in the abdomen. Intestinal lymphangiectasia is either present at birth or acquired as a side effect of another disorder, such as pancreatitis.

See also PANCREATITIS.

Lymphangitis (lim fan jī′tis) is inflammation of the lymphatic vessels. It occurs, to a certain extent, with lymphadenitis. It may also be caused by a serious infection of the skin, such as a septic wound, in which red lines can be seen in the skin running from the wound to the nearest lymph nodes. This is a serious sign and requires urgent medical treatment.

See also BLOOD POISONING; LYMPHADENITIS.

Lymphatic leukemia. *See* LEUKEMIA.

Lymphatic system (lim fat′ik) is a network of thin-walled vessels found throughout the body. They drain fluid (lymph) from between the body cells into the bloodstream. The lymph vessels contain small valves, similar to those in veins, which prevent the backflow of lymph.

Rounded bean-shaped structures, called lymph nodes, are situated at frequent intervals along the lymph vessels. Major lymph nodes occur in the groin, armpits, and neck and alongside the aorta and inferior vena cava in the chest and abdomen.

Most of the lymph vessels eventually converge to form the thoracic duct, a major lymph vessel that runs alongside the descending aorta. The thoracic duct connects with the left subclavian vein (a main branch of the superior vena cava) at a point above and slightly to the left of the heart.

Lymphatic vessels are important to the mechanism by which fats are processed by the body. Vessels draining the small intestine collect the digested fat and pass it directly into the main blood circulation, bypassing the liver.

See also LYMPH; LYMPH NODE

The lymphatic system

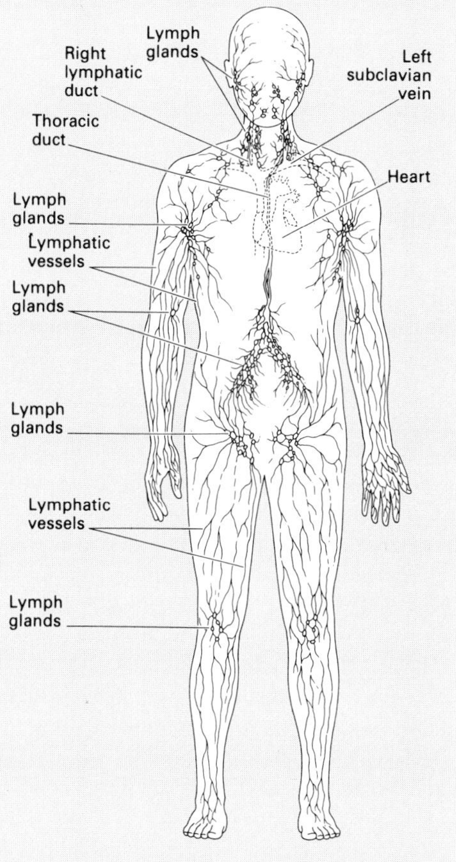

The **lymphatic system** is a body-wide network of vessels that drain fluid (lymph) from body cells into the bloodstream.

Lymphedema (lim fi dē′mə) is a chronic edema (swelling caused by excess fluid retention) of the extremities. It may be either primary or secondary.

The primary type is either present at birth (congenital lymphedema, also called Milroy's disease); or may occur in adolescent girls and young women (lymphedema praecox); or in middle age (lymphedema tarda). It is caused by hyperplasia (increase) of the lymph vessels and is more common in women than in men. *See also* MILROY'S DISEASE.

Secondary lymphedema is usually the result of infection; malignancy blocking the lymphatic system; or lack of lymph vessels after surgery, for example, lymphedema of the arm after radical mastectomy.

Lymphedema is aggravated in hot weather, when the limb is allowed to hang down unsupported so that the lymph collects in the extremity, and before menstruation.

Treatment consists of elevating the foot of the bed slightly when resting or sleeping to improve lymph drainage; wearing a tight stocking or bandage; and taking precautions against skin infections because any resultant scarring may be increased by the swelling. Operations to remove the swollen tissues are seldom successful.

Diuretics may be of some help in lessening the edema; spicy, salty foods should be avoided, since they increase thirst and, therefore, fluid intake into the body.

See also LYMPH; LYMPHATIC SYSTEM.

Lymph gland. *See* LYMPH NODE.

Lymph node (nōd) is a small bean-shaped structure that forms part of the lymphatic system. Lymph nodes are found throughout the body, particularly in places where lymph vessels unite.

The lymph nodes have three main functions: (1) to filter out and destroy foreign substances, such as bacteria and dust; (2) to produce some of the white blood cells called lymphocytes; and (3) to produce antibodies to help in the body's immune system.

Specialized lymphoid tissue, similar to lymph nodes, includes the tonsils, adenoids, appendix, spleen, and areas of the body such as the Peyer's patches in the wall of the small intestine.

See also LYMPH; LYMPHATIC SYSTEM.

Lymphocyte (lim'fə sīt) is one type of white blood cell. Lymphocytes are made in the lymph nodes, bone marrow, and thymus gland. They are concerned with the formation of antibodies and are major components in the body's immune system.

See also BLOOD CELL, WHITE; IMMUNITY; LEUKEMIA.

Lymphocytopenia (lim fō sī tə pē'nē ə) is an abnormally smaller number of lymphocytes, due to disease, infection, or cancer.

See also LYMPHOCYTE.

Lymphogranuloma venereum (lim fō gran yə lō'mə və nir'ē əm), LGV, is a sexually transmitted disease caused by chlamydia, organisms related to those that cause psittacosis and trachoma. Symptoms include enlargement of the lymph nodes in the groin.

See also SEXUALLY TRANSMITTED DISEASE.

Lymphoid system (lim'foid) is the collection of tissues in the body consisting of the thymus, marrow of the bone, spleen, lymph nodes, and other lymphoid tissues.

See also LYMPH NODE; LYMPHOID TISSUE; SPLEEN; THYMUS.

Lymphoid tissue (lim'foid) is the tissue that forms most of the lymph nodes and the thymus gland. It consists of connective tissue containing lymphocytes.

See also LYMPH NODE; LYMPHOCYTE; THYMUS.

Lymphoma (lim fō'mə) is any form of growth connected with lymphoid tissue. A growth of this kind occurs, for example, with Hodgkin's disease.

See also HODGKIN'S DISEASE; LYMPHOSARCOMA.

Lymphosarcoma (lim fō sär kō mə) is a kind of malignant (cancerous) growth connected with lymphoid tissue. The symptoms are very similar to those of lymphatic leukemia.

See also LEUKEMIA.

Lysergic acid diethylamide (lī sėr'jik as'id dī eth ə lam'īd), commonly known as LSD, is a drug that, even in minute doses, produces disturbances in the autonomic nervous system and the brain. It may produce apprehension, hallucinations, and various states of anxiety and depression. Persons who take LSD claim that it may also produce elation and heightened perception.

One possible result of taking LSD is a flashback. This is an episode in which an unpleasantness, experienced while on LSD, is later reproduced when the person has not taken the drug, with all the upsetting symptoms of the original experience. For example, a person on LSD may become frightened in a crowd, and he or she may later feel exactly the same when in a crowd again, even though the drug had not been taken.

LSD is not an addictive drug. But experimenting with it is dangerous, especially for those who are not mentally or emotionally stable. Long-term damage can occur. Some LSD takers have developed a persistent psychosis.

LSD has been used medically in psychological research into various forms of mental illness, such as psychotic disorders, as well as in the treatment of chronic alcoholism.

See also DRUG ADDICTION; HALLUCINOGEN.

Lysosome (li'sə sōm) is a part of the cell containing the enzyme lysozyme, which is involved in the process of digestion within the cell.

See also CELL.

Lysozyme (lī'sə zīm) is an enzyme that is capable of destroying some types of bacteria. It is found in certain blood cells, including monocytes and neutrophils, and is usually present in egg white and most body fluids.

See also BLOOD CELL, WHITE; LYSOSOME.

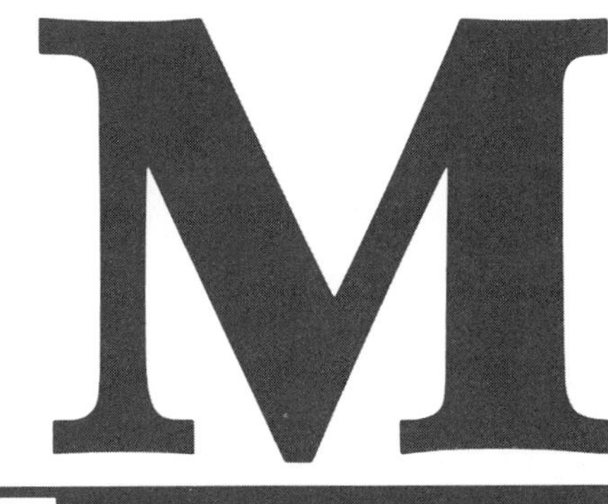

Macula (mak′yə lə) is a spot or a flat blemish on the skin. The term macula often refers to the area of the retina (macula retinae) where vision is sharpest. The macula retinae has the highest concentration of nerve endings in the eye.

See *also* MACULAR DEGENERATION.

Macular degeneration (mak′yə lər) is an eye disorder caused by the degeneration of the retinal macula, the area of the eye where vision is the sharpest. It is a major cause of vision impairment among the elderly. The disorder hampers central vision, but peripheral vision is unimpaired. Macular degeneration is painless; vision impairment may be slow or rapid. There is no known cause. One type of macular degeneration can be partially controlled by laser treatments.

See *also* MACULA.

Madura foot. See MADUROMYCOSIS.

Maduromycosis (mə dü rō mī kō′sis) is a chronic fungus infection that occurs most commonly when fungi spores enter a wound in the foot.

Magnesia, milk of (mag nē′shə). Milk of magnesia is a suspension of magnesium hydroxide in water. It is used as a mild laxative or antacid.

See *also* ANTACID; LAXATIVE.

Magnesium sulfate (mag nē′shē əm sul′fāt), commonly known as Epsom salts, is generally used as a laxative and, when dissolved in water, as a soaking solution.

See *also* LAXATIVE.

Magnesium trisilicate (mag nē′shē əm trī sil′ə kit) is a chemical compound of magnesium oxide, silicon dioxide, and water. It is used as an antacid in various preparations for treating indigestion.

Magnetic resonance imaging (mag net′ik rez′ə nəns im′ij ing), MRI, is part of a relatively new breed of imaging techniques or scanners that enable medical professionals to see deep within the human body in a noninvasive way, that is, without entering the body or breaking the skin.

The system consists of a series of powerful electromagnets in the shape of a large tube, which surrounds the patient, enveloping him or her in a powerful magnetic field.

The system enables medical professionals to see inside the body by making use of the body's natural chemistry. Since the body contains abundant amounts of hydrogen, an element that has prominent magnetic qualities, the scanner is able to excite the protons of the hydrogen atoms in such a way that they transmit faint radio signals. The signals are then read by a computer and converted into a very detailed image.

The advantage of MRI over past imaging techniques is that by using magnetism instead of X rays, MRI avoids exposing patients to ionizing radiation.

Maidenhead. See HYMEN.

Malabsorption syndrome (mal ab sôrp′shən) is a group of disorders involving impaired intestinal absorption of dietary nutrients resulting in loss of nutrients through the stool. Symptoms include anorexia, weight loss, bloating, cramps, bone pain, abnormal stools, and diarrhea. Anemia, weakness, and fatigue may also result due to loss of vitamins and minerals.

Many conditions can cause malabsorption, including a digestive enzyme defect, celiac disease, tropical sprue, cystic fibrosis, or a lymphatic obstruction. Treatment is determined by the underlying cause.

See *also* CELIAC DISEASE; MALNUTRITION; SPRUE.

Malaise (ma lāz′) is a vague feeling of weakness and fatigue, often indicating the onset of an illness.

Malaria (ma lăr′ē ə) is a serious disease caused when a parasitic single-celled organism, called *Plasmodium*, enters

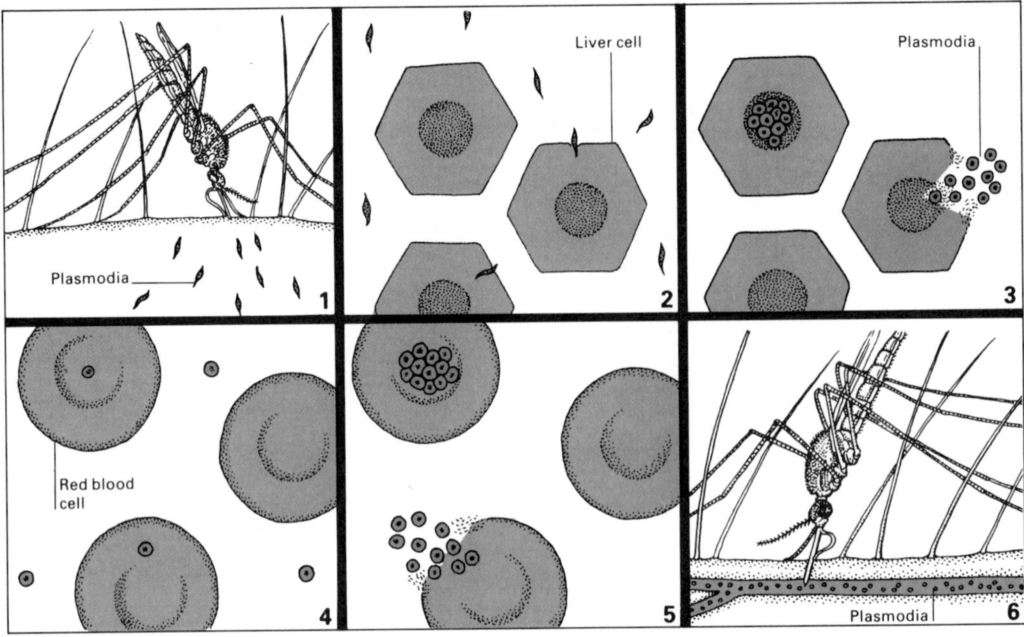

The life cycle of the malaria parasite

An infected mosquito injects *Plasmodia* with its bite (1). Each *Plasmodium* then invades a liver cell and multiplies (2). The cell then bursts, releasing a new form of *Plasmodia* (3). Each new *Plasmodium* then enters a red blood cell and multiplies (4). The cell then ruptures, and *Plasmodia* invades more red blood cells (5). Some *Plasmodia* develop into a form that infects other mosquitoes (6).

the red blood cells. It is transmitted by the *Anopheles* mosquito. The most severe form of malaria is called malignant tertian malaria (because in many cases the symptoms recur every three days). It is caused by the parasite *Plasmodium falciparum*. The other three, milder forms of malaria are caused by *P. vivax*, *P. ovale*, and *P. malariae*.

Mosquitoes carrying malaria are found in tropical and subtropical climates. Therefore, a person who is planning to travel in such regions should contact a physician. The physician can inform the patient if malaria is endemic in the region, and if so, the physician can prescribe medication to reduce the risk of contracting the disease.

Q: *What are the symptoms of malaria?*

A: After an incubation period of two to five weeks, there is a sudden attack of shivering followed by a high fever of at least 104°F (40°C). This is often accompanied by confusion, headache, and vomiting that lasts for several hours. These symptoms may occur at intervals of two to three days, depending on the type of malaria, and, if the disease is not treated, they will recur at irregular intervals for many years.

Q: *How is malaria diagnosed and treated?*

A: The diagnosis is made by examination of a blood sample, which reveals the presence of malarial parasites.

Initial treatment is with the drug chloroquine. Unfortunately, *P. falciparum*, the most dangerous cause of malaria, is often resistant to chloroquine and many other drugs.

See also CHLOROQUINE.

Male pattern baldness. *See* BALDNESS.

Malignancy (mə lig′nən sē) describes any condition or disorder that is dangerous and has a tendency to become worse. For example, a cancer is a malignant growth. The opposite of malignant is benign.

Malleus (mal′ē əs) is one of the three small ossicles or bones in the middle ear. It is shaped somewhat like a hammer.

See also INCUS; STAPES.

Mallory-Weiss syndrome (mal′ō rē-wīs) is a tear in the mucous membrane where the esophagus (gullet) meets the stomach. This results in massive bleeding. It is usually caused by prolonged vomiting or retching. Surgery is often necessary to stop the bleeding.

Malnutrition (mal nü trish′ən) describes the physical deterioration of the body caused by an inadequate or inappropriate diet or by disorders in which the body fails to absorb nutrients.

See also ANOREXIA NERVOSA; KWASHIORKOR; MARASMUS; NUTRITION; SPRUE.

Malocclusion (mal ə klü′zhən) is the failure of the teeth of the upper and lower jaws to meet correctly. It may cause problems with biting and chewing but can usually be corrected with a brace on the teeth and proper orthodontic care.

See also DENTAL DISORDERS; ORTHODONTICS; TOOTH.

Malpractice insurance. See INSURANCE, MALPRACTICE.

Malpresentation (mal prez en tā'shən), or malposition, describes any abnormal position of a fetus in the uterus, possibly making natural childbirth difficult. The normal position of the fetus during labor is with the head downward in the mother's pelvis, and the back of the head (occiput) angled toward the front.

See also CESAREAN SECTION; PREGNANCY AND CHILDBIRTH.

Mammary glands (mam'ər ē), or breasts, are special glands that enlarge and develop on the chest of mature females. They are present but undeveloped in males. The glands contain lobules or sacs that secrete milk. The milk travels through ducts into the nipple of the breast where it is released for feeding the infant.

See also BREAST; LACTATION.

Mammogram (mam'ə gram) is an X-ray film of the breast tissue. A mammogram is commonly used to detect breast cancer in its early stages. Current medical recommendations are for all women to obtain a baseline mammogram between the ages of 35 and 40, to be followed by a mammogram every other year between the ages of 40 and 49, and annually after the age of 50. Women at high risk for breast cancer may need mammograms earlier in life or at more frequent intervals.

See also CANCER; THERMOGRAM.

Mammography. See MAMMOGRAM.

Mammoplasty (mam'ō plas tē) is an operation to reconstruct a breast after removal of a tumor or to change the size and shape of the breasts. In reduction mammoplasty, the breasts are made smaller by removing some tissue. To increase the size of the breasts, an immovable fluid-filled bag is implanted behind each breast.

See also SURGERY, COSMETIC.

Mandible (man'də bəl) is the lower jawbone.

See also JAW.

Mandibular joint syndrome (mandib'yə lər) is the degeneration of the joint in the lower jaw, resulting in pain and limited jaw movement.

See also TEMPOROMANDIBULAR JOINT DYSFUNCTION.

Mania (mā'nē ə) is a form of mental disorder characterized by emotional excitement and lack of self-control, often resulting in rapid, irregular speech and violent behavior.

See also DEPRESSION; MANIC-DEPRESSIVE ILLNESS.

Manic-depressive illness, or bipolar disorder, is a psychiatric disorder characterized by severe swings in mood from mania to depression. One mood phase may be predominant, phases may alternate, or they may be present at the same time.

Q: *How is manic-depressive illness treated?*

A: In severe forms of the disorder hospitalization is necessary, particularly in the depression that follows a manic phase. The patient's remorse at this time is so great that suicide may occur.

The controlled use of the medication lithium carbonate or lithium citrate often prevents recurrences of mania. When combined with an antidepressant drug, given on maintenance therapy, they help to lessen the mood swings of manic-depressive illness.

See also DEPRESSION; LITHIUM; MANIA.

Mantoux test (man tü') is a test for tuberculosis in which old tuberculin in a diluted mixture is injected between the layers of the skin. A positive reaction generally indicates that the person has been exposed to the disease and has developed an immunological response. A negative reaction normally indicates a lack of immune response; this usually suggests that the person has not been exposed to tuberculosis.

See also TINE TEST.

MAO inhibitor (monoamine oxidase inhibitor) is a drug that is used in the treatment of selected atypical depressions, particularly those unresponsive to other antidepressant drugs. Great care must be taken, however, to avoid adverse effects.

Q: *What adverse reactions can occur with the use of MAO inhibitors?*

A: Monoamine oxidase is an enzyme contained in the body that metabolizes and renders ineffective agents such as adrenaline, norepinephrine, and similar substances. MAO inhibitors slow the rate of metabolism of such substances and allow them to accumulate in the blood and tissues. Thus, in a patient taking an MAO inhibitor, any drug or food that contains adrenaline-like substances or that stimulates the body to form adrenaline may cause a sudden and dramatic rise in blood pressure. This results in a severe headache and the danger of rupturing a blood vessel, which in turn, may lead to a stroke. For this reason, a psychiatrist may be wary of prescribing such drugs to a patient with a history of stroke, high blood pressure, or heart or liver disease. Occasionally, however, an MAO inhibitor causes low blood pressure, fainting, and loss of consciousness to occur.

Other side effects include dry mouth, insomnia, nausea, dysuria (painful urination), and constipation.

Q: *What foods and drugs should a patient avoid if taking MAO inhibitors?*

A: Foods high in tyramine (a derivative of the amino acid tyrosine), such as aged cheeses, red wine, pickled herring, beer, and yogurt, are likely to interact with MAO inhibitors, causing a severe hypertensive episode. Therefore, patients taking MAO inhibitors should not consume any drug or food without first consulting a physician.

Marasmus (mə raz′məs) is a severe form of malnutrition and progressive emaciation usually occurring in young children, often in the first year of life. Marasmus is caused by an inadequate intake of both protein and calories. This is different than the form of malnutrition known as kwashiorkor, in which there is inadequate protein intake, but sufficient calories are ingested.

See also KWASHIORKOR.

Marfan syndrome (mär fän′) is a congenital and hereditary condition associated with skeletal, ocular (eye), and cardiovascular abnormalities. It is characterized by elongated bones, long, spider-like limbs, and other musculoskeletal disturbances. Alterations of the cardiovascular system, for example, dilatation of the ascending aorta, may occur, as well as eye disorders, such as dislocation of the lens. Treatment generally has not been successful and is thus limited to management of the associated problems.

Marijuana (mar ə wä′nə), also known as cannabis, is a drug made from the dried leaves or flowers of the hemp plant. It is usually smoked in cigarettes and is regarded as only mildly addictive. Other names for marijuana include hashish, grass, and pot. The possession or use of marijuana is illegal in most Western countries.

Q: *What are the effects of "taking" marijuana?*

A: Mild drowsiness is sometimes accompanied by an increased awareness of color, sounds, or taste, which fluctuates in accordance with complex mood changes. Occasionally, there may be the desire for increased physical activity and a feeling of immense cheerfulness.

Many persons who regularly smoke marijuana tend to become apathetic and may have difficulty in concentrating. Physical inertia is commonly accompanied by altered appetite, loss of weight, and a general lack of concern about physical appearance. Some individuals, however, experience few side effects.

Q: *Is there any harm in smoking marijuana?*

A: When marijuana is smoked infrequently by an otherwise well-adjusted individual there appears to

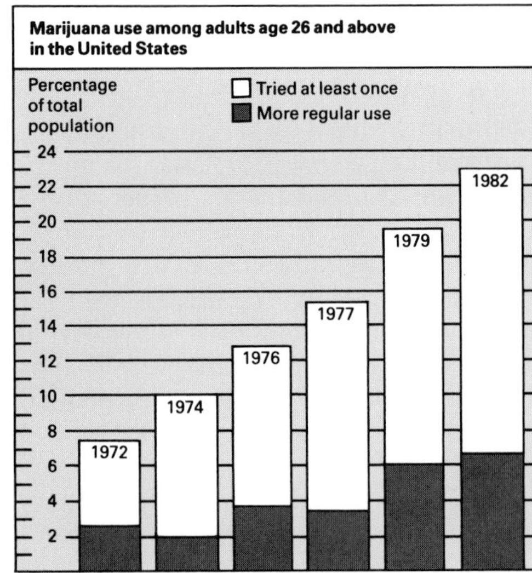

Of those who use **marijuana,** about one-third smoke it regularly and two-thirds infrequently.

be little harm. Marijuana may, however, be hazardous to the fetus and so should be avoided by pregnant women.

Continued, frequent use of marijuana, however, produces physical changes, and sometimes, a true state of addiction. Physical changes that may result include loss of weight, loss of sex drive, a reduced sperm count, and respiratory and cardiac disturbances.

Q: *Can the use of marijuana lead to other, more serious forms of drug abuse?*

A: An adolescent who experiments with marijuana even once has at least an eight percent risk of becoming a daily smoker. It is unlikely that an adolescent will try cocaine or hallucinogens without prior experimentation with marijuana.

See also DRUG ABUSE.

Marrow (mar′ō) is the soft, central portion of the bone. There are two types of marrow: red marrow, where blood elements are formed, and yellow marrow, where the majority of the marrow cavity is occupied by fat cells.

See also BONE.

Masochism (mas′ə kiz əm) is a psychiatric term for a feeling of sexual satisfaction derived from being hurt. It is named for the Austrian novelist von Sacher-Masoch. Masochism is manifested in many minor ways, for example, lovers' bites. In its more severe forms, however, such as whipping, it can cause physical harm and suffering. A physician may recommend psychiatric counseling.

See also SADISM.

Massage (mə säzh′) is a therapeutic treatment in which the muscles are rubbed and manipulated for the relief of local pain and for relaxation. It is often used to soothe sore or tense muscles. Massage also helps to increase the muscle tone after a long illness. The person who gives the massage should be well-trained and have a knowledge of human anatomy.

Mastectomy (mas tek′tə mē) is an operation to remove a breast. A partial mastectomy is the removal of one section of the breast; simple mastectomy is the removal of the whole breast; and radical mastectomy is the removal of the breast as well as some of the underlying muscle and the lymph nodes in the armpit. At present, radical mastectomy has been generally replaced by the modified radical mastectomy, in which the underlying muscle is not removed. There are fewer postoperative complications with this procedure and the results are more cosmetically appealing.

Q: *Why is a mastectomy performed?*

A: The operation is performed to remove breast tumors. Simple and radical mastectomies are performed as treatments for breast cancer, where the tumor is malignant and there is a danger of cancerous cells spreading to other parts of the body.

Q: *Is any further treatment given for breast cancer?*

A: Yes, sometimes, but this depends on the type and extent of the cancer. If the cancer is localized in the breast tissue, further treatment may not be required. Radiotherapy and chemotherapy are often used in conjunction with the operation if the cancer is more advanced.

Q: *What problems may occur after a mastectomy?*

A: Because fluid may gather under the wound, drainage tubes are normally left in place for a few days. Weakness and swelling of the arm may occur following a radical mastectomy. In addition to the physical discomfort associated with the operation, a woman may also face major psychological problems as a result of her change in body image. Frequently, a talk with another woman who has had the same operation can be most helpful. The woman's husband or partner is often also given counseling. Family and friends' understanding and reassurance will help to restore the woman's confidence.

Mastectomy, radical (mas tek′tə mē). Radical mastectomy is a surgical removal of the breast, some of the underlying chest muscles, and all of the lymph nodes in the armpit. This procedure is now rarely done; it has been replaced by the modified radical mastectomy, in which chest muscles are not removed. By leaving the underlying muscles, the modified radical mastectomy produces fewer complications for the patient.

See also MASTECTOMY.

Mastitis (mas tī′tis) is inflammation of the breast. It may be acute or chronic.

Q: *What causes acute mastitis?*

A: Acute mastitis is caused by an infection, which occurs most commonly during lactation after childbirth, when the breast is swollen with milk. Infection usually enters through a cracked nipple.

Q: *How is acute mastitis treated?*

A: If possible, breast-feeding should be continued, because this keeps the breast ducts clear. Firm bandaging of the breast and a reduction in the amount of fluid consumed help to reduce any excessive swelling (engorgement). A physician may prescribe antibiotic drugs and painkillers until the infection is under control. Application of warm compresses may also help.

Occasionally, these treatments fail and an abscess starts to form. In such cases, breast-feeding must be stopped and the abscess incised and drained.

Q: *What is chronic mastitis?*

A: Chronic mastitis is not an infection. It is caused by hormones in the body affecting the breast tissues, making them swollen and tender. Chronic mastitis occurs quite commonly just before a menstrual period. In women who suffer from premenstrual tension, it can last from several days to two weeks. Chronic mastitis frequently occurs in women who are approaching menopause. This form of the disorder ceases after menopause is complete.

Q: *How is chronic mastitis treated?*

A: A firm, well-fitting brassiere may be all that is necessary. If the discomfort persists, fluid-removing (diuretic) pills may be helpful. The regular use of hormones is sometimes necessary.

Mastoid (mas′toid) is a part of the temporal bone that is located behind the ear. The mastoid is filled with air cells arranged like a honeycomb that communicate with the middle ear.

See also MASTOIDITIS.

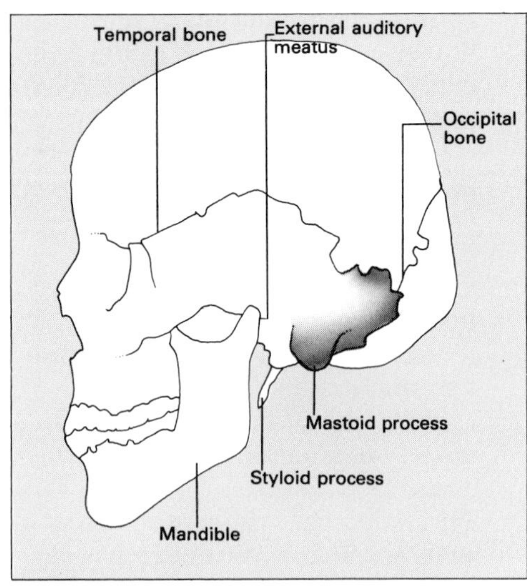

Mastoid is a part of the temporal bone that protrudes downward just behind and below the ear.

Mastoiditis (mas toi dī′tis) is an infection of the mastoid bone, located behind the ear. It is usually caused by the spread of an infection from the middle ear. The symptoms include fever, a throbbing earache, ringing in the ears, and reduced hearing. In some patients, the bone behind the ear may hurt, and the ear may discharge pus.

Treatment with antibiotic drugs cures most patients. Early treatment is essential to prevent damage to the mastoid bone. If bone damage has already occurred or if the infection does not respond to antibiotics, part of the mastoid bone may be surgically removed.

Masturbation (mas tər bā′shən) is the stimulation of one's own genitals to produce an orgasm.

Q: *Why do people masturbate?*

A: Masturbation is a normal activity when it reduces sexual tension when sexual intercourse is not possible or desirable. Small children are normally curious and explore their genital area. This exploration is normal, and the child should not be punished or shamed. Masturbation normally occurs during adolescence, both with boys and girls. Full sexual maturity and regular sexual intercourse reduce the need for, and the frequency of, masturbation. Masturbation continues, however, as a common outlet for sexual tension.

Q: *Is masturbation harmful?*

A: Masturbation is not harmful. There is absolutely no evidence to support theories that it causes physical problems. The anxiety and feelings of guilt aroused because a person feels that he or she is doing something wrong are much greater problems.

See also SEXUAL PROBLEMS.

Maxilla (mak sil′ə) is the upper jawbone. *See also* JAW.

Measles (mē′zelz), also known as rubeola, is a highly contagious viral disease that causes fever and a characteristic rash. It occurs most commonly before adolescence. One attack usually confers immunity for life. The incubation period varies between 8 and 14 days. Measles is contagious from approximately 4 days before until 5 days after the rash appears.

Q: *What are the symptoms of measles?*

A: The initial symptoms include fever, which may reach 104°F (40°C); a sore throat; red eyes; coughing; and a runny nose. These symptoms usually last for about 4 days. About 2 days before the rash breaks out, small white spots (Koplik's spots) may appear inside the mouth and eyelids. These usually fade when the rash appears. The characteristic rash of measles is blotchy and orange-red in color. It usually appears first behind the ears, then spreads to the face and neck. About 24 hours after its first appearance, the rash has usually affected the whole body. During the next 3 or 4 days, the rash and fever gradually disappear, although the cough may persist for an additional 10 to 14 days.

Q: *How is measles treated?*

A: There is no cure for measles. Treatment is directed at reducing the fever, preventing any complications from developing, and making the patient comfortable. The fever and cough may be helped with acetaminophen or similar drugs, a cough mixture, steam inhalations, and a vaporizer.

Q: *Can measles be prevented?*

A: Yes. A vaccine of a mild form of the measles virus will protect 97 percent of children against the disease. They should be vaccinated at the age of 12 to 15 months and again at 10 to 12 years of age.

Meckel's diverticulum. *See* DIVERTICULUM, MECKEL'S.

Meconium (mə kō′nē əm) is the greenish-brown, thick feces that an infant passes in the first few days following birth. It consists mainly of the bile and cell debris that a fetus ingests while in the uterus.

Medical bathing. *See* BATHS, MEDICINAL.

Medical education is the process by which a physician is trained. Only a limited number of applicants are accepted into medical schools each year. A four-year baccalaureate degree is required; the undergraduate curriculum generally should include special premedical courses in the sciences.

Medical school consists of four years of study involving preclinical training, composed of classes and book study, and clinical training, in which students observe and care for patients.

Following graduation from medical school, most physicians serve as hospital interns for a year, examining patients and prescribing treatment under the supervision of experienced physicians. The physician must train for two or more additional years as a hospital resident in a particular field of specialization. Examinations are required for a physician to become licensed to practice medicine and be certified in his or her specialty.

Medical education includes the study of anatomy and other basic medical sciences.

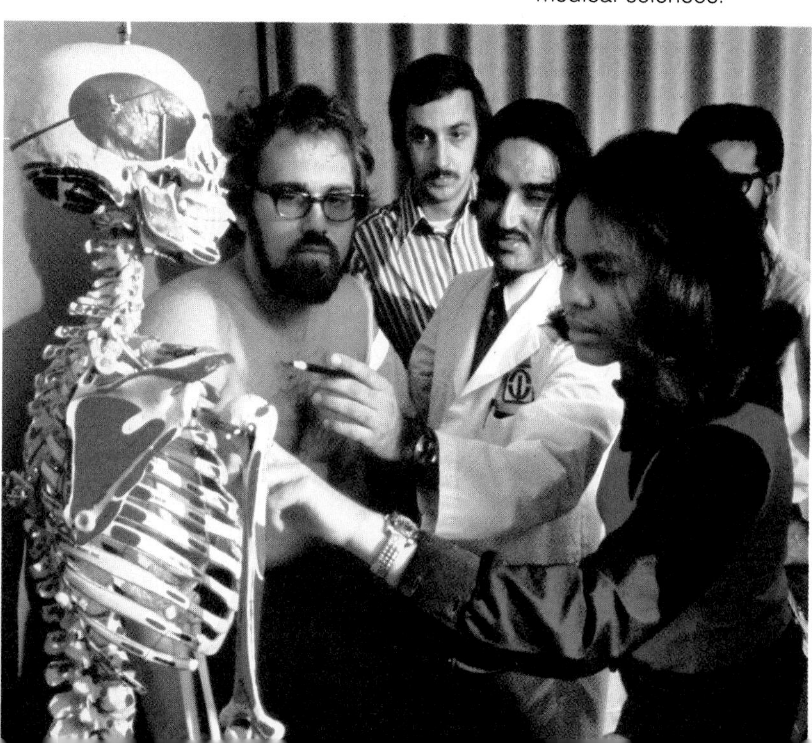

Medical ethics refer to the professional guidelines of a physician. These guidelines include the doctrine of serving patients in a caring and knowledgeable fashion, and such matters as charging reasonable fees and respecting a patient's confidence.

Modern medicine's ability to prolong life has raised ethical questions, such as those surrounding euthanasia (mercy killing) and turning off a life-support system in the case of a terminal disease.

Medical expenses and insurance are paid for by a variety of public and private means. Employed people most often obtain health insurance through their employer. There are also several public programs for financing the health care of the elderly, the disabled, the poor, the unemployed, and military personnel.

Q: *What points should be considered in choosing a private health plan?*

A: Since there are many types of health plans and different methods of payment (detailed below), it is generally a good idea to ask friends or people whose advice can be trusted which plan they are covered by, how they pay, and what medical services are provided. In this way, a general comparison of plans can be made, with some indication of advantages or disadvantages in regard to personal circumstances. Information about various plans is given below. Most health maintenance organizations are glad to provide more when contacted.

Any agreement form should be studied carefully. All the details should be fully understood by the person who is to sign. It is also preferable that other persons covered by the same agreement (if there are any) should be aware of the details. In particular, it is essential to know exactly what services are included or excluded, how the appropriate charges are made, and what the out-of-pocket costs are likely to be.

Q: *What are the different kinds of payment plans?*

A: Payment is made directly in one or more of these ways:

(1) Exclusion or maximum plan. The patient pays for those services received that are specifically excluded from the health plan coverage. Voluntary services, such as cosmetic surgery, for example, are usually excluded. There may be a maximum limit on the number of days covered for hospitalization. The patient is then responsible for all charges over the maximum.

(2) Deductible plan. The patient may be required to pay a certain amount toward the medical bills before the health insurance makes a contribution.

(3) Cost-sharing plan. The patient pays a portion of the cost of each service or of some of the services received. When payment is a fixed dollar amount per unit of service, it is called a co-payment; when it is a percentage of the charges, it is called coinsurance. A standard guideline called UCR (usual, customary, and reasonable charges) is one kind of cost sharing. Everything that exceeds the UCR amount is paid by the patient.

These three types of payment, plus the enrollment fee or the contribution to the premium, make up the out-of-pocket costs for the health plan member.

Q: *What are the different health plans available?*

A: There are three general types: service plans, indemnity plans, and health maintenance organization (HMO) plans.

(1) Service plans are run by two nonprofit organizations, Blue Cross and Blue Shield. They pay hospital and professional charges directly to providers on behalf of their members. A coinsurance amount is usually paid by the member and a "deductible" may also be required before the service plan makes payments.

(2) Commercial indemnity plans are offered by insurance companies. They pay a fixed sum on behalf of the patient toward a visit by a physician, surgeon's fees, hospital charges, and other medical expenses. The insured person is responsible for all charges in excess of these indemnity amounts.

To supplement service and indemnity plans, insurance companies offer what are called major medical plans that cover large medical bills in excess of the limits in the basic plans. They may also cover some of the services not included in a basic plan or a hospitalization plan.

(3) Health maintenance organization (HMO) plans use the same organization to pay for and provide medical services. These are often called "prepaid" plans. The provider organization receives a fixed amount periodically (the member enrollment fee) and, in return, provides comprehensive care to members. There are both group practices and individual practices within HMO's. There are no "deductibles" and no "maximums" on covered services in HMO's. Some studies have shown that the total costs per person (premium plus out-of-pocket costs) are lower for those in an HMO plan than for those who use a fee-for-service, cost-reimbursement system.

Health-care alliances and insurer-physician plans are among the new organizations similar to HMO. They are also based on prepaid premiums for comprehensive care.

In plans offered with employment, agreements between employers and employees vary regarding how much of the premium or enrollment fee is paid by the employer and how much by the employee. The amount an employer pays to obtain a health plan for an employee is not counted as the employee's taxable income. Since the mid-1970's, an increasing number of employers have offered a choice of health plans.

Q: *What public medical care programs exist?*

A: The two largest are Medicare and Medicaid.

Medicare is a two-part system providing insurance for a physician's services and hospitalization for citizens who have reached 65 years of age. Because the insurance pays less than half the costs of all health-care services provided, many people eligible for Medicare buy additional private health insurance.

Medicaid is a combined federal and state-administered program that pays for medical care for welfare recipients in such categories as families with dependent children, the blind, and the disabled. Eligibility and benefits vary from state to state.

Medical specialists are medical professionals who have knowledge, education, and training in a particular field of medicine. The vast amount of medical knowledge gained from advanced research in recent years has led to increasing specialization among medical personnel. Technological developments have contributed to this trend.

There are physicians who specialize in primary care. This includes family physicians, general pediatricians, and general internists. These primary-care specialists provide most of the general health care for the population. Other specialists provide care in a specific area and most often serve as consultants. Specialists take certification examinations to become "board-certified" in their specialties.

The current medical situation has not diminished the need for primary-care physicians, for whom there is an increasing demand. Patient needs usually can not be categorized as neatly as the distinct branches of medicine covered by some specialists. In addition, the knowledge of a patient's medical history that is possessed by a primary-care physician is essential for the diagnosis and treatment of many disorders. In most cases, the primary-care physician will diagnose and manage the problem. In certain situations, the primary-care physician may refer the patient to a particular consultant specialist for a difficult or unusual problem.

The following table lists some types of medical specialists and their areas of expertise.

Speciality	*Area of expertise*
Allergist	Treatment of allergies
Anesthesiologist	Administration of anesthetics for surgery
Cardiologist	Diseases of the heart and circulatory system

Speciality	*Area of expertise*
Chest Physician (Pulmonary Specialist)	Diseases of the lungs and chest
Dermatologist	Diseases of skin, hair, and nails
Emergency Medicine Specialist	Emergency treatment of acute illnesses and injuries
Epidemiologist	Causes, transmission, and control of infectious diseases
Family Physician	Ongoing health care for persons of all ages
Gastroenterologist	Diseases of the digestive system
General Surgeon	Surgical treatment of diseases of the abdomen, breast, and other areas
Gynecologist	Diseases of the female reproductive organs
Hematologist	Diseases of the blood, bone marrow, and lymph tissues
Internist	Nonsurgical treatment of diseases of the internal organs
Nephrologist	Diseases of the kidney
Neurologist	Diseases of the brain and nervous system
Neurosurgeon	Surgical treatment of diseases of the brain and spinal cord
Obstetrician	Health care for pregnancy, labor, and childbirth
Oncologist	Treatment of cancer
Ophthalmologist	Diseases of the eye
Orthopedist	Diseases of the bones, joints, and muscles
Otolaryngologist	Diseases of the ear, nose, throat, and neck
Pathologist	Study of biopsy specimens and body fluids
Pediatrician	Health care of infants, children, and adolescents
Physiatrist	Rehabilitation of patients following illness or injury
Plastic Surgeon	Cosmetic surgery and surgical reconstruction
Podiatrist	Disorders of the foot
Proctologist	Diseases of the anus, rectum, and colon
Psychiatrist	Treatment of mental disorders
Radiologist	Study of X ray and ultrasound
Rheumatologist	Treatment of rheumatic diseases
Urologist	Diseases of the urinary tract and the male reproductive organs
Vascular Surgeon	Surgical treatment of diseases of blood vessels

Medical test is an examination that ascertains the state of a person's general physical health or confirms a provisional diagnosis. At right and on the following page is a list of some medical tests. For more information, see the individual entry for each test in this encyclopedia.

See also HEALTH TESTS, ROUTINE; HOSPITALIZATION: ADULTS.

Amniocentesis	Gastroscopy
Angiogram	Glucose tolerance test
Aortogram	Intelligence quotient (IQ)
Arteriogram	Ishihara's test
Audiogram	Laryngoscopy
Barium (study)	Lung function test
Basal metabolic rate	Mammogram
Biopsy	Mantoux test

Blood count, complete	Myelogram
Bronchogram	Phonocardiogram
Cervical smear	Pregnancy test
Cholangiogram, intravenous	Pyelogram, intravenous
Cholecystogram, oral	Rinne's test
Computerized axial tomography scanner (CAT)	Schick test
Culture (test)	Sedimentation rate
Cystogram	Sonography
Cystoscopy	Spinal tap
Echocardiogram	TSH (thyroid function) test
Echogram	Tuberculin test
Electrocardiogram (EKG)	Urinalysis
Electroencephalogram (EEG)	Venogram
Electromyogram (EMG)	Wassermann test
Endoscopy	Widal's test
Gastrointestinal series (GI series)	

Medicine, administration of. *See* NURSING THE SICK.

Medicine chest is where first-aid equipment for the emergency treatment of injuries and illnesses should be kept. The kitchen is where household accidents most commonly occur. Most kitchens also have direct access to the yard, where accidents to children are also common. In or near the kitchen, therefore, is the most advisable place in which to keep the home medicine chest.

Keep all first-aid equipment out of reach of children, in a box or cupboard with a childproof lock. A first-aid box should be labeled clearly and put in a place that is easily accessible to adults. Replace supplies as necessary. *See illustrations on pages 553–556 for contents of a home medicine chest.*

Label all prescribed medicines with an expiration date and check them regularly. Flush outdated medicines down the toilet. Keep only basic medicines.

Mediterranean anemia. *See* THALASSEMIA.

Mediterranean fever is another name for brucellosis.

See also BRUCELLOSIS.

Home medicine chest contents

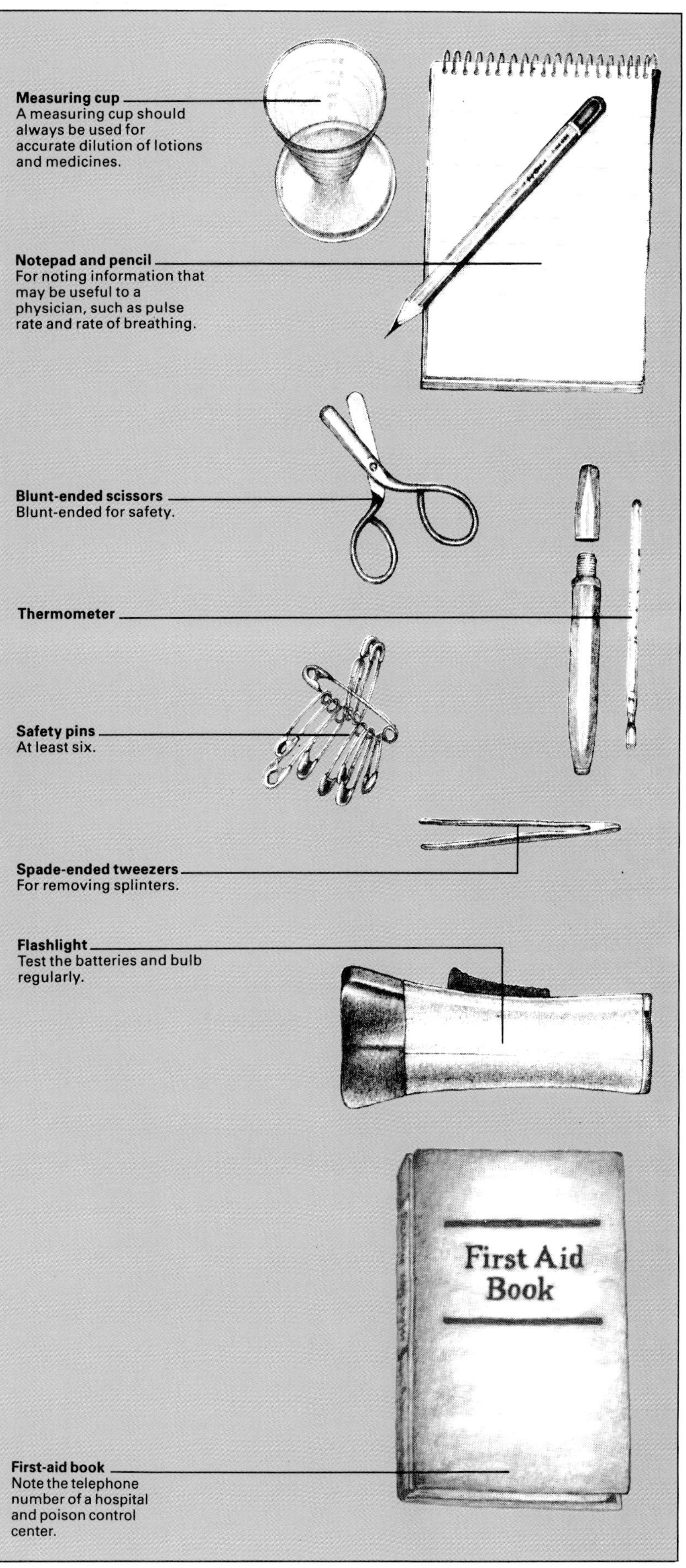
Measuring cup
A measuring cup should always be used for accurate dilution of lotions and medicines.
Notepad and pencil
For noting information that may be useful to a physician, such as pulse rate and rate of breathing.
Blunt-ended scissors
Blunt-ended for safety.
Thermometer
Safety pins
At least six.
Spade-ended tweezers
For removing splinters.
Flashlight
Test the batteries and bulb regularly.
First Aid Book
First-aid book
Note the telephone number of a hospital and poison control center.

Home medicine chest contents

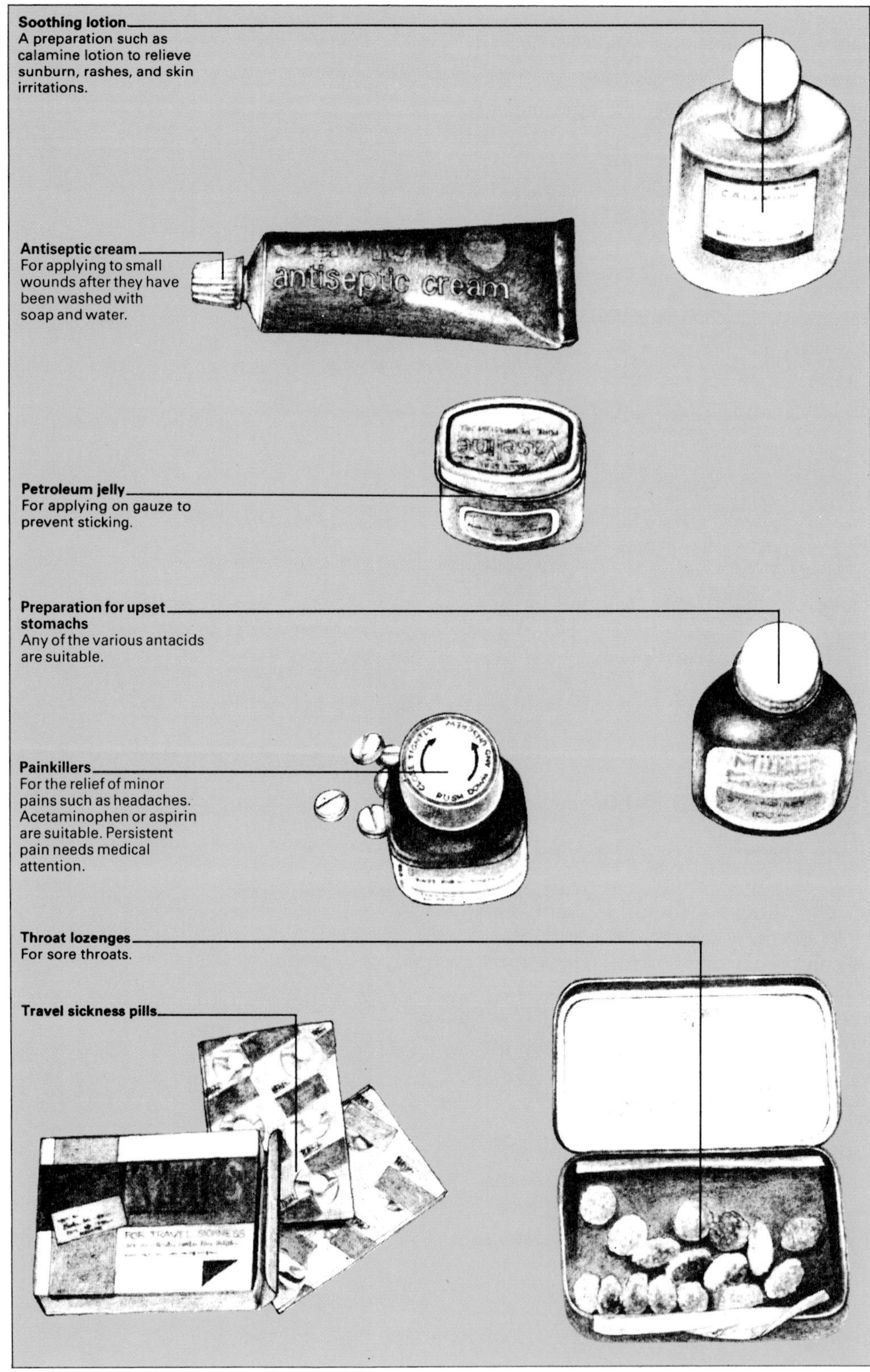

Soothing lotion
A preparation such as calamine lotion to relieve sunburn, rashes, and skin irritations.
Antiseptic cream
For applying to small wounds after they have been washed with soap and water.
antiseptic cream
Petroleum jelly
For applying on gauze to prevent sticking.
Preparation for upset stomachs
Any of the various antacids are suitable.
Painkillers
For the relief of minor pains such as headaches. Acetaminophen or aspirin are suitable. Persistent pain needs medical attention.
Throat lozenges
For sore throats.
Travel sickness pills
FOR TRAVEL SICKNESS

Home medicine chest contents

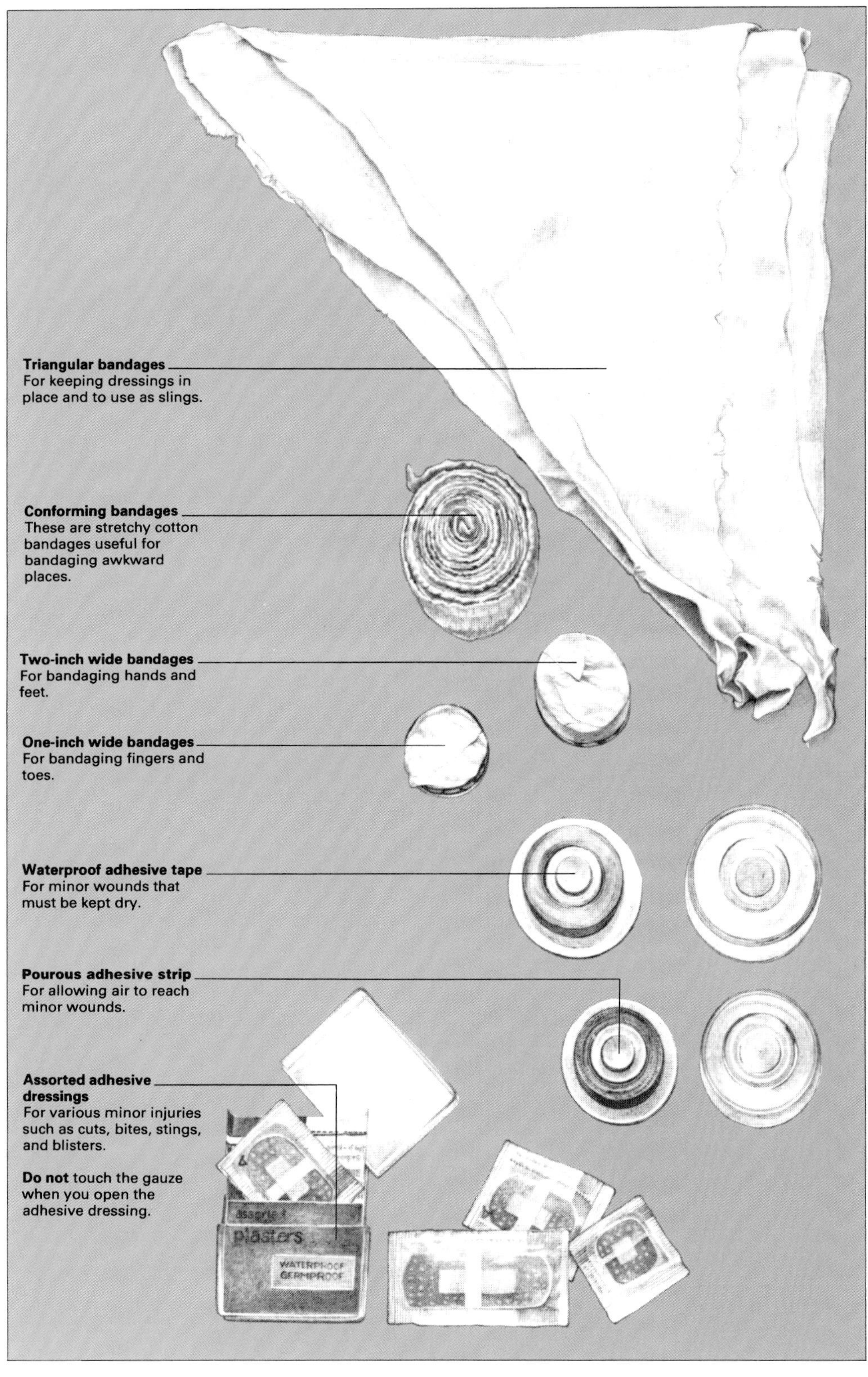
Triangular bandages
For keeping dressings in place and to use as slings.
Conforming bandages
These are stretchy cotton bandages useful for bandaging awkward places.
Two-inch wide bandages
For bandaging hands and feet.
One-inch wide bandages
For bandaging fingers and toes.
Waterproof adhesive tape
For minor wounds that must be kept dry.
Pourous adhesive strip
For allowing air to reach minor wounds.
Assorted adhesive dressings
For various minor injuries such as cuts, bites, stings, and blisters.
Do not touch the gauze when you open the adhesive dressing.
plasters
WATERPROOF
GERMPROOF

Home medicine chest contents

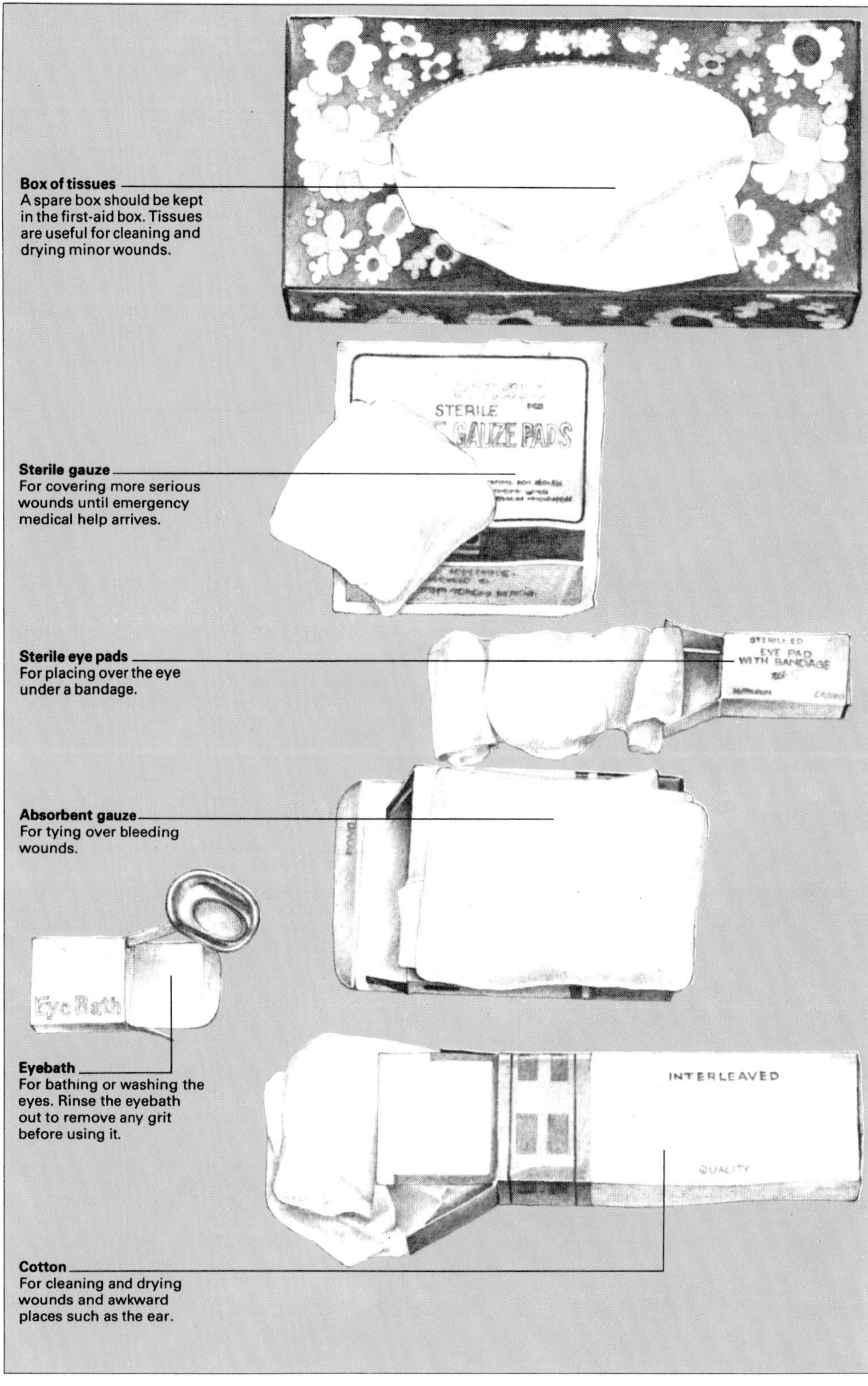

Box of tissues
A spare box should be kept in the first-aid box. Tissues are useful for cleaning and drying minor wounds.
STERILE
GAUZE PADS
Sterile gauze
For covering more serious wounds until emergency medical help arrives.
EYE PAD
WITH BANDAGE
Sterile eye pads
For placing over the eye under a bandage.
Absorbent gauze
For tying over bleeding wounds.
Eye Bath
Eyebath
For bathing or washing the eyes. Rinse the eyebath out to remove any grit before using it.
INTERLEAVED
QUALITY
Cotton
For cleaning and drying wounds and awkward places such as the ear.

Medulla (mə dəl′ə) is the inner portion of a body structure, such as bone. The outer part of a body structure is called the cortex.

Medulla oblongata (mə də′lə äb lông gät′ə) is the bottom part of the three parts of the brainstem. It is situated between the spinal cord and the pons. The medulla oblongata is an essential part of the brain. It contains the cardiac, vasomotor, and respiratory centers of the brian.

See also BRAIN.

Megacolon (meg ə kō′lən) is an extremely enlarged colon that usually results from Hirschsprung's disease, which is a congenital abnormality of the large intestine. Rarely, a megacolon may be caused by chronic constipation or by damage to the intestinal wall, as may occur with ulcerative colitis and diverticulitis.

See also COLITIS, ULCERATIVE; DIVERTICULITIS; HIRSCHSPRUNG'S DISEASE.

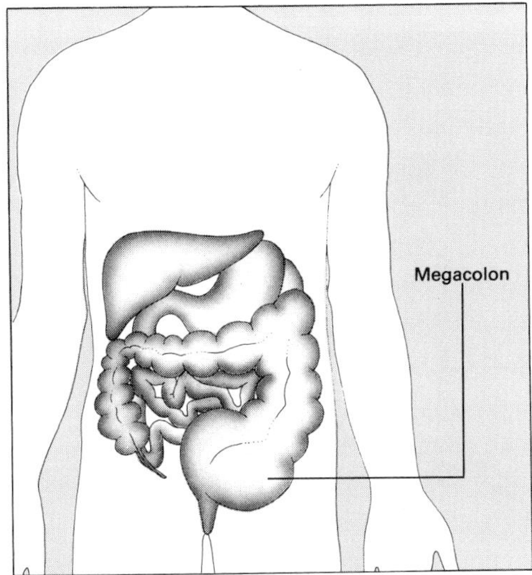

A **megacolon** usually occurs in the descending section of the large intestine, just above the rectum.

Megaloblast (meg′ə lō blast) is a large, immature type of cell that is found in the bone marrow. It forms abnormal red blood cells, particularly those associated with pernicious anemia.

See also ANEMIA, PERNICIOUS.

Megalomania (meg ə lō mā′nē ə) is an unrealistic and unshakable belief that one is of great importance, usually associated with the conviction that others do not recognize this importance. It is also known as delusion of grandeur.

Meibomian cyst. *See* CHALAZION.

Melancholia (mel ən kō′lē ə) is a term that in earlier years was synonymous with depression. Although the term is no longer commonly used, it refers to the feelings of sadness and the inability to experience happiness or enjoyment that usually accompany a depressive period.

See also DEPRESSION.

Melanin (mel′ə nin) is the dark pigment that is found in the skin, hair, and the choroid of the eye.

See also CHLOASMA; CHOROID; MELANOMA; MELASMA.

Melanoma (mel ə nō′mə) is a malignant (cancerous) tumor formed from a pigment cell (melanocyte) in the skin. Most melanomas arise from melanocytes in normal skin; a few may develop from pigmented moles. Melanomas are extremely rare in children. Persons who have been exposed to strong sunlight throughout their lives and fair-skinned persons with light colored eyes are more likely to develop melanomas than others. Pigmented growths on the legs, particularly in women, under the nails, on the palms of the hands and soles of the feet, or on the mucous membranes inside the mouth are particularly likely to become malignant. Melanomas may also occur in the pigmented choroid layer of the eyeball.

Q: *What are the symptoms of a melanoma?*

A: Most melanomas do not produce any specific symptoms, especially when they are in the early stages of development. For this reason, a physician should be consulted when any lesion, whether pigmented or not, forms a scab, bleeds, becomes surrounded by a reddened or inflamed area, becomes larger, or changes color.

Q: *How is a melanoma treated?*

A: It is usually necessary for the melanoma to be surgically removed. If the melanoma has spread, it may also be necessary to remove any lymph glands that have been affected.

Chemotherapy may be used if a melanoma is situated on a limb. Cytotoxic drugs are usually injected into an artery to give a high concentration of the drug in the affected area. By the time the drug has reached the rest of the body, it has been greatly diluted; this method keeps any adverse effects to a minimum. Cytotoxic drugs are usually more effective than radiotherapy. *See also* CYTOTOXIC DRUG.

Q: *How can melanomas be prevented?*

A: Since the major cause of melanoma is excessive sun exposure, sunbathing should be avoided; wearing protective clothing and using sun blocking applications is advisable, especially for fair-skinnned people.

Melasma (me laz'mə) is pigmentation of the skin in which brown patches occur on the forehead and cheeks. It affects some women who take contraceptive pills or who are pregnant. In such women, the condition is called chloasma. Melasma is increased by sunlight. The skin patches usually fade naturally when the woman stops taking the contraceptive pills or after childbirth.

See also CHLOASMA.

Melena (me le'nə) are feces that are black and tar-like. The condition is caused by the action of the intestinal enzymes on blood and is usually the result of bleeding in the upper gastrointestinal tract. Melena is often a symptom of peptic ulcer.

See also ULCER, PEPTIC.

Melioidosis (me lē oi dō'sis) is a rare infectious disease caused by the bacteria *Pseudomonas pseudomallei.* It is acquired by direct contact with infected animals. Melioidosis occurs most commonly in Southeast Asia and is generally not transmissible by humans. The acute form is characterized by pneumonia-like symptoms. With chronic melioidosis, abscesses often develop in the skin or any organ of the body, and osteomyelitis is often present.

See also OSTEOMYELITIS.

Membrane (mem'brān) is a thin tissue layer that covers the surface of an organ, lines the inside of a tube or cavity, or separates one organ from another.

Memory disorder is a condition that causes either the temporary or permanent impairment of the memory function. Memory impairment frequently occurs as a sign of dementia and may be caused by brain tumors, chronic alcohol abuse, cerebral arteriosclerosis, or Alzheimer's disease. Memory disorders are often progressive, with a patient's mental capacity deteriorating over a period of time.

See also ALZHEIMER'S DISEASE; AMNESIA; DEMENTIA; KORSAKOFF'S SYNDROME.

Menarche (mə när'kē) is the onset of menstruation at puberty.

See also MENSTRUATION.

Ménière's disease (mā nyārz') is a disorder of the inner ear arising from changes in the pressure of fluid within the inner ear balance receptors (semicircular canals, utricle and saccule). Symptoms include attacks of severe dizziness (vertigo), nausea, vomiting, tinnitus, and fluctuating hearing loss in the affected ear.

There is no single treatment that is effective in all cases. Several different drugs are used to treat Ménière's disease. The most suitable for a particular case may only be found after trying several drugs. Antinausea drugs may be given during an acute attack; other drugs may reduce the frequency of attacks.

See also TINNITUS.

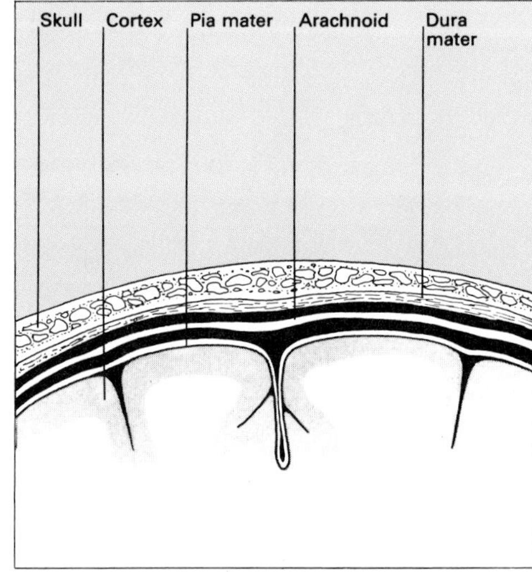

Meninges are three membranes that surround the brain: the pia mater, the dura mater, and the arachnoid.

Meninges (mə nin'jēz) are the three membranes that cover the surface of the brain and spinal cord. They are the pia mater; the arachnoid; and the dura mater.

See also HEMATOMA, SUBDURAL; HEMORRHAGE, SUBARACHNOID; MENINGIOMA; MENINGITIS.

Meningioma (mə nin jē ō′mə) is a tumor that arises from the meninges, usually those around the brain and most commonly those above the cerebellum. Multiple meningiomas may occur in von Recklinghausen's disease. They are usually benign (noncancerous) but may occasionally form a sarcoma.

See also CEREBELLUM; MENINGES; SARCOMA; VON RECKLINGHAUSEN'S DISEASE.

Meningitis (men in jī′tis) is inflammation of the membranes (meninges) that cover the brain and the spinal cord. The symptoms of meningitis usually appear suddenly (acute meningitis), but in some forms of the disorder, the onset of symptoms may be gradual. If untreated, acute meningitis is rapidly fatal.

Q: *What are the symptoms of meningitis?*

A: Acute meningitis is often preceded by a minor, influenza-like infection or by a sore throat. After one or two days, there is a sudden onset of a severe headache, vomiting, fever, stiff neck, and mental confusion. In severe cases, the patient goes into a coma. The patient may also be unable to straighten the leg after bending it at the hip joint (Kernig's sign) and may be abnormally sensitive to light (photophobia). Some infections that cause meningitis, such as meningococcal meningitis, may produce skin rashes. In small children, meningitis may cause irritability, lethargy, and a loss of appetite.

If the onset of meningitis is gradual, the symptoms are similar to those of the acute form, but develop over one or two weeks.

Q: *What causes meningitis?*

A: Meningitis may be caused by a wide variety of viral, fungal, protozoan, or bacterial infections.

Q: *How is meningitis treated?*

A: The treatment of meningitis depends upon the cause. Meningitis may be fatal if treatment is not started in the early stages; immediate hospitalization is necessary. A lumbar (spinal) puncture is then performed and the cerebrospinal fluid examined to determine the cause of the meningitis.

Most patients with acute bacterial meningitis respond well to treatment with powerful antibiotics. Intravenous fluids may also be necessary if the patient is dehydrated.

The treatment of protozoan and viral meningitis depends upon the symptoms. Patients with viral meningitis usually recover, but they may be extremely ill during the early stages of the disorder.

In some cases, meningitis may cause residual injury to the nervous system, such as deafness.

See also KERNIG'S SIGN; PHOTOPHOBIA.

Meningocele (mə ning′gō sēl), also known as neural tube defect, is a saclike protrusion of the meninges through a congenital defect in the skull or vertebral column. The protrusion forms a cyst filled with cerebrospinal fluid. It is now possible to test for meningocele early in pregnancy by testing the maternal blood or amniotic fluid.

See also MENINGES.

Meniscus (mə nis′kəs) is a thin, crescent-shaped cartilage that is attached to the upper end of the shinbone (tibia) within the knee joint. There are two menisci: the lateral meniscus and the medial meniscus. Collectively, they are called the semilunar cartilages.

The most common disorder that affects the meniscus is tearing of the cartilage. It is a common athletic injury and usually occurs when the knee is twisted violently while in a half-bent position. There is usually pain as soon as the cartilage is torn. The victim often falls down and is unable to straighten the leg. The following day the knee is usually swollen and pain-

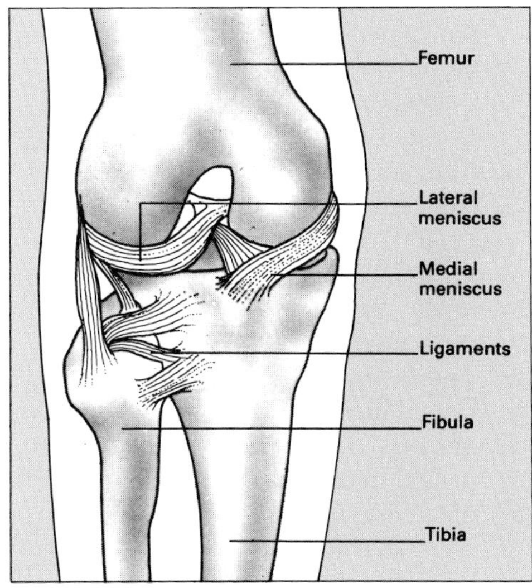

Meniscus, a type of cartilage composed of strong fiber, is an important part of the mechanism by which the knee is locked to produce a strong, straight lower limb.

ful. The swelling may disappear after resting the knee for one or two weeks. When normal activity is resumed, the knee may give way or may suddenly lock so that the leg can not be straightened normally. The usual treatment is to remove the cartilage surgically (meniscectomy).

See also KNEE.

Menopause (men′ə pôz) is the end of menstruation. By popular usage, however, the term has come to be synonymous with female climacteric (that combination of physical and psychological changes that take place during menopause).

Q: *At what age does menopause usually occur?*

A: Natural menopause occurs most commonly between the ages of 45 and 55 years but it may occur earlier or later without there being any abnormality. As a general rule, the younger a woman was when she began to menstruate, the older she will be at the start of menopause.

Menstruation ceases at any age after the surgical removal of the uterus (hysterectomy). The symptoms of menopause occur only if both ovaries as well as the uterus are removed and menopause has not already taken place naturally.

Q: *How does menstruation cease?*

A: This varies greatly from woman to woman. Some women menstruate normally and regularly, then stop relatively abruptly. In most women, menstruation becomes irregular during menopause. The periods themselves may be either shorter or longer than usual, and the interval between them may vary from about 2 weeks to 10 weeks. The periods may be heavy or light.

Any bleeding that occurs more than six months after the last period, even if it seems like a normal period, should be regarded as abnormal and reported to a physician.

Q: *What are the symptoms associated with menopause?*

A: The most common symptoms are hot flashes, sweating, palpitations, depression, irregular menstruation, fatigue, headache, and sleeping difficulties.

Q: *Do all women suffer from menopausal symptoms?*

A: No. In a few women the symptoms are absent or extremely mild. Most women do have some symptoms, although many do not consider the problems serious enough to consult a physician. It is often difficult to be sure that the symptoms are associated with menopause and not with other problems. For example, headaches are common at any age, and depression may have various other causes.

Q: *Why do menopausal symptoms occur?*

A: The symptoms are caused by hormonal changes that occur gradually over several years. In a woman of childbearing age, the ovaries secrete the estrogen hormones in response to follicle-stimulating hormone (FSH) from the pituitary gland. At the approach of menopause, the ovaries become less responsive to FSH and secrete less estrogen. As a result, the pituitary gland produces more FSH to try to maintain estrogen levels.

As a direct result of these hormonal changes, ovulation becomes infrequent, periods become irregular and menopause finally occurs. However, the pituitary still secretes large amounts of FSH. The resulting low estrogen imbalance affects the blood vessels in the skin, causing them to dilate. This in turn produces the hot flashes, sweating, palpitations, and headaches. *See also* FOLLICLE-STIMULATING HORMONE.

The hormonal changes also cause the breasts and uterus to become smaller after menopause. The lining of the vagina becomes thinner and drier, and the muscles that support the uterus become weaker, so that a prolapse may occur. *See also* PROLAPSE.

Q: *How can the symptoms of menopause be treated?*

A: Medical treatment is not always necessary, however estrogen replacement therapy to decrease the symptoms and prevent osteoporosis is recommended for many women. A physician may be able to help by explaining what happens during menopause and by dispelling the anxieties that a woman may have about loss of femininity and the expectation of years of depression and unhappiness.

Q: *What other changes may occur after menopause?*

A: Apart from gradual reduction in size of the breasts and uterus, the vagina and the vulva also change. These changes may cause discomfort and pain during sexual intercourse. If this occurs, estrogen-containing suppositories or creams, used regularly, restore the thickness and moistness of the vaginal lining.

Q: *Should a woman still have regular gynecological examinations after menopause?*

A: Yes. Regular gynecological examinations, including a cervical smear test, are as important after menopause as before it.

See *also* CERVICAL SMEAR.

Q: *Is there any change in attitudes toward sex after menopause?*

A: This varies among individual women. Most women do not notice any change in their sex drive. Some find that their sex drive is increased after menopause, when the risk of an unwanted pregnancy has definitely disappeared. However, women who become depressed find that often their sex drive is reduced. This is usually caused by the depression rather than by menopause itself.

Q: *What form of contraception should be used during menopause?*

A: A physician should be consulted about contraception during menopause. Contraceptive pills are inadvisable for women over the age of 40 years. Barrier methods, such as condoms, spermicidal foams, or a diaphragm with a spermicidal cream or jelly, probably give the best protection. Contraceptive measures should be used for at least six months and sometimes up to one year after menopause until it is certain that periods have finally stopped and that the woman is no longer fertile. See *also* CONTRACEPTION.

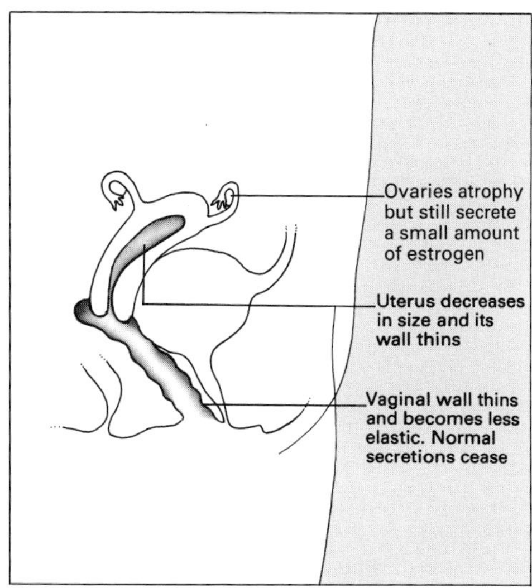
Ovaries atrophy but still secrete a small amount of estrogen
Uterus decreases in size and its wall thins
Vaginal wall thins and becomes less elastic. Normal secretions cease

After **menopause,** hormonal changes cause the breasts and uterus to become smaller. The lining of the vagina becomes thinner and drier, and the muscles that support the uterus become weaker. These changes in the vagina and vulva may cause discomfort and pain during sexual intercourse. Suppositories or creams that contain estrogen can restore the thickness and moistness of the vaginal lining.

Menorrhagia (men ə rā′jē ə) is the medical term for heavy periods; that is, regular menstruation that involves greater than normal blood flow and that usually lasts longer than normal.

See *also* MENSTRUAL PROBLEMS.

Menstrual cramps.

See DYSMENORRHEA.

Menstrual problems (men′strů əl) may occur at any time between menarche (when periods first begin) and menopause (when they end).

During puberty, many girls have irregular periods. As a menstrual rhythm becomes established, problems become less common; the absence of periods (amenorrhea) is usually a sign of pregnancy or of a psychological problem. See *also* AMENORRHEA.

The most common problem during the early years of menstruation is painful menstruation, also known as dysmenorrhea. In later years there may be feelings of irritation and depression, breast tenderness, and ankle swelling caused by premenstrual syndrome. There may also be fluid retention for a few days prior to menstruation. See *also* DYSMENORRHEA; PREMENSTRUAL SYNDROME.

Bleeding between periods may occur at any time, but is most common during the years before menopause. If it persists, a physician should be con-

Menstrual problems occur for a variety of reasons and can usually be easily identified and treated by a physician.

Menstrual problems	Associated symptoms
Amenorrhea	Absence of menstruation. Commonly due to pregnancy, menopause, anemia, and emotional disturbance.
Dysmenorrhea	Painful menstruation. Due in many cases to an obstructed cervix.
Menorrhagia	Prolonged or unusually heavy periods. Result of fibroids of the uterus or pelvic congestion.
Metrorrhagia	Bleeding between periods. Possibility of uterine fibroids or cancer of the uterus.

sulted. Heavy periods, called menorrhagia, or irregular periods, called metrorrhagia, also commonly occur. A threatened miscarriage may simulate a menstrual problem when in fact it is caused by a pregnancy. *See also* ABORTION, SPONTANEOUS; MENORRHAGIA; METRORRHAGIA.

Q: *What conditions cause abnormal menstrual bleeding?*

A: Heavy periods may be caused by various conditions that affect the uterus, such as endometriosis, endometritis, fibroids, or salpingitis. Occasionally, general disorders, such as hypothyroidism or thyrotoxicosis, cirrhosis of the liver, and blood disorders involving a reduction in clotting ability, may cause abnormal menstrual bleeding. More frequently, heavy periods are associated with the hormone imbalance related to menopause or, less frequently, to an ovarian cyst. *See also* BLOOD DISORDERS; CIRRHOSIS; CYST, OVARIAN; HYPOTHYROIDISM; THYROTOXICOSIS.

Q: *How is abnormal menstruation treated?*

A: Treatment depends on the cause. A woman experiencing this problem should consult a physician. A diagnosis will be made after physical and gynecological examinations. If necessary, it will include a cervical smear test and a vaginal swab to discover if any infection is present. A pregnancy test reveals if pregnancy is the cause of lack of menstruation.

If no physical cause can be found for the absence of menstruation, a hormonal disturbance may be the cause. The physician may prescribe a regular course of synthetic hormones. This usually produces menstruation, followed by normal periods when the hormone treatment is stopped. *See also* ESTROGEN REPLACEMENT THERAPY.

Q: *What are other treatments if diagnosis is uncertain or hormone therapy is unsuccessful?*

A: A diagnostic D and C (dilatation and curettage) is a simple and minor operation that allows a general gynecological examination as well as a microscopic examination of the lining of the womb. Often this simple operation is in itself sufficient to return menstruation to normal. The woman does not need to remain hospitalized for more than a day.

If abnormal bleeding continues, either because of hormonal disturbance, fibroids, or cancer, a hysterectomy (surgical removal of the uterus) may have to be performed. Since a hysterectomy creates artificial premature menopause (cessation of periods) with possible attendant problems (if a radical hysterectomy is performed with removal of the ovaries), it is becoming a less common surgical procedure than previously. *See also* HYSTERECTOMY; MENOPAUSE.

Menstruation (men strü ā'shən) is the shedding of the lining of the uterus (endometrium) that occurs regularly in women between menarche (the beginning of menstrual periods) and menopause (the end of periods). It produces vaginal bleeding that lasts for 3 to 7 days and occurs every 24 to 34 days—the length of the menstrual cycle. About halfway through the cycle, an egg is released from an ovary to travel along a fallopian tube to the uterus. This process is called ovulation. *See also* OVULATION.

Q: *How is the length of a menstrual cycle calculated?*

A: The menstrual cycle is the time between the first day of one period and the first day of the next, including the days when bleeding occurs.

Q: *Are all menstrual cycles the same?*

A: No. The average cycle is 28 days, but some women have a cycle that is consistently longer or shorter than that. Additionally, each woman's cycle can vary in length from month to month.

Q: *Is menstruation always the same?*

A: Like the menstrual cycle, the period may have slight variations in individual women. Bleeding is usually heavier in the first day or two and then becomes lighter for the next two or three days.

Q: *How does the body control menstruation?*

A: Regularity of menstruation is a complex balance between the levels of hormones produced by the ovaries (estrogens and progesterone) and those produced by the pituitary gland at the base of the brain, the follicle-stimulating hormone (FSH) and the luteinizing hormone (LH). FSH stimulates the ovary to produce estrogen in the first half of the menstrual cycle. Estrogen causes a thickening of the lining of the uterus. In mid-cycle, a sudden increase in LH causes ovulation, and progesterone alters the nature of the uterus lining in preparation for a fertilized egg.

Fertilization produces an embryo that stimulates another hormone to maintain the uterus lining. If fertilization does not take place, the uterus lining is shed as the menstrual flow and the cycle of events begins all over again.

Q: *How are the hormones from the pituitary gland involved in menstruation?*

A: As the production of estrogen increases from the ovaries, its rising concentration diminishes the level of FSH from the pituitary gland by a mechanism known as "feedback." The pituitary gland then releases LH, controlled by feedback of progesterone from the ovaries.

The feedback of the various hormones is detected by the hypothalamus in the brain. The hypothalamus can also be affected by other factors, such as emotions, anxiety, or depression, and the effects of other hormones in the bloodstream. *See also* HYPOTHALAMUS.

Q: *Why do menarche and menopause occur?*

A: The onset of menstruation is associated with the hormonal changes of puberty, and the final end of menstruation is caused by aging of the ovaries. In neither case is the exact mechanism fully understood.

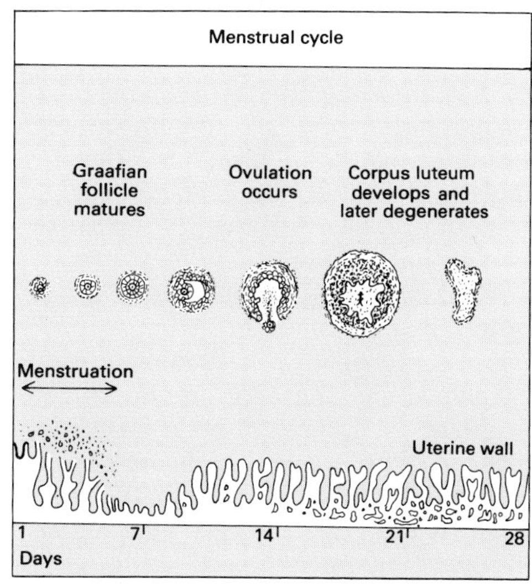

Menstruation usually occurs during the first five days of the menstrual cycle.

Q: *What care should a woman take during menstruation?*

A: There is no need to restrict any activities during menstruation unless the blood flow is extremely heavy. Absorbent pads (sanitary napkins) or internal tampons may be worn. Sanitary napkins are more obtrusive and may cause vulval soreness, but they are more absorbent than tampons. Tampons left in the vagina for a long time may produce offensive discharge because of vaginitis and may also predispose the wearer to toxic shock syndrome. There is no need to curtail sexual activity during menstruation, except for reasons of personal preference. Menstrual blood has no harmful effects on the woman or anything with which it may come into contact. *See also* TOXIC SHOCK SYNDROME.

Q: *At what age may tampons be used?*

A: Any girl who is menstruating may use tampons; if she is not sexually active, she may prefer to use a smaller, more slender tampon. It is often advisable to attempt to insert the first tampon when she is not menstruating, because the technique is sometimes difficult to learn.

See also CORPUS LUTEUM; GRAAFIAN FOLLICLE; MENOPAUSE; MENSTRUAL PROBLEMS; OVULATION.

Mental health is fundamental for personal happiness, including the ability to develop close friendships and intimate relationships and to gain satisfaction from work, hobbies, and other interests. Mental fitness is just as important a factor in overall health as is physical well-being.

Mental illness, in one form or another, is quite common. A large number of a physician's daily consultations involve some mental or emotional problem. At any one time, a large percentage of all hospital beds are occupied by patients with psychiatric disorders. At least one in every ten persons at some time in life needs treatment for emotional problems.

Given the right combination of past experiences, current stresses, and genetic predispositions, anyone can experience psychiatric symptoms. Mental health experts do not know the specific causes of all types of mental illness. Some mental disorders have physical causes, such as brain injuries, nutritional deficiencies, and poisons; others have psychological causes. *See also* MENTAL ILLNESS.

Stress, however, seems to play a major role in triggering emotional problems. Such stress could result, for example, from anxiety about personal relationships, finances, or work. Successfully managing stress may help prevent some forms of mental illness.

However, the decisions and problems that arise unexpectedly usually cause the most stress — a sick child, an accident, a depressed friend or family member, and other similar situations. It is not possible to avoid these types of stress, so the better equipped a person is to cope with stress, the more likely he or she is to remain mentally fit.

Coping with the Stresses of Life

Many of the factors that help a person handle the ordinary stresses of life can simply involve a common-sense approach to daily activities: getting enough sleep each night; setting aside time for relaxation; avoiding overwork; discussing problems with family or friends; and cultivating a confident, positive mental attitude.

The amount of sleep required varies from person to person and, even in the same person, from night to night. It is important to have a steady and sufficient amount of sleep if you are to avoid chronic fatigue and exhaustion.

Another major factor in promoting mental health is having a circle of family members and friends on whom an individual can rely for psychological support or financial aid in times of trouble. The security of such a support group can eliminate or greatly reduce anxiety about how to handle problems.

When a problem does arise, discussing it with a family member or friend is often enough to put the problem into its proper perspective. By the same token, a person can attain great satisfaction and feelings of self-worth from supporting another in time of stress, acting as an adviser, helper, or just a good listener.

The more secure a person feels, the more likely he or she is to be mentally healthy. The groundwork for emotional security is laid in childhood. Children need affection, support, understanding of their problems and fears, and a sense of being wanted in the home. Children are often troubled by ordinary fears, such as the dark, or by special circumstances, such as moving to a new house, attending a new school, witnessing an accident or other violent event, experiencing a death in the family, or having to be hospitalized. Children need at least one adult on whom they feel they can rely. The child who grows up in a loving, trusting family environment has the best chance of becoming a mentally healthy adult with a confident, positive outlook on life.

Routine, Boredom, and Change. Setting up a daily routine is an unconscious way of avoiding mental stress. Tasks done through habit cause the minimum amount of difficulty. At the same time, too much routine creates boredom, which in itself can be fatiguing and create stress. As in any other aspect of life, people vary widely in their need for routine in any form without realizing that they do. In fact, most people automatically combine routine with change and stimulation in the right proportions to maintain their own mental fitness.

A certain amount of change from the daily routine is essential for mental well-being. But major life changes can create a great deal of stress. The loss of a loved one, the birth of a child, a new job or home, marriage or divorce, even a change in diet are all sources of added stress. If several major life changes occur within a one-year period, chances of incurring some type of mental or even physical illness are greatly increased. A person experiencing such major changes should make special efforts to protect his or her mental health by getting enough rest and relaxation.

Taking a Vacation. For most people, vacations are the greatest change from daily routine. Some people gain the most rest and enjoyment from vacations that allow them to pursue favorite pastime activities, such as fishing, sunbathing, boating, hiking, and other sports. Others use vacation time to see new parts of the world, shop, sample different kinds of food, and enjoy foreign cultures.

While vacations are generally beneficial to mental health, they usually require organization and travel. And this can produce varying amounts of mental stress.

Driving a car over a long distance can cause both physical and mental stress, especially if the driver attempts to meet a deadline. With air, ship, bus, or train transport available, the main cause of anxiety is arriving at the airport, harbor, or station on time. The actual traveling itself is less stressful. However, in every form of transport there may be peaks of anxiety, for example, during take-off and landing and in turbulence in an airplane. Rail travel seems to be the most relaxing way of going from one place to another. Travel on board ship is unique in that passengers' stress levels generally change with the weather.

Gaining the most benefit from a vacation requires planning and an effort to remain in a calm, unhurried state of mind. On a car journey, motorists should prepare themselves to be late if the unexpected, such as a flat tire or traffic jam, occurs. Other travelers should be prepared to accept delays in flight, train, or bus schedules.

Planning the details of a vacation early will eliminate the strain of handling last-minute preparations. Vacationers should have tickets, passports, visas, and room reservations well in advance and should make lists of clothing and other items needed for the journey.

Persons who travel by air from one time zone to another that has a difference of more than four hours will still be physically and mentally geared to the original time zone. This is called jet lag. A traveler may require several days to adjust, depending on how great is the time difference between zones. The effects of jet lag can be reduced by planning to arrive in the new zone during the evening. Meetings and business discussion should then take place only after a night's rest, if not sleep. If all business discussions can be arranged for times that correspond with working hours in the original "day," then little or no adaptation is necessary. *See also* JET LAG.

An alternative kind of vacation is to enjoy leisure at home in known and nonstressful surroundings. Such a vacation can be used as a time for making new resolutions and for finally sorting out problems that may have seemed too difficult while other day-to-day routines and stresses were in the way.

Relieving Mental Tension. In the daily routine of life, it is not always easy to achieve a proper balance between work and leisure. Many people find it difficult to relax physically and mentally without making a definite effort. The thoughts of the day just ending or worries about events to come — fears, pleasures, embarrassments, and triumphs — create a state of tension that makes relaxation difficult.

There are dozens of techniques to relieve excessive tension, some from the ancient East, others from the modern West. What constitutes an effective method of relaxing depends largely on personal preference. A technique that works well for one individual might not work at all for another. Many factors enter into choosing a relaxation technique, such as the amount of time and discipline needed. Some techniques can be learned by the individual alone; others require more formal instruction.

Many people have found that various forms of meditation relieve tension. In general, meditation involves focusing on a thought, word, phrase, or object to calm the mind. Some meditation techniques also involve breathing exercises. Scientists have found that during meditation the body undergoes physical changes, such as slower heartbeat or lower blood pressure, which indicate a state of deep relaxation.

One of the more popular forms of meditation is transcendental meditation (TM). Those who practice TM sit quietly for 15 to 20 minutes twice each day and repeat a mantra, or word from the Hindu scriptures. TM is taught by instructors who select a personal mantra for each individual.

Some people find that simply envisioning peaceful or pleasant scenes helps relieve tension. Many books explaining other meditation and thought control techniques have been written and are widely available in bookshops and libraries.

Another relaxation technique popular in the Western world is yoga, the Hindu system of mental and physical exercise. It is wise to learn yoga from an expert instructor because many books on yoga describe some difficult yoga postures that may cause injury to a beginner.

Other Eastern systems that have been modified and adapted in the West to promote relaxation and peace of mind include some of the Japanese martial arts and the Chinese exercise, tai chi.

Because there appears to be a direct connection between mental and muscular tension, some scientists have experimented with relieving mental tension by relaxing the muscles. Using a system called progressive relaxation, a person alternately tenses and relaxes various muscles to become more aware of the degrees of tension and relaxation that they can achieve. A similar technique, called autogenic training, involves suggestions that various parts of the body are warm, heavy, and relaxed. These relaxation techniques can be learned from a therapist or from popularly available books or recordings.

One of the newest relaxation techniques involves biofeedback. Researchers have found that biofeedback is useful in relaxing muscles, lowering blood pressure, and increasing the long, slow brain waves called alpha waves. Electronic sensors are placed on the skin to monitor bodily conditions, such as skin temperature, muscle tension, and brain waves. Once a person receives feedback indicating excessive tension (for example, seeing on a monitor that his or her brain waves have changed), he or she can direct the body to correct this condition. Because the sensitive electronic equipment involved must be calibrated carefully and the electrodes placed precisely, it is advisable that this technique be practiced under the supervision of a biofeedback expert if the technique is to be successful.

Many people find inner calm and peace through sincere religious beliefs. For them, prayer and worship produce a state of profound joy and contentment that contributes greatly to their mental well-being. A strong religious faith can also help a person cope with the various crises that arise in life. Even those who do not have religious beliefs often have some kind of faith, perhaps in a particular philosophy of life, that helps contribute to emotional stability and provides underlying mental strength.

Onset of Mental Problems

Everyone, on occasion, experiences the unpleasant emotions of anger, frustration, sadness, mild depression, worry, loneliness, and uncertainty. This is normal. Sometimes, these feelings persist for long periods of time or grow more intense. This could be a sign that mental or emotional problems are developing. These feelings could stem from a specific cause, but often there seems to be no apparent reason.

Other indications of mental problems include alcoholism, drug abuse, suicidal thoughts or actions, irrational fears, sexual difficulties, obsessive thoughts, and compulsions to perform the same acts repeatedly.

Sometimes problems arise within a family that can best be remedied with outside help. These may include a troubled child, difficulties involving household finances, and sexual problems.

Treatment for Problems. Mental problems can be treated with drugs, psychotherapy, or both. Some forms of therapy probe a person's past experiences to uncover connections with present feelings and behavior. Other forms concentrate on changing thought patterns or behavior, without going through the longer process of looking for the cause. Some people prefer individual counseling; others prefer group therapy, in which the group members share and discuss their feelings and problems. Family therapy that includes all family members can be helpful in identifying and correcting maladaptive family patterns that are contributing to an individual's problems.

Persons feeling in need of such professional help should contact a local mental health center or ask their pastor or family physician for a referral. In addition, many communities have specialized services for problems, such as alcoholism and drug abuse, and for the mental and emotional needs of the elderly.

Seeking Professional Help. Many people benefit from discussing their problem with the family physician and having an examination to determine whether there is an underlying physical cause. Others may seek advice from members of the clergy, many of whom have received training in family counseling. Sometimes, the service of a marriage counselor, psychiatrist, psychologist, social worker, or psychiatric nurse can provide the most help toward relieving anxiety, fear, and tension.

Schools often have social workers to help with the problems of children. Many communities also have crisis "hotlines" that troubled individuals can use to call for immediate advice on how to handle problems or where to get further help.

Just as important to mental well-being as maintaining good habits of rest and relaxation is knowing when help is needed and a willingness to seek it.

Mental illness refers to a broad range of psychiatric disorders that reflect a deviation from normal thought and behavioral patterns. Mental illness is a relative term; it does not, in and of itself, reflect the seriousness of an individual's problems. Certain psychiatric disorders, such as schizophrenia, are serious conditions that may require hospitalization and long-term treatment. Individuals who fall into other categories of mental disorders, such as anxiety disorders, may be relatively well-functioning and require only brief counseling. Some persons diagnosed with a psychiatric disorder will not require formal therapy to function adequately.

Because the normal range of behavior is so wide, it is often difficult to make a specific diagnosis; psychiatry is not an exact science, and cultural norms must be taken into consideration when looking at an individual's behavior. Individuals in all age ranges can experience psychiatric problems. As more is learned about these problems, treatment is becoming more effective, and the stigma of seeking help has been lessened.

Q: *What types of mental illness may occur?*

A: There are several different ways of classifying mental illness, none of which is completely satisfactory. One of the most widely used systems of classification is the DSM (Diagnostic and Statistical Manual of Mental Disorders). The current version divides mental disorders into the following major categories: substance use disorders (alcohol/drug abuse or addiction); schizophrenic disorders; paranoid disorders; affective disorders (depression; mania; manic-depressive illness); anxiety disorders; somatoform disorders; personality disorders; psychosexual disorders; and disorders of infancy, childhood, and adolescence. Each of these categories is subdivided into several subtypes. *See also* ALCOHOL ABUSE; ANXIETY; DEPRESSION; DRUG ABUSE; SCHIZOPHRENIA.

Q: *What causes mental illness?*

A: Different types of emotional disor-

Some types of **mental illness** can be treated through group therapy.

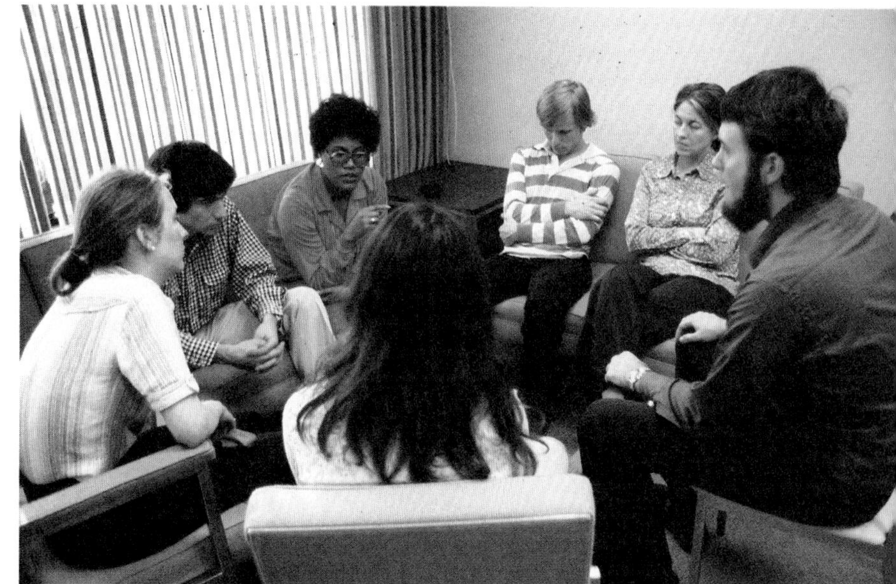

ders probably result from different causes. There is increasing evidence that some psychiatric disorders are inherited and/or involve biochemical imbalances. For example, schizophrenia, alcoholism, and some types of affective and anxiety disorders are hereditary.

It is also clear that an individual's upbringing can predispose him or her to psychological problems. For example, severe loss during childhood may lead to subsequent difficulties. Also physical, sexual, or emotional abuse, neglect, or significant family dysfunction may not provide an individual with good coping skills and a positive self-image. For many psychiatric disorders, a combination of genetic predispositions, maladaptive patterns during one's upbringing, and current stresses combine to cause emotional problems. A thorough medical evaluation should always be undertaken to rule out a physical condition causing psychiatric symptoms, such as hyperthyroidism.

Q: *How is mental illness treated?*

A: There is a wide range of treatment methods depending on the particular psychological problem. Treatment for psychotic disorders, such as schizophrenia, will usually involve antipsychotic medication and hospitalization. Many such individuals will require long-term outpatient follow-up with periodic rehospitalization. Most other psychiatric disorders can be treated on an outpatient basis, unless the individual is a danger to self or others or simply can not function at a particular point in time. Medications, such as antidepressants or minor tranquilizers, may be instrumental in the outpatient management of some disorders, particularly depression and anxiety. Some persons will benefit from long-term psychotherapy, whereas others require minimal counseling to learn more effective ways of managing their lives. Counseling is offered by psychiatrists, psychologists, and social workers, as well as other mental health professionals. Therefore, it may be helpful for the patient to contact his or her physician, local hospital, or mental health agency for referrals to aid him or her in selecting a therapist, especially since a good relationship between the patient and the therapist is vital to the success of the therapy. Support groups can be very effective for a wide variety of problems, such as alcohol/drug abuse, gambling, and coping with death, divorce, and illness.

Mentally retarded, care of. The very first issue in the care of the mentally retarded child is the recognition that a problem exists. If the child has an associated physical problem, such as epilepsy, heart disease, or blindness, the diagnosis may be suspected quite early in life.

If, however, the child appears physically normal, a mental disability may not be obvious in the first few months of life. It is only as the child fails to develop normally in several areas that the parents may become concerned. Once a handicap has been confirmed, many parents blame themselves for their child's condition. Unintentionally insensitive remarks by family members or friends often increases this sense of guilt. It is important for parents to realize that mental handicaps can afflict any family. Prolonged guilt, or blaming oneself, will interfere with the care of the child and can lead to a frustrating cycle of guilt and anger.

Family problems may also arise when all of the parents' attention is focused on the handicapped child. It may be difficult for parents with a handicapped child to spend enough time with other children in the family. Often, siblings are too young to understand what is happening and feel that one child is a "favorite." This may cause resentment toward the handicapped child. It should also be emphasized that parents should take time for themselves, as well, and attend to their own personal needs. Issues of anger, guilt, depression, fatigue, and frustration need to be discussed by the family in an open, honest manner.

Most parents decide to care for the mentally retarded child themselves.

Raising a developmentally delayed child is challenging and very difficult at times. The child may not learn to sit, crawl, walk, or acquire bowel or bladder control until much later than normal. Thus, while the mentally retarded child can learn, the process is often a slow one. The parents must persevere and praise each of the child's accomplishments. What each child can accomplish will vary greatly, depending on many factors. The mentally retarded child should undergo a thorough intellectual assessment to help parents focus their efforts on helping the child to achieve his or her maximum potential.

Many parents of mentally retarded children find that a regular daily routine is reassuring to the child. Thus, while normal children might find an orderly schedule to be rigid and confining, such a schedule may be a source of security for the retarded child.

Depending on the severity of the handicap, the parents must decide what type of school setting is best for their child. Many retarded children benefit from the company of normal children, and most educators now feel that keeping the child "sheltered" in separate schools is probably not helpful. Every school district is required by law to provide services to mentally handicapped students within the regular schools, so that this option should be available throughout the country. Some children, however, feel more at ease in an environment with other handicapped children and may do better in a special school. Learning and education specialists, psychologists, and the child's physician can usually assist the parents with this decision. In fact, because of the number of problems involved in the care of the mentally retarded child, parents should try to assemble such a supportive "team" to help assist in decision-making and care of the child. Family and friends can and should be included in this team, as they can help by giving the parents a well-earned rest. Social service agencies are also available to provide assistance. As the child grows up, he or she can go to special holiday camps that have trained staff who can fulfill special needs of mentally handicapped children.

The parents of a mentally handicapped child have to cope with all of the usual problems of child rearing as well. Thus, each stage in the retarded child's development may bring with it a new and unique set of issues. Puberty may trigger issues of sexuality and aggression. Later, adolescence may bring with it issues of work and conflict between independence and dependence.

Many mentally retarded persons learn to do simple jobs and support themselves independently. They can work with other handicapped persons and feel secure in a comfortable working routine. Sheltered workshops often provide such an environment. The responsibility of parents of a handicapped child is to prepare him or her for as independent a life as possible, and to give the child the opportunity to develop to his or her fullest capacity. The role parents play in caring for a handicapped child will determine largely the extent to which he or she realizes his or her potential capabilities in life. Any decision must be based on the effect of the handicapped child on the rest of the family and on advice from the child's physician and other professionals. As the parents become older, questions will arise as to who will provide care for the retarded child in the future. Again, the need for support and professional advice whenever problems arise is most important.

See also MENTAL RETARDATION.

Mental retardation (re tär dā′shən) is subnormal intelligence. It may be caused by lack of brain development or by brain damage from injury or illness.

Q: *What causes mental retardation?*

A: In most cases, the cause is unknown, but the normal variation in intelligence that occurs in the population can produce persons with below average as well as above average intelligence. Several rare inherited disorders, such as phenylketonuria, Tay-Sachs disease, and von Recklinghausen's disease may cause mental retardation. *See also* PHENYLKETONURIA; TAY-SACHS DISEASE; VON RECKLINGHAUSEN'S DISEASE.

Chromosomal abnormalities (of which Down's syndrome is the

most common) and prenatal infection (such as rubella and toxoplasmosis) may also result in brain damage. Various disorders, such as preeclampsia and placenta previa, may reduce the blood flow to the developing fetus. This may produce a mild form of fetal malnutrition that may affect development of the brain. *See also* DOWN'S SYNDROME; PREECLAMPSIA; RUBELLA; TOXOPLASMOSIS.

Brain damage may occur at birth. It may, for example, be caused by asphyxia or hemolytic disease of the newborn. Premature babies, especially if their birth weight is less than 3 pounds (1.5kg), are more likely to be mentally retarded during infancy and childhood. Such brain damage may be caused by a serious head injury; a serious infection, such as meningitis; or poisoning, especially with heavy metals such as lead. Chronic malnutrition, such as kwashiorkor, can also prevent normal brain development, thereby reducing intelligence. *See also* ASPHYXIA; HEMOLYTIC DISEASE OF THE NEWBORN; KWASHIORKOR.

In many cases of mild mental retardation, social and economic factors can be more significant than medical causes. These factors include poverty, social isolation, and cultural deprivation during early childhood. The majority of retarded individuals falls within the category of mild mental retardation. In cases of severe retardation, the primary factors are usually physical.

Q: ***How is mental retardation assessed?***

A: In some cases, mental retardation may be detected at birth or soon afterward. For example, Down's syndrome is usually apparent at birth. However, mental retardation, particularly if it is mild, is often detected first by the parents, who may notice that their child has problems with feeding, lacks normal responses, such as smiling, or is slow in learning to crawl or walk. In such cases, the parents should consult a pediatrician who will examine the baby to try to find a cause. The examination usually includes a full neurological investigation, sometimes with an electroencephalogram (EEG), skull X rays, hearing tests, and vision tests. From these, a pediatrician may be able to give the parents an

What is meant by "retarded"

Mental retardation is subaverage intellectual development, usually measured by an IQ (Intelligence Quotient) test. Parents may worry that an IQ test will prevent their mentally retarded child from going to a normal school. However, children are not assessed on the basis of an IQ test alone. The test reveals one facet of the child's makeup, but the complete diagnosis doesn't depend on it.

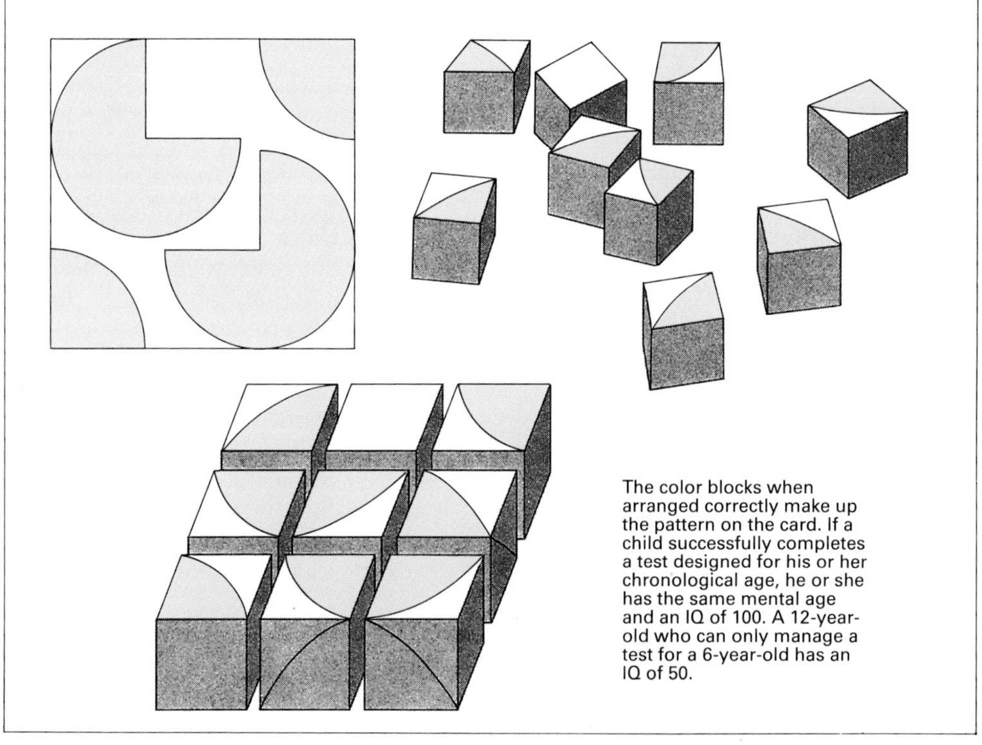

The color blocks when arranged correctly make up the pattern on the card. If a child successfully completes a test designed for his or her chronological age, he or she has the same mental age and an IQ of 100. A 12-year-old who can only manage a test for a 6-year-old has an IQ of 50.

indication of the degree of the child's retardation and the problems that they may encounter. Many parents find it difficult to accept that their child may be mentally retarded. Even if they suspect that this may be the case, they refrain from seeking expert confirmation. Professional advice, however, is essential if the child's learning potential is to be developed as fully as possible; it will also help the parents to cope with the strain and responsibility of bringing up a mentally retarded child.

An accurate assessment of an infant's intelligence is impossible. When the child is about three years old, an intelligence test may be given. This can give a reasonable indication of the severity of mental retardation, which may help the parents to plan for the child's future. Usually, multiple assessments with several instruments are done during the child's development to provide the broadest picture of the child's capabilities and skills in all areas of functioning. Thus, close follow-up with the child and the family is important.

Mental retardation is generally classified as mild, moderate, or severe. Individuals are assessed according to their degree of subnormality and their potential for learning social, occupational, and academic skills.

Children with mild retardation (with an intelligence quotient in the range of 50-70) can usually be taught to do simple mathematics, to read and write, and to perform uncomplicated tasks. Those with severe retardation may have difficulties with speech, coordination, bladder control, and bowel control. The most severely retarded seldom learn to walk and usually remain incontinent, needing lifelong supervision. *See also* INTELLIGENCE QUOTIENT.

Q: ***Can mental retardation be prevented?***

A: In some cases, it is possible to prevent mental retardation. At present, however, it is not possible to prevent most cases of mental retardation. If any inherited disorder has occurred in the family of either of the potential parents, a genetic counselor may be able to give advice about the likelihood of retardation in their children. Some chromosomal abnormalities can be detected by testing fluid from the uterus during pregnancy (amniocentesis). If this indicates that the baby will be retarded, the parents will have time to examine their options regarding the pregnancy.

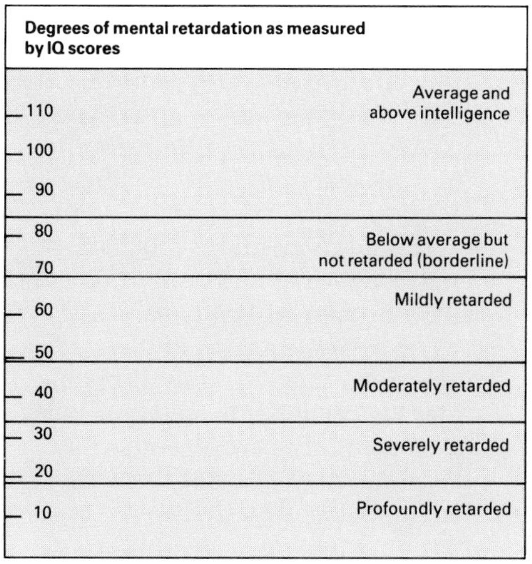

The possibility of brain damage in an infant can be reduced by stopping smoking, drinking, and drugs before and during pregnancy, by skilled prenatal care, and by following a healthy diet during pregnancy.

Tests for phenylketonuria are performed routinely within a day or two of birth. If these are positive, a special diet will prevent brain damage. Early diagnosis and treatment of hypothyroidism prevents cretinism. *See also* HYPOTHYROIDISM; PHENYLKETONURIA.

Q: ***Are there other problems that are associated with mental retardation?***

A: Yes. Cerebral palsy and epilepsy, which are also caused by brain damage, often occur in the mentally retarded. The drugs that are used to control epilepsy may further impair mental functioning because of their sedative effects.

It is more difficult to teach mentally retarded persons about safety

Degrees of mental retardation as measured by IQ scores

IQ score	Degree
110, 100, 90	Average and above intelligence
80, 70	Below average but not retarded (borderline)
60, 50	Mildly retarded
40	Moderately retarded
30, 20	Severely retarded
10	Profoundly retarded

An IQ test can measure the degrees of **mental retardation** and provide a partial assessment of a child's mental ability.

precautions, and so they tend to be more accident-prone.

Q: *How can the mentally retarded be helped?*

A: Skill, patience, and understanding from the parents, pediatricians, and educators who specialize in teaching the mentally retarded can enable retarded children to be educated to their fullest capabilities.

The severely retarded often have other disorders, such as spina bifida, hydrocephalus, cerebral palsy, or congenital heart disease. Such disorders may prevent them from being educated to the fullest extent, and they may need lifelong hospitalization. *See also* CEREBRAL PALSY; HEART DISEASE, CONGENITAL; HYDROCEPHALUS; SPINA BIFIDA.

Home care of the mentally retarded is extremely demanding on other members of the family, even with the support and encouragement of relatives and friends. Societies that have a special interest in a particular disorder can often give expert advice and may be able to put parents in contact with others who have similarly retarded children. Attention to the family's emotional needs can be just as important as treating the retarded child. *See also* MENTALLY RETARDED, CARE OF.

Mercury (mėr'kyər ē) is a liquid, metallic element that is commonly used in thermometers and other measuring instruments. Some mercury compounds are still used in antiseptics and eye ointments.

Q: *Is mercury poisonous?*

A: Small amounts of liquid mercury, such as that found in a thermometer, are not especially dangerous, because the element if ingested is poorly absorbed by the gastrointestinal tract. However, mercury compounds, known as mercury salts, and mercury vapor are toxic, particularly the vapor, which is very readily absorbed through the lungs. It affects the brain very quickly and is retained in the kidneys, resulting in renal failure.

Q: *How do people get mercury poisoning?*

A: Acute mercury poisoning may result from accidental (or deliberate, in the case of suicide attempts) ingestion of mercury salts. Chronic mercury poisoning usually results from exposure to mercury in the workplace or ingestion of mercury from foods contaminated by industrial pollution or chemical treatment. A pollution-related outbreak occurred in Minamata Bay, Japan, where several hundred people suffered irreversible damage or death from eating contaminated fish. Symptoms of acute mercury poisoning include diarrhea, vomiting, and kidney failure. Symptoms of chronic poisoning include tremors, albuminaria, paralysis, and mental disturbances.

Mescaline (mes'kə lēn) is an alkaloid that is the active hallucinogenic substance of the peyote cactus *(Lophophora williamsii)*, which grows in parts of Mexico and the southwestern United States. The drug is usually taken in capsule form. The effects of mescaline are similar to those of LSD and include visual and auditory hallucinations, distortions of time sense, feelings of anxiety or even persecution, and feelings of elation. Not all of these effects necessarily occur because the reaction to mescaline varies considerably among individuals, as well as in the same person at different times. A user's personality, the setting, and the dose all affect the experience.

See also DRUG ABUSE; DRUG ADDICTION; HALLUCINOGEN.

Mesentery (mes'ən ter ē) is a membrane-like fold of tissue attached to the back of the abdominal wall. It supports the intestines and contains the blood vessels, nerves, and parts of the lymphatic system that connect with the intestines.

Mesoderm (mes'ə dėrm) is the middle layer of cells formed during the development of the embryo. Muscles, bones, the circulatory system and connective tissues are some of the body parts derived from the mesoderm.

See also ECTODERM; ENDODERM; MESOMORPH.

Mesomorph (mes'ə môrf) is a person with a body structure derived principally from the mesodermal layer of the embryo. Such a person is a muscular, physical type, with a predominance of bone and muscle.

The mesomorph is one of three hypothetical body types used to explain certain aspects of personality, ectomorph and endomorph being the other two.

See also ECTOMORPH; ENDOMORPH; MESODERM.

Metabolism (mə tab′ə liz əm) is the sum of all the chemical and physical processes that occur within the body. It includes the repair and replacement of dead or damaged tissues and the production of energy.

Metabolism involves two basic processes: anabolism and catabolism. Anabolism is the synthesis of complex substances from simpler ones, which occurs during the growth of body tissues. Catabolism is the reverse process, the breakdown of complex substances into simpler substances. The "basal metabolic rate" (BMR) is a measure, expressed in calories, of the body's energy expenditure when at complete rest.

See also BASAL METABOLIC RATE.

Metacarpal (met ə kär′pəl) is any one of the five bones that form the structure of the palm of the hand.

See also HAND.

Metastasis (mə tas′tə sis) is the spread of a disease from one part of the body to another. The term usually refers to the spread of cancer, although metastasis may also occur in some infections, such as endocarditis and tuberculosis.

In cancer patients, cells that have separated from a primary tumor may spread through the lymphatic system into the veins or, more rarely, into an artery. These cells (metastases) may also spread across the surface of a structure, such as the peritoneum lining of the abdomen or the pleura surrounding the lungs. Occasionally, metastases result from surgery and may be found in the scar of the wound through which a tumor has been removed.

See also CANCER.

Metatarsal (met ə tär′sel) is any one of the five bones that form the main part of the arch of the foot.

See also FOOT; METATARSALGIA.

Metatarsalgia (met ə tär sal′jē ə) is pain in the instep area. The most common cause is a form of flatfoot in which the arch between the bases of the big and little toes is deformed and the heads of the metatarsal bones rest on the ground. This pressure on the bones produces pain, causes the skin to thicken, and may eventually cause the toes to curl.

Metatarsalgia may also be caused by a stress fracture, which can occur after prolonged walking or running. Resting the injured foot and wearing a soft-soled shoe is usually the only treatment required. Prolonged physiotherapy to strengthen the underlying muscles may be effective in patients under the age of 40 years. But if the pain is severe, it may be necessary to wear a cast for about one month.

Methadone® (meth′ə dōn) is a synthetic painkiller similar to morphine. It may be used as a potent narcotic-like analgesic for cancer patients and in the treatment of heroin addiction. Methadone is used in the treatment of heroin addiction because it blocks the effects of heroin withdrawal; although methadone itself is addictive, it is thought to be easier to withdraw from than is heroin. The use of methadone in heroin addicts decreases the risk of AIDS from intravenous injection of heroin, as well as the risk from contaminated heroin. Use of methadone in heroin withdrawal should be under expert medical supervision.

See also DRUG ADDICTION; HEROIN.

Methamphetamine (meth am fet′ə mēn) is a stimulant drug that has effects similar to those of amphetamine.

See also AMPHETAMINE.

Methemoglobin (met hē mə glō′bin) is a compound form of hemoglobin that prevents the hemoglobin in red blood cells from carrying adequate amounts of oxygen to the body tissues. The presence of methemoglobin usually results from poisoning with aniline dyes, potassium chlorate, or various other chemicals, including nitrites in drinking water. But it may also result from a hereditary deficiency of the substance that helps convert methemoglobin to hemoglobin.

See also HEMOGLOBIN.

Methyl alcohol. *See* ALCOHOL.

Metrorrhagia (mē trə rā′jē ə) is the medical term for bleeding from the uterus at times other than menstruation, possibly resulting from uterine lesions. It may also be a sign of cervical cancer.

See also MENORRHAGIA; MENSTRUAL PROBLEMS.

Microbe (mī′krōb) is a microscopic living organism. The term is often applied to any organism that causes disease, such as bacteria, viruses, or fungi.

See also GERM.

Microcephaly (mī krō sef′ə lē) is a congenital condition characterized by a disproportionately small head in relation to the rest of the body. The abnormally small head, present at birth, is usually associated with mental retardation.

Microscopy (mī kros′kə pē) is the observation and examination of minute structures using a microscope. Light microscopy refers to the use of a standard microscope, in which lenses magnify an image. Other kinds of microscopy exist, however, including electron microscopy, immunofluorescent microscopy, and television microscopy.

Microsurgery (mī krō sėr′jər ē) is any surgical technique that requires the use of a microscope and specially adapted hand-held instruments. It is used for operations that require extreme delicacy, as in surgery of the ears, the eyes, or the brain.

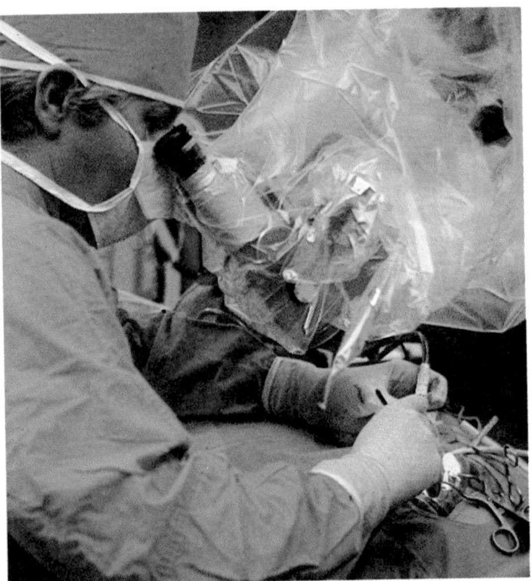

The surgeon shown here is performing **microsurgery** on a patient's ear.

Micturition (mik chə rish′ən) is the medical term for the act of passing urine.

See also BLADDER DISORDERS; URINE.

Middle ear. See EAR.

Midwife (mid′wīf), or nurse-midwife, is a person skilled and educated in caring for, and assisting, women in normal pregnancy, during labor and delivery, and following childbirth. Nurse-midwives are now becoming more common on many hospital staffs.

See also PREGNANCY AND CHILDBIRTH.

Migraine (mī′grān) is a recurring severe headache, often affecting only one side of the head and accompanied by a variety of other symptoms. It occurs more commonly in women than in men and usually first appears between the ages of 10 and 20 years. Although many people use the word "migraine" to describe any severe headache, this is not correct. Migraines are a specific type of headache caused by changes in the blood vessels that supply the brain.

Q: *What are the symptoms of migraine?*

A: In classic migraine headaches, a group of premonitory symptoms, known as an "aura," precedes the actual headache. These symptoms vary, but may include visual disturbances with irregular, flashing patterns of light (scotoma); temporary blindness in one half of the visual field (hemianopia); or double vision (diplopia) because of eye muscle weakness. Sometimes, there is also weakness or loss of sensation in a limb (hemiparesis), a strange taste or odor, tingling, vertigo, or a feeling that part of the body is distorted in size or shape.

The symptoms may last a few minutes and disappear before the beginning of the typical throbbing pain. It should be noted, however, that many people with migraines have so-called "common migraines," in which there is little or no aura present before the onset of the headache.

The headache in both types of migraine is frequently accompanied by nausea and vomiting, aversion to light (photophobia), and sensitivity to noise. The headache may last several hours, or even a day or two, before disappearing and allowing the individual to fall asleep and then to awake refreshed. Migraine attacks may occur daily or as infrequently as once every few months.

Q: *What causes migraine?*

A: The cause is not known, though about half of all migraine sufferers have another member of the family who has similar headaches. Sometimes, there is an association with certain foods, such as chocolate, cheese, or cured meats, suggesting an allergy. The initial symptoms result from a narrowing of the blood vessels that supply the brain, followed by an expansion that produces the headache.

Q: *Does migraine last for life?*

A: Usually, migraine becomes less frequent with increasing age and is relatively uncommon after the age of 50. Some persons, however, continue to suffer from migraine into old age.

Q: *Can migraine occur in young children?*

A: Yes. A child may not complain of a headache, but suffer from recurrent attacks of malaise accompanied by nausea and vomiting. The child may be able to describe the first symptoms of distorted vision and flashing lights, which can be extremely frightening if neither the child nor the parents understand what is happening.

Q: *Can anything increase the likelihood of migraine?*

A: Yes. Apart from certain foods that may cause migraine in some individuals, there are other factors that may bring on the symptoms. Many women experience a migraine a day or two before menstruation, when the headache is associated with premenstrual tension. Some people develop a migraine when they are under emotional stress or after a period of stress, typically during the weekend. Bright lights or loud noises may also trigger an attack. Some people find that particular wines can produce a migraine, probably because of a combination of alcohol and other wine ingredients.

Q: *Why does alcohol cause migraine?*

A: It is not known why alcohol causes migraine. But there is a particular kind of migraine, sometimes called a cluster headache, in which a one-sided headache is accompanied by a runny nose and a sore, reddened eye on the affected side. Several attacks occur within a few days and then there is a prolonged period without headaches. This type of migraine is more common in middle-aged men and may be triggered by alcohol. *See also* HEADACHE, CLUSTER.

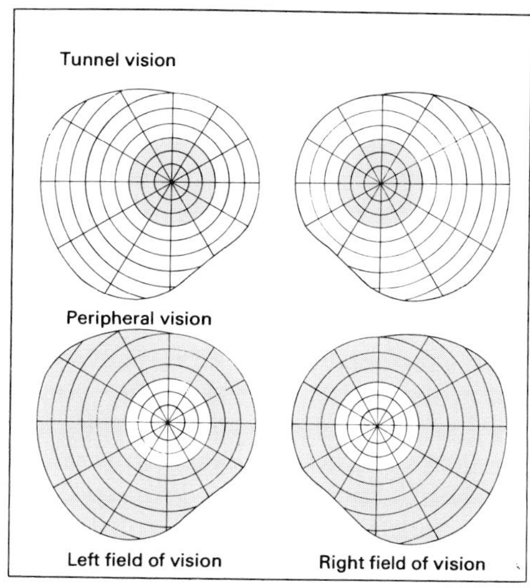

Migraine may cause visual disturbances, such as tunnel and peripheral vision. (Shaded section indicates area of vision.)

Q: *How is migraine treated?*

A: Drug therapy has now been proven effective in the treatment of migraine. If the headaches are infrequent, the drug of choice is ergotamine tartrate, which is used for pain relief. It may be given in various forms: rectally in the form of a suppository; by inhalation; by injection; or by absorption underneath the tongue.

Propranolol is sometimes prescribed for patients with frequent attacks. It cuts down the frequency, severity, and duration of migraine attacks. The drug should be administered only under a physician's careful guidance. A new group of drugs, known as calcium channel blockers, are also used in the treatment of migraines. *See also* CALCIUM CHANNEL BLOCKER.

Relaxation therapy, such as biofeedback, wherein instruments teach a person how to control the symptoms of migraine, is also a helpful treatment.

Q: *Can migraine be prevented?*

A: Migraine sufferers should learn to keep track of factors and conditions that normally precede their attack. Steps can then be taken in the future to prevent similar attacks. This procedure can be simple, such as learning to avoid certain foods or drinks, or it can be more difficult, such as trying to reduce tension and anxiety and just relaxing.

See also HEADACHE.

Miliaria (mil ē âr′ē ə) is a fine, red rash on the body, especially round the waist and in the bends of the knees and elbows. It is especially common in infants.

See also PRICKLY HEAT.

Milk is the secretion from the female breast that feeds a newborn baby. Human breast milk contains the right balance of ingredients, such as water, organic substances, antibodies, enzymes, and mineral salts, for the infant's well-being, although human milk varies in quantities of nutritive ingredients week by week during lactation. Processed cow's milk, although not as nutritious, is an acceptable substitute once a child has reached the age of one year. Prior to that age a specially processed formula, derived from cow's milk, is the only acceptable substitute. Untreated cow's milk should never be fed to babies.

See also BABY CARE; LACTATION.

Milk of magnesia. *See* MAGNESIA, MILK OF.

Milk teeth are the first, temporary set of teeth to appear. They are also called deciduous teeth. The teeth are present, hidden in the jaws, in a newborn baby. They begin to grow through the gums by the end of the first year. A child has 20 milk teeth.

See also TOOTH.

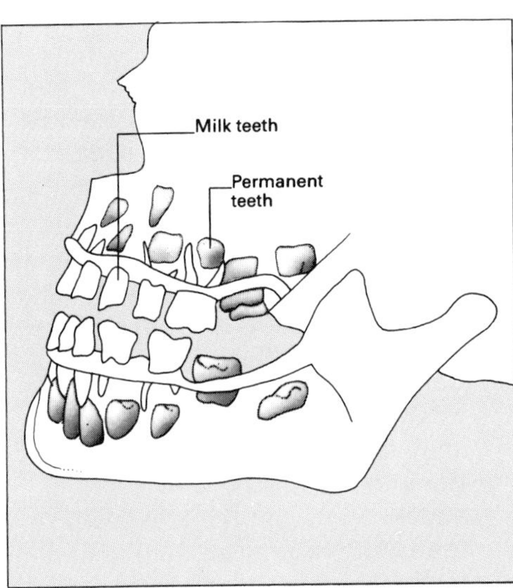

Milk teeth begin to be replaced by permanent teeth when a child is about six years old.

Milroy's disease (mil′roiz) is a congenital form of hereditary lymphedema, primarily affecting the legs. It is caused by chronic obstruction of the lymphatic system, whose vessels are either underdeveloped or incomplete. Other areas of the body, such as the arms, face, and trunk, may also be involved. It is also known as congenital lymphedema.

See also EDEMA; LYMPH; LYMPHATIC SYSTEM; LYMPHEDEMA.

Minamata disease (min ə mä′tə) is mercury poisoning named after Minamata Bay in Japan, where several hundred people suffered irreversible brain damage or death after eating fish contaminated with mercury.

See also MERCURY.

Mineral is an inorganic element or compound. Minerals in the diet are important to good health. Various elements are essential parts of body cells, including calcium, chlorine, copper, fluorine, iodine, iron, magnesium, manganese, phosphorus, potassium, zinc, and sodium. The chief mineral salts in the body are chlorides and phosphates. Some minerals are incorporated into body tissues; others are excreted. For this reason, a balanced diet must contain the correct amounts of various essential minerals.

See also NUTRITION.

Mineral oil (liquid petrolatum) is a preparation of light petroleum oils sometimes used in medicine. The oil is used on the skin and as a lubricant for catheters (tubes passed into the body to inject or remove fluid) and surgical instruments. Taken internally, mineral oil acts as a laxative; because mineral oil can be extremely toxic if accidentally aspirated into the lungs, physicians generally recommend other preparations in the treatment of constipation.

See also CONSTIPATION.

Miotic (mī ot′ik) is any substance that makes the pupil of the eye constrict. Pilocarpine is a miotic.

Mirror writing is writing formed from right to left (instead of left to right), so that it appears normal when seen reflected in a mirror. Mirror writing commonly occurs in left-handed children who are attempting to write with their right hand. Learning problems can be avoided if the trait is recognized and help is obtained for the child.

See also LEARNING DISABILITY.

Miscarriage (mis kar′ij) is the spontaneous or accidental termination of pregnancy without outside intervention prior to the twentieth week of gestation before the embryo or fetus can live independently of its mother. The usual reason for a miscarriage is a defect in the embryo or fetus that prevents its natural development. This defect may be inherited, caused by an exposure of the mother to medications or radiation, or result from infectious illness. The first symptom of a threatened miscarriage in a pregnant woman is vaginal bleeding; this requires immediate medical attention. A miscarriage is most likely to occur in the second, third, or fourth month of pregnancy.

The medical term for a miscarriage in the early months of pregnancy is *spontaneous abortion*. Expulsion of a fetus from the uterus after approximately the twentieth week of pregnancy is known as a *stillbirth*, if the fetus is dead, and as a *premature birth*, if the fetus is alive.

Mite (mīt) is a minute arachnid related to the spider. Mites belong to the animal order *Acarina*, which includes a great number of different species, among them chiggers and ticks. Mites may exist on the skin or in the hair as parasites and can transmit disease.

See also RICKETTSIA; SCABIES.

Mitochondria (mī tə kon′drē ə) are one of the several kinds of tiny structures, called organelles, located in the cytoplasm of cells. Hundreds of mitochondria may be found in one cell. They are the power producers of the cell. Through various chemical processes, mitochondria provide almost all the energy a cell needs to live and function. Mitochondria are self-replicating and are also known as chondriosomes.

See also CELL.

Mitral valve disease (mī′trəl) refers to one of several disorders of the heart valve between the upper chamber (atrium) and the lower chamber (ventricle) on the left side of the heart. The opening in the valve may be narrower than normal (mitral stenosis) or wider than normal (mitral incompetence). Commonly, these conditions result from scarring caused by rheumatic fever, or rarely, they may be present at birth. *See also* RHEUMATIC FEVER.

Q: ***What are the symptoms of mitral stenosis?***

A: The first symptoms are usually shortness of breath during exercise and, sometimes, episodes of breathlessness at night because the lungs become congested with blood. The symptoms begin gradually, as it takes many years for the scarring to take place. As scarring worsens, the symptoms become more severe so that acute breathlessness may occur on the slightest exertion, and there may be signs of heart failure because of back pressure of blood into the right side of the heart. Signs include a bluish tinge to the lips (cyanosis) and swollen ankles.

Many patients develop a rapid irregular heartbeat called atrial fibrillation. Sometimes, the shortness of breath is accompanied by coughing attacks that may produce bloodstained sputum (hemoptysis). *See also* FIBRILLATION.

Q: ***What is the treatment for mitral stenosis?***

A: A physician may prescribe diuretic drugs and some compound of digitalis to help control the heart failure. If atrial fibrillation has recently occurred, beta-blocking drugs or a controlled electric shock (cardioversion) may restore normal heart rhythm. *See also* CARDIOVERSION.

Moderately severe or severe mitral stenosis may be treated by surgery. The valve can be enlarged by cutting the scarred tissue (commissurotomy) or replaced with an artificial valve or one obtained from a pig's heart.

Q: ***What are the symptoms of mitral incompetence and how is it treated?***

A: The symptoms are less severe than those of mitral stenosis, but increasing fatigue and shortness of breath commonly occur. Usually, drug treatment with diuretics and digoxin is sufficient to control the symptoms. However, if this fails, the damaged valve can be replaced by surgery, as in mitral stenosis.

Mitral valve prolapse (mī′trəl) is the condition in which one or both of the cusps of the mitral valve slip out of position, resulting in an incomplete closure of the left atrium during contraction of the heart. It is a fairly common disorder, and most patients have no symptoms. Some patients may experience such symptoms as chest pain, palpitations, and fatigue. Mitral valve prolapse sometimes accompanies the rare Marfan syndrome. Treatment includes medication before dental work or surgery to prevent subacute bacterial endocarditis; sometimes, drugs are needed to control the palpitations.

See *also* ENDOCARDITIS; MARFAN SYNDROME.

Molar (mō′lər) is a broad tooth at the back of the mouth used for chewing and grinding. An adult has 12 molar teeth, with 3 upper and 3 lower molars on each side of the mouth. The back 4 molars are also known as wisdom teeth.

See *also* TOOTH.

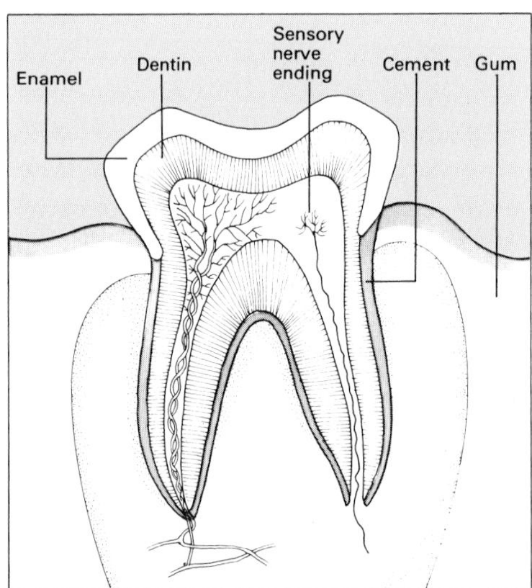

Molar is a large, deep-rooted tooth at the back of the jaw used for chewing and grinding.

Molar, impacted (mō′lər, im pak′tid). An impacted molar is a molar tooth that is prevented from emerging normally because of its wedged position between another tooth and the jawbone. The wisdom tooth, or third molar, is the tooth most often impacted.

See *also* TOOTH, WISDOM.

Mole (mōl) is a colored area or spot on the skin. Moles may be flat or raised and vary in size and color or pigmentation. Some moles are covered with hair.

Moles are formed from cells containing the dark pigment melanin. Some may be present at birth, although many develop during childhood or adolescence. A mole that is present at birth is usually called a birthmark.

Q: *Do moles require treatment?*

A: Treatment is not necessary unless the mole is disfiguring, such as a large hairy mole on the face. Treatment may also be necessary if the mole is situated where clothing irritates it, such as around the waist, possibly resulting in infection and inflammation. Moles can usually be removed via plastic surgery under a local anesthetic.

Q: *Can moles become cancerous?*

A: Yes, but this is rare. A mole that changes in size, color, or shape should be examined by a physician. Bleeding moles may be malignant (cancerous), and they should be reported to a physician at once.

See *also* MELANOMA.

Mole, hydatidiform (mōl, hī də tid′ə fôrm). A hydatidiform mole is a usually benign (noncancerous) growth within the uterus that may develop in early pregnancy. A pregnant woman may experience bleeding similar to that from a threatened miscarriage. The bleeding tends to continue and may result in the spontaneous loss of a mass of small, grape-like tissue from the uterus.

Q: *What is the treatment for a hydatidiform mole?*

A: If the growth is not spontaneously expelled, the obstetrician induces early labor through the administration of the drug oxytocin, followed a few days later by a dilatation and curettage surgical procedure.

See *also* DILATATION AND CURETTAGE; MISCARRIAGE.

Molluscum contagiosum (mə lus′kəm kən tā jē ō′səm) is a viral infection of the skin. The infection is characterized by small, raised, flesh-colored lesions that have a central dimple.

Molluscum fibrosum. See VON RECKLINGHAUSEN'S DISEASE.

Mongolism. See DOWN'S SYNDROME.

Moniliasis. See CANDIDIASIS.

Monoamine oxidase inhibitor. See MAO INHIBITOR.

Monocyte (mon′ə sīt) is a type of white blood cell that has a single nucleus and a relatively large amount of surrounding cytoplasm.

See *also* BLOOD CELL, WHITE.

Mononucleosis (mon ə nü klē ō′sis), also called infectious mononucleosis and glandular fever, is an infectious illness caused by a herpes virus (Epstein-Barr virus). It is spread by saliva and nasal secretions and is sometimes known as the "kissing disease." Most common in persons between 15 and 25 years of age, mononucleosis is only mildly infectious. But the crowded conditions of a school classroom, for example, favor the spread of the disease through airborne droplet infection. Once infected, however, an individual is permanently immune to the illness.

Q: *What are the symptoms of mononucleosis?*

A: About a month after contracting the disease, the patient has a period of increasing fatigue and lethargy and a slight fever that lasts for 7 to 10 days. This is followed by a sore throat, similar to tonsillitis, with a high fever and generalized enlargement of the lymph nodes in the neck. Often, the spleen also becomes enlarged. There may be a faint, pink rash over the body. The acute phase of the illness lasts for 7 to 10 days. The fever then subsides slowly with rapid improvement of the sore throat. *See also* LYMPH NODE.

The acute phase of the illness is followed by several weeks of lethargy and vague discomfort, often accompanied by depression and a feeling of fatigue after any form of mental or physical effort. During this time a relapse may occur, particularly if the patient attempts too much too soon. In a few cases, inflammation of the liver (hepatitis) may occur as a complication of mononucleosis and can delay recovery even further.

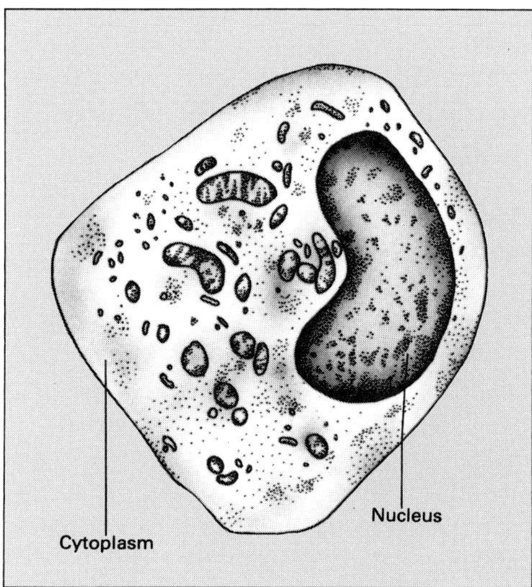

The largest of the white blood cells is the **monocyte,** comprising about 3 to 8 percent of the total number of white blood cells.

Q: *How is mononucleosis diagnosed and treated?*

A: An examination of the white blood cells and a special blood test confirm the diagnosis and eliminate common conditions with similar symptoms, such as tonsillitis, Vincent's infection, and toxoplasmosis. *See also* TONSILLITIS; TOXOPLASMOSIS; VINCENT'S INFECTION.

There is no cure for mononucleosis. It should be treated with ample bed rest, painkilling drugs, and mouthwashes for the sore throat. Rest and avoidance of exercise, while the spleen is enlarged, is important. Antibiotics are of little help, unless a secondary bacterial infection occurs. Ampicillin may produce a rash in patients with mononucleosis.

Mononucleosis, infectious. *See* MONONUCLEOSIS.

Monoplegia (mon ə plē'jē ə) is paralysis of one limb.

See also PARALYSIS.

Monosodium glutamate (mon ə sō'dē əm glü'tə māt), also known as MSG, is the sodium salt of glutamic acid. It is used to enhance the flavor of foods.

MSG is often used in Chinese cooking and is suspected to be the cause of Chinese restaurant syndrome. This is a condition characterized by dizziness, headache, chest pain, and tingling or burning sensation of the skin.

Morbidity (môr bid'ə tē) is the state or condition of being afflicted with disease. The term is also used to describe the proportion of sick people in a particular community.

See also MORTALITY.

Morbilli. *See* MEASLES.

Morning sickness affects about 50 percent of women in early pregnancy. They experience nausea and vomiting, from about the sixth through the twelfth week of pregnancy. A headache often occurs with morning sickness, along with a feeling of dizziness and exhaustion. The symptoms usually occur in the morning, but may be present at any time during the day.

Q: *What causes morning sickness?*

A: The cause of morning sickness is not fully understood. It may result from an increased sensitivity of the vomiting center in the brain, caused by the hormonal activity of early pregnancy. These hormones also have an effect on the gastrointestinal tract, so that the movement of feces along the colon is slowed down. As a result, some food and gastric secretions remain in the stomach in the morning.

Q: *How is morning sickness treated?*

A: Many women find that nausea can be prevented by eating frequent, small, bland meals and avoiding an empty stomach. Eating soda crackers before rising may be helpful. In severe cases, a physician may prescribe an antinausea drug to be taken before going to bed. B-complex vitamins may also be prescribed.

See also PREGNANCY AND CHILDBIRTH.

Moro reflex (môr′ō), or startle reflex, is an infant's normal reflex to a sudden stimulus, such as a loud noise. The infant will flex the legs, throw the arms outward, and then bring them together in an embrace position.

Morphine (môr′fēn) is an alkaloid drug derived from the opium poppy. It is a powerful narcotic analgesic (painkiller) and cough suppressant. Morphine relieves anxiety and induces contentment in patients suffering from severe pain. It is also used in the treatment of such conditions as acute heart failure and shock. Prolonged use of morphine can result in psychological and physical dependence.

Generally, morphine is injected in order to produce a predictable and rapid result. The drug is often prescribed for persons with terminal cancer. When morphine is prescribed to be taken orally, it is given in high dosage because of its slow and poor absorption by the intestine.

Morphine should be prescribed cautiously for the elderly or the very young because persons in those age groups are particularly sensitive to the drug's respiratory depressant effects. Morphine may also be dangerous to those who have lung disease, such as asthma, because of the same depressant effect on breathing.

See also ALKALOID; METHADONE; OPIATE.

Mortality (môr tal′ə tē) is the state of being subject to death. It is also a term used to refer to the rate of death per unit of population.

See also MORBIDITY.

Mosquito (mə skē′tō) is a bloodsucking insect. It can carry parasites that cause diseases in human beings. There are many species of mosquitoes. Those of the *Anopheles* group carry malaria. The *Aedes* mosquito carries yellow fever and dengue fever, as well as viruses that cause encephalitis in some tropical countries. The *Culex* mosquito carries a form of filaria that causes elephantiasis.

See also DENGUE; ELEPHANTIASIS; ENCEPHALITIS; MALARIA; YELLOW FEVER.

Motion sickness is nausea and vomiting caused by repeated movements in any combination of directions, as in a car, boat, or train. Motion sickness may be preceded by sweating, headache, and fatigue. It is more common in children and often disappears with age as the organ of balance (the semicircular canals within the ear) becomes less sensitive to movement. Airsickness, carsickness, and seasickness are all examples of motion sickness. It may be caused by any form of transport, as well as by amusement rides, such as carousels and roller-coasters.

See also MOTION SICKNESS: TREATMENT.

Motion sickness: treatment. If you suffer from motion sickness, you should take antinauseant drugs the night before the journey and again on the morning of the journey. Antinauseant drugs may cause drowsiness and should not be taken if you intend to drive a car. If you are taking regular medication for other disorders, consult a physician before the journey, because the drugs may interact with some antinauseants.

A light meal should be eaten about one-half hour before the journey because an empty stomach may increase the feeling of nausea. During the journey, you should lie down with the head braced. Avoid reading. You should remain in a part of the vehicle with the least movement, such as the center of a boat or near the wings of an airplane. If this is not possible, it sometimes helps to look at the horizon or a stationary point within the vehicle. Small amounts of food and drink should be taken at regular intervals. Alcohol should be avoided.

Motor describes any body structure that is concerned with movement. For example, a motor nerve carries the "instructions" that make a muscle move.

Motorcycle safety. Motorcyclists are more vulnerable on the road than drivers of cars because a motorcycle is less visible to other road users and provides less protection in the event of an accident. Car drivers often do not notice motorcyclists until they are very close and may allow them little room when passing. For this reason, motorcyclists should drive cautiously, take special care of their equipment, and wear conspicuous and protective clothing.

Motorcyclists can increase their safety by practicing correct riding techniques. Give clear, positive hand signals before turning right or left in busy traffic. Never assume that because you can see other drivers, they can see you. Use your headlights and horn to make sure that other road users are aware of your presence.

Many techniques can be learned only by experience and should be practiced on quiet roads before they are attempted on main highways or in heavy traffic. These techniques include controlled, progressive braking on wet or slippery roads; leaning into the bend combined with the correct use of gears and brakes when rounding a corner; and allowing for airstreams when overtaking another vehicle.

Motorcyclists should choose their clothing and protective equipment carefully. The helmet is especially important. Many states in the United States require that a motorcyclist wear a helmet while riding. Whichever type you buy—fiberglass or polycarbonate, full-face or open-face—make sure that it fits correctly.

Try on a helmet and fasten the straps; if you can wriggle out of it, it is the wrong size. If a visor is fitted to the helmet, remember it is dangerous to ride with a visor open. This may expose you to eye damage from particles in the air and also lift the helmet. Replace the visor when it becomes scratched. Wash your helmet in water only, and never allow it to come into contact with gasoline, grease, or other organic solvents. Also, do not paint your helmet or stick tape or transfers on it. This can damage the shell structure, and the helmet may then shatter on even slight impact. Check the straps regularly to see that they do not become worn or frayed. Helmets that get heavy use should be replaced every three years. Otherwise, they should be replaced every five years. Never reuse a helmet that has been involved in an accident or dropped, because many helmets are designed to absorb a single impact only. All other items of clothing should be conspicuous and provide long-term protection against the weather. Leather is the most suitable material for comfort and warmth.

If you are buying a motorcycle, safety should be a more important consideration than speed. Choose a machine of reasonable size and power, one that you will be able to ride with confidence. Inspect the motorcycle carefully before committing yourself to buying it, especially if you are buying it secondhand. Get an expert to advise you and to help you check the condition of the tires, the brakes, the wheel and steering bearings, the chain, the exhaust, the suspension, the lights, and the engine. For your own safety, you should learn

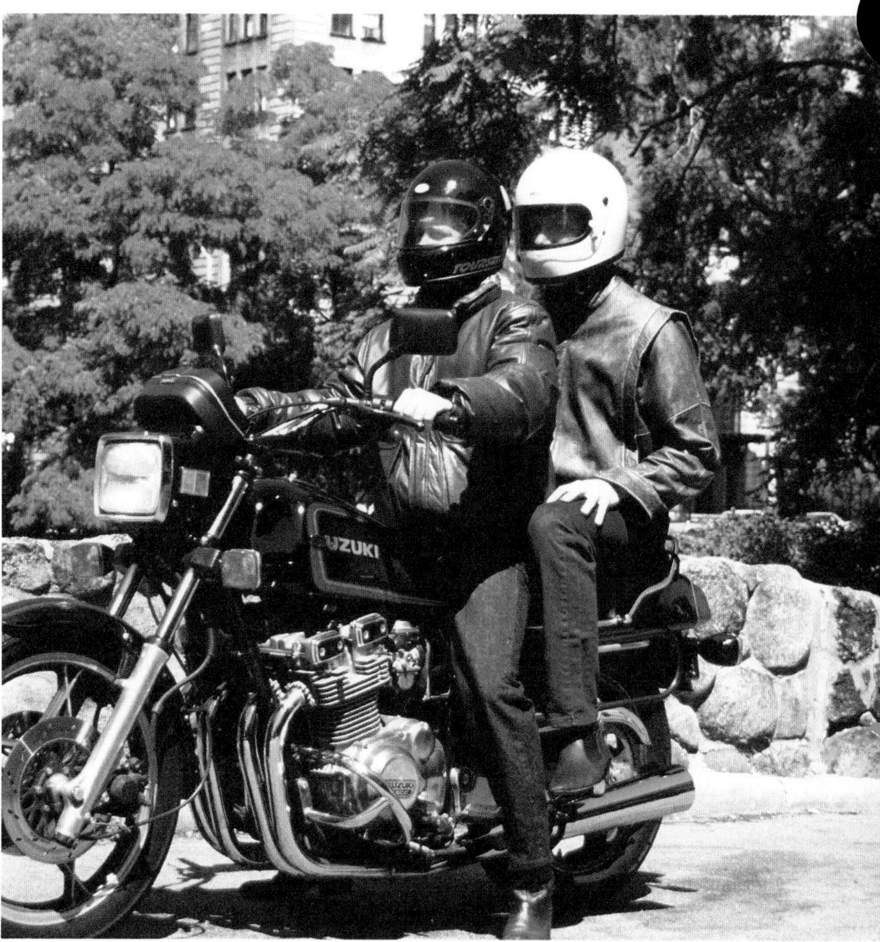

In addition to proper driving techniques and a smoothly-running machine, the wearing of appropriate clothing also enhances **motorcycle safety.** This includes helmets for protecting the head in case of accident, leather jackets for warmth and comfort, long pants to shield the legs from exposure to wind and sun, and boots, which provide better foot protection than sandals or low-cut shoes.

how a motorcycle works and how to maintain all the parts in good running order.

Motor neuron disease (nůr′on) is a group of similar disorders of unknown origin that cause degeneration of the nerve cells in the spinal cord or brain and affect muscle activity. There is increasing muscle weakness and wasting, usually beginning in the hands and feet and spreading to involve the shoulders and buttocks. It usually affects adults in late middle age.

The type of motor neuron disease, called amyotrophic lateral sclerosis, is usually fatal within 3 years, while a person with progressive muscular atrophy may live for as long as 20 years. The condition known as progressive bulbar palsy affects the throat muscles and causes difficulty in talking, chewing, and swallowing. Death from pneumonia often occurs within a year or two.

There is no effective treatment for motor neuron disease, although physiotherapy may help to maintain mobility.

See also AMYOTROPHIC LATERAL SCLEROSIS; BULBAR PARALYSIS; MUSCULAR ATROPHY, PROGRESSIVE.

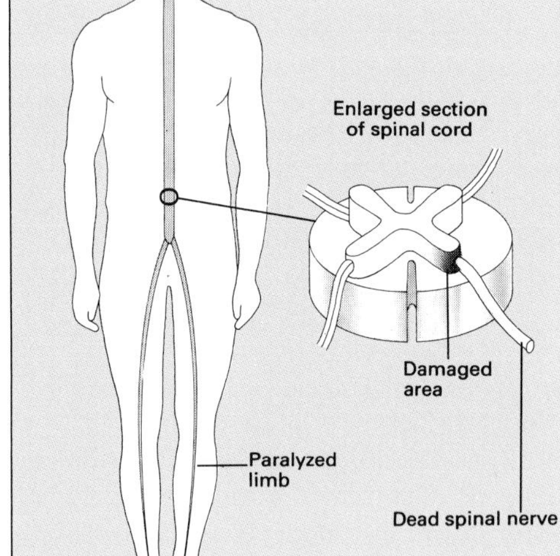

Motor neuron disease affects the spinal nerves and results in leg paralysis.

Mountain sickness. *See* ALTITUDE SICKNESS.

Mouth is formed by the bone structure of the jaws. The upper part is formed by the upper jawbone (maxilla) and the lower part by the lower jawbone (mandible). The entrance to the mouth is surrounded by the skin and muscles that form the lips. The interior contains the gums, palate, teeth, and tongue. The mucous membrane, the soft skin lining the mouth, is kept moist by the secretions of the salivary glands and heals rapidly if damaged.

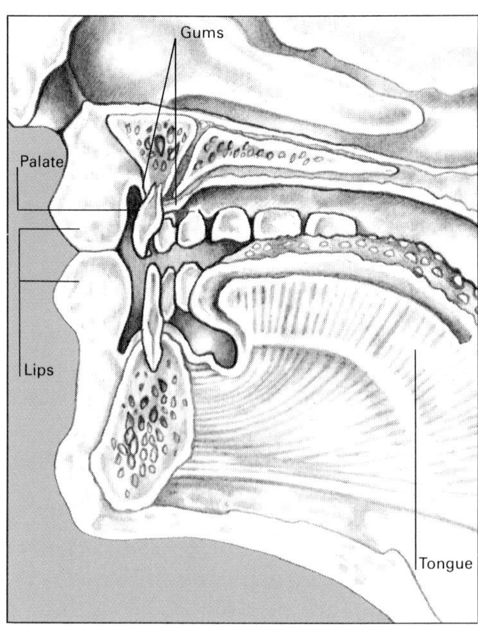

The **mouth** is formed by the upper jawbone (maxilla) and by the lower jawbone (mandible).

See also CANKER SORE; CHEILITIS; CHEILOSIS; CLEFT PALATE; DENTAL DISORDERS; GINGIVITIS; GUM; HARELIP; LIP; PALATE; SALIVARY GLAND; STOMATITIS; TONGUE; TOOTH.

Mouth breathing is breathing through the mouth when the nose is blocked, perhaps as a result of an infection, such as a cold, or an injury to the nose, for example, a fracture. In children, mouth breathing is often caused by swollen adenoids. *See also* ADENOID.

Mouth breathing may cause snoring and disturbed sleep. The mouth may also become dry, which increases the probability of gum infection. Normal breathing is resumed when the cause disappears.

Mouth-to-mouth resuscitation (ri sus ə tā′shən) is a form of artificial respiration in which the victim's lungs are inflated with air exhaled by the rescuer.

See also ARTIFICIAL RESPIRATION.

Mouth ulcer (ul′sər) is any open sore that affects the mucous membrane that lines the inside of the mouth.

See also CANKER SORE; HAND-FOOT-AND-MOUTH DISEASE; STOMATITIS.

MRI. *See* MAGNETIC RESONANCE IMAGING.

MS. *See* MULTIPLE SCLEROSIS.

Mucopurulent (myü kō pyůr'ə lənt) describes a discharge from the body that contains both mucus and pus. Examples of the discharge include mucus from the nose, sputum from the lungs, or fluid from the anus when disorders involve inflammation of the colon or rectum, such as ulcerative colitis and diverticular disease.

See also MUCUS; PUS; SPUTUM.

Mucous (myü'kəs) is the adjective form of the word mucus, as in mucous membrane, or a combining word form meaning "composed of mucus," as in fibromucous.

See also MUCUS.

Mucous colitis. *See* IRRITABLE BOWEL SYNDROME.

Mucous membrane (myü'kəs) is a thin layer of cells containing glands that secrete a sticky fluid called mucus. Mucous membranes line the internal passages and cavities of the body, such as the bladder, bronchial tubes, intestine, mouth, and vagina. *See also* MUCUS.

Mucus (myü'kəs) is a moist, sticky substance that is continually secreted by glands within any of the body's mucous membranes. Mucus acts as a protective barrier.

See also MUCOUS MEMBRANE.

Multipara (mul tip'ər ə) is the medical term for a woman who has had 2 or more pregnancies that lasted for more than 20 weeks. A grand multipara is a woman with 4 or more pregnancies.

See also NULLIPARA.

Multiphasic health testing laboratory (mul ti fā'sik) is a specially designed building with automated chemical analyzers, electronic computers, and other instruments. In a few hours, dozens of medical tests can be performed. The information from these and other measurements is fed into computers that quickly prepare and print reports for the physician.

Such tests should not be performed indiscriminately. Specific laboratory tests should only be ordered after a careful consideration of a patient's medical history and a physical examination by a physician or other health professional.

Multiple personality, or split personality, is an abnormal, fragmented mental condition that is characterized by a sudden change of identity and unpredictable alternation between two or more subpersonalities.

See also MENTAL ILLNESS.

Multiple sclerosis (mul'tə pəl skli rō' sis), also known as MS or demyelinating disease, is a disorder of the brain and spinal cord in which a degeneration of the fatty myelin sheath that surrounds nerve fibers occurs, leading to a short-circuiting of nerve impulses. This results in a great variety of symptoms, sometimes followed by recovery or marked improvement. Further damage may occur at irregular intervals over many years, causing increasing disability in some, but not all, patients.

The cause of multiple sclerosis is not known, but it may be associated with some kind of altered immunity to a virus infection.

Q: *What are the symptoms of multiple sclerosis?*

A: The first symptoms usually occur between the ages of 20 and 40. The onset is usually gradual and may include slight, temporary weakness in one arm or leg; tingling or numbness in a limb or on one side of the face; double vision (diplopia) because of weakness of an eye muscle; blurred vision (amblyopia); or, frequently, pain in one eye because of neuritis affecting the optic nerve (retrobulbar neuritis). Other symptoms that may occur at the same time or in later attacks include incontinence of urine, unsteady gait (ataxia), vertigo, and sometimes, emotional disturbance with sudden tears or laughter, depression or cheerfulness. *See also* ATAXIA; NEURITIS, RETROBULBAR; VERTIGO.

As the disorder progresses, these symptoms recur along with various others that involve the nervous system. They tend to last longer and may not disappear completely, so that the patient may be left with a limp, a hesitation in speech, or a flickering movement of the eye.

Some patients are never disabled by their symptoms, but in others, the symptoms may be severe enough to confine them to bed and make them unable to walk or maintain bladder control. As the disorder progresses, recovery from each attack is less complete. The

Multilple sclerosis is a progressive degeneration of nervous tissue, causing a variety of symptoms.

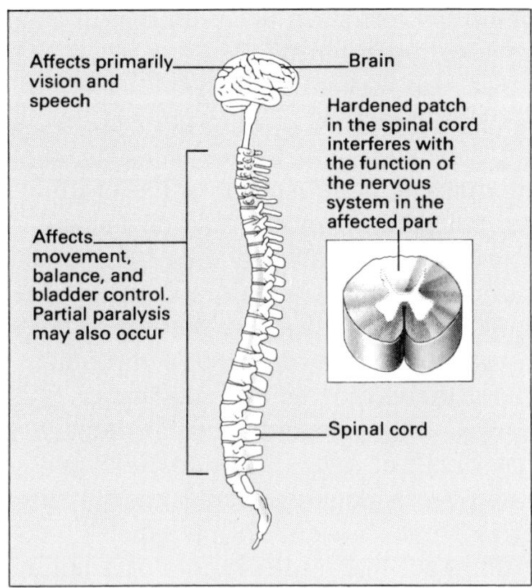
Affects primarily vision and speech
Brain
Hardened patch in the spinal cord interferes with the function of the nervous system in the affected part
Affects movement, balance, and bladder control. Partial paralysis may also occur
Spinal cord

patient may be left with stiff limbs, often accompanied by intermittent, painful spasms of the muscles. Eventually, urinary or lung infections may occur, and one of these complications may cause death.

Q: *Is the progression of the disease always the same?*

A: A few patients have a rapid, progressive disease with frequent relapses that lead to death within one or two years. Others may have only one or two minor problems followed by complete, spontaneous recovery without further trouble. Most patients, however, have recurring symptoms for 15 to 25 years and may then stabilize.

Q: *What is the treatment for MS?*

A: Until recent years, there was no treatment for the disorder. Researchers are now using a combination of ACTH, a pituitary hormone used to reduce inflammation, and Cytoxan®, an anticancer drug, to treat MS. Those patients injected with the Cytoxan-ACTH have either improved or shown no further signs of deterioration. The treatment is, however, still highly experimental. *See also* ADRENOCORTICOTROPIC HORMONE.

Patients are generally encouraged to lead as normal a life as possible, avoiding overwork, however. Massage or physical therapy of weakened limbs is often used to make patients more comfortable.

See also NERVOUS SYSTEM.

Mumps (mumpz), also called epidemic parotitis or infective parotitis, is a virus infection that causes painful inflammation and swelling of the salivary glands. Mumps is most common among children, but it may also affect adults. *See also* SALIVARY GLAND.

Q: *How long is the incubation period for mumps and for how long is it contagious?*

A: The incubation period is between 15 and 25 days, usually 21 days. The disease is infectious for about 2 days before the swelling appears and about 3 days after the swelling goes down.

Q: *What are the symptoms of mumps?*

A: There is usually an initial period of one to two days of headache, malaise, and fever. This stage is followed by a sudden rise in temperature to about 104°F (40°C), which accompanies the onset of painful swelling of the salivary glands. The parotid glands in front of the ears are the glands most commonly involved in the early stage, but swelling may spread to the glands under the jaw. The swollen glands are tender to touch and may cause difficulty opening the mouth. The extent of the swelling may vary from day to day. Only one side may be affected. The acute stage of the illness usually lasts five to six days, with a gradual reduction in the swelling as the patient improves.

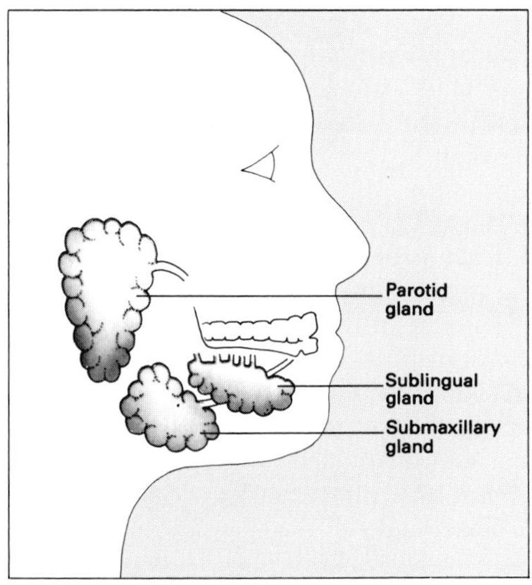
Parotid gland
Sublingual gland
Submaxillary gland

Mumps causes painful swelling and inflammation of the parotid, sublingual, and submaxillary glands. The swollen salivary glands may make swallowing more difficult.

Mumps in adults may cause inflammation of the testicles in men, which may lead to sterility, or inflammation of the ovaries in women.

Q: *What is the treatment for mumps?*

A: There is no cure for mumps. Therapy is directed toward making the patient comfortable, reducing fever, and ensuring adequate fluid intake. Painkilling and sedative drugs may be prescribed.

Q: *Can mumps be prevented?*

A: Yes. A vaccine containing a mild, living virus is available. It should be used to immunize children at the age of 12 to 15 months and repeated at 10 to 12 years of age. In the United States, it is commonly combined with measles and rubella (German measles) vaccine. Occasionally, mumps vaccine produces a mild illness. It is not certain whether immunity lasts for life, but the vaccine seems to protect about 95 percent of children.

Munchausen's syndrome (mun chô′ zənz), also called pathomimicry, is a mental disorder in which the patient persuades physicians that he or she has a real physical disease, when no disease is actually present. The disorder is named for Baron Karl F. H. von Munchausen, who was known for his tall tales of courage and skill on the battlefield, none of which were true.

Patients with Munchausen's syndrome are skilled at mimicking the physical signs and symptoms of a disorder, such as myocardial infarction, appendicitis, and cerebral tumor. Such pretended complaints may lead to hospitalization and multiple tests to try to determine the cause of the "disorder." The desire for medication and attention is a definite decision on the part of the patient, who may be unaware of his or her underlying need for sympathy and care.

See also HYPOCHONDRIASIS.

Murmur. *See* HEART MURMUR.

Muscle is a tissue composed of fibers that can contract and relax to produce movement in a part of the body. There are three kinds of muscles: striated, smooth, and cardiac.

Striated muscles are typically those muscles under voluntary control, such as the muscles of the arms and legs.

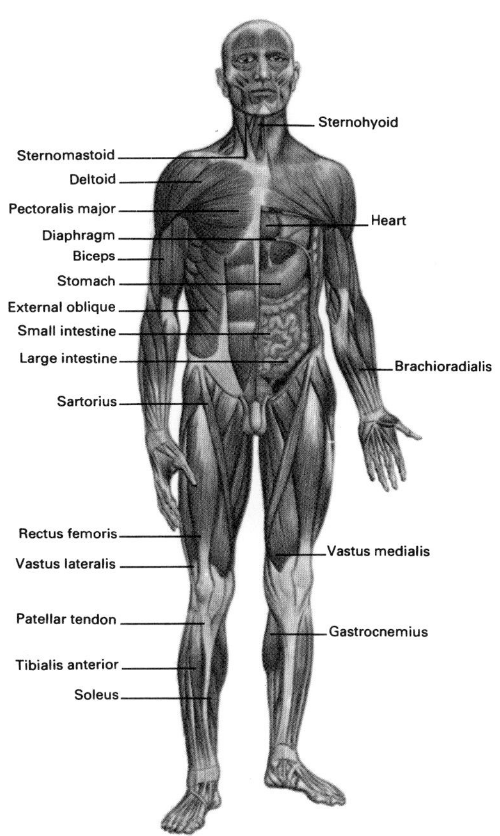

Body muscles layered over the skeleton are consciously controlled. Muscles of the heart and internal organs act without conscious control.

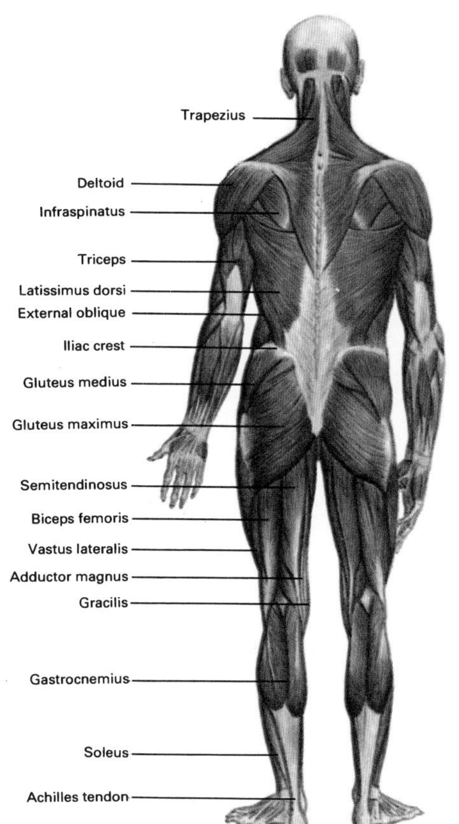

The voluntary muscles are active even when the body is standing still. Their contractions are needed to bear the body's weight and counteract gravity.

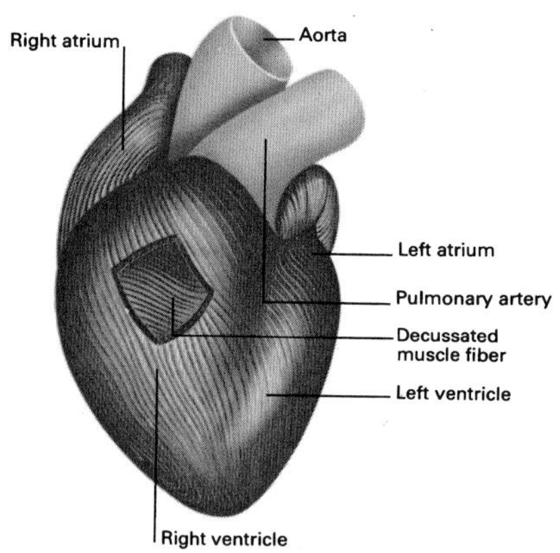

The muscles of the heart are bound spirally around the upper and lower chambers (atria and ventricles) and contract rhythmically to maintain the heartbeat.

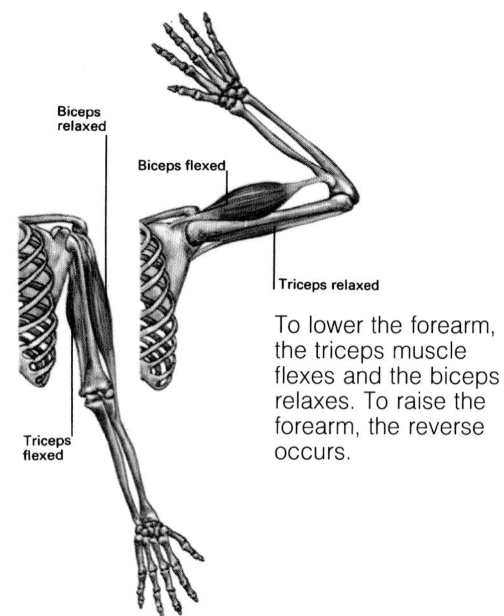

To lower the forearm, the triceps muscle flexes and the biceps relaxes. To raise the forearm, the reverse occurs.

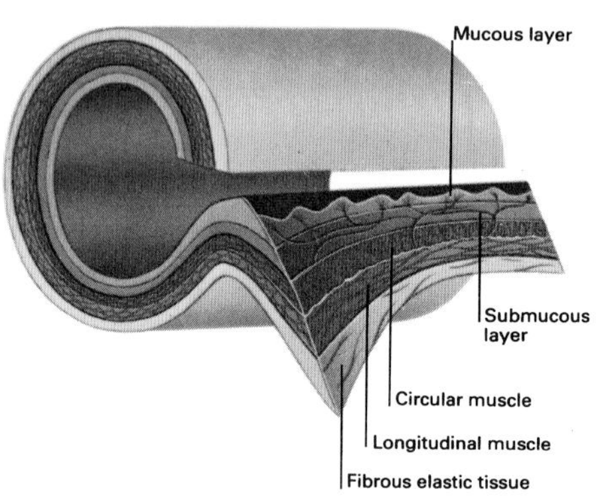

The gullet (esophagus) wall contains longitudinal and circular muscle layers that help propel food to the stomach.

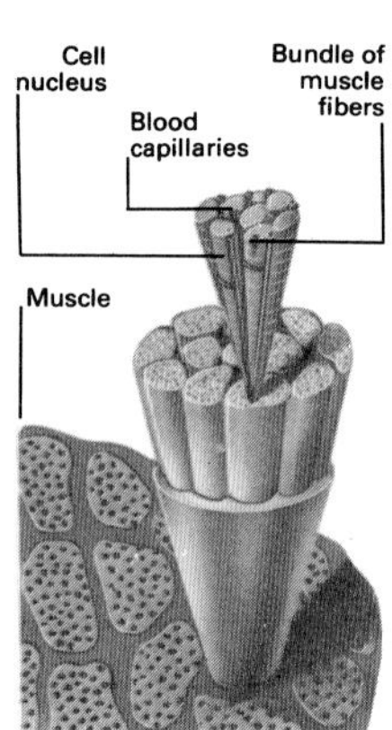

Voluntary muscle is made up of bundles of fibers. The fibers are divided into myofibrils that contain strands of the proteins actin and myosin. Actin and myosin slide over one another to make the muscle contract.

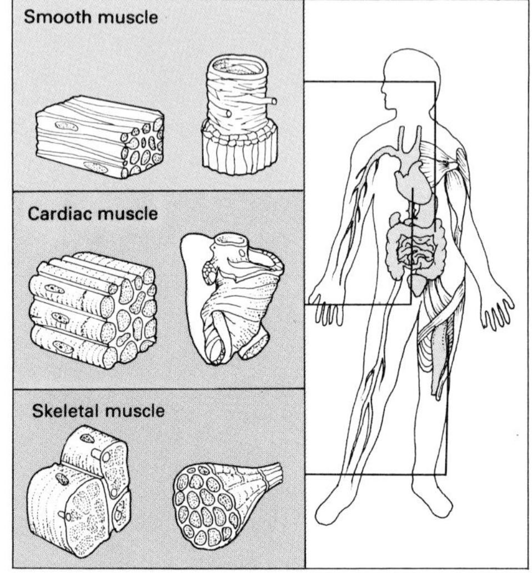

Muscle may be smooth (involuntary), cardiac (the heart), or striated (skeletal).

Smooth muscles can be found in arteries, bronchioles, the gastrointestinal tract, and other organs. They are generally not under voluntary control. The cardiac muscle is the muscle of the heart.

See also MUSCLE DISORDERS.

Muscle disorders include diseases or disorders that affect the muscles. Each of the following disorders has a separate entry in this encyclopedia: amyotrophic lateral sclerosis; Cushing's syndrome; Friedreich's ataxia; hyperthyroidism (thyrotoxicosis); hypothyroidism; muscle, pulled; muscular atrophy, progressive; muscular dystrophy; myalgia; myasthenia gravis; myocarditis; myositis; myotonia congenita; and tetany.

Muscle, pulled. Pulled muscle, also known as a strained muscle, is a common term for a muscle that has been slightly damaged by a sudden rupture of fibers within the muscle tissue. The pulled muscle causes pain and stiffness that gradually improves over a number of days.

See also SPRAINS AND STRAINS: TREATMENT; STRAIN.

Muscle, pulled: treatment. *See* SPRAINS AND STRAINS: TREATMENT.

Muscle relaxant drug is a drug that relaxes the central skeletal muscles by acting on the central nervous system to decrease muscle contraction. Neuromuscular blocking drugs paralyze skeletal muscles and are used in general anesthesia to produce complete relaxation of the muscles during surgery. Antispasmodic drugs relieve painful muscle spasms that sometimes occur in spastic conditions, such as those following a stroke, in some muscle and rheumatic disorders, and in some skeletal muscle disorders.

See also ANESTHETIC.

Muscular atrophy, progressive (at′rə fē). Progressive muscular atrophy is a form of motor neuron disease in which there is a gradual wasting of the muscles due to degeneration of the spinal cord. The exact cause of the condition is unknown, although in many cases, it seems to be genetically determined. The disorder is characterized by muscular weakness that progressively worsens over a period of several years.

See also MOTOR NEURON DISEASE.

Muscular dystrophy (dis′trə fē) is the name of a group of chronic, hereditary disorders, characterized by progressive degeneration and malfunction of voluntary muscles.

The most common and severe type is Duchenne muscular dystrophy. It typically occurs in boys between the ages of three and six. In this type, the disease progresses rapidly, and few survive their early 20's. Other forms include limb-girdle, Becker, facioscapulohumeral, and myotonic. In these types, progression of the disease is generally slow.

There is no known treatment that will arrest or reverse the dystrophy process, but medical management, such as the use of orthopedic devices and physical therapy, can increase mobility, maximize independence in daily activities, and ease the patient's discomfort. In forms that progress slowly, corrective surgery might be considered to help maintain limb function.

Mutation (myü tā′shən) is a sudden change in some characteristic. In genetics, mutation describes a permanent change in one of the genes of a chromosome, which may then be transmitted to future generations.

See also GENETIC ENGINEERING.

Mute (myüt) describes someone who is unable or unwilling to speak. A person who is deaf from birth may never acquire the ability to speak. A person may also lose the ability to speak following a stroke or disease or injury to the vocal cords. The condition may also be rarely caused by a subconscious response to emotional problems.

The condition of being mute has no correlation with a person's intelligence. Thus, the old use of the word "dumb" for someone who is mute is both insensitive and incorrect.

See also APHASIA.

Myalgia (mī al′jə) is pain in a muscle. Such pain may occur after excessive physical exercise. Myalgia may also develop during any acute viral illness and is an indication of mild inflammation of the muscles (myositis). It is frequently associated with inflammation of fibrous tissue (fibrositis).

The pain is usually made worse by movement and the muscles are frequently tender. Treatment with mild painkilling drugs and the application of heat is usually effective.

See also RHEUMATIC DISEASE.

Myasthenia gravis (mī əs thē′nē ə gräv′is) is a disorder affecting the nerve impulses that control the movement of muscles. It is a form of autoimmune disease. The muscles become weak, although temporary recovery slowly takes place if affected muscles are rested. *See also* AUTOIMMUNE DISEASE.

Q: *What are the symptoms of myasthenia gravis?*

A: The onset is often sudden, producing a drooping eyelid (ptosis) and double vision (diplopia) because of weakened eye muscles. These symptoms may be accompanied by difficulty in swallowing or speaking. Weakness of a limb may occur, particularly after the limb has been moved. On some days, the symptoms may not be noticeable, whereas on others they may become severe. Occasionally, the muscles involved in breathing become affected, producing the risk of asphyxiation. *See also* ASPHYXIA.

Q: *How is myasthenia gravis diagnosed and treated?*

A: A physician may suspect the presence of myasthenia gravis if a patient complains of muscle weakness after exercise. The diagnosis can be confirmed by the drastic improvement that takes place after use of a drug that helps to improve nerve transmission to the muscles.

There are several treatments available for myasthenia gravis: medications that improve nerve transmission to the muscles; corticosteroid medications; drugs that suppress the immune system; surgical removal of the thymus; and replacement of the patient's blood plasma. Selection of the proper treatment requires careful evaluation and close follow-up care. *See also* CORTICOSTEROID; THYMUS.

Mycobacteria (mī kō bak tir′ē ə) are a group of microorganisms, two of which cause leprosy and tuberculosis.

See also LEPROSY; TUBERCULOSIS.

Mycosis (mī kō′sis) is an infection caused by a fungus, such as actinomycosis and blastomycosis.

See also FUNGAL INFECTION.

Mydriatic (mid rē at′ik) describes any substance that makes the pupil of the eye dilate. Atropine and cocaine are mydriatics.

See also ATROPINE; COCAINE.

Myelin sheath (mī′ə lin shēth) is a tubular structure composed of a fatty substance (myelin) that wraps around many of the body's nerves.

Myelitis, acute transverse (mī ə lī′tis). Acute transverse myelitis is a disorder of the spinal cord characterized by inflammation of the gray and white matter in adjacent spinal cord segments. It is a severe and rapidly developing condition that affects both sensory and motor nerves.

Myelocele (mī′ə lō sēl) is an abnormal opening in the lowest part of the spine that exposes the underlying spinal cord. Myelocele is the most serious form of spina bifida.

See also SPINA BIFIDA.

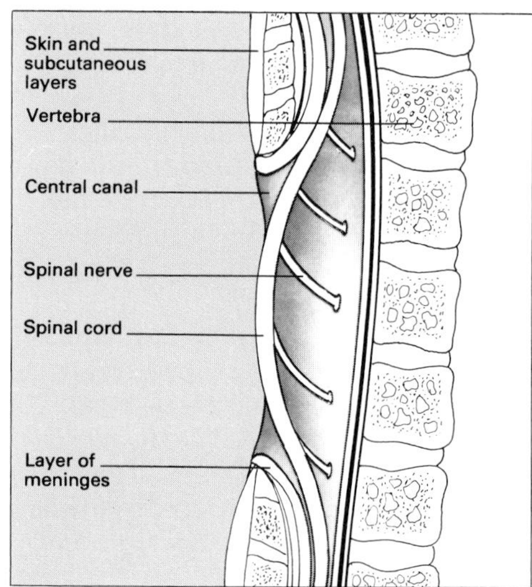

Myelocele is a condition is which the spinal cord protrudes through the skin. This is caused by incomplete development of vertebrae, usually in the lumbar or sacral regions.

Myelofibrosis (mī ə lō fī brō′sis) is the replacement of bone marrow by fibroblastic cells or fibrous tissue. It is characterized by the development of blood cells in the liver and spleen. The development of blood cells (hematopoiesis) normally occurs in the bone marrow. Myelofibrosis is the primary form of the disorder myeloid metaplasia, which may be associated with leukemia or carcinoma.

Myelogram (mī′ə lō gram) is an X-ray film of the spinal cord, produced after a dye is injected into the spinal fluid around the spinal cord. This injection creates a silhouette of structures in the spinal cord. A myelogram is used in the diagnosis of spinal tumors, herniated disks, and other spinal disorders.

Myeloid leukemia. *See* LEUKEMIA.

Myeloma (mī ə lō′mə) is a malignant (cancerous) tumor of the bone marrow. The tumor usually occurs first in one bone, but soon spreads to many other bones (multiple myeloma or myelomatosis). The bones of the skull, ribs, spine, and pelvis are usually involved, although myelomas may occur in any bone. Myelomatosis is most common in the elderly.

Q: *What are the symptoms of multiple myeloma?*

A: Backache or pain in the affected bone is a common symptom, although fatigue and shortness of breath caused by anemia may be noticed first. The patient's resistance to infection is lowered, allowing chest and urinary infections to develop. The tumors weaken the bones, and fractures commonly occur.

Q: *How is multiple myeloma diagnosed and treated?*

A: Many patients with myelomatosis produce an abnormal type of gamma globulin (Bence Jones protein) that can be detected in the urine. The presence of this protein, anemia, and a high ESR (erythrocyte sedimentation rate) all suggest multiple myeloma. The diagnosis can be confirmed by a bone marrow biopsy, in which a sample of bone marrow is examined using a microscope. *See also* BLOOD CELL, RED.

Treatment with chemotherapy, corticosteroids, and radiotherapy may greatly prolong the patient's life, but the disease is eventually fatal. Treatment of secondary infection with antibiotics and blood transfusion for severe anemia improve the patient's general health and vitality. *See also* CHEMOTHERAPY; CORTICOSTEROID; RADIOTHERAPY.

Myocardial infarction. *See* HEART ATTACK.

Myocarditis (mī ō kär dī'tis) is inflammation of the heart muscle. The symptoms at first are often vague and mild. Fatigue, shortness of breath, and sometimes palpitations (rapid, irregular heart beat) occur. Heart failure may develop, and sometimes blood clots form in the heart. Pieces of the clots (emboli) may travel in the blood circulation to other parts of the body and cause strokes or sudden obstruction of an artery to a limb, resulting in gangrene, the decay and death of tissue.

Q: *What causes myocarditis?*

A: Various infections can affect the heart muscle, either directly or by producing toxins that affect it, such as those from diphtheria. Many other conditions, such as disseminated lupus erythematosus and rheumatic fever, can also involve the heart. *See also* DIPHTHERIA; LUPUS ERYTHEMATOSUS; RHEUMATIC FEVER.

Various chemicals and some drugs, particularly those used in the treatment of cancer, can damage the heart muscle.

Q: *How is myocarditis diagnosed and treated?*

A: A physician makes an initial diagnosis from the symptoms and confirms it with an electrocardiogram (EKG) and other heart investigations. Treatment is directed at the cause, once it has been discovered. The patient must have complete rest and may require oxygen. Corticosteroid drugs might be helpful, but must be used with caution. *See also* CORTICOSTEROID; ELECTROCARDIOGRAM.

Myoclonus (mī ō klō'nəs) is a brief spasm of muscular contraction that may involve a group of muscles, a single muscle, or only a number of muscle fibers. Often, the contractions occur rhythmically, producing a regular twitching of the affected muscle. If myoclonus involves several muscles, it may be sufficiently violent to cause the person to fall over. The treatment depends on the cause. There is a variety of antispasmodic drugs that may help to reduce the likelihood of myoclonus.

Myoma (mī ō'mə) is a tumor on the uterine muscle. Most myomas are benign (noncancerous), although a few may become malignant (cancerous).

Myopathy (mī äp'ə thē) is any muscular disorder that results in weakness and degeneration of the muscle tissue that is not caused by a defect in the nervous system. The muscular dystrophies are classified as myopathic disorders.

See also MUSCULAR DYSTROPHY.

Myopia (mī ō'pē ə) is the medical term for nearsightedness, a visual defect in which distant objects can not be seen clearly. It occurs because light entering the eye is focused in front of the retina instead of on it. Distant objects are out of focus because either the lens of the eye is too curved, bending the light rays too much or the eyeball is too long, a condition that seems to be inherited. Close objects can be seen sharply, and even in old age, nearsighted people may be able to read easily without glasses.

Myopia can be corrected with contact lenses or by wearing eyeglasses with concave (converging) lenses.

See also CONTACT LENS; EYEGLASSES.

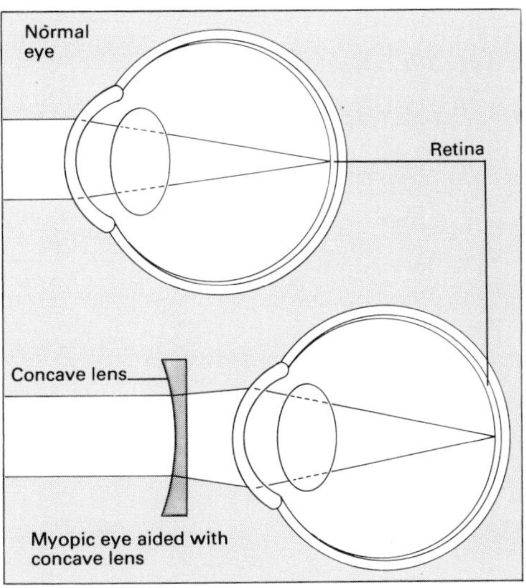

Myopia can be corrected through the use of a concave lens that refracts light and focuses it on the retina.

Myositis (mī ə sī'tis) is inflammation of the muscle tissues. It may be caused by injury, infection, exposure to cold, or parasitic infestation.

Myositis ossificans (mī ə sī'tis ä sif'ə kanz) is a rare muscle disease characterized by bony deposits or replacement of muscle tissue by bone. It generally begins in childhood. There is no cure for the disease.

Myotonia congenita (mī ə tō'nē ə kän jen'i tə), also called Thomsen's disease, is a rare, inherited muscular disorder in which muscles relax slowly after contraction. This causes stiff movements, for example, difficulty in relaxing the grip after shaking hands. The throat muscles may be affected, causing difficulty in speaking or swallowing. There is no cure, but drug treatment can control the disorder.

Myringotomy (mi ring got'ə mē), or tympanotomy, is surgical perforation of the eardrum, usually performed under a general anesthetic, when the middle ear is filled with thick mucus (glue ear). Glue ear may occur following unsuccessful or incomplete antibiotic treatment for otitis media and may cause deafness.

See also MASTOIDITIS.

Myxedema (mik se dē'mə) is a severe form of hypothyroidism characterized by swelling of the face, particularly the lips, nose, and around the eyes. The hands and the feet also swell.

See also HYPOTHYROIDISM.

Myxovirus (mik sə vī'rəs) is a family of viruses usually transmitted by air-borne droplets. It includes those that cause mumps and influenza.

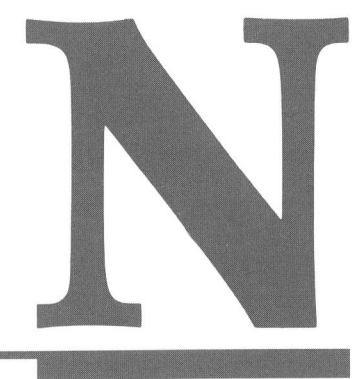

Nail (nāl) is the hard semitransparent tissue that covers the upper surfaces of the fingers and toes. Nails are dead tissue, without nerves or a blood supply. They are a modification of skin and grow from a groove that is overlapped by a fold of the skin, the nailfold. The semicircular whitish area near the base of the nail is called the lunula.

See also KERATIN; NAIL CARE; NAIL DISORDERS.

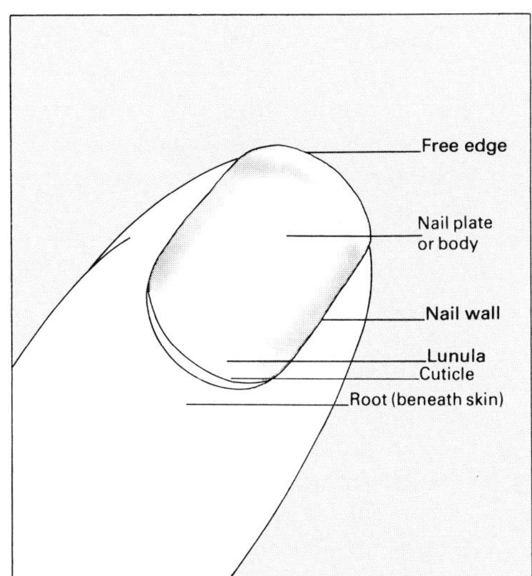

Nail is dead, hard tissue on the fingers and toes. The semicircular, paler area near the base of each nail is called the lunula.

Nail care. Fingernails grow at an average rate of about one-fiftieth of an inch (0.05mm) per week; toenails grow at about one-fourth this rate. Nails can be damaged by any change in the body, for example, insufficient diet or a serious illness. However, some disorders, such as an ingrown toenail, can be avoided with proper care of the nails.

Routine Nail Care. The nails should be cut every two to three weeks. The correct way to cut a nail is with small snips along the contour. Toenails should be cut straight across. After cutting, the nails should be shaped with a nail file. File in one direction only, to prevent the nails from splitting.

Nail polish encourages the layers of keratin, which is the primary component of the nail body, to split. Persons who use polish regularly should leave a small area at the base of the nail free, remove the polish completely every six days, and leave the nail bare on the seventh.

See also NAIL DISORDERS.

Nail disorders. Damage to the fingernails or toenails can be caused either by improper nail care or by an underlying illness. For example, an ingrown toenail is often caused by improper clipping of the nails, while clubbing, in which the ends of the fingers and fingernails become rounded, may be the sign of a serious heart or lung disorder. In other instances, nail deformity may be caused by insufficiencies in the diet, such as an iron deficiency. *See also* CLUBBING; KOILONYCHIA.

Ridging or grooving on the nails is evidence of altered nail growth due to illness or damage to the nail bed. The nail bed may become infected with tinea or monilia (both fungal diseases), causing deformity of the nail with discoloration and splitting. The nails of psoriasis patients are frequently pitted and often split easily. A similar condition may be seen in patients with rheumatoid arthritis. Nails can also be damaged by certain hormonal deficiencies. Bitten fingernails may be a sign of anxiety.

See also NAIL CARE; PARONYCHIA; TOENAIL, INGROWN.

Narcolepsy (när′kə lep sē) is an uncommon sleep disorder characterized by sudden and uncontrollable attacks of sleep at unexpected and irregular intervals. The attacks may last minutes or hours and vary in frequency from a few to many in a single day. The cause is unknown, although some patients have a family history of the disease. Narcolepsy usually begins in adolescence or young adulthood and continues throughout life. Narcoleptic people sometimes suffer from a sudden loss of muscle tone (cataplexy) that causes the victim to fall to the floor without losing consciousness. Stimulant drugs, such as amphetamines, may help prevent the sleeping attacks. MAO inhibitors and imipramine have also been used successfully in the treatment of narcolepsy, but they should not be combined with amphetamines.

See also SLEEP DISORDERS.

Narcotic (när kot′ik), or narcotic analgesic, is a substance that reduces perceptions of pain and produces a state of stupor or drowsiness. The term refers to the naturally occurring opiates, morphine and codeine; derivatives of these substances, including heroin; and totally synthetic compounds that produce similar effects. The term narcotic, when properly applied, does not include sedatives or hypnotics such as barbiturates.

Prolonged use of narcotic drugs may be habit-forming. An overdose may cause death.

See also CODEINE; DRUG; DRUG ADDICTION; HEROIN; MORPHINE.

Nares (nār′ēz) is the medical name for the nostrils, the external openings of the nose.

Nasal (nā′zəl) describes anything pertaining to the nose.

See also NOSE.

Nasogastric tube (nā zo gas′trik) is any tube passed into the stomach via the nose. It may be used to remove gastric secretions or food or to introduce medicine, fluids, or food.

Nasopharynx (nā zō far′ingks), or upper pharynx, is the small space above the soft palate at the back of the roof of the mouth, that connects the nasal cavities with the throat. Also known as the postnasal space, it contains the adenoids and the openings of the two Eustachian or auditory tubes that lead to the ears. During swallowing, the nasopharynx is closed by the muscles of the soft palate.

See also OROPHARYNX; PHARYNX.

National Institutes of Health (NIH) is an agency within the United States Department of Health and Human Services that classifies and distributes biological and medical information. NIH conducts and supports a wide range of biomedical research and training within 11 major areas: (1) aging; (2) allergy and infectious diseases; (3) digestive and kidney diseases, arthritis, and diabetes; (4) cancer; (5) child health and human development; (6) dental research; (7) environmental health sciences; (8) eye; (9) general medical sciences; (10) heart, lung, and blood; and (11) neurological and communicative disorders and stroke.

Natural childbirth. *See* CHILDBIRTH, NATURAL.

Naturopathy (nā chə rop′ə thē) is a therapeutic system in which natural agents, such as fresh air, exercise, and massage, are preferred to drugs or surgery. Conventional drugs are not used. A naturopath may treat a patient through the use of a diet of natural foods, herbal medicines, hydrotherapy, or other natural remedies. This form of therapy is considered unorthodox and unproven by the medical establishment.

Nausea (nô′shə) is the sensation of feeling sick in the stomach. It is often followed by vomiting. In nausea, the muscles of the stomach wall slow or stop their movement. This slows or stops digestion of the contents of the stomach. If vomiting takes place, most of the substances in the stomach will be expelled.

Q: *What causes nausea?*

A: Nausea may be caused by a variety of conditions, including seasickness and other forms of motion sickness. Digestive disorders, particularly acute or chronic gastritis, may be accompanied by nausea. A physical or emotional shock or food poisoning may also cause nausea. It is also frequently a symptom of early pregnancy. *See also* GASTRITIS; MORNING SICKNESS; MOTION SICKNESS.

Q: *How is nausea treated?*

A: The treatment of nausea depends on the cause. A severely nauseated person may be more comfortable lying down in a quiet place, possibly with head and shoulders raised. Anyone with persistent nausea should consult a physician.

Navel. *See* UMBILICAL CORD.

Nearsightedness. *See* MYOPIA.

Neck is any narrow region between two parts of an organ or body, although the

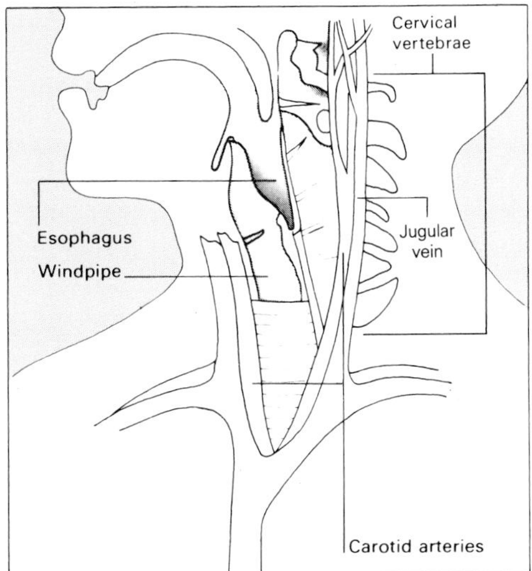

The seven cervical vertebrae of the **neck** support the head. The neck contains major arteries and veins, the esophagus, and the windpipe.

term usually applies to the part of the body between the shoulders and the head.

The neck is a flexible structure that supports the head and contains major blood vessels and separate tubes for air and food. The seven bones in the neck, called cervical vertebrae, form the upper part of the spine. The two top cervical vertebrae, the atlas and axis, are able to pivot, thus allowing rotation of the head.

Strong muscles on each side of the spine partially protect the structures in the front part of the neck. These structures include the esophagus, the trachea (windpipe), and the larynx (voice box). The carotid arteries and jugular veins in the neck carry blood to and from the head and brain. There is also a series of lymph nodes that guard against the entry of infection from the throat. The thyroid gland, just below the larynx in front of the trachea, produces hormones that control the body's metabolism.

See also NECK, STIFF.

Neck disorders. *See* DISK, HERNIATED; NECK, STIFF.

Neck, stiff. A stiff neck is a condition characterized by limited mobility of the neck as a result of an acute or chronic muscle disorder. Osteoarthritis, osteoporosis, and degenerative disks also can cause discomfort in the neck. A stiff neck may occur as a result of trauma to the muscles in the cervical region or as a result of torticollis (wryneck), in which the muscles of one side of the neck constrict, inclining the head toward that side.

Q: *What causes a stiff neck?*

A: A common cause of a stiff neck is a twisting or whiplash injury suffered from jerking the neck too hard, as in a car accident or a sports injury. It may also occur after sleeping with the neck in an awkward position. A stiff neck can also be caused by a spasm of the neck muscles or by a fibrotic inflammation (especially in the elderly). The most serious cause of a stiff neck is meningitis, although other symptoms, such as fever, headache, sensitivity to light, and vomiting, are usually more prominent.

Q: *How is stiff neck treated?*

A: Treatment depends on the cause of the disorder. If the stiffness is caused by an injury, then heat, massage, and traction may be required. Painkilling drugs and antirheumatic drugs (if swelling is present) may also be prescribed. Early evaluation and diagnosis before treatment is important because the stiffness may result from a herniated disk or other abnormality in which manipulation may cause further damage or delay in recovery.

See also DISK, HERNIATED.

Necrosis (ne krō′sis) is the death of a small area of tissue within an organ. It may occur as a result of an accident, such as a burn, or of a disease, such as tuberculosis. Necrosis often follows obstruction of an artery that supplies a particular area of tissue, as in gangrene.

See also GANGRENE.

Neisseria (nīs se′rē ə) is a group of bacteria that includes the organisms that cause gonorrhea and one of the common forms of bacterial meningitis.

Nematode (nem′ə tōd) is a type of parasitic roundworm.

See also ROUNDWORM.

Neonatal (nē ō nā′təl) describes the period of time immediately after birth and lasting through the first four weeks of an infant's life.

See also PRENATAL.

Neoplasm (nē′ō plaz əm) is the medical name for any abnormal new growth, but in common usage, it is frequently used to refer to a tumor. Physicians distinguish between malignant (cancerous) neoplasms and benign (noncancerous) neoplasms.

See also CANCER; TUMOR.

Nephrectomy (ni frek'tə mē) is an operation to remove a diseased kidney. A partial nephrectomy is performed when only part of the kidney is diseased.

A nephrectomy may be necessary if there is a kidney tumor such as hypernephroma; if the kidney is severely damaged by disease, for example, hydronephrosis or a calculus (stone); or following an accident in which the kidney is badly damaged. The remaining kidney is usually able to compensate for the loss of the other and can maintain normal urine output by itself.

See also CALCULUS; HYDRONEPHROSIS; HYPERNEPHROMA.

Nephritis (ni frī'tis) is a general term for any inflammation or infection of the kidney. The condition may involve the kidney's filtration unit (glomerulus), producing glomerulonephritis. Nephritis may also involve the spaces within the kidney, causing problems in reabsorption of water and salts (interstitial nephritis). Inflammation affecting the drainage area of the kidney, with damage to the kidney, pelvis, and surrounding tissue, leads to pyelonephritis.

See also GLOMERULONEPHRITIS; NEPHROTIC SYNDROME; PYELONEPHRITIS.

Nephritis is inflammation or infection of any part of the kidney, which contains innumerable microscopic nephrons. Each nephron consists of the renal corpuscle (the glomerulus of capillaries in Bowman's capsule), the loops of Henle, and the renal tubules.

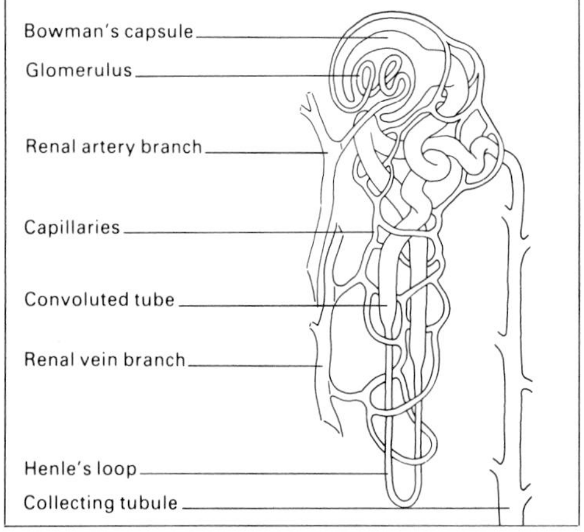

Nephrolithiasis (nef rə li thī'ə sis) is the presence of stones (calculi) in the kidney.

Q: *Why do kidney stones form?*

A: Stones may form if there is obstruction of the normal urine flow, as in hydronephrosis. They may result from an excess of certain chemicals in the bloodstream, such as uric acid in gout and calcium in parathyroid gland disorders, or from certain hereditary disorders.

Q: *What are kidney stones made of?*

A: There are three common forms of stones: those formed from uric acid; those made of calcium oxalate; and mixed stones composed of calcium, magnesium, and ammonium phosphates.

Q: *What are the symptoms of nephrolithiasis?*

A: Often, there are no symptoms until the stone moves from its initial position. Rarely, stones can form in the kidney (staghorn calculi), causing kidney damage without any obvious symptoms.

When a stone moves from the pelvis of the kidney into the ureter (the tube that carries urine to the bladder), there are severe spasms (renal colic) of pain from the lower back to the groin, with vomiting and sweating. There may also be blood in the urine (hematuria).

Q: *How is nephrolithiasis diagnosed and treated?*

A: A history of pain and hematuria suggests a stone, and its presence can usually be detected by an X ray. An intravenous pyelogram (IVP) reveals where the stone is causing an obstruction. *See also* PYELOGRAM, INTRAVENOUS.

A small stone may eventually pass down the ureter and out through the bladder. But large stones either remain in the kidney (and may have to be removed surgically) or become stuck in the ureter. A special instrument can be used to extract the stones during cystoscopy (an examination of the bladder). If this measure fails, surgery has to be done to remove the stone. A new therapy, called lithotripsy, involves a machine called a lithotriptor that sends sound waves into the body to break up stones; these are then easily passed out of the body. This procedure saves the patient from undergoing surgery. *See also* LITHOTRIPSY.

An acute attack of pain requires urgent treatment with strong painkilling and antispasmodic drugs prescribed by a physician. Large quantities of fluid should be drunk, because this helps the stone to pass down the ureter. All the urine that is passed must be filtered through a fine cloth so that the stone can be seen. It is usual to have an X ray a few weeks later to make certain that a second stone has not stuck in the ureter.

Q: *Apart from pain, what are the dangers of a kidney stone?*

A: The stone may obstruct urine flow and cause hydronephrosis or frequent attacks of pyelonephritis (inflammation of kidney substance).

Q: *Why do some people develop stones more easily than others?*

A: Apart from the reasons already mentioned, stones may develop from drinking water with a high concentration of salts. Stones occur more commonly in hot climates as the urine is more concentrated. It is necessary for people in tropical countries to drink plenty of fluids.

See also CALCULUS; HYDRONEPHROSIS; PYELONEPHRITIS.

Nephron (nef′ron) is the basic unit within the kidney that serves to filter waste matter from the blood. There are over one million such units in the average kidney. Each nephron includes Bowman's capsule, a hairpin loop, the glomerulus, and the distal and proximal tubule.

See also KIDNEY.

Nephrosis (ni frō′sis) is any disorder of the kidney that is caused by a degenerative process other than infections, for example, hydronephrosis (obstructed outflow) and the nephrotic syndrome (degenerative kidney change). It may also occur with amyloidosis (enlarged kidney) and some forms of poisoning.

See also AMYLOIDOSIS; HYDRONEPHROSIS; NEPHROTIC SYNDROME.

Nephrostomy (ni frost′ə mē) is an operation in which a catheter is inserted into the kidney pelvis in order to drain urine. A nephrostomy is usually performed because the ureter is blocked by a stone (calculus) or a tumor.

Nephrotic syndrome (ni frot′ik) is an abnormal kidney condition marked by excess protein in the blood, disturbances of body fats, and edema (swelling of the body tissues). Other symptoms include fatigue, weakness, and loss of appetite. A physical examination may reveal a sudden or slow accumulation of fluid in the tissues of the arms and legs.

Q: *What causes nephrotic syndrome?*

A: Acute or chronic glomerulonephritis may result in the disorder. Also, any abnormality that causes an increase in the pressure of blood in the veins leaving the kidney produces congestion in the kidney tissue. This can happen in heart failure or following a thrombosis in the renal vein.

Nephrotic syndrome may be a result of some systemic disease, such as amyloidosis (enlarged kidney), diabetes mellitus, malaria, or myeloma (bone marrow tumor). It may also be caused by an allergic reaction to drug treatment. In rare cases, the disorder may be present at birth or occur spontaneously in early childhood. *See also* AMYLOIDOSIS; DIABETES MELLITUS; GLOMERULONEPHRITIS; MALARIA; MYELOMA; SERUM SICKNESS.

Q: *What is the treatment for nephrotic syndrome?*

A: Nephrotic syndrome requires careful and skilled attention from a specialist in kidney disease. The more serious cases make treatment difficult, and the outcome may be fatal. Corticosteroid drugs are particularly useful in one type of nephrotic syndrome that commonly affects children. Chemotherapy is sometimes effective in certain other types. Diuretic drugs to increase the urine flow help reduce the swelling of edema, but do not treat the underlying causes.

See also NEPHRITIS.

Nephrotomy (ni frot′ə mē) is a surgical incision into the kidney. It is sometimes done as part of the treatment for a kidney stone.

See also NEPHROLITHIASIS.

Nerve is an element of the central or peripheral nervous system that carries impulses, especially of sensation and motion, from the brain or spinal cord to the eyes, ears, muscles, glands, and other parts of the body. Nerves consist of bundles of fibers covered with a sheath of connective tissue and sometimes by a layer of fatty cells (myelin). Nerve impulses are transmitted by a weak electrical current that results from chemical changes taking place

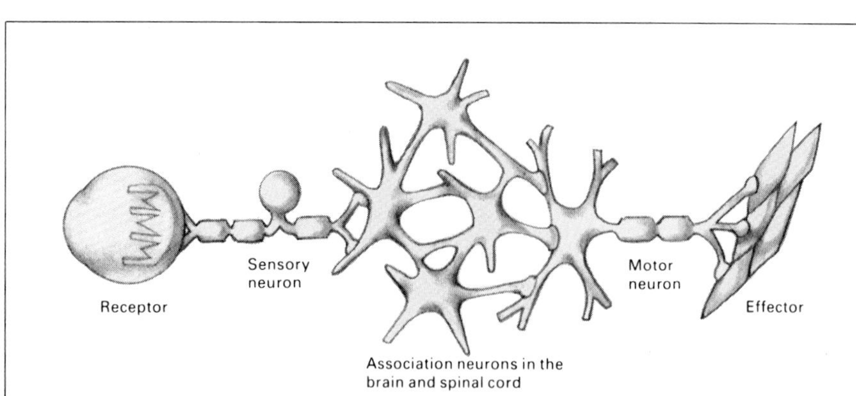

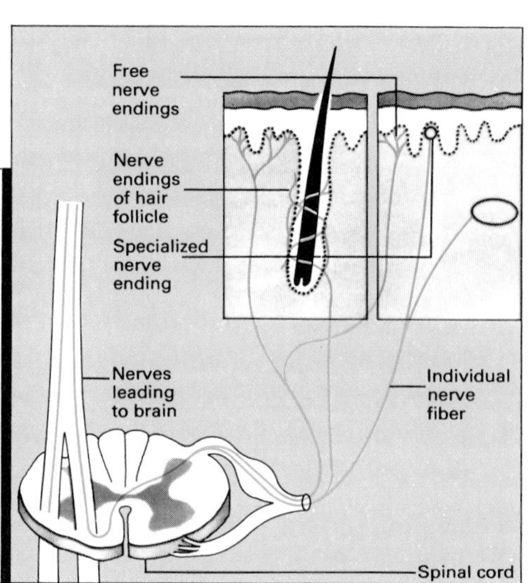

Nerves are a collection of bundled fibers that carry impulses throughout the body. The impulses are transmitted by an electrical current that results from chemical changes that take place through the nerve wall.

through the nerve wall. The final transmission, from one nerve to another or from a nerve to another structure is carried out by a chemical reaction via substances known as neurotransmitters.

Sensory nerves collect information from the body and transmit it in the form of electrical impulses to the central nervous system for action. Other nerves pick up the impulses at nerve junctions (synapses) and trigger appropriate responses. For example, specialized nerve endings in the skin may detect a sensation, such as cold, and pass the information to the brain. The brain may react by causing other nerves to stimulate shivering.

Motor nerves cause movement through the action of muscles. A reaction to intense heat, for example, causes the brain to stimulate motor nerves that cause the part of the body to be jerked away from the source of heat.

The main nerves are named according to the regions to which they branch off. There are 12 pairs of cranial nerves and 31 pairs of spinal nerves. The spinal nerves consist of 8 pairs of cervical nerves, 12 pairs of thoracic nerves, 5 pairs of lumbar nerves, 5 pairs of sacral nerves, and 1 pair of coccygeal nerves.

See also NERVOUS SYSTEM; NERVOUS SYSTEM, AUTONOMIC.

Nerve disorders. *See* NEUROLOGICAL DISORDERS.

Nervous breakdown is an informal, nonspecific term used to describe any psychiatric condition that renders a person unable to function on a day-to-day basis. For example, two people may use the term to refer to two such different conditions as severe depression and schizophrenia.

The term does not, therefore, apply specifically to a particular disorder, but rather typifies the effect of the disorder on a given individual.

See also MENTAL ILLNESS.

Nervous disease. *See* MENTAL ILLNESS; NEUROLOGICAL DISORDERS.

Nervous system is a network of billions of interconnected nerve cells (neurons) that receive stimuli, coordinate this sensory information, and cause the body to respond appropriately. The individual nerve cells transmit messages by means of a complicated electrochemical process.

The nervous system is comprised of two main divisions: the central nervous system (CNS), which consists of the brain and the spinal cord; and the peripheral nervous system (PNS), which consists of spinal nerves and cranial nerves that link the CNS with the body's receptors and effectors.

Q: *What are receptors and effectors?*

A: The receptors include the various sensory cells and sense organs, whose function is to sense and respond to various types of stimulation. For example, eyes respond to light, and ears respond to sound.

The effectors are all of the parts

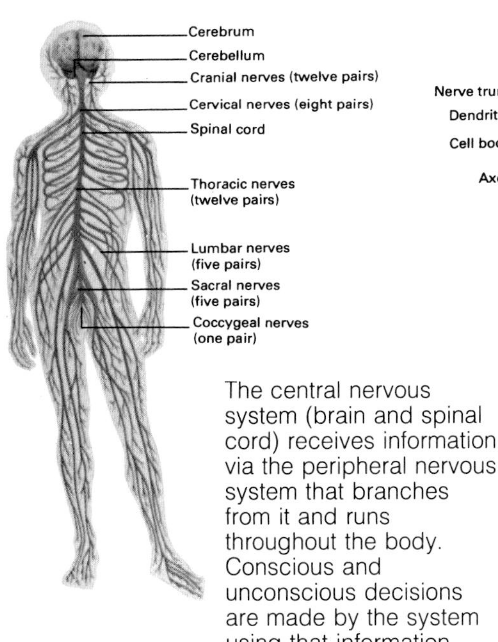

The central nervous system (brain and spinal cord) receives information via the peripheral nervous system that branches from it and runs throughout the body. Conscious and unconscious decisions are made by the system using that information.

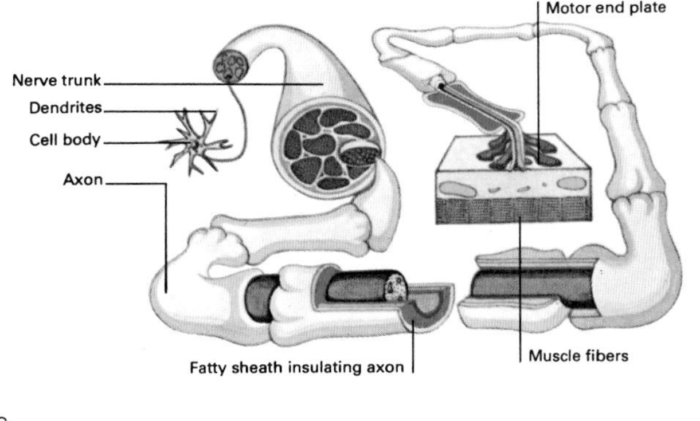

A nerve cell consists of a cell body and a long axon contained in a fatty sheath. The dendrites of the cell body receive impulses that are transmitted via the axon to muscle fibers.

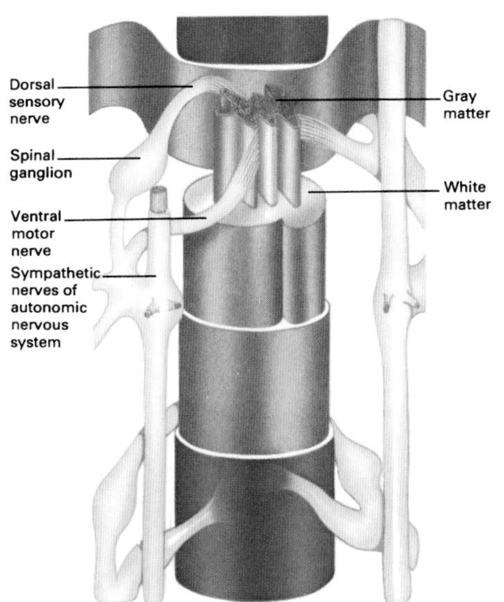

Sensory nerves bring messages to the gray matter in the spinal cord; white matter relays messages to and from the brain; and the motor nerves carry instructions for action to parts of the body.

of the body, such as muscles and glands, that respond to nerve impulse instructions from the CNS.

Q: *What are the functions of the CNS?*

A: The CNS integrates the information from the PNS and sends instructions to various parts of the body so that appropriate responses are made to continually changing conditions. The brain is also involved in the processes of thinking, learning, memory, and intelligence.

Q: *What are the functions of the PNS?*

A: The PNS signals changes in the environment, as registered by the receptors, to the CNS. The instructions from the CNS to different parts of the body are also carried by the PNS.

Anatomically, the autonomic nervous system (ANS) is part of the PNS. However, in terms of function, the ANS can be considered as a separate system. The ANS is concerned with controlling the body's involuntary activities, such as the beating of the heart, intestinal movements, and sweating. The actions of the ANS can be modified by the CNS, but it also has a degree of independence. *See also* NERVOUS SYSTEM, AUTONOMIC.

Nervous system, autonomic (ô tə nom'ik). The autonomic nervous system is the part of the nervous system that controls involuntary functions in the body. These functions include gland activity, contraction of involuntary (smooth) muscles, and the action of the heart. Within the autonomic nervous system, there are two divisions: the sympathetic system and the parasympathetic system.

Q: *What functions does the sympathetic system control?*

A: The sympathetic system controls those activities that prepare the body for sudden activity. These include increasing the blood pressure and heart rate (sending blood to the muscles), increasing glucose production by the liver, reducing the secretion of saliva, causing the erection of hairs on the skin, and causing dilation of the pupils of the eyes. *See also* NERVOUS SYSTEM, SYMPATHETIC.

Q: ***What functions does the parasympathetic system control?***

A: The parasympathetic system produces effects that are sometimes opposite to those of the sympathetic system. It is responsible for a reduction in blood pressure and the slowing of the heart rate, contraction of the pupils of the eyes, copious secretion of saliva, and increased activity in the stomach and intestines. *See also* NERVOUS SYSTEM, PARASYMPATHETIC.

Nervous system, central. The central nervous system (CNS) is the part of the nervous system consisting of the brain and spinal cord. The CNS receives information from nerve cells located throughout the body, analyzes that information, and then sends instructions via the nerve cells to the various parts of the body so that an appropriate response is taken to the original information.

See also NERVOUS SYSTEM; NERVOUS SYSTEM, PERIPHERAL.

Nervous system, parasympathetic (par ə sim pə thet′ik). The parasympathetic nervous system is one of the two divisions of the autonomic nervous system, the other division being the sympathetic nervous system. Parasympathetic nerve fibers occur in some of the cranial nerves of the brain and in the sacral nerves of the lower end of the spinal cord. Parasympathetic nerves connect with many parts of the body, including the eyes, the internal organs, and the intestines. The effects of the parasympathetic nervous system include constriction of the pupils, slowing of the heart rate, contraction of the bladder, increase in the rate of digestion, and constriction of the air passages (bronchi). The parasympathetic nervous system effectively calms the body down again, after the sympathetic nervous system has speeded up its responses.

See also NERVOUS SYSTEM, AUTONOMIC; NERVOUS SYSTEM, SYMPATHETIC.

Nervous system, peripheral (pə rif′ər əl). The peripheral nervous system consists of the nerves and ganglia outside the brain and spinal cord. The peripheral nervous system spreads out from the brain and spinal cord all over the body, carrying information to and from the central nervous system.

See also GANGLION; NERVOUS SYSTEM; NERVOUS SYSTEM, CENTRAL.

Nervous system, sympathetic (sim pə thet′ik). The sympathetic nervous system is part of the autonomic nervous system. It operates in conjunction with the parasympathetic nervous system. The sympathetic nervous system prepares the body for action by dilating the pupils of the eyes, cooling the skin, and raising the blood pressure and pulse rate. The blood is diverted from the intestines to the skeletal muscles, and the adrenal glands are stimulated to produce the hormone epinephrine, which enhances these actions.

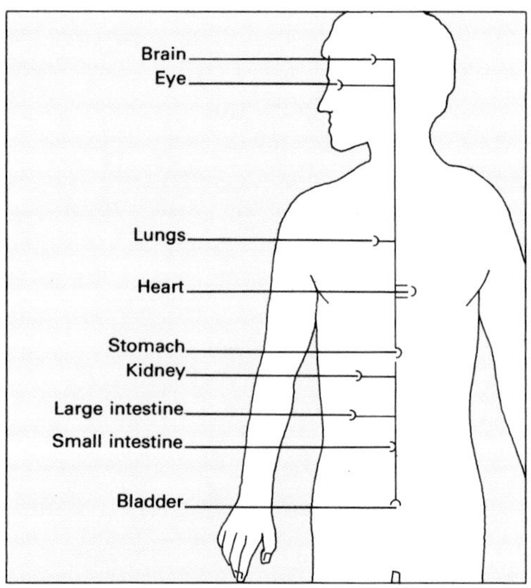

The **sympathetic nervous system** prepares the body for instant activity by increasing blood pressure and pulse rate and decreasing gastrointestinal activity.

The smooth muscle in the bronchi relaxes, allowing more air to enter the lungs; muscular movement in the intestines slows down; and sweating occurs.

All of this activity increases the basic metabolic rate of the body, increasing the use of glucose released from the liver, and prepares the body for instant physical and mental activity.

See also NERVOUS SYSTEM; NERVOUS SYSTEM, AUTONOMIC; NERVOUS SYSTEM, PARASYMPATHETIC.

Nettle rash. *See* HIVES.

Neuralgia (nu̇ ral′jə) is a pain, usually sharp, along the course of a nerve. Neuralgia can affect any portion of the body. For example, pressure on the neck, such as from a herniated disk in the neck, may produce continuous pain in the arms and shoulders. Neuralgia may also occur as a result of the inflammation that accompanies shingles (herpes zoster). The pain may persist in the trunk area after the shingles attack has ended, due to scarring around the nerve endings. This condition is known as postherpetic neuralgia. Trigeminal neuralgia is a rare and acute form of the disorder involving severe spasms of pain in the nerve endings of the face. Another form of neuralgia affects the nerve endings in the head, creating severe migraines. *See also* HEADACHE, CLUSTER; NEURALGIA, TRIGEMINAL.

Q: ***How is neuralgia treated?***

A: Treatment is directed at finding the cause, which may be difficult because some causes are not well understood. Painkilling and muscle relaxant drugs frequently give relief until the cause can be identified and treated. If drugs are not effective, some types of neuralgia may be treated surgically.

Neuralgia, trigeminal (nů ral′jə, trī jem′ə nəl). Trigeminal neuralgia, or tic douloureux, is a disorder of the trigeminal nerve, a facial nerve that is essential for chewing as well as to sensory and motor functions of the face. The disorder occurs most commonly in the elderly; its cause is unknown.

Q: ***What are the symptoms of trigeminal neuralgia?***

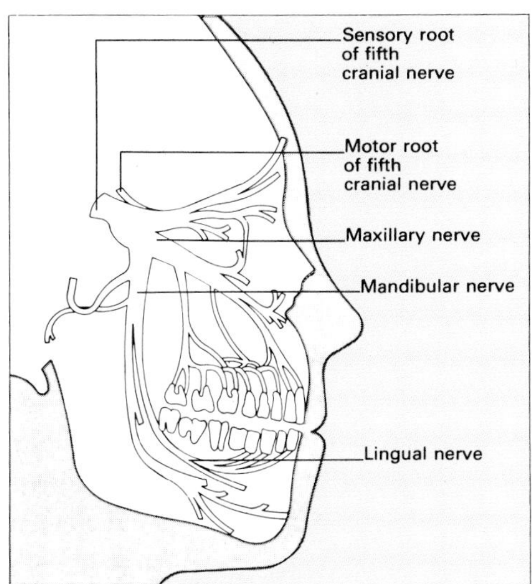

Trigeminal neuralgia can affect any part of the face supplied by the fifth cranial nerve. Attacks consist of brief spasms of intense pain.

A: The disorder is characterized by a brief, intense pain along one side of the face. This pain is often triggered by a light touch or by activities such as cleaning the teeth or chewing. Although these attacks of pain are brief, they tend to recur unless the disorder is successfully treated.

Q: ***How is trigeminal neuralgia treated?***

A: Treatment with some anticonvulsant drugs, such as carbamazepine and phenytoin, or with antimigraine drugs is often effective. If such treatment is not successful, a physician may recommend a surgical operation to cut the trigeminal nerve.

Neurasthenia (nůr əs thē′nē ə) is a neurotic disorder in which a person feels lethargic, complaining of a lack of energy and loss of appetite. The condition is often accompanied by weight loss, insomnia, fatigue, and a feeling of inadequacy. Neurasthenia is usually a sign of mental depression, but it may also signal the onset of any chronic illness. A physician may suggest psychotherapeutic counseling for the patient.

See also DEPRESSION; MENTAL ILLNESS.

Neuritis (nů rī′tis) is the inflammation of a nerve. If neuritis affects more than one nerve, the condition is called polyneuritis.

See also POLYNEURITIS.

Neuritis, retrobulbar (nů rī′tis, ret rə bul′bər). Retrobulbar neuritis is an inflammation of the part of the optic nerve that is within the eye socket. It may be caused by the spread of infection from the sinuses, bleeding into the nerve from an injury, a generalized illness, such as multiple sclerosis or diabetes mellitus, or infections of the nervous system, such as polyneuritis and encephalitis. Often, however, there is no apparent cause for the condition. *See also* DIABETES MELLITUS; ENCEPHALITIS; MULTIPLE SCLEROSIS; POLYNEURITIS.

Q: ***What are the symptoms of retrobulbar neuritis?***

A: The main symptoms are a rapid and progressive loss of vision, pain when the eye is moved, and a headache. The condition usually affects only one eye. There may be a spontaneous, almost complete recovery. However, further attacks are common.

Q: *How is retrobulbar neuritis treated?*

A: An ophthalmologist should be consulted so that the underlying cause can be diagnosed and treated. Generally, retrobulbar neuritis is treated with corticosteroid drugs.

Neuroblastoma (nůr ə blas tō′mə) is a highly malignant cancer of the sympathetic nervous system in which embryonic nerve cells are affected. The disorder is most prevalent in young children, usually beginning in the adrenal gland. Symptoms vary according to the location of the tumor and may include an abdominal growth and anemia. Neuroblastoma is a grave, often fatal, disorder. Surgery or chemotherapy are often successful in eradicating the tumor, especially if undertaken before the tumor spreads. In rare cases, the tumor regresses spontaneously.

See also CANCER.

Neurodermatitis. *See* LICHEN SIMPLEX CHRONICUS.

Neurofibroma (nůr ō fī brō′mə) is the swelling of a peripheral nerve, caused by a thickening of the nerve sheath or connective tissue. If a neurofibroma occurs in soft tissue, such as that of the mouth or stomach, there may be only slight discomfort. But neurofibromas that develop on nerves radiating from the skull or spine, or on nerves adjacent to bones, may cause loss of sensation or paralysis as a result of pressure on the nerve.

See also VON RECKLINGHAUSEN'S DISEASE.

Nucleus
Axon
Neurofibroma
Motor end plate

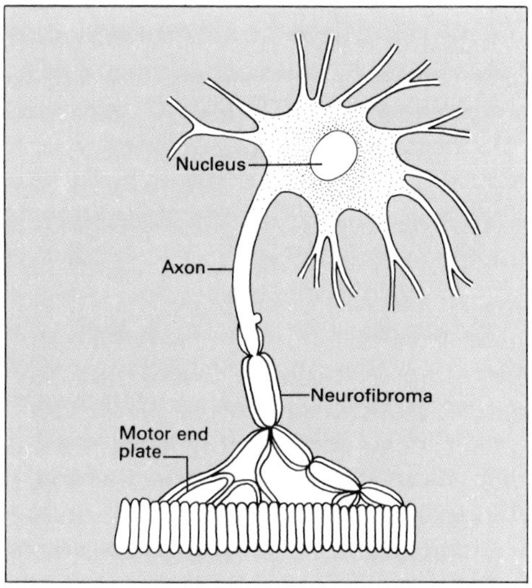

Neurofibroma is a swelling of a peripheral nerve that is caused by thickening of the nerve sheath or connective tissue. Neurofibromas located on nerves radiating from the brain, spine, or bones can cause paralysis.

Neurofibromatosis (nůr ō fī brō mə tō′sis) is a disorder in which pigmented areas form on the skin. It is associated with multiple neurofibromas (fibrous tumors).

See also NEUROFIBROMA; VON RECKLINGHAUSEN'S DISEASE.

Neuroglia (nů rog′lē ə) is the connective or supporting tissue between nerve cells within the central nervous system of the brain and spinal cord.

Neurological disorders (nůr ə loj′ə kəl) are disorders that affect the nervous system. The following table lists some disorders affecting the nervous system according to their location in the body. All of these disorders have a separate article in this encyclopedia.

Structure	*Disorder*
Meninges (membranes surrounding the brain and spinal cord)	Meningioma (a tumor of the meninges)
	Meningitis (inflammation of the meninges)
	Spina bifida (a congenital defect of the spinal canal)
Central nervous system (brain and spinal cord)	Alzheimer's disease
	Brain disorders
	Encephalitis (inflammation of the brain)
	Encephalopathy (any brain abnormality)
	Epilepsy
	Glioma (tumor of supporting cells of the brain)
	Hemorrhage, extradural (external bleeding around the brain)
	Hemorrhage, cerebral
	Hemorrhage, subarachnoid (bleeding into the meninges)
	Hydrocephalus (build-up of fluid within the brain)
	Korsakoff's syndrome (generalized brain dysfunction)
	Microcephaly (incomplete brain development)
	Migraine
	Motor neuron disease (degeneration of brain cells)
	Poliomyelitis
	Stroke
	Syringomyelia (cavity formation in spinal cord)
	Tabes dorsalis (brain dysfunction due to syphilis)
Peripheral nervous system	Bell's palsy (facial paralysis)
	Neurofibroma (a tumor of the connective tissue of a nerve)

Polyneuritis (inflammation of several nerves)
Retrobulbar neuritis (inflammation of the optic nerve)
Trigeminal neuralgia (facial pain)
Von Recklinghausen's disease (multiple tumors of the nerve sheaths)

Neurology (nu̇ rol′ə jē) is the field of medicine concerned with the study of the nervous system and its diseases. A specialist in this branch of medicine is called a neurologist.

Neuroma (nu̇ rō′mə) is a benign (noncancerous) tumor that is made up of nerve cells. A mature nerve cell can not reproduce and so can not form a tumor. The connective tissue (neuroglia) that supports the nerve cells, however, can form tumors.

Some neuromas occur singly; others may be found throughout the body, characterized by pigmented patches on the skin. This condition is called von Recklinghausen's disease.

See also VON RECKLINGHAUSEN'S DISEASE.

Neuron (nu̇r′on) is one of the basic cells of which the brain, spinal cord, and nerves are composed. Different neurons conduct impulses toward the brain and spinal cord, within the brain or spinal cord, or away from the brain and spinal cord toward the muscles and other body tissues. Each neuron consists of a cell body containing the nucleus, several branching processes (dendrites), and at least one long nerve fiber called an axon. A thin membrane surrounds the entire neuron. The dendrites and axon differ from neuron to neuron, according to the function of the neuron.

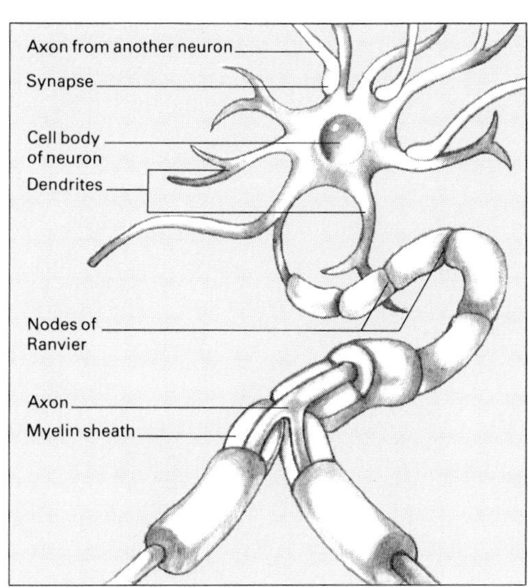

Neurons, basic cells of the brain, spinal cord, and nerves, consist of a cell body containing a nucleus, dendrites, and an axon.

Neuronitis, vestibular (nu̇ ron ī′tis, ves tib′yə lər). Vestibular neuronitis is a disorder characterized by periodic attacks of severe dizziness (vertigo). These attacks may be accompanied by sharp, stabbing pains in the inner ear. The disorder is contagious and is thought to be caused by a virus that inflames a nerve or nerve cell along the spine. There is no loss of hearing. The disorder gradually disappears on its own.

Neuropathic joint disease. *See* JOINT, CHARCOT'S.

Neuropathy (nu̇ rop′ə thē) is a general term for any disorder of the peripheral nerves, such as those of the autonomic nervous system, which regulates the involuntary functions of the body. Common causes of neuropathy include diabetes mellitus, alcoholism, and lead poisoning. Patients with neuropathic disorders often experience a "pins and needles" sensation known as paresthesia. Treatment of neuropathy depends on its underlying cause.

See also NERVOUS SYSTEM, PERIPHERAL; PARESTHESIA.

Neurosis (nu̇ rō′sis) is an obsolete term describing a variety of emotional disorders, such as anxiety problems and personality disorders. This term is best replaced with more specific terms, such as anxiety attack or problems of daily living.

See also MENTAL ILLNESS.

Neurosurgery (nu̇r ō sėr′jər ē) is the branch of surgery that deals with disorders of the nervous system.

Neutropenia (nu̇ trō pē′nē ə) is a decrease in the number of neutrophils, the most common type of white blood cell. The condition most commonly results from a viral infection, but may also be caused by alcoholism or occur as a side effect to drug treatment.

See also AGRANULOCYTOSIS.

Nevus. *See* MOLE.

Niacin (nī′ə sin), or nicotinic acid, is the chemical name for one of the B-complex vitamins. Niacin has been effectively used to treat hypercholesterolemia, a condition characterized by abnormally high cholesterol levels in the blood, and tinnitus, a condition characterized by ringing heard in one or both ears. A side effect of using niacin is flushing, in which the face and neck develop a reddish color.

See also VITAMIN.

Nicotinamide (nik ə tin′ə mīd), more commonly referred to as niacinamide, is a derivative of niacin and as such is one of the B-complex vitamins.

See also NIACIN; VITAMIN.

Night blindness is an eye disorder in which vision is abnormally impaired in dim light or at night. It is caused by a deficiency of visual purple (rhodopsin) in the light-sensitive rod cells of the retina at the back of the eye. Night blindness most commonly occurs as a result of retinitis pigmentosa, a degenerative condition of the retina. Visual purple may also decrease if there is a dietary deficiency of vitamin A—its principal component. Another cause may be the slow regeneration of visual purple after exposure to bright lights, which causes the supply of visual purple to be depleted. Night blindness may also occur in other eye disorders, such as choroidoretinitis and glaucoma.

Night blindness caused by vitamin A deficiency can be treated with therapeutic dosages of the vitamin, sometimes in the form of halibut liver oil. Some types of damage to the retina, such as retinitis pigmentosa, are usually irreversible.

Nightmare (nīt′mār) is any frightening dream. Nightmares are most common in young children.

Nightmares may occur in adults who are depressed or anxious about something. Such nightmares are often accompanied by the physical signs of fear, such as palpitations and sweating, and may awaken the individual. Antidepressant drugs may help those whose nightmares result from depression.

Nightmares may also result from a traumatic experience, such as a serious accident or a death in the family.

See also NIGHT TERROR.

Night sweat is profuse sweating during sleep. It is common in children and normal when caused by vigorous activity before going to bed. Most cases are harmless and require only fewer blankets and a change of night clothes.

Night sweats, in both adults and children, may also be caused by a chronic disease in which the body temperature rises during the night and falls during the following morning. Some diseases that may cause night sweats include tuberculosis, brucellosis, malaria, and lymphoma. The treatment of night sweats depends upon the cause. If night sweats persist, it is advisable to consult a physician.

Night terror, or sleep terror disorder, is a sleep disorder in which a child or adult wakes up screaming and frightened. Dreams cannot be recalled, and there is usually no memory of the episode. These usually occur earlier in the night.

Nightmares differ from night terrors in that they can be remembered, cause a milder reaction, and occur in the latter part of the night.

In children, night terrors are not usually associated with emotional problems. Adults with night terrors, however, frequently experience other psychological problems. A psychological evaluation should be sought.

See also NIGHTMARE.

Nipple (nip′əl) is the raised area in the center of the breast. It is surrounded by a disk-shaped pigmented area called the areola. In a woman, about 20 milk ducts join in the nipple, and it is from these that milk is secreted by a nursing mother. *See also* LACTATION.

Any bleeding from the nipple may indicate breast cancer and so should be

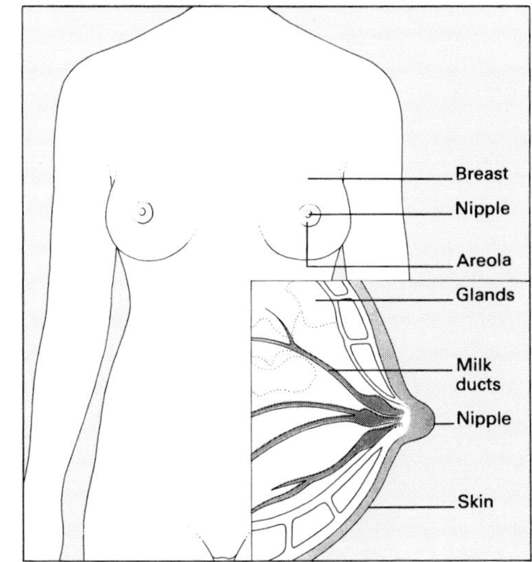

The **nipple** is surrounded by the pigmented areola and is the outlet for the milk ducts of each breast.

discussed immediately with a physician. Skin diseases can also affect the nipple. The most serious of these is a moist, red eczema called Paget's disease of the nipple.

See also PAGET'S DISEASE OF THE NIPPLE.

Nipple discharge (nip'əl) is the secretion of fluid by a woman's breast. It is a common condition among pregnant women and mothers after giving birth and before lactation begins. The discharge is a thin, yellow fluid called colostrum.

Nipple discharges by other women may be a sign of an endocrinologic disorder, in which an excess of hormonal secretions, such as prolactin, stimulates a discharge through the nipples; breast cancer, in which the discharge may contain blood; various infectious diseases; or fibrocystic disease, in which benign cysts are also present in the breasts.

See also ENDOCRINE GLAND; LACTATION; PROLACTIN.

Nit (nit) is the egg of a louse. Nits may be seen as small white spots on the hair of an infested person.

See also LICE.

Nitrate (nī'trāt) is a salt of nitric acid. Some nitrates, such as glyceryl trinitrate, cause the blood vessels to dilate and are used to treat the heart condition angina pectoris. Others, such as potassium nitrate (saltpeter), are used as food preservatives.

Nitroglycerin (nī trə glis'ər in) in medicine is a drug that helps expand blood vessels, thereby increasing the flow of blood to the heart. It is used primarily in the treatment of angina pectoris, an acute chest pain caused by a temporary drop in the amount of blood reaching the heart muscle. Possible side effects include a drop in blood pressure, headache, and dizziness. In the event of any sudden, acute chest pain, a physician should be contacted immediately, as the pain could signify a severe cardiac problem.

See also TRANSDERMAL INFUSION OF MEDICATION.

Nitrous oxide (nī'trəs ok'sīd) is a colorless gas with a faint, characteristic odor. It is used as a general anesthetic in minor operations. In combination with another anesthetic, nitrous oxide can be used for major surgery. Recovery from nitrous-oxide anesthesia is often accompanied by a period of confusion, during which time the patient alternates between tears and laughter. For this reason, nitrous oxide is commonly called laughing gas.

Nocardiosis (nō kär dē ō'sis) is a rare, sometimes fatal, infection caused by the bacterium *Nocardia asteroides*. In most cases, the microorganism infects the lungs. Less commonly, it then spreads via the bloodstream to other parts of the body, including the brain and subcutaneous tissue (tissue beneath the skin). The disease is characterized by the formation of abscesses in infected tissue and pneumonia-like symptoms, including fever, cough, chills, and chest pains. Treatment includes drainage of the abscesses and the use of the antibacterial drug sulfonamide.

Nocturia (nok tėr'ē ə) is the need to pass urine at night. It is differentiated medically from involuntary urination at night (nocturnal enuresis).

Nocturia commonly occurs in the elderly because the kidneys are less able to concentrate urine, and it becomes necessary to empty the bladder once or twice a night. In pregnant women, nocturia results when the enlarged uterus presses on the bladder.

Nocturia may also be a symptom of an enlarged prostate (benign prostatic hypertrophy); diabetes mellitus; or a kidney disorder, such as chronic nephritis, nephrotic syndrome, or pyelonephritis. Nocturia often occurs in heart failure or liver disease when there is edema (fluid retention).

Treatment depends on the cause. Assessment may involve kidney function measurements and other tests.

Nocturnal emission (nok tėr'nəl i mish'ən), or wet dream, is the involuntary ejection of semen during sleep. It is a normal, healthy occurrence brought about by the accumulation of semen in a male who does not have sexual intercourse or does not masturbate. During adolescence, a nocturnal emission is usually associated with an erotic dream.

Nocturnal enuresis. *See* BED-WETTING.

Nodule (noj'ül) is a growth of tissue, usually in the form of a small knot or swelling. A nodule may be symptomatic of a disorder, such as when a small lump appears on the skin above an arthritic joint. Nodules may also be internal, involving organs such as the liver or lung. As a rule, nodules that change in size, even if not painful, should be seen by a physician. Nodules or lumps on the breast should always be seen by a physician, even if they do not change in size.

Nonspecific urethritis. *See* URETHRITIS, NONSPECIFIC.

Nonsteroidal anti-inflammatory drug (non stə roi′dəl), or NSAID, is a painkilling and anti-inflammatory agent that works by inhibiting the synthesis of prostaglandin. Prostaglandin is a hormone-like substance that is found in most body tissues and that is believed to be a vital ingredient in the body's perception of pain and in the development of inflammation. NSAID's, including aspirin, are often used in the treatment of osteoarthritis (degenerative joint disease), rheumatoid arthritis, and a variety of other rheumatic and nonrheumatic disorders. Newer NSAID's are increasingly being used in place of aspirin because it is believed they cause fewer gastrointestinal problems than aspirin. However, newer NSAID's can also cause other harmful side effects, including kidney and liver damage and allergic reactions.

See also ACETAMINOPHEN; ASPIRIN.

Noradrenaline (nôr ə dren′ə lin) is another name for the hormone norepinephrine.

See also NOREPINEPHRINE.

Norepinephrine (nôr ep ə nef′rin) is a hormone that is secreted by the sympathetic nervous system. Produced at nerve endings, it is the main chemical transmitter from sympathetic nerves to smooth muscle, the heart muscle, and the glands. It is also produced by the central part (medulla) of the adrenal glands, from which it passes into the bloodstream. Norepinephrine is a hormone that prepares the body for "fight or flight" in situations of stress. Circulating in the blood, it constricts the blood vessels and so reduces the blood flow to the brain, intestine, liver, and kidneys; relaxes the pupils of the eyes; and soothes movement of the smooth muscle of the intestine. When given in a large dose, norepinephine acts to stimulate the release of glucose from the liver, causing a rise in the blood sugar level.

Norepinephrine can be released by stimulating the nerves or by the action of drugs such as levarterenol. It is given by intravenous infusion to treat shock.

See also HORMONE; NERVOUS SYSTEM, SYMPATHETIC; PHEOCHROMOCYTOMA.

Nose, an external protrusion in the center of the face, is used for breathing and is the organ primarily associated with the sense of smell. It extends as far as the nasopharynx at the upper, back part of the throat. The nose has an internal portion that extends backwards as two channels through the front of the skull. The channels are separated from each other by a thin partition bone called the nasal septum.

The external nose is formed by two small nasal bones, which can be felt at the bridge of the nose, and by pliable cartilage covered with more flexible areas of skin that form the flare of the nostrils.

Q: *What are the functions of the nose?*

A: In addition to serving as a passageway for air both to and from the lungs, the nose has several protective functions. The hairs at the entrance of the nose filter out large dust particles and the adenoids at the back of the nose combat disease organisms. The mucous membrane lining the nose warms and humidifies the air before it passes into the throat. And at the top of the nose, adjacent to the frontal sinuses, sensitive endings of the olfactory nerve detect smells. In addition, the cavities of the nose and sinuses help to give the voice its characteristic resonance.

Q: *What disorders may affect the nose?*

A: The common cold is the most usual infection that affects the nose, although an allergy such as hay fever or vasomotor rhinitis may be another cause of a runny nose. A nosebleed may occur spontaneously or following infection or an accident. Chronic nasal infections produce nasal mucus and a postnasal drip. The skin on the surface of the nose may become swollen and reddened, a condition known as rhinophyma.

A blow to the front of the face may break the nose bones and damage the cartilage. Often, the structures return to their natural positions after healing and, pro-

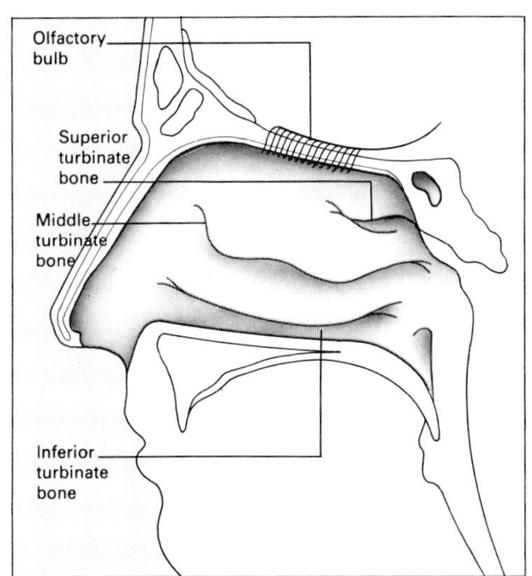

At the top of the **nose,** adjacent to the frontal sinuses, sensitive endings of the olfactory nerve detect smells.

vided that the nasal septum is straight, no permanent damage results. If, however, the nose is deformed, it should be surgically reset in the correct position. Sometimes, the nasal septum is deformed either as a result of a congenital anomaly or following an accident.

Occasionally, small, soft swellings called polyps occur in the nose, causing obstruction to one or both nostrils. These swellings may result from an allergy or a chronic infection. They can usually be removed under local anesthetic.

It is usual for the sense of smell to deteriorate with age and to be lost entirely whenever the nose is blocked because of infection, injury, or on the rare occasions when a foreign body is pushed into a nostril. Smoking may also reduce the sense of smell.

See also SINUS; SINUSITIS.

Nosebleed is bleeding from one or both nostrils. Possible causes include an accident; an infection, such as the common cold; a blood disorder, such as leukemia or hemophilia; repeated picking of the nose with the fingernails; or hypertension (high blood pressure).

Spontaneous nosebleeds in the elderly may be associated with deterioration of the blood vessels. This is a result of arteriosclerosis and is not linked with hypertension, as is commonly believed. Spontaneous nosebleeds are also common at puberty, particularly in boys, when they are thought to be

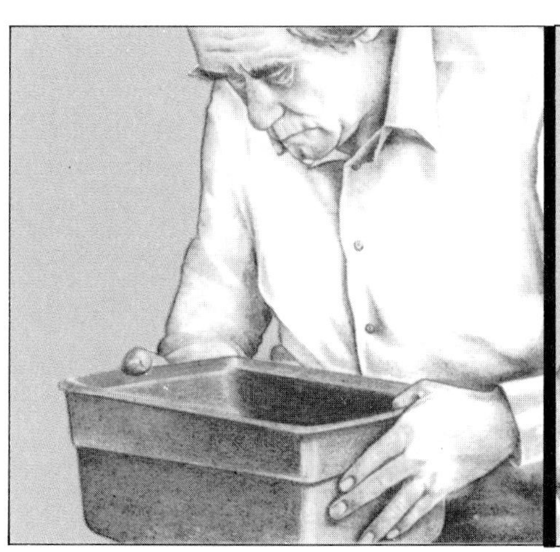

Nosebleeds occur for many different reasons, including illness, infections, accidents, and local irritation. When a nosebleed occurs, have the victim sit down with his or her head tilted forward over a bowl. Place a gauze pad in each nostril, and instruct the victim to breathe through the mouth and avoid swallowing the blood from the nose.

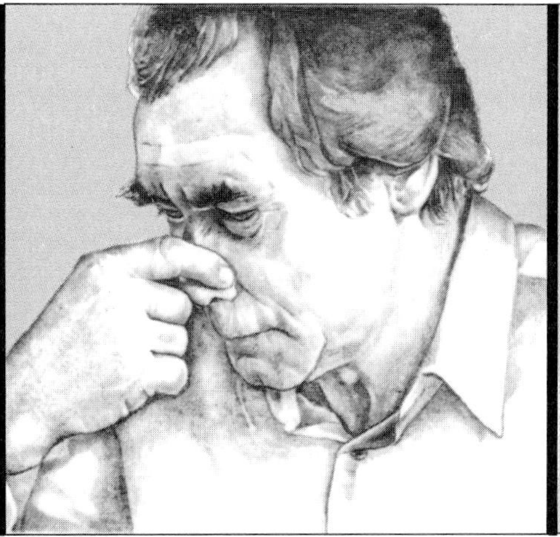

Firmly pinch, or have the victim pinch, the soft part of the nose just below the bone for about 10 minutes or until the bleeding stops. Instruct the victim not to blow the nose for several hours following the nosebleed. If bleeding has not stopped within 30 minutes, summon emergency medical aid. Loss of blood may become serious.

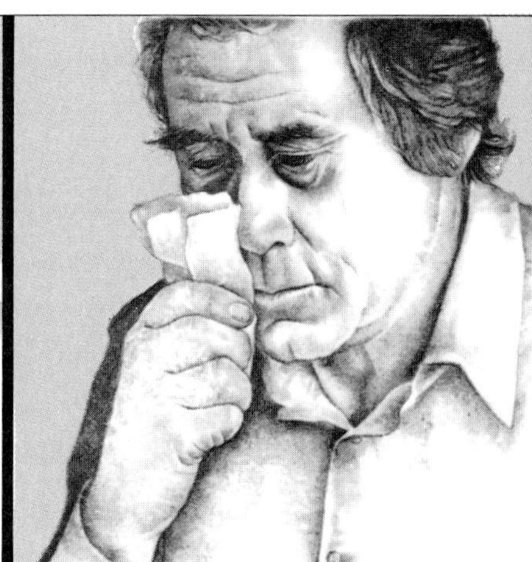

An icepack can be applied to the bridge of the nose to reduce the flow of blood down the nostril. An icepack can also be applied to the side of the nose that is bleeding.

If bleeding does not stop or reoccurs and if nosebleeds happen frequently without apparent cause, a physician should be consulted. Cauterization may be necessary.

caused by an expansion of the blood vessels in the nose from the stimulus of the sex hormones. Drying of the mucous membrane within the nose, such as may occur during the winter months, can also increase the incidence of nosebleeds.

See also NOSEBLEED: TREATMENT.

Nosebleed: treatment. Ruptured blood vessels are the cause of most nosebleeds. Bleeding may occur due to injury, sneezing, blowing, or picking. A nosebleed may also be caused by an infection, allergy, tumor, arteriosclerosis, skull fracture, or various blood disorders. In addition, nosebleeds may occur as a result of taking anticoagulant drugs. If this happens, the drug should be stopped and the dose adjusted by a physician.

A physician should be consulted if nosebleeds occur without obvious cause, especially if the nosebleeds are frequent. Nosebleeds resulting from a possible broken nose or a skull fracture require immediate medical attention.

Treatment. Place the victim in a sitting position with the head tilted forward over a bowl. Firmly pinch the soft part of the nose just below the bone for about 10 minutes or until the bleeding stops. An ice pack placed on the bridge of the nose helps to reduce the pain, swelling, and blood flow.

See illustrations on page 605.

If the nosebleed is caused by a ruptured blood vessel, a physician may be able to cauterize (burn) it with chemicals or electricity, thereby stopping the bleeding. If this is not possible, the nose can be packed with a special gauze for a day or two. It is rarely necessary to do more than this, although occasionally the victim needs a transfusion or additional blood vessel surgery to stop the bleeding.

Nosedrops: administration. Place two pillows under the patient's shoulders so that the head is tilted backward. The further back the head rests, the more effective is the treatment. Insert the end of the dropper into one nostril and release the prescribed number of drops. Instruct the patient to sniff gently. Repeat with the other nostril. The patient should stay in position with the head back for about one minute. Wipe away any excess fluid with cotton.

Nose, foreign body in: treatment. Children often stuff small objects such as beans or crayons into their nose.

Treatment: If the object is easily seen in the nostril and small tweezers are available, try removing the object with the tweezers. If this is not possible, have the person hold the unobstructed nostril closed and blow hard through the nose. If the person is too young to cooperate, hold the unobstructed nostril closed and "puff" air into the child's mouth. If these remedies prove unsuccessful, take the patient to a physician.

Nose, runny. A runny nose is a discharge from one or both nostrils. It results from any condition that causes inflammation of the lining of the nose (rhinitis). The most common cause is the common cold, although it may also be caused by an allergy or sinusitis. A runny nose following a head injury may be a sign of a fractured skull in which the cerebrospinal fluid leaks into the nose. The fluid may then become infected, and the condition can result in meningitis. In the case of a persistent discharge from one or both nostrils, especially if pus or blood are detected, a physician should be contacted.

See also NOSEBLEED; SINUSITIS.

Nose, stuffy. A stuffy nose is a popular term for the blockage of one or both nostrils, resulting in difficulty in breathing. It is common in nasal infections that cause inflammation of the nose, but may also be caused by a polyp (a small growth on a mucous membrane) or a deviated nasal septum.

See also COLD; POLYP; SEPTUM, DEVIATED.

Nosocomial infection (nos ə kō′mē əl) is an infection acquired during hospitalization. These infections are of special concern because they are usually resistant to many antibiotics. The diseases a patient can accidentally acquire in the hospital include infections of the urinary tract, hepatitis, and pneumonia.

See also HOSPITAL.

Nostril (nos′trəl) is one of the two external openings of the nose.

See also NOSE.

Nuclear medicine (nü′klē ər) is the branch of medicine that involves the use of radioisotopes in the study, diagnosis, and treatment of various diseases, as in the field of cancer research and treatment.

See also ISOTOPE; RADIOISOTOPE IMAGING.

Nucleolus (nü klē′ə ləs) is a small, usually round structure within the nucleus of a cell. It contains a high concentration of ribonucleic acid, a chemical compound vital in the making of proteins and in genetic transmission.

See also CELL; RIBONUCLEIC ACID.

Nucleus (nü′klē əs) is a central point around which matter is concentrated. For example, every body cell has a nucleus, which contains chromosomes and various other minute structures.

The term nucleus is also used to describe a collection of nerve cells within the brain.

See also CELL; CHROMOSOME.

Nucleus pulposus (nü′klē əs pəl pō′sis) is the central part of an intervertebral disk, which is part of the spine. It is surrounded by a ring of tough, fibrous cartilage. At birth, the nucleus pulposus is a soft, jelly-like material, but with increasing age this material is gradually replaced with fibrocartilage from the surrounding ring and thus loses much of its elastic quality.

See also DISK, HERNIATED; VERTEBRA.

Nullipara (nə lip′ər ə) is the medical term for a woman who has never given birth. The term covers women whose pregnancies have been terminated naturally or under medical supervision.

Numbness (num′nis) is complete or partial loss of sensation in an area of skin.

There are many conditions that may cause numbness, and most of them involve the nervous system. Intense cold produces numbness of the hands, feet, and other skin areas, particularly in persons with poor peripheral circulation. Numbness may also be a symptom of an acute emotional disturbance, such as hysteria.

Q: *What are the neurological causes of numbness?*

A: Neurological causes of numbness include pressure on a nerve, such as the sciatica nerve along the back of the leg; spondylosis (a degenerative condition of the spine); carpal tunnel syndrome (a disorder of the wrist); and polyneuritis. Numbness may also result from disorders of the central nervous system, such as a stroke, multiple sclerosis, syringomyelia (a disorder of the spinal cord), tabes dorsalis, or locomotor ataxia (a disorder of the nervous system). Numbness may also be caused by a deficiency of vitamin B_{12}, resulting in polyneuritis and degeneration of the spinal cord.

Q: *How is numbness treated?*

A: The treatment depends on a correct diagnosis of the cause. This can be made only by a physician, who should be consulted when any numbness persists.

See also POLYNEURITIS.

Nurse, licensed practical. A licensed practical nurse (LPN), also called a licensed vocational nurse (LVN), is a professional nurse, who is licensed to administer patient care under the supervision of a doctor or a registered nurse.

An LPN usually studies practical nursing and direct patient care for two years at a public school or a private school operated by a hospital, health agency, junior college, or university. The course combines classroom study with practical experience. The graduate must then pass a state board examination to be licensed as an LPN.

Practical nurses may work in hospitals, private homes, nursing homes, public health agencies, and physicians' offices.

See also HOSPITAL; NURSE, REGISTERED.

Nurse practitioner is a professional nurse who has had additional training in a certain area of specialized practice. For example, some nurse practitioners specialize in geriatrics and others in pediatrics. Nurse practitioners perform many tasks that were previously done only by physicians. These nurses give physical examinations, diagnose and treat minor illnesses, and advise patients on health problems. By administering much of the routine health care, nurse practitioners free physicians to treat patients suffering from more serious ailments. Most nurse practitioners work in private clinics or physicians' offices or in a group practice with physicians or other nurse practitioners.

See also NURSE, REGISTERED.

Nurse, public health. Public health nurses usually help care for large groups of persons outside hospitals. Most of these nurses work for government or private agencies.

Visiting nurses are public health nurses. So are the nurses employed by city, county, or state health departments. The public health nurse may go into homes to care for patients who have just returned from hospitals. One of the main functions of the public health nurse is often to teach patients with chronic illness how to care for themselves. He or she teaches patients and their families about proper diet, personal hygiene, and other ways of preventing illness. Often, the public health nurse is concerned with the health of the people of the area in which he or she works. He or she may also take part in community projects, such as immunization programs.

See also NURSE, LICENSED PRACTICAL.

Nurse, registered. A registered nurse (RN) is a professional nurse, who is licensed to practice nursing and may use the initials R.N. after his or her name.

A registered nurse completes a four- or five-year baccalaureate program at a college or university, graduating with a bachelor of science degree, or an approved three-year diploma program. After obtaining the necessary training, the nursing school graduate must pass the National Council Licensure Examination (NCLEX-RN). The nurse is then licensed by the state to practice nursing as a registered nurse.

Most RN's are employed in hospitals, where they work with physicians and other medical personnel in various ways. They may be members of a surgical team or a physical therapy team. They may administer blood transfusions or injections. They may keep track of a patient's recovery, observing any changes in physical condition, mental attitude, or reaction to drugs or other treatment. With added education, they may become nurse practitioners, specializing in a particular kind of nursing, for example, in the care of newborn babies or heart patients.

See also HOSPITAL; NURSE, LICENSED PRACTICAL; NURSE PRACTITIONER.

Nursing the chronically ill. We are not all born nurses, and caring for the sick does not come easily to everyone. However, compassion for someone is the essential quality in the care and attention that you give your patient. Like love in all its forms, there are times of irritation and frustration and times of contentment and happiness.

Personal hygiene is important. It is essential to have clean hands and short nails to prevent scratching. If you have

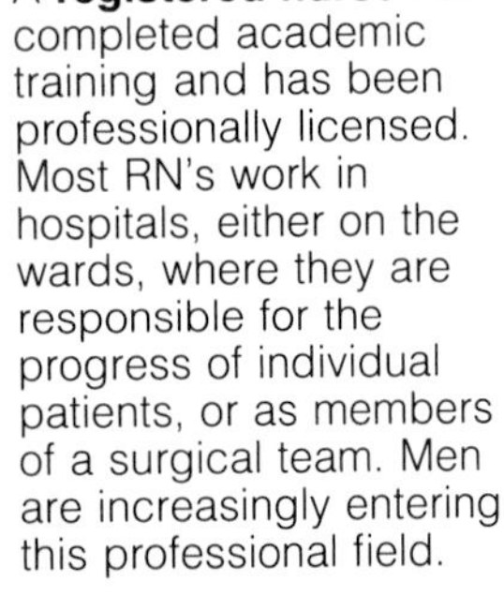

A **registered nurse** has completed academic training and has been professionally licensed. Most RN's work in hospitals, either on the wards, where they are responsible for the progress of individual patients, or as members of a surgical team. Men are increasingly entering this professional field.

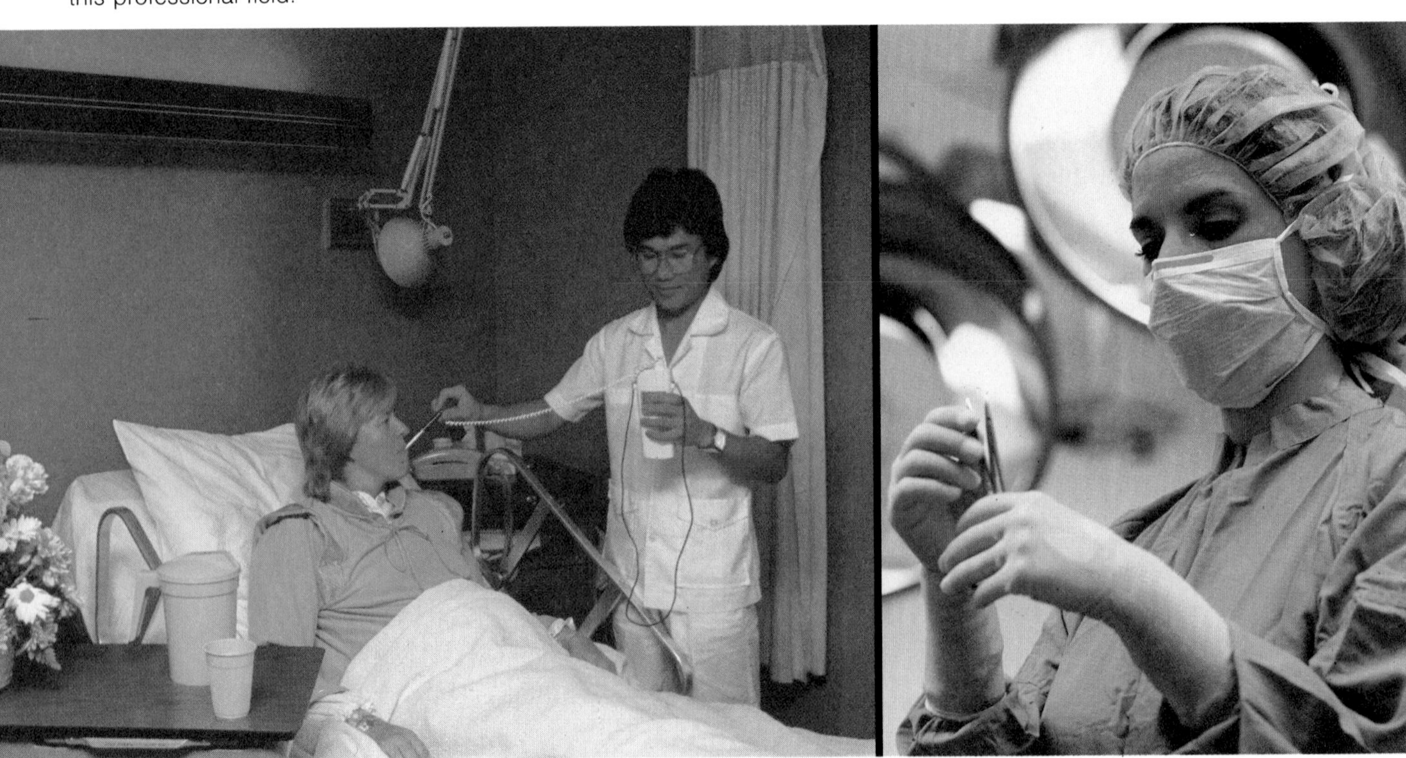

long hair, tie it back to prevent it dropping across your face and into the patient's eyes when moving him or her. Sharp rings, other jewelry, and watches should be removed from your hands and wrists. They not only scratch, but may become entangled in the bed linens or soaked by water.

You may find it more comfortable to keep a special pair of old, rubber-soled, low-heeled shoes in the sickroom. Such shoes are less likely to slip if the soles get wet.

It is important to follow the physicians directions for administering the prescribed medications. This includes exactly when and how they should be given. If you do not understand, ask your physician again. This is essential. Do not guess and give medicines because you think they are needed.

The best way of working out a routine of looking after a chronically ill patient is through discussions with the family physician. Remember that not only the patient's needs, but also your own have to be considered. Prepare the sickroom. For detailed instructions, refer to the appropriate section in NURSING THE SICK.

If the patient is incontinent, or likely to be so, the mattress must be protected with plastic sheeting and covered with an easily removable drawsheet. Incontinence pads must be readily available. It is important to remember to offer the bed pan or commode every three or four hours as this may prevent further incontinence. Bed bathing, or washing, should be done in the morning, as incontinence and perspiration during the night leave the patient's skin moist and vulnerable to ulceration. If a patient is entirely confined to bed, the pressure areas on the buttocks, heels, and elbows should be thoroughly rubbed with alcohol and powdered twice a day. Part of your daily routine must include care of your patient's hair, teeth—even false ones—and nails. A little makeup for a female patient helps her morale as well as yours. Prepare food attractively, and serve it in small portions. Fluids are essential and can be of different varieties, coffee, fruit juice, or milk. All the above subjects are more thoroughly discussed in the entry NURSING THE SICK.

A patient who is inactive may have two additional problems. The first is constipation, which may be helped by a high-roughage diet, occasional laxatives, or suppositories. The second problem can arise if your patient has a good appetite and gains weight. This can make nursing more difficult and should be avoided by leaving carbohydrates, such as sugar, out of the patient's diet and increasing the bulk with fruits and vegetables, which also help to prevent constipation.

Visitors not only help to share in the care of the patient, but also to boost his or her morale. They can talk about old times, the family, and future plans for grandchildren, as well as discussing friends at work. This acts as a stimulus, provided the visit does not last too long leaving the patient overtired. You need tact to end a visit before this point is reached. It is usually wise to warn the visitor that the physician only allows visits to be a certain length of time. This gives you the chance to intrude without making the visitor feel that he or she is being sent away.

Unless the patient is completely bedridden, a wheelchair gives some degree of mobility and allows him or her to be moved from one room to another, out into the garden, or sometimes, for a drive in the car. This may tire the patient, but the stimulus is good for morale. The sickroom can be thoroughly

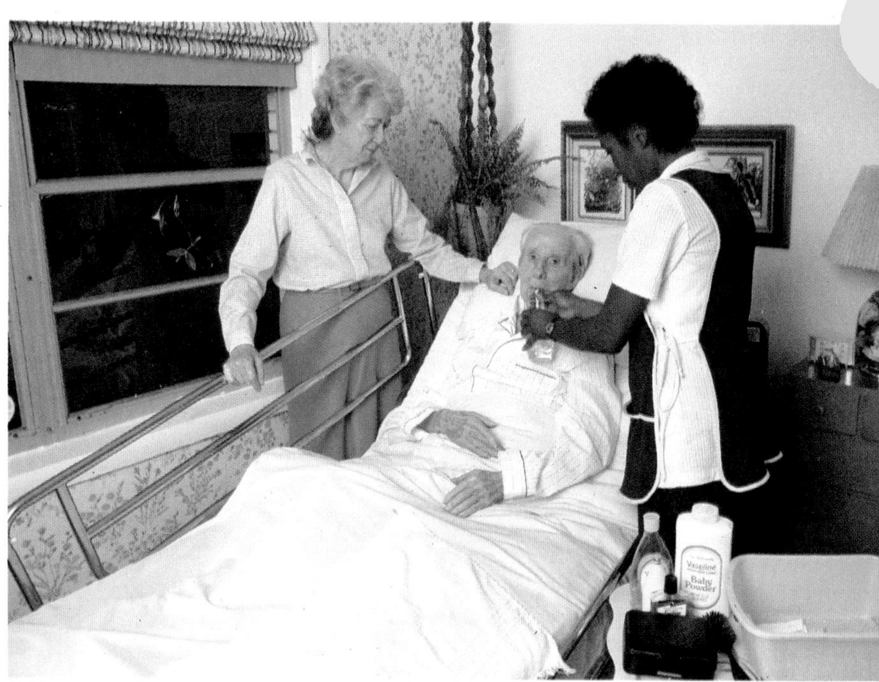

Long-term **nursing of the chronically ill patient,** however much he or she may be loved by the caregiver, can be a great emotional strain. It is very important to seek additional help, either from other family members or from trained nursing help, to relieve the caregiver and to ensure that the patient feels adequately cared for.

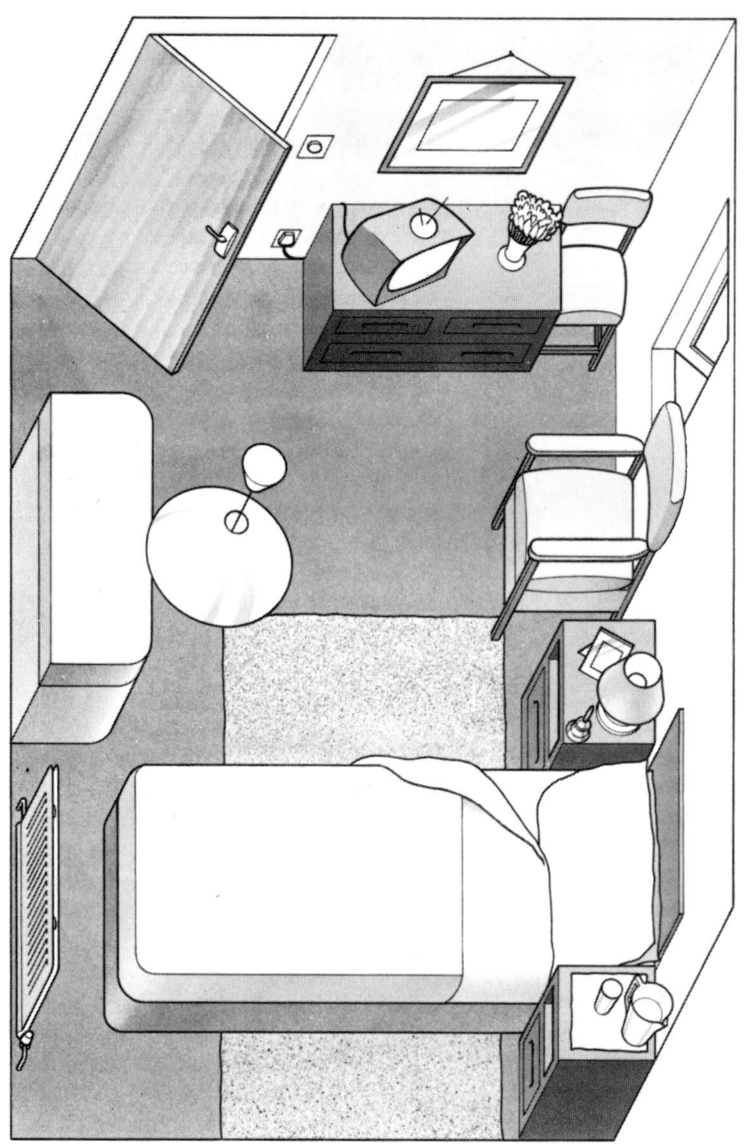

The bedroom

The bedroom should contain the necessary equipment and material to meet the needs of the chronically ill patient. The bed should have a firm mattress and be at the correct height, which is low enough to make getting in and out easy, yet high enough not to cause difficuly to a family member bending over the patient. If the patient is incontinent, or might become so, the mattress should be covered with plastic sheeting. Generally, the most practical position for a bed is such that a person can approach from either side. But when the patient is senile or in a confused state, it is sometimes better to have one side of the bed against a wall; this does tend to make bedmaking difficult, however.

There should be two chairs fairly close to the bed. One should be specially comfortable, for the patient's use when he or she is able to get out of bed. The other chair is for visitors, and for use in holding bedclothes and pillows when stripping and remaking the bed.

A commode can be useful if the patient is able to move to it.

There should also be a chest of drawers or a cupboard of about waist height in which to store essential equipment, such as spare linen. The top can be used as a working surface by members of the family, and by the physician.

cleaned while the patient is out, and the caring relative can have a rest.

Household pets, a favorite dog or cat, can give great pleasure to the chronically ill. Their companionship is undemanding and removes the feeling of loneliness that so often burdens someone who spends most of his or her time in one room.

The overall responsibility for the patient's care usually falls on a single family member. The rest of the family can help in various ways. Someone can do the shopping, another may prepare food to be kept in the freezer, and another can take responsibility for exercising and looking after the dog. Even children in the house can help by carrying trays, getting books, or helping with bedmaking. Involvement of the whole family makes everyone realize they are part of a team and prevents the patient from being too much of a burden to one person. It also gives the family a feeling of responsibility to each other and to the patient.

Relatives and friends often share the work to give the immediate family time off: time to go to the hairdresser; time to walk and think; time to be alone; time to visit with friends, away from the surroundings of the home without the feeling of always being "on call"; time to rest and sleep if tired from disturbed nights.

If you are going out, it is useful to write down exactly what needs to be done and when, so that a different person can become acquainted with the patient's routine. Even details about the

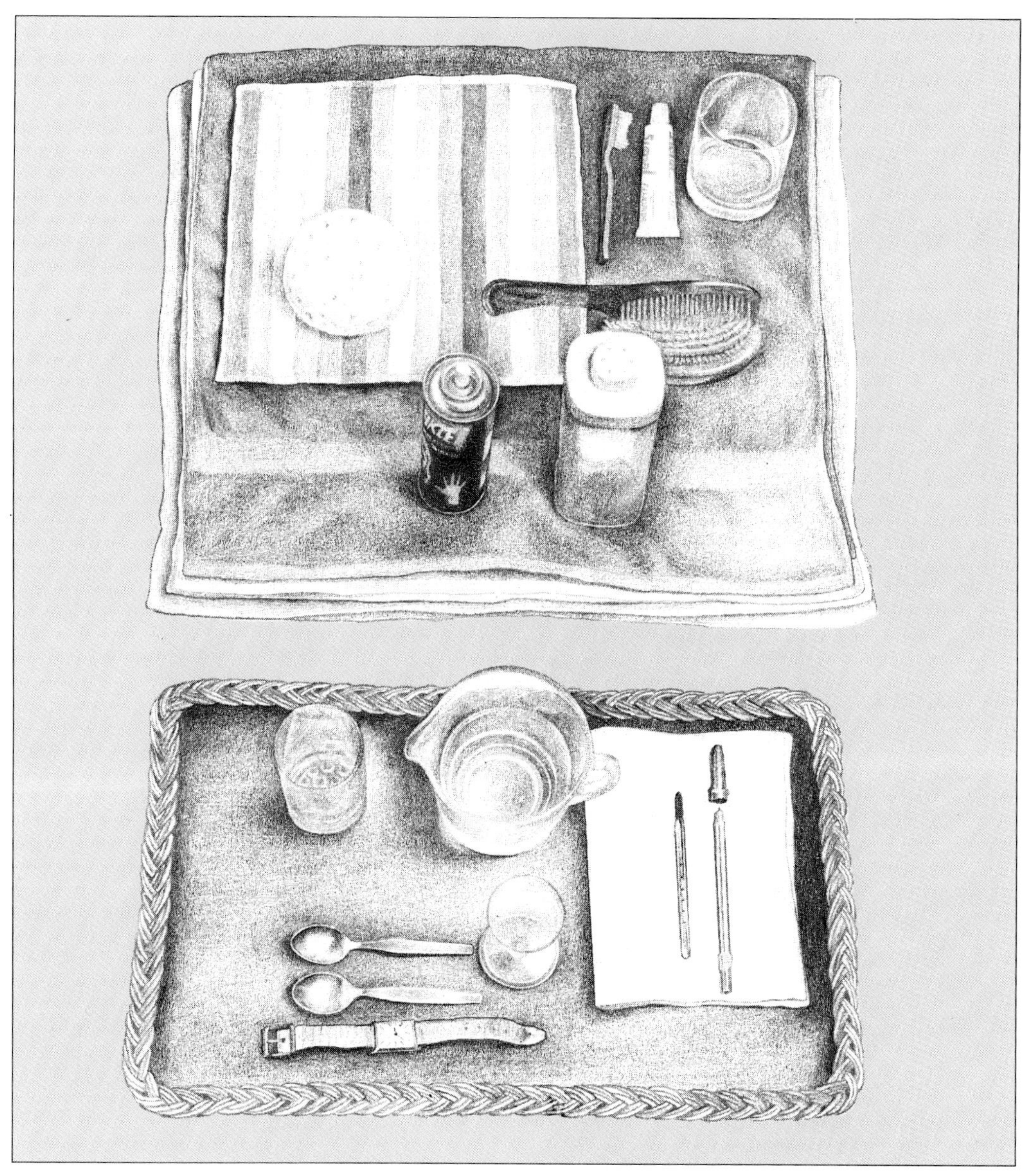

Beside the bed
Somewhere close to the bed, space must be found for the means by which a patient can take pride in his or her own appearance. It is also important to have the articles and materials used for bodily hygiene near the patient. Even if patients can not attend to their own hygiene, the materials are then convenient for those who assist the patient.

If they are physically able, patients generally prefer to wash themselves. For this purpose, at least two facecloths or sponges are required, with soap, talcum powder, and deodorant. For drying, there should be two or three bathtowels for the body, and a soft towel for the face. To keep teeth clean, a toothbrush, toothpaste, and a small mug or bowl, should be provided, with denture brush and denture bath if necessary. For hair grooming, there should be a hairbrush, a comb, and a mirror.

Medical equipment that should be kept on hand includes: a clinical thermometer; a medicine glass and one or two teaspoons; a clock or watch that records seconds (for use in taking the pulse); and a small napkin.

It is also useful to have a container for dirty clothing, a box of tissues, and a wastepaper basket.

way pillows are arranged in bed are important to the patient who may feel that this is essential for comfort and sleep.

Sometimes, when dealing with a long-term invalid, arrangements must be made for the one caring for the patient to have a complete change and holiday. Another member of the family can take over, after a day or two in the house to see how things are done. If this is not possible, your physician can make arrangements for a temporary stay in the hospital for the patient. If this is going to happen, it is essential to explain everything to the patient, who may momentarily feel frightened and deserted. He or she should realize the need for this change. If the patient is being moved to the hospital, a preliminary visit by a member of the family enables the nurse to discover any problems that may have to be faced and the details of the routine that has been established at home. This helps the nursing staff to look after the patient in a way to which he or she has become accustomed. In addition, the relative can tell the patient about the hospital and the staff. This acts as a preliminary introduction. If the change has been a success, further arrangements can be made from time to time, which give the family the assurance that outside help is available and acceptable when it is necessary.

As time goes by, the patient becomes used to his or her daily routine. Any changes that are made may cause him or her distress, so they should be ex-

Hygiene

Persons who are confined to bed still need to wash frequently, and a good wash and brushing of teeth can do much to improve a patient's morale. If there is no built-in washstand in the bedroom, some attempt must be made to provide hot and cold water. The most convenient way to maintain a hot water supply is to use a thermos bottle, although pouring may be difficult in bed. An alternative is a large enamel pitcher. Both containers may be refilled when necessary. Cold water can be provided in a light plastic bucket or pitcher, preferably with a lip or spout and a handle. All such vessels should be stood on a flat surface no higher than the patient's mattress.

The patient should be provided with a large plastic bowl to wash in. It should be made of the more inflexible plastic, and should be at least 6 inches (15cm) deep to stop water from splashing out.

A smaller bowl is also useful for holding the patient's dentures.

Urination and defecation can be both difficult and embarrassing for a bedridden patient. The family should respect the patient's need for privacy to carry out such bodily functions. Bedpans should generally be kept and carried under cloths. The toilet paper should be kept out of the sight of visitors. Frequent washing and sterilization are essential for all equipment of this kind.

Space may also be needed in the bedroom for medical equipment such as bandages and dressings.

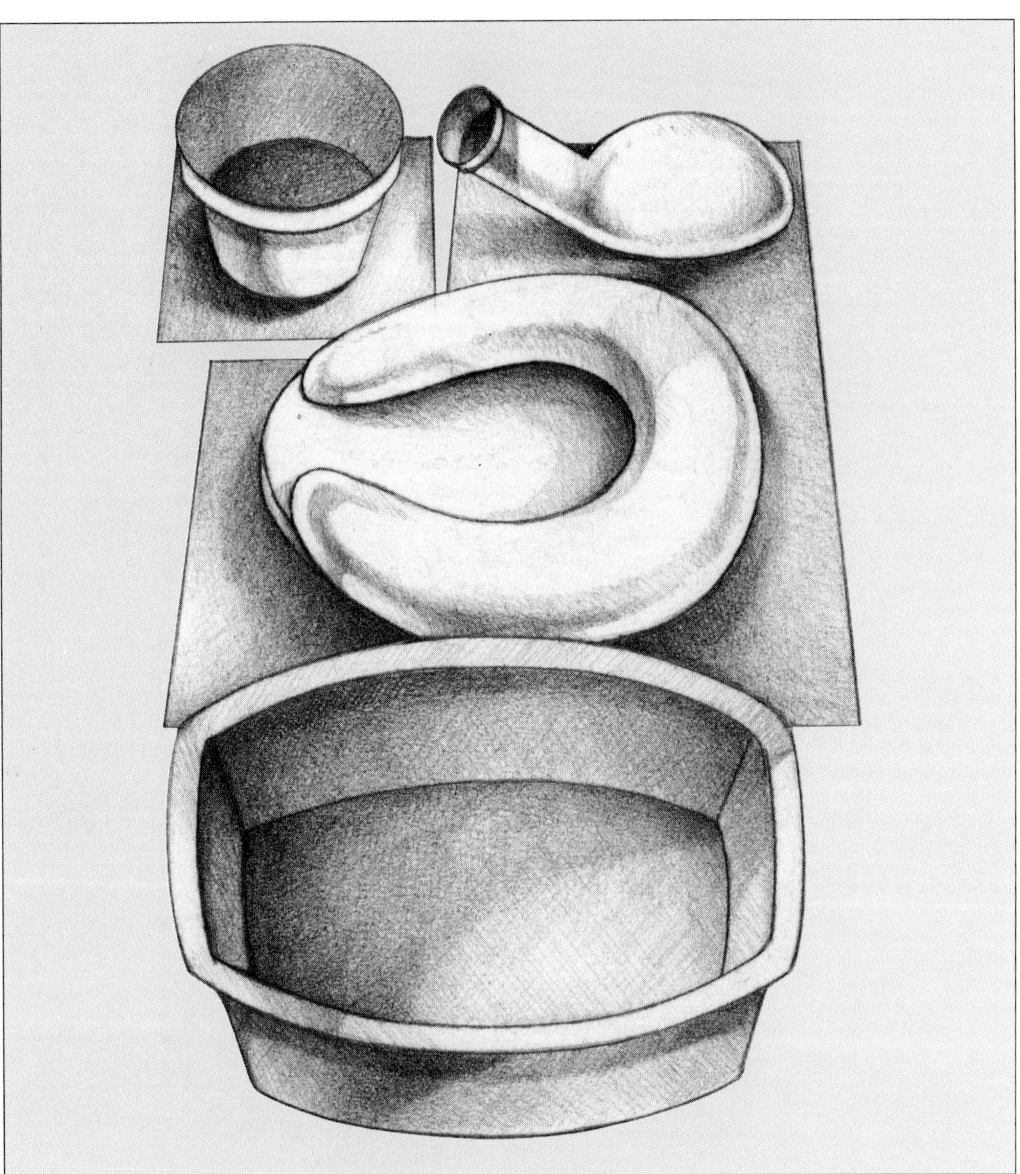

plained before they occur. For example, lunch may be earlier than usual because of the expected visit of the physician or a relative.

Smoking in the sickroom should be forbidden. The smell of stale cigarette smoke is unpleasant, unless the patient smokes. This is always a problem and a source of anxiety. A dropped cigarette may burn the bed linen or the patient or start a fire. There is no easy answer to this.

Apart from the obvious hazards of smoking there are some other things that are dangerous. Never use a hot-water bottle. It may leak and cause burns. A sedated patient may not feel the burning heat of a bottle against his or her leg. A tray containing very hot fluids should not be balanced on the patient's legs because it may easily overturn. A light located above the patient's head must be securely fixed to the wall, or the patient may pull it down while feeling for the switch. If you cannot secure the light, change the position of the bed. A bed on casters may move if the patient tries to get out of bed. Instead of supporting him or her, the bed could slide away, allowing the patient to fall, even if you are helping. Always be sure the bed is secure and that the carpet on the floor can not slip.

The comfort of the patient is your main concern. Patients with heart and chest problems are usually helped by sitting upright with plenty of pillows arranged behind the back and head. Of-

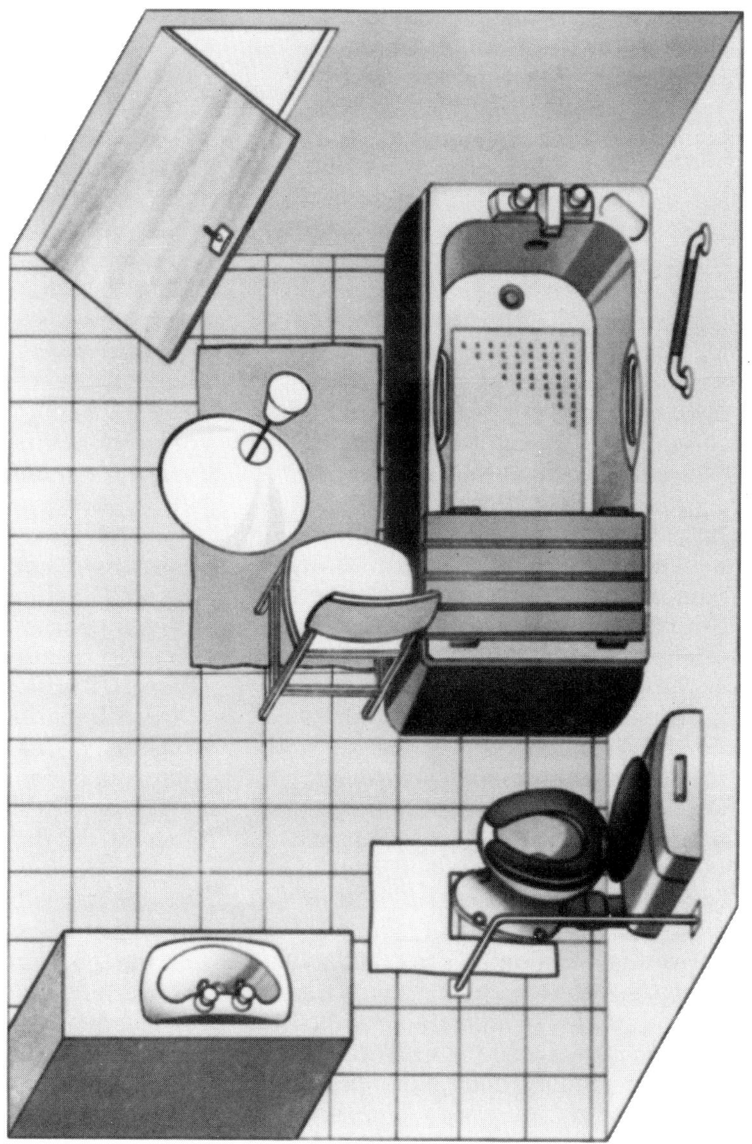

The bathroom
Of all the rooms in a house, the bathroom is the one in which most ingenuity and care has to be exercised to make it safe for a chronically ill patient. There are many simple improvements that can be made or purchased.

The light switch should be by the door. There should be rails on each side of the bathtub and on the wall slightly above the bathtub. A rubber mat with suction cups beneath provides a secure footing. A seat alongside the bath makes getting in and out much easier. A short plank from a nearby chair may help a patient to reach the bath surface.

The toilet should have a lever or a push-bar rather than a suspended chain. If necessary, the height of the seat can be altered by adding specially-shaped pieces of wood. A rail alongside helps the patient to sit down and to get up. Here too, a rubber mat provides a nonslip surface for the feet.

It is more practical for the washbasin to have a flat surface surrounding it.

The door of the bathroom should never be locked when an unsteady person is taking a bath, and make sure a responsible person knows when the patient is in the bathroom.

Some audible, non-electrical means of alarm can also be useful.

ten, a small cushion or pillow behind the patient's head gives additional support to the neck and allows these muscles to relax. The patient may have a tendency to slide down the bed. You can prevent this by tucking a box, suitcase, or pillow, rolled in a sheet, firmly under the mattress, at the foot of the bed. This allows the patient to push gently with his or her feet to maintain his or her position and, at the same time, exercise the calf muscles, preventing deep vein thrombosis. If necessary the end of the bed can be raised on wooden blocks or large books. For more detailed information, see NURSING THE SICK.

The patient's morale depends on your care and attention. If you are overtired you may find yourself less able to help. It is for this reason that you need time away from the patient to rest and recover. Even a short time away refreshes you and helps you remain cheerful.

The patient gets great comfort from listening to your voice telling him or her about the family, the outside world, and neighborhood news. It is not always necessary for the patient to talk to you. Some families are more musical than others, and humming or singing old, familiar songs gives the patient pleasure and brings back memories. A radio, a record player, a television, or books often give pleasure and help pass the time. Flowers in the room and a favorite picture, positioned so that it can easily be seen, are restful and give the patient enjoyment. Photographs of the family can be placed on the bed table. All these things are simply and easily done and help to make the invalid's life cheerful and less monotonous.

Nighttime is a particular problem for the chronically sick. The patient needs a telephone or some other means of communication. Open doors may not be sufficient to hear what is happening in the sickroom. Last thing in the evening, make sure the patient has emptied his or her bladder and has taken the necessary medicines. Tidy the bed and make the patient comfortable. Leave a shaded light in the room to help prevent the patient from being confused in the night if he or she wakes up. The confusion could be due to the illness, drugs, or the dark. Confusion is greatly reduced if the patient recognizes familiar surroundings. Usually, however, an invalid feels sufficiently secure at home to have a reasonably good night's sleep.

The rewards of nursing a chronically ill patient are often difficult to appreciate. The forced changes in your family and personal life are often difficult to accept. They are easier to sacrifice if the patient is someone you love, who returns this affection by showing his or her appreciation and thanks.

Providing care is much more difficult to do when the patient is confused, irritable, demanding, and unable or unwilling to show any gratitude for your help. This is the most testing of all relationships, and you can only survive with sufficient outside help to allow you to escape occasionally.

Sometimes, the burden is too much, and you must be prepared to take outside advice from friends, family, and physician if both you and your patient are suffering. There is no shame in admitting that you have undertaken an impossible task, because you have the justification that you have tried. Often, however, the care of a patient in your own home is an immensely satisfying, though tiring, job. You have shared in a human experience that gives you a deeper understanding of other people's problems, fears, and troubles. You know that you have done a job well.

Depression and Anxiety are two of the most common emotional disorders. Anxiety may be realistic, stemming from worries about a dying parent or an alcoholic spouse. Sympathy, understanding, and help from relatives and friends are very important.

Anxiety coupled with depression may be unrealistic. Fears may be associated with mood changes, chemical imbalances, alcoholism, or an inability to cope with stress. You can help by being reassuring and trying to find practical answers to a problem. Decision-making is always difficult for someone who is depressed. Your assistance may make life easier, even if it is only in keeping the anxious person company. If it is a neighbor who is depressed, frequent visits from you may help. *See also* ANXIETY.

Severe depression may lead to a state of complete hopelessness and suicidal despair. Suicidal talk is a serious symptom and must not be ignored. Professional help is mandatory. A psychiatrist can recommend psychotherapy, treatment with antidepressant drugs, or, occasionally, hospitalization. Your role is one of friendship and understanding toward the patient. Unfortunately, the depressed patient may feel that he or she has failed and let you down. His or her sense of inadequacy is thereby increased. It is important that you let the patient feel that your friendship outweighs any of the burdens that he or she places upon you. This human warmth is a lifeline that gives the patient hope of recovery. *See also* DEPRESSION.

Hysteria, as commonly understood, is an emotional outburst, whose severity is out of proportion to the situation that triggers it. The symptoms can take many physical forms, for example, pain in the neck, head, or stomach; uncontrollable laughing or crying; choking sensations; dimness of vision; inability to urinate; or even dizziness and fainting. Your firmness, sympathy, and support are necessary. If you can help the hysteric person to face up to the situation, the patient can build up confidence and increase his or her ability to cope with the next problem when it occurs. Occasionally, holding the patient's arms firmly in your hands and talking slowly, quietly, and with emphasis are necessary to bring symptoms under control and to calm down the hysterical person. Hysteria, as a psychiatric condition, is quite different from the type of hysteria discussed here. *See also* HYSTERIA.

Mental Instability is difficult to define. Even physicians disagree on the range of normal human behavior. Some specialists accept behavior that others would consider to be definitely abnormal. Instability may be considered to be a disorder of the patient's normal thought processes, so that conclusions are reached that do not fit in with the facts of the situation and the reactions of the individual do not follow any apparent logical pattern.

Some patients have fixed delusions. In this form of instability, the patient is convinced that some underlying force is working against him or her, for example, that men in gray topcoats are agents of a secret enemy and must be avoided. These beliefs modify the patient's behavior so that he or she avoids the particular "enemy," but behaves normally in all other respects. This is a form of paranoia.

The patient with more serious paranoia may hear unexplained voices, receive messages and instructions, and see visions of things that the rest of us can not see. Whatever the age of the individual, these symptoms must not be ignored. The paranoia may be a symptom of schizophrenia or drug addiction. You must avoid conflict with the patient's views; to him or her, they are very real. You should talk to the relatives about the problem or, if it is a member of your own family, discuss it with a psychiatrist. It is important to try and get the patient to accept medical help. Sometimes, the patient is aware that he or she is confused, and this makes it easier for you to persuade him or her to seek help. Often, the problem is more difficult. A direct confrontation may produce a physical reaction and violence. You must be careful and ensure that help is at hand. The patient may treat you with suspicion if you disagree with him or her, so you have to be subtle in your approach. If you fail, do not try again, unless you feel the patient to be a danger to himself or herself or to others. If you feel this is the case, then you must get help from a psychiatrist or, if necessary, the police. The patient may be so ill that he or she needs to be hospitalized. This decision is not taken by you and depends on psychiatric and medical advice. *See also* MANIA; MANIC-DEPRESSIVE ILLNESS.

Mania is another form of mental disorder. This occurs when an overactive mind overflows with enthusiasm, and ideas replace one another so quickly that there is often no time to carry them out. The patient is convinced he or she can change the world. The excessive enthusiasm ultimately leads to physical fatigue and confusion, but the patient cannot tolerate any frustrations or attempts to deflect him or her from his or her desires. The patient may react violently if you try to hinder his or her intentions. It is safer to gently deflect the patient from the ideas, while apparently agreeing with his or her intentions. This gives the ideas a chance to spontaneously change and a new course of action to start. It is important not to become personally involved in these schemes. In an extreme form, the patient's loss of judgment, physical exhaustion, and confusion need to be treated by hospitalization and sedation. Only the psychiatrist can help. *See also* MANIA; MANIC-DEPRESSIVE ILLNESS.

When you are dealing with a mentally disturbed patient, it is important not to get hurt. Try to ensure that you are not alone and that the patient is not between you and the door. Be prepared to leave quickly and, if necessary, move a chair between yourself and the patient as you escape from the room. There is no point in being brave and getting hurt. It is more sensible to admit that you can not help any further and to summon professional help as soon as possible.

Confusion, like mental instability, is difficult to define. It is not the same as dementia, which is a mental deterioration due to age and/or gradual changes in the brain tissue, resulting from disease. Confusion and dementia may occur together. Confusion usually affects recent memory and is of fairly rapid onset. The patient loses a sense of time and place. He or she feels agitated and sometimes has hallucinations, hears voices, or feels that he or she does not really exist.

If the patient is confused, he or she needs a friend or relative to stay, to prevent him or her from coming to any harm. Sit the patient down, preferably in familiar surroundings, and talk quietly about familiar things. Reassure the patient in a calm voice that everything is all right and that you can help. Ask someone else to contact a physician or make arrangements to take the patient to the physician.

Confusion can be a symptom of physical illness, such as the onset of diabetes, pneumonia, or heart failure, which reduces the oxygen content of the blood reaching the brain. It may be caused by alcohol, drugs, concussion from an accident, or a stroke. A physician must make a diagnosis before treatment of the cause of the confusion can begin.

Elderly people may become confused only at night. This may result from mental strain or from various physiologic factors, such as sleeping pills, slight anemia, or an inefficient heart.

A permanently confused patient is probably suffering from dementia.

Dementia is a major problem in old age, affecting about 20 percent of the elderly aged 85 or over. An older person can still lead an independent life if he or she is simply absent-minded and forgetful. But in a serious form of permanent confusion, the patient loses all sense of time, feels there is no need for meals, can not remember how to dress or wash, is occasionally incontinent, and fails to recognize relatives or friends. Alzheimer's disease is the leading cause of dementia among the elderly, though not the sole cause. Dementia can also be caused by various other disorders, which affect people of any age, though this is rare. *See also* ALZHEIMER'S DISEASE; DEMENTIA.

The family often has great difficulty in persuading the patient that the time has come to live with the family or to move into a home for the aged. Although the patient's confusion is increased by a move, it has to be made. Your physician is an ally to the family and a friend to the ailing relative.

A demented patient at home alone is constantly at risk. He or she could fall and break a bone; fall into a fire; get burned while lighting a cigarette or cooking; become undernourished from failing to eat; get skin problems from failing to keep clean; feel constantly persecuted from the imagined voices and persons that populate a disorganized mind.

The problems you and your family must deal with are how to keep the patient safe, nourished, and clean, as well as how to control any agitation and disturbance in the patient's mind.

Set aside a room with carpets that do not slip and a bed that is against a wall, to prevent the patient from falling out on at least one side. A chair can be pushed firmly against the open side of the bed after the patient has been put to bed. A comfortable arm chair is essential, and a bed table can be placed across the chair to prevent the patient from getting out without help. The furniture in the room should be simple, preferably containing some of the things from the patient's own home, with his or her favorite pictures on the wall. If the room is upstairs, it is advisable to have a gate on the staircase. Make sure that the lock on the bathroom door can be opened from the outside. If not, remove the lock altogether.

Although the progress of the dementia usually can not be prevented, a normal, healthy diet with plenty of fresh fruit and additional vitamins helps to maintain the patient's general health and well-being. The physician may prescribe a tranquilizer to be taken last thing at night, to ensure a good sleep for the patient and the family.

A strict routine helps the patient to achieve a comfortable rhythm to his or her life. Meals, washing, and visits to the bathroom should be at regular times. However irritated you may feel, talk to the patient in a calm voice. It produces better results than shouting. Even when you are in the room tidying or bedmaking, use a gentle voice to tell the patient about neighbors, visits by the children, and other potential disturbances. Such casual conversation may help keep the patient in touch with normal life.

Care of the patient is likely to be long-term, so you will need your own time off. Relatives and friends may help out on a daily basis, but, occasionally, you need a vacation. Ideally, someone should take over your work in the home, as the patient is almost always made worse by a move to the hospital and the change of routine, then worse again on the return home. However, if it is not possible to arrange for someone to come in, you must accept the patient's increased confusion on his or her return, in order to get your vacation.

Eventually, the elderly patient is unable to get out of bed, get dressed, or go to the bathroom. Occasional incontinence becomes chronic. The patient's skin may ulcerate and form bedsores. The problems of home-nursing a chronically ill patient are aggravated by the dementia. You may feel you can not cope any longer because of exhaustion, the upheaval of family life, and most of all, the physical inability to move and help your relative. You need to talk to your physician, who will then make arrangements for the patient to be hospitalized. Your physician can also put you in contact with an Alzheimer's support group, which exists in most major urban areas in the United States.

Nursing the sick. The aim of this entry is to explain how to take care of a patient in a well-organized and nurturing way at home, with a minimum of disruption to family life.

Nursing skills take time to acquire. With the step-by-step illustrations of basic nursing techniques presented here, even an inexperienced person can soon learn essential routines. What may be lacking in professionalism, however, can be compensated for with will, thorough organization, and affection. The spirit in which the task is approached can make all the difference between drudgery and the satisfaction that comes from doing a worthwhile job.

The task of home nursing must often be combined with family and career commitments. Some families share the caring, however, which lightens the burden for everyone and can also make life more interesting for the patient. It also has the advantage of teaching compassion to the younger members of the family.

With planning, much climbing up and down stairs can be eliminated. Good organization means saving time and energy. For this reason here are some pointers on how to choose the room most suitable for use as a sick room.

A number of factors are taken into account. Is the position of the room convenient for the family? Is the room near the bathroom? Is it well-heated and ventilated? Is it the most practical room for the season of the year? But at the same time, of course, the patient should not be isolated from the rest of the family just because the room has all the other advantages.

Furnishing the room also requires careful thought. For example, the bed should be high enough so that it is convenient for the patient to get in and out of, yet not inconvenient for the family and visitors who have to bend over the patient. Other qualifications for various items of furniture are discussed, taking into account how they are to be used by patient, nurse, and visitors.

Safety is another important factor when planning living space for someone who is ill or physically disabled. An ordinary bathroom can present many potential hazards; instructions are given for making the bathroom both safe and easy for the patient to use.

Physicians agree that boosting the patient's morale is an important part of nursing. The bored patient has time to linger on unhappy thoughts, which may lead to depression or to excessive demands on the family. Some advice is given on how to keep the patient cheerfully occupied by encouraging an interest in family matters, personal appearance, and hobbies.

Just as the patient needs to be kept cheerful, so do those in attendance need to be refreshed from time to time by a change of surroundings. Relatives and friends should be called upon to substitute.

Many parents have experienced how exhausting it can be to nurse a child who is bedridden with some common complaint. There is always the comfort, however, of knowing that the illness will run a known course and that recovery is assured within a certain time. *See also* NURSING THE SICK CHILD.

The problems are much more complex with patients who are chronically ill. It can often be very discouraging to care for such a patient, often an elderly parent suffering from increasing immobility.

The seemingly never-ending chores of bedmaking, washing and feeding, offering the bedpan, administering medicines, turning the patient to prevent bedsores, and so many other necessary actions become less burdensome when carried out in as professional a way as possible. The illustrations in this section show how to accomplish these tasks skillfully. *See also* NURSING THE CHRONICALLY ILL.

One common problem in nursing the chronically ill is ensuring that enough nourishment is taken. Loss of appetite is usual during illness and the patient may have to be encouraged to eat. The basic requirements of a well-balanced diet, a suggested dietary timetable, and other special diets are discussed in the entry DIET, SPECIAL.

Making the patient as independent as possible of physical help should be a prime aim. Accordingly, ideas are included here for devising simple aids to walking or general mobility, with the emphasis on safety. Some useful gadgets are also mentioned to help the chronically-ill person cope with daily life.

The patient needing perhaps the most loving care is the one who is either mentally confused or retarded. The senility of old age and the more common and less severe forms of mental illness are discussed in the entry NURSING THE CHRONICALLY ILL. The problems arising in the care of a retarded child are discussed in the entry MENTALLY RETARDED, CARE OF.

There may come a time when the care of such a person is beyond the capabilities or endurance of the family. The family physician may then recommend hospitalization or special care in a place that can provide professional attention. The family should not regard this as defeat, but make every effort to continue to maintain links with the patient by frequent visiting.

Finally, for a discussion on the care of the dying and the death of a loved one, *see* DYING, CARE OF THE.

The Sickroom

The choice of any one room as a sick room requires some consideration. Many factors should be taken into account, and it may not be enough just to put the sick person in what is usually a bedroom. A room that best fills all the needs should become the sickroom.

The room should, of course, be pleasant for the sick person, but should also be in a position of maximum convenience for the rest of the family. In a house of two or more stories, the ground floor is usually by far the most practical choice for a sickroom, especially if there is a downstairs bathroom. It may also be preferable for the patient, because no stairs intervene between him or her and the center of family life. Not having to go up and down stairs is convenient for the family when carrying trays and other articles to and from the patient.

On the other hand, if the only bathroom is upstairs, the most practical situation for the sickroom may also be upstairs, depending on the individual patient. Another consideration is that a room upstairs may provide more peaceful, less stressful, and more therapeutic surroundings. It is also generally easier to arrange for a more pleasing view through a window from an upstairs room.

Ventilation of the sickroom is of great importance. Sick people need fresh air. A small window, or part of a large one, should be kept open at most times, as long as the patient is not in a draft. In summer, the room should be kept comfortably cool. In winter, the room temperature should be maintained at a constant warmth for a sedentary individual.

An electric humidifier or small bowl of cold water placed in front of a heating duct helps to keep the humidity at a healthful level.

The sickroom should be pleasant and homey to the patient. There should be favorite pictures, furniture, and other articles. Some form of entertainment should be provided, such as radio or television, which can be switched on and off from the bed.

In cases where the patient has difficulty in moving, aids such as rails and flat surfaces are extremely useful in the sick room. The room in which they are most needed, however, is the bathroom.

The sickroom should contain not only the means for maintaining the patient's physical comfort, but also enough aids and items to keep the patient cheerful and occupied.

The room should be well lit. It should be possible for at least one lamp in the room to be dimmed, or shaded, from the patient at night.

Because a bedridden patient needs to have many things within reach at all times, it is generally more practical to place a bedside table or a locker on each side of the bed. These can hold the usual bedside lamp, radio, tray with pitcher and glass, bowl of fruit or candy, clock, and a favorite photograph or picture.

A bedside lamp is of great importance, since a patient may want to spend time reading. A lamp that is easily adjusted to the desired height and direction is the most suitable. The lamp should be within easy reach of the patient and should be heavy enough at its base so as not to be easily toppled.

It is also advisable to have an alarm bell, an intercom system, or some other audible means of summoning help in emergencies.

There should be an adequate supply of bed linens, not just blankets for warmth, but enough sheets and pillowcases, in case there is an accident in bed, resulting from incontinence or an upset breakfast tray. Where incontinence is to be expected, drawsheets and at least one waterproof sheet are also necessary (see "Bedmaking," page 621). Diapers or disposable undergarments may also be helpful.

Much of the equipment now used in sickrooms is disposable. But other items, made of glass, metal, or ceramics, should be thoroughly washed after use. And if the patient has an infectious illness, such equipment should be washed, placed in water that is brought to boil, and boiled for at least five minutes.

The patient's attitude toward the surroundings can affect his or her well-being. If possible, there should be something either in the room or visible through a window that is of great interest to the patient. The patient's interest should also be encouraged in the rest of the family and its daily life. An occasional change of scenery within the room, such as new flowers or drapes, is recommended.

Bedmaking

The most important piece of furniture in the sickroom is, of course, the bed. It is essential that the bed is firm to lie on. A sagging bed provides poor support for the back and tires the patient. To make a sagging bed firm, simply place a board between the bedsprings and the mattress. Make sure, too, that the mattress is firm and well-sprung. Patients who suffer from back problems will certainly need a firm bed. A physician can give advice about this.

Choose bed linen with care. Polyester sheets are easy to launder, but are not as absorbent as sheets made from cotton or linen. Cotton flannel sheets have a slightly raised nap and so they are warmer than sheets made from other materials. It is advisable to always have an adequate supply of bed linen available. Woolen blankets are warm, but the patient may find them to be too heavy. Cellular blankets of cotton or Dacron are lighter than woolen ones and are also easier to wash. The patient may require three or four blankets on the bed. Patients who suffer from painful joints or poor circulation may prefer the lightness of a comforter to the weight of blankets. It is advisable to have no fewer than four pillows available for a sickbed. Additional pillows may be needed to support the patient and relieve fatigue at various points, such as the elbows and arms or under the knees.

To make up the bed, the mattress should first be protected with a waterproof sheeting, such as polyethylene. Place a blanket over this to provide a soft and warm surface for the patient. Place the sheets on the bed and keep the right (nap) side of each sheet innermost. (A waterproof sheet and a drawsheet placed over the bottom sheet saves unnecessary changing of linen if the patient is likely to soil the bed frequently.) Place the blankets on the bed and cover them with an attractive, cheerful looking bed spread. When the bed has been made up, give the bed linen a slight upward tug over the area of the patient's feet so as to allow plenty of freedom of movement. Remember that elderly patients feel the cold easily, and may prefer to keep a shawl or light blanket between them and the sheets.

When sitting up in bed, the patient will need a minimum of four pillows for support. See accompanying illustrations.

Sitting up in bed

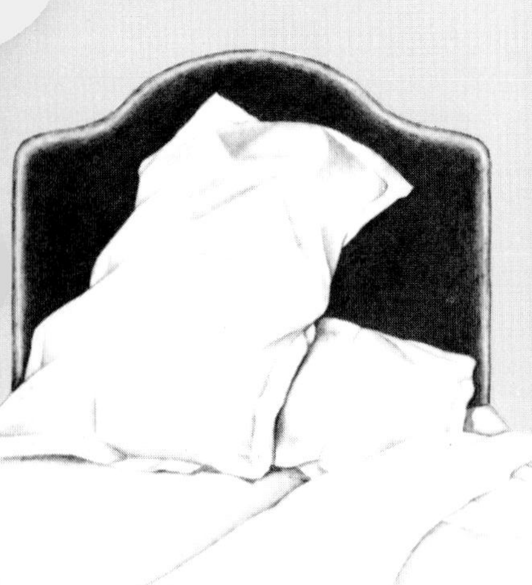

The armchair position provides the most comfortable and practical arrangement of pillows for those who like to sit upright in bed. A minimum of four pillows will be needed. Place a fairly solid pillow horizontally at the head of the bed. Position another pillow vertically on top of this and slanted to one side. Prop a third pillow vertically and angled from the other side.

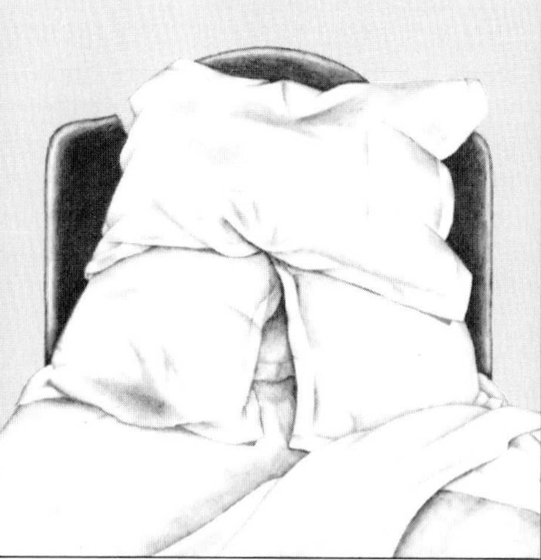

On top of this triangular shape place the fourth soft pillow for the head. Adjust extra pillows for taller patients. The two vertical pillows support the small of the back and make an especially comfortable arrangement for the patient who has trouble breathing; it helps to keep the shoulders back and the lungs unconstricted.

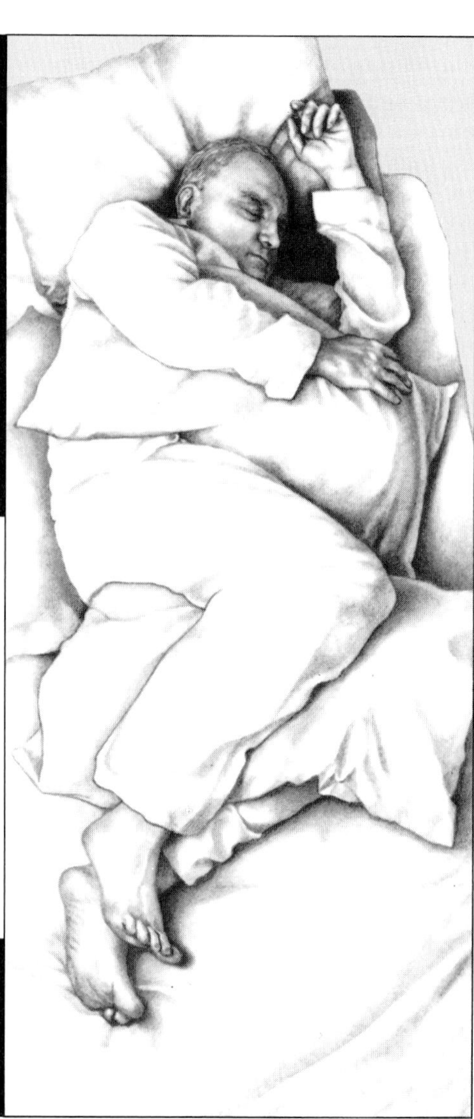

A patient who is unable to sit up in bed may like to lie on one side with just two pillows to support the head. Place a third pillow in the small of the patient's back to provide support and to prevent the patient from rolling backward. Now place another pillow between the patient's legs for general comfort as well as to prevent any soreness. Place another pillow under the patient's free arm. This is a good position for any patient unable to lie on the back or one who is paralyzed.

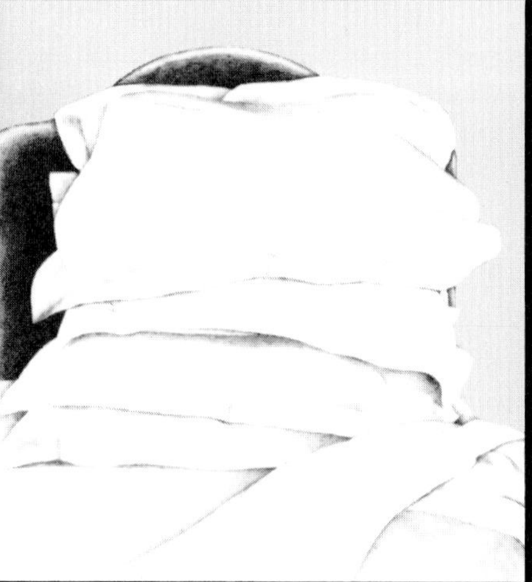

Alternatively, the pillows can be arranged in an upright position. Stack four or more pillows, depending on the patient's height, on top of each other. As many as six or seven may have to be used for total comfort. The firmest pillow is placed at the bottom of the pile, and the softest one is placed at the top to cushion the head of the patient.

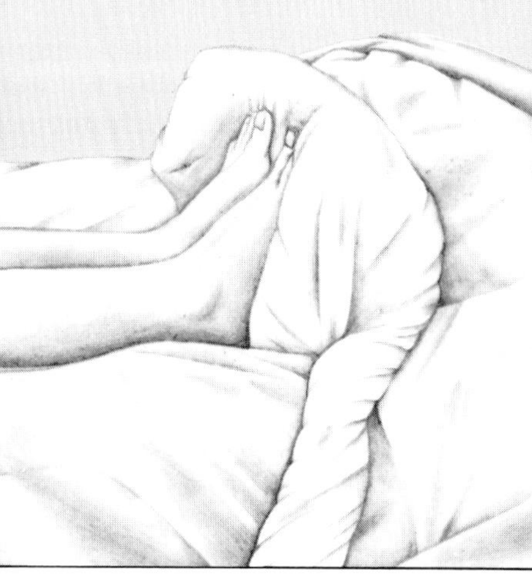

Frail or elderly people have a tendency to slip down in the bed. A footrest may help prevent this. Form one by rolling a firm pillow in a sheet, twisting the ends firmly around it. Place the pillow at the patient's feet, and tuck in the ends of the sheet under the mattress. Alternatively, raise the foot of the bed a few inches onto a pile of books or telephone directories.

Bedmaking

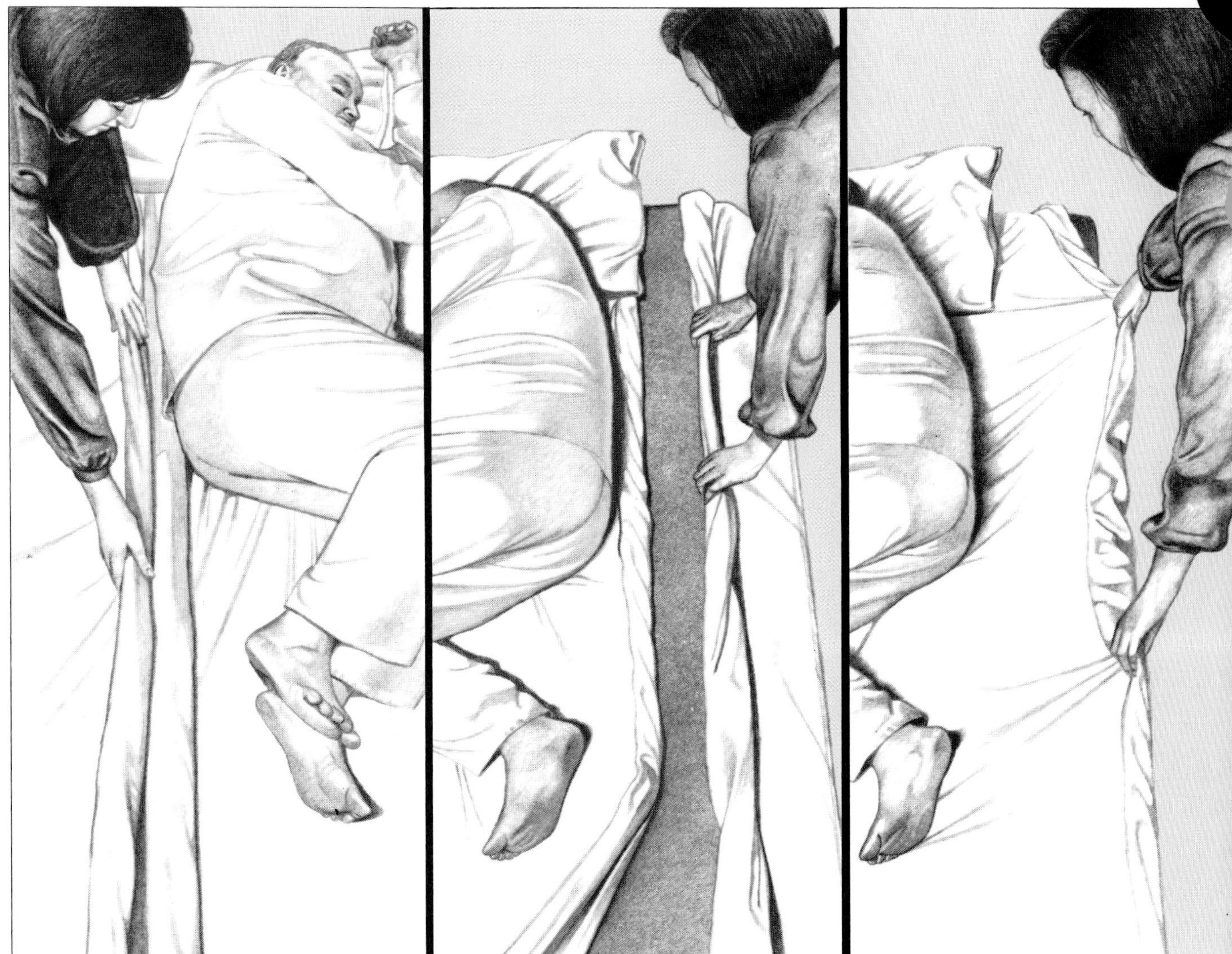

Roll a clean sheet lengthwise in half. Roll the patient to the edge of the bed; roll the dirty sheet up to the patient; lay the clean sheet next to it, unroll and tuck in.

Move the patient's pillow before rolling the patient the other way over both sheets onto the clean half. Remove the dirty one completely.

Unroll the clean sheet to the other side of the bed, and draw taut. Tuck it in on all sides. If necessary change other bedlinen, and reposition the pillows.

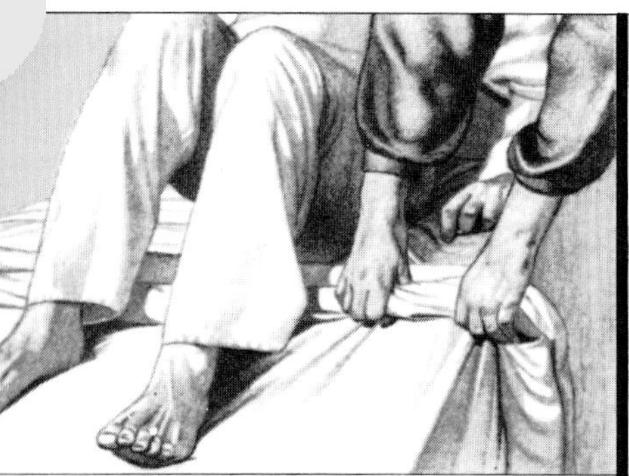

Sometimes one has to change the bed from bottom to top by placing both rolls of sheeting under the patient's knees.

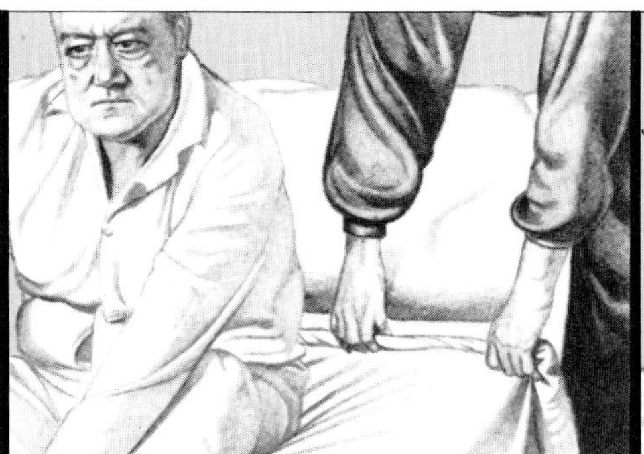

Help the patient move down in the bed, and roll both sheets higher up the bed.

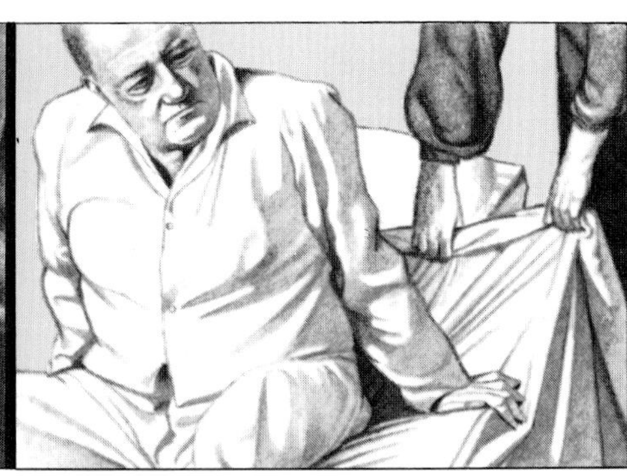

Remove the dirty sheet, and draw the clean one taut. This method is good with heart patients.

Pressure Points

One of the most important aspects of nursing the patient at home is, without doubt, the prevention of bedsores. This is even more essential when caring for a patient confined to bed for any length of time. Frequent repositioning is the most important and effective way to prevent bedsores.

The first warning sign that the skin is under stress is a slight local reddening of the skin. At this stage, good nursing care can prevent a bedsore from developing. The importance of changing the position of the patient every two hours can not be emphasized enough. If this procedure is not carried out, the skin is more likely to break, leaving the underlying flesh exposed and open to infection. A physician or qualified nurse should be consulted immediately, so that appropriate treatment can be given without delay.

Protective heel-pads or elbow-pads may be useful. To make one, take a piece of foam rubber about 1 inch (2.5 cm) thick and cut out 2 strips, each 10 inches by 4 inches (25 by 10cm), long enough to reach around the patient's ankle or heel. Attach Velcro or tape to the ends to act as a fastening. Other methods include the use of sheepskins and foam rubber rings (*see* "Comfort in Bed," page 624).

When turning a patient, apply gentle massage to the area which has been subjected to pressure. Careful rubbing with the palm of the hand helps to stimulate the blood supply to the skin.

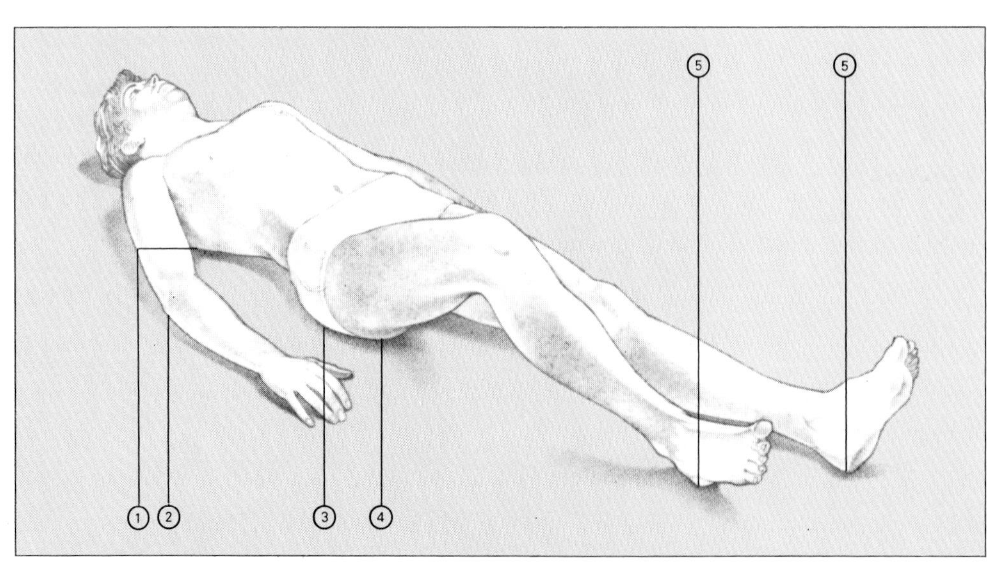

Pressure sores form in immobile patients, especially older people, because the weight of the body causes pressure on the skin, depriving it of normal blood circulation. The parts of the body most susceptible to pressure sores are (1) the shoulder blades at the top of the back; (2) the elbows; (3) the sacrum, lower in the back; (4) the buttocks; and (5) the heels.

Prevention of bedsores

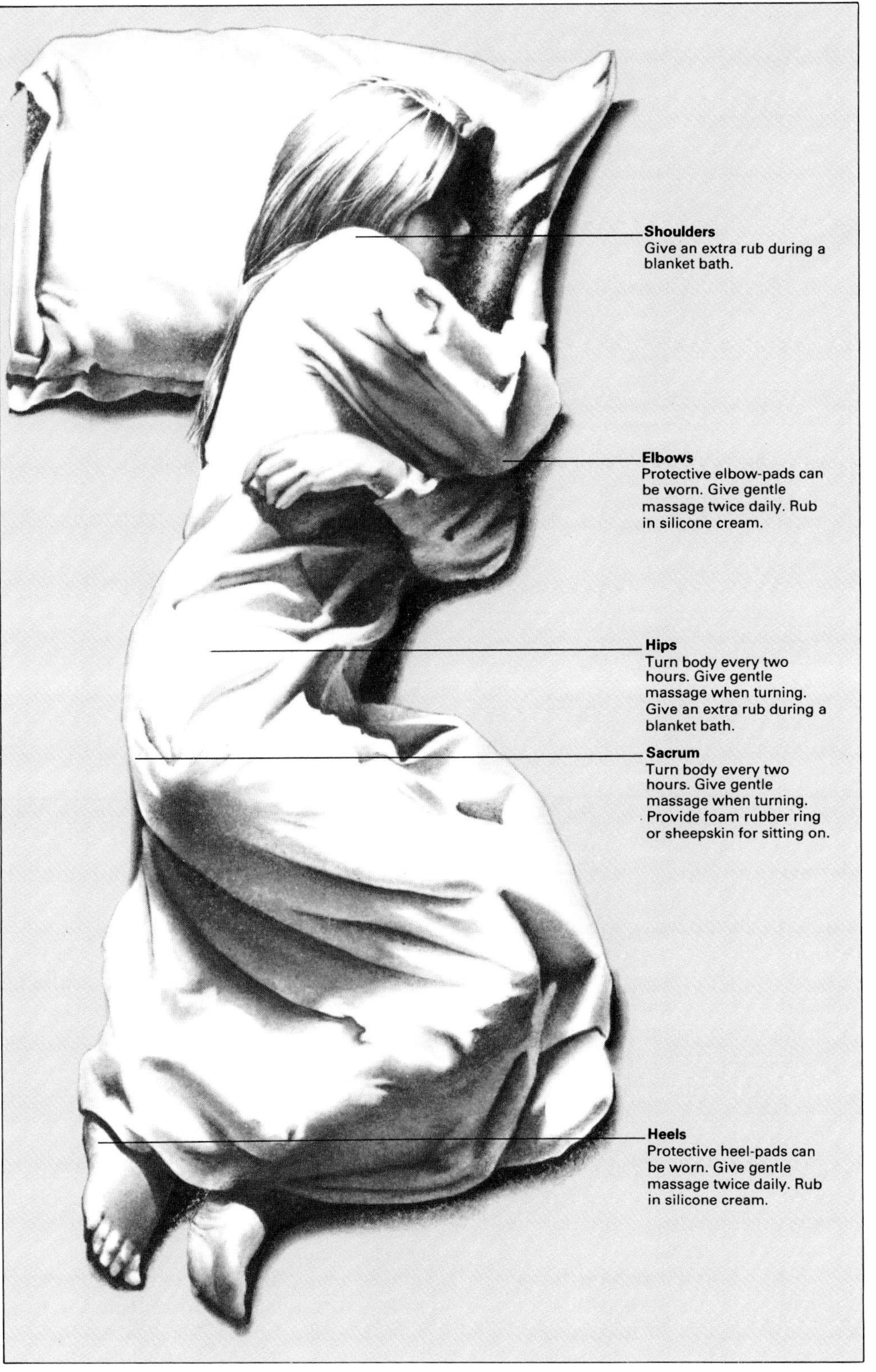
Shoulders
Give an extra rub during a blanket bath.
Elbows
Protective elbow-pads can be worn. Give gentle massage twice daily. Rub in silicone cream.
Hips
Turn body every two hours. Give gentle massage when turning. Give an extra rub during a blanket bath.
Sacrum
Turn body every two hours. Give gentle massage when turning. Provide foam rubber ring or sheepskin for sitting on.
Heels
Protective heel-pads can be worn. Give gentle massage twice daily. Rub in silicone cream.

Comfort in bed

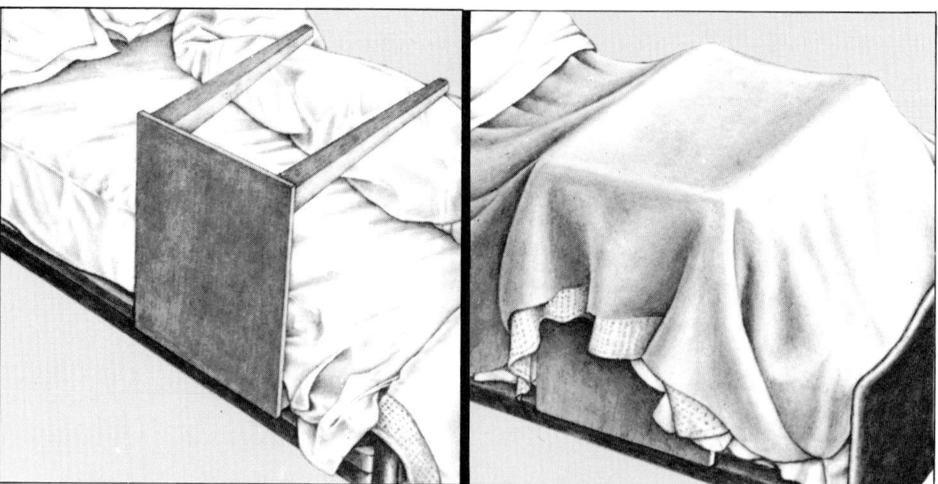

A patient sometimes needs the weight of the bedlinen to be removed from the feet or legs. This is important with patients with varicose ulcers. A frame can be made by using a stiff cardboard carton or a small wooden table. Turn either on its side and slip a side of the carton or the legs of the table under the mattress. The exposed legs of the table will bear the weight of the sheets.

Lift the bedlinen up and over the top of the improvised frame. If possible, tuck it in. The most usual position for the frame is over the feet, but, if the patient has pain in the legs, position the frame accordingly. This procedure removes the bedlinen from contact with the patient's legs. Elderly patients, who feel the cold easily, may like the extra warmth and comfort of a light blanket over the feet.

Sprinkle on some talcum powder at the same time. This will be a pleasant freshener for the patient, as well as lessening the friction of your hands against the skin. Alternatively, you can use any one of a number of lotions. A simple and inexpensive lotion can be easily made using equal parts of rubbing alcohol and glycerin (glycerol).

Apply a little lotion to the palm of the hand. Massage should be firm but gentle, so as to move the top layers of tissue over those underneath. This helps to get the blood moving again. Too heavy and grinding a pressure will simply break the skin.

Every day, when the patient has a sponge bath, pay particular attention to the pressure areas. Rub these areas twice a day to prevent any soreness from appearing.

When coping with an incontinent patient, it is important that you wash all urine off the skin. Any remaining urine may cause irritation, which can speed up the formation of bedsores and encourage infection. A barrier cream helps to give adequate protection.

A little silicone cream (not as greasy as petroleum jelly) is particularly good for dealing with drier areas of skin, such as the elbows or heels.

Comfort in Bed

There are a number of devices available on the market that have been designed specifically with the comfort of the bedridden patient in mind.

Bedsores are one of the main causes of discomfort for anyone who has to spend a great length of time confined to bed (*see* "Pressure points," page 622). The discomfort is likely to be increased if the patient is either extremely overweight or underweight. A sheepskin placed beneath the patient's body can help enormously in preventing the formation of bedsores. Placed with the fleecy side up, a sheepskin provides a soft springy surface for the patient to lie on. The woolliness of a sheepskin's fiber allows for circulation of air, which evaporates any excess moisture. Another virtue of a sheepskin is that it can absorb an appreciable amount of water before it feels damp. Natural sheepskins are far better than imitation ones, but imitation sheepskins are eas-

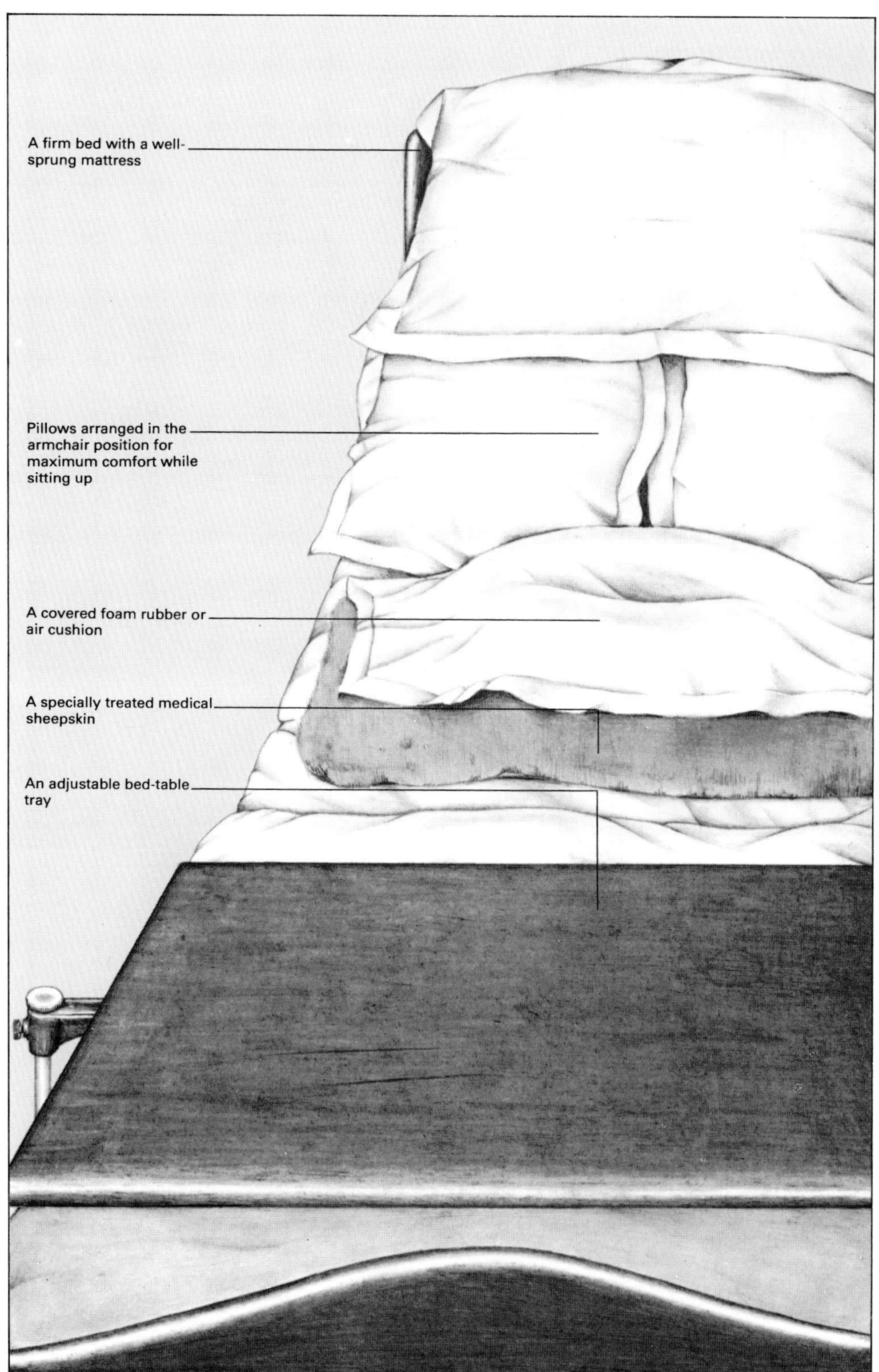

Comfort in bed

Certain items can greatly increase the comfort of a bedridden patient. The bed itself should have a firm, well-sprung mattress. A number of pillows of varying softness are used to give support in the armchair position, as well as support for the neck and head.

A circular foam rubber or air cushion relieves discomfort when sitting upright. A sheepskin pad provides a soft, springy surface for the patient to lie on; natural ones absorb moisture easily as well. A free-standing bed table should be adjustable, both as regards height and angle.

Turning a patient

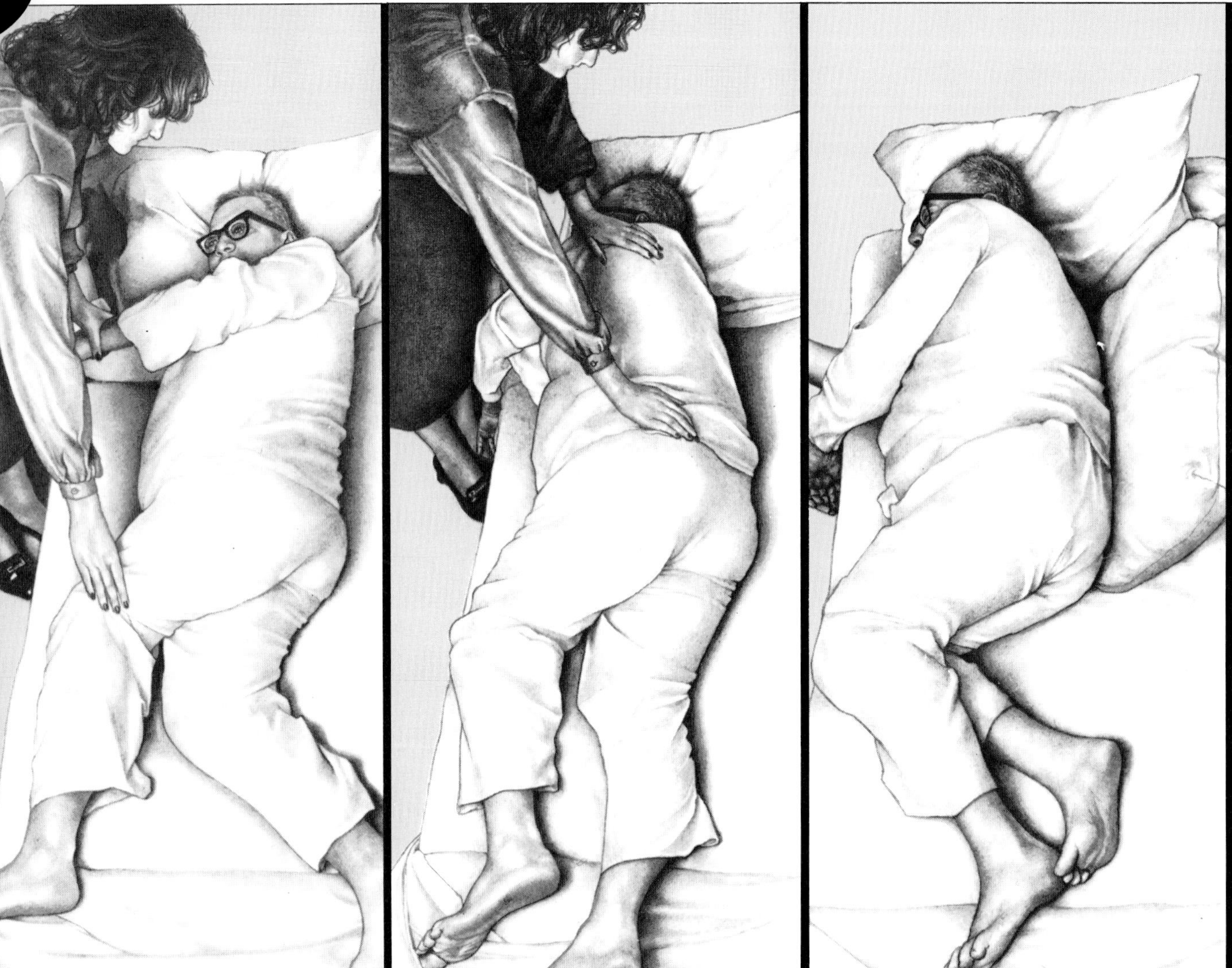

1 A patient who is confined to bed should change position every two hours to avoid the risk of developing bedsores. Gain the patient's cooperation by explaining how you plan to turn him or her. If you are alone, turn the patient in the following manner. Remove all the top bedding and all pillows except one. To turn a patient to the right side, gently ease the patient's head, shoulders and hips to the left side of the bed by supporting the body with your hands and forearms. Turn the patient's head to his or her right. Bring the patient's left arm across to meet the right arm, and the left leg across the right one.

2 Remain on the same side of the bed. Place your left hand on the patient's left shoulder blade, and the other hand just above his or her buttocks. Gently pull the patient up and over onto the side of the body. Use pillows to secure the patient's position. Move the pillow across the bed to support the patient's head. Any movements the patient is able to make alone should be encouraged, since praise will help his or her morale enormously, and this in itself speeds up the recovery period. Use this as an opportunity to talk with and to the patient, and to listen to any concerns or queries he or she may have.

3 The patient is now lying on his or her right side. Place a pillow in the small of the back to prevent the body from rolling backward again. A patient with sufficient strength can help at this point by holding onto the side of the bed while you move around to the other side. Some elderly people feel vulnerable and are afraid of falling off the bed if left unprotected. Reassure the patient before moving; you can also place some piece of furniture next to the bed to act as a barrier. Obviously, if there are two of you working together, you can stand one on either side of the bed; additionally, two people can complete the process much more quickly and easily than one.

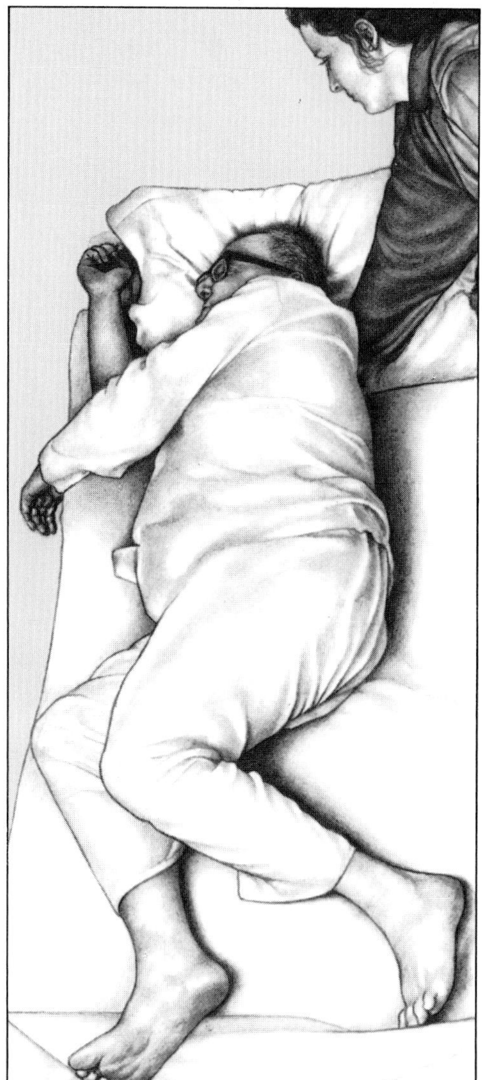

4 Standing at the other side of the bed, you should gently push the top of the patient's left shoulder and the left hip towards the other side of the bed. At the same time, gently pull the right shoulder towards you, lifting slightly to prevent friction. The patient's upper leg should be bent slightly and extended to a comfortable position. The lower leg should be bent more forward and upward so as to prevent the trunk from rolling over. Reposition the head pillow so as to make the patient as comfortable as possible.

To turn the patient from the back to the left, follow the above directions, substituting left for right.

Always check the room's temperature before starting to turn the patient, so that he or she does not catch cold.

ier to wash and quicker to dry. Whichever type you decide on, buy two. The patient will then always have one to lie on.

Some patients may prefer to use either an air mattress or a waterbed. One air mattress that is especially effective in preventing bedsores is the ripple bed, which has an electrical device that constantly changes the pressure of air in the mattress. The changes in air pressure within the bands of the mattress cause a gentle rippling beneath the patient's body and a continual shifting of the patient's weight.

Patients who are able to sit up in bed may prefer to sit on a foam rubber ring or a ring-shaped air cushion, either of which removes pressure from the buttocks. To make your own foam rubber ring, use a piece of foam rubber about 3 to 4 inches (7 to 10cm) thick, and cut a hole out of it to suit the size of the patient. Then cover it with a pillowcase. An air cushion can be inflated or deflated in size according to individual preference, but is seldom as comfortable as a foam rubber ring.

A free-standing adjustable bed table can be of great benefit to patients who are able to sit up in bed. The bed table is designed so that its foot can be slipped under the side of the bed and the table's top placed directly in front of the patient. The table's top can be raised or lowered and its angle altered from the horizontal to the perpendicular, if required. Patients can use the table not only at mealtimes, but also for doing jigsaw puzzles, for reading books, or for drawing or writing. All of these activities can make a long-term confinement to bed more tolerable.

Lifting a Patient

A patient should always be encouraged to do whatever possible alone and unaided by anyone else. This is good for the patient's morale and gives the bedridden patient a welcome sense of independence.

Using the pull strap as described in the accompanying illustration, the patient can sit up without your help. This leaves your two hands free for washing the patient's back or brushing the hair. The pull strap also enables a patient to move more freely within the bed than might otherwise be possible. If the pa-

Lifting the patient

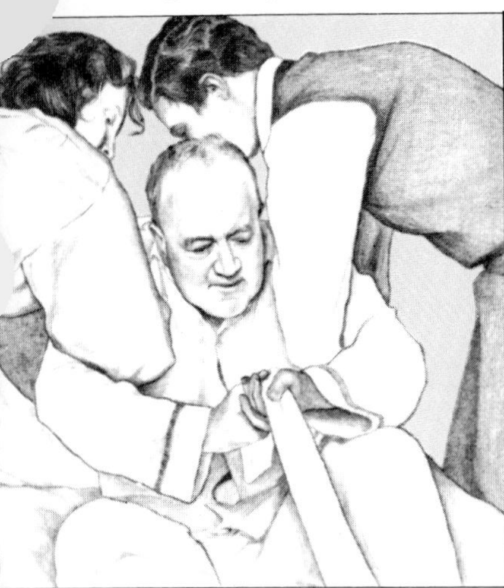

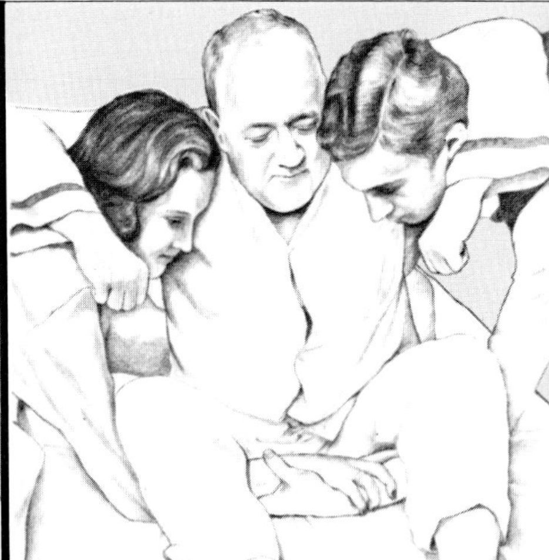

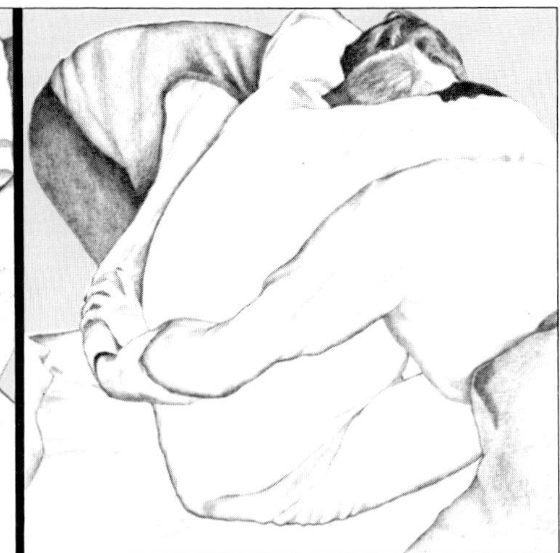

1 If the patient cannot lift himself, two people are needed. Stand on each side of the patient, facing the head of the bed. Both should slip a hand under the patient's arm, using the other hand to support the back. Help the patient into a sitting position by both lifting simultaneously. If possible, have the patient help by pulling on a pull strap.

2 You can now move the patient forward or backward. You should each stand on either side of the patient, facing each other. Bend your knees in preparation for lifting the patient. Now, each of you should put the arm that is nearer to the foot of the bed under the patient's thighs; grasp hold of your colleague's elbow so that your forearms are locked together.

3 Put the other arm as low down the patient's back towards the buttocks as it will go. The lower the arm is, the easier it is to lift the patient. Lock forearms with the person who is helping you by gripping each other's elbows. Moving together, lift the patient and move in the desired direction. The patient can help by pushing down with his or her feet.

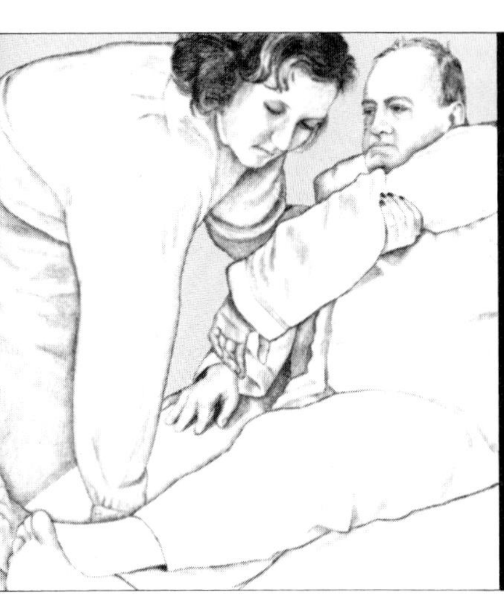

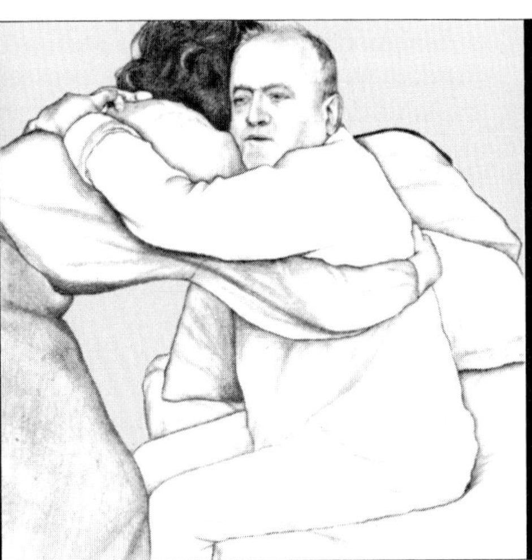

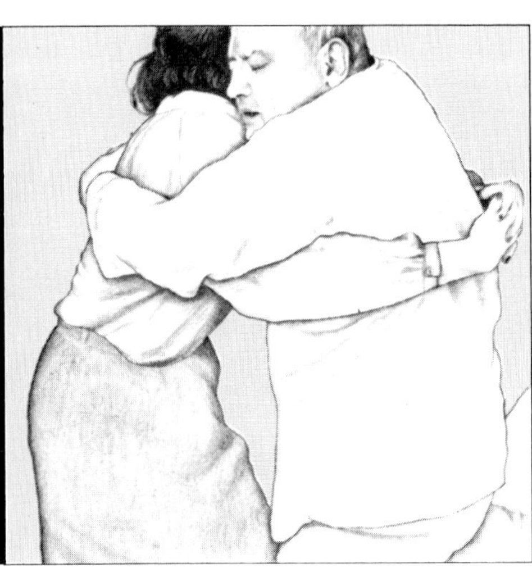

4 A patient may wish to use the toilet, but may need help getting out of bed. One person can easily provide that help. Use one hand to lift the patient's legs round the edge of the bed to bring the patient into the sitting position. Pass your other hand and arm around the patient's upper arm to provide support for him or her.

5 Bend your knees and place them securely on each side of the patient's knees. Your knees should always be bent when doing any sort of lifting to prevent backstrain. Ask the patient to clasp hands around your neck or around the top of your back. Meanwhile, nestle your head into the patient's shoulder and clasp your hands around the patient's back, holding the patient tightly to you.

6 With a gentle rocking motion, backward and forward, count one, two, three. On the count of four, come up, with each of you holding on to the other, and move on to the commode. Keep your knees bent while doing this so as to take the weight of the patient's body more easily. To get the patient back into bed again, repeat the process in reverse order, keeping your knees bent when you lift the patient.

Sponge bath

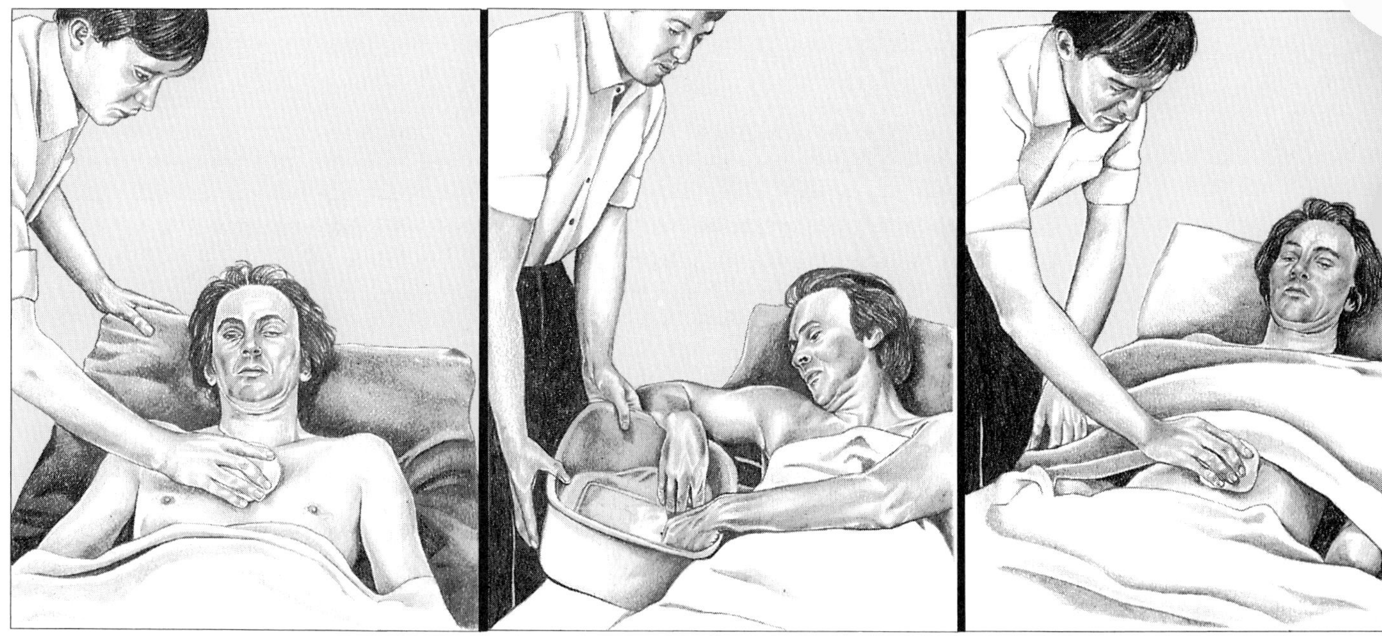

1 Start with the face, neck, and ears. The patient may be well enough to do this unaided. Pat the skin dry with a soft towel.

2 Wash and dry the chest and arms. Let the patient dip the hands in the bowl of water to rinse off any soap.

3 Keep the chest and lower parts of the body covered while you wash the patient's abdomen. Do not forget the navel.

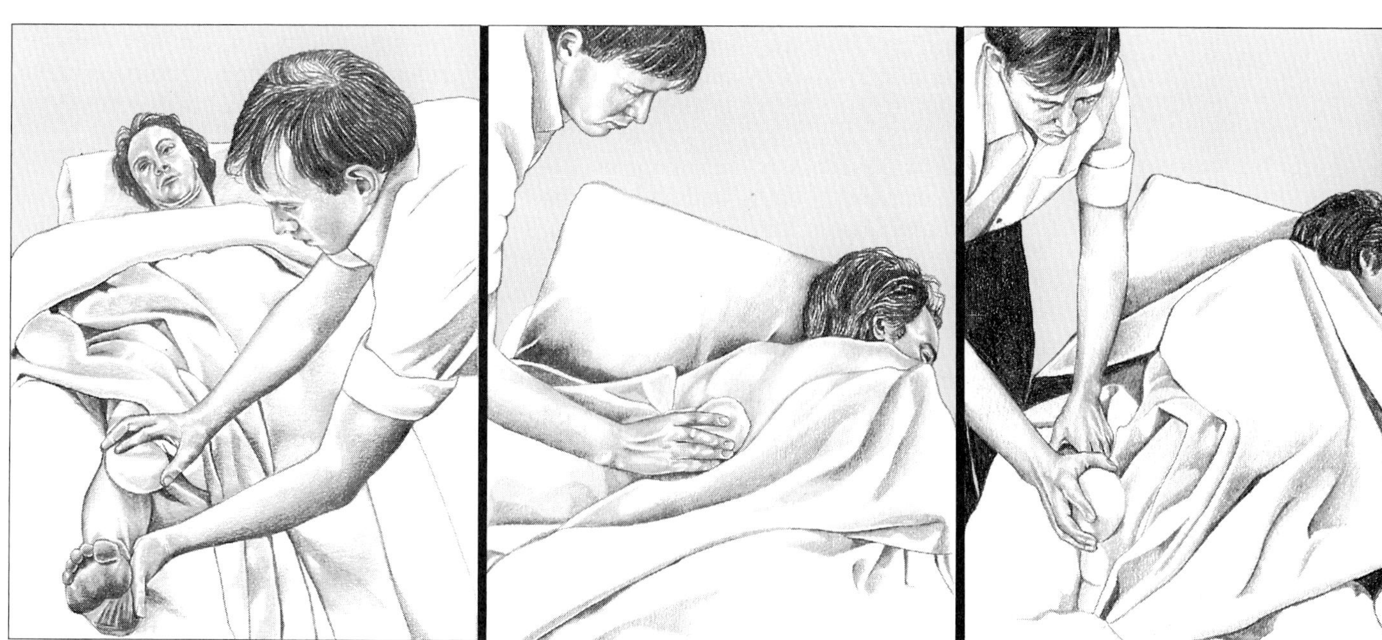

4 Wash the legs, one at a time, paying particular attention to the area between the toes. Cut the toenails if they need it.

5 Turn the patient onto one side, then the other, to do the upper half of the back. Alternatively, get the patient to sit up.

6 Lastly, wash the lower part of the back. Most patients prefer to wash their genitals themselves.

tient has a physical disability, however, a pull strap is unlikely to be of use. Indeed, it may require two people to lift a helpless patient up or down in the bed.

One person, working alone, can easily help a patient out of bed. When not in bed, the patient should wear night clothes, a robe, socks, and slippers. You should prepare an armchair for the patient by placing a blanket across it and a pillow for the patient's head. Wrap a blanket around the patient's body, and provide a footstool to keep the feet off the floor and away from drafts. If you should decide to use a heater in the room, make sure that the patient is not positioned too close to it. Ensure that everything the patient might need is within reach. If it is the patient's first time out of bed, do not leave the patient up for too long.

Sponge Bath

A patient who is lying in bed all day needs to wash just as often as an active, healthy person. For a bedridden patient, a sponge bath can be extremely refreshing. Ideally, a sponge bath should be given every day. But if this is not possible, the patient should be bathed at least every other day.

Remember that the patient may feel that he or she is putting you to a great deal of unnecessary trouble or may feel embarrassed at being bathed by someone else. Your calm and efficient manner can do much to reassure the patient that this is not so, and the patient may come to enjoy the routine.

Equipment needed includes a pitcher of hot water; a fairly large bowl; a bucket; soap; two washcloths, one for the face and one for the body; talcum powder; a small, soft towel for the face; and plenty of larger towels, for drying the patient and for placing under each part of the body as it is being washed.

Shut all the windows and make sure that the room is warm. It may be better if the patient is first accompanied to the toilet or is given a bedpan, to avoid interrupting the sponge bath.

Undress the patient and remove the top bed linens. Place an old towel or blanket on the bed underneath the patient and a blanket on top to keep the patient warm. If the patient is comfortable lying flat, arrange two pillows for the head. If not, wash the patient in the sitting position.

Expose only one part of the patient's body at a time, as it is being washed. Change the washing water halfway through the routine, after washing the legs and before starting on the back.

A sponge bath is a good opportunity to massage any potentially sore areas of the body, such as the shoulder blades, base of the spine, and hips. While soaping, give these areas a few extra gentle rubs. If the patient's elbows and heels are dry, rub them with a nongreasy cream.

Always dry the patient's body carefully before putting the night clothes back on. Pay particular attention to any crevices or cracks, because these can get sore if left moist. For a female patient, do not forget the areas underneath the breasts and, in fat people, the groin area at the top of the legs. When the patient is completely dry, dust on some talcum powder.

Brush the patient's teeth, and brush and comb the hair. Perhaps the patient would like to use a deodorant, and a woman might want to apply lipstick or a dab of perfume. All these will contribute toward the patient's general sense of well-being. Finally, remake the bed, with clean sheets if necessary.

Helping a Patient Into the Bathtub

The first bath after a long illness can greatly boost a patient's morale. The fact that it is being attempted at all is a sure sign that the patient is recovering.

Prepare the bathroom beforehand. Close the windows to keep out any drafts and fill the bathtub halfway with warm water. The temperature should not be hotter than normal body temperature 98.6°F (37°C). Test the temperature of the water with your elbow; the water should feel comfortably warm.

Equipment needed includes soap, two washcloths (one for the face and one for the body), a face towel, and two body towels.

If the patient has difficulty getting into the bathtub, place an upright chair of roughly the same height alongside the bathtub. Drape one towel over the back of the chair and one on the seat.

Patients who are unable to lie down may miss the pleasant sensation of warm water splashing around the shoulders. Do this for them by splash-

Helping a patient into the bathtub

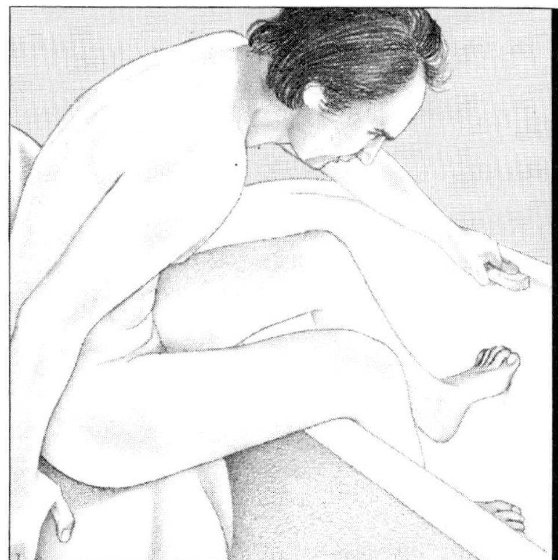

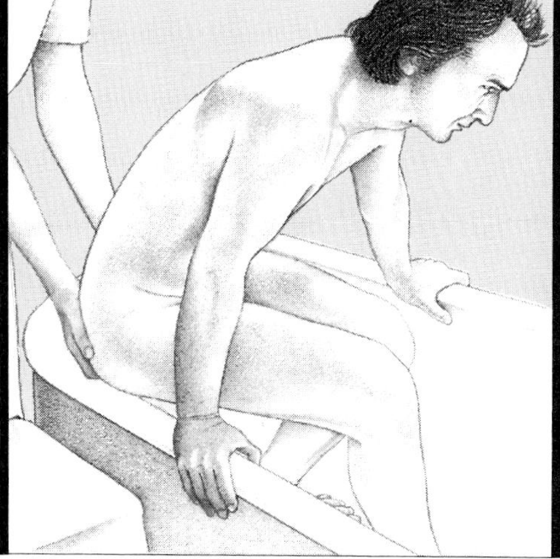

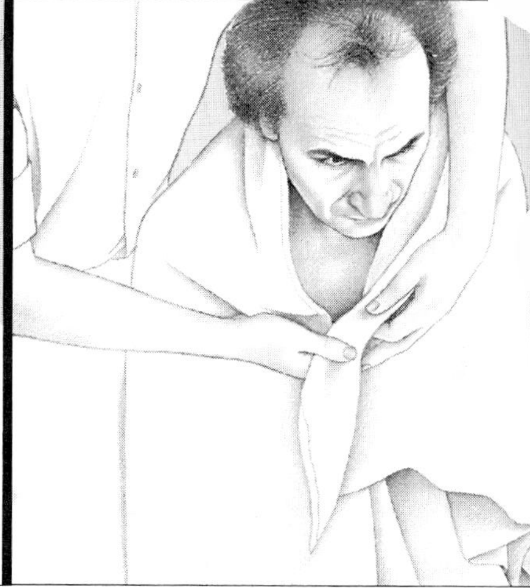

1 Help the patient to get into the bathtub by lifting the legs together up and over the side. The patient should be well enough to be able to pull himself or herself forward on the bathrail, placing the free hand on the edge of the tub for support. A nonslip mat in the bottom of the tub may give confidence to a person who is afraid of falling.

2 Some patients, especially the elderly, may have difficulty in lowering themselves into a sitting position. They can be helped by placing both hands on the buttocks. A bath seat in the bottom of the tub is also a great aid. You can improvise by using a low stool or a wooden block.

3 Help the patient out of the tub by guiding him or her onto the chair beside the tub, which should already have towels draped over it. Wrap the towel from the back of the chair around the patient's body and shoulders, leaving the other one for sitting on. It is pleasant for the patient if the towels have been warmed beforehand.

Hairwashing in bed

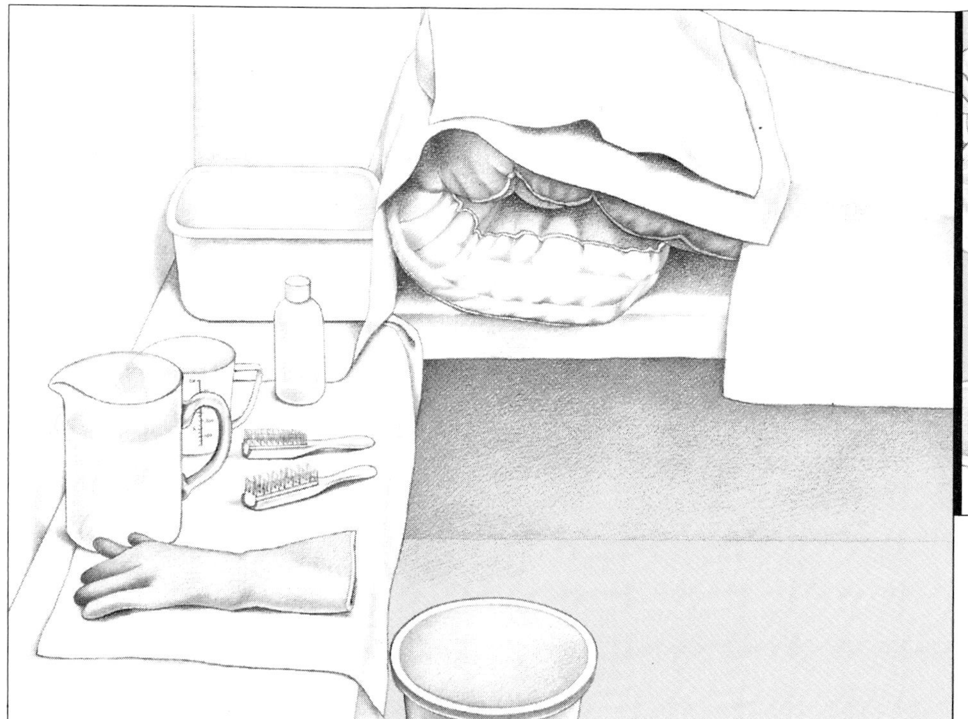

Sit the patient upright, and roll the top of the mattress under on itself. Protect the bedding with plastic sheeting. Put a plastic cape and a towel around the patient's shoulders, and have him or her lie down so the head is above the washbowl.

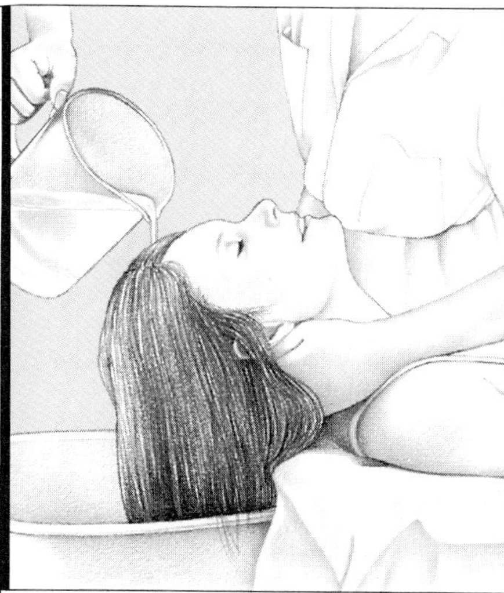

Support the patient's neck with one hand, and wash the patient's hair with the other. Use water from the small pitcher to wet the hair. Pour on the shampoo and rub it in. Comb the shampoo gently into the hair. Rinse and repeat. After the final rinse, dry the hair with a warm towel. Finish off using an electric hairdrier.

ing water on the shoulders using cupped hands.

Make sure the patient is dried thoroughly before accompanying him or her to the bedroom. Keep the patient covered and warm at all times.

Hairwashing in Bed

Care of a bedridden patient's hair is important. The hair should be combed or brushed at least twice a day. If necessary, use a dry shampoo to combat grease. Washing the hair with water and liquid shampoo is not difficult and can be a good boost to the patient's morale.

Ensure that the top of the bed is near an electric socket into which the hairdryer can be plugged. Ask the patient to move toward the foot of the bed, giving help if needed. Sit the patient upright and roll the top of the mattress under itself. If this is not possible, use several firm pillows or rolled blankets.

Place one or two pillows on the end of the mattress, so that the top of the patient's back is well supported.

Put rubber sheeting over the springs of the bed to protect them, and cover the bed linens with plastic sheeting and a towel. Put a plastic cape and a towel around the patient's shoulders, and get the patient to lie back so that the head can hang down over a bowl placed underneath it.

Other equipment needed includes two pitchers, a large one containing a supply of warm water and a small one to work with; a bucket, in which to pour used water; shampoo; a brush and comb; towels; and a hairdryer. A female patient may also need rollers to set her hair.

Feeding in Bed

To prepare a patient for a meal, make sure the pillows are comfortable behind his or her back when the patient is in the sitting position. If there is a bed table tray, place it in front of the patient. Adjust it to the appropriate height and angle for the patient to eat comfortably.

A bedridden patient may have a poor appetite. Careful presentation of food can help to overcome this. Make use of attractive table linen and tableware. The simplest foods can be brightened up considerably with a sprig of parsley or a slice of lemon to add color and decoration. A bouquet of flowers, or

Feeding in bed

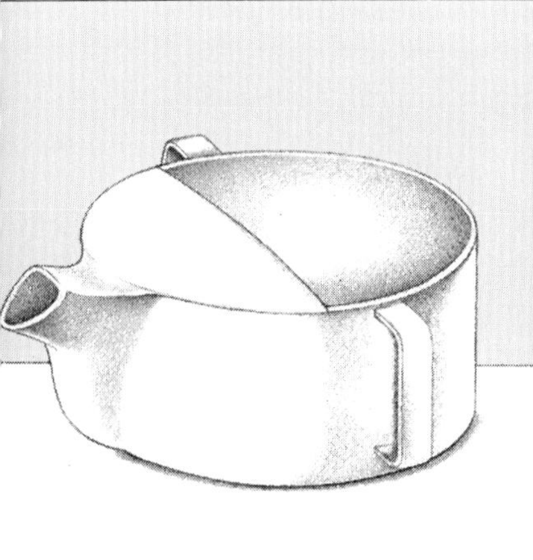

1 The feeding cup is a useful utensil for the patient who is unable to cope alone with feeding. It is easier to use than an ordinary cup because it is light and has a spout-like opening. This allows a greater control over the flow of liquid. The handles on each side of the cup allow the patient to hold the cup if able to do so. The handles also make it easier for you to pour.

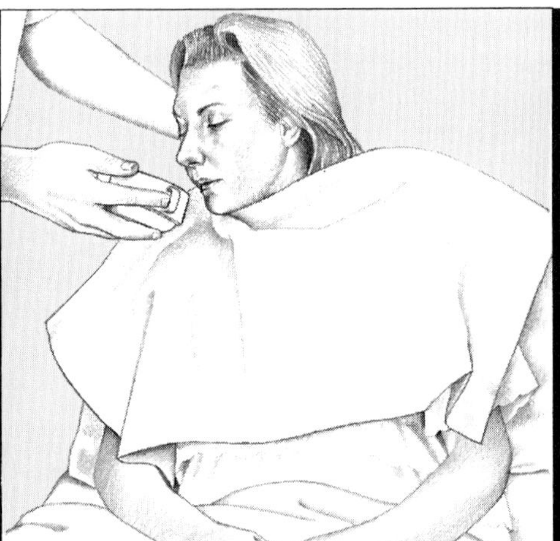

2 If possible, prop the patient up in a sitting position. Lay a napkin over the patient's night clothes in case of spillage. Check the temperature of the liquid. It should be neither too hot nor too tepid. Support the patient's neck with one hand, tilt the cup with your other hand, and gently pour into the patient's mouth. The cup is useful in giving the patient nutritious soups, as well as tea and coffee.

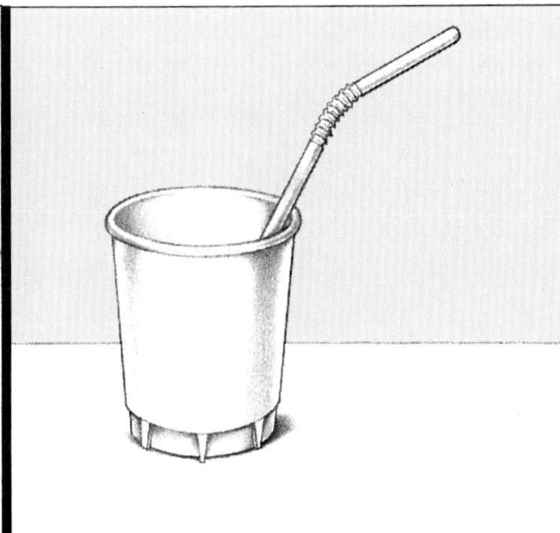

3 Often, a feeding cup is not available just when you need it most. One practical alternative is to let the patient drink through a flexible straw. Ordinary drinking straws are not satisfactory unless the patient can incline the head towards the straw.

Flexible straws can be purchased at most drugstores and are best used with a slim cup or flask to prevent the straw from slipping out.

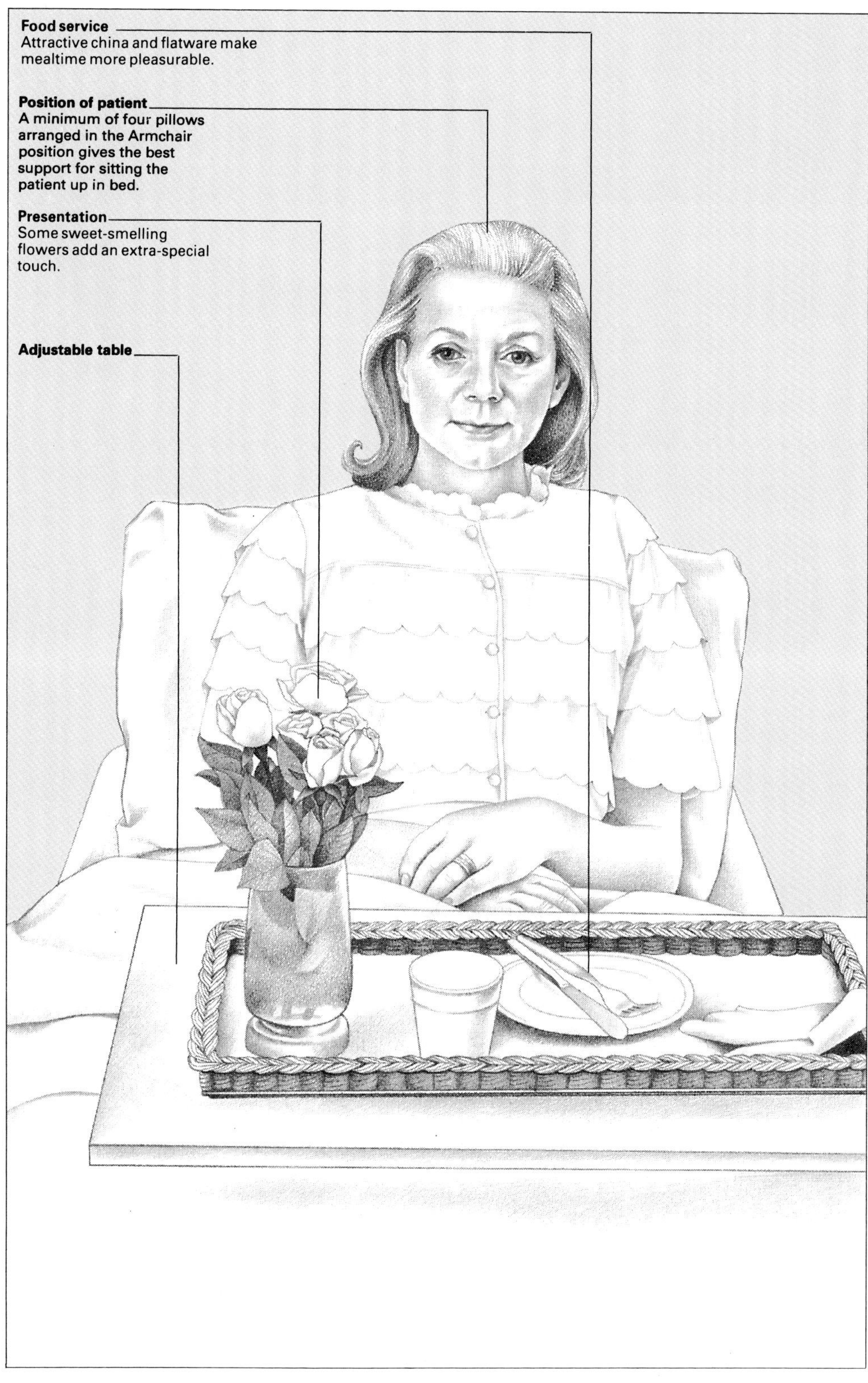
Food service
Attractive china and flatware make mealtime more pleasurable.
Position of patient
A minimum of four pillows arranged in the Armchair position gives the best support for sitting the patient up in bed.
Presentation
Some sweet-smelling flowers add an extra-special touch.
Adjustable table

Taking temperature and pulse

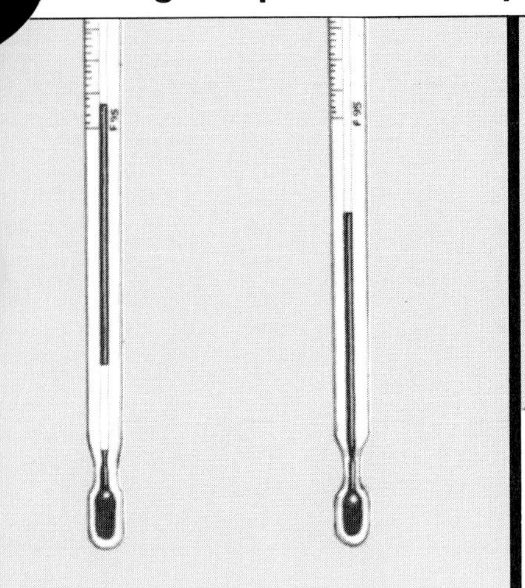

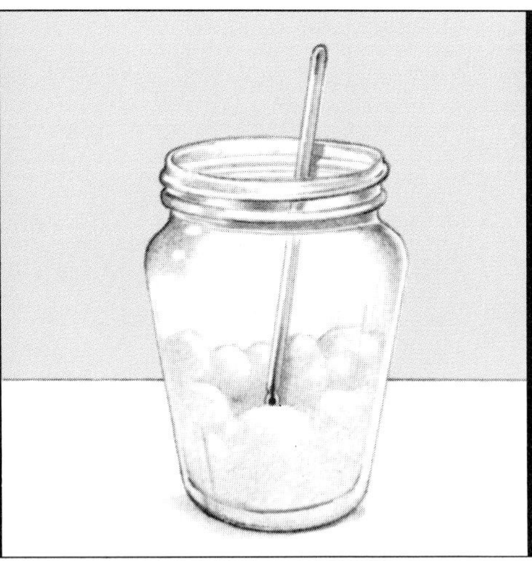

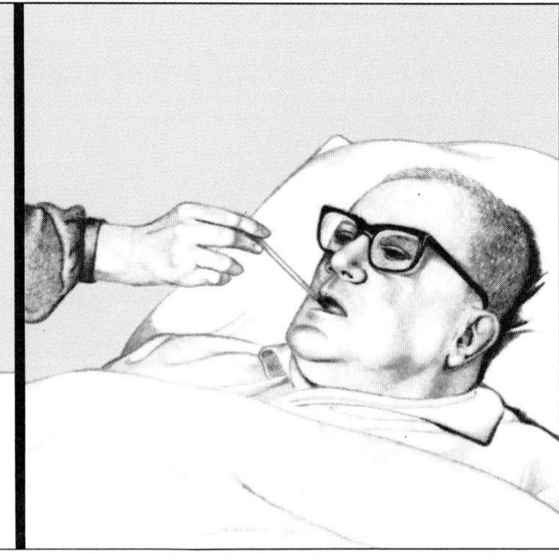

1 Before taking the patient's temperature, you must ensure that the mercury ribbon in the thermometer is well below the "normal" mark of 98.6°F (37°C). To do this, you hold the thermometer at the opposite end to the bulb firmly between the finger and thumb. Give the thermometer two or three sharp flicks of the wrist. Check the new reading, repeating the flicking action if necessary.

2 During the period over which you use a clinical thermometer, keep it in a jar with a wad of absorbent cotton at the bottom.

After you have used the thermometer, rinse it thoroughly under tepid running water, then with a disinfectant, dry it, and replace it in the jar. Never rinse the thermometer under hot water. The mercury may expand too much and break the bulb.

3 Check that the patient has not had a hot or cold drink or a smoke within the last half hour. Place the bulb of the thermometer under the patient's tongue. Ask the patient to close the lips (but not the teeth) gently around the stem of the thermometer. Leave the thermometer in place at least one minute. Remove the thermometer and record the reading.

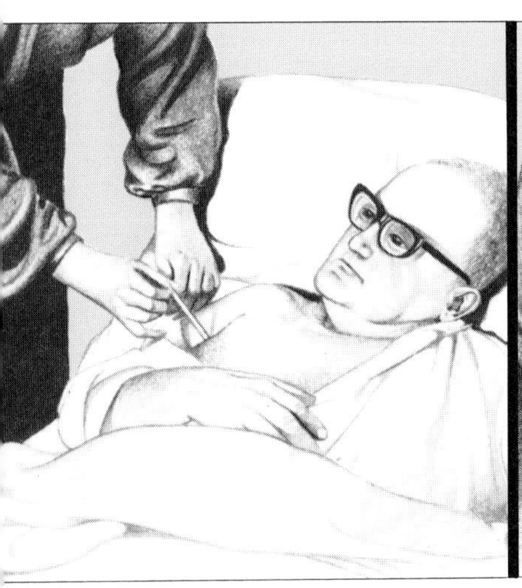

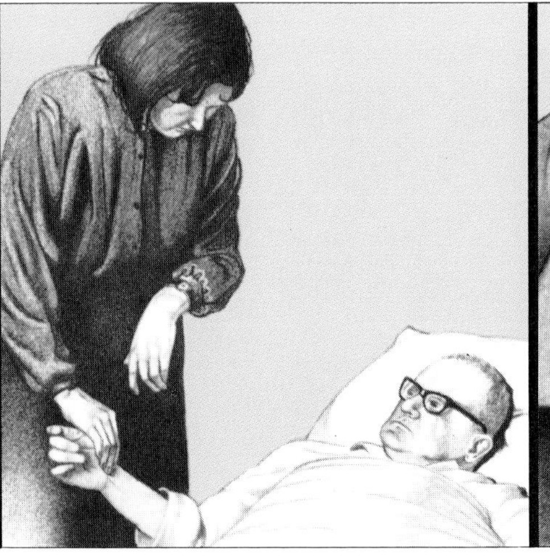

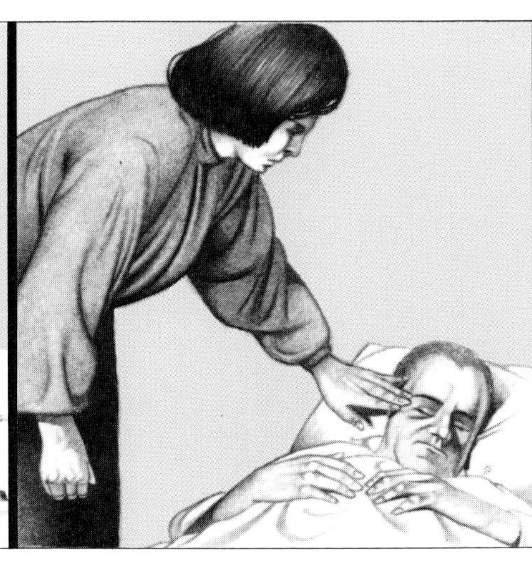

4 An alternative method is to lift up the patient's arm and slip the thermometer under it, so that the bulb rests in the armpit. Bring the patient's arm across the chest to ensure that the thermometer stays securely in place. Leave the thermometer in position for at least three minutes. Remove it and record the reading. A subaxillary temperature is about 1°F lower than a sublingual temperature.

5 You can feel a pulse wherever an artery lies across a bone. The usual place to take a patient's pulse is at the wrist. Place the first and second fingers of your hand gently on the patient's wrist at the base of the thumb. After a few moments you should feel the beats of the pulse. Count the number of beats during one full minute by watching the second hand of a clock or wrist watch.

6 If the patient is asleep or whenever the wrist is not readily accessible, simply place two fingers lightly on the patient's temples and take the pulse reading. The most accurate reading is obtained by counting the beats over a full minute. You should avoid taking the pulse for a shorter time and multiplying the number of beats by a factor to get the result.

even a single bloom picked from the garden and placed in a vase, provides a delightful finishing touch.

Serve only small helpings of food. Too large a helping heaped onto a plate may take away the appetite of the sick or elderly. If the patient is still hungry after the meal, a further portion can always be given. The patient may enjoy helping to plan the menu, and he or she may welcome the opportunity to be useful.

The food must be fresh and served at the right temperature. Preparing food at home does not mean you can ignore the strictest rules of a good restaurant; hot food should always be served hot and cold food served cold.

Taking Temperature, Pulse, and Respiration Rate

The average human body temperature in health, taken from under the tongue, registers 98.6°F (37°C) on the thermometer. Both the mercury thermometer and the newer digital thermometer are available at drugstores. They can be easily cleaned with prepackaged alcohol sponges.

Taking the temperature from under the tongue gives the most accurate reading. However, this method is not suitable for babies or for senile or confused patients. A reading taken from under the arm (subaxillary) is a suitable method for the elderly and senile. Alternatively, a reading can be taken by placing the thermometer in the patient's rectum. This may be necessary when a patient is unable to have the thermometer placed under the tongue (sublingually) because of, say, inflammation of the mouth. A rectal temperature reading is usually taken from children under age four.

Never use a long-tipped mercury thermometer for taking a rectal temperature. Use only the short-tipped, stubby type of mercury thermometer with a bulb the same diameter as the stem. Lubricate the thermometer bulb with petroleum jelly before inserting it about an inch into the rectum. Hold the thermometer in place for one minute. Remove the thermometer and record the reading. A rectal temperature is about 1°F higher than a sublingual temperature.

The average adult pulse rate varies from 68 to 74 beats per minute at rest. In men, the normal pulse rate is 70 to 72 beats a minute; in women, 78 to 82; in infants and children, still higher, 100 to 120. A baby's pulse rate is much higher, about 120 to 140 beats per minute at rest. The pulse of a twelve-year-old is 80 beats per minute at rest.

Having taken the patient's pulse, you should keep hold of the wrist and observe the patient's respiration rate. Do not let the patient know what you are monitoring. The patient's awareness could cause a subconscious reaction that would change the rate of breathing. One respiration consists of one complete inhalation and exhalation. Count the respirations for a full minute. For a healthy adult, the total is 16 to 22 respirations per minute; for a baby it is 30 to 50. A twelve-year-old's respiratory rate is the same as an adult's.

It is important that you write down the daily readings of the patient's temperature, pulse rate, and respiration rate. A temperature chart can be bought from the drugstore to help you do this more efficiently. The physician may want you to keep a record of other bodily functions, such as how often the patient moves the bowels or how much fluid intake and output there is. When the patient's illness has passed and a thermometer is no longer needed, swab it in disinfectant before finally putting it away.

Medicines

Wash your hands before administering any medicines. Always check the instructions on the container before use, whether pills or liquids are being given.

If the medicine is liquid, thoroughly shake the container. When pouring liquid from a medicine bottle, always hold the bottle with the label uppermost to prevent the label from becoming stained with the medicine and thereby illegible. Hold a medicine glass at eye level in order to measure the prescribed amount exactly.

If the medicine is in tablet form, give the patient a glass of water to drink to make swallowing the tablets easier. Children, in particular, and some elderly people may find a tablet difficult to swallow even with a drink of water. In these circumstances, crush the tablet between two spoons. If necessary, disguise the powder by mixing it with food, such as applesauce, before giving it to the patient. Wash the medicine glass or spoon after use.

Be sure to always follow accurately the instructions given on the medicine container. For example, when specifically directed to give tablets only before meals, do not give them at any other time. If a medicine has to be given at four-hour or six-hour intervals, keep to the times as closely as possible, without unnecessarily disturbing natural sleep patterns. If the medicine has to be given three times a day, breakfast, lunch, and supper times provide an easy timetable to follow.

Once such a pattern has been established, make it a routine and keep to it. A routine encourages calm acceptance by the patient and is easier for you to remember. Such a timetable also ensures that a balanced concentration of the drug is maintained in the bloodstream.

Always make sure, personally, that the patient takes the medicine. Do not assume, for example, that it will be taken after you have left the room.

All medicines should be kept outside the sickroom, preferably in a locked and childproof cupboard.

Use of Bedpans and Drawsheets

When giving a bedpan or urinal, allow the patient as much privacy as possible. Most persons will prefer to be left on their own.

The bedpan or urinal should be carried to and from the patient covered with a clean towel. A urinal should be placed in position for a helpless or confused patient.

A bedpan should be warm and dry. Warm it with running water from a hot faucet, and dry it thoroughly. Raise the patient's buttocks with one hand, while gently slipping the bedpan underneath with the other. Two persons are needed to give a bedpan to a helpless patient. Take care not to graze the patient's skin. Provide a supply of soft toilet paper, and give assistance only if specifically requested.

Remove the bedpan or urinal and cover it immediately with a towel. Give the patient a bowl of water, some soap, and a towel with which to wash the hands.

Observe the contents of the bedpan or urinal before emptying it down the toilet. Rinse the bedpan thoroughly under running water, and clean under the rim with a toilet bowl cleaner, which should be kept for this purpose in a pitcher of disinfectant.

The physician may prescribe glycerin suppositories or an enema for a patient who is having bowel difficulties.

To insert a suppository use a pair of thin rubber gloves. Lubricate the suppository with petroleum jelly. Use the first finger to insert the suppository into the rectum as far as it will go. This may be embarrassing to the patient, so remain calm and be efficient. Tell the patient that the longer it is kept in, the more effective it will be.

An enema comes in the form of a plastic sachet with a nozzle attached. Immerse the sachet in a bowl of hot water for ten minutes to warm the contents. Lubricate the nozzle with petroleum jelly and insert it slowly about three inches into the rectum, while gently squeezing out the sachet's contents. The enema should be retained for as long as possible.

Retention is made easier if the foot of the bed is raised slightly. It also helps if the patient can be distracted in some way. Let the patient lie on the back while listening to the radio or reading a book.

When retention is no longer possible, help the patient out onto a commode or provide a bedpan. Provide toilet paper, followed by a bowl of water and soap for washing.

The patient should then be left in peace and quiet. Having an enema can be exhausting, particularly for an elderly person.

Elderly persons suffering from incontinence often feel distressed and degraded by it. Getting annoyed with them only aggravates the problem. The home nurse should make the situation as easy and comfortable as possible for the patient. Often, incontinence can be prevented altogether by giving the patient a bedpan regularly every two hours.

An incontinent patient should always have a protective waterproof

Use of bedpans and drawsheets

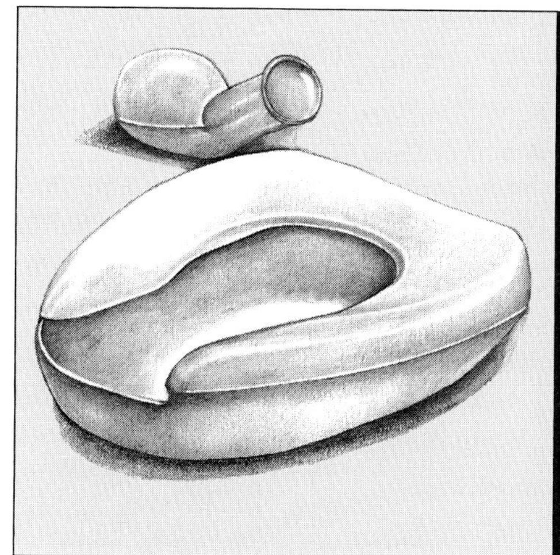

For some patients, it is necessary to keep a record of the intake and output of fluids. Keep two separate measuring pitchers, one to measure the volume of fluids before the patient drinks them, the other for measuring the volume of urine. Some urinals have a measuring scale down one side. The liquid from a bedpan, however, has to be separated out.

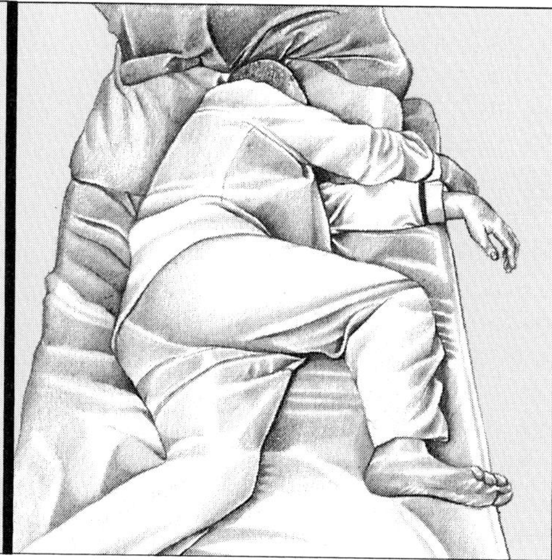

Enemas and suppositories should be given to a patient when he or she is lying on one side. This position provides easy access to the rectal area. Encourage the patient to empty the bladder beforehand. Place an old towel under the buttocks, and keep the patient warm with a blanket, leaving a minimum of skin exposed while the enema is administered. Encourage the patient to relax, and to retain the enema as long as possible.

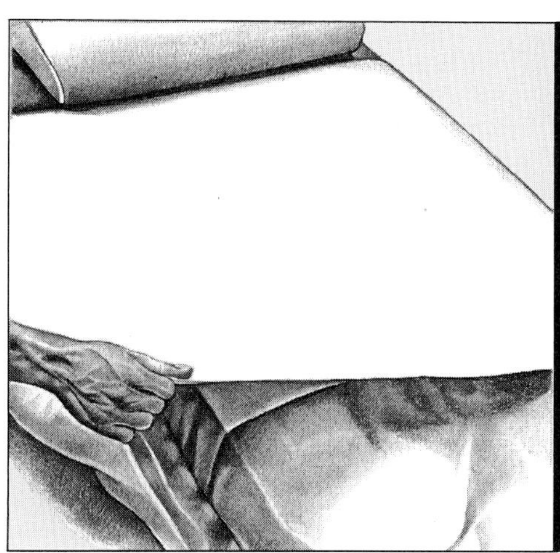

1 When nursing an incontinent patient, first place a plastic sheet across the bed over the bottom sheet, and tuck it in. Take the drawsheet (an old sheet torn in half is ideal for this) and tuck it in under the mattress at one side of the bed. Take the other end of the sheet to the other side of the bed, and tuck in only the end so that a large fold hangs down. Tuck in the whole of the remaining length of fold.

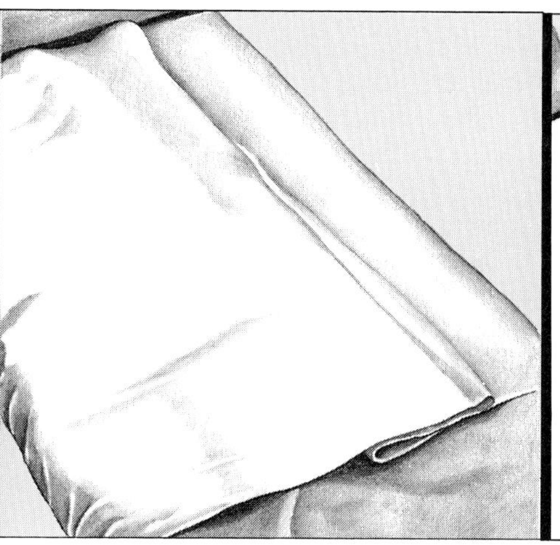

2 If the drawsheet becomes damp or if the patient feels hot and wants to lie on a cooler piece of sheet, the large fold can be untucked and some of it moved across the bed as necessary. When the required amount has been moved across, tuck what remains of the large fold back underneath the mattress for future use. (A badly soiled sheet, however, will have to be removed.)

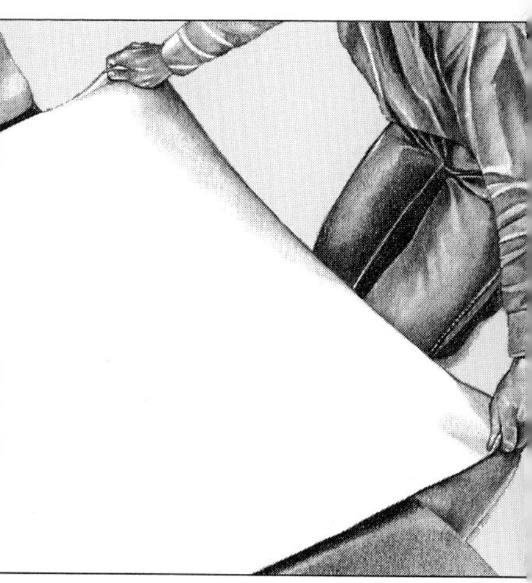

3 From the other side of the bed pull the new piece of sheet taut. Tuck the used piece underneath the mattress on this side of the bed. If the slack in the drawsheet is always moved in the same direction, it is possible to get four clean pieces of sheet. If not soiled, it can be moved back in the other direction.

sheet placed over the mattress of the bed. Disposable incontinence pads, with a waterproof backing and absorbent top, can be bought at most drugstores.

The patient should use nightclothes that are easy to wash and dry. A nightdress can be split down the back and fitted with Velcro® along its length. This enables it to be opened out if it becomes wet.

Urine is a skin irritant and so should not be left in contact with it for any length of time. Change the patient's bedclothes and wash and dry the skin as soon as possible, applying a barrier cream, if recommended by the physician.

To avoid frequently changing bed linen, make up the bed with a drawsheet. This is a long narrow sheet placed across the bed under the area of the patient's buttocks.

Aids and Devices

Reimbursement for medical aids and devices is possible. Medicare will cover their costs, if there is a physician's prescription for them. The American Cancer Society also donates some items, including special belts for home use by cancer patients.

Walking Aids include canes, walking frames, elbow crutches, and long crutches. It is important that walking aids are the right height for the patient who is using them. The use of any at the wrong height can lead to neck or shoulder tension. Long crutches should not be so high that they push upward under the patient's armpits. Most of the body's weight should be supported by the hand grips attached to each crutch and carried by the arms and hands.

Rails and handles fixed at strategic places around the home can be an enormous help for those who have difficulty in walking and moving independently. Whenever possible, a handrail should be placed on both sides of the stairs. Grab rails should be secured wherever a person has to get up or sit down, for example, next to the lavatory, beside the bath, by an armchair in the living room, and next to the bed.

A wheelchair should be chosen with great care. When in the sitting position, the patient should be able to relax the arms comfortably on the armrests. The armrests may also be used to push the body up into the standing position. The back should be well supported and the feet placed flat on the footrest. Sitting down for long periods of time can lead to discomfort in the pelvic area. To help prevent this, an effective cushion can be made by cutting a circular hole in a piece of foam rubber.

Moving about the home in a wheelchair is made considerably easier if steps are replaced by slopes or ramps. A short slope can be made by placing triangular wooden blocks against a step. Ramps can be bought or improvised. They consist of two tracks for the wheels of the wheelchair to run along. The ramp is placed between the upper and lower levels of a step, thus allowing the patient to move up the step by his or her own efforts.

Make sure that the home has no potential hazards for the patient. Loose furniture fittings can be extremely dangerous; they should be securely attached. Check also that carpets are well tacked down. Keep a fire screen in front of an open fire, and do not position seats close to radiators. A flashlight kept at the patient's bedside may be useful at night or during a power failure.

Personal Aids and devices give a physically disabled patient or an elderly person a new independence that is essential for morale. However, overuse of such aids can sometimes retard recovery. In some cases, the patient should be encouraged to make an effort, in order that his or her condition may improve. Always check with a physician before providing a patient with an aid device.

Dressing and undressing can be extremely difficult if there are many zippers and buttons on clothing. A stick with a hook at the end is a simply made tool that can be used to pull a zipper to which a loop has been attached. Alternatively, replace all zippers and buttons with Velcro fastenings, preferably sewn into the front of clothing.

People who wear eyeglasses may like to keep them on a cord around the neck. This ensures that they remain at hand and are not mislaid.

A long mirror in the bedroom or bathroom is always useful for checking that clothes have been fastened cor-

Walking aids

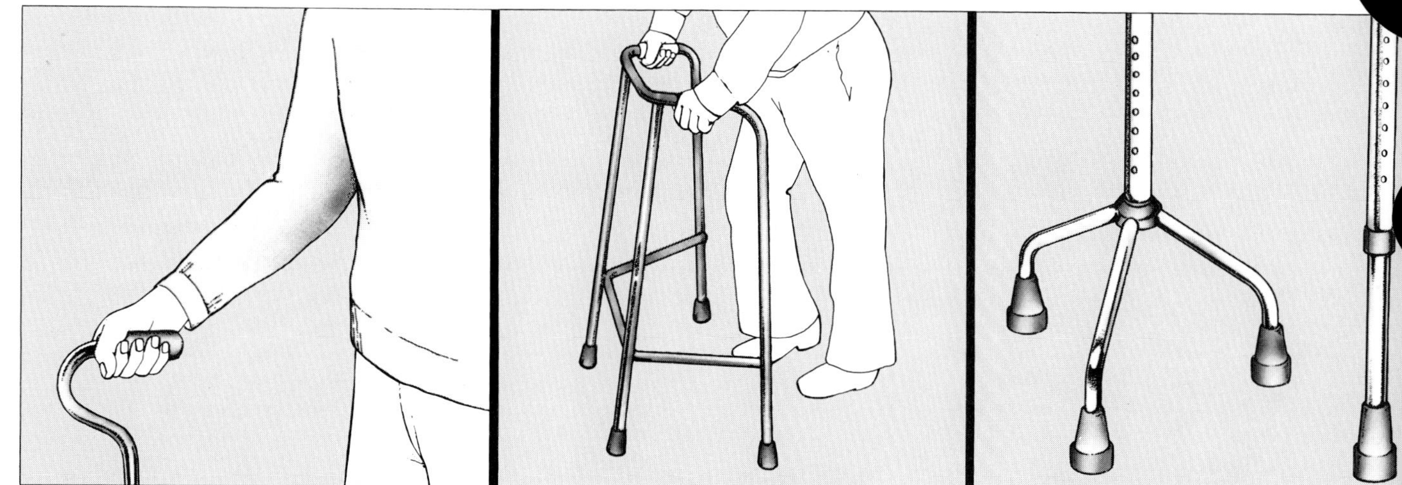

To calculate the correct height for a cane, the patient should hold his or her arm by the side of the body, with the arm loosely bent at an angle of about 160°. Measure the distance from the palm of the hand to the floor. This measurement should allow for the rubber grip (ferrule) at the bottom of the cane. Wooden canes can be cut to the right length. Most metal canes are adjustable.

A walker of the right height can provide a great deal of stable support. As with all walking aids, great care should be taken to ensure that it is the right height. If a walker is too high, it causes a hunching of the shoulders, which in turn leads to tension around the neck area. If it is too low, the patient is forced to stoop unnecessarily, putting strain on the muscles of the back.

All walking aids should have a large rubber ferrule at the end to prevent slipping. A ferrule can be purchased separately and is essential. This is important on a hard, resistant surface, such as linoleum or wood. A cane with three legs at its base provides greater stability and support than does an ordinary cane.

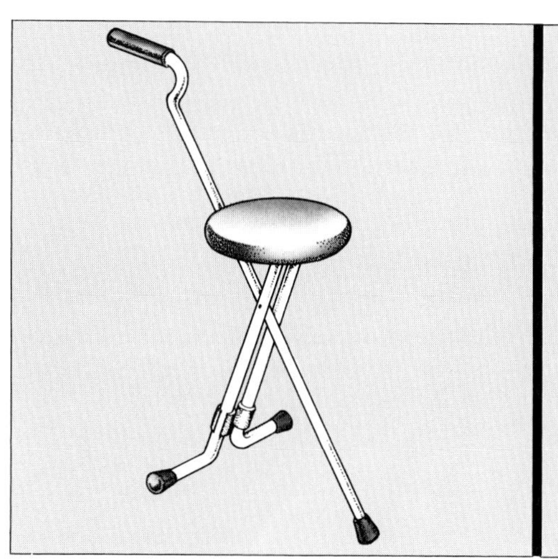

The seat cane is a combination of a cane and a hinged seat. The actual seat must be strong enough to be both secure and comfortable for the patient. Yet the whole device can be folded up. It is lightweight, so that it can be carried and used like an ordinary cane. The seat cane encourages a patient to be mobile, by allowing rest to be taken when required.

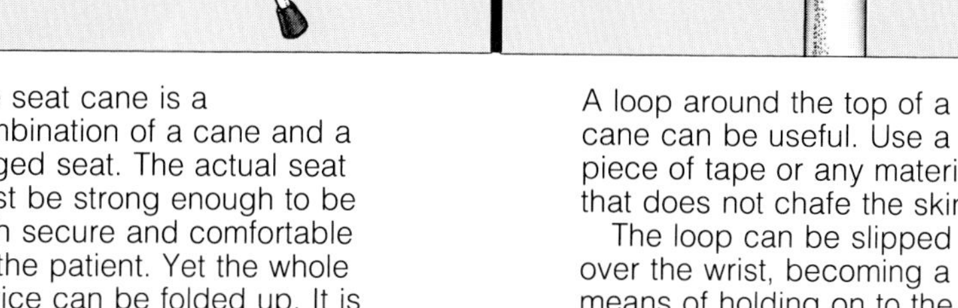

A loop around the top of a cane can be useful. Use a piece of tape or any material that does not chafe the skin.

The loop can be slipped over the wrist, becoming a means of holding on to the cane when both hands are needed for some other purpose, especially when climbing stairs. The loop can also be used for hanging up the cane when it is not needed.

Clips to hold a cane can be attached to various pieces of furniture or wherever it is convenient, for example, on the edge of a table or on a wall. Clips are most commonly required in the kitchen, next to a favorite armchair in the living room, next to the bed, and in the bathroom, one near the bath and another close to the toilet. A clip can also be attached to a wheelchair.

Domestic aids

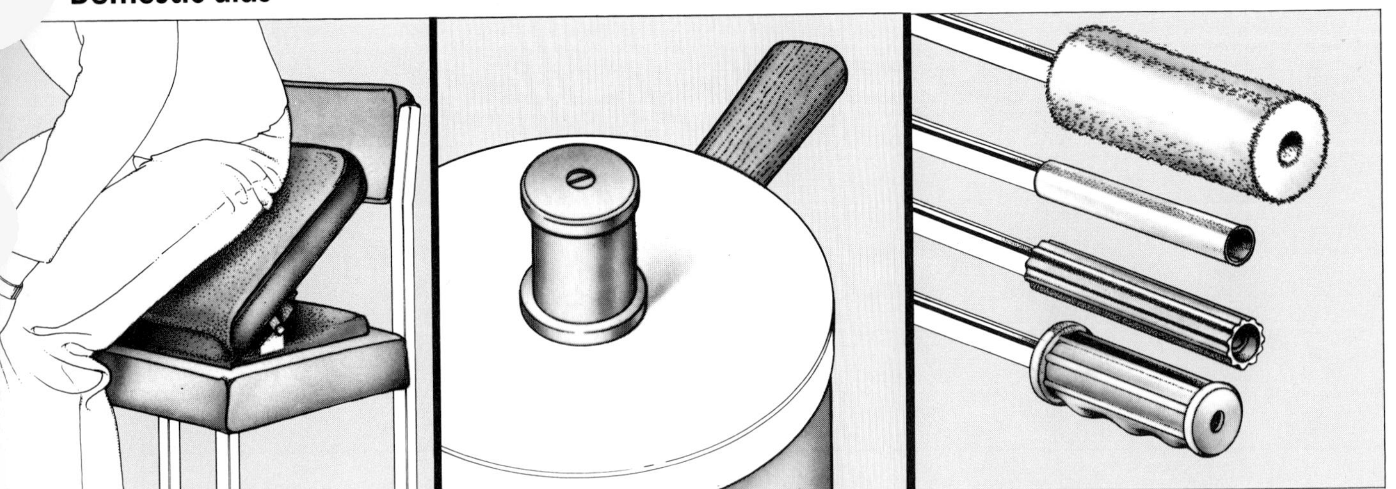

The tip-up chair can be a great help if a person has difficulty rising to the standing position. Springs attached to the seat raise it up at the back when the person sitting on it leans forward in preparation for standing. The seat thus acts as a lever. It is also possible to obtain these chairs with armrests, which help a disabled person to sit down and stand up.

Lids of pots and pans may be difficult to lift off if the knob is rather small. A knob can usually be unscrewed quite easily and a thread spool or larger block of wood put in its place. Buy only pots and pans with handles that do not conduct heat. When arranging a kitchen it may be preferable for the stove to be placed close to the sink, so that dirty pans can be transferred easily.

Handles can be enlarged according to requirements and using a variety of different materials. The illustration shows, from top to bottom: a paint roll cover, aluminum tubing, a piece of garden hose, and a bicycle handle grip. To enlarge the handle of a telephone, wrap a piece of foam rubber around it and tie it securely in position with a bandage.

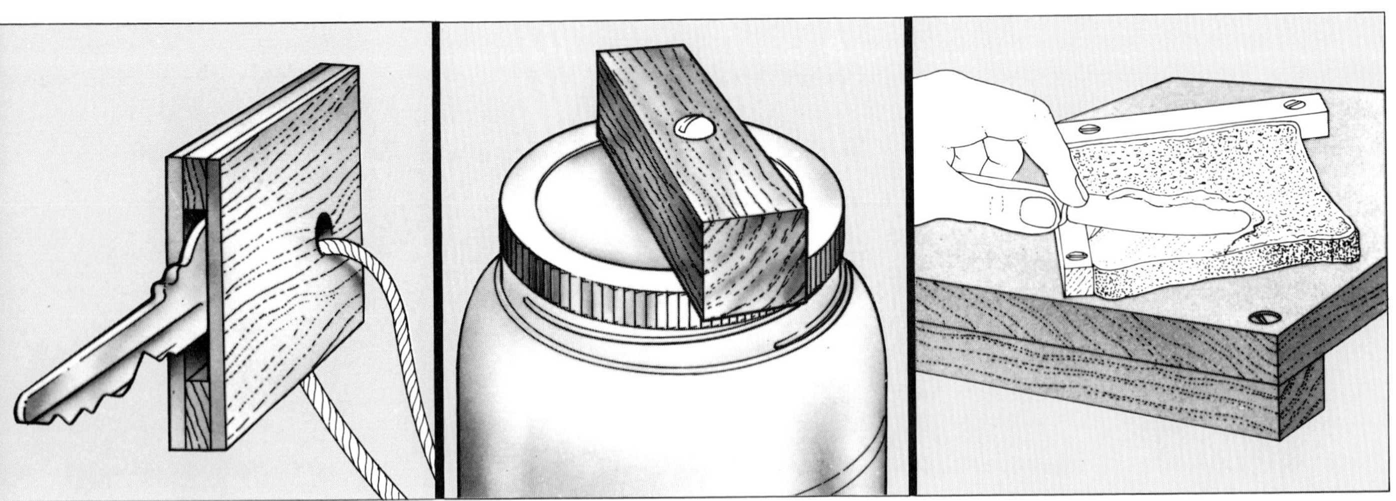

A key can be enlarged by enclosing its "head" in a piece of cork or wood. It is then readily locatable in a bag or pocket and is easier to turn in the lock. If the lock on a door has become frozen in cold weather and the key cannot be inserted, an effective way of freeing the lock is to heat the key using matches or a cigarette lighter. The heat of the key should unfreeze the lock.

Unscrewing the lid of a jar can be a difficult task for a patient with arthritic hands. A block of wood screwed on to the top of the lid will provide something substantial to hold on to. Alternatively, screw two strips of serrated metal in a "V" -shape under the surface of a table or under a wall cupboard. Slide the lid between the two pieces of metal until tight against both, then turn the jar.

A wooden choppingboard can be held firmly in place if an extra piece of wood is fixed on the underside of one end of it. This ensures that it will not slip forward when being used. Two wedges of wood placed in a "V"-shape on the top of the board can also prevent anything on its surface from slipping. For example, a piece of bread can be pushed up against it while being spread with butter.

Personal aids

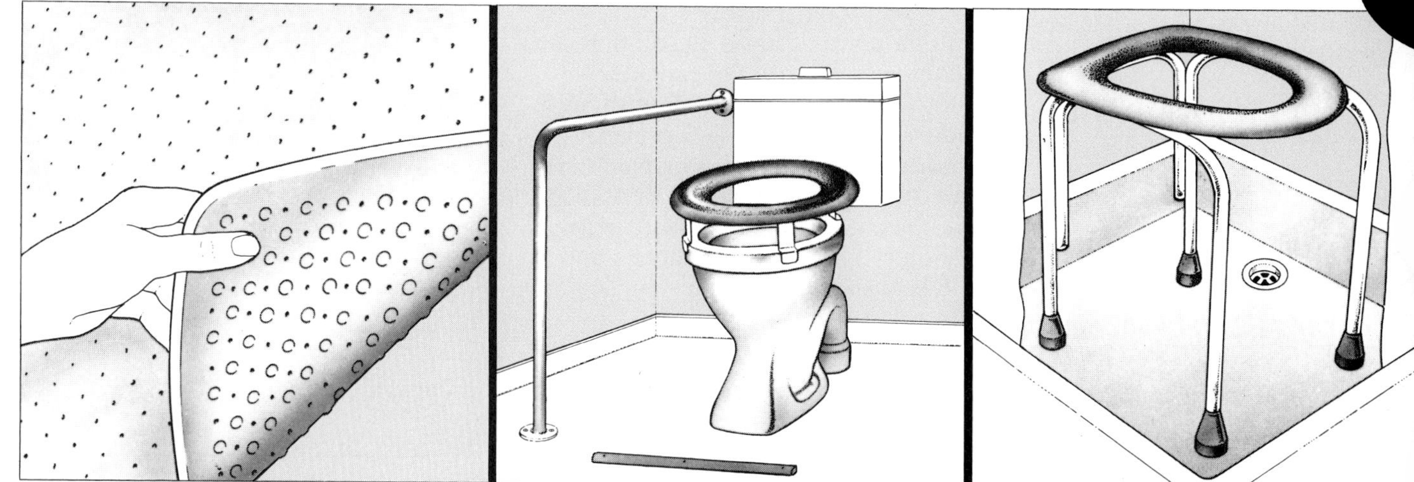

A rubber mat with suction cups on its underside gives added security to unsure walkers. One can be placed wherever there is a likelihood of the feet slipping, especially in the bottom of the bathtub or in front of the toilet or a chair. Patients who are likely to be unsteady should always wear shoes that give firm support. Soft-soled shoes should be avoided, however comfortable.

An elevated toilet seat can help a patient who has difficulty in rising from the sitting position. A strong rail secured by the side of the toilet can also be a great help. To prevent the feet slipping when standing up, put a safety mat in front of the toilet, or screw a wooden wedge into the floor. The door can be left unlocked, if help might be needed, and an "occupied" tag hung on the outside.

For patients who like to use a shower, a shower seat may be necessary. Ensure that this is the right height, so that the patient is able to stand up and sit down without difficulty. A magnetic soap clip or a piece of soap on a rope may be useful to prevent the soap from slipping out of reach.

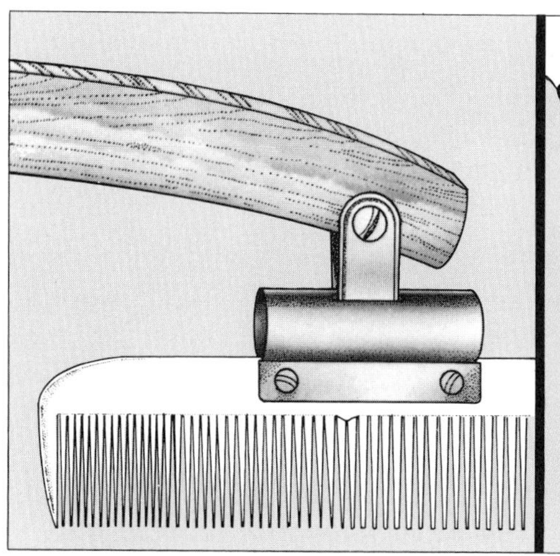

A long-handled comb can be simply devised using an old wooden coat hanger. Remove the metal hook from the top. Screw a spring clip into one end of the hanger and attach the comb as shown in the illustration. Aids like this can give a patient an enormous feeling of independence. It can be demoralizing to ask other people to do such a simple and personal thing as to comb one's hair.

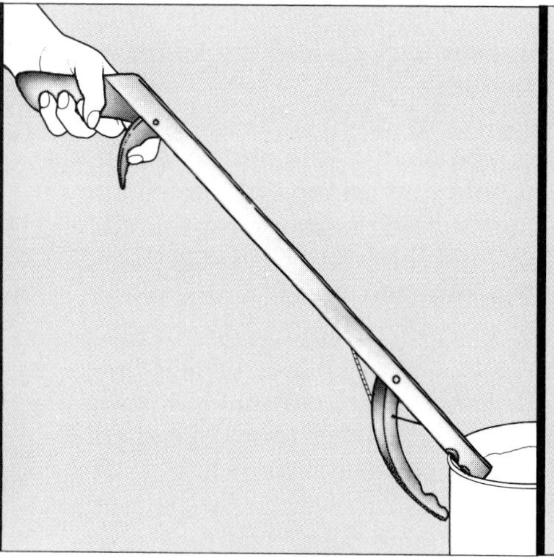

The device illustrated acts as an extended hand. It is particularly useful for people who have difficulty bending over or reaching up. With it, they can pick things up off the floor or take things down from shelves. It should not be used to such an extent that a patient becomes unnecessarily lazy. Designs range from the simple to the sophisticated; some even have magnetic attachments.

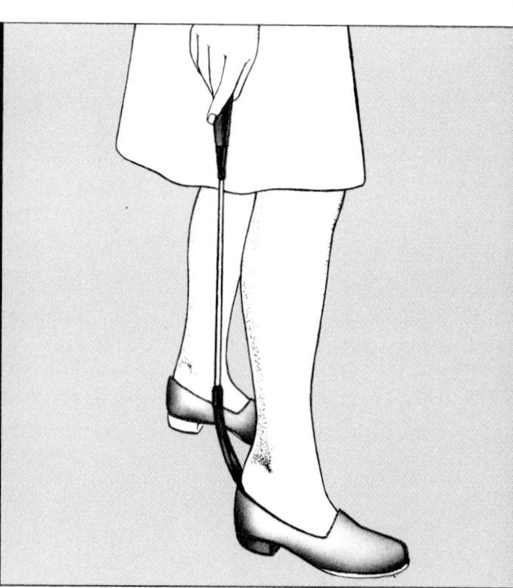

A shoehorn with a long handle can help considerably in putting on a pair of shoes. Some shoehorns have a flexible spring attached near the end, so that the foot can be slipped into the shoe from practically any angle. Patients with laced shoes may also find it useful to have elastic shoelaces. This makes the shoe enlarge around the foot as the shoe is being put on, without having to untie and tie the laces.

rectly and for practicing correct posture. Attach the hand towel in the bathroom to a piece of loose elastic that can be hung over a hook. This enables the towel to be pulled and used, without it having to be unhooked and replaced.

Domestic Aids. Life can be made easier for anyone with physical disabilities if the objects around the house, especially those used in daily chores, are adapted to suit that person's particular needs and capabilities.

Working surfaces should always be at the correct height, so that the patient's shoulders do not have to be hunched. If a seat is needed, its height should also be measured with care. In the kitchen, suction cups can be attached to the table or counter in order to hold articles such as a bowl or plate, freeing at least one hand for other duties.

Another extremely useful item in the kitchen is a large funnel, which can be used when pouring liquids into containers. It is particularly useful when pouring out hot liquids.

An automatic electric kettle that switches itself off when the water is boiling is appreciated in any home. It will be especially useful to a person who has to move slowly. Such a device can prevent the kitchen from getting steamed up and the kettle from boiling dry.

Finally, an apron with several pockets can be handy. It is one way of keeping a hold on various little items and prevents having to move continually around the room searching for them.

Nursing the sick child. A sick child needs the same comfortable environment and special diet as does a sick adult. However, in caring for a sick child, you will need to make a special effort to encourage him or her to take medicines and to relieve the patient's boredom. Some childhood disorders, such as chicken pox, can not be treated with drugs, and it then becomes even more important to be able to relieve the symptoms with careful home nursing.

Before you give any medicine, try to relax and assume that the child will like it. Most medicines for children nowadays have a pleasant taste. However, if you start apologizing and explaining why the medicine is necessary, the child will anticipate an

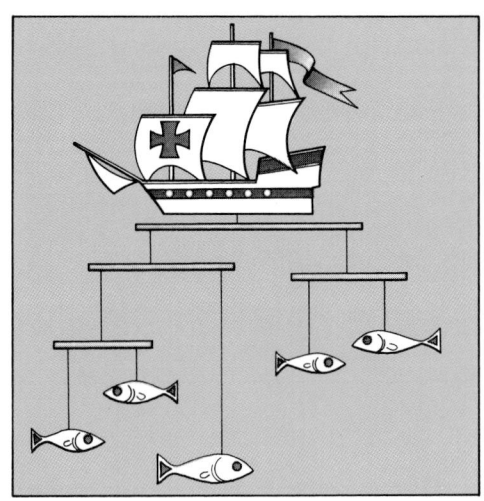

Mobiles are easy for a bedridden child to make and fun to wach when completed and hung over the bed. A child can paste pictures from magazines onto cardboard before cutting them out. Together you can make more complicated objects to hang on the mobile: cotton-reel animals, origami shapes, ribbon, cooking foil shapes, and wool pompons.

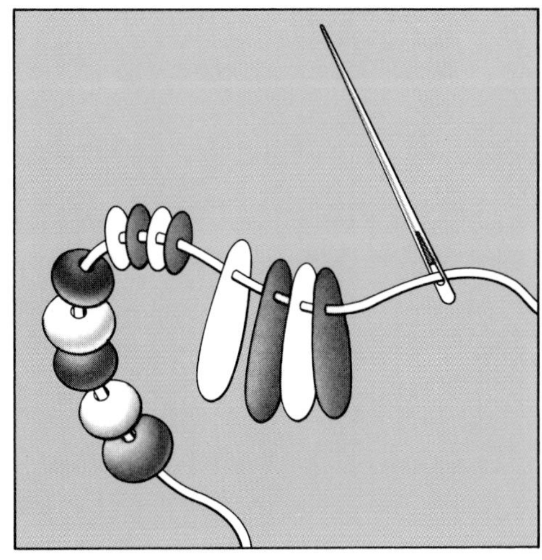

Bead stringing can amuse a convalescent child who does not feel overenergetic. Give the child a blunt darning needle and some thick cotton thread. Strings of beads can be made out of the dried pits of apples, oranges, lemons, and melons. Large seeds such as sunflower seeds and lentils can be used and even painted before stringing. Small colored buttons also work well.

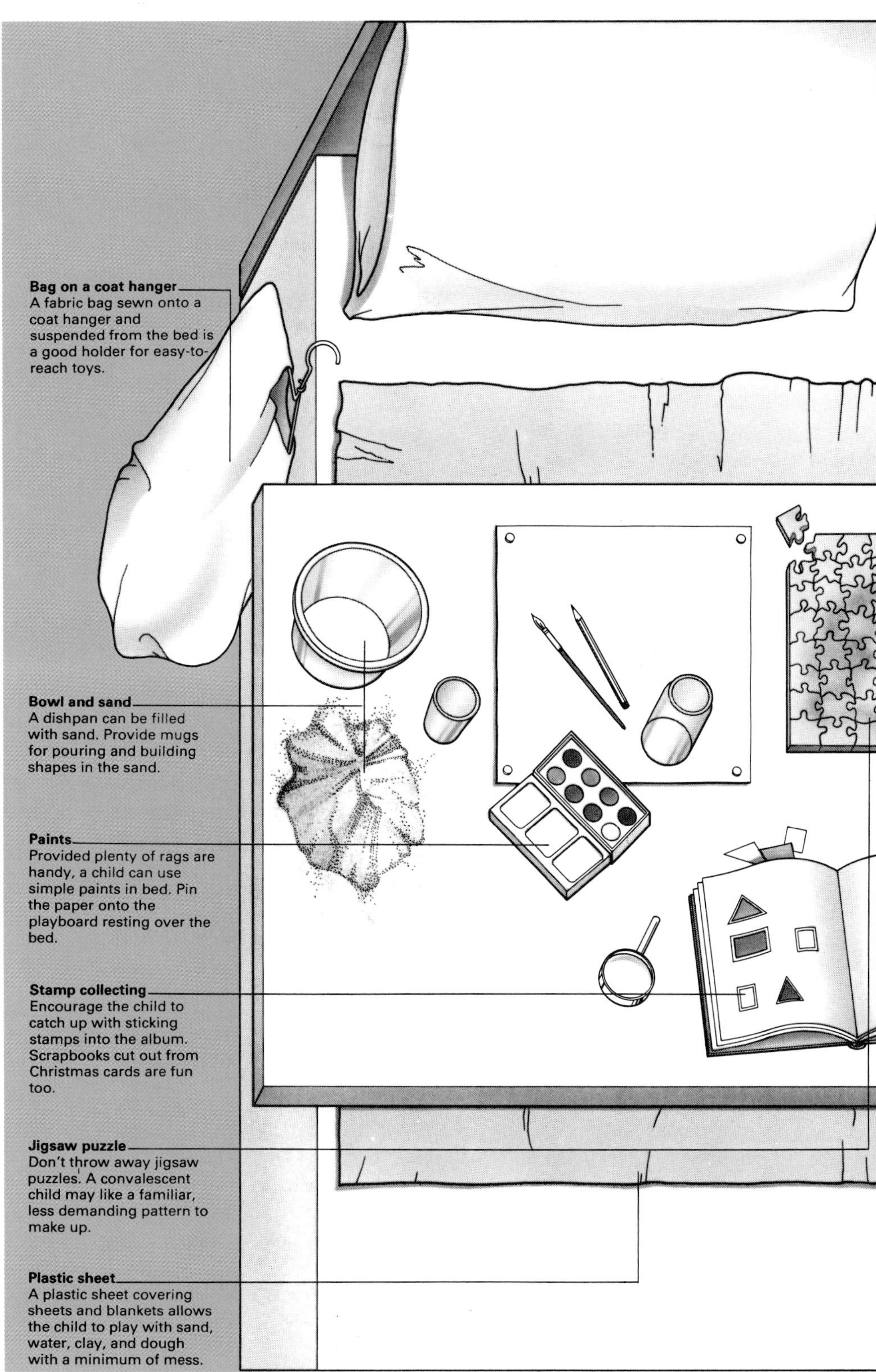

Bag on a coat hanger
A fabric bag sewn onto a coat hanger and suspended from the bed is a good holder for easy-to-reach toys.
Bowl and sand
A dishpan can be filled with sand. Provide mugs for pouring and building shapes in the sand.
Paints
Provided plenty of rags are handy, a child can use simple paints in bed. Pin the paper onto the playboard resting over the bed.
Stamp collecting
Encourage the child to catch up with sticking stamps into the album. Scrapbooks cut out from Christmas cards are fun too.
Jigsaw puzzle
Don't throw away jigsaw puzzles. A convalescent child may like a familiar, less demanding pattern to make up.
Plastic sheet
A plastic sheet covering sheets and blankets allows the child to play with sand, water, clay, and dough with a minimum of mess.

A recuperating child, or a child who is not seriously ill, becomes easily bored lying in bed and needs to be amused. The caregiver should plan to read to the child or play games with the patient, but there will be times when the child will have to amuse himself or herself. Potentially messy activities, such as painting or playing with soap bubbles or sand, can still be pursued if the bedlinen is first protected with plastic sheeting. A piece of wood or a low, folding table acts as a playboard, and loose, small items can be kept within easy reach in a fabric bag attached to the bed.

unpleasant taste and will expect not to like it.

If your child refuses to take the dose, try to mix it with a drink. It is best to use an unfamiliar drink, such as grape or apple juice, because most children notice immediately any change in the taste of familiar drinks.

Tablets can be crushed and mixed with the first spoonful of any food with a strong taste, such as stewed fruit. Any medicine with a bitter taste can be mixed with something sweet, such as jelly or honey. If the medicine is in the form of a capsule, put it into soft food, such as chopped bananas. Always remember to keep any medication out of reach of children, and to throw it away once the illness is over.

A comforting eyewash may be made from a quart of lukewarm water containing a teaspoonful of baking soda (sodium bicarbonate). This is particularly soothing for the child with eyes that are crusted, as for example in measles. Whenever you are bathing eyes, be sure to use a fresh piece of cotton for each eye to prevent spreading infection from one eye to the other.

A child with spots that itch, as for example in chicken pox, runs a risk of infecting the spots by scratching them. The itching can be relieved somewhat by bathing the child in a solution of two cups of baking soda to a large tubful of water. Dabbing the spots with calamine lotion often helps. To avoid infection, keep the child's fingernails short and wash his or her hands several times a day.

With some childhood illnesses, such as measles and mumps, the mouth can get sore and dry. This can be alleviated by using mouthwash frequently. If your child has a stuffy nose, you can occasionally administer medicine to constrict the nasal tissues, such as Neo-Synephrine®. Consult the label for the weaker dosage for children. However, avoid any prolonged use of such medicine, as this may lead to even worse congestion.

See also NURSING THE SICK.

Nutrition (nü trish′ən) is the sum total of the processes of eating, digesting, and assimilating food to maintain growth and health. Nutrition is also the science involved with the study of foods and their relationship to health. *See also* DIET.

The Process

Simple elements in the earth and the surrounding air, such as carbon dioxide, water, minerals, and salts, provide energy for plants to grow, respire, and reproduce. These simple elements are converted into complex food materials, which can subsequently be broken down for energy. Humans can not convert these simple elements into energy, so they have to ingest complex food materials, either directly from plants or from other animals that have previously ingested plants.

In humans, the complex materials are broken down during the process of digestion, then absorbed as nutrients for use in three main ways: (1) the food components can be oxidized and used as energy; (2) the components may be used to build, repair, or maintain body tissue; or (3) they may be used to regulate body processes.

A well-balanced diet must provide proteins, fats, and carbohydrates in the correct proportions; trace elements, such as vitamins and mineral salts; and fluids and roughage. These must be consumed in adequate quantities to provide energy and must be adjusted to suit individual variables such as age, sex, physical build, and level of activity. For example, an active adolescent boy needs a different diet than a 70-year-old woman; and the dietary requirements of a 130-pound secretary are different than those of a 200-pound coal miner. An intake of less than 1,500 calories a day for a working person will result in weight loss and wasting, because the body has to oxidize food stored in the tissues to provide energy. However, if a person eats more than he or she requires for energy, the body stores the excess initially as glycogen in the liver, and then as fat in the fat cells beneath the skin. A person who weighs 20 percent or more above the norm for his or her height, age, and bone structure is termed obese, and his or her health may suffer. (For further information, see "Obesity," page 649).

Nutrients

Nutrients are the nourishing elements within foodstuffs and as such are classified into five main groups: (1) proteins, (2) carbohydrates, (3) fats, (4) minerals, and (5) vitamins.

Proteins. Every living cell contains protein, complex chemical compounds that break down into amino acids during digestion. These are absorbed into the bloodstream and transported to different parts of the body, where they are then reformed into different types of protein. The human body can synthesize some amino acids (nonessential amino acids), but there are ten that have to be ingested (essential amino acids) from proteins in the diet. Essential amino acids include lysine that is found in bread, methionine that is found in beans, and many others. Very young babies need two extra essential amino acids, arginine and histidine. *See also* AMINO ACID.

Proteins are essential for the constant repair and replacement of the body tissues. For example, proteins are vital ingredients in skin-cell multiplication, hair and nail growth, and gradual replacement of degenerated bone cells. The proteins responsible for digestion are known as enzymes. Some of the body's hormones are proteins, and antibodies are proteins that group in response to foreign proteins (antigens) that invade the body and cause a range of diseases from chicken pox to hay fever. *See also* ANTIGEN.

Extra proteins are particularly important during times of growth in childhood or for pregnant women who are building the bodies of their new babies. Similarly, a woman who is breast-feeding her baby needs extra protein to make milk.

After a serious illness a person must eat a high protein diet to regain the protein lost during fever. Similarly, a person who has been involved in a surgical operation or an accident resulting in multiple injuries needs extra protein to build scar tissue and bone during the convalescent period. *See also* PROTEIN.

Protein in Food. Proteins are present in small quantities in nearly every type of food. In Western society a majority of the protein intake comes from meat, fish, and dairy products.

About 20 percent of the protein in the American diet comes from bread, and about 5 percent from potatoes. Even foods such as lettuce or mushrooms contain up to 2 percent protein.

A great deal of research has gone into finding alternative sources of protein food, because animal protein is expensive to produce—the cost is prohibitive for many underdeveloped countries, which rely on bean proteins to supplement their diets. For example, lentils combined with rice have a well-balanced content of protein and carbohydrate, although the vitamin content is fairly low. If land is used for grazing and raising cattle for beef, 30 acres are needed to produce the same amount of protein yielded by 1 acre of soya bean crop.

A good diet should consist of around 12 percent protein. But in prosperous countries nearly everybody eats double the amount of protein necessary to stay healthy. The danger of not reaching a minimum level (under 6 percent) does exist, however, because a person who eats a highly refined carbohydrate diet, consisting of mostly white sugars, candies, and fats, may habitually avoid foods that contain even small amounts of protein, like fruit and vegetables.

If a person eats more protein than the body needs for growth and repair, some of it can be converted into carbohydrates and stored as glycogen. But most of it is broken down into its simple chemical compounds and excreted by the kidneys as urea.

The percentage of protein present in certain kinds of food has no influence on the quality of the protein. For example, a hen's egg contains 12 percent

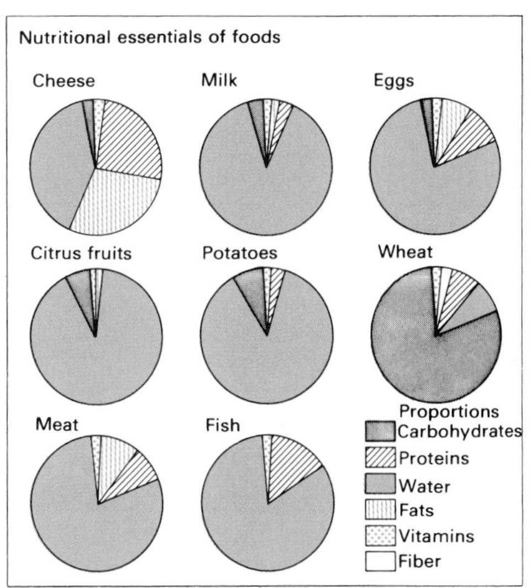

Every type of food contains different proportions of nutrients. A well-balanced diet includes many different kinds of foods to provide the body with sufficient quantities of the essential nutrients.

protein, but that protein can supply the human body with all the essential amino acids, whereas a piece of cod consisting of over 17 percent protein does not contain all of the essential amino acids. Therefore, it is necessary to obtain the missing amino acids from other sources of protein. The only factor that is important is that a person varies the sources of protein and does not depend on one food for the total protein intake.

Carbohydrates are principally energy providers. This energy can be measured in calories. Every activity that a person indulges in can be analyzed as calories spent. If the balance between calories consumed and calories expended is unequal, a person either stores the excess as fat beneath the skin and puts on weight or begins to use up existing stores for energy and loses weight. *See also* CALORIE.

Carbohydrates include sugars and starches. Foods such as potatoes, bread, pastas, cereals, jams, and honey are rich in carbohydrates. About half of a person's average diet consists of carbohydrates—a third of this is actually sugar itself, which is pure carbohydrate. For further information, *see* "Sugar," page 648. Other foods in the carbohydrate group, the starchy foods, also contain many other important nutrients. Potatoes, for instance, are high in vitamin C and contain proteins. A quarter of these are in the skin, so an unpeeled boiled potato or a baked potato is more nutritious than a roasted or mashed potato. Fried potatoes, however, retain much of their vitamin content because cooking time is short. Bread is also rich in carbohydrates, but brown bread also contains proteins, iron, fat, and vitamins. Even white bread often has added calcium, iron, and vitamins. *See also* CARBOHYDRATE.

Fats and oils are also measured in calories and are a more concentrated form of energy than carbohydrates, although their chemical makeup is similar. Animal fats consist mainly of saturated fat and are hard at room temperature, whereas vegetable oils and fish oils consist mainly of polyunsaturated and monounsaturated fats and are liquid at room temperature. Saturated fats have been associated with heart disease and certain cancers. Many authorities believe that the average diet in the United States contains a higher proportion of meat and dairy products than the body was designed to cope with. It is sensible, therefore, to cut down on the amount of animal fats consumed. *See also* FATS.

The chart below shows the average number of calories that a person requires daily, and also shows how this figure varies depending on the person's age. The number of calories needed depends on the amount of energy expended during the day. This can be calculated from the chart on the right, which shows different normal activities and the energy output of each. The amount of energy expended also depends, to some extent, on physical build, sex, and even disposition: a person who does everything vigorously and with enthusiasm is likely to use up more energy in these activities than the person who does the same things half-heartedly. Also, sportsmen or sportswomen and manual laborers tend to use, and therefore require, more calories each day than the average person to whom these charts relate.

Average daily energy requirement at different ages

Age (years)	2	4	8	12	16	22	30	40	60	70+
Requirement (calories)	1250	1500	2000	2500	2900	3100	2800	2700	2600	2400

Energy requirements
Energy expended during ordinary daily activities

	cals/ minute	cals/ hour	Approximate time required to use up 100 calories
Sleeping	1.1	66	1hr 30mins
Light activity, seated	1.4	84	1hr 10mins
Standing	1.6	96	1hr
Light activity, standing	3.0	180	30mins
Driving a car	3.0	180	30mins
Light activity, moving	4.8	288	20mins
Walking	5.5	330	18mins
Medium activity	6.5	390	15mins
Heavy activity	7.6	456	12mins
Running	10.0	600	10 mins

Cholesterol is a fatty substance manufactured in the liver. The body uses it to make membranes and steroid hormones. High levels of cholesterol in the blood (greater than 230 mg/dl) may be associated with arteriosclerosis, so it may be sensible to restrict dietary cholesterol in hopes of minimizing plasma cholesterol and thus heart disease. *See also* ARTERIOSCLEROSIS; CHOLESTEROL.

Minerals. Calcium and phosphorus are considered the major minerals because the body needs these in fairly large quantities. Both elements are essential for the formation of teeth and bone. Milk and cheese are rich in calcium, as is "hard" water. A pregnant woman should drink an extra pint of milk a day to provide herself and her baby with sufficient calcium and phosphorus for developing bones. The body does, however, need vitamin D in order to absorb the calcium. Unfortunately, the milling of white flour removes much calcium, but many companies now fortify white bread during the manufacturing process in order to raise the vitamin D level. Phosphorus occurs in nearly all foods, and therefore, deficiencies of it are rare.

Many other minerals, such as iron and sulfur, are needed by the body. These are known as the trace elements because they are needed only in tiny amounts. If a person is eating a well-balanced diet, he or she is consuming enough of the trace elements. Liver is rich in iron, eggs are rich in sulfur and iron, and salt contains sodium and chlorine. Fish also provides sulfur, as does cabbage and poultry—fish also provides iodine. Other minerals, such as fluorine, zinc, copper, chromium, manganese, and magnesium, are present in a variety of foods. *See also* MINERAL.

Vitamins, unlike minerals, are chemical compounds that have no energy value, but act as catalysts. That is, they are responsible for the start and completion of certain essential chemical processes in the body. But like some trace minerals, the body only needs the smallest amount of them; anything over that amount is excreted by the kidneys. It is therefore not usually necessary to take multivitamin tablets or fortified tonics. In some cases it may even be dangerous, because overdoses of vitamins A and D can cause illness and even death.

The importance of essential vitamins was only discovered this century, and it was assumed that there were four varieties—A, B, C, and D. Since then, research has shown that there are many other varieties.

Vitamin A group includes retinol and carotene. These vitamins are present in fresh green vegetables, milk and butter, liver, and cod-liver oil. Animals obtain most of their vitamin A from carotene (yellow pigment in vegetables such as carrots). A diet that is deficient in vitamin A reduces a person's resistance to diseases, particularly ones that infect the body through the skin. The linings of the throat and bronchial tubes deteriorate; the skin becomes dry and scaly; and the cornea of the eye may also become affected, causing chronic conjunctivitis. A person's ability to see in the dark rapidly deteriorates. *See also* CAROTENE; CONJUNCTIVITIS.

Vitamin B. There are at present seven known varieties of vitamin B. This group plays an important part in the release of energy from carbohydrates, fats, and proteins. Thiamine (B_1) occurs in yeast, liver, pork, and whole-grain cereal; riboflavin (B_2) also appears in liver and yeast, but meat and milk contain it as well; pyridoxine (B_6) is present in almost all foods, and cyanocobalamin (B_{12}) occurs in nearly all animal food. Folic acid, important for development of red blood cells, is present in fresh green vegetables, fruit, dried yeast, and liver. Vitamin B deficiency diseases include beriberi and other digestive disturbances. A victim will also suffer from loss of appetite, wasting, and swelling of the hands and feet. Pellagra is a deficiency of one of the B vitamins known as nicotinic acid or niacin. The victim suffers from diarrhea and vomiting, skin disorders, and mental disorders. The disorder is sometimes a complication of chronic alcoholism. *See also* BERIBERI; PELLAGRA.

Vitamin C (ascorbic acid) is present in citrus fruits, such as oranges and lemons, but it also occurs in nuts and fresh vegetables. It is destroyed during cooking. A diet without vitamin C results in the disorder called scurvy, characterized by weakness, hemorrhaging under the skin and around the gums, slow wound healing, and various skin eruptions. If the diesase is not treated with vitamin C doses, death quickly follows. *See also* SCURVY.

Vitamin D, also called calciferol, can be made by the body when ultraviolet rays are absorbed through the skin. Other sources of vitamin D are cream, egg yolk, and cod-liver oil. A lack of it results in rickets in children, and osteomalacia in adults. The bones weaken and soften, and the ends swell. However, it is *not* recommended that supplemental vitamin D be taken to try to prevent osteoporosis. *See also* OSTEOMALACIA; OSTEOPOROSIS; RICKETS.

Vitamin E, or tocopherol, is present in vegetable oils.

Vitamin K, known as menadione, is present in green vegetables, particularly spinach and cabbage. An inability to absorb it produces blood disorders. Vitamins A, D, E, and K are considered fat-soluble vitamins. Because of this property, there is a greater danger of toxicity from an overdose than there is with other vitamins.

There are a few other vitamins, such as biotin and pantothenic acid, that occur in many different foods.

Dietary Fiber

Dietary fiber is the indigestible remains of plant food that pass through the large bowel. This consists mostly of cellulose (the substance that makes cell walls of plants), lignin, hemicellulose, and pectin.

Fiber is often classified as "soluble" or "insoluble." Insoluble fiber (found in wheat) is associated with "transit time," or how long it takes food to travel through the intestines. This fiber will bind water and thus increase stool size, frequency, and ease of bowel movement. Soluble fiber (found in oat bran, legumes, and fruit) has been associated with lowering plasma cholesterol. In order to optimize the benefits of these fibers, a varied diet including plenty of fresh vegetables, fruits, beans, and cereal products is recommended.

Too much fiber may cause stomach aches and may deplete certain minerals. Unfortunately, Western society now favors foods, such as bread, made from refined flour and eats a greater proportion of meat than vegetables. This low-fiber diet leads to constipation, which can cause straining and lead to hemorrhoids. It may also lead to diverticular disease in which small pouches on the bowel wall become inflamed. *See also* APPENDIX IV.

Fluids

Body function depends on fluids. Cell protoplasm is fluid, and within cells, all essential chemical reactions and exchanges occur. Fluid lubricates the food as it is chewed and digested, helping the flow of digestive juices and enzymes. Fluids make up most of the blood volume in the form of plasma, and through this medium, oxygen, foods, and wastes, such as carbon dioxide, are carried around the body. In fact, an average human body contains up to 72 pints (34.2L) of fluid. The kidneys keep the body's fluid level constant, but during the summer or at times when a person perspires heavily (for example, during physical exercise), it is important to drink an adequate amount of fluid in any form to replace the loss. The only exception is alcohol, because this tends to act as a diuretic and to encourage the kidneys to excrete more fluid than normal, dehydrating the body further. If you do want to drink alcohol when you are thirsty, it should be backed up by at least two pints of nonalcoholic liquid. Mild dehydration over a long period of time can result in constipation and even the development of kidney stones. Without fluid a person dies within a few days.

Sugar

Sugar is instant energy, but apart from that it contains no other nutritional properties. Sugar occurs naturally in many foods, so added sugars are an unnecessary danger that may result in obesity. They raise the level of triglycerides in the blood. Excesses of glucose have been associated with coronary heart disease. Sugar also raises the level of uric acid in the blood, and this has been associated with gout.

There are various forms of sugars. Brown sugars contain more minerals than white sugar. Honey is composed of fructose and glucose, which the human body can use without digesting further. Syrups and molasses contain less calories because they contain more water, but if they are used as sugar substitutes, more is needed to obtain the same amount of sweetness. Recently, much controversy has surrounded the manufacture and safety of synthetic sweeteners—one variety has been completely banned, but others are still available. It is far safer to cut down sugar intake in tea, coffee, cakes, and cookies. In most cases, the palate quickly adjusts to a less sweet diet.

Nutritional Disorders

Nutritional disorders are caused either by a deficiency of the correct nutrients in a diet or by a failure of the body to assimilate the correct nutrients. There also can be too much of a nutrient in the diet, such as an excess of carbohydrates, which results in obesity.

It is probable that conditions such as appendicitis, constipation, diverticulitis disease, and irritable bowel syndrome are aggravated by a diet rich in refined carbohydrates and containing little vegetable fiber. It can not be emphasized enough that roughage is an important ingredient of any balanced diet. A diet rich in saturated fats causes an increase in the levels of cholesterol and fats in the blood, exposing the person to the risks of atherosclerosis. *See also* APPENDICITIS; CONSTIPATION; DIVERTICULITIS; IRRITABLE BOWEL SYNDROME.

Many people who drink too much alcohol, eat too little food. Alcohol is a common substitute for energy foods and is the cause of many health problems. In some parts of the world, people drink large quantities of herbal tea that can cause cirrhosis and liver cancer.

Nutritional disorders can also result from fad or crash diets, voluntary or psychological refusal to eat some or all foods, or from an increased intake of food. Children in underdeveloped countries, who eat a diet that contains adequate calories but is deficient in protein, develop a disease known as kwashiorkor. In many such cases, the protein deficiency is accompanied by a deficiency of vitamins. *See also* ANOREXIA NERVOSA; BULIMIA; KWASHIORKOR; MALNUTRITION.

Medical Causes of nutritional disorders include liver disease (cirrhosis), malabsorption from the intestine because of conditions such as Crohn's disease (inflammation of the ileum), and sprue (malabsorption). Other medical causes include genetic anomalies (such as phenylketonuria) and disorders that sometimes develop following gastrointestinal surgery, during which part of the intestine is removed or bypassed (such as gastroenterostomy). *See also* CIRRHOSIS; CROHN'S DISEASE; GASTROENTEROSTOMY; PHENYLKETONURIA; SPRUE.

Symptoms. The symptoms depend on which nutrient the body lacks. For example, lack of iron produces anemia and nail deformity (koilonychia); lack of calcium causes bone softening (osteomalacia); and deficiencies of protein, carbohydrate, and fat may result in weight loss. *See also* ANEMIA; KOILONYCHIA; OSTEOMALACIA.

Treatment. When there is no underlying medical problem, nutritional disorders can usually be cured or prevented by eating a varied, well-balanced diet. A health professional can help in planning an appropriate diet, if necessary.

When a nutritional disorder is well advanced and serious, it may be necessary to hospitalize a patient and supply that person with a diet of nutrient concentrates administered either through a gastric tube or intravenously.

Obesity. About 40 percent of the people in the United States are obese, and many more are overweight. It is easy to slip from being overweight to being obese. (*See* "Contents of selected foods" chart, page 650, for relevant figures.) The chance of dying before the age of 60 is 30 percent higher if a person is 10 percent overweight, and 150 percent higher if 20 percent overweight. Obese people run a high risk of coronary diseases. An obese person may develop diabetes, is likely to suffer from varicose veins and hemorrhoids, and by putting an unnatural load on joints can develop arthritis at an early age. An obese person may suffer from skin irritation in the folds of fat and is likely to develop breathing difficulties in later life.

Obesity is seldom caused by a glandular disorder. Obesity is usually caused by a person eating more than he or she is using up in energy. An obese person must reduce his or her caloric intake to a level below what the body needs, forcing it to use the excess stored in the tissues. Since obesity is a medical condition, it is wise to consult

Contents of selected foods

	Water %	Carbohydrate %	Fat %	Protein %	Fiber %
Meat					
Beefsteak	64	0	17	18	0
Liver	64	0	16	19	0
Pork	64	0	18	17	0
Chicken	63	0	16	20	0
Duck	53	0	30	16	0
Turkey	63	0	16	20	0
Cod	81	0	0.5	17.5	0
Mackerel	68	0	13.5	17.5	0
Dairy Products					
Butter	16	0.5	83	0.5	0
Cheese	40	2	29	25	0
Egg	74	1	12	12	0
Milk	87	4.5	4	3.5	0
Vegetables					
Broccoli	90	5	0.5	3.5	1
Cabbage	90	5	0.5	3.5	1
Carrot	89	8	0	1.5	1
Celery	93	3	0.5	2.5	1
Kidney bean	12	55	2	24	4.5
Lettuce	94	3	0.5	1.5	1
Mushroom	92	0	0.5	2	5.5
Onion	90	7	0	1.5	1
Pea	81	11	0.5	6	1.5
Potato	80	17	0	2	0.5
Tomato	95	3	0	0.5	1
Nuts and Cereals					
Almond	5	16	59	16	2
Barley	12	75	1.5	8	1.5
Corn	12	55	7	22	4
Peanut	5	16	59	16	2
Rice	12	77	1	7	1
Wheat	10	70	3	13.5	1.5
Fruit					
Apple	84	13	0.5	0.5	2
Banana	80	18	0.5	0.5	1
Grape	81	17.5	0.5	0.5	0.5
Grapefruit	88	10	0.5	1	0.5
Melon	93	5.5	0.5	0.5	0.5
Orange	88	10	0.5	1	0.5
Pear	84	13	0.5	0.5	2
Plum	85	13	0.5	1	0.5
Raisin	23	68	1	3	3
Strawberry	87	8	1	1	3

Vitamins and minerals

Food	Vitamin A	Thiamine	Riboflavin	Niacin	Vitamin C	Vitamin D	Iron	Calcium
Meat								
Beefsteak			●	●			●	
Liver	●	●	●	●	●	●	●	
Pork		●	●	●				
Chicken				●				
Duck				●			●	
Turkey			●	●			●	
Cod				●				
Mackerel	●		●	●		●	●	
Dairy produce								
Butter	●					●		
Cheese	●			●	●			●
Egg	●	●	●	●		●	●	●
Milk	●		●					●
Vegetables								
Broccoli	●		●		●		●	●
Cabbage	●				●			
Carrot	●				●			
Celery					●			
Kidney bean				●	●			
Lettuce	●				●			
Mushroom			●	●				
Onion					●			
Pea		●		●	●		●	
Potato		●			●			
Tomato	●				●			
Nuts and cereals								
Almond		●	●	●			●	●
Barley				●				
Corn								
Peanut		●	●				●	●
Rice				●				
Wheat		●		●			●	●
Fruit								
Apple					●			
Banana					●			
Grape					●			
Grapefruit					●			
Melon	●				●			
Orange		●			●			
Pear					●			
Plum					●			
Raisin							●	●
Strawberry					●			

Vitamins act as a catalyst in the proper functioning of the body's chemical processes. Inadequate intake of the necessary vitamins will result in nutritional disorders. Calcium and iron are needed in large quantities by the body for bone formation and healthy blood. Other minerals are needed in minimal quantities, and are therefore known as trace minerals. This chart shows the vitamin and mineral quantities in sample foods.

a physician who can recommend a carefully controlled diet that maintains all the essential nutrients. Without carbohydrates, for example, the body metabolizes proteins to use as energy—fats will be used for energy after three to four days. Excess ingestion of amino acids (broken-down protein) will be converted to fat. *See also* DIET, SPECIAL; WEIGHT PROBLEM; APPENDIX IV.

Nutritional disorders. *See* NUTRITION.

Nymphomania (nimf ə mā'nē ə) is an abnormally excessive desire in females for sexual intercourse. It may sometimes be associated with an inadequate personality development. Such a personality is unable to sustain a deep, lasting commitment and is able only to support superficial and transient relationships.

As with any compulsive behavioral pattern, this degree of sexual desire may be difficult to control. The sufferer may retain little self-control and feel powerless. Support groups for "sex addicts" now exist. They are based on the principles of groups such as Alcoholics Anonymous.

Nystagmus (nis tag'məs) is a disorder that involves involuntary eye movement. The eyes move rapidly and constantly from side to side or, less commonly, up and down or rotationally.

Q: *What causes nystagmus?*

A: Congenital nystagmus is usually the result of an inherited defect in the central nervous system. It often affects albinos. Nystagmus that occurs later in life may be the result of chronic eye strain. It can be an indication of a disorder of the organ of balance (such as labyrinthitis or Ménière's disease) or of the center in the brain associated with balance (caused by, for example, a brain tumor or a stroke). Other causes include motion sickness, drugs such as alcohol or barbiturates, and multiple sclerosis.

Q: *How is nystagmus treated?*

A: The treatment is directed at the cause, although there is no real treatment for congenital nystagmus.

See also LABYRINTHITIS; MÉNIÈRE'S DISEASE; MULTIPLE SCLEROSIS.

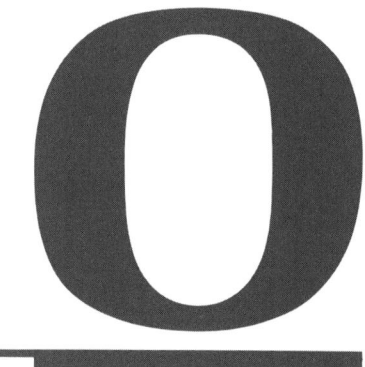

Obesity (ō bē′sə tē) is the condition of being overweight because of excess body fat. Strictly, the term obesity is used to denote a body weight that is 20 percent or more over the ideal weight as determined from the life insurance statistics for a person's age, build, sex, and height. The degree of obesity can be determined by measuring the thickness of the fat over the muscles of the back of the upper arm.

See also DIET, SPECIAL; NUTRITION; WEIGHT PROBLEM.

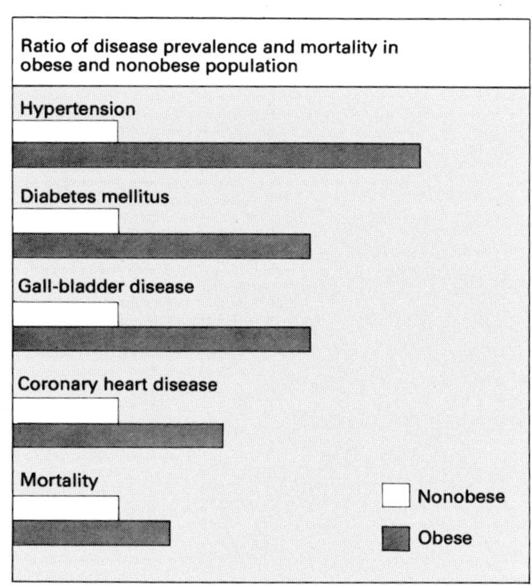

Obesity can seriously increase the incidence of certain diseases.

Obsession (əb sesh′ən) is a recurrent thought, image, or impulse that causes an individual significant anxiety, but can not be ignored or suppressed. These intrusive and uncontrollable thoughts and urges seem alien or unacceptable to the individual. Common obsessions include thoughts of violence, contamination, and doubt. These are different from the sometimes excessive worrying people might do when bothered by specific, real situations.

When a person's life becomes impaired by such obsessions, the usual psychiatric diagnosis is obsessive-compulsive disorder. It is the rarest form of anxiety disorder and very difficult to treat. A combination of medication and behavior modification is the most effective therapy. A careful evaluation is necessary to rule out other psychiatric problems, such as depression or alcohol/drug abuse.

See also ANXIETY; BEHAVIOR THERAPY.

Obstetrics (ob stet′riks) is the branch of medicine that is concerned with pregnancy, labor, and the period just after childbirth. Obstetricians also specialize in gynecology, which is the branch of medicine that is concerned with diseases of the female genital tract.

See also PREGNANCY AND CHILDBIRTH; PUERPERIUM.

Obstruction (əb struk′shən) is a blockage of an internal structure. If obstruction occurs in a muscular organ, colic-like discomfort is often the primary symptom because the muscles contract in an attempt to overcome the obstruction. A blood vessel may become blocked with an embolus or thrombosis. Obstruction of urine may be caused by a calculus (stone) or by various prostate disorders. The gall bladder may also become obstructed by a stone.

See also CHOLELITHIASIS; GANGRENE; HYDROCEPHALUS; INTESTINAL OBSTRUCTION; PROSTATE DISORDERS.

Occlusion (ə klü′zhən) is the state of being closed. This may be normal, as in the occlusion of the small gaps, called fontanels, in the skull of a baby, which occurs by the age of two years. An occlusion may also be abnormal, for example, when it is caused by an obstruction. Occlusion also refers to the way in which the teeth of the upper and the lower jaw fit together when the jaws are closed. (See illustration, page 654.)

See also MALOCCLUSION; OBSTRUCTION.

Occlusion of the upper and lower teeth ensures an efficient and strong bite.

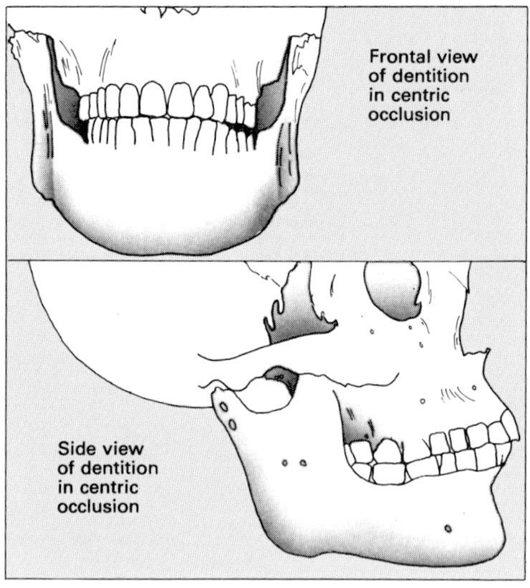

Occult blood (ə kult′) is blood that comes from an unspecified source, with signs and symptoms that are obscure and difficult to detect. For example, minor bleeding in the intestines may not produce any obvious changes in the feces, but a simple chemical test on the feces can detect the occult (hidden) blood. This test is extremely sensitive, and to guarantee accuracy, the patient must not clean his or her teeth for at least a day before the test or eat meat or other foods that contain blood.

It is important for people, 40 and older, to take this test on an annual basis.

Occupational hazard is any aspect of a person's work that may cause harm. Many occupations or ways of life carry the risk of particular diseases or disorders.

See also ALCOHOLISM; ANTHRAX; ASBESTOSIS; BACK PAIN; BENDS; BLACK LUNG; BRUCELLOSIS; BURSITIS, PREPATELLAR; BYSSINOSIS; CANCER; DEAFNESS; ELBOW, TENNIS; LEPTOSPIROSIS; MENISCUS; MERCURY (poisoning); OCCUPATIONAL MEDICINE; OSHA; PNEUMOCONIOSIS; PSITTACOSIS; RADIATION; RINGWORM; STRESS; WRITER'S CRAMP.

Occupational medicine is a branch of medicine concerned with the prevention, detection, and treatment of disorders that are related to the workplace. Occupational medicine is growing rapidly and is playing a leadership role in overall health promotion for workers.

Workers and managers in various industries are discovering that exposure to noxious chemicals and other substances can represent a health hazard. For example, the coal industry has undergone changes due to the finding that black lung disease is caused, in large part, by contact with coal dust. Workplaces are now being required by "right-to-know" laws to notify workers of potential work-related health hazards.

Occupational Safety and Health Administration. *See* OSHA.

Occupational therapy. *See* THERAPY, OCCUPATIONAL.

Odontitis. *See* PULPITIS.

Odynophagia (ō din ō fā′jē ə) is pain associated with swallowing. Difficulty with swallowing (dysphagia) may or may not be present. It may be caused by destruction of the mucous membrane, infection, chemicals, or motor disorders of the esophagus.

Oedipus complex (ed′ə pəs) is a psychoanalytical term for the sexual love of a son for his mother, often accompanied by feelings of jealousy toward the father. The female counterpart is the Electra complex.

See also COMPLEX; ELECTRA COMPLEX.

Olecranon (ō lek′rə non) is that part of the bone of the forearm (ulna) that sticks out at the back of the elbow. With the bone of the upper arm (humerus), the olecranon forms part of the elbow joint.

See also ELBOW.

Olfactory (ol fak′tər ē) signifies anything relating to the sense of smell.

See also SMELL, SENSE OF.

Olfactory bulb (ol fak′tər ē) is the enlarged end of the olfactory lobe, the portion of the brain responsible for the sense of smell. The olfactory nerve begins at this point.

See also NOSE.

Olfactory tract. *See* NOSE.

Oliguria (ol i gu′rē ə) is the excretion of abnormally small amounts of urine. It may occur as the result of a high fever, poisoning, or shock, or it may accompany excessive fluid loss from sweating, vomiting, or diarrhea. Oliguria may also be a symptom of a kidney disorder, such as nephritis, pyelonephritis, or uremia. If oliguria is present, a physician should be consulted.

See also KIDNEY DISEASE.

Omentum (ō men′təm) is a loose fold of the membrane (peritoneum) that hangs from the stomach and covers the front of the intestines. It protects the intestines and helps to seal any damage to the intestinal wall, thus helping to prevent infection.

Onchocerciasis (ong kō sėr sī'ə sis) is infestation with the parasitic worm *Onchocerca volvulus*. It occurs in regions of Africa, Mexico, and South America. The larvae of the worms are transmitted by the bite of infected black flies of the genus *Simulium*.

See also WORM.

Oncology (ong kol'ə jē) is the branch of medicine concerned with treatment of malignant tumors. It involves the development of improved surgical techniques, radiotherapy, and chemotherapy for the treatment of malignancies.

See also TUMOR.

Onychia (ō nik'ē ə) is inflammation of the nail bed.

See also PARONYCHIA.

Onychomycosis (on ə kō mī kō'sis) is a fungus disease of the nails, characterized by thickened, brittle, white nails. One form of onychomycosis is caused by the *Trichophyton* species of fungus and usually affects the toenails. The treatment is specific and prolonged.

See also RINGWORM.

Oophorectomy (ō ə fə rek'tə mē) is the surgical removal of an ovary. It is usually performed when there is a cyst or a tumor in the ovary. It may also be necessary if a fertilized ovum has become implanted on the ovary. If there is a benign cyst in the ovary, a partial oophorectomy may be performed. *See also* PREGNANCY, ECTOPIC.

When a woman over 45 years of age has a hysterectomy, both ovaries are usually removed. This is called a bilateral oophorectomy. A bilateral oophorectomy may also be performed as part of the treatment for breast cancer. In such cases, it is performed only when a physician considers that a reduction in the amount of estrogens (sex hormones produced by the ovaries) will slow the growth of the cancer.

See also HYSTERECTOMY; OVARY.

Oophoritis (ō ə fə rī'tis) is inflammation of an ovary. It may be caused by mumps or by virus organisms. It may be secondarily related to salpingitis (inflammation of the fallopian tubes) or an infection of the pelvis, such as appendicitis. The symptoms of oophoritis are pain and perhaps excessive menstruation. If associated with salpingitis, there is abnormal vaginal bleeding in about one-third of all cases. Most patients respond to treatment with antibiotics, but severe cases may require surgery.

See also OVARY.

Ophthalmia (of thal'mē ə) is any inflammation of the eye. Ophthalmia neonatorum affects newborns; the conjunctivae (membranes covering the eyeball and lining the inside of the eyelid) are contaminated during passage through the birth canal, usually because the mother has gonorrhea. Early treatment with antibiotic drugs can prevent the onset of blindness. All children receive preventive treatment following birth.

Sympathetic ophthalmia is inflammation of one eye as a reaction to injury of the other eye. This disorder is rare, and it can usually be treated with drugs. In certain cases, the injured eye must be removed to prevent blindness in the inflamed eye.

Electric ophthalmia is caused by prolonged exposure to intense light. Symptoms are pain, sensitivity to light, and excessive watering of the eyes.

See also CONJUNCTIVITIS; EYE DISORDERS; TRACHOMA.

Ophthalmic (of thal'mik) describes anything pertaining to the eye.

Ophthalmology (of thal mol'ə jē) is the branch of medicine dealing with the structure, functions, and diseases of the eye.

Ophthalmoplegia (of thal mō plē'jē ə) is paralysis of some or all of the muscles of the eye. It may affect one or both eyes and may come on gradually

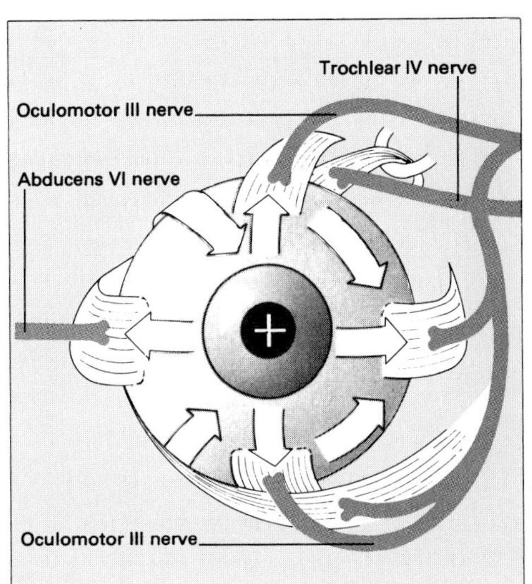

Ophthalmoplegia is a paralysis of some or all of the muscles of the eye. The condition can be caused by migraine, myasthenia gravis, thiamine deficiency, multiple sclerosis, or by polyneuritis. It can also be caused by pressure on nerves that supply the optic muscles.

or occur suddenly. External ophthalmoplegia is paralysis of the muscles on the outside of the eye that control movement of the eyeball. Internal ophthalmoplegia makes the pupil and lens flexible.

Q: *What causes ophthalmoplegia?*

A: Ophthalmoplegia may occur temporarily with migraine or the neuromuscular disorder, myasthenia gravis. It may also occur in an advanced or acute stage of thiamine (vitamin B_1) deficiency or with polyneuritis, particularly when associated with diabetes mellitus. It can also be caused by pressure on nerves that supply the optic muscles, whether from an aneurysm, brain tumor, or brain infection, such as meningitis. Ophthalmoplegia can also occur with multiple sclerosis. External ophthalmoplegia is a result of hyperthyroidism (thyrotoxicosis). Fatty tissues in the eye socket swell and press on the eyeball, which makes the eye bulge outward and eventually paralyzes the eye muscles.

Q: *What are the symptoms of ophthalmoplegia?*

A: Ophthalmoplegia in one eye causes double vision (diplopia), because the affected eye is immobile while the other eye is free to move. Internal ophthalmoplegia impairs vision because the pupil is unable to react to variations in the amount of light reaching the eye, and the lens is unable to focus at different distances.

Q: *How is ophthalmoplegia treated?*

A: The cause of the condition must be found and treated. However, if only one eye is affected, temporary relief from the distress of double vision can be obtained by wearing a patch over the paralyzed eye.

Ophthalmoscope (of thal′mə skōp) is an instrument for examining the eye. It has lenses of differing focal lengths, an internal mirror, and a light that shines a bright beam through the patient's pupil. Using an ophthalmoscope, a physician can examine the anterior chamber (containing the pupil and lens); the posterior chamber (containing the vitreous humor); and the retina, optic nerve, and the eye's network of blood vessels. The diagnosis of specific eye disorders and some physical conditions can be facilitated by the use of this instrument.

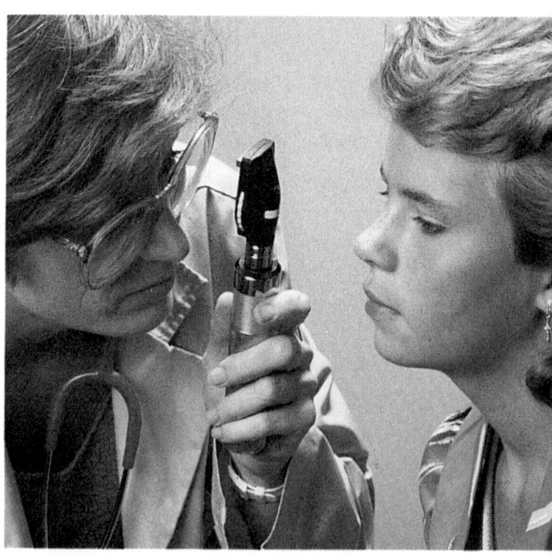

Through the use of an **ophthalmoscope,** a physician can examine the interior of the eye and diagnose eye disorders.

Opiate (ō′pē it) is any drug that contains opium or one of its derivatives—morphine or codeine.

Opisthotonus (op is thot′ə nəs) is a severe form of body spasm in which the back, head, and legs arch backward. It is a symptom of strychnine poisoning and severe forms of tetanus.

See also STRYCHNINE; TETANUS.

Opium (ō′pē əm) is the dried secretion from the unripe seed pods of the opium poppy *(Papaver somniferum)*. It has a bitter taste and a characteristic smell. Opium contains more than 20 alkaloid drugs, including morphine, codeine, and papaverine. The effects of opium are similar to those of morphine and, like morphine, it produces physical dependence. Heroin is a semisynthetic derivative of opium. The use of opium and its derivatives, morphine and codeine, is strictly controlled by law.

See also DRUG ADDICTION.

Opportunistic infection (op ər tü nis′tik) is an infection caused by normally harmless microorganisms in a host body, whose resistance has been lowered by such diseases as cancer, diabetes mellitus, or as the result of surgical procedures. An opportunistic infection is likely to occur if broad-spectrum antibiotics and/or antimicrobial drugs are used. The use of these drugs alters the natural balance of the microorganisms within the body. This allows the microorganisms to flourish, which often results in superinfection. A superinfection is an invasion of the body by microorganisms that are resistant to antibiotics. Nosocomial infections are those acquired during the patient's stay in the hospital. The sources of such infections include inadequately sterilized equipment, the patient's own body, and/or the hospital staff. Nosocomial infections are generally quite serious and resistant to antibodies.

Aplastic anemia, Hodgkin's disease, leukemia, and myeloma are characteristic of diseases that decrease the immune resistance of the host. Serious infections from *Candida, Staphylococcus,* and *Aspergillus* frequently occur. Corticosteroids and cytotoxic drugs also increase the susceptibility of the tissues to infection by lowering their resistance.

The use of broad-spectrum antibiotics and antimicrobial drugs, which may eventually result in infection, should be avoided if possible. The microorganisms of opportunistic infections are usually resistant to treatment with antibiotics. Treatment with antibiotics, therefore, tends only to control the symptoms of the infection, but does not cure the underlying cause.

See also ASPERGILLOSIS; CANDIDIASIS; FUNGAL INFECTION; STAPHYLOCOCCUS.

Optic (op'tik) describes anything concerned with the eye or vision.

Optician (op tish'ən) is a person who prepares lenses and fits glasses and contact lenses for patients as prescribed by an ophthalmologist or an optometrist.

See also OPHTHALMOLOGY.

Optic nerve. See EYE.

Oral (ôr'əl) describes anything pertaining to the mouth.

See also MOUTH.

Oral cholecystogram. See CHOLECYSTOGRAM, ORAL.

Oral contraception. See CONTRACEPTIVE, ORAL.

Oral surgery is surgery performed on the mouth. It may be performed by a dental surgeon to treat diseased or impacted teeth, gum disorders, or disorders of the underlying bone. Oral surgery is sometimes necessary in the treatment of a malocclusion.

An otolaryngologist specializes in disorders of the ear, nose, and throat and may perform oral surgery to treat cancer of the jaw, mouth, or tongue. Some disorders of the salivary glands, such as tumors or stones, may also require oral surgery. Fractures of the jaw and face usually require surgery.

See also MALOCCLUSION.

Orbit (ôr'bit) is the bony socket that surrounds and protects the eye. The socket is considerably larger than the eye and is filled with fatty tissue that cushions the eyeball and enables it to move freely. The six muscles that move the eye are attached to the orbit at one end and to the outer coat of the eyeball at the other. There is a hole at the back of the orbit through which the optic nerve and blood vessels pass.

See also EYE.

Orbit, blowout fracture of (ôr'bit). Blowout fracture of the orbit is a fracture of the orbital wall. It may cause entrapment of one or more of the external muscles of the eye. If this occurs, double vision results.

See also ORBIT.

Orchiectomy (ôr kə ek'tə mē), or orchidectomy, is the surgical removal of one or both testicles. It may be necessary if there is a tumor of the testicle, if the testicle has become twisted, or if the testicle is undescended. Bilateral orchiectomy (removal of both testicles) may be necessary for the treatment of prostate cancer. Testicles may be replaced with a synthetic substitute for cosmetic purposes.

See also CRYPTORCHIDISM; TESTIS.

Orchiopexy (ôr kē ō pek'sē) is the surgical restoration of an undescended testicle to its place in the scrotum. In some forms of this operation, the testicle and the scrotum are temporarily attached to the inner side of the thigh to ensure the descent is permanent.

See also SCROTUM; TESTIS.

Orchitis (ôr ki'tis) is inflammation of the testicles. It occurs most commonly as a complication of mumps, but it may also be caused by injury to the testicles or by the spread of infection from elsewhere in the body, such as occurs in epididymitis. One or both testicles may become enlarged and extremely pain-

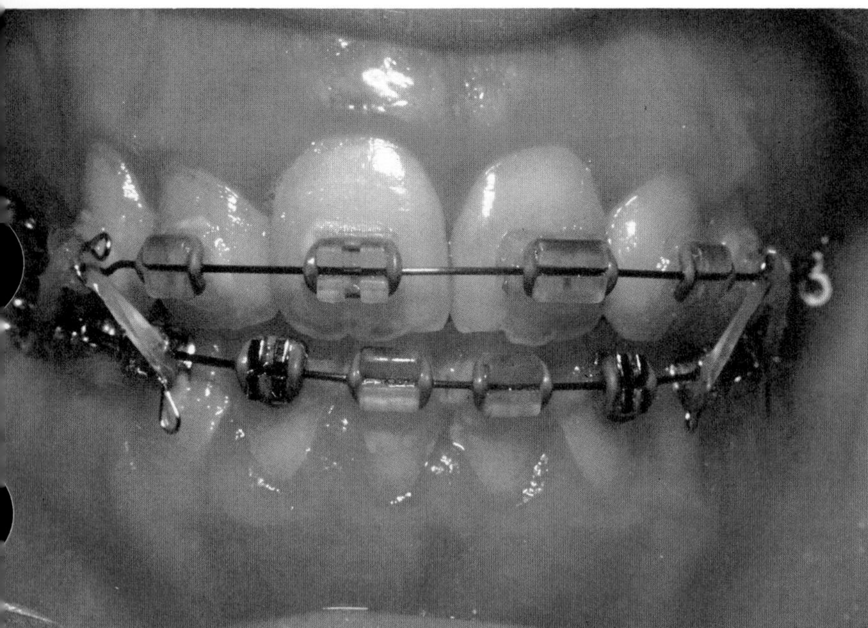

Orthodontic treatment may include the use of braces with plastic brackets to help adjust the movement of the teeth.

ful. Fever, nausea, and vomiting may also occur. These symptoms may be relieved by the application of ice packs and the use of painkillers. The scrotum should also be placed on an absorbent cotton pad, which should be supported by adhesive tape stretched between the thighs. The inflammation usually subsides within a few days.

See also EPIDIDYMITIS; MUMPS; SCROTUM; TESTIS.

Organ transplant. *See* TRANSPLANT SURGERY.

Orgasm (ôr′gaz əm) is a pleasurable sexual climax. In men, it is accompanied by the ejaculation of semen and by rhythmic contractions of muscles in the genital area. In women, orgasm is accompanied by contractions of the vagina.

An orgasm does not necessarily always occur during sexual intercourse. Continual failure to attain orgasm may be caused by psychological factors. Failure to achieve orgasm in the female does not mean that the woman is frigid. Chronic failure to achieve orgasm in the male is an abnormal condition requiring consultation with a physician.

See also SEXUAL INTERCOURSE.

Ornithosis. *See* PSITTACOSIS.

Oropharynx (ôr ə far′ingks) is one of the three divisions of the pharynx, the other two being the nasopharynx and the laryngeal pharynx. Also called the oral part of the pharynx, it extends from the soft palate, behind the mouth, to just above the hyoid bone. Below it are the palatine and lingual tonsils.

See also PHARYNX.

Orthodontics (ôr thə don′tiks) is the branch of dentistry that is concerned with the prevention and correction of abnormally positioned teeth. Orthodontic treatment is usually performed during childhood, when the jaw is still developing and when the gradual restraint of certain teeth can prevent development of a malocclusion.

See also DENTAL DISORDERS; MALOCCLUSION.

Orthodontist (ôr thə don′tist) is a dentist who specializes in the straightening or repositioning of the teeth.

See also ORTHODONTICS.

Orthopedics (ôr thə pē′diks) is the branch of medicine concerned with treating disorders of the bones and joints. Orthopedic surgery is the surgical prevention or correction of bone deformities. Orthopedics also includes the study and treatment of rheumatic disorders and disorders of muscles or nerves that may aggravate or cause orthopedic conditions.

See also BONE DISORDERS.

Orthopnea (ôr thop′nē ə) is the sensation of shortness of breath or difficulty breathing when in a horizontal position. When the patient assumes a vertical sitting or standing position, breathing becomes much easier.

Orthoptics (ôr thop′tiks) is a technique used to correct defects in the muscles that control the alignment of the eyes. It involves a set of eye exercises to coordinate the movements of the two eyes. Orthoptic training is beneficial in the treatment of strabismus (squint).

See also STRABISMUS.

Orthosis (ôr thō′sis) is an orthopedic appliance or apparatus used to support, align, prevent, or correct deformities or to improve the function of movable parts of the body.

Orthotic (ôr thot′ic) describes anything to do with orthotics, the use or application of orthoses to protect, to restore, or to improve functioning of the movable parts of the body.

See also ORTHOSIS; ORTHOTICS.

Orthotics (ôr thot′iks) is the field of knowledge related to the rehabilitation of injured or impaired joints or muscles through the use of an artificial support, known as an orthosis, when the affected bodily part itself is still present.

Osgood-Schlatter disease (oz′ gůd-shlat′tėr) is a common form of osteochondrosis seen in athletic adolescents. It is characterized by a painful swelling of the tibial tubercle, which is a bony outgrowth on the top of the shinbone just below the knee. This disorder is caused by chronic irritation or overuse of the quadriceps muscle, resulting in separation or inflammation of the tubercle. Pain and swelling are increased by any activity and exercise that stretches the leg.

Treatment includes the prevention of additional irritation during healing, which may necessitate the immobilization of the knee in a cast or complete bed rest. Any bone fragments found after healing will have to be surgically removed. The prognosis for Osgood-Schlatter disease is good, with remission usually occurring by age 18.

See also KNEE; KNEE DISORDERS; OSTEOCHONDROSIS.

OSHA (Occupational Safety and Health Administration) was established by Congress in 1970 ". . . to assure so far as possible every working man and woman in the nation safe and healthful working conditions and to preserve our human resources."

Among other things, the federal agency encourages both employers and employees to reduce hazards in the workplace; supports research; establishes training programs; sets and enforces standards; and analyzes and evaluates occupational health and safety programs of states.

Ossicle (os′ə kəl) is any small bone. The term usually refers to one of the three small bones in the middle ear: the malleus, incus, or stapes.

See also EAR.

Ossification (os ə fə kā′shən) is the formation of bone. It occurs normally during the development of a fetus, when bone is formed and replaces cartilage. It continues during childhood. The final stage in bone formation, the ossification of the growing ends of bones, occurs during adolescence.

Abnormal ossification may develop within tissues that have been damaged, particularly in muscles, ligaments, and sometimes tendons. Bone formation may occasionally occur in a frozen shoulder (a form of tendinitis) in the muscle of the shoulder blade, but is more frequent in metabolic disorders associated with raised calcium levels in the blood.

See also OSTEOGENESIS IMPERFECTA; SHOULDER, FROZEN.

Osteitis (os tē ī′tis) is inflammation of any bone. It causes periostitis, a swelling and local tenderness of the periosteum, the membrane that surrounds the bone. For practical purposes, osteitis and osteomyelitis can be considered to have the same causes and treatment.

See also OSTEOMYELITIS; PERIOSTEUM; PERIOSTITIS.

Osteitis deformans. *See* PAGET'S DISEASE OF BONE.

Osteoarthritis (os tē ō är thrī′tis) is a very common, chronic disorder involving the joints. It is a degenerative change in the joints and should properly be called osteoarthrosis, since it is not caused by inflammation. The degenerative changes take place because of the rubbing of the joint surfaces, causing a wearing away and disintegration of the tissues.

There is usually some additional factor that speeds up this process. The factors include unusual stresses on the joint, such as those resulting from obesity or bowleg; disorders that damage the joint cartilage, such as rheumatoid arthritis and osteochondritis (bone and cartilage inflammation); or damage to the joint surfaces from a fracture or torn cartilage. Other factors are disorders of the joint, such as congenital dislocation of the hip, and the slowing

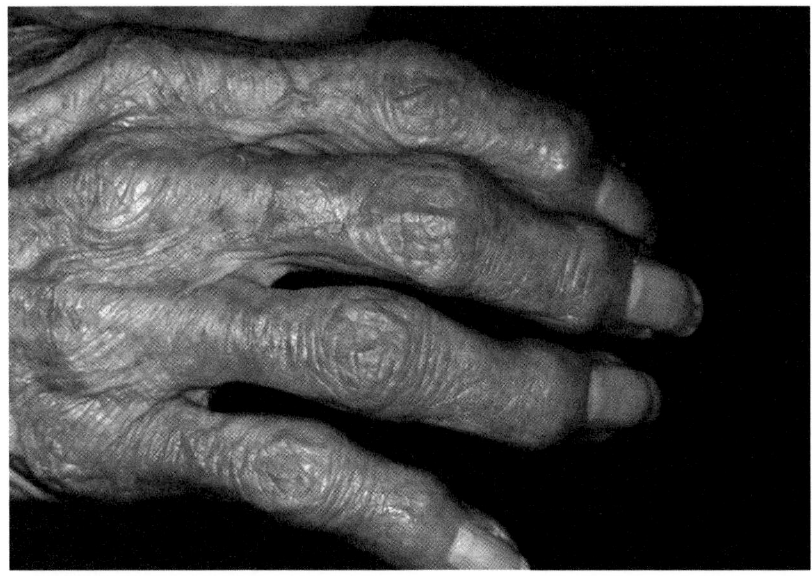

The effects of **osteoarthritis** are shown in this photograph of an arthritic hand. The finger and knuckle joints have degenerated.

down in old age of the normal repair processes.

Q: *Which joints are most likely to be affected by osteoarthritis?*

A: The joints that carry the body's weight are most likely to develop osteoarthritis. For example, repeated injuries to an athlete's hips, knees, or ankles are likely to result in osteoarthritis in those joints in later life. Repeated attacks of gout or of septic arthritis can also cause osteoarthritis.

Q: *What happens to the joint in osteoarthritis?*

A: The slippery cartilage that lines the joint surface is gradually worn away, exposing the underlying bone. The bone becomes smooth and its edges rough, with small areas of bony formation, known as osteophytes. The surrounding ligaments and membranes also become thickened because of the recurrent slight strains that occur in an osteoarthritic joint.

Q: *What are the symptoms of osteoarthritis?*

A: There is gradually increasing pain, with restriction of movement. The amount of pain varies from time to time; additional strains or unexpected movements make the condition worse. In most joints, this process is accompanied by a grating that can frequently be heard and usually felt. The joints may feel particularly stiff when getting up in the morning or after sitting for any length of time.

Q: *How is osteoarthritis diagnosed?*

A: A physician makes the diagnosis after an examination of the joint and confirming X rays. Swellings adjacent to the end joints of the fingers (Heberden's nodes) are common.

Q: *What is the treatment for osteoarthritis?*

A: Osteoarthritis is increasingly common with age. Treatment is directed toward improving general health and maintaining as normal a lifestyle as possible. The patient should lose weight, if necessary, and perform exercises designed to strengthen surrounding muscles and maintain movement of the joint when it is not bearing weight.

Total pain relief for osteoarthritis is rarely achieved. During the initial stages, aspirin or some other painkiller may be prescribed. Various antirheumatic drugs, such as Indocin®, Feldene®, and Clinoril®, may be used, but these sometimes produce gastric ulceration and, in rare cases, blood disorders. Milder antirheumatic drugs, such as ibuprofen, may also be prescribed. Heating pads may provide relief if a joint has become acutely painful. Frequent rest can help, too. If necessary, canes, crutches, or walking frames can be used.

Q: *Does surgery help in osteoarthritis?*

A: Yes. Several surgical procedures may be helpful for joints that are severely damaged. Arthrodesis, an operation to fuse the joint in one position, can be done to prevent further pain.

Other operations include removing some of the membranes around the joint or forming a new joint, as is done in treatment for hallux valgus deformities.

In recent years, total replacement of a joint has become possible by the insertion of a plastic and metal artificial joint. Hip replacement surgery is now widely available with good success; artificial joints have also been used in finger and knee joints.

See also ARTHRITIS, RHEUMATOID; ARTHRODESIS; GOUT; HEBERDEN'S NODES; OSTEOCHONDRITIS.

Osteoarthropathy (os tē ō är throp′ə thē) is any disease of the joints and bones. Usually, the joints become damaged as a result of some other disorder. For example, nerves in the joints, which normally give a sense of position and are responsible for the sensation of pain, may be affected by inflammation (peripheral neuritis).

Common causes of such conditions include tabes dorsalis (damage to the lower spinal cord); neuritis associated with diabetes mellitus; and syringomyelia, another spinal cord disease. Atherosclerosis of the arteries supplying the bone may cause destruction of the bone, especially at the hip joints. Repeated damage results in a thickening or enlargement of the joints, instability of movement, and osteoarthritis of the joint.

Chronic hypertrophic pulmonary osteoarthropathy is the medical term for clubbing of the fingers and toes in persons with chronic lung or heart disease.

See also CLUBBING; NEURITIS; OSTEOARTHRITIS.

Osteoarthrosis. *See* OSTEOARTHRITIS.

Osteochondritis (os tē ō kon drī'tis) is inflammation of bone and cartilage. In most cases, it leads to degeneration of these tissues. There are two forms of the disorder, osteochondritis dissecans and osteochondritis deformans juvenilis. Their causes are not known.

Q: *What are the symptoms of osteochondritis dissecans and how is it treated?*

A: The disorder usually affects young adults, who have recurrent attacks of mild pain, usually in the knee joint. Fluid in the area may increase, followed by sudden and recurrent locking of the joint.

The blood supply to the local bone and cartilage is most probably affected and causes a piece of cartilage and underlying bone to break off and move into the joint. This loose fragment causes the sudden locking and resulting pain.

The condition is usually diagnosed late. Bone and cartilage may heal if the joint is kept in a cast for eight to ten weeks. But an operation to remove the fragment is the best form of treatment.

Q: *What are the symptoms of osteochondritis deformans juvenilis and how is it treated?*

A: This disorder, also known as Perthes' disease, occurs in children. It usually affects the thoracic spine, the top of the thighbone (femur), the wrist, and the foot. The bone becomes softened and may easily be deformed by pressure or accident. The usual symptom is pain over the bone, and the damage can be seen via X ray. The disorder is relatively harmless, but may ultimately lead to osteoarthritis of the joint.

If the condition is diagnosed early, the joint can be rested in a cast so that further deformity does not occur. This is particularly important when the condition affects the hip joint.

See also OSTEOCHONDROSIS; PERTHES' DISEASE.

Osteochondroma (os tē ō kon drō'mə) is the most common of the benign (noncancerous) bone tumors. The condition is usually seen in young people between 10 and 20 years of age and may manifest itself with single or multiple tumors. The tendency to have multiple osteochondromas may be hereditary.

See also OSTEOMA.

Osteochondrosis (os tē ō kon drō'sis) is an abnormal condition of bone and cartilage formation in children. It involves temporary degeneration of tissue due to inadequate blood supply, followed by spontaneous regeneration.

See also OSGOOD-SCHLATTER DISEASE; OSTEOCHONDRITIS; PERTHES' DISEASE.

Osteogenesis imperfecta (os tē ə jən' ə sis im per fek'ta), also called fragilitas ossium or brittle bones, is an inherited disorder in which the bones are abnormally brittle and may break easily, often causing deformities. The condition may be associated with a blue coloration of the whites of the eyes and with chronic, progressive deafness.

A child with osteogenesis imperfecta usually dies early in life, shortly after birth. Those who do survive are usually physically deformed, but develop normally mentally, as long as there is no incidence of head trauma.

Osteology (os tē ol'ə jē) is the study of the structure and function of bones. It also involves the study of all the diseases and disorders that affect bones.

Osteoma (os tē ō'mə) is a benign (noncancerous) tumor of bone. It usually forms on the skull or long bones. Most osteomas cause local thickening of bone and do not produce any symptoms. They can be left alone or removed if they are unsightly or obstruct a blood vessel. But an osteoid osteoma, a rare benign tumor of bone, can cause severe and deep pain. It is treated by surgical removal of the tumor, which gives immediate relief from pain.

See also OSTEOCHONDROMA.

Osteomalacia (os tē ō mə lā'shə) is a softening of the bones in an adult, similar to rickets in children. In persons with osteomalacia, the basic structure of the bone remains unaltered.

Q: *What are the symptoms of osteomalacia?*

A: Common symptoms are aching and painful bones, as well as fractures. Softened bones may also bend under the weight of the body.

Q: *What causes osteomalacia?*

A: Osteomalacia is also called adult rickets because it usually results from a lack of vitamin D and calcium in the diet. Other causes include kidney failure and intestinal disorders.

Q: *How is osteomalacia diagnosed and treated?*

A: Diagnosis depends on bone X rays and blood tests to determine calcium and phosphorus levels. The possibility of conditions with similar symptoms, such as osteoporosis, hyperparathyroidism, and Cushing's syndrome, must first be eliminated.

See also OSTEOPOROSIS; RICKETS.

Osteomyelitis (os tē ō mī ə lī'tis), or osteitis, is an inflammation of bone, especially of the marrow. It is usually caused by a bacterial infection.

There are two kinds of osteomyelitis, acute and chronic. Children most commonly suffer from acute osteomyelitis. Chronic osteomyelitis usually follows an acute attack and rarely occurs on its own. It can, however, be caused by tuberculosis.

Q: *Why does acute osteomyelitis occur?*

A: In acute osteomyelitis, bacteria may be carried via the bloodstream from another area of infection to the bone. It may be the result of a septic tooth, a boil, or an ear infection. The infection can also reach the bone through an injury, such as an open fracture. There is frequently a history of recent minor injury or knocks to the affected bone. The growing end of the bone is the area most frequently infected.

Q: *What are the symptoms of acute osteomyelitis?*

A: Children may have several days of fever and general illness before suffering from local bone pain. In both adults and children, bone pain is followed by a sudden increase in temperature, sometimes with vomiting, and local tenderness of the bone, with painful movement of nearby joints. Swelling occurs and the skin becomes red.

Q: *How is acute osteomyelitis diagnosed and treated?*

A: X rays seldom help diagnosis in the early stages, but a white blood cell count shows the type of response the body is making to acute infection. A bone scan will confirm the diagnosis of osteomyelitis in the early stages of the disease, enabling a physician to begin treatment immediately. Massive doses of antibiotics, usually one of the penicillin drugs, are given for at least six weeks. An orthopedic surgeon may perform a bone biopsy to see if an abscess has formed on the bone. If an abscess is found, antibiotics are given and surgery is performed to remove the abscess. If pus has formed, it is sometimes necessary to drain the bone by drilling holes in it.

Q: *What are the symptoms and treatment of chronic osteomyelitis?*

A: The usual symptom is pain. The bone abscess usually discharges pus through the skin, although sometimes only pain and swelling occur over the bone and the patient has a mild fever. An X ray confirms the diagnosis and surgery is performed to remove any fragments of dead bone that may encourage continued infection. Complete cleansing of the area is

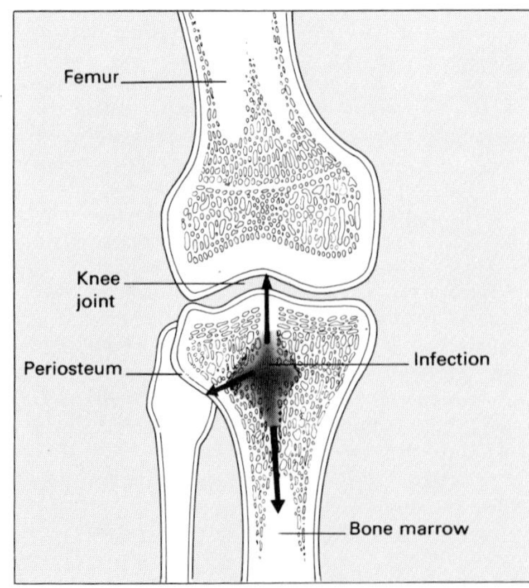

Osteomyelitis is an infection of the bone and bone marrow that can spread to the periosteum membrane, which covers the bone.

generally required. This is followed by antibiotic therapy.

Q: *What other forms of osteomyelitis may occur?*

A: Tuberculosis may spread to bone, primarily in the spine, producing a "cold" abscess in which there is painful swelling without heat or redness to the skin. The patient usually experiences a slight fever, loss of weight, and general malaise. The diagnosis is confirmed by a combination of X rays, blood tests, Mantoux test (a test for tuberculosis infection), and the examination of pus from the abscess.

Treatment consists of antitubercular drugs, possible splinting of the bone, and an operation to remove the abscess.

It is important that a search be carried out for other possible areas of tubercular infection, especially in the lungs and kidneys. Persons who have had contact with the patient, particularly children, must be examined to prevent spread of the disorder.

Osteopathy (os tē op′ə thē) is a system of medical practice that in addition to the traditional approaches to health care emphasizes the importance of the neuromusculoskeletal system in health and disease. The neuromusculoskeletal system includes the nervous system and the muscles and bones with their connecting tendons and ligaments.

Osteopathic physicians are trained to treat a wide variety of medical and surgical conditions and, when indicated, utilize various types of manipulative techniques on the muscles, tendons and bones.

Osteoporosis (os tē ō pə rō′sis) is a disorder in which both calcium salts and bone fabric are depleted. It is different from osteomalacia, in which only calcium is lost from the bone.

Normal bone consists of two layers, a compact, outer layer (cortical bone) and a porous, inner layer (trabecular bone). Osteoporosis attacks bones containing a large percentage of trabecular bone, including the vertebral column, the hips, and the wrist. The bones affected by osteoporosis are more fragile and prone to fracture.

Q: *What are the symptoms of osteoporosis?*

A: There may be no symptoms, but

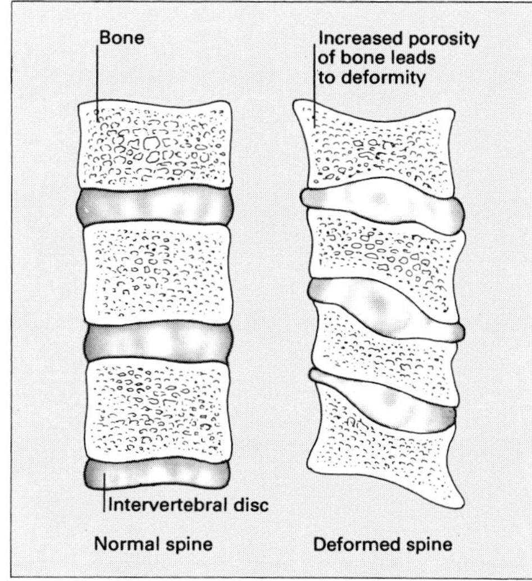

the individual may lose height because of a collapse of the vertebrae and suffer from increasing kyphosis (bending forward of the spine). There may also be a vague, generalized backache because the vertebrae, in becoming thinner, tend to compress the surrounding nerves. Bones fracture more easily, causing acute pain. Such severe pain is caused by a compression fracture of one of the vertebrae, commonly in the mid-spine. Other bones, such as the hip, may fracture more easily than usual in the elderly.

Q: *What causes osteoporosis?*

A: The cause is not precisely known. After about the age of 30, the body normally loses bone mass at a slow rate. In women, this rate of bone loss accelerates significantly after menopause. The presence of certain diseases, such as Cushing's syndrome (overactivity of the adrenal glands) and hyperparathyroidism (overactivity of the parathyroid glands), can further encourage osteoporosis.

Q: *How is osteoporosis diagnosed and treated?*

A: Osteoporosis is usually asymptomatic. Over many years a person may become shorter, with his or her back increasingly hunched forward. Ultimately, the person may experience severe back pain and require the use of a back brace for support.

A diagnosis of osteoporosis is usually confirmed by the person's

Osteoporosis weakens the bone and leads to deformities in weight-bearing bones, such as those in the spine.

physical appearance, the use of X rays to reveal that the bones are less dense than normal, and photodensitometry. Unfortunately, by the time these changes are observed, the bones have already lost over one-third of their original density. *See also* PHOTODENSITOMETRY.

Although the rate of bone loss can be dramatically slowed, there is no treatment at present that can reverse osteoporosis or increase bone strength.

Q: *Can osteoporosis be prevented?*

A: Yes. The best preventive steps are regular exercise; not smoking; adequate calcium in the diet (at least 3-4 glasses of milk per day, or the equivalent); and avoidance of fad diets and rapid weight loss. The best time to start these preventive measures is in the teen years, literally decades before osteoporosis occurs.

Physicians may prescribe calcium supplements, vitamin D, or female sex hormones (estrogens) to prevent osteoporosis, especially in women after menopause. Estrogens are particularly effective in preventing osteoporosis, but they may be harmful and therefore require close medical supervision. It is thought that estrogen treatment must be continued for many years, and possibly the rest of the woman's life, in order to maintain the beneficial effects. For these reasons, estrogens are not appropriate for every woman and should generally be taken only by women at increased risk for osteoporosis.

Osteosarcoma (os tē ō sär kō'mə) is a malignant (cancerous) bone tumor that usually arises on either side of the knee joint or on the upper end of the armbone. The disorder is most common in the first 20 years of life, but may occur at any age with Paget's disease of bone, in which the bones become thickened and soft.

Q: *What are the symptoms of osteosarcoma?*

A: There is local pain and swelling with an increased sensation of warmth, similar to that accompanying osteomyelitis (infection and inflammation of bone).

Q: *How is an osteosarcoma treated?*

A: Intensive radiotherapy is usually attempted first. If this fails, amputation of the affected limb must be considered. This operation is followed by chemotherapy to combat the spread of the tumor to the lungs and other tissues. These modern forms of medical treatment have improved life expectancy considerably. In the past, osteosarcoma was generally fatal.

See also OSTEOMA; PAGET'S DISEASE OF BONE.

Osteotomy (os tē o'tə mē) is an operation in which a bone is cut, enabling a surgeon to reposition it. An osteotomy may be performed to lengthen or shorten a leg, to correct bowed or bent legs, or to reset a fracture.

An osteotomy may be carried out in hip operations to alter the position of the thighbone and can be of help in the treatment of osteoarthritis of the hip. Total replacement of the hip joint with an artificial joint, however, is often more effective.

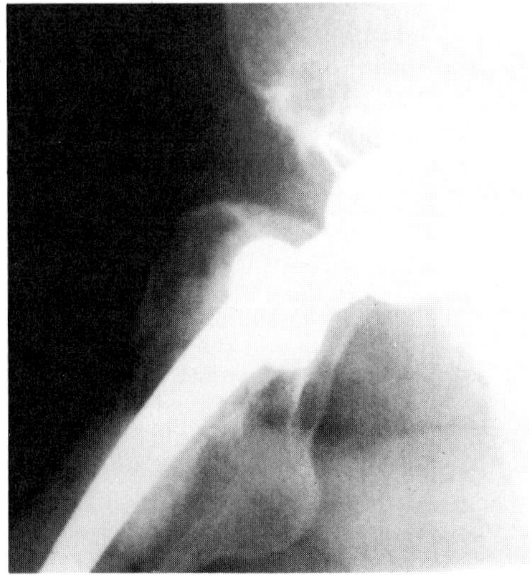

Osteotomy is a surgical procedure used to implant an artificial hip joint (white area) into the thighbone (white protrusion).

Otalgia. *See* EARACHE.

Otic preparation (ō'tik) is a substance used in the treatment of various ear conditions, such as otitis externa (inflammation of the outer ear).

Otitis (ō tī'tis) is inflammation of the ear. Inflammation of the outer ear is called otitis externa; inflammation of the middle ear is otitis media; and inflammation of the inner ear is called labyrinthitis. Infection of the external ear flap (pinna) may be caused by otitis externa or by any skin disorder.

Q: *What are the symptoms of otitis externa?*

A: The symptoms include itching, pain in the ear, a slight discharge, and deafness. Occasionally, the infection is localized and a boil forms. This condition is called furunculosis.

Q: *What causes otitis externa?*

A: It is often caused by a combination of bacterial and fungal infections. Such infections may result from scratching the ear, swimming, or excessive sweating. Otitis externa is more common in persons with eczema (an inflammation of the skin) and in those with diabetes mellitus.

Q: *How is otitis externa treated?*

A: The dead skin, pus, and wax should be removed by a physician. Antibiotics and antifungal preparations may be prescribed to treat the infection. In some cases, it may be necessary to pack special dressings into the ear until the infection is cured.

Q: *How can otitis externa be prevented?*

A: The ears should be kept dry by wearing earplugs when swimming. A physician may also advise the use of certain ear preparations after swimming. The ears should not be scratched.

Q: *What are the symptoms of otitis media?*

A: The main symptoms are severe earache, deafness, and fever. There is an accumulation of pus in the middle ear that may build up to such an extent that the eardrum ruptures, thereby releasing the pus and relieving the earache. Young children may also have diarrhea, abdominal pain, and vomiting.

Q: *What causes otitis media?*

A: It is most commonly caused by the spread of infection from the back of the nose, along the Eustachian tube, and into the middle ear. This may occur with the common cold, tonsillitis, or any infection that affects the upper part of the respiratory system, such as influenza, measles, or whooping cough. Less commonly, otitis media may be caused by sudden pressure changes, such as barotrauma, or by an infection, such as sinusitis. It may also occur after a tonsillectomy or following rupture of the eardrum.

As a result of infection, there is increased secretion from the membranes that line the middle ear. These secretions and the swollen membranes block the Eustachian tube and cause an increase in pressure, resulting in earache.

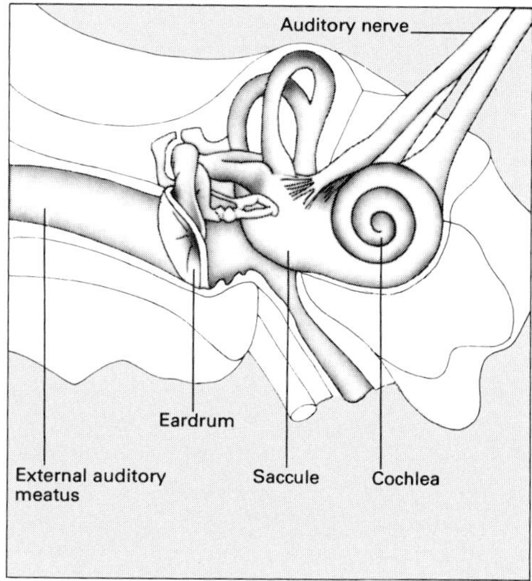

Otitis can affect any part of the ear, producing inflammation, swelling, and possible deafness.

Q: *How is otitis media treated?*

A: In the early stages of otitis media, before the eardrum has burst, antibiotics are usually effective. A physician may also prescribe painkillers and nose drops to relieve the congestion at the lower end of the Eustachian tube. Antihistamine, taken in the form of tablets, may help to relieve blockage. Occasionally, it may be necessary to open the eardrum surgically (myringotomy).

If the eardrum has ruptured or been surgically opened and is discharging pus, the ear should be kept clean and dry until the eardrum has healed.

Q: *Can otitis media cause any complications?*

A: Yes. The infection may spread to the mastoid portion of the bone, causing mastoiditis. Occasionally, treatment kills the infection, but the pus may be unable to escape because the Eustachian tube is blocked. Such obstructions may be caused by enlarged adenoids and may result in continued deafness. In adults, this condition may be treated by passing a tube into the nose and gently blowing clear the Eustachian tube. In children, it is usually treated with a myringotomy and the insertion of a drainage tube. If the obstruction is not treated, some degree of permanent hearing loss may result.

Q: *What precautions should be taken in connection with otitis media?*

A: Any minor respiratory infection may result in otitis media, particularly in children whose adenoids and tonsils become swollen. A physician may recommend that the adenoids be surgically removed (adenoidectomy).

A child who is recovering from otitis media should not be allowed to swim until a physician has given permission. It is also advisable to have the child's hearing tested after the condition has been treated to make sure that there is no residual deafness.

See also LABYRINTHITIS.

Otolaryngology. *See* OTORHINOLARYNGOLOGY.

Otology (ō tol′ə jē) is the branch of medicine concerned with the ear and the diagnosis and treatment of its diseases.

Otomycosis (ō to mī kō′sis) is a fungal infection of the outer ear. The condition may be associated with the fungal infection, candidiasis, or aspergillosis, a mold infection. Otomycosis is a form of otitis externa and is common following swimming or working in hot, humid conditions.

See also OTITIS.

Otorhinolaryngology (ō tə rī nō lar ing gol′ə jē), or otolaryngology, is the branch of medicine that is concerned with the diseases of the ear, nose, and throat and their treatment.

Otorrhea (ō to rē′ə) is a discharge from the ear. It may be caused by inflammation of the external ear (otitis externa) or by a perforated eardrum. Any ear discharge should be reported to a physician.

See also OTITIS.

Otosclerosis (ō tə skli rō′sis) is a disorder of the middle ear that leads to progressive deafness. It is one of the main causes of deafness in young adults. Otosclerosis is caused by the gradual build-up of extra bony tissue around one of the small bones (the stapes) in the middle ear. As a result, the stapes can not vibrate, thereby preventing the transmission of sound from the eardrum to the inner ear. In some persons with otosclerosis, there is a family history of deafness. Otosclerosis usually affects one ear before the other, but eventually both ears become affected.
See also DEAFNESS.

Q: *What are the symptoms of otosclerosis?*

A: The major symptom is progressive deafness. There may also be noises in the ear (tinnitus), and the whites of the eyes may be slightly blue in some patients. Progression of the symptoms may become worse during pregnancy.

Q: *How is otosclerosis treated?*

A: Surgery is usually the most effective treatment. Fenestration, which is an operation to make an artificial opening into the inner ear, has largely been replaced by stapedectomy, in which the fixed stapes bone is replaced. This operation usually restores normal hearing. However, the patient should avoid exposure to loud noises because the sound vibrations may damage the inner ear, since the protective action of the stapedius (middle ear muscle) is lost.

Otoscope (ō′tə skōp) is an instrument for examining the ear. It provides a light source that enables the ear canal and the eardrum to be examined.

Outer ear. *See* EAR.

Outpatient is a person receiving medical or surgical treatment in a hospital but not staying overnight. Due to escalating inpatient health care costs, hundreds of different operations, from cataract removal to hernia repair, are now being done on a one-day, outpatient basis. The typical patient may be a little doubtful at first about the wisdom of receiving surgery on an outpatient basis, but for most procedures this approach is quite safe. In addition, it avoids the cost and the possible risks of a hospital stay.

See also NOSOCOMIAL INFECTION.

Ovariectomy. *See* OOPHORECTOMY.

Ovaritis. *See* OOPHORITIS.

Ovary (ō′vər ē) is a female organ that produces ova (eggs) and sex hormones.

The two ovaries, each about the size of a walnut, lie on each side of, and usually slightly behind, the uterus. They are attached to the uterus and the inner walls of the abdomen by ligaments, which give them a mobility that many other internal organs do not have. This mobility may allow one or both ovaries to take up a slightly different position.

The surface of each ovary is covered by a layer of connective tissue called the tunica albuginea. Inside, the ovary is composed of many thousands of cells, which have the potential to form ova, and a firm structure of connective tissue. Before puberty, the ovaries are small and soft. During the child-bearing years, the ovaries are smooth and firm. After menopause, they shrink in size.

The ends of the fallopian tubes, with their long, finger-like extensions, overhang the ovaries. In a woman of child-bearing age, the fallopian tubes collect an ovum (egg) every month when it is released.

Q: *How many ova does an ovary produce?*

A: The ovaries produce one mature egg each month throughout the fertile life of a woman, beginning at menarche (the start of menstrual periods) and ending at menopause (the end of periods). During this time, the ovarian tissue is under the regular rhythmical control of hormones from the pituitary gland at the base of the brain. *See also* MENSTRUATION; OVULATION.

Q: *What disorders can affect an ovary?*

A: Inflammation of the ovaries (oophoritis) usually accompanies salpingitis (infection of the fallopian tubes), but may also result from mumps.

Tumors of the ovary are frequently cysts and occur in women over 35 years of age. About 95 percent of these tumors are benign (noncancerous). In younger women, a follicle may sometimes develop into a cyst and be discovered during a routine gynecological examination. It is usually worth waiting to see if the cyst is still present after menstruation. In women nearing menopause, an ovarian tumor or cyst is more likely to be malignant.

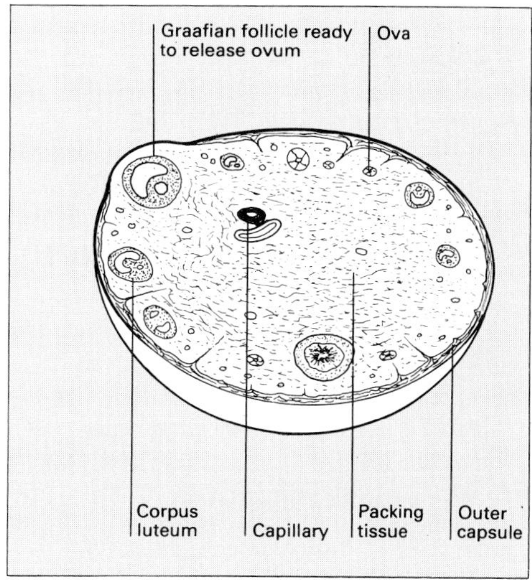

Q: *What symptoms are caused by an ovarian tumor or cyst?*

A: Frequently, there are no symptoms, unless the tumor has grown so large that it causes abdominal swelling or presses on the bladder to cause frequent passing of urine.

Ovarian tumors are commonly discovered during a routine gynecological examination. They seldom cause pain unless they twist or are malignant (cancerous) the cancer having already spread to involve adjacent tissues.

Cysts can be caused by an imbalance of the hormones from the pituitary gland, so that the ovary is subjected to a constant abnormal stimulus. This may produce a condition in which there is infertility, infrequent menstruation, and an abnormal growth of body hair (Stein-Leventhal syndrome).

Q: *How is an ovarian tumor treated?*

A: An examination of the inside of the abdomen with a lighted tube (laparoscopy), an X ray, ultrasound scanning, or exploratory surgery may be done to confirm the presence of an ovarian tumor. Such examinations may confirm that the tumor is neither a fibroid (a benign tumor of connective tissue) nor a swelling of a fallopian tube that sometimes follows salpingitis. A special blood test, CA 125, may indicate the presence of a malignant ovarian tumor.

If an ovarian tumor is found, the ovary is generally totally or par-

An **ovary** produces many ova (eggs), one of which is released during the middle of each menstrual cycle.

tially surgically removed (oophorectomy).

Q: *Can ovarian tumors or cysts produce complications?*

A: Yes. A cyst may occur in early pregnancy because of an increase in the size of the corpus luteum (a small structure in the ovary) and this may occasionally remain, causing problems of obstruction later in pregnancy.

A tumor can cause the ovary to twist on its ligaments, resulting in severe abdominal pain. There may also be abdominal pain if the cyst ruptures or if there is bleeding into the cyst.

Overweight. *See* WEIGHT PROBLEM.

Ovulation (ō vyə lā'shən) is the release of a mature ovum (egg) from an ovary. It occurs about every 4 weeks in the middle of the menstrual cycle, approximately 14 days before the start of the next menstrual period. After ovulation, the ovum passes along a fallopian tube to the uterus.

The development of an ovum is under hormonal control. A follicle-stimulating hormone (FSH) from the pituitary gland stimulates the ovum to mature within the ovary. On approximately the fourteenth day of the menstrual cycle, there is a sudden increase in the amount of luteinizing hormone (LH), and ovulation occurs.

See also MENSTRUATION.

Ovum (ō'vəm) is a mature female reproductive cell, also known as an egg. Ova are formed in the ovaries, pass down the fallopian tubes, and then enter the uterus. Usually, one ovum matures each month, although not necessarily in alternate ovaries. During sexual intercourse, if a sperm fertilizes the ovum, it develops into an embryo. If the ovum is not fertilized, it degenerates and passes out of the body at menstruation.

See also OVARY.

Oxycephalic (ok sē se fal'ik) describes the shape of a skull in which the top part appears unusually high and pointed. A newborn baby's head is often slightly pointed because of the molding of the skull during childbirth, but it returns to a normal shape within a few weeks.

An oxycephalic skull may also occur as a congenital anomaly, which can be associated with syndactyly (webbing of the fingers) or other abnormalities. The anomaly is caused by the skull bones joining together earlier than normal. It can be corrected surgically to prevent the possible development of mental retardation or blindness.

See also SYNDACTYLY.

Oxygen (ok'sə jən) is an odorless, colorless gas that makes up about 20 percent of normal air. It is an essential component for respiration in humans and animals.

See also OXYGEN THERAPY; RESPIRATION.

Oxygen tank (ok'sə jən) is a machine that holds and distributes oxygen to patients suffering from respiratory problems. The tank can be of therapeutic use to patients suffering from chronic lung disease and abnormal heartbeats and pulse rates—conditions often associated with a lack of oxygen.

Oxygen tent (ok'sə jən) is a pliable, plastic sheet held by a frame above and below the mattress to produce an enclosed atmosphere. Humidified oxygen is blown into the tent, and the patient moves without restriction in an atmosphere containing a much higher proportion of oxygen than normal.

Oxygen tents are no longer widely used. Physicians, however, continue to employ them for the treatment of croup (an acute breathing disorder) in children.

See also CROUP.

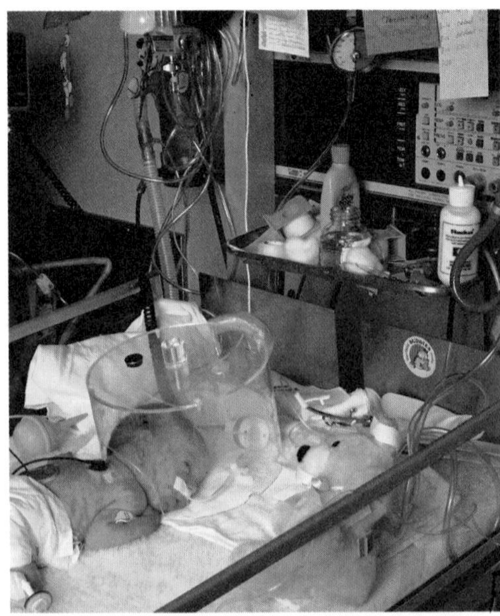

An **oxygen tent** is sometimes used in the treatment of an infant with an acute respiratory tract infection.

Oxygen therapy (ok′sə jən) is the administration of oxygen to patients. Oxygen gas is supplied from a cylinder that has a valve to allow the release of oxygen at low pressure.

Q: *What disorders are treated using oxygen therapy?*

A: Any condition that causes decreased transfer of oxygen to the blood in the lungs may be helped by oxygen therapy. These conditions include heart failure; reduced circulation, as occurs in acute shock and heart attack; pneumonia; and chronic bronchitis with emphysema. Oxygen is often given to newborn babies to assist their respiration in the first few minutes after birth.

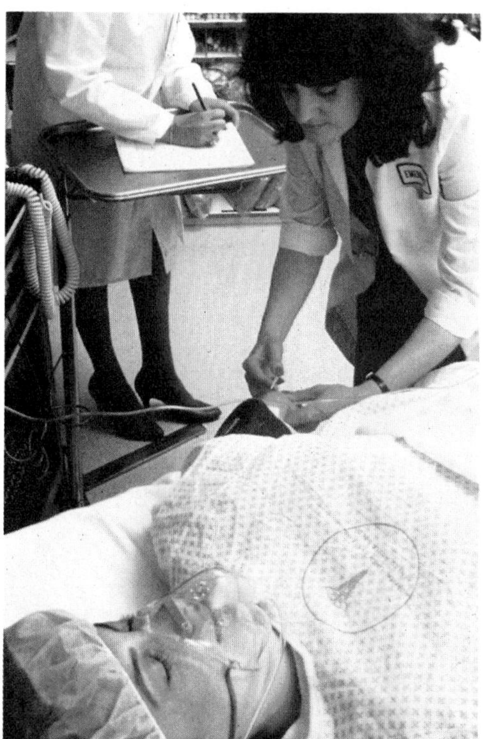

Oxygen therapy is often administered immediately prior to surgery via a mask that is placed over a patient's nose and mouth.

Q: *How is oxygen therapy given?*

A: Oxygen is commonly given through a mask that fits over the patient's nose and mouth. An alternative and more comfortable way is to administer oxygen through small plastic tubes inserted into each nostril.

Hyperbaric or high-pressure oxygen therapy is administered in centers that have a special chamber in which oxygen pressure can be increased to about three times normal. It is used in the treatment of gas gangrene, carbon monoxide poisoning, and in radiotherapy treatment for cancer.

Q: *Are there any other situations in which oxygen is used?*

A: Yes. Oxygen is administered routinely in most operations as an aid to anesthesia. It enables the anesthetist to give a larger dose of an anesthetic gas, such as nitrous oxide, without the risk of anoxia (lack of oxygen).

Q: *Are there hazards in using oxygen?*

A: Under medical control there are few hazards. However, the condition of retrolental fibroplasia in premature infants is caused by high oxygen concentration. Also, oxygen toxicity is a hazard for both adults and children when a high concentration of oxygen prevents the correct ventilation of the lungs.

Oxyhemoglobin (ok si hē mə glō′bin) is a combination of hemoglobin (the oxygen-carrying protein in blood) and oxygen. Hemoglobin combines with oxygen in the lungs, and the resultant oxyhemoglobin carries oxygen to the tissues. Oxyhemoglobin gives the bright red color to arterial blood.

See also BLOOD CELL, RED.

Oxytocin (ok si tō′sin) is a hormone that is produced in women by the hypothalamus in the brain and is stored in the rear lobe of the pituitary gland. It stimulates the uterus to contract during childbirth and also stimulates the breasts to produce milk (lactation). A baby sucking at the nipple causes oxytocin to be released automatically, which in turn increases lactation.

Oxytocin can be synthesized. Synthetic oxytocin may be given intravenously to induce labor. This is usually done only when labor is unusually slow. Administration of the drug is carefully supervised by an obstetrician. Induction of labor by this method is usually a safe procedure if carried out by an experienced obstetrician. Rarely, however, labor may not begin, or, if too much oxytocin is given, the contractions of the uterus may be too strong and may endanger the baby.

Oxyuriasis. *See* ENTEROBIASIS.

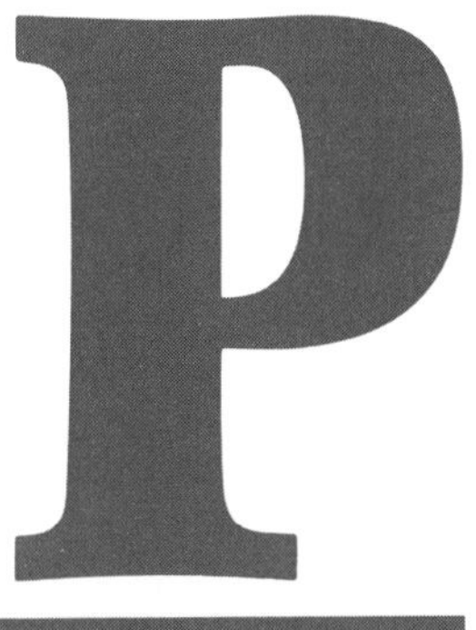

Pacemaker, artificial (pās′mā kər). An artificial pacemaker is an electronic device that produces an electrical current to stimulate regular contractions of the heart muscle. The pacemaker's generator and batteries are placed under the skin, usually in the right chest wall, and wires are passed to the heart.

A pacemaker may be used temporarily during heart surgery; following a cardiac infarction, when an irregular heartbeat is causing episodes of dizziness or faintness; and in some forms of heartblock when the heart's own electrical current is not being conducted normally.

Pacemaker, natural (pās′mā kər). A natural pacemaker is the specialized heart tissue, near the top wall of the right auricle, that sends out the rhythmic impulses that regulate the contractions of the heart. One part of this system, the sinoatrial or S-A node, has the job of starting each heartbeat, setting the pace, and causing the contraction of the heart muscle. It has been called the "pacemaker" of the heart.

Pacifier. See BABY CARE.

Paget's disease of bone (paj′its), or osteitis deformans, is a bone disorder of unknown cause in which there is a slow progressive thickeniong of several bones, most often the pelvis, the lower limbs, and the skull. Elderly persons are most commonly affected. Paget's disease of bone is not related to Paget's disease of the nipple.

Q: *What are the symptoms of Paget's disease?*

A: There may be thickening of the skull, and the leg bones may bend because of gradual softening as well as thickening. Pain may be noticed in the legs. The diagnosis is commonly made during a routine examination of an elderly person or from the X-ray examination of some other condition.

Q: *What is the treatment for Paget's disease?*

A: Paget's disease is local and frequently asymptomatic, therefore treatment is not necessary in many cases. Anti-inflammatory drugs, such as aspirin and indomethacin, are useful for relief of pain. If given in large enough doses, these drugs may also lessen the disease activity.

Drugs such as calcitonin and disodium etidronate help to suppress bone loss and subsequently produce a decrease in bone formation and pain. Cytotoxic drugs may be given to patients with a severe case of the disease or who show no response to other treatments.

Patients with Paget's disease involving the hip that have not received satisfactory relief from drug therapy may benefit from total hip replacement.

Q: *Are there any complications of Paget's disease?*

A: Yes. Bones affected by Paget's disease fracture more easily than others and, rarely, form osteosarcomas.

See also BONE DISORDERS; MYELOMA; OSTEOPOROSIS; OSTEOSARCOMA.

Paget's disease of the nipple (paj′its) is a rare type of cancer of the mammary ducts. It begins superficially in the ducts, causing the nipple to become red and crust-like. If the condition is discovered and treated before it penetrates beyond the ducts, the survival rate is very high. Therefore, any crust or rash on the nipple should receive immediate medical attention. The treatment is the same as for other types of breast cancer.

See also CANCER.

Pain is a sensation of physical discomfort, mental anguish, or suffering caused by aggravation of the sensory nerves. Pain is most often a symptom of injury, inflammation, or pressure.

Many pains can be relieved with commercial preparations. However, if a pain persists, a physician should be consulted. Most severe pains can be treated with regulated doses of strong analgesics (painkilling drugs). Chronic pain, however, generally does not respond to even very potent analgesics. Chronic pain can be found in some patients with cancer, diabetes, and other illnesses, and requires a comprehensive approach that includes medication, physical rehabilitation, and psychological support.

See also ANESTHETIC; COLIC; HEADACHE; HYPERESTHESIA; HYPESTHESIA; MIGRAINE; TIC DOULOUREUX.

Painkilling drug. *See* ANALGESIC.

Pain, referred. Referred pain is an acute sensation felt at a body location other than the location of the diseased or injured part of the body actually causing the pain. The pain of a heart attack, for example, may be referred to the jaw.

Palate (pal'it) is the roof of the mouth. It consists of two parts. The front part, the hard palate, is made up of the base of the two upper jawbones (maxillae) and the palatal bones of the skull. The back part, the soft palate, is fleshy and forms, at its midline, a small projection (the uvula). The soft palate consists of muscle. The whole palate is covered with a mucous membrane.

See also CLEFT PALATE.

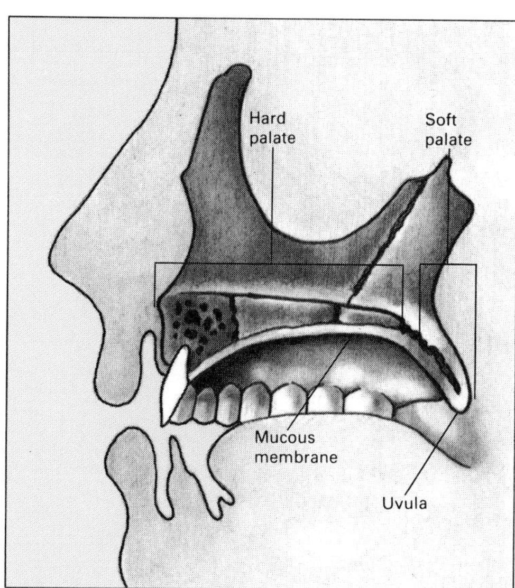

Palate, the roof of the mouth, is composed of hard, bony tissue in front, and soft, muscular tissue in back.

Palate, cleft. *See* CLEFT PALATE.

Paleness. *See* PALLOR.

Palliative (pal'ē ā tiv) is a drug or a treatment that relieves the symptoms of a condition without producing a cure. An example of palliative therapy is the use of radiotherapy to treat an inoperable lung cancer.

Pallor (pal'ər), or paleness, is a lack of normal skin color. It may result from fatigue, cold, low blood pressure (hypotension), or constriction of the blood vessels in the skin. Pallor may also be a symptom of various disorders, such as anemia, Cushing's syndrome, and hypothyroidism. The pallor of those who are ill is usually caused by the loss of the slight skin pigmentation that normally develops from exposure to the wind and the sun.

Palm is the front part of the hand that extends from the wrist to the bases of the fingers.

See also HAND.

Palpation (pal pā'shən) is a diagnostic technique in which the hands are used to make a physical examination of a part of the body. An example of this method is self-palpation of the breasts, which is recommended to women as a way of detecting a lump in the breast while it is still in the early stages of development and therefore easier to treat. A breast self-examination should be conducted once a month, 7 to 10 days after the onset of menstruation. Any irregularities in texture or consistency should be reported to a physician.

See also BREAST EXAMINATION.

Palpitation (pal pə tā'shən) is a rapid, violent, regular or irregular heartbeat. Palpitations are most commonly caused by anxiety, fear, excessive smoking, or by drinking too much coffee. They may also be caused by heart disease, anemia, and hyperthyroidism. Patients experiencing palpitations should consult a physician.

See also HEART DISEASE.

Palsy (pôl'zē) is the lessening or loss of power to feel, to move, or to control motion in some part of the body. It is a condition of some medical disorders.

See also BELL'S PALSY; CEREBRAL PALSY; PARALYSIS; PARKINSON'S DISEASE.

Pancreas (pan'krē əs) is a large, soft, irregular gland about 5 to 6 inches (12-15cm) long. It is located on the back wall of the abdomen, behind the stom-

The **pancreas** produces enzymes essential for digestion. These enzymes flow through the pancreatic duct into the duodenum portion of the small intestine.

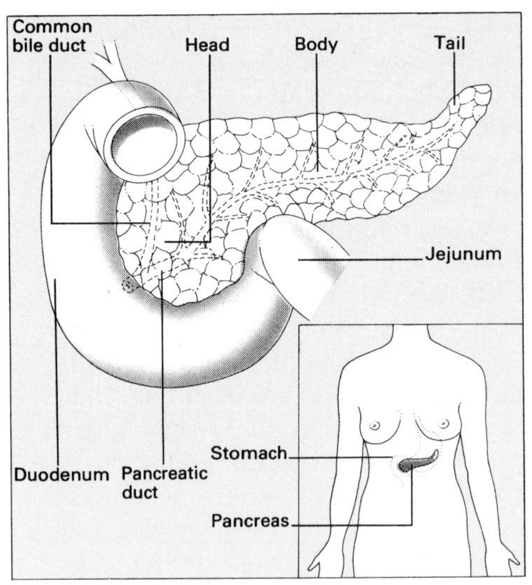

ach, and extends horizontally from the duodenum to the spleen. The area next to the duodenum is the thickest part of the pancreas and is commonly called the head. The pancreas tapers through the middle part, the body, before ending at the thinnest part, the tail, adjacent to the spleen. The pancreas has a large blood supply, mainly from the splenic artery, as well as many nerves from the autonomic nervous system.

Two ducts, the main pancreatic and accessory pancreatic ducts, join together and leave the head of the pancreas to join with the common bile duct just before it penetrates the duodenal wall, forming the ampulla of Vater, protruding into the duodenum.

Q: *What are the functions of the pancreas?*

A: The main part of the gland produces enzymes essential for digestion. Also lying within the structure of the pancreas are many microscopic areas, the islets of Langerhans, which are part of an endocrine gland that manufactures the hormones insulin and glucagon. Lack of insulin and/or excess glucagon can result in diabetes mellitus.

Pancreatic juice contains enzymes, activated by intestinal juice, that digest proteins, carbohydrates, and fats. The pancreatic enzymes trypsin and chymotrypsin digest protein; amylase digests starches and other carbohydrates; and lipase changes fats into glycerol and fatty acids. Pancreatic juices are produced partly in response to nervous stimulation, but mainly as a reaction to hormone secretion in the upper part of the small intestine. This hormone secretion is activated, in turn, by the presence of food in the stomach.

See also CYSTIC FIBROSIS; DIABETES MELLITUS; INSULIN.

Pancreatin (pan′krē ə tin) is a preparation made from the pancreatic enzymes of animals. Pancreatin tablets are prescribed for patients who are unable to digest food properly because of an insufficient amount of natural pancreatic secretions. This deficit may be caused by disorders of the pancreas, for example, cystic fibrosis or pancreatitis.

See also CYSTIC FIBROSIS; PANCREATITIS.

Pancreatitis (pan krē ə tī′tis) is an inflammation of the pancreas. It may be acute or chronic.

Q: *What are the symptoms of acute pancreatitis?*

A: The symptoms usually include severe upper abdominal pain, often accompanied by backache, vomiting, and fever with the onset of shock. The pain may continue for several days or even weeks before gradually lessening. Concentration of the enzyme amylase is frequently increased in the blood and this, along with a high white blood cell count, usually suggests acute pancreatitis.

Q: *What causes acute pancreatitis?*

A: The main cause of acute pancreatitis in the United States is alcoholism. Infection of the gall bladder and bile ducts (cholecystitis) is another frequent cause. Acute pancreatitis also can be associated with the passage of a gallstone into the duodenum, causing a temporary blockage of the pancreatic duct and back pressure of the enzymes. The pancreatic cells may be damaged and become inflamed. This may occur after abdominal surgery, particularly on the stomach or gall bladder. Viral infections, especially mumps, may infrequently trigger an attack of acute pancreatitis.

Q: *How is acute pancreatitis treated?*
A: Treatment includes intravenous infusions, evacuation of the stomach, and large doses of painkilling drugs, until the condition improves. Disturbances in the salts, particularly calcium, is probable, so calcium may be added to the infusion. Insulin may have to be given if there is an acute onset of diabetes mellitus. Antibiotics may be administered if there is evidence of bacterial infection.

Acute pancreatitis may recur or chronic pancreatitis may develop. It can also be fatal. This is especially true in hemorrhagic pancreatitis, which is fatal in 90 percent of all cases.

Q: *What are the symptoms of chronic pancreatitis?*
A: The main symptom is either intermittent or continuous upper abdominal pain of varying intensity, often accompanied by backache. During the moments when pain is most severe, there may be nausea and vomiting. Continued symptoms, caused by increasing damage to the pancreas, reduce the output of the digestive enzymes. This may result in the malabsorption of food, with excessive fat in the feces (steatorrhea). Some patients develop diabetes mellitus.

Q: *What causes chronic pancreatitis?*
A: Chronic pancreatitis may occur as a milder form of acute pancreatitis. It is also associated with chronic cholecystitis or, less commonly, cancer in the pancreatic duct.

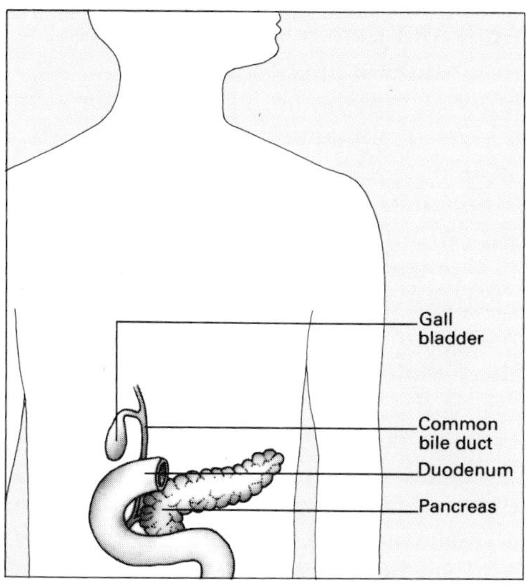

Pancreatitis is frequently associated with an infection of the gall bladder and the common bile duct.

Q: *How is chronic pancreatitis treated?*
A: Treatment may include removal of the gall bladder (cholecystectomy) if gallstones are thought to be the cause. Most importantly, the patient must avoid drinking alcohol. Abstention usually is followed by loss of pain and improvement in general health. A low-fat diet may be necessary, and pancreatin may be given to help digestion. Vitamin supplements, especially of folic acid and vitamins A, D, B_{12}, and K, are particularly important if malabsorption is taking place.

See also PANCREATIN.

Pandemic (pan dem′ik) describes any disease, such as malaria, that affects many people over a large region or continent. A disease that is pandemic is more widespread than one that is epidemic.

See also EPIDEMIC.

Panencephalitis, subacute sclerosing (pan en sef əl ī′tis, sub ə kyüt′ skler ōz′ing). Subacute sclerosing panencephalitis (SSPE) is an inflammation of the brain. It is a rare childhood disease, usually affecting boys under 12 years of age. The condition is believed to be caused by a slowly developing measles virus, which follows recovery from a previous measles infection. Immunosuppressants, interferon inducers, and antiviral drugs are used in treatment, but the recovery rate from SSPE is very low.

Panic (pan′ik) is an irrational fear affecting an individual or a whole group of persons, so that they lose control of their rational faculties. It is characterized by extreme anxiety or even terror.

See also PANIC ATTACK.

Panic attack (pan′ik), also known as anxiety attack, is an uncontrollable and sudden reaction, both psychological and biological, characterized by intense anxiety or terror and various physical symptoms. These latter usually include a combination of shortness of breath, excessive perspiration, trembling throughout the body, dizziness, draining of color from the face, stomach cramps, and a feeling of impending doom.

The attacks vary in duration and frequency, depending on the individual. They usually occur outside the home in places such as stores and restaurants and while driving. If the condition is untreated, the sufferer can develop a fear of leaving the home (agoraphobia). Treatment often involves medication to relieve the anxiety symptoms along with therapy aimed at helping patients cope with anxiety and stress in their lives. A thorough medical evaluation is necessary to rule out other psychiatric problems, such as depression.

See also DEPRESSION.

Panophthalmitis (pan of thal mī′tis) is an inflammation of the entire eye. It can be a complication of any serious eye disorder, such as choroiditis, or result from infection following an eye injury. Panophthalmitis is a painful condition that requires immediate treatment or blindness may result.

Papilla (pa pil′ə) is a small protuberance from the surface of a tissue. Papillae occur in many parts of the body. They are particularly numerous on the surface of the tongue, where specialized papillae contain the taste buds.

Papilledema (pap ə lə dē′mə) is an eye disorder in which the optic nerve is swollen and inflamed at the point where it joins the eye. The causes include raised pressure within the brain, sometimes triggered by a tumor or infection; retrobulbar neuritis (inflamed optic nerve), which can be caused by multiple sclerosis; and diffused edema (swelling) of the retina involving the optic nerve, which can be caused by severe hypertension (high blood pressure).

Treatment of papilledema is directed at the cause.

Q: *What are the symptoms of papilledema?*

A: Blurred vision is the most common symptom. There may be fleeting loss or dimming of vision (amaurosis fugax) occurring for up to 10 minutes. The vision defects are warning signs of partial blindness that may follow rapidly, sometimes within 24 hours. Without treatment, the patient's vision deteriorates rapidly.

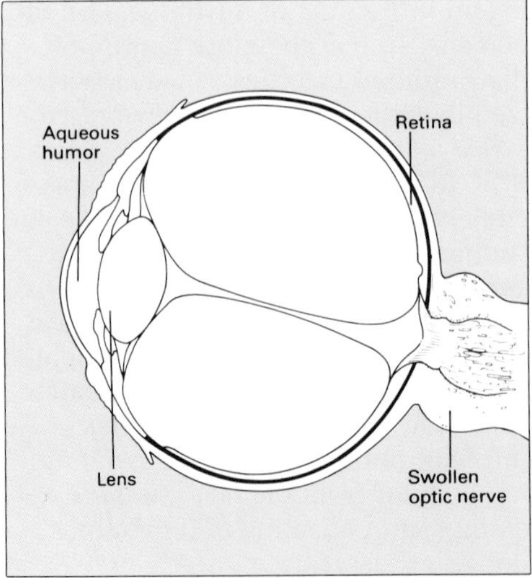

Papilledema is swelling and inflammation of the optic nerve where the nerve enters the eyeball.

Papillitis (pap i lī′tis) is an inflammation of a portion of the optic nerve. It may be caused by an infarction of all or part of the optic nerve head, by tumors, by chemicals, by meningitis, or by syphilis. The only symptom, loss of vision, varies from a small scotoma (blind spot on the retina) to total blindness, usually occurring one to two days after the onset of inflammation. A significant cause of papillitis in patients over the age of 60 is giant cell arteritis (inflammation of the arteries). Typically these elderly patients experience headaches and fatigue; sometimes the papillitis can spread quickly to the other eye, causing bilateral blindness. With prompt treatment or spontaneous remission, vision is frequently restored. Otherwise, optic atrophy occurs, with accompanying loss of vision. Treatment of papillitis includes application of corticosteroid hormones.

See also ARTERITIS, TEMPORAL.

Papilloma (pap ə lō′mə) is a benign (noncancerous) growth of the skin or mucous membrane, usually covered by a layer of thickened epidermis. Warts and corns are papillomas.

See also CORN; WART.

Pap smear test, or Papanicolaou test, is a procedure for detecting and diagnosing malignant (cancerous) and premalignant (precancerous) conditions of the female genital tract. The site of the test is the cervix, which is the small circular opening of the cervical canal that leads to the uterus. The cervix is the visible part of the uterus and is not a separate organ. The normal cervix is pink and covered with scale-like squamous cells. The cervical canal is lined with cells that are tall and narrow, called columnar cells. Columnar cells become inflamed more easily than the squamous cells. The area where the two kinds of cells come together is called the T-zone or transition zone. The T-zone is the area where the squamous cells are constantly replacing the columnar cells. Abnormal cells are most likely to develop in the T-zone.

The Pap test is a simple procedure done in the physician's office. It involves the use of a speculum, an instrument that allows the doctor to view the cervix easily. There is no pain, just mild discomfort from the insertion of the speculum. The doctor, using a cotton applicator, takes a sample of cells from the inside of the cervix and smears them on a slide. A second sample of cells is taken from the T-zone, using a small wooden spatula, and placed on another slide. Both slides are stained and sent to the laboratory. Pathologists, physicians trained in the microscopic examination of cells (cytology), review the slides for evidence of abnormal precancerous cells (dysplasia). Over a period of several years, mild dysplasia may progress to severe dysplasia and then to carcinoma *in situ*, or very early cancer. In the past, these stages of abnormal development were identified as classes II-V. (Class I referred to a normal Pap smear.) At present, however, most pathologists prefer to use a more definitive verbal description of their findings.

The advancement of modern diagnostic procedures has made it possible to detect and treat precancerous conditions, such as dysplasia, 5 to 10 years before cancer actually develops. The medical procedures include biopsy, cone biopsy, endocervical curettage, and cryosurgery. By treating dysplasia, cervical cancer is now almost completely preventable.

Q: *How often should a woman have a Pap smear test?*

A: The frequency of the Pap smear test can vary from every six months to every three years depending on a woman's risk factors. These factors include age at the time of first sexual intercourse; multiple sex partners; history of herpes infection or venereal warts; or previously abnormal Pap smears. Many physicians recommend an annual Pap smear test from the time a woman becomes 21 years old or becomes sexually active.

See also CANCER; CARCINOMA IN SITU.

Papule (pap′yül) is a small, solid, raised spot on the skin.

See also RASH.

Paracentesis (par ə sen tē′sis) is a minor surgical procedure in which a needle is passed into a body cavity, such as the abdomen, to remove fluid. It is usually performed under a local anesthetic for diagnostic purposes or for the removal of excess fluid.

Paragonimiasis (par ə gon i mī′ə sis) is infestation with small parasitic flukes (flatworms) of the genus *Paragonimus*, which form cysts in the lungs. Humans become infested by eating raw or undercooked crabs that contain larval flukes. Once ingested, the larval flukes penetrate the intestinal wall and then continue through the diaphragm to invade the lungs. In the lungs the larval flukes grow into mature adults and produce eggs. Some of the larval flukes may mature in other parts of the body, such as the abdomen or the brain.

Q: *What are the symptoms of paragonimiasis?*

A: The major symptoms include persistent spitting of blood, breathlessness, and chest pains. There may also be clubbing of the fingers. In the comparatively rare cases of infestation of the brain, there may be epilepsy and varying degrees of paralysis.

Q: *How is paragonimiasis treated?*

A: Treatment with drugs that kill the flukes is usually effective, but surgery may be needed to remove some of the adult flukes.

See also FLUKE.

Paralysis (pa ral′ə sis) is the temporary or permanent loss of the ability to move either a limb or the whole body, usually also accompanied by a loss of sensation. Paralysis is generally the result of muscle or nerve disturbance.

Q: *How does nerve disturbance cause paralysis?*

A: Most paralysis is caused by damage to a peripheral nerve or to the central nervous system. The results of damage to a peripheral nerve are different from those due to damage to the central nervous system, brain, and spinal cord.

Paralysis may result from the destruction of the anterior nerve roots in the spinal cord.

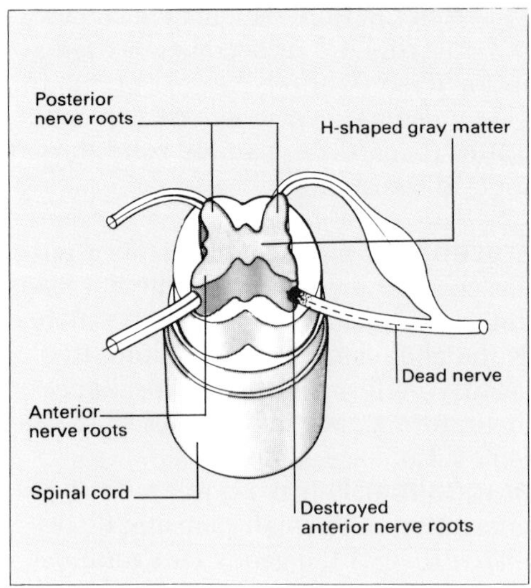

Damage to a peripheral nerve can cause complete loss of the ability to move a particular muscle or muscles, and a consequent wasting away. Damage to the central nervous system produces weakness or loss of the use of a group of muscles, such as those of the arm or leg, but no wasting. The affected muscles may make the limb feel stiff when moved. This is known as spasticity.

Q: *How is paralysis treated?*

A: Treatment depends on the cause and can be started only when a physician has made a definite diagnosis.

Physiotherapy can be employed to treat muscles that can still move, to maintain a full range of movement of joints, and to prevent stiffness. This may be helped by the use of electrical equipment, such as ultrasound, high-frequency heat treatment, hydrotherapy pools, and neuromuscular facilitation techniques.

Paralysis of speech may require speech therapy, but if swallowing is involved, a tracheotomy, the insertion of a tube into the windpipe, may be necessary.

Peripheral nerve injuries can be helped by nerve transplants, orthopedic operations to immobilize a joint (arthrodesis), or the transplant of the tendon of a working muscle to aid paralyzed muscles.

See also BABINSKI'S REFLEX; BULBAR PARALYSIS; CEREBRAL PALSY; DYSARTHRIA; HEMIPARESIS; MENINGIOMA; MOTOR NEURON DISEASE; MULTIPLE SCLEROSIS; MUSCLE; MYASTHENIA GRAVIS; NEUROLOGICAL DISORDERS; NEUROMA; POLIOMYELITIS; POLYNEURITIS; STROKE; SYRINGOMYELIA.

Paralytic ileus (par ə lit′ik il′ē əs) is a form of intestinal obstruction caused by paralysis of the muscles of the intestinal wall. It is a failure of the normal muscular contractions (peristalsis) to pass food along inside the intestine. The abdomen becomes swollen, and this condition results in symptoms of constipation, abdominal pain, and vomiting.

Q: *What conditions produce a paralytic ileus?*

A: A paralytic ileus most commonly occurs as a result of disturbance to abdominal nerves and tissue. It can also occur with peritonitis and severe chemical upsets, such as those coinciding with kidney failure, diabetic coma, and extreme loss of body potassium salts. It may also be the result of a disturbance to the autonomic nervous system associated with an injury to the spine or treatment to prevent spasms or combat hypertension (high blood pressure).

Q: *How is a paralytic ileus treated?*

A: Hospitalization is necessary. The patient's stomach is emptied to prevent further vomiting. The patient is then given intravenous fluids to supply necessary salts, water, and glucose. After two to three days, peristalsis restarts and the patient can sip fluid before returning to a normal diet within the next three or four days.

See also ILEUS.

Paramedic (par ə med′ik) is a trained medical worker who substitutes for a physician in certain situations. Most paramedics handle routine medical duties, giving physicians more time with patients who need specialized care. Some paramedics, called Emergency Medical Technician-Paramedics (EMT-paramedics) give emergency medical aid if a physician is not available.

EMT-paramedics give emergency care chiefly to accident victims and to persons stricken by sudden illnesses. Two or more EMT-paramedics usually work together as a team called a Mobile Intensive Care Unit (MICU). They use ambulances that carry a wide range of drugs and medical equipment.

Before treating a victim, EMT-paramedics use a two-way radio to contact a physician at a nearby hospital. They report the extent of any injuries and other information about the victim's condition. For victims of a heart attack, EMT-paramedics have an instrument that can send the physician an electrocardiogram to describe heart activity. Such basic information helps the physician determine the proper treatment. In serious cases, EMT-paramedics continue to treat the victim on the way to the hospital.

Paranoia. *See* MENTAL ILLNESS.

Paraphimosis (par ə fī mō'sis) is a condition in which the foreskin of the penis is retracted and can not be returned to its normal position. It occurs when the foreskin is inflamed (balanitis) and thereby constricts the normal circulation of blood. As a result, the bulbous end of the penis (*glans penis*) becomes swollen and painful.

Q: *How is paraphimosis treated?*

A: With the patient under a general anesthetic, the foreskin usually can be pulled back into position quite easily. However, it is probably best if the surgeon performs a circumcision to prevent the condition from recurring.

See also BALANITIS; CIRCUMCISION; PHIMOSIS.

Paraplegia (par ə plē'jē ə) is paralysis of the lower half of the body. It is usually caused by injury, damage, or disease of the spinal cord.

See also PARALYSIS.

Parasite (par'ə sīt) is any organism that lives at the expense of another (host) organism. Ectoparasites, such as lice, fleas, and mites, live on the outside of their hosts. Endoparasites, such as flukes and intestinal worms, live within their hosts. Some parasites carry or cause disease.

See also FLEA; FLUKE; LICE; PARASITICIDE; WORM.

Parasiticide (par ə sit'ə sīd) is a substance, such as a chemical compound or another agent, that kills parasites.

In order to kill parasites that live on the outside of their hosts (ectoparasites), such as scabies and lice, gamma benzene hexachloride is usually used. It is available in a variety of medical shampoos and other chemical solutions. Instructions, however, should be carefully adhered to. Overuse of the solution may result in temporarily dry and itchy skin or even in genital dermatitis. This medication should not be used by infants or pregnant women. Other parasiticides can be safely used by these patients.

In order to kill parasites that live within their hosts (endoparasites), such as roundworms, tapeworms, protozoa, and flukes, various oral drugs are available, including mebendazole, paromomycin, and metronidazole. However, there are some tapeworms, against which no drugs are effective. These parasites are usually removed by surgery.

See also KWELL; PARASITE.

Parasympathetic nervous system. *See* NERVOUS SYSTEM, PARASYMPATHETIC.

Parathormone (par ə thôr'mōn) is the hormone produced by the parathyroid glands. It controls the level of calcium in the blood and, indirectly, reduces the level of phosphate. It works by releasing calcium from the bones, increasing calcium absorption from food in the intestine, and reducing calcium excretion by the kidneys. At the same time, the excretion of phosphate from the body is also increased. The rise in the calcium level reduces the secretion of parathormone. This "feedback" mechanism has the effect of maintaining a constant level of calcium in the blood.

See also PARATHYROID GLAND.

Parathyroid gland (par ə thī'roid) is an organ that secretes parathormone, the hormone that controls the level of calcium in the blood. The four parathyroid glands are embedded, two on each side, in the thyroid gland tissue located in the lower part of the front of the neck.

Q: *Can anything go wrong with the parathyroid glands?*

A: Yes. Lack of parathormone (hypoparathyroidism) often occurs if the parathyroid glands are accidentally damaged or removed during a partial thyroidectomy. More rarely, the parathyroid glands fail to secrete parathormone, or there may be resistance of the body tissues to the stimulating action of parathormone. Excessive secretion of para-

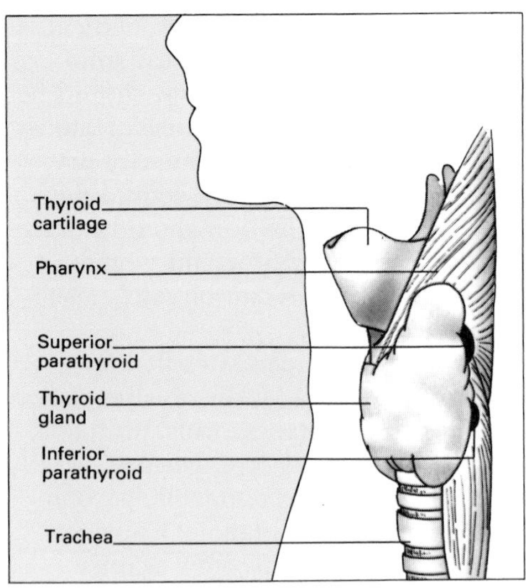

Parathyroid glands are embedded within the tissue of the thyroid gland in the throat.

thormone (hyperparathyroidism) may also occur for no obvious reason.

Q: *What are the symptoms of hypoparathryroidism?*

A: Lack of parathormone leads to an abnormally low level of calcium in the blood (hypocalcemia). The major symptom is the twitching and spasm of muscles (tetany).

Q: *What are the symptoms of hyperparathyroidism?*

A: Excess production of parathormone (hyperparathyroidism) leads to a high level of calcium in the blood and a serious drainage of calcium from the bones. Symptoms include weakness, nausea, and constipation. These symptoms may be accompanied by thirst and the frequent passing of urine.

Kidney stones (nephrolithiasis) are also a common complication. Bones may lose minerals and later develop cysts if the disease progresses without treatment.

Q: *How is hyperparathyroidism treated?*

A: After a careful assessment and diagnosis has been made by a physician, a surgeon may be asked to operate and remove the parathyroid gland.

Paratyphoid (par ə tī′foid) is a form of intestinal (enteric) fever that is caused by certain bacteria of the genus *Salmonella*. The disease resembles typhoid fever but its symptoms, including headache and constipation, are usually milder.

See also TYPHOID FEVER.

Paresis (pə rē′sis) is weakness of the muscles. It may be caused by damage to the central nervous system.

See also PARALYSIS.

Paresthesia (par əs thē′zhə) is an abnormal sensation of prickling, numbness, or itching of the skin, commonly known as a feeling of "pins and needles." These sensations are commonly experienced when a limb "falls asleep" or when a person hyperventilates. In these instances the paresthesia may last only a few minutes. Sometimes, however, paresthesia may be chronic or the result of an underlying medical disorder, such as diabetes mellitus, hypothyroidism (underactivity of the thyroid gland), alcoholism, or neurologic disease.

Parietal (pə rī′ə təl) describes the two bones that form the sides and roof of the skull. Parietal also describes the wall of a body cavity.

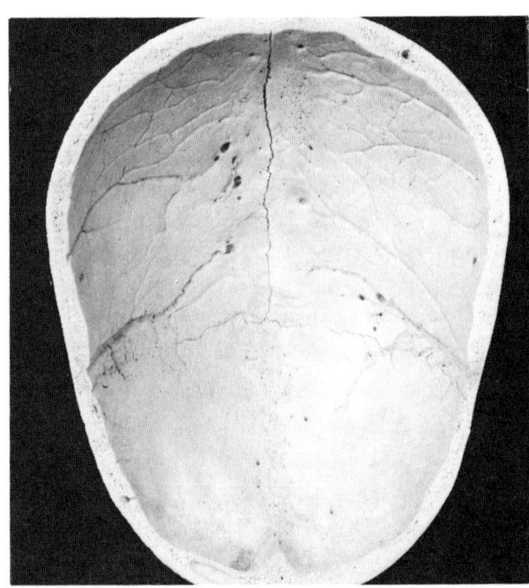

Parietal bones are the two bones that form the sides and roof of part of the skull (cranium).

Parietal lobe (pə rī′ə təl lōb) is the middle section of each hemisphere of the brain. The lobes are situated between the frontal and the occipital lobes, directly inside the parietal bones, which form the roof and sides of the skull.

See also BRAIN.

Parkinson's disease (pär′kin sənz) is a chronic disorder of the nervous system characterized by tremors, slow movements, and generalized body rigidity. It occurs most commonly in the middle-aged and elderly. Parkinsonism is the term that denotes the symptoms of Parkinson's disease.

The cause of Parkinson's disease itself is not known, although Parkinsonism may be caused by several factors. In some patients, Parkinsonism is thought to be caused by arteriosclerosis, in which there is degeneration of the brain cells that control body movements. Parkinsonism also may be caused by encephalitis (inflammation of the brain); a brain tumor; brain damage; or poisoning, either from drugs, such as the tranquilizer reserpine, from metallic chemical elements, such as manganese, or from poisonous gases, such as carbon monoxide.

Q: *What are the symptoms of Parkinson's disease?*

A: The onset of symptoms is usually gradual, and the disease progresses slowly. The initial symptoms include an occasional trembling of one hand and increasing clumsiness of the same arm. As the disorder progresses, both sides of the body become affected, movements become slow and stiff, the face assumes a blank expression because of rigid face muscles, and the patient may drool. Speech may also become impaired. Dementia, or deterioration of thought processes, is frequently seen in Parkinson's disease. It is important to distinguish between patients who appear confused because of rigid face, drooling, and slurred speech and those patients who actually suffer dementia.

In the later stages, there may be continual hand tremors and movement of the fingers; the arms may be held in a bent position, and the body may be bent forward in a permanent stoop. The patient may also walk slowly with shuffling steps and then start to run to prevent falling forward. This characteristic gait is called festination. The patient's handwriting may become small and illegible, and speech may become slurred and unintelligible.

Q: *How is Parkinson's disease treated?*

A: There is as yet no cure, but the symptoms can be controlled in many cases. Drug treatment with levodopa (L-dopa), particularly when combined with carbidopa, can control the symptoms in some patients and enable them to resume a normal life for several years. Some patients respond to treatment with the drug amantadine, either by itself or in combination with L-dopa.

If treatment with L-dopa or amantadine is ineffective, atropine-like drugs may be used. These drugs tend to cause adverse side effects, such as constipation, dry mouth, and retention of urine.

Research is currently underway in the use of MAO inhibitors as a treatment for Parkinson's patients. It is believed that MAO inhibitors retard the progression of Parkinson's disease by blocking the production of the MAO enzyme. Approval has recently been granted by the U.S. Federal Drug Administration to test MAO inhibitors on the victims of Parkinson's disease.

Because Parkinson's disease is a chronic illness, treatment should also include an excercise program.

See also LEVODOPA; MAO INHIBITOR.

Paronychia (par ə nik′ē ə) is an inflammation of the skin that surrounds a nail. The affected area becomes red and swollen and may discharge pus. Acute paronychia is usually caused by a bacterial infection. Chronic paronychia occurs most commonly in those who have their hands in water for long periods of time. It is usually caused by candidiasis, which is a fungal infection. Chronic paronychia may damage the nail bed, which may result in distorted, ridged nails.

Q: *How is paronychia treated?*

A: The treatment of acute paronychia usually involves a combination of antibiotics and minor surgery, in which the inflamed area is drained of pus. Chronic paronychia may be treated with antifungal creams. It is advisable to keep hands dry by wearing rubber gloves when hands are in water.

Parotid gland. See SALIVARY GLAND.

Parotitis (par ə tī′tis) is an inflammation of one or both parotid glands, the salivary glands located in the cheeks, in front of the earlobes. It is most commonly caused by mumps but may occur with any virus infection of the salivary glands. It also can be caused by a bacterial infection resulting from a stone in the salivary duct (sialolithiasis) or by mouth infections (stomatitis), particularly in elderly patients who are seriously ill and dehydrated. Chronic swelling of the parotid gland is often seen in persons suffering from alcoholism.

See also SALIVARY GLAND.

Paroxysm (par′ək siz əm) is a sudden attack of a disease or an increase in the severity of its symptoms. For example, paroxysmal atrial tachycardia is the sudden onset of an episode of very rapid heart beats.

The term paroxysm is also used to denote a sudden spasm or convulsion.

Paroxysmal tachycardia. *See* TACHYCARDIA, PAROXYSMAL.

Parrot fever. *See* PSITTACOSIS.

Parturition (pär tů rish′ən) is a term for the process of childbirth.

See also PREGNANCY AND CHILDBIRTH.

Patch test (pach) is a skin test that is used to identify the specific cause of an allergy. In a patch test, a small amount of the suspected causative agent (allergen) is applied to the skin and covered with adhesive tape. Another patch without allergen on it, the control patch, is also attached to the skin. Both patches are removed after a specified period of time. If the skin is red and swollen under the suspect patch, and the skin is not abnormal under the control patch, the patient is probably allergic to that particular allergen.

See also ALLERGY.

Patella (pə tel′ə), or kneecap, is a small, disk-shaped bone about 2 inches (5cm) in diameter located in the tendon of the quadriceps femoris muscle in front of the knee joint. The inner surface forms the front of the knee joint and is covered by cartilage.

Q: *What disorders can affect the patella?*

A: Softening of the cartilage (chondromalacia) may occur in young adults, causing an aching pain deep in the knee, which is made worse by walking. Exercise of the quadriceps muscle is usually helpful in the treatment of chondromalacia. *See also* CHONDROMALACIA.

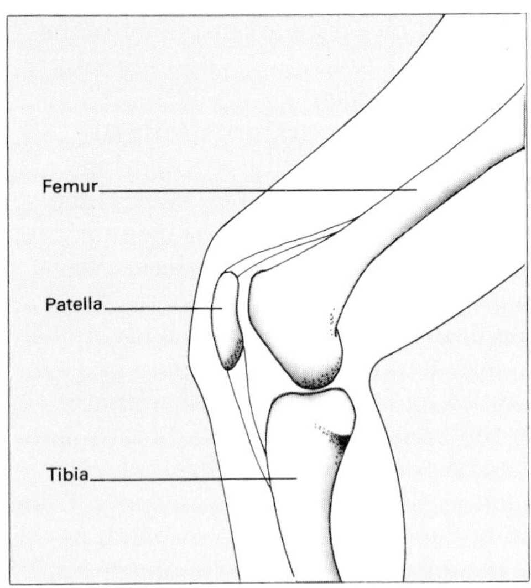

Patella is the movable cap of bone that protects the joint at the knee.

Recurrent dislocation of the patella usually begins in adolescence if the individual keeps the knee slightly bent for too long and the patella slips sideways, causing severe pain and an inability to straighten the leg. The patella usually can be relocated without a general anesthetic. If the dislocations continue, the likelihood of developing osteoarthritis of the knee later in life increases.

The tendon of the patella also can rupture, usually because of some violent exercise, and requires surgery to stitch it back into place. In the same way, a fracture of the patella may occur. Treatment depends in part on the severity of the fracture and in part on the age of the patient.

See also OSTEOARTHRITIS.

Patent ductus arteriosus (pa′tent duk′tus är tir ē ō′səs) is an abnormal opening of the fetal blood vessel, the ductus arteriosus, that connects the aorta with the left pulmonary artery. The condition, which is primarily found in premature infants, occurs when the ductus arteriosus fails to close after birth.

Normally the ductus arteriosus becomes a fibrous cord, the ligamentum arteriosum, in the weeks immediately following birth. When the ductus arteriosus remains open, however, arterial blood recirculates through the lungs and back through the left side of the heart, causing both the lungs and heart to work harder.

If the condition is not naturally resolved, surgery is indicated. If left untreated, this condition can lead to congestive heart failure and pulmonary vascular disease.

See also DUCTUS ARTERIOSUS; HEART DISEASE, CONGENITAL.

Pathogen (path′ə jen) is any organism or substance that is capable of causing a disease.

Pathognomonic (pə thog nə mon′ik) describes anything that is characteristic of a particular disease and helps a physician make a diagnosis of that disease.

Pathology (pə thol′ə jē) is the study of the causes and nature of diseases, especially the structural and functional changes brought about by diseases.

Pathology, forensic. *See* FORENSIC MEDICINE.

Patient care. *See* NURSING THE SICK.

Patient, lifting of. *See* NURSING THE SICK.

Patient/physician relationship. The patient-physician relationship is not easy to describe, and its importance is both underrated and exaggerated. The main requirement of any physician is that he or she is competent and that the patient's problem is skillfully treated. For minor ailments this may be all that some persons need from a physician. Feeling at ease with him or her may be less important.

Confidence. There are situations, however, when trust and confidence in a physician is of great importance. That is the best reason for associating the whole family with a regular physician. If a condition is discovered that is, or may be, serious, decisions will have to be made about a course of treatment. For example, the discovery of a lump in the breast may indicate cancer, which raises the possibility of a surgical operation. The patient must have confidence in the physician's decision and should feel enough at ease with the physician to be able to ask questions.

Most people, at some time in their lives, undergo a period of emotional stress. It may be an illness, such as depression; a sexual problem; anxiety or tension at work; family strife; or any of the problems created by modern living. When confronted by such situations, most people prefer to confide in a physician whose judgment and advice they can trust. It is important that the patient feels able to discuss sensitive or embarrassing matters.

Having a regular physician who knows the family well, means that many problems can be dealt with over the telephone. If the physician is familiar with the patient's problems, this can be an efficient method of consultation. For example, a patient with an acute infection may not need to visit the office and risk spreading the infection to other patients. Instead, the physician can discuss the problem as well as possible treatment in a telephone call. The physician can also renew drug prescriptions by telephone. If the patient has called in advance, the physician can telephone the pharmacy and arrange for the prescription to be ready for collection.

Annual Checkup. Although the annual checkup has been strongly encouraged in the past, this is impractical, costly, and seldom followed by most persons. By having a regular primary physician, a person can have his or her physical exam and screening lab tests done a little at a time. For example, if one physician is responsible for a family's primary care, a person can have his or her blood pressure checked when he or she brings his or her spouse to the doctor, or have a heart and lung exam when he or she comes in for a cold. In addition, a person is most likely to stick to a health-promoting regime—such as a diet or exercise—if he or she has an ongoing relationship with his or her physician.

House Calls. Few physicians make house calls, and most are frequently unable to meet a patient taken to the hospital in an emergency. Telephone consultation between the family physician and the physician in the emergency room, however, can ensure that the patient receives proper attention and treatment.

The subject of house calls is a sensitive one in physician-patient relationships. It is argued by a physician that a better examination can be conducted in an office, where simple tests may be performed immediately, than in the patient's home. If a person is too sick to visit the physician's office, then he or she should probably be taken to a hospital anyway. On the other hand, it is an ordeal for some patients, especially the elderly, to make the journey to and from the physician's office. In addition, a house call can give the physician valuable information about the patient's diet, safety, and health needs; this information can literally not be obtained any other way; it is especially important in the care of the elderly.

A physician who makes house calls is not necessarily better than one who does not. This merely indicates a difference in the style of practice among physicians.

When to Call or Visit. If a visit to the physician seems necessary, there is no danger to the patient from exposure to inclement weather, even if there is a fever, as long as clothing is adequate. However, a telephone call to the physician may eliminate the need for an office visit.

Symptoms such as sudden and severe central chest pain require skilled emergency help and quick transportation to a hospital. To wait for a physician to arrive or to call for an appointment would be foolish and possibly dangerous. Sick children are usually better taken care of at the physician's office.

The First Visit. It is helpful to have your thoughts organized before you see the physician for the first time. If possible, it is an advantage if the first visit is for something other than an emergency. This gives you a chance to be more objective in appraising the service given.

Some practices make use of the physician's assistant or a trained nurse to take the patient's history and run routine tests. The assistant may also arrange for X rays or other special tests before the patient sees the physician. In general, however, no X rays or blood tests should be ordered until after the patient has been evaluated by the physician; the indiscriminate use of "routine" laboratory tests is costly, unscientific, and ignores important differences between individuals.

A patient may also be asked to answer some questions using a medical computer. The machine asks a set series of questions, which the physician can expand upon during the patient's first visit. Patients often find it easier to give yes and no answers to the machine about embarrassing topics. But if patients object to responding to the machine, they can of course refuse and speak directly to the doctor.

When you see the physician, try to present your symptoms in as concise and accurate a way as possible. If you are particularly concerned about something, mention it.

It is often necessary for the physician to ask questions that may not seem to be related to your symptoms. Even if the questions seem unnecessary, it is important to answer them accurately. What may seem trivial to you might sound much more important to the physician trying to make a diagnosis, and the reverse is also true.

Next, an examination is needed. Do not make judgments based on the length of the examination, but more on its relevance. If you have a cough, for example, it is reasonable to expect the physician to examine your chest before an X ray is ordered. The symptoms may be enough for the physician to reach a firm conclusion, prescribe some medication, and complete the whole procedure without the use of invasive tests or X rays. On the other hand, in some cases, a diagnosis will not be possible without X rays.

The next stage after the examination has been completed is when and how the physician explains the problem and proposed course of treatment to the patient. This is the key element in physician-patient communication. A patient must understand why the physician has recommended a certain course of action; what medication has been prescribed and why; how long the medication is needed; and if and when the prescription should be renewed.

If the patient understands everything after explanation, this is a big plus in the physician's favor. If certain details are still unclear to the patient, but questions are answered openly, that should count equally in the physician's favor, because it is impossible to communicate clearly with everybody all of the time. However, failure to answer reasonable queries, or a show of resentment at being asked to do so, is not an encouraging characteristic in a physician.

In answering your questions, a physician may sometimes use technical language or jargon with which you are unfamiliar. Most physicians do this quite unintentionally, using terms that are clear and commonplace to them. Do not hesitate to ask your physician to speak in layman's terms or to repeat an explanation.

If you know you are allergic to any particular drug, you should always mention it, and you should also mention any medication you may be taking, including the contraceptive pill. If you ever visit a hospital without your physician in attendance, the hospital staff must be given the same information.

Legally, a physician is obliged to tell the patient all the possible side effects of a drug. This is known as informed consent. Some physicians give the patient a list of possible side effects. The companies that supply drugs often distribute such lists to physicians. If you are worried or alarmed by the possible side effects, talk it over with the physician who can explain why the benefits of the drug outweigh possible side effects.

A patient who suffers from a chronic (long-lasting) problem must understand the probable course of the illness. For instance, if he or she suffers from high blood pressure, and suddenly develops severe headaches, the patient must know that this is a serious symptom. The patient should feel free to telephone the physician at any time.

Neither should a patient hesitate to telephone the physician if he or she suspects an unexpected side effect from a drug. The dosage of the drug may need to be altered or a different drug substituted.

Physicians vary greatly in technique and personality. If the physician makes an overall good impression, if you like the physician and feel at ease, then your choice is probably correct.

The Case for a Family Physician. There is an increasing demand in the United States for physicians who are able to look after most, if not all, family members. A variety of titles are in common use for these physicians, such as general practitioner or primary-care physician. This type of physician offers many advantages. He or she is familiar with the entire family, and this is particularly helpful in a number of situations: pregnancy, child care, chronic illness, stress, emotional illness, terminal care, and many others. It is important that the physician's temperament suits the family, who must feel comfortable with the physician and trust his or her decisions and advice. Successful medical care depends on mutual respect and trust, and if this does not exist the patient should look for another physician.

If a physician belongs to a group practice or health maintenance organization (HMO), this offers some advantages. Group practices and HMO's are made up of several physicians, usually each with a different medical specialty. While the family may have a regular physician, if that physician is part of a group practice or HMO, family members may see other physicians in the practice about specific complaints.

The Hospital. Most physicians have hospital privileges. This means that the physician's qualifications and experience have been approved by a hospital and that he or she has been granted permission to be directly responsible for patients admitted to that hospital.

If a patient consults a regular physician about a specific complaint the physician may arrange hospitalization and treat the patient personally. Depending on the complexity of the medical illness, the family physician may consult one or more specialists. The family physician will then follow the patient's progress throughout hospital care and coordinate all aspects of the hospital care, including the planning of care following the hospitalization.

The family physician usually goes to the hospital daily to see what progress his or her patients are making. If a specialist feels that a second opinion is needed, the family physician will be informed and in turn discuss the situation with the patient.

If a person does not have a regular physician and is taken to a hospital for any reason, such as a traffic accident, a physician on duty at the hospital's emergency room will see the patient on arrival. The emergency room physician will treat any urgent problems. If the nature of the illness or injury requires hospitalization or continued care, the hospital assigns a staff physician to the patient.

See also PHYSICIAN CHOICE.

Patient, turning of. *See* NURSING THE SICK.

Pectoral (pek′tər əl) refers to the chest.

See also ANGINA PECTORIS; CHEST.

PCP. *See* PHENCYCLIDINE.

Pediatrics (pē dē at′riks) is the branch of medicine concerned with the growth, development, and diseases of children.

Pediculosis pubis (pi dik yə lō′sis pyü′bis), commonly known as crabs, is an infestation of the pubic hair area by the crab louse. In more severe cases, crabs may spread to the hair of eyebrows, eyelashes, armpits or beard and even to the body surface of hairy individuals. Crabs are usually acquired through sexual contact or, sometimes, from toilet seats or by contact with infested clothing or bedding.

Q: *What are the signs of crab lice?*

A: Intense itching in the pubic area is usually the first sign of the presence of crabs. Prolonged scratching may result in a secondary infection if the skin is broken. Although crabs are large, resembling dandruff flakes, they are difficult to see. More easily spotted are the nits (eggs) near the base of the hairs. Another sign of the infestation is the presence of tiny dark brown specks on underwear.

Q: *How are crab lice treated?*

A: Various lotions are available without a prescription. Several applications are necessary over a period of days. Dead lice and nits should then be combed out with a fine-toothed comb. To prevent reinfestation by nits that may have survived, a further application should be made several days or a week after the initial ones. If crabs have infested the eyebrows and eyelashes, forceps usually have to be used to remove them.

All bedding and clothing should be sterilized by hot water, 150°F (66°C) or higher for 5 minutes, or by dry cleaning. Combs, brushes and headwear also have to be disinfected.

See also KWELL; LICE.

There are three main types of lice that infest human beings: the two varieties of *Pediculus humanus,* which live in the hair or on the body, and the crab louse, **Pediculosis pubis,** which lives in pubic hair. Various lotions are available without a prescription to treat an infestation of *Pediculosis pubis.*

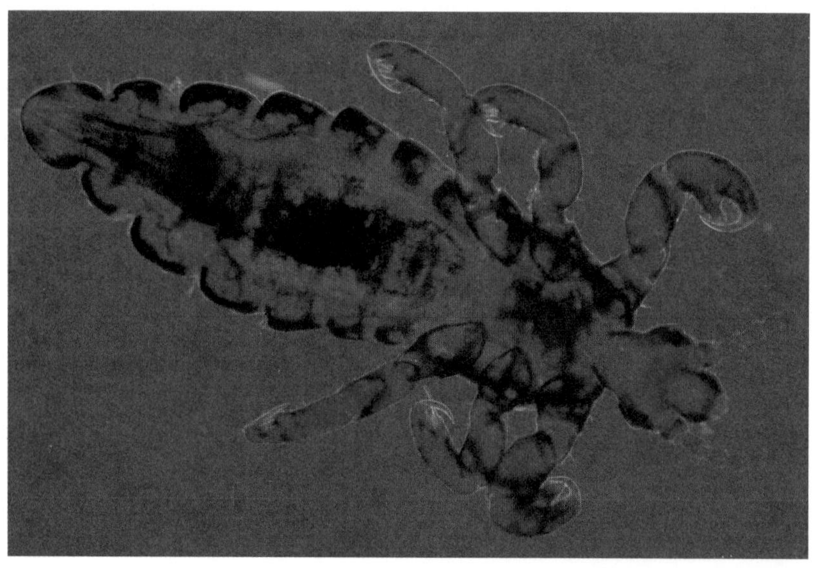

Pellagra (pə lag′rə) is a vitamin deficiency disease caused by a lack of niacin, an element found in the B-complex vitamins. Pellagra most commonly occurs in those whose staple diet is corn. Pellagra also may result from alcoholism; cirrhosis of the liver; and malabsorption of food, which is often caused by chronic diarrhea.

Q: *What are the symptoms of pellagra?*

A: Initial symptoms include a smooth, red tongue, a sore mouth, and ulceration of the inside of the cheeks. The skin on the neck, chest, and back of the hands may become brown and scaly. Often there is nausea, vomiting, and diarrhea. There may also be insomnia, depression, confusion, and rapid changes of mood. Long-standing pellagra can result in dementia and death.

Q: *How is pellagra treated?*

A: Pellagra is treated via a nutritionally balanced diet with niacin supplements.

Pelvic girdle (pel′vik gėr′dəl) is the bony arch made where the hipbone, sacrum, and coccyx meet to form the pelvis.

See also PELVIS.

Pelvic inflammatory disease. *See* ENDOMETRITIS; SALPINGITIS.

Pelvimetry (pel vim′ə trē) is the measurement of the size of a woman's pelvis, to determine if the pelvis is wide enough for normal childbirth.

Pelvis (pel′vis) is a basin-shaped cavity. There are two such cavities in the body. The pelvis of the kidney collects urine and funnels it into the ureter, the

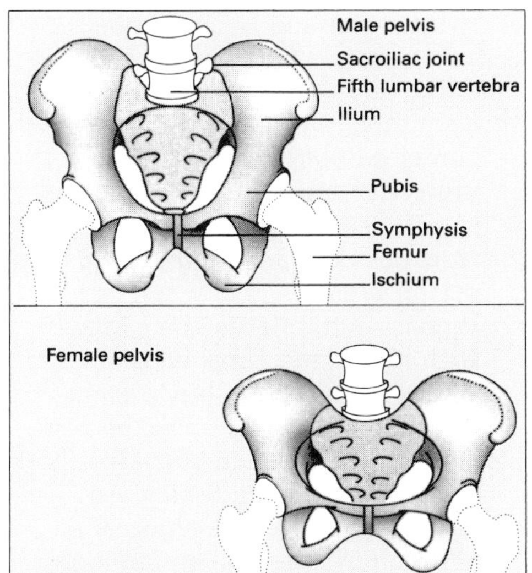

The **pelvis** of a woman is flatter and broader than a man's and has a larger central cavity to accommodate childbirth.

tube that leads to the bladder. The term pelvis usually refers to the bones in the lower part of the torso that support the spine and connect to the legs at the hip joints.

The pelvis consists of two hipbones, each composed of the pubis, ilium, and ischium. These join in front at the pubic bone *(symphysis pubis)* and are attached at the back to the sacrum, the lower backbone, by the two sacroiliac joints. The coccyx, a small bone at the lower end of the spinal column, is attached to the sacrum.

The wide wings of the two hipbones form the upper extremities of the pelvis and are known as the false pelvis. They sweep down to a narrower part called the true pelvis. The pelvis of the female is wider than that of the male, and the entrance to the true pelvis is usually circular in shape to accommodate the birth of a child.

Q: *What structures does the pelvis contain?*

A: The side walls of the pelvis contain muscles that help movement of the thighs. The bottom of the pelvis is made up of ligaments and muscles (the pelvic floor) that support the bladder and rectum and, in a female, the vagina and uterus. The false pelvis supports the large and small intestine, which intertwine above the contents of the true pelvis.

See also HIPBONE; SACRUM.

Pemphigoid, bullous (pem′fə goid bůl′əs). Bullous pemphigoid is a chronic skin condition, much like pemphigus, in which large blisters erupt over various parts of the body. The disorder affects mainly the elderly; it is not considered as serious as pemphigus. Treatment usually involves the use of corticosteroid drugs.

See also PEMPHIGUS.

Pemphigus (pem fī′gəs) is a disease of the skin, characterized by successive outbreaks of large, fluid-filled blisters. It can result from a type of impetigo caused by a staphylococcal infection.

In adults there are two rare forms of pemphigus that may be a form of autoimmune disease. They produce blisters in the mouth and on exposed mucous membrane, as well as on the skin.

It is difficult to distinguish between pemphigus, a disease of middle-aged adults, and a similar disorder called pemphigoid, which occurs mainly in the elderly and produces itching of the skin followed by blistering.

In infants, impetigo caused by a staphylococcal infection may be associated with small fluid-filled blisters. This condition is not related to pemphigus, however.

Q: *How are pemphigus and pemphigoid treated?*

A: Pemphigus that is due to impetigo is treated with antibiotics. The general treatment for other forms of pemphigus and pemphigoid is corticosteroids, which relieve and control the symptoms. Both diseases are, at present, incurable.

See also AUTOIMMUNE DISEASE; IMPETIGO.

Penicillin (pen ə sil′in) is one of a group of antibiotics that were once extracted from molds of the genus *Penicillium*, but are now synthesized. The basic penicillin is called penicillin G.

Overuse of penicillins can result in their becoming ineffective because of the development of resistant bacterial strains. However, penicillin G is still effective against many of the common bacterial infections, and it can be modified to produce a number of more effective penicillins, such as ampicillin, methicillin, oxacillin and, didoxacillin. Some of these derivatives are effective against a wider range of organisms than is penicillin G, and some are effective against bacteria that have developed a resistance to penicillin G.

Q: *How do penicillins work?*

A: The penicillins work mainly by killing bacteria while the bacteria are multiplying, but penicillins also inhibit the growth of bacteria to some extent.

Q: *Can the penicillins produce adverse side effects?*

A: Yes. All of the penicillins carry the risk of producing allergic reactions. However, these usually do not occur until a patient has had at least two treatments of penicillin. An allergic reaction may produce skin rashes, swelling of the throat, fever, and swelling of the joints. Rarely, anaphylaxis may occur, which may be fatal.

People who are allergic to one type of penicillin are allergic to all types, and often to a similar group of antibiotics, the cephalosporins. Such people should warn their physicians so that other antibiotics are prescribed instead. It is also advisable that people allergic to penicillin wear a medical identification tag.

See also SHOCK, ANAPHYLACTIC.

Penicillin V (pen ə sil′in vē) is a semisynthetic form of ordinary penicillin (penicillin G). It is marketed under many brand names, including Pen-Vee K®, V-Cillin K®, Veetids®, and SK-Penicillin VK®. Like the other forms of penicillin, penicillin V is effective against a wide range of bacterial infections. It is more resistant to acid in the stomach than penicillin G; it is, thus, more effective when taken orally.

The drug has few side effects, but it should not be taken by persons who are sensitive to other forms of penicillin.

See also ANTIBIOTIC; PENICILLIN.

Penis (pē′nis) is an external, male reproductive organ. Both semen and urine leave the body through the penis. The penis is shaped somewhat like a finger and is attached at its base to the pelvic bone by connective tissues.

Q: *How is the penis constructed?*

A: The urethra, the tube for the passage of urine or semen, is surrounded by special tissue. It ends in an external swelling called the glans. The urethra lies on top of two tubular and honeycombed areas of erectile tissue. The glans at the end of the penis is particularly sensitive and, in an uncircumcised penis, is covered by a protective foreskin. *See also* FORESKIN.

Q: *How does the penis function as a sexual organ?*

A: When erectile tissue is engorged with blood, the penis becomes erect and hard. The blood is unable to drain out through the veins because they are temporarily closed by special muscles. An erection results from physical or psychological sexual stimulation, which enables the male to insert the erect penis into the female's vagina during sexual intercourse. It is at the stage of greatest sexual excitement (orgasm) that the semen is released into the vagina.

An erection ceases when the veins open, so that the blood is able to flow back into the general circulation of the body.

Q: *What disorders can affect the penis?*

A: Inflammation of the glans (balanitis) may cause narrowing of the foreskin (phimosis) or cause it to act in a constrictive manner if it is pulled back (paraphimosis). *See also* BALANITIS; PHIMOSIS.

Venereal diseases, such as syphilis or chancroid, form ulcers, or chancres, on the skin of the penis; other venereal diseases, such as gonorrhea, cause infections of the urethra (urethritis). *See also* GONORRHEA; SYPHILIS; URETHRITIS, NONSPECIFIC.

Small cysts (sebaceous cysts) may form on the skin of the penis and occasionally cancer can occur. On rare occasions, erections may be prolonged and painful (priapism).

Q: *How is cancer of the penis recognized and treated?*

A: Cancer of the penis occurs most commonly in elderly males who have not been circumcised and whose low standard of personal hygiene has caused repeated mild attacks of balanitis. A small ulcer that bleeds easily is the first sign that cancer may be present.

Cancer of the penis is treated either by amputating the end of the penis or by radiotherapy.

See also CIRCUMCISION.

Pep pill is a street term for a drug that contains amphetamine. Pep pills produce a feeling of well-being and excitement, but are addictive.

See also AMPHETAMINE; DRUG ADDICTION; METHAMPHETAMINE; STIMULANT.

Pepsin (pep'sin) is an enzyme that starts the digestion of proteins in the stomach by breaking down the large protein molecules into smaller molecules, called peptides. In the small intestine, the peptides are further broken down by other enzymes into molecules (amino acids) that are small enough to be used by the body.

See also AMINO ACID; DIGESTION; ENZYME.

Peptic ulcer. *See* ULCER, PEPTIC.

Percussion (pər kush'ən) is a diagnostic procedure in which a physician places a finger over the part of the body to be examined and taps it sharply with a finger of the other hand. Different sounds are made, depending on whether the physician is tapping over a solid structure, a fluid-filled structure, or a hollow, air-filled cavity. The different sounds enable a physician to determine the size, position, and consistency of underlying body structures.

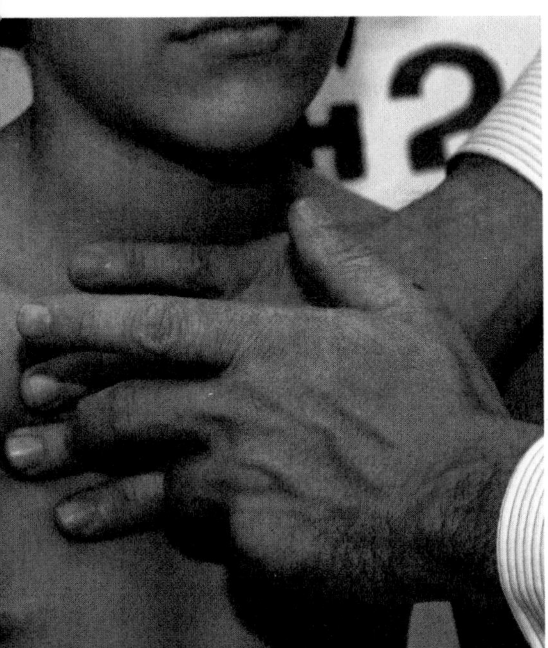

Percussion is a hands-on procedure commonly used in examinations of the heart and lungs.

Percutaneous biopsy (pėr kyü tā'nē əs bī'op sē) is the removal of body fluid or tissue for clinical examination. The biopsy is performed through the skin by means of a needle.

See also BIOPSY.

Perforation (pėr fə rā'shən) is either a hole that is made in a part of the body or the process of making such a hole as part of a surgical procedure.

Perfusion (pər fyü'zhən) is a technique in which fluid is passed through a blood vessel or a part of the body, either for investigating or for treating a disorder. Occasionally, the terms perfusion and infusion are used interchangeably.

See also INFUSION.

Periarteritis nodosa (per ē är tə rī' təs nə dō'sə) is a rare, potentially fatal inflammation of the small arteries. It often results in arterial thrombosis and death of the surrounding tissue. The cause of periarteritis nodosa is not known. Periarteritis nodosa usually occurs in persons between the ages of 25 and 50 years and is more common in men than in women.

Q: *What are the symptoms of periarteritis nodosa?*

A: The symptoms of this disorder are extremely variable. The most common symptoms include fever, recurrent abdominal pain, weight loss, peripheral neuritis, asthma, hypertension, edema, and fatigue. The muscles and joints may ache, and nodules and ulcers may appear on the skin. The kidneys also may be affected.

Q: *How is periarteritis nodosa treated?*

A: There is, as yet, no cure for this disorder, which is fatal in most cases. However, the symptoms can be controlled, and life can be prolonged by treatment with large doses of corticosteroids.

See also CORTICOSTEROID.

Pericardial tamponade (per ə kär'dē əl tam pon ād') is a potentially life-threatening condition in which fluid accumulates in the sac enclosing the heart (pericardium), causing pressure on the heart. The fluid build-up may result from a wound, which ruptures blood vessels in the heart muscle, or from an inflammation of the pericardium. The fluid may be removed by means of a needle with a suction syringe, inserted through a surgical puncture.

See also PERICARDITIS; PERICARDIUM.

Pericarditis (per ə kär dī′tis) is an inflammation of the membranous sac that surrounds the heart (pericardium). A wide variety of disorders may cause pericarditis. Most commonly, it is due to a viral infection. Sometimes bacteria or tuberculosis may cause the disorder. It can also be associated with rheumatoid arthritis, systemic lupus erythematosus, and uremia. It may also occur as a complication of cancer of adjacent structures, such as the lungs or esophagus. Often, however, no definite cause can be identified. *See also* ARTHRITIS, RHEUMATOID; LUPUS ERYTHEMATOSUS; TUBERCULOSIS; UREMIA.

Q: ***What are the symptoms of pericarditis and how is it treated?***

A: In most cases, there is pain in the center of the chest, which may vary in intensity and may be worsened by movement or coughing. Other common symptoms of pericarditis include fever, breathlessness, coughing, and rapid pulse rate. The treatment of pericarditis is directed toward the underlying cause. In the early stages of the disorder, painkillers are usually prescribed. Antibiotics may be necessary if pericarditis is caused by an infection. Various other treatments may be necessary if complications develop.

Q: ***Can pericarditis cause complications?***

A: Yes. The most common complication is an accumulation of fluid in the pericardium (pericardial tamponade). This causes pressure on the heart and a rapid pulse rate. One type of pericarditis, called constrictive pericarditis, causes scarring and thickening of the pericardium. This may result in progressive heart failure, with increasing breathlessness, enlargement of the liver, and an accumulation of fluid in bodily tissues and cavities (edema).

See also PERICARDIAL TAMPONADE; PERICARDIUM.

Pericardium (per ə kär′dē əm) is the structure that surrounds the heart. It consists of two layers, between which is a small amount of fluid. This fluid enables the heart to beat almost without friction. The inner layer of the pericardium is soft and membranous. The outer layer is thicker and fibrous and helps protect the heart.

Perimetry (pə rim′ə trē) is a method of examining the area that the eye can see (visual field) when it is focused on a central point. This point is marked in the middle of a blank, curved screen. A small light or disk is moved inward from many points on the edge of the screen. The point at which a person first sees the small light or disk is noted. Connecting the points defines the edge of his or her peripheral vision. Visual fields can be made smaller by glaucoma, stroke, or other neurological illnesses.

See also GLAUCOMA; PERIPHERAL.

Perinatal medicine (per ə nā′təl) concerns medical treatment just before and after childbirth, encompassing approximately the last 7 weeks of gestation and the first 28 days following birth.

See also PREGNANCY AND CHILDBIRTH.

Perinephric (per ə nef′rik) describes the tissues that surround the kidney.

See also KIDNEY.

Perineum (per ə nē′əm) is the area between the anus and the lower edge of the pubis at the front of the pelvis. In a female, it includes the opening of the vagina and the surrounding vulva, as well as the firm fibrous tissue area between the back of the vagina and the anal opening. In a male, the perineum is the small area of fibrous tissue behind the pouch that contains the testicles (scrotum).

Period. *See* MENSTRUATION.

Periodontal disease (per ē ə don′təl) is any disorder affecting the tissue surrounding the teeth. Periodontal disease usually begins as gingivitis, an inflammation of the gums. If untreated, gingivitis may progress to periodontitis, a condition in which the gums and underlying bone become more severely infected. The teeth ultimately may become loose and fall out due to loss of supporting bone.

The most common cause of periodontal disease is the accumulation of dental plaque as a result of poor dental hygiene. Other contributing factors include tartar formation, systemic disturbances, such as diabetes mellitus, or an allergic reaction. Any periodontal abnormality should be brought to the immediate attention of a dentist.

Periodontal disease is responsible for more tooth loss in adults than any other cause. It is the most common serious dental disorder today.

See also GINGIVITIS; PERIODONTITIS; TOOTH CARE.

Periodontitis (per ē ō don tī'tis) is a gum condition in which the mucous membrane, gums, and underlying bone become infected. The teeth ultimately become loose and usually fall out.

Q: *What is the cause of periodontitis?*

A: The condition most often develops as a result of dental plaque due to poor oral hygiene, especially insufficient flossing between the teeth and under the gums. Lack of regular professional care is a secondary cause.

Q: *What are the symptoms of periodontitis?*

A: In addition to loose teeth, the gums are swollen, inflamed, and bleed upon brushing. There is often a discharge of pus from around one or more of the teeth. The breath smells foul, and pockets form between the teeth and gums.

Q: *Why do so many people lose teeth from periodontitis?*

A: Many people ignore or are unaware of the early symptoms of the disease and it tends to be painless. Thus, the loss of bone support to the teeth may progress prior to one's awareness of the disease. If left untreated, there is loss of underlying bone, and the teeth ultimately fall out.

Q: *How is the condition treated?*

A: Most therapy is directed at plaque control and reducing pocket depth to a cleansible level. Swollen, bleeding tissue usually responds best to cleaning, but tough, fibrous scar tissue often has to be trimmed away surgically. In the most severe cases involving bone loss, it is frequently necessary to reshape the rough underlying bone. Improved oral hygiene, with daily brushing and flossing of the teeth and gums, and regular dental visits are necessary to avoid a recurrence of the condition.

See also GINGIVITIS; PERIODONTAL DISEASE; TOOTH CARE.

Period pain. *See* DYSMENORRHEA.

Periosteum (per ē os'tē əm) is a thin, fibrous membrane that covers all bone surfaces, except at the joints. It consists of a dense outer layer containing nerves and blood vessels and an inner layer made up of cells that help to form new bone. The periosteum plays an essential part in the nutrition of the bones.

See also BONE.

Periostitis (per e os tī'tis) is an inflammation of the membrane that covers the bone (periosteum). It may occur during the healing of a fractured bone, but it is usually caused by a bone infection, such as osteomyelitis, or rarely, syphilis.

See also OSTEOMYELITIS; PERIOSTEUM.

Peripheral (pə rif'ər əl) means situated at the outer part of an organ or structure. Peripheral vision refers to the outer limits of a person's visual field.

Peripheral nervous system. *See* NERVOUS SYSTEM, PERIPHERAL.

Peristalsis (per ə stal'sis) is a series of involuntary muscle contractions that move food along the intestines. In the stomach, peristalsis produces a churning action that aids digestion. Occasionally, reverse peristalsis may occur, causing vomiting.

See also DIGESTIVE SYSTEM; VOMITING.

Peritoneal dialysis (per ə tə nē'əl dī al'ə sis) is a procedure used to remove poisonous (toxic) substances and other waste matter from the body or to correct a fluid imbalance in the body. Both these functions are normally performed by the kidneys. The procedure is performed by passing chemical solutions through the peritoneal cavity, a small space between the layers of the peritoneum, the membrane lining the abdominal cavity.

Peritoneal dialysis may be part of the continual treatment of patients with kidney failure.

See also KIDNEY DIALYSIS; PERITONEUM.

Peritoneum (per ə tə nē'əm) is the membrane that lines the abdominal cavity and surrounds the abdominal organs, such as the intestines, liver, spleen, uterus, and bladder. In some places it forms the mesentery, which supports the intestines. The peritoneum is richly supplied with blood vessels and nerves and produces a fluid that lubricates the abdominal organs.

See also ABDOMEN; MESENTERY.

The **peritoneum** is the thin membrane that lines the walls of the abdomen and surrounds the organs within the abdomen.

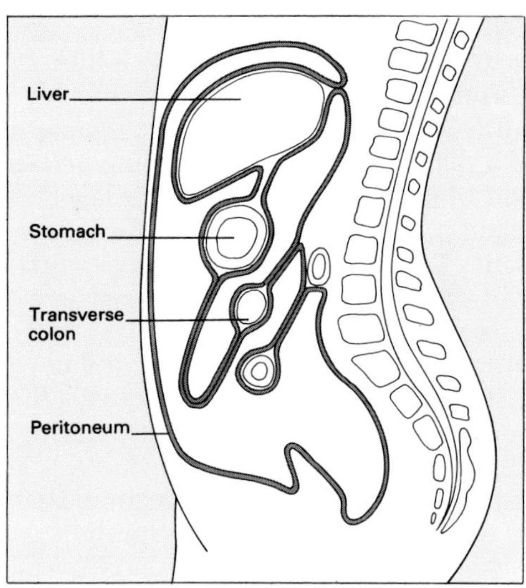

Peritonitis (per ə tə nī'tis) is an inflammation of the peritoneum, the membrane that lines the abdominal cavity and covers the abdominal organs. It usually accompanies an infection. Rarely, it may occur with conditions such as rheumatoid arthritis, systemic lupus erythematosus, or pancreatitis. *See also* ARTHRITIS, RHEUMATOID; LUPUS ERYTHEMATOSUS; PANCREATITIS.

Q: *What causes peritonitis?*

A: Peritonitis is most commonly caused by infection of an abdominal organ, such as appendicitis, perforation of a peptic ulcer, or an inflamed appendix. It may also be associated with inflammation of the fallopian tubes (salpingitis) or follow an abdominal operation.

Q: *What are the symptoms of peritonitis?*

A: The chief symptom is severe, generalized abdominal pain. If the diaphragm is irritated, the person may complain of aching shoulders ("referred pain"). Usually there is a fever, accompanied by rapid pulse rate. Vomiting often occurs as the result of the onset of a paralytic ileus. *See also* PAIN, REFERRED; PARALYTIC ILEUS.

Q: *How is peritonitis treated?*

A: The patient is hospitalized and treatment begins with intravenous antibiotics and other drugs, which are used to treat any infection and to control pain. Emptying of the stomach through a nasogastric tube is sometimes needed. A surgical operation is required if appendicitis or a ruptured peptic ulcer is found.

Q: *Are there any complications of peritonitis?*

A: Yes. If treatment is not started immediately, death may result. An abscess may form under the diaphragm, or in the pelvis as a result of salpingitis. Both conditions may require surgical draining after the initial stage of peritonitis has settled. Scarring and adhesions of abdominal organs are also complications of peritonitis.

Peritonsillar abscess. *See* ABSCESS, PERITONSILLAR.

Pernicious anemia. *See* ANEMIA, PERNICIOUS.

Personality disorder. *See* MENTAL ILLNESS.

Perspiration (pėr spə rā'shən) is the production of sweat by the sweat glands. The main ingredients of sweat are sodium chloride (common salt), potassium salts, urea, and lactic acid. *See also* LACTIC ACID; UREA.

In cold weather, perspiration is minimal. In extreme heat, about 3 pints (1.5l) of sweat may be lost each hour. Persons who have become acclimatized to heat may lose up to 8.5 pints (4l) per hour. It takes about 6 weeks to become acclimatized. During this period, the sweat glands gradually increase the amount of sweat and decrease the amount of salts in the sweat, thereby preserving salts in the body.

Q: *How do the sweat glands work?*

A: A sweat gland consists of a coiled

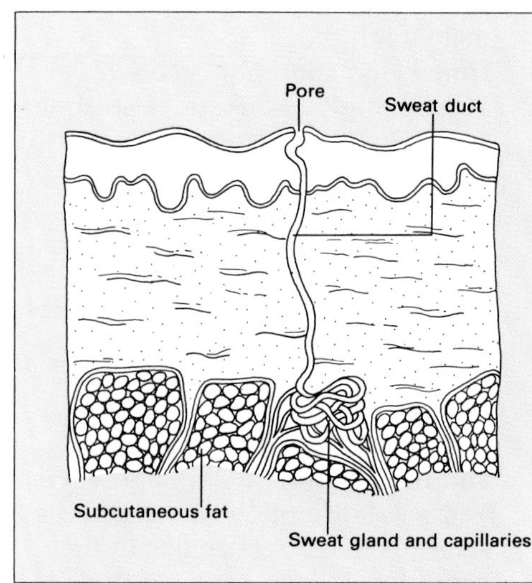

Perspiration is produced by sweat glands in the skin and is secreted through pores.

structure that lies deep within the skin and a duct that passes through the skin layers to the surface. The coiled structure is well supplied with blood by capillaries. It absorbs fluid from the capillaries and surrounding cells and passes this to the surface through the duct. Some of the salts are reabsorbed in the duct. But when sweating is profuse, large amounts of salts may be lost.

The sweat glands are controlled by the autonomic nervous system. This is connected to the hypothalamus in the brain, which is part of the body's heat-regulating mechanism. Sweating is also influenced by adrenaline and norepinephrine, hormones that cause the cold sweats of fear. *See also* HYPOTHALAMUS; NERVOUS SYSTEM, AUTONOMIC.

Q: *What are the functions of perspiration?*

A: The main function of perspiration is to cool the body by evaporation. The other function of perspiration is the elimination of waste products, such as urea. However, the amount of body wastes lost through sweating is small.

Q: *What conditions may affect perspiration?*

A: Perspiration may cease completely in the final stages of heatstroke. This is caused by a breakdown of the body's heat-regulating mechanism. Without emergency treatment at this stage, the person may die. *See also* HEATSTROKE, FIRST AID.

Increased sweating may occur with fever and in conditions that raise the metabolic rate, such as hyperthyroidism. Cystic fibrosis causes an excessive concentration of salts in perspiration.

Some people sweat excessively, particularly from the soles of the feet, palms of the hands, and the armpits. This condition is known as hyperhidrosis and may be aggravated by stress. Bromhidrosis is a condition in which the sweat has an unpleasant odor. This is caused by the action of bacteria in breaking down dead skin cells.

See also BODY ODOR.

Perthes' disease (per'tēz) is a chronic disorder of children, in which the head of the femur (the ball part of the ball-and-socket hip joint) becomes inflamed and deformed because of an inadequate blood supply to the developing bone. The cause of the disorder is not known. It is most common in boys between 5 and 10 years old and usually affects only one of the hip joints. Movement of the affected joint may be limited, resulting in a limp. There may also be pain in the thigh and groin.

Q: *How is Perthes' disease treated?*

A: Most forms of treatment involve reducing the pressure on the affected joint. This may necessitate the wearing of caliper splints for up to two years, while natural healing takes place. Children with Perthes' disease are likely to develop osteoarthritis in the affected hip when they reach adulthood.

See also OSTEOARTHRITIS.

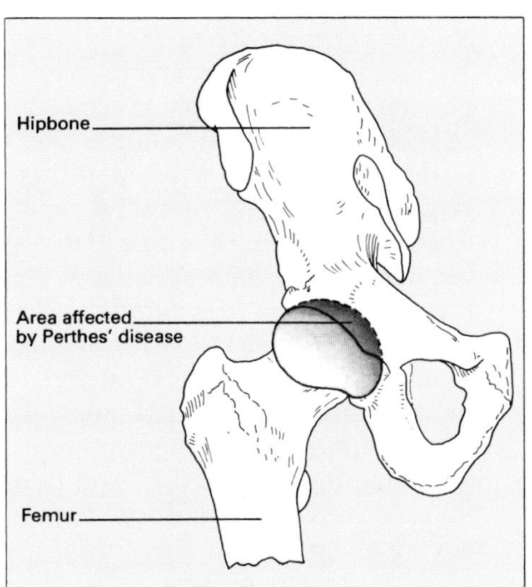

Perthes' disease disrupts the blood supply to the head of the femur, causing inflammation and deformity of the bone.

Pertussis (pər tus'is), or whooping cough, is a disease of the respiratory tract. The infection is caused by the microorganism *Bordetella pertussis* and is transmitted by droplets in the air from an infected person. The disease most commonly occurs in infancy. The incubation period is 10 to 21 days. The infectious period starts at the onset of symptoms and lasts for approximately two weeks.

Q: *What are the symptoms of whooping cough?*

A: The symptoms are divided into three stages. In the first, or catarrhal stage, the patient develops common cold symptoms, including a slight fever, sneezing, rhinitis, irritability, loss of appetite (anorexia), and a dry cough. The cough increases in violence after two weeks and becomes a series of short coughs, followed by a long dragging in of air, during which the "whoop" is heard.

During the second, or paroxysmal, stage, vomiting commonly follows coughing. Severe coughing can cause hemorrhage of the membranes in the nose and eyes. Mental retardation can result from cerebral hemorrhage, as can spastic paralysis. Complications from pneumonia may lead to bronchiectasis and emphysema in later life.

The third stage, the decline, begins after four weeks. The coughing episodes subside and food intake improves. Recovery may last several months.

Q: *How is pertussis treated?*

A: The antibiotic erythromycin may prevent the onset of paroxysmal coughing if given early in the catarrhal stage. If not arrested at this stage, isolation and normal cough treatment combined with sedatives for sleep are recommended.

Q: *Can pertussis be prevented?*

A: Yes. A vaccine of killed *Bordetella pertussis* organisms must be given to an infant, in three doses, usually in combination with the diptheria and tetanus vaccines (DPT), at two, four, and six months of age. Boosters are given at 15 to 16 months and 4 to 6 years of age.

In recent years, some parents have become reluctant to give their children the pertussis vaccine for fear of complications. In extremely rare cases (less than 1 in 100,000) the vaccine may cause neurologic problems in children. There is no question, however, that not vaccinating children and, thus, risking an outbreak of pertussis far exceeds the minimal dangers of the pertussis vaccine. Newer pertussis vaccines with fewer side effects are being developed, but these are not available for use as yet.

Whooping cough is uncommon in later life, and it is rarely dangerous to an adult. The main danger is the possibility that the disease may spread to an infant.

See also DPT VACCINE.

Pes cavus (pēz kā'vəs), or clawfoot, is a condition in which the arches of the feet are abnormally high. The condition may be inherited. In most cases, however, there is no apparent cause. Other causes that have been identified include various muscular and neurological disorders, such as spina bifida or poliomyelitis in early infancy.

Q: *What are the symptoms of pes cavus?*

A: There are often no symptoms. However, pes cavus causes the weight of the body to be borne on the front part of the feet. This may cause clawing of the heads of the metatarsal bones. This in turn may lead to the formation of calluses over the metatarsals and corns on the toes.

Q: *How is pes cavus treated?*

A: Most cases require podiatric treatment and the wearing of pads under the metatarsal heads. If these measures are ineffective, surgery may be necessary

See also METATARSAL.

Pes planus. *See* FLATFOOT.

Petechia (pə tek'ē ə) is a small red spot in the skin caused by a tiny hemorrhage of a blood capillary.

See also CAPILLARY.

Petit mal (pə tē má') is a form of epilepsy in which there is a momentary loss of awareness, but no convulsions. The preferred term is "absence seizure."

See also EPILEPSY.

Petroleum jelly (pə trō'lē əm) is used in medicine to prevent dressings from sticking to the skin. It is also used as a base for various ointments.

Pets and disease. *See* ANIMALS AND DISEASE.

PETT. *See* POSITRON EMISSION TRANSAXIAL TOMOGRAPHY.

Peyer's patch (pī'ərz) is a collection of lymph nodules that occur mainly in the ileum of the small intestine.

See also LYMPHATIC SYSTEM.

Phagocytosis (fag ə sī tō'sis) is the absorption or destruction of harmful material, such as disease-causing bacteria or cell debris, by phagocytes. Phagocytes are a type of white blood cell present in body fluids and tissues.

See also BLOOD CELL, WHITE.

Phalanx (fā'langks) is the term given to any one of the bones of the fingers or toes. The thumbs and big toes each have two phalanges; the other fingers and toes each have three.

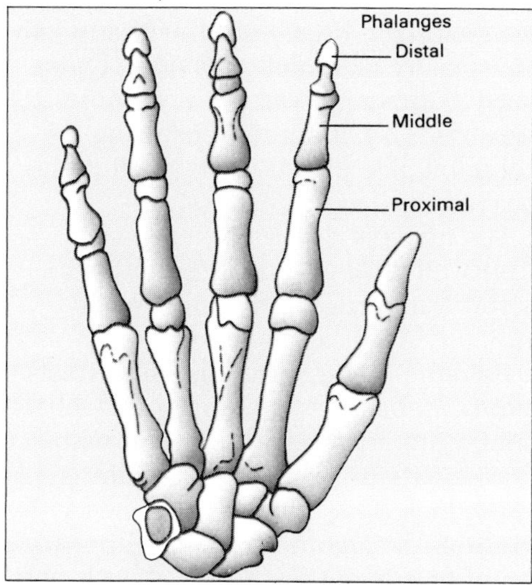

Phalanx is any of the bones of the fingers and toes. There are 14 such bones that form the fingers of each hand.

Phallus (fal'əs) is another term for the penis.

See also PENIS.

Phantom limb (fan'təm) is the illusion that a limb is still present after it has been amputated. This condition is not psychological in origin. Rather, it is the result of sensory centers in the brain remaining intact, although there has been partial or full loss of a limb. Thus, the brain interprets nerve signals from the area of amputation as if the limb were still present. This condition may respond to treatment with tranquilizers and antidepressant drugs. It is a common symptom following an amputation, but usually disappears within a few months.

Pharmacology (fär mə kol'ə jē) is the study of the effects of drugs on the living processes of all cells. Clinical pharmacology is the study of drugs that are useful in the prevention, diagnosis, and treatment of human disease.

Pharmacopeia (fär mə kə pē'ə) is an official compendium of drugs that contains information on their preparation, effect, and dosages and legal requirements of purity, strength, and quality.

Pharyngectomy (far in jek'tə mē) is an operation to remove the pharynx, usually in the treatment of cancer. The operation involves not only the removal of the pharynx, but also its reconstruction using other tissues. This is a complex procedure that often requires several operations to complete.

See also CANCER; PHARYNX.

Pharyngitis (far in jī'tis) is an inflammation of the pharynx. It is one of the most common of all disorders. Usually it comes on suddenly (acute pharyngitis), although some persons have a persistent form of the disorder (chronic pharyngitis), which may be caused by smoking, drinking, or postnasal drip. The symptoms of pharyngitis include a sore throat and discomfort or pain on swallowing. Acute pharyngitis may be caused by the common cold, laryngitis, stomatitis, glandular fever, tonsillitis, or sinusitis. *See also* POSTNASAL DRIP.

Q: ***What causes acute pharyngitis?***

A: Acute pharyngitis is most commonly caused by a common cold virus. In such cases, only the symptoms are treated. Antibiotics are ineffective. However, if the cause is the streptococcal bacterium, the infection is known as strep throat. Other bacterial causes include gonorrhea and mycoplasma. Acute pharyngitis is sometimes associated with inflammation of the larynx (laryngitis), inflammation of the mouth (stomatitis), infectious mononucleosis (glandular fever), tonsillitis, or nasal conditions, such as sinusitis. In rare cases, diphtheria or leukemia may be the cause. *See also* THROAT, STREP.

Q: ***Are there any particular problems associated with acute pharyngitis?***

A: No, there are no problems other than those associated with any infection of the back of the throat and nose, such as laryngitis and otitis media (inflammation of the middle ear).

Q: ***Why do some people continually suffer from a chronic sore throat and discomfort on swallowing?***

A: Chronic pharyngitis, like chronic laryngitis, may occur in those who smoke too many cigarettes or drink too much alcohol. It may also be caused by postnasal drip resulting from chronic nasal or sinus inflammation. Frequently, a definite cause can not be found.

The condition can often be cleared up by improved oral hygiene, giving up smoking, and the use of antiseptic gargles. If the chronic inflammation is caused by respiratory tract allergies, the sore throat may clear up when the allergies are properly controlled.

Pharynx (far′îngks) is the part of the throat situated behind the arch at the back of the mouth. The pharynx connects the mouth, nose, and larynx. It includes the nasopharynx, the space just above the soft palate that joins with the back of the nose and contains the adenoids and openings of the Eustachian tubes; the oropharynx, containing the tonsils and the back of the tongue; and the laryngeal pharynx, the back of the throat.

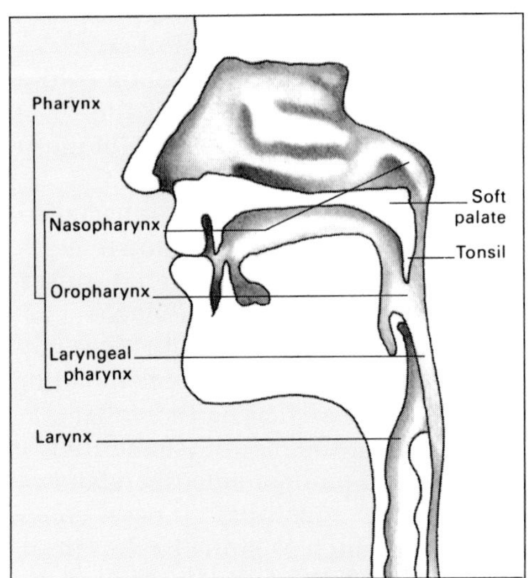

The **pharynx,** consisting of the nasopharynx, oropharynx, and laryngeal pharynx, serves as a passageway for air from the nasal cavity to the larynx.

Q: *What conditions may affect the pharynx?*

A: Infection may cause inflammation (pharyngitis). The pharynx may also be involved in mononucleosis tonsillitis, and adenoid problems. More rarely, Vincent's angina, syphilis, or diphtheria may cause inflammation, and occasionally, it may result from cancer.

See also NASOPHARYNX; OROPHARYNX; PHARYNGITIS.

Phencyclidine (fen sik′lə dēn) is an intravenous, general anesthetic drug commonly used in veterinary medicine. It was originally made as an anesthetic for humans. However, it is considered unsuitable because of its adverse side effects, such as hallucinations, agitation, and nightmares. It poses a major health hazard because of street drug abuse.

Phencyclidine, or PCP, is also known as angel dust. A major psychiatric hazard of PCP abuse is a psychotic state characterized by extraordinary strength and bizarre criminal behavior. Hypertensive episodes, cardiac arrythmias, seizures, and abnormal posturing are common side effects. PCP street use peaked in the early 1980's.

See also DRUG ABUSE.

Phenobarbital (fē nō bär′bə tôl) is a barbiturate drug used mainly as an anticonvulsant and as a sedative.

Patients undergoing long-term treatment can become tolerant to phenobarbital. Care must be taken when withdrawing its use, particularly with epileptics. It should be prescribed with caution for the elderly. Combining alcohol or any depressant drug with phenobarbital may produce serious central nervous system depression, possibly leading to coma, respiratory failure, or death.

See also BARBITURATE.

Phenol (fē′nol) is another name for carbolic acid.

See also CARBOLIC ACID.

Phenylketonuria (fen əl kē tə nyůr′ē ə), PKU, is an inherited disease characterized by the body's inability to properly metabolize phenylalanine. Normally the enzyme phenylalanine hydroxylase breaks down phenylalanine into amino acids. In about one in 16,000 infants, this enzyme is missing. The chief symptom of the disorder is mental retardation. Other neurological symptoms include seizures and psychotic episodes. A child with PKU is likely to have lighter hair and lighter skin than other family members.

Q: *How is phenylketonuria diagnosed?*

A: Since symptoms of PKU are not readily apparent at birth, a PKU blood test (Guthrie's test) is performed on all infants. This test is normally performed on infants several days after birth and is required by state laws. If PKU is detected, further blood tests are taken. If PKU is diagnosed in a child, a special diet that limits the intake of phenylalanine is prescribed. Milk substitutes are part of this diet. If treatment is started immediately after birth, the damaging symptoms of the disorder can probably be avoided. In adulthood, it may be possible for a patient to revert to a normal diet.

Pheochromocytoma (fē ō krō mō sī tō′ mə) is a tumor of the central part (medulla) of the adrenal glands. The adrenal gland medulla secretes the hormones adrenaline and norepinephrine. A pheochromocytoma causes excessive amounts of these hormones to be produced. The cause of pheochromocytomas is not known, but the tendency to develop them may be inherited in association with other rare hereditary disorders, such as von Recklinghausen's disease.

Q: *What are the symptoms of a pheochromocytoma?*

A: The excessive amounts of adrenaline and norepinephrine cause attacks of palpitations, nausea, and severe headaches. These may be accompanied by a feeling of great anxiety. The patient also may be pale and sweating, the pulse may be rapid, and the blood pressure is usually high and fluctuates widely. These attacks may occur at any time, or they may be triggered by emotional stress, a change of posture, or pressure on the abdomen.

It may be necessary to perform urine tests and to take X rays for the diagnosis of a pheochromocytoma. There are usually no indications of the condition, apart from hypertension (high blood pressure) unless the patient is examined during an attack.

Q: *How is a pheochromocytoma treated?*

A: The tumor is surgically removed only after the patient's hormone levels have been controlled with drugs.

See also ADRENALINE; NOREPINEPHRINE.

Phimosis (fī mō′sis) is a condition in which the foreskin (prepuce) of the penis is so tight that it can not be easily pulled back over the tip (glans).

Q: *What problems occur with phimosis?*

A: During urination, the foreskin can be seen to bulge. The stream of urine is narrow and comes out slowly. In serious cases, the back pressure of the urine may damage the kidneys (hydronephrosis).

Q: *What causes phimosis?*

A: At birth, the foreskin and tip of the penis are joined together. Separation of the two parts occurs gradually during the first three to four years of a child's life. Repeated attempts to forcibly pull back the foreskin before it is ready may cause phimosis where none had existed before. The condition may also be caused by repeated infections.

Q: *What is the treatment for phimosis?*

A: The condition usually is prevented and corrected by circumcision.

See also BALANITIS; CIRCUMCISION.

Phlebitis (fli bī′tis) is an inflammation of a vein.

See also THROMBOSIS, VENOUS.

Phlebolith (fleb′ə lith) is a chalky stone (calculus) in a vein. It results from a blood clot (thrombus) that has been present for so long that it has become calcified. It seldom causes symptoms and does not usually require treatment.

Phlebothrombosis. *See* THROMBOSIS, VENOUS.

Phlebotomus (fle bot′ō məs) is a genus of bloodsucking flies. Some species transmit infections to humans; for example, *Phlebotomus sergenti* is one of the species that transmits leishmaniasis.

See also LEISHMANIASIS.

Phlebotomy (fli bot′ə mē) is an incision or needle puncture of a vein in order to withdraw blood, either for therapeutic purposes or to collect blood, as at a blood bank.

Phelgm (flem) is thick mucus that is secreted by the mucous membranes of the nose, throat, and other respiratory passages. Phlegm discharges often accompany a cold or other respiratory disorders.

See also COLD; MUCUS.

Phobia (fō′bē ə) is a persistent, strong fear of a certain object or situation. Common phobias include fear of crowds, darkness, heights, and such animals as cats, snakes, or spiders. Most phobias do not significantly interfere with one's life and do not require treatment. However, some phobias, such as agoraphobia (fear of open spaces) and social phobias, may severely limit a person's life. Such phobic individuals may spend much time worrying about their fears and may be too frightened to carry out normal activities. Psychologists and psychiatrists classify phobias as an anxiety disorder.

Behavioral therapy holds that a phobia is a learned response and can therefore be unlearned. Therapists using behavioral treatments often employ techniques that involve gradually exposing the phobic individual to whatever is feared. The exposure may take place in real life or in the person's imagination. For example, claustrophobic patients may imagine themselves in smaller and smaller rooms until they can visualize a tiny space without anxiety. The gradualness of the exposure is considered important in making the treatment effective and relatively painless. A popular technique called systematic desensitization combines gradual exposure with relaxation or other experiences to reduce anxiety.

Many therapists who treat phobias conduct group therapy in addition to individual treatment. Group therapy enables phobic patients to talk with others who have the same fears and to learn from one another. Some therapists also use hypnosis to help phobic patients face their fears. In some cases, particularly agoraphobia, medication may be helpful as an adjunct to therapy.

Some of the special names for particular phobias include acrophobia (fear of heights), agoraphobia (fear of open spaces), claustrophobia (fear of being closed in), ailurophobia (fear of cats), ophidiophobia (fear of snakes), arachnophobia (fear of spiders), hydrophobia (fear of water), mysophobia (fear of dirt or germs), and triakaidekaphobia (fear of the number 13).

See also ANXIETY; GROUP THERAPY.

Phonocardiogram (fō nō kär′dē ə gram) is a graphic recording of heart sounds obtained through the use of a device that incorporates several microphones placed on a patient's chest (cardiograph). A phonocardiogram is used in the diagnosis of heart diseases.

Photodensitometry (fō tō den sə tom′ ə trē) is the study of photographic negatives in order to ascertain the density of a substance. An image is taken of the biological substance through the use of a photoelectric cell. It is used today to screen patients for osteoporosis.

See also OSTEOPOROSIS.

Photophobia (fō tō fō′bē ə) is an abnormal visual sensitivity to bright light. It is a symptom of migraine, high fever, measles, rubella (German measles) and can occur with any form of acute brain infection, such as meningitis or encephalitis. Photophobia may accompany any infection of the eye, such as iritis.

See also PHOTOSENSITIVITY.

Photosensitivity (fō tō sen sə tiv′ə tē) is excessive susceptibility of the skin to sunlight, caused by a medical disorder, for example, albinism. It may also be triggered by the use of certain drugs, such as tetracycline or calcium cyclamate.

See also ALBINISM; PHOTOPHOBIA.

Phototherapy, ultraviolet (fō tō ther′ə pē, ul trə vī′ə lit). Ultraviolet phototherapy is treatment by means of ultraviolet radiation (the invisible part of the spectrum of light whose rays have wavelengths shorter than the violet end of the visible spectrum and longer than X rays). It can be used in treating rickets and various skin disorders, such as acne, bedsores, and psoriasis. Under the name of photochemotherapy, it is also used in conjunction with chemotherapy, to enhance the effect of a particular drug.

See also CHEMOTHERAPY; RADIATION.

Phthisis (thī′sis) is any progressive, wasting disease of the body, especially tuberculosis of the lungs.

See also WASTING.

Physiatrist (fiz ē at′rist) is a physician who tests the physical functioning and oversees the physical rehabilitation of a patient.

See also PHYSICAL MEDICINE AND REHABILITATION.

Physical fitness. *See* EXERCISE.

Physical medicine and rehabilitation, also known as physiatrics, is the branch of medicine concerned with helping physically injured patients recover bodily functions. The partial or complete impairment of such functions is usually due to disease, congenital disorder, or trauma suffered by the neuromuscular (nerves and muscles) system of the body. Causes for physical impairment range from injuries sustained in athletics and home and auto accidents, to strokes, heart attacks, arthritis, and respiratory illnesses.

A physiatrist may employ one or a combination of physical therapy techniques to foster recovery. These techniques include moderate exercise, massage, hydrotherapy, and the application of mild electricity combined with drug therapy and the prescription of such devices as braces, wheelchairs, and electronic aids. When needed, special surgical procedures are also prescribed. The specific course of treatment depends on the nature and severity of the injury or disorder and the patient's age and general physical condition.

The goal of physical rehabilitation is always to restore normal use of bodily functions as quickly as possible. In some cases, such as in injuries to the spinal cord, complete restoration may be impossible. Nevertheless, proper therapy can help to rehabilitate partially paralyzed muscles in the arms and legs and to restore control over bladder, bowel, and sexual functions.

Physical medicine and rehabilitation can play a vital role in treating persons suffering from rheumatoid arthritis and other chronic pain disorders and in treating those recovering from heart attacks and strokes. In cases of rheumatoid arthritis, heat, medications, and splints are often applied to affected body areas to relieve muscle spasms and reduce stiffness. Passive range-of-motion exercises can help minimize or even prevent loss of joint motion.

Programs of exercise conditioning are often prescribed for heart attack patients. This conditioning not only hastens a patient's return to normal functioning, but also lessens the likelihood of subsequent attacks.

Early rehabilitation programs for stroke victims brighten the prospects for functional improvement and lessen possible complications that can develop from remaining in bed. Limited mobility exercises have proven effective in reducing circulatory complications and thereby minimizing muscle atrophy.

Physician choice. Choosing a new physican is often made necessary by the relocation of a family or the retirement or death of a family physician. Another reason for choosing a new physician is dissatisfaction with the medical care you have been receiving.

There are several ways that a new physician may be found. Ask the new

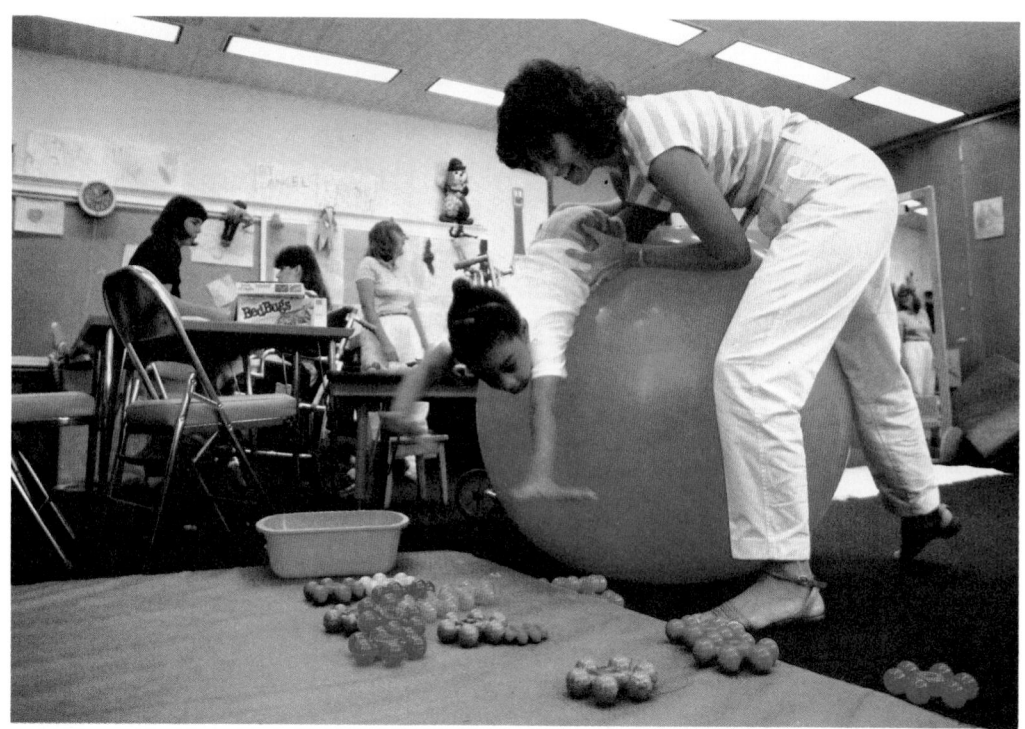

Physical medicine and rehabilitation includes the use of a variety of techniques to help injured patients restore normal bodily functions. Playful activity is one technique. Here, a therapist utilizes a large inflated ball to help a young patient improve her eye-hand coordination.

neighbors or people with whom you work about local physicians. Another way to obtain a recommendation is to call the local medical society. It will provide a list of physicians and their specialties.

Once you have received a recommendation, there are a number of things to find out from the receptionist at the office. Ask the following questions: Does the physician have a specialty? Is the physician willing to look after all members of the family? What are the physician's office hours? Is there X-ray and laboratory test equipment in the office? Is the physician taking new patients? How long should a patient expect to wait for an appointment? In addition, ask for the physician's list of fees, which should include the cost of an annual checkup and a first consultation. Tell the receptionist how you intend to pay and what kind of medical insurance you have.

Another factor that you may want to consider when choosing a new physician is whether or not the physician makes house calls. This may be important if a member of the family is handicapped by age or illness and can not travel to the physician's office.

New patients are usually advised to have a detailed physical examination during their first visit. Your medical records can be sent by your previous physician's office to the new physician. However, it is important to note that medical records are confidential and can not be released to anyone without your consent, unless requested by a court of law as a means of collecting legal evidence. The new physician may get some useful information from your medical records. However, most physicians prefer to see the patient and run through a checkup and medical history themselves in order to make a personal assessment of general health.

The general atmosphere and attitude of the receptionist, nurse, and office usually reflect the character of the physician. When choosing a new physician, it is important that you and your family feel comfortable with the office and the physician's staff.

A Male or Female Physician. People often wonder about whether to select a male or female physician. There is no simple answer. The only thing that should be emphasized is that competence is the most important requirement. Confidence will usually follow, whatever the sex of your physician. Male and female physicians can be equally competent. You owe it to yourself to examine carefully the reason for your choice of a physician. It would be unfortunate to deny yourself the service of a good, competent physician merely on the grounds of his or her sex.

Dissatisfaction. What can you do if you are not satisfied with your medical care? As an outpatient, you can look for another physician, which has been previously discussed in this article.

As an inpatient, you may express dissatisfaction to a variety of persons or ask a member of your family to complain. First, the physician in charge of the patient should be told of the grievance. The family can ask for another physician to take over. If the family does not request another physician, but asks for the current one to be dismissed, the hospital has a legal obligation to provide adequate care during the hospital stay. This includes finding another physician. The head nurse on the unit, a resident physician, or the patient representative, if the hospital has one, are all there to deal with this kind of situation. If you or your family are still unable to get satisfaction, you should ask to see the chief of the department (for instance, surgery or medicine), or the hospital administrator. Finally, you or your family can take the problem up with a lawyer.

In an emergency the same considerations apply, but time may be short. In this case, it may be better to request a second opinion rather than to discharge the attending physician immediately.

Before making the change, be sure that the reasons have been stated clearly and logically. Reasonable grounds for a change include repeated failures by the physician to respond to requests for information; lack of courtesy or consideration; or the use of too many medications without adequate explanation.

Payment. In certain circumstances, visits to a physician's office must be paid for by the patient. How much is paid depends on a number of factors. A visit for a minor complaint such as a cold, a headache, or a stomach upset, does not take long, and most routine visits to a family physician do not cost very much.

Many patients now join health maintenance organizations (HMO'S) and pay a monthly fee that covers medical expenses, both in the hospital and in the office. *See also* HEALTH MAINTENANCE ORGANIZATION.

There are also many prepayment plans and insurance plans available now, and you should choose the one that fits your own needs. If you have a health insurance policy, make yourself familiar with the items covered by the policy and, equally important, items that are not covered. For example, most policies cover injuries and emergency treatment. However, some pay for care received at the hospital emergency room, but not for care administered in a physician's office even though the latter may be less expensive.

Health insurance policies cover most, if not all, of the costs incurred during inpatient treatment. In the past, this has led to many questionable admissions to the hospital because of the attitude that "the insurance will cover the bills." An effort is currently being made to cut down on such unnecessary admissions.

The cost of malpractice insurance for health care professionals in the United States is very high, and this cost is part of the physician's fee. A specialist in a branch of medicine such as plastic surgery has a far higher malpractice insurance premium than a generalist. A general practitioner is sometimes unwilling to carry out even minor surgery in the office because of the malpractice implications and higher rates he or she may have to pay.

Finally, always carry with you a notification of insurance, or other payment arrangements, in case you are involved in an accident and taken to the emergency room without your physician in attendance.

See also MEDICAL EXPENSES AND INSURANCE.

Physician/patient relationship. *See* PATIENT/PHYSICIAN RELATIONSHIP.

Physiology (fiz′ē ol′ə jē) is the study of the functions of the cells, tissues, and organs of a living organism. It is closely associated with anatomy, which deals mainly with the structure rather than the function of living organisms.

Physiotherapy (fiz ē ō ther′ə pē), or physical therapy, is the use of rehabilitation techniques such as exercise, massage, heat, and hydrotherapy in the treatment of physically impaired patients.

Physiotherapy is helpful in treating many diseases, such as lung and heart diseases, and various types of paralysis and muscle weaknesses, such as those caused by strokes and multiple sclerosis. It is also an important part of the rehabilitative process for persons who have sustained fractures and other injuries, or have undergone amputations. With the aid of physiotherapy, a disabled person may lead a useful and productive life.

A physiotherapist may utilize various treatment combinations in order to improve a patient's joint and muscle function, or develop training for the purpose of improving physical performance that has been reduced by either injury or disease. The use of heat-producing equipment, for example, helps relieve pain, improves circulation, and relaxes muscles. Cold, when used soon after injury, lessens pain and swelling. Ultrasound aids in the treatment of inflamed joints, muscles, and nerves. Exercise helps to maintain an improved body function and increases muscle tone, strength, and endurance.

See also DIATHERMY; PHYSICAL MEDICINE AND REHABILITATION; ULTRASOUND.

Pica (pī′kə) is the craving to eat substances not considered food, such as chalk, earth, and clay. Pregnant women sometimes suffer from pica, as do some undernourished children. Pica may also be a symptom of mental illness or iron deficiency anemia.

See also ANEMIA, IRON DEFICIENCY.

PID. *See* PELVIC INFLAMMATORY DISEASE.

Pigeon breast is the protrusion of the breastbone (sternum), caused either by a congenital structural abnormality or a respiratory illness during childhood. It rarely requires corrective surgery.

Pigeon-toed (toeing in) describes the condition in which a person walks with the feet turned inward. Most infants begin walking in this way because it aids balance. If there is no improvement after six months, the child's physician should be consulted.

Pigmentation disorder (pig mən tā′ shən), known medically as hypopigmentation, is a reduction in the production of melanin, a black or dark brown pigment that occurs naturally in the hair, skin, and eyes. Albinism (a congenital pallor of the skin), vitiligo (total or partial covering of the skin with pale, ivory-white spots), and the common, colorless scar are all examples of pigmentation disorders.

See also ALBINO; VITILIGO.

Piles. *See* HEMORRHOID.

"Pill," the. *See* CONTRACEPTIVE, ORAL.

Pilonidal sinus. *See* SINUS, PILONIDAL.

Pimple (pim'pəl) is a small, inflamed swelling on the skin. Pimples may or may not contain pus.

See also ACNE.

Pineal body (pin'ē əl), or gland, is a small, somewhat cone-shaped structure situated in the center of the brain. It secretes various chemical substances, such as melatonin (a hormone) and is thought to play a role in the body's neuroendocrine system.

See also BRAIN; ENDOCRINE SYSTEM.

Pink disease (pingk), or acrodynia, is a disorder, especially of very young children, characterized by redness of the skin and lesions on the hands and feet. Its cause is unknown, although the disease is usually associated with the eating of mercury compounds. These compounds once appeared in some baby teething powders, which have now been withdrawn from the market.

See also MERCURY.

Pinkeye (pingk'ī) is a contagious disease that causes inflammation and soreness of the membrane that lines the eyelid and covers the eyeball. It is a form of conjunctivitis, which is caused by a bacterial or viral infection. A crusty discharge in the morning is characteristic of pinkeye.

See also CONJUNCTIVITIS.

Pinna (pin'ə), or auricle, is the visible external part of the ear. It consists of felxible cartilage and skin.

See also EAR.

Pins and needles is a sensation of tingling that may be associated with a nerve or circulatory disorder.

See also PARESTHESIA.

Pinta (pin'tə) is a chronic skin infection that is caused by the spiral-shaped bacterium *Treponema carateum*, which is similar to teh bacterium that causes syphilis and yaws. It is found only in remote areas of tropical Latin America. Pinta is transmitted by physical contact. After an incubation period of between one and three weeks, a small nodule appears on the skin. This gradually enlarges and becomes surrounded by other nodules. The lymph nodes in the affected area may also swell. Within the next several months blue patches develop, usually on the face and the limbs. These patches gradually fade, leaving scars. Pinta can usually be cured with penicillin.

Pinworm (pin'wėrm) is a small, parasitic worm, *Enterobius vermicularis*, that infects the large intestine and rectum. The condition is usually without symptoms, but itching may occur around the anus due to the presence of worm eggs. Pinworm infestation is especially prevalent among young children as a result of the children scratching around the anus and then putting their hands into their mouths, reintroducing the parasitic worm. Pinworms cause pruritis, which often causes children to wake up at night crying. Pinworm is easily treated with oral medication. The patient's bedding should be washed, and other family members should be treated if the infection is recurrent.

See also PRURITUS.

Pipe smoking. *See* SMOKING OF TOBACCO.

Pitocin® (pi tō'sin) is the brand name for oxytocin, a female hormone that is synthesized in the hypothalamus of the brain and stored in the posterior pituitary gland. Oxytocic agents stimulate contraction of the muscles of the uterus. Pitocin is primarily used, when indicated, to start or enhance labor. It is also used to decrease bleeding after delivery of a baby. A nasal spray containing oxytocin is used to assist "letdown" of milk from the breasts.

See also OXYTOCIN.

Pituitary gland (pi tü'ə ter ē), or hypophysis, is a small gland about the size of a pea, situated at the base of the brain; it is larger in women than in men. The pituitary gland is connected by a short stalk to the hypothalamus, which helps regulate body temperature, blood pressure, fluid balance, weight, and appetite. The gland is protected by a circle of bone, called the pituitary fossa, in the center of the skull just behind the point at which the two optic nerves join.

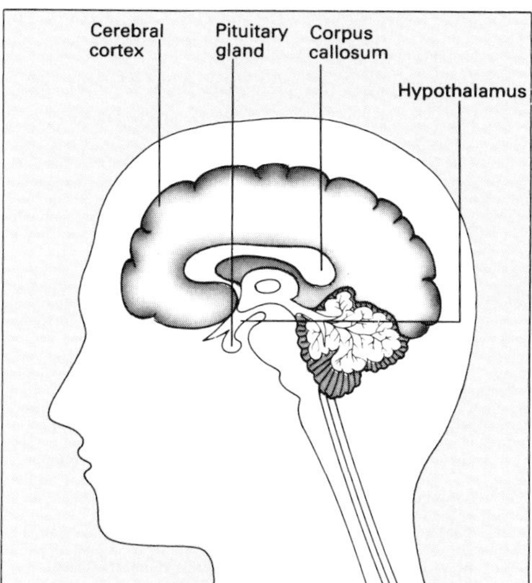

The **pituitary gland** is situated at the base of the brain and controls hormonal secretions into the bloodstream.

The pituitary gland is made up of two parts, the anterior or front lobe and the smaller posterior or rear lobe.

Q: *How does the pituitary anterior lobe function?*

A: This is the most important of the glands that secrete hormones directly into the bloodstream. It produces hormones that stimulate other endocrine glands to manufacture their individual hormones. The level of these hormones is carefully regulated by special areas in the hypothalamus that are sensitive to the blood level of a variety of hormones and accordingly regulate the pituitary gland, sending chemical messages down the connecting stalk.

Q: *What hormones does the anterior pituitary lobe produce?*

A: The anterior lobe produces a number of hormones. They are thyroid stimulating hormones (TSH) to control the production of the thyroid gland hormones, thyroxine and triiodothyronine; adrenocorticotropic hormone (ACTH) to stimulate the cortex of the adrenal gland to produce hydrocortisone and other corticosteroids; follicle-stimulating hormone (FSH) and luteinizing hormone (LH) that control the testes and ovaries; growth hormones (GH) that maintain normal growth until adult life; and prolactin, which helps induce lactation. *See also* CORTICOSTEROID; PROLACTIN; THYROXINE.

Q: *How does the posterior lobe of the pituitary gland function?*

A: The hypothalamus produces the two hormones oxytocin and vasopressin (antidiuretic hormone). These are stored in the cells of the pituitary's posterior lobe. The production of these hormones is carefully monitored by the same kind of "feedback" system that works in the anterior pituitary lobe.

Q: *What do vasopressin and oxytocin control?*

A: Vasopressin controls the excretion of water by the kidneys. An increase in vasopressin causes an increased reabsorption of water by the kidney tubules. A lack of vasopressin results in diabetes insipidus.

Oxytocin stimulates the pregnant uterus to contract.

See also ACROMEGALY; ADDISON'S DISEASE; CUSHING'S SYNDROME; DWARFISM; GIGANTISM; HYPOPITUITARISM; HYPOTHYROIDISM; INFERTILITY.

Pityriasis rosea (pit′ə rī ə sis rō′se ə) is a common skin disease that starts with a slightly oval, pink, scaly area on the skin, known as a herald lesion, which is about one inch in diameter. It develops into a rash of discreet oval plaques on the torso, but rarely on the face or other exposed parts of the body. The condition causes mild itching, and the rash usually persists for six to eight weeks before disappearing spontaneously. The disease is not thought to be contagious. Its peak incidence is in the spring and fall.

Pivot joint. *See* JOINT.

PKU. *See* PHENYLKETONURIA.

Placebo (plə sē′bō) is a pill, preparation, or treatment that is given to a person as medicine, but which actually contains no active medical ingredients. Placebos are sometimes given for psychological effect, especially to satisfy a patient who needs no additional medication (placebo effect). Placebos are also used as controls in testing the effectiveness of new medicines.

Placenta (plə sen′tə) is the specialized organ by which the fetus is attached to the inner wall of the uterus and nourished. A developing fetus is completely dependent on the placenta for its nourishment.

The **placenta** nourishes the developing fetus. It is linked to the fetus through the umbilical cord.

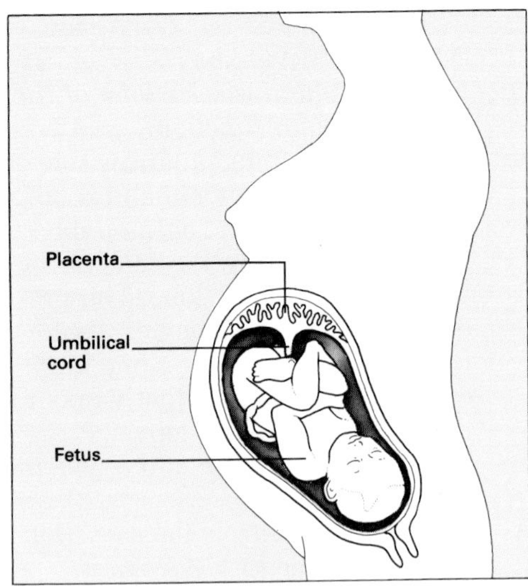

The disk-shaped placenta is made up of 20 to 40 smaller areas, called cotyledons. One side of the placenta is connected to the wall of the mother's uterus; the other side is connected with the membrane containing the amniotic fluid that surrounds the embryo or fetus. The umbilical cord provides a direct link between the placenta and the developing baby.

By the time the fully developed fetus is ready to be born, the placenta weighs about one-sixth the weight of the infant and measures about 9 to 10 inches (22.5–25cm) across. The placenta is expelled shortly after the birth of the baby as part of the afterbirth.

Q: *How does the placenta work?*

A: The mother's blood flows through the uterine wall and an exchange of the substances that the fetus needs (such as food and oxygen) and those that have to be excreted (such as carbon dioxide and urea) takes place between the placenta and the uterine wall through a thin film of cells. Thus, there is no direct contact between the fetal and maternal blood circulations.

Q: *What abnormalities can affect the placenta?*

A: The umbilical cord may be attached to one side of the placenta, instead of to its center. Or one or more of the cotyledons may lie apart from the main body of the placenta. There also can be abnormalities of the cord or of the shape of the placenta.

Sometimes, the placenta is situated in front of the fetus so that the exit from the womb is partly or completely blocked. This is known as a placenta previa, and it is a serious complication of pregnancy. In most cases of placenta previa it is necessary to perform a Cesarean section. *See also* CESAREAN SECTION.

Q: *Are there any conditions that may damage the placenta?*

A: Yes. Conditions in the mother, such as high blood pressure, chronic nephritis, diabetes mellitus, and preeclampsia (toxemia of pregnancy), damage the blood vessels and reduce the efficiency of the placenta. This increases the risk of intrauterine death of the fetus and reduces the rate at which the fetus grows.

Recent research has shown that maternal smoking also damages the placenta, resulting in smaller-than-average babies who have a greater chance of early death.

Q: *What happens to the placenta before and during normal labor?*

A: There is some deterioration in the way the placenta functions during the last two weeks of pregnancy. This is probably a factor in causing the onset of labor.

Once labor has started, the mother's blood supply to the placenta stops during contractions of the womb and returns when the muscles relax. During the final minutes of labor, the restricted blood flow probably causes a slight increase in the carbon dioxide level in the fetal bloodstream. This acts as an additional stimulus for the baby to start breathing through the lungs immediately after birth.

The placenta is delivered in the third stage of labor. It should be examined to make sure that it is complete. If a piece of placenta is left in the womb, it can cause a postpartum hemorrhage.

See also PREGNANCY AND CHILDBIRTH.

Plague (plāg) is a severe, potentially fatal infection that is caused by the bacterium *Yersinia pestis* (also called *Pasteurella pestis*). It occurs primarily in wild rodents (rats, mice, squirrels) but can be transmitted to humans. There are two main forms of plague that affect humans: bubonic plague, which results from the bite of an infected animal flea; and primary pneumonic plague, which results from inhaling droplets breathed by infected people. Both forms of plague are now rare.

Q: *What are the symptoms of bubonic plague?*

A: After a variable incubation period, which is usually between two and five days, there is a sudden onset of repeated shivering attacks, and the patient's body temperature rises to over 104°F (40°C). The lymph nodes become swollen and painful (buboes), and the patient may become delirious. The death rate in untreated patients is higher than 50 percent, with most deaths occurring within about 5 days.

Q: *What are the symptoms of primary pneumonic plague?*

A: After an incubation period of about two days, there is a sudden onset of high fever, chills, and headache. There may also be increasing breathlessness and coughing with foamy, bloodstained sputum. Most untreated patients die within about two days.

Q: *How is plague treated?*

A: Immediate treatment can be life-saving. Both forms of plague are treated with large doses of antibiotics, such as streptomycin, tetracycline, sulfa, or chloramphenicol. The patient must be isolated to prevent the spread of infection. Prompt treatment usually alleviates the symptoms rapidly and enables most patients to survive the infection.

Q: *How can plague be prevented?*

A: Prevention is based on rodent control and the use of insect repellents to reduce the incidence of flea bites. All persons traveling to India or southeast Asia should be immunized against plague. Anybody who has been in contact with an infected person should be treated with antibiotics immediately.

Plantar neuroma (plan′tər nü rō′mə) is a tumor composed of nerve cells and fibers on the sole of the foot.

Plantar reflex (plan′tər) is the normal contraction of the big toe and other toes when the outer side of the sole is stroked, causing it to point down. This reflex indicates that the nervous system is reacting normally. The opposite response is called the Babinski reflex, a pointing up of the big toe and flaring of the other toes when the outer side of the sole is stroked. The lack of a plantar reflex and the presence of the Babinski reflex may indicate a disorder of the nervous system. This response is normal in healthy infants of less than two years of age, because the corticospinal tract of the nervous system has not yet fully developed.

See also BABINSKI'S REFLEX.

Plantar wart. *See* WART, PLANTAR.

Plants, dangerous. *See* POISONING: FIRST AID.

Plaque (plak) has three medical meanings: (1) as a skin complaint, it is a group of eruptions that form a plate or patch on top of the skin; (2) plaque as a dental disorder is an accumulation of somewhat hard bacterial material on the teeth that can cause gum disorders, such as gingivitis and pyorrhea; (3) plaque also refers to fatty deposits in blood vessels (atherosclerosis).

See also ATHEROSCLEROSIS; GINGIVITIS; PYORRHEA.

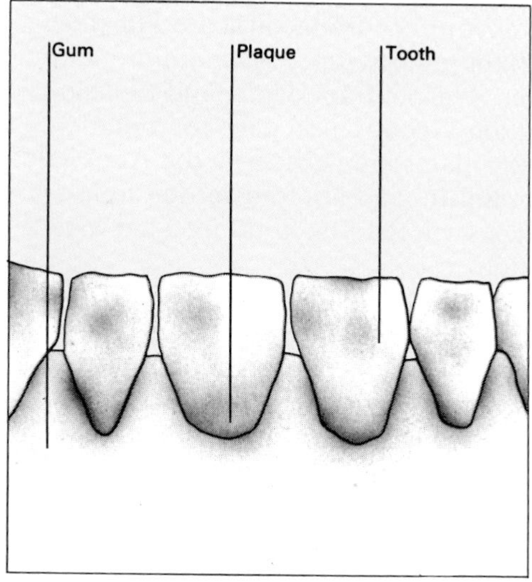

In dentistry, **plaque** refers to an accumulation of hard material on teeth. Dental plaque can cause such disorders as gingivitis and pyorrhea.

Plasma (plaz′mə) is the fluid part of the blood in which the blood cells and the platelets are suspended. It consists of water in which many chemicals are dissolved, including proteins, salts, sugars, nitrogenous wastes, and carbon dioxide. Plasma is different from serum, which is the fluid that remains when blood has clotted; serum is plasma without fibrinogen and the other components of a blood clot.

Plasma is the main medium for the transportation of substances throughout the body. It carries nutritive substances to the body structures and removes their waste products. Plasma also makes possible chemical communications within the body by transporting hormones.

Plasma may be given by transfusions to patients who have lost serum through burns. It also may be used to treat shock or disorders in which protein is lost from the body, such as ascites and nephrosis.

See also PLASMA FRACTIONS; SERUM.

Plasma fractions (plas′mə) are the different proteins that can be extracted from the blood plasma and used to treat various disorders. For example, gamma globulin can give temporary protection against some diseases, such as measles; antihemophilic globulin may be used to prevent bleeding in hemophiliacs; and albumin may be used in the treatment of nephrosis and liver cirrhosis.

See also ALBUMIN; GAMMA GLOBULIN.

Plasmodium (plaz mō′dē əm) is a genus of protozoa, certain species of which cause malaria. The species that are known to cause malaria are *Plasmodium falciparum, Plasmodium malariae, Plasmodium ovale,* and *Plasmodium vivax.* These parasitic microorganisms are carried by the Anopheles mosquito and are transmitted to humans via the bite of an infected mosquito.

See also PROTOZOA.

Plaster of Paris is a form of gypsum that when mixed with water forms a paste that hardens quickly. It can be applied to cotton bandages and used as a cast to immobilize fractured limbs.

Plastic surgery (plas′tik) is the replacement, alteration, or restoration of a visible part of the body through the use of corrective surgery. It is used to treat certain physical deformities caused either by injury or birth defects. For example, transplanting healthy skin tissue to an area covered with damaged tissue is a form of reconstructive surgery widely used in the treatment of severe burns.

See also SURGERY, COSMETIC; TRANSPLANT SURGERY.

Platelet (plāt′lit), or thrombocyte, is one of the many disc-shaped structures that float in blood plasma and are crucial to the clotting process. Platelets are formed by the fragmentation of large cells called megakaryocytes in the bone marrow.

See also BLOOD; PLASMA.

Plating (plāt′ing) is the application of bacteria onto a culture dish in order to reproduce and study them. Plating also refers to a surgical technique in which a metal plate is screwed onto a fractured bone.

Play, child's. *See* CHILD.

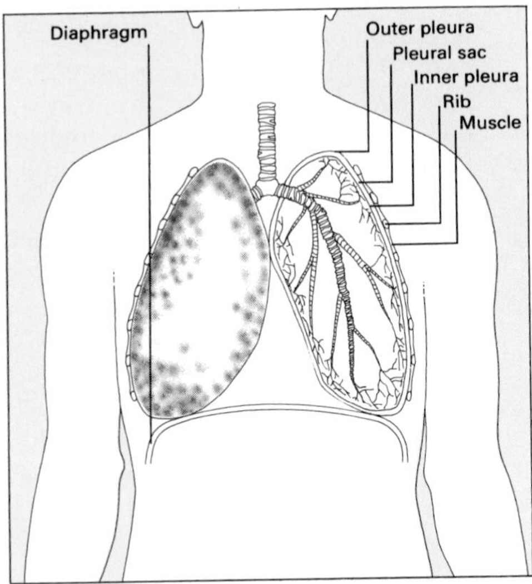

Pleura is a membrane that folds around each lung and lines the inside of the thorax (chest cavity).

Pleura (plůr′ə) is the membrane that surrounds each lung and lines the internal surface of the chest cavity. There are two pleurae, one around each lung. Each pleura consists of two layers: the parietal layer, which lines the chest cavity; and the visceral layer, which covers the surface of the lung. The space between the layers is known as the pleural cavity. It contains a small amount of fluid that lubricates the two layers, thereby facilitating the movements of the lung during breathing.

See also EMPYEMA; HEMOTHORAX; PARACENTESIS; PLEURISY; PNEUMOTHORAX.

Pleural effusion (plůr′əl i fyü′zhən) is a build-up of fluid in the pleura, the membrane that surrounds each lung and lines the chest cavity. It is caused by a fluid discharge from a pleural inflammation, such as may occur in association with a tumor or infection. It may also be commonly seen in congestive heart failure and other noninflammatory conditions. Symptoms may include chest pain, fever, and a cough.

Treatment may include the draining of the pleural effusion for diagnostic and therapeutic reasons.

See also PLEURA; PLEURISY.

Pleurisy (plủr'ə sē) is the inflammation of the pleura, a membrane that lines the inside of the chest and covers the lungs. Normally, the two surfaces of the membrane are moist and allow the lungs to move smoothly over the chest wall when a person breathes. When the pleura is inflamed, the surfaces become dry and rough and rub together. This condition, known as dry pleurisy, causes intense pain, which is made worse by coughing or deep breathing. *See also* PLEURA.

As the condition develops, the pain usually ceases because fluid forms in the pleural cavity and separates the inflamed surfaces of the pleura. If a large amount of fluid forms (wet pleurisy or pleural effusion), the underlying lung may collapse, causing breathlessness.

Q: *What causes pleurisy?*

A: Usually, pleurisy is caused by an infection of the pleura or of the underlying lung, as may occur with pneumonia. Pleurisy may also be caused by a pulmonary infarction; the spread of disease from elsewhere in the body, such as cancer; or a generalized disease, such as kidney failure. *See also* UREMIA.

Q: *How is pleurisy treated?*

A: Treatment is directed toward the underlying cause. Initially, painkillers and anti-inflammatory drugs may be given and, if the patient has a fever, antibiotics may be prescribed. When a specific diagnosis has been made, the appropriate treatment can be given, such as anticoagulants for a pulmonary infarction.

Q: *Can pleurisy cause complications?*

A: Yes. Injury to the pleura or lung cancer may cause bleeding into the pleural cavity (hemothorax). Pleurisy that is caused by infection may result in an accumulation of pus in the pleural cavity (empyema). This may require antibiotic treatment or surgical drainage. Pleural effusions that are caused by cancer tend to recur. They may need treatment with cytotoxic drugs. *See also* PLEURAL EFFUSION.

Pleurodynia (plủr ə din'ē ə) is a virus infection causing painful inflammation of the muscles of the diaphragm and the chest. Pleurodynia often causes sharp chest pains that are similar to, but which are not caused by, pleurisy. Pleurodynia may be caused by fibrositis.

See FIBROSITIS; PLEURISY; PLEURODYNIA, EPIDEMIC.

Pleurodynia, epidemic (plủr ə din'ē ə). Epidemic pleurodynia is a disease, most common in children, caused by the Group B coxsackie viruses. It is characterized by severe pain in the lower chest, muscle pain, fever, sore throat, and frequent headaches. Symptoms usually clear up in two to four days without treatment. Relapses may occur within a few days or weeks. In uncomplicated cases, epidemic pleurodynia is not serious. It is also called epidemic myalgia or devil's grip.

See also COXSACKIE VIRUS; PLEURODYNIA.

Plexus (plek'səs) is a network of nerve fibers, blood vessels, or lymphatic vessels. The solar plexus is a collection of nerves that lies behind the stomach.

Plumbism. *See* LEAD POISONING.

PMS. *See* PREMENSTRUAL SYNDROME.

Pneumococcal polysaccharide vaccine (nü mə kok'əl pol ē sak'ə rīd) is used against diseases caused by streptococcus pneumonia. The vaccine contains 23 of 83 types of pneumococcal bacteria. This formulation includes at least 85 percent of all bacteria responsible for pneumococcal diseases. When administered, it may cause mild erythema and pain at the injection site. A second dose may cause severe reactions. The vaccine should be given only once.

Q: *Who should receive the pneumococcal polysaccharide vaccine?*

A: The vaccine should be given to high-risk children and adults, such as those with sickle cell disease, the elderly, and persons with chronic debilitating diseases or with immunologic defects.

Pneumoconiosis (nü mə kō nē ō'sis) is a general term for any chronic lung disease caused by the inhalation of dust particles. It is usually caused by environmental or occupational factors, such as the inhalation of coal dust particles during coal mining. There are three main types of pneumoconiosis. (1) Simple pneumoconiosis results from the deposition of inert dust in the lungs and is apparently harmless. For example, iron, tin, and carbon dust do not seem to cause any adverse effects. (2) Irritant dusts, such as silica and asbestos, can cause silicosis or asbestosis. These diseases cause scarring and gradual destruction of the lung tissue. (3) Organic dusts may cause a form of allergic reaction. For example, byssinosis is caused by cotton fiber dust, and bagassosis is caused by sugar cane residue.

Q: *What are the symptoms of pneumoconiosis?*

A: Simple pneumoconiosis seldom produces symptoms. Coal dust, however, may cause scarring and destruction of lung tissue similar to that caused by silica and asbestos.

Pneumoconiosis that results from irritant dusts may cause increasing breathlessness, coughing, and spitting of blood. Asbestosis may develop into lung cancer.

The main symptom of pneumoconiosis that is caused by organic dusts is asthma. In some cases, this may be complicated with bronchitis.

Q: *How is pneumoconiosis treated?*

A: There is no cure for this condition. It is essential that a person change jobs or living environment at the first suspicion of pneumoconiosis. It is impossible to remove the dust particles once they have reached the lungs, and lung deterioration is likely to continue for some time after a person has stopped inhaling the dust. Dust suppression and regular medical examinations are essential.

See also ASBESTOSIS; BAGASSOSIS; BLACK LUNG; BYSSINOSIS; SILICOSIS.

Pneumocystis carinii pneumonia (nü mō sis'tis cär in'nē nü mōn'yə), or pneumocystosis, is a parasitic lung ailment caused by the organism *Pneumocystis carinii,* most often seen in individuals suffering from severely depressed immune systems, particularly those individuals suffering from acquired immune deficiency syndrome (AIDS). The symptoms include high fever, rapid and shallow breathing, coughing, and discoloration of the skin due to lack of oxygen intake. The disease may appear sporadically; however, without early detection and appropriate treatment, its fatality rate is nearly 100 percent. Various drugs, including trimethoprim-sulfamethoxazole and pentamidine, are often used to treat the illness.

See also ACQUIRED IMMUNE DEFICIENCY SYNDROME.

Pneumonectomy (nü mə nek'tə mē) is the surgical removal of a lung. A partial pneumonectomy, which also is known as a lobectomy, is the removal of a section of a lung. A pneumonectomy is most commonly performed in the treatment of lung cancer. A partial pneumonectomy may be necessary in some cases of tuberculosis, bronchiectasis, or a lung abscess.

See also BRONCHIECTASIS; TUBERCULOSIS.

Pneumonia (nü mōn'yə) is inflammation of the lungs, usually caused by a bacterial, viral, or fungal infection or from inhaled matter. If infection spreads down the bronchioles, it is known as bronchopneumonia. If only one lung is inflamed, it is called lobar pneumonia. *See also* BRONCHOPNEUMONIA.

Before the development of antibiotic drugs in the 1940's, pneumonia killed about one-third of its victims. Today, with proper medical treatment, over 95 percent of all patients recover. But pneumonia still ranks as a leading cause of death in the United States.

Q: *How does a pneumonia inflammation develop?*

A: In most cases, a person gets pneumonia by inhaling small droplets that contain harmful viruses or bacteria. These droplets are sprayed into the air when an infected person coughs or sneezes. Many cases of pneumonia result when bacteria normally present in the mouth, nose, and throat invade the lungs. The body's defense mechanisms ordinarily prevent these bacteria from reaching the lungs, but if the defenses weaken enough, severe pneumonia may develop. Such infections occur most often among patients hospitalized for some other serious illness. Conditions that increase the risk of pneumonia include emphysema, heart disease, alcoholism, and other diseases that weaken the body's resistance to infection. Children and the elderly also have a greater chance of getting pneumonia.

A wide variety of viruses cause pneumonia, including some of the same ones responsible for influenza and other respiratory infections. Many types of bacteria also cause pneumonia; most cases of bacterial pneumonia result from the bacteria *pneumococci,* also know as *Streptococcus pneumoniae.*

In the lungs, microbes that cause pneumonia lodge in the air sacs, where the blood normally exchanges carbon dioxide for oxygen. There they multiply rapidly, and the air sacs soon fill with fluid and white blood cells produced by the body to fight infection.

Q: ***What are the symptoms of pneumonia?***

A: In bacterial pneumonia, the patient develops the symptoms of a cold followed by a sudden shivering attack, sputum that is often bloody, and a high fever (104°F; 40°C) with rapid respiration and pulse rate. The patient feels pain on one side of the chest. Vomiting and diarrhea may occur; confusion is common.

In other forms of pneumonia, especially among elderly patients, the symptoms develop slowly, with clear evidence of bronchitis and a worsening cough, often with bloodstained sputum. Headache, muscle aches, and cyanosis (blue-tinged lips because of poorly oxygenated blood) are common. Progress depends on the individual's resistance to the type of infection. In elderly or weak patients, death is possible. Children or babies show few symptoms suggesting a chest infection. But the child is obviously ill and may collapse.

Q: ***How is pneumonia diagnosed and treated?***

A: Diagnosis follows a physician's examination and, usually, a chest X ray. A specimen of the sputum is examined and cultured to identify the infective organism. Sometimes, a white blood cell count may help to determine whether the infection is caused by bacteria or by a virus.

Antibiotics are used in the treatment of bacterial and fungal infections.

Breathing exercises and percussion to shake the chest wall encourage the patient to cough up sputum. If the sputum is thick and sticky, steam inhalations may also help. A seriously ill patient may need oxygen therapy. Painkilling drugs are prescribed if the patient has pleurisy. *See also* PLEURISY.

Most patients suffering from mild forms of pneumonia can be treated at home with rest, antibiotics, and breathing exercises.

Pneumonia, bronchial. *See* BRONCHOPNEUMONIA.

Pneumonitis (nü mə nī'təs) is any one of a number of acute inflammations of the lungs, such as pneumonia and pneumoconiosis.

See PNEUMOCONIOSIS; PNEUMONIA.

Pneumothorax (nü mō thôr'aks) is the presence of air or gas in the pleural cavity, the space between the lungs and the chest wall. The condition prevents the normal expansion of the lungs, thereby impairing breathing. It may result in a collapsed lung. *See also* LUNG, COLLAPSED.

Q: ***What causes a pneumothorax?***

A: The most common cause of a pneumothorax is a penetrating injury of the chest wall. This is known as a traumatic pneumothorax. Rarely, injury may cause a life-threatening form of traumatic pneumothorax in which a flap of tissue acts as a valve that allows air to be drawn into the chest, but not to be blown out again. The pressure within the chest rises rapidly and causes both lungs to collapse. This condition is known as a tension pneumothorax.

A spontaneous pneumothorax is caused by air leaking from the lungs. This may be the result of an underlying disease, such as emphysema, or of a congenital weakness of the lungs.

Pneumothorax may also be produced artificially, as by the surgical introduction of a needle into the pleural cavity to collapse a lung in the treatment of pulmonary tuberculosis. *See also* EMPHYSEMA.

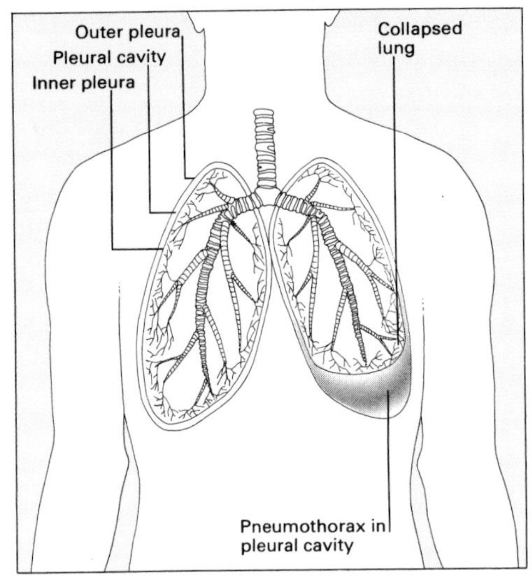

Pneumothorax is an accumulation of air or gas in the pleural cavity, which may cause the lung to collaspe.

Q: *What are the symptoms of pneumothorax?*

A: The symptoms of pneumothorax vary widely, depending on the cause of the disorder. The main symptoms of a traumatic pneumothorax are breathlessness and severe chest pains. A tension pneumothorax causes extreme breathing difficulty and may be rapidly fatal.

The symptoms of a spontaneous pneumothorax range from slight breathlessness on exertion to the sudden onset of severe chest pains and extreme breathing difficulty.

Q: *How is a pneumothorax treated?*

A: A patient with a traumatic pneumothorax requires hospitalization so that the air in the pleural cavity can be removed by insertion of a needle into the chest wall. Then the injury is treated. A tension pneumothorax requires emergency medical treatment; the rapid removal of air from the pleural cavity may be lifesaving.

Most patients with a small, spontaneous pneumothorax do not require treatment because the air is gradually reabsorbed. Occasionally, the condition may recur, in which case surgery may be necessary.

Pockmark is a small scar left after the healing of a pustule.

See also PUSTULE.

Podagra. See GOUT.

Poisoning (poi′zən ing) is the toxic condition caused by the ingestion, inhalation, or absorption of any substance that damages the body or prevents its normal functioning.

Poisoning: first aid. For emergency treatment of poisoning, call the area poison center, a hospital, or your physician immediately. If possible, tell the physician the exact name of the poison. The following emergency steps may be taken if no other advice is available.

Swallowed Poison. If the poison is a corrosive agent, such as lye, acids, or rust remover, or a petroleum product, such as gasoline, *do not* make the victim vomit. If the victim can swallow and is conscious, give the victim water and milk and wait for emergency medical attention to arrive. If the poison is not a corrosive or petroleum product, try to make the victim vomit by giving syrup of ipecac and water. Ipecac can be bought without a prescription and should be part of a home first-aid kit. If spontaneous vomiting does not occur, try touching the back end of his or her throat with the blunt end of a spoon or your finger. When vomiting begins, place the victim face down with the head lower than the hips. Save the poison container for the physician to inspect. *Never* induce vomiting in an unconscious victim.

Inhaled Poison. Carry the victim to fresh air; *do not* let him or her walk. Loosen any tight-fitting clothing, and wrap the victim in a blanket to prevent chills. Do not give any kind of alcohol. If breathing stops, apply artificial respiration. *See also* ARTIFICIAL RESPIRATION.

Poison in the Eye. Hold the victim's eyes open, and keep washing them with running water until medical assistance arrives. *Do not* apply any chemicals.

Poison on the Skin and Chemical Burns. Remove the victim's clothing if necessary. Drench and wash the skin with water. When the poison is removed, cover the victim with loose, clean cloth. Do not use ointment or other first aid for treatment of burns.

Precautions. (1) Many household products, such as domestic bleach and paint, are poisonous. Keep all household chemicals out of the reach of children. (2) Pesticides and herbicides are not only poisonous if swallowed, they can also cause damage if absorbed through the skin. Be extremely careful when handling these substances. Wear protective clothing. If any chemical is spilled on the skin, wash it off immediately. (3) Most cases of poisoning

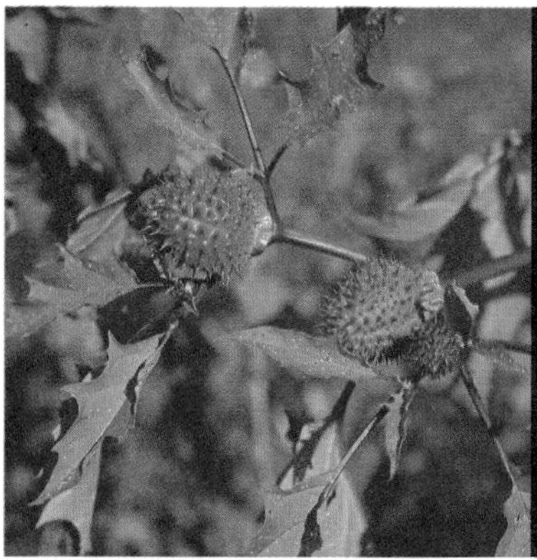

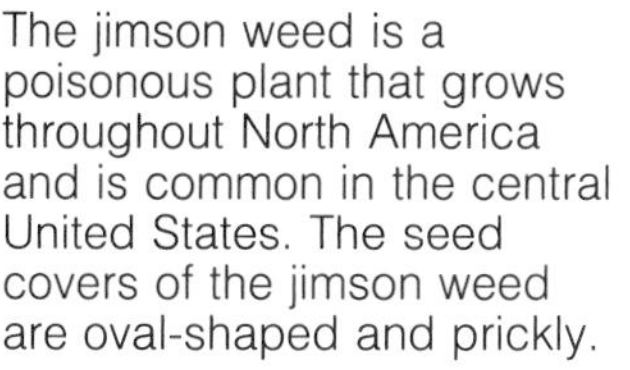

The jimson weed is a poisonous plant that grows throughout North America and is common in the central United States. The seed covers of the jimson weed are oval-shaped and prickly.

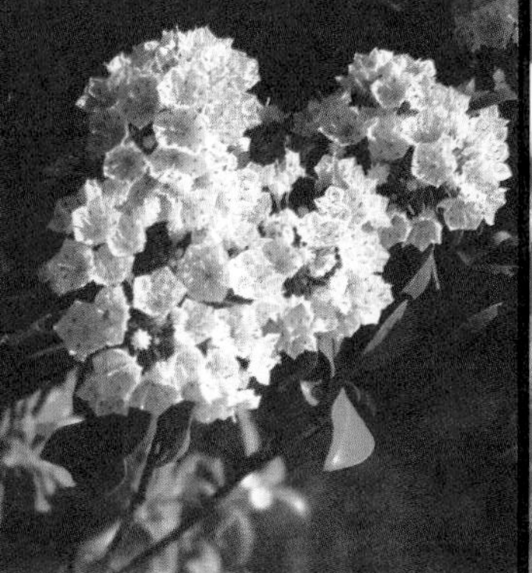

The mountain laurel, which grows in eastern North America, has poisonous leaves and berries. Its pink or white flowers may have purple markings.

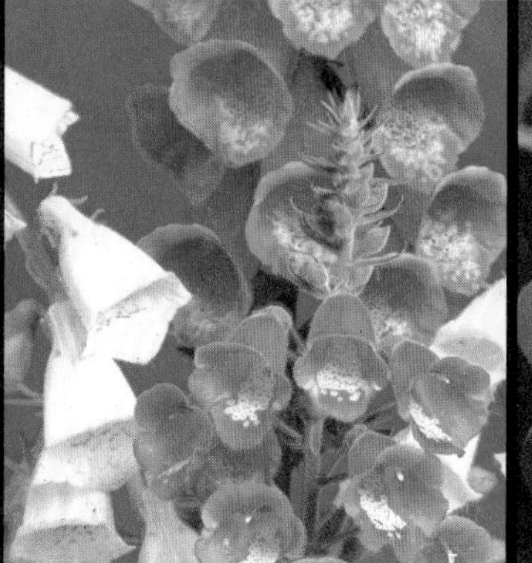

The leaves of the purple foxglove contain digitalis, a powerful poison that can be fatal when ingested in quantity. Minute amounts of digitalis are used to treat some heart diseases.

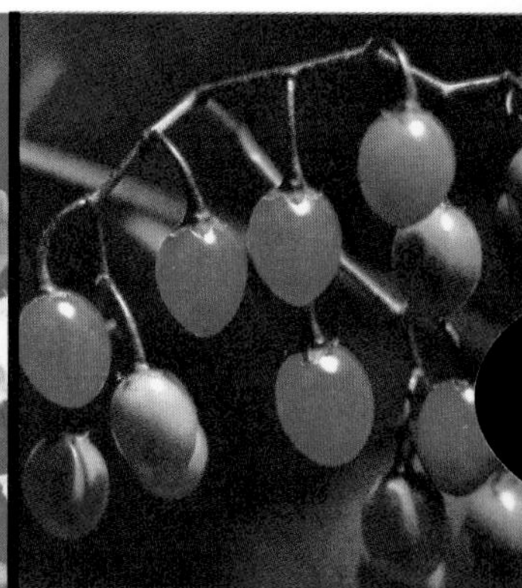

The deadly nightshade plant (belladonna) has drooping, bell-shaped flowers. The berries from the plant may be fatal if ingested.

through inhalation occur from breathing automobile exhaust fumes. Be careful when in the vicinity of a car that has its motor on. Never leave a car with its motor running in a closed garage. (4) Some plants and mushrooms are poisonous. Do not eat any wild vegetation unless you are certain it is harmless. If a person has ingested or touched a poisonous plant, see discussion on dangerous plants later in this article.

Dangerous Plants. Although only a few common plants are dangerous, no plant should be eaten unless you are certain it is harmless. Poisoning from plant substances now ranks number one among childhood ingestion of poison. This applies especially to mushrooms and toadstools, because harmless and poisonous varieties are similar. Some plants contain substances that are harmful only to those who are allergic to them. Initial contact with a poisonous plant does not give immunity, but rather increases susceptibility. The symptoms of poisoning depend on both the amount of poison ingested and the individual's reaction to the poison.

Action. If the victim has eaten a poisonous plant or mushroom, summon emergency medical aid immediately. If the victim has been in contact with a poisonous plant, like poison ivy, ensure that your hands are protected before removing the victim's contaminated clothing. Do not touch other parts of the victim's body, especially the eyes. Wash the affected area several times with soap and water. Calamine lotion may be applied.

If the Victim Is Conscious. Ask which plant was eaten. Induce vomiting by giving the patient a glass of syrup of ipecac. Save any vomit for medical analysis. *Do not* induce vomiting if the patient is unconscious.

Give the patient milk or water to drink in order to dilute the poison left in the body.

If the Victim is Unconscious. Place the victim in the recovery position, as described in FAINTING: FIRST AID. *Do not* leave the victim alone. *Do not* give the victim food or drink or induce vomiting. *See also* UNCONSCIOUSNESS: TREATMENT.

If the victim stops breathing, give artificial resuscitation. For instructions, *see* ARTIFICIAL RESPIRATION.

Poison Ivy and Poison Oak. After a person has touched a poison ivy or poison oak plant, it usually takes some time for the oily resin to penetrate and irritate the skin. Before this happens, it is wise to wash the skin thoroughly several times with soap and water. Care should be taken not to touch any other parts of the body, for even tiny amounts of the oily substance can cause irritation.

If symptoms of poisoning develop, the blisters and irritated skin can be treated with dressings of calamine lotion, Epsom salts, or bicarbonate of soda. A vaccine has been developed to prevent the rash, but this is only effec-

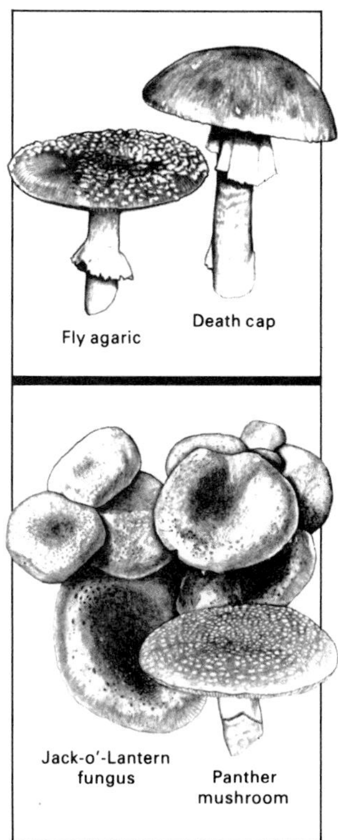

Although most toxic mushrooms are not fatal if eaten, a few species, such as the fly agaric, death cap, and panther, can cause death.

Table of dangerous plants

Name	*Poisonous parts*	*Symptoms of poisoning*
Aconite	Roots; leaves; seeds.	Nausea; vomiting; slow pulse; burning sensation in the mouth, throat, and skin; collapse.
Baneberry	Roots; sap; berries.	Vomiting; rapid pulse; diarrhea.
Bittersweet	Leaves; berries.	Burning sensation in the mouth; dizziness; weakness; convulsions.
Blood root	Stem; roots.	Burning sensation in the mouth and stomach; nausea; vomiting; slow heart rate; coma.
Castor bean	Beans; seeds.	Diarrhea; vomiting; abdominal cramp; convulsions; collapse.
Daphne	Bark; leaves; berries.	Burning sensation in the mouth and stomach; severe cramp.
Deadly nightshade (belladonna)	Roots; leaves; seeds.	Dry mouth; dilation of the pupils; irregular heartbeat; nausea; vomiting; coma.
Foxglove	Leaves; seeds.	Dizziness; nausea; vomiting; slow pulse.
Hellebore	Roots; leaves; seeds.	Salivation; abdominal pain; clammy skin; coma.
Jequirity bean	Seeds.	Vomiting; diarrhea; chills; convulsions; heart failure.
Jimson weed	Roots; seeds; leaves.	Pupil dilation; dry mouth; irregular heartbeat; vomiting; coma.
Larkspur	Leaves; seeds.	Tingling sensation in the mouth; agitation; severe depression.
Lily of the valley	Roots; leaves; fruit.	Irregular pulse; nausea; vomiting; dizziness.
Manchineel	Fruit; sap.	Sap causes burning of the skin; bleeding of the eyes. Fruit causes vomiting; diarrhea; burning sensation in the mouth and throat.
Mountain laurel	All parts are poisonous.	Salivation; tingling sensation in the skin; vomiting; convulsions; paralysis; coma.
Poison hemlock	Leaves; fruit.	Burning sensation in the mouth; slow pulse; paralysis; coma.
Poison ivy, oak, and sumac	All parts are poisonous; leaves irritate the skin.	Redness and blistering of skin; burning sensation; severe itching.
Pokeweed	All parts are poisonous.	Vomiting; drowsiness; impaired vision; coma.
Water hemlock	All parts are poisonous.	Stomach cramp; vomiting; excitation; irregular breathing; frothing; convulsions.
Yew	Roots.	Abdominal pain; nausea; vomiting; diarrhea; difficulty in breathing.

Poisoning and dangerous chemicals

Poison and sources	*Symptoms*	*Treatment*
Benzene, toluene, and xylene These substances are present in many commercial solvents and domestic paint removers. Poisoning may occur after ingestion or inhalation.	Burning sensation in the mouth leading to vomiting; chest pains; coughing; and dizziness. In later stages, lack of coordination; confusion; stupor; and coma. Death is usually from respiratory or heart failure.	Remove the victim from the source of poisoning. Carefully remove the victim's clothing if contaminated. Arrange for hospitalization of the victim. If the victim is unconscious, put in the recovery position.* If the victim stops breathing, give artificial respiration.** If the victim's heart stops, apply external cardiac compression.***
Carbon monoxide The most common source of carbon monoxide is automobile fumes. Poisoning may occur following inhalation.	The victim may be hyperactive. There may also be mild headache; irritability; fatigue; vomiting; confusion; lack of coordination; transient fainting fits with convulsions; and incontinence. Death is usually from respiratory failure.	Remove the victim from the source of poisoning. Arrange for hospitalization of the victim. If the victim is unconscious, put in the recovery position.* If the victim stops breathing, give artificial respiration.**
Carbon tetrachloride Carbon tetrachloride is present in many solvents used for removing grease. Poisoning may occur following inhalation or ingestion.	There may be vomiting; headache; dizziness; confusion; convulsions; difficulty breathing; and coma. Death is usually from respiratory or heart failure.	Remove the victim from the source of poisoning. Carefully remove the victim's clothing if it is contaminated. Arrange for hospitalization of the victim. If the victim is unconscious, put in the recovery position.* If the victim stops breathing, give artificial respiration.** If the victim's heart stops, apply external cardiac compression.***
Chlorate compounds Chlorate compounds occur in some mouthwashes and weedkillers. Poisoning may occur following ingestion.	There may be vomiting; diarrhea; blood in the urine; jaundice; delirium; convulsions; and coma. Death is usually from kidney failure.	Arrange for hospitalization of the victim. If the victim is conscious, give large drinks of water. If the victim is unconscious, put in the recovery position.* If the victim stops breathing, give artificial respiration.**
Corrosives Strong acids, such as battery acid; strong alkalis, such as caustic soda; strong antiseptics; and tincture of iodine. Poisoning may occur following ingestion.	There may be burns around the lips and mouth; intense pain in the mouth, throat, and stomach; vomiting, sometimes with blood; shock; and difficulty breathing. Death is usually from respiratory failure.	Arrange for hospitalization of the victim. If the corrosive has been spilled on the skin, place the affected area under running water for at least 10 minutes, then treat the injury as an ordinary burn. *See* BURNS AND SCALDS: FIRST AID. If the victim is conscious, give small drinks of water. If the victim is unconscious, put in the recovery position.* If the victim stops breathing, give artificial respiration.**

*For instructions, *see* FAINTING: FIRST AID.
**For instructions, *see* ARTIFICIAL RESPIRATION.
***For instructions, *see* HEART ATTACK: FIRST AID.

Poison and sources	*Symptoms*	*Treatment*
Kerosene and petroleum distillates These substances are present in many domestic cleaning fluids, paint thinners, and polishes. Poisoning may occur following ingestion or inhalation.	Mild poisoning may produce a state similar to drunkenness. Severe poisoning may cause pain in the mouth, throat, and stomach; vomiting; diarrhea; headache; blurred vision; agitation; lack of coordination; delirium; convulsions; and coma. Death is usually from respiratory failure.	Remove the victim from the source of poisoning. Carefully remove all of the victim's contaminated clothing. Arrange for hospitalization of the victim. If the victim is unconscious, put in the recovery position.* If the victim stops breathing, give artificial respiration.**
Metaldehyde Metaldehyde is present in slug and snail poison. Poisoning may occur following ingestion.	There may be nausea; vomiting; exaggerated reflexes; convulsions; and difficulty breathing. Death is usually from circulatory failure.	Arrange for hospitalization of the victim. If the victim is conscious, induce vomiting, as described earlier in this article. If the victim is unconscious, put in the recovery position.* If the victim stops breathing, give artificial respiration.** If the victim's heart stops, apply external cardiac compression.***
Naphthalene Naphthalene is present in moth balls and air fresheners. Poisoning may occur following ingestion or contact.	There may be abdominal pain; vomiting; diarrhea; difficulty breathing; delirium; convulsions; and coma. Death is usually from liver or kidney failure.	Arrange for hospitalization of the victim. If the victim is conscious, give sodium bicarbonate in water. If the victim is unconscious, put in the recovery position.* If the victim stops breathing, give artificial respiration.**
Organophosphorous compounds These substances are present in many insecticides. Poisoning may occur following ingestion, inhalation, or absorption through the skin.	There may be increased salivation; vomiting; abdominal pain; diarrhea; pinpoint pupils; difficulty breathing; convulsions; and coma. Death is usually from respiratory failure.	Carefully remove all of the victim's contaminated clothing. Arrange for hospitalization of the victim. If the victim is conscious, induce vomiting, as described earlier in this article. If the victim is unconscious, put in the recovery position.* If the victim stops breathing, give artificial respiration.**
Oxalic acid Oxalic acid is present in some bleaches and metal cleaners. Poisoning may occur following ingestion.	There may be pain in the mouth; vomiting; thirst; twitching; convulsions; and coma. Death is usually from heart failure.	Arrange for hospitalization of the victim. If the victim in conscious, give milk of magnesia or ordinary milk to drink. If the victim is unconscious, put in the recovery position.* If the victim's heart stops, apply external cardiac compression.***

*For instructions, *see* FAINTING: FIRST AID.
**For instructions, *see* ARTIFICIAL RESPIRATION.
***For instructions, *see* HEART ATTACK: FIRST AID.

Poison and sources	*Symptoms*	*Treatment*
Phenol and cresol These substances are present in many strong antiseptics. Poisoning may occur following ingestion, inhalation, or absorption through the skin.	If inhaled or absorbed, there may be difficulty breathing and unconsciousness. If ingested, there may also be burning of the mouth and throat and vomiting. Death is usually from respiratory failure.	Remove the victim from the source of poisoning. Carefully remove all of the victim's clothing. Arrange for hospitalization of the victim. If the victim is unconscious, put in the recovery position.* If the victim stops breathing, give artificial respiration.**
Phosphorus Phosphorus is present in some rat poisons. Poisoning may occur following ingestion.	There may be some burning of the mouth; a smell of garlic on the breath; vomiting; diarrhea; delirium; and coma.	Arrange for hospitalization of the victim. If the victim is unconscious, put in the recovery position.* If the victim stops breathing, give artificial respiration.**
Sodium hypochlorite Sodium hypochlorite is present in domestic bleach. Poisoning may occur following ingestion.	There may be vomiting; pain and inflammation of the mouth and throat; difficulty breathing; delirium; and coma.	Arrange for hospitalization of the victim. If the victim is unconscious, put in the recovery position.* If the victim stops breathing, give artificial respiration.**

*For instructions, *see* FAINTING: FIRST AID.
**For instructions, *see* ARTIFICIAL RESPIRATION.
***For instructions, *see* HEART ATTACK: FIRST AID.

tive if administered before exposure to the plant.

Food Poisoning. Serious diseases can be contracted from infected food and water. You should avoid unwashed fruit, precooked foods, and unsterilized water. Bottled drinking water can be bought in many countries. If in any doubt about the water, use sterilizing tablets or boil the water first. You should always wash your hands before handling food.

The symptoms of food poisoning include diarrhea, vomiting, headache, and fever. If any of these symptoms persist for more than 12 hours, consult a physician.

Poisoning, ptomaine (tō′mān). Ptomaine poisoning is an old term for a type of food poisoning that was thought to be caused by the bacterial decomposition of proteins forming ptomaine (a poison). It was later discovered that the digestive processes usually destroy ptomaine before poisoning can occur and that such food poisoning is usually caused by bacteria or their toxins.

See also FOOD POISONING.

Poison ivy is a climbing vine that produces an oily resin (urushiol) that causes a painful rash on most people if they touch the plant. Poison ivy is very common in the forests and fields of North America. For symptoms and treatment of the poison ivy rash, *see* POISONING: FIRST AID.

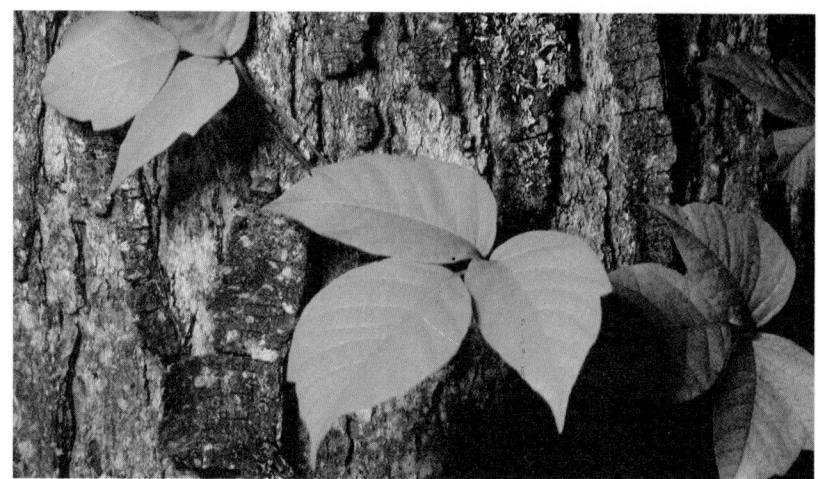

The **poison ivy** plant has green, compound leaves of three leaflets each. It is abundant in the forests and fields of the United States.

Poison ivy: first aid. *See* POISONING: FIRST AID.

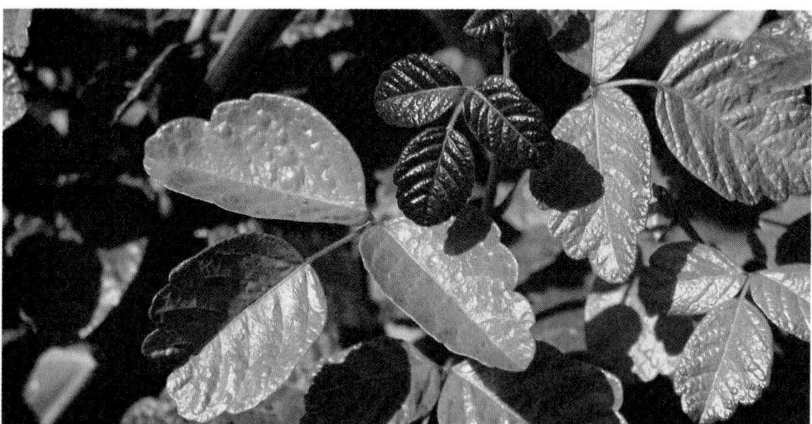

Poison oak, a shrub similar to poison ivy, is especially plentiful in the western United States.

Poison oak is any of several types of bushy shrubs that produce an oily resin causing a painful allergic rash on most people who touch the plant. Poison oak is prevalent in North America. The symptoms of the rash and its treatment are similar to those of poison ivy.

See also POISONING: FIRST AID.

Poison oak: first aid. *See* POISONING: FIRST AID.

Polio (pō′lē ō) is the common term for poliomyelitis.

See also POLIOMYELITIS.

Poliomyelitis (pō lē ō mī ə lī′tis), also known as infantile paralysis or polio, is an inflammation of the brain and spinal cord. The disease is caused by any of three polio viruses that attack the grey matter of the brain and spinal cord. Poliomyelitis occurs throughout the world. Epidemics of poliomyelitis can occur, but the risk of an epidemic is lessened by improved sanitation and eliminated by immunization of children with oral vaccine. *See also* VACCINE.

Q: *What causes poliomyelitis?*

A: Most experts believe that the virus enters the body through the nose and mouth and is carried to the intestines. Then the virus travels along the nerve fibers or is carried by the bloodstream to the central nervous system. There, the virus enters nerve cells and alters them. The virus damages or kills the cells. Paralysis results when many cells are destroyed.

Scientists usually call the three kinds of polio viruses types I, II, and III. Both the Salk and Sabin vaccines protect against all types of polio viruses.

Q: *How long does poliomyelitis take to develop and what are its symptoms?*

A: The polio virus does not always cause disease, and 95 percent of affected individuals remain without symptoms. In those it does effect, there is an incubation period of three days or more, followed by a feverish illness. A sore throat and headaches develop over a period of one to two (and occasionally five) weeks. Most people recover after this stage of abortive or nonparalytic poliomyelitis without further symptoms. One-tenth-of-one percent, however, suddenly develop severe headaches, fever, muscle pains, and neck stiffness, suggestive of meningitis. There is a tingling sensation in the limbs, increased weakness, and paralysis.

Bulbar and respiratory poliomyelitis may be fatal. Many patients suffering from paralysis during the illness regain most, or all, movement in time, but in severe cases paralysis may remain. Some residual paralysis does remain in one-third of all survivors.

Q: *How is poliomyelitis treated?*

A: Mild cases require bed rest. Severe cases need isolation and complete bed rest, with slight sedation and painkilling drugs. With respiratory paralysis, artificial respirators and a tracheostomy are necessary. A physiotherapist regularly moves the patient's joints to prevent stiffness. Extra fluids are given to prevent dehydration. The patient may have to be fed through a tube into the stomach, and a catheter is needed if the bladder is paralyzed. *See also* TRACHEOSTOMY.

Poliomyelitis is much easier to prevent than to treat. Infants should be given 3 doses of oral Sabin, live, attenuated virus vaccine (OPV), with boosters at 18 months, 5 years, and when recommended by a physician. Epidemic poliomyelitis is unlikely in vaccinated communities.

Pollen (pol′ən) is the powder-like substance produced by male flowers to fertilize other plants. Pollen produces an allergic reaction in some people.

See also ALLERGY.

Pollinosis (pol ə nō′sis) is another name for hay fever.

See also HAY FEVER.

Polyarteritis nodosa (pol ē är tə rī′təs nō dō′sah) is a rare disorder characterized by widespread inflammation of the small arteries. It is a form of periarteritis nodosa, with similar symptoms and treatment.

See also PERIARTERITIS NODOSA.

Polyarthritis (pol ē är thrī′tis) is an inflammatory condition that affects several joints at the same time.

See also ARTHRITIS; ARTHRITIS, RHEUMATOID; OSTEOARTHRITIS.

Polycystic kidney (pol ē sis′tik) is a congenital anomaly characterized by the formation of cysts in the kidney. The cysts act to enlarge the kidney, while at the same time reducing its effectiveness. Polycystic kidney is inherited, with several members of the same family sometimes having the disorder.

There are two forms of the disease, the infantile form and the adult form. The infantile form is much rarer than the adult form and also more severe. Kidney failure usually leads to an early death. The adult form usually does not manifest itself until a person is about 30 years old. Symptoms include blood in the urine (hematuria), hypertension (high blood pressure), kidney infection, and pain in the lumbar region (the lower back). The disease is progressive, and a patient usually becomes uremic within several years after the beginning of symptoms. Unless dialysis or a kidney transplant is undertaken, death occurs about 20 years after the onset of symptoms. *See also* UREMIA.

Due to the hereditary nature of the disease, genetic counseling is suggested for those in a family in which one or more members have been diagnosed with the disorder.

See also GENETIC COUNSELING.

Polycythemia (pol ē sī thē′mē ə) is an excess of red blood cells. It may be a normal temporary response to a lack of oxygen in the blood (hypoxia), as may occur as a result of heart disease or a continued exposure to high altitudes. Polycythemia may also be symptomatic of a disease of the bone marrow, as occurs with polycythemia vera. In polycythemia vera, the number of red cells and the total volume of blood increases gradually over several years. The cause of polycythemia vera is not known. The disorder can not be cured. However, by removing blood regularly (phlebotomy) or with drug treatment, the disease can be controlled.

See also BLOOD CELL, RED.

Polydactylism (pol ē dak′tə liz əm) is an anomaly characterized by extra digits on the hands or feet.

Polymorph (pol′ē môrf) is an abbreviation of polymorphonuclear leukocyte, a type of white blood cell, which has a nucleus with two or more lobes.

See also BLOOD CELL, WHITE.

Polymyalgia rheumatica (pol ē mī al′jē ə rü mat′ik ə) is a rare form of rheumatic disease that affects the elderly, usually those over 60 years of age. It is more common in women than in men. Polymyalgia rheumatica is characterized by pain and stiffness in the neck, shoulders, and back. There may also be a persistent headache. Patients often feel unwell, but rarely are seriously ill. The cause of the condition is unknown, but it is thought to result from a type of arterial inflammation. A persistent headache can also be a sign of temporal arteritis, inflammation of the arteries, a dangerous condition that results in blindness.

Treatment with corticosteroid drugs is often rapidly effective. It not only relieves the muscle pains, but also prevents damage to the eyesight. Treatment usually must be continued for several months.

See also RHEUMATIC DISEASE.

Polymyositis (pol ē mī ō sī′tis) is a disease characterized by the inflammation of many muscles. It is often a degenerative condition, accompanied by an accumulation of fluid in the muscle tissue, pain, and sweating. Its cause is unknown.

Polyneuritis (pol ē nů rī′tis) is damage to, or inflammation of, the nerves. Damage to one nerve (mononeuritis) or to several nerves in more than one area (mononeuritis multiplex) are closely related disorders.

Polyneuritis may be caused by injury, autoimmune problems, viral infection, toxic poisoning, industrial poisoning, vitamin B_{12} deficiency, alcoholism, diabetes mellitus, or cancer of the lung. Symptoms may be mild, producing tingling or altered sensation in the affected area, or severe, affecting respiration. In most cases of polyneuritis, patients make a complete and spontaneous recovery, although some may require physiotherapy, corticosteroid treatment, or surgery.

Polyp (pol′ip) is a growth or tumor on a mucous membrane. It may contain a stalk. Polyps are usually benign (noncancerous). They may occur anywhere in the body, but are most common in the nose, the cervix of the womb, within the uterine cavity, and in the colon.

Polyps within the colon or large intestine may become malignant. A condition in which there are many intestinal polyps (familial polyposis) commonly develops into cancer.

See also POLYPOSIS, FAMILIAL; TUMOR.

Polyposis, familial (pol ē pō′sis fə mil′yəl). Familial polyposis is a rare, inherited disorder in which the rectum and colon are covered with multiple polyps. Unless a total proctocolectomy (surgical removal of the rectum and colon) is performed, the condition usually results in cancer by the time a patient is 40 years old. Other complications of the disorder include rectal bleeding and possible polyp infection. Due to the hereditary nature of familial polyposis, both the patient and his or her family should be monitored closely.

See also POLYP.

Polyuria (pol ē yůr′ē ə) is the frequent passing of excessive amounts of urine. It is a typical symptom of diabetes and kidney disease, such as chronic Nephritis.

See also DIABETES MELLITUS; KIDNEY DISEASE.

Pompholyx (pom′fo liks), or dyshidrosis, is a skin eruption of highly irritating blisters on the hands and feet. The cause is usually unknown, although a fungus or allergen may be responsible. The condition lasts for one to two weeks, but commonly recurs.

The blisters break into small open sores that gradually heal. Treatment with soothing corticosteroid creams reduces the irritation until natural healing takes place. It is important to keep the area clean and dry to prevent secondary infection.

Pore (pôr) is a very small opening in the skin that allows matter to pass through. Sweat passes through the pores.

See also SKIN.

Porphyria (pôr fir′ē ə) is a group of metabolic disorders characterized by excessive secretions of porphyrins in blood-forming tissue or the liver. Porphyrins are nitrogen-containing organic compounds that are needed to unite with iron and the protein globin to form hemoglobin.

There are two main types of porphyria, the one that occurs in the red blood cells formed in bone marrow and the one that occurs in the liver.

Q: *What are the symptoms of porphyria?*

A: The symptoms occur most commonly in children and may be very severe. They include blisters, red teeth, and purple or pink urine. If the skin is exposed to the sun, the blister formations may progress to a stage of scarring. The condition may be fatal, but in its mildest form the patient needs only to avoid sunlight.

Q: *What are the symptoms of porphyria in the liver?*

A: There may be severe abdominal pain, vomiting, and abdominal swelling. These may be accompanied by any form of neurological disorder, such as epileptic seizures. Heavy alcohol consumption is also sometimes associated with porphyria.

Q: *How is porphyria treated?*

A: Children with porphyria must avoid sunlight. In adults, the precipitating cause, usually drugs, must be discovered and avoided. Relatives of a person with porphyria should also be examined. Treatment with painkilling drugs is usually necessary, and dietary treatment is also recommended.

Portacaval shunt. *See* SHUNT, PORTACAVAL.

Portal vein. *See* VEIN.

Port-wine stain (pôrt′-wīn), or port-wine mark, is a flat, purplish-red birthmark formed by abnormal blood vessels. It most often appears on the back of the head or the face.

See also BIRTHMARK.

Positron emission transaxial tomography (poz′ə tron i mish′ən tranz ak′sē əl tə mog′rə fē), abbreviated PETT, is one of a relatively new breed of imaging techniques or scanners. With PETT, trace amounts of radioisotopes are injected into the organ under study. The radioisotopes emit positrons, which collide with electrons, forming gamma rays. A computer records the location of the gamma rays, plots the source of the radiation, and creates an image of the organ on a video screen. Such scans can detect early warning signs of diseases. In the case of the heart, for example, a PETT scan could reveal an inadequate supply of blood in the tissues or a partial blockage in the coronary artery. Many persons are alive today because their diseases were detected early by a PETT scan.

See also TOMOGRAPHY.

Postnasal cavity (pōst nā′zəl kav′ə tē) is the hollow structure located behind the nose.

See also NOSE.

Postnasal drip (pōst nā′zəl) is a condition in which mucus from the back of the nasopharynx drips down the back of the throat. Postnasal drip may be caused by sinusitis or other inflammatory disorders. Symptoms include the intermittent blocking of one or both nostrils and an unpleasant taste caused by the mucus going down the throat.

Treatment includes nasal drops or nasal sprays and possible use of antibiotics. Continued use of nasal drops or sprays may only aggravate the condition, so they should not be used for a prolonged period without medical supervision.

See also HAY FEVER.

Postoperative disorder (pōst op′ə rā tiv) is a medical complication that arises following surgery. Monitoring of a patient's vital signs, which is a normal part of postoperative care, is important in avoiding or limiting medical problems. However, complications, such as an error in medication, may occur.

See also SURGERY.

Postpartum (pōst pär′təm) describes anything concerning a new mother that occurs after childbirth.

See also POSTPARTUM BLUES; POSTPARTUM DEPRESSION.

Postpartum "blues" (pōst pär′təm) are experienced by many mothers after childbirth. Generally described as a mild feeling of being "let down," the condition lasts from a few days to weeks or months.

Postpartum "blues" are characterized by some weeping, slight irritability, difficulty in sleeping, and loss of appetite—all possibly linked to hormonal activity. Another contributing factor may be anxiety regarding the care of a newborn child and the inevitable changes that must occur. The condition usually improves by itself without medication or treatment. Family support is helpful in dealing with postpartum "blues."

See also POSTPARTUM DEPRESSION.

Postpartum depression (pōst pär′təm) afflicts about 3 percent of women following childbirth. In some cases, it may be indicative of preexisting psychological difficulties that have been aggravated by the physical and psychological stresses of the pregnancy and delivery. In other cases, the hormonal changes occurring after delivery may cause a biochemical imbalance in susceptible individuals, producing the depression.

The condition is characterized by feelings of hopelessness and despondency, mood swings, insomnia, and an inability to cope with normal situations. There is a high level of anxiety concerning the baby, difficulty in caring for the infant, and a feeling of guilt about not loving it enough. Postpartum depression often requires antidepressant medication to correct a biochemical imbalance and possibly also counseling.

See also POSTPARTUM "BLUES."

Posttraumatic (pōst trô mat′ik) describes any medical condition that occurs as a result of, or following, an injury.

Postural drainage (pos′chər əl) is a type of positioning used by physiotherapists, respiratory therapists, and surgeons to place a patient in such a way that gravity assists in the drainage of a congested area, especially in the drainage of secretions from the lungs and bronchial tubes. The process of postural drainage often calls for the use of pillows to elevate portions of the body.

Postural hypotension (pos′ chər əl hī pə ten′shən) is the lowering of the blood pressure that occurs when a person stands up. Blood pressure normally dips when a person stands up, but an acute drop in blood pressure, as may occur when a bedridden patient stands up after a long period of lying down, might cause loss of consciousness.

Potassium (pə tas′ē əm) is a metallic, chemical element that is abundant in the earth's crust. Potassium salts play a vital role in metabolism, the process by which humans change food into energy and new tissue. For example, potassium helps enzymes speed up several chemical reactions in the liver and muscles. It is essential for nerve transmission and contraction of muscles, including the heart. Potassium also combines with sodium to contribute to the normal flow of water between the body fluids and the cells of the body. A daily diet that includes fruit, vegetables, meat, and whole grains supplies enough potassium for the normal needs of the human body. High blood pressure medications causing excessive urinating often result in a low potassium level.

See also MINERAL.

Pott's disease (pots) is tuberculosis of the spine. It is a grave disorder that produces destruction of a vertebra by tuberculous osteitis (inflammation of the bone). Collapse of a vertebra results in the compression of the spinal cord and nerves. Pott's disease gives the individual the typical hunchback appearance of kyphosis. Paralysis may also occur.

Treatment includes arresting the destruction of tissue with antituberculosis drugs, relieving the spinal cord from pressure, bed rest, adequate diet, and careful exercise.

See also KYPHOSIS.

Pott's fracture (pots) is a fracture of the ankle. The break usually involves the tibia (shinbone) or fibula (the second of the two long bones in the lower leg), or both. The ankle joint is often dislocated, and the ligaments are torn.

Pott's fracture is a fairly common injury. It is usually treated by manipulating, under general anesthesia, the fractured bone into the correct position and immobilizing the ankle in a plaster cast. With severe fractures, the broken bones are operated on.

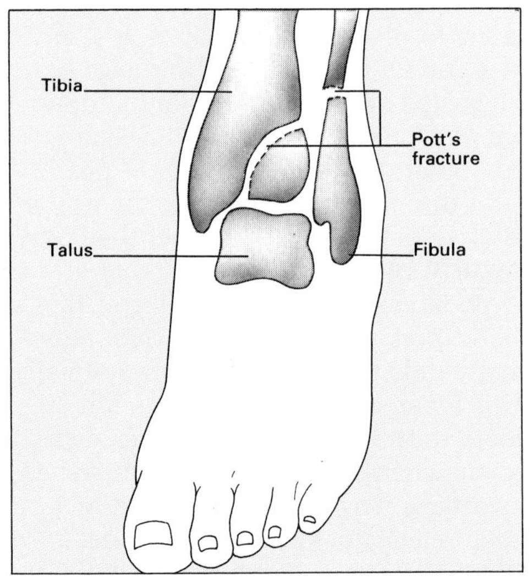

Pott's fracture is an ankle fracture that is often caused by a violent backward jerk of the foot and ankle.

Precocious puberty. *See* PUBERTY, PRECOCIOUS.

Prednisone (pred'nə sōn) is a steroid hormone, used in treating arthritis, inflammatory diseases, asthma, and certain allergies. Prednisone and another corticosteroid drug, prednisolone, are synthetic preparations that act similarly to the naturally occurring steroid hormone cortisol, which is formed by the adrenal glands.

Prolonged use of prednisone, especially at high dosage, causes undesirable side effects. These include a typical moon face and acne; an increase in body fat; loss of calcium from the bones (osteoporosis); a tendency to develop diabetes mellitus; a higher risk of developing a peptic ulcer; reduced resistance to infection; and thin skin, which heals more slowly than normal skin. If prednisone has been taken for a long period of time, the dosage must be reduced slowly, until the adrenal glands start producing cortisol again.

See also CORTICOSTEROID DRUG.

Preeclampsia (prē ek lamp'sē ə) is a condition that sometimes occurs late in pregnancy. Symptoms include high blood pressure; swelling (edema) of the legs, hands and, to a lesser extent, the face; and protein in the urine (albuminuria). It is sometimes called toxemia of pregnancy, although there is no evidence to suggest that it is caused by a toxin. In fact, the cause of preeclampsia is not known. But the condition is more likely to occur in women who already have hypertension (high blood pressure), who suffer from chronic nephritis, or who are expecting their first baby. *See also* EDEMA; PROTEINURIA.

Q: *How is preeclampsia treated?*

A: In the very early stages, the patient is instructed to take additional rest. She is advised not to lie on her back because this causes the uterus to press on the blood vessels that supply it. She is given mild sedatives and a strict diet plan emphasizing high protein and normal salt intake to prevent any further weight gain.

If these measures are not successful, the woman may be admitted to the hospital.

Q: *What complications may occur with preeclampsia and how are they treated?*

A: The most serious complication is eclampsia, in which convulsions and coma may occur in the woman. The more common complications are those that affect the fetus. The blood supply to the uterus is reduced, and fetal growth is slowed. There is an increased likelihood of intrauterine death.

If severe preeclampsia occurs after the thirty-sixth week of pregnancy, induction of labor or a Cesarean section may be performed.

See also ECLAMPSIA.

Pregnancy and childbirth (preg'nən sē). Although pregnancies naturally vary in duration, a normal pregnancy lasts from conception to delivery. In women with "normal" 28-day menstrual cycles, pregnancies last 280 days from the first day of the last normal period to delivery.

Q: *Can a woman always be sure that her estimated date of delivery is correct?*

A: No. A woman whose periods have always been irregular is unlikely to reach an accurate date for delivery based on calculation. This is because the date of ovulation, and thus fertilization, probably occurred about two weeks before a period was due.

It is possible for bleeding to occur during pregnancy. However, this bleeding may make a woman think she has menstruated and become pregnant a month later than was actually the case.

Q: *What are early symptoms of pregnancy?*

A: Often, the earliest sign is the absence of a period (amenorrhea). This may be accompanied by a feeling of heaviness in the breasts, slight nausea the first thing in the mornings (morning sickness), and frequency of urination.

Q: *What tests and examinations are carried out to confirm pregnancy?*

A: A pregnancy test can be performed using a sample of urine, after the period has been overdue for eight days. If this is positive, it is relatively certain that the woman is pregnant. If the test is negative, it should be repeated in a week's time. From about two weeks after a missed period onward, an ultrasound examination of the uterus can definitely verify pregnancy by showing the gestational sac and the developing fetus. *See also* PREGNANCY TEST; PREGNANCY TESTING KIT.

Once the period is more than two weeks overdue, a gentle vaginal examination usually reveals an enlargement of the uterus. This, combined with other symptoms suggestive of pregnancy, may con-

Jan.	1	2	3	4	5	6	7	8	9	10	11	12	13	14	15	16	17	18	19	20	21	22	23	24	25	26	27	28	29	30	31	Jan.
Oct.	8	9	10	11	12	13	14	15	16	17	18	19	20	21	22	23	24	25	26	27	28	29	30	31	(1	2	3	4	5	6	7	Nov.
Feb.	1	2	3	4	5	6	7	8	9	10	11	12	13	14	15	16	17	18	19	20	21	22	23	24	25	26	27	28				Feb.
Nov.	8	9	10	11	12	13	14	15	16	17	18	19	20	21	22	23	24	25	26	27	28	29	30	(1	2	3	4	5				Dec.
Mar.	1	2	3	4	5	6	7	8	9	10	11	12	13	14	15	16	17	18	19	20	21	22	23	24	25	26	27	28	29	30	31	Mar.
Dec.	6	7	8	9	10	11	12	13	14	15	16	17	18	19	20	21	22	23	24	25	26	27	28	29	30	31	(1	2	3	4	5	Jan.
April	1	2	3	4	5	6	7	8	9	10	11	12	13	14	15	16	17	18	19	20	21	22	23	24	25	26	27	28	29	30		April
Jan.	6	7	8	9	10	11	12	13	14	15	16	17	18	19	20	21	22	23	24	25	26	27	28	29	30	31	(1	2	3	4		Feb.
May	1	2	3	4	5	6	7	8	9	10	11	12	13	14	15	16	17	18	19	20	21	22	23	24	25	26	27	28	29	30	31	May
Feb.	5	6	7	8	9	10	11	12	13	14	15	16	17	18	19	20	21	22	23	24	25	26	27	28	(1	2	3	4	5	6	7	Mar.
June	1	2	3	4	5	6	7	8	9	10	11	12	13	14	15	16	17	18	19	20	21	22	23	24	25	26	27	28	29	30		June
Mar.	8	9	10	11	12	13	14	15	16	17	18	19	20	21	22	23	24	25	26	27	28	29	30	31	(1	2	3	4	5	6		April
July	1	2	3	4	5	6	7	8	9	10	11	12	13	14	15	16	17	18	19	20	21	22	23	24	25	26	27	28	29	30	31	July
April	7	8	9	10	11	12	13	14	15	16	17	18	19	20	21	22	23	24	25	26	27	28	29	30	(1	2	3	4	5	6	7	May
Aug.	1	2	3	4	5	6	7	8	9	10	11	12	13	14	15	16	17	18	19	20	21	22	23	24	25	26	27	28	29	30	31	Aug.
May	8	9	10	11	12	13	14	15	16	17	18	19	20	21	22	23	24	25	26	27	28	29	30	31	(1	2	3	4	5	6	7	June
Sept.	1	2	3	4	5	6	7	8	9	10	11	12	13	14	15	16	17	18	19	20	21	22	23	24	25	26	27	28	29	30		Sept.
June	8	9	10	11	12	13	14	15	16	17	18	19	20	21	22	23	24	25	26	27	28	29	30	(1	2	3	4	5	6	7		July
Oct.	1	2	3	4	5	6	7	8	9	10	11	12	13	14	15	16	17	18	19	20	21	22	23	24	25	26	27	28	29	30	31	Oct.
July	8	9	10	11	12	13	14	15	16	17	18	19	20	21	22	23	24	25	26	27	28	29	30	31	(1	2	3	4	5	6	7	Aug.
Nov.	1	2	3	4	5	6	7	8	9	10	11	12	13	14	15	16	17	18	19	20	21	22	23	24	25	26	27	28	29	30		Nov.
Aug.	8	9	10	11	12	13	14	15	16	17	18	19	20	21	22	23	24	25	26	27	28	29	30	31	(1	2	3	4	5	6		Sept.
Dec.	1	2	3	4	5	6	7	8	9	10	11	12	13	14	15	16	17	18	19	20	21	22	23	24	25	26	27	28	29	30	31	Dec.
Sept.	7	8	9	10	11	12	13	14	15	16	17	18	19	20	21	22	23	24	25	26	27	28	29	30	(1	2	3	4	5	6	7	Oct.

The estimated date of childbirth can be calculated from the first day of the woman's last menstrual period. Find the latter date (in light type) and the delivery date is below it (in heavy type).

firm pregnancy without a pregnancy test.

Q: ***How are the common problems of early pregnancy treated?***

A: Morning sickness affects about 50 percent of women. For the more severe condition (hyperemesis gravidarum), a physician may prescribe antinauseant drugs to be taken at night. Frequent small meals and dry foods, such as crackers, help to control mild nausea. Breast tenderness is relieved by wearing a firm brassiere that gives good support.

Q: ***What information is required, and what examinations and tests are carried out by the obstetrician?***

A: It is most important for the woman to give the full history of any previous pregnancies or abortions she may have had.

She will also be asked about any illnesses or disorders she may have had. Chronic nephritis, diabetes mellitus, high blood pressure, and rheumatic valve disease of the heart all can cause problems during pregnancy. If there is a family history of diabetes mellitus, there is a possibility that the patient could develop mild diabetes while under the stress of pregnancy. *See also* DIABETES MELLITUS; HYPERTENSION; NEPHRITIS; RHEUMATIC DISEASE.

A complete physical examination includes weighing, breast examination, blood pressure test, urine test, cervical smear, and vaginal examination. At each subsequent visit, blood pressure, weight, and urine are monitored, and the obstetrician checks the ankles for signs of edema. The growth of the uterus is checked each visit after the fourteenth week of pregnancy. The obstetrician can check this by feeling the abdomen. *See also* EDEMA.

Finally, some laboratory tests are made on a sample of the woman's blood. The blood group and rhesus (Rh) factor are determined, and tests are made for anemia and syphilis. The blood should also be tested for antirubella (the antibody for German measles) and other antibodies. *See also* ANEMIA; RUBELLA; SYPHILIS.

The obstetrician usually discusses the findings of the examinations and tests with the patient, to reassure her that the pregnancy is normal and to emphasize the importance of regular prenatal checkups. At first, these are generally given on a monthly basis, unless there is some abnormality present. But later in pregnancy the visits become more frequent, usually occurring every two weeks from the twenty-eighth week of pregnancy, and weekly from the thirty-sixth until delivery.

Q: ***Should a woman in early pregnancy keep to a special diet and carry out routine exercise?***

A: Unless she suffers from a condition that demands special attention (such as obesity or diabetes mellitus), diet and exercise are dictated by common sense.

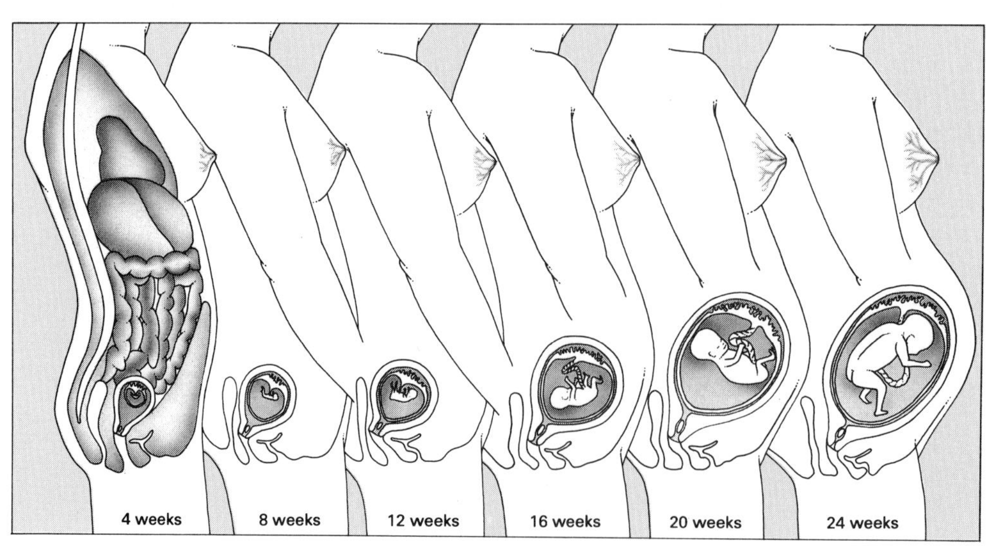

The first 6 months of pregnancy: At about 4 weeks the fetus's heart has developed, and by 8 weeks the fetus has begun to develop nearly all its body organs. After week 12 the mother's breasts enlarge and the abdomen swells as the fetus continues to grow.

Q: *May sexual intercourse continue throughout pregnancy?*

A: Yes. In general, if the course of pregnancy is normal, intercourse may take place as usual. If there is a history of spontaneous abortion, however, the obstetrician probably will advise avoiding intercourse during the first three months, around each time when a period would normally have occurred. *See also* ABORTION, SPONTANEOUS.

Q: *What tests and examinations may be carried out during the middle three months of pregnancy?*

A: Using ultrasonic equipment, the obstetrician usually can detect fetal life without known danger for either the mother or fetus. Ultrasound may continue to be used if there are any problems, such as the possibility of twins. *See also* ULTRASOUND.

Amniocentesis involves taking a sample of fluid from around the fetus by inserting a needle into the uterus, under local anesthetic. This procedure may be carried out if there is any possibility of a congenital fetal abnormality, such as Down's syndrome. It also can detect some developmental disorders of the nervous system, as well as other abnormalities. *See also* AMNIOCENTESIS; DOWN'S SYNDROME.

Q: *What is "quickening," and at what stage can it be felt?*

A: Quickening describes the first movements of the fetus in the uterus felt by the mother. A woman undergoing her first pregnancy usually feels it between the eighteenth and twentieth weeks. In subsequent pregnancies, however, when the mother is aware of what to expect, she may feel it about two weeks earlier.

Q: *What are the common problems of the latter half of pregnancy?*

A: Many minor problems may affect a woman as pregnancy progresses, although few are serious.

(1) *Backache.* This is extremely common because the ligaments that normally hold the joints in place are affected by hormones, which cause the ligaments to become more stretched and relaxed.

The woman is advised to wear low-heeled shoes and to place a firm board under her mattress (or under her side of it). Muscle strengthening exercises and instruction on how to hold the body properly help to relieve backache. Occasionally, it is necessary to wear a lumbar support corset.

(2) *Headaches.* A common symptom, these may be associated with fatigue and the additional stress and anxiety placed upon a woman during pregnancy. They are generally not serious and seldom need more than simple treatment.

(3) *Constipation.* This is a common complaint throughout pregnancy, caused by the production of the hormone progesterone. This hormone has a relaxing effect on the intestinal tract. The condition often is improved by adding increased bulk to the diet, such as

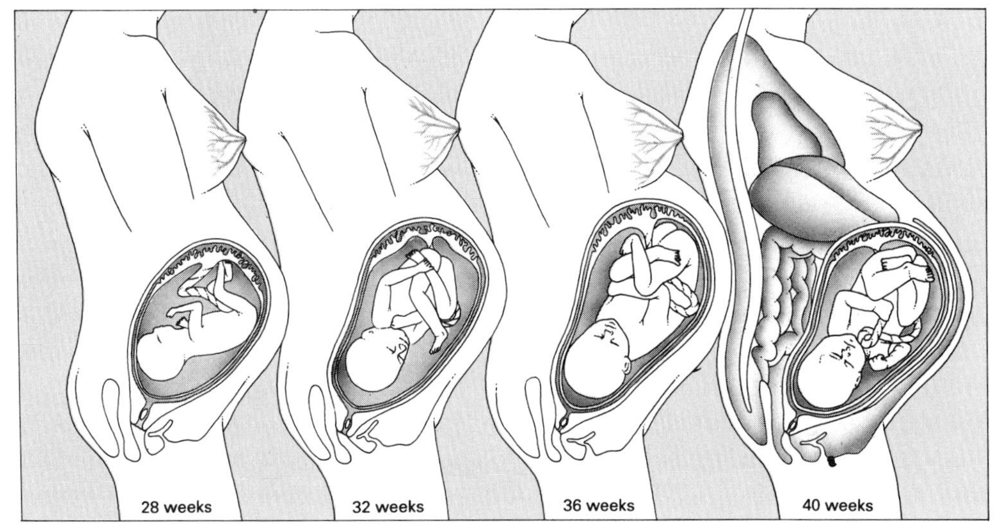

The latter months of pregnancy: At about 28 weeks the fetus usually settles in the uterus with the head pointing downward. During the next several weeks the uterus continues to enlarge, until about 2 weeks before delivery when it "lightens."

bran and fresh vegetables, as well as by drinking additional fluids. *See also* PROGESTERONE.

(4) *Increased Frequency of Urination.* This occurs not only in the early days of pregnancy, but also toward the end because of increased pressure on the bladder.

Painless increase in urination is seldom anything to worry about. If there is any discomfort, however, it should be reported to the obstetrician because urinary infections, such as cystitis, can occur during pregnancy. *See also* CYSTITIS.

(5) *Heartburn.* The production of the hormone progesterone during pregnancy causes relaxation of the muscle at the lower end of the esophagus. This allows the normal acid contents of the stomach to pass back into the esophagus.

The symptoms can be improved by taking frequent small meals and by avoiding a large meal before going to bed. Antacid medicines often can help, as can raising the head and shoulders at night.

(6) *Ankle Swelling.* This is a common symptom caused by the effect of progesterone on the blood vessels, as well as by the pressure and weight of the pregnant uterus on the veins that carry blood from the legs. Varicose veins may aggravate the condition.

To treat swollen ankles, the feet should be raised above the level of the pelvis as often as possible during the day, and the foot of the bed should be raised at night.

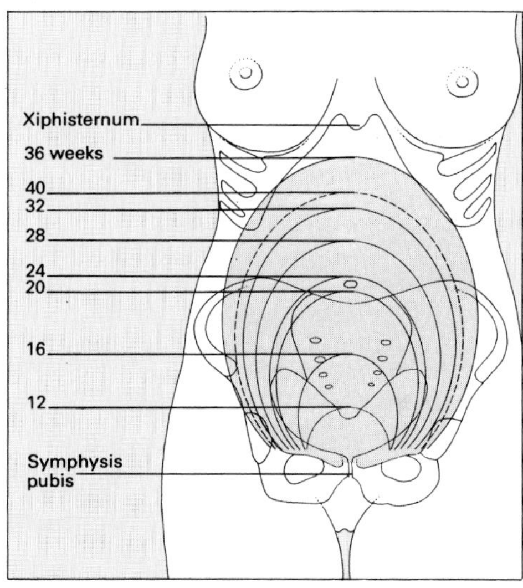

The uterus expands steadily during pregnancy, reaching its greatest size at about week 36.

(7) *Varicose Veins and Hemorrhoids.* Varicose veins may occur as a result of increased pressure within the veins of the legs. The enlarged uterus presses down on the veins of the pelvis and obstructs the blood flow from the legs to the heart. Hemorrhoids (piles) is a similar condition, usually caused by the pressure set up in the anal area by the straining action of constipation.

During pregnancy, women with varicose veins should wear elastic stockings. Hemorrhoids can be relieved with ointments and by taking preventive measures against constipation. *See also* HEMORRHOID; VARICOSE VEIN.

(8) *Insomnia.* Sleeplessness commonly occurs in the last few weeks of pregnancy. Insomnia may be caused by the enlarged abdomen, backache, or vigorous fetal movements. If necessary, the obstetrician may prescribe a mild sedative. *See also* INSOMNIA; SLEEP DISORDERS.

(9) *Palpitations and Sweating.* These symptoms are similar to those experienced during menopause and are caused by the effects of the hormones on the mother's body during pregnancy. They are seldom severe. *See also* MENOPAUSE.

Q: ***What regimen of diet and exercise should be followed in the latter half of pregnancy?***

A: During the second half of pregnancy, the mother should pay particular attention to diet. The fetus requires increased nourishment, but the woman must avoid excessive weight gain.

First-class proteins (such as those in eggs, milk, fish, and meat), together with vegetable proteins, are particularly important.

Energy requirements are supplied mainly by carbohydrates in the diet. These should be adjusted to fit in with the protein and the small amount of fat that make up the remainder of the diet.

Fresh fruit and vegetables are an essential part of the diet because they supply vitamins and the bulk that helps to prevent constipation. The obstetrician often prescribes small doses of supplementary vitamins and iron.

Milk contains protein, calcium, and phosphorus, the minerals responsible for bone formation. But milk is not essential as long as the diet includes meat and cheese.

Regular exercise is an essential part of maintaining good health. Routine prenatal exercises are an essential part of maintaining physical and psychological well-being.

Q: *When should a pregnant woman start attending prenatal classes?*

A: The timing depends on the recommendation of the individual obstetrician, but it is usual to defer prenatal classes until the last 3 months of pregnancy. Usually, a series of 8 to 12 weekly classes are attended by the same group of prospective parents. They are told about the normal development of the fetus, the progress of pregnancy, and the stages of labor.

The class is also shown exercises to strengthen the back and pelvic muscles, as well as special methods of breathing that may be of assistance during the various stages of labor. The women are asked to practice these exercises at home.

At least one class is devoted to the care of the newborn baby, how to bathe and dress the baby, as well as how to change a diaper. Often a mother who had just had a baby returns to the class to demonstrate baby care, bringing her own infant with her.

It is usual, at some point during prenatal classes, to discuss the problems that may arise in labor and the kind of action that the obstetrician may take.

Q: *What is "lightening," and when can it be expected to occur?*

A: Lightening is the sensation of increased physical comfort that is experienced when the fetus has descended into the lower part of the uterus in the pelvic cavity, thus relieving pressure on the upper abdominal area. It usually occurs at about the thirty-sixth week; however, in women who have had babies before, it may not occur until labor starts.

Q: *What special tests or examinations are carried out by the obstetrician during the last three months of pregnancy?*

A: Provided the pregnancy is developing normally, the only special tests needed are a reassessment of the level of hemoglobin in the blood to check for anemia, a repetition of the antibody test for the Rh (rhesus) factor, and sometimes a test of the urine to ensure that there is no

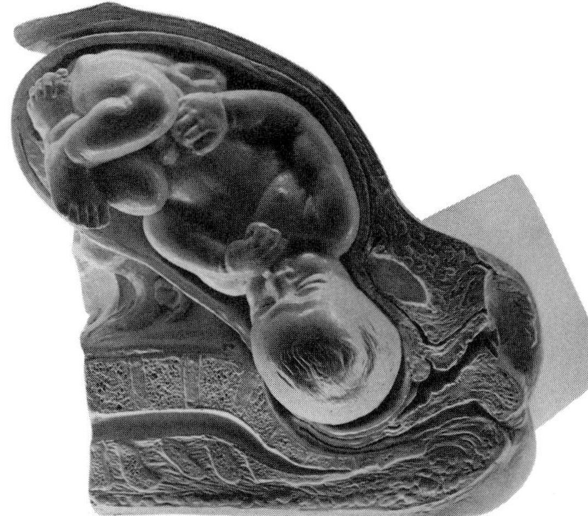

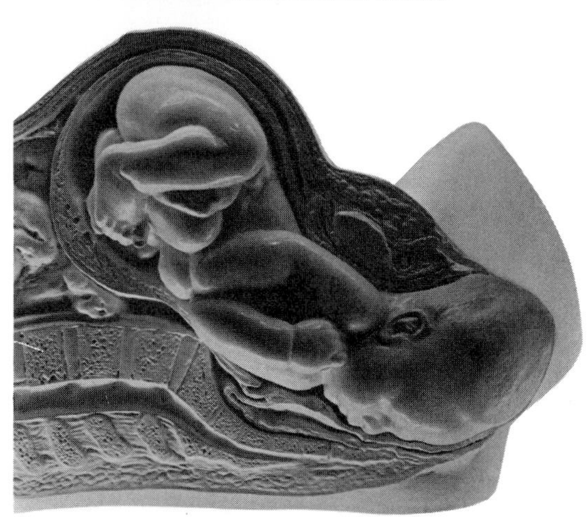

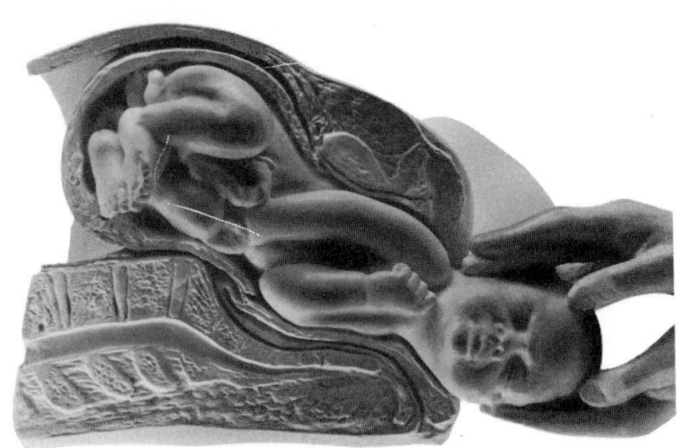

The birth process, called *labor*, results from muscle action forcing the baby out of the uterus. At the beginning of labor, (1) the head of the baby points toward the opening of the uterus. As the muscles contract, the head turns and (2) passes through the vagina. The baby is born (3) when its head comes out of the vagina.

infection. The obstetrician usually performs an internal, gynecological examination at about the thirty-seventh week of pregnancy. This is done to assess the size of the pelvis to ensure that there is enough room for the fetus to be born. *See also* RH FACTOR.

Q: *Why may pregnancy end prematurely, and is this a problem?*

A: In many cases the cause of premature birth is not known. Factors that may contribute to prematurity include preeclampsia, twins, and prepartum hemorrhage. If premature rupture of the membranes occurs, without the onset of labor, it usually is advisable to keep the woman resting in bed until at least the thirty-sixth week of pregnancy, when labor can be induced. *See also* PREECLAMPSIA.

The main problem of premature labor is that it produces an immature baby who will require specialized care.

Q: *What are the problems associated with prolonged pregnancy?*

A: There is a gradual deterioration in the placenta toward the end of pregnancy. Even at 42 weeks, however, the placenta is still capable of providing a mature fetus with all the nourishment it needs. But there is a greater likelihood of fetal death occuring, so the obstetrician usually induces labor if the woman is considered to be more than two weeks overdue, and if the circumstances are favorable for induction.

Q: *Is infection serious during pregnancy?*

A: Rubella (German measles) is a serious infection when contracted by a woman in early pregnancy. It greatly increases the risk of congenital anomalies in the fetus. Infection with a type of herpes virus may be fatal to the fetus. Any infections should be reported to the obstetrician.

Q: *What is the onset of labor?*

A: During the final two or three weeks, the woman may notice the occasional, irregular, but firm contraction of her uterus. The abdomen hardens, but no discomfort is felt. If this is confused with the actual onset of labor, it is termed a false labor. Labor commences when regular, powerful contractions occur every 20 to 30 minutes, accompanied by a dull ache in the lower abdomen and back.

Sometimes there is a "show" of blood and mucus from the vagina as the plug of mucus that blocks the cervix during pregnancy breaks apart and the cervix starts to open.

Rupture of the membranes (bag of waters), followed by a rush of clear fluid from the vagina, occasionally may be the first sign of labor.

As soon as the contractions are occurring every 10 to 15 minutes, or the membranes have ruptured, the woman should go to the hospital. She should take a suitcase that has already been packed with some clothing for the baby and a nightgown, robe, and nursing brassiere, as well as cosmetic articles for herself.

Q: *What occurs during labor, and how can the mother help?*

A: Labor is divided into three stages. The first stage continues, with regular contractions of increasing frequency, until the cervix of the uterus is fully open (dilated). The second stage includes the passage of the baby through the pelvis, until it is delivered. The third stage is the expulsion of the placenta and membranes from the uterus.

The first stage of labor varies greatly in duration, but commonly takes between 5 and 10 hours. It is shorter in women who have previously had a baby.

At first, contractions may occur only every 20 to 30 minutes, each one lasting for 10 to 15 seconds. As the contractions become more frequent and longer in duration, the cervix progressively dilates. It is during these contractions that the breathing methods, learned in the prenatal classes, are useful. Usually during this first stage of labor, the membranes rupture.

Eventually the contractions occur every two to three minutes, and the woman feels the urge to push. This sensation may be accompanied by a dull, deep backache. This is the beginning of the second stage of labor. The second stage is one of hard, physical effort with contractions coming every 1 to 2 minutes, and each one lasting at least 30 seconds. The second stage seldom continues longer than two hours and is frequently over in less than an hour. Before it commences, the obstetrician usually carries out a careful, sterile gynecological examination to ensure that the cervix is fully dilated and to assess the position of the fetal head.

During the second stage of labor the fetal head is pushed down into the mother's pelvis. When it reaches the pelvic floor, the back of the head rotates round to the front of the pelvis. The fetus's chin is pressed down onto its chest. As the fetus extends the head from this bent position upward, the mother's vulva is extended and stretched open. The head is "crowned" at the moment when the vulva is stretched round the greatest circumference of the fetal head.

During this stage, the mother can help by taking a deep breath prior to the contraction and forcibly trying to expel the baby through the pelvis by "bearing down" during the contraction. It is most comfortable if she can keep her knees bent and her head and shoulders raised. This exercise and position is taught in the prenatal and natural childbirth classes.

As the fetal head is crowned, the obstetrician may decide to cut the skin at the back of the vulva (episiotomy) so that the fetal head can be delivered more easily. This keeps the vagina from tearing. Once the head comes through, the rest of the body follows quite rapidly.

Just after being born, the baby's mouth is sucked clear of mucus, so that breathing can take place easily, and the eyes are cleaned. The umbilical cord is clamped, tied, and cut, and the baby is wrapped in a towel. The baby often is handed to the mother so that she can enjoy her first moments with her child.

The third stage of labor usually is over within 30 minutes. Contraction of the uterus is helped by the administration of oxytocin, which is given to the mother after the baby is delivered. There is slight vaginal bleeding as the obstetrician gently maneuvers the placenta out of the womb. All that is required of the mother at this stage is a final, gentle push.

While waiting for the placenta to be expelled, the obstetrician may inject a local anesthetic, stitch up the episiotomy, and repair any minor damage to the vagina that has occurred during delivery of the baby.

Q: *What can the woman's partner do to help during labor?*

A: During the first stage of labor, which may last some hours, he can accompany his partner while she walks up and down in her room or the corridor of the hospital. During contractions, he can apply gentle but firm pressure with his hands to her back, as well as remind her to breathe correctly. In the second stage, while in the delivery room, he can provide encouragement to his partner. He also can help to support her neck and legs when she is trying to expel the fetus.

Q: *How can pain be reduced during labor?*

A: Painkilling drugs can be given during labor if requested. An injection of either a local or a spinal anesthetic causes only slight discomfort and allows the woman to remain fully conscious throughout labor. A skilled anesthesiologist is required to carry out this procedure. Occasionally, quite severe headaches may occur for two or three days after delivery. From time to time, general anesthesia is needed during labor. *See also* ANESTHETIC.

Q: *What can the obstetrician do if labor is not normal?*

A: Sometimes, the obstetrician decides, before labor commences, that a normal delivery would be too risky. This may occur with a placenta previa, in which the placenta blocks the passage of delivery, with abnormalities of the pelvis or, sometimes, if the woman has previously had a Cesarean section. In such cases, the obstetrician performs a Cesarean just before the baby is due.

Sometimes, problems occur once labor has already started, such as fetal distress or prolonged labor. To deal with these problems, the obstetrician either performs a Cesarean, if labor is still in the first stage, or helps the delivery by carefully applying forceps around the baby's head. In this way, the baby is gently, firmly, and steadily pulled out.

A malpresentation requires repositioning of the baby's head by internal manipulation. This can be done either by the hand or, more usually, with a pair of special forceps. *See also* MALPRESENTATION.

Q: ***Are there any dangers involved in the use of forceps?***

A: There is a slight chance that the fetus will be damaged or bruised as a result of pressure exerted by the forceps. The risks of fetal damage should be weighed against the risks of not using additional methods to help a difficult delivery.

Q: ***How long is it necessary to stay in the hospital?***

A: This depends on the obstetrician's advice as to whether both the mother and the baby are well enough to return home. If the pregnancy has been normal, the mother and child are well, and lactation is established, discharge from the hospital can often take place within 48 hours of delivery.

Q: ***What can the mother do to help in her physical recovery after labor?***

A: It is usual to allow 24 hours of rest after labor. Following her obstetrician's advice, the mother can help to get her figure back to normal with exercises to strengthen the muscles of the pelvis, abdomen, and back. Care should be taken not to do these too strenuously at first. The ligaments of the joints are still soft, and excessive exercise could cause joint strains.

Q: ***Why is it sometimes necessary to induce labor artificially, and how is it done?***

A: Labor is induced if either the health or life of the mother or fetus is at risk. It may be recommended for a variety of reasons: preeclampsia; a pregnancy that has continued for more than a week or 10 days past the expected date of delivery; a placenta previa, in which the placenta is obstructing the passage of delivery; a maternal problem, such as diabetes mellitus; or Rh incompatibility of the blood, which could lead to hemolytic disease of the newborn. *See also* HEMOLYTIC DISEASE OF THE NEWBORN; PREECLAMPSIA.

Generally, oxytocin is given to the woman intravenously. Labor usually starts within a few hours. Artificial rupture of the membranes that surround the fetus (amniotomy) may also aid induction of labor. The procedure is carefully monitored, and an induced labor should follow the pattern of a normal labor.

Q: ***Are there any things that a woman should avoid during pregnancy and the puerperium?***

A: Yes. All drugs, even aspirin, must be avoided during early pregnancy unless they have been prescribed by a physician. This is primarily to reduce the chances of congenital malformation in the fetus. The use of alcohol, cocaine, heroin, and/or marijuana can have detrimental effects on the developing fetus and on the nursing infant. Drug addiction must be stopped and abstinence maintained from the beginning of pregnancy through the period of lactation.

Mothers who smoke cigarettes are more likely to go into premature labor than those who do not. Their babies also tend to be born smaller than average, greatly increasing the chances of the baby dying.

Some drugs may adversely affect the mother. For example, many commonly used drugs aggravate the symptoms of heartburn during the latter months of pregnancy and should be avoided.

See also BABY; BABY CARE; CHILD BIRTH, NATURAL.

Pregnancy and childbirth: emergency delivery. See CHILDBIRTH: EMERGENCY DELIVERY.

Pregnancy, ectopic (preg'nən sē, ek top'ik). Ectopic pregnancy, or extrauterine pregnancy, occurs when a fertilized ovum, instead of passing along the fallopian tube from the ovary and implanting in the lining of the uterus, implants in the tube itself or, rarely, on the ovary, cervix, or in the abdomen. Such a pregnancy seldom lasts more than two months; usually the fallopian tube then bursts. Occasionally, the embryo dies and is absorbed, although there have been cases in which a fetus has survived long enough to be born by Cesarean section. Ectopic pregnancy may be caused by infection of the fallopian tube (salpingitis) or any other condition that might block the tubes, or if an IUD is used for contraception.

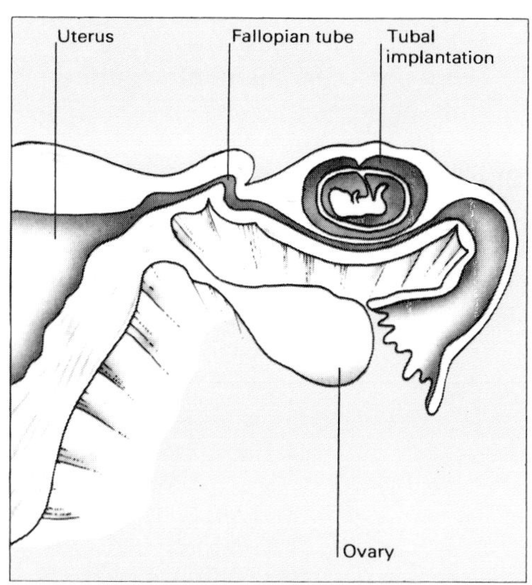

An **ectopic pregnancy** can occur anywhere outside the uterus—a common site is in the fallopian tube itself.

Q: *What are the symptoms of ectopic pregnancy?*

A: In its early stages, it may be impossible to distinguish between a normal and an ectopic pregnancy. Later, there may be a sudden onset of severe abdominal pain and loss of blood from the vagina, caused by abnormal uterine bleeding and bursting of the fallopian tube. The bleeding causes shock and collapse.

Q: *How is an ectopic pregnancy treated?*

A: If the embryo is detected before the tube ruptures, the fallopian tube can be preserved after the products of conception are surgically removed. When the fallopian tube ruptures, immediate hospitalization is necessary; the entire tube has to be removed. Ectopic pregnancy is usually fatal without surgical intervention.

Q: *Can a woman conceive after having had an ectopic pregnancy?*

A: Yes, further pregnancies are usually possible if one healthy fallopian tube remains. Expert medical advice should be sought.

See also PREGNANCY AND CHILDBIRTH.

Pregnancy, false (preg'nən sē). False pregnancy (pseudocyesis) is a condition in which a patient shows most of the outward, physical signs and symptoms of pregnancy, but is not pregnant. Among these signs are an enlarged abdomen, absence of menstruation, morning sickness, and weight gain. False pregnancy is thought to have an emotional origin, which causes the pituitary gland to be affected in the same way as during a real pregnancy. It occurs in women with a strong desire to have a child or in those who are anxious not to conceive. It can also be caused by malfunctioning of the endocrine system. The condition has also been reported in men.

Q: *Is there any treatment for a false pregnancy?*

A: Psychiatric help may be useful. When the patient is asleep or under hypnosis, the enlargement of the abdomen disappears.

Pregnancy test (preg'nən sē) is a urine test to confirm whether or not a woman is pregnant. It is about 95 percent accurate in women whose periods are 2 to 3 weeks overdue. Most tests will not register a reliable result until the period is at least 8 days overdue. More recently, tests have been devised to detect pregnancy earlier.

See also PREGNANCY TESTING KIT.

Pregnancy testing kit (preg'nən sē) is a device that enables a woman to determine whether or not she is pregnant by means of a simple, self-administered test in her own house. A common type of kit uses a chemical solution that detects the presence of human chorionic gonadotropin (HCG), a hormone present in the urine of pregnant women.

The user simply places a few drops of her urine in a test tube. If a dark ring forms after the prescribed amount of time, the woman can be reasonably sure she is pregnant.

Negative results with such kits should be viewed with somewhat more caution, particularly if the user is taking antidepressant drugs, having irregular or infrequent periods, or nearing menopause. Pregnancy testing kits may be purchased at drug stores without a prescription.

Pregnancy, tubal. *See* PREGNANCY, ECTOPIC.

Premarin® (prem′ə rin) is a preparation of natural estrogens (female sex hormones) obtained from the urine of pregnant mares. Available in tablet form, as a vaginal cream, or as an injection, it is used primarily in hormone replacement therapy during and after menopause. *See also* ESTROGEN REPLACEMENT THERAPY.

If possible, Premarin should not be given to pregnant women or to women with histories of thrombosis, uterine fibroids, or cancer of the uterus or breast. Side effects of the systemic administration of the drug include nausea, breast fullness and tenderness, and water retention (edema).

Premature birth. *See* BIRTH, PREMATURE.

Premature ejaculation. *See* EJACULATION, PREMATURE.

Premedication (prē med ə kā′shən) is a drug or combination of drugs that is given to a patient before a general anesthetic. It produces a state of mild drowsiness and dries the secretions in the mouth and the bronchi, the main airways to the lungs.

Premenstrual syndrome (prē men′strů əl) consists of various symptoms that, in some women, occur regularly for several days before each menstrual period. Symptoms vary in severity and include irritability, depression, fatigue, headaches, breast tenderness, and a feeling of abdominal swelling. There may also be a runny nose, asthma, migraine, and backache. Premenstrual syndrome can also make women anxious, intolerant, and prone to accidents.

Q: *What causes premenstrual syndrome?*

A: The cause is thought to be a hormonal disturbance, accompanied by retention of water within the body tissues.

Q: *Can premenstrual syndrome aggravate any other problems?*

A: Yes. Depression, from causes other than premenstrual syndrome, tends to be increased. Women who suffer from epilepsy may have convulsions only during this time. Interpersonal relationships may be strained at this time, due to increased irritability.

Q: *What treatments can help premenstrual syndrome?*

A: A physician may prescribe a diuretic (water-removing) drug to relieve bloating. Proper nutrition and regular aerobic exercise are often helpful.

If these simple treatments are not successful, hormone preparations of estrogens or progesterone may give relief from all the symptoms. In some cases, a physician may prescribe the contraceptive pill.

See also MENSTRUATION.

Premolar (prē mō′lər) is a bicuspid tooth, which is well adapted for grinding food. There are two pairs of premolars in each jaw, located between the canine teeth and the molars.

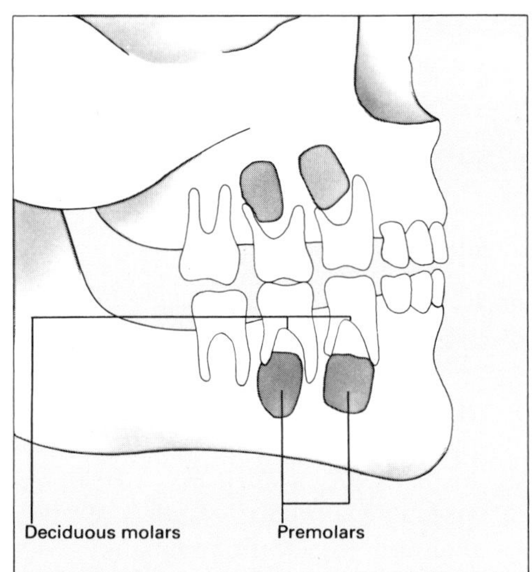

The **premolars** emerge during early childhood, replacing the deciduous molars.

Prenatal (prē nā′təl) means before birth and refers to the care given to the expectant mother and her baby from the time that conception has been confirmed by a pregnancy test until the start of labor. Such care is now considered to be as important as the delivery itself.

See also PREGNANCY AND CHILDBIRTH.

Prepatellar bursitis. *See* BURSITIS, PREPATELLAR.

Prepuce. *See* FORESKIN.

Presbyopia (prez bē ō'pē ə) is farsightedness that occurs as a normal process of aging. As a person becomes older, the lens of the eye loses its elasticity, so that the muscles that adjust it become less effective. Distant vision remains unaltered, but the ability of the eye to focus on close objects is impaired. Eyeglasses usually correct the condition.

Presentation (prez ən tā'shən) is an obstetric term used to indicate which part of a fetus is positioned lowest in the uterus, just above the cervix. The position of the baby's body is called the "lie."

The normal presentation is occipital, meaning that the back of the head is just above the cervix.

See also MALPRESENTATION; PREGNANCY AND CHILDBIRTH.

Preventive medicine is the branch of medicine that pertains to the prevention of disease or to its early diagnosis, so as to lessen the severity of the disorder. Preventive medicine is carried out at all levels of the health profession and includes such areas as health education and vaccination programs.

In its broadest sense, preventive medicine also includes such disciplines as physiatry, in which physically impaired patients undertake a rehabilitation program to recover bodily functions and prevent further physical deterioration.

There are three levels of preventive health care. (1) Primary prevention is concerned with preventing susceptible individuals from developing a particular disorder; examples include dietary modification for children with a family history of heart disease and use of car seats to prevent injury. (2) Secondary prevention is the identification and early treatment of asymptomatic disease; examples include Pap smears for cervical cancer and mammograms for breast lumps. (3) Tertiary prevention is the limiting of further disease or disability in patients with chronic disorder; examples include cardiac rehabilitation following heart attack and respiratory therapy for emphysema.

Priapism (prī'ə piz əm) is a persistent, painful erection of the penis without sexual stimulus. It is caused by blockage of the veins that carry blood from the penis. Sometimes, blood can be extracted from the penis. Anticoagulant drugs may also help.

Prickly heat (prik'lē), or miliaria, is an intensely irritating, fine red rash. The irritation is caused by the body's inability to produce sweat because the sweat glands have become blocked by dead skin cells.

Calamine lotion may give some relief, and light cotton clothing should be worn.

Primary care is comprehensive, ongoing health care for individuals and their families. It includes care for acute illnesses, chronic problems, and preventive care. Family physicians, general pediatricians, and general internists are major providers of primary care.

Primary-care providers are usually the first professionals consulted in the case of an injury or illness. They diagnose the most common disorders and prescribe or provide appropriate treatment. If a case is complicated or severe, the primary-care provider may consult another health professional with specialized expertise in that area. In these cases, the primary-care provider usually stays involved with any subsequent diagnosis or treatment. *See also* MEDICAL SPECIALISTS.

Primary care can be provided in a variety of settings, including a physician's office, a health clinic, at home by means of a house call, or in the hospital or nursing home.

Prion (prē'on) is a protein particle approximately 100 times smaller than a normal virus. It was first isolated from the brain of sheep infected with scrapie, which is a virus disease of sheep that attacks the nervous system, usually causing death. Prion is thought to be the cause of scrapie and other degenerative diseases of the nervous system.

Procaine hydrochloride (prō kān' hī drə klôr'īd) is one of the safest and least toxic local anesthetics. However, excessive amounts of procaine or an allergy to it may be associated with lowered blood pressure, possibly fatal cardiac arrest, and seizures.

See also ANESTHETIC.

Procidentia. *See* PROLAPSE.

Proctalgia (prok tal′jē ə) is pain in the anal region without obvious cause. Proctalgia fugax is an intermittent pain in the anal region, commonly occuring at night.

Proctitis (prok tī′tis) is inflammation of the rectum and anus. The main symptoms are pain in the rectal region and a frequent desire to pass feces. Defecation is painful and may be accompanied by diarrhea and the passing of blood and mucus. This is often followed by tenesmus (spasm of the local muscles) and pain. The symptoms may be controlled with antispasmodic and painkilling drugs. Hospitalization may be necessary for thorough investigations; sometimes, steroid enemas are necessary.

Proctology (prok tol′ə jē) is a medical specialty concerned with disorders of the anus, rectum, and colon.

Proctoscope (prok′tə skōp) is a metal or plastic tubular endoscope, often containing a light, that is used to examine the rectum.

See also ENDOSCOPY.

Prodromal (prod′rə məl) means any early, minor symptom or sign of disease that occurs before the onset of the actual condition.

Progeria (prō jir′ē ə), which means "prematurely old" in Greek, is an extremely rare disorder that causes premature aging in children. Affected individuals appear normal at birth but soon develop the typical symptoms of progeria: a wrinkled skin, stooped posture, and a "plucked bird" facial appearance, with prominent eyes, beaked nose, and loss of hair, eyebrows, and eyelashes.

Victims usually die before the age of 20, often of circulatory problems, such as heart attacks or atherosclerosis. The cause of the disorder is not known, and there is no effective cure. It is also known as Hutchinson-Gilford syndrome.

Progesterone (prō jes′tə rōn) is a female sex hormone produced by the corpus luteum in an ovary during the second half of the menstrual cycle. It prepares the lining of the uterus for the reception of a fertilized ovum (egg). Preparations called progestins have similar effects to progesterone. They are used in some contraceptive pills and to treat some menstrual disorders.

See also ESTROGEN; MENSTRUATION.

Progressive muscular atrophy. *See* MUSCULAR ATROPHY, PROGRESSIVE.

Prolactin (prō lak′tin) is a hormone that is produced by the front lobe of the pituitary gland in women. It stimulates the glands in the breasts (mammary glands), thereby initiating milk production (lactation) at the end of pregnancy and sustaining it after childbirth. Prolactin has this effect only when certain hormones, such as estrogen, progesterone, and oxytocin, are also present.

See also ESTROGEN; OXYTOCIN; PITUITARY GLAND; PROGESTERONE.

Prolapse (prō laps′) is an abnormal, downward displacement of a part of the body. Examples include prolapse of the rectum, in which the membranes that line the rectum protrude through the anus; and prolapse of the uterus, in which the supporting ligaments become so weak that the uterus is displaced into the vagina. Prolapse of the rectum is relatively uncommon and may be the result of an underlying disorder or a congenital abnormality.

Q: *How is prolapse of the rectum treated?*

A: This is seldom a problem when it occurs in infants, providing a physician is consulted. By applying gentle pressure to the protruding tissue, it generally can be pushed back inside, and the condition usually is self-correcting in a matter of weeks.

In the elderly, prolapse of the rectum is a more serious matter. If it recurs frequently or if it is not possible to push it back, an operation may have to be done to remove the surplus membranes. Alternatively, a circle of wire or nylon can be placed around the anus to tighten the opening.

Q: *Why does prolapse of the uterus occur?*

A: The cause is a gradual slackening of the ligaments that support the walls of the vagina and uterus. This usually happens because the ligaments are stretched during childbirth; they also become weakened after menopause because of lack of hormone production. Although prolapse of the vagina may occur without prolapse of the uterus, the two usually occur together.

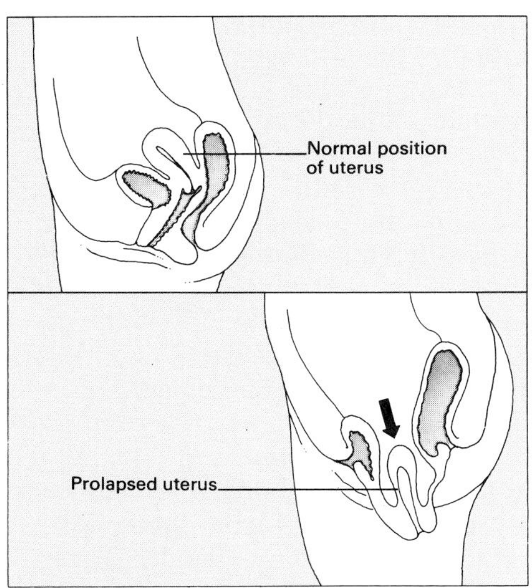

A **prolapse** of the uterus may occur when the ligaments that support the uterus are weakened, displacing the uterus into the vagina.

Q: *What are the symptoms of prolapse of the uterus?*
A: The main symptom is a sensation of "something falling out of the vagina." This is sometimes accompanied by a deep ache in the lower abdomen. If the prolapse is severe, the neck of the uterus (cervix) sticks out of the vagina, between the labia; this is known as a procidentia.

Other symptoms include incontinence of urine on coughing, laughing, or lifting weights (stress incontinence); and, occasionally, difficulty in defecating. The prolapse may be accompanied by a vaginal discharge.

Q: *How is a prolapse of the uterus treated?*
A: The best treatment is a surgical operation to shorten the ligaments that support the uterus and to stitch the top of the vagina back into a firm position. This operation is usually accompanied by removal of the uterus, or part of the cervix, or both.

If an operation cannot be performed, a plastic ring (pessary) can be inserted into the vagina to hold the uterus in place.

Q: *Is there any way in which a woman can prevent a prolapse of the uterus from occurring?*
A: Yes. Care during childbirth is essential so that the second stage of the labor does not last too long. After childbirth, the woman should strengthen the muscles and ligaments surrounding the uterus by doing postnatal exercises, as recommended by a physiotherapist.

See also PREGNANCY AND CHILDBIRTH.

Prolapse, mitral valve. *See* MITRAL VALVE PROLAPSE.

Prone (prōn) is the position of the body when lying face downward.

Prophylactic (prō fə lak'tik) is any agent that is used to prevent disease, for example, immunization in childhood or the use of antimalarial drugs.

The term prophylactic also describes any chemical or physical device used to reduce the risk of contracting a venereal disease, such as a condom.

See also CONDOM.

Proptosis (prop tō'sis) is a forward bulge, especially of the eye. It is usually a symptom of exophthalmos, but it may also occur if there is a tumor in the eye or in the eye socket.

See also EXOPHTHALMOS.

Prostaglandin (pros tə glan'dən) is any one of a group of hormones found in many tissues of the body. They have widely diverse actions including vasodilatation, stimulation of uterine muscle contraction, inhibition of gastric acid secretion, and platelet aggregation. Various chemical derivatives are under investigation for medical use (in effecting abortions and in peptic ulcer disease, myocardial infarction, and peripheral vascular disorders).

Prostatectomy (pros tə tek'tə mē) is an operation to remove the prostate gland, usually because it is enlarged, but also to treat cancer of the prostate gland. Prostatectomy always results in sterility, but most men are still able to have sexual intercourse.

See also PROSTATIC HYPERTROPHY.

Prostate disorders (pros' tāt) generally cause difficulties with urination, because the prostate gland surrounds the urethra (the tube that carries urine from the bladder). A gradual enlargement of the prostate gland (prostatic hypertrophy) normally occurs with increasing age. But enlargement may also be caused by cancer of the prostate. Inflammation of the prostate (prostatitis), caused by an infection, tends to occur in younger men.

Q: *What symptoms occur with prostate problems?*

A: The symptoms caused by prostatic hypertrophy, prostatitis, and cancer are all similar. There is increased frequency of passing urine, combined with a feeling that the bladder is not empty, even immediately after urination. Sometimes, there is extreme urgency as well as slight discomfort on passing urine (dysuria) or, alternatively, the patient is unable to pass urine even when he has the opportunity. Usually, he has to urinate several times at night (nocturia), and occasionally, there is blood in the urine (hematuria).

Sometimes, the patient can not pass urine at all. This may occur gradually over a matter of a few weeks (chronic retention), with backflow of excess urine leading to kidney failure (uremia). Or it may occur suddenly, as a painful, acute retention of urine. Any form of retention needs urgent medical treatment.

Q: *How are prostate problems treated?*

A: Treatment depends on the cause.

See also CANCER; PROSTATE GLAND; PROSTATIC HYPERTROPHY; PROSTATITIS.

Prostate gland (pros′tāt) is a walnut-sized organ that is part of the male urinogenital system. It lies beneath the bladder and surrounds the urethra, the tube that carries urine from the bladder. The prostate gland produces secretions that maintain the vitality of sperm.

See also SPERM.

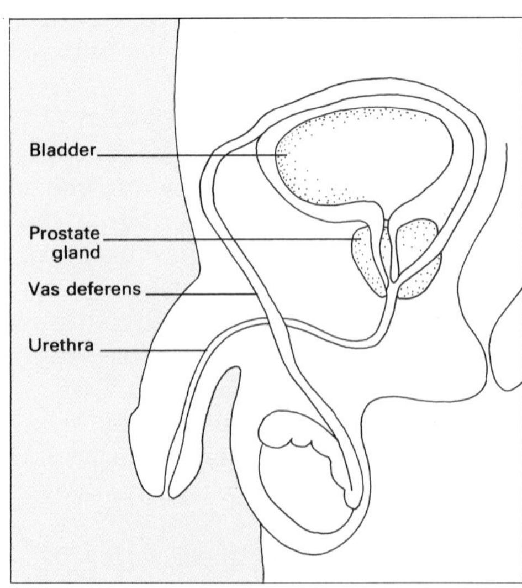

An enlarged **prostate gland** impedes urination by constricting the urethra, cutting the flow of urine from the bladder.

Prostatic hypertrophy (pros tat′ik hī pėr′trə fē), also called prostatomegaly, is an increase in the size of the prostate gland. It normally occurs in men over the age of 50 years and slowly, but steadily, worsens, so as to cause the minor symptoms of prostate problems. This condition is known as prostatic hypertrophy and often needs no treatment. But if the symptoms become severe or are caused by cancer, medical treatment is necessary.

Q: *Can complications arise from prostatic hypertrophy?*

A: Yes. Complications arise from back pressure of the urine and poor drainage from the bladder. These may result in (1) retention of urine and bleeding from a dilated vein, which causes blood in the urine (hematuria); (2) the formation of bladder stones (calculi); and (3) damage to the kidney, causing hydronephrosis and uremia. *See also* HYDRONEPHROSIS; UREMIA.

Q: *How is prostatic hypertrophy treated?*

A: Surgical removal of the prostate gland (prostatectomy) is the only way of curing the symptoms. Occasionally, it may be necessary to reduce the pressure caused by retention of urine by catheterizing the patient for a few days before the operation. He may require treatment for kidney failure, and his general health may need to be improved as well. *See also* PROSTATECTOMY.

Q: *What is the treatment for prostatic hypertrophy caused by cancer?*

A: In the early stages of the disorder, an operation to remove the prostate gland often cures the condition. In later stages, particularly if the man is elderly and the cancer has spread, treatment with female hormones (estrogens) often is effective. It can prevent further spread and development for many years, as well as reduce the size of the gland and lessen the symptoms.

Prostatitis (pros tə tī′tis) is inflammation of the prostate gland. It may occur as the result of a venereal disease, nonspecific urethritis, or infection spreading from the intestine, or it may develop after an examination of the inside of the bladder (cystoscopy).

Prostatitis causes symptoms similar

to those of other prostate problems. Painful and frequent passing of urine (dysuria) is a common symptom if the infection is acute.

Prolonged treatment with antibiotics may be necessary, and the patient usually is advised to avoid sexual intercourse until the infection is cured.

See also URETHRITIS, NONSPECIFIC.

Prostatomegaly. *See* PROSTATIC HYPERTROPHY.

Prosthesis (pros'thə sis) is the medical term for the replacement of any part of the body by an artificial substitute. Some external prostheses are used for purely cosmetic reasons.

See also REPLACEMENT SURGERY.

Prostration (pros trā'shən) is a dangerous state of physical and mental exhaustion that occurs as a result of excessive fatigue, heatstroke, or illness. The victim should be placed in the recovery position, as described in FAINTING: FIRST AID. Someone should remain with the victim until professional medical help arrives. It is essential to find the cause of prostration so that appropriate treatment can be given.

Protein (prō'tēn) is a class of complex nitrogenous compounds composed of amino acids.

Human proteins are formed in the body from amino acids derived from the digestion of protein-containing foods or from amino acids manufactured by the body.

Proteins are formed from about 20 different amino acids, and the body is able to synthesize most of these. A total of eight essential amino acids cannot be made by the body, and so they must be obtained from the diet. These essentail amino acids occur in a wide variety of foods, including grains, seeds, and vegetables, as well as meat, fish, and dairy products.

Hemoglobin, a complex protein, is responsible for carrying oxygen to all cells. Enzymes are also complex proteins and are necessary for metabolism.

See also AMINO ACID; NUTRITION.

Proteinuria (prō tə nůr'ē ə) is the existence of protein in the urine, which is usually in the form of albumin, a protein that is soluble in water and can be coagulated by heat. Proteinuria can be a sign of kidney disease or failure. Strenuous exercise can also cause proteinuria.

Prothrombin (prō throm'bin) is a protein substance that is an essential factor in the clotting of blood. When bleeding takes place, prothrombin is changed by a complex series of reactions into the insoluble protein thrombin. Anticoagulant drugs depress the formation of prothrombin in the liver and reduce the ability of the blood to clot.

Modern materials and designs enable advanced **prosthetic** (artificial) feet to flex almost naturally. A plastic keel inside the Seattle Foot, *below left,* acts as a spring, bending upward and downward at the ankle. Moving parts inside the Mauch Hydraulic ankle, *below right,* adjust their flexing action automatically when the wearer walks on a sloping surface.

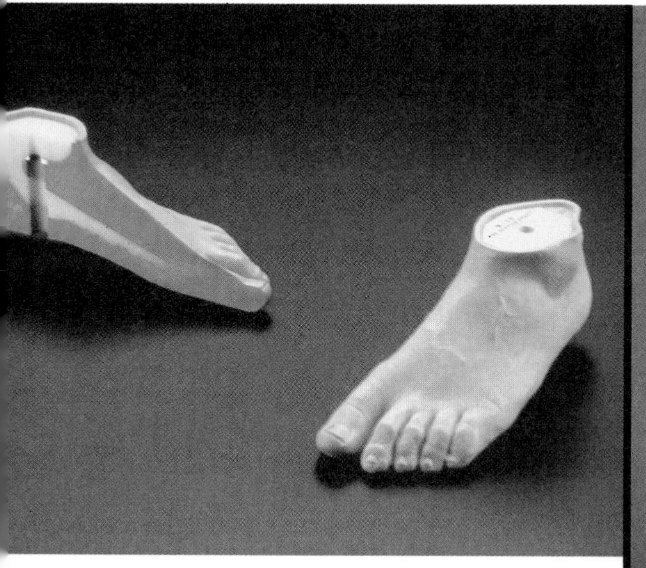

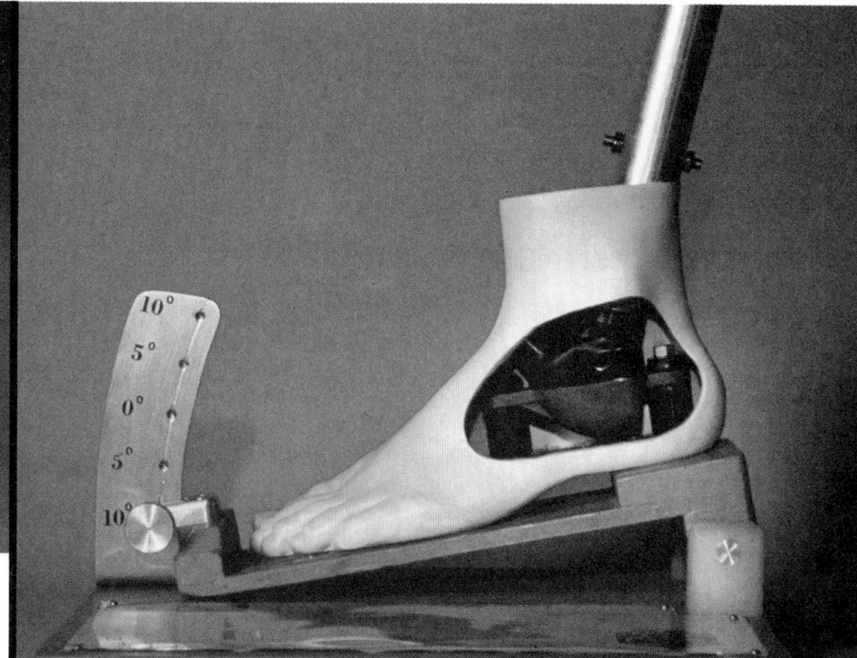

Protozoa (prō tə zō'ə) are the simplest single-celled organisms to be classified as animal. Some species can cause infectious diseases in human beings.

Proximal (prok'sə məl) describes a part of the body that is closer than some other part to a central point. The part that is farther away is referred to as being distal.

Prurigo (prü rī'gō) is a skin condition in a patient who has been suffering from severe itching (pruritus). Small, firm lumps appear on areas of the skin associated with crusting and sometimes obvious scratch marks.

Pruritus (prü rī'təs) is intense itching that frequently leads to infection from the scratching of the skin. Allergies, infections, and jaundice are causes of pruritus. Treatment of pruritus is directed at the cause. Topical applications of alcohol and corticosteroids may relieve some of the symptoms.

Pseudocyesis (sü dō sī ē'sis) is the medical term for a false pregnancy.

See also PREGNANCY, FALSE.

Pseudogout (sü'dō gout), or chondrocalcinosis, is an arthritic condition affecting the joints of people over 50 years of age. Characterized by deposits of calcium in the joints, pseudogout is treated with anti-inflammatory drugs.

Pseudomonas (sü də mon'as) is a group of bacteria. *Pseudomonas aeruginosa* can infect human beings, causing pneumonia, endocarditis, or urinary infections. Treatment of pseudomonas infections is often difficult. Few antibiotics are capable of killing the bacteria.

Pseudotumor cerebri (sü dō tü'môr ser'ə brē) is a disorder caused by edema, an abnormal accumulation of fluid, in the brain. It is characterized by an increase in pressure and pain in the head, vomiting, nausea, and an absence of any neurological problems.

Psittacosis (sit ə kō'sis), also called ornithosis and parrot fever, is a rare form of pneumonia caused by a microorganism *(Chlamydia psittaci)* carried by birds. It is usually caught by inhaling dust from feces or feathers of infected birds. The disorder is infectious and can be transmitted from one person to another by means of airborne droplets (produced by coughing).

Q: *What are the symptoms of psittacosis?*

A: The infection usually takes between one and three weeks to develop and may begin suddenly or slowly as an influenza-like illness with fever, aching muscles, and malaise accompanied by a cough. The cough produces a small amount of sputum that may become bloodstained as the illness progresses.

Without treatment, the illness lasts for about two weeks, with a gradual improvement followed by a further month of malaise, weakness, and often mild depression.

Usually, the disorder is fairly mild, but occasionally it can be severe and even fatal in the elderly, if untreated.

Q: *How is psittacosis treated?*

A: The tetracycline group of antibiotics are usually used in treatment, producing a rapid improvement within two days. The patient should be kept isolated in bed until the fever has subsided. Strong cough mixtures, oxygen, and other forms of treatment for pneumonia may be given.

Psoriasis (sə rī'ə sis) is a chronic skin condition that is found in about 1 percent of the population. The cause is unknown, but heredity probably is the most important factor; children of an affected parent have a one in four chance of developing the condition. Psoriasis may appear for the first time soon after a streptococcal throat infection. The condition usually occurs in persons between the ages of 10 and 25 and, although it may disappear for short periods of time, long periods of remission are rare.

Q: *What are the symptoms of psoriasis?*

A: A typical lesion of psoriasis is an oval, slightly raised area covered with dry, silvery scales overlying a red area of skin. The size, extent, and distribution of the lesions vary considerably. They may be scattered all over the body, including the scalp, or there may be only one or two rather large lesions, with normal skin elsewhere on the body. The pattern of distribution may be influenced by hormonal changes that occur at puberty, at menopause, or during pregnancy.

Some drugs, such as chloroquine, aggravate the condition. The lesions can join together into ex-

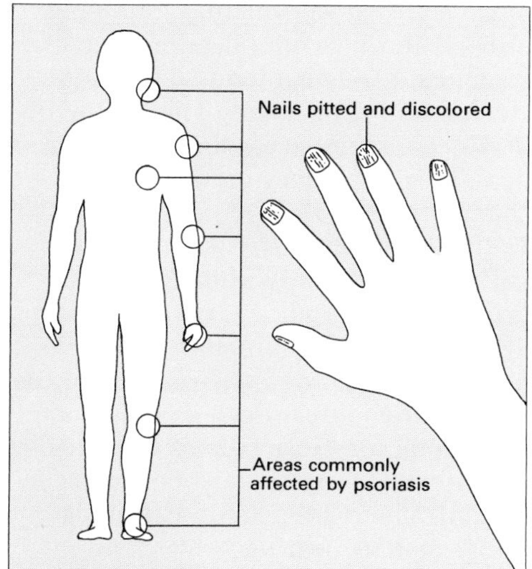

Psoriasis lesions, dry, silvery scales overlying a red area of skin, may be distributed over a wide area of the body.

tensive areas of scaling skin. Lesions on the scalp do not affect hair growth, and it is unusual for the lesions anywhere on the body to cause more than the mildest irritation.

The condition is often improved by sunlight, and it is noticeable that psoriasis is more common in temperate regions than in the tropics.

Q: *Are there any complications with psoriasis?*

A: Yes. In about a quarter of the patients, the fingernails become pitted, ridged, or discolored. The nails may also break much more easily than normal.

A form of arthritis sometimes occurs in patients suffering from psoriasis. Any joint may be affected, but commonly it is those of the fingers and lower spine. This produces a condition similar to a mild form of rheumatoid arthritis.

Q: *What is the treatment for psoriasis?*

A: Most physicians start by prescribing a simple regimen of ointments, such as those containing coal tar and salicylic acid. If these prove ineffective, the drug anthralin may help, but anthralin may stain the skin brown and cause allergies. Psoriasis of the scalp may be treated with various shampoos and creams to separate the scaly skin from the hair.

For more severe cases, corticosteroid creams are applied under a layer of polyethylene at night. This treatment is generally successful for a short time. The use of cytotoxic drugs is sometimes advisable in patients who have extensive and severe psoriasis. This treatment should be given only under the close supervision of a dermatologist.

Ultraviolet light is of benefit to patients with psoriasis, and treatments involving sunlight or artificial ultraviolet light produce an improvement. Recently, a new form of treatment has been instituted using psoralens, drugs that encourage the skin to peel. The administration of psoralens is followed by courses of exposure to ultraviolet light (PUVA treatment).

Due to the nature of psoriasis, some patients become extremely depressed and may require medical treatment, for example antidepressant drugs.

Psychiatry (si kī′ə trē) is the medical specialty that deals with mental illness and emotional disorders. A psychiatrist holds an M.D. degree, having completed medical school prior to undergoing additional training of at least three years, specializing in the treatment of psychiatric disorders.

Psychoanalysis (si ko ə nal′ə sis) is a method, devised by Sigmund Freud, of treating emotional problems. It attempts to uncover the unconscious

During **psychoanalysis,** a therapist helps the patient to understand the underlying reasons for feelings and behavior.

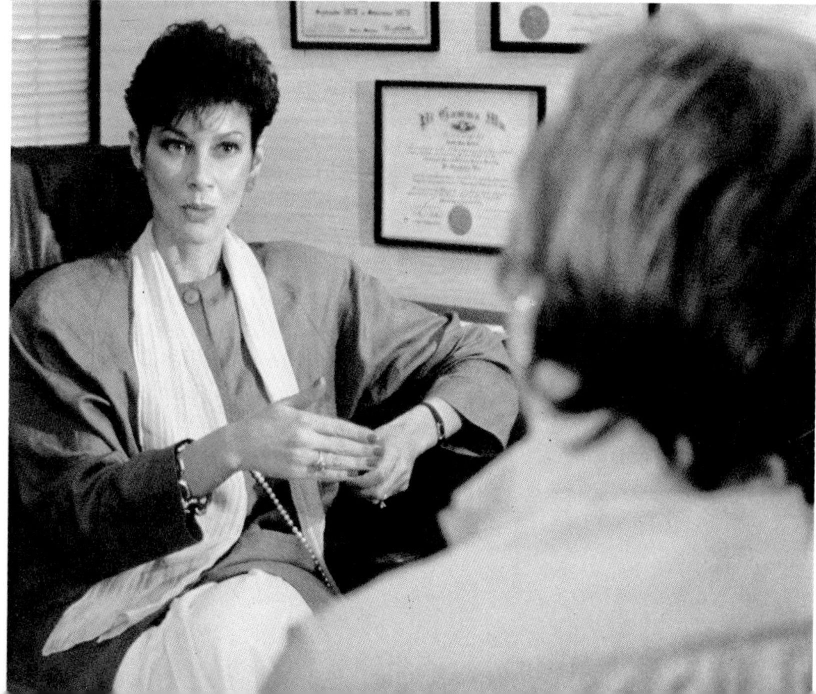

conflicts underlying abnormal behavior. There is a strong emphasis on childhood experiences in explaining adult behavior. Freud believed that patients unconsciously employ different defense mechanisms to repress childhood anxieties and conflicts that are too threatening for them to face.

The therapist's role is to help the patient achieve insight into these intrapsychic conflicts rather than to attempt to directly eliminate the problematic behavior. Psychoanalysis relies on techniques such as free association and dream analysis and tends to involve long-term therapy. Psychoanalytic therapists usually receive specialized training in psychoanalysis.

See also EGO; ID; SUPEREGO.

Psychology (sī kol'ə jē) is the study of behavior. Human psychology attempts to measure development, change, normality, and abnormality. A psychologist is trained to make these comparative assessments and to apply principles of behavioral change to modify maladaptive behavior.

There are various subspecialties within the field of psychology. Child or educational psychologists assess the mental and emotional development of children, their intelligence, and social development. Analytical psychologists investigate the workings of the human mind through psychoanalysis. Psychologists often specialize in several areas of expertise, such as marriage counseling, child therapy, and psychosomatic disorders.

See also PSYCHOSOMATIC DISORDER.

Psychomotor seizure (sī kō mō'tər), or a complex partial seizure, is an episode of altered consciousness sometimes accompanied by automatic behavior caused by discharge of excessive electrical energy in the brain.

See also EPILEPSY.

Psychoneurosis. *See* NEUROSIS.

Psychopathy (sī kop'ə thē) is a type of personality disorder, also referred to as antisocial personality or sociopathy. There is a long history of antisocial behavior in which the rights of others are violated. Such individuals usually show instability in jobs and relationships. Early childhood signs include lying, stealing, fighting, and truancy. Some psychopaths will end up in jail for criminal acts. They tend to be impulsive and have difficulty following projects through from beginning to end. Psychopaths have a tendency towards alcohol and drug abuse. They show little sincere remorse for their behavior; thus, they have poor motivation to change.

Psychopharmacology (sī kō fär mə kol'ə jē) is the study of the effects of drugs on the mind.

Psychosis (sī kō'sis) refers to a severe psychiatric disorder, such as one of the schizophrenic disorders, in which an individual may lose contact with reality and suffer severe personality degeneration. There are usually hallucinations, such as hearing voices, and delusions, such as an unshakeable, unfounded belief that one is being persecuted.

Hospitalization is often necessary as well as antipsychotic medication. Despite their severity, psychoses can be short-lived with a good chance for recovery. Some individuals, on the other hand, may require long-term medication and follow-up to control their psychotic behavior. A thorough evaluation is necessary to rule out physical causes, such as brain tumors or alcohol or drug abuse, that may underlie the psychosis.

Psychosomatic disorder (sī kō sō mat'ik) is a bodily disorder related to, and sometimes caused by, mental or emotional disturbances. Typical psychosomatic disorders might include headache, certain types of ulcers, and hypertension.

Psychotherapy. *See* MENTAL ILLNESS.

Ptomaine poisoning. *See* POISONING, PTOMAINE.

Ptosis (tō'sis) is the dropping or drooping of an organ such as the stomach (gastroptosis), kidney (nephroptosis) or, especially, the upper eyelid. Stretched ligaments, obesity, or lack of muscle tone are usually responsible.

Q: *What causes ptosis of the eyelid?*

A: Ptosis of the eyelid may be a minor congenital anomaly, but the most common causes are a cyst, infection, muscle disorders, and paralysis of the nerves to the eyelid muscles.

Q: *Can ptosis be treated?*

A: Abdominal ptosis can sometimes be treated by wearing a surgical belt which helps to strengthen the abdominal muscles. Ptosis of the eyelid improves with treatment of the underlying cause. In some cases, surgery may be done to elevate the drooping lid.

Puberty (pyü'bər tē) is the period between childhood and adolescence when hormonal body changes produce development of the secondary sexual characteristics.

See also ADOLESCENCE; SEXUAL CHARACTERISTICS, SECONDARY.

Puberty, precocious (pyü'bər tē pri kō'shəs). Precocious puberty is the premature development of secondary sexual characteristics.

See also ADOLESCENCE; SEXUAL CHARACTERISTICS, SECONDARY.

Pubic lice. *See* PEDICULOSIS PUBIS.

Pubis (pyü'bis), also called the pubic bone or os pubis, is the smallest of the three bones that together make up the hipbone, the other two being the ilium and the ischium. The midline joint, made up of strong ligaments and a disk of fibrocartilage, is known as the pubic symphysis. Toward the end of pregnancy, the cartilage in a woman's pubis softens to allow the birth canal to widen for childbirth.

See also HIPBONE; ILIUM; ISCHIUM; PELVIS.

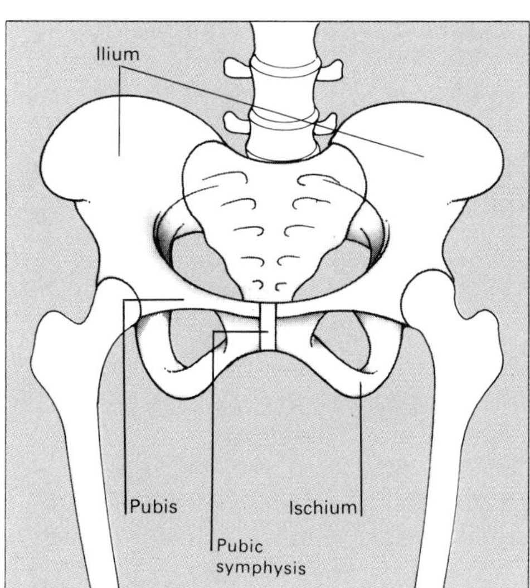

The **pubis** joins with the ilium and the ischium to form the innominate bone (hipbone).

Public health nurse. *See* NURSE, PUBLIC HEALTH.

Puerperal fever (pyü ėr'pər əl), also called childbed fever or postpartum fever, is any fever causing a temperature of 100.4°F (38°C) or over that lasts for more than 24 hours within the first 10 days after a woman has had a baby.

Puerperal fever used to be a common cause of maternal death after childbirth. Infection caused by streptococcus bacteria was spread by unsanitary techniques once used by physicians. Now, puerperal fever is rare because of high standards of hygiene in maternity wards.

Q: *What causes puerperal fever?*

A: The most common causes of fever following childbirth are infections of the genital tract and of the urinary system, especially the bladder. Breast infections, pelvic abscesses, and blood clots in the leg can also cause fevers.

Q: ***How is puerperal fever diagnosed and treated?***

A: After a careful examination, an obstetrician uses a swab to take a sample from the vagina and submits this and a specimen of urine for bacteriological tests. A blood test to detect anemia and the reaction of white blood cells to bacterial infection is taken. The patient is usually isolated to prevent the spread of infection to other patients.

Once the tests have been made, treatment with antibiotic drugs usually lasts for at least a week, or until the patient's condition improves.

Puerperium (pyü ər pir'ē əm) is the recovery time after the delivery of a baby. This period is generally considered to end with the obstetrician's postnatal examination at about six weeks.

Q: ***What particular care should a mother take during puerperium?***

A: During puerperium, a healthy mother and baby have to deal with each other, for the first time, as individuals. If the woman has never been a mother before, she is naturally anxious about handling, washing, and feeding the baby. It is during this time that experts can help to build up her confidence by showing her how to do things in the correct way, and by reassuring her that the baby's crying is not necessarily caused by hunger or stress. The reassurance helps a great deal toward the woman's recovery.

During the first 24 hours, it is often advisable to rest in bed. After this time, however, the woman is encouraged to get up and walk around. This helps to prevent deep vein thrombosis.

Routine care includes observations of the lochia (vaginal discharge) as well as vulval swabbing with antiseptic solutions to keep the area clean and to aid the healing of any lacerations or cuts. If there are any stitches in the perineum, these may cause discomfort, and a rubber ring can give greater comfort when sitting.

There may be problems with passing urine in the first 24 hours, caused by swelling around the urethra (exit tube from the bladder) as a result of labor. Occasionally, it is necessary to introduce a catheter into the bladder in order to release the urine. It is also often necessary to give laxatives to encourage normal working of the bowels.

A transient depression, in which tears mix with laughter, commonly occurs a few days after delivery. These are known as the "blues" and usually pass within 24 to 48 hours. They result from the combination of excitement, fatigue, and anxiety that is mixed with the happiness of having a baby. *See also* POSTPARTUM "BLUES."

Q: ***Are there any serious conditions that may develop during the puerperium?***

A: Yes. Occasionally, a woman who has had preeclampsia develops the more serious condition of eclampsia. This can usually be prevented by careful obstetric care. *See also* ECLAMPSIA; PREECLAMPSIA.

Puerperal fever occurs in about 2 percent of women during the 10 days after delivery. *See also* PUERPERAL FEVER.

Depression may occasionally become increasingly severe and, in 5 to 10 percent of women, may require medical treatment. Increasing fatigue and a feeling of futility, combined with despair at her own imagined inadequacy in dealing with the baby, are usually sufficient signs for the mother or her partner to discuss the matter with the obstetrician. Occasionally, a true psychotic illness occurs that necessitates admission to the hospital. *See also* POSTPARTUM DEPRESSION.

A postpartum hemorrhage is a serious complication that may occur because of infection of the genital tract or retention of part of the placenta in the womb. This requires urgent treatment in the hospital. *See also* HEMORRHAGE, POSTPARTUM.

Q: ***What physical changes take place in the mother during the puerperium?***

A: During this time, lactation begins and the mother's body undergoes considerable change. First, a large amount of extracellular fluid is lost, followed by a gradual tightening of the ligaments and tendons that have become softened by the effect of hormones on the body during pregnancy. The uterus gradually becomes smaller and produces noticeably less lochia, which also changes in color. The mother becomes aware that she is returning to her original weight and shape.

Q: ***May sexual intercourse be resumed during the puerperium?***

A: Deep sexual intercourse must not be resumed within the first month of puerperium to avoid the possibility of introducing infection into the genital tract. Contraception should consist of condoms and contraceptive creams until the postnatal examination by the obstetrician, when some other form of contraception may be recommended.

See also CONTRACEPTION.

Pulled muscle. *See* MUSCLE, PULLED.

Pulmonary (pul′mə ner ē) describes anything having to do with the lungs.

See also LUNG.

Pulmonary disease, chronic obstructive (pul′mə ner ē). Chronic obstructive pulmonary disease is a disorder of the lungs in which the airways become blocked or narrower, making it more difficult to move air through them. Emphysema, asthma, and chronic bronchitis are examples of chronic obstructive pulmonary diseases.

See also ASTHMA; BRONCHITIS; EMPHYSEMA.

Pulmonary function test. *See* LUNG FUNCTION TEST.

Pulpitis (pu̇l pi′tis) is the inflammation of the pulp of a tooth, usually caused by infection of the central cavity. Pulpitis is usually painful when acute, but may be asymptomatic if it occurs over a long period of time. All forms of pulpitis, with the exception of transient hyperemic pulpitis, are usually irreversible and result in pulp necrosis unless they are treated in time.

Pulse (puls) is the rhythmical expansion and contraction of an artery that can be felt near the surface of the body. The rate and regularity of the pulse is an indication of the pumping action of the heart and varies with age and activity. The pulse rate of a young baby may be as high as 120 to 140 beats per minute; for a resting adult it is about 70 beats per minute. A trained athlete at the extreme of physical effort may have a pulse rate of up to 180 beats per minute, with a resting pulse rate of less than 60 beats per minute.

Irregularities of the pulse may occur in even a healthy young person when the rate varies slightly with breathing (sinus arrhythmia) or occasionally misses a beat.

Ectopic beat (missed beat) occurs more frequently in persons who smoke or those who have some underlying form of heart disease. Rapid pulse rates are known as tachycardia and slow pulse rates as bradycardia. Totally irregular pulse rates are usually caused by atrial fibrillation.

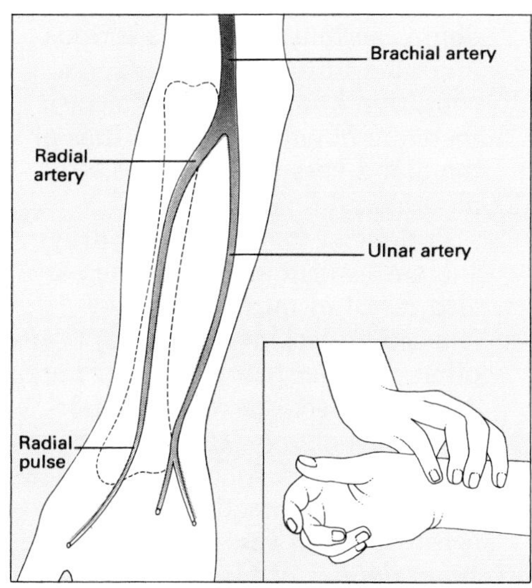

Pulse is taken by pressing the artery onto the radius bone just above the wrist.

See also BRADYCARDIA; ECTOPIC BEATS; FIBRILLATION; PULSE, TAKING OF; TACHYCARDIA.

Pulse, taking of. You can feel a pulse wherever an artery lies across a bone. The usual place to take a patient's pulse is at the wrist. Place the first and second fingers of your hand gently on the patient's wrist about 1 inch (2.5cm) above the base of the thumb. After a few seconds, you should feel the beats of the pulse through the radial artery. Count the number of beats during one full minute by watching the second hand of a clock or wristwatch.

An alternative place to take the pulse is just in front of the ear, where the temporal artery passes to the forehead. Patients who have collapsed from shock or undergone cardiac arrest do not have detectable pulses in these locations. The only place that a pulse can then be felt is over the carotid artery where it passes up the neck next to the Adam's apple.

See also PULSE.

Punch-drunk (punch′drungk) is an imprecise term used to describe a form of chronic brain damage usually caused by repeated minor injuries to the head. The repeated damage produces multiple concussions, minor hemorrhages, and loss of brain substance that results in a gradual physical and mental deterioration.

Q: ***What symptoms are shown by a person who is punch drunk?***

A: The condition develops gradually with slurring speech, staggering gait, and dementia. There is a lack of tolerance for alcohol and an underlying belligerence that may be easily triggered.

Pupil (pyü′pəl) is the circular opening in the center of the colored area (iris) of the eye. Light enters the eye by means of the pupil and passes through the lens to the back of the eye (retina). The pupil contracts in bright light and when the eye is focusing on a near object. It dilates in dim light, when the eye is focusing on a distant object, and at times of excitement or emotion. The ability of the pupil to change size is known as the pupil reflex. The size of the pupil is controlled by muscles in the iris, which are supplied by nerves in the autonomic nervous system. An abnormal pupil reflex can indicate a neurological disorder.

Q: *Why does the pupil appear black?*
A: The pupil seems black because light that passes through it to the retina is not reflected back.

Q: *What can go wrong with the pupil?*
A: Disorders that affect the iris, such as iritis, can make the pupil irregular in shape. If iritis causes the iris to stick to the lens, pupil reflex is absent. Constriction of the pupil may be caused by old age, oversensitivity to light (photophobia), Horner's syndrome, or drugs. Dilation of the pupil may be caused by blindness or poor sight, fever, glaucoma, paralysis of the nerve that controls eye movements (oculomotor nerve paralysis), or drugs, such as cocaine. Argyll-Robertson pupil is failure of the pupil to adjust to the intensity of light. Adie's syndrome is a congenital anomaly in which one pupil contracts or dilates more slowly than the other. *See also* ARGYLL-ROBERTSON PUPIL; GLAUCOMA; HORNER'S SYNDROME; IRITIS; PHOTOPHOBIA.

Q: *How are pupil disorders treated?*
A: Most disorders of the pupil improve with treatment of the underlying cause. Miotic drugs, such as pilocarpine and physostigmine, constrict the pupil; mydriatic drugs, such as atropine and homatropine, act as pupil dilators.

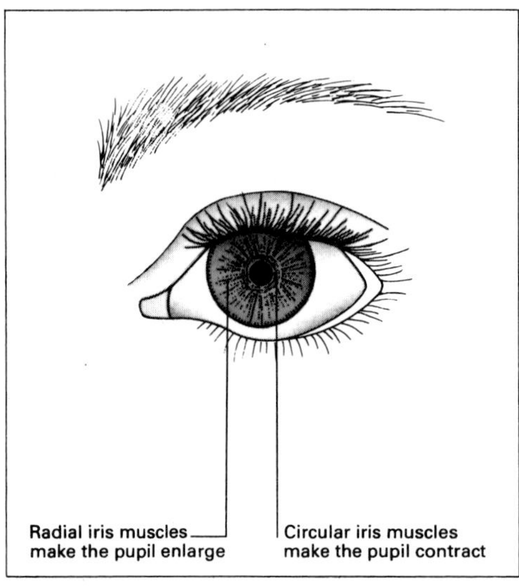

The **pupil** becomes larger or smaller as the iris muscles relax or contract.

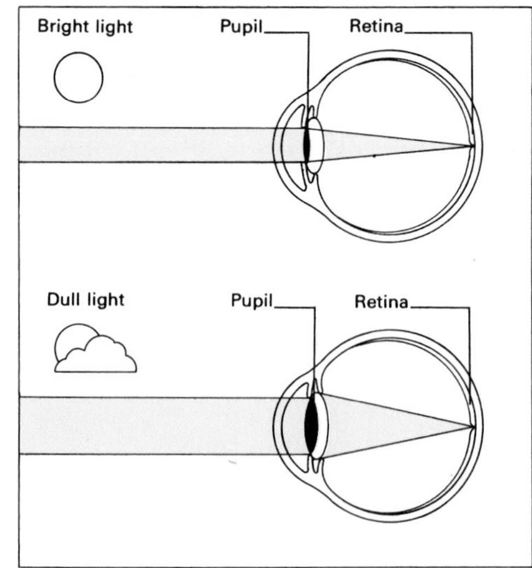

The **pupil reflex** automatically adjusts the size of the pupil and thereby regulates the amount of light entering the lens of the eye.

Pupil reflex (pyü′pəl) is constriction of the pupil of the eye in response to light or in focusing on a near object.

Purgative (pėr′gə tiv) is any substance that increases bowel movement.
See also LAXATIVE.

Purpura (pėr′pyür ə) is a skin discoloration caused by bleeding (hemorrhage) under the skin. A small hemorrhage is called a petechia and a large one, as in a bruise, is called an ecchymosis. Purpura may result from fragility of the blood vessels.

Q: *What causes fragility of the blood vessels?*
A: Fragility of the blood vessels usually is inherited, although it seldom is serious. In a more serious inherited form of the disorder, a condition known as telangiectasia, there are obvious abnormalities of the blood vessels in the lips, mouth, and fingers.

Prolonged treatment with drugs such as aspirin and cortisone may also result in purpura. Scurvy (caused by lack of vitamin C) is another disorder that causes purpura. A rare, but serious, cause of purpura is an allergy (Henoch-Schönlein purpura), which may follow a streptococcal infection that damages the blood vessels.

Q: *What defects of blood clotting cause purpura?*
A: Various clotting defects can cause purpura. They include hemophilia,

thrombocytopenia (deficiency of platelets in the blood that help coagulation), and liver disorders in which the level of prothrombin (a protein necessary for blood clotting) is lowered. Drugs may also cause clotting defects. Examples include heparin or warfarin (used in the treatment of rheumatoid or arthritic disorders).

Q: *What are the symptoms of purpura and how are they treated?*

A: There may be purple or reddish spots on the skin. Other symptoms may vary from very minor bleeding under the skin to major areas of bruising and hemorrhage into tissues, such as the pleural membranes surrounding the lungs, the back of the eye, or the intestines. Repeated bleeding may cause anemia.

Treatment of purpura must depend on the accurate diagnosis of the cause. Serious conditions, such as allergic purpura, need urgent hospitalization, with specialized investigation and care.

Purulent. *See* PUS.

Pus is the thick liquid produced by inflammation in abscesses and other infected areas. It contains white blood cells, cellular debris, and fluid. The white blood cells gather in the area to fight infection; the fluid drains from the damaged tissue.

Pustule (pus′chül) is a small, pus-containing area just under the skin.

Pyelitis (pī ə lī′tis) is an infection of the pelvis of the kidney.

See also KIDNEY; PYELONEPHRITIS.

Pyelogram (pī′ə lə gram) is an X ray of the kidneys made with special iodine-containing dyes, which are opaque to X rays. There are two main methods of obtaining a pyelogram: intravenous pyelography (IVP) and retrograde pyelography. In retrograde pyelography, a small tube is inserted into one or both of the ureters using a cystoscope. The dye is then forced along the tube to the kidneys.

See also CYSTOSCOPY; PYELOGRAM, INTRAVENOUS.

Pyelogram, intravenous (pī′ə lə gram, in trə vē′nəs). Intravenous pyelogram (IVP) is a special X ray of the kidneys and the urinary system taken after an intravenous injection of an iodine salt that contains a radiopaque solution.

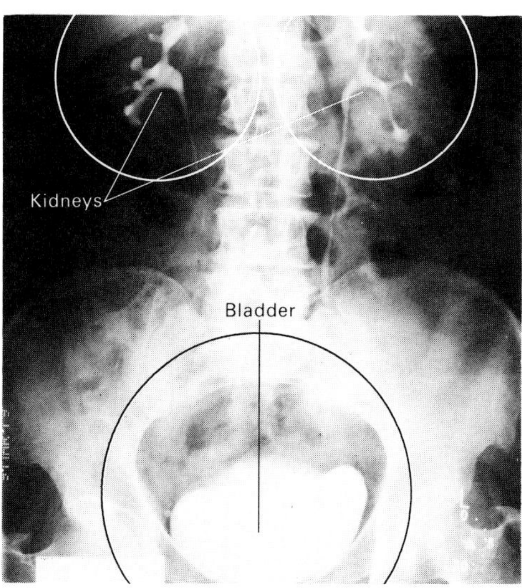

A **pyelogram** is an X ray of the kidneys taken after the injection of a radiopaque dye.

Pyelonephritis (pī ə lō nē frī′tis) is an inflammation of the kidney and the renal pelvis, which is the hollow cone into which urine flows from the kidney. The onset of pyelonephritis may be sudden (acute pyelonephritis) or gradual (chronic pyelonephritis).

Acute pyelonephritis is usually caused by the spread of infection from the bladder. Occasionally, it may be caused by the spread of infection through the bloodstream. Chronic pyelonephritis is caused by destruction and scarring of the kidney tissue as a result of an untreated bacterial infection. Both forms of pyelonephritis are associated with an obstruction to the flow of urine.

Q: *What are the symptoms of acute pyelonephritis?*

A: Usually, there is a sudden onset of pain in the lower back, fever with chills, nausea, and vomiting. Urination may be painful (dysuria) and more frequent than usual. *See also* DYSURIA.

Q: *How is acute pyelonephritis treated?*

A: Acute pyelonephritis is treated with antibiotics and an increased fluid intake. Surgery may be necessary if an obstruction is present.

Occasionally, the treatment eliminates the symptoms without destroying the infection. Such a symptomless infection is rare in men.

Q: *What are the symptoms of chronic pyelonephritis?*

A: The disorder progresses over several years with recurrent attacks of acute pyelonephritis. Usually, there are no symptoms between attacks. These attacks may cause high blood pressure and eventually kidney failure, with uremia and a large output of urine. *See also* HYPERTENSION; UREMIA.

Q: *How is chronic pyelonephritis treated?*

A: Treatment involves removal of any obstruction, which may require surgery and a prolonged course of antibiotics. Treatment for high blood pressure and uremia may also be necessary.

Pyemia (pī ē′mē ə) is a serious condition in which septicemia (blood poisoning) occurs from a pus-forming area and produces multiple abscesses throughout the body.

Q: *What are the symptoms of pyemia?*

A: The symptoms of pyemia are violent shivering because of sudden chill with high rises in temperature, followed by sweating. Frequently, jaundice develops, as well as abscesses in various areas of the body, such as the liver, lungs, and kidneys.

Q: *How is pyemia treated?*

A: The development of pyemia requires urgent hospitalization with full investigations to find the cause. Large doses of antibiotics must be given for some weeks to ensure recovery. Abscesses may have to be lanced.

See also BLOOD POISONING.

Pyloric stenosis (pī lôr′ik sti nō′sis) is a narrowing of the exit (pylorus) from the stomach to the duodenum, causing a partial obstruction. It is also known as pyloric obstruction.

Q: *What causes pyloric stenosis?*

A: Congenital hypertrophic pyloric stenosis occurs in about 1 in 500 babies. It is 400 percent more frequent in boys than girls and is a genetic malformation.

Pyloric stenosis in adults is caused by spasm of the pyloric muscle. This is commonly associated with a peptic ulcer, often because of the scarring from repeated ulceration.

Q: *What are the symptoms of congenital hypertrophic pyloric stenosis?*

A: The symptoms usually start in the second week of life with occasional vomiting after feeding. But, within a few days, there is vomiting after every feeding. It is termed projectile vomiting, because the milk is ejected out of the mouth with a characteristic violence. The baby is constipated and hungry and rapidly becomes dehydrated if the vomiting continues.

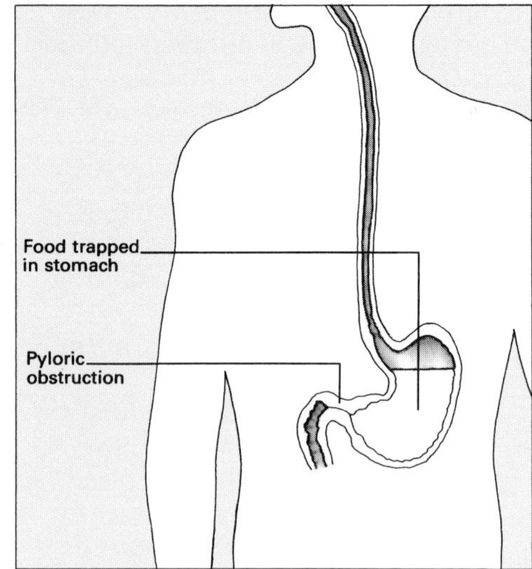

Pyloric stenosis is a thickening of the pylorus portion of the stomach, causing an obstruction.

Q: *How is congenital hypertrophic pyloric stenosis treated?*

A: The usual treatment is an operation that is performed after the baby has been given intravenous fluids to correct any dehydration and to replace salts that may have been lost. The thickened muscle around the pylorus is cut to prevent it from going into spasm.

Pyloroplasty (pī lôr′ə plas tē) is an operation to relieve the obstruction of pyloric stenosis by cutting through the pyloric muscle.

See also PYLORIC STENOSIS.

Pylorospasm (pī lôr′ə spaz əm) is a spasm of the pyloric muscle at the exit from the stomach, causing the symptoms of pyloric stenosis.

See also PYLORIC STENOSIS.

Pylorus (pī lôr′əs) is the narrow exit from the stomach into the duodenum. It contains a circular muscle called a sphincter. The pyloric sphincter helps to control the gradual emptying of the stomach.

See also DIGESTIVE SYSTEM.

Pyogenic (pī ə jen′ik) is any condition that produces pus.

See also PUS.

Pyorrhea (pi ō rē′ə) is a discharge of pus from any part of the body, such as from a boil. The term is most commonly applied to a discharge of pus from the gums.

Pyrexia. *See* FEVER.

Pyridoxine (pir ə dok′sēn), vitamin B_6, is essential to the body for the formation of proteins from amino acids. It is found in many foods, particularly eggs, cereals, meat, and fish. Pregnant women and those taking contraceptive pills need more vitamin B_6 than usual.

Pyrogen (pī′rə jen) is any substance that produces a fever.

Pyrosis. *See* HEARTBURN.

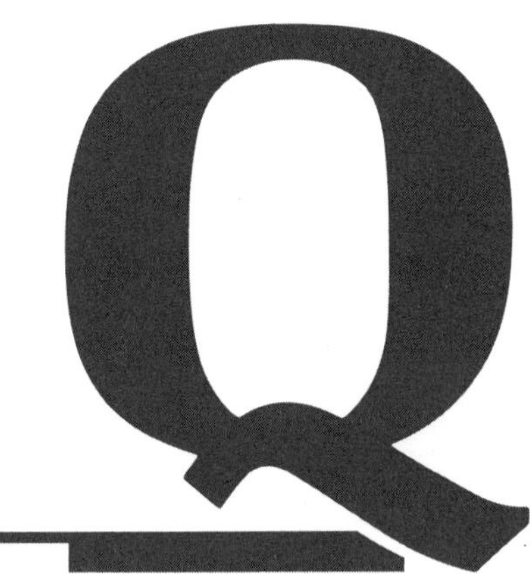

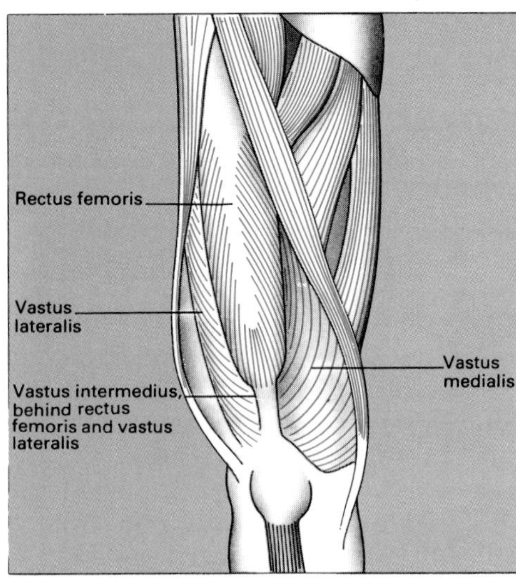

Quadriceps femoris is the strong muscle in the thigh composed of a group of four muscles that share a common tendon.

Q fever is an infectious disease caused by the microorganism *Coxiella burnetti,* which is a form of rickettsia. Q fever commonly occurs in sheep and cattle. Humans usually become infected by inhaling droplets from the milk, urine, or feces of infected animals. The placenta of infected animals is particularly infectious. Rarely, the infection is transmitted by a tick bite or from handling wild animals. *See also* RICKETTSIA.

Q: *What are the symptoms of Q fever?*

A: After an incubation period of 9 to 28 days, there is a sudden onset of fever, severe headache, shivering, muscle pains, and often chest pains. A dry cough may develop after about a week. The fever may rise to about 104°F (40°C) and usually lasts for one to three weeks. Complications, such as pneumonitis, hepatitis, and endocarditis, may also develop. Despite the severity of the disease, death is rare, even in untreated patients. *See also* ENDOCARDITIS; HEPATITIS; PNEUMONITIS.

Q: *How is Q fever treated?*

A: The disease is treated with antibiotics, usually tetracycline.

Quadriceps (kwod′rə seps) is a muscle with four heads. The term is usually applied to the quadriceps femoris, the large muscle in front of the thighbone. It consists of a group of four muscles that share a common lower tendon. This tendon surrounds the kneecap (patella) and is attached to the front of the tibia (shinbone). Contraction of the quadriceps femoris straightens the lower leg.

Quadriplegia (kwod rə plē′jē ə) is paralysis of all four limbs.

See also PARALYSIS.

Quarantine (kwôr′ən tēn) is a period of isolation from public contact, after exposure to an infectious disease, so that the infection does not spread. The length of the quarantine period varies according to the incubation period of the infection. For example, the incubation period of mumps varies between 10 and 28 days. The quarantine period is 28 days after the time of last contact with an infected person.

Total isolation of potentially infected persons is rarely necessary. In most cases of common infectious diseases, only a patient who actually contracts the disease is advised to remain at home, avoiding work, school, and other public situations, until he or she is no longer contagious. Because of widespread use of immunizations and other public health measures, strict quarantine is seldom needed anymore.

In certain uncommon circumstances, all people coming into contact with an infectious disease, such as typhoid, may need to be quarantined with the patient.

A distinction is made between quarantine and isolation. At times, some patients may require isolation *not* to

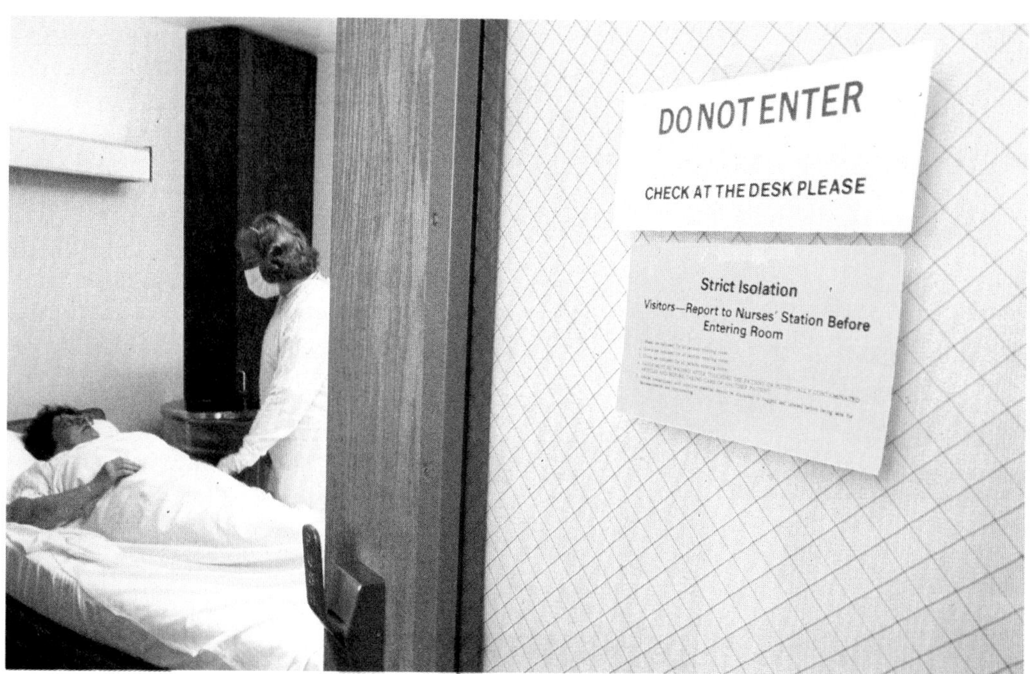

A patient may be put in **quarantine** to keep an infectious disease from spreading throughout a community or district.

prevent them from spreading their disease but to protect them from illnesses that others may be carrying. This type of isolation is used with patients with suppressed immune systems, such as AIDS victims or people undergoing cancer chemotherapy.

See also INFECTIOUS DISEASE.

Quickening (kwik′ə ning) is the term used to describe a mother's awareness of her unborn baby's first movements. It usually occurs sometime between the eighteenth and twentieth weeks of pregnancy. Women who have already had a child usually experience quickening earlier than those who have never been pregnant before.

See also PREGNANCY AND CHILDBIRTH.

Quinine (kwī′nīn) is a bitter, white, crystalline alkaloid substance obtained from the bark of the cinchona tree. It is effective against malaria, but in the prevention of the disease, quinine has largely been replaced by synthetic antimalarial drugs. However, it is still used to treat malaria in areas where strains of malaria have developed that are resistant to the synthetic drugs. Quinine is also used to treat night leg-muscle cramps in the elderly.

Excessive doses of quinine may cause headaches, vomiting, noises in the ears (tinnitus), and visual disturbances that may result in blindness. This collection of symptoms is known as cinchonism.

See also MALARIA.

Quinsy. *See* ABSCESS, PERITONSILLAR.

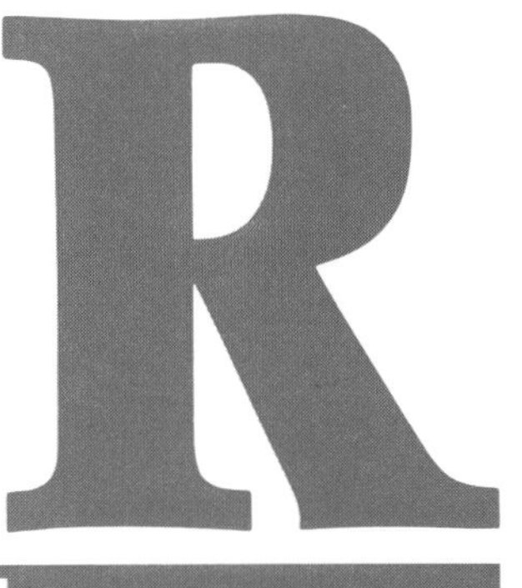

Rabbit fever is an infectious disorder that is transmitted by the bite of an infected bloodsucking insect or tick. It is known medically as tularemia.

See also TULAREMIA.

Rabies (rā′bēz) is a viral infection transmitted to humans and certain other mammals by the saliva of an infected animal. Infection is through a bite or by skin or mucous membrane contact with infected saliva. The incubation period of the disorder can be as short as ten days or as long as one year; the usual time is one to two months. Death usually follows within a week if the condition is not treated promptly. Immunization is available for persons particularly at risk.

Q: *What animals commonly carry rabies?*

A: Most current cases of rabies are the result of bites from infected bats, foxes, skunks, and cats. The domestic dog is a relatively rare source of the disease, in large part because of the enforcement of animal control ordinances.

Q: *How can you tell if an animal has rabies?*

A: The animal, even if a wild animal, behaves abnormally, often without fear of humans. Usually, it is extremely agitated and vicious, but this behavior is followed by gradual paralysis, which makes the animal move slowly. Infected nocturnal animals may be active during daylight.

Q: *What are the symptoms of rabies in humans?*

A: The first symptoms are fever, depression, and increasing restlessness that turns into uncontrollable excitement. There is agitation in which painful spasms of the throat muscles occur, accompanied by excessive saliva, which froths and flows down the chin. Drinking even a sip of water produces spasms of the swallowing muscles, followed by saliva flow, hence the archaic name hydrophobia (meaning "fear of water").

If rabies is not treated promptly, death, from a combination of asphyxia, generalized paralysis, and exhaustion, usually occurs within a week.

Q: *How is rabies treated?*

A: No real treatment or cure for rabies exists once symptoms begin to appear. Even with aggressive medical care and mechanical artificial respiration, only three persons have ever been known to survive rabies. Thus, the best treatment is careful medical assessment of a person following any animal bite.

If rabies is suspected in an animal that has bitten a person, an attempt should be made to capture the animal as soon as possible. If the need for special preventive immunizations is seen, the patient will be hospitalized to receive injections of immune globulin to provide temporary protection; an active antirabies vaccine, which uses killed rabies virus, is then administered in a series of five injections over a one-month period.

Rabies is not spread from human to humans. No one has ever contracted rabies by handling a person with the infection.

Radiation (rā dē ā′shən) is any form of electromagnetic energy wave or any stream of ions (electrically charged atoms or molecules) or subatomic particles. Therefore, although radiation commonly means ionizing radiation, the term also includes heat, light, magnetism, and sound, as well as X rays.

The different types of radiation have both therapeutic and harmful effects. Solar radiation—light from the sun—can damage the skin and cause skin cancer; at the same time, phototherapy is the use of ultraviolet light to treat skin diseases. The use of ionizing radiation is widespread in medicine. X rays are used both in diagnosing diseases and treating certain kinds of cancers. Yet, radiation sickness can result from extreme exposure to ionizing radiation. Infrared heat and shortwave diathermy are other forms of radiation that are used by physiotherapists to treat problems of the musculoskeletal system, the muscles and bones of the body. *See also* DIATHERMY; PHOTOTHERAPY, ULTRAVIOLET; RADIATION, IONIZING; RADIATION SICKNESS.

Physicians also use the word radiation to describe pain or discomfort that is felt in a site other than the area of the problem. For example, the pain associated with a heart attack often radiates down the victim's left arm.

Radiation, ionizing (rā dē ā′shən, ī′ən ī zing). Ionizing radiation is any radiation that causes substances to break up into ions (charged atoms or molecules). Gamma rays and X rays are two examples of ionizing radiation.

See also RADIATION.

Radiation sickness (rā dē ā′shən) is an illness caused by overexposure to ionizing radiation from radioactive substances, such as radium and uranium, or from X rays. The symptoms depend mainly on the total dosage of radiation and the duration of exposure. Acute radiation sickness results from the absorption of a high dose of radiation over a short time. Delayed radiation sickness results from repeated or prolonged exposure to low doses of radiation. Adequate precautions can prevent the danger of radiation sickness in persons who might be exposed to the dangers of radiation in their work. *See also* RADIATION.

Q: *What are the symptoms of acute radiation sickness?*

A: The initial symptoms usually appear within a few hours of exposure and include nausea, vomiting, diarrhea, and burns. At a later stage, there may be conjunctivitis (inflammation of a membrane of the eye), loss of hair, disorientation, a staggering gait, and convulsions. Anemia and a severe, often fatal form of gastroenteritis (inflammation of the stomach and intestinal lining) may also develop. The body's immune system may be affected, thereby making the person vulnerable to infection.

Radiation may damage the fetus in a pregnant woman. This may result in a miscarriage, or the fetus may suffer from any of a variety of congenital anomalies, such as mental retardation or skull damage.

Q: *What are the symptoms of delayed radiation sickness?*

A: There may be cataracts, hypothyroidism, and a reduction in fertility. Persons who have been exposed to low levels of radiation for a long time have an increased likelihood of developing cancer and leukemia.

See also RADIATION.

Radical mastectomy. *See* MASTECTOMY, RADICAL.

Radiculitis (ra dik yə lī′təs) is a form of neuritis in which there is inflammation of the spinal nerve roots in the spinal canal.

See also DISK, HERNIATED; NEURITIS.

Radiography (rā dē og′rə fē) is the use of radiation, usually X rays, for studying the internal structures of the body as an aid to diagnosis. The X rays are recorded on photographic plates, or they may be projected "live" on a fluoroscope or a television screen, so that a

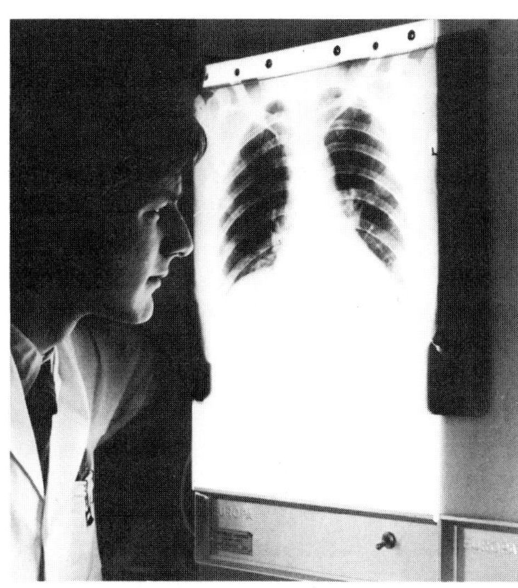

Radiography is the use of radiation, usually in the form of X rays, to study the internal structure of the body. It is an important tool in the diagnosis of various illnesses.

physician can study the movement of various structures within the body. Other X-ray images are recorded and analyzed using computers; CAT (computerized axial tomography) scans are the best-known example of this.

Although radiography has long been associated with the use of X-ray radiation, radiologists can also use sound waves in the form of ultrasound, as well as magnetism in the form of magnetic resonance imaging, to create images.

See also COMPUTERIZED AXIAL TOMOGRAPHY SCANNER; MAGNETIC RESONANCE IMAGING; RADIOTHERAPY; ULTRASOUND.

Radioisotope imaging (rā dē ō ī'sə tōp im'ij ing) is a branch of nuclear medicine in which a visual representation of the body is used to show the quantity of radioactive material in the body and where it is distributed. Radioisotope imaging is used to diagnose a variety of problems, including tumors, thyroid disease, and cardiac disease.

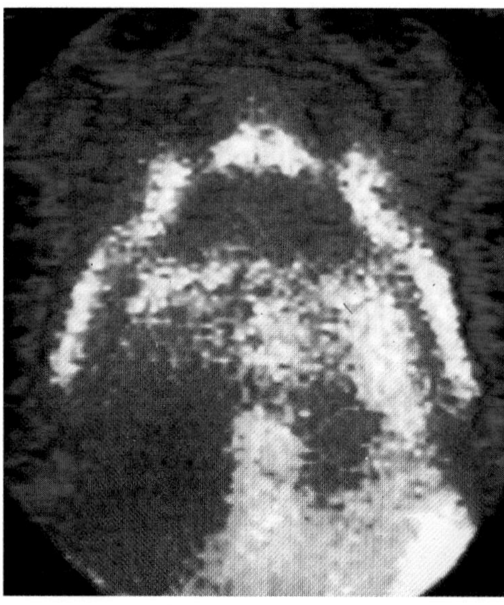

Radioisotope imaging is used as a diagnostic device to scan parts of the body, such as the pelvis, and to determine the quantity of radioactive material present.

Radiology (rā dē ol'ə jē) is the branch of medicine that involves radiography and radiotherapy.

See also RADIOGRAPHY; RADIOTHERAPY.

Radiotherapy (ra dē ō ther'ə pē) is the treatment of disorders using radiation. The machinery used is similar to X-ray equipment, but it contains a source of high-energy radiation, such as radium or a radioactive isotope of cobalt. An injection of a strong radioactive isotope is another technique of radiotherapy.

Q: *What conditions can be treated by radiotherapy and is the treatment effective?*

A: Radiotherapy is most widely used in the treatment of many different types of cancer. It is often used in conjunction with surgery or cytotoxic drugs.

Radium (rā'dē əm) is a rare, naturally-occurring radioactive element. It produces alpha, beta, and gamma rays, which can be used in radiotherapy.

See also RADIOTHERAPY.

Radius (rā'dē əs) is the outer of the two bones of the forearm; it forms part of the elbow joint and the wrist joint. It rotates around the other forearm bone, the ulna, allowing the hand to rotate at the wrist.

See also COLLES' FRACTURE.

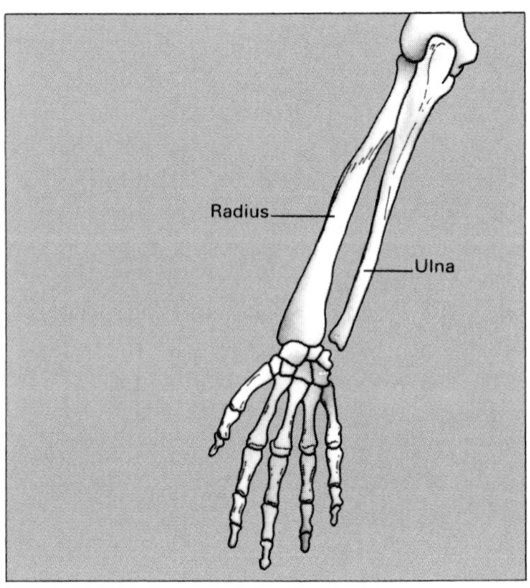

The **radius** is one of the two bones of the forearm. The ulna, the inner bone, is parallel to the radius, the outer bone.

Rale (räl) is the abnormal sound heard by a physician when listening to air passing into or out of a damaged lung. The sound arises from the air sacs in the lungs called alveoli. Some describe rales as crackles; others liken it to the sound made when rubbing hairs together next to one's ear. Rales are heard when the lungs fill with fluid or develop stiffness or scarring.

Ranula (ran'yə lə) is a small cyst under the tongue, commonly caused by the blockage of a salivary duct. Although not serious, a ranula should be examined and treated by a physician.

Rape (rāp) is the illegal sexual penetration of any body orifice, or opening, without consent. Although referred to as a "sex crime" in the past, rape is now classified as a crime of violence.

Statistics on rape are elusive because most incidents of rape are unreported. It is estimated that only 10 to 20 percent of all rapes are reported. In 50 percent of rape cases, the victim knows the assailant. One in four women will be the victim of some form of sexual assault. Males as well as females can be raped, although among males rape is usually confined to children and teenagers. Among boys up to the age of 18, it is estimated that 1 in 9 will be the victim of sexual assault. In general, however, rape is a crime committed against women.

A rape victim should go or be taken to a rape treatment center or emergency room as soon as possible after the attack has taken place. Ideally, these facilities are staffed with personnel who have had experience with rape victims and have been specially trained to be sensitive to the particular nature of the trauma. Most cities have rape hotlines, rape victims' advocacy organizations, and other agencies that can refer victims to the nearest appropriate facility. Some will send one of their own counselors to be with the victim throughout the medical exam and police questioning and then accompany the victim home.

Rape victims should undergo a thorough examination to assess physical injury. In the course of this process, steps can be taken, if indicated, to prevent pregnancy or sexually transmitted disease. The examining physician will also be responsible for gathering physical evidence, such as sperm, blood, and hair, for use by legal authorities.

Some rape victims will need subsequent therapy for "rape trauma syndrome," a condition that is very similar to "post-traumatic stress syndrome." There are three phases in the syndrome. In the initial or crisis phase, the victim may experience guilt, shame, humiliation, loss of appetite, fatigue, headaches, sleepiness, nausea, vomiting, and flashbacks. The victim may also have difficulty concentrating and completing everyday tasks.

In the second, or latency phase of the syndrome, the victim may use denial to mask feelings still present from the first phase. This denial may also be accompanied by behavior that is out of character, such as promiscuity, loss of interest in sex, or running away (especially in younger victims).

In the third phase of "rape trauma syndrome," the victim acknowledges what has happened, may want to talk about it, and regains control of her or his life. The successful outcome of the third stage depends heavily on the strength of the victim's ego, the support of friends, and the manner in which she or he was initially treated as a victim.

Rash is a temporary discoloration or eruption of the skin, usually caused by an allergy, but it may also be a sign of an underlying disease.

See also ALLERGY.

Ratbite fever, or ratbite disease, is a bacterial infection caused by the bite of a rat or other infected animal. It is characterized by fever, ulceration, and enlargement of the local lymph nodes. Penicillin is effective in treating the infection.

See also ANIMALS AND DISEASE.

Raynaud's phenomenon (rā nōz′ fə nom′ə non) is a spasm of the superficial blood vessels, especially those of the digits, the fingers and toes. The digits become cold and pale. Attacks may last from a few minutes to several hours and are usually precipitated by cold or emotional upset. In severe cases, ulcers and gangrene on the fingers are possible. *See also* GANGRENE.

Often, the cause of Raynaud's phenomenon is unknown. Sometimes, it is a complication of such other conditions as vascular disease, trauma, or disease of the endocrine glands or central nervous system. Therapy includes analgesics, avoiding cold and emotional upset, keeping the body warm, psychotherapy, treatment of any underlying disorders, or, if the condition is severe, sympathectomy.

See also SYMPATHECTOMY.

RBC. *See* BLOOD CELL, RED.

Recessive (ri ses′iv) is a term used to describe certain genes in heredity. Such genes do not express themselves as a trait unless both genes in the pair are specific for that trait.

See also DOMINANT.

Recommended Dietary Allowance (RDA) is the amount of nutrients that population groups should consume over a period of time.

See *also* APPENDIX IV.

Recovery position. See FAINTING: FIRST AID.

Rectal disorders (rek'təl) are conditions affecting the rectum, which include amebic dysentery, schistosomiasis, and ulcerative colitis.

The rectum may undergo a prolapse, in which its internal mucous membranes become detached from the underlying wall and protrude from the anus. This usually corrects itself in infants, but in adults an operation is usually necessary.

Tumors of the rectum may be either benign (noncancerous) or malignant (cancerous). Such tumors are similar to those elsewhere in the colon and often produce bleeding, rectal pain, and spasmodic anal contractions.

See *also* CANCER; COLITIS, ULCERATIVE; DYSENTERY, AMEBIC; SCHISTOSOMIASIS.

Rectal fissure (rek'təl fish'ər), also known as anal fissure, is a tear in the mucous membranes that line the anus. It may extend into the lower part of the rectum and commonly accompanies constipation.

See *also* CONSTIPATION; FISSURE.

Rectocele (rek'tə sēl) is relaxation of the tissues that support the rectum so that it forms a type of hernia into the rear wall of the vagina. A rectocele occurs with prolapse of the uterus. It may be accompanied by a similar prolapse of the front wall of the vagina and may involve the bladder and urethra, causing stress incontinence (the inability to retain urine). The symptoms and treatment are those associated with prolapse.

See *also* PROLAPSE.

Rectum (rek'təm) is the final portion of the large intestine, extending through the pelvis from the end of the colon to the anus. Situated in front of the sacrum and behind the bladder, the rectum is about 5 inches (12.7cm) long. The upper part is covered by the peritoneum, the membrane that lines the abdominal cavity, and the lower part is supported by the muscles and ligaments of the pelvic floor.

The desire to defecate is caused by the feeling that occurs when feces are passed from the colon into the rectum. Failure to defecate reduces the desire to do so; chronic constipation may then develop.

See *also* RECTAL DISORDERS.

Red blood cell. See BLOOD CELL, RED.

Red eye is a condition in which there are brilliant red streaks across the white of the eye. Occasionally, the entire white of the eye is affected. Red eye is usually painless and is caused by bleeding under the conjunctiva (a subconjunctival hemorrhage). A subconjunctival hemorrhage may occur following vigorous nose blowing. Red eye may also occur in more serious conditions, such as pink eye, iritis, and glaucoma.

See *also* GLAUCOMA; IRITIS; PINKEYE.

Referred pain. See PAIN, REFERRED.

Reflex (rē'fleks) is an involuntary muscular response to a stimulus, also known as a reflex action. The automatic muscular response is triggered by a short nerve pathway between the point of stimulation and the responding muscle, without the involvement of the brain. For example, a person who touches something hot immediately recoils and pulls his or her hand away from the source of heat, even before the brain registers the discomfort. A more commonly known example is the knee jerk reflex, produced in a test that is part of a physician's basic examination of the nervous system. See *also* KNEE JERK.

A conditioned reflex is any reflex not inborn or inherited. Often associated with the Russian scientist Pavlov, who trained dogs to salivate at the sound of a bell, a conditioned reflex is learned by pairing a behavior with a specific stimulus. For example, a child may see the doctor only for shots, which may cause anxiety and fright. The doctor becomes associated with this fear response, so that any time the child thinks about seeing the doctor, he or she exhibits a conditioned fear reflex.

Reflux (rē'fluks) is the abnormal backward flow of a fluid, as of blood or urine.

Refraction (ri frak'shən) is the process of turning or bending light waves when they pass from one medium to another of a different density. Many eye disorders are due to refractive errors, in which the lens fails to focus images onto the retina.

See *also* EYE DISORDERS.

Refractory (ri frak'tər ē) means failing to respond or responding slowly to treatment.

Registered nurse. *See* NURSE, REGISTERED.

Regression (ri gresh'ən) in medicine is a return to an earlier stage of a disorder, which could be favorable or unfavorable. Biologically, filial regression is a return to the normal or average in inherited conditions. Psychologically, regression is a return to an earlier developmental level in the face of stress or psychological conflict. It is considered a type of unconscious psychological defense mechanism to avoid dealing directly with the conflict.

Regurgitation (rē gėr jə tā'shən) is a backflow of fluid. The term usually applies to the backflow of food from the stomach to the mouth, usually because of eating too quickly with insufficient chewing. Various disorders of the esophagus can also cause regurgitation.

Regurgitation also describes the backflow of blood in the heart, caused by damage or diseased heart valves, which may lead to heart failure.

Reiter's disease (rī'tərz), or syndrome, is a group of three disorders—nonspecific urethritis, conjunctivitis, and arthritis. It sometimes follows a period of diarrhea or, more commonly, sexual contact. The cause is unknown and there is no specific treatment. The disorder is more common among men than among women.

See also ARTHRITIS; CONJUNCTIVITIS; URETHRITIS, NONSPECIFIC.

Rejection (ri jek'shən) in medicine is the body's resistance to or destruction of a foreign tissue or organ. For example, the body may reject a transplanted organ, such as a liver. The process of rejection may take place over a period of days, or it may be immediate.

See also TRANSPLANT SURGERY.

Relapse (ri laps') is the return of the symptoms of a disorder after an apparent recovery.

Relapsing fever (ri lap'sing), also known as recurrent fever or tick fever, is a disease carried by ticks and lice. The patient has a high fever for about 10 days; the temperature then returns to normal. However, a relapse follows in a day or two. This pattern is repeated until immunity is built up by the patient.

Q: *What causes relapsing fever?*

A: The disorder is caused by spirochete organisms of the species *Borrelia*, which can be transmitted from infected animals to humans by ticks. The ticks are commonly found in the western United States, West Africa, and various tropical and subtropical regions of the world. *See also* LYME DISEASE.

Q: *What are the symptoms of relapsing fever?*

A: After an incubation period averaging seven days, the patient has shivering attacks, headache, high fever, rapid heartbeat, vomiting, muscle and joint pain, and a skin rash. Delirium may occur. The fever rises to a peak during the following 5 to 10 days and then suddenly falls.

After a short period of a day or two, a relapse occurs, often accompanied by jaundice, and the pattern of symptoms is repeated, but without the rash. Most cases respond to treatment with antibiotic drugs.

Relaxant (ri lak'sənt) is any agent that causes mental or physical relaxation. Physiotherapy often includes relaxation exercises, as do most prenatal classes. A simple hot bath can also relax tense muscles.

Special groups of drugs can be prescribed, usually with painkillers, to relax muscles after an injury or an operation. During surgery, similar drugs are used to produce complete muscle paralysis, which helps the surgeon while operating.

Remission (ri mish'ən) is a period during the course of an illness during which a patient's symptoms become less severe or may even disappear completely.

Renal (rē'nəl) refers to anything having to do with, or shaped like, a kidney.

See also KIDNEY.

Renal calculus (rē'nəl kal'kyə ləs) is a stone forming in the kidney.

See also CALCULUS; NEPHROLITHIASIS.

Renal cortex (rē'nəl kôr'teks) is the soft outer layer of the kidney. It contains about one million microscopic filters called nephrons, which aid in the processing of body waste.

See also KIDNEY; NEPHRON.

Renal medulla (rē'nəl mi dul'ə) is the inner portion of the kidney. It contains nephrons, microscopic units which serve to filter the blood.

See also NEPHRON.

Renal pelvis (rē′nəl pel′vis) is the hollow structure at the center of the kidney that serves to collect urine before the urine is passed out of the kidney through the ureter.

See also KIDNEY.

Renin (rē′nin) is a hormone that is released by the kidney to maintain normal blood pressure. Elevated renin levels are found in certain types of hypertension (high blood pressure).

See also HYPERTENSION.

Rennin (ren′in) is an enzyme produced in a baby's stomach that curdles milk, aiding in its digestion.

Replacement surgery (ri plās′mənt) is the replacement of diseased or damaged body parts with natural or artificial substitutes. Materials used range from plastic and metal parts to donated human tissue. Most parts of the body, such as the arteries, eyes, joints, and nerves, can thus receive some form of treatment.

See also TRANSPLANT SURGERY.

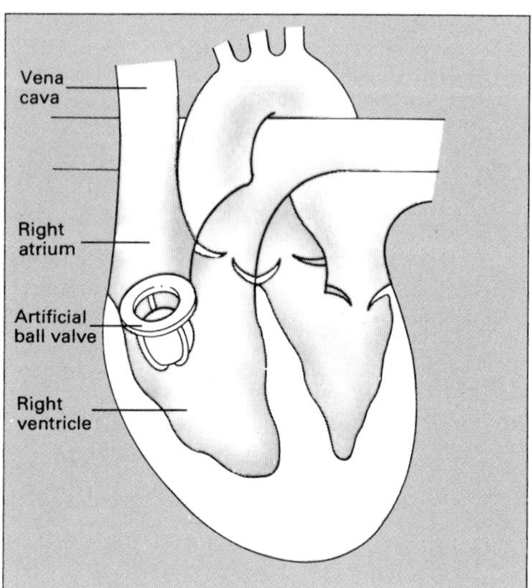

Replacement surgery may be performed to replace a damaged heart valve with an artificial ball valve.

Reportable disease (ri pôrt′ə bəl) is a disease that must be reported to a community health officer, who can then take action to control the spread of the disease. Diseases that must be reported vary from region to region and include many of the infectious diseases.

See also INFECTIOUS DISEASE.

Repression (ri presh′ən) is a psychiatric term used to describe the transfer of unpleasant or painful memories, as well as unacceptable desires, from the conscious to the unconscious mind. It is an unconscious defense mechanism used to avoid dealing directly with conflict and stress.

See also PHOBIA; STRESS.

Reproduction, human (rē prə duk′ shən). Human reproduction is the process by which offspring are produced. The biological purpose of the sex organs is the reproduction of the human race. To make this possible, a male's reproductive system must be able to make sex cells (sperm) and place them inside the female. The female's reproductive system must be able to release mature female sex cells (eggs or ova).

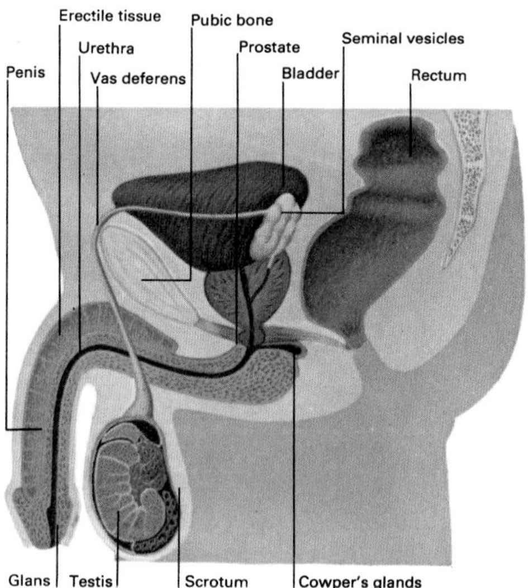

In the male, sperm are made in the testes. During intercourse, they pass along the vas deferens and the urethra in the penis. Seminal vesicles, prostate, and Cowper's glands make fluids that combine with the sperm to form semen.

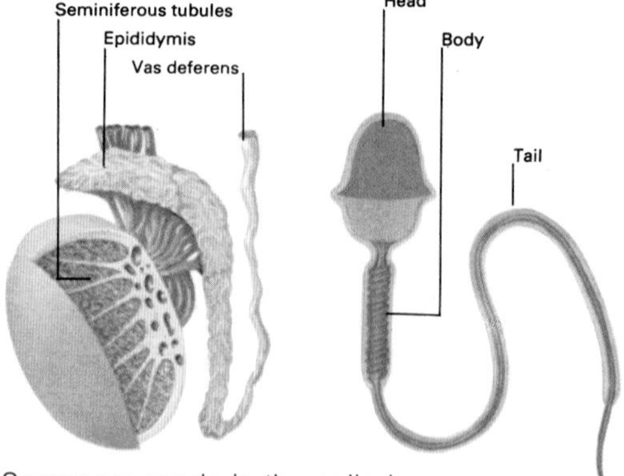

Sperm are made in the coiled seminiferous tubules of the testis, then stored in the adjoining epididymis until coitus (sexual intercourse). The microscopic sperm has a head containing genetic material, a "body" that provides energy, and a whiplash tail for movement.

The sperm enter and fertilize the eggs, and the developing fetus is nurtured within the female until it is born.

In a mature man, sperm are made in the two testes (testicles). The testes are suspended in a sac, the scrotum, outside the body. The scrotum lies behind the penis, the organ sensitive to sexual arousal through which the sperm are transmitted to the female. Sperm are made continuously in the testes and stored in the seminal vesicles, two small structures next to the prostate gland. During sexual intercourse, some 250 million tadpole-like sperm are ejaculated from the penis, together with secretions from several sex glands, including the prostate gland and the seminal vesicles. The mixture of sperm and fluids is known as semen. *See also* SEMEN.

All of the reproductive organs of the female are internal. Eggs are produced in a pair of organs, the ovaries. The ovaries are connected by the fallopian tubes to the uterus, the site of fetus development. The uterus leads through a narrow opening (the cervix) into the vagina, the cavity into which the penis is placed during intercourse. Surrounding the entrance to the vagina, on the outside of the body, are two pairs of skin folds. The larger pair (labia majora) lie outside the smaller (labia minora). Behind these folds is the clitoris, an organ of sexual arousal.

Puberty, the start of sexual development, begins in boys at the age of 12 or 13. The hypothalamus in the base of the brain stimulates the pituitary gland to secrete two hormones. These hormones act on the testes to make them

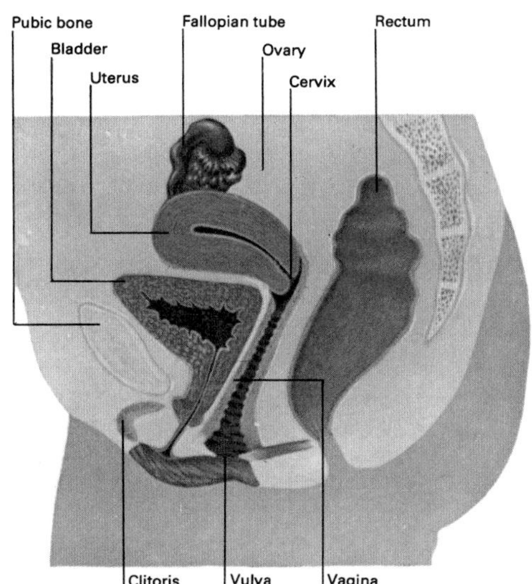

In the female, ova (eggs) are made in the ovaries and move through the fallopian tubes to the uterus, where they will develop if fertilized. During intercourse, the male penis is placed in the vagina.

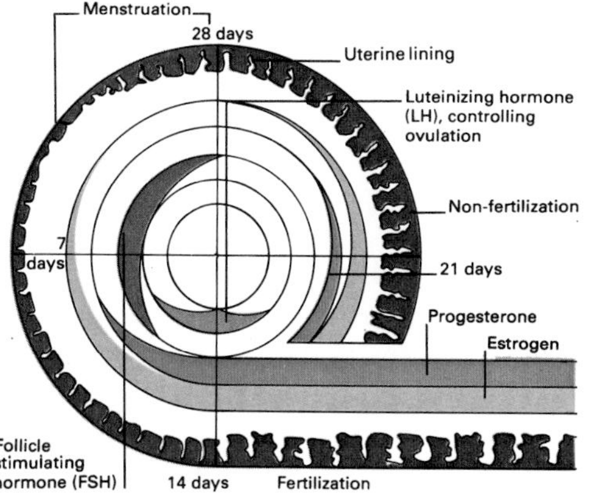

Hormones regulate the menstrual cycle. The ovum (egg) matures under FSH influence, estrogen starts the build-up of the uterine lining, and LH controls the release of the egg. Progesterone completes the uterine lining. If the egg is not fertilized, hormone production stops and menstruation occurs.

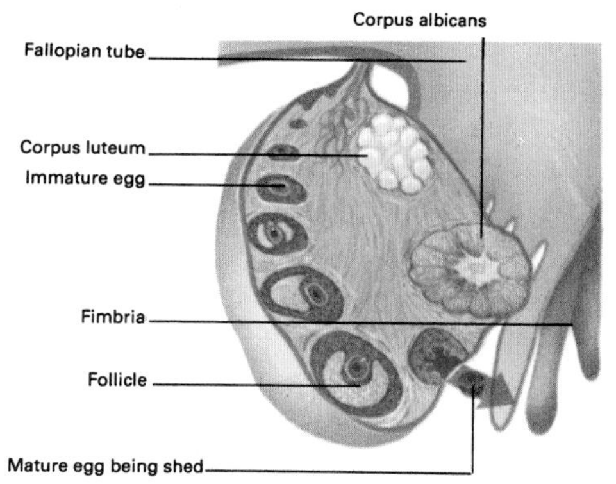

The ovaries contain thousands of immature eggs. After a girl reaches puberty, one egg ripens and is shed each month, leaving a corpus luteum, which produces hormones essential to the early stages of pregnancy. Fertilization usually occurs in the fimbria of the fallopian tubes.

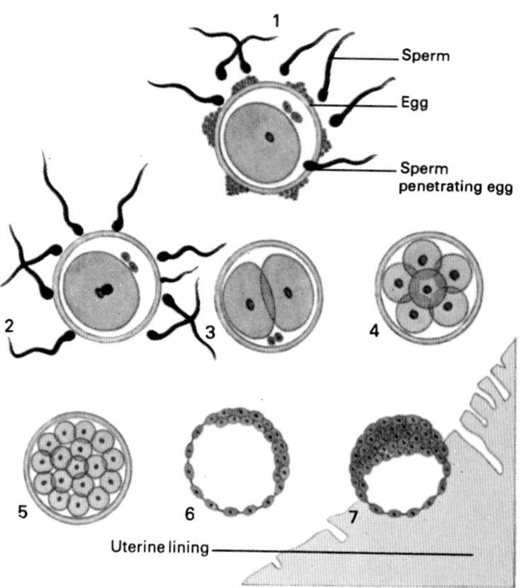

After fertilization (1), the egg divides and multiplies (2-5) to form a ball of cells. A fluid-filled cavity then develops inside the structure (6), which enters the uterine lining (7) a week after fertilization. When implanted in the uterine lining, the structure develops into the embryo.

release male hormones (androgens), the most important of which is testosterone. This hormone brings about the enlargement of the sex organs, the start of sperm production, and the appearance of secondary sexual characteristics. Among these characteristics are the growth of hair on the body and face, the deepening of the voice, and the increased development of bones and muscles. Male maturation is usually complete by the age of 20.

Girls start to mature sexually about two years earlier than boys. The pituitary gland, under the influence of the hypothalamus, secretes hormones that act on the ovaries and stimulate them to produce the hormones estrogen and progesterone. Estrogen brings about enlargement of the sex organs and controls the development of the female secondary sexual characteristics. These characteristics include the growth of the breasts, the widening of the hips, and the appearance of hair in the armpits and pubic region. The whole body grows rapidly, and maturity is usually reached by the age of 16. *See also* ESTROGEN; PROGESTERONE.

A girl experiences her first menstrual period at about the same time as ovulation begins. Menstruation, a bleeding from the uterus, takes place about every 28 days and lasts for 4 or 5 days. It is closely controlled by hormones. In the ovary each egg develops in a sac called a follicle. As the egg is prepared for release, the follicle produces the hormone estrogen, which starts the build-up of the lining of the uterus in preparation for receiving a fertilized egg. Once the egg has left the ovary, the empty follicle secretes more estrogen plus a second hormone progesterone. Together, estrogen and progesterone aid further in the thickening of the lining of the uterus. If the egg is not fertilized, the follicle degenerates, hormone output ceases, and the lining of the uterus is shed during the menstrual period. If the egg is fertilized, it makes yet another hormone that preserves the lining of the uterus in order to nurture the embryo until birth. *See also* MENSTRUATION; OVULATION.

In a man, the production of sex hormones and sperm continues through maturity for the rest of his life, although there is a gradual decline from the age of 40 onward. In a woman, however, ovulation becomes less frequent as she becomes older and the ovaries become less responsive to the pituitary hormones. Eventually, the ovaries do not respond at all and menstruation ceases (menopause). This commonly occurs during a woman's mid-40's.

Resection (ri sek'shən) is the removal of a part of an organ or a bone. Usually, it means that the remaining undamaged sections are joined together.

Reserpine (res'ər pin) is the principal alkaloid obtained from the root of the rauwolfia plant. It was once widely used in the treatment of hypertension (high blood pressure).

Residency (rez'ə dən sē) is a period of time (usually three to six years) that a physician spends in a medical facility as on-the-job training. During this period, a physician is trained in one of the medical specialities.

Resolution (rez ə lü'shən) has two medical meanings: the ability of the eye to distinguish between two separate but close objects; and a return to normalcy or an improvement of any process that caused symptoms or observed physical changes.

Respiration (res pə rā'shən), or breathing, is the process by which oxygen from the air is exchanged for carbon dioxide from the body tissues. The process of breathing involves the inhaling of air into the lungs and the carrying of the oxygen from that air to the body tissues via the bloodstream. In the various body tissues, the oxygen is absorbed, and carbon dioxide and water vapor are expelled into the bloodstream, returned to the lungs, and exhaled.

See also LUNG; RESPIRATORY SYSTEM.

Respirator (res'pə rā tər) is an apparatus used to purify the air a person inhales. It may be a simple gauze mask or a complex piece of machinery that extracts dust and gases from the air in a building.

A respirator is also a machine that is used to aid or maintain breathing. It is commonly used during general anesthesia when the patient's breathing muscles have been paralyzed by muscle relaxant drugs.

Respiratory disorders. *See* LUNG DISORDERS.

Respiratory distress syndrome, adult (res′pər ə tôr ē). Adult respiratory distress syndrome (ARDS) is an acute lung disease in which respiratory failure is accompanied by swelling and hemorrhaging within lung tissue. The condition may be associated with low blood pressure, the aspiration of toxic substances into the lungs, or a respiratory infection, such as pneumonia. ARDS is rapidly fatal. Even with prompt medical attention, it has a high mortality rate.

Respiratory distress syndrome of the newborn (res′pər ə tôr ē), also called hyaline membrane disease, is a lung disorder of the newborn, particularly of premature babies. Other predisposing factors include poorly controlled diabetes mellitus in the mother and maternal hemorrhage before the onset of labor.

Q: *What causes respiratory distress syndrome?*

A: The condition may be caused by a failure of the immature lung in the fetus to produce a substance that prevents the lung from collapsing once air has been inhaled immediately after birth. In a premature baby, areas of the lung may remain collapsed. These areas become inflamed, producing an abnormal membrane called a hyaline membrane. Provided the baby can survive a few days, the necessary substance that keeps the lungs open is produced, and the baby survives.

Q: *What are the symptoms of respiratory distress syndrome?*

A: Usually, the symptoms begin immediately after birth, although they may not be apparent for two or three hours. Symptoms include rapid breathing, often with an expiratory grunt, a bluish tinge to the lips (cyanosis), and sometimes respiratory arrest.

Q: *How is respiratory distress syndrome treated?*

A: Treatment is carried out in a neonatal special care unit or a neonatal intensive care unit, depending on the severity of the condition. Mild cases may be treated with supplemental oxygen; severe cases may be treated with mechanical ventilation.

Respiratory stimulant (res′pər ə tôr ē) is a drug or other substance used to stimulate the physical action of breathing. In cases of acute respiratory failure, for example, as can occur during surgery, it is possible to use such stimulants until mechanical methods are begun.

Respiratory syncytial virus. *See* VIRUS, RESPIRATORY SYNCYTIAL.

Respiratory system (res′pər ə tôr ē) is the network of organs and passages by which air is taken into the lungs and carbon dioxide and oxygen are exchanged within the body.

Breathing. Air enters the respiratory system through the mouth and nose, where it is warmed and moistened. Air breathed in through the nose is filtered by the coarse hairs that line the nostrils, which trap large dust particles. Smaller particles are trapped in a sticky fluid (mucus) produced by the cells lining the passage between nose and mouth. This mucus is continuously moved away by the beating of minute hair-like projections (cilia).

From the mouth, air travels through the throat (pharynx), voicebox (larynx), and windpipe (trachea). At the entry to the windpipe is a flap, the epiglottis, which closes to prevent choking when food is swallowed. At its base, the windpipe divides into two tubes or bronchi, and one bronchus enters each lung. Both windpipe and bronchi are stiffened by rings of cartilage. As in the nose, the windpipe and bronchi produce dust-trapping mucus and have cilia to move this mucus up to the mouth.

Within each lung, the bronchi split successively into smaller bronchi and then into many thousands of even narrower tubes called bronchioles. The bronchioles branch through the lungs and lead into millions of air sacs (alveoli) of the lung tissue. It is in the air sacs that gases are exchanged. Each air sac is meshed with small blood vessels (capillaries) carrying blood containing carbon dioxide and water from the heart. Oxygen breathed in from the air passes into the blood and, in return, carbon dioxide and water vapor are released into the air sacs of the lungs to be breathed out. The blood in the capillaries, now rich in oxygen, flows into

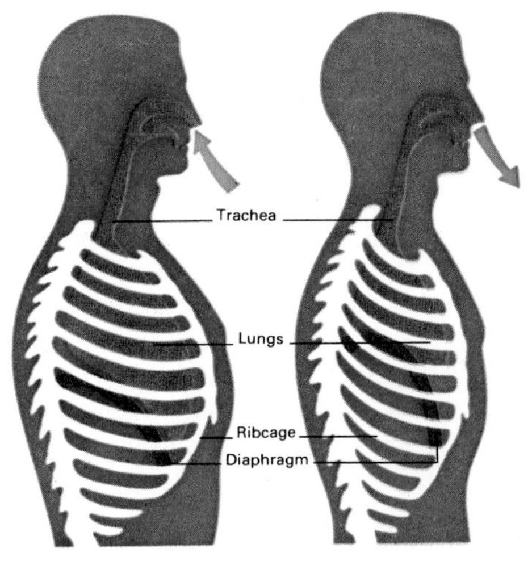

During inhalation, air is drawn in as the ribcage expands and the diaphragm contracts. During exhalation, the lungs recoil, the diaphragm relaxes, and the ribcage subsides.

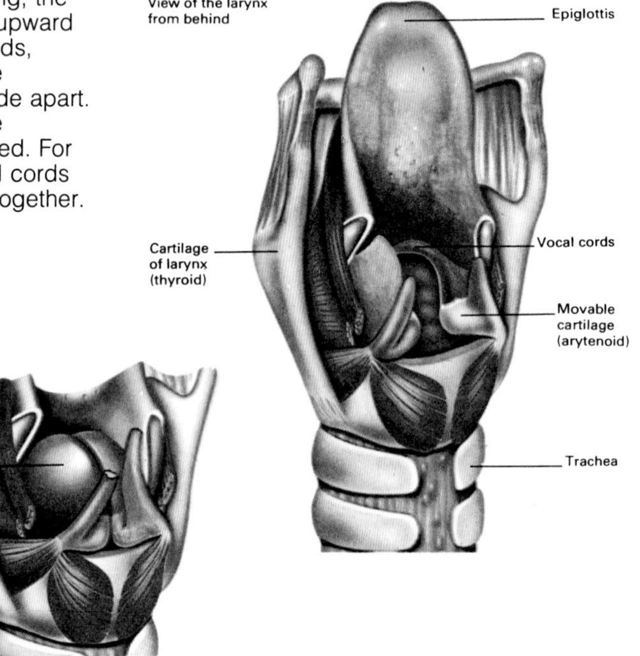

In normal breathing, the epiglottis is held upward and the vocal cords, joined to movable cartilages, are wide apart. In swallowing, the epiglottis is lowered. For speech, the vocal cords are drawn close together.

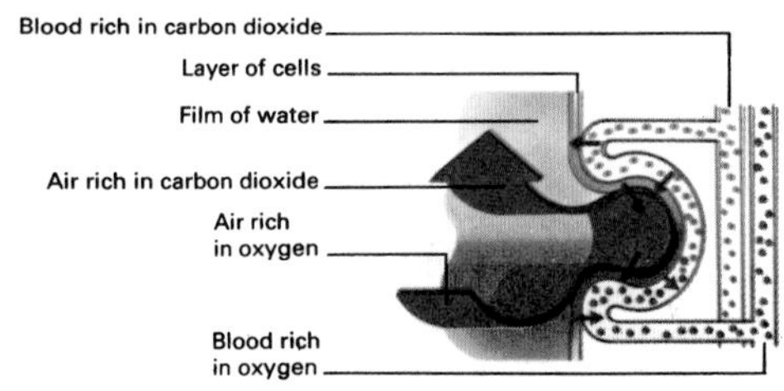

In the alveoli, gases are dissolved in water, then transported across a single layer of cells between alveoli and capillaries.

the pulmonary vein and back to the heart for redistribution.

The lungs are housed in a bony cage made up of the ribs, breastbone, and backbone. The floor of the cage is formed by a sheet of muscle called the diaphragm. When a person breathes in, the muscles of the diaphragm contract, pulling the diaphragm downward. At the same time, the ribcage is pulled up and out by the contraction of the muscles between the ribs, and air rushes in. When a person breathes out, the diaphragm and rib muscles relax and the chest subsides.

Respiration takes place 10 to 15 times a minute and is normally controlled unconsciously by a collection of cells in the brain called the respiratory center. After air has been breathed out, carbon dioxide builds up again in the bloodstream. The cells in the respiratory center are extremely sensitive to carbon dioxide concentrations. When the carbon dioxide in the blood reaches a certain level, messages are sent from the respiratory center to the diaphragm and rib muscles that trigger contraction. This once more initiates breathing in. As the lungs expand during inhalation, cells (stretch receptors) in the lung walls send signals back to the respiratory center. The center responds by instructing the muscles of ribs and diaphragm to relax so that exhaling takes place.

Respiration is not always a quiet process. The presence of many dust particles in the nose can trigger sneezing. Irritants or too much mucus in the windpipe and bronchi cause coughing.

Speech is also a special sort of "noisy" breathing. The sounds of speech are produced in the voicebox (larynx) and molded into words in the mouth.

The larynx consists of a box of cartilage. Across the inside of the box are flap-like structures, the vocal cords. The cords move by the action of muscles attached to the cartilages of the larynx. During normal breathing, the vocal cords are held apart. For speech, the cords are pulled together after a breath in; during breathing out, the air is, thus, forced between the cords, making them vibrate. The tighter the cords are pulled together, the higher is the pitch of the sound produced. For loud

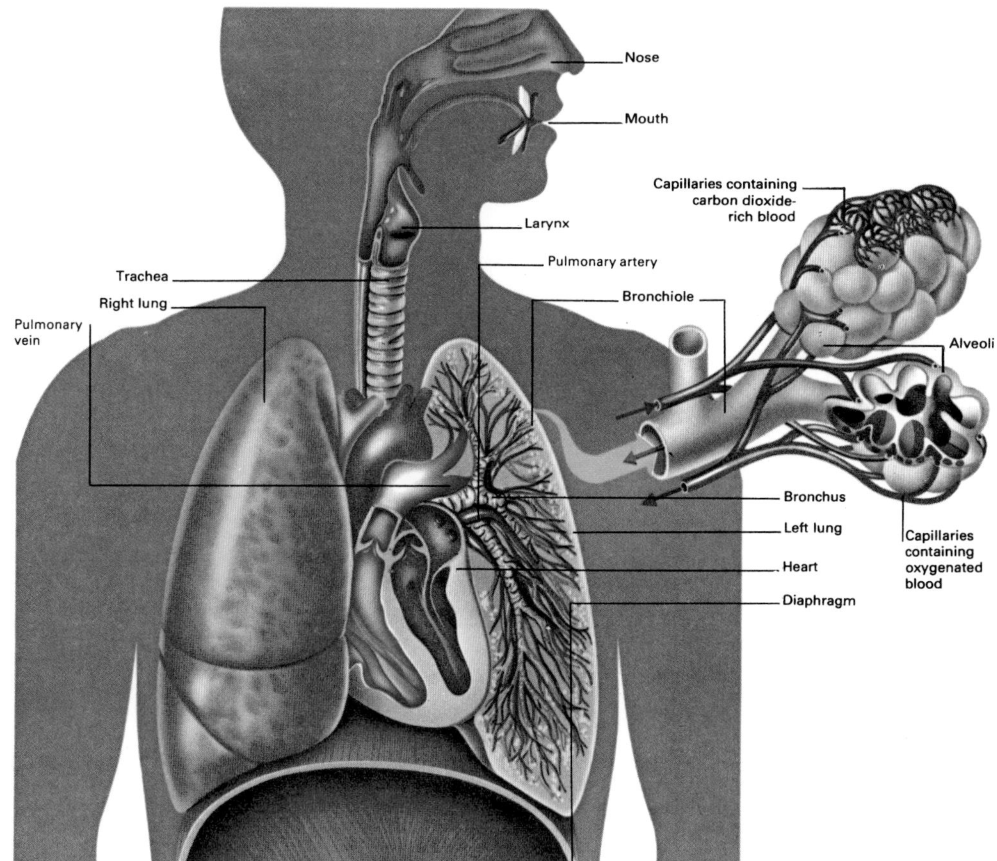

On breathing in, air is drawn down the trachea and into the bronchi. In each lung, the bronchi branch into bronchioles, which lead into the alveoli. Here, the carbon dioxide in blood brought from the heart in the pulmonary artery is exchanged for oxygen. Oxygenated blood returns to the heart in the pulmonary vein.

sounds, the air is forced through the cords faster than it is for soft sounds. The movements of the lips and of the tongue against the teeth and roof of the mouth achieve articulation. The resonance of spoken sounds and the characteristics of every individual voice are created by the cavities of the sinuses, nose, throat, and chest.

Respiratory tract (res′pər ə tôr ē) is another term for respiratory system.

See also RESPIRATORY SYSTEM.

Respiratory tract infection, upper (res′pər ə tôr ē). An upper respiratory tract infection is a viral or bacterial infection involving the body's air passages, including the nose, throat, and trachea. *See also* RESPIRATORY TRACT, UPPER.

The most frequent upper tract infection is the common cold; others include laryngitis and tonsillitis. Treatment depends on the nature of the infection. However, since most of these illnesses are caused by viruses, rest is usually one of the major features of any cure.

Respiratory tract, upper (res′pər ə tôr ē). The upper respiratory tract is one of two parts of the respiratory system. It includes the mouth, nose, nasal cavity, pharynx, larynx, and trachea. The upper tract serves to bring air to and from the lungs.

See also RESPIRATORY SYSTEM; RESPIRATORY TRACT INFECTION, UPPER.

Rest and relaxation. *See* STRESS MANAGEMENT.

Restless leg syndrome is a common complaint of the elderly in which there is a feeling of general discomfort that compels a person to move his or her legs, sometimes almost involuntarily, when sitting at rest or lying down.

The condition may be associated with iron-deficiency anemia, varicose veins, or polyneuritis. It may follow a partial gastrectomy or surgical removal of a section of the stomach. Tranquilizers, such as the phenothiazines, used in the treatment of mental illness may also be an aggravating factor.

Resuscitation (ri sus ə tā′shən) is any one of various methods used to restore breathing and heart action.

See also ARTIFICIAL RESPIRATION; CARDIOPULMONARY RESUSCITATION.

Retention (ri ten′shən) generally refers to the inability to pass urine. The term is also used to describe a method of keeping false teeth in their correct position. Retention is also a psychological term meaning the ability to remember.

Q: *What causes urinary retention?*

A: Retention may result if normal sensations from the bladder are disturbed by drugs.

Physical causes of retention include multiple sclerosis, stroke, bladder disorders, and prostate problems. Treatment is directed at the underlying cause of the disorder.

Reticulum (ri tik′yə ləm) is a network, such as the network of microscopic tubules in muscle tissue that aids in metabolism.

Retina (ret′ə nə) is the light-sensitive area at the back of the eyeball. It consists of a layer of cells called rods and cones. Rod cells are sensitive to various intensities of light, and cone cells are sensitive to color.

See also EYE; RETINA, DETACHED; RETINITIS.

The **retina** receives light stimuli through the lens and transmits the image to the brain via the optic nerve. The expansion or contraction of the iris regulates the amount of light that reaches the retina.

Retina, detached (ret′ə nə, di tacht′). A detached retina is the separation of the retina in the eye from its vascular base, the choroid. It causes partial loss of vision. The symptoms include "floating" specks and transient flashes of light, followed later by a shadow in front of the eye. *See also* EYE; RETINA.

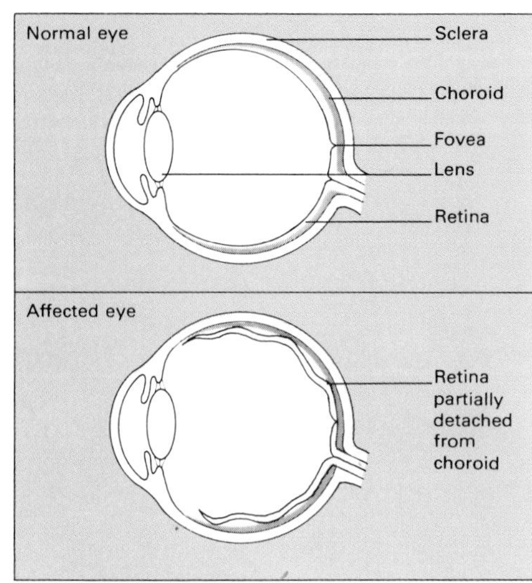

A **detached retina** is the partial or total separation of the retina from the choroid of the eye.

Q: *How is detachment caused?*

A: Detachment results from a hole in the retina that allows fluid to leak through and separate the retina from the choroid. The hole usually results from degenerative changes in the retina, most common in nearsighted people, or from a blow to the eye. Detachment may also be caused by a tumor or disease in the eye.

Q: *What is the treatment?*

A: Various surgical techniques, including the use of laser beams, are used to reseal the retina to the choroid.

Retinitis (ret ə nī′tis) is inflammation of the retina, the light-sensitive surface inside the back of the eye. Retinitis is a symptom of a wide variety of conditions, including tuberculosis, kidney disease, arteriosclerosis, syphilis, eclampsia (convulsions during pregnancy), leukemia, prenatal toxoplasmosis, hypertension, diabetes mellitus, and nervous system degeneration. Retinitis may also be caused by damage to the retina through excessive exposure to light (photoretinitis). Other forms of retinitis, such as retinitis pigmentosa and retinitis proliferans, may be caused by an inherited disorder or by scarring following repeated retinal hemorrhages.

See also RETINITIS PIGMENTOSA.

Retinitis pigmentosa (ret ə nī′tis pig men tō′sə) is a degenerative condition of the retina of unknown cause. Degeneration of the light-sensitive rod cells in the retina occurs first, and night blindness is generally the first symptom. This usually begins in early adult life. The color sensitive cone cells become involved more gradually, daytime vision deteriorates, and the field of vision is slowly reduced from the edges inward, a condition know as telescopic vision. *See also* RETINITIS.

Q: *How is retinitis pigmentosa treated?*

A: There is as yet no definitive treatment for the condition.

Retrobulbar neuritis. *See* NEURITIS, RETROBULBAR.

Reye's syndrome (rāz) is a rare childhood disease, which is fatal in 10 to 40 percent of cases. It affects the liver and central nervous system and usually develops while the child is recovering from a mild viral infection, such as influenza or chickenpox.

Symptoms include repeated vomiting and such mental disturbances as lethargy, mild amnesia, and disorientation. In severe cases, the child falls into a coma and dies.

Aspirin has been proven to be a factor in the development of Reye's syndrome. It is therefore recommended that aspirin not be used to treat any febrile (feverish) illness in children.

Treatment is basically supportive—making the patient comfortable, giving intravenous feeding if necessary, and monitoring blood chemistry and treating any imbalances. Those children who recover do so without ill effects.

Rhesus factor. See RH FACTOR.

Rheumatic disease (rü mat′ik) stems from a wide group of disorders. They include various forms of arthritis and various inflammatory disorders of muscles and ligaments. Symptoms of most rheumatic diseases include muscle stiffness, aching, and sometimes, joint pain. Continued discomfort requires investigation by a physician.

Q: *How are rheumatic diseases treated?*

A: Drugs based on aspirin are used when the complaint is mild. Various anti-inflammatory drugs may also be prescribed. Sometimes, in extremely painful cases, a local anesthetic and a corticosteroid drug are injected directly into the area of pain to relieve the immediate local symptoms.

Heat, shortwave diathermy, or ultrasonic treatment are often given by physiotherapists as short-term relief.

The following table lists rheumatic disorders and related diseases. Each has a separate article in this encyclopedia.

Rheumatic type	*Related disease*
Arthritis of unknown cause	Arthritis, rheumatoid
	Osteoarthropathy
	Psoriasis
	Reiter's disease
	Spondylitis, anxylosing
Osteoarthritis	Osteoarthritis
Metabolic arthritis	Acromegaly
	Gout
	Hemophilia
	Hyperthyroidism
	Hypothyroidism
	Osteomalacia
	Scurvy
	Sickle cell anemia
Cartilage disorders	Chondromalacia
	Disk, herniated
	Osteochondritis
Generalized diseases often involving joints	Colitis, ulcerative
	Crohn's disease
	Sarcoidosis
Rheumatic fever	Rheumatic fever

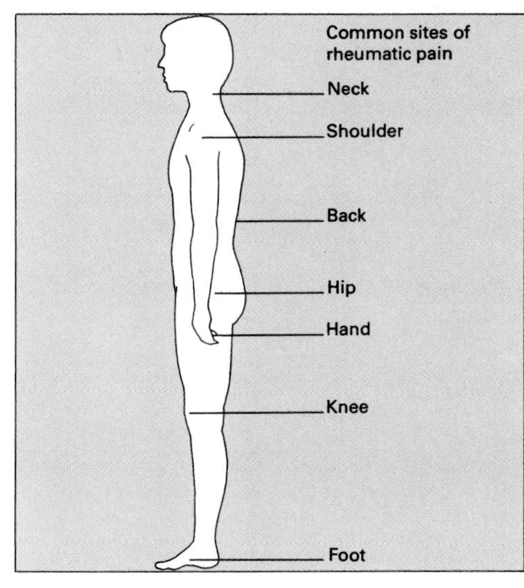

Rheumatic disease is commonly characterized by stiffness, pain, and inflammation in muscles and joints.

Rheumatic type	*Related disease*
Disorders of connective tissue	Allergy (particularly to drugs)
	Lupus erythematosus
	Polyarteritis nodosa
	Polymyalgia rheumatica
	Scleroderma
Rheumatism	Backache
	Bursitis
	Capsulitis
	Carpal tunnel syndrome
	Fever
	Fibrositis
	Myalgia
	Myositis
	Polyneuritis
	Tendinitis
	Torticollis
Miscellaneous	Parkinson's disease
	Various psychological disorders

Rheumatic fever (rü mat′ik) is a form of allergic reaction by the body to a particular kind of streptococcal infection. The infection usually occurs with tonsillitis or pharyngitis (inflammation of the mucous membrane of the pharynx). Rheumatic fever causes damage to the body's tissues, and this damage is most serious when it involves the tissues of the heart. But rheumatic fever-related damage can also involve the central nervous system, the joints, skin, and subcutaneous tissues.

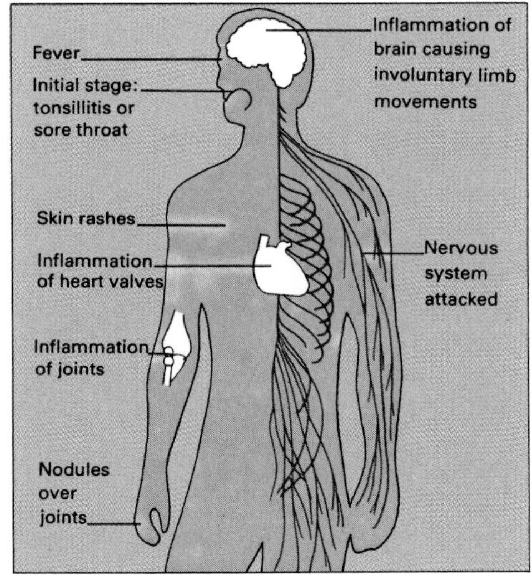

Rheumatic fever begins with a throat infection, but progressively causes other symptoms, including fever, rashes, and various inflammations.

Rheumatic fever most commonly occurs in children between the ages of 5 and 15 years, but it may also affect young adults. The incidence of rheumatic fever has declined significantly in the past three decades as the result of recognition and treatment of streptococcal infections.

Q: *What are the symptoms of rheumatic fever?*

A: Usually, the patient has had tonsillitis or a severe sore throat. This may have improved by the time the symptoms of rheumatic fever appear, which is usually about two weeks later. The most common symptom of rheumatic fever is a form of arthritis in which the joints become tender, swollen, and red.

Typically, as the swelling of one joint seems to settle, another joint becomes swollen and inflamed. The patient appears unwell, flushed, and has a moderate fever.

Less commonly, symptoms of breathlessness, fever, or mid-chest pain, due to underlying rheumatic pericarditis, cause the patient to consult a physician. It is then that the physician, when examining the heart, detects the abnormal murmurs produced by inflammation of the heart valves.

Another possible, but less common, symptom is chorea, an inflammation of the brain, which causes the victim to twist and turn the limbs involuntarily, become clumsy and irritable, and have facial contortions. The sufferer may also grunt and have difficulty speaking normally. *See also* CHOREA.

Q: *What other symptoms may occur with rheumatic fever?*

A: Painless nodules may develop under the skin, particularly over the surface of the large joints, such as the knee and elbow. Transient rashes are also common, but seldom last for more than a day or two.

Abdominal pains are a common occurrence in young children and are probably caused by a combination of a swollen liver, slight heart failure, and inflammation of the lymph nodes behind the peritoneum, the membrane that lines the abdominal cavity.

Q: *What is the progress of rheumatic fever?*

A: Usually, the fever and joint pains subside within two or three weeks. A patient with chorea may take some months before losing all the symptoms. Skin rashes usually disappear by the end of the fever, and any nodules around the joints gradually become smaller and disappear in a matter of weeks.

The only permanent damage that can be caused by rheumatic fever is to the heart valves. Any pericarditis or rheumatic myocarditis disappears, but scarring occurs on the lining of the heart (endocardium), causing distortion of the heart valves and eventually resulting in valvular disease of the heart. *See also* MYOCARDITIS; PERICARDITIS.

However, at least half of all patients who develop the cardiac form of rheumatic fever make a recovery without any valve damage.

Q: *How is rheumatic fever treated?*

A: The most effective and still the basic form of therapy is acetaminophen. In patients with arthritis, the inflamed joints are rested, often in splints padded with cotton. Corticosteroid drugs are usually prescribed if acetaminophen is found to be ineffective. For those patients with heart involvement, bed rest is essential until the acute stages of the illness have passed.

It is essential that all patients with rheumatic fever be given antibiotics, preferably penicillin, to kill any residual streptococcal infection.

Q: *For how long should rheumatic fever be treated?*

A: Because the diagnosis is usually made while the patient is in the hospital, treatment is started immediately, and the patient is allowed to return home only when symptoms have improved to such a degree that relatively normal activity can take place. Continued treatment with acetaminophen is necessary for some weeks or months. Antibiotic treatment should be continued for some years. Any patient who has had rheumatic fever, particularly if the heart has been involved, must have precautionary antibiotics before dental surgery.

Q: *Can a patient have a second attack of rheumatic fever?*

A: Yes. At present, a second attack of rheumatic fever is much less common because the continued daily use of antibiotics prevents further streptococcal infections. Some physicians recommend the use of antibiotics at the onset of any acute throat infection occurring in anyone who has had rheumatic fever. This may further reduce the chances of another attack.

Rheumatism (rü'mə tiz əm) is a general term for any condition that is characterized by stiffness and pain in the muscles and joints.

See also RHEUMATIC DISEASE.

Rheumatoid arthritis. *See* ARTHRITIS, RHEUMATOID.

Rh factor (rhesus factor) is the basis of the Rh system of blood groups, which is independent of the ABO system. The Rh factor was first discovered in the blood of the rhesus monkey.

Eighty-five percent of the population is Rh positive. Persons without the Rh factor are Rh negative. If Rh positive blood is transfused into an Rh negative person, rhesus antibodies (agglutinins) are formed. There is no adverse reaction the first time this occurs. But subsequent transfusions of Rh positive blood will result in a transfusion reaction in which the red blood cells of the Rh negative person are destroyed. For this reason, it is essential that blood is grouped for A, B, O, and Rh factors before a transfusion is made.

Hemolytic disease of the newborn results from the incompatability of an Rh positive fetus and an Rh negative mother.

See also BLOOD GROUP; BLOOD TRANSFUSION; HEMOLYTIC DISEASE OF THE NEWBORN.

Rhinitis (rī nī'tis) is inflammation of the mucous membrane that lines the nose, producing a watery discharge. It may be caused by an infection, such as the common cold, or by an allergy, such as hay fever; or the cause may be unknown, for example, as with vasomotor rhinitis. Persistent inflammation may result in gross swelling of the mucous membrane and the formation of a polyp.

See also COLD; HAY FEVER; POLYP; RHINITIS, VASOMOTOR.

Rhinitis, vasomotor (rī nī′tis, vas ō mō′tər). Vasomotor rhinitis is a condition affecting the mucous membranes that line the nose. It causes symptoms of runny nose, sneezing, postnasal drip, and occasionally headache. The symptoms are similar to those of hay fever, but no allergic cause can be found.

Q: *What causes vasomotor rhinitis?*

A: In most cases, there is no obvious cause. Sometimes, anxiety, changes in room temperature, or hormonal changes associated with adolescence, menstruation, or menopause may be factors.

Occasionally, a similar condition occurs in a person who has been overusing nasal sprays or drops.

Q: *How is vasomotor rhinitis treated?*

A: Treatment is difficult. The symptoms are thought to be caused partly by overactivity of the parasympathetic nervous system, so loss of weight, regular exercise, and the stopping of smoking may all help.

Treatment of corticosteroid nasal sprays is effective in some cases.

Rhinophyma (rī nə fi′mə) is a form of rosacea in which there is swelling of the sebaceous (wax-producing) glands in the skin, which causes them to become large, red, and misshapen. Antibiotics given at an early stage may be effective in treating the disorder.

See also ROSACEA.

Rhinoplasty (rī′nə plas tē) is plastic surgery of the nose to correct its shape.

See also SEPTUM, DEVIATED; SUBMUCOUS RESECTION.

Rhinorrhea (rī nə rē′ə) is the medical term for a thin, watery discharge from the nose.

See also NOSE, RUNNY.

Rhonchus. *See* RALE.

Rhythm method (rith′əm) is a form of contraception in which the woman abstains from sexual intercourse on the days when she is likely to be fertile. The method is generally considered to be a poor contraceptive method, because of the high rate of pregnancies that occur during its use. However, the use of other techniques, such as basal body temperature and examination of cervical mucus, can help a woman predict and determine her fertile days with much greater accuracy, thus avoiding conception more successfully.

See also CONTRACEPTION; OVULATION; TEMPERATURE.

Rib is one of the 12 pairs of thin, curved bones that form the wall of the chest and surround the lungs and heart. The movement of the ribcage and the diaphragm controls the flow of air into and out of the lungs.

The ribs are joined at the back to the thoracic vertebrae of the spine. The upper seven pairs are called the true ribs, because they are connected in front to the breastbone (sternum). The remaining five pairs of ribs are called the false ribs. The eighth, ninth, and tenth pairs of ribs are connected to the breastbone by cartilage.

Q: *What is a cervical rib?*

A: It is an additional rib, joined to the seventh cervical vertebra in the neck. A cervical rib may cause pressure on the nerves and blood vessels serving the arm and produce symptoms of neuralgia or Raynaud's phenomenon. Surgical removal of the rib cures the symptoms.

Q: *Can the ribs be broken?*

A: Yes. A fracture is the most com-

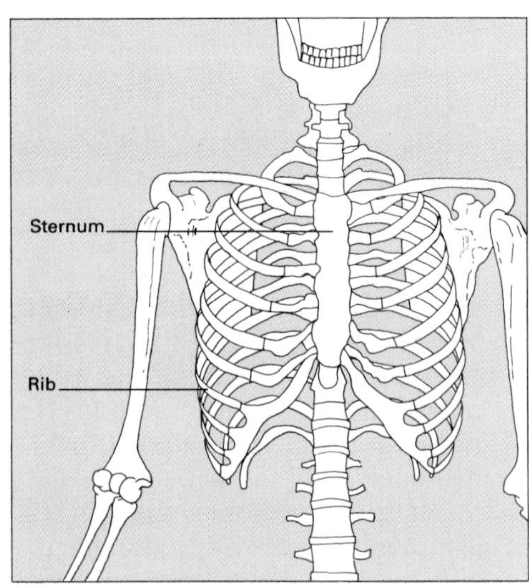

A **rib** is 1 of 24 bones forming a protective cage for the chest cavity. The 11th and 12th pairs are called floating ribs.

mon injury to a rib. It is most likely to occur in the middle ribs. Although painful, a broken rib is seldom serious. The usual treatment is to give the patient painkilling drugs. However, sometimes a surgeon will inject the area of the fracture with a local anesthetic.

A complete fracture sometimes pierces the chest wall. This causes air or gas to collect in the chest cavity (pneumothorax) or allows bloody fluid to accumulate (hemothorax). Hospital treatment and surgery are necessary if either condition occurs.

See also HEMOTHORAX; NEURALGIA; PNEUMOTHROAX; RAYNAUD'S PHENOMENON.

Ribcage (rib'kāj) is the skeletal structure formed by the ribs that serves to protect the heart and lungs.

Rib fracture: first aid. *See* FRACTURE: FIRST AID.

Riboflavin (rī'bō flā vin), or vitamin B_2, is a water-soluble vitamin of the B-complex group. It is found in many foods, particularly beef, fish, liver, kidney, leafy green vegetables, milk, and milk products, such as yogurt.

Riboflavin is essential for the production of energy in the body. Deficiency results in eye disorders, forms of dermatitis, and cheilosis (in which there are small sores at the corners of the mouth).

See also CHEILOSIS; VITAMIN.

Ribonucleic acid (rī bo nü klē'ik) is commonly known as RNA. Found in both the nucleus and the cytoplasm of cells, RNA is a nucleic acid that carries out DNA's instructions for protein production. It resembles DNA chemically, but there are two major differences.

The sugar in RNA is ribose instead of deoxyribose, and RNA contains the base uracil (U) instead of thymine. Like thymine, uracil will pair only with the base adenine. RNA's other three bases—adenine, cytosine, and guanine—and the phosphate unit are identical to those in DNA. For a more complete discussion, *see* DEOXYRIBONUCLEIC ACID.

The process of protein production begins with the blueprint supplied by DNA in the cell's nucleus. RNA copies that blueprint in the following manner. A part of the DNA molecule unwinds and splits. One of the halves then serves as a mold for lining up the RNA bases. Free bases, with their sugars and phosphates, attach to the exposed DNA bases. For example, the RNA bases AUCGAU attach to the DNA bases TAGCTA. An RNA strand is formed, and it is a reverse copy of the DNA master plan.

This messenger RNA (mRNA), which may consist of hundreds of bases, peels off the DNA mold and carries the instructions for making a protein to the ribosomes in the cytoplasm. The bases of the DNA molecule rejoin, the ladder rewinds, and the master plan is again locked away.

How messenger RNA is formed

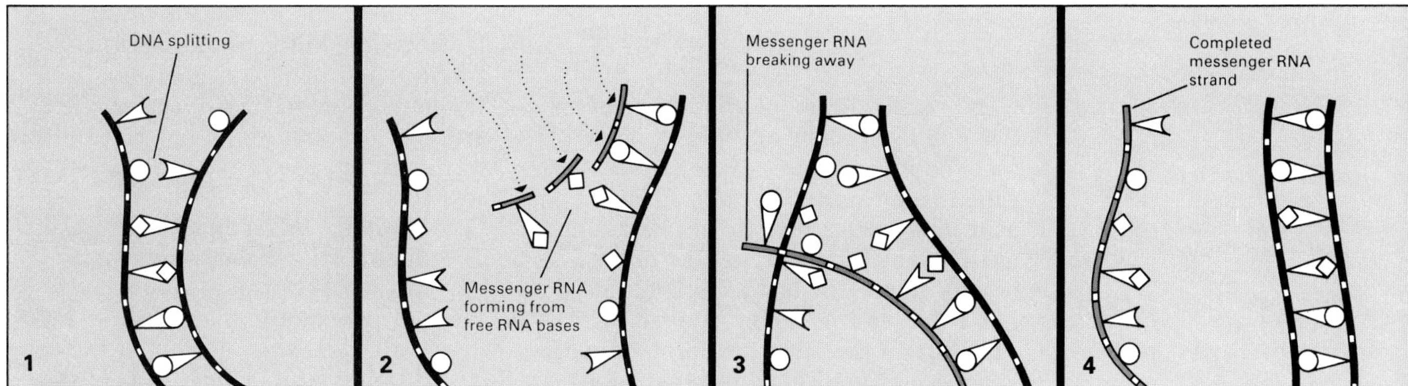

(1) When RNA copies DNA's blueprint for making a protein, the DNA ladder first splits lengthwise through its bases. One half of the ladder then serves as a mold to form messenger RNA. (2) Free RNA bases, with their attached sugars and phosphates, match up with the exposed DNA bases. A strand of messenger RNA thus begins to form. (3) As messenger RNA forms, it becomes a reverse copy of the DNA blueprint, and begins to peel off the DNA mold. As it breaks away, the bases of the DNA ladder start to rejoin. (4) The completed strand of messenger RNA leaves the nucleus and goes to the ribosomes. There, it will serve as a mold on which amino acids will be linked into a protein chain.

Meanwhile, a ribosome moves along the mRNA "reading" the information coded on it. The mRNA acts as a template (mold) to line up the amino acids in the exact order called for by the DNA of the genes. The amino acids are linked together one by one to form the polypeptide chain, the main component of a protein molecule.

Another type of RNA, called transfer RNA (tRNA), collects the amino acids in the cytoplasm and brings them to the mRNA. There is at least one tRNA molecule for each kind of amino acid. The specific tRNA and the correct amino acid are brought together with the help of adenosine triphosphate (the "electricity" that runs the cell's activities) and an enzyme designed for the job.

When a particular protein is to be made, the messenger RNA goes from the nucleus to a ribosome in the cytoplasm, where it lines up amino acids in the proper order. Another type of RNA, transfer RNA, collects amino acids in the cytoplasm.

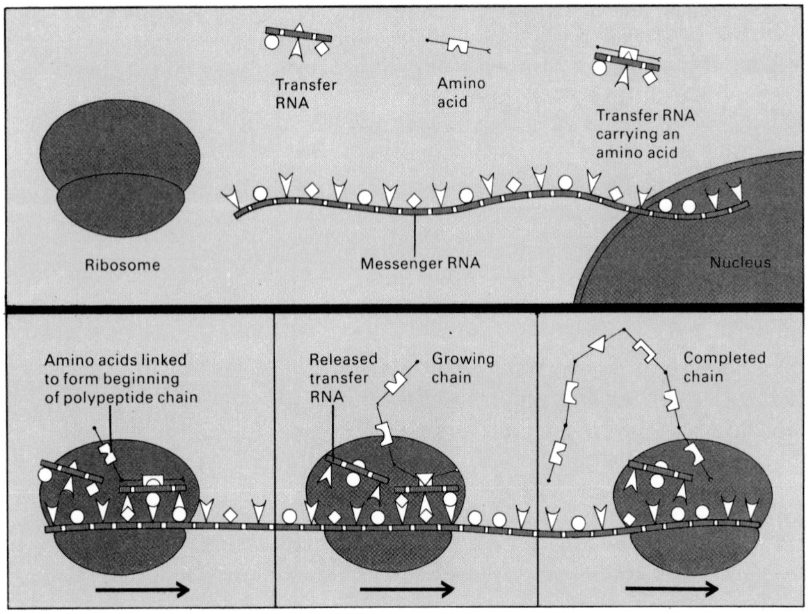

The Ribosome moves along the messenger RNA. The appropriate kinds of transfer RNA, carrying their amino acids, line up with the messenger RNA in the ribosome. The amino acids link together, and the transfer RNA is released, *left.* As the ribosome moves down the messenger RNA, a polypeptide chain forms, *center.* The final segment of messenger RNA, *right,* signals that the chain is complete.

At any one time, the ribosome covers two coding segments of mRNA. Each of these coding segments, which are called codons, specifies one amino acid. The correct tRNA, with its amino acid attached, lines up on the first codon of the mRNA template. After a second tRNA and its amino acids have lined up on the other codon, the two amino acids are linked together. The first tRNA is then set free to collect more amino acids.

The second tRNA holds the growing polypeptide chain to the ribosome. The ribosome then moves one codon further down the mRNA. The appropriate tRNA, with its attached amino acid, lines up on this codon. The amino acid is joined to the first two amino acids, and the second tRNA is now set free.

The ribosome moves one position further, covering the next codon on the messenger RNA template. This process continues until the ribosome has passed over the entire length of the mRNA. The last codon on the mRNA does not code for an amino acid. It signals that the chain is complete. The finished polypeptide chain is then released.

In this case, the protein is now complete. In most proteins that consist of more than one polypeptide chain, the chains are manufactured separately; they then combine to make the protein. The finished protein then starts to do its particular job. Some proteins are used inside the cell. Others, such as hormones and digestive enzymes, are released from the cell to do their work.

See also CELL; DEOXYRIBONUCLEIC ACID; PROTEIN; RIBOSOME.

Ribosome (rī′bə sōm) is a small, round particle made up mostly of ribonucleic acid (RNA). Ribosomes are found in the cytoplasm of cells and produce protein and enzymes.

See also RIBONUCLEIC ACID.

Rickets (rik′its) is a bone disease of children that is caused by a lack of vitamin D. Vitamin D deficiency may also occur in adults where it causes osteomalacia. Vitamin D is formed in the skin when it is exposed to sunlight. It may also be obtained from some foods, such as fish and eggs. Lack of vitamin D affects the kidneys and disrupts the calcium and phosphorus metabolism in the body. This in turn affects the deposition of calcium in the bones, resulting in deformity. *See also* CALCIUM; OSTEOMALACIA; VITAMIN.

Q: *What are the symptoms of rickets?*

A: Infants with rickets are usually restless, grow more slowly than normal, and do not crawl or walk until older than normal. If the condition continues, the ends of the long bones become enlarged. When the infant starts to walk, the legs may bend, resulting in either bowlegs or knock-knees. The chest may also be deformed, producing a pi-

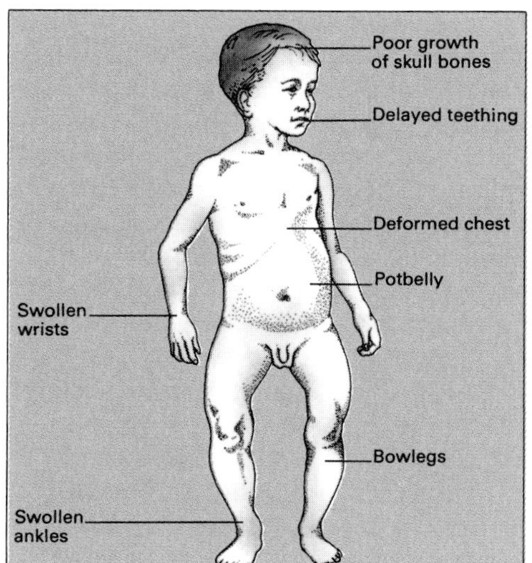

Rickets affects bone formation, producing a variety of symptoms in children.

geon breast, and small knobs may develop on the ends of the ribs. Occasionally, there may be spasms (tetany) due to the low level of calcium in the body. *See also* TETANY.

Q: *How is rickets treated?*

A: Rickets is treated by giving a concentrated supply of vitamin D in addition to an adequate diet. Calcium supplements may also be prescribed to help restore the normal calcium metabolism. Any deformities usually disappear if the condition is treated in the early stages.

Rickettsia (ri ket'sē ə) is a group of microorganisms that have characteristics of both bacteria and viruses. Rickettsia cause many diseases and are usually transmitted by parasites, such as fleas, lice, mites, and ticks. Rickettsial diseases tend to be of sudden onset and produce various symptoms, which are usually the result of blockage of the blood vessels by the rickettsia.

There are four main groups of rickettsial disease: the typhus group; the spotted fever group, including Rocky Mountain spotted fever and rickettsialpox; Q fever; and trench fever, which is transmitted by lice and causes an illness that is similar to a mild form of Rocky Mountain spotted fever.

See also Q FEVER; RICKETTSIALPOX; ROCKY MOUNTAIN SPOTTED FEVER; TRENCH FEVER; TYPHUS.

Rickettsialpox (ri ket'sē əl pox) is an infectious disease caused by the bacteria *Rickettsia akari*, which often infest mice. The disease is transmitted to humans via mites, which travel from the mice to human skin. Symptoms are usually mild and include lesions and a rash resembling chickenpox. Treatment is usually unnecessary. The disease, which is also known as Kew Gardens spotted fever, may be prevented by eliminating house mice.

See also MITE.

Right-handedness is the natural tendency to use the right hand, in preference to the left, in the performance of tasks.

See also LEFT-HANDEDNESS.

Rigor (rig'ər) is a sudden attack of shivering with a high fever, followed by excessive perspiration. It is most commonly associated with the onset of an acute infectious illness, such as malaria or pneumonia.

Rigor mortis (rig'ər môr'tis) is the stiffening of the body after death. It may last for several hours before the body becomes relaxed again.

Ringing ear. *See* TINNITUS.

Ring stuck on finger: treatment. *See* FINGER, RING STUCK ON: TREATMENT.

Ringworm (ring'wėrm) is an infection of the skin caused by a fungus from the group called dermatophytes. The three main types of these fungi are *Epidermophyton, Microsporum,* and *Trichophyton*. Typically, they produce raised reddened rings or scaling of the skin as they feed on the dead skin tissue (epidermis) and affect the live tissue underneath. The infection is also known as *tinea*.

Q: *What areas of the body are likely to be affected by ringworm?*

A: The feet may pick up the fungus *Trichophyton* in public places such as swimming pools or locker rooms. This form of the infection is known as athlete's foot (tinea pedis). Sometimes, it develops into a secondary infection that causes the tissues of the feet, including the toenails, to develop a gnarled, thickened appearance. *See also* ATHLETE'S FOOT.

Ringworm of the nails (tinea unguium) is commonly caused by either the *Epidermophyton* or *Trichophyton* fungus. Jock itch is a skin infection caused by the fungus *Epidermophyton* in combination with hot weather and tight underwear and/or obesity. Ringworm of the scalp (tinea capitis) is usually caused by the fungi *Microsporum*, and sometimes a variety of *Trichophyton*. *See also* JOCK ITCH.

Q: *How is ringworm treated?*

A: A number of antifungal creams can be used to treat ringworm of the body, athlete's foot, and jock itch.

Ringworm is a contagious disease, so it is important that the patient be isolated as much as possible from other members of the family. Careful personal hygiene and drying of the body after bathing should prevent ringworm.

See also HYGIENE.

Rinne's test (rin'nēz) is a hearing test in which a vibrating tuning fork is placed, alternately, with its prongs near the auditory canal of the ear (air conduction), then with its base on the bone behind the ear (bone conduction). Normally, the sound is heard for some time longer when the tuning fork is placed near the auditory canal. This is a positive result. In conductive deafness, the sound is heard longer through the bone. The test is usually used in conjunction with the Weber test.

See also DEAFNESS; WEBER'S TEST.

Rio Grande fever (rē'ō grən'dā) is a local name for brucellosis.

See also BRUCELLOSIS.

Risk factor. *See* CANCER.

Ritalin® (rit'ə lin) is the trade name for methylphenidate hydrochloride, a drug that stimulates the central nervous system. When drug therapy is indicated, Ritalin is often used in the treatment of children diagnosed as being severely hyperactive (an attention deficit disorder). It may also be useful in treating people with narcolepsy.

Side effects of Ritalin may include nervousness, loss of appetite, and difficulty in sleeping. Patients may also become dizzy, have headaches, and have a fast heart rate. Prolonged use of the drug may lead to psychological dependence. This has not however been reported in children.

See also ATTENTION DEFICIT DISORDER; HYPERACTIVITY; NARCOLEPSY.

R.N. *See* NURSE, REGISTERED.

RNA. *See* RIBONUCLEIC ACID.

Rocky Mountain spotted fever is an infectious rickettsial disease caused by the microorganism *Rickettsia rickettsii*, which is transmitted by ticks. It is most commonly seen in the United States in the southeastern and south central states; it is rare in the Rocky Mountains.

Q: *What are the symptoms of Rocky Mountain spotted fever?*

A: After an incubation period of about one week, there is the sudden onset of a severe headache, muscle pains, and a high fever. Within four days, a rash appears on the arms and legs and spreads rapidly to the rest of the body. Areas of the rash may coalesce and ulcerate. A dry, unproductive cough may also develop. In severe cases, the patient becomes delirious or comatose. The fever lasts between two and three weeks.

If untreated, various complications may develop, such as pneumonia, brain damage, and heart damage.

Q: *How is Rocky Mountain spotted fever treated?*

A: Immediate treatment with antibiotics, such as tetracycline, usually produces a rapid improvement. Hospitalization may be necessary in severe cases.

A vaccine against Rocky Mountain spotted fever is available, but it is necessary only for those who frequently encounter ticks in high-risk areas.

Rod is one of the microscopic sensory cells in the retina of the eye that is sensitive to light.

The term *rod* is also used by physicians to describe bacteria that are long and narrow in shape. Such bacteria are usually classified as bacilli.

See also BACILLUS; EYE.

Rodent ulcer. *See* CARCINOMA, BASAL CELL.

Roentgenogram (rent'gə nə gram), or radiograph, is an X-ray photograph produced by roentgenography.

See also ROENTGENOGRAPHY.

Roentgenography (rent gə nog'rə fē), or radiography, is the process of photographing internal body organs or tissue by use of X rays.

Romberg's sign (rom'bergz) is the inability to maintain balance when the feet are together and the eyes are shut. If the sense of balance is disturbed, as may occur with diabetes, B_{12} deficiency, hypothyroidism, or tabes dorsalis (a syphilitic infection of the nerves), the person sways and may fall.

Root canal (rüt kə nal') is a passage in the root of a tooth through which nerves and vessels pass to the pulp. Root canal surgery is performed when the pulp of a tooth has died or becomes infected because of caries (decay) or trauma; it must, therefore, be removed to avoid an abscess and/or a toothache. During root canal surgery, a dentist removes the pulp and fills the empty space, usually with a rubber-like substance called gutta-percha.

Rosacea (rō zā'shē ə), also called acne rosacea, is a skin inflammation associated with disorders of the sebaceous (oil-secreting) glands in the skin. It usually affects the forehead, cheeks, nose, and chin. Rosacea is often seen in alcoholics. *See also* ACNE.

Q: *What are the symptoms of rosacea?*

A: The chief symptom is frequent flushing of the skin, with residual redness. The sebaceous glands produce acne-like lumps, giving the skin a rough, reddish appearance. There are also symptoms of seborrheic dermatitis with scurf (dandruff) on the scalp, as well as inflammation of the eyelids.

Q: *How is rosacea treated?*

A: Tetracycline drugs and other broad-spectrum antibiotics usually are effective. Corticosteroid creams should not be used because they may damage the skin. Solutions containing sulfur may be beneficial.

See also ANTIBIOTIC; SEBORRHEA.

Roseola (rō zē'ə lə), also known as exanthema subitum, is a disease of young children. The cause is not known, but it is thought to be a viral infection.

Q: *What are the symptoms of roseola?*

A: After an incubation period of four to seven days, there is the sudden onset of high fever, which may reach 105°F (40.5°C). The fever usually lasts for three or four days, then disappears suddenly, and a pink rash appears. This occurs mainly on the body, but the limbs and face may also be mildly affected. The rash usually disappears within two days.

Q: *How is roseola treated?*

A: Acetaminophen may be prescribed to reduce the fever. Further treatment is usually unnecessary once the fever has abated.

Rotator cuff (rō tā'tor kŭf) is the part of the shoulder that enables the arm to be pulled away from the side of the body. The rotator cuff is made up of four muscles and their four tendons. Overuse of the rotator cuff can lead to degeneration and tearing of the tendon(s). This produces pain and weakness of the shoulder. Larger tears may need surgical repair.

Roughage (ruf'ij), or dietary fiber, is the indigestible matter present in whole grain, root vegetables, and fruits. Roughage aids digestion and serves as a natural laxative.

See also NUTRITION; DIGESTIVE SYSTEM.

Roundworm (round'wėrm), also called nematode worm, is one of a group of parasitic worms. Roundworm infestations incude ascariasis, enterobiasis, ankylostomiasis, strongyloidiasis, and trichuriasis.

Ascariasis is an infestation of the small intestine with the giant intestinal roundworm *Ascaris lumbricoides*. The infestation seldom causes symptoms. In some cases, there may be abdominal pain, fever, and coughing. Rarely, roundworms may block the bile or pancreatic ducts, causing jaundice or pancreatitis. The appendix may also become blocked. Treatment with drugs, such as piperazine, is usually effective.

Enterobiasis is an infestation with *Enterobius vermicularis*. These roundworms are commonly known as pinworms or seat worms. Treatment with piperazine is usually effective. *See also* ENTEROBIASIS.

Ankylostomiasis is infestation with hookworms (*Ankylostoma duodenale* and *Necator americanus*). It may cause a skin rash, a cough, anemia due to loss of blood, and occasionally abdominal pain. In children, infestation with a large number of worms may cause malnourishment. Treatment with bephenium hydroxynaphthoate or thiabendazole is usually effective. *See also* ANKYLOSTOMIASIS.

Strongyloidiasis is due to an infestation with the threadworm (*Strongyloides stercoralis*). Symptoms are divided into three stages: a pruritic, or itchy, red rash on the skin is followed by migration of the worms through the lungs to the intestine, producing abdominal pain and diarrhea. Thiabendazole usually offers effective treatment. *See also* STRONGYLOIDES.

Trichuriasis is infestation with the whipworm (*Trichuris trichiura*), which lives in the intestine. Trichuriasis may not produce symptoms. Occasionally, there may be abdominal pain on the right side and bloodstained diarrhea. In children, prolapse of the rectum may occur. Trichuriasis is often difficult to cure, but drugs such as mebendazole may be effective. *See also* PROLAPSE; TRICHURIASIS.

Rubella (rü bel'ə), or German measles, is an infectious viral disease that produces a rash. The incubation period of rubella varies between two and three weeks. The patient can transmit the virus during a period from one week before the appearance of the rash to five days after its onset. Quarantine is usually three weeks.

Q: ***What are the symptoms of rubella?***

A: Initial symptoms include drowsiness, headache, fever, and a sore throat. There may be swelling of the lymph nodes behind the ears and down the side of the neck.

The eruption of a rash of small pink and red spots follows, and the patient's temperature rises to about 101°F (38°C). The rash spreads from the face down the whole body and usually lasts between two and four days.

Q: ***How is rubella treated?***

A: There is no cure for rubella; treatment is directed toward alleviating the symptoms. Treatment includes rest, a liquid diet, and acetaminophen for the fever.

Q: ***What complications may occur with rubella?***

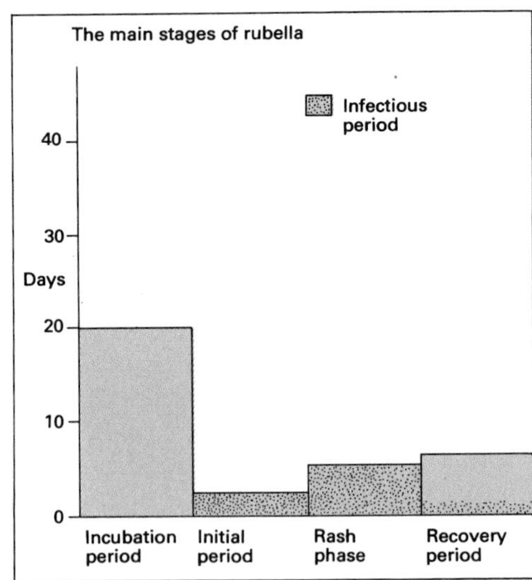

Rubella is infectious before and during the rash phase, and is slightly infectious during recovery.

A: Rubella is particularly dangerous to an unborn child if the mother is in the first three months of pregnancy when she becomes ill, because it may cause congenital anomalies. Rarely, a form of encephalitis (inflammation of the brain) may develop.

Q: ***What should a pregnant woman do if she is exposed to rubella?***

A: She should consult a physician immediately. The physician may test her blood for rubella antibodies, which, if present, will prevent the infection and, therefore, any risk to the unborn child. If the blood is low in antibodies, further tests are needed to see whether an infection has occurred, with the possibility that the child has been affected.

Q: ***Can rubella be prevented?***

A: Yes. Rubella vaccine, combined with mumps and measles vaccines, is given to children aged 15 months and a booster is given at 10 to 12 years of age.

Rubeola (rü bē'ō lə) is the medical term for measles.

See also MEASLES.

Running nose. See NOSE, RUNNY.

Rupture. See HERNIA.

Rupture: first aid. See HERNIA, STRANGULATED: FIRST AID.

S

Sabin's vaccine (sā'binz) is a vaccine against poliomyelitis. It is a preparation of one or a combination of the three poliomyelitis viruses, which have been modified so that they confer immunity and only rarely cause illness or symptoms. These modified viruses are referred to as "attenuated" (weakened). The Sabin's vaccine is taken orally and is considered to be the most effective form of poliomyelitis immunization. For these reasons, it has generally replaced the Salk vaccine as the prevention for polio in the United States.

See also POLIOMYELITIS; SALK VACCINE; VACCINE.

Saccharin (sak'ər in) is a very sweet, white crystalline substance obtained from coal tar and used as a low-calorie substitute for sugar. A pellet of it has as much sweetening power as several hundred times its weight in cane sugar.

Saccule (sak'yül) is a little sac or bag, also known as sacculus. The lungs contain air saccules, and there is a membranous saccule in the labyrinth of the inner ear.

Sacroiliac (sā krō il'ē ak) is the area of the body related to the sacroiliac joint that connects with the two large ilium bones on each side of the sacrum at the base of the spine. Strong ligaments surround the joint; these can become strained, causing backache and pain related to the movement of the joint. Inflammation of the sacroiliac joint is a symptom of ankylosing spondylitis and other rheumatic diseases of the joints.

See also SPONDYLITIS, ANKYLOSING; SACRUM.

Sacrum (sā'krəm) is a triangular bone that forms the dorsal (rear) part of the pelvis. It binds the two hip bones together and transmits the weight of the body from the spine to the pelvis.

The sacrum is made up of five sacral vertebrae, which are fused together to form a single bone. At the lower end it forms a joint with the coccyx. The upper end is joined to the fifth lumbar vertebra with an intervening disk. On each side are the sacroiliac joints with the two ilium bones of the pelvis.

Spondylolisthesis, a condition in which the lumbar vertebra tends to slip forward onto the sacrum, may occur. The result is chronic backache.

See also SPONDYLOLISTHESIS.

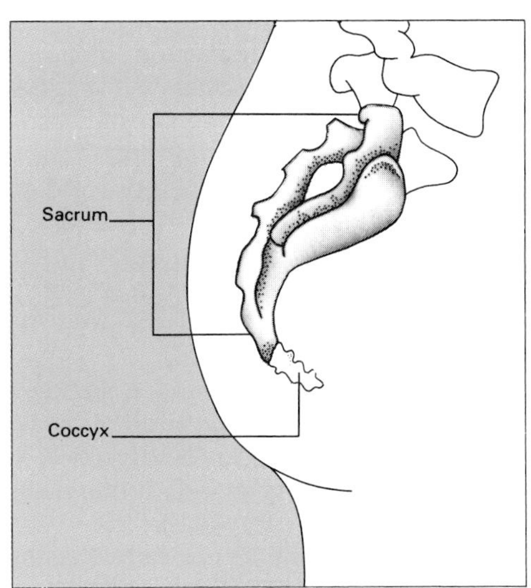

The **sacrum** is a triangular shaped bone composed of five fused vertebrae located at the lower end of the spine, just above the coccyx bone.

Saddle joint. *See* JOINT.

Sadism (sā'diz əm) is a sexual practice in which individuals achieve sexual excitement by inflicting physical pain upon others. In some individuals, sadism is the preferred or exclusive mode of achieving sexual enjoyment. This more extreme form of sexual activity contrasts with normal love play in which sexual partners may inflict slight pain upon each other, such as by light scratching or biting.

See also MASOCHISM.

Sailing safety. *See* WATER SPORTS SAFETY.

Saint Vitus's dance (vī'tə siz) is another name for Sydenham's chorea, a symptom of rheumatic fever.

See also CHOREA; RHEUMATIC FEVER.

Salicylate (sal′ə sil āt) is a salt of salicylic acid. Salicylates have painkilling, anti-inflammatory, and fever-reducing properties. The most common compound of salicylic acid is acetylsalicylic acid (aspirin). Sodium salicylate is sometimes used as an alternative to aspirin.

See also ASPIRIN.

Saline (sā′līn) commonly refers to a solution containing salt (sodium chloride). Physiological saline is a solution of sodium chloride that is of the same concentration as the body fluids (isotonic). This solution may be given by intravenous infusion to replace salt that is lost either during surgery or as a result of shock.

Saliva (sə lī′və) is a watery, slightly alkaline fluid that is secreted by the salivary and mucous glands in the mouth. Saliva helps to keep the mouth clean, lubricates food, and makes possible taste, since the sensory nerves for taste respond only to dissolved substances. It contains various salts and the enzyme ptyalin that begins the process of the digestion of starch. Salivation occurs as a reflex response to either the presence of food in the mouth or the anticipation of food.

See also SALIVARY GLAND.

Salivary gland (sal′ə ver ē) is a gland located in the mouth that produces saliva and thereby aids in the digestion of food. The salivary glands include the two parotid glands located in the cheeks, in front of and just below each ear; the two submandibular and the two sublingual glands located mainly on the floor of the mouth, beneath the tongue; and the buccal glands in the mucous membranes of the cheeks and lips. The salivary glands can be adversely affected by viral infection (such as mumps), bacterial infection, small stones in the salivary ducts, or cancer.

See also GLAND; SALIVA.

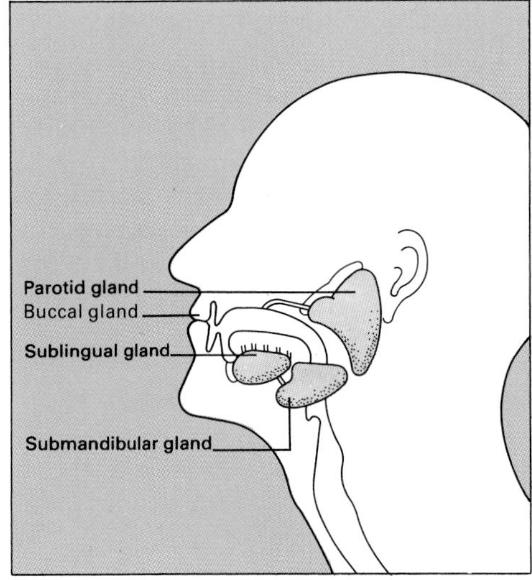

Salivary glands secrete saliva to moisten the mouth and help begin the digestion of food.

Salk vaccine (sôk) is a vaccine against poliomyelitis, developed by Jonas Salk. It contains three types of inactive poliomyelitis virus, which are administered by injection. Salk vaccine was the first successful immunizing vaccine to counteract polio. It has now been largely superseded by the orally administered Sabin's vaccine.

See also POLIOMYELITIS; SABIN'S VACCINE; VACCINE.

Salmonella (sal mə nel′ə) is a genus of rod-shaped bacteria, some species of which can cause disease in humans. The most serious salmonella bacteria may cause typhoid and paratyphoid fevers. However, the term is generally used to refer to the species that causes salmonella gastroenteritis, which may vary from a mild to a severe, and occasionally fatal, form of food poisoning.
See also TYPHOID FEVER; PARATYPHOID.

Q: *What are the symptoms of salmonella gastroenteritis?*

A: The symptoms may vary from mild abdominal pain with occasional diarrhea to extremely severe vomiting and persistent bloody diarrhea. They usually occur within two days of eating contaminated food. The severe form may result in shock due to fluid loss, requiring immediate hospitalization. In some cases, a fever develops, but this rarely lasts for more than a day.

Occasionally, the infection may spread into the bloodstream (septicemia) and cause localized abscesses in other parts of the body. Fatalities from salmonella gastroenteritis are usually confined to the young, the elderly, and those who already have a serious underlying physical disorder.

Q: *How is salmonella gastroenteritis treated?*

A: Treatment is directed toward alleviating the symptoms and includes plenty of fluids, a bland diet, and antispasmodic drugs to relieve abdominal cramps. Generally, antibiotic drugs are not prescribed because they may prolong the course of the illness. However, antibiotics become necessary if the patient develops septicemia.

If a large amount of fluid has been lost by vomiting and diarrhea, the patient may be given fluids intravenously to replace the lost fluid. If the patient has localized abscesses, surgery may also be necessary.

See also FOOD POISONING.

Salpingectomy (sal pin jek'tə mē) is the surgical removal of one or both fallopian tubes (oviducts), often performed to excise a tumor or cervical cyst. One tube may have to be removed because of an ectopic pregnancy. Both tubes may have to be removed if chronic abdominal pain occurs due to salpingitis. The operation is also performed as a means of sterilization.

See also PREGNANCY, ECTOPIC; SALPINGITIS; STERILIZATION.

Salpingitis (sal pin jī'tis) is inflammation of the fallopian tubes. It may affect only one tube, but usually both are involved. The surrounding tissues and the ovaries may also become infected and inflamed. *See also* FALLOPIAN TUBE.

Salpingitis is most commonly caused by the spread of infection following sexual intercourse. The venereal diseases gonorrhea and chlamydia are the two most common causes of salpingitis. It may also occur following childbirth, an abortion, or sometimes after the insertion of an IUD (intrauterine device). Rarely, salpingitis occurs in young girls and adolescents as a result of tuberculosis. *See also* SEXUALLY TRANSMITTED DISEASE.

Q: *What are the symptoms of salpingitis?*

A: Acute salpingitis occurs suddenly and produces severe abdominal pain, a purulent vaginal discharge, fever, and, occasionally, vomiting. Chronic salpingitis may occur after treatment for the acute form of the disease. With chronic salpingitis, there may be a dull abdominal ache, irregular and painful periods, and pain while having sexual intercourse. Many women also feel vaguely ill, with backache, fatigue, and weight loss.

Q: *How is salpingitis treated?*

A: Immediate treatment with antibiotics cures infection and prevents possible sterility. Severe cases may need hospitalization.

Chronic salpingitis is difficult to treat because the fallopian tubes may become scarred and blocked. A long course of antibiotics is usually prescribed. The patient may also be advised to abstain from sexual intercourse for several weeks.

The sexual partner of a woman with salpingitis should also be examined and, if necessary, treated. Failure to do so is a major cause of recurrent infections.

San Joaquin fever. *See* COCCIDIOIDOMYCOSIS.

Saphenous vein. *See* VEIN.

Sarcoidosis (sär koi dō'sis) is a condition of unknown origin in which areas of scar tissue are formed in many parts of the body, most commonly in the lungs, liver, eyes, skin, and lymphatic system. It is also known as sarcoid.

Q: *What are the symptoms of sarcoidosis?*

A: Frequently, there are no symptoms at all. Diagnosis is often made from a routine chest X ray or a physical examination in which the patient's lymph nodes are found to be enlarged. Some patients, however, have symptoms of fever, vague muscle aching, joint pains, and skin lesions (erythema nodosum). The liver may become affected in a minor way, and rarely, cardiac involvement may result in heart failure.

Q: *How is sarcoidosis treated?*

A: The aim of treatment is to prevent further damage to body tissue. If the patient has no symptoms and there is no evidence of damage, regular examination is all that is necessary. Corticosteroid drug treatment may have to be given for several years in patients with severe symptoms.

Sarcoma (sär kō'mə) is a malignant (cancerous) tumor formed from connective tissue, such as cartilage, bone, or muscle. The usual treatment for sarcoma is surgical removal, often followed by radiotherapy or, in the case of bone tumors (Ewing's sarcoma), by a combination of radiotherapy and multiple-drug chemotherapy.

See also CANCER; TUMOR.

Scab (skab) is a protective layer of dried serum and blood that often forms over a sore or a wound. The tissues beneath the scab, thus protected, are allowed to heal. The scab falls off when healing is complete.

See also SCRAPES AND ABRASIONS: TREATMENT.

Scabicide (skā'bi sīd) is a drug used in the treatment of scabies. Crotamiton and gamma benzene hexachloride are commonly used scabicides.

See also SCABIES.

Scabies (skā'bēz) is a contagious skin infection, caused by the itch mite *Sarcoptes scabiei.* The female mite burrows beneath the skin, lays eggs, and forms tunnel-like nests. The eggs, in turn, produce larvae that mature and mate. The victim's body suffers an allergic reaction to the mite in the form of an extremely itchy rash. The rash is restricted to areas in which the mite burrows, such as the hands, fingers, wrists, pubic areas, inner thighs and, sometimes, the soles of the feet.

Q: *What are the symptoms of scabies?*

A: For the first month following contact, there are no symptoms. During this period, the eggs of the mite hatch and develop into adults. The female lays several eggs a day for several weeks, so that by the end of the month many more females have burrowed beneath the skin. Localized rash and intense itching then occurs as an allergic reaction.

Q: *How is scabies treated?*

A: The patient takes a bath and is painted over the whole body surface (excluding the eyes, nose, and mouth) with scabicides. This treatment is repeated twice at daily intervals. A physician may prescribe antihistamine drugs to relieve the allergic reaction. Usually, the patient's family has to be treated as well, because the infection spreads very easily.

Scald (skôld) is a burn on the skin caused by hot vapor or liquid.

See also BURNS AND SCALDS: FIRST AID.

Scalded skin syndrome (skôld'əd), known medically as toxic epidermal necrolysis (TEN), is a serious skin disorder in which the skin becomes inflamed and blistered, coming off sometimes in large sections. If untreated, the syndrome causes a dangerous loss of tissue fluid and can lead to potentially fatal complications.

In infants, it is usually caused by a staphylococcal infection and can be treated with appropriate antibiotics. In adults, it most often results from an adverse drug reaction and requires immediate hospitalization, where the patient is treated as for severe burns.

Scald: first aid. *See* BURNS AND SCALDS: FIRST AID.

Scale (skāl) is a small, thin piece of skin. It is normal for the body to shed scales of dead skin in small amounts. Excessive shedding may be a sign of a skin disorder, such as psoriasis, eczema, or seborrhea.

See also ECZEMA; PSORIASIS; SEBORRHEA.

Scalene node biopsy (skā lēn' nōd bī'op sē) is a diagnostic procedure in which an enlarged lymph node from behind the scalene muscles in the neck is surgically removed and then examined microscopically. In the past, scalene node biopsy was frequently used to diagnose lung masses, because of the relative ease of the procedure. Now, however, other techniques, such as bronchoscopy, are much more widely used.

See also BRONCHOSCOPY.

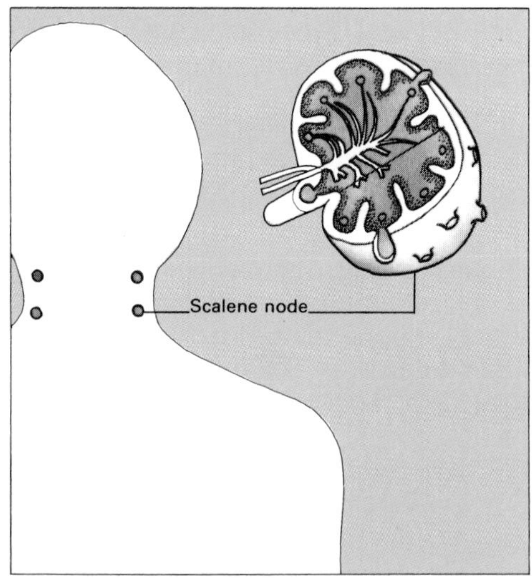

A **scalene node biopsy** is the diagnostic examination of a lymph node removed from the neck.

Scalp (skalp) is a part of the covering of the skull consisting of hair, skin, and underlying layers of muscle and fibrous tissue (fascia).

Scaphoid (skaf′oid) is a small, irregularly-shaped bone in each wrist (carpus) and ankle (tarsus). In the wrist, it is jointed to the radius bone in the forearm and is one of the bones most likely to be fractured in a fall onto the outstretched hand. This fracture can be difficult to diagnose by X ray and is referred to as a navicular fracture.

See also SKELETON.

Scapula (skap′yə lə), or shoulder blade, is one of a pair of flat triangular bones that, together with the upper bone of the arm (humerus), forms the shoulder joint. The ball-and-socket joint at the shoulder allows a wide range of movements, activated by muscles at the front and back of the chest wall, as well as those from the scapula.

See also SKELETON.

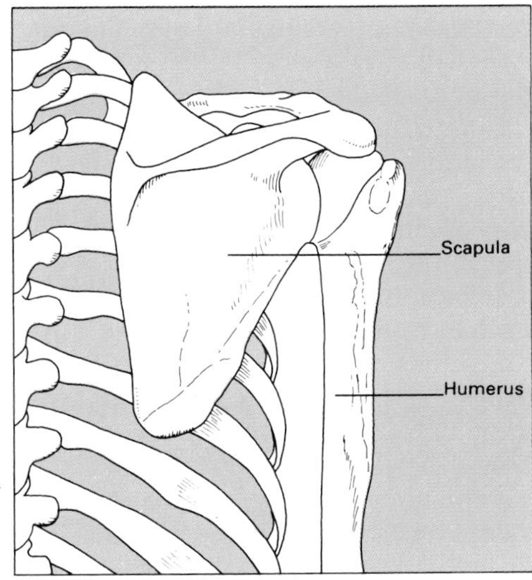

The **scapula** is a flat, triangular bone that forms the posterior portion of the shoulder.

Scar (skär), known medically as cicatrix, is a mark left by a healed wound, burn, or incision. It is composed of tough fibrous tissue.

Scar tissue inside the body seldom causes any problems. But adhesions (long strips of scar tissue) in the abdomen may distort the intestine and lead to intestinal obstruction.

Scar tissue on the skin may become abnormally thickened, raised, or red. This is known as a keloid scar. Most unsightly scars can be removed or treated by plastic surgery.

See also INTESTINAL OBSTRUCTION; KELOID.

Scarlatina (skär lə tē′nə) is another name for scarlet fever.

See also SCARLET FEVER.

Scarlet fever (skär′lit), or scarlatina, is an infectious disease caused by bacteria called group A beta-hemolytic streptococci. It may develop after a sore throat or acute tonsillitis. Scarlet fever can be spread by contaminated food or by infected droplets in the air.

The symptoms usually take from one to three days to appear. The patient is contagious while the bacteria are still in the nose and throat, which may be for two or three weeks. Some persons become carriers of the infection for several months.

Q: *What are the symptoms of scarlet fever?*

A: There is usually a sudden fever and a sore throat. There may also be vomiting, diarrhea, and a severe headache. About one or two days after infection, a rash of small, red spots appears, initially on the neck and chest, then spreading rapidly to the rest of the body and limbs. The rash is very fine and feels like sandpaper. Typically, the face is flushed, with a pale area around the mouth. The surface of the tongue is coated with small, red spots protruding from a milky white background, giving the tongue a strawberry-like appearance. The rash usually lasts for three or four days, after which the other symptoms gradually disappear.

Q: *How is scarlet fever treated?*

A: Penicillin or other antibiotics are usually given for 10 days, even for mild cases of the disease. The full course recommended by a physician must be completed to prevent complications from developing. If scarlet fever is not properly treated, the patient may develop the more serious condition of rheumatic fever. Acetaminophen may also be prescribed to relieve the fever, headache, and sore throat. It is usually advisable for other members of the family to be treated with antibiotics so that the infection does not spread.

See also RHEUMATIC FEVER.

Schick test (shik) is a method of testing immunity to diphtheria. A small amount of diphtheria toxin is injected into the skin. If immunity to diphtheria is not present, a small, red, inflamed area develops on the skin. The Schick test is rarely used anymore.

See also DIPHTHERIA.

Schistosomiasis (shis tə sō mī'ə sis), also known as bilharziasis, is a parasitic disease that occurs mostly in Africa, South America, and the Far East. It can be caught by swimming in infected water.

The worm responsible for schistosomiasis is a species of fluke (*Schistosoma*), which uses freshwater snails and humans as hosts in its life cycle.

The symptoms are fever, cough, muscle pains, blood in the urine, and skin irritation.

Schistosomiasis is difficult to treat, but a variety of therapeutic drugs are available. Surgery may be needed if internal organs, such as the bladder or rectum, are severely scarred.

See also FLUKE.

Schizoid personality (skit'soid) is a psychological term that describes a personality type characterized by emotional coldness, an absence of warm feeling for others, and an inability to develop close friendships. Individuals with this disorder show little or no desire for social involvement. They appear reserved, withdrawn, and seclusive and are often described as "loners." Schizoid persons may be unable to verbally express anger, preferring to keep their feelings to themselves. Although a schizoid personality may lead to schizophrenia, many schizoid individuals can function reasonably well.

See also MENTAL ILLNESS; SCHIZOPHRENIA.

Schizophrenia (skit sə frē'nē ə) is a severe mental disease characterized by unpredictable disturbances in thinking. It refers to the characteristic schizophrenic behavior of withdrawing from reality and thinking in illogical, confused patterns. The term does not mean that a victim has more than one personality, but that there is a split or incongruence between thought and emotional content.

Schizophrenia ranks as one of the most common mental disorders. It affects about 1 percent of the population. About 75 percent of all cases develop the disease between the ages of 15 and 25. While the incidence is low, the disease tends to be chronic, causing a major disruption of the victim's life. Recent studies have shown that more individuals with schizophrenia make a partial or complete recovery than was previously thought. Schizophrenics often suffer disturbances in mood and behavior. Some patients seem to feel no emotions, but others may display inappropriate emotions, such as laughing at sad situations. Some schizophrenics withdraw from their family and friends. Others develop extreme delusions and suffer additionally from hallucinations, most commonly the hearing of voices.

Physicians do not know the cause of schizophrenia. However, there is increasing evidence that the disease results from an inherited defect involving certain brain chemicals. These chemicals, called *neurotransmitters*, enable the nerve cells of the brain to communicate with one another. Schizophrenics may be born with a defect that causes certain brain cells to release excess amounts of *dopamine,* a neurotransmitter.

Before the 1950's, most schizophrenics had to remain in mental hospitals. Since then, scientists have developed drugs that block the action of dopamine on certain nerve cells. In most cases, these drugs do not cure schizophrenia, but they may reduce the symptoms so that many patients can leave the hospital. In addition, psychotherapy can help prepare patients for life outside the hospital. But even with drug treatment and psychotherapy, some schizophrenics must remain hospitalized for much of their lives.

See also DOPAMINE; MENTAL ILLNESS.

School phobia (fō'bē ə) is an anxiety disorder of childhood and adolescence, characterized by an intense fear of going to school. Such children may be overdependent on their parents, shy, and emotionally immature. School phobia often reflects other problems in the child's family, such as parental alcoholism, marital conflict, anxiety, or depression. The child may develop numerous physical complaints in order to stay home. In contrast to normal school anxieties, which tend to alleviate with time, school phobia often requires psychotherapy. The longer the time away from school, the worse the problem often becomes. It is, therefore, important to treat it aggressively.

See also PHOBIA.

Sciatica (sī at′ə kə) is pain along the course of the sciatic nerve, which serves the buttock and the back of the thigh and leg. Onset may be sudden or gradual. Sciatica is usually caused by pressure on the sciatic nerve, which may be the result of a herniated disk, osteoarthritis of the spine, congenital anomalies of the spine, such as spondylolisthesis, or tumors of the spinal canal.

See also DISK, HERNIATED; OSTEOARTHRITIS; SPONDYLOLISTHESIS.

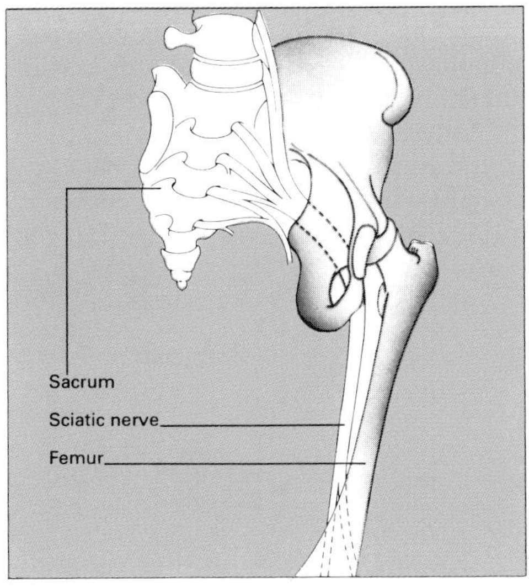

Sciatica is pain along the path of the sciatic nerve and its branches in the hip, thigh, and leg.

Scintiscan (sin′ti skan) is a diagnostic test that produces an image of a bodily organ or organs by injecting a patient with a radioactive substance. The substance then concentrates itself in the organ. The scintillations (radioactive emissions) are then photographed, and a picture, the scintiscan, of the outline and function of the organ under study is obtained.

Scirrhus (skir′əs) is a hard, cancerous tumor caused by the abnormal growth of muscle or other fibrous tissue.

See also TUMOR.

Sclera (sklir′ə) is the white, fibrous outer coat of the eyeball. It forms the visible white of the eye and surrounds the optic nerve at the back of the eyeball.

See also EYE.

Scleritis (skli rī′tis) is inflammation of the sclera of the eyeball, sometimes associated with rheumatic disorders. The condition is serious, and a physician should be consulted.

See also SCLERA.

Scleroderma (sklir ə dėr′mə) is an uncommon, progressive disease that involves the blood vessels and fibrous tissue of the skin, eyes, joints, and internal organs, particularly the lungs, kidneys, and intestines. The cause of scleroderma is not known. It is more common in women than men, and most cases occur during middle age.

Q: *What are the symptoms of scleroderma?*

A: The symptoms usually develop gradually. Initially, the fingers and toes become pale and painful when cold (Raynaud's phenomenon). There may also be pain in the joints, swelling of the hands, and muscle weakness. If the lungs or the heart are affected, pleurisy, pericarditis, or heart failure may occur. The skin commonly becomes very tight over the face and fingers. *See also* PERICARDITIS; PLEURISY; RAYNAUD'S PHENOMENON.

Q: *How is scleroderma treated?*

A: There is no specific treatment. Scleroderma may occur in a mild form that is compatible with a long life, but it usually causes early death because of the involvement of the internal organs. However, in many cases the symptoms can be alleviated. Corticosteroid drugs may be prescribed to reduce the pain and swelling in the joints. Physiotherapy may help to preserve muscle strength.

Sclerosing agent (skli rōs′ing) is any substance, such as salt, that causes sclerosis, a hardening of a tissue or a part of the body. These agents may also be used in the unusual situation in which a physician wants such sclerosis to occur. For example, when a patient repeatedly collects fluid around the outside of the lungs, a sclerosing agent may be injected into the space to prevent further recurrences.

Sclerosis (skli rō'sis) is the hardening of any body structure, often caused by inflammation and the resultant scarring of body tissue.

See also ARTERIOSCLEROSIS; MULTIPLE SCLEROSIS.

Scolex (skō'leks) is the head-like end of a tapeworm, containing small hooks or suckers, by which the worm attaches itself to the intestinal wall.

See also TAPEWORM.

Scoliosis (skō lē ō'sis) is curvature of the spine to one side; it most often occurs during childhood. Scoliosis may be caused by an alteration in the position of the underlying bones or by a reaction of the spinal muscles, both of which make the spine temporarily change position.

Treatment depends on the cause and severity. Most cases of scoliosis show no symptoms and do not require therapy. Severe cases can cause problems of chronic back pain, as well as shortness of breath due to the effects on both lungs and heart. These cases require surgery.

The best prevention of structural disorders of the spine is prompt detection of scoliosis, especially in early adolescence. If diagnosed early, measures can be taken to prevent severe deformity.

Scotoma (skə tō'mə) is a loss of part of the field of vision, often experienced as a blind spot. Causes include a lesion within the eyeball, choroiditis, or hemorrhage. Treatment depends on the cause.

See also CHOROIDITIS; EYE DISORDERS.

Scrapes and abrasions: treatment. Scrapes and abrasions are superficial injuries to the skin and mucous membranes. Although scrapes and abrasions are relatively minor injuries, like all open wounds they are painful and highly susceptible to infection. Following an abrasion or scrape, a physician should be consulted about antitetanus injections.

If dust and grit are left in the wound, scars may form on the skin. Any foreign matter should be removed before the wound has healed.

Action. Clean the abrasion with soap and water, and rinse thoroughly. Examine the victim for other injuries. If the victim has other injuries or extensive abrasions, summon medical aid. *Do not* remove any scabs that may form over the injury. They will fall off when the wound has healed. If scabs are removed before the wound has fully healed, the abrasion may begin to bleed again.

Treatment for scrapes and abrasions

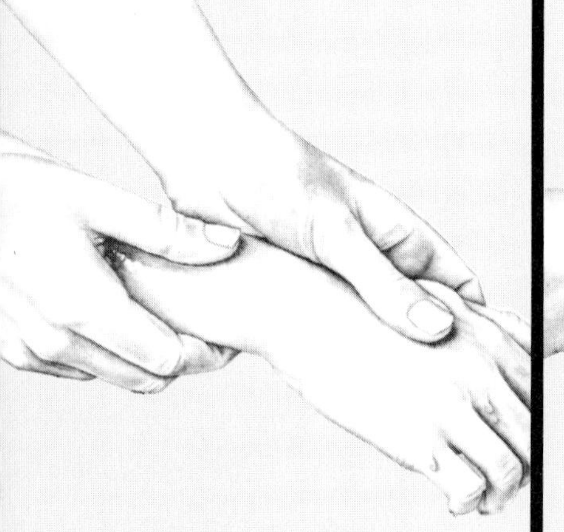

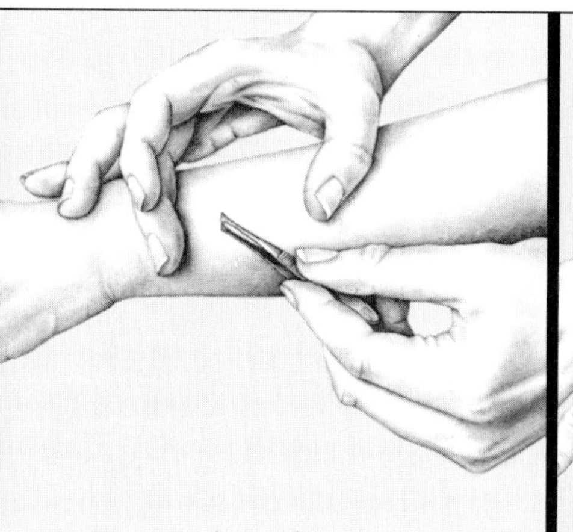

1 Wash the wound with soap and water, rinse it thoroughly, and dry the area. *Do not* cover the wound unless it is bleeding or is in a place where the victim's clothing will rub it. Minor wounds heal better if left exposed to the air. If the wound becomes inflamed and painful, or exudes pus, consult a physician.

2 Any pieces of grit lying loose in the wound can be removed with a pair of sterilized tweezers. *Do not* dig deeply into the wound. If there is a lot of grit in the wound or if the grit is too deeply embedded to be removed easily, dress and bandage the wound, and seek medical attention. *Do not* apply any lotions or ointments.

3 If the wound is bleeding, place a clean dressing over the wound. Apply firm pressure over the dressing until the bleeding stops, and then carefully remove the dressing. If the bleeding is severe, try to control it, and make sure medical aid has been summoned. For information on controlling bleeding, *see* BLEEDING: FIRST AID.

Scratch dermatitis. *See* DERMATITIS.

Scrofula (skrof'yə lə) is a term formerly used to describe tuberculosis of the lymph nodes.

See also LYMPH NODE.

Scrotum (skrō'təm) is the bag of skin that contains testicles, epididymides, and part of the spermatic cords. The skin of the scrotum contains muscles that can raise or lower the testicles, thereby keeping them at the optimum temperature for sperm production.

Any skin condition may affect the scrotum. The most common disorders are a sebaceous cyst and tinea cruris.

See also CYST, SEBACEOUS; EPIDIDYMIS; JOCK ITCH; TESTIS.

Scurvy (skėr'vē) is a deficiency that is caused by a lack of vitamin C (ascorbic acid) in a person's diet. Vitamin C is essential for the maintenance of the normal structure of the connective tissues. Vitamin C deficiency results in weakening of the blood capillaries, with subsequent bleeding, and defects of the bones.

Fresh vegetables and fruits should be eaten regularly to prevent scurvy.

Q: *What are the symptoms of scurvy?*

A: Scurvy in infants may cause irritability, fever, loss of appetite, and failure to gain weight. The infant may keep his or her limbs motionless because of pain caused by bleeding under the periosteum (the tissue layer covering the bones). The infant may also be anemic.

In adults, there may be a delay of 3 to 12 months after the onset of severe vitamin C deficiency before any symptoms appear. Initially, there may be lethargy, irritability, weight loss, and aching of the joints. As the disease develops, there may be bleeding under the skin, particularly under the nails; the gums swell and bleed; bruising may occur spontaneously; and wounds may not heal.

Q: *How is scurvy treated?*

A: Treatment involves the administration of large amounts of vitamin C until the symptoms have disappeared. In addition to a balanced diet, vitamin C supplements may also be necessary for several months after the symptoms have disappeared.

Seasickness. *See* MOTION SICKNESS; MOTION SICKNESS: TREATMENT.

Seat belt. *See* AUTOMOBILE SAFETY.

Sebaceous cyst. *See* CYST, SEBACEOUS.

Sebaceous gland (si bā'shəs gland) is one of several types of glands located in the skin. Sebaceous glands occur most commonly in association with hair follicles, as on the face and scalp and in the genital area. These glands produce sebum, a greasy secretion that conditions the skin.

See also SEBUM.

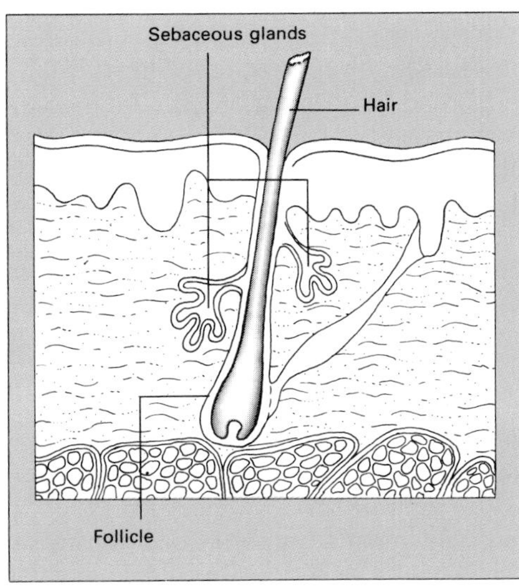

Sebaceous glands are situated in the inner layer of skin, around the hair follicles.

Seborrhea (seb ə rē'ə) is a skin disorder caused by overactivity of the sebaceous glands. It results in dandruff (scaling of the skin of the scalp), often accompanied by blepharitis (scaling and redness of the eyelids) and slight oiliness of the face. In infants, the crusting of the scalp (cradle cap) is a form of seborrhea. Seborrhea is not serious and tends to occur more in winter than in summer.

Q: *How is seborrhea treated?*

A: Various commercial shampoos, some containing selenium, are available. These should be used two or three times a week. Scalp solutions containing corticosteroid drugs may be prescribed to control the condition until there is improvement. An infant's scalp needs only regular washing with shampoo.

See also BABY CARE; BLEPHARITIS; DANDRUFF; SEBACEOUS GLAND.

Sebum (sē'bəm) is a thick, slightly oily secretion that is produced by the sebaceous glands in the skin.

See also SEBACEOUS GLAND.

Secretion (si krē′shən) is the release of any substance produced by body cells. For example, hormones are secreted into the bloodstream, and saliva is secreted into the salivary ducts.

Sedative (sed′ə tiv) is a drug used to reduce excitement or irritability. In small doses, sedatives, such as barbiturates, usually calm a patient; larger doses may produce sleep.

See also BARBITURATE; HYPNOTIC; TRANQUILIZER.

Sedimentation rate (sed ə men ta′shən), or erythrocyte sedimentation rate (ESR), is a type of blood test. It is performed by placing blood containing an anticoagulant in a long, narrow glass tube and observing the speed at which the red blood cells settle and form a sediment at the bottom.

Abnormally slow sedimentation rates occur in the presence of any serious infection, malignancy, or inflammatory disorder. The test does not diagnose any particular disorder, but indicates that one might be present.

Seizure (sē′zhər) is the sudden onset of a condition or illness. The term is, however, most commonly used to mean a convulsion or a nonconvulsive episode of epilepsy, but can also refer to the rigor (shivering attack) that may accompany the start of an acute feverish illness, such as malaria.

See also CONVULSION; EPILEPSY.

Semen (sē′mən) is the thick, creamy secretion discharged by the penis during ejaculation. It consists of sperm and the fluids secreted by the prostate gland, seminal vesicles, certain epithelial cells, and other glands.

See also PROSTATE GLAND; SEMINAL VESICLE; SPERM.

Semicircular canal (sem ē sėr′kyə lər) is one of the three fluid-filled tubes that form part of the inner ear. They are arranged at right angles to each other, one for each plane of movement. The canals are the body's major organs of balance. Disorders that affect the semicircular canals, such as labyrinthitis and Ménière's disease, usually cause vertigo and disturb the patient's balance.

See also BALANCE; LABYRINTHITIS; MÉNIÈRE'S DISEASE.

Seminal vesicle (sem′ə nəl ves′ə kəl) is either one of two glands, situated at the back of the bladder. These glandular sacs secrete a thick fluid that combines with the sperm from the testes and with other secretions to form the semen.

See also SEMEN; SPERM.

Seminiferous tubule (sem ə nif′ər əs tü′byül) is any one of the long, coiled small tubes of the testes that produce and convey semen.

See also SEMEN; TESTIS.

Seminoma (sem ə nō′mə) is the most common form of cancer of the testis. It usually occurs in males between the ages of 30 and 40.

See also CANCER.

Senescence (sə nes′əns) is the process of growing old. Although often used to refer to the later stages, when aging causes a failure of the normal functioning of the body, senescence is a normal process for all living organisms.

See also SENILITY.

Senility (sə nil′ə tē), like senescence, refers to the aging process of the body and mind. It is commonly associated with the mental deterioration associated with people of advanced age. Although many people have mental impairment in advanced age as a result of Alzheimer's disease or strokes, the majority live with no mental impairment whatsoever.

Separation anxiety (sep ə rā′shən ang zī′ə te) is a syndrome in which a child or adolescent experiences great, or excessive anxiety upon separation from his or her parents or from familiar surroundings. The anxiety may build to the point of panic or anxiety attacks. Children with this disorder feel uncomfortable away from the safety of their home. They may develop physical complaints, such as stomachaches, in order to stay at home. Such children may develop multiple fears.

School phobia is an example of a separation anxiety. This condition may reflect problems elsewhere in the family, such as parental alcoholism, depression, anxiety, or marital conflict. Psychological evaluation and therapy is usually indicated.

See also ANXIETY; PANIC; PANIC ATTACK; SCHOOL PHOBIA.

Sepsis (sep′sis) is the presence in the body or bloodstream of disease-producing microorganisms, such as bacteria or viruses. Contamination of the bloodstream (septicemia) is sometimes called blood poisoning.

Other symptoms of sepsis may include fever, chills, headache, general weakness, and possible shock. Infection may spread to other parts of the body. Treatment includes bedrest and intravenous antibiotics.

See also ABSCESS; BLOOD POISONING.

Septal defect (sep'təl) is a hole or some other defect in a septum or membranous wall dividing an organ or structure. Usually, the term refers to a birth defect in which there is a weakness or hole in the septum between the two sides of the heart. *See also* HEART DISEASE, CONGENITAL.

Septal defects of the heart may be accompanied by other congenital anomalies of the valves, which can be repaired by heart surgery. These conditions may have dramatic symptoms or may have no symptoms. The diagnosis may be suspected by a physician's examination and confirmed by cardiac catheterization. This test can be carried out even on small infants.

See also CARDIAC CATHETERIZATION.

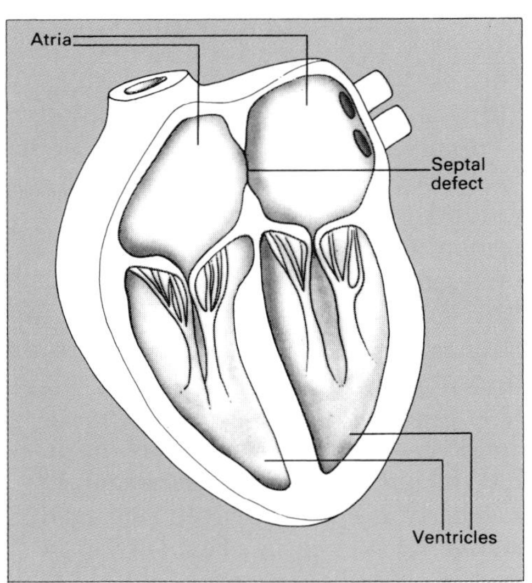

The most common type of **septal defect** is in the membranous wall separating the two atria of the heart.

Septic (sep'tik) is any condition that produces pus and is caused by sepsis.

See also SEPSIS.

Septicemia (sep tə sē'mē ə) is sepsis occurring in the blood.

See also BLOOD POISONING; SEPSIS.

Septum (sep'təm) is a thin layer of membranous tissue that forms a dividing wall between the two parts of an organ. There are septa between layers of muscle, between various parts of the brain, and between the two halves of the scrotum. Most commonly, the term refers to the division between the two halves of the heart, the atrial septum and the ventricular septum. A septum is also present between the two halves of the nose, formed partly by cartilage and partly by bone.

See also SEPTAL DEFECT; SEPTUM, DEVIATED.

Septum, deviated (sep'təm, dē'vē āt id). A deviated septum is a condition in which the partition in the nose (the septum) is displaced so that it partly blocks one or both nasal passages. Deviation is usually caused by a broken nose, but it may be congenital or occur for no obvious reason. One nostril may be smaller than the other, with symptoms of snoring, headaches, recurring nose bleeds, difficulty in breathing, mucus, and recurrent sinusitis.

When a deviated septum causes chronic or acute symptoms, a physician may recommend an operation called a submucous resection. The deformed part of the septum is removed, and the nose is packed with gauze for a few days while it heals. Otherwise, an operation called a septoplasty may be required, to rebuild the septum.

See also NOSE; SUBMUCOUS RESECTION.

Serology (si rol'ə jē) is the clinical study of blood serum and the investigation of immunity to disease.

See also IMMUNITY.

Serotonin (sir'ō tō nən), also known as 5-hydroxytryptamine (5-HT), is a chemical widely found in the animal and plant kingdoms. Most serotonin is synthesized from tryptophan in the cells of mammals. It stimulates smooth muscle contraction of the intestine; in low doses, it dilates blood vessels in skeletal muscles; and in higher doses, it constricts blood vessels.

Serotonin functions as a neurotransmitter in the brain and is present in platelets and enterochromaffin cells.

Some 5-HT antagonists are employed as drugs that are useful in the treatment of hypertension (high blood pressure), migraine, and skin allergies.

See also TRYPTOPHAN.

Serum (sir′əm) is the clear, fluid part of the blood that is left after a clot forms. Serum is similar to plasma (the total liquid part of the blood) except that serum does not contain fibrinogen, a substance that causes clotting. Serum from persons or animals that are immune to a particular disease (antiserum) can be injected into a patient to confer temporary, passive immunity.

Q: *Are there any possible dangers from the use of an antiserum?*

A: Yes. Until recently, many antisera were prepared from animals, and these often produced an allergic reaction known as serum sickness. Now, however, many antisera are prepared from humans, which greatly reduces the likelihood of serum sickness. Human serum can, of course, carry viruses, such as those that cause AIDS or hepatitis. Fortunately, routine screening of serum for those infectious agents prevents this complication from occurring.

See also SERUM SICKNESS.

Serum sickness (sir′əm) is a form of allergic reaction that may occur two to three weeks after the injection of an antiserum prepared from animal serum. Such an antiserum contains antibodies to specific diseases. Many drugs, including penicillin, occasionally produce a condition indistinguishable from serum sickness. *See also* SERUM.

Q: *What are the symptoms of serum sickness?*

A: A skin rash and intense irritation (urticaria) are usually the first signs. These are commonly accompanied by joint stiffness, swelling, and a mild fever that lasts several days. Frequently, lymph nodes enlarge, particularly near the site of the injection, causing a generalized aching.

In severe forms of serum sickness, the heart muscles may be involved (myocarditis); very rarely the kidneys are affected. Kidney involvement causes a form of nephritis, with ankle swelling and high blood pressure. Occasionally, polyneuritis occurs, and recovery from this form of the disorder is seldom complete. However, most patients with serum sickness make a rapid and complete recovery within four weeks. *See also* NEPHRITIS; POLYNEURITIS.

Q: *How is serum sickness treated?*

A: Treatment depends on the severity of the symptoms. Injections of antihistamines followed by doses of antihistamines by mouth usually control the irritation and joint stiffness. If these measures fail, corticosteroid drugs may be given to decrease the symptoms. Drug treatment is usually continued until the symptoms cease.

Sex and health. Sexuality is part of every person's life. Good health helps to maintain libido (sexual drive), and a satisfactory sex life helps keep a person's mental and physical health in good form.

Sexuality at Different Ages

When a baby reaches the age of about one year, he or she begins to explore the genitals. Once out of diapers, some babies may begin massaging the genitals and occasionally seem to reach some kind of climax. It is important that parents do not stop the child from doing this; babies usually stop handling the genitals after a few months. Only at the onset of puberty might a child start to again handle the genitals.

Parents should answer any questions the child asks on the subject during childhood. Few children are interested in more than a few details at a time. Such questions represent the child's natural need for factual knowledge, and parents should approach the subject unemotionally and informatively. A parent's answer to such questions should be direct and in simple terms that the child can easily understand.

Puberty is a time of rapid physical change when a child's sexual interest awakens. By the time the child has reached this age, subjects such as menstruation, ovulation, fertilization, and nocturnal emission of semen should have been discussed. Contraception also should have been mentioned by the age of puberty. *See also* CONTRACEPTION; MENSTRUATION; NOCTURNAL EMISSION.

A year or two before the onset of menstruation, it is normal for the vagina to produce a slight discharge. As long as the discharge causes no irritation and does not smell, it is nothing to worry about. When a girl first begins to menstruate, the periods may be irregular and occur once every two or three months before settling into a regular rhythm. *See also* MENSTRUATION.

If a boy knows about nocturnal emission he will not feel guilty and ashamed about it when it happens. There is normally a long interval between the first "wet dream" and the second. The dreams that cause nocturnal emission are usually symbolic rather than obviously sexual. *See also* NOCTURNAL EMISSION.

Masturbation is a way of releasing a build-up of sexual tension in the adolescent who does not have regular sexual intercourse. Whether an adolescent masturbates several times a night, or not at all, may depend on the individual's upbringing, temperament, or perhaps only on the way in which emotional and physical energy has been used during the day. Punishment or ridicule for masturbation may lead to long-term sexual difficulties. *See also* MASTURBATION.

Sexual drive, or libido, is at its height during a person's early twenties. However, many factors can interfere with a person's libido, such as fatigue and stress. Some women find that premenstrual tension also reduces their libido. If such disruption causes problems, the woman should discuss the situation with a physician who may prescribe medication to relieve some of the premenstrual symptoms. *See also* LIBIDO.

Other women find that the contraceptive pill can also reduce libido. The reduction may happen very gradually, but as soon as it becomes a problem this situation too should be discussed with a physician or gynecologist, who may suggest a different type of contraceptive pill or contraceptive device.

By middle age, the rhythm of sexual activity has usually settled into a pattern for the persons concerned. Although there is still a great range of variations, the immediate urgency and frequency has usually gone. Some men may find that prostate gland problems stimulate their sex drive, but reduce their performance. *See also* PROSTATE DISORDERS.

Menopause does not mean the end of a woman's sexual life. Many women find instead that once released from the burden of contraception, they can indulge in sex with renewed vigor. But without the regular stimulation of the menstrual cycle, the vagina can shrink in size and become dry. Intercourse is advantageous because it keeps the vagina moist and supple. If dryness is causing concern, a physician may recommend ointments or suppositories.

A woman's partner should be understanding and helpful during menopause. Some women find that the night sweats make sharing a double bed impossible. If sex life has not been very good before menopause, a woman may use it as an excuse to stop intercourse altogether after menopause. But a satisfactory sex life in early adulthood usually continues into old age. *See also* MENOPAUSE.

Although sexual intercourse continues for some persons until they are well into their eighties, there is usually a great reduction in frequency. However, the close physical contact of another loving person is a warm and satisfying compensation.

Sex Drive (libido) varies among different people and varies at different ages. Opportunity to indulge in sexual intercourse also affects libido. A couple who can have intercourse whenever they feel like it may experience less urgency than a couple who must take advantage of a chance the moment it is presented.

A woman's libido varies during her menstrual cycle and often reaches its height at midcycle, at the time of ovulation, and again during menstruation, possibly because the flow of menstrual blood slightly stimulates the vagina. If two persons' sexual arousal and satisfaction seem persistently incompatible, they may choose to discuss the subject with a sex counselor or a psychologist. *See also* SEX THERAPY.

The frequency of intercourse varies greatly from couple to couple. Some partners may have intercourse two or three times a day, while others may be satisfied with two or three times a month. Similarly, a practice that one couple finds natural may repel another couple. The important thing is that both partners communicate and respect each other's needs.

Health Concerns

Sexually Transmitted Disease. The most common risk associated with sexual intercourse is sexually transmitted disease. Some sexually transmitted diseases can be contracted without sexual contact, although this is uncommon.

Nonspecific urethritis (NSU) is an inflammation of the urethra by an organism other than gonorrhea. Most often this organism is chlamydia and will respond to specific antibiotic therapy. Symptoms usually appear only in the man and include a watery discharge from the penis and pain during urination. Symptoms in a woman are uncommon, but when present include burning with urination and urethral irritation. Chlamydia can cause pelvic inflammatory disease, a severe complication that can be painful and lead to sterility. *See also* URETHRITIS, NONSPECIFIC.

Gonorrhea produces symptoms similar to, but more severe than NSU. The symptoms are evident in the man and may also be present in the woman. A woman may experience pain during urination and may have a vaginal discharge. It is a serious disease if left untreated, and can lead to sterility. Treatment is usually with antibiotic drugs. The completion of treatment is strongly advised. *See also* GONORRHEA.

Trichomoniasis usually produces symptoms only in a woman. The organism that infects the vagina is most commonly, but not always, transmitted sexually. Symptoms include a smelly and irritating vaginal discharge. Men occasionally suffer from a corresponding irritation in the penis. Drug therapy is effective, if both partners are treated.

Syphilis is a potentially fatal sexually transmitted disease, although the final, most harmful stages are now rarely seen because of the availability of antibiotics. The first symptom of syphilis is a painless ulcer on the genitals, around the anus, or sometimes around the mouth. The ulcer heals in two or three weeks. About six weeks later, a fever and a generalized rash appear. A person who detects any of these symptoms should quickly seek medical help. Although syphilis is easily cured with antibiotics, it is still serious. Later, syphilis can cause disease in a variety of organs, including the heart and brain. *See also* SYPHILIS.

Candidiasis or moniliasis or thrush, is a fairly common fungal infection that can be transmitted through sexual intercourse. As an infection of the vagina, candidiasis appears when some other agent upsets the normal bacterial balance in the intestine, from where the infection spreads. It is also common in diabetics or when taking broad-spectrum antibiotics, the contraceptive pill, and during pregnancy, because of the associated hormonal changes. Symptoms include vaginal itching and a white, curd-like discharge. The infection can be controlled with fungicidal suppositories or cream. A man may get a corresponding irritation on the penis. *See also* CANDIDIASIS.

Cystitis is inflammation of the bladder. One form, so-called "honeymoon" cystitis, can be caused by sexual intercourse. Symptoms affect both men and women, although women experience symptoms much more commonly; these include a burning sensation during urination, increasing frequency of urination, and sometimes incontinence. Although the condition is uncomfortable and distressing, antibiotic treatment is generally swift and successful. *See also* CYSTITIS.

Anytime a person detects symptoms of a genitourinary disorder, it is extremely important that three rules are followed: (1) tell the partner (or partners); (2) consult a physician as soon as possible; and (3) complete a course of treatment. *See also* ACQUIRED IMMUNE DEFICIENCY SYNDROME; SEXUALLY TRANSMITTED DISEASE.

Cervical Cancer. Every female who has passed the age of puberty should have a regular Pap smear test. A physician can advise the woman how often the test should be carried out. A smear test can indicate signs of cervical cancer as early as 10 years before serious symptoms appear.

Prolonged hormone replacement therapy (HRT) during menopause is associated with a higher risk of uterine cancer. A woman going through menopause who experiences unpleasant symptoms, such as hot flashes, night sweats, and depression, may use estrogen replacement therapy. HRT should be used with care, and a gynecologist can advise whether HRT should be carried out with a withdrawal period every month or two, or whether it should be accompanied by annual or biannual examinations of cells from the uterus. *See also* CANCER; PAP SMEAR TEST.

Drugs. The drug treatment of some disorders may reduce libido. Such treatments include those for high blood pressure and hormone disorders, as well as treatments involving some tranquilizing drugs. Other drugs can have a profound effect on libido; for example, marijuana smoking over a prolonged period of time gradually reduces libido.

Social drugs, such as alcohol, reduce the many inhibitions on sexual behavior, but frequently hamper a man's ability to achieve satisfactory intercourse. *See also* DRUG ABUSE.

Obesity. A person who is overweight commonly finds libido is reduced. A loss of weight eliminates many physical difficulties during intercourse and increases the person's sex drive and stamina.

Illness. Most illnesses are accompanied by a reduction in libido. This reverses when the person returns to normal health. In most illnesses, a person's common sense is the best guide to follow as to when intercourse is safe. After a serious disorder such as a heart attack, a return to normal sexual intercourse is encouraged, but the timing should be discussed with a physician. The exertion involved in sexual intercourse is comparable to climbing two flights of stairs.

Contraception

For most women, pregnancy is a healthy and happy state. But for others, a pregnancy may be unwanted, physically unpleasant, and damaging to mental health. The consequences of such a pregnancy may be extremely serious. Yet, many people still find the subject of contraception impossible to mention to a partner until too late. Some fall back on amateurish alternatives, such as douching after intercourse or using the withdrawal method. (Douching does not work because however soon after intercourse it is done, the man's sperm, ejaculated

Methods of contraception

Oral contraceptive
Contains synthetic estrogens and progesterones that stop ovulation. A pill is taken daily for 21 days of a 28-day cycle. Virtually 100 percent reliable.

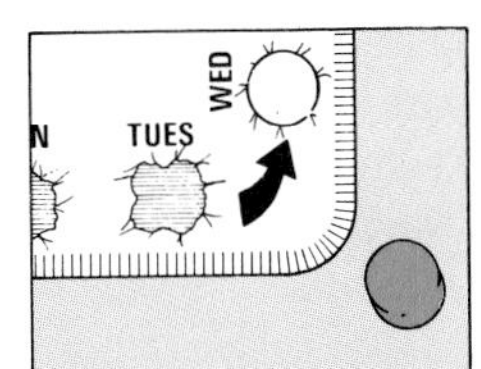

Condom
Thin rubber sheath placed over erect penis before intercourse. Reliable if used correctly with a spermicidal jelly. Helps reduce the transmission of venereal disease.

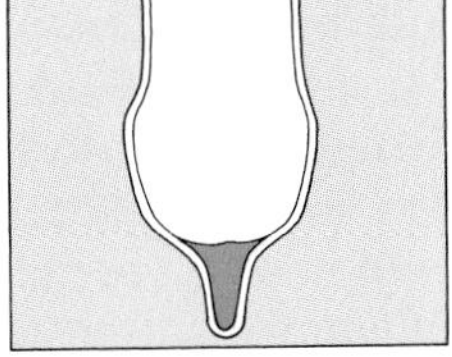

Intrauterine device (IUD)
Serious pelvic infections and infertility in many IUD users have brought about the withdrawal of most IUD's from the United States market.

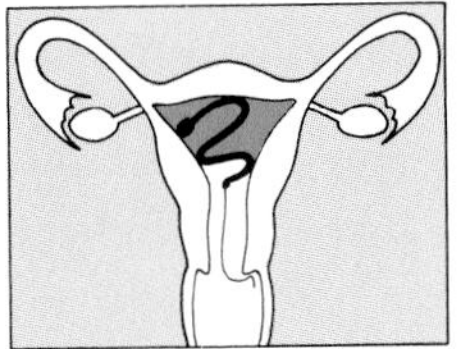

Diaphragm and chemical
Thin rubber cap filled with spermicidal jelly and inserted over the neck of the uterus before intercourse. Afterwards, left in place for eight hours. Very reliable if used correctly.

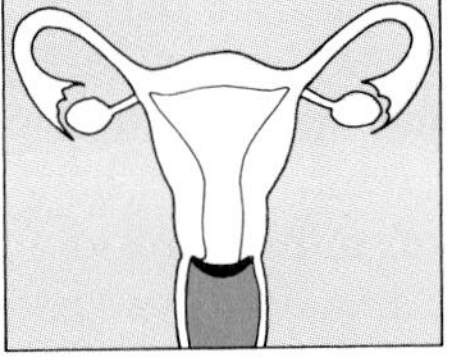

Spermicides
Jelly, cream, or foam introduced into the vagina before intercourse. Unreliable unless used in conjunction with a diaphragm or condom.

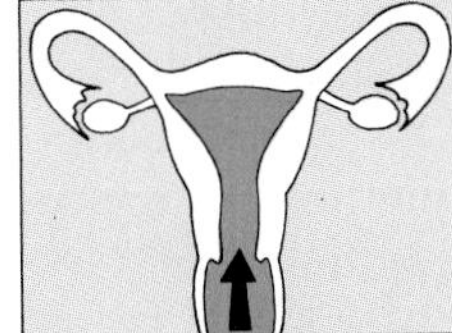

Rhythm method
Abstinence from sexual intercourse for a 10-day period in the middle of the 28-day cycle. Unreliable because monthly cycles vary.

	1	2	3	4
5	6	7	8	9
10	11	12	13	14
15	16	17	18	19

Sterilization
Vasectomy in the male, tubal ligation in the female. Tube carrying germ cells (vas deferens in the man, fallopian tube in the woman) cut surgically. Almost 100 percent effective. Should be considered permanent.

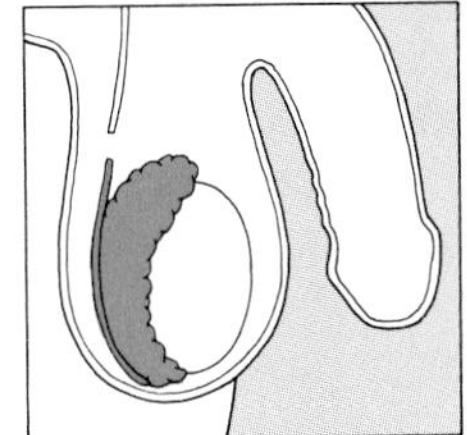

deep inside the vagina, has already entered the uterus. Not only is withdrawal emotionally unsatisfactory, but sperm can escape from the penis before ejaculation.)

Family planning clinics and personal physicians offer helpful and confidential advice about contraception. It is important to stress that despite commonly held myths, pregnancy can occur from any episode of intercourse, including the first; and pregnancy can occur no matter what position is used in intercourse. To reliably prevent pregnancy, contraception must be practiced consistently and correctly.

Unwanted pregnancies may also occur following the birth of a first baby and during menopause. A woman who has just had a baby should never assume that breast-feeding or the absence of menstruation means she is infertile. If the couple does not want another pregnancy immediately, they should arrange some form of contraception. (If the woman had been using a diaphragm before, she should have it refitted, because the shape of the vagina and cervix may change following labor.) A woman going through menopause must wait at least one year after the last menstruation until she can forego methods of contraception.

See also CONTRACEPTION.

Sex education is instruction about sex and human sexuality. Traditionally, children are supposed to receive information about sex from their mothers and fathers. Parents, however, do not always instruct their children on the subject. Youngsters are then left to learn about sex from their friends, from television or the movies, or from other sources. This often leads to incorrect information about sexual practices, birth control, prevention of the spread of venereal disease, proper hygiene, etc.

Educators and mental health professionals have long believed that sex education should be taught in schools by properly trained teachers. This would ensure all children receiving correct and complete information about sex. Opponents argue that children need moral guidance, based on religious principles, as well as knowledge about sex. They contend that only parents can provide this guidance.

Sex education programs vary greatly from one school to another. In the earliest years, children learn about sex as a part of reproduction in plants and animals. They are taught that males differ from females and that both are needed to produce offspring. At the same time, teachers try to correct any false ideas about sex that the children may have learned.

As the children approach puberty, they are taught about menstruation, nocturnal emissions, and the changes that will take place in their bodies. They also study reproduction in human beings and how the male and female reproductive systems work.

As the interest in sex increases during puberty, young adolescents are taught about the responsibilities of boy-girl relationships and dating. They should learn about birth control and venereal disease. It is extremely important that they become aware of AIDS and how it is spread. *See also* ACQUIRED IMMUNE DEFICIENCY SYNDROME.

In high school, students learn more about the social and psychological aspects of sex. Marriage and the family are discussed, along with such subjects as abortion, homosexuality, and prostitution.

Studies have shown that sex education actually causes teenagers to defer initial sexual contacts probably because they are more aware of the risk of pregnancy and sexually transmitted diseases.

While school-based sex education is extremely helpful, it is not intended to, nor does it function as, a substitute for family discussion of these subjects.

See also ABORTION; ADOLESCENCE; CONTRACEPTION; HOMOSEXUALITY; MENSTRUATION; NOCTURNAL EMISSION; REPRODUCTION, HUMAN; SEX AND HEALTH; SEXUALLY TRANSMITTED DISEASE.

Sex gland is a type of gland that produces the cells necessary for human reproduction and the various sex hormones. The male sex gland is the testis, which produces spermatozoa and the hormone, testosterone. The female sex gland is the ovary, which produces the ovum and the hormones, estrogen and progesterone.

See also REPRODUCTION, HUMAN.

Sex hormone (hor′mōn) is one of the hormones produced by the gonads: the ovaries in females and the testicles (testes) in males. The production of sex hormones is under the control of the

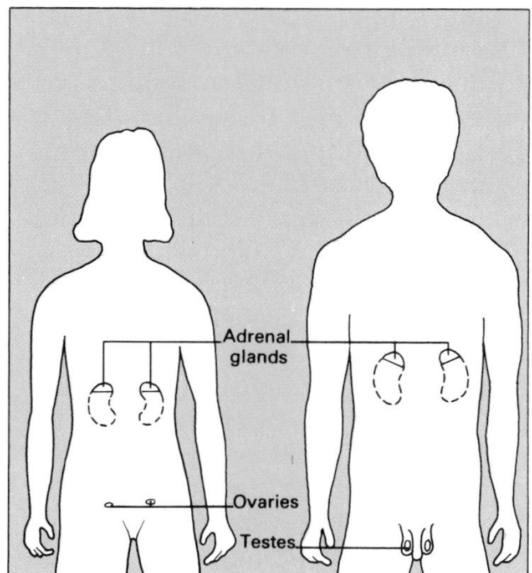

Sex hormones are produced by the ovaries in women, by the testes in men, and by adrenal glands in both sexes.

pituitary gland at the base of the brain. The main hormones produced by the ovaries are estrogens and progesterone; the testes produce testosterone. Small amounts of sex hormones are also produced by the adrenal glands.

See also ESTROGEN; HORMONE; PROGESTERONE; TESTOSTERONE.

Sex therapy is treatment of sexual problems: for example, impotence (inability of an adult male to achieve or maintain erection); frigidity (in an adult female, the inability to achieve orgasm); premature ejaculation; or low sex drive. The techniques involved include counseling, psychotherapy, behavior modification, and marital therapy. When possible, both partners usually attend therapy. There are generally good success rates in treating sexual problems by these techniques.

Legitimate sex therapy has nothing to do with surrogates or other paid sexual partners.

See also EJACULATION, PREMATURE; FRIGIDITY; SEXUAL PROBLEMS.

Sexual characteristics, primary. Primary sexual characteristics identify a baby as being male or female. The sex is denoted by the baby's reproductive organs, or genitals. In males, both the penis and the scrotum containing the testicles are on the outside. In females, the vulva and the vagina are also on the outside, but the uterus and the ovaries are inside the body. All the sex organs, except for the ovaries, are dormant until puberty, when they go through rapid and concentrated development.

See also REPRODUCTION, HUMAN; SEXUAL CHARACTERISTICS, SECONDARY.

Sexual characteristics, secondary. Secondary sexual characteristics develop in a two to six year period, called puberty, during early adolescence; the average span of puberty is four years. *See also* PUBERTY.

In females, secondary sexual characteristics include development of the breasts, widening of the hips, rapid growth of the uterus, and the appearance of hair on the underarms and around the vulva. Menstruation, a monthly discharge of blood and tissue from the vagina, also begins during puberty. *See also* MENSTRUATION.

In males, secondary sexual characteristics include rapid growth in the size of the testes and the penis; an increase in the size of the larynx, which deepens the voice and gives the familiar "Adam's apple" look to the front of the neck; and the appearance of facial, axillary (underarm), pubic, and body hair.

In both males and females, there is also increased glandular activity. The apocrine glands, located in the underarms, the anus, the genitals, and the breasts, become active at this time, giving off their characteristic odors. The sebaceous glands increase their production of sebum, an oily substance that lubricates the skin and sometimes leads to the familiar acne problems of adolescence.

Sexual intercourse, also known as coitus, is the physical act of sexual union between a man and woman. It begins with the insertion of the man's penis into the woman's vagina and the beginning of physical movements, partly voluntary and partly reflex. The act usually ends with the male orgasm and ejaculation of semen and may be accompanied by the female orgasm.

Sexually transmitted disease is a communicable disease usually transmitted via sexual intercourse or close body contact. Despite improvements in diagnosis and treatment incidence of sexually transmitted diseases, commonly referred to as venereal diseases, has risen over the last several years. Gonorrhea is probably the most common form of venereal disease, with over 200 million people worldwide estimated to be infected annually. Other sexually transmitted diseases include acquired immune deficiency syndrome (AIDS); chancroid; chlamydia; gardnerella vaginalis; granuloma inguinale; herpes genitalis; lymphogranuloma venereum; nonspecific urethritis; scabies; syphilis; trichomonas vaginalis; and venereal warts. Each of the diseases mentioned above has its own entry in this encyclopedia; refer to the individual entry for specifics on symptoms and treatment.

Q: *What should a person do who may have a sexually transmitted disease?*

A: It is imporant to consult a physician or go to a clinic. A specific diagnosis of a sexually transmitted disease may require a physical examination and samples of any penile or vaginal discharge. Blood tests to detect the presence of antibodies to syphilis may also be performed.

If the patient has a sexually transmitted disease, appropriate treatment is needed. In the case of syphilis, the patient must regularly attend a clinic, usually every two weeks at first, then once a month for six months. This is necessary to ensure that the disease has been cured and that more than one sexually transmitted disease was not contracted at the same time.

Q: *Should a patient with a sexually transmitted disease take any other precautions?*

A: Yes. It is essential to abstain from sexual intercourse until it is certain that the infection has been cured. All sexual partners of an infected person should receive medical attention.

Q: *Can a sexually transmitted disease be cured?*

A: Many forms of sexually transmitted disease can be cured with antibiotics. However, persons with herpes genitalis must wait for the condition to improve naturally. At this time, AIDS is incurable.

In order to improve the chances of successful treatment, it is essential that the patient's disease be correctly diagnosed early on. Persons who suspect that they have the symptoms of a sexually transmitted disease should consult a health professional as soon as possible.

Q: *Can sexually transmitted diseases be prevented?*

A: Complete sexual abstinence is usually the only way to completely avoid the risk of becoming infected. Proper hygiene and monogamous sexual relationships greatly diminish the chance of infection. The use of a condom may help reduce the likelihood of catching a sexually transmitted disease for both men and women.

Q: *Is it possible to immunize against a sexually transmitted disease?*

A: No. There are currently no vaccines that are effective against any form of sexually transmitted disease.

Sexual organ is any one of the bodily organs associated with reproduction. In the female, the sexual organs include the uterus, the ovaries, the vulva, and the vagina. In the male, the sexual organs are the penis and the testes.

See also REPRODUCTION, HUMAN.

Sexual problems. Healthy sexuality depends on age, vocation, culture, personal disposition, and physical and psychological attitudes towards sex. Feelings of sexuality begin in infancy and develop along with physical, social, psychological, and instinctive characteristics, all of them unique to a particular individual.

Sexual problems may arise because of a physical disorder, a psychological disturbance during growth and development, or disturbances in relationships with another person or persons. The causes are varied and complex.

Q: *What are the most common reasons for sexual problems?*

A: Most common sexual problems are not related to severe physical or psychological problems. They often arise due to difficulties in the relationship between the two people concerned. There is often failure to understand each other's needs and desires. This, combined with feelings of guilt or anxiety, can cause sexual difficulties. Often, there is conflict elsewhere in the relationship that spills over into the sexual relationship. Also, stress from outside of the relationship or

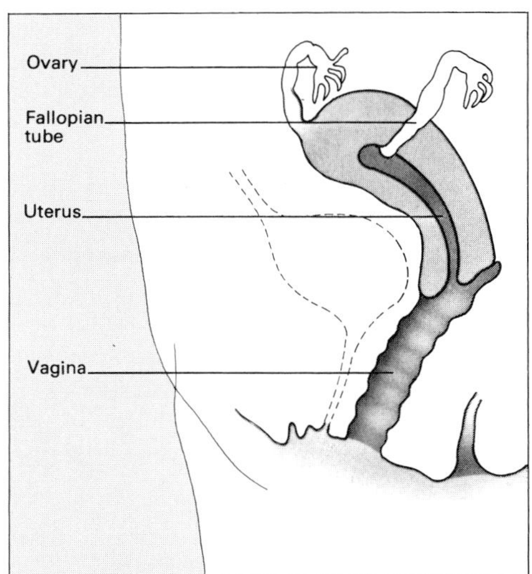

Sexual problems in women may be caused by a physical disorder such as vaginitis (inflammation of the vagina).

problems due to past sexual experiences may lead to sexual problems.

Simple lack of knowledge often is a problem, either in not understanding what is physically or psychologically normal or in being inexperienced with sexual matters.

Q: *What kind of sexual difficulties can arise from psychological problems?*

A: Impotence, although it can be caused by physical problems, is most commonly due to psychological causes. Often, the original episode of impotence results from stress, physical exhaustion, or having had too much alcohol to drink. This can then lead to anxiety that can interfere with subsequent sexual encounters, causing further failure, and so on, until failure becomes the general rule.

Premature ejaculation is a common problem. This occurs when ejaculation occurs before or almost immediately after insertion of the penis into the vagina. Commonly, this occurs due to anxiety, inexperience, or extreme arousal. This can result in the man feeling that he has failed, and the woman feeling unsatisfied and frustrated.

Vaginismus occurs when the woman's vaginal muscles go into spasm and prevent penetration by the man's penis. In contrast, frigidity occurs when the female has difficulty becoming aroused. Both of these can arise from stress, fear, or unpleasant past sexual experiences.

Q: *How are such disorders treated?*

A: The key to treating such problems often lies in removing the source of stress that is interfering. It is very important that the couple involved communicate both their worries and their needs to each other. Also, concentrating on mutual pleasure and not worrying about achieving a goal, such as orgasm, often relaxes the situation so that worries about sexual performance are eliminated. More time should be given to preintercourse love play. This is relaxing and allows more time for the degree of physical arousal necessary for a mutually satisfying sexual relationship.

Q: *What other sexual problems have a psychological basis?*

A: More uncommon problems can arise from severe emotional problems or the failure of normal sexual development. Such problems as fetishism (sexual arousal due to an inanimate object or specific parts of the body, such as the feet), sadism, and masochism are much more difficult to treat and require expert psychological counseling. *See also* MASOCHISM; SADISM.

Q: *What physical disorders cause sexual problems?*

A: Painful intercourse (dyspareunia) can be caused by many problems, including a tight hymen, vaginitis (inflammation of the vagina), or pelvic inflammatory disease. Often, dyspareunia is caused by insufficient vaginal lubrication, which may simply require longer foreplay. After menopause, lack of vaginal secretions is a common problem, and lubricants or estrogen-containing vaginal creams may help.

Painful intercourse in the man may be caused by balanitis, an infection of the penis. Impotence may arise from a variety of disorders, including diabetes mellitus and arteriosclerosis.

Alcohol, street drugs, and some prescription medications can also interfere with sexual function.

Sexual problems in men may be caused by a physical disorder, such as balanitis (inflammation of the penis).

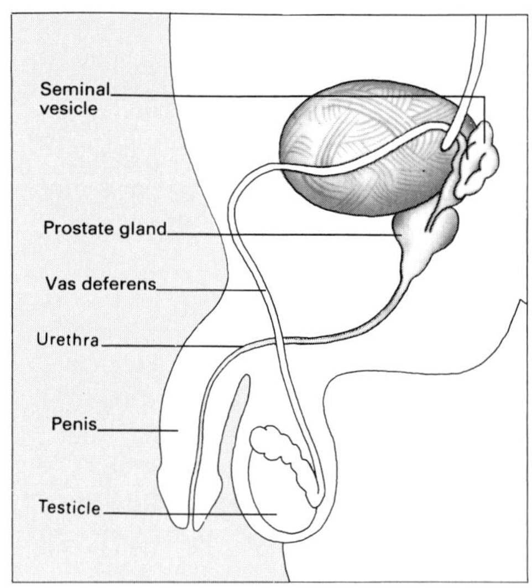

Less commonly, disorders can be present from birth, such as hypospadias, in which the urethral opening can be malpositioned on the penis, or hermaphroditism, in which a person is born with some of the sexual characteristics of both sexes.

If any physical problem, such as pain, persistently interferes with sexual relations, this may point to a serious problem, and a physician should be consulted.

Q: *Can excessive sex drive be a problem?*

A: Yes, although what is meant by excessive must be carefully explored. There is a wide range in the amount of sexual activity that is considered normal. The amount of sexual activity desired by the two people involved in a relationship may differ, but this does not necessarily mean that either partner has an excessive or underactive sex drive. Sex drive that is truly excessive, to the extent that it starts to interfere with the conduct of everyday life, can be associated with psychiatric disorders, such as nymphomania.

Q: *What sexual problems occur in adolescence?*

A: The sexual problems of adolescence usually center on sexual ignorance, fear of venereal disease, and anxiety about sexual success. Masturbation is a common form of sexual outlet that may induce fears and anxieties. Many adolescents also go through a phase when they have homosexual feelings and may fear that the feeling is going to be permanent. *See also* HOMOSEXUALITY; MASTURBATION.

Such problems can be helped by discussion with parents and by routine education about the basic biological facts of life in the classroom. A good counselor at school can often help an adolescent to resolve his or her problems, sexual or otherwise.

Q: *What sexual problems occur in the elderly?*

A: Sexual intercourse may continue into old age provided the partners are healthy. The most common problems arise after an illness or operation; the break from regular sexual intercourse may be sufficient to stop it completely. This may not be a problem to the person who has had the illness, but it may create frustration in the healthy partner.

The best way to deal with this situation is frank discussion between the partners in the hope that either sexual intercourse will be resumed or the less fit partner will realize that some form of sexual stimulation is still necessary.

If regular intercourse has been maintained, there are seldom any problems, apart from a slight dryness of the vagina after menopause. Lubricant jellies or a cream containing estrogens can be prescribed by a gynecologist.

Q: *Who is the best person to help someone with sexual problems?*

A: There are now many trained people who have knowledge of sexual problems and of ways of dealing with them. The family physician may be sympathetic and helpful, but often considers that he or she is not sufficiently trained to help with more than minor sexual problems. The physician may, therefore, recommend someone who is specially trained.

Sheehan's syndrome (shē′əns) is a condition in which there is a drop in the production of a mother's pituitary hormone as a result of shock or hemorrhage following childbirth. This is caused by thrombosis (clot) of the blood vessels supplying the pituitary gland, which causes the tissues to die. Prolactin, the milk-stimulating hormone, is not produced, and breast-feeding can not take place.

See also PITUITARY GLAND; PROLACTIN.

Shigella (shi gel'ə) is a genus of rod-shaped bacteria that are closely related to salmonella; they can cause diseases of the intestine, such as bacillary dysentery. The bacteria are spread by infected feces, contaminated food, or flies.

See also DYSENTERY; SHIGELLOSIS.

Shigellosis (shi gə lō'sis), also called bacillary dysentery, is an acute intestinal infection causing diarrhea, fever, and abdominal pain. Hospitalization and isolation are required.

Shingles (shing'gelz), known medically as herpes zoster, is an acute inflammatory infection of part of the peripheral nervous system that produces painful blisters on the skin over the sites of nerves. It is most common in adults, especially in those who are 50 or older, although it is also found in children.

Shingles occurs only in persons who have previously had chickenpox. The chickenpox virus, *varicella zoster,* can lie dormant for many years in the nerves of a patient. If the virus is reactivated, it causes shingles. A person who has never had chickenpox can catch the disease from someone with shingles.

Q: *What are the symptoms of shingles?*

A: The patient feels generally unwell, often with a headache, fever, chills, and moderate to severe pain in the area where the infection is active. After three to five days, a red rash appears, which rapidly develops into the clear blisters typical of shingles. As new blisters erupt, the old ones form pus and then scabs, which fall off between 7 and 10 days later. The blisters appear on the area supplied by the nerves and may cover any part of the body. The chest is a common site for the blisters. They usually appear more on one side of the body than on the other.

It is common for the affected area to be sensitive to touch, and the patient often suffers severe pain. As the blisters heal, the central part of the affected area may be without sensation at all.

Q: *How is shingles treated?*

A: In most cases, the infection is not severe and can be treated with painkilling drugs and a soothing lotion, such as calamine lotion. Even after the blisters resolve, there may be some persistent weakness for a few days or weeks.

Painkilling medications are often required during the acute phase. Corticosteroid medications may also be prescribed for older patients to reduce the risk of developing postherpetic neuralgia. This is a condition that is characterized by continued shooting pain along the path of the nerves, even after the acute attack of shingles is over. Treatment can be difficult, and the pain severe.

Shivering (shiv'ər ing) is an uncontrollable trembling caused by rapid, involuntary muscle contractions, which produce a large amount of heat. It may be a response to cold, emotional shock, or fear. Extremely severe shivering is known as rigor.

See also RIGOR.

Shock (shok) is a condition in which inadequate blood flow in the body's tissue results in physical failure or collapse, together with an extreme drop in blood pressure. Shock can result in unconsciousness and may be fatal. It may be caused by severe heart attack, allergic reaction, loss of blood, or infection. Shock is characterized by pallor of the skin, weak and rapid pulse, and an irregular breathing rate.

Shock has nothing to do with emotional stress, although people will often speak of being "in shock" over a stressful event.

See also SHOCK, ANAPHYLACTIC; SHOCK: TREATMENT.

Shock, anaphylactic (shok, an ə fə lak'tik). Anaphylactic shock is the sudden, severe reaction to the introduction into the body of any substance to which the body is hypersensitive. It may, for example, follow the injection of a drug or the sting of an insect. Initially, anaphylactic shock victims feel faint and become pale. The victim's breathing then becomes wheezy, his or her throat may swell inside, and the blood pressure starts to fall. The person may vomit and have no control over bowel movements. The victim may then collapse; this may be followed by death. These symptoms can occur in rapid succession.

Q: *What is the treatment for anaphylactic shock?*

A: Emergency treatment is essential, and the patient should be hospitalized as soon as possible. Treatment includes injections of epinephrine, intravenous fluids, antihistamines, corticosteroids, and oxygen. The type of aerosol medication that asthmatics use may be helpful in easing the victim's breathing until skilled help arrives.

See also ANTIHISTAMINE; CORTICOSTEROID; EPINEPHRINE.

Shock, electric. *See* ELECTRIC SHOCK: FIRST AID.

Shock, lung. *See* RESPIRATORY DISTRESS SYNDROME, ADULT.

Shock therapy. *See* ELECTROCONVULSIVE THERAPY.

Shock: treatment. A victim in shock may appear fearful, light-headed, weak, and extremely thirsty. In some cases, the victim may feel nauseous. The victim's skin appears pale and feels cold and damp. The pulse is rapid and breathing is quick and shallow or deep and irregular. It is best to treat a seriously injured person for shock even if these symptoms are not present. The treatment will help prevent a person from going into shock.

Shock often accompanies severe injuries, burns, hemorrhage, heart attack, infection, poisoning, respiratory failure, and an overdose of insulin or other substances. The severity of shock depends on the gravity of the cause and an individual's reactions to it. Reactions may vary from a feeling of weakness to collapse and subsequent death.

Action. Do not move the victim unnecessarily, especially if there is a possibility that the person has been seriously injured.

In most cases, a person in shock should be laid on his or her back with legs slightly raised. An individual in shock resulting from heart trouble should be placed in a semireclining position. If the victim is unconscious or likely to vomit, place the victim in the recovery position, if injuries permit. *See also* FAINTING: FIRST AID; UNCONSCIOUSNESS: TREATMENT.

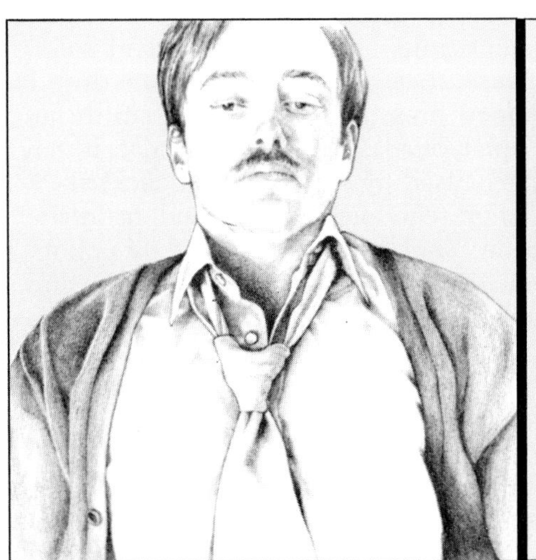

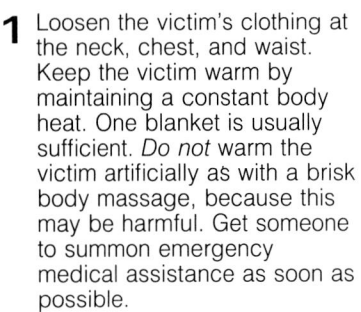

1 Loosen the victim's clothing at the neck, chest, and waist. Keep the victim warm by maintaining a constant body heat. One blanket is usually sufficient. *Do not* warm the victim artificially as with a brisk body massage, because this may be harmful. Get someone to summon emergency medical assistance as soon as possible.

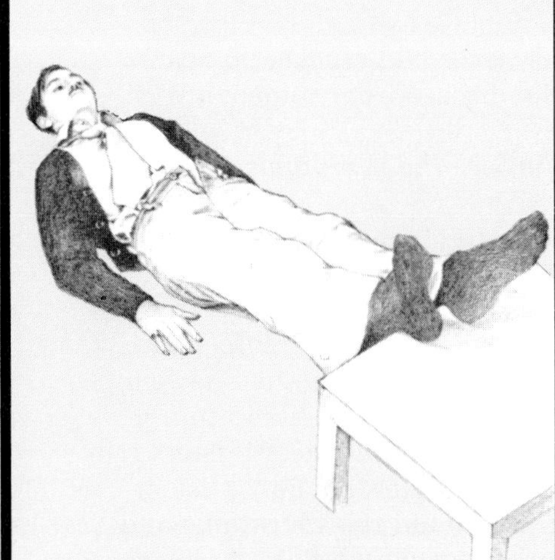

2 If the victim is conscious, lay him or her face up with the legs raised. If there is any injury to the victim's head, chest, or abdomen, the victim's shoulders should be raised slightly and supported. Turn the victim's head slightly to one side.

Do not give the victim any food or drink if there may be an injury to the head or abdomen; if the victim is unconscious, vomiting, or convulsing; or if medical help will arrive within one hour. If the victim complains of thirst, moisten the lips with water.

Do not leave the victim alone. Ask somebody else to summon emergency medical aid. Keep a close check on the victim's breathing and heartbeat at all times. If the victim has stopped breathing, give artificial respiration. If the victim's heart has stopped, apply external cardiac compression. If the shock has been caused by a burn, use appropriate treatment. *See also* ARTIFICIAL RESPIRATION; BURNS AND SCALDS: FIRST AID; HEART ATTACK: FIRST AID.

If the shock has been caused by an insulin overdose and the victim is conscious, give any food or drink that contains sugar. Artificial sweeteners will not help.

Shortness of breath. *See* BREATHLESSNESS.

Shoulder (shōl′dər) is the junction of the arm and the trunk. The ball-and-socket shoulder joint is located between the humerus (upper arm bone) and scapula (shoulder blade). It is held in place by strong ligaments and supported by the clavicle. The shoulder muscles control a wide range of movement.

Q: *What disorders can affect the shoulder?*

A: Dislocation of the shoulder joint is the most common complaint. It mainly results from weakness of the ligaments, although it is also common in certain contact sports. Repeated shoulder dislocation may need surgical treatment to tighten the ligaments.

The shoulder joint can be affected by any joint disorders, such as osteoarthritis and rheumatic conditions.

Pain in the shoulder may be the result of inflammation of the shoulder membrane, ligaments, or tendon. Pain may also be referred to the shoulder; that is, a pain that is felt in the shoulder but is really caused by a problem elsewhere in the body. This may occur with angina, pleurisy, or gall bladder disease.

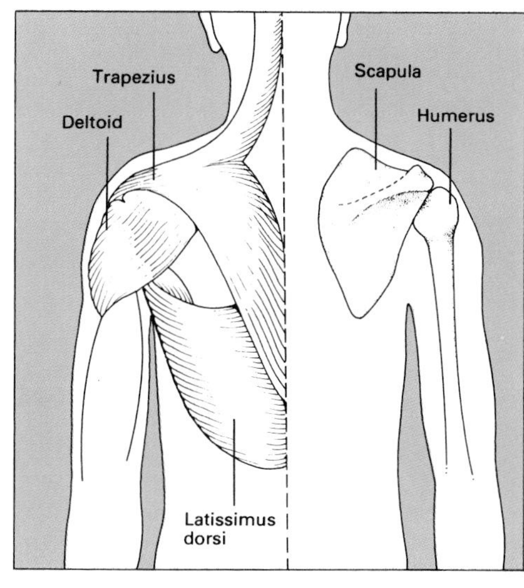

The **shoulder** joint between the humerus and the scapula is moved by three main muscles: the trapezius, the deltoid, and the latissimus dorsi.

See also ANGINA PECTORIS; GALL BLADDER; PLEURISY; SHOULDER, FROZEN.

Shoulder blade. *See* SCAPULA.

Shoulder fracture: first aid. *See* FRACTURE: FIRST AID.

Shoulder, frozen (shōl′dər, frō′zən). Frozen shoulder, or adhesive capsulitis, is characterized by pain and stiffness in the shoulder with a resulting limitation of normal shoulder movements. It is caused by inflammation of the joint capsule. This usually follows an injury or strain, although sometimes the cause may not be known. Prolonged immobilization of the shoulder joint may precede this problem.

Usually, the stiffness and pain become gradually worse over a period of weeks. The pain then disappears, but the stiffness remains, with slow improvement over the next 6 to 12 months. If the patient does not maintain some movement of the shoulder with gentle exercise, the damage can become permanent. In such cases, the frozen shoulder has extremely limited movement and is quite incapacitating.

Q: *What is the treatment for frozen shoulder?*

A: Prevention is the best treatment. An arm may have to be kept in a sling to reduce the pain, but some movement should always be maintained and a graduated exercise program should be followed to increase mobility. Injection of a corticosteroid drug into the joint may produce some improvement. When the shoulder does not improve with more conservative treatment,

Frozen shoulder is an inflammation of the shoulder joint capsule, causing stiffness in the shoulder.

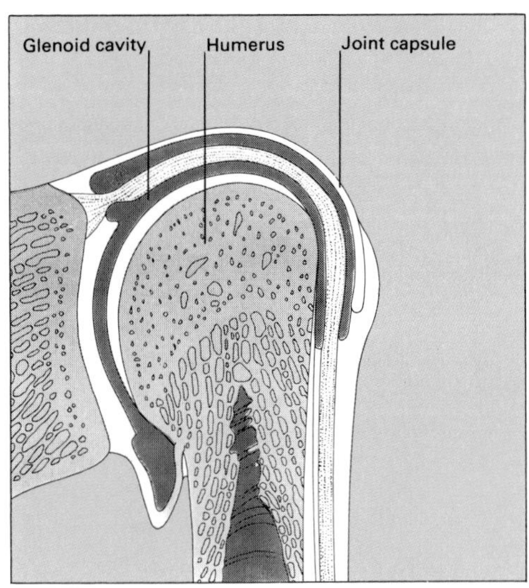

the physician may consider manipulation of the shoulder under a general anesthetic.

Shower seat. *See* NURSING THE SICK.

Shunt (shunt) is an abnormal junction between two body passages that allows the contents of one to pass to the other, by-passing the normal channel. The term usually refers to a junction between two blood vessels, such as an arteriovenous shunt operation in which an artery is connected directly to a vein, by-passing the capillary network.

See also SHUNT, PORTACAVAL.

Shunt, portacaval (shunt, por tə kā′vəl). Portacaval shunt is a surgically-produced junction between the hepatic portal vein and the inferior vena cava. It is performed in order to improve the flow of blood through the portal vein to the vena cava in disorders where blood flow through the liver is impeded, such as cirrhosis.

See also VENA CAVA.

Sialolithiasis (sī ə lō li thī′ə sis) is the presence of a stone (calculus) in the duct of a salivary gland. It prevents the escape of saliva, which accumulates in the affected gland and causes it to swell.

The stone is made of calcium salts and can usually be detected by an X ray. But in some cases, a special radiopaque dye may have to be injected into the duct to reveal the presence of the stone.

Q: *What are the symptoms of sialolithiasis?*

A: Painful swelling of one salivary gland occurs when eating. The swelling settles when the meal ends, only to begin again at the next meal.

Q: *How is sialolithiasis treated?*

A: In some cases the stone escapes spontaneously, and no treatment is required. Usually, however, a minor operation is necessary to remove the stone.

See also CALCULUS; SALIVARY GLAND.

Siamese twins (sī ə mēz′ twinz) are equally developed, identical twins (formed from a single egg) that are still joined at birth, most commonly at the hip, chest, or head. Siamese twins are known medically as conjoined twins. They are extremely rare and often difficult to deliver; a Cesarean section is usually necessary.

The likelihood of both twins surviving a surgical separation is greatest when only superficial tissues are shared.

See also TWINS.

Sickle cell anemia (sik′əl sel ə nē′mē ə) is a hereditary, chronic form of anemia characterized by the presence of abnormal, sickle-shaped red blood cells. It occurs most commonly in black people, but can also occur in Hispanics and others.

Sickle cell anemia results from a condition in which a person's red blood cells carry almost exclusively an abnormal type of hemoglobin, called Hemoglobin S. For this to occur, the person must have received a Hemoglobin S gene from each parent. If a person has received a Hemoglobin S gene from only one parent, and a normal hemoglobin gene from the other, that person is said to have *sickle trait.*

Persons with sickle trait rarely have problems and, unless tested, may be unaware that they carry the gene. A few people with sickle trait have problems at high altitudes, where there is less oxygen. The important issue for people with sickle trait is that, if two persons with sickle trait marry, there is a one in four chance of a child being born with sickle cell anemia.

In sickle cell anemia, the abnormal cells are unable to pass through the capillary blood vessels, leading to widespread thrombosis (clotting). This clotting clogs blood vessels and thereby interferes with the flow of blood, depriving the body tissues of oxygen and

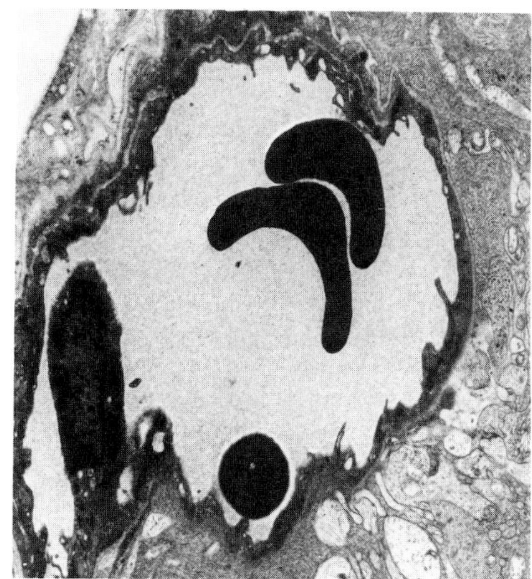

Sickle cell anemia is a hereditary form of anemia in which the normally round red blood cells become sickle-shaped.

causing a painful attack called a crisis. A sickle cell crisis may last several days.

Sickle cell anemia may injure almost all parts of the body, especially the bones, central nervous system, liver, lungs, and the spleen. Some victims suffer blindness, convulsions, paralysis, or loss of speech. Many die in childhood, and few live past the age of 40.

Q: *How is sickle cell anemia treated?*

A: Until 1970, physicians knew no way to prevent sickle cell crisis. Since then, researchers have found that several chemical compounds, including urea, carbamyl phosphate, and sodium cyanate, can reverse the sickling process. However, these drugs can have serious side effects and, under some testing procedures, have not proved as effective as researchers originally hoped. Researchers are experimenting with these and other drugs in an effort to find a safe, effective treatment. Currently, blood transfusions are usually given only when the anemia is severe enough to cause serious illness.

Q: *Can sickle cell disease be prevented?*

A: Since sickle cell anemia is an inherited disease, only the offspring of two persons with sickle cell anemia and/or sickle trait can develop the condition. Persons at high risk for being carriers (having sickle trait) may wish to be tested for the trait before having children. If they test positive, they should discuss the risks of producing a child with sickle cell anemia with their physician or genetic counselor.

See also ANEMIA; GENETIC COUNSELING.

Sick room. See NURSING THE SICK.

Siderosis (sid ə rō′sis) is a lung condition caused by the inhalation of iron particles. It is usually caused by breathing in dust or fumes containing iron.

The term siderosis also refers to any condition causing excess iron build-up in body tissue. The iron build-up is itself usually benign, but it may be associated with a disease such as thalassemia.

See also THALASSEMIA.

SIDS. *See* SUDDEN INFANT DEATH SYNDROME.

Sigmoidoscopy, flexible (sig moi dos′kō pē, flek′sə bəl). Flexible sigmoidoscopy is the examination of the rectum, the descending portion of the colon, and the sigmoid colon (the S-shaped lower part of the colon that connects the other two). It is performed using a sigmoidoscope, a lighted tube that is much more flexible than the rigid proctoscope or colonoscope and causes much less discomfort to the patient. Because of its flexibility, the sigmoidoscope allows the physician to examine a much greater area of the colon than do other instruments. Flexible sigmoidoscopes come in lengths of 14 and 24 inches (35 and 60cm).

Q: *Why is a sigmoidoscopy performed?*

A: A sigmoidoscopy may be done in a routine examination, particularly in patients over the age of 40, to exclude any local disease or cancer of the rectum and sigmoid colon, or in the investigation of tropical diseases, such as amebiasis and schistosomiasis, and in conditions such as ulcerative colitis and Crohn's disease. It is often performed to evaluate the colon if blood is found in the stool. *See also* AMEBIASIS; COLITIS, ULCERATIVE; CROHN'S DISEASE; SCHISTOSOMIASIS.

A small piece of tissue may be taken (biopsy). A sigmoidoscopy is commonly performed before a barium enema.

See also BARIUM ENEMA; COLONOSCOPY.

Silicosis (sil ə kō'sis) is a form of pneumoconiosis caused by inhaling silica, which is found in sand and many types of rocks. It is an occupational hazard of coal miners, quarry workers, and stone workers, as well as anyone who is exposed to silica dust. The fine particles of silica cause scarring within the lungs, impairing lung function and causing increasing shortness of breath. Usually, prolonged exposure (20 to 30 years) is needed before symptoms manifest themselves.

Over a period of years, a person with silicosis suffers frequent attacks of chronic bronchitis that increase the development of the chronic pulmonary disorder, emphysema. There is also an increased incidence of tuberculosis and spontaneous pneumothorax, a collection of air in the pleural cavity. Death may result from pneumonia or heart failure.

There is no cure for silicosis, but it is fairly easy to prevent if proper silica dust-control methods are adopted.

See also EMPHYSEMA; PNEUMOCONIOSIS; PNEUMOTHORAX.

Singer's nodule. *See* VOCAL CORD NODULE.

Singultus (sing gul'tus) is another name for hiccup.

See also HICCUPS.

Sinus (sī'nəs) is a cavity, usually filled with air or blood. There are many sinuses throughout the body. The term usually refers to the cavities in the bone behind the nose. These air-filled sinuses reduce the weight of the skull and act as resonant chambers for the voice. They also serve to warm inhaled air.

Sinus is also the medical term for a drainage channel formed from an abscess to the surface of the skin or to an internal organ.

See also SINUSITIS.

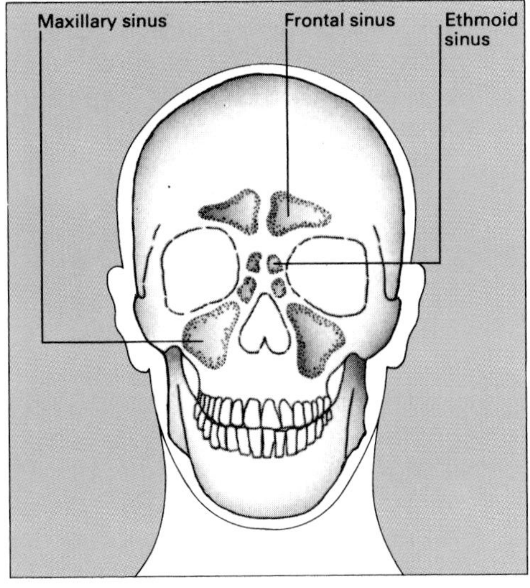

Sinus usually refers to one of the air cavities in the bones of the skull. These sinuses connect with the nasal cavity.

Sinusitis (sī nə sī'tis) is inflammation of the mucous membranes that line the sinuses of the skull (the cavities within the skull bones that open into the nose). Acute sinusitis may be caused by a nasal infection (rhinitis) in which the sinuses become blocked, by the common cold, or by any feverish respiratory illness, such as influenza. Acute sinusitis may also be caused by a dental abscess, a fracture of a bone in the face, or sudden pressure changes. Chronic sinusitis may be caused by an allergy, such as hay fever; repeated attacks of acute sinusitis; or inadequate treatment of acute sinusitis combined with nasal obstruction, as may occur with a polyp, a deviated nasal septum, or chronic dental infections. *See also* BAROTRAUMA.

Q: *What are the symptoms of sinusitis?*

A: The area over the affected sinus may be painful and tender, and there is usually a severe headache. The nose may be blocked on the affected side, causing the patient to breathe through the mouth. Thick mucus may drain from the nostril. The patient may also have a fever, chills, cough, and a sore throat.

Q: *How is sinusitis treated?*

A: Painkilling drugs, such as acetaminophen, may help to relieve the pain. Inhaled steam may help to open the sinuses and help to promote drainage of mucus that has accumulated within the affected sinus. A physician may also prescribe antibiotics and advise rest. In cases of recurrent or severe infection, sinus X rays may be used. In severe cases, surgery may be necessary to drain and wash out the infected sinus.

See also CALDWELL-LUC OPERATION.

Sinus, pilonidal (si'nəs pī lə nī'dəl). Pilonidal sinus is a common disorder that occurs most frequently in hairy young males. The affected area is a tiny opening or multiple openings in the lower back above the crack between the buttocks. Obstruction of the sinus opening by broken-off hair may result in infection and the formation of a cyst.

Q: *How is an infected pilonidal sinus treated?*

A: The infection is allowed to subside. The infected tissue often requires surgical drainage and ultimately removal of the sinus tract. This eliminates the cause of the recurrent infection in most cases.

Skeletal muscle (skel′ə təl) is muscle connected to a bone, also called striated muscle.

See also MUSCLE.

Skeleton (skel′ə tən) is the strong, flexible, bony framework that supports the body and protects the internal organs. The skeleton also provides the framework that allows for body movement. It houses bone marrow; stores elements, such as sodium, calcium, and phosphorus; and releases these elements to the blood.

An adult skeleton consists of about 206 bones, divided into 2 groups, the axial skeleton and the appendicular skeleton. Both men and women have the same average number of bones and the same basic skeletal structure. However, a man's skeleton has broader shoulders and a longer ribcage, while a woman's skeleton has a wider pelvic opening, to make childbirth easier.

Q: *How is the skeleton formed?*

A: In a developing fetus, the skeleton is composed of soft cartilage that hardens partially before birth. This skeletal development is aided by the calcium intake of the pregnant woman.

The skeleton develops rapidly during childhood and into adolescence. A baby's skeleton has about 350 bones, but many of these fuse (join) during the normal growth process, so that an adult over the age of 25 has a total of 206 bones.

In middle age, bone destruction begins to outpace bone development. This rate of bone destruction continues to increase as a person ages, sometimes leading to bone disorders, such as osteoporosis.

See also BONE DISORDERS.

Q: *What is the axial skeleton?*

A: The axial skeleton is the main supporting framework of the body. It consists of the skull, spine, and ribcage. The spine consists of 7 cervical, 12 thoracic, and 5 lumbar vertebrae. The 5 sacral vertebrae and the 4 bones of the coccyx at the base of the spine are joined together to make a solid bone at the back of the pelvis. The thorax is composed of 12 pairs of ribs, joined at the back to the thoracic vertebrae; the upper 10 pairs are joined by cartilage at the front to the breastbone (sternum). Some persons have an extra rib or an extra vertebra.

Q: *What is the appendicular skeleton?*

A: The appendicular skeleton consists of the limbs. The upper limbs are

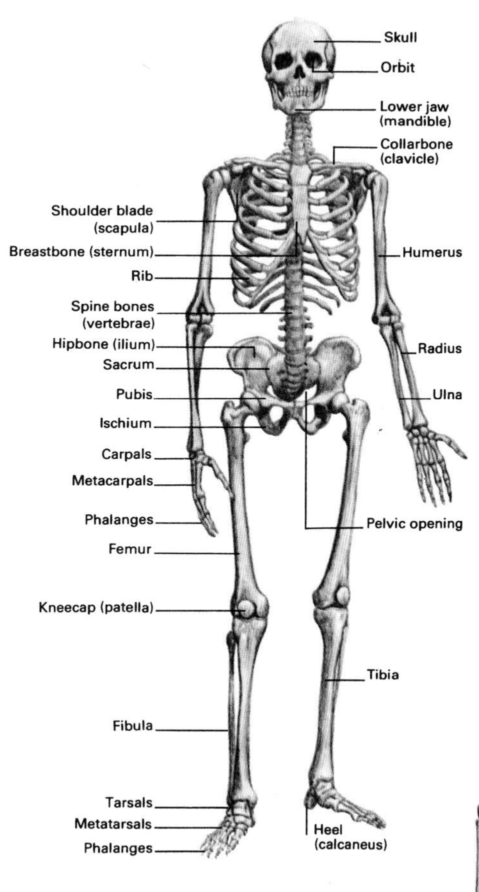

A man's skeleton, *left,* has broader shoulders, longer ribcage, and a smaller pelvic opening than that of a woman. A baby's skeleton has 350 bones, but many of these fuse to give an adult a total of 206 bones.

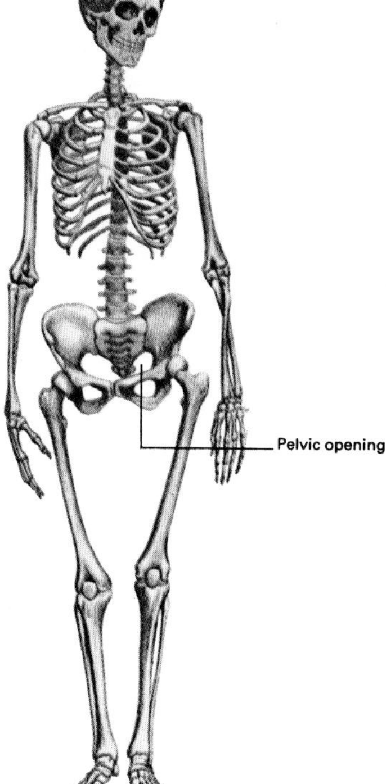

A woman's skeleton, *right,* has the same bone complement as a man's, but its wider pelvic opening assists childbirth.

composed of the shoulder girdles, each of which consists of a collarbone and a shoulder blade, as well as the bones of the arms and hands.

The lower limbs consist of the pelvis, which includes the sacrum, the coccyx, and the hipbones, and the bones of the legs and feet.

Q: *What types of bones are there in the skeleton?*

A: The skeleton is made up of four different types of bone: (1) long bones, such as the tibia and fibula in the leg, and phalanges in the fingers and toes; (2) short bones, such as the carpal in the wrist and the tarsal in the ankle; (3) flat bones, such as the ribs, scapula, and some of the bones in the skull; (4) irregular bones, such as the vertebrae (backbone) and the mandible (lower jawbone).

Q: *How does the skeleton protect the internal organs, and what are some of the other functions of the skeletal structure?*

A: The 22 skull bones form a protective vault for the brain and sockets for the eyes, ears, and organs of smell. The only skull bone that can move is the lower jaw. Teeth are embedded in this bone and in the upper jaw.

Beneath the skull is a total of 34 vertebrae, which make up the spine (backbone) and encase the spinal cord. Toward the base of the spine, 5 vertebrae are fused together to form the sacrum, with the 4 fused bones of the coccyx beneath them. The 24 curved rib bones are attached to the spine. At the front of the body, the top 10 rib pairs are attached to the breastbone (sternum). The ribcage protects the heart, lungs, and large blood vessels; it moves in and out during breathing.

Lying over the upper part of the ribcage at the back of the body are the shoulder blades (scapulae). The collarbones (clavicles) link the shoulder blades with the breastbone and give support to the

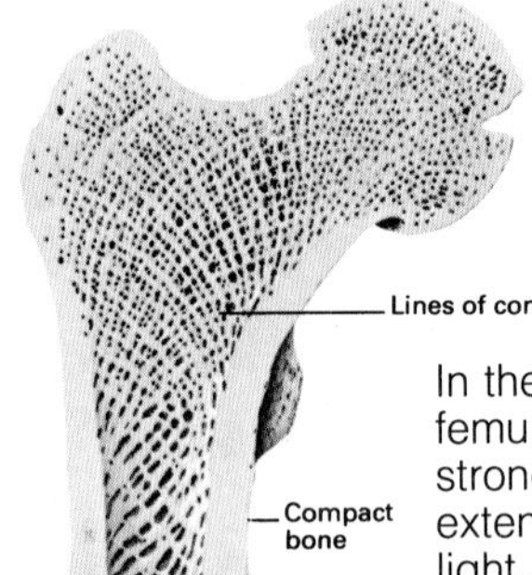

In the head of the femur, *left,* lines of strong, compact bone extend through the light, spongy bone along lines of maximum stress.

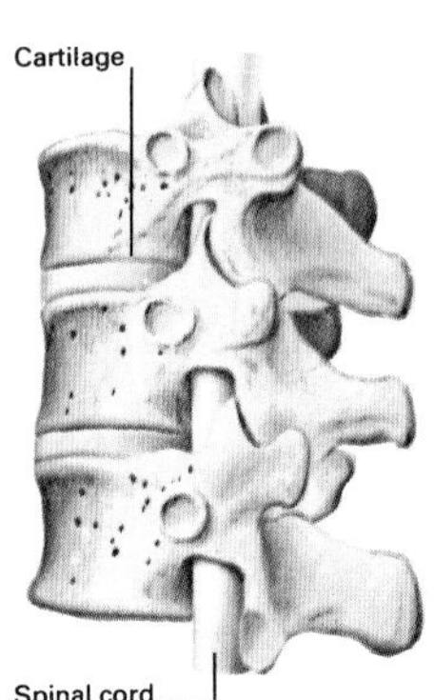

The disks of cartilage between the vertebrae, *left,* aid movement and resist compression.

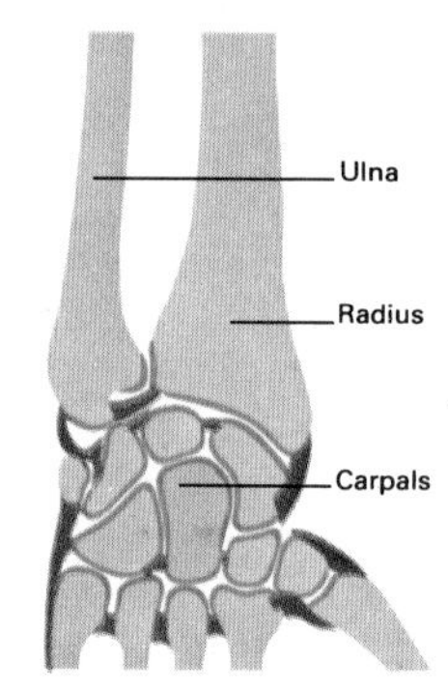

The surfaces of the carpal bones, *right,* slide over one another at the gliding joints.

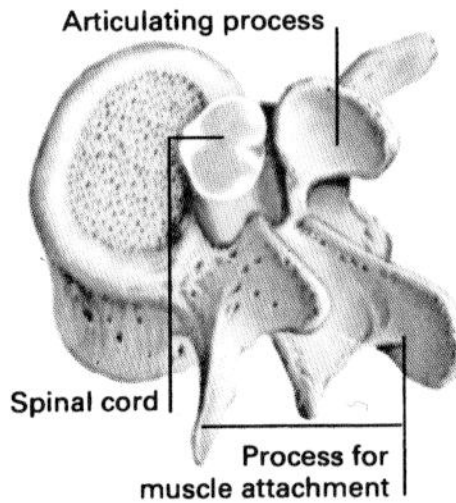

A vertebra, *left,* allows minimal movement and is shaped for muscular attachment.

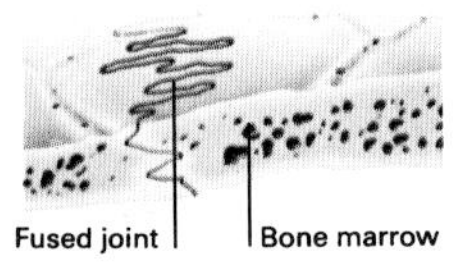

The flat bones of the skull, *left,* are connected by fused, unmovable joints.

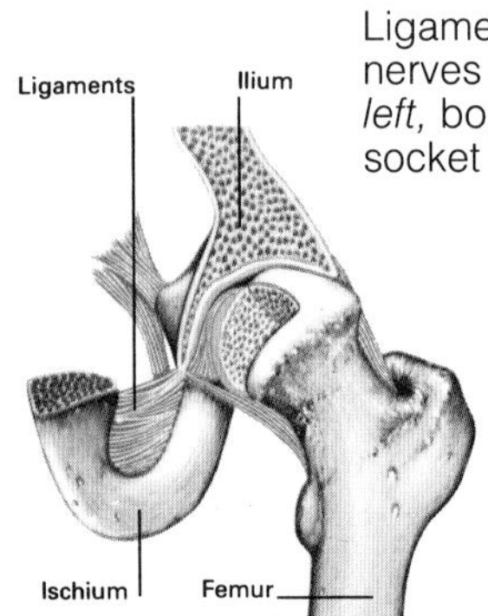

Ligaments, carrying nerves and blood vessels, *left,* bond the ball-and-socket joint of the hip.

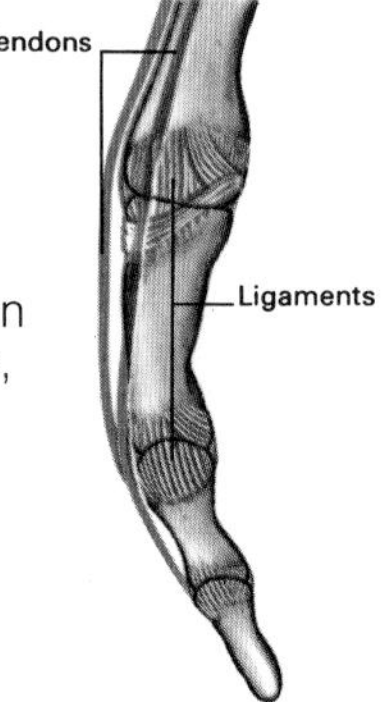

The hinge joints between the bones of the fingers, *right,* bound with ligaments, allow movement only in one plane.

shoulders. The upper arm bone (humerus) fits into a socket in the shoulder blade.

The bones of the arms and shoulder girdle are designed for dexterity. In contrast, those of the pelvic girdle and legs are constructed for weight-bearing and walking. The pelvic girdle also houses and supports the organs of the lower abdomen. It is made up of the sacrum, the coccyx, and the two hipbones. Each hipbone is composed of three fused bones: the ilium, the pubis, and the ischium. The ilia are attached to each side of the sacrum, and the two pubic bones are joined at the front of the pelvic girdle. On each side, the ischium unites the ilium with the pubis. The upper leg bone (femur) is socketed into a cavity at the junction of these three bones.

Joined to the strong upper bones of each limb are paired parallel bones—the radius and ulna in the forearm, the tibia and fibula in the lower leg. The wrist and the ankle are composed of a number of small bones, carpals in the wrist and tarsals in the ankle. The framework of the hand is made up of metacarpals; the foot is composed of metatarsals. The fingers and toes are constructed of bones called phalanges, those of the fingers being much longer than those of the toes.

Q: *How does the skeleton allow for body movement?*

A: Movements of the skeleton are made possible by the joints formed wherever two bones meet. The joints that allow most freedom of action are those at the shoulder and hip. Here a ball at the end of the limb bone fits into a socket on the girdle. At knee and elbow, hinge joints permit the limbs to bend in one direction only. The elbow also has a pivot joint enabling the arm to twist.

Other mobile joints include the ellipsoid joints between the hand's phalanges and metacarpals, which permit circular movement. The saddle joint of the thumb enables the thumb to touch each finger in turn.

Some joints are designed for only restricted motion or none at all. Disks of cartilage between the vertebrae permit only slight movement of the spine. The fused jigsaw-like joints between the skull bones eliminate all movement; their purpose is protection rather than mobility.

The detailed structure of each joint depends on the job it has to do. Wherever freedom of movement is possible, the ends of each bone are capped with cartilage to cut down friction. A freely movable joint is lubricated with liquid produced by the capsule surrounding it. A large joint, such as the knee, also has a fluid-filled cavity (bursa) to the front that acts as a shock absorber. Joint strength is enhanced by ligaments and by tendons, which are extensions of the muscles whose action makes joints move.

Skeleton, appendicular. *See* SKELETON.

Skeleton, axial. *See* SKELETON.

Skiing safety. *See* WINTER SPORTS SAFETY.

Skin is the tough, membranous tissue that covers the body. It is the largest organ in the body. The skin acts as a waterproof covering, a defense against damage and infection, a regulator of body temperature, and a sensory organ.

Specialized areas of the skin constitute particular organs. For example, the female breast is composed of about 20 modified sweat glands, and the nails are developed from a special layer of hard keratin (a tough protein substance) that grows over the outer skin at the ends of the fingers and toes.

Certain areas of the skin, such as the scalp, armpits, and pubic areas, are more thickly covered with hair than others. A finer growth of hair, called vellus hair or lanugo, covers the rest of the body, except for the soles of the feet and the palms of the hands.

Q: *What is the structure of the skin?*

A: The skin has three layers of tissue: (1) epidermis, the outermost layer; (2) dermis, the middle layer; and (3) subcutaneous tissue, the innermost layer. The most superficial portion of the skin consists of dead cells that break away continually. This happens as the underlying layer of epidermis grows outward. Pigment-producing cells (melanocytes) are in the deep layer of the epidermis. Beneath the epidermis,

The **skin** contains cells with many different functions. For example, the epidermis waterproofs and the dermis and muscle layers support tissue. In addition, hairs and sweat glands aid temperature control; fat cells insulate and store fuel; and sensory cells detect touch, temperature, pressure, and pain.

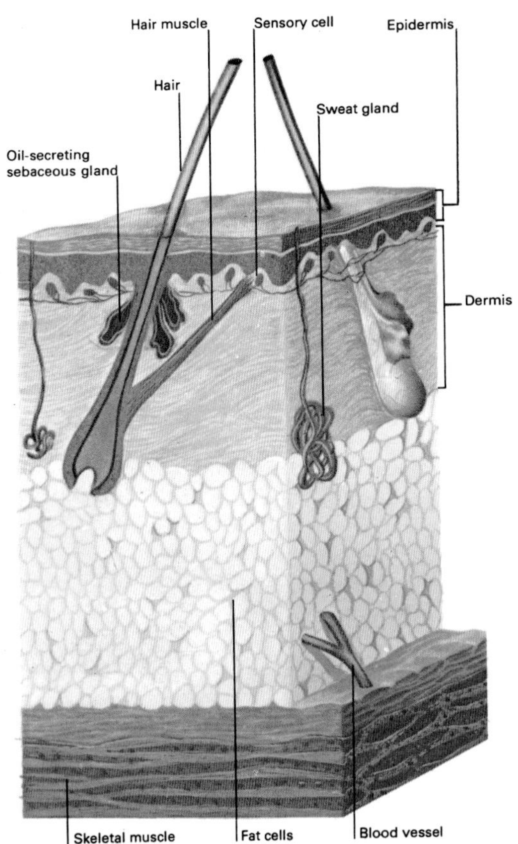

the dermis consists of supporting connective tissue, blood and lymph vessels, nerve endings, and hair follicles. Subcutaneous tissue consists mainly of connective tissue, blood vessels, and cells that store fat.

In addition to these three layers of tissue, the skin includes the hair, nails, and certain glands.

See also SKIN CARE; SKIN DISORDERS.

Skin care. The skin is the largest organ of the body. It has three main functions: (1) to protect the tissues beneath from injury, from invasion by bacteria, from drying out, and from ultraviolet light damage; (2) to inform the body of changes in environment through a network of specialized nerve sense organs; and (3) to keep the temperature of the body constant. Some areas of the body are covered with specialized skin, for example, the palms of the hands or the soles of the feet.

The skin contains specialized glands. There are three main types. (1) Eccrine glands secrete a salty sweat containing some of the body's waste products. The secretions have a mild antiseptic quality. (2) Sebaceous glands secrete sebum, an oily substance that prevents the skin from drying out. (3) Apocrine glands, which are another kind of sweat gland, develop only in hairy areas at puberty and produce a pungent odor caused by bacterial activity on the glands' secretions.

The skin is vulnerable to many different kinds of disorders, but misuse or inadequate care of the skin can encourage or aggravate problems. Skin conditions can be classified as those that (1) arise from outside invasion by microorganisms; (2) are caused by bacteria already present on the skin; and (3) are self-inflicted.

Preventing Invasion from Outside Sources. The skin can be infected by a virus or a fungus. Infections, such as pityriasis rosea, are difficult to avoid. But an adult is unlikely to suffer a second attack, and provided the skin is not broken down by scratching, the disease remits spontaneously within a few weeks, leaving a clear skin. *See also* PITYRIASIS ROSEA.

A fungal infection can be contracted easily if an area of skin is too moist. For example, fungal infections of the nail bed are common among persons who constantly have their hands submerged in water. *See also* FUNGAL INFECTION.

Attention must be paid to creases and folds in the skin, especially in hot weather. It is essential to wash and thoroughly dry creases beneath the arms, in the groin, or under the breasts each day. A light dusting of talcum powder helps to keep the area dry. If this is not done regularly, a condition known as intertrigo may develop. This produces red, inflamed areas of skin that are susceptible to fungal infections, particularly in obese persons. *See also* INTERTRIGO.

Maintaining the Bacteria Balance. The skin is covered with bacteria. Most of them are harmless, and some benefit the body in its fight against infection. However, if the balance of bacteria is altered, infection can set in. This commonly occurs following interference with the body's natural defense system. For example, vaginal douching or the use of broad-spectrum antibiotics can change the bacteria balance in the vagina and encourage candidiasis (thrush). *See also* ANTIBIOTIC; TETRACYCLINE; CANDIDIASIS.

Boils. Another example of harmful interference with the body's natural defenses often occurs during home treatment of boils. A boil is a deep infection of a hair follicle. It is frequently caused by staphylococci. Redness and swelling developing around the site of infection is the body's defense mechanism working to isolate and kill the infection. If the boil is squeezed, the staphylococci can spread to another follicle and start a crop of boils. It should be covered with a bandage and left alone. Soaking with warm water may help a boil to drain on its own. *See also* BOIL: TREATMENT.

Similarly, a sty developing on an eyelid should not be rubbed or scratched, however irritating it is. The infection can be carried to the other eye by the fingers. A physician may prescribe antibiotic treatment. *See also* STY.

Impetigo. Impetigo is caused by either a streptococcal or staphylococcal infection. Impetigo can occur as a complication of another skin disorder. It enters through abrasions caused by scratching. To prevent it occurring, a person must never scratch skin made vulnerable by an irritating skin condition. If a member of a household catches impetigo, that person's towels and clothing must be isolated and washed separately to prevent it spreading through the household. Medical treatment must be sought immediately. *See also* IMPETIGO.

How the Sun Affects the Skin. A limited amount of sun is beneficial to the skin. Acne vulgaris often improves when exposed to ultraviolet rays, and the skin manufactures vitamin D from sunlight. Overexposure, however, can lead to serious burning, and prolonged exposure reduces the skin's elasticity, resulting in premature aging of the skin. Prolonged exposure over many years may produce skin cancer.

Specialized cells in the skin produce a protective pigment, known as melanin. The pigment protects the skin's underlying tissues from ultraviolet rays and also determines the skin's color. The amount of damage done to the skin by exposure to sunlight depends on skin type and intensity and duration of exposure.

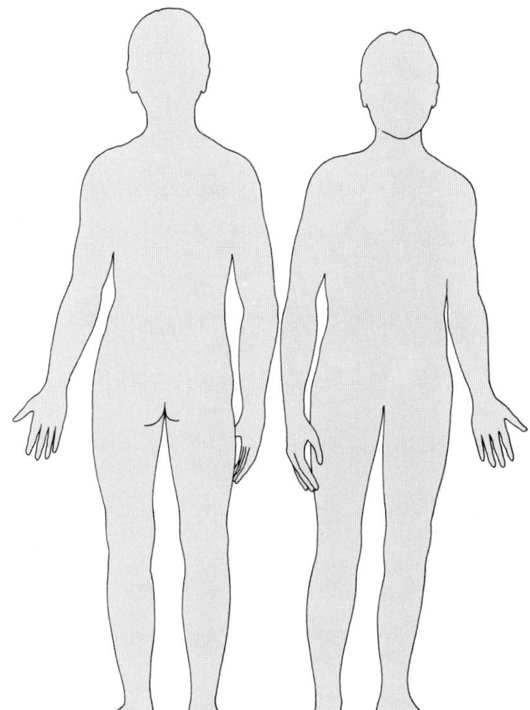

Skin care is the maintenance of the largest, and one of the most complex, organs of the body. Skin covers a total area of about 17 square feet ($1.5m^2$) in an average-sized person, and weighs about 6 pounds (2.7kg). It is very elastic, but gradually loses the ability to return to its original tension with increasing age. Some parts of the body are covered with specialized skin. For example, the palms of the hands and the soles of the feet are cornified. This type of skin contains no hair follicles and hardly any skin pigment (melanin).

Fair-skinned persons with a tendency to freckle are vulnerable to sunburn because their skin produces less melanin. Dark skin contains more pigment and is usually thicker than fair skin. At the beginning of the summer months, fair-skinned persons should limit sunbathing to a few minutes a day. The sun is at its hottest at midday; therefore, it is safer to sunbathe in the morning or evening. As the skin tans, the length of time in the sun may be increased. Each person achieves an amount of suntan that is related to genetic factors as well as to the degree of exposure. Any tanning or sun exposure can damage skin and should be minimized by the use of protective clothing and sunscreens.

Protection against the sun is essential for everyone, especially fair-skinned persons. However, even medium- to dark-skinned individuals can get sunburned. Areas such as the back of the neck are particularly vulnerable. A person who burns easily must apply sun block lotion to any exposed areas, including the tops of the ears, the backs of the hands, and the soles of the feet, before lying in the sun. If a person is walking on sand or snow in bright sunshine, sun block lotions must be applied beneath the eyebrows, under the nose and chin, and beneath the earlobes to protect the skin from reflected sunlight. Lotion must be reapplied, particularly after swimming. Sun blocks with a solar protective factor (SPF) of 15 or more are most effective. *See also* SUNBURN; SUNBURN: TREATMENT.

Dry Skin. Sebum is secreted onto the skin to prevent moisture loss from the underlying tissues. Sebum production varies from person to person, but frequent washing with soaps or detergents can dry out the skin and leave it rough and flaking. The skin on the hands is particularly susceptible to damage. Frequent use of moisturizing lotion helps to minimize dryness. Persons using any kind of chemical or soap powder must wear protective gloves. Continual use of even a mild household cleaner may suddenly produce an acute allergy. Irritation can cause itching, and scratching can open the skin to infection. Children have scanty sebum secretion and, therefore, dry, sensitive skin. Only mild soaps and shampoos should be used for children and older persons to avoid overly dry skin.

Skin Problems. The skin has an abundant blood supply. In fact, almost one-third of the blood pumped from the heart reaches the skin. If the blood supply is cut off for more than a few hours through pressure, the tissue dies. This can occur in elderly, bedridden persons, resulting in bedsores. Persons suffering from disorders such as diabetes are particularly susceptible to this kind of skin damage and must take special care.

Scab formation is a normal part of healing. A scab is formed from blood, serum, and clotting factors, such as platelets and fibrin. Scabs must never be picked at. Otherwise, the healing process is delayed, and infection may be introduced into the open wound. Scarring is more likely to occur. *See also* SCRAPES AND ABRASIONS: TREATMENT.

Diet has some influence on the condition of the skin. In extreme cases, vitamin deficiency leads to skin disorders. A deficiency of vitamin C causes scurvy.

See also SKIN; SKIN DISORDERS.

Skin disorders. As the largest organ in the body, the skin is susceptible to a variety of disorders, with a wide range of symptoms and severity. This article concerns minor skin disorders, such as dry skin. For a discussion of other skin disorders, refer to separate articles listed under the name of the disorder.

The majority of minor skin disorders are the result of various forms of lesions, dry or moist skin, or skin that itches. A combination of these symptoms is quite common.

Dry skin is helped by increasing the room humidity using a room or central humidifier. Showers or baths should be short and infrequent using water that is not too hot. Itching is particularly distressing; clothes made from artificial fibers often aggravate the complaint. In many instances itching is made worse or is brought on by too frequent bathing. Antihistamine drugs are moderately effective, and a change to natural fibers can help.

Both corticosteroid and antibiotic creams and local anesthetics should be used with caution and only on medical advice, because they have side effects and they can be dangerous if used for the wrong condition. Corticosteroids prevent the normal biological reaction to infection, thus an infection may spread. Antibiotics should be used only if the condition is a bacterial infection; used for any length of time, they can cause skin sensitivity.

See also SKIN; SKIN CARE.

Skin graft is a procedure in which layers of skin are transferred surgically, either from one part of a patient's body to another part or from one person to another. Skin grafts are of two main types: (1) a full-thickness graft, usually employed for only small areas of skin; and (2) a Thiersch's, or split-skin, graft, a thinner layer of skin taken from a healthy part of the patient's body.

For a full-thickness graft, surgeons leave one end of a flap of skin attached to the donor (healthy) area, and the free end attached to the area to be grafted. This allows the blood supply to continue while the graft and its blood supply is becoming established. When the graft has taken, the end still attached to the donor area may be removed and stitched to the recipient area. This is known as a pedicle graft.

In patients with severe burns, it may not be possible to take sufficient skin from donor areas of the patient's body. Temporary grafting, using skin from a cadaver or even that of a pig, can give protection while the patient recovers from the burn.

See also GRAFT.

Skull. *See* CRANIUM.

Sleep is a period during which a person rests body and mind. Sleep restores energy to the body, particularly to the brain and nervous system. Most adults sleep from seven to eight-and-one-half hours every night. Persons who go without their normal amount of sleep lack concentration and become quick-tempered. Extreme sleep deprivation (two days or more without sleep) can result in hallucinations.

A person's sleeping patterns develop gradually. Newborn babies sleep for periods throughout the day and night. By the age of two or three months, many babies have learned to sleep through the night, though they nap for periods during the day. By the age of four, most children have given up daytime naps. Four-year-olds average from 10 to 14 hours of sleep a night and ten-year-olds average from 9 to 12 hours.

Most adults need slightly less sleep as they grow older. A person who slept 8 hours a night at 30 years of age may need only 7 hours of sleep at age 60.

Normal sleep consists of two types. The first is known as slow-wave sleep, because during it there is reduced electrical activity in the brain. It is also known as non-REM (rapid eye movement) sleep, because the eyes do not move rapidly during this phase. During slow-wave sleep, there is a decrease in the basal metabolic rate, blood pressure, and respiratory rate so that the person is relaxed.

The second type of sleep is known as paradoxical or REM sleep, because of the rapid eye movements that take place behind the closed eyelids. Also during this phase, dreaming takes place and the heartbeat and respiration become irregular, but there is no limb movement. An electroencephalogram shows electrical brain activity similar to that which occurs when a person is awake.

There is a period of normal wakefulness as a person falls asleep, followed by a state of relaxation that becomes light sleep, before the body enters the phase of slow-wave (non-REM) sleep. Slow-wave sleep initially lasts about two hours before the first episode of REM sleep begins. Sleep then alternates between periods of non-REM sleep and REM sleep; the latter periods last 10 to 20 minutes and occur every hour-and-a-half until the person awakes.

REM sleep is now known to be essential, because waking a person repeatedly at the beginning of each period of REM sleep produces depression, anxiety, and fatigue out of proportion to the amount of sleep that has been lost. Dreaming is a necessary part of normal sleep and is also probably necessary for the well-being of the mind. Everyone dreams, even if he or she can not remember the dreams on waking.

See also DREAM; INSOMNIA; SLEEP DISORDERS.

Sleep apnea (ap nē′ə) is a temporary suspension of breathing during sleep, sometimes occurring periodically. Sleep apnea is caused by a variety of problems, including severe obesity.

In some cases, surgery may be necessary to correct an airway obstruction that is causing the apneic spells. In severe cases of obstructive sleep apnea, the patient may need to have a tracheostomy to be able to breathe while sleeping.

See also TRACHEOSTOMY.

Sleep disorders. Insomnia (difficulty falling or staying asleep) is the most common sleep problem and one that causes great distress. But other sleep problems commonly occur, particularly in children. *See also* INSOMNIA.

Q: *What sleep problems occur in children?*

A: Sleep problems may be associated with behavior problems in children. For example, a child may refuse to settle down at night and may constantly get up or make excuses about some minor discomfort. Such a child is often worried about something and needs a set ritual, without overexcitement, at bedtime.

Another problem is the young child, usually between the age three and five, who wakes in the early hours of the morning. A solution that can be tried by the parents is to stop afternoon naps and

Sleep disorders may occur if the depth of sleep and pattern of rapid eye movement (REM) are disturbed.

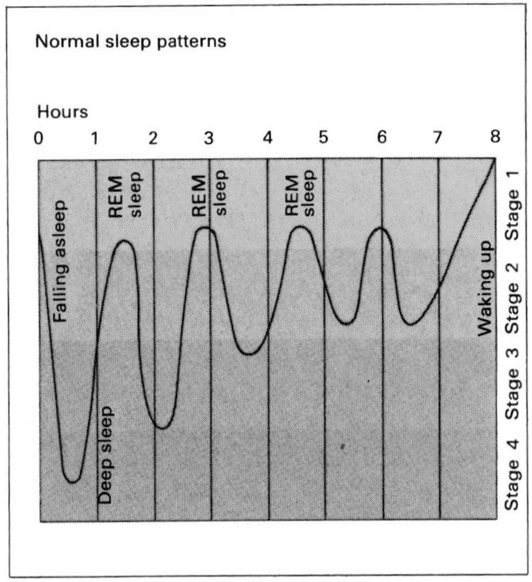

put the child to bed later in the evening.

Sleepwalking and sleeptalking are two conditions that are common in childhood and tend to improve with the approach of puberty. They do not usually reflect psychological difficulties. In addition, nightmares and night terrors can be quite disturbing, but tend to improve with time. *See also* NIGHTMARE; NIGHT TERROR; SLEEPTALKING; SLEEPWALKING.

Q: *Can excessive amounts of sleep be a serious symptom?*

A: Hypersomnia, as it is sometimes called, may develop after serious illnesses during the convalescent period. It may also be a result of anemia or depression and sometimes occurs in adolescence as normal behavior. Daytime sleepiness can, however, be a symptom of narcolepsy, in which the person suddenly falls asleep for 10 to 15 minutes (sleep attacks). Many narcoleptics also experience episodes of muscular weakness (cataplexy) lasting for only seconds while remaining awake. Cataplexy ranges from mild weakness to full paralysis. *See also* NARCOLEPSY.

Daytime sleepiness may also be the result of sleep apnea, which can be a potentially serious medical problem. Individuals with sleep apnea suffer from recurrent episodes of apnea (cessation of breathing lasting 10 seconds or longer) during a night's sleep. They tend to snore loudly and have restless sleep. *See also* SLEEP APNEA.

Q: *How can sleep problems be treated?*

A: A full understanding of how the sleep disorder occurs is most important to the physician, although diagnostic tests may be of help. An evaluation in a sleep laboratory may be needed for more complicated sleep problems.

Difficulty falling or staying asleep may reflect anxiety, stress, or simply a bad habit. Relaxation training may be helpful. Counseling may be indicated if there is significant stress or psychological conflict. Consistently waking up early in the morning and daytime sleepiness are often symptoms of depression, which should be treated. Narcolepsy does not have a full cure, but small doses of amphetamines may be helpful for the hypersomniac. Sleep apnea requires medical attention, sometimes surgery. In some cases of insomnia, a short trial of sleep medication may be beneficial.

Problems may be caused by the repeated or chronic use of sedative and hypnotic drugs in the treatment of insomnia, especially since these medications can also be addictive. Although it is not known exactly how these drugs work, it seems that there is a reduction in the length and number of periods of REM sleep under their influence. This can cause mild depression for reasons that are not fully understood. When the drugs are stopped, sleep may be disturbed for 10 to 14 days. REM sleep increases, and the person feels that the insomnia is worse than before. After about two weeks, natural sleep patterns return.

Another problem with sleep-inducing drugs is the slight daytime sedation that may occur, which reduces a person's reaction time. This is particularly relevant when driving an automobile, using machinery or, most important of all, taking alcohol. Alcohol in combination with barbiturates, for example, is dangerous and can be fatal. This is especially important since it is not unusual for individuals with insomnia to use alcohol to fall asleep. Eventually, alcohol actually disrupts sleep patterns, leading to poor quality of sleep. It may also lead to alcohol dependency.

See also SLEEP.

Sleeping sickness, or African trypanosomiasis, is a disorder caused by protozoans called trypanosomes. The disease is common in tropical and subtropical regions of Africa and causes fever, inflammation of the brain, sleepiness, weariness, and usually death. The protozoans are carried by the tsetse fly and enter the blood of a human through the bite of an infected fly. Therapy is available for the disease if it is diagnosed at an early stage of the disorder, before the brain is affected.

Sleeplessness. See INSOMNIA; SLEEP DISORDERS.

Sleeptalking is a common occurrence in children. It may consist of no more than a few grunts or an occasional word, or it may be a whole sentence. It is even possible to hold a brief conversation with a sleeptalker. Sleeptalking is probably the result of a vivid dream or a nightmare.

Sleep terror disorder. *See* NIGHT TERROR.

Sleep, twilight. Twilight sleep is a condition of impaired consciousness that is produced by a combination of painkilling drugs and inhaled anesthetic gases. This used to be utilized during childbirth, but it has been replaced by better methods of pain control.

See also PREGNANCY AND CHILDBIRTH.

Sleepwalking, or somnambulism, is most common between the ages of 4 and 14 and more frequent in boys than girls. It seldom lasts for more than about one-half-hour and is more likely to occur when the person is sleeping in a strange room.

The individual may appear normal and can perform complex movements, such as opening and shutting doors and walking down stairs. The eyes may be closed or open and may appear to be looking at something.

The sleepwalker may grunt or speak, but returns to bed with no memory of the episode in the morning.

Q: *Is it dangerous to wake someone who is sleepwalking?*

A: No. However, it is better not to try because the sleepwalker may be frightened upon waking. It is best to attempt to lead the sleepwalker back to bed.

Q: *Why does sleepwalking occur?*

A: The cause is not known. It is associated with the dreaming stage of sleep or with underlying fears and anxieties.

Slimming. *See* WEIGHT PROBLEM.

Slipped disk. *See* DISK, HERNIATED.

Slow virus. *See* VIRUS, SLOW.

Small intestine. *See* INTESTINE, SMALL.

Smallpox (smôl′poks), a highly contagious viral infection, was the first disease eradicated via vaccination. The last known cases of naturally-occurring smallpox were isolated in 1977; in 1980, the World Health Organization (WHO), an agency of the United Nations, announced that smallpox had been eliminated.

Throughout history, smallpox had killed hundreds of millions of people and scarred and blinded millions more.

Smallpox was caused by a virus that spread from person to person through the air. A smallpox victim expelled droplets containing the virus from the nose and mouth. Another person inhaled the droplets and became infected. In most cases, symptoms appeared in the new victim 10 to 12 days later. The person developed aches and a high fever. Two to four days later, a rash appeared on the face and spread to other parts of the body. The rash resembled thousands of small pimples. During the next week, the pimples became larger and filled with pus. Scabs formed over the pimples and fell off three or four weeks later, leaving scars.

There was no treatment for smallpox, of which the most serious form killed about 20 percent of its victims. Those who survived were permanently scarred, and many were blind. Survivors were immune after one attack.

Smallpox was once so common that almost everyone had it at some time. During the Middle Ages, smallpox epidemics frequently swept across Asia, Africa, and Europe. In some wars, more soldiers died from smallpox than in combat. Europeans brought the disease to America, and millions of Indians died as a result of it.

In 1796, Edward Jenner, an English physician, developed the first vaccine—one that prevented smallpox. Its use quickly spread to other parts of the world. During the 1800's, many countries passed laws requiring vaccination. But the disease continued to exist almost everywhere until the 1940's, when it was eliminated in Europe and North America. For many years, most children in the United States were vaccinated as infants and then revaccinated about every five years. In 1971, United States government health officials ended routine vaccinations except for persons traveling to or from countries where smallpox still existed.

In 1967, the WHO began a program to eradicate smallpox. At that time, the disease infected more than 30 countries in Africa, Asia, and South America. Over 700 physicians, nurses, scientists, and other personnel from WHO joined about 200,000 health workers in the infected countries to fight the disease. They formed vaccination teams that traveled from village to village and searched from home to home for smallpox cases. The victims were isolated, and everyone who had been in contact with them was vaccinated.

See also VACCINATION.

Smear (smir) is a small amount of body tissue or other substance spread on a slide for microscopic examination.

See also PAP SMEAR TEST.

Smegma (smeg′mə) is a thick, greasy secretion produced by the sebaceous glands under the foreskin of the penis. If the end of the penis is not kept clean, smegma is thought to be a factor in causing cancer of the penis in uncircumcised males.

See also CIRCUMCISION.

Smell, sense of. Sense of smell is the ability to detect odors. The organ of smell consists of a group of sensitive cells situated in the upper part of the nasal cavity, which is connected to the brain by the olfactory nerve. The sense of smell is not well developed in humans. It is limited to the sensation of seven basic odors and their combinations. It is, however, an important contributory factor to the sense of taste. Like the sense of taste, it becomes less acute as a person becomes older.

Inflammation or blockage of the nasal passages, as with a common cold, dulls the sense of smell. The sense is also less acute in persons who smoke. A skull fracture can destroy the sense of smell completely (anosmia).

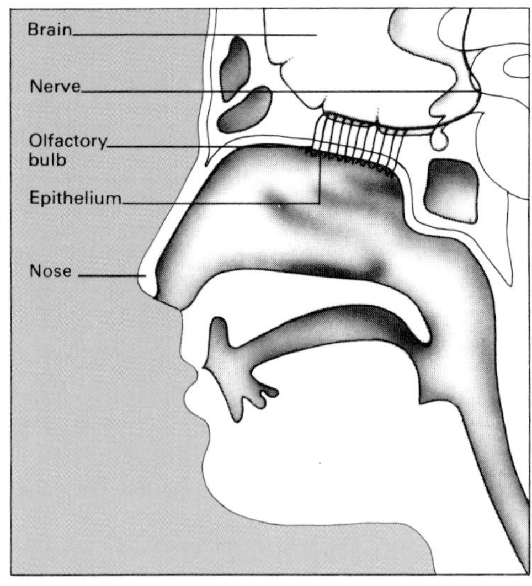

Smell stimuli enter the nose and pass through the olfactory bulb up to the brain.

See also ANOSMIA; TASTE.

Smoke inhalation: first aid. The inhaling of smoke can result in serious lung damage, caused by excessive amounts of toxic by-products from the burning of fuels. Smoke sometimes contains finely divided solid particles suspended in the air or noxious fumes, which can injure the lungs.

Excessive breathing of smoke may lead to inflammation of the lungs, asphyxiation, physical trauma, or pulmonary edema (the build-up of fluid in the lungs). Smoke inhalation is especially dangerous for persons suffering from chronic respiratory or cardiac disease.

Treatment. It is imperative to immediately remove the victim from the smoke-filled area. If not too much smoke has been inhaled, long, deep breaths of fresh air are sufficient to stop any coughing and clear the lungs.

If there is continued coughing or even choking, breathlessness, singed nasal hairs, irritation, pain, or raspy sounds while breathing, then a physician should be consulted as soon as possible. For severe cases of smoke inhalation, hospitalization may be required in order to administer humidified oxygen, intravenous fluids, or bronchial dilators (drugs that widen the airway to the lungs). Observation in the hospital may continue up to 2 days, since pulmonary edema sometimes develops 48 hours after smoke inhalation.

Smoking of marijuana. *See* MARIJUANA.

Smoking of tobacco, in cigarettes, cigars, or a pipe, is a habit that meets many of the criteria that define an addiction. For some smokers, it provides a relief from anxiety and tension; but for others, it becomes a physical and psychological burden. Cigar and pipe smoking, although they present some hazards to health, are thought to be less dangerous to health than cigarette smoking.

Cigarette smoking damages the lungs, blood vessels, and, to a lesser extent, other organs, such as the heart.

Cancer of the lung is a serious health hazard; the peak of its incidence in men occurs in the 55 to 65 age group (when 1 in 7 deaths results from lung cancer). Approximately 2 out of every 5 heavy smokers die before the age of 65. In women who smoke, the highest mortality rate occurs 10 years earlier than in men, and 1 death in 3 caused by lung cancer will be that of a woman. *See also* CANCER.

People who smoke not only damage their own health, but also harm others. For instance, a pregnant woman who smokes harms her unborn child; children exposed to smoke have more respiratory illnesses; a person who suffers from heart disease may be adversely affected by other persons' smoke; and people who live or work in smoky environments have an increased risk of developing respiratory ailments. In the last several years, many governmental agencies and private companies have instituted policies that limit or ban smoking in public areas.

Although the sale of cigarettes to persons below the age of 18 is not allowed in the United States and other countries, tobacco remains one of the most easily obtained addictive drugs.

Q: *What are the harmful substances in tobacco and what do they do?*

A: There are four main groups of dangerous substances in tobacco smoke. Nicotine is the substance that causes addiction. It stimulates the release of epinephrine and other substances in the body that cause an increase in pulse rate, a rise in blood pressure, and a narrowing of the blood vessels in the skin. Epinephrine also causes an increase in fatty substances in the blood and makes blood platelets (factors in blood clotting) stickier and therefore more likely to form blood clots.

Carbon monoxide is a poisonous gas produced by the incomplete burning of tobacco. In the lungs, it combines with hemoglobin in the

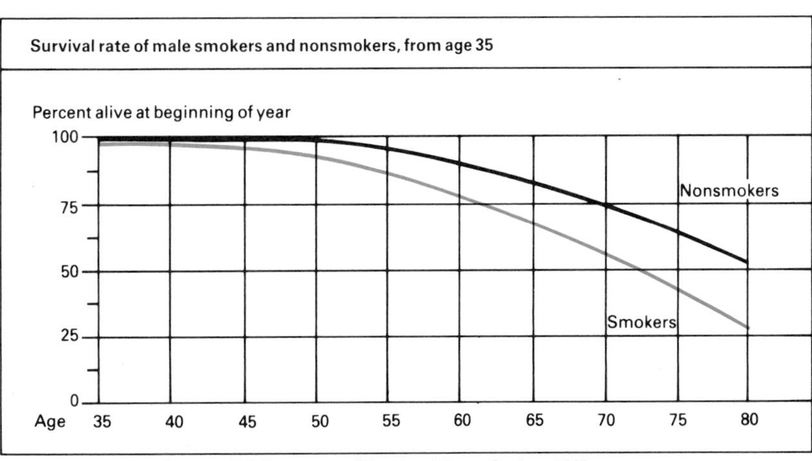

From Smoking Tobacco & Health: U.S. Department of Health and Human Services, 1987

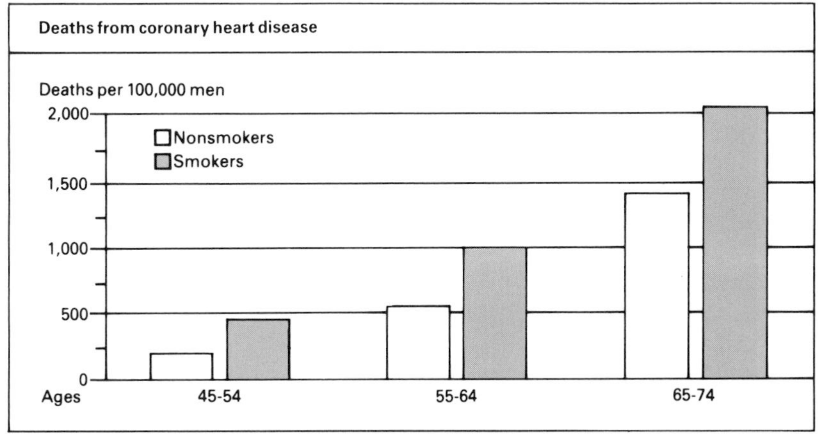

From Smoking Tobacco & Health: U.S. Department of Health and Human Services, 1987

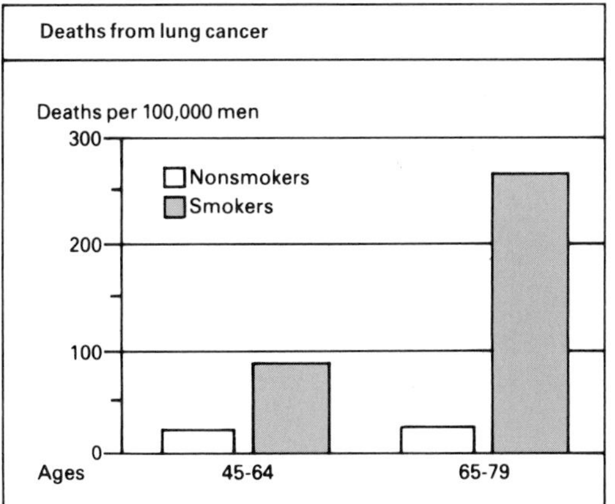

From Smoking Tobacco & Health: U.S. Department of Health and Human Services, 1987

About 2 out of every 5 heavy smokers die before the age of 65. However, if a person stops the **smoking of tobacco,** the likelihood of disease diminishes.

blood and thus prevents the hemoglobin from carrying its full quota of oxygen throughout the circulation. It reduces a person's physical fitness and also acts as a poison.

Various substances in tobacco irritate the lining of the bronchi, inducing spasm and increasing bronchial secretions. At the same time, these irritants damage cells that usually sweep the secretions out of the lungs. This increases the likelihood of developing bronchitis.

Cancer-producing substances are present in the tar in cigarette smoke.

Q: *Is there any way of reducing the dangers of cigarette smoking?*

A: Yes. Obviously, the best way of avoiding the dangers of cigarette smoking is to give up the habit. If this seems impossible, the smoker can use brands with low nicotine and tar content. Cigarettes, preferably with filters, should be smoked to a long and not a short stub. The greatest concentration of tar and other irritants is in the stub of the cigarette. Removing the cigarette from the mouth between puffs helps to reduce the amount of smoke that is inhaled.

Q: *What effect does smoking during pregnancy have on the fetus?*

A: Babies born to mothers who smoke are 5-13 ounces (140-364g) lighter on average than those born to mothers who do not smoke. Also, pregnant women who smoke are more likely to have a miscarriage, a stillborn baby, or an infant that dies soon after birth. Twice as many premature babies are born to smoking mothers than to mothers who do not smoke. There is also evidence to suggest that by the age of 11 the children of mothers who smoked more than 10 cigarettes a day during pregnancy are slightly shorter and slightly below the average in reading, mathematics, and general ability than are the children of nonsmoking mothers.

Q: *What are the effects of smoking on the lungs?*

A: There are two main effects of smoking on the lungs. Chronic bronchitis and, eventually, emphysema commonly occur in heavy

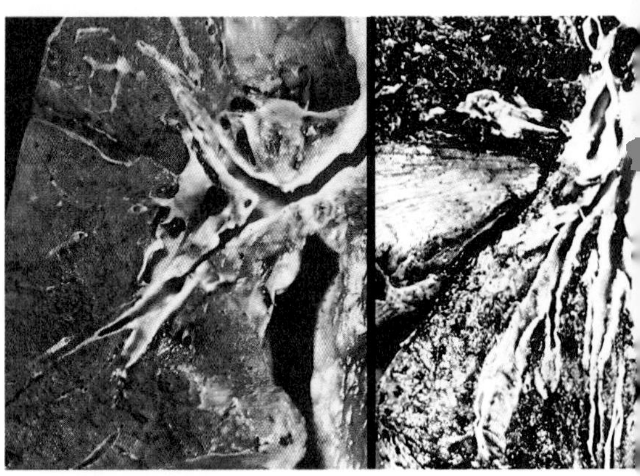

A healthy lung, *left,* is elastic and dark pink, with unobstructed airways. A lung damaged by **smoking of tobacco,** *right,* is flabby and blackened, with scarred and blocked airways.

smokers, and a morning cough, which clears the bronchi, is a common feature of all smokers. Early lung damage can be detected by pulmonary function tests before there is any obvious shortness of breath.

Among persons who smoke a pack of cigarettes a day, lung cancer occurs 20 times more frequently than in nonsmokers. The risk is increased in those who smoke high tar cigarettes, who inhale deeply, and who began smoking in adolescence. *See also* BRONCHITIS; EMPHYSEMA.

Q: *Can smoking cause other cancers of the body?*

A: Yes. There are more cancers of the bladder and pancreas in smokers than in nonsmokers. Cancer of the mouth, tongue, larynx, and esophagus are also more common in smokers of all kinds of tobacco, including pipe smokers and cigar smokers.

Q: *Can smoking affect the heart?*

A: Cigarette smoking increases the likelihood of arteriosclerosis, and there is twice the risk of coronary thrombosis than in those who do not smoke. The risk of developing other blood vessel disorders is also increased.

Q: *What other diseases are more likely to occur in smokers?*

A: Dental disorders, gingivitis, and other infections of the gums occur more commonly in smokers. Smokers are also more likely to develop tuberculosis, probably because the damaging effect of the irritants in tobacco lowers the resistance of the lungs to this type of infection.

Although smoking does not cause peptic ulcers, the continued habit prevents them from healing. Consequently, complications are more common and mortality from perforated ulcers is greater.

Q: *What are the benefits from stopping smoking?*

A: Within a few days or weeks, there is an improvement in the sense of taste and smell, a gradual reduction in the amount of morning coughing, and less shortness of breath during exercise.

Although lung damage, such as that caused by chronic bronchitis and emphysema, can not be reversed once it has occurred, its progress is arrested.

However, the greatest long-term benefit is the steady decrease in the chances of getting cancer. If a person who stops smoking cigarettes lives for 10 years, his chance of developing lung cancer is no more than for someone who has never smoked.

Smooth muscle. *See* MUSCLE.

Snakebite (snāk′bīt) is a wound that results from the bite of a snake; a snakebite can be poisonous or nonpoisonous.

Poisonous snakebites vary in effect from species to species. Some poisons (venoms) cause mainly tissue damage; others principally affect the nerves; and some cause destruction of blood cells and act as an anticoagulant. It is usually impossible to tell from the marks of a bite which species of snake has bitten a person. If possible, the snake should be killed, because this provides the positive identification which is important in subsequent treatment. If the snake is known to be nonpoisonous, the bite should be treated as a wound and washed thoroughly with soap and water.

Q: *What are the symptoms of poisonous snakebite?*

A: The symptoms depend on the species of snake, but usually there is a severe local pain starting soon after the bite, accompanied by swelling of the area, discoloration of the skin, and blisters.

Nausea, vomiting, and a slight fever often occur, but danger signals are tingling, numbness, and weakness in the face; fainting; breathlessness; and blood in the urine, sputum, or vomit. Sometimes, there is severe abdominal or chest pain. Some snakebites result in convulsions and kidney failure.

Death may result within a few hours in untreated cases, usually after the nervous system becomes involved, causing convulsions and muscular weakness. Death may also occur within several days if the damage is mainly to the tissues or from bleeding. Bleeding can cause anemia or fatal cerebral or intestinal hemorrhage.

Q: *What are the main ways of treating snakebite poisoning?*

A: The venom must be prevented from spreading through the body. The victim should stay as motionless as possible. If the bitten part is an arm or a leg, let it hang down.

In severe cases, antivenin can be given by means of an injection into a muscle or by diluted intravenous infusion. Some persons have an allergic reaction to antivenins. Hospitalization is essential in severe cases.

See also BITES AND STINGS: FIRST AID.

Snakebite: first aid. *See* BITES AND STINGS: FIRST AID.

Sneezing is a sudden, involuntary expulsion of air from the nose and mouth, resulting from irritation of the nose. A sneeze may be caused by dust, pollen, or the common cold. A sneeze

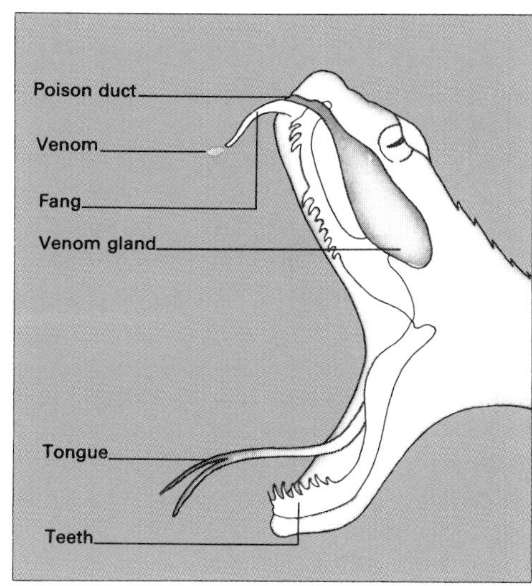

The venom in a poisonous **snakebite** is transmitted via a groove in the fang as the snake bites.

may project infected droplets into the air, so a sneeze should be blocked by a handkerchief or by the hand.

Snellen's chart (snel'ənz) is a chart of letters of decreasing size used to test a person's eyesight; it is one of several charts so used.

See also EYEGLASSES.

Snoring (snôr'ing) is a rough, broken sound made during sleep. Almost everyone snores occasionally, but men usually snore more often than women and children. Snoring occurs when air rushing through the mouth vibrates the soft palate, the soft tissue in the roof of the mouth near the throat. This vibration produces the snoring sound. As the soft palate vibrates, the lips, cheeks, and nostrils may also vibrate, making the snoring louder.

Snoring may be habitual, or it may result from an underlying condition that blocks the nose, such as swollen adenoids, mucus, a deviated nasal septum, or a nasal polyp.

Snow blindness is temporary or partial blindness caused when the eyes are directly exposed to the sun's ultraviolet light reflected off snow or ice. It can also occur from exposure to arc welding flames, high-voltage electric sparks, and artificial sun lamps. The ultraviolet light causes severe eye pain and photophobia. In most cases, snow blindness disappears when a person rests the eyes and remains indoors. However, prolonged exposure to reflected light can lead to solar retinopathy, a disorder that may result in some permanent loss of vision. Wearing sunglasses or dark-colored goggles helps prevent snow blindness.

Social and Rehabilitation Service (SRS) is an agency of the United States government. It has five major divisions. (1) The Rehabilitation Services Administration administers programs that aid physically and mentally handicapped persons. (2) The Community Services Administration administers the agency's service program for children and adults. (3) The Administration on Aging administers programs that help the elderly. (4) The Medical Services Administration is responsible for Medicare and other medical assistance programs that are administered by state and local communities. (5) The Assistance Payments Administration handles payments involved in public aid programs.

Sodium (sō'dē əm) is a metallic chemical element. Its salts, particularly the chloride, form the principal salts within the body. Most people get sufficient sodium in the food they eat, such as foods high in protein and some vegetables, such as celery. Many Americans consume a diet that is too high in salt content. In individuals predisposed to high blood pressure, excessive salt intake may worsen the condition.

Q: *What happens if the body's level of sodium is incorrect?*

A: Any condition that causes excessive loss of sodium from the body, such as severe vomiting and diarrhea, kidney disease, a disorder of the adrenal glands (Addison's disease), or excessive use of diuretic drugs, produces signs of dehydration and shock. Less commonly, lack of sodium occurs in the body fluids because of diabetes insipidus or excessive sweating.

An excess of sodium may occur when a patient is recovering from acute kidney failure (when there is an imbalance of sodium and water). This may lead to symptoms of mental confusion, thirst, and high blood pressure.

See also ADDISON'S DISEASE; DIABETES INSIPIDUS; KIDNEY DISEASE; SODIUM-FREE DIET.

Sodium bicarbonate (sō'dē əm bī-kär'bə nit) is a white, odorless, crystalline salt powder that is used medically as an antacid to neutralize the stomach's acid secretions and in weak solutions as intravenous infusions in the treatment of certain disorders. It should not be taken by people with kidney disease or bleeding ulcers. Heart problems may also rule out its use. Side effects of sodium bicarbonate may include swelling of the stomach and abnormal body electrolyte levels.

Sodium bicarbonate is also commercially available as baking soda, one of the ingredients of baking powder.

Sodium-free diet (sō'dē əm), also called a low-salt or low-sodium diet, is the restriction of a person's intake of sodium chloride. Other compounds containing chloride are also limited, including monosodium glutamate, sodium sulfate, and baking powder or soda (sodium bicarbonate).

The sodium-free diet is prescribed for persons suffering from hypertension, kidney or liver disease, or edema (the retention of bodily fluids). The seriousness of the condition defines the degree of the sodium restriction. Corticosteroid therapy also necessitates a sodium-free diet. *See also* CORTICOSTEROID DRUG.

Foods that are not recommended for persons on a low-salt diet include most canned and frozen foods; pork products such as ham and bacon; frankfurters, luncheon meats, and sausages; all shellfish; breads or cereals containing salt; cheese and salted butter or margarine; and certain vegetables, including celery, carrots, beets, sauerkraut, and spinach. Some drugs (alkalizers, laxatives, and sedatives) and water filtered through a water softener also contain sodium and should be avoided.

Foods permitted on the diet include skimmed milk and eggs; beef, veal, pork, lamb, and poultry; fish; fresh fruits; and vegetables, including salad ingredients, potatoes, asparagus, broccoli, peas, and green beans. Many low-sodium foods are available commercially; the consumer should read the product labels to ascertain sodium content.

See also DIET, SPECIAL; SODIUM.

Soft palate. *See* PALATE.

Soft sore is a common name for chancroid.

See also CHANCROID.

Solar plexus (sō'lər plek'səs) is a network of nerves behind the stomach.

See also PLEXUS.

Somatization disorder (sō ma ti za'shen) occurs when a patient complains of frequent physical symptoms that have no apparent physical cause. Because the patient converts mental experiences or anxiety into bodily symptoms, these vary tremendously depending on the individual and his or her state of mind. It is most commonly found in adolescent and young adult women.

Some of the more common symptoms include painful or irregular menstruation, pain during intercourse, paralysis, temporary blindness, and distress of the gastrointestinal tract. The condition is closely related to hypochondriasis, a disorder characterized by an undue concern for the state of one's health. Another related condition is Briquet's syndrome, which is pulmonary distress caused by a hysterical paralysis of the diaphragm.

See also HYPOCHONDRIASIS.

Somatotype (sō'mə tə tīp) is a general classification of human body types within which certain distinct types are arranged. For example, an ectomorph is tall and thin with poorly developed muscles; an endomorph is short and rounded; and a mesomorph is muscular and well-built.

Somnambulism. *See* SLEEPWALKING.

Sonography (sə nog'rə fē) is a diagnostic technique in which high-frequency sound (ultrasound) is used to obtain a picture of the internal body structures, such as the heart and liver.

See also ULTRASOUND.

Sore is any tender or painful lesion or ulcer on the skin, especially in the mouth or throat.

See also BEDSORE; CANKER SORE; THROAT, SORE.

Sore throat. *See* THROAT, SORE.

Spare part surgery is any form of surgery that uses artificial parts to replace diseased or injured parts of a patient's body.

See also REPLACEMENT SURGERY; TRANSPLANT SURGERY.

Spasm (spaz'əm) is a sudden involuntary contraction of a muscle or group of muscles, usually accompanied by pain and movement.

See also CHOREA; COLIC; SPASTIC; TETANY.

Spasms: treatment. *See* CRAMPS AND SPASMS: TREATMENT.

Spastic (spas'tik) describes a condition in which a recurrent muscular contraction occurs. This condition is present in neurological disorders that affect the brain, such as those that follow a stroke, or in cerebral palsy resulting from congenital brain damage.

Spastic colon. *See* IRRITABLE BOWEL SYNDROME.

Specialists, medical. *See* MEDICAL SPECIALISTS.

Specimens, collection of (spes'ə mənz). Collection of specimens refers to the gathering of samples of body fluids, tissues, or pus in order to isolate and identify an infection or disease-causing agent.

Spectacles. *See* EYEGLASSES.

Speculum (spek'yə ləm) is a surgical instrument used for examining the interior of the body, usually through one of the normal openings such as the ear, nose, rectum, or vagina.

Speech (spēch) is the act of speaking. The average child learns to speak by imitating other people. It is important that a child hear proper speech. Parents should note any speech difficulties, such as lisping or stuttering. If such difficulties occur, parents should discuss the problem with their family physician who may perform evaluative tests or refer the family to a speech pathologist.

See also SPEECH DEFECT; SPEECH DEVELOPMENT.

Speech defect includes any condition that results in a failure to speak normally. Most speech defects are first detected in childhood, when a baby fails to begin talking at the usual age. *See also* SPEECH DEVELOPMENT.

The most common cause of delayed speaking is probably some form of mental retardation, but hearing problems, ranging from complete deafness to impaired hearing of certain tones, can also cause difficulty in learning to speak. A rare cause of failure to speak is the psychological condition autism. *See also* AUTISM.

Q: *Are there any other conditions that may cause failure to develop normal speech?*

A: Yes. Children with cerebral palsy or a cleft palate have difficulty in pronouncing words clearly. *See also* CLEFT PALATE; CEREBRAL PALSY.

Some children, who are in other ways normal and intelligent, develop a kind of word deafness. Sounds are not understood, although they are heard, and this results in disordered speech. Stuttering or stammering, however, may also sometimes be the result of severe emotional disturbances. *See also* STUTTERING.

Q: *When should a parent become concerned about speech defects in a child?*

A: A parent who notices that a baby is not reacting to sounds (by moving the eyes or head) between the ages of four and six months should discuss the matter with a physician, because the infant may have a hearing problem. If an infant of eight to nine months is not able to repeat sounds, then a thorough assessment is needed.

The age at which a child learns to speak varies. On the average, a child of two-and-one-half should be able to understand simple speech and speak reasonably well, using phrases and short sentences.

A child who is not speaking by the age of two-and-one half, but who is in other ways developing normally, may have some problems and a physician should be consulted.

Q: *How can speech defects in children be treated?*

A: Treatment of speech defects depends on the cause. Speech defects that are the result of temporary and permanent conductive deafness may be overcome by the use of a hearing aid. Lisping or stuttering can often be improved if the child is encouraged by the family to speak slowly and correctly. More complicated speech problems, such as the use of incorrect words (dysphasia), may require help from a speech therapist. Autistic children require special training. *See also* DYSPHASIA.

Q: *What speech disorders occur in adults?*

A: Once speech has been learned, the onset of deafness has no effect on the ability to speak. Loss of speech (aphasia) may occur after any form of brain damage that involves the speech area of the brain. Recovery may be complete, or it may leave some degree of dysphasia. *See also* APHASIA.

Aphonia, the inability to speak, may occur if the laryngeal muscles are paralyzed or destroyed. Dysarthria, speech that is correct but altered, may be the result of muscular or neurological disorders, such as Parkinson's disease. *See also* APHONIA; DYSARTHRIA.

Q: *How can speech defects in adults be treated?*

A: Treatment depends on the cause. Cancer of the larynx may require surgery to remove the larynx. As a result, the patient may be taught esophageal speech. Drug treatment can sometimes help speech problems in neurological or muscular disorders. A speech therapist can help a patient with dysphasia following a stroke. *See also* SPEECH, ESOPHAGEAL.

Speech development refers to the learning process by which a child learns to speak. At 18 months of age, a toddler has a vocabulary of 10 to 20 words. By 3 years of age, the vocabulary has increased to about 900 words. It is very important that a child hear proper speech, since he or she learns primarily by imitating. If difficulties occur, such as lisping or stuttering, a competent authority on speech problems should be consulted.

See also CHILD; SPEECH DEFECT.

Speech, esophageal (ē sə faj′ē əl). Esophageal speech is a method of producing understandable speech by vibrating air in the esophagus instead of the voice box (larynx). It is sometimes used after the surgical removal of the larynx.

See also ESOPHAGUS.

Sperm (spėrm) is the male sex cell, known also as a spermatozoon. It is produced in the testicles and ejaculated in semen. After sexual intercourse, fertilization may occur if a sperm from the male combines with an ovum (egg) from the female. The sperm and ovum each contain half the normal number of chromosomes that are required to form a single cell.

Infertility in men may be caused by an absence of sperm, sometimes resulting from a blockage of the vas deferens between the testicle and the prostate gland. Other causes of infertility include the failure to produce sperm and a deficiency of healthy sperm.

Infection of the reproductive tract and prostatitis (inflammation of the prostate gland) cause defective sperm. Other factors influencing the development of defective sperm include obesity, smoking, drinking alcohol, and serious illness. Sperm production takes place only if the temperature of the testicles is two degrees below that of the rest of the body. Underwear that is too tight may hold the testicles too close to the body, thus raising their temperature and hampering production of sperm.

See also REPRODUCTION, HUMAN.

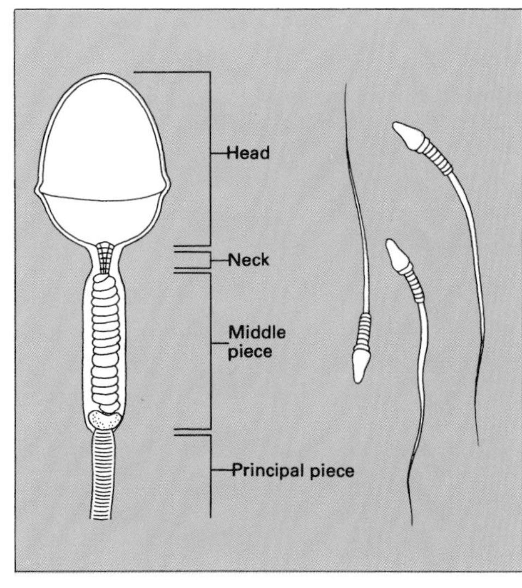

Sperm is the microscopic male gamete that fertilizes the female gamete, the ovum. A typical sperm cell has a head, neck, and a long thread-like tail.

Spermatic cord (spėr mat′ik) is the cord by which the testicle is suspended within the scrotum, enclosing the vas deferens, the blood vessels, and the nerves serving the testicle. The spermatic cord extends to the groin, with the left spermatic cord usually longer than the right. This results in the left testicle usually hanging lower than the right within the scrotum.

See also TESTIS; VAS DEFERENS.

Spermatocele (spėr′mə tə sēl) is a cyst in the epididymis that contains spermatic fluid. It is usually painless and does not require medical treatment.

See also CYST; EPIDIDYMIS.

Spermicide (spėr′mə sīd) is a substance that kills sperm. It is usually used in contraceptive creams and jellies.

See also CONTRACEPTION.

Sphincter (sfingk′tər) is a ring of muscle that closes or constricts an opening or passage in the body when the muscle contracts.

Sphygmomanometer (sfig mō mə nom′ə tər) is an instrument that measures blood pressure. A rubber cuff is placed around the upper arm, or sometimes the thigh, and inflated with air to pressure greater than that of the blood in the arteries. This temporarily stops the flow of blood. The air pressure is then gradually released while a stethoscope is used over the artery to listen for the sound of the pulse as the blood starts to flow again. When this sound is heard, the air pressure in the cuff equals the upper blood pressure,

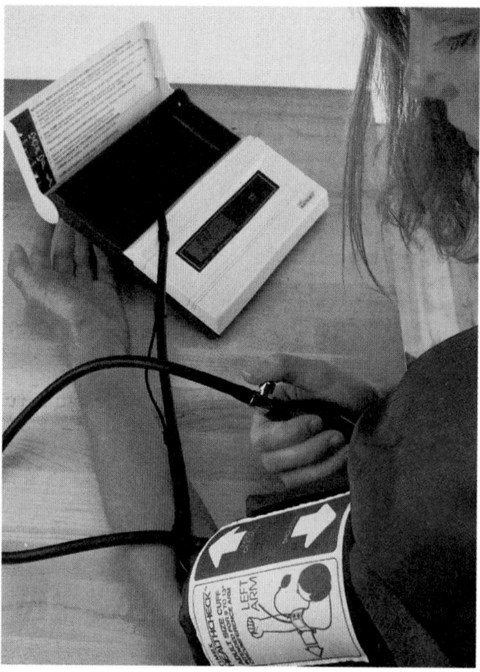

A **sphygmomanometer** is an instrument for measuring blood pressure.

known as the systolic blood pressure. The pressure is further reduced in the cuff until the sounds disappear. This is known as the diastolic pressure. The measurement of blood pressure is expressed in millimeters of mercury.

See also BLOOD PRESSURE.

Spina bifida (spī'nə bīf'ə də) is a congenital anomaly of the spine in which one or more vertebral segments are incompletely developed. The defect may extend over a number of vertebrae, usually in the lumbar or sacral regions. Spina bifida occurs in about 1 or 2 births out of 100.

The disorder is classified as either *spina bifida occulta,* which has few outward signs except sometimes a congenital anomaly, such as a clubfoot, or as *spina bifida cystica,* which is also a defect of the central nervous system, with a sac protruding from the spine. This sac may contain either membranes (a condition called meningocele), the spinal cord (myelocele) or both (myelomeningocele). If the protruding sac is damaged, meningeal infection or death may result. Additionally, spina bifida is commonly associated with hydrocephalus. *See also* CLUBFOOT; HYDROCEPHALUS.

Spina bifida occulta seldom produces neurological symptoms. But in cases where the spinal cord is involved, the patient's legs may be paralyzed, and urinary and fecal incontinence is common.

Q: *What is the treatment for spina bifida?*

A: Immediate surgery is necessary in cases where there is a protruding sac and, therefore, risk of meningitis. This is avoided by surgery to cover the exposed area with skin.

Q: *Can spina bifida be detected in a fetus before birth?*

A: Spina bifida can be detected by checking the mother's blood for a high level of alpha fetoprotein. The disorder can also be detected by measuring the amount of this protein in the amniotic fluid surrounding the fetus by means of the procedure known as amniocentesis. If the fetus is found to have spina bifida, the parents may choose to terminate the pregnancy.

See also AMNIOCENTESIS; CHORIONIC VILLUS BIOPSY.

Spinal cord (spī'nəl) is the part of the central nervous system that extends along the spinal column from the base of the brain to the second lumbar vertebra in the small of the back. The spinal cord is covered by the three membranes (pia, dura, and arachnoid) that make up the meninges and is lubricated by cerebrospinal fluid.

The spinal cord is composed of 31 bundles of nerves formed of sensory and motor fibers that carry impulses from the brain and relay messages from various parts of the body back to the brain. At the lower end of the spinal cord is the cauda equina, a fan-shaped network of nerves running in the spinal canal and supplying the lumbar, sacral, and coccygeal nerves that serve the lower part of the body.

See also NERVOUS SYSTEM.

Spinal curvature (spī'nəl kėr'və chůr) is any abnormal shape of the spine. A normal spine appears straight when viewed from the front. When viewed from the side, it has an elongated double S-shape, with four curves.

When viewed from the front, an abnormal sideways curvature of the spine is called scoliosis. Lordosis is an increased curvature of the lumbar spine, and kyphosis is an increased curvature of the thoracic spine.

See also KYPHOSIS; LORDOSIS; SCOLIOSIS.

Spinal fluid. See CEREBROSPINAL FLUID.

Spinal puncture. See SPINAL TAP.

Spinal tap (spī'nəl), also called lumbar puncture or spinal puncture, is the insertion of a long needle into the spinal cavity to extract cerebrospinal fluid, usually for purposes of diagnosis.

See also CEREBROSPINAL FLUID.

Spine (spīn), also called the spinal column or backbone, is a part of the axial skeleton (head and trunk). It is made up of 7 cervical (neck) vertebrae; 12 thoracic (chest) vertebrae; 5 lumbar (lower back) vertebrae; and the sacrum and coccyx.

The vertebrae are separated by tough, intervertebral disks of fibrocartilage and held together by ligaments. In addition, there are muscles that extend up and down, supporting the spine and the body and producing movement. Some of these muscles extend up to the back and side of the skull to help to support the head.

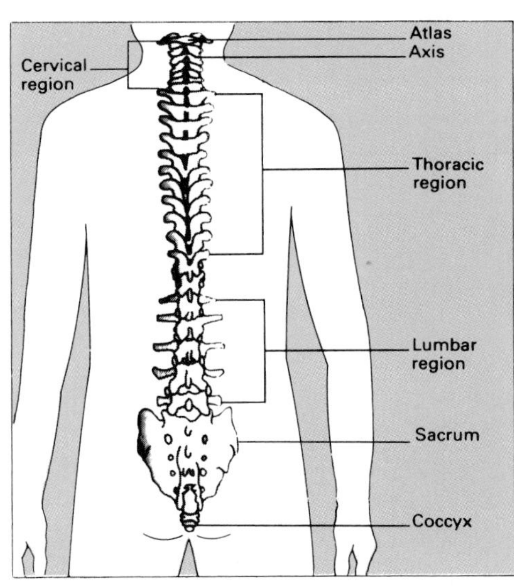

The **spine** consists of 33 vertebrae that encase and protect the spinal cord and nerves.

Q: *What disorders may affect the spine?*

A: Many spinal disorders cause pain in the back. Spondylolisthesis, a common cause of lower back pain, affects the joint between the fifth lumbar vertebra and the sacrum. Fusion of the small joint between the sacrum and the coccyx can cause stiffness in this region, particularly in the elderly.

Congenital anomalies of the spine may include additional vertebrae, usually in the lumbar region; half vertebrae in the thoracic spine; fusing of the fifth lumbar vertebra with the sacrum; or the opposite effect, in which the first sacral vertebra is separated from the rest of the sacrum.

Certain malignant tumors may metastasize (spread) to the vertebrae, causing pain and sometimes fractures.

See also BACKACHE; DISK, HERNIATED; SKELETON; SPINA BIFIDA; SPINAL CURVATURE; SPONDYLOLISTHESIS; VERTEBRA.

Spine fracture: first aid See FRACTURE: FIRST AID.

Spirochete (spī'rə kēt) is a spiral-shaped bacterium. Syphilis, for example, is caused by a spirochete.

See also BACTERIA.

Spirometer (spī rom'ə tər) is an instrument for measuring the capacity of the lungs by measuring the volume of air that is breathed in and out of the lungs and the speed with which the air is exhaled. The patient breathes through a tube connected to the spirometer, which records the data on paper.

See also LUNG FUNCTION TEST.

Splanchnic (splangk'nik) describes anything concerned with the intestines or internal organs, such as the liver and spleen.

Splayfoot (splā'fu̇t) is another term for flatfoot (pes planus).

See also FLATFOOT.

Spleen (splēn) is an abdominal organ that stores blood and plays a part in the body's immune system. It is about the size of an adult's fist and varies in weight between 5 ounces (140g) and 10 ounces (280g), depending on the amount of blood it contains. It lies in the upper left part of the abdominal cavity, above and behind the stomach, and is protected by the lower ribs. It has a large blood supply through the splenic artery. If the body experiences severe blood loss, the spleen can produce 12-19 fluid ounces (360-570ml) of blood in less than a minute.

The spleen is composed of sponge-like tissue (splenic pulp), consisting of white lymphoid tissue scattered throughout the reddish mass that makes up the basic substance of the spleen.

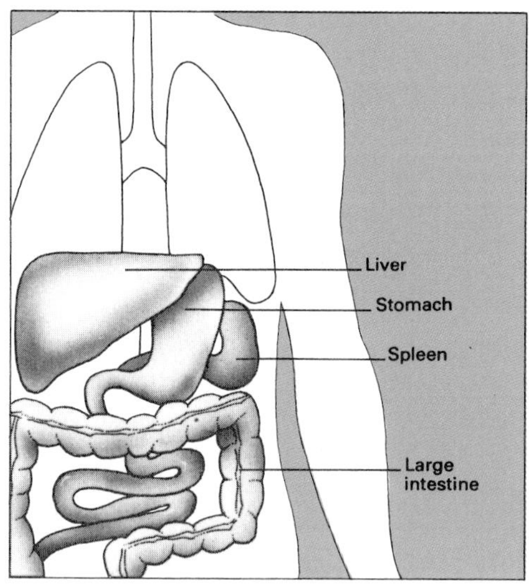

The **spleen,** which lies to the left of the stomach, stores blood and helps filter foreign substances from the blood.

The white pulp produces lymphocytes (white blood cells) and the red pulp stores excess red blood cells and filters out any damaged cells, debris, and bacteria in the circulation.

See also SPLEEN DISORDERS.

Spleen disorders (splēn). The most common disorder is enlargement of the spleen (splenomegaly), which may have various causes. Spleen enlargement occurs in forms of chronic hemolytic anemia, such as sickle cell anemia; malignant conditions of the lymphatic system, such as Hodgkin's disease, leukemia, and polycythemia vera; in cirrhosis of the liver, when there is an increase in venous pressure; in various inflammatory diseases, such as mononucleosis, hepatitis, malaria, brucellosis, and kala-azar; and in conditions such as sarcoidosis. All the above-mentioned disorders have separate entries in this encyclopedia.

If the spleen is damaged by injury, such as a blow to the abdomen in an automobile accident, it can be surgically removed (splenectomy) in an adult with little or no effect on the patient's general health. The spleen can also sometimes be repaired if the injury is small. A patient who has a splenectomy is at risk for a pneumococcal bacterial infection and should receive a pneumococcal vaccine.

Splenectomy (spli nek'tə mē) is the surgical removal of the spleen. There may be various reasons for this operation, including rupture of the spleen; enlargement of the spleen, often accompanying cirrhosis of the liver; varicose veins in the esophagus that cause internal bleeding; and certain malignancies.

See also SPLEEN.

Splenomegaly (splē nō meg'ə lē) is an enlargement of the spleen. It can be caused by a variety of disorders, such as Hodgkin's disease and cirrhosis of the liver.

See also SPLEEN; SPLEEN DISORDERS.

Splint (splint) is a device that is used to immobilize and support an injured part of the body, usually a fractured limb.

See also FRACTURE: FIRST AID.

Splinter (splin'tər) is a slender piece of wood, metal, or similar material embedded in the layers of the skin. It can also be a fragment from a fractured bone.

See also SPLINTER: TREATMENT.

Splinter: treatment. Do not attempt to remove a large splinter or one that is deeply embedded and is not protruding from the skin. In these instances, consult a physician.

If the splinter is small and is protruding from the skin, grasp the end of the splinter with a pair of tweezers and carefully pull out the splinter. Apply an antiseptic, such as hydrogen peroxide, over the wound.

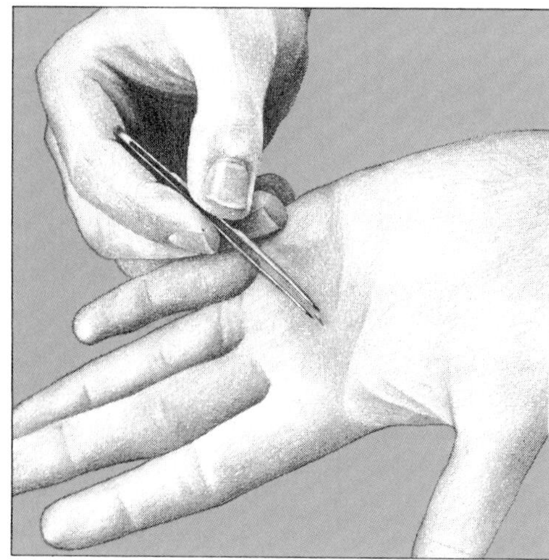

If a small **splinter** is protruding from the skin, carefully remove it with a pair of tweezers.

Spondylitis (spon də lī'tis) is inflammation of the vertebrae. The most common form is ankylosing spondylitis, which is a rheumatic disorder. There are various possible causes, including tuberculosis of the vertebrae.

Symptoms of spondylitis include back pain, pain on movement, a stiff back, and occasionally a fever. Diagnosis is confirmed by an X ray, white blood cell count, and raised erythrocyte sedimentation rate (ESR). Treatment usually involves rest, spinal support, and therapy specifically directed at the cause of the inflammation. Occasionally, surgery may be necessary to drain any abscess of the bone, in order to prevent pressure on the spinal cord or nerves.

See also SEDIMENTATION RATE; SPONDYLITIS, ANKYLOSING.

Spondylitis, ankylosing (spon də lī'tis, ang kə lō'zing). Ankylosing spondylitis, also known as bamboo spine, is a condition in which the bones of the spine (vertebrae) fuse together. This causes stiffness, and the spine can become bowed. Early symptoms are backache and stiffness in the morning. Ankylosing spondylitis occurs more often in men than in women and usually starts early in adult life. The symptoms gradually worsen, but pain need not be continuous. The patient's eyes often become inflamed (iritis) and the joints can become swollen and tender (arthritis). The cause of ankylosing spondylitis is not known.

Q: *Can treatment arrest the progress of ankylosing spondylitis?*

A: Yes, but only to the extent that a physician can reduce the pain and stiffness associated with the disorder. Anti-inflammatory drugs are prescribed and, if the pain and stiffness are severe enough, radiotherapy may be used. Exercises are essential to keep the spine mobile and straight. Physiotherapy (including breathing exercises) is an important aspect of treatment.

Spondylolisthesis (spon di lō lis'the sis) is a deformity of the spine in which one vertebra slides forward over the top of another. It can occur in the neck or in the lumbar spine (lower back).

Q: *What are the symptoms of spondylolisthesis?*

A: The main symptoms of spondylolisthesis in the neck are weakness and pain in the arms caused by compression of the spinal cord. Later symptoms are paralysis in the lower part of the body, with accompanying disorders of the bowel and bladder.

Spondylolisthesis in the lumbar spine is one of the causes of backache and sciatica. *See also* SCIATICA.

Q: *How is spondylolisthesis treated?*

A: Treatment of spondylolisthesis in the neck depends on the severity of the condition. Often, the initial treatment is traction, which can only be applied to a patient in bed. A metal frame is attached to the head and weights are attached to stretch the neck. Following this treatment, a neck cast may be necessary for some months. Sometimes an operation is required to place the vertebrae back into the correct position.

There is no need to treat spondylolisthesis of the lumbar region unless the symptoms are severe. If they are, a surgical corset and muscle-strengthening exercises may be sufficient. Patients with spondylolisthesis should avoid heavy lifting.

See also DISK, HERNIATED.

Spondylosis (spon di lō'sis) is osteoarthritis that affects the spine. It involves a degeneration of the joints, frequently accompanied by a breakdown of the intervertebral disks. *See also* OSTEOARTHRITIS.

Spondylosis in the neck usually affects the lowest three vertebrae. It causes aching and stiffness in the back of the neck and a grating sound when turning the neck. The patient may also have a headache at the back of the head. Spondylosis of the lower spine most commonly occurs in people who have done heavy manual labor or who have a history of either injury or degenerative changes following a herniated disk or osteochondritis (inflammation of bone and cartilage). Backache with muscle spasm is the usual symptom. The condition may cause pressure on local nerves, resulting in pain in the legs or around the ribs.

Q: *Does spondylosis always produce symptoms?*

A: No. X-ray examination of the spine shows many of the characteristics of spondylosis in people as they get older, but symptoms need not occur. Symptoms may occur, however, if there is some minor injury to the spine, such as that caused by a fall or sudden twist.

Q: *How is spondylosis treated?*
A: Treatment depends on the severity of the symptoms. Anti-inflammatory drugs are usually helpful, but sometimes temporary immobilization of the spine in a neck splint or spinal brace is necessary. Physiotherapy, with heat and massage, may be an additional form of treatment.

See also DISK, HERNIATED.

Spondylosis, cervical (spon di lō'sis, sėr'və kəl). Cervical spondylosis is an arthritic condition of the upper spine and neck, which tends to become worse with time. A stiff neck may be the only symptom, although pressure on nearby nerves may cause pain and weakness in the arm and hand. Cervical spondylosis is most commonly part of the normal aging process. It can begin earlier in life as the result of back injuries, such as those sustained playing football or riding a horse.

Q: *How is cervical spondylosis treated?*
A: Heat applied locally to the affected area, massage, physiotherapy, and anti-inflammatory drugs may be utilized in treating the condition. If these are not successful, it may be necessary to immobilize the neck in a surgical collar.

Sponge, contraceptive (spunj, kon trə sep'tiv). A contraceptive sponge is a sponge that has been saturated with a spermicide. The woman inserts it into her vagina prior to intercourse, pushing the sponge up against the cervix. Here the sponge continuously releases the spermicide for up to 24 hours. No additional applications of spermicide are necessary.

As is the case with a contraceptive diaphragm, a sponge requires no fitting and may be purchased without a prescription. Tests show it to be about 85 percent effective, and side effects have been few and minor. Proper use is extremely important. A physician should be consulted before this method of birth control is employed.

See also CONTRACEPTION; SPERMICIDE.

Spore (spôr) is the reproductive cell of a primitive organism, such as a fungus or bacterium. It is usually protected by a thick membrane, which makes it resistant to the effects of heat, chemicals, and dehydration. As a result, prolonged boiling or intense heat is usually required to kill spores.

Sport and exercise. *See* EXERCISE.

Sports injuries occur under a variety of circumstances, their frequency and severity depending on the physical demands of each individual sport and on the fitness, stamina, and strength of the individual participant. Many of the injuries occur because of repeated movements of or stresses on particular joints, bones, and muscles. Training for a particular sport is aimed at increasing the stamina and strength of the participant in line with the stresses to be met. A physical examination prior to an athletic undertaking is essential.

A primary requirement before a person takes part in any sport is physical fitness. This requires the slow development of physical capacity in all areas so that it is possible for the body to withstand the initial strain of training. Too much exercise, too soon, can produce muscle and ligament strain, inflamed tendons (tendinitis) inflamed bursae (bursitis), and other injuries.

Stamina implies an increase in reserve capacity, especially of the heart and the lungs. During an athletic undertaking, the heart has to pump blood at an increased rate and the lungs have to take in oxygen more rapidly. Strength develops by building muscle power through a slow process of using muscles a little harder over a period of

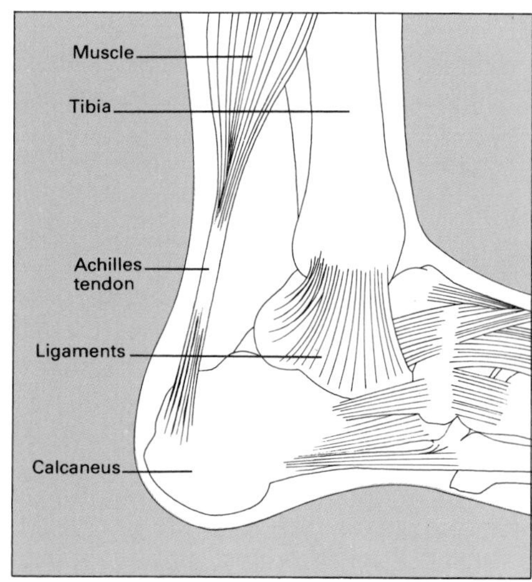

A **sports injury,** such as the rupture of the achilles tendon, may occur if a person makes a sudden turn during a sporting event.

time. When an individual has progressed to a required level of physical fitness, he or she is less likely to suffer injury and, if injured, is more likely to heal quickly.

See also SPORTS MEDICINE.

Sports medicine is a field that provides health care for physically active people. Its main purpose is to minimize the risk of injury and to treat effectively injuries that do occur. Sports medicine draws on the knowledge of many specialists, including physicians, athletic trainers, physiologists, kinesiologists and physical educators. These experts aid in determining the kind of training needed to help athletes perform to their highest capabilities, without injury. Sports medicine has led to improved diagnosis and treatment of common problems, such as knee injuries and muscle strains, which affect the general public as well as athletes.

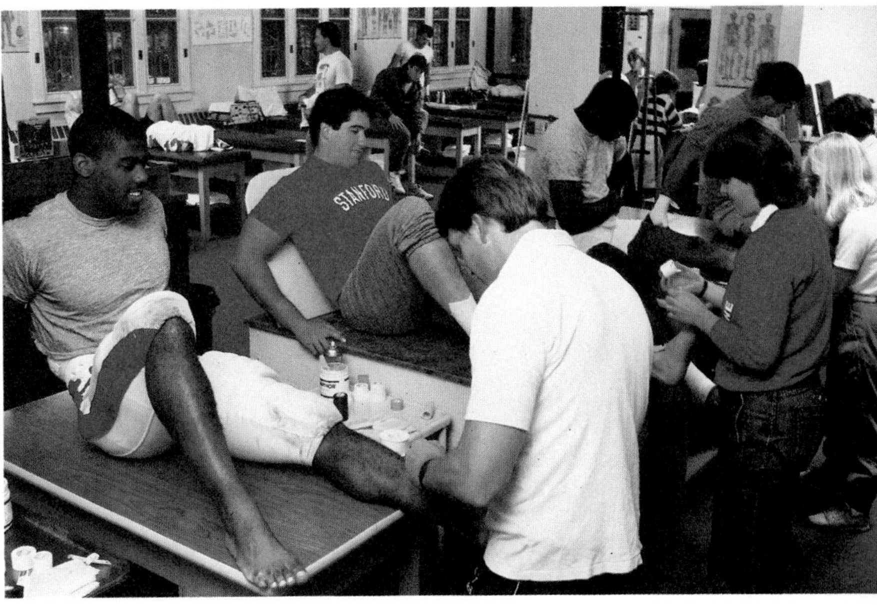

Athletic trainers perform a preventive aspect of **sports medicine** by taping the ankles of football players prior to competition.

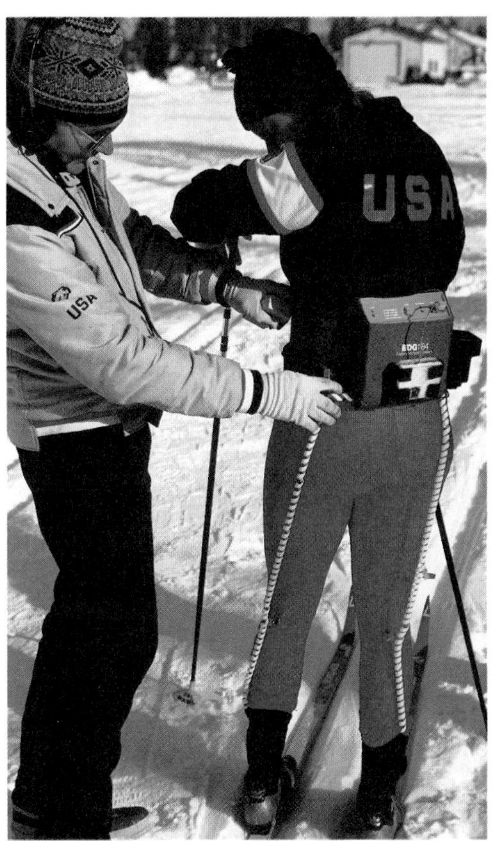

Sports medicine includes the use of sophisticated equipment, such as a device that records how much pressure the feet receive during cross-country skiing.

Sprain (sprān) is an injury to a joint in which some of the ligaments are severely stretched or even partly torn, producing swelling, pain, and tenderness. These symptoms are usually temporary and disappear when the joint is rested. A severe sprain may need expert splinting and bandaging.

See also MUSCLE, PULLED; SPRAINS AND STRAINS: TREATMENT.

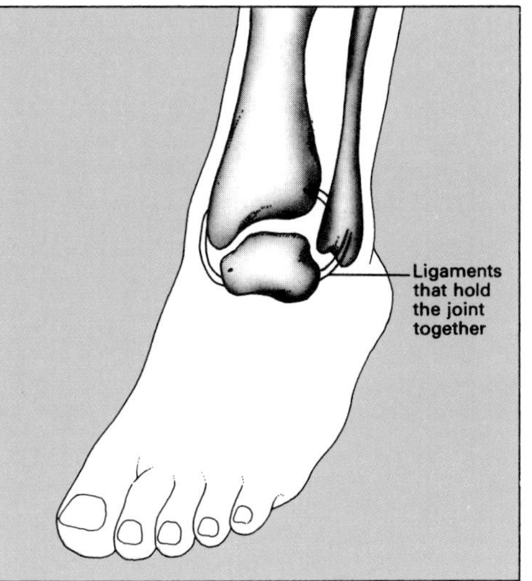

An ankle **sprain** is painful because the surrounding fibers and ligaments become stretched or torn.

Sprains and strains: treatment. A sprain is an injury to the ligaments that surround a joint. The ligaments hold the joint in position, but may be stretched or torn. Sprains most often occur in the ankle, knee, finger, wrist, shoulder, or spine.

Sprains and strains: treatment

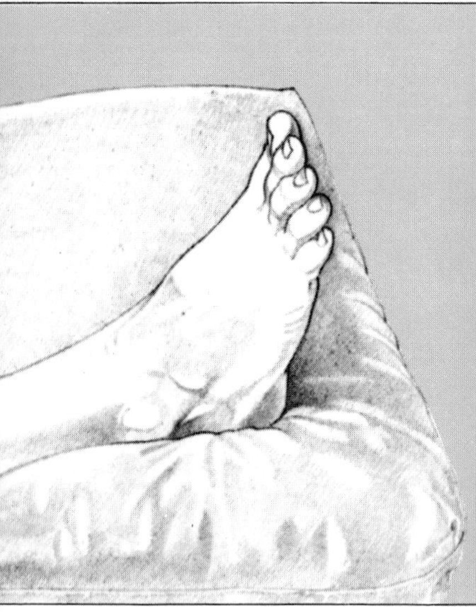

1 If the victim has a sprain, elevate and support the joint with pillows in the most comfortable position. Carefully remove the clothing around the joint.

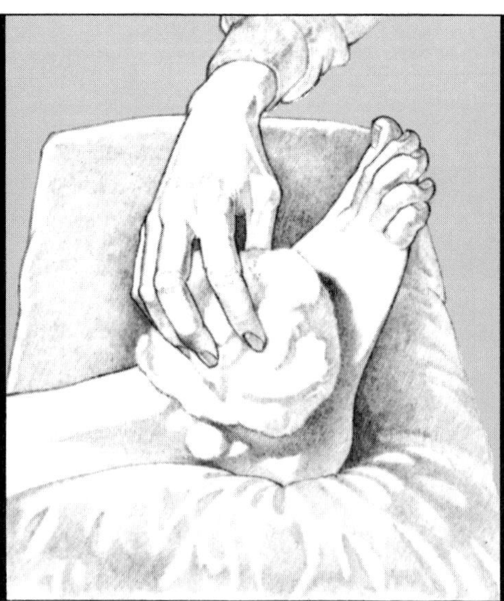

2 Apply an ice pack to the affected joint for several minutes every hour. This eases the pain and minimizes the swelling. A cold, wet cloth may be used instead of an ice pack. *Do not* immerse the joint in iced water.

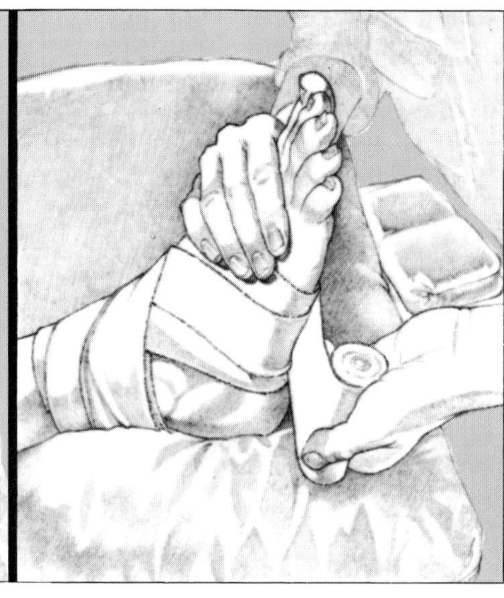

3 Immobilize the joint by surrounding it with a layer of cotton, keeping it in place with a bandage. If the joint begins to swell, loosen the bandage.

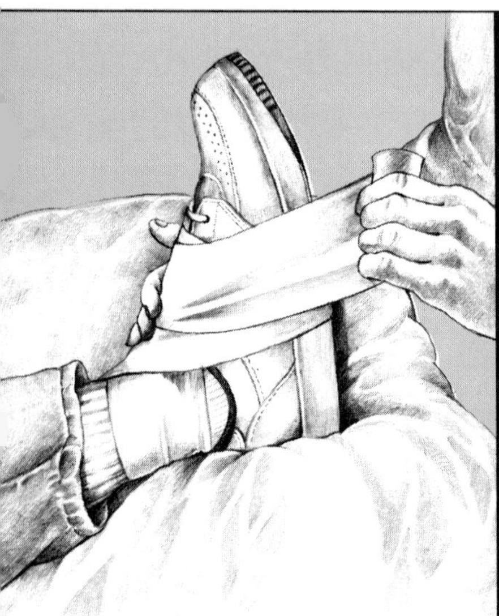

4 If an ankle sprain occurs outdoors, *do not* remove the victim's shoe. Give ankle support by applying a figure-eight bandage over the shoe.

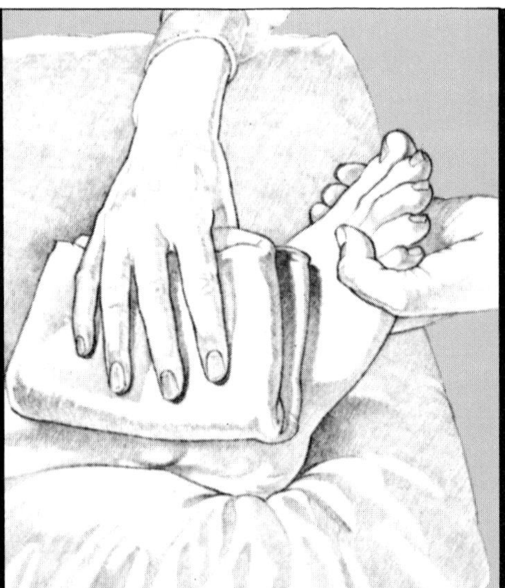

5 If the victim has strained a muscle, intermittently apply ice packs at first. After a day or two, discontinue treatment with ice packs and apply local heat with massage. A heat lamp or heating pad is a suitable way of relieving the pain. A hot bath also helps.

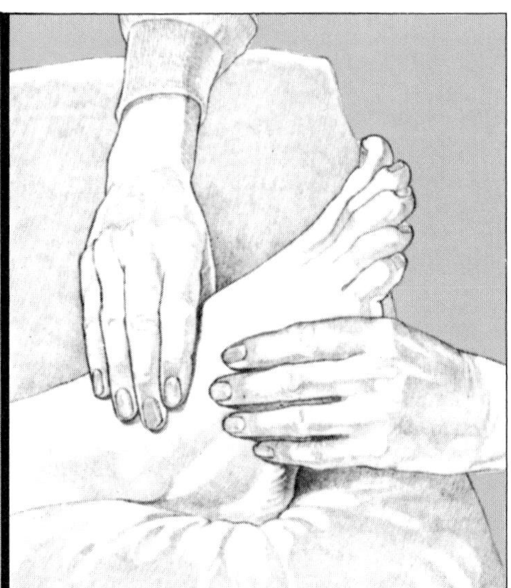

6 Gentle massage of the strained muscle may help to relieve the pain. Any strain that causes severe pain should be examined by a physician.

A strain, known also as a pulled muscle, is an injury to a muscle in which the muscle fibers are torn or stretched. It is a less serious injury than a sprain. The area most often affected by a strain is the lower back. This injury is usually caused by incorrectly lifting heavy objects.

With a severe sprain, the joint usually swells rapidly. Several hours after the initial injury bruising may appear. There is pain, especially on movement. The major symptom of a strain is a sharp pain at the time of injury. The muscle may feel stiff and the pain may become worse.

Treatment. The symptoms of both sprains and strains resemble those of a fracture and need medical attention. *See also* FRACTURE: FIRST AID.

With any sprain or strain, the injured part should be moved as little as possible. Do not allow the victim to walk if there is any injury to any part of the leg. A severe sprain may need expert splinting and bandaging.

Sprue (sprü) is an intestinal disorder characterized by impaired absorption of food, particularly fats, in the small intestine. It is common in the tropics but also occurs in temperate countries, where it is known as idiopathic or nontropical sprue.

Q: *What causes sprue?*

A: There are many disorders that may cause sprue. The disorders include celiac disease in infants and pancreatitis, in which there is an insufficient secretion of the pancreatic enzymes that chemically break down food. Sprue may be caused by any condition that interferes with normal intestinal cell activity, for example, the metabolic disorder amyloidosis. Sprue may also develop following irradiation treatment, worm infections, blockage of the lymphatic system from heart failure, or an operation in which part of the stomach or small intestine has been removed. Tropical sprue is thought to be caused by infection. *See also* CELIAC DISEASE; IRRADIATION.

Q: *What are the symptoms of sprue?*

A: The patient usually appears unwell, is underweight, and has a dry, pale skin. Soreness at the corners of the mouth (cheilosis) and a red tongue are present because of vitamin B deficiency. There may be clubbing of the fingers and swelling (edema) of the ankles. The abdomen may also swell. The patient may complain of weakness, fatigue, and frequent muscle cramps. Bruising may occur easily, and diarrhea, with large, pale, fatty stools that float, may be present.

Q: *How is sprue treated?*

A: Treatment depends on the cause. Celiac disease is treated with a gluten-free diet and the avoidance of all wheat and rye protein. Pancreatic enzymes can be given orally if there is a deficiency of the enzyme. Patients with pancreatitis must avoid alcohol. *See also* DIET, SPECIAL; GLUTEN.

Sputum (spyü'təm) is the material that is coughed up from the windpipe, bronchi, and lungs. A small amount of clear mucus is normally produced by the lungs each day. This is swept through the windpipe (trachea) and over the larynx by the hair-like cells that keep the lungs free of dust and other particles. The amount of clear sputum increases in any minor respiratory infection.

Thick yellow sputum may be caused by a bacterial infection. If yellow sputum is present, a physician should be consulted.

Bloodstained sputum may be an indication of a burst blood vessel in the lungs or an underlying condition, such as severe infection or cancer. It requires prompt medical attention.

Squint. *See* STRABISMUS.

Stammering. *See* STUTTERING.

Stapedectomy (stā pə dek'tə mē) is an operation to remove the stapes (one of the small bones in the middle ear). The stapes is replaced with a plastic or metal equivalent, which transmits sounds to the oval window of the inner ear.

Stapedectomy is indicated in the treatment of deafness due to otosclerosis.

Stapes (stā'pēz) is the innermost of the three small bones in the middle ear (the other two being the incus and the malleus). The stapes transmits sound vibrations to the oval window of the inner ear.

See also EAR; OTITIS; OTOSCLEROSIS.

Staphylococcus (staf ə lə kok′əs) is one of a group of bacteria that grow in clumps or clusters and, on microscopic examination, appear like bunches of grapes. Staphylococci are extremely common microorganisms that cause boils and other forms of skin infection characterized by pus. They also cause pneumonia and other infections. Staphylococci may also contaminate food and cause food poisoning.

Some staphylococci produce enzymes (penicillinase) that inactivate some penicillins. For this reason, physicians take particular care when treating staphylococcal infections.

See also BACTERIA.

Startle reflex (stär′təl), also known as Moro's reflex, is the reflex reaction in infants under the age of three months to sudden movement or loud noise. The startle reflex can be seen if a baby is gently lifted a short way from a bed and then released, or if the bed is jostled while the baby lies on it. The infant throws his or her arms outward and then moves them slowly inward in a grasping movement as the legs are stretched out. This is usually accompanied by a cry.

A symmetrical movement is an indication that the central nervous system is functioning normally. An asymmetrical movement, in which one arm or leg seems to lag behind the other, may suggest a problem such as a birth injury to the collarbone or nerves of the arm or, in some cases, damage to the brain.

Starvation (stär vā′shən) is the physical change that the human body undergoes with lack of calories. Provided fluids are available, a person can usually survive without food for six to eight weeks before finally dying.

In infants, starvation or protein-energy malnutrition may cause marasmus or kwashiorkor.

See also KWASHIORKOR; MARASMUS.

Steatorrhea (stē ə tə rē′ə) is excessive fat in the feces. It usually indicates a failure of fat absorption in the small intestine and commonly occurs in sprue. The condition may also accompany severe jaundice or chronic pancreatitis.

See also JAUNDICE; PANCREATITIS; SPRUE.

Stelazine® (stel′ə zēn) is a drug that is classified as a neuroleptic and is prescribed in the treatment of psychotic illnesses, such as schizophrenia. Because Stelazine is a sedative, it should be used with care when driving an automobile or when using moving machinery. Stelazine is capable of causing abnormal movement disorders, especially when used for prolonged periods of time or in high doses.

See also SEDATIVE.

Stenosis (sti nō′sis) is a narrowing of a duct or tube within the body. It may develop in various places, such as at a heart valve (aortic or mitral stenosis); at the exit of the stomach, from spasm of the muscle (pyloric stenosis); or in the duct of a salivary gland, following infection or the passage of a small stone. Stenosis may also develop in the carotid artery in the neck or in the arteries of the leg, producing symptoms of reduced blood flow, such as transient ischemic attacks or intermittent claudication.

See also CLAUDICATION, INTERMITTENT; ISCHEMIA; STROKE.

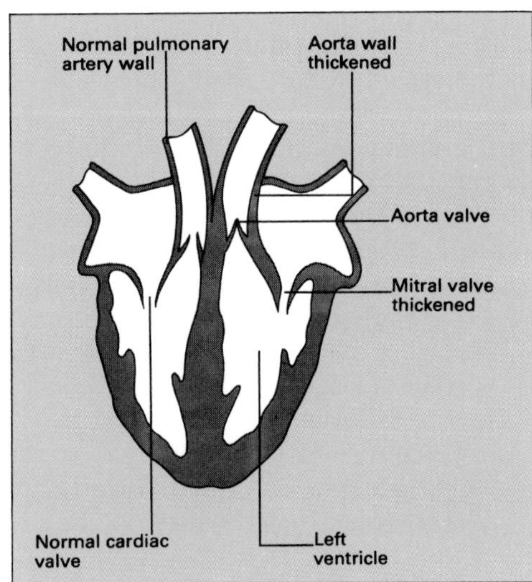

A **stenosis** is a contraction of a passage in a body structure, such as may occur in the aorta or mitral valve.

Sterility (stə ril′ə tē) is the inability to produce offspring. Sterility also refers to the state of being free from living microorganisms, such as bacteria and viruses.

See also INFERTILITY; STERILIZATION.

Sterilization (ster ə lə zā′shən) is any method by which various microorganisms, such as bacteria and viruses, are killed. Forms of sterilization include boiling, dry heat, exposure to steam at high pressure, exposure to various gases or liquids, or exposure to radioactivity. The method used depends on the material to be sterilized.

Sterilization is also the term used to describe an operation to make a man or woman infertile.

Q: *How is a man sterilized?*

A: A man can be sterilized by having a vasectomy, a simple operation that can be performed under a local anesthetic, usually taking less than half an hour. Each vas deferens (the duct that carries sperm from the testicle) is cut and the ends tied. *See also* VASECTOMY.

Q: *How is a woman sterilized?*

A: There are two procedures that can be used to sterilize a woman, salpingectomy or tubal ligation. Salpingectomy is the surgical removal of both fallopian tubes. Tubal ligation is the alteration of the fallopian tubes, usually by cutting them and tying off the ends. The operations are normally performed by means of an abdominal incision, under a general anesthetic. The woman may have to remain hospitalized for two or three days. A tubal ligation can also be performed using a laparoscope. *See also* SALPINGECTOMY; STERILIZATION, LAPAROSCOPIC; TUBAL LIGATION.

Q: *Can sterilization be reversed in men or women?*

A: Yes, but the chances of success are small. Both the ends of a fallopian tube (if not removed during a salpingectomy) or a vas deferens can be rejoined by careful, skilled surgery. Even so, the likelihood of an egg or sperm getting through and producing a pregnancy is low.

Sterilization, laparoscopic (ster ə lə zā'shən, lap ə rə skop'ik). Laparoscopic sterilization is a surgical technique in which a woman's fallopian tubes are altered so as to block passage of the male's sperm to the ovum, thus preventing conception.

This is accomplished by cutting or destroying a portion of the tube with electric current and then sealing the ends, or by using a metal or plastic clip or a rubber band to block the tubes. This procedure is performed using an instrument called a laparoscope inserted through a small incision at the umbilicus (navel).

This sterilization procedure may be performed under local anesthetic. Only a short hospital stay is required, and it is often performed on an ambulatory basis ("one day" surgery), in which the patient is released from the hospital the same day as surgery. Sterilization of this nature may also be performed via an abdominal incision.

It must be noted that laparoscopic sterilization procedures are not 100 percent effective.

See also LAPAROSCOPY; STERILIZATION.

Sternum (stėr'nəm), or breastbone, is a flat, dagger-shaped bone that forms the front, middle part of the chest wall. It is about seven inches (17cm) long in men, five inches (13cm) long in women, and one-and-one-half inches (4cm) across at its widest part.

The sternum is made up of three segments: the widest, top part (the manubrium), also known as the handle; the body of the sternum; and the tip (the xiphoid process or xiphisternum). In children, the three parts of the sternum are jointed. In adults they are fused to form one continuous bone.

Anomalies of the sternum may produce a protuberant, pigeon-chested appearance or a sunken, funnel-chested appearance. These relatively common anomalies do not usually cause any major problems.

See also PIGEON BREAST.

Steroid (ster'oid) is a class of chemical compounds. The term is commonly applied to the corticosteroid hormones produced by the adrenal glands. Other steroids include the reproductive hormones progesterone, estrogen, and testosterone, as well as bile salts and cholesterol.

See also CHOLESTEROL; CORTICOSTEROID; ESTROGEN; PROGESTERONE; TESTOSTERONE.

Steroid, anabolic (ster'oid, an ə bol'ik). Anabolic steroids are any of a number of compounds, produced either synthetically or derived from the male hormone testosterone. They help stimulate skeletal muscle development and growth and are also responsible for the development and maintenance of secondary sexual characteristics. *See also* SEXUAL CHARACTERISTICS, SECONDARY.

Anabolic steroids are used by some athletes who claim that they improve muscle strength and endurance, a claim disputed by most physicians and medical scientists. The use of anabolic steroids in competitive sports remains controversial and is illegal. Possible side effects of usage include liver damage and the appearance of male physical characteristics in females. The steroids may also depress blood concentrations of testosterone, resulting in decreased testicle size and sperm production.

Anabolic steroids are sometimes prescribed to treat certain types of anemia and advanced breast cancer. They are also used for replacement therapy in certain hormone deficiency states. *See also* ANEMIA; CANCER; ESTROGEN REPLACEMENT THERAPY.

Stethoscope (steth'ə skōp) is an instrument for listening to the internal sounds of the body. The medical term for such listening is "auscultation."

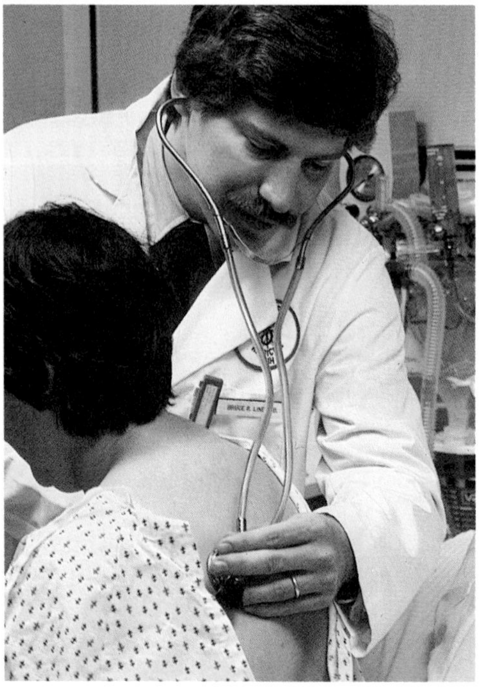

A **stethoscope** can pick up sound from the front or the back of a patient's chest.

Stevens-Johnson syndrome is a rare skin disorder in which there are painful blisters in the throat and mouth, the conjunctiva of the eyes, and the anal region. It is a severe form of erythema multiforme, which causes red skin lesions shaped like rings or targets. Other reddish nodules and sometimes blisters may appear on the arms and legs. Blisters in the throat may be so painful as to prevent swallowing. The syndrome is often caused by an adverse drug reaction. Treatment with corticosteroid drugs may be necessary.

See also CONJUNCTIVA; ERYTHEMA MULTIFORME.

Stiff neck. See NECK, STIFF.

Stiffness (stif'nəs) is a common symptom of disorders of the muscles and joints. It can be accompanied by aching pain. Use of the hands or feet in the affected limb can often lessen the stiffness. Otherwise, anti-inflammatory drugs or massage will relieve the pain. Recurrent morning stiffness is a characteristic of rheumatoid arthritis.

See also ARTHRITIS, RHEUMATOID; MASSAGE.

Stigma (stig'mə) is any physical mark on the body characteristic of a particular disorder.

Stillbirth (stil'bėrth) is the birth of a dead fetus after 20 weeks of pregnancy. It can result from various disorders, such as congenital anomalies in the fetus, hemolytic diseases of the newborn, placental insufficiency, or maternal disorders, such as diabetes mellitus or heart disease.

See also MISCARRIAGE.

Still's disease (stilz) is a juvenile form of rheumatoid arthritis. Initial symptoms include a sudden, high fever, vague rashes that appear and disappear all over the body, and enlargement of the lymph glands and spleen. The fever may continue for several weeks before any joint pain occurs, or the joints may become swollen and tender within a few days.

Anti-inflammatory drugs are usually prescribed until spontaneous improvement occurs. Corticosteroids may be given to treat severe cases. Physiotherapy and a diet containing additional protein, calcium, and vitamins help to speed recovery.

See also ARTHRITIS, RHEUMATOID.

Stimulant (stim'yə lənt) is a drug or other agent that increases the activity of an organ or other part of the body.

See also AMPHETAMINE.

Sting is the damage and pain caused by contact with the poison from a plant or insect.

Sting: first aid. See BITES AND STINGS: FIRST AID.

Stirrup (stėr'əp) is a U-shaped cup to support the feet during a gynecological examination. Stirrup (stapes) is also the name of one of the three tiny bones in the middle ear.

See also EAR; STAPES.

Stitch (stich) is a term popularly used to refer to a severe pain in the abdomen, usually under the ribcage, that occurs with physical exertion. It is caused by a cramp in the muscles of the abdominal wall.

In surgical practice, the term stitch is equivalent to suture.

See also SUTURE.

Stitch: treatment. A stitch is a cramp-like pain in the abdomen that is caused by a spasm of the diaphragm. It occurs most commonly during exercise, particularly in those persons who are not in good physical condition.

Lay the victim down and gently rub the affected part of the abdomen. *Do not* start to exercise again for at least fifteen minutes after pain has gone.

Stokes-Adams syndrome (stōks'-ad'əmz) is a form of heartblock. The normal electrical impulses that regulate the heartbeat are blocked. The heart first stops contracting and then continues at a much slower rate than normal. The rate may spontaneously return to normal. Stokes-Adams syndrome is characterized by a sudden loss of consciousness, sometimes with immediate recovery, but often followed by a period of faintness, dizziness, and nausea when the patient tries to sit up. The length of these episodes may vary from periods as short as a few seconds to a few minutes. Occasionally, a complete heartblock may persist.

An artificial pacemaker is the most effective form of treatment, although drug treatment may sometimes be used. Stokes-Adams syndrome is most common in the elderly and is associated with coronary heart disease.

See also HEARTBLOCK; PACEMAKER, ARTIFICIAL; PACEMAKER, NATURAL.

Stoma (stō'mə) is either a small opening, such as a skin pore; a surgically created opening, such as the abdominal incision made during a colostomy; or a small surgical opening created between two internal organs, such as between the stomach and small intestine (gastroenterostomy).

See also COLOSTOMY; GASTROENTEROSTOMY.

Stomach (stum'ək) is the muscular storage organ of the intestinal tract. It lies in the upper part of the abdomen, under the liver, and below the left part of the diaphragm.

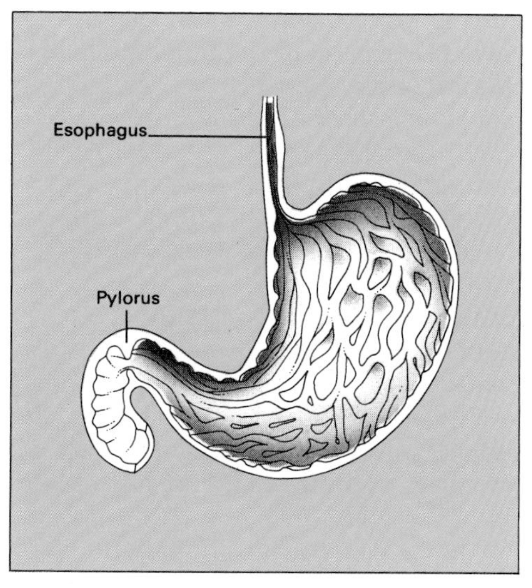

Food enters the **stomach** through the esophagus and leaves, partially digested, through the pylorus.

Food and liquid from the mouth enter the stomach from the esophagus (gullet). The stomach can hold up to 3 pints (1.5l) of fluid.

The three chief activities of the stomach are contracting and squeezing the food it contains: digestion and sterilization of the food by gastric secretions; and intermittent and gradual release of the contents into the duodenum, where digestion continues. The stomach is also able to absorb some substances, such as water, glucose, and alcohol. This explains the rapid effects of these, when they are ingested.

The stomach is composed of three layers of muscle covered with a membrane (the peritoneum). The inner surface is lined with a mucous membrane that secretes gastric juices. The lower and narrow end of the stomach is formed of tough muscle fiber ending in the pyloric sphincter, which controls the exit to the duodenum.

See also DIGESTIVE SYSTEM.

Stomachache (stum'ək āk) is a vague feeling of upper abdominal discomfort, often accompanied by a swelling of the stomach. It is one of the symptoms of indigestion.

See also ABDOMINAL PAIN; INDIGESTION.

Stomach disorders (stum'ək). There are many disorders that may directly involve the stomach. *See also* BELCHING; CANCER; FOOD POISONING; GASTRITIS; GASTROENTERITIS; HYPERCHLORHYDRIA; ULCER.

Many other disorders primarily involve other parts of the body, but can also affect the stomach.

See also ABDOMINAL PAIN; BLOOD, VOMITING OF; COLIC; COLIC, BILIARY; DIARRHEA; FLATULENCE; HYPEREMESIS; INDIGESTION; MOTION SICKNESS; NAUSEA; STENOSIS; PYLOROSPASM; VOMITING.

Stomach, foreign objects in: treatment. Small, rounded objects, such as stones and coins, are often swallowed by children and are rarely harmful. The child's feces should be examined for several days until the object has passed out of the body.

If you suspect that an ingested object is poisonous or sharp, consult a physician immediately. *Do not* attempt to make the person vomit.

Stomatitis (stō mə tī'tis) is inflammation of the mouth. It may be caused by a local disorder in the mouth, or it can occur as the result of generalized disease of the body.

A physician or dentist should be consulted to obtain treatment for the cause of the problem. The mouth must be kept clean with mouthwashes, and any deposits must be cleaned off the teeth and lips. Dehydration may have reduced the amount of salivation, and plenty of fluids should be consumed.

Infection of the salivary glands may occur with stomatitis.

See also SALIVARY GLAND.

Stone. *See* CALCULUS.

Stool (stül) is the common name for feces.

See also FECES.

Strabismus (strə biz'məs), also called a squint, is a condition in which the axes of the eyes are not parallel even when a person is looking at a distant object. It is usually the result of an imbalance in the movement of the two eyes caused by poor muscle control. The attempt to coordinate vision when one eye has better sight than the other (amblyopia) or when one eye has farsightedness (hyperopia) is also called strabismus. In convergent strabismus (crosseye), the axes of the eyes converge; in divergent strabismus (walleye) they diverge.

Q: *What symptoms may develop with strabismus?*

A: If only the unaffected eye is used, the other eye may get worse, and defective vision or blindness may occur in that eye. Paralytic strabismus, caused by paralysis of an eye muscle, results in double vision (diplopia). This may be accompanied by giddiness, vertigo, difficulty in focusing on close objects, and a tendency to incline the head to one side.

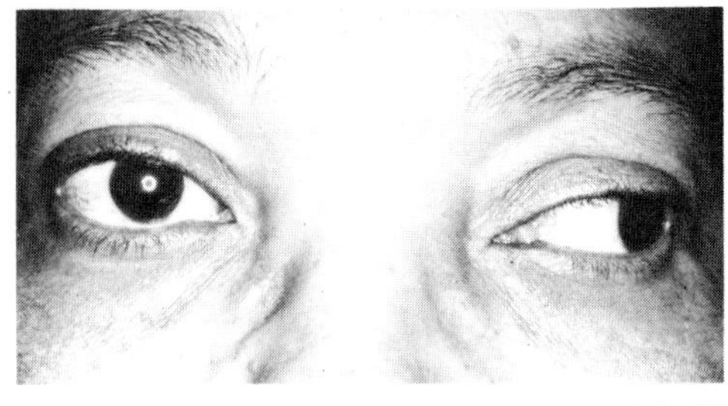

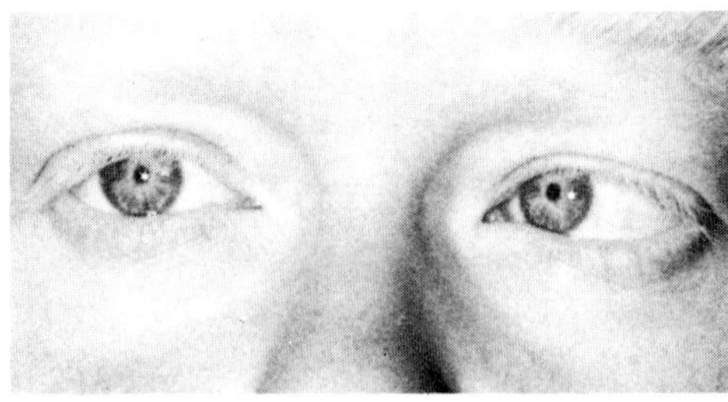

Strabismus is usually caused by the inability of the eye muscles to coordinate eye movements.

Q: *What is the treatment for strabismus?*

A: Depending on an ophthalmic surgeon's assessment of the condition, strabismus can be corrected with eyeglasses or training exercises (orthoptics). If these methods fail or if the amount of ocular deviation is very large, an operation may be carried out to tighten the affected muscle. Treatment of a child with strabismus should begin as soon as the condition is diagnosed, in order to prevent vision loss.

See also AMBLYOPIA; FARSIGHTEDNESS; VISION, DOUBLE.

Strain (strān) is a term that is used to describe either an emotional or a physical disorder.

An emotional strain causes symptoms of fatigue, anxiety, and sometimes depression. This may result in irritability, difficulty in sleeping, and loss of weight.

Physical strain can cause tearing of muscle fibers, resulting in local pain and stiffness. It is less serious than a sprain, which may involve tearing of the ligaments around a joint. Rest, analgesic drugs, physiotherapy, infrared heat treatment, or gentle exercise help a muscle strain to heal.

See also SPRAINS AND STRAINS: TREATMENT; STRESS.

Strain: treatment. *See* SPRAINS AND STRAINS: TREATMENT.

Strangulation (strang gyə lā′shən) is the constriction of a tube or passage within the body, which may prevent adequate blood flow to the affected part. It may result in partial or complete obstruction of the affected part. Strangulation is one of the causes of intestinal obstruction.

See also INTESTINAL OBSTRUCTION.

Strawberry mark. *See* HEMANGIOMA, CAPILLARY.

Strep throat. *See* THROAT, STREP.

Streptococcus (strep tə kok′əs) is a genus of bacteria that grows in straight strings or chains, as seen under a microscope. Many streptococci are harmless, normally found in the body without causing any disorder. Some types, however, cause conditions such as sore throat, tonsillitis, impetigo, erysipelas, and puerperal fever. Others may infect wounds. *See also* ERYSIPELAS; IMPETIGO; PUERPERAL FEVER; THROAT, SORE; TONSILLITIS.

Q: *Can streptococcal infections have complications?*

A: Yes. Infection by streptococcus may be followed by an allergic reaction involving other tissues of the body. This can lead to disorders such as acute nephritis, rheumatic fever, chorea, and scarlet fever. *See also* CHOREA; NEPHRITIS; RHEUMATIC FEVER; SCARLET FEVER.

Q: *How are streptococcal infections treated?*

A: Almost all streptococcal infections respond to penicillin. This treatment usually produces a cure if used for at least 10 days. Persons allergic to penicillin are given erythromycin or other drugs effective against streptococci.

See also ERYTHROMYCIN; PENICILLIN.

Streptokinase (strep tō kī nās′) is a nonenzymatic protein that loosens or dissolves blood clots, pus, and other waste matter associated with infections. It is derived from secretions of a particular strain of the streptococcal bacteria. Streptokinase is used medically to treat heart attacks, deep vein thrombosis, and pulmonary embolism.

See also EMBOLISM; THROMBOSIS, VENOUS; STREPTOCOCCUS.

Streptomycin (strep tə mī′sin) is a powerful antibiotic of the aminoglycoside group. It is obtained from a group of microorganisms named *Streptomyces*. It is used in the treatment of tuberculosis, typhoid fever, and certain other bacterial infections. Side effects include possible kidney damage, deafness, and weakness in the muscles. As with any antibiotic, allergic reactions are also possible.

Stress is a physical and psychological reaction to excessive stimulus. It is considered by some experts to be a psychological disorder caused by constant mental strain; but it is also a physiological response.

Physical stress on various parts of the body can cause damage. For example, repeated minor injuries to a bone, such as one in the leg or foot of a runner, may cause a stress fracture in that bone.

Psychological stress, to a minor degree, is necessary for normal alertness and awareness, but excessive stress can have the opposite effect. The most common cause of psychological stress is fatigue, and a state of stress may be aggravated by a physical illness or by a mental disorder such as depression. *See also* DEPRESSION.

Q: *What are the symptoms of stress?*

A: Symptoms of stress vary. Some people appear on the outside to be calm, but are inwardly in turmoil; others panic. Some people experi-

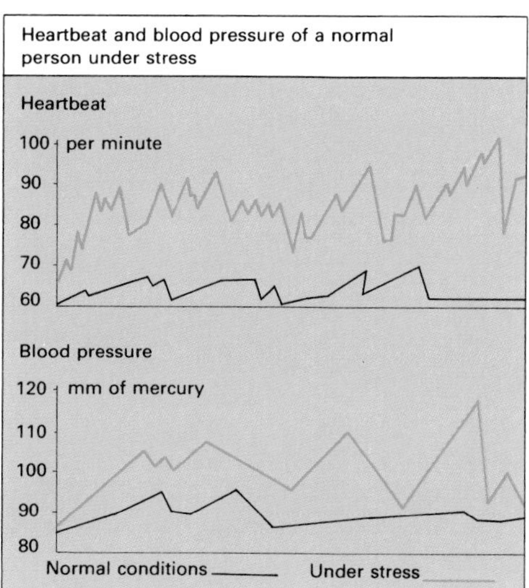

Stress can be measured in terms of specific physiological responses to external factors.

Adult stress chart

This chart assigns numerical values to various life events. Studies indicate that a person who accumulates 150 to 300 points within a 12-month period has a 50 percent chance of coming down with an illness requiring hospitalization. A 12-month score of 300 points raises the risk of serious illness to 90 percent.

Event	*Value*
1. Death of spouse	100
2. Divorce	73
3. Marital separation	65
4. Jail term	63
5. Death of close family member	63
6. Personal injury, illness	53
7. Marriage	50
8. Dismissed from job	47
9. Marital reconciliation	45
10. Retirement	45
11. Change in health of family member	44
12. Pregnancy	39
13. Sex difficulties	39
14. Gain of new family member	39
15. Business readjustment	39
16. Change in financial state	38
17. Death of close friend	37
18. Change to different line of work	36
19. Change in number of arguments with spouse	35
20. Mortgage over $10,000	31
21. Foreclosure of mortgage or loan	30
22. Change in responsibilities at work	29
23. Son or daughter leaving home	29
24. Trouble with in-laws	29
25. Outstanding personal achievement	28
26. Wife begins or stops work	26
27. Begin or end school	26
28. Change in living conditions	25
29. Revision of personal habits	24
30. Trouble with boss	23
31. Change in work hours or conditions	20
32. Change of residence	20
33. Change of school	20
34. Change of recreation	19
35. Change of church activities	19
36. Change of social activities	18
37. Mortgage or loan less than $10,000	17
38. Change in sleeping habits	16
39. Change in number of family get-togethers	15
40. Change in eating habits	15
41. Vacation	13
42. Christmas	12
43. Minor violation of law	11

Reprinted with permission of *Journal of Psychosomatic Research*, Holmes, T.H., and Rahe, R.H., "The Social Readjustment Rating Scale," copyright 1967, Pergamon Press, Ltd.

ence great discomfort in acute stress; they become hot and sweaty, have a rapid heartbeat, or even vomit or faint. Others experience sleep difficulty, headaches, stomachaches, chest pains, or tearfulness. *See also* ANXIETY; PANIC ATTACK.

Q: *What physical disorders can stress produce?*

A: Disorders produced by stress vary greatly, but there are many disorders that can be triggered or made worse by psychological stress, particularly when it is combined with anxiety or depression. Asthma and migraine are likely to occur more frequently with stress. Stress can also be a factor in causing peptic ulcer, irritable bowel syndrome, and ulcerative colitis.

In some people, the onset of hyperthyroidism (overactivity of the thyroid gland) is associated with a period of stress. Neurodermatitis, a skin condition accompanied by intense irritation, is often a stress disorder. Hyperhidrosis, or excessive sweating, is thought to be affected by stress.

Heavy, prolonged menstrual periods (menorrhagia) occur in some women as a result of continued stress, and in younger women may even lead to a cessation of periods (amenorrhea).

Q: *How is stress treated?*

A: A person who suspects that he or she is suffering from stress should consult a physician. The physician will be able to decide whether external stress is the main factor or whether the condition is caused by depression or a phobic anxiety state. The physician will also be able to give medication or advice that may help to relieve the symptoms of stress. External stress is most safely and effectively treated by stress reduction; by relaxation training; and by changing one's attitude toward whatever is causing the stress. Support from family or friends is important in reducing stress levels. A referral to a mental health professional may be indicated to learn more effective coping techniques, such as relaxation training, or to be counseled on long-standing problems that are affecting one's ability to cope with stress.

See also STRESS MANAGEMENT.

Stress incontinence (in kon′tə nəns) is the inability to prevent loss of urine during physical stress, such as coughing, laughing, or sudden movement. It may be caused by a structural abnormality, such as a prolapse of the uterus. In such cases, the uterus may pull the bladder from its normal position and weaken the muscle that closes the bladder. Women who suffer from stress incontinence should consult a physician to determine the cause and the appropriate treatment.

Conservative treatment may include Kegel's exercises to strengthen the pelvic muscles surrounding the urethra, as well as topical estrogen therapy for women past menopause. If these measures fail, surgery may be needed.

See also PROLAPSE.

Stress management is the understanding of stress and its symptoms, and the performing of activities that increase relaxation and, therefore, reduce stress.

Fatigue is a signal for rest and relaxation. The changes in the body that produce fatigue are not fully understood. A person naturally feels tired at the end of a stressful day or after heavy physical exercise. A violently stressful situation, a car crash for instance, produces severe fatigue a few minutes after the event, even if the person is not injured by the accident. If a person does not rest and sleep properly, important faculties such as concentration and reflexes are impaired.

Fatigue also changes a person's ability to cope with stress. In some per-

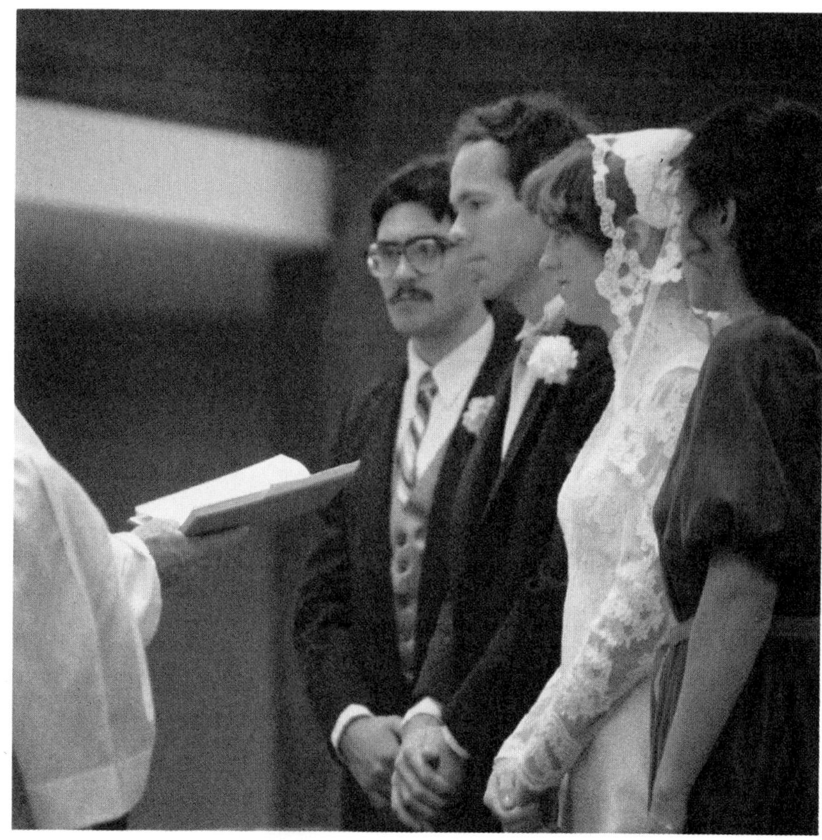

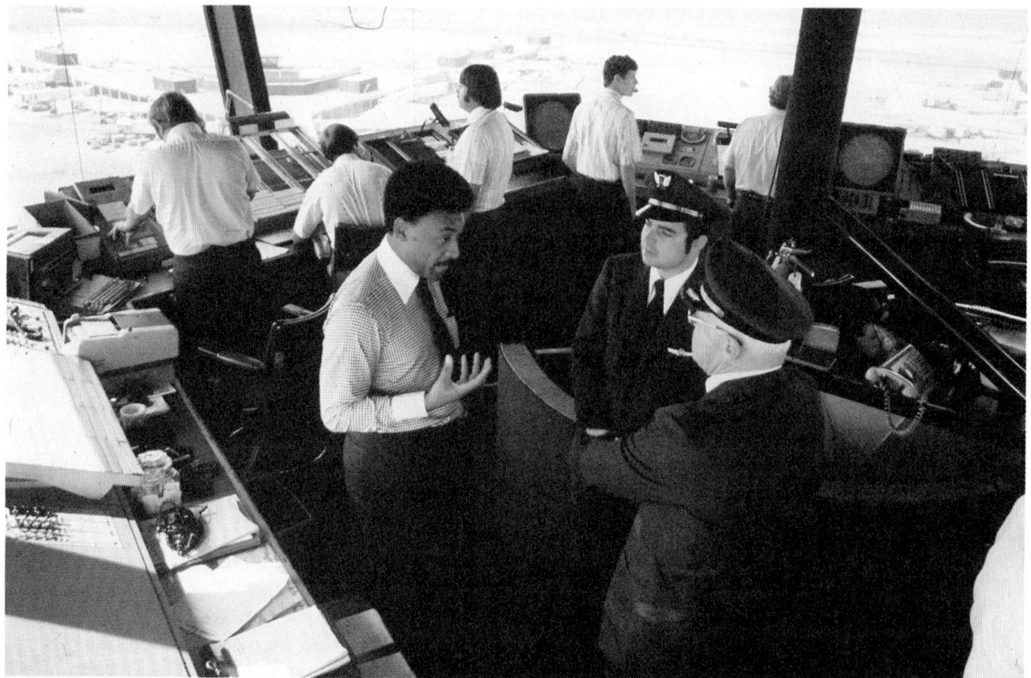

Two stimuli that can produce **stress** include a wedding, *above,* which signals a major change in lifestyle for most people, and air traffic control, *left,* a type of work in which a small mistake can be the difference between life and death for many people.

sons, stress contributes to disorders like diarrhea, migraine, skin eruptions, and even asthma. Also, many authorities believe that stress may have a direct link with high blood pressure and coronary heart disease. If a person pushes himself or herself to the limits of fatigue, he or she is unable to deal adequately with stress, and health suffers.

Coping with Stress

Rest and Relaxation. A relaxed person is better equipped to cope with the pressures of everyday living. Many people find it difficult to relax and need to be taught relaxation techniques in order to stop wasting energy on needless activity.

Relaxing is a skill. Physical relaxation is best obtained after a period of intense activity, such as a sports game or jogging. This principle applies to relaxation exercises that help a person to be aware of the tone of the body muscles. It is easy to feel when a muscle is tensed for activity, but difficult to feel when it is fully relaxed. Relaxation exercises systematically tense the muscles throughout the body, starting at the toes and working upward toward the head. Then there is a conscious "letting go" or relaxing of the muscles. The person can then begin to distinguish between a tense muscle and a relaxed one. It is at this point that a person can start, after much practice, to "automatically" relax.

Deep breathing with the diaphragm is also a good way to help relaxation. Lie or sit down comfortably. Place the hands on the abdomen just below the rib cage. Slowly inhale through the nostrils, and feel the diaphragm descending and pulling the fingers open. Feel the chest expansion spread upward to the shoulders. Hold the breath for a few seconds, and then slowly exhale through the nostrils. At the end of the exhalation, concentrate on the rib and shoulder muscles in their relaxed state. Many people find that four or five deep breaths prepare them for any stressful situation. Diaphragmatic breathing is a relaxation skill that can be performed throughout the day. It lowers the heart rate as it increases the oxygen intake of the body.

Some people find that meditation and professional relaxation exercises (for example, yoga) are two methods of successful deep relaxation. This enables the person to dismiss all other thoughts from the mind.

Relaxation is often taught in prenatal classes. In the early months of pregnancy, fatigue may increase feelings of nausea. Most obstetricians recommend

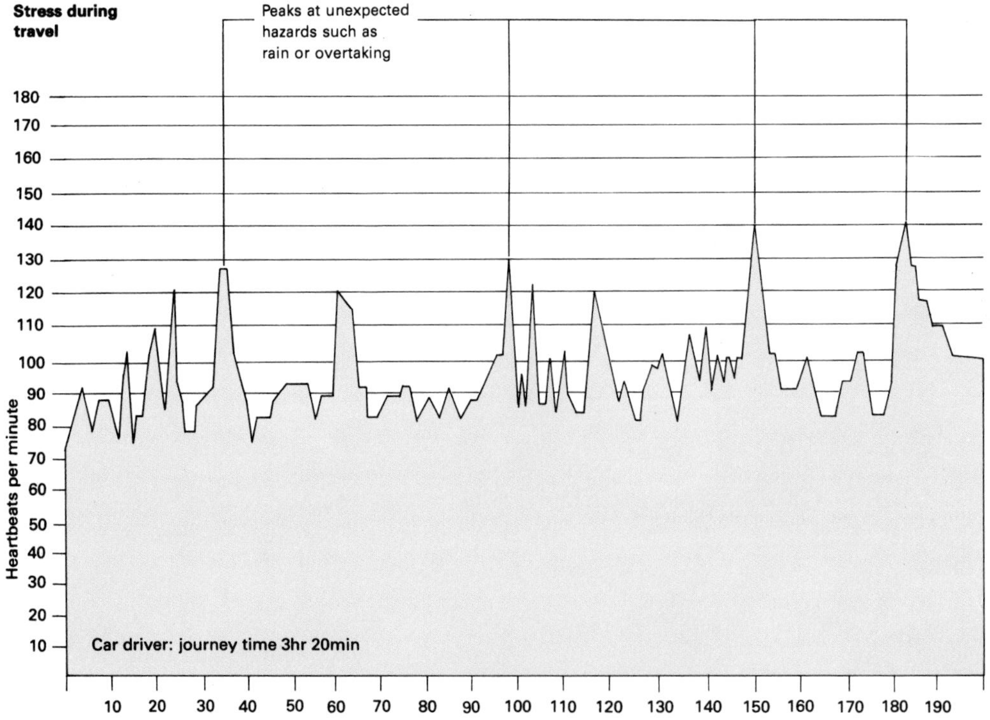

a rest period of two hours a day, preferably after lunch.

The aim of relaxation and deep breathing during childbirth is to conserve the woman's energy for effective muscle control throughout labor. Many women continue relaxation and breathing exercises after the baby is born. A new mother should take every opportunity during the daytime to rest and relax while the baby sleeps. This enables her to make up for some of the sleep that may have been lost earlier.

Chronic fatigue produced by the monotony of many kinds of work can be cured only by a long relaxation period. A vacation should be at least two weeks long, because it takes two to three days for a person to recover from acute fatigue, aggravated by traveling and organizing the vacation, and another week to overcome chronic fatigue. It is only after about 10 days that the benefits of a vacation take effect.

Intercontinental travelers often suffer from jet lag because of the change of time zone. A person must have a period of rest on arrival and should postpone all important decisions until after a night's sleep.

It is also important to rest after a meal. Digestion requires additional blood flow through the intestine after a meal. Physical activity disrupts digestion because the blood is concentrated in the muscles for exercise. The main meals of each day should be followed by a half hour of physical relaxation.

Sleep. Although most persons spend a third of each 24-hour day asleep, no one fully understands why the body has to sleep. Without sleep a person begins to hallucinate, and mental faculties quickly deteriorate.

When a person is asleep, body metabolism is slower, and breathing rate and heart rate both drop. Body temperature also drops, and there is a reduction in muscle tone.

Sleep occurs in several stages. About three-quarters of sleep time is spent in deep sleep. An electroencephalogram during this period indicates slow waves of brain activity. However, there are several periods throughout the night when the waves of brain activity become very active. The eyes move from side to side beneath the eyelids. This is known as rapid eye movement, or REM. During these periods the person is dreaming.

Sleep requirements vary from person to person and from age to age. A newborn baby may need as much as 21 hours of sleep per day. A growing child needs more sleep than an adult, and parents should try to establish a pattern of regular bedtimes for children. Many

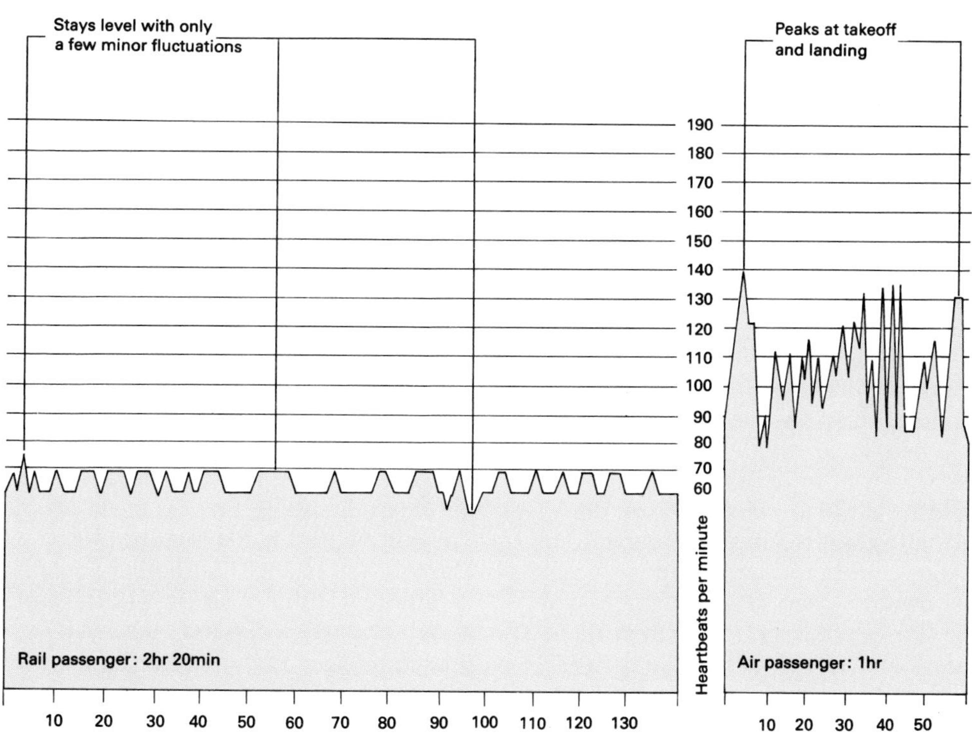

young children wake up early in the morning. Although this is annoying for the rest of the family, it is normal. Make sure that the child has plenty of toys within easy reach to play with until the rest of the household is awake. Children often need a nap during the day. Most young children sleep during the afternoon, but some prefer to go back to sleep after breakfast. Allow the child to set his or her own time for a nap.

A major problem for the parent of an adolescent is trying to encourage the adolescent to get enough sleep. Periods of intense physical and emotional activity are interspersed with periods of extreme lethargy, which are often due to physical and mental fatigue. Sleep rhythms are also broken by the adolescent's need to maintain an active social life. Parents should encourage an adolescent to sleep at least seven hours a night.

Elderly persons tend to require less sleep than an active adult but they make up for sleep lost during the night by napping during the day. *See also* SLEEP.

Insomnia is a much misused word. Throughout a night's sleep a person is drifting from deep to shallow sleep, and often wakes up. Most people can not remember how many times they have awakened during the night. But if a person is sure he or she is an "insomniac," a short period of wakefulness may be prolonged with worry.

There are several different types of insomnia. Difficulty falling asleep may be due to anxiety or stress. Early morning awakening is often associated with depression. Inability to remain asleep may result from drug or alcohol abuse.

Sleeping difficulties are often a sign of stress, worry, and depression. A person should not resort to sleeping pills to solve the problem. Other ways of promoting sleep include taking exercise before bed, for example, a short walk; drinking warm milk (tea and coffee should be avoided); and relaxing the mind with light reading. If a person awakens during the night and is unable to get back to sleep, it is preferable that he or she read a book rather then lie in the dark and worry. Often, the distraction of going to the kitchen to get a drink helps a person fall asleep when he or she returns to bed.

Chronic insomnia may have a physical or psychological cause, and in such cases medical advice should be sought. A mental health professional can usually find the underlying reason and prescribe appropriate treatment.

See also INSOMNIA.

Staying Mentally Fit

Mental and emotional health is fundamental for personal happiness, including the ability to develop close friendships and intimate relationships and to gain satisfaction from work, hobbies, and other interests. Mental fitness is just as important a factor in overall health as is physical well-being.

Yet mental illness, in one form or another, is quite common. Many of a physician's daily consultations involve some mental or emotional problem. At any one time, a large percentage of all hospital beds are occupied by those who have emotional problems. One in every ten persons at some time during his or her life needs treatment in a hospital for a mental disorder.

Given the right combination of past experiences and current stresses, anyone can develop psychiatric difficulty, but mental-health experts do not know the specific causes of all types of mental illness. Some mental disorders have physical causes, such as brain injuries, nutritional deficiencies, and poisons; others have psychological causes.

Stress, however, seems to play a major role in triggering emotional problems. Such stress could result, for example, from anxiety about personal relationships, finances, or work. Avoiding excessive stress may prevent some forms of mental illness.

However, the decisions and problems that arise unexpectedly usually cause the most stress—a sick child, an accident, a depressed friend or family member, and other similar situations. It is not possible to avoid these types of stress, so the better equipped a person is to cope, the more likely he or she is to remain mentally fit.

Coping with the Stresses of Life. Many of the factors that help a person handle the ordinary stresses of life can simply involve a common-sense approach to daily activities: getting enough sleep each night; setting aside time for relaxation; avoiding overwork;

discussing problems with family or friends; and cultivating a confident, positive mental attitude.

The amount of sleep required varies from person to person, and even in the same person from night to night. It is important to have a steady and sufficient amount of sleep if you are to avoid chronic fatigue and exhaustion. The amount of sleep needed to feel rested and refreshed indicates how many hours of sleep an individual requires. If insufficient sleep is obtained one night, the next sleep period should be longer to make up for it. It is better to go to bed earlier on the next night rather than to wake up later on the following day.

Another major factor in promoting mental health is having a circle of family members and friends on whom an individual can rely for psychological support or financial aid in times of trouble. The security of such a support group can eliminate or greatly reduce anxiety.

When a problem does arise, discussing it with a family member or friend is often enough to put the problem into its proper perspective. By the same token, a person can attain great satisfaction and feelings of self-worth from supporting another in time of stress, acting as an adviser, helper, or just a good listener.

The more secure a person feels, the more likely he or she is to be mentally healthy. The groundwork for emotional security is laid in childhood. Children need affection, support, understanding of their problems and fears, and a sense of being wanted in the home. Children are often troubled by ordinary fears, such as the dark, or by special circumstances, such as moving to a new house, attending a new school, witnessing an accident or other violent event, experiencing a death in the family, or having to be hospitalized. Children need at least one adult on whom they feel they can rely. The child who grows up in a loving, trusting family environment has the best chance of becoming a mentally healthy adult with a confident, positive outlook on life.

Routine, Boredom, and Change. Setting up a daily routine is an unconscious way of avoiding mental stress. Tasks done through habit cause the minimum amount of difficulty. At the same time, too much routine creates boredom, which in itself can be fatiguing and create stress. As in any other aspect of life, people vary widely in their need for routine in any form without realizing that they do. In fact, most people unconsciously combine routine with change and stimulation in the right proportions to maintain their own mental fitness. If the daily routine is changed, an allowance for additional rest and relaxation should be made until the initial weariness has gone. Changes in routine that are known to be unnecessary generally seem to be more tiring.

A certain amount of change from the daily routine is essential for mental well-being, but major life changes can create a great deal of stress. The loss of a loved one, a new job or home, marriage or divorce, even a change in diet are all sources of added stress. If several major life changes occur within a one-year period, chances of incurring some type of mental, even physical illness, are greatly increased. A person experiencing such major changes should make special efforts to protect his or her mental health by getting enough rest and relaxation.

Taking a Vacation. For most people, vacations are the greatest change from daily routine. Some people gain the most rest and enjoyment from vacations that allow them to pursue favorite pastime activities, such as fishing, sunbathing, boating, hiking, and other sports. Others use vacation time to see new parts of the world, shop, sample different kinds of food, and enjoy foreign cultures.

While vacations are generally beneficial to mental health, they usually require organization and travel, and this can produce varying amounts of mental stress.

Driving a car over a long distance can cause both physical and mental stress, especially if the driver attempts to meet a deadline. With air, ship, bus, or train transport available, the main cause of anxiety can be arriving at the airport, harbor, or station on time. The actual traveling itself is less stressful. However, in every form of transport there may be peaks of anxiety, for example, during take-off and landing and in turbulence in an airplane. Rail travel seems to be the most relaxing way of going from one place to another. Travel on board ship is unique in that passengers' stress levels generally change with the weather. The charts on pages 828 and 829 give some indication of the average stresses experienced on a journey of the same distance using different forms of transport.

Gaining the most benefit from a vacation requires planning and the ability to remain in a calm, unhurried state of mind. On a car journey, motorists should prepare themselves to be late if the unexpected, such as a flat tire or a traffic jam, occurs. Other travelers should be prepared to accept delays in flight, train, or bus schedules.

Planning the details of a vacation early will eliminate the strain of handling last-minute preparations. Vacationers should have tickets, passports, visas, and room reservations well in advance and should make lists of clothing and other items needed for the journey. International travelers must obtain any necessary immunizations or medications and take proper precautions, to protect themselves from infectious diseases present in the countries of destination.

Persons who travel by air from one time zone to another, with a time difference of more than four hours, will still be physically and mentally geared to the original time zone. This is called jet lag. A traveler may require several days to adjust, depending on how great is the time difference between zones. The effects of jet lag can be reduced by organizing the arrival in the new zone during the evening. Meetings and business discussion should then take place only after a night's rest, if not sleep. If all business discussions can be arranged for times that correspond with working hours in the original "day," then little or no adaptation at all is necessary. *See also* JET LAG; JET LAG: TREATMENT.

An alternative kind of vacation is to enjoy leisure at home in known and nonstressful surroundings. Such a vacation can be used as a time for making new resolutions and for finally sorting out problems that may have seemed too difficult while other day-to-day routines and stresses were in the way.

Relieving Mental Tension. In the daily routine of life, it is not always easy to achieve a proper balance between work and leisure. Many people find it difficult to relax physically and mentally without making a definite effort. The thoughts of the day just ending or worries about events to come—fears, pleasures, embarrassments, and triumphs—create a state of tension that makes relaxation impossible.

There are dozens of techniques to relieve excessive tension, some from the ancient East, others from the modern West. What constitutes an effective method of relaxing depends largely on personal preference. A technique that works well for one individual might not work at all for another. Many factors enter into choosing a relaxation technique, such as the amount of time and discipline needed. Some techniques can be learned by the individual alone, others require more formal instruction.

Many people have found that various forms of meditation relieve tension. In general, meditation involves focusing on a thought, word, phrase, or object to calm the mind. Some meditation techniques also involve breathing exercises. Scientists have found that during meditation the body undergoes physical changes, such as slower heartbeat or lower blood pressure, which indicate a state of deep relaxation.

Some people find that simply envisioning peaceful or pleasant scenes helps relieve tension. Many books explaining other meditation and thought control techniques have been written and are widely available in bookstores and libraries.

Other Eastern systems that have been modified and adapted in the West to promote relaxation and peace of mind include some of the Japanese martial arts and the Chinese exercise, tai chi, as well as transcendental meditation and yoga.

Because there appears to be a direct connection between mental and muscular tension, some scientists have experimented with relieving mental tension by relaxing the muscles. Using a system called "progressive relaxation," a person alternately tenses and relaxes various muscles to become more aware of the degrees of tension and relaxation that he or she can achieve. A similar technique, called "autogenic training," involves suggestions that various parts of the body are warm, heavy, and relaxed. These types of relaxation techniques are best learned from a therapist.

One of the newest relaxation techniques involves biofeedback. Researchers have found that biofeedback is useful in relaxing muscles, lowering blood pressure, and increasing the long, slow brain waves called alpha waves. Electronic sensors are placed on the skin to monitor bodily conditions, such as skin temperature, muscle tension, and brain waves. Once a person receives feedback on a monitor that his or her brain waves have changed, indicating excessive tension, he or she can direct the body to correct this condition. Because the sensitive electronic equipment involved must be calibrated carefully and the electrodes placed precisely, it is advisable that this technique be practiced under the supervision of a biofeedback expert if the technique is to be successful.

Many people find inner calm and peace through sincere religious beliefs. For them, prayer and worship produce a state of profound joy and contentment that contributes greatly to their mental well-being. A strong religious faith can also help a person cope with the various crises that arise in life. Even those who do not have religious beliefs often have some kind of faith, perhaps in a particular philosophy of life, that helps contribute to emotional stability and provides underlying mental strength.

Onset of Mental Problems. Everyone, on occasion, experiences the unpleasant emotions of anger, frustration, sadness, mild depression, worry, loneliness, and uncertainty. This is normal. Sometimes, these feelings persist for long periods of time or grow more intense. This could be a sign that mental or emotional problems are developing. These feelings could stem from a specific cause, but often there seems to be no apparent reason.

Other indications of mental problems include alcoholism, drug abuse, suicidal thoughts or actions, irrational fears, sexual difficulties, obsessive thoughts, and compulsions to perform the same acts repeatedly.

Sometimes, problems arise within a family that can best be remedied with outside help. These may include a troubled child, marital difficulties involving household finances, and sexual problems.

Treatment for Mental Problems. Mental problems can be treated with drugs, psychotherapy, or both. Some therapists probe a person's past experiences to uncover connections with present feelings and behavior. Others concentrate on changing thought patterns or behavior, without going through the longer process of looking for the cause. Some people prefer individual counseling, others prefer group therapy, in which the group members share and discuss their feelings and problems. A special type of counseling is also available for all members of a family. *See also* BEHAVIOR THERAPY; FAMILY THERAPY; PSYCHOANALYSIS.

Persons feeling in need of such professional help should contact a local mental-health center or ask their religious leader or family physician for a referral. In addition, many communities have specialized services for problems such as alcoholism and drug abuse and for the mental and emotional needs of the elderly.

Seeking Professional Help. Many people benefit from discussing their problems with the family physician and having an examination to determine whether there is an underlying physical cause. Others may seek advice from their priests, ministers, or rabbis, many of whom have received training in family counseling. Sometimes the service of a marriage counselor, psychiatrist, psychologist, social worker, or psychiatric nurse can provide the most help toward relieving anxiety, fear, and tension.

Schools often have social workers to help with the problems of children. Many communities also have crisis "hotlines" that troubled individuals can call for immediate advice on how to handle problems or where to get additional help.

Just as important to mental well-being as maintaining good habits of rest and relaxation is knowing when help is needed.

See also MENTAL HEALTH.

"Stress test" is a test that measures the functioning of the cardiopulmonary and the respiratory systems of the body. The patient is hooked up to an ECG and then walks on a treadmill or rides a stationary bicycle. Functions, such as consumption of oxygen by the lungs and the change in the heartbeat, are carefully monitored, as the amount of physical stress is slowly increased.

See also ELECTROCARDIOGRAM; THALLIUM STRESS TEST.

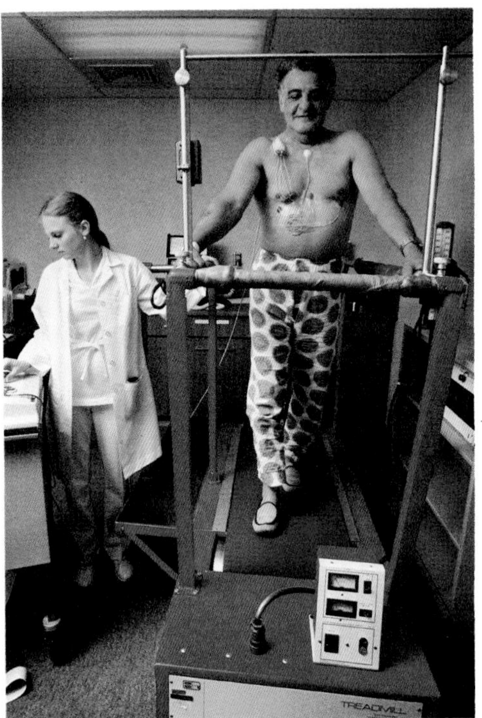

To perform a **stress test,** a patient walks on a treadmill while an ECG (electrocardiogram) measures various body functions.

Stretch marks, or striae, are the streaks, usually several inches in length, that commonly appear on the abdomen, thighs, and breasts of women who are or have been pregnant. The marks are normal, the result of skin tension due to hormonal activity.

Stretch marks can also be caused by obesity or other conditions that stretch the skin.

Stricture (strik′chər) is an abnormal narrowing of a duct or passage within the body. It may be caused by inflammation; injury, with subsequent scarring of the tissues; a muscle spasm; or pressure, as from a growth or tumor. Strictures may also be caused by a congenital anomaly, such as Hirschsprung's disease.

See also HIRSCHSPRUNG'S DISEASE; STENOSIS.

Stridor (strī′dər) is a high-pitched rasping sound produced by partial obstruction of the vocal cords. It is a common condition in children with croup. Stridor may also be produced by inflammation or tumors of the larynx or vocal cords.

Stroke (strōk), also known as apoplexy, is a stoppage of the blood supply to part of the brain. The blockage can have one of three causes: (1) a blood clot, from somewhere else in the body (embolus), obstructing an artery; (2) clotting within an artery (cerebral thrombosis); or (3) the bursting of a blood vessel (cerebral hemorrhage). A stroke may be a relatively minor occurrence, and temporary strokes that are followed by complete recovery also occur.

Transient, temporary strokes may occur as a result of disturbances in blood flow to the brain. This may be caused by constriction of the carotid and vertebral arteries in the neck by patches of arteriosclerosis in their walls. These constrictions reduce the blood supply so that a slight drop in blood pressure, from any cause, may produce a stroke. This is particularly likely to occur in an elderly person and may be the result of illness, coronary thrombosis, or cardiac irregularities such as atrial fibrillation, as well as anemia, sudden blood loss, or pressure on the neck from a tight collar. Temporary strokes may also occur from small emboli, usually blood clots, that form on the arteriosclerotic areas of the arteries, or sometimes from damaged heart valves that have been caused by subacute endocarditis. These small particles cause a momentary blockage of a small artery in the brain, which produces symptoms that disappear without loss of consciousness.

Q: *What are the symptoms of a stroke?*

A: The symptoms depend on the area of the brain that is involved. In an acute stroke, breathing is difficult, and there is paralysis of part of the body, often affecting one whole side of the body, including the face, torso, and one leg and arm. The skin feels clammy to the touch, and speech may be affected. Loss of consciousness may occur extremely rapidly. Occasionally a

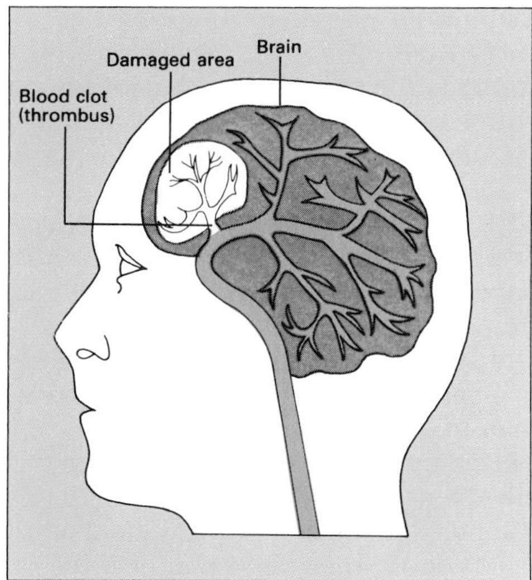

A **stroke** is caused by a blood clot that stops the blood supply from reaching an area of the brain, or the rupture of a blood vessel in the brain.

patient may remain conscious, but confused. A temporary stroke may produce all the symptoms of a severe stroke, but the person usually recovers completely after a short time.

Q: *What can be done to help someone who has a stroke?*

A: An ambulance must be called immediately. Keep the patient quiet and warm (with a rug or blanket), either sitting up or lying down with the head and shoulders raised. An unconscious patient should be placed in the recovery position. The patient should not be moved until professional help arrives, unless it is essential. Give no food or drink, and keep the head and neck cool. *See also* FAINTING: FIRST AID.

Q: *What is the hospital treatment for stroke patients?*

A: Careful nursing is necessary, including constant exercise of the limbs, to prevent stiffening or shrinking of the muscles. Many routine actions (such as walking and sitting down) may have to be learned again. This is the task of a physiotherapist. A speech therapist helps the patient to speak normally again. Recovery from a stroke is never speedy because retraining, a long and slow process, may take several months or even years.

It is rare that the cause of a stroke can be actively treated. Anticoagulants will make a cerebral hemorrhage worse, therefore they can only be given if the physician considers that a slowly progressing stroke is due to cerebral thrombosis. Occasionally a neurosurgeon will operate if an aneurysm has been found to be the cause of subarachnoid hemorrhage or, less commonly, to remove a large clot following a cerebral hemorrhage. Rarely, hemorrhage occurs underneath (subdural) or outside (epidural) the dural layers that surround the brain. These hemorrhages can be diagnosed by the appropriate neurological investigations and can be treated surgically. *See also* ANEURYSM.

Q: *What are the patient's chances of making a full recovery from a stroke?*

A: Each case must be judged on the severity of its symptoms. In the most severe cases, patients fail to regain consciousness at all and die shortly after an attack.

Many patients return to normal health, however, with only a slight speech defect and perhaps some awkwardness in walking or handling objects. In some cases, people are left paralyzed on one side (hemiplegia), with a speech disorder (aphasia) and an inability to control bladder and bowel functions (incontinence).

Q: *Can strokes be prevented?*

A: In the majority of people there is no way of preventing a stroke. Exceptions incude those with arteriosclerosis, who may be helped by regular doses of aspirin or other anticoagulants under the supervision of a physician, and people with high blood pressure or diabetes in whom these conditions can be controlled. Transient strokes are often a warning that a major stroke will occur. If the cause, such as a constriction in a carotid artery, can be found, an operation to remove the affected part of the artery may be a cure. Control of cardiac irregularities is necessary to prevent a sudden drop in blood pressure, and damage to the heart valves from endocarditis must be treated at once. *See also* ENDOCARDITIS.

The majority of strokes occur in elderly people and are the consequence of arteriosclerosis, which can not be treated effectively once it has occurred.

Stroke patient, aids for. *See* NURSING THE SICK.

Strongyloides (stron ji̦ loi'dēs) is a genus of roundworms, one species of which, *Strongyloides stercoralis*, is a common intestinal parasite in people who live in hot climates. Infestation with this roundworm, which is also known as the threadworm, is called strongyloidiasis.

There may be no symptoms if the infestation is light. But migration of larvae through the lungs usually produces a cough. Heavy infestations may also cause abdominal pain, vomiting, and diarrhea.

In most cases, drug treatment with thiabendazole is effective. It is advisable to have regular drug treatment in areas where the parasite is common.

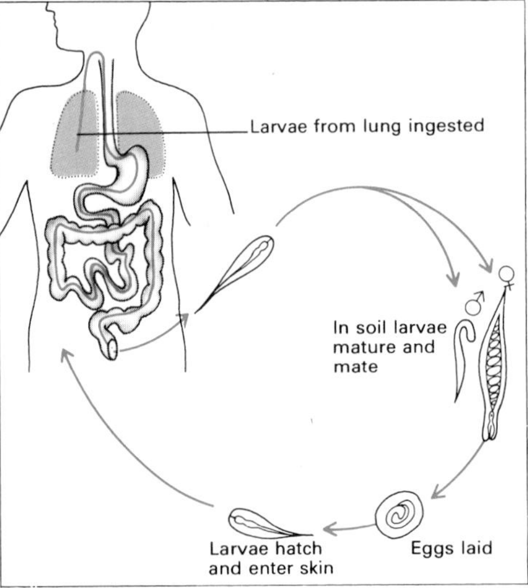

Strongyloides is a roundworm that enters the bloodstream after penetrating intact skin.

Strychnine (strik'nin) is a poisonous alkaloid obtained from the seeds of the tree *Nux-vomica*. Strychnine poisoning causes extreme activity of the central nervous system, leading to repeated muscle spasms (convulsions) that may end in death. Treatment of strychnine poisoning is the immediate washing out of the victim's stomach, supporting the victim's respiration as needed, and the administration of diazepam to relax the muscle spasms.

Stuffy nose. *See* NOSE, STUFFY.

Stupor (stü'pər) is a state of semicoma, with suppression of the senses and of the normal thought processes.

See also COMA.

Stuttering (stut'ər ing), or stammering, is a speech disorder in which speech is faltering or hesitant, and the initial sounds of words are repeated. It usually starts between the ages of two and five years and is more common in boys than in girls. In many children, it is caused by psychological factors and may be aggravated by parental anxiety. If there is no sign of improvement after the child is seven years old, or if the stuttering gets worse, a speech therapist should be consulted.

Sty (stī), medically known as a hordeolum, is an abscess of a sebaceous (grease-producing) gland on or under the eyelid. It is caused by a bacterial infection and is commonly associated with blepharitis (inflammation of the eyelid).

The symptoms of a sty include swelling, redness, and pain. When the sty bursts, there is relief from pain and an immediate improvement.

Treatment is to bathe the sty with a clean cloth soaked repeatedly in hot water.

See also BLEPHARITIS.

Styptic (stip'tik) is a substance, such as alcohol, silver nitrate, or alum, that stops bleeding by its astringent action.

Subacute bacterial endocarditis. *See* ENDOCARDITIS, BACTERIAL.

Subarachnoid (sub ə rak'noid) refers to the space between the arachnoid and the pia mater. These are the second and third meninges (membranes) covering the brain and spinal cord.

See also MENINGES.

Subarachnoid hemorrhage. *See* HEMORRHAGE, SUBARACHNOID.

Subclavian (sub klā'vē ən) describes anything that lies beneath the clavicle (collarbone).

See also CLAVICLE.

Subconjunctival hemorrhage. *See* HEMORRHAGE, SUBCONJUNCTIVAL.

Subconscious (sub kon'shəs) describes mental activity that occurs just beneath the levels of normal conscious awareness. Psychoanalysts define it as a level between the conscious and the unconscious.

Subcutaneous (sub kyü tā'nē əs) means beneath the skin and above the underlying layers of tissue, such as muscle. The subcutaneous layer contains fat and connective tissue and varies in thickness in different parts of the body.

See also SKIN.

Subdural hematoma. *See* HEMATOMA, SUBDURAL.

Sublingual gland (sub ling'gwəl) is the smallest of the salivary glands. There are two sublingual glands located between the side of the tongue and the jawbone, one on each side of the face.

See also SALIVARY GLAND.

Subluxation (sub luk sā'shən) is a partial or incomplete dislocation. It may occur in a joint or in the lens of the eye.

See also DISLOCATION.

Submandibular gland (sub man dib'ye lər) is one of the salivary glands. There are two submandibular glands, one on each side of the mouth under the jawbone and below the back teeth.

See also SALIVARY GLAND.

Submaxillary gland (sub mak'sə ler ē) is another name for the submandibular gland.

See also SUBMANDIBULAR GLAND.

Submucous resection (sub myü'kəs ri sek'shən) is a common operation on the nose, carried out under a local or general anesthetic, to correct a deviated nasal septum. The operation removes the deformed part of the nasal septum (the cartilage and bone that divide the nostrils), allowing the two layers of mucous membrane to take up a straight position along the midline.

See also SEPTUM, DEVIATED.

Succus entericus (suk'əs en ter'i kus) is the secretion of the glands that line the small intestine. It contains various enzymes essential for the digestion of food.

See also DIGESTIVE SYSTEM.

Sudden infant death syndrome (SIDS), also known as cot death and crib death, is thought to be a respiratory illness that usually affects infants under the age of six months.

Q: *Are some babies more likely than others to succumb to SIDS?*

A: Such deaths are more likely to occur in families living in crowded conditions, during the winter months, and in bottle-fed infants. SIDS is more common at night than in daytime. Boys of low birth weight succumb more often than do girls under similar conditions.

Q: *What causes SIDS?*

A: During sleep, the respiration of all infants is irregular, with brief periods when breathing stops completely. But if respiration stops for longer than 15 or 20 seconds, death can occur.

In most cases SIDS can not be prevented, because obvious warning symptoms have not yet been discovered. Apnea monitors to detect cessation of breathing may be used at home for high-risk infants, such as premature babies. *See also* APNEA.

In all cases of SIDS, it is the parents who suffer grief and shock, often blaming themselves. The family needs social and psychological support at this time. Help can be provided by the pediatrician, the family's physician, and family counselors. The family can also be helped by their religious adviser, or by contacting the National Sudden Infant Death Syndrome Foundation, which can give immediate counseling and support.

Suffocation (suf ə kā'shən), or asphyxiation, is the result of blockage of the air passage or a reduction or absence of oxygen in the air breathed in.

Brain damage, due to shortage of oxygen, occurs within five minutes if the condition is not treated. Treatment is to clear the airway, if it is obstructed, and give artificial respiration.

See also ARTIFICIAL RESPIRATION.

Suffocation: first aid. *See* ARTIFICIAL RESPIRATION.

Sugar is a sweet-tasting carbohydrate, present in many foods. The sugar commonly used to sweeten food is sucrose, but there are many other sugars. They are either simple monosaccharides (such as dextrose, glucose, and fructose) or disaccharides (such as sucrose, maltose, and lactose).

Sugars are a readily available source of energy and can be broken down by the body to form glucose (blood sugar). Glucose can be reconstructed by the liver and body cells into various other forms of carbohydrates.

Excess intake of sugar contributes to dental caries and obesity and may be a contributory factor in arteriosclerosis.

See also CARBOHYDRATE; GLUCOSE; INSULIN.

Suicide (sü'ə sīd) is the taking of one's own life. It is a common cause of death between the ages of 15 and 40, second only to accidents. However the suicide rate is even higher among the elderly. Attempted suicide is responsible for about 20 percent of all emergency hospital admissions.

In the last few years, teenage suicide has increased significantly. Stress, pressure to succeed, and the use of drugs are among the factors contributing to the increase. Recently the phenomenon of "cluster" and "imitation" suicides has occurred. Research indicates that there is some correlation between television coverage of suicides and the number of suicides following the airing of the programs. Young people who suffer very low self-esteem may feel that, by committing suicide, they will attain importance or significance as a result of the sensationalizing of a behavior which is really motivated by fear and anxiety.

Q: *Why do people try to commit suicide?*

A: Suicide is most common in patients with emotional disorders, such as clinical depression, alcoholism, or schizophrenia, when these disorders are complicated by depressive features. There may be a history of antisocial behavior, delinquency, alcoholism, poor school attendance, poor work record, depression, loneliness, or indications of problems with social relationships. Many persons who attempt suicide do not really want to kill themselves at all. Their attempts are desperate acts to draw attention to their plight.

Hopelessness, usually caused by depression or other forms of mental illness, has been shown to be the most common reason for suicide. In the case of young people, especially, great stress or shame sometimes creates a perception of hopelessness, which leads them to attempt suicide. They feel overwhelmed by a situation, which actually is a temporary stress, which could probably be resolved with help and support.

Q: *How can suicide be prevented?*

A: Seek professional help, if it is thought that a person is likely to commit suicide. If there is time, seek help from the family physician. Alternatively, there are many social or religious groups that specialize in helping the suicidal individual.

A physician may suggest psychotherapy or prescribe antidepressant drugs. Seriously depressed persons

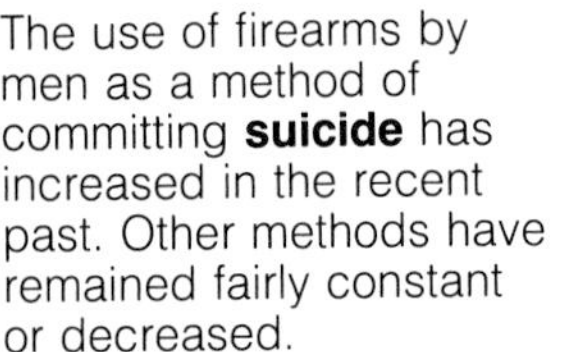

The use of firearms by men as a method of committing **suicide** has increased in the recent past. Other methods have remained fairly constant or decreased.

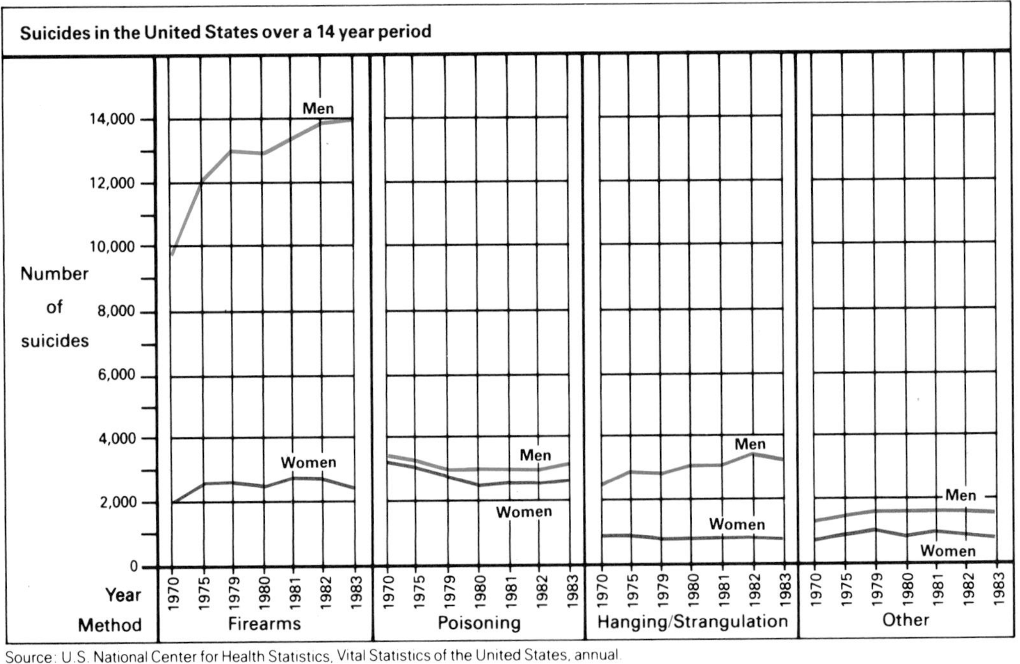

should, however, be hospitalized immediately for observation.

Q: *What should be done if someone has already attempted suicide?*

A: Get the suicide victim to the hospital as quickly as possible. In the meantime, give appropriate first aid. Collect and keep any empty bottles, and look for a suicide note.

If a person telephones to say that he or she has attempted suicide, find out the exact location and address, keep the person talking, and get someone else to call for the police and other emergency aid. Continue talking until help arrives.

Sulfa drug (sul′fə) is an antibacterial drug. There are several related types that are used in the treatment of infection. Sulfonamide is an example of one type.

Possible side effects of sulfa drugs include nausea, diarrhea, vomiting, skin rashes, decreased white blood cell count, and very rarely, Stevens-Johnson syndrome. Careful monitoring of sulfa drugs reduces the likelihood of this happening. *See also* STEVENS-JOHNSON SYNDROME.

Sulfite (sul′fīt) is an inorganic salt or compound of sulfurous acid. Some patients with asthma are quite sensitive to sulfites; an acute asthmatic attack can be triggered by these agents. Since sulfites are used commonly as preservatives in many drugs, appropriate labeling has become necessary. Sulfites are also present in foods, for example, salads; therefore, the sensitive patient must be careful about food selection as well.

Sulfite oxidase is a substance that helps oxidize sulfite to sulfate in the cystoplasm of cells.

Sulfone (sul′fon) is a group of drugs used in the treatment of leprosy and dermatitis herpetiformis. Only the sulfone, dapsone, is available in the United States.

Sunburn occurs after exposure to ultraviolet light. Mild sunburn usually occurs a few hours after exposure as red skin, which eventually peels. Severe sunburn, however, results in extreme pain, swelling, and blistering a few days after excessive exposure, accompanied by fever, weakness, and symptoms of shock. The blisters are second-degree burns and may become infected. *See also* SUNBURN: TREATMENT.

Q: *How is sunburn prevented?*

A: Since everyone is vulnerable to sunburn, everyone, particularly those with fair skins, should take precautions when in the sun. Sunbathing should be avoided during the middle of the day, when the sun's rays are at their strongest, and limited during the remainder of the day. Twenty minutes in the morning and twenty minutes in the evening is enough sun exposure. In addition, sunscreen lotions containing PABA (p-aminobenzoic acid) should be applied regularly for their protective effect. A sunscreen with protective factor of at least 15 provides the best protection.

Q: *Are there any long-term hazards of sunburn?*

A: Yes. Constant exposure to sunlight damages the skin and causes wrinkles. It also alters the skin structure, producing warty lumps called keratosis, which may ultimately form basal cell carcinoma, or cancer of the skin. Malignant melanoma may be the result of severe sun damage to skin.

See also CARCINOMA, BASAL CELL; KERATOSIS; MELANOMA.

Sunburn: treatment. Sunburn is an inflammation of the skin caused by excessive exposure to ultraviolet rays. In mild cases of sunburn, the radiation causes the skin to become red, but with severe sunburn, blisters may form. Later the burned skin flakes off in scales.

A person suffering from a large or severe sunburn may suffer from headaches, dizziness, fever, vomiting, rash, and shock. Sunburn can be avoided by limiting exposure to the sun, avoiding midday sun, and by using a sunscreen that contains PABA (p-aminobenzoic acid). Sunscreens are numerically rated for effectiveness, with a protective factor of at least 15 being the most effective.

Action. Get the victim into the shade immediately. Cool the burned area with cold water or an ice pack. Immersion in a tub of cool water is soothing. The first-aid treatment for sunburn is the same as that for other burns. Anti-inflammatory pain medicine, for example, aspirin or Ibuprofen®, can be

Sunburn: treatment

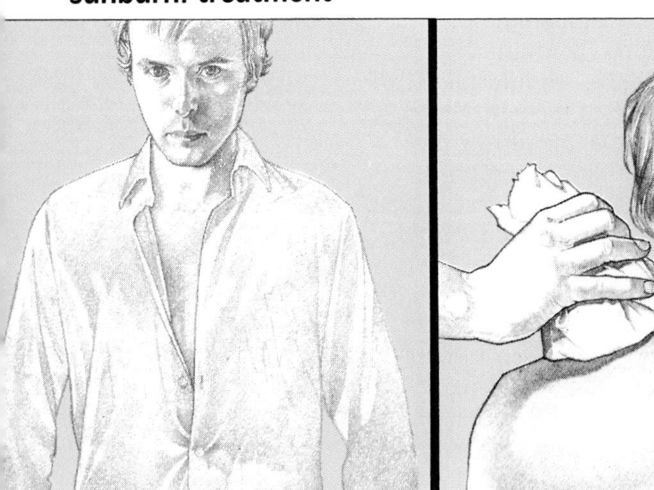

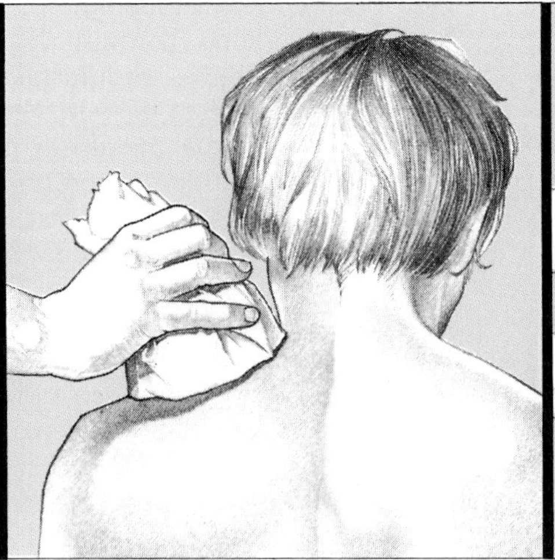

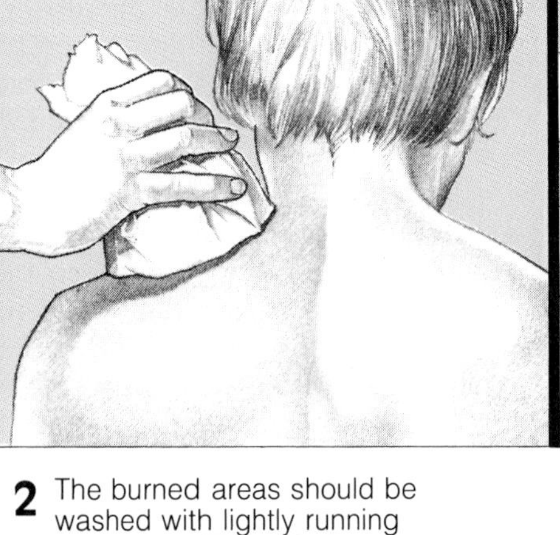

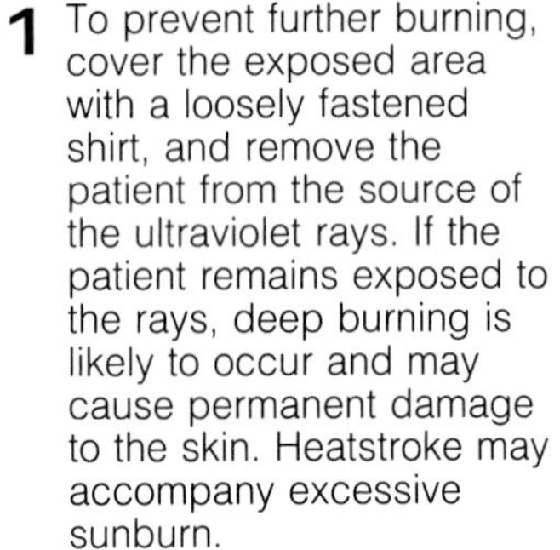

1 To prevent further burning, cover the exposed area with a loosely fastened shirt, and remove the patient from the source of the ultraviolet rays. If the patient remains exposed to the rays, deep burning is likely to occur and may cause permanent damage to the skin. Heatstroke may accompany excessive sunburn.

2 The burned areas should be washed with lightly running cold water. The pain from burns on the shoulders and upper regions can be relieved with a cold compress, such as one made from crushed ice in a plastic bag that is covered with soft, cotton material. If the burn is severe, medical attention should be sought.

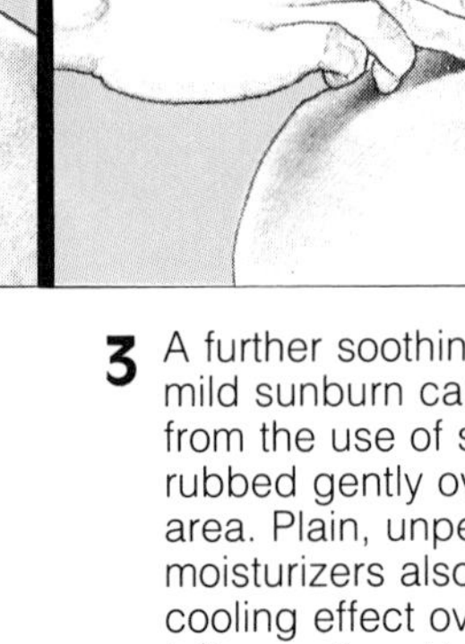

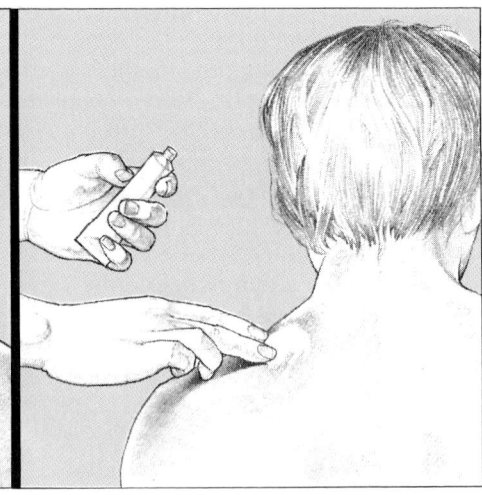

3 A further soothing effect for mild sunburn can be obtained from the use of sunburn lotion rubbed gently over the burned area. Plain, unperfumed moisturizers also have a cooling effect over the area of inflammation. Never use creams or moisturizers until after the skin has been cooled with ice water. Do not cover the area, but leave it exposed to the air. Let blisters heal naturally.

given. *See also* BURNS AND SCALDS: FIRST AID.

If the burn is severe or extensive, or the victim experiences a strong reaction to exposure, treat the victim for shock. Seek medical help immediately. *See also* SHOCK: TREATMENT.

Sundowning (sun′dou ning) is a condition affecting elderly patients in which mental and physical acuity decrease at the end of the day. The condition is characterized by varying degrees of disorientation and hearing and seeing difficulties. It frequently occurs during hospitalization which adds to the problem of unfamiliar surroundings.

Sunstroke is a form of heatstroke that is caused by overexposure to the sun.

See also HEATSTROKE.

Sunstroke: first aid. *See* HEATSTROKE: FIRST AID.

Superego (sü pər ē′gō) is a psychoanalytic term that describes the part of a person's psyche that determines right or wrong conduct, the conscience. The superego, comprising rules governing conduct, morality, and ethics, controls the expression or repression of the drives of the id by the ego. The superego is shaped by one's parents, caretakers, and teachers.

See also EGO; ID.

Superfluous hair. *See* HIRSUTISM.

Supine (sü pīn′) describes the position of lying on the back with the face upward.

Suppository (sə poz′ə tôr ē) is a cone-shaped or cylindrical medication that is inserted into the rectum or vagina, either for therapeutic or for contraceptive purposes. Suppositories usually consist of glycerin or cocoa butter that contain medication and liquefy at body temperature.

Suppuration (sup yə rā′shən) is the formation and discharge of pus. It may occur when an abscess or a wound becomes infected with pyogenic (pus-forming) microorganisms.

See also PUS.

Suprapubic (sü prə pyü′bik) defines the area above the pubic bone in the pelvis. The suprapubic region is the lowest area of the abdomen.

Suprarenal gland. *See* ADRENAL GLAND.

Surgery (sėr′jər ē) is the branch of medicine that treats disorders by surgical operation. For example, a surgeon can remove a diseased part of the body, correct deformities, repair injuries, or carry out internal examinations.

There are many different specialties within surgery, but every surgeon is trained in certain basic techniques and skills before starting further specialized training.

Kinds of Surgery

Some surgeons specialize in dealing with certain age groups, such as children (pediatric surgery), or particular conditions, such as cancer, when the surgeon is part of a team including other physicians and radiotherapists. Common specialties include general surgery, abdominal surgery, surgery of the gastrointestinal tract, trauma surgery or the immediate treatment on emergency hospital admission, cardiac surgery or treatment of heart conditions, and cosmetic surgery, which is really a subspecialty of plastic surgery. Other specialist areas include dental surgery, which includes faciomaxillary surgery, used in the treatment of teeth and damage to facial bones; genitourinary surgery for treatment of urinary disorders and male genital problems; gynecological surgery, treatment of disorders of the female reproductive system; and neurosurgery, treatment of the brain and nervous system.

There is also obstetric surgery, the specialty of dealing with childbirth; ophthalmic surgery, treatment of eye disorders; orthopedic surgery, treatment of bone and joint disorders; otorhinolaryngological surgery (ENT), treatment of ear, nose, and throat disorders; and plastic surgery, to reform and replace damaged tissues.

There are three other common specialties: rectal surgery, a subspecialty of genital surgery; thoracic surgery, treatment of the chest, particularly the lungs; and vascular surgery, treatment of the peripheral blood vessels.

Specialized Surgical Techniques. Some surgeons may perform microsurgery, using a microscope. Eye surgeons may also use laser beams in the treatment of certain disorders. Cryosurgery, a freezing technique, can be used in eye surgery, as well as in surgery on other parts of the body. Cautery, or the use of heat or chemicals to destroy tissue, is another surgical technique. In

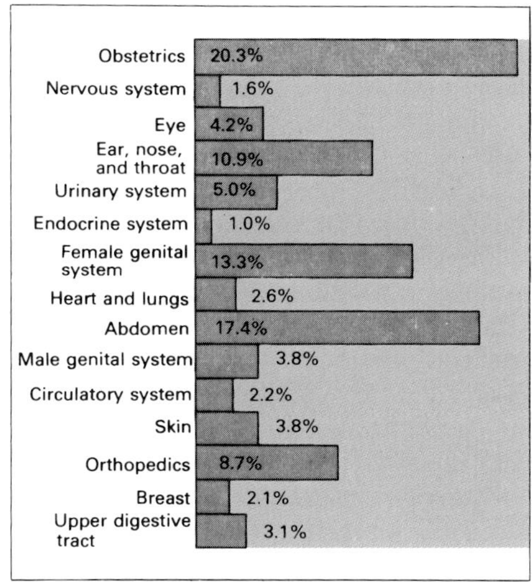

The areas of the body most often subject to **surgery** are listed, *left,* as percentages of the total number of surgeries.

replacement surgery, damaged body tissues, such as arthritic joints or damaged heart valves, may be replaced by artificial ones.

Bloodless surgery is a technique used to prevent excessive bleeding in the limbs. This technique must be performed within a certain time to prevent tissue death. The patient is anesthetized and the limb tightly bandaged, squeezing the blood out from the hand or foot upward, and then a tourniquet is left in place. This stops blood from entering the limb and makes surgery easier. The tourniquet must be released after about 30 minutes.

In heart surgery, special kinds of drugs are used to protect the heart muscle (myocardium), including cold solutions (perfusion hypothermia). An extracorporeal circulation (heart-lung machine) has been developed by using a pump oxygenator to supply the brain and other parts with oxygen-carrying blood and to reduce the patient's blood temperature.

Before Surgery

Surgery may be necessary for many reasons. It may offer a patient the only chance of survival in an emergency or slow down the rate of a progressive disease, such as cancer. Surgery may be performed to improve the quality of a patient's life, as in a total hip replacement. It may be done to improve a patient cosmetically. Surgery may also be performed as a diagnostic aid, for instance, the removal of a mole or enlarged gland to test for malignancy. It may be performed to remove some obstruction or disturbance of normal bodily function, such as a gall bladder containing stones.

Your physician and the attending surgeon will explain exactly why the operation is being performed, how it will be done, the chances of success, and any possible side effects or complications.

If after a full discussion you are still doubtful whether the operation is necessary, you may obtain a second opinion from another surgeon. This does not reflect badly on the first surgeon. If it relieves your anxiety, it makes the surgeon's job easier. If at all possible, talk to a person who has already had the same operation. Advice is especially helpful when surgery is going to result in a permanent alteration, such as a colostomy or the removal of a breast. Special organizations are run by patients who have had such operations.

Minor surgery can frequently be performed in the physician's office under local anesthetic. Operations such as the incision of an abscess or the suturing of a wound do not require the facilities of a hospital.

Nevertheless, it is usually advisable to have even minor operations performed in an operating room of a hospital. You can then have access to professional care during the recovery phase. Operations such as removal of benign breast lesions, dilatation and curettage, and many dental operations are performed on a day admission basis.

Hospitalization. Having found out the facts and agreed to the operation, you are admitted to the hospital. You will have to fill out an admission form and a consent form. These forms are illustrated in the entry HOSPITALIZATION: ADULT.

The consent form states that you agree to the operation and that the details of the operation have been explained. The form also gives the surgeon permission to carry out any further procedure necessary if there is an unexpected complication. Permission for an operation can be given by you, if you are over the age of consent, or by a parent or guardian, if you are under this age.

If the patient is unconscious or mentally ill, consent must be obtained from the nearest relative or legal guardian. A surgeon may also be faced with an unconscious patient who is in need of urgent treatment and for whom permission can not be obtained. This may be because the identity of the patient is not known or the next of kin is not available. In this situation, the surgeon has to make every effort to find someone who can give permission. If no one is available, the surgeon is under a moral, if not legal, duty to undertake any lifesaving surgery.

The day before surgery, an anesthesiologist will visit you to check the condition of your heart and lungs and ask if you have any allergies to drugs, adhesives, or other medications. A patient who is a heavy smoker may have to spend an extra day or two doing breathing exercises to try and eliminate mucus from the bronchial tubes and to help decrease the risk of pulmonary complications. Many surgeons ask their patients to stop smoking for at least two weeks before surgery. Some other tests may also be done, as described in the entry on HOSPITALIZATION: ADULTS.

For 12 hours before the operation you will not be allowed to eat or drink. If someone mistakenly offers you something, refuse it. The stomach must be empty before the anesthetic is given, because if there is anything in it, you may vomit during the operation and inhale the vomit.

Asepsis (the absence of infection) is essential to prevent microorganisms from entering your body. This is achieved by careful sterilization of all surgical instruments and by the wearing of masks and special sterile clothing by the medical staff. Your skin must also be sterilized.

The area of the incision is shaved, and shortly before you go to the operating room, it may be cleaned with an antiseptic soap and covered with a sterile dressing. After you are anesthetized, the area is cleaned again with antiseptics immediately before the first incision is made.

About an hour before you are taken to the operating room, you will be given an injection that makes you drowsy and dry in the mouth. This is called a "premed", an abbreviation for preoperative medication. It is a combination of drugs that calms you and dries up the secretions of saliva and mucus. The nurse makes sure you have removed all jewelry, including rings and earrings, as well as dentures and nail polish.

Before you are given the premed, a canvas undersheet may be put on your bed. This enables the orderlies to slide stretcher poles through the canvas and lift the stretcher and patient onto the gurney.

The orderlies then wheel you down to the operating room. A nurse from your floor accompanies you and then hands you over to an operating room nurse.

Anesthesia. Most major surgical operations are performed under a general anesthetic. Before this is given to you, the anesthesiologist injects intravenous anesthetic into a vein on the back of your hand. He or she may press on the vein before inserting the needle to make the vein stand out. While the anesthetic is slowly injected, the anesthesiologist may ask you to count. As the drug begins to take effect, your concentration will fail.

A piece of metal may be strapped to your leg, either before or just after you are given the anesthetic. It is part of the diathermy equipment that is used during the operation. The diathermy equipment produces a high frequency electrical current that is grounded through the metal. This enables the surgeon to electrically stop any bleeding of vessels exposed by the incision.

Everyone who has an operation has an intravenous line put into a vein in the arm. It is inserted prior to surgery and strapped to your wrist to prevent movement of the needle. The intravenous line serves several purposes. Fluid can be infused through the vein to prevent dehydration. If a transfusion is quickly needed, the line for administration is already set up. Also, the same line can be used for giving intravenous medication to relax the muscles or, in an emergency, to control the heart rate or stimulate the heartbeat. It is quicker to inject directly into the tubing of the intravenous lines than try to find a vein, which might be least prominent in an emergency.

The Surgical Operation

During the operation the anesthesiologist keeps a constant check on your pulse rate, blood pressure, and breathing. The anesthesiologist is also responsible for any blood transfusions or intravenous injections that may be necessary.

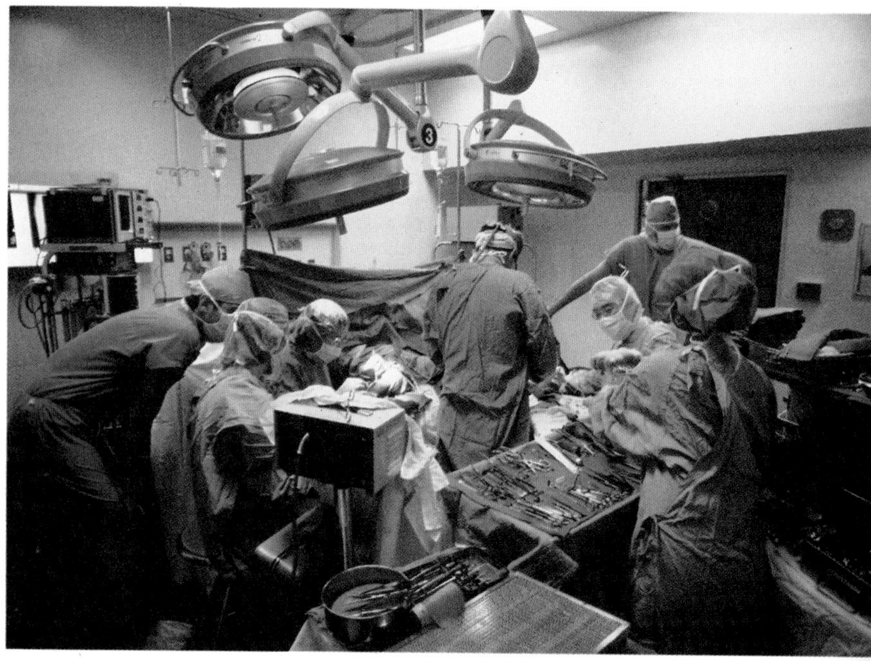

A surgeon and an assistant perform **surgery,** while nurses supply them with surgical instruments. An anesthesiologist is also part of the surgical team.

All the apparatus used during the operation is carefully checked beforehand, and all the gauze sponges are carefully counted before and after the incision is closed.

When the operation is complete, the surgeon closes the incision. From the patient's point of view, one of the most important things is a neat scar, but the surgeon must always have sufficient room to perform the operation effectively. Because of this, the scar may be larger than the patient expected. Initially the surgeon stitches the underlying tissues with sutures that are eventually absorbed by the body tissues and uses a similar type of material to sew the layer of connective tissue beneath the skin. Finally, the surgeon joins the edges of the skin together. This is done with either nonabsorbable thread stitches or staples.

If the incision is in an area under a great deal of pressure, for instance, a large abdominal incision, the surgeon may insert large-tension stitches to support the skin stitches, particularly if the patient has a chest problem and may strain the incision by coughing. Clips tend to mark the skin less than stitiches, but can not be used if the area of the incision is under great tension.

It is sometimes necessary to leave a drain in the incision to allow blood and other secretions to escape, either into the dressing or into a special bottle. The drain is either a tube or a piece of plastic or rubber. This is normal procedure following an operation such as a cholecystectomy.

If an incision has hardly any pressure exerted on it, for example, on the face, the surgeon can use butterfly sutures. These are pieces of adhesive tape, shaped like a butterfly, that are stuck onto the skin to hold it together. The incision is supported by the dissolving stitches in the deep tissue layer. The butterfly sutures have only to exert a slight pressure to keep the skin edges together until the skin heals. This method leaves no stitch marks at all. Another type of suture that leaves the skin free of stitch marks is the subcutaneous suture. A thread is run alternately through the fat layer and up into the skin layer.

After Surgery

After the operation, you will be taken to the recovery room where you will be monitored until you wake up from the anesthetic. A nurse will talk to you to help you regain consciousness. You will be kept under close observation before you wake up. Your pulse, respiration, and blood pressure will be recorded at frequent intervals. The nurse will ask if you have any pain and, if necessary, he or she will give you an injection of a painkilling drug. You will be kept in the recovery room until you are fully awake and your pulse, temperature, blood pressure, and breathing are all stable. Some people feel nauseated after the anesthetic and may even vomit, although this is increasingly uncommon with modern anesthetics. The nurse will watch for any indications of potentially serious postoperative complications, such as shock, bleeding, or discharge from the incision and amount of drainage.

You will be taken from the recovery room to the intensive care unit or your room. Again, a nurse will attend you during the journey. If you are taken to the intensive care unit, it does not indicate that something has gone wrong during the operation or that you are in any danger. After certain operations, careful monitoring is essential. This is easier to do in the intensive care unit with special equipment than in a room on a regular nursing unit.

After a major abdominal operation, the patient is usually given an intravenous infusion of fluids or blood into the vein of one arm. A nasogastric tube may have been passed through one nostril and into the stomach to keep it empty of fluid. In addition to a dressing over the wound, a drain (frequently a tube) may extend from it to a suction bottle. This prevents the collection of blood or serous fluid in the operation area. In patients who have gynecological or genitourinary operations, a catheter into the bladder is usually left in place. This is connected to a collection bag at the side of the bed.

As soon as the intestine is starting to work again, the patient is allowed to have sips of liquid and the nasogastric tube and intravenous infusion are removed.

Post-operative Problems. Immediately after the operation, the main danger is a sudden hemorrhage from the operated area, producing shock. A common problem in the immediate recovery period following all abdominal operations is paralytic ileus, or failure of the intestine to work. Continued paralytic ileus may result in abdominal swelling that opens the wound or the area of operation in the intestine. Breakdown or bursting of any wound may occur if the patient is ill or debilitated.

Patients stay in a surgical recovery room in order to facilitate close monitoring of their vital signs, while the anesthesia used during **surgery** wears off.

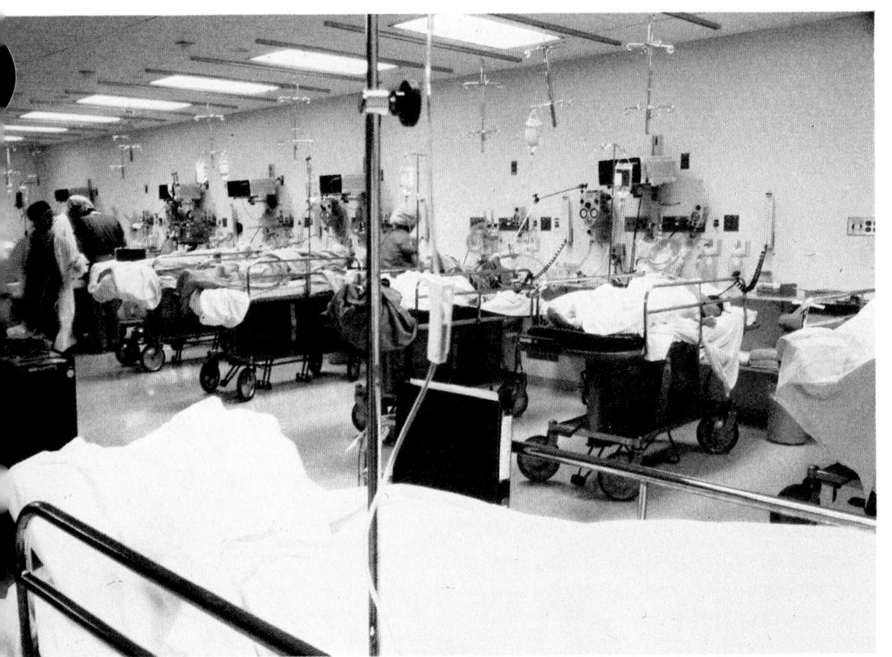

Lung infections, such as pneumonia, and urinary retention are common problems. A serious problem that can occur suddenly and unexpectedly is a pulmonary embolus from a blood clot formed in a deep vein, usually in the legs or pelvis.

Wound infections may develop from the cause of the original operation, such as in appendicitis. They sometimes also occur, despite all precautions, during the operation.

Late complications of any operation may occur from the scar tissue or adhesions that are formed. In the abdomen, these may cause obstruction.

Pain Relief. A patient is naturally concerned about postoperative pain. It is impossible to predict how much pain a patient will have, because awareness of pain and tolerance of pain vary from person to person. Powerful narcotics relieve pain efficiently and are given to most patients for the first four or five days after major surgery. The attending surgeon during the preparation for surgery should have given you some idea of what to expect in terms of soreness. However, in the unlikely event of him or her not doing so, you should ask, because if you know what to expect, you will find it easier to cope with your aftercare and will not be unduly anxious about the type of discomfort that is normal for your operation.

Painkilling drugs sometimes suppress a patient's urge to empty the bladder. This is more common in men than women and may cause problems with passing urine.

Intravenous Lines. If you have had surgery involving the digestive tract, you will not be able to eat for several days. You will have to rely on an intravenous line for nutrition. It may also be necessary to remove the secretions in your stomach and intestines with a tube that passes down one nostril to the stomach.

After an abdominal operation, the intestines tend to lose their normal function temporarily. Instead of continually contracting and relaxing to pass on the contents, they become inactive. This is why you may not be allowed foods or fluids by mouth. The attending surgeon will listen to the abdomen with a stethoscope because it is possible to hear sounds of returning function. It is common for the return of intestinal movement to be accompanied by several hours of uncomfortable swelling which is relieved by passing flatus. This may be followed by several loose bowel movements. The nurse will want to know when you first pass gas after the operation.

Breathing Exercises. After any type of surgery under a general anesthetic and particularly if the operation involves the chest or abdomen, it is difficult to take deep breaths or to cough. The air is distributed to the lungs by a system of tubes which subdivide into increasingly smaller tubes, ending in balloon-shaped alveoli. The tubes produce mucus, which forms a thin, sticky coating that traps tiny particles of dust or bacteria. The mucus is constantly moved toward the larger tubes and coughed up. If you can not take a deep breath, then the mucus accumulates in the base of the lungs, blocking the smaller tubes. Once this has happened, the area of blocked lung collapses and becomes highly susceptible to infection. For this reason, a respiratory therapist will visit you after your operation to help you to breathe deeply and cough up any sputum. You will be given adequate pain relief and shown how to make the coughing less painful. It is important to continue with these breathing and coughing exercises.

Muscular Exercises. It is essential to keep the circulation in the legs moving to prevent deep vein thrombosis and possible embolism. Before the operation, a physiotherapist will teach you exercises, such as bending the knees or forcefully contracting the leg muscles.

Convalescence. After the first day or two, you will begin to feel better, and the drains and intravenous lines will usually be removed. You will be encouraged to sit in the chair by the bed as much as possible and go for short walks around the floor.

In modern post-operative care, every effort is made to get the patient out of bed and moving around as soon as possible. This practice has proved to be beneficial to the patient because it has reduced the occurrence of complications, such as lung infection, lung collapse, thrombophlebitis (clotting in the

Post-surgical exercise

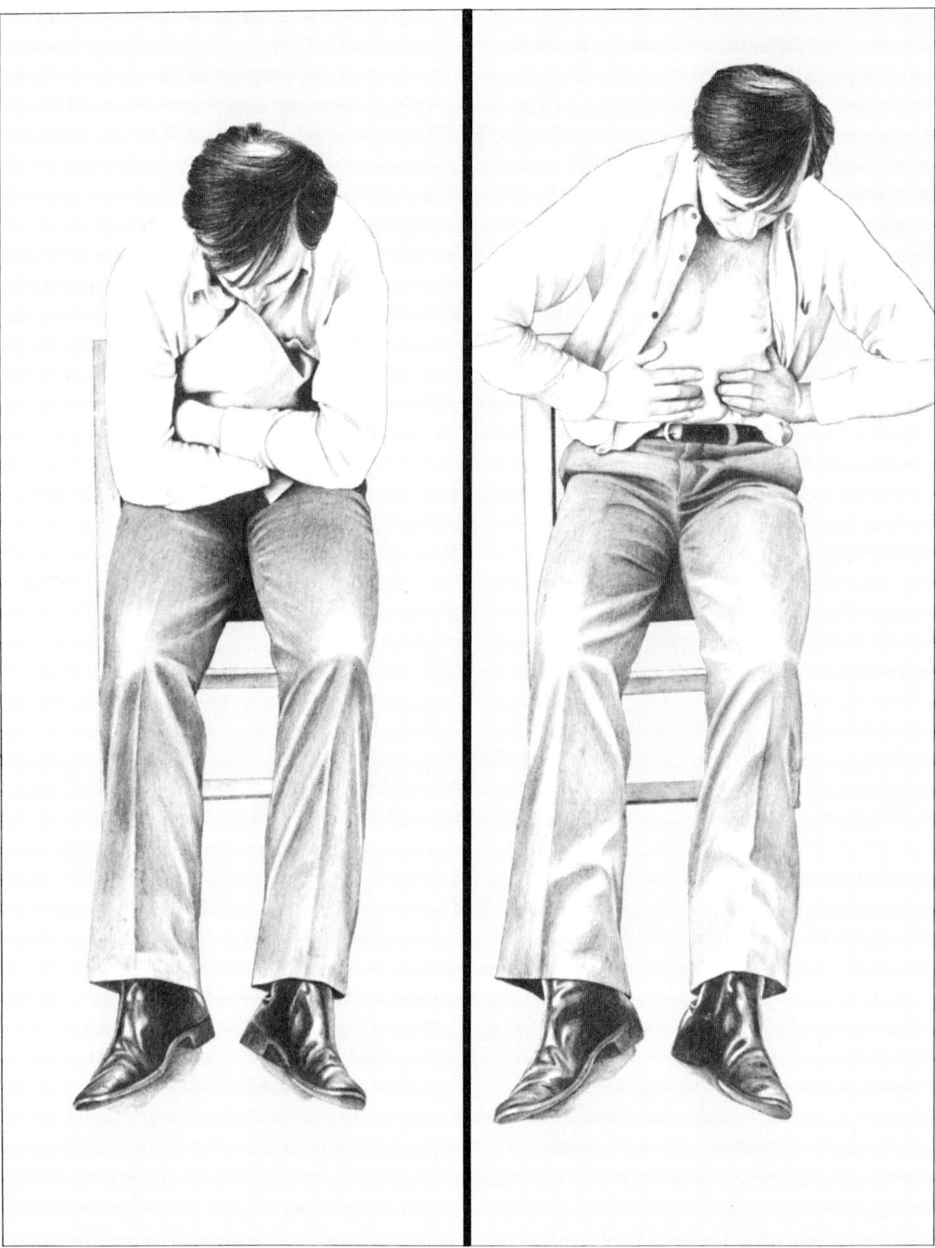

It is important for a patient's post-surgical recovery that he or she should start breathing exercises as soon as possible. The respiratory therapists encourage the patient to cough as much as possible. If the patient has undergone a large abdominal operation this can be difficult. The exercises are made easier if the patient holds a pillow tightly against the stomach while he or she is breathing deeply.

Patients often feel that the incision is not strong enough to take the strain of a cough. This is untrue, but because the incision is uncomfortable, a patient needs more confidence before he or she is able to cough deeply. In order to give the patient confidence, the therapist often instructs him or her to reduce tension on the incision by pressing on each side of the stitches. The patient can then take a deep breath and cough.

veins), and emboli (movement of clots to the heart or lungs).

Skin stitches and clips are usually removed after 8 to 10 days. On a large abdominal scar, every second stitch is removed on one day, and the rest are removed a day or two later. The stitch is cut below the knot and pulled out with a pair of forceps. It is no more uncomfortable than having a hair plucked out. To remove clips, the nurse uses a special pair of forceps that are placed under the clip and squeezed to open it. Again, the discomfort is minimal. Butterfly sutures are removed like a piece of adhesive tape.

The scar is cleaned with an antiseptic solution and re-covered with an ordinary dressing. A deep scar does not fade completely for up to a year, although by the time the stitches come out, the wound is stable enough for normal daily activities. At first the scar is a raised, red line, but as the line fades to white, the swelling slowly reduces and the scar shrinks. You may experience a slight tingling sensation or numbness in the skin surrounding the scar, but this usually disappears after a few months.

If you have had tension sutures placed by the wound, these are removed usually a few days after the stitches in your skin. The tension stitches are clipped on one side and pulled through on the other side.

Once the sutures are removed, you are usually ready to go home. After some operations, it is possible to return home before the stitches are removed. Ask the attending surgeon what activities you are allowed to do at home and when it is safe to resume normal activities. For some operations the patient is given a written list of instructions to follow.

While you are in the hospital there are a number of milestones that help you gauge your rate of recovery: the first time you walk to the bathroom unaided, the first walk outside your room, or the first time you can cough without pain. Many patients find that once they arrive home and are in familiar surroundings, they realize they have a long way before they are completely back to normal. A patient may feel weak after walking up a few steps, and many people suffer from depression during the first days at home. It is important to realize your limitations. If you have any worries about your rate of progress, the best person to talk to is your family physician or surgeon. Remember to always get your surgeon's permission before returning to work.

Surgery, cosmetic (sėr′jər ē, koz met′ik). Cosmetic surgery is a form of surgery done to improve a person's appearance. It is a branch of plastic surgery.

Q: *Why do people have cosmetic surgery?*

A: Usually, they are distressed or dissatisifed by their natural face or figure, or they have been involved in a disfiguring accident. Skillful surgery can alleviate mental as well as physical anguish, giving or restoring confidence to those who would otherwise avoid normal contacts.

Q: *What kinds of cosmetic repairs can be made?*

A: Almost any kind is possible. A cleft lip may be closed; a hand made immobile by scars can be restored to function; injuries to the face, from car accidents or industrial accidents, can be repaired by sculpting and realigning the delicate bones. In such cases, wires and splints are used to reconstruct facial features, and flaps of muscle fill the vacant spaces left by bone that has been destroyed or removed. Bone grafts may also be used.

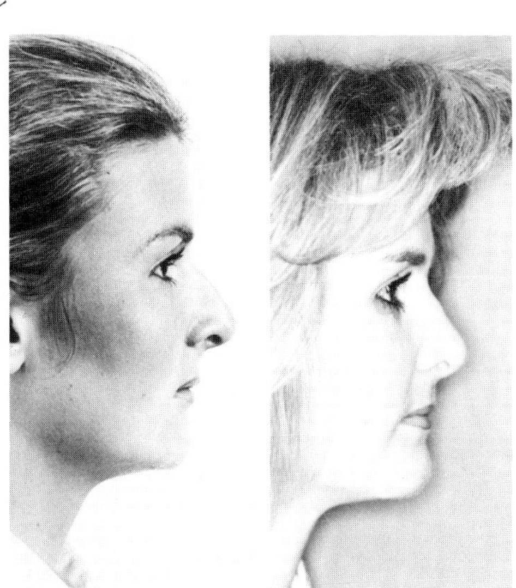

Cosmetic surgery performed on the nose (left) may result in a smaller nose with a better shape (right).

Women who are dissatisfied with the shape or size of their breasts can have them altered by mammoplasty. Some physicians, however, question the safeness of such techniques. *See also* MAMMOPLASTY.

Q: *What other methods of cosmetic surgery are there?*

A: Skin grafts are sometimes made to cover large raw areas, as in severe burns, and to serve as an efficient dressing to protect the raw area from infection and loss of body fluid. A thin layer of skin is surgically removed from one part of the body and laid over the injured area, where the skin cells are soon nourished by the tiny blood vessels of the injured area. *See also* SKIN GRAFT.

Pitting of the skin, caused by acne or smallpox for example, may be treated by a dermatologist with surgical planing, often called dermabrasion. In this method, a local anesthetic is given, and the doctor uses a rapidly rotating wire brush to remove the pitted surface of the skin. Healing takes place beneath a scab in a little more than a week. The new skin that forms is usually a great improvement over the scarred and pitted one. Wrinkles, if they are not deep, may also be removed or made less conspicuous in this way.

Another method used is cryotherapy, in which the skin is frozen with solid carbon dioxide. This produces peeling of old, scarred, or wrinkled skin.

Q: *Can scars result from cosmetic surgery operations?*

A: Every surgical operation leaves a scar, but its size depends partly on the skill of the surgeon and partly on the healing properties of the individual.

See also PLASTIC SURGERY.

Surgery, exploratory (sėr′jər ē, ek splôr′ə tôr ē). Exploratory surgery is a surgical procedure that is performed to aid the precise diagnosis of a disorder. It is performed when there is no time for conventional diagnostic testing or when conventional diagnostic methods have failed to reveal a disorder.

Suture (sü′chər) is the technique of uniting parts of the body by stitching them together. The term has several other meanings, including the material with which a wound is stitched together or the stitch that is left after the wound has been sutured. A suture is also a joint between two bones formed by fibrous tissues, as between the bones of the skull.

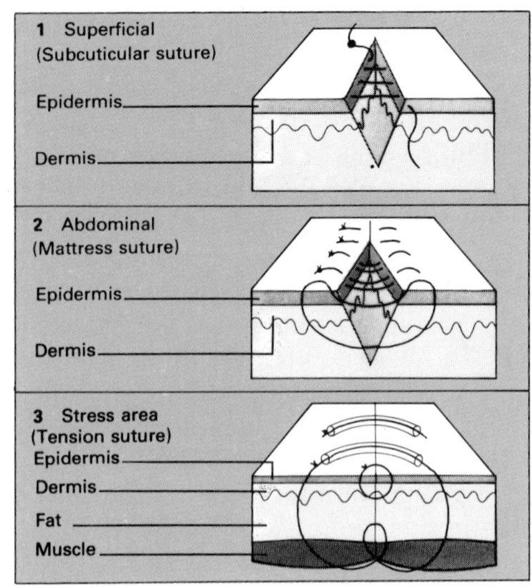

There are several types of **sutures** used to close incisions, such as (1) superficial, (2) abdominal, and (3) stress area.

The materials most commonly used for surgical sutures are nylon and other synthetic fibers, but steel wire may also be used for additional strength. Some sutures are made of materials such as catgut or synthetic substances that are slowly dissolved by the body. The tissues are finally held together by scar formation.

Swab (swob) is a piece of cotton that is used to collect pus or suppurating fluid for bacteriological culture and examination. The term also refers to the gauze used by a surgeon to soak up blood and body secretions when cleaning a wound during an operation.

Swaddling. *See* BABY CARE.

Swallowing (swol′ō ing) is the movement of food from the mouth, through the pharynx, into the upper part of the esophagus, and down to the stomach. It is a complex, coordinated movement of various muscles. The tongue forces the food backward and the glottis closes, blocking the windpipe and preventing food from passing into the lungs. The food passes along the esophagus by peristalsis, a series of waves of muscular contractions.

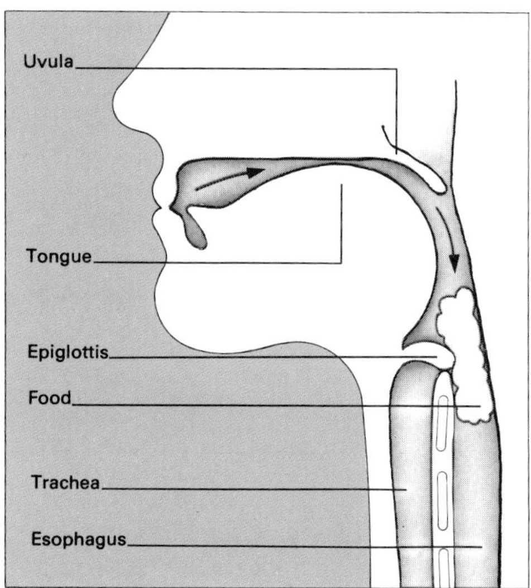

Swallowing closes the epiglottis over the trachea (windpipe), thereby preventing food from entering the trachea.

Q: *What disorders cause difficulty in swallowing?*
A: Difficulty in swallowing is known medically as dysphagia. It may be caused by a disorder of the throat, or it may be a symptom of a more general disease.
Q: *What disorders of the throat produce dysphagia?*
A: A common cause is a foreign body, such as a bone or the pit or the seed of a fruit, that blocks the esophagus and prevents swallowing. If the pharynx becomes infected, it results in pain as well as dysphagia. Tonsillitis and quinsy are examples of such infection.

Achalasia, a lack of the normal muscle coordination of swallowing, can produce dysphagia.

Occasionally, cancer of the pharynx, larynx, or esophagus is the cause of problems while swallowing. *See also* ABSCESS, PERITONSILLAR; ACHALASIA; TONSILLITIS.
Q: *What general diseases cause dysphagia?*
A: It may be caused by a muscle disorder, such as myasthenia gravis; a neurological disorder, such as stroke or poliomyelitis; or an infection, such as diphtheria, which causes both muscle weakness and nerve damage. Sometimes, iron deficiency anemia can be associated with dysphagia.
Q: *How is dysphagia treated?*
A: The treatment of dysphagia depends on the cause, which must be diagnosed by a physician.

Swallowing foreign objects: treatment. *See* STOMACH, FOREIGN OBJECTS IN: TREATMENT.

Sweat. *See* PERSPIRATION.

Swelling (swel′ing) is an abnormal enlargement of any part of the body.

See also EDEMA.

Swimming safety. *See* WATER SPORTS SAFETY.

Sydenham's chorea. *See* CHOREA.

Sympathectomy (sim pə thek′tə mē) is an operation in which the nerves of the sympathetic nervous system are inactivated, either by surgically cutting them or by destroying them chemically.

Sympathectomy may be performed on the sympathetic nerves in the neck to relieve the symptoms of Raynaud's phenomenon. It may also be done in the lumbar region to improve the blood circulation to the legs. This may be used to treat intermittent claudication or gangrene of the feet.

See also CLAUDICATION, INTERMITTENT; GANGRENE; NERVOUS SYSTEM, SYMPATHETIC; RAYNAUD'S PHENOMENON.

Sympathetic nervous system. *See* NERVOUS SYSTEM, SYMPATHETIC.

Symphysis (sim′fə sis) is a cartilage joint between two bones. An example is the joint between the two bones at the front of the pelvis (pubic symphysis).

Symptom (simp′təm) is a disruption of the normal functioning of the body that a patient notices, which may indicate an underlying disorder.

See also SYNDROME.

Syncope (sing′kə pē) is a sudden, temporary loss of consciousness that is caused by an inadequate flow of blood to the brain. It is the medical term for a faint.

See also FAINTING.

Syndactyly (sin dak′tə lē) is webbing between the fingers and toes. In most cases, the condition is inherited and usually affects both hands or both feet. Certain congenital chromosomal disorders cause syndactyly. Syndactyly of the toes does not require treatment. Syndactyly of the fingers can usually be corrected by surgery.

See also CONGENITAL ANOMALY.

Syndrome (sin′drōm) is a group of signs and symptoms that collectively indicate a particular disease or disorder.

Synovitis (sin ə vī′tis) is inflammation of the synovial membrane, the layer of smooth, slippery cartilage that lines the joints, surrounds tendons, and forms protective bags over bony protuberances (bursae).

Synovitis may be caused by injury to a joint, infection, or by various joint disorders, such as arthritis. The affected joint becomes swollen and painful, especially when the joint is moved. Treatment is directed toward the underlying cause.

See also ARTHRITIS; BURSITIS; CAPSULITIS; TENOSYNOVITIS.

Syphilis (sif′ə lis), also known in the past as lues, is a contagious sexually transmitted disease that is caused by infection with spiral-shaped bacteria called *Treponema pallidum.* It can affect any tissue in the body, causing a wide variety of symptoms and complications.

The infection can enter the body through the mucous membranes, such as the vagina and male urethra, or through cuts in the skin. It is usually transmitted by sexual intercourse. The infection can also pass through the placenta to a fetus, causing syphilis in the unborn child.

Preliminary diagnosis of syphilis is made by such blood tests as VDRL (Venereal Disease Research Laboratory) or RPR (Rapid Plasma Reagin) tests. These are the tests usually performed as premarital blood tests. Confirmation of a preliminary diagnosis is usually made by a test called FTA-ABS (Fluorescent Treponemal Antibody-Absorbed).

After infection, there is an incubation period before any symptoms appear. This may vary from a week to three months, but is usually about three or four weeks. Then the disease progresses through three stages, known as primary, secondary, and tertiary syphilis.

Q: *What are the symptoms of primary syphilis?*

A: A small red spot appears at the site of infection and ulcerates to form a chancre that has a hard base. The chancre is usually painless and does not bleed, but, when cut, exudes a clear fluid that contains the syphilis bacteria, which is contagious. The local lymph glands may become swollen. The chancre usually occurs on the penis, anus, or rectum in men and on the vulva, cervix, or anal area in women. Occasionally, the chancre may appear on the lips, tongue, or even the tonsils.

The chancre heals spontaneously in about one or two months, often leaving a scar. In a few cases, there is no chancre, and the disease passes directly to secondary syphilis.

Q: *What are the symptoms of secondary syphilis?*

A: The symptoms of secondary syphilis usually appear about two months after infection. There is generalized illness, with fever, headache, tiredness, aching of limbs, and a rash. Flat ulcers with raised edges often form in the mouth, vulva, penis, or rectum at the junction of the mucous membranes and the skin. These ulcers are known as condylomata lata and are extremely infectious.

Secondary syphilis may also cause enlargement of the liver, spleen, and lymph glands. This stage of the disease may persist for several months before the symptoms disappear. It is followed by a latent stage, after which tertiary syphilis may develop.

Q: *What are the symptoms of tertiary syphilis?*

A: It may take as long as 20 years before tertiary syphilis develops, or it

Syphilis is characterized by different symptoms at various stages of its development.

Characteristic symptoms of syphilis	
Primary stage 2 to 4 weeks	Chancres appear on lip, tongue, nipples, or genitals. Painless swelling of lymph glands near genitals.
Secondary stage 6 weeks	Mild rash appears. Eruption of skin, reddish brown coppery spots, recurring possibly at a later stage.
Latency period	No obvious symptoms
Tertiary stage up to 20 years later	Heart, blood vessels, and central nervous system may be involved. Insanity and various types of psychoses may develop.

may never occur. It may affect any part of the body and may simulate almost any disease. Tertiary syphilis is much rarer now because of antibiotic therapy of early syphilis.

Tertiary syphilis may affect the central nervous system (neurosyphilis) or the heart and blood vessels (cardiovascular syphilis), or it may produce swelling in the skin, bones, and intestinal organs (benign tertiary syphilis).

Neurosyphilis may cause general weakness in the patient, with delusions, personality deterioration, and insanity, or it may cause tabes dorsalis in which the normal reflexes are lost. If the spinal cord is affected, there may be sudden paralysis of the legs and either urinary retention or incontinence. *See also* TABES DORSALIS.

Cardiovascular syphilis damages the aorta, causing it to become dilated (aneurysm). This swelling may compress adjacent organs, resulting in difficulty in swallowing, difficulty in talking, or collapse of part of the lungs. The aneurysm may rupture, causing sudden death. The heart valves may also be damaged, causing angina pectoris or heart failure.

Benign tertiary syphilis is characterized by the formation of gummas, which are swollen areas of soft, scar-like tissue. They may affect any part of the body, but usually produce only minor symptoms caused by localized swelling. *See also* GUMMA.

Q: *How is syphilis treated?*

A: Penicillin is effective in treating all stages of syphilis. Primary and secondary syphilis can be completely cured, but tertiary syphilis can only by arrested because the tissue damage can not be restored. Other drugs are available for penicillin-allergic patients.

It is important for the patient to have regular medical checkups to ensure that the treatment has been effective. The sexual contacts of the patient should be traced and, if necessary, treated for syphilis.

See also SEXUALLY TRANSMITTED DISEASE.

Syringe (sə rinj′) is an instrument for injecting fluids into the body or for washing out cavities or wounds. A hypodermic syringe consists of a glass or plastic tube, a fine nozzle, and a tightly-fitting plunger. A needle is attached to the nozzle, and the complete assemblage is sterilized before use.

An irrigating syringe has a large rubber bulb instead of a plunger. It is used to wash out wax from the ears and to cleanse wounds and body cavities.

See also INJECTION.

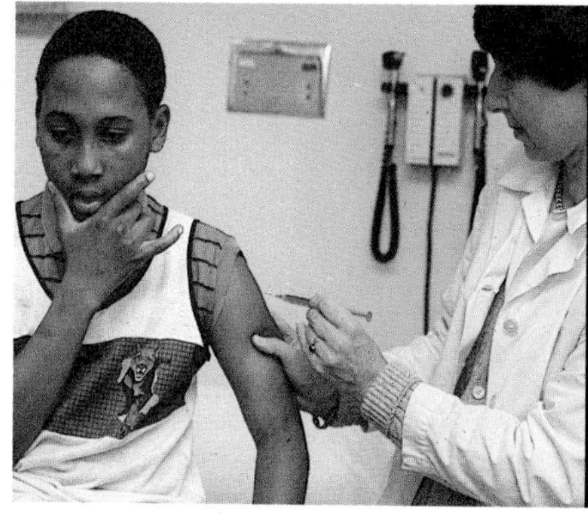

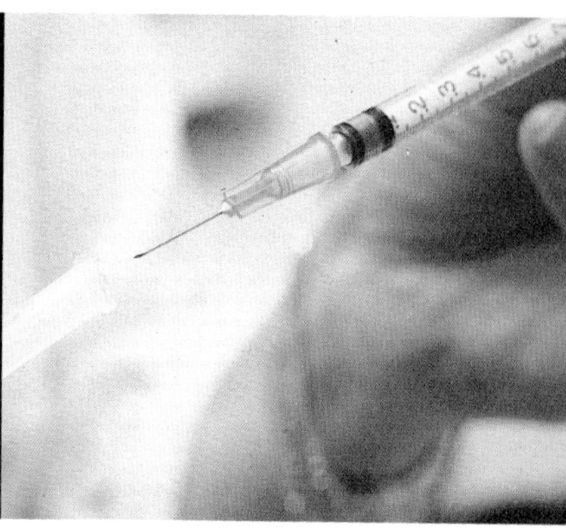

A **syringe** is used for injecting or withdrawing fluids into or out of the body.

Syringomyelia (sə ring gō mī ē′lē ə) is a rare congenital anomaly of the spinal cord or the lower part of the brain involving the central canal. Cavities slowly form in the substance of the cord in the region of the lower neck, but do not produce symptoms until late adolescence or early adulthood.

Q: *What are the symptoms of syringomyelia?*

A: There is a gradual loss of sensation in the shoulders, hands, and arms, accompanied by weakness of the legs, as the disorder slowly progresses. If the lower part of the brain is involved, dizziness and problems with speech and swallowing may occur.

The condition slowly progresses over many years, causing increasing loss of sensation and paralysis, first of the legs and later of the rest of the body.

Q: *What is the treatment for syringomyelia?*

A: There is no effective form of treatment. Surgery has been attempted and may, in very few cases, be successful.

Systole (sis′tə lē) is the contraction of the heart muscle that causes the forceful ejection of blood into the arterial system.

See also BLOOD PRESSURE; DIASTOLE.

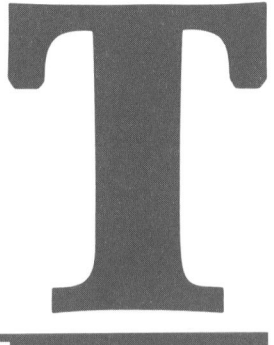

Tabes dorsalis (tā'bēz dôr sā'lis), also known as locomotor ataxia, is a syphilitic infection of the nerves in which there is progressive degeneration of the nerve fibers of the spinal cord. Tabes dorsalis may not develop until 10 or 20 years after the original infection and is more common in men than in women. Although quite common in the past, the condition is rarely seen anymore.

The initial and most characteristic symptom is an intense stabbing pain in the legs; this is known as a lightning pain. There may also be a loss of sensation in the limbs and a lack of awareness of their position.

As the disease progresses, the patient may walk unsteadily, with a typical high-stepping gait. There may also be a loss of sensation in the bladder, causing retention of urine and, eventually, incontinence. In the late stages of the disease, there may be lightning pains in the abdomen and vomiting.

Tabes dorsalis is prevented by early diagnosis and treatment of syphilis. Once tabes dorsalis develops, a more prolonged course of antibiotic therapy is needed.

See also SYPHILIS.

Tablet (tab'lit) is a form of solid medication, different from a capsule (a soluble container enclosing oral medication). Tablets are often disk-shaped, though size and shape can vary. They are generally intended to be swallowed whole, but some tablets can be chewed or dissolved in the mouth.

See also CAPSULE.

Tachycardia (tak ə kär'dē ə) is a rapid heart rate of more than 100 beats a minute when the patient is at rest. Tachycardia may be caused by excessive exercise; an emotional response, such as fear; or an increase in the metabolic rate, which may occur with hyperthyroidism (hyperactivity of the thyroid gland), fever, or infection. Tachycardia may also result from anemia, hemorrhage, a heart disorder, or the use of certain drugs.

See also ARRHYTHMIA; BRADYCARDIA.

Tachycardia, paroxysmal atrial (tak ə kär'dē ə, par ək siz'məl ā'trē əl). Paroxysmal atrial tachycardia is a sudden increase in the heart rate to 150-200 beats a minute for no apparent reason. The average rate during an attack is around 180 beats per minute. Normally, the heart beats about 70 times per minute. A large quantity of urine may be passed after the attack.

Q: *What causes paroxysmal atrial tachycardia?*

A: Frequently, the cause is not known, but the origin seems to lie with a sudden increase in the number of electrical stimuli starting the atrium of the heart, producing a rapid, regular contraction of the ventricles. This may occur in young people without any sign of heart disease. In the elderly, the cause of the attack is usually arte-

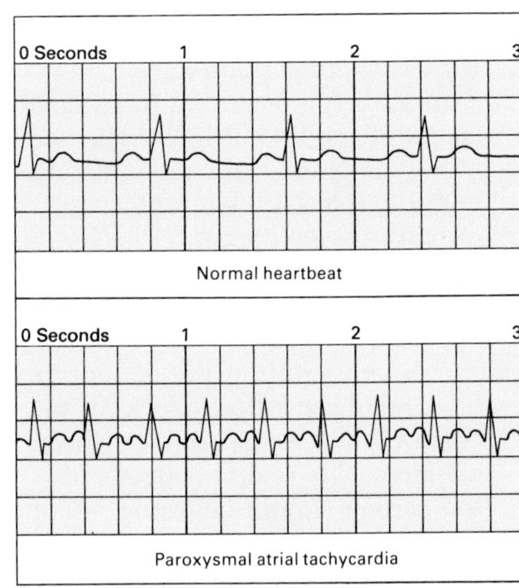

Paroxysmal atrial tachycardia can increase a normal heartbeat of about 70 beats per minute to about 180 beats per minute.

riosclerosis (hardening of the arteries). *See also* ARTERIOSCLEROSIS.

Q: *How is paroxysmal atrial tachycardia treated?*

A: An acute attack should be treated by a physician, and hospitalization may be necessary. Frequently, drug therapy may be needed to prevent or stop attacks. Some patients are taught to hold their breath while trying to expel air; this may stop an attack.

See also TACHYCARDIA.

Tagamet® (tag′ə met) is a preparation of the drug cimetidine, a histamine H_2-receptor antagonist. It is often used in the treatment of peptic ulcer disease.

See also HISTAMINE H_2-RECEPTOR ANTAGONISTS; ULCER, PEPTIC.

Talipes (tal′ə pēz) is the medical term for any one of the several clubfoot deformities, which are characterized by a twisting of the foot to the inside or the outside.

See also CLUBFOOT.

Talus (tā′ləs), or ankle bone, is one of the seven tarsal bones of the foot. It articulates with the lower ends of the tibia and fibula bones to form part of the ankle joint.

See also ANKLE; FOOT.

Tapeworm (tāp′wėrm), also called cestode, is a parasitic worm shaped like a long, flat piece of tape. Three main species of tapeworm infest human beings: *Taenia saginata* (beef tapeworm); *Taenia solium* (pork tapeworm); and *Diphyllobothrium latum* (fish tapeworm). Occasionally, another species of tapeworm, *Echinococcus granulosus*, may infest people, causing cysts to form in the liver.

The adult worms live in the human intestine. At one end of the worm is a head (scolex) with small hooks that attach to the intestinal wall. Behind the scolex are hundreds of segments in which eggs develop. The segments break off, pass out of the body in the feces, and are eaten by the primary host (cattle, hogs, or fish). The worm eggs hatch into larvae in the primary host. The larvae penetrate the intestinal wall and are carried by the blood circulation to the muscles, where they form cysts.

People become infested when they eat undercooked meat. The cysts mature into adult worms in the human intestine, thereby perpetuating the cycle.

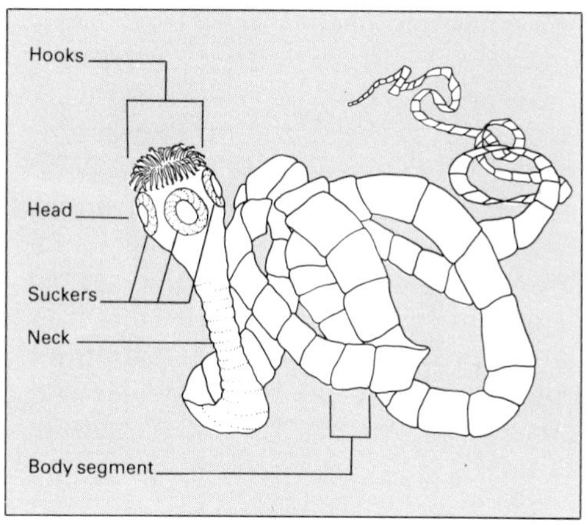

A **tapeworm,** growing inside the host's intestine, can range in length from 1 inch to 100 feet.

Q: *What are the symptoms of an infestation with tapeworms?*

A: The most common symptom is the presence of tapeworm segments in the feces. If a person is heavily infested, there may also be abdominal pain, diarrhea, and loss of weight.

Q: *How are tapeworm infestations treated?*

A: In most cases, treatment with worm-killing drugs, such as niclosamide, is effective. Tapeworm infestation can be prevented by thoroughly cooking all meat and fish.

See also CYSTICERCOSIS; WORM.

Target cell is an abnormal red blood cell deficient in hemoglobin or with an excess of membrane. Under a microscope, target cells appear as thin cells with a center dot of hemoglobin. They can be found in the blood after a splenectomy (surgical removal of the spleen) or in individuals with anemia, hemoglobin C disease, or thalassemia.

See also ANEMIA; HEMOGLOBIN; THALASSEMIA.

Tarsal (tär′səl) refers to any one of the bones of the ankle and foot.

See also FOOT; TARSUS.

Tarsus (tär′səs) is the back of the foot between the metatarsal bones and the tibia and fibula bones. The tarsus consists of seven tarsal bones. One of these, the talus, forms part of the ankle joint. *See also* ANKLE; TALUS.

Tarsus also refers to any one of the plates of cartilage forming the eyelids.

Tartar (tär′tər) is a deposit on the teeth that consists of calcium salts and the remains of food. If the layer of tartar is allowed to accumulate, it may irritate the gums and cause gingivitis or periodontitis.

See also GINGIVITIS; PERIODONTITIS.

Taste (tāst) is the sensation that is obtained when specialized sensory nerve endings on the front, back, and sides of the tongue (the taste buds) detect soluble substances. The taste buds can register four fundamental tastes, either singly or in combination: sweet, bitter, sour, and salty. The sense of taste can be affected by a disorder of the mouth or nose.

See also TASTE BUD.

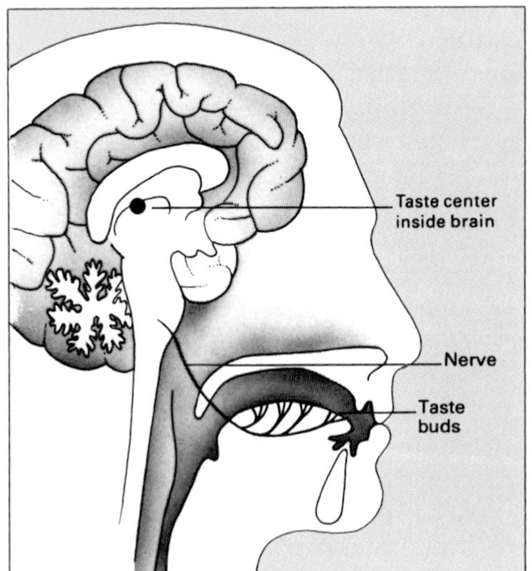

Taste stimuli are received by the taste buds on the tongue and transmitted to the taste center in the brain.

Taste bud, or gustatory organ, is a sensory nerve ending on the outer surface of the tongue. Taste buds detect tastes and send impulses to the cortex and thalamus of the brain, where the perception of taste occurs. Adults have approximately 9,000 taste buds.

See also TASTE.

Tay-Sachs disease (tā'-saks) is an inherited disorder in which there is a deficiency of a specific enzyme that breaks down fatty substances called lipids in the nervous system. The lipids accumulate in the brain cells, which gradually degenerate. The disease is transmitted genetically as a result of both the mother's and the father's recessive chromosomes and is far more common in families of Eastern European Jewish descent than in others.

Q: *What are the symptoms of Tay-Sachs disease?*

A: An affected child appears to be normal for the first few months following birth. But as the brain cells degenerate, there is a gradual onset of spasticity, convulsions, blindness, and a progressive loss of physical and mental abilities. Tay-Sachs disease is invariably fatal; the child usually dies before the age of four years.

Q: *Can Tay-Sachs disease be prevented?*

A: Yes. All potentially affected parents should obtain genetic counseling. Screening blood tests can be performed that can identify carriers of Tay-Sachs disease. Ideally, such tests are performed prior to a couple conceiving a child.

It is also possible to detect the disorder in a fetus by using amniocentesis, the withdrawing of amniotic fluid from around the fetus for diagnostic purposes. Further information is available from the Tay-Sachs Foundation.

TB is an abbreviation for tuberculosis.

See also TUBERCULOSIS.

T cell. *See* BLOOD CELL, WHITE.

Tear (tir) is a watery, slightly alkaline secretion that protects and lubricates the eyes. Tears contain salt and also an antibacterial enzyme (lysozyme) that prevents the eye from becoming infected. Tears are secreted by the lacrimal glands around the eyes.

See also LACRIMAL APPARATUS; LYSOZYME.

Teeth. *See* TOOTH.

Teeth, Hutchinson's (huch'ən sunz). Hutchinson's teeth is a congenital anomaly in which the permanent incisor teeth (the teeth at the front of the mouth) are narrow and notched. It is usually a sign of congenital syphilis.

See also SYPHILIS.

Teething (te'thing) is the natural process by which a baby's teeth erupt through the gums. Teething may cause excessive drooling, rubbing of the gums on hard objects, difficulty sleeping, and general irritability. In most babies, there is no need for any specific treatment for teething.

See also BABY CARE.

Telangiectasia (tə lan jē ek tā'zhə) is a disorder in which the small blood vessels become abnormally dilated, producing a type of angioma (a benign tumor usually composed of blood vessels). Telangiectases usually occur as red spots on the face and thighs. They are more common in the elderly, in people who have been continually exposed to the sun, and in people with varicose veins. In most cases, the cause of the disorder is unknown.

Temperature (tem′pər ə chər) is a measurement of the amount of heat in an object. The normal body temperature of a healthy person (taken with a thermometer placed under the tongue) is about 98.6°F (37°C), but even in a healthy person this varies slightly during the course of the day. It is lowest early in the morning and highest later in the afternoon. The temperature taken in the rectum is more accurate, but tends to be about 1°F (0.5°C) higher than the oral temperature. The least accurate temperature is that taken in the armpit or groin.

Q: *What can cause variations in normal body temperature?*

A: An unexpected variation in body temperature may be a sign of illness or may merely reflect normal changes taking place in the body. Children have a wider temperature range, so a physically active day may raise their temperatures a degree or so above normal without any sign of illness.

Between puberty and menopause, women experience a rise in body temperature midway through the menstrual cycle, when ovulation takes place. This higher temperature continues as the basic normal one until menstruation. Such temperature measurement can be used to time the occurrence of ovulation and improve the chances of conception in a woman who wants to have a baby.

See also FEVER; HYPOTHERMIA; TEMPERATURE, TAKING OF.

Temperature, taking of. When taken orally, the average body temperature of a healthy, resting person is 98.6°F (37°C). Taking the temperature by placing the thermometer under the tongue (sublingually) for about five minutes is the most common method. While the thermometer is in place, the person should not breathe through the mouth. However, this method may not be suitable for babies, senile or confused patients, or other persons. A reading taken from under the arm (subaxillary) is suitable for many senile or confused patients. Alternatively, a reading can be taken by placing the thermometer in the person's rectum. This may be necessary when a patient is unable to have

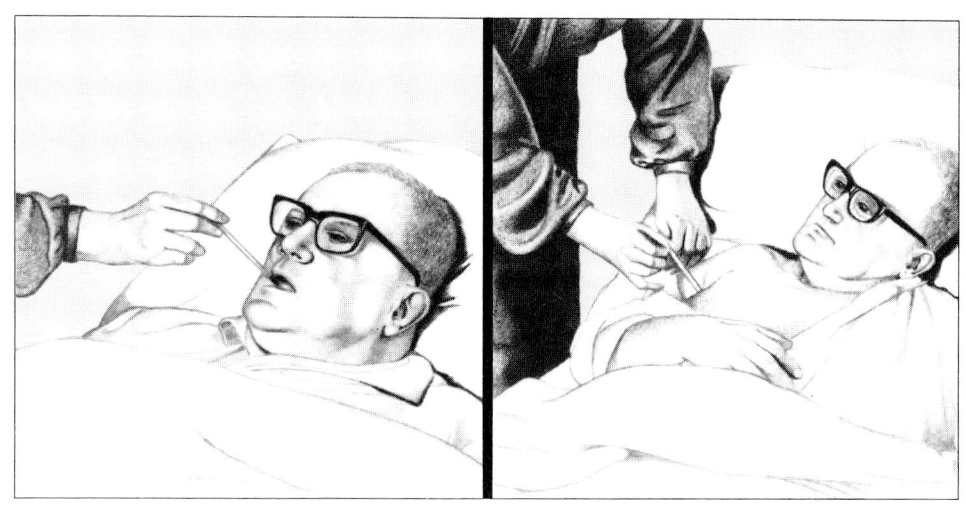

To take an oral (sublingual) temperature reading, check that the patient has not had a hot or cold drink, or a smoke, within the last half hour. Place the bulb of the thermometer under the patient's tongue. Ask the patient to close the lips (but not the teeth) gently around the stem of the thermometer. After at least one minute, remove it and record the reading.

To take a subaxillary temperature reading, slip the thermometer under the patient's arm, so that the bulb rests in the armpit. Bring the patient's arm across the chest to ensure that the thermometer stays securely in place. After at least three minutes, remove it and record the reading. A subaxillary temperature is about 1°F (0.5°C) lower than a sublingual temperature.

the thermometer placed under the tongue because of an inflammation of the mouth or other disorder. A rectal temperature reading is usually taken from children under the age of four. The temperature taken in the rectum is the most accurate, but tends to be about 1°F (0.5°C) higher than the oral temperature.

Never use a long-tipped mercury thermometer for taking a rectal temperature; use only the short-tipped, stubby type of thermometer with a bulb the same diameter as the stem. Lubricate the thermometer bulb with petroleum jelly before inserting it approximately 1 inch (2.5cm) into the rectum. Hold the thermometer in place for about 2 minutes. Remove the thermometer and record the temperature reading. After taking the temperature, clean the thermometer with soap and cool water.

The current advances in thermometers include reasonably priced and readily available digital thermometers. They are safe, practical, and easy to read. Digital thermometers can be used for taking a young child's temperature once the child will allow it to remain in place under the tongue. The digital thermometer may also be used for taking the temperature under the arm. A digital thermometer may be cleaned by washing it with soap and hot water or by swabbing it with an alcohol disinfectant.

It is important that you record the daily readings of a patient's temperature. A temperature chart can be purchased from the drugstore to help you do this more efficiently.

When the patient's illness has passed and a thermometer is no longer needed, swab it with alcohol or other disinfectant before finally putting it away.

Temper tantrum (tan'trəm) is a fit of bad temper exhibited for the purpose of getting what one wants. It is a common occurrence during childhood, when the child is trying to assert his or her individuality. Temper tantrums usually last only a minute or two, but may recur if the child is unable to get what he or she wants.

Q: *How should a child with temper tantrums be treated?*

A: Parents should be firm and consistent in attitude toward the child. It is advisable for them not to show anxiety and stress during a temper tantrum. If possible, the tantrum should be ignored and the child allowed to misbehave if no harm is being done. It is best not to try and reason with the child during the tantrum or to punish him or her. Once the tantrum is over and the child is acting more appropriately, the parent can once again interact with the child. If parents are consistent in their approach to tantrums, the tantrums will usually decline over time without the need for further intervention.

Temporal arteritis. *See* ARTERITIS, TEMPORAL.

Temporal lobe epilepsy. *See* EPILEPSY, TEMPORAL LOBE.

Temporomandibular joint dysfunction (tem pə rō man̍ dib'ü lar), TMJ, is a condition often characterized by facial pain, tenderness of the chewing muscles, lower jaw dysfunction, and pain and/or "clicking" sounds in the joint of the jaw. Prior trauma has been implicated in many cases of TMJ.

Hot, moist applications and muscle relaxants or analgesics (painkillers) are helpful in treating the symptoms of the dysfunction, but are not curative. Persons with TMJ should avoid chewy food and clenching and grinding of the teeth. Definitive treatment usually involves the use of a bite repositioning appliance to alleviate the symptoms, followed by the correction of the bite through surgery or other means.

Tendinitis (ten də nī'tis) is inflammation of a tendon. It is usually accompanied by tenosynovitis (inflammation of the membrane around a tendon). Treatment may include rest and corticosteroid therapy.

See also TENOSYNOVITIS.

Tendon (ten'dən) is the thick, strong, inelastic band of fibrous tissue that attaches a muscle to a bone. A tendon may be strained by excessive use or, occasionally, ruptured. A tendon and its surrounding synovial membrane may also become inflamed (tenosynovitis).

See also TENDINITIS; TENOSYNOVITIS.

Tenesmus (ti nez'məs) is painful, ineffective straining to urinate (vesical tenesmus) or defecate (rectal tenesmus). Vesical tenesmus may be a symptom of cystitis, a bladder stone, or disorders of the prostate gland in which the flow of urine is obstructed. Rectal tenesmus may be a symptom of constipation, an anal fissure, an anal fistula, an anal abscess, or, rarely, cancer of the rectum.

See also CONSTIPATION; RECTAL DISORDERS; URINARY DISORDERS.

Tennis elbow. *See* ELBOW, TENNIS.

Tenosynovitis (ten ō sin ə vī'tis) is an inflammation of the synovial membrane that surrounds a tendon. It is often accompanied by inflammation of the underlying tendon (tendinitis). The cause of tenosynovitis is not known, but it may result from strenuous exercise; infection from an overlying wound; or from various diseases, such as rheumatoid arthritis, gout, or Reiter's disease.

See also SYNOVITIS; TENDINITIS.

Tension relief. *See* STRESS MANAGEMENT.

Teratoma (ter ə tō'mə) is a usually malignant tumor that consists of several different types of tissue, such as skin, hair, teeth, and bone, none of which originates in the area in which the tumor occurs. Teratomas occur most frequently in the ovaries or testes; treatment requires surgical removal, followed by radiotherapy and chemotherapy.

Termination (tėr mə nā'shən) means the end of an event. It commonly refers to the termination of a pregnancy (abortion).

See also ABORTION.

Testicle. *See* TESTIS.

Testicle, undescended (tes'tə kəl). Undescended testicle is a condition in which a testis remains in the abdomen at birth instead of descending into the scrotum. For a more complete discussion of this condition, *see* CRYPTORCHIDISM.

Testis (tes'tis) is one of the two primary male reproductive organs (gonads) that lie in the scrotum. Each testis is about 1.5 inches (4cm) long.

Q: *What are the functions of the testes?*

A: After puberty, the testes produce the male hormone testosterone and the reproductive cells (sperm). From the testes, the sperm pass along special ducts to the epididymis. The epididymis leads to the vas deferens, through which the sperm are carried to the seminal vesicles where they are stored. *See also* REPRODUCTION, HUMAN; SCROTUM.

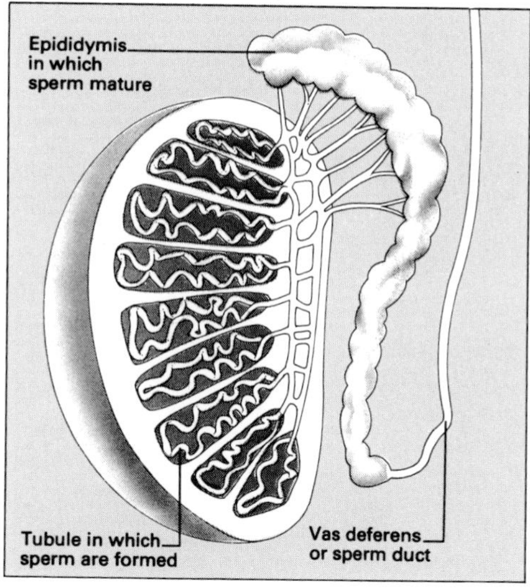

The **testis** produces sperm in its tubules. The sperm later mature in the epididymis.

Q: *What conditions affect the testes?*

A: A testis may not reach the correct position after passing out of the abdomen and into the scrotum. This condition is known as an undescended testicle or cryptorchidism. Excessive fluid may accumulate in the small bag next to a testis in a condition known as hydrocele. The testes may also become infected and inflamed (orchitis), which may lead eventually to sterility. Mumps is the most common cause of orchitis. Occasionally, cancer of the testes (seminoma) may develop.

Test meal is a standardized meal that is given to test the gastric secretion of the stomach. A test meal may be used in the diagnosis of various gastrointestinal disorders. Modern methods of testing acid secretion are usually done without giving a test meal.

Testosterone (tes tos'tə rōn) is the male sex hormone produced principally by the testes. The amount of testosterone produced is controlled by the follicle-stimulating hormone (FSH) and luteinizing hormone (LH), both of which are secreted by the front lobe of the pituitary gland. At the onset of puberty, there is an increase in the production of testosterone, particularly in boys. *See also* TESTIS.

Q: *What are the effects of testosterone?*

A: Testosterone stimulates the development of male secondary sexual characteristics. These include facial and pubic hair; enlargement of the larynx, which produces deep-

Testosterone stimulates the development of the male secondary sexual characteristics during puberty.

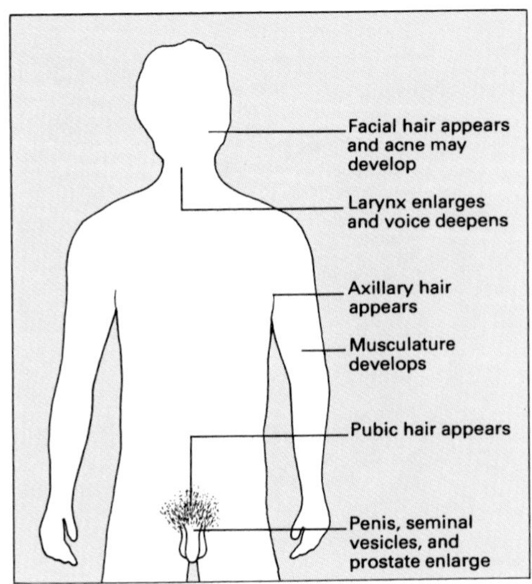

ening of the voice; enlargement of the penis and testes; alteration of body shape; and an increase in muscle strength. Testosterone is also thought to influence the development of balding.

Although women produce only a small amount of testosterone, it occasionally affects hair growth after menopause. Rarely, overproduction of testosterone by the adrenal glands may result in the development of male secondary sexual characteristics in women.

See also SEXUAL CHARACTERISTICS, SECONDARY; VIRILISM.

Tests and testing. *See* MEDICAL TEST.

Tests, hospital admission. *See* HOSPITALIZATION: ADULTS.

Tetanus (tet′ə nəs), also known as lockjaw, is caused by the toxin of the bacterium *Clostridium tetani.*

The bacteria are usually found in soil and animal feces. Thus, barnyards and fields fertilized with manure are often highly contaminated. The bacteria can remain alive for many years in the form of spores. The microorganisms grow in dead or damaged tissue that does not have an adequate blood supply and therefore has a low oxygen level. Infection may result from any wound that is contaminated by infected soil.

Q: *What are the symptoms of tetanus?*

A: There is an incubation period that may vary between 4 and 14 days, but can last as long as 7 weeks. The initial symptoms include stiffness of the jaw, slight difficulty in swallowing, restlessness, and stiffness of the arms, legs, and neck.

As the disease progresses, the patient may run a fever and may have difficulty opening the mouth (trismus or lockjaw). This may be accompanied by stiffness of the facial muscles, which may contract to produce a characteristic fixed grin. As the stiffness of the muscles increases, there may be painful convulsions, which may be fatal.

Q: *How is tetanus treated?*

A: Hospitalization is necessary. A tracheostomy, a temporary opening in the windpipe, may be performed, and the patient may be given mechanical artificial respiration to aid breathing. An intravenous infusion may also be necessary to correct the patient's fluid balance. Antitoxin in the form of gamma globulin is given to reduce the effect of the toxin. Muscle relaxant drugs will reduce the muscle spasms, and drugs that cause complete paralysis may be used when the patient is maintained on artificial respiration. However, death is still common despite these measures.

Q: *Can tetanus be prevented?*

A: Yes. An attack of tetanus itself does not confer immunity, but tetanus can be prevented by vaccination. After the childhood series of immunizations, adults should receive a tetanus booster shot once every 10 years to prevent the disease.

See also IMMUNIZATION.

Tetany (tet′ə nē) is a spasm of the muscles producing contractions in the hands, feet, and face. Sometimes, flexing of the arms and legs with cramplike pain, may occur. Occasionally, seizures may occur.

Tetany may result from an abnormally low concentration of calcium in the blood (hypocalcemia). Temporary hypocalcemia may be caused by hyperventilation (resulting from temporary lowering of calcium when carbon dioxide is lost from the body). Prolonged hypocalcemia may be caused by a deficiency of the parathyroid hormones. Vitamin D deficiency may also cause tetany. *See also* HYPOCALCEMIA.

Q: *How is tetany treated?*

A: If tetany is caused by hyperventilation, the patient should breathe into a paper bag. This normalizes the carbon dioxide concentration of the blood. Tetany that is caused by prolonged hypocalcemia may be treated with intravenous injections of calcium salts. Tetany resulting from vitamin D deficiency disappears when the deficiency is corrected.

Tetracycline (tet′rə sī klin) is a group of antibiotics that is produced by certain species of the fungus *Streptomyces.* Tetracycline drugs are effective against many bacterial infections. They are commonly prescribed to treat urinary infections, streptococcal infections, pneumonia, brucellosis, and rickettsial diseases, such as typhus. Tetracyclines may also be used to treat bacterial infections in patients who are sensitive to penicillin. Bacteria may become resistant to tetracyclines, but this does not usually occur during a short course of treatment.

Q: *Can tetracyclines produce adverse side effects?*

A: Yes. Treatment with tetracyclines may produce nausea, vomiting, and diarrhea. Allergic reactions are extremely rare. Prolonged treatment may lead to candidiasis and deficiency of the B vitamins. Occasionally, the skin may become abnormally sensitive to light. In children, tetracyclines may discolor the teeth and form drug deposits in the bones. For this reason, tetracycline should not be given to children under the age of 10 or to pregnant women.

See also ANTIBIOTIC; PENICILLIN.

Tetraplegia (tet rə plē′jē ə), also known as quadriplegia, is paralysis of all four limbs.

See also PARALYSIS.

Thalamus (thal′ə məs) is a collection of nerve cells that is situated above the hypothalamus and is part of the forebrain. There are two thalami, one on each side of the midline of the brain. The thalami act as coordinating centers for nerve impulses from all the senses. The impulses are then relayed to the appropriate areas in the cerebral cortex, where they are consciously perceived.

See also BRAIN; HYPOTHALAMUS.

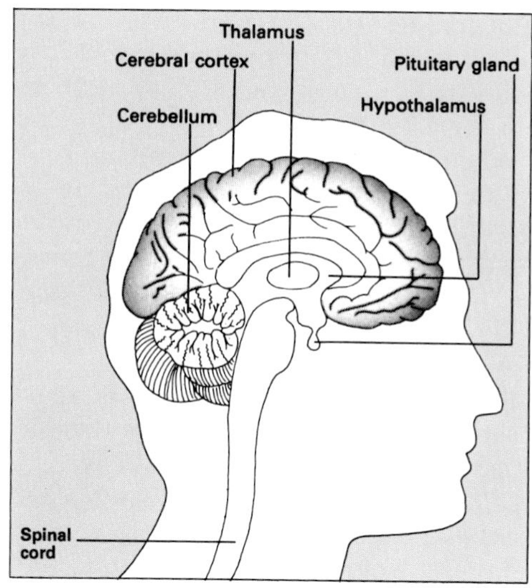

The **thalamus** is an oblong mass of grey matter in the posterior portion of the forebrain, from which nerve fibers pass to the sensory parts of the cerebral cortex.

Thalassemia (thal ə sē′mē ə) is the name given to a group of hemolytic anemias, which are disorders that affect the red blood cells. Cooley's anemia and Mediterranean anemia are types of thalassemia.

Q: *What are the symptoms of thalassemia?*

A: Symptoms of thalassemia usually occur only in those who have inherited an abnormal gene from both parents; this is called thalassemia major, or Cooley's anemia. When only one gene is inherited (thalassemia minor), there are usually no symptoms, but the individual is a carrier of the disease.

The symptoms of thalassemia major vary in severity. The common symptoms include breathlessness, pallor, and fatigue. There may also be jaundice, leg ulcers, enlargement of the spleen, and the formation of gallstones. The skull bones may thicken, and other bones may fracture easily.

Iron that is released from damaged red blood cells is deposited in the tissues (hemosiderosis), which may damage the heart muscle and ultimately result in heart failure.

Q: *How is thalassemia treated?*

A: There is no treatment required for thalassemia minor. For thalassemia major, blood transfusions are necessary but will ultimately result in iron overload. Most other treatments are ineffective.

See also ANEMIA; SIDEROSIS.

Thalidomide® (thə lid′ə mīd) is a sedative drug that was prescribed extensively in Europe during the late 1950's and early 1960's.

When taken by pregnant women, thalidomide was found to cause fetal deformities, especially of the limbs, and the drug was withdrawn from the market. It was also discovered that thalidomide caused a permanent form of peripheral neuritis.

Thallium stress test (thal′ē əm) is a nuclear scan used to supplement a regular stress electrocardiogram (or "stress test"). As the patient is exercising, a radioactive isotope is injected into a vein. The isotope completely enters only normal heart muscle cells. If a section of heart muscle is dead or not receiving an adequate blood supply, the isotope is not absorbed and that part of the heart does not produce an image on the X-ray scan.

After the exercise is completed and the patient has rested, another X-ray scan is taken. In this scan, the heart muscle that was previously not receiving enough blood will not appear normal. By comparing the two scans, a physician can determine if there is an area of the heart that has coronary artery disease and is at risk of developing a heart attack.

See also ELECTROCARDIOGRAM; HEART DISEASE, CORONARY; ISOTOPE; "STRESS" TEST.

Therapy. *See* PHYSICAL MEDICINE AND REHABILITATION; PSYCHOANALYSIS.

Therapy, occupational (ther′ə pē, ok yə pā′shə nəl). Occupational therapy involves the use of purposeful activities to treat persons disabled by injury, illness, emotional problems, or aging. Physically disabled individuals are helped to use their bodies more effectively; mentally disabled individuals are helped to overcome emotional problems. The major focus of occupational therapy is to help patients develop the skills necessary for performing specific activities of daily living: eating, dressing, bathing, as well as homemaking and recreational skills. These tasks help maximize independence, prevent disability, and maintain health. Activities are planned and supervised by a registered therapist.

Thermogram (thėr′mə gram) is a record of the infrared heat waves that are emitted by the body. It gives a visual display of the hot and cold areas of the whole body. The technique of obtaining a thermogram is known as thermography; it involves photographing or scanning the body with a special television camera that is sensitive to heat.

Thermography is sometimes useful in detecting breast cancer because the tumor is slightly hotter than the surrounding body tissues. Unfortunately, this test is too insensitive and, therefore, not always reliable for the screening of breast cancer. It may also be used to study the flow of blood throughout the body.

Thermometer (thər mom′ə tər) is an instrument for measuring temperature. It usually consists of a liquid-filled glass tube marked in degrees of Celsius or Fahrenheit. The liquid, usually mercury, expands or contracts with changes in temperature. A clinical thermometer is used to measure body temperature.

See also TEMPERATURE.

Thiamine (thī′ə min) is a vitamin (vitamin B_1) that occurs naturally in such foods as dried yeast, wheat germ, liver, legumes, and whole grains. Thiamine is essential for the normal metabolism of fats and carbohydrates, and also the functioning of nerves and heart muscle. Thiamine deficiency may result from an inadequate diet; impaired absorption of nutrients, as may occur with sprue or alcoholism; or increased bodily demands, which may result from hyperthyroidism or pregnancy. Thiamine deficiency may cause beriberi or Korsakoff's syndrome.

See also BERIBERI; KORSAKOFF'S SYNDROME; VITAMIN.

Thigh (thī) is the section of the leg between the hip and the knee.

Thigh fracture: first aid. *See* FRACTURE: FIRST AID.

Thirst (thėrst) is the desire for fluid, especially water. The sensation of thirst is caused by, among many other factors, an increase in sodium concentration in the blood and by loss of potassium from the body cells.

Thirst may be a symptom of various conditions, such as hemorrhage, profuse sweating, vomiting, diarrhea, or excessive urination, as in diabetes mellitus or diabetes insipidus. Patients with heart failure may suffer from extreme thirst, but if they drink too much water, edema of the legs may develop.

See also DIABETES; EDEMA.

Thoracic duct (thô ras′ik) is the largest lymphatic vessel in the body, joined to the superior vena cava. It extends from the second lumbar vertebra up to the root of the neck. It conveys lymph from the whole body except for the upper right quadrant of the body, which is served by the right lymphatic duct.

See also LYMPHATIC SYSTEM.

Thoracic surgery (thô ras′ik) is any operative procedure performed on the thorax or chest.

Thoracoplasty (thôr′ə kō plas tē) is a surgical operation in which several ribs are removed. The chest wall then collapses onto the underlying diseased lung, causing the lung itself to collapse. This operation was frequently used in the treatment of tuberculosis, but is rarely necessary now because of the modern antitubercular drugs.

See also TUBERCULOSIS.

Thoracotomy (thôr ə kot′ə mē) is any surgical operation that involves opening the chest wall.

Thorax (thôr′aks), or chest, is the part of the trunk between the neck and the abdomen. It is enclosed by the thoracic spine at the back, ribs on either side, the breastbone (sternum) in front, and the diaphragm muscle at the bottom.

The thorax contains the two lungs, the heart, the main blood vessels (the aorta, the pulmonary artery, their branches, the venae cavae, and the pulmonary veins), and the esophagus (gullet). Other structures include the thoracic duct, the thymus, the sympathetic ganglia and nerves, and the pleura (the membrane surrounding the lungs). The central part of the thorax that contains the heart and esophagus is the mediastinum.

The muscles of the thorax include the intercostal muscles between the ribs and the muscles that attach the shoulder bone (scapula), the collarbone (clavicle), and the bone of the upper arm (humerus) to the chest wall.

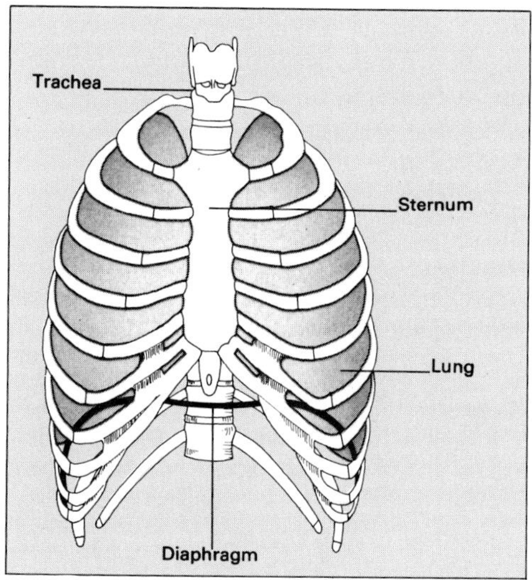

The **thorax** (chest) is the portion of the body from the trachea to the diaphragm, including the heart and the lungs.

Thorazine® (thôr′ə zēn) is a preparation of the drug chlorpromazine hydrochloride. It is used primarily as an antipsychotic. It can also be used to treat unmanageable vomiting.

Threadworm (thred′wėrm) is a small, parasitic nematode worm that infests the intestine. Some authorities use this term to refer to the worm *Enterobius vermicularis;* others use it to refer to the worm *Strongyloides stercoralis.*

See also ENTEROBIASIS; STRONGYLOIDES.

Throat (thrōt) is the common name for the pharynx and the fauces, the opening that leads from the back of the mouth into the pharynx. The front part of the neck is also referred to as the throat.

See also PHARYNX.

Throat abscess. *See* ABSCESS, THROAT.

Throat, lump in. A lump in the throat is a symptom of many disorders, such as a mild throat infection and laryngitis. It is often accompanied by inflammation of the throat and slight discomfort on swallowing. A lump in the throat may also be caused by pressure on the throat from an enlarged thyroid gland (goiter) or from swollen lymph glands. Emotional states may cause the sensation of a lump in the throat that varies in severity, and this condition is known as globus hystericus.

If the sensation of a lump in the throat persists, a physician should be consulted.

See also GLOBUS HYSTERICUS.

Throat, sore. A sore throat is a symptom of many disorders, including a cold, diphtheria, influenza, laryngitis, measles, mononucleosis, pharyngitis, and tonsillitis. (Each of these disorders has a separate entry in this encyclopedia.) A sore throat may also be caused by heavy smoking.

Temporary relief may be obtained by taking medicated throat lozenges, aspirin, or acetaminophen. It is also advisable to stop smoking, to drink plenty of fluids, and to eat soft foods. A physician should be consulted if a sore throat persists; there may be a serious underlying illness.

Some sore throats are the result of streptococcal pharyngitis. Although the sore throat will resolve itself even without treatment, antibiotics are prescribed to prevent complications of the strep infection, such as scarlet fever, rheumatic fever, or glomerulonephritis.

See also GLOMERULONEPHRITIS; RHEUMATIC FEVER; SCARLET FEVER.

Throat, strep (strep). Strep throat, or streptococcal sore throat, is an infection of the throat and tonsils characterized by a sore throat, fever, chills, swollen tonsils and lymph nodes in the neck, and in some cases, nausea and vomiting. The disorder occurs primarily in children and is spread via droplets of moisture sprayed from the nose and mouth of infected persons. Strep throat is caused by bacterium from the species *Streptococcus*. Treatment usually involves administering penicillin.

See also STREPTOCOCCUS.

Thromboangiitis obliterans (throm bō an jē ī'tis ə blit'ə rənz), also known as Buerger's disease, is a chronic disease of the blood vessels, usually in the legs, in which there is a narrowing of the arteries and veins.

See also BUERGER'S DISEASE.

Thrombocytopenia (throm bə sī tə pē' nē ə) is a decrease in the normal number of platelets (thrombocytes), which are the particles in the blood that are essential for clotting. The condition may result from decreased platelet production, caused by leukemia, cancer, drugs, aplastic anemia, or irradiation. Thrombocytopenia may also result from increased platelet destruction, which may be caused by drugs, such as sulfonamides, or poisons. Injuries and burns may cause the body to use platelets faster than they can be replaced, which may cause a temporary platelet deficiency. Another frequent cause is idiopathic thrombocytopenic purpura (ITP), which is a disease in which platelets are destroyed by an autoimmune process; the cause of this process is usually unknown.

Q: *What are the symptoms of thrombocytopenia?*

A: The main symptom is bleeding, which may occur in any part of the body. Usually, bleeding occurs just below the skin, producing bruises and small hemorrhages (petechiae). Anemia may result from excessive bleeding.

Q: *How is thrombocytopenia treated?*

A: Treatment is directed toward the underlying cause. Transfusions of platelets may be given until the treatment takes effect or until the patient recovers naturally. In patients with thrombocytopenic purpura, treatment with corticosteroid drugs may be effective. In severe cases, removal of the spleen may be necessary.

Thrombolysis (throm bol'i sis) is the destruction of a blood clot (thrombus) by means of an intravenous infusion of enzymes that dissolve the thrombus. The technique involves a continuous infusion of enzymes into a vein for at least two days. This is followed by treatment with anticoagulant drugs to prevent further blood clots from forming. Thrombolysis may cause adverse tissue reactions.

See also ANTICOAGULANT.

Thrombophlebitis. *See* THROMBOSIS, VENOUS.

Thrombosis (throm bō'sis) is the formation of a blood clot (thrombus) in an artery or vein. When a thrombus becomes detached from its original site of formation, it is called an embolus.

See also EMBOLISM; STROKE; THROMBOSIS, VENOUS.

Thrombosis, cerebral (throm bō'sis sə rē'brəl). A cerebral thrombosis is the formation of a blood clot in any blood vessel of the brain.

Thrombosis, coronary (throm bō'sis, kor'ə ner ē). A coronary thrombosis is the formation of a blood clot blocking a coronary artery, often resulting in myocardial infarction (heart attack) and death.

See also HEART ATTACK.

Thrombosis, venous (throm bō'sis, vē'nəs). Venous thrombosis is the formation of a blood clot (thrombus) in a vein. Clotting that is associated with

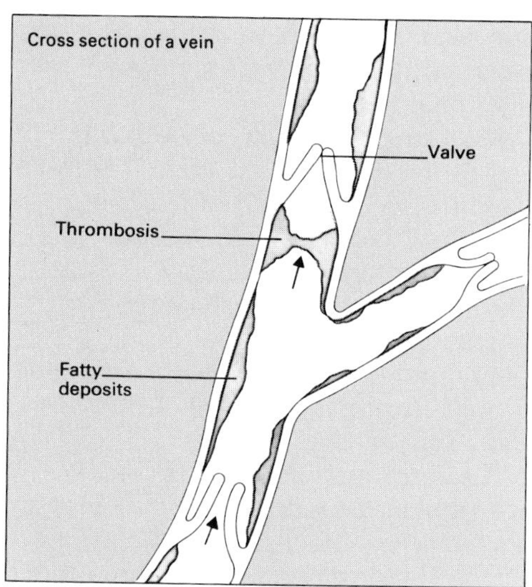

A **venous thrombosis** is more likely to occur near a valve where the blood can clot more easily, due to the slower flow of blood.

inflammation of a vein (phlebitis) is known as thrombophlebitis; clotting that occurs without venous inflammation is called phlebothrombosis.

Q: *What causes venous thrombosis?*

A: Venous thrombosis may be caused by any of several factors. It may result from damage to the wall of a vein caused by injury, infection, or some form of autoimmune disorder, in which the body reacts against itself, causing venous inflammation. Sometimes, thrombosis may develop because of the combination of an increase in the clotting factors within the blood and slowing of the normal blood circulation. The use of hormones, particularly estrogen, may predispose a person to blood clotting. Pregnancy and prolonged bed rest are both associated with venous thrombosis.

Q: *What are the symptoms of venous thrombosis?*

A: Symptoms vary according to whether a superficial or deep vein is involved. The most common type of venous thrombosis is associated with superficial veins. With varicose veins, a combination of poor blood circulation, mild skin inflammation and, sometimes, ulceration may cause thrombophlebitis of the leg. This may result in local tenderness and swelling of the vein, and redness and swelling of the nearby skin. If a deep vein has thrombosed, the symptoms may include swelling of the ankles, slight tenderness when the calf is pressed, and discomfort when the foot is pulled upward; the calf may be swollen, red in appearance, and warm to the touch. Deep vein thrombosis in areas other than the leg may be impossible to detect, and the diagnosis of deep vein thrombosis may require special techniques such as X rays of the veins, ultrasound techniques, and a blood count of the number of platelets. *See also* VENOGRAM.

Q: *Can venous thrombosis cause complications?*

A: Yes. The most serious complication occurs when a piece of the blood clot breaks off to form an embolus. This is potentially fatal. Emboli, however, are relatively rare compared with the number of deep vein thromboses. The long-term consequence of deep vein thrombosis is usually degeneration of the valves in the affected veins. This may result in swelling of the ankles and skin disorders, such as dermatitis and ulcers. *See also* EMBOLISM.

Superficial venous thrombosis seldom causes serious complications.

Q: *How is venous thrombosis treated?*

A: If a deep thrombosis is diagnosed, hospital treatment with anticoagulant (commonly known as "blood thinning") therapy is required. Initially, injections of heparin are usually given. Later, other anticoagulant drugs are administered orally.

Anticoagulant treatment may need to be continued from two to six months. If an embolus develops, surgery may be necessary to tie off the affected vein.

Superficial venous thrombosis is usually treated with painkillers, heat, elevation of the affected limb, and bandaging of the leg to reduce swelling.

If ankle swelling or other complications develop after deep vein thrombosis, the patient should wear elastic support stockings during waking hours for his or her lifetime.

Q: *Can venous thrombosis be prevented?*

A: Yes. Some persons are more likely than others to develop venous thrombosis. Those at risk include the elderly; those with diabetes; those with blood disorders, such as polycythemia vera; women who take contraceptive pills that contain estrogens; persons with a history of thrombosis; and patients who have undergone gynecological surgery. In such cases, anticoagulant treatment may be necessary before any surgery is performed. This may prevent venous thrombosis from occurring.

Before surgery is performed, the patient should do special calf and leg exercises. After surgery, he or she should resume physical activity as soon as possible. Such measures reduce the likelihood of venous thrombosis.

See also BLOOD CLOT; BUDD-CHIARI SYNDROME.

Thrombus (throm′bəs) is a blood clot in a blood vessel.

See also BLOOD CLOT; THROMBOSIS, VENOUS.

Thrush (thrush) is an infection of the mouth tissues caused by the fungus *Candida albicans*. It is commonly seen in young babies and in patients who are using inhaled steroid medications.

See also CANDIDIASIS.

Thumb is the first digit of the hand. It contains only two bones (phalanges), unlike the fingers, which have three.

See also HAND.

Thumb fracture: first aid. *See* FRACTURE: FIRST AID.

Thumb-sucking is a common habit in almost all babies and children. It occurs as frequently in breast-fed babies as in bottle-fed babies. Thumb-sucking becomes less frequent after the age of 3 years and seldom continues after the age of 10.

Excessive thumb-sucking may cause blistering of the thumb, which may lead to skin infection. Continual thumb-sucking may also affect the alignment of the front teeth.

Usually, it is safe to let a child suck his or her thumb. In fact, if there are no other significant problems, ignoring the behavior is probably the best strategy. But, if problems such as skin damage or dental deformity develop, the child should be gently persuaded to stop. The child should not be punished or ridiculed. Persistent thumb-sucking in older children may be a sign of an emotional problem.

Thymus (thī′məs) is an organ that is part of the lymphatic system. It is located in the upper part of the chest cavity just behind the breastbone (sternum). It is composed largely of cells similar to lymphocytes. The thymus grows rapidly during fetal development, gradually until puberty, and then shrinks during adult years of life. *See also* LYMPHOCYTE.

The full function of the thymus is not known. It produces lymphocytes, a type of white blood cell, and plays a part in the development of immunity.

Q: *What disorders may affect the thymus?*

A: Disorders of the thymus are uncommon. Rarely, children are born without a thymus or with a defective one. This produces a defect in immunity, and the child suffers from repeated infections. Tumors of the thymus are also rare, but many patients with myasthenia gravis have thymic tumors and may improve when the tumor is removed. Most thymic tumors are benign (noncancerous).

See also MYASTHENIA GRAVIS.

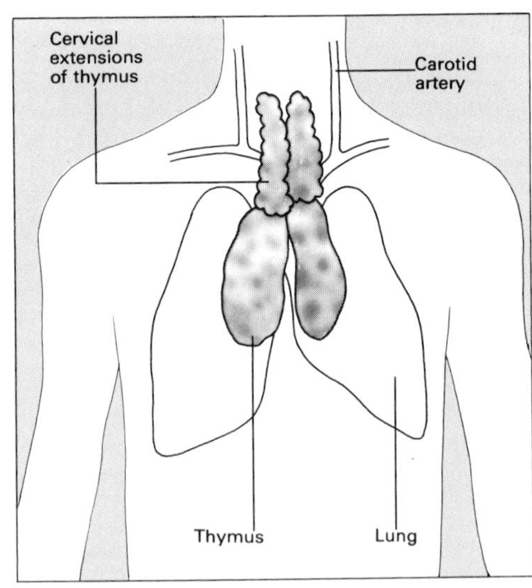

The **thymus** produces lymphocytes and helps in the development of the body's natural immunity during infancy and childhood.

Thyroidectomy (thī roi dek′tə mē) is the surgical removal of part or all of the thyroid gland. A medical thyroidectomy is the destruction of part or all of the thyroid gland by the use of drugs.

A thyroidectomy may be performed to treat overactivity of the thyroid gland (hyperthyroidism) or to remove nodules that form in or on the gland. It may be necessary to remove part of the thyroid gland if it becomes greatly enlarged (goiter) and obstructs breathing. *See also* GOITER; HYPERTHYROIDISM.

Q: ***Are there any hazards associated with a thyroidectomy?***

A: Yes, but these are rare. During surgery, great care has to be taken not to remove the four parathyroid glands or to cut the nerves to the vocal cords. Removal of the parathyroid glands may cause hypocalcemia and tetany. If one of the nerves to the vocal cords is cut, hoarseness may result; if both nerves are cut, the person's voice will be of markedly decreased intensity, and breathing will be impaired. If too much of the thyroid gland is removed, hypothyroidism eventually develops, and replacement of the deficient thyroid hormones will be necessary.

See also HYPOCALCEMIA; HYPOTHYROIDISM; TETANY; THYROID GLAND.

Thyroid gland (thī′roid) is an endocrine gland in the front of the neck. It consists of two lobes, one on each side of the Adam's apple, which are joined across the front of the windpipe, just below the voice box.

The thyroid gland secretes two main hormones, thyroxine and triiodothyronine, into the bloodstream. These hormones stimulate all the cells in the body. The thyroid gland also secretes a hormone (calcitonin) that reduces the concentration of calcium in the blood.

The production of thyroid hormones is controlled by the thyroid stimulating hormone (TSH), which is secreted by the pituitary gland. This control is modified by the hypothalamus, which detects thyroid hormone levels in the blood and influences the secretion of TSH.

Q: ***What disorders affect the thyroid gland?***

A: The thyroid gland may become enlarged (goiter) because of a deficiency of iodine. It can also become overactive (hyperthyroidism) or underactive (hypothyroidism). Nodules may form in the thyroid gland and cause hyperthyroidism.

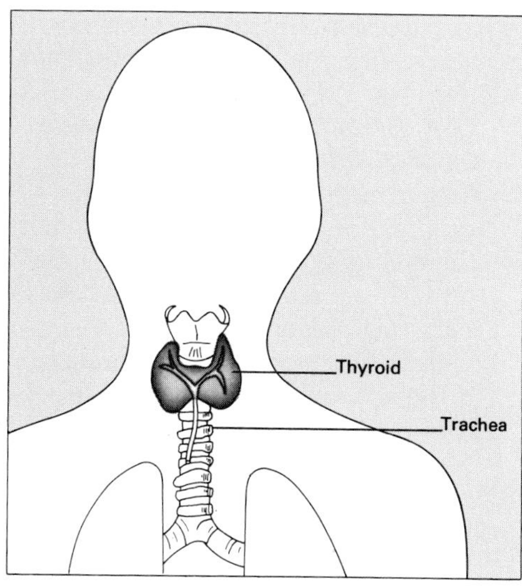

The **thyroid gland** is located below the Adam's apple and folds around the trachea.

These may be either benign or malignant (cancerous). *See also* GOITER; HYPERTHYROIDISM; HYPOTHYROIDISM.

Occasionally, the thyroid gland may become inflamed (thyroiditis) as a result of infection. If chronic, thyroiditis may be associated with autoimmune disease (Hashimoto's thyroiditis).

See also THYROIDITIS, HASHIMOTO'S.

Thyroiditis, Hashimoto's (thī roi dī′tis, hä shi mō′tōz). Hashimoto's thyroiditis is an inflammation of the thyroid gland caused by an increase in the fibrous tissue and an infiltration of white blood cells; this is due to an autoimmune process in which the body produces antibodies to thyroid tissue. The condition is more common in women than in men and usually develops during early middle age. The symptoms, which develop slowly, include difficulty swallowing, enlargement of the thyroid gland, occasionally anemia, enlargement of the thymus, lethargy, loss of appetite, underactivity of the thyroid gland, and eventually myxedema.

See also MYXEDEMA; THYROID GLAND.

Thyroid preparations (thī′roid) are drugs that are used to treat disorders of the thyroid gland, such as simple goiter, hypothyroidism (underproduction of thyroid hormones), hyperthyroidism (overproduction of thyroid hormones), and thyroiditis (inflammation of the thyroid gland). *See also* GOITER; HYPERTHYROIDISM; HYPOTHYROIDISM.

Thyroid preparations are available as extracts of thyroid glands from animals, which are less preferable, or as synthetic preparations of thyroxine or triiodothyronine. *See also* THYROXINE.

Q: ***Can thyroid preparations produce adverse side effects?***

A: Yes. Overdosage of any thyroid preparation causes thyrotoxicosis. Signs and symptoms may include rapid heart rate, palpitations, chest pain, nervousness, insomnia, weight loss, and heat intolerance. If the appropriate amount of thyroid hormone is provided for replacement, no adverse reactions occur. A physician should carefully monitor the level of thyroid hormone in the blood when these preparations are used. *See also* THYROTOXICOSIS.

Thyrotoxicosis (thī rō tok sə kō′sis), also known as Graves' disease, is a disorder caused by the overproduction of thyroid hormones by the thyroid gland (hyperthyroidism). *See also* THYROID GLAND.

Often, the cause is not known. There seems to be a breakdown in the normal balance of the feedback mechanism from the pituitary gland that produces thyroid stimulating hormone (TSH), so that an excessive amount of TSH causes overproduction of thyroid hormones. Rarely, the thyroid gland grows a benign tumor, and this can also cause an overproduction of thyroid hormones.

Occasionally, thyrotoxicosis starts after an emotional shock or prolonged period of anxiety. It may sometimes occur at the onset of Hashimoto's thyroiditis. *See also* THYROIDITIS, HASHIMOTO'S.

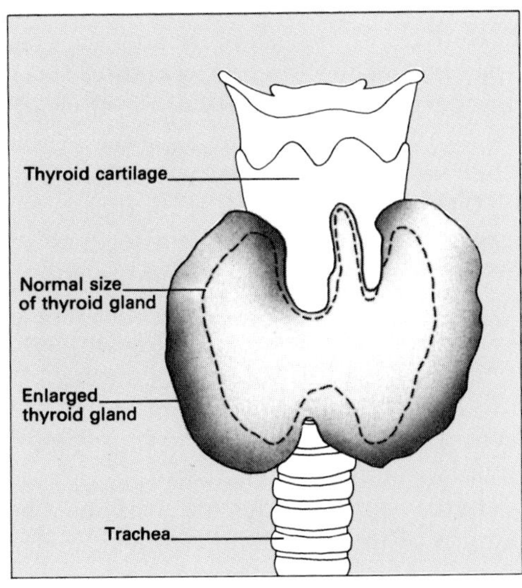

Thyrotoxicosis results from overactivity of the thyroid gland, which may become enlarged.

Q: ***What are the symptoms of thyrotoxicosis?***

A: The symptoms include sweating, nervousness, fatigue, insomnia, sensitivity to heat, hunger, loss of weight, diarrhea, trembling hands, and bulging of the eyes (exophthalmos). Often, there is a slight swelling in the neck, just below the Adam's apple, because of enlargement of the thyroid gland. In older persons, there may also be depression, atrial fibrillation, and heart failure. *See also* FIBRILLATION.

Q: ***How is thyrotoxicosis treated?***

A: While the condition is being diagnosed, drugs (beta blockers) may be prescribed to control the symptoms. Once the diagnosis has been confirmed, there are three possible forms of treatment. The most suitable depends on expert medical advice.

Drugs that reduce thyroid activity are usually effective. Alternatively, the patient may undergo surgery to remove part of the thyroid gland or any active nodule in the gland.

Radioactive iodine treatment is simple and effective. Both surgery and radioactive iodine treatment tend to be followed, some years later, by diminished production of the thyroid hormones. *See also* HYPOTHYROIDISM.

Q: ***Are there any complications of thyrotoxicosis?***

A: Yes. Occasionally, the symptoms of thyrotoxicosis suddenly become much worse in a condition called a thyroid crisis, which may be brought on by acute anxiety, childbirth, or an operation. Thyrotoxicosis can develop into a fatal condition, with fever, rapid heartbeat, and worsening of all the other symptoms. This requires urgent hospital treatment.

A more common complication is that caused by protuberance of the eyes (exophthalmos). Such eye problems sometimes become worse after treatment for thyrotoxicosis and result in swelling of the eyelids and tissues behind the eyeball. This condition requires skilled care to prevent eye infection. Another possible complication is ophthalmoplegia (paralysis of the nerves of the eye) that results in double vision (diplopia). This condition tends to improve on its own.

Thyroxine (thī rok'sēn) is one of the two principal hormones that are secreted by the thyroid gland; the other main thyroid hormone is triiodothyronine.

The effect of both hormones is similar: they increase the metabolic rate of the body cells. Preparations of these hormones may be given to treat thyroid gland deficiency disorders, such as hypothyroidism.

See also THYROID GLAND.

Tibia (tib'ē ə), also known as the shinbone, is the innermost and larger of the two bones of the lower leg. The fibula is the smaller outer bone.

The upper end of the tibia forms the knee joint with the femur and is covered by two semicircular cartilages (menisci). The lower end of the tibia forms the ankle joint with the fibula and the talus bone.

See also LEG.

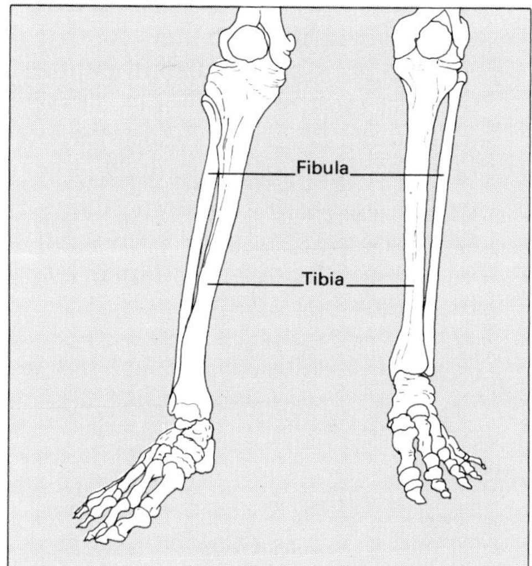

The **tibia** is the inner and thicker of the two bones of the lower leg.

Tic (tik) is an habitual, involuntary spasm or twitch that usually affects the face, neck, or shoulder muscles.

Tics often become more frequent when a person is under emotional stress, and disappear during sleep. For this reason, they are thought to be of psychological origin.

Childhood tics usually disappear spontaneously. But tics in adults may resist treatment. Psychotherapy may help some people, but it is not always successful.

See also CHOREA.

Tic douloureux, (tik' dü lü rü'), also known as trigeminal neuralgia, is a nervous disorder that causes severe facial pain. A tic, or facial spasm is not present in most cases.

See also NEURALGIA, TRIGEMINAL.

Tick (tik) is a small, tough-skinned parasite that is related to mites and spiders. Ticks often attach themselves to the skin of humans and animals and suck their blood. Soft-bodied ticks (*Argasidae*) may transmit the spiral-shaped bacteria that cause relapsing fever. Hard-bodied ticks (*Ixodidae*) may transmit the rickettsial bacteria that cause African tick typhus, Rocky Mountain spotted fever, and Q fever. Ticks have been found to transmit Lyme disease to humans and may also play a part in the transmission of tularemia.

Some species of ticks can cause tick paralysis. This condition is characterized by lethargy, muscle weakness, loss of coordination, and paralysis, which may affect the respiratory muscles. Removal of the tick usually leads to rapid recovery. It is advisable to have these species of ticks removed by a medical professional, as tick paralysis can be fatal, and ticks may be difficult to locate.

Q: ***How should a tick be removed?***

A: Do not try to pull the tick out forcibly; this may cause its toothed beak to break off and remain inside the skin, resulting in a sore. The best method is to place a drop of alcohol or nail polish on the tick, wait several minutes, and then carefully remove the tick using tweezers. Wash the affected area of skin thoroughly with soap and water.

See also LYME DISEASE; Q FEVER; RELAPSING FEVER; ROCKY MOUNTAIN SPOTTED FEVER; TULAREMIA.

Tietze's syndrome (tēt'sēz) is a rheumatic disorder that is characterized by pain and tenderness on the front of the chest, with the pain sometimes spreading to the arm, shoulder, or neck. The radiating pain is similar to that associated with coronary artery disease. The underlying cause of Tietze's syndrome is not known; the pain is the result of the swelling of the rib cartilages where they join the breastbone. It occurs many times following open-heart surgery. The disorder usually disappears spontaneously within about eight weeks.

See also HEART DISEASE, CORONARY.

Tinea (tin′ē ə), or ringworm, is any of several skin diseases caused by a group of fungi and characterized by itching and lesions. Athlete's foot (tinea pedis) and jock itch (tinea cruris) are forms of this infection.

See also ATHLETE'S FOOT; JOCK ITCH; RINGWORM; TINEA VERSICOLOR.

Tinea cruris. *See* JOCK ITCH.

Tinea versicolor (tin′ē ə vėr′sə kul ər) is a mild fungal skin infection that produces small, pale, itchy patches on the shoulders and upper arms. Selenium soap or shampoo usually cures the condition.

Tine test (tīn) is a skin test for tuberculosis. It is performed using an instrument with several prongs (tines) that penetrate the skin and introduce a solution of dead tuberculosis organisms (tuberculin). This test is not as sensitive as the Mantoux test.

See also MANTOUX TEST; TUBERCULIN TEST.

Tinnitus (ti nī′təs) is the subjective sensation of noise in one or both ears, without there being any external sound. It may be experienced as a buzzing, ringing, hissing, or roaring noise, or as a series of more complex sounds. Tinnitus may be continuous or intermittent and is usually associated with varying degrees of deafness.

Any disorder of the ear may cause tinnitus, such as wax in the outer ear, Ménière's disease, otosclerosis, and otitis. It may also result from a head injury, nerve disorders, arteriosclerosis, smoking, and drugs, such as aspirin or antibiotics.

Objective tinnitus also occurs, but much less frequently. It is usually associated with vascular formations close to the ear or in the neck.

A person with tinnitus may find sleeping especially difficult. Background noise, made by a fan or a radio turned between stations so as to produce soft, static noise, will often mask the tinnitus and make the person more comfortable.

See also MÉNIÈRE'S DISEASE; OTITIS; OTOSCLEROSIS.

Tobacco smoking. *See* SMOKING OF TOBACCO.

Tocopherol (tō kof′ə rōl) is a general term for vitamin E (alpha tocopherol) or several compounds that are chemically related to vitamin E. Vitamin E plays a vital role in the metabolism of polyunsaturated fats in the body cells; it also appears to be necessary for the production of hemoglobin. It occurs naturally in wheat germ and other food products, but can be produced artificially.

See also VITAMIN.

Toe is any of the digits of the foot. Each toe has a protective nail at the end. The big toe (hallux) has two phalangeal bones; the other four toes each have three phalangeal bones. Movement of the toes is controlled by muscles in the foot and leg.

The toes help to distribute the weight of the body evenly along the heads of the main bones of the foot (the metatarsal bones). The toes also help to balance the body.

Q: *What disorders can affect the toes?*

A: Various generalized bone and joint disorders may affect the toes, such as osteoarthritis, rheumatoid arthritis, and gout, which usually affects the first joint of the big toe. These disorders may cause deformities of the toes, such as hallux valgus, hallux rigidus, and hammertoe. Rarely, a child may be born with more than the normal number of toes (polydactylism).

See also FOOT; HALLUX RIGIDUS; HALLUX VALGUS; HAMMERTOE.

Toe fracture: first aid. *See* FRACTURE: FIRST AID.

Toenail. *See* NAIL.

Toenail, ingrown. An ingrown toenail is a toenail that has a tendency to grow into the adjacent soft skin tissue, producing infection and inflammation. This condition most commonly develops on the big toe from a combination of factors, including tight shoes; the tendency to cut the nail in a semicircular shape; and, in many people, having nails with an inverted U shape rather than a flat surface, so that the edges point down into the toe.

Q: *What is the treatment for an ingrown toenail?*

A: Treatment includes wearing wider, round-toed shoes to remove pressure from the nail. In addition, the toenail should be cut straight across and not in a curve. Regular cleaning of the toenail helps to reduce minor infection, and a small plug of cotton, soaked in rubbing alcohol, can be used as an antiseptic.

If these simple measures fail to control the infection and inflammation, or if a chronic infection (paronychia) develops, then antibiotic creams and lotions may be tried. If infection still persists, a minor surgical operation may be performed to remove the side of the nail and part of the skin of the toe.

Toilet seat, elevated. *See* NURSING THE SICK.

Toilet training. *See* BABY CARE.

Tomogram (tō'mə gram) is an X-ray image made via tomography.

See also TOMOGRAPHY.

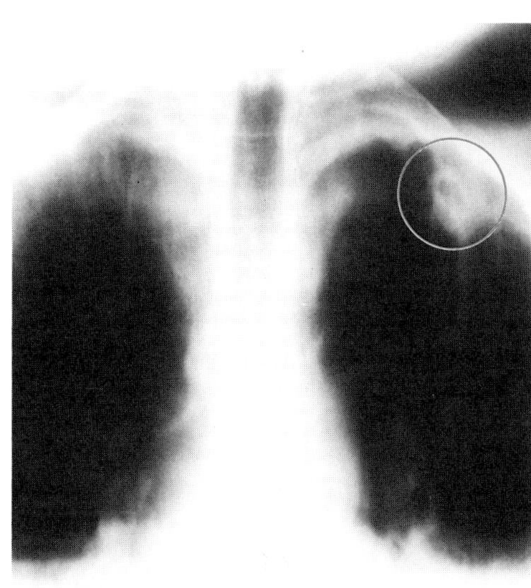

A **tomogram** is a selective X ray that photographs a particular layer of tissue, while blurring out images of other layers.

Tomography (tə mog'rə fē) is X-ray photography that focuses on a structure in a certain layer of tissue in the body, while images of structures in other layers of tissue are not recorded. The process utilizes a special technique in which the X-ray apparatus is rotated around the patient while the X-ray picture is taken.

See also COMPUTERIZED AXIAL TOMOGRAPHY SCANNER; POSITRON EMISSION TRANSAXIAL TOMOGRAPHY.

Tongue (tung) is the movable muscular organ that lies partly on the floor of the mouth and partly in the pharynx. It is attached to the hyoid bone above the larynx, the base of the skull below the ears, and the lower jaw.

The tongue is the main organ of taste. Its surface is covered with a special mucous membrane that contains numerous taste buds. The tongue also manipulates food and helps in the production of normal speech.

Q: *What disorders can affect the tongue?*

A: The most common disorder is inflammation of the tongue (glossitis). Ulcers may form as a result of rubbing against broken teeth or the spread of a mouth ulcer (canker sore).

An ulcer or a lump on the tongue may be caused by cancer; it occurs most commonly in those who smoke. Cancer of the tongue is generally treated by surgical removal of the cancer.

Q: *Why may the tongue become discolored or furred?*

A: Discoloration or furring of the tongue is not always a sign of disease. It may result from smoking, a course of antibiotics, indigestion, a respiratory infection, or tonsillitis.

A bright red tongue may be a symptom of a vitamin B deficiency, either pellagra or pernicious anemia. A black tongue is often due to excessive smoking, but it may also appear for no apparent reason, then disappear spontaneously.

See also ANEMIA, PERNICIOUS; CANKER SORE; GLOSSITIS; PELLAGRA.

Tongue, hairy (tung, hār'ē). Hairy tongue is a formation of dark pigmentation on the tongue. It may be either the result of fever or a side effect of antibiotics. The condition is harmless and gradually disappears on its own. Heavy smoking stains the tongue dark brown; this may be mistaken for hairy tongue.

Tonic (ton'ik) is the medical term for a continuous muscle contraction, as opposed to clonic contractions, in which the muscles alternately contract and relax.

Tonic also refers to a preparation that is supposed to give strength or invigorate the body.

Tonsil (ton′səl) is an almond-shaped mass of sponge-like lymphoid tissue. The two palatine tonsils are situated at the entrance to the pharynx, one on each side, below the soft palate and above the base of the tongue. The lingual tonsil is a similar mass of lymphoid tissue that is situated on the back of the tongue and which, with the adenoids and palatine tonsils, forms a ring of lymphoid tissue that protects the entrance to the throat. The tonsils and adenoids grow smaller as children grow older.

Q: *What are the functions of the tonsils?*

A: The tonsils apparently have two functions: they trap and destroy microorganisms that enter the throat, and they play a part in the body's immune system by producing antibodies.

Q: *What disorders may affect the tonsils?*

A: The most common disorders that affect the tonsils are tonsillitis and infectious mononucleosis. Abscesses may form around the tonsils, and cancer of the tonsil also occurs.

See also MONONUCLEOSIS; TONSILLITIS.

Tonsillectomy (ton sə lek′tə mē) is the surgical removal of the palatine tonsils. The adenoids are often removed (adenoidectomy) at the same time. The tonsils are not usually removed unless the patient has suffered several attacks of severe tonsillitis or a peritonsillar abscess; if there is airway obstruction; or if there is a suspicion of cancer. A physician may also recommend a tonsillectomy if a complication, such as peritonsillar abscess, develops from tonsillitis or if the tonsils are so large that they obstruct breathing.

Q: *Can a tonsillectomy cause complications?*

A: Yes. However, these are rare. Middle ear infections, such as otitis media, may occur, but the most serious complication is hemorrhage. For this reason, it is advisable to stay in the hospital until the surgeon is certain the area is healing well.

Q: *What happens at the operation, and how long is it necessary to stay in the hospital?*

A: For four hours before the operation the patient must not eat or drink. Two hours later a sedative is given. Generally, a parent is allowed to stay with a young patient until the anesthesiologist is ready to inject an anesthetic into a vein in the arm.

After the operation, the child is sleepy for several hours, but apart from some bloodstained saliva there should be no complications. The next day the child may complain of a sore throat. This is controlled with acetaminophen, ice drinks, ice cream, and gelatin, which can be consumed without too much discomfort. In most cases, the patient returns home within a few days.

See also TONSIL; TONSILLITIS.

Tonsillitis (ton sə lī′tis) is an inflammation of the tonsils. It may be caused by a viral infection or infection with streptococcal bacteria. Tonsillitis occurs most commonly during early childhood.

Q: *What are the symptoms of tonsillitis?*

A: Tonsillitis is characterized by a sore throat, difficulty in swallowing, headache, swollen glands, and high fever. In very young children, the main symptoms may be abdominal pain, vomiting, and diarrhea.

Q: *How is tonsillitis treated?*

A: The treatment of viral tonsillitis is directed toward relieving the symptoms. It is not usually necessary to remove the tonsils surgically (tonsillectomy) unless tonsillitis recurs or complications arise.

Tonsillitis that is caused by streptococcal infection is treated with antibiotics, usually penicillin or erythromycin, for a full 10 days to eradicate the infection. An analgesic may also be prescribed to relieve the pain. The patient should eat soft foods and drink plenty of fluids to prevent dehydration.

Q: *What complications can result from tonsillitis caused by streptococcus?*

A: The body's immune system may react to the streptococcal organism, causing rheumatic fever. The infection may also spread to surrounding tissues, producing a peritonsillar abscess. *See also* ABSCESS, PERITONSILLAR; RHEUMATIC FEVER.

Tooth (tüth) is any of the hard, bone-like structures in the mouth, used for biting and chewing. Adults normally have an average of 32 teeth, 16 in each jaw. Children have 20 deciduous, or milk teeth, which gradually fall out and are replaced, one by one, by the permanent adult teeth.

The outer layer of a tooth consists of hard, white enamel. Under the enamel is dentin, which is an ivory-like substance. Dentin forms the major part of a tooth. In the center of a tooth is a soft pulp layer, which contains blood vessels, nerves, and odontoblasts (cells that can form more dentin if a tooth is damaged).

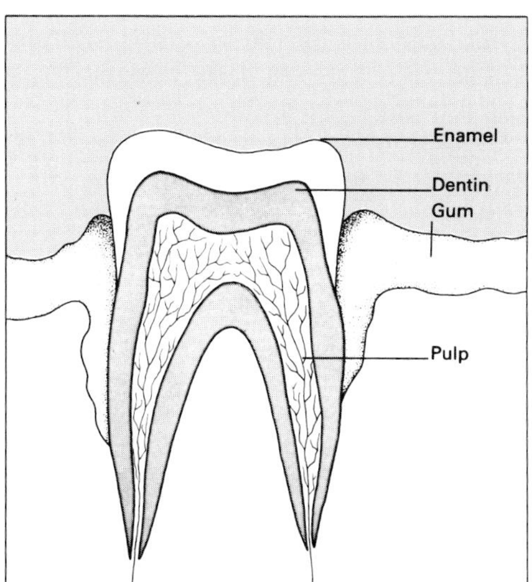

A **tooth** extends from the crown, or visible part above the gums, to the root, which extends into the bone of the jaw.

Q: *What are the functions of the teeth?*

A: There are four different types of teeth: incisors, canines, premolars, and molars. The incisors are used for cutting; the canines are used for gripping and tearing; and the back teeth, the premolars and molars, are used for grinding and chewing.

Q: *How should teeth be cared for?*

A: The teeth can be kept healthy by careful diet, with as little sugar as possible, regular brushing after meals, daily dental flossing, and semiannual visits to the dentist.

See also DENTAL DISORDERS; TOOTH CARE; TOOTH DECAY.

Toothache (tüth'āk) is pain in a tooth or in the area around a tooth. It can be a symptom of almost any dental disorder but is most commonly caused by caries. Other common causes of toothache include gingivitis, periodontitis, and an abscess at the root of the tooth.

Q: *How is toothache treated?*

A: A dentist should be consulted as soon as possible so that the underlying cause can be treated. Pain-killing drugs, such as aspirin, acetaminophen or ibuprofen, may give temporary relief.

See also GINGIVITIS; PERIODONTITIS; TOOTHACHE: TREATMENT; TOOTH DECAY.

Toothache: treatment. Toothache is a symptom of many dental disorders, but most often of tooth decay, in which the outer layers of the tooth are eaten away and the nerve is exposed. A filling that is too close to the pulp of the tooth may also cause toothache, especially after eating or drinking hot, cold, or sweet substances. Occasionally, toothache may be caused by a disorder in

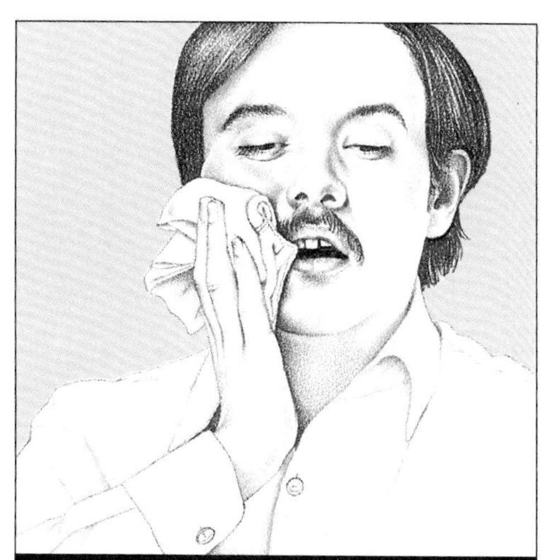

A warm towel held against the cheek may sometimes relieve the pain of a toothache, until a dentist can be consulted. If the jaw is swollen, intermittent use of an ice pack is recommended.

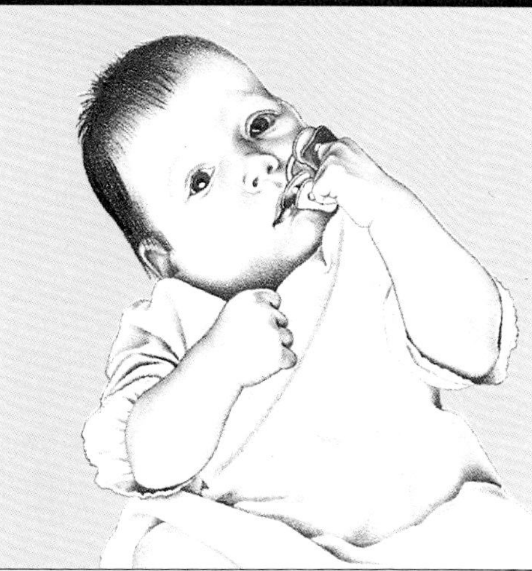

Chewing on a teething biscuit or ring helps relieve an infant's discomfort during teething.

another part of the body, such as an ear or sinus infection. A gumboil, an abscess caused by infection of the pulp of the tooth, causes swelling and extreme pain in the affected tooth. *See also* GUMBOIL.

There are several ways of reducing the likelihood of dental decay and, therefore, of toothache: (1) regular brushing and use of dental floss; (2) regular visits to the dentist; and (3) reducing the amount of sugar in the diet. *See also* TOOTH CARE.

Action. Although pain may subside for awhile, a toothache or gumboil should be treated by a dentist as soon as possible. In the event of a gumboil, there may be an escape of pus. Take care not to swallow any of this pus.

Painkillers such as acetaminophen or aspirin may help. *Do not* exceed the recommended dosage, no matter how painful the toothache is. *Do not* put a pain-relieving tablet directly on an affected tooth. The position of the tablet can not lessen the toothache, and the drug may be harmful to the gum. *Do not* eat or drink hot, cold, or sweet substances. Gently wash out a cavity with mouthwash.

Tooth, broken: treatment. Try to avoid touching the tooth with the tongue. Make an emergency filling by placing a piece of gauze soaked in oil of cloves over the broken tooth; the oil of cloves helps relieve the pain. Place another piece of gauze inside the cheek; this will help prevent the tooth from damaging the inside of the cheek.

If the tooth has been knocked out of the mouth, immediately retrieve it and wrap it in clean tissue; a dentist can sometimes put the tooth back into place. A dentist should be consulted as soon as possible.

Tooth care. To keep teeth and gums healthy you should eat a nourishing and varied diet, follow a strict routine of oral hygiene, and visit the dentist every six months. Children should be encouraged to adopt this routine from the age of two.

The teeth cut and grind the food in the first part of digestion. The more use the teeth have, the stronger and healthier they remain. A varied diet gives teeth tough and crisp food to chew as well as soft food, and the gums are stimulated at the same time.

Deficiency diseases are comparatively rare in modern society but when they occur, the teeth are one of the first areas to be affected. If local drinking water is low in fluoride, a mineral that is essential for the formation of healthy teeth, your teeth and your children's teeth may be more susceptible to decay. Supplemental fluoride may be recommended by the physician or dentist. *See also* FLUORIDE.

A diet low in vitamin D also makes the teeth less resistant to decay. The condition is common in young children or in dark-skinned persons living in northern climates, where the exposure to sunlight is not sufficient for the skin to manufacture the usual amount of vitamin D. A pregnant woman may also suffer from lack of the vitamin. Vitamin D is abundant in sea fish; it is also added to most pasteurized milk.

Daily Routine. Teeth should be brushed twice a day, or better still, after each meal. Choose a toothbrush with a small head to reach well back into the mouth. The bristles should be soft and long to ensure that the gum and tooth can be cleaned with one flicking sweep of the brush, as shown in the accompanying illustrations.

Tooth Decay. Poor tooth-cleaning habits encourage tooth decay for a number of reasons. Bacteria are always present in the mouth. But when food becomes trapped between the teeth, the bacteria break it down and form a harmful acid capable of softening the enamel and eroding the teeth. The film of saliva, bacteria, and food particles is known as plaque. If this remains on the teeth, calcium salts begin to form and build up a hard, chalky deposit around the teeth known as tartar. Although careful cleaning and flossing can remove the particles of food that encourage plaque, no amount of cleaning can remove tartar. Once it is there, the dentist or hygienist has to scale the teeth to get rid of it.

The Gums. The gums also suffer from poor cleaning habits. A healthy gum should come to a fine point between each tooth, and look moist and pink. If the gum margin is rounded, red, and slightly puffy it means that the early stages of gum disease (gingivitis) may have begun. The puffiness of the gums means you are not cleaning your

Proper care of teeth

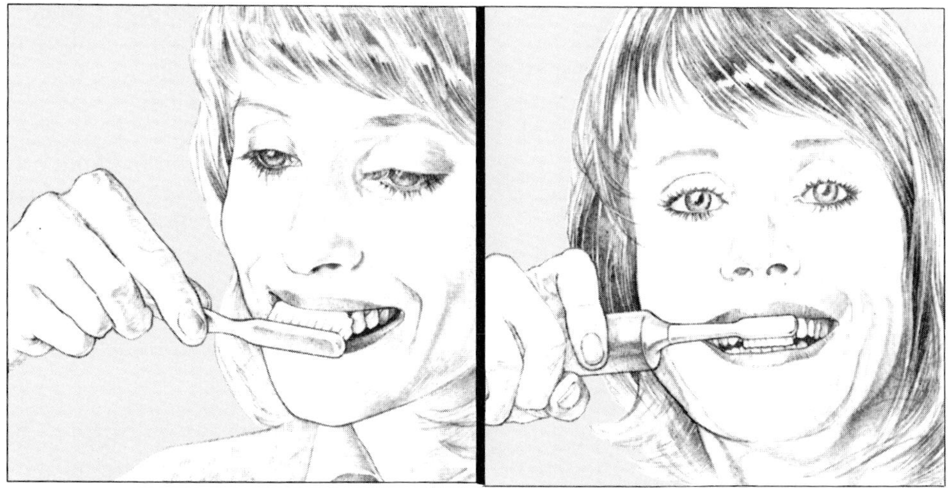

Correct brushing

Using a small, soft brush with rounded ends, lay the side of the bristles at a 45° angle and brush in a circular motion 10 or more cycles per tooth. Brush carefully behind the teeth as well. The brushing routine should take at least 5 minutes a session, with preferably 3 sessions a day, although 2 are regarded as adequate. Change the brush every 2 months, or whenever wear is obvious.

Electric toothbrush

An electric toothbrush is an efficient tooth cleaner. It brushes the teeth in the correct manner and massages the gums if laid gently on them. Children enjoy the novelty of electric toothbrushes, and introducing one into the family often encourages children to brush their teeth more often. The brush attachments should be changed every two months.

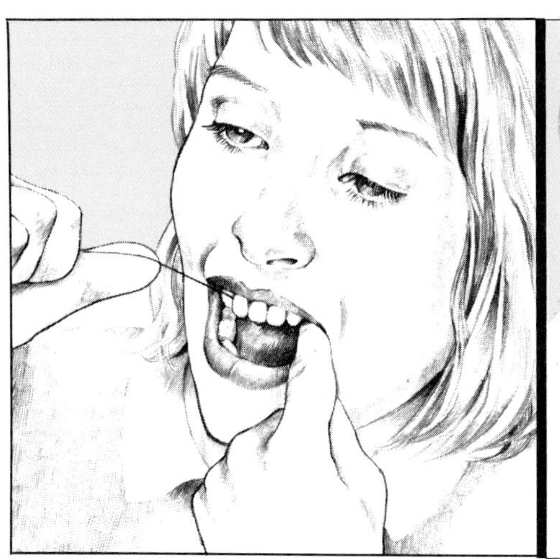

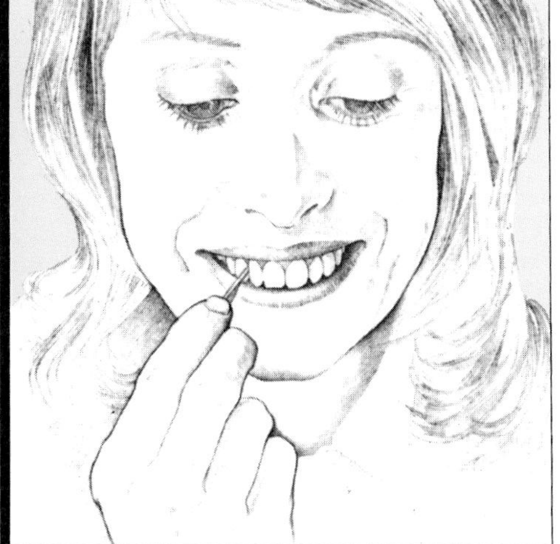

Dental floss

Dental floss is made of a strong thread that is either waxed or unwaxed; the unwaxed floss is preferred. Use it every day, preferably at night. Cut off a long piece of floss, wrap each end several times around the middle fingers, and run the center portion over the tip of the index fingers. With a gentle sawing action, move the floss down between each tooth in turn, and stroke the surface of each tooth below the gum line.

Toothpick

A toothpick is useful for removing large pieces of debris from the teeth, but is not as efficient as floss for cleaning between each tooth. It is, however, more convenient for use in the daytime. Do not force the toothpick down between the teeth, because this can damage the gum.Work the pick downward with a gentle massaging or rubbing motion. The pick can be made of wood or plastic.

teeth correctly, and the gums are reacting to the build-up of plaque and tartar.

Puffy gum margins may also occur during pregnancy because of hormonal changes in the mother's body. Step up the oral hygiene during pregnancy, and see your hygienist as often as every three months.

Gingivitis can lead to acute infection of the gum and produce a painful boil or abscess called a gumboil. This can even cause the gum to recede permanently. Once the root is exposed, infection can enter and penetrate into the bony tooth socket, loosening the teeth. This can eventually lead to tooth loss.

The Dentist. When you visit the dentist, he or she can detect signs of decay or gum disease before any permanent damage is done. The dentist may X-ray the teeth because decay among the back teeth can be seen more easily on an X ray. The dentist also checks that existing fillings are not leaking or damaged in any way. If a filling needs replacing, the dentist drills away the old filling and any affected tooth material and refills the tooth.

The Orthodontist. During the preteen years, a child's permanent teeth are emerging and settling down into position. Irregularities are common—there may be gaps between the teeth, or the teeth may be overcrowded and overlapping. The dentist may refer a child to an orthodontist, who takes a series of X rays before correcting the irregularities with braces or similar equipment. Braces should not be uncomfortable, but the child must be especially careful about cleaning the teeth.

Tooth decay, also known as dental caries, is disintegration of a tooth due to bacterial action. Tooth decay begins with the formation of jelly-like plaque on the surface enamel of the teeth. Bacteria in the plaque produce acid, which erodes the enamel and exposes the underlying dentin. The acid may also irritate the gums and cause gingivitis. If the decay is not stopped by dental treatment, it spreads to the central pulp and eventually reaches the root canals. Bacteria may penetrate the decayed teeth and produce a dental abscess, which may cause toothache.

Q: *How is tooth decay treated?*

A: Tooth decay requires professional dental treatment. If the decay is relatively minor, the damaged area of the tooth is drilled out, then filled with a special metal amalgam. Severely decayed teeth may need to be extracted.

Q: *How may tooth decay be prevented?*

A: Tooth decay may be prevented by a correct diet and good dental hygiene. The teeth should be cleaned thoroughly with a toothbrush after every meal. Dental floss should also be used daily to remove plaque and food from between the teeth.

See also TOOTH CARE.

Toothpaste (tüth'pāst) is a form of dentifrice paste that consists of a mild abrasive, a detergent, and, usually, flavoring and coloring. Fluoride is added to many toothpastes to help prevent decay. Good dental hygiene depends more upon correct brushing than the type of toothpaste used.

Tooth, wisdom. Wisdom teeth are the last molars on each side of the upper and lower jaw. These third molars ordinarily appear between the ages of 17 and 25.

If the jaw is not large enough to accommodate them, the wisdom teeth may become impacted, causing pain and other dental problems. When this happens, the teeth are usually extracted by an oral surgeon.

Tophus (tō'fəs) is a lumpy deposit consisting of the salts of uric acid. It is found in the ears and joints of some persons with gout.

See also GOUT.

Torn cartilage. *See* CARTILAGE; MENISCUS.

Torpor (tôr'pər) is an abnormal state of lethargy, listlessness, and dullness.

Torticollis (tôr tə kol'is), or wryneck, is a muscular disorder in which the neck is twisted and the head turned to one side.

See also NECK, STIFF.

Touch, sense of. The sense of touch is the sense by which pressure on the skin is perceived. There are many thousands of sensory nerve endings throughout the surface of the skin that detect different levels of pressure and vibration. Some of the nerve endings are concentrated in particular parts of the body, such as the fingertips and lips. The nerve endings send impulses to the brain, where they are deciphered into various touch sensations.

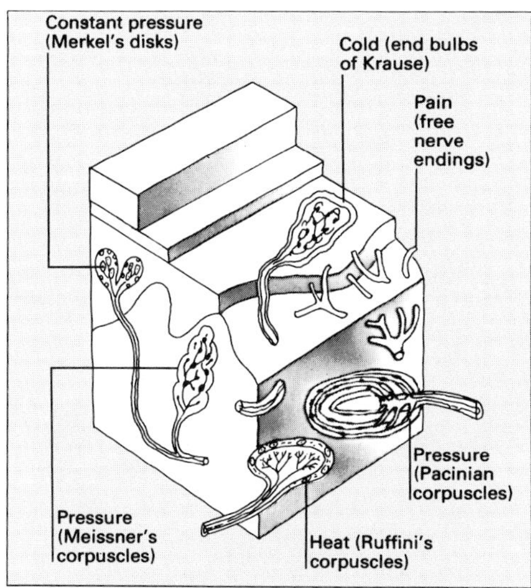

The **sense of touch** involves specialized nerves (seen here in a cut-away view of a section of skin), which relay touch sensations to the brain.

Tourette's syndrome (tü retz'). Gilles de la Tourette's syndrome is a nervous disorder characterized by spasms of the facial muscles, shoulders, and extremities. It is accompanied by grunts and other noises; it usually begins in late childhood and is found mostly in males. In adolescence, the condition usually worsens, with the person involuntarily using obscene language. Treatment with haloperidol or other dopamine antagonists has been proven successful. The disorder is thought to be caused by a chemical imbalance.

Tourniquet (tůr'nə ket) is a constricting band that is placed around a limb to stop hemorrhaging.

It is extremely dangerous for an unskilled person to use a tourniquet in the treatment of severe bleeding. If the tourniquet is applied too long, the tissues in the limb die, and the limb may need to be amputated. A tourniquet, therefore, should be used only as a last resort to control life-threatening bleeding.

See also BLEEDING: FIRST AID.

Toxemia (tok sē'mē ə) is a type of blood poisoning caused by toxins (metabolized poisons), especially toxins produced by pathogenic bacteria that enter the bloodstream from a local lesion and are distributed throughout the body. Toxemia may also refer to a serious complication of pregnancy known as eclampsia or preeclampsia.

See also ECLAMPSIA; PREECLAMPSIA; TOXIN.

Toxic (tok'sik) is a condition having to do with, or caused by, a toxin or poison.

See also TOXIN.

Toxicology (tok sə kol'ə jē) is the science that deals with poisons. This includes the detection of poisons, the effects of poisons, and the treatment of poisonous conditions.

See also POISONING.

Toxic shock syndrome (tok'sik shok) is an acute illness caused by the toxin-producing bacteria *Staphylococcus aureus.* The onset of the syndrome, first discovered in 1978, is characterized by high fever, severe vomiting, explosive diarrhea, and a vivid skin rash on the palms and soles of the feet. The severity of the disease can range from mild to fatal. In severe cases, loss of body fluids produces a sudden drop in blood pressure, precipitating shock.

Q: *What causes the growth of the toxin-producing bacteria?*

A: The cause is not fully understood. Researchers have, however, found that a link exists between the use of superabsorbent tampons and the growth of the bacteria. Approximately 1 percent of all menstruating women carry the bacteria in their vaginas during their menstrual periods. The superabsorbent tampons may create an environment highly conducive to the growth of the infection. Frequent changing of tampons decreases the risk of toxic shock. Not all toxic shock syndrome victims, however, are menstruating women. The disease has been found in children, postmenopausal women, and men. *Staphylococcus aureus* is sometimes found in women after childbirth; it is ordinarily found anywhere on the skin and is capable of entering the body through a boil, an internal sore, or a postsurgical wound.

Q: *How is toxic shock treated?*

A: Methods of treatment vary because of the extreme variation in the severity of the disease. Antibiotics and the intravenous introduction of large amounts of fluids are usually administered. The earlier the condition is treated, the better the prognosis for recovery.

Toxin (tok'sən) is any poison formed by an animal or plant organism as a product of its metabolism. For example, venom is the toxin of snakes. The term usually refers to poisons that are produced by bacteria.

Many bacterial toxins can cause diseases, such as bacterial dysentery, diphtheria, food poisoning, and tetanus. The body reacts to some toxins by producing antitoxins, which are antibodies. It is possible to immunize individuals against certain diseases, such as tetanus or diphtheria, by administering inactivated toxins to stimulate the production of antibodies.

See also ANTIBODY; ANTITOXIN; ANTIVENIN.

Toxocariasis (tok sō kār i'ə sis) is a parasitic disease that is caused by infestation with the larvae of either of two species of roundworm, *Toxocara canis* or *Toxocara cati*. The adult worms live in the intestines of dogs and cats. The worms produce eggs, which are discharged in the feces.

Toxocariasis occurs most commonly in children, as a result of ingestion of soil contaminated with the eggs. The eggs hatch into larvae in the intestine, penetrate the intestinal wall, and then spread throughout the body in the bloodstream. The larvae can affect most tissues in the body.

Q: *What are the symptoms of toxocariasis?*

A: The symptoms include fever, coughing or wheezing, and, occasionally, a skin rash. The liver and spleen may be enlarged, and there may be inflammation of the back of the eye. The larvae may affect the lungs, causing pneumonia. The disease is usually mild and rarely causes prolonged illness.

Q: *How is toxocariasis treated?*

A: The use of medication is seldom necessary; the disease usually disappears on its own. Housepets should be regularly checked for worms as a means of preventing toxocariasis.

See also ROUNDWORM.

Toxoid (tok'soid) is a bacterial toxin that has been modified by chemical treatment so that it has lost its poisonous properties, but can still stimulate the formation of antibodies. Injections of toxoids can induce immunity against various diseases, such as diphtheria and tetanus.

See also IMMUNIZATION; TOXIN.

Toxoplasmosis (tok sə plaz mō'sis) is infection with the parasitic protozoan *Toxoplasma gondii*. This microorganism can infect any warm-blooded animal, but it requires a member of the cat family as its main host. In cats, the microorganism produces infectious cysts (oocysts), which are shed in the cat's feces. In other animals, the microorganisms form cysts in the muscles. Humans become infected by exposure to oocysts in cat feces or by eating undercooked meat that contains the muscle cysts. The microorganisms then reproduce within the body cells. But, as immunity develops, reproduction stops, and the parasites form cysts in the body tissues. The microorganisms can also cross the placenta and infect an unborn child (congenital toxoplasmosis).

Q: *What are the symptoms of toxoplasmosis?*

A: In most cases, toxoplasmosis does not produce any symptoms. When symptoms do occur, they include slight fever, tiredness, muscle pains, and enlargement of the lymph nodes.

At birth, the symptoms may be severe and rapidly fatal. Alternatively, symptoms may be absent at birth but may develop within a few months. In such cases, there may be choroiditis, which may lead to blindness, jaundice, skin rashes, and enlargement of the spleen and liver. There may also be brain damage.

Q: *How is toxoplasmosis treated?*

A: Drug treatment with a combination of pyrimethamine (an antimalarial drug) and sulfonamides is usually effective when the toxoplasmosis organisms are reproducing. There is no effective treatment for destroying organisms in the cyst stage. However, toxoplasmosis is rarely fatal in adults.

Q: *How can toxoplasmosis be avoided?*

A: Meats should be properly cooked to destroy any cysts. Pregnant women should avoid handling cat litter-box materials, as cysts can be inhaled from the dust.

Trachea (trā'kē ə), or windpipe, is the cylinder-shaped tube that extends from the voice box (larynx) to a point above the heart, where it divides into two tubes (bronchi) that lead to the lungs. The trachea is composed of C-shaped cartilage rings, which are held together by fibrous tissue. It is lined with a layer of mucous membrane.

Food and liquid are both prevented from entering the trachea by a hinged flap of tissue (epiglottis) that diverts the food from the back of the tongue toward the esophagus.

Tracheitis (trā kē ī′tis) is an inflammation of the trachea (windpipe). It is commonly associated with an infection of the larynx (laryngitis) or bronchial tubes (bronchitis).

See also BRONCHITIS; LARYNGITIS.

Tracheostomy (trā kē ost′ə mē) is the surgical creation of an opening in the front of the trachea (windpipe) to relieve an obstruction and maintain a clear airway, by means of a silicone tube placed in the hole.

A tracheostomy may be performed as part of the treatment of a patient who has sustained a mouth or chest injury or who has undergone a major operation, such as lung surgery.

Tracheotomy (trā kē ot′ə mē) is a surgical incision that is made into the trachea (windpipe).

See also TRACHEOSTOMY.

Trachoma (trə kō′mə) is a chronic infection of the thin membrane that covers the front of the eye (conjunctiva). It is the most common cause of blindness in tropical countries.

Trachoma is caused by infection with the microorganism *Chlamydia trachomatis*. It is highly infectious and is usually transmitted either directly by rubbing the eyes with infected hands or, in warm climates where sanitation and personal hygiene is poor, by flies that feed on ocular discharge.

Q: *What are the symptoms of trachoma?*

A: After an incubation period of about 10 days, the symptoms of severe conjunctivitis appear, with sore, watering eyes and abnormal sensitivity to light (photophobia). *See also* CONJUNCTIVITIS.

The symptoms gradually disappear but leave the conjunctiva red, inflamed, and covered with small lumps. These lumps eventually scar, causing blurring of vision and finally blindness. The scarring may also affect the eyelids, causing the edges to turn inward.

Q: *How is trachoma treated?*

A: Treatment with antibiotics is usually effective. Early diagnosis and treatment by an ophthalmic surgeon is essential in preventing scarring and possible blindness. If scarring and blindness have already taken place, a corneal graft operation may be necessary.

Traction (trak′shən) is the act of pulling or drawing. This is the method by which a baby may be delivered with forceps, a fracture reduced, or a fracture reduction maintained. Weight traction is a system of weights and pulleys that are attached to a fractured limb so that the broken bones remain in the correct position. Traction is also used in manipulative and osteopathic treatment.

Traction is a method of treatment that holds bones in position by using weights and pulleys.

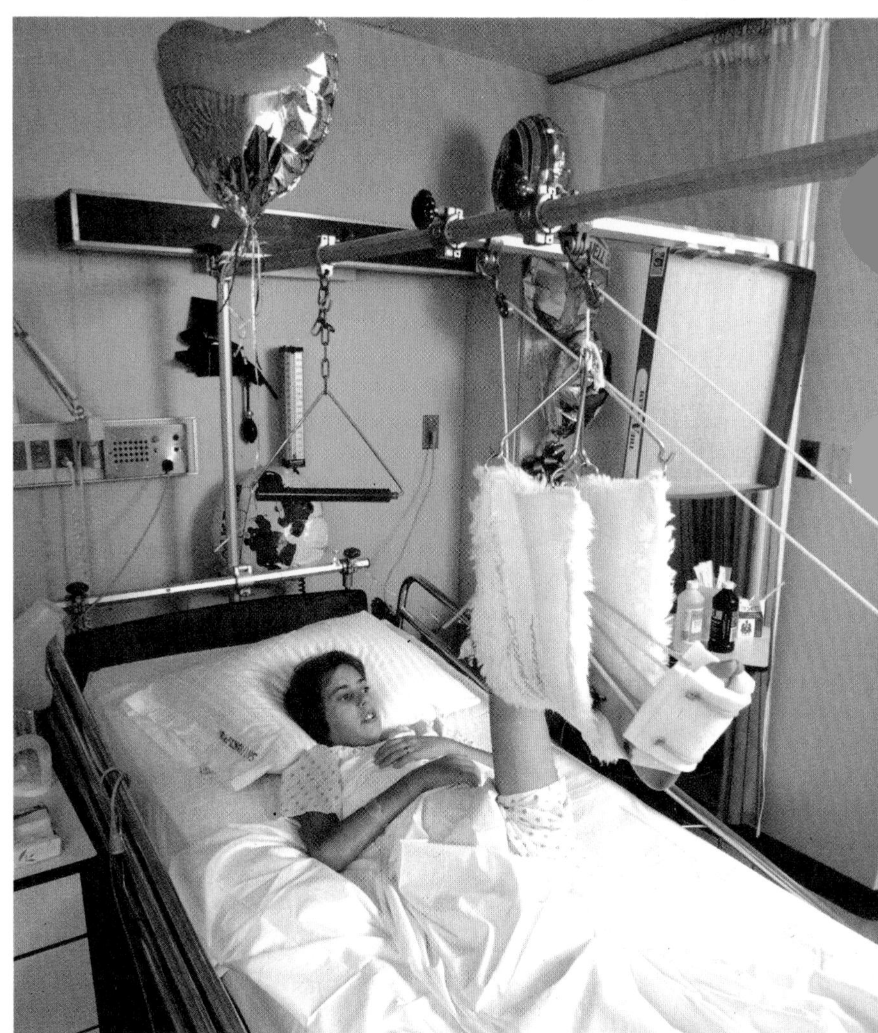

Tranquilizer (trang'kwə lī zər) is a drug used to reduce mental stress without disturbing normal mental activities. There are two main groups of tranquilizing drugs, minor tranquilizers and major tranquilizers. The minor tranquilizers are used to treat acute anxiety. They may also be combined with antidepressant drugs to treat patients who are both anxious and depressed. The major tranquilizers are used to treat psychotic mental illnesses, such as schizophrenia.

Q: *What are the different types of minor tranquilizers?*

A: The benzodiazepine drugs are the most commonly prescribed minor tranquilizers. They produce four main effects: sedation, alleviation of anxiety, prevention of convulsions, and muscle relaxation.

Various other drugs are also used as minor tranquilizers, such as hydroxyzine and loxapine.

Q: *Can minor tranquilizers produce adverse side effects?*

A: Yes. The main side effects include dizziness, drowsiness, and lack of coordination. Care should be taken when driving or operating machinery, and alcohol should be avoided. Minor tranquilizers may produce physical and psychological dependence during a course of treatment lasting longer than four months, so their use is limited.

Q: *What are the different types of major tranquilizers?*

A: The major tranquilizers include the phenothiazines, thioxanthene derivatives, and butyrophenones. The phenothiazines are the most commonly prescribed of these drugs. All the groups of major tranquilizers produce similar effects, which include sedation, relaxation of the muscles, reduction of aggression, and prevention of nausea.

The major tranquilizers are extremely effective in controlling the symptoms of serious mental illnesses. Their use has enabled many patients to lead relatively normal lives.

Q: *Can major tranquilizers produce adverse side effects?*

A: Yes. Patients who are highly sensitive to these drugs may develop skin rashes and jaundice. The production of hormones may also be affected, which may cause irregular menstruation. Large doses may cause trembling and muscle rigidity. Prolonged use may in some cases cause abnormal involuntary movements of the face and limbs.

Transcutaneous electric nerve stimulation (trans kyü tā'nē əs), TENS, is the application of skin electrodes to nerve endings in order to limit the sensation of pain. The electrodes transmit mild electrical impulses that act to block the transmission of pain signals to the brain. There are no known side effects to this treatment, and it is often effective for certain types of chronic pain, especially low back pain.

See also ELECTRODE.

Transdermal infusion of medication (trans dėr'məl in fyü'zhən) is a technique for applying medication in which a gel-like strip of material is placed on the skin. The medication is then absorbed into the skin at a constant rate. This technique is often used in the administration of estrogen, nitroglycerin, and scopolamine (a belladonna alkaloid).

See also ESTROGEN; NITROGLYCERIN.

Transference (trans fėr'əns), in psychoanalysis, is a revival of emotions previously experienced and repressed, as toward a parent, with a new person as the object. During psychoanalytic therapy, a psychiatrist or other physician who is treating a person may become the object of the patient's repressed emotions.

Transfusion (trans fyü'zhən) is the infusion of blood or blood components, such as plasma, into the veins of a person.

See also BLOOD TRANSFUSION.

Transfusion reaction (trans fyü'zhən) is a dangerous condition that occurs when the blood of a donor is incompatible with the blood of the recipient. Such reactions are rare when the blood types of the donor and the recipient are properly cross-matched before the blood transfusion. The severity of transfusion reactions varies greatly. The onset of the reaction is usually rapid, with fever and chills, breathlessness, chest pain, severe headache, rapid pulse, and vomiting. In occasional cases, a patient may lapse into a state of shock within about 60 minutes.

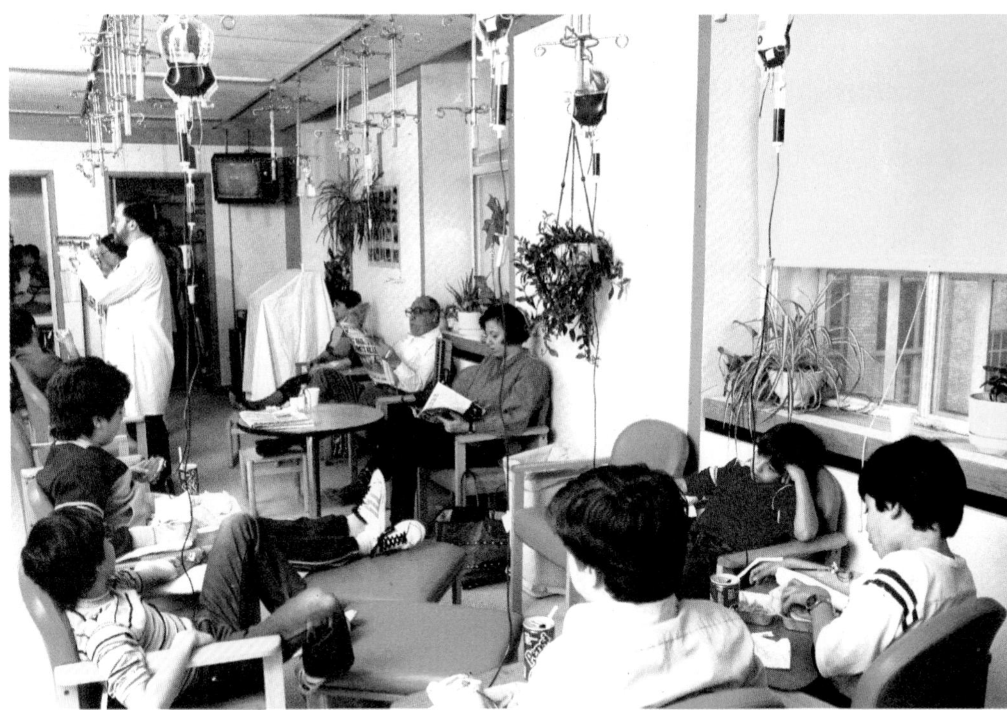

During a **transfusion,** the blood flows through a plastic tube and into the patient's vein.

Q: *What causes a transfusion reaction?*

A: A transfusion reaction is caused by an incompatability between the blood of the donor and that of the recipient. The recipient possesses antibodies that destroy the red blood cells of the transfused blood. This reaction may cause jaundice and disorders of the kidneys, which may become blocked, resulting in hemoglobin in the urine and kidney failure.

In most cases, such complications are temporary and are usually followed by a complete recovery.

See also BLOOD TRANSFUSION.

Transplant surgery (trans′plant) is the transfer of a tissue or an organ from one person to another, or from one site to another in the same person. The problem with transplantation is that the body has the tendency to treat the new organ as a foreign substance and destroy or reject it.

Q: *When is transplant surgery performed?*

A: Transplant surgery is performed when it is considered the most effective form of treatment. For example, a kidney transplant may be performed to stop the need for regular kidney dialysis. Corneal transplants may be performed to restore the sight of a person with severe corneal scarring. Heart valves may be transplanted to treat valvular heart disease. Diseased blood vessels may be replaced to treat arteriosclerosis. The technique has been performed successfully with tendons, nerves, bones, and skin.

Transplants between different people have been performed with the heart, liver, kidneys, and bone marrow. Other organs, such as the lungs, fallopian tubes, and pancreas, have also been transplanted, but such transplants are still experimental.

Q: *Are transplant operations successful?*

A: There is no guarantee that a transplant operation will be successful. The success rate depends to some extent on the tissue being transplanted.

Seventy percent of patients with heart and kidney transplants survive for at least two years after the operation. Fifty percent of all liver transplant patients survive on an average of two years.

Q: *Why is not transplant surgery always successful?*

A: The relatively few transplantations that fail do so because of tissue rejection. Every person, unless he or she is an identical twin, has a unique set of proteins in the body (tissue type), similar to a fingerprint. The better the match between tissue types of the transplanted organ and the recipient, the lower the chances of rejection. Identical twins have the same tissue type, so rejection is extremely unlikely. *See also* REJECTION.

Q: *Can rejection be prevented?*

A: Yes, although the prevention is not always successful. Several drugs reduce the ability of the transplant recipient to produce antibodies (which could attack the new organ and reject it) by suppressing the immune system of the recipient. These drugs are called immunosuppressive drugs. *See also* IMMUNOSUPPRESSIVE DRUG.

Because these drugs suppress the immune system, they also prevent the body from reacting to infection so that even the mildest infection may be fatal. However, new immunosuppressive drugs are being developed, and rejection is becoming less of a problem.

Q: *Which transplants need immunosuppressive drug treatment?*

A: Kidney, heart, and liver transplants usually require immunosuppressive treatment for several years. The dosage is reduced slowly when a physician is satisfied that rejection is unlikely. The drug cyclosporine has greatly reduced the incidence of organ rejection.

Q: *Which transplants do not need immunosuppressive drug treatment?*

A: Corneal, tendon, and heart valve transplants can be performed without the problem of rejection. Transplantation of blood vessels is usually successful without drug treatment because the transplanted tissues are from the patient's own body.

Q: *What happens if the transplanted organ is rejected?*

A: The result of rejection depends, to some extent, on the organ that has been transplanted. If a vital organ, such as the heart or liver, is rejected, the patient usually dies unless another transplant can be performed. Most kidney transplant patients can be kept alive by kidney dialysis until another kidney is available for transplantation.

Transporting an injured person. *See* FIRST-AID FUNDAMENTALS.

Transvestism (trans ves'tiz əm) refers to dressing in the clothing of the opposite sex (cross-dressing) as a means of obtaining sexual excitement on a recurrent and persistent basis. Interference with the cross-dressing results in intense frustration. Cross-dressing usually begins in childhood or adolescence; it may start with just one article of clothing and then broaden. The basic sexual preference is heterosexual.

Trauma (trô'mə) is the medical term for an injury. It usually refers to a physical injury, but may also refer to a psychological shock.

Traveler's diarrhea. *See* DIARRHEA, TRAVELER'S.

Travel sickness. *See* MOTION SICKNESS.

Trematode (trem'ə tōd), or fluke, is any of a species of parasitic flatworms that requires a member of the snail family as an intermediate host before entering and causing various organ infections in humans.

See also FLUKE; SCHISTOSOMIASIS.

Trembling. *See* TREMOR.

Tremor (trem'ər) is an involuntary quivering of the muscles. There are several different types of tremor. A coarse tremor is one in which the movements are slow. A fine tremor produces rapid movements. An intention tremor appears only when voluntary movements are attempted. Tremors may be present all the time, or they may occur irregularly.

Tremors may be associated with shivering, excitement, or fear. They may also be a symptom of a more serious underlying disorder. Tremors may be caused by acute anxiety, alcoholism, poisoning, overactivity of the thyroid gland, or failure of the liver or kidneys. Other underlying causes of tremors include neurological disorders, such as Parkinson's disease, multiple sclerosis, Huntington's chorea, syphilis of the brain, and Friedreich's ataxia, which is degeneration of the spinal cord. Some otherwise healthy persons have a tremor that is hereditary (familial tremor).

See also TIC.

Trench fever is an infectious fever caused by the organism rickettsia and transmitted by lice.

See also LICE; RICKETTSIA.

Trench foot is a condition resembling frostbite of the foot.

See also FOOT, IMMERSION.

Trench mouth is a painful ulceration of the mucous membranes of the mouth and throat.

See also VINCENT'S INFECTION.

Trephine (tri fīn') is a small, cylindrical saw that is used to make a circular hole in the skull, thereby exposing the brain for surgery.

Treponema (trep ə nē'mə) is a genus of spiral-shaped bacteria. Many of these bacteria cause various diseases, such as pinta and syphilis.

See also BACTERIA; PINTA; SYPHILIS.

Triage system. *See* HOSPITAL.

Trichiasis (tri kī'ə sis) is a condition in which the eyelashes grow inward and rub against the cornea of the eye. This causes irritation, watering of the eyes, and a feeling of a foreign body in the eye.

Trichiasis may result from various eye disorders, such as trachoma, inflammation of the eyelids (blepharitis), or entropion, in which the eyelids turn inward. It is treated by removing the inturned eyelash or by surgical outturning of the eyelids.

Trichinosis (trik ə nō'sis) is a disorder that is caused by the parasitic roundworm *Trichinella spiralis*. Persons become infected by eating raw or undercooked pork that contains cysts of the parasite. The cysts break open in the stomach and release larvae, which penetrate the wall of the small intestine, mature into adult males and females, and mate. After mating, the female worms discharge larvae which spread to the muscles and form small cysts that eventually calcify.

Q: *What are the symptoms of trichinosis?*

A: The symptoms vary according to the number of infecting larvae. Diarrhea, nausea, and vomiting may occur within a few days of infection. About two weeks later, there may be swelling of the eyelids, inflammation of the membrane covering the eye (conjunctivitis), and abnormal sensitivity to light (photophobia). These symptoms may be followed by aching of the muscles, intermittent fever, and increasing weakness.

Q: *How is trichinosis treated?*

A: Treatment with thiabendazole is usually effective. Corticosteroid drugs may also be necessary to prevent an allergic reaction to the infection.

Trichinosis can be prevented by thoroughly cooking all pork.

See also ROUNDWORM.

Trichomonas vaginalis (trik ō mo'nəs vaj i nal'əs) is a parasitic protozoan that is found in the vagina and in the male urethra. It seldom causes any symptoms in men, but the protozoan may be transmitted to sexual partners. In women, it usually causes symptoms only after it has been disturbed by sexual intercourse, menstruation, or, rarely, vaginal surgery. The protozoan may cause vaginitis, with an irritant vaginal discharge and painful urination.

Treatment with drugs, such as metronidazole, is usually effective. The patient's sexual partner should also be treated.

See also PROTOZOA; VAGINITIS.

Trichotillomania. *See* HAIR PULLING.

Trichuriasis (trik u rī'ə sis) is an infestation with the parasitic roundworm *Trichuris trichiura* (whipworm). It results from eating food that is contaminated with the worm's eggs. The eggs hatch into larvae in the small intestine and migrate to the large intestine. By the time the larvae have reached the colon, they have matured into adult roundworms. The adults attach themselves to the lining of the colon and produce more eggs, which pass out of the body in the feces.

Q: *What are the symptoms of trichuriasis?*

A: Symptoms usually appear only with heavy infestations. In such cases, there may be abdominal pain and diarrhea. Extremely heavy infestations, particularly in children, may cause intestinal bleeding, anemia, weight loss, and rectal prolapse, the protrusion of a part of the rectum through the anus.

Q: *How is trichuriasis treated?*

A: Treatment with mebendazole is usually effective.

See also ROUNDWORM.

Trigeminal neuralgia. *See* NEURALGIA, TRIGEMINAL.

Triglyceride (trī glis′ə rīd) is a type of lipid that is formed from a combination of fatty acids and glycerol. Most animal and vegetable fats are triglycerides, but because those of animal origin are saturated fats, a diet high in animal fats has been implicated in various disorders.

The relationship between triglycerides, cholesterol, and lipoproteins is complex, but there is evidence to associate high levels of these three substances in the blood with an increased incidence of arteriosclerosis.

Excessive animal fat in the diet causes a long-term increase in the concentration of triglycerides and cholesterol in the blood. A high triglyceride blood concentration may also be associated with alcoholism, diabetes mellitus, the nephrotic syndrome (a kidney disorder), and hypothyroidism (decreased activity of the thyroid gland).

Regular exercise and diet that is low in animal fats can help to reduce the level of triglycerides in the blood.

See also CHOLESTEROL; GLYCEROL; FATS; LIPOPROTEIN.

Trismus (triz′məs) is a spasm of the jaw muscles causing difficulty in opening the jaws. It may be caused by a fracture or dislocation of the jaw, a severe throat infection, or irritation of the nerves that control the jaw muscles, as occurs with tetanus.

See also JAW; TETANUS.

Trisomy 13 (trī′ sō mē) is a congenital defect that causes anatomic defects of the brain; cleft palate; cleft lip; and other physical and mental problems. It occurs in about 1 in 5,000 births and most patients die before the age of six months.

Trisomy 18 (trī′ sō mē) is a congenital defect caused by the presence of an additional chromosome 18. There are a number of physical and cardiovascular defects. Trisomy 18 occurs in about 1 in 3,000 births. Survival beyond a few months is rare.

Trisomy 21. *See* DOWN'S SYNDROME.

Tropical disease (trop′ə kel) is a disease that occurs almost exclusively in tropical climates. This is mainly because the organisms that cause the diseases are able to survive only in tropical conditions; the diseases are transmitted by insects or animals found only in the tropics; and poor sanitation and health care are common in the tropics.

Travelers can be immunized against some tropical diseases. The use of insect repellents may help to prevent insect-borne diseases. Careful personal hygiene can usually prevent diseases transmitted by body contact.

Air travel has introduced some tropical diseases to temperate climates where such diseases do not usually occur. Any fever or disorder that occurs within two months of returning from the tropics should be reported to a physician immediately.

Tropical sore (trop′ə kel), also known as a Delhi boil and an Oriental sore, is a skin ulcer that is caused by an infection with parasitic microorganisms of the genus *Leishmania.*

See also LEISHMANIASIS.

Truss (trus) is a device that is used to hold a hernia (rupture) in place. A truss is usually used only when surgical treatment of a hernia is not possible.

See also HERNIA.

Trypanosomiasis (trip ə nō sō mī′ə sis) is a term for any of several related diseases that are caused by parasitic protozoa of the genus *Trypanosoma.*

See also CHAGAS' DISEASE; PROTOZOA; SLEEPING SICKNESS.

Trypsin (trip′sən) is an enzyme, produced by the pancreas, that digests proteins in the small intestine.

See also ENZYME; PANCREAS.

Tryptophan (trip′tə fan) is a colorless, solid, essential amino acid, formed from proteins by the digestive action of the enzyme, trypsin. Until recently it was being used as a safe, nonhabit-forming medication to promote sleep. The use of L-Tryptophan was discontinued by the Food and Drug Administration in late 1989 because of reports that it caused severe illness in some, characterized by muscle pain; weakness; swelling of the arms and legs; fever; and skin rash.

See also AMINO ACID; DIGESTIVE SYSTEM; TRYPSIN.

Tsetse fly (tset′sē) is a bloodsucking insect that transmits sleeping sickness.

See also SLEEPING SICKNESS.

TSH test is performed to assess the activity of the thyroid gland. It involves measuring the concentration of thyroid-stimulating hormone (TSH) in the blood serum. TSH, which is secreted by the pituitary gland, stimulates the thyroid gland to produce hormones. Any change in the level of TSH in the blood signifies a malfunctioning of the thyroid gland.

See also HYPERTHYROIDISM; HYPOTHYROIDISM; THYROID GLAND.

Tubal ligation (tü'bəl lī gā'shən) is a female sterilization procedure in which the fallopian tubes are surgically cut and tied, or blocked by means of suture or clip, in order to prevent conception. After the operation, the ovum (egg) can no longer reach the uterus (womb). The operation is safe, but complications such as a hemorrhage or an infection can occasionally occur.

See also STERILIZATION.

Tubal pregnancy. *See* PREGNANCY, ECTOPIC.

Tubectomy. *See* STERILIZATION, LAPAROSCOPIC.

Tuberculin test (tü bėr'kyə lin) is a skin test to determine whether a person has ever been infected with tuberculosis or related bacteria. A small amount of tuberculin, which is a preparation made from dead tuberculosis bacteria, is injected into the skin. A swelling indicates previous infection with tuberculosis or immunization with BCG vaccine. A tuberculin test does not reveal whether the person has active tuberculosis.

See also BCG VACCINE; MANTOUX TEST; TINE TEST; TUBERCULOSIS.

Tuberculosis (tü bėr kyə lō'sis) is an infectious disease that is usually caused by the bacteria *Mycobacterium tuberculosis.*

Infection may result from inhalation of minute droplets of infected sputum or, less commonly, from drinking infected milk. If the infected person is not immune, the bacteria grow freely within the body and spread from the lungs to other parts of the body.

Eventually, the patient develops immunity and the bacteria stop spreading. They become surrounded by scar tissue and do not cause further tissue damage.

At a later stage, the protective layer of scar tissue may break down. This may be due to the development of another disorder; a reduction in immunity, which may occur with old age; the use of corticosteroid drugs; or malignant diseases, such as leukemia and Hodgkin's disease.

Symptoms of tuberculosis occur when the body's immunity does not develop fast enough to prevent the infection from spreading to various parts of the body or when immunity is interrupted by old age or certain drugs or diseases. The symptoms of tuberculosis in children usually differ from those in adults.

Q: *What are the symptoms of tuberculosis?*

A: There is often a period of many months before symptoms appear. In most cases, the infection primarily involves the top of one of the lungs, although it may spread to other parts of the body. The initial symptoms include tiredness, weight loss, fever during the evening, and profuse sweating at night.

As the infection progresses, the patient begins to cough up blood-stained sputum, which may be infectious. If a large area of the lung is affected, pleurisy may develop, causing breathlessness and chest pain. *See also* PLEURISY.

In some patients, particularly the elderly and those with silicosis (a lung infection), the progress of the disease is extremely slow and is accompanied by a large amount of lung scarring. In such cases, the main symptoms are usually breathlessness and coughing. In children, fever, weight loss, and swelling of lymph glands occur frequently with tuberculosis.

Q: *What other organs can be affected by tuberculosis?*

A: Any organ may be occasionally affected. Meninges (the membranes covering the brain and spinal cord), the kidneys, and bone are the most frequently affected areas after the lungs.

Q: *How is tuberculosis diagnosed?*

A: Active tuberculosis may be diagnosed with X rays and examination of the sputum for the tuberculosis bacteria. Various tests such as the tuberculin test may be used to test for previous exposure to tuberculosis. *See also* TUBERCULIN TEST.

In children, X rays are usually not helpful. The physician must obtain a history and administer the tuberculin test to determine if there has been exposure to tuberculosis.

Tuberculosis of the spine, also known as Pott's disease, destroys affected vertebrae. This results in compression of the spinal cord and nerves. The victim, thus, appears to be hunchbacked.

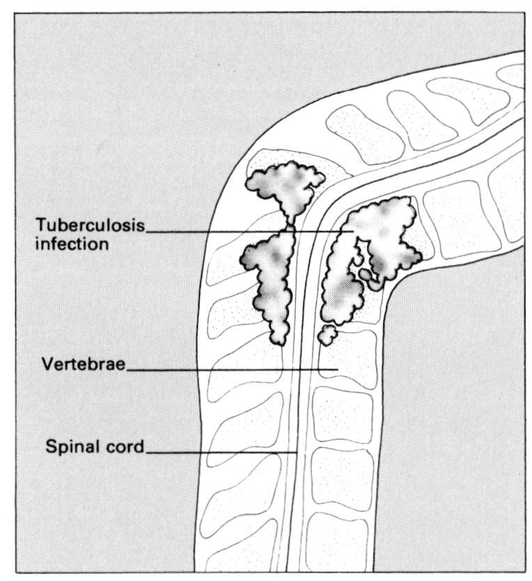

Q: *How is tuberculosis treated?*

A: Most patients respond quickly to treatment with various drugs. Patients who are seriously ill may require hospitalization for two or three months.

Drugs are prescribed until the patient improves with antibiotic treatment. The treatment should be continued for approximately 18 months. The drugs most commonly used are isoniazid (INH) in combination with rifampin or ethambutol.

Tuberculous meningitis requires specialized treatment. Early diagnosis is extremely important.

Q: *Can tuberculosis be prevented?*

A: Yes. A physician may decide that certain persons who have been exposed to tuberculosis should take isoniazid (INH) as a precautionary measure.

In some cases, the BCG vaccine, which can create immunity to tuberculosis, may be given. This vaccine, however, has not been found appropriate for the population in general. *See also* BCG VACCINE.

Important to the control of tuberculosis is that diseased persons be identified quickly so that they can be isolated from others and treated.

Q: *What precautions should be taken by persons who have been in contact with tuberculosis?*

A: Those who have been in contact with an infectious case of tuberculosis should be examined for infection by a physician and, in most cases, have their skin tested.

"Tubes tied." *See* TUBAL LIGATION.

Tularemia (tü lə rē′mē ə), also known as rabbit fever, is an infectious disease that is caused by the bacterium *Francisella tularensis*. The bacteria can penetrate unbroken skin, and most cases of tularemia result from handling infected wild animals, particularly rabbits. Occasionally, infection may result from eating undercooked meat from a diseased animal or from the bite of an infected tick.

Q: *What are the symptoms of tularemia?*

A: After an incubation period of about one week, there is a sudden onset of high fever, headache, nausea, vomiting, and extreme weakness. A day or two later, an inflamed nodule appears at the site of the infection. The nodule ulcerates rapidly, and additional ulcers may appear near the mouth or eye. The lymph glands around the site of infection may become swollen; they may also ulcerate and discharge pus.

The patient may develop a skin rash or pneumonia at any time during the illness, which usually lasts three or four weeks.

Q: *How is tularemia treated?*

A: Treatment with streptomycin or tetracycline is effective in most cases. The patient should undergo the full course of treatment to prevent a relapse.

Tumor (tü′mər) is any swelling of the body tissues, such as an abscess, cyst, or a tissue growth. The term usually refers to a spontaneous new growth (neoplasm), which may be either malignant (cancerous) or benign (noncancerous). A malignant tumor is a neoplasm that grows and spreads throughout the body. A benign tumor is a neoplasm that does not spread or infiltrate other tissues of the body.

At the first sign of a swelling, an individual should see his or her family physician to determine if the tumor is malignant or benign. Early treatment of a malignant tumor can stop the extensive damage that is likely to occur.

See also ABSCESS; CANCER; CARCINOMA; CYST; SARCOMA.

Turner's syndrome (tėr′nėrz) is a chromosome anomaly of females in which 1 of the 2 X chromosomes is absent, so that there are 45, instead of the normal

46, chromosomes. *See also* CHROMOSOME.

A person with Turner's syndrome has the physical appearance of an immature female. The characteristic signs include short stature, webbing of the neck, multiple birthmarks, and underdeveloped or absent ovaries. There may be swelling of the hands and feet during infancy. Some patients have congenital heart defects, and a few are mentally retarded. At puberty, the breasts fail to develop normally, and menstruation does not occur.

There is no effective treatment for Turner's syndrome until the patient reaches puberty. After puberty, estrogen and progesterone drugs can be given to replace the deficiency of ovarian hormones. Normal secondary sexual characteristics should then develop and menstrual periods may occur. The individual, however, remains sterile.

See also SEXUAL CHARACTERISTICS, SECONDARY.

Turning a patient. *See* NURSING THE SICK.

Twilight sleep. *See* SLEEP, TWILIGHT.

Twins may be identical (monozygotic or monovular) or fraternal (dizygotic or binovular). Identical twins look exactly alike and are always of the same sex. Fraternal twins may look no more alike than any two siblings, and they may be of different sexes.

Identical twins result from the fertilization of a single egg that later divides into two eggs. The eggs share a single placenta and in rare cases may be born as Siamese twins, a partial joining of the two infants that occurs when the single egg does not divide completely. Besides looking alike, identical twins also carry identical genes.

Fraternal twins result when two separate eggs, usually released simultaneously, are fertilized by two separate spermatozoa. They have either a separate placenta within the womb or a fused placenta, and each develops independently of the other.

When twins are of the same sex, it is not always apparent at birth whether they are identical or fraternal. To make this determination with certainty, a microscopic examination of the placenta and the membranes is sometimes conducted, or blood studies are done on the twins when they reach the age of approximately six months.

Twins occur in about 1 of every 80 or 90 pregnancies. The frequency varies somewhat from one country to another. About two-thirds of twins are fraternal. Fraternal twins are more common in families with a history of twins, in mothers who are older than average, among mothers who have had more than the average number of babies, and among black women.

Preeclampsia, anemia, and premature labor occur more commonly with twin births. However, the main problem of a twin pregnancy is delivery. The first baby usually causes little difficulty, but the second may be in the wrong posi-

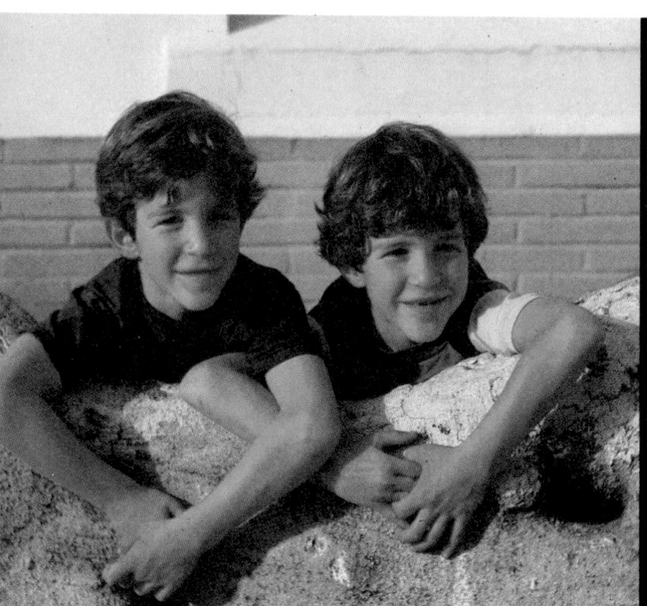

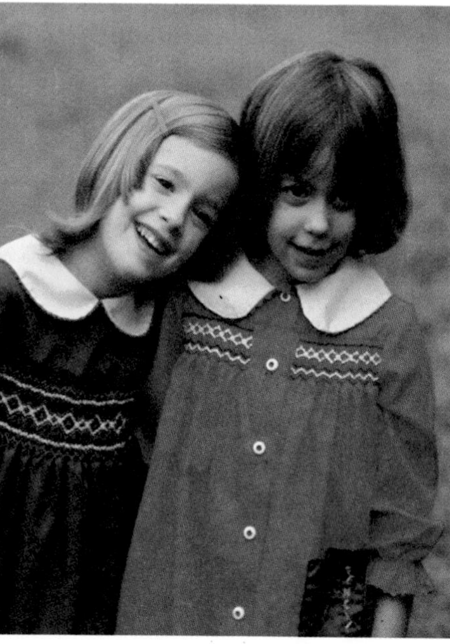

Twins may be either identical, *left*, or fraternal, *right*.

tion and may require turning for a normal delivery.

Due to problems of preeclampsia and prematurity, there is a greater incidence of infant mortality in twin pregnancy during the latter half of pregnancy, during labor, or within a few days of birth. There is also a greater risk of hemorrhage in the mother after birth.

Risks can be reduced by early detection of twins. Rapid uterine enlargement is an indication. It can easily be confirmed by diagnostic ultrasound as early as 9 or 10 weeks.

See also PREECLAMPSIA.

Twitching (twich'ing) is an involuntary muscle contraction that produces a small, spasmodic jerking movement. It may occur as a tic, as restless legs, or as a symptom of tetany. Twitching may be a symptom of various neurological disorders, but occasional twitching in a healthy person is not serious.

See also TETANY; TIC.

Tylenol with codeine® (tī'le nəl with kō'dēn) is a preparation of acetaminophen and codeine. It is prescribed to relieve moderate pain.

The most common side effects of this drug are stomach upset and constipation. An overdose of Tylenol with codeine may produce vomiting, lightheadedness, and liver damage, which may lead to liver failure. The codeine is also habit-forming.

See also ACETAMINOPHEN; CODEINE.

Tympanic membrane (tim pan'ik mem'brān), or eardrum, is the thin sheet of tissue that forms the separation between the middle ear and the external ear. It vibrates with sound waves and transmits the vibration to the malleus, the first ossicle (tiny bone) in the middle ear.

See also EAR.

Tympanometry (tim pah nom' e trē) is a measurement of the ability of the eardrum to absorb sound waves. If the ear is infected (otitis media) or if there is fluid behind the eardrum, the absorption of sound waves is significantly decreased.

See also EAR; OTITIS.

Typhoid fever (tī'foid), also known as enteric fever, is an intestinal disease that is caused by infection with the bacterium *Salmonella typhi*. Typhoid is the most serious of the salmonella infections. Similar, but milder infections with other salmonella bacteria cause paratyphoid fever. *See also* PARATYPHOID.

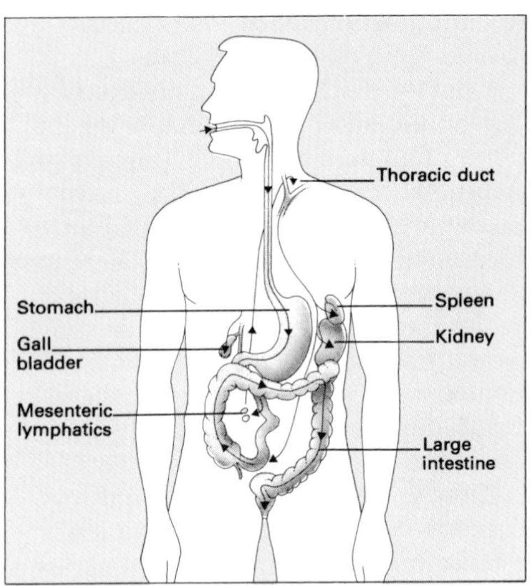

Typhoid fever bacteria enter the body through the mouth and then infect the blood via the thoracic duct.

Most cases of typhoid result from eating infected food or from drinking contaminated water. Food and water may become contaminated by direct contact with the urine or feces of an infected person. Flies may carry the infection from feces to food. When the bacteria have been ingested, they penetrate the small intestine and spread throughout the body in the bloodstream.

Q: *What are the symptoms of typhoid?*

A: After an incubation period of about one or two weeks, there is a gradual onset of headache, loss of appetite, fatigue, and constipation.

During the following week, the patient's temperature rises gradually to about 104°F (40°C). This is accompanied by abdominal pain, nosebleeds, and slow pulse rate. Pale, rose-colored spots may appear on the chest and abdomen; they usually last for about three or four days.

The high fever usually lasts for about a week, and the patient may become delirious. Diarrhea may develop toward the end of the second week, by which time the fever starts to disappear. In most cases, the fever disappears completely by the end of the third week.

Q: *Can typhoid cause complications?*

A: Yes. Pneumonia is the most common complication. More serious complications may occur in patients who develop diarrhea. In such cases, the intestine may ulcerate and bleed. Severe bleeding from an ulcer may lead to anemia or may even be fatal. Perforation of the ulcer may cause peritonitis. Relapses occasionally occur, but they are usually minor.

Q. *How is typhoid diagnosed and treated?*

A: A positive diagnosis may require a blood count of the number of white blood cells, and blood tests to detect the typhoid bacteria (Widal's test) and the presence of antibodies. The patient's urine and feces may be tested for the typhoid bacteria.

Typhoid is usually treated with antibiotics. Chloramphenicol is generally the most effective antibiotic, but bacterial strains have developed that are resistant to it. In such cases, ampicillin or trimethoprim-sulfamethoxazole drugs may be prescribed.

In addition to drug therapy, the patient may require intravenous infusions of fluid to prevent dehydration. Patients with perforation or hemorrhage of the intestine may need an emergency operation to repair the ulcerated area. If the patient suffers a relapse, an additional course of antibiotics is usually necessary.

It is essential that all patients who have had typhoid should have at least six specimens of feces cultured and examined to ensure that the bacteria have been killed. Until this has been done, the patient should not be allowed to handle food and should take great care with personal hygiene.

Q: *What is a carrier of typhoid?*

A: A typhoid carrier is a person who has made a complete recovery from the disease, but who continues to excrete typhoid bacteria in the urine and feces. Such persons can transmit the infection to others.

Q: *Can typhoid be prevented?*

A: No. But it is possible to reduce the likelihood of infection. All drinking water should be purified, if necessary by boiling. Milk should be pasteurized. Carriers of typhoid should not be allowed to handle food. Immunization with typhoid vaccine gives partial protection against infection and may reduce the severity of the symptoms in those who contract typhoid.

See also IMMUNIZATION; SALMONELLA.

Typhus (tī′fəs) is a general term for any of several related diseases caused by various species of *Rickettsia,* which are microorganisms that resemble both bacteria and viruses.

The typhus group is generally considered to consist of a range of similar diseases, including epidemic typhus, endemic typhus, and scrub typhus. Some authorities consider Rocky Mountain spotted fever and Q fever to be forms of typhus. Although these diseases are also caused by *Rickettsia,* they are usually classified as forms of spotted fever.

Epidemic typhus is caused by *Rickettsia prowazekii.* The infection may result from contamination of a bite puncture by the human body louse or from inhalation of louse feces. Endemic typhus is caused by *Rickettsia typhi,* which is transmitted by fleas from infected rats or mice. Scrub typhus is caused by *Rickettsia tsutsugamushi,* which is transmitted by a mite that normally lives on rodents.

Q: *What are the symptoms of epidemic typhus?*

A: After an incubation period between 10 and 14 days, there is a sudden onset of a severe headache and fever. The fever rises to about

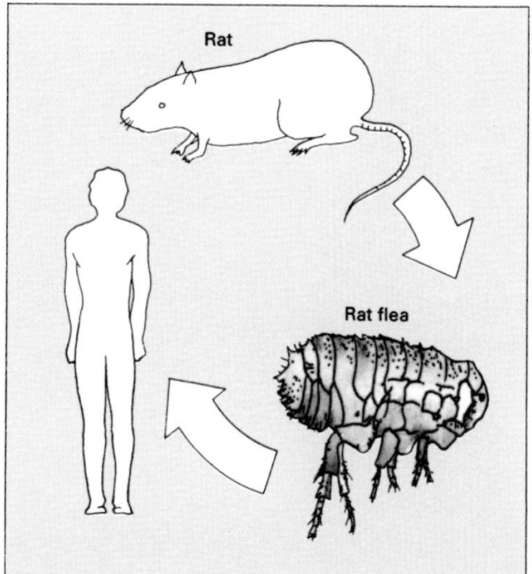

Endemic **typhus** is transmitted by fleas that infest rats and then bite humans.

104°F (40°C) and usually lasts for about two weeks. Between four and six days after the onset of symptoms, pink spots appear on all parts of the body except the face, hands, and feet. The spots may darken as a result of bruising. The patient may also vomit and be in a state of delirium or shock. Epidemic typhus has a high mortality rate, particularly among untreated patients. Rarely will the symptoms of epidemic typhus recur, without the patient being reinfected. This is called Brill-Zinsser disease.

Q: *What are the symptoms of endemic typhus?*

A: The symptoms of endemic typhus are similar to those of epidemic typhus, but are usually much milder. The mortality rate is low.

Q: *What are the symptoms of scrub typhus?*

A: The symptoms are similar to those of epidemic typhus, but scrub typhus may also cause a red nodule at the site of the mite bite. The nodule ulcerates and forms a black scab (eschar). A skin rash and cough may also develop. The rash is usually less clearly defined than the rash of epidemic typhus. Some patients may also develop complications, such as pneumonia and, rarely, inflammation of the heart muscle (myocarditis).

Q: *How is typhus treated?*

A: For all forms of typhus, treatment with antibiotics is usually effective. Patients who are seriously ill may also require hospitalization and treatment with intravenous infusions of fluid.

Q: *Can typhus be prevented?*

A: Yes. Effective vaccines are available against epidemic and endemic typhus, but not against scrub typhus.

The control of mites, lice, and rodents are also effective preventive measures. It is advisable to use insecticides and mite-repellent creams when visiting areas in which typhus is common.

See also RICKETTSIA.

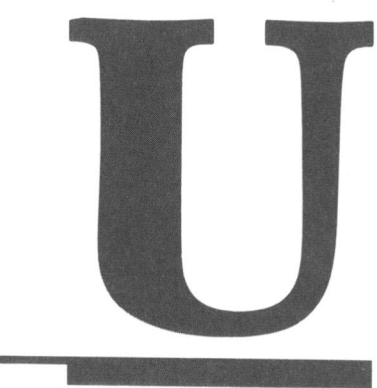

Ulcer (ul'sər) is an open sore that may occur on the skin or the internal mucous membranes of the body. For example, an ulcer may develop inside the mouth (canker sore, or aphthous ulcer), around the lips (cold sore), on the cornea of the eye, or in the stomach and duodenum (peptic ulcer).

Q: *What causes ulcers?*

A: The cause depends on the type of ulcer. Ulcers may be caused by relatively minor disorders, such as a burn or abrasion. They may also result from more serious disorders. For example, ulcerative colitis produces ulceration of the colon, and syphilis produces a chancre. Cancer may produce an ulcer in almost any part of the body.

Ulcers are particularly likely to develop in parts of the body where there is poor blood circulation, which may be caused by varicose veins. Reduced sensation in a particular part of the body may be caused by various neurological diseases and may also lead to ulceration.

See also BEDSORE; CANKER SORE; CARCINOMA, BASAL CELL; COLD SORE; COLITIS, ULCERATIVE; ULCER, PEPTIC.

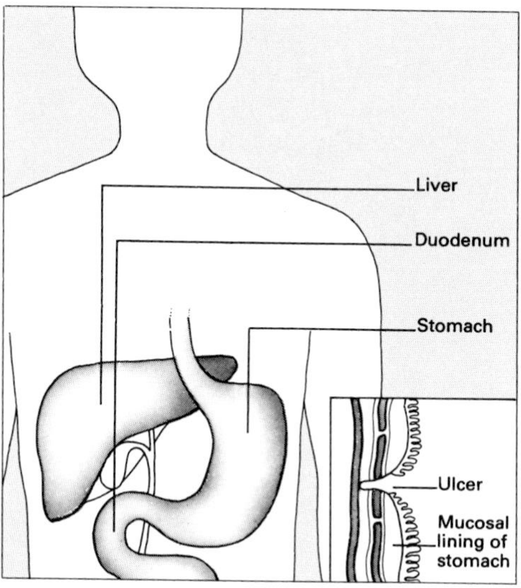

A **peptic ulcer** may occur in the mucosal lining of the stomach or in the duodenum portion of the small intestine.

Ulcer, aphthous (af'thəs). An aphthous ulcer is a small whitish sore, usually in the mouth, that is commonly called a canker sore.

See also CANKER SORE.

Ulcerative colitis. *See* COLITIS, ULCERATIVE.

Ulcerative proctitis. *See* PROCTITIS.

Ulcer, decubitus. *See* BEDSORE.

Ulcer, gastric (gas'trik). A gastric ulcer is the ulceration of an area of the stomach lining.

See also ULCER, PEPTIC.

Ulcer, peptic (pep'tik). A peptic ulcer is an eroded area in the lining of the stomach (gastric ulcer) or in the first part of the duodenum (duodenal ulcer). Peptic ulcers are caused by the combined action of pepsin and hydrochloric acid in the digestive juices of the stomach. They are more common in men than in women.

Q: *Why do peptic ulcers occur?*

A: Acute peptic ulcers occur suddenly and are usually the result of an excess of alcohol, aspirin, or other drugs.

Sometimes, they are called "stress ulcers" because they are considered to be related to periods of intense physical stress, such as those occurring with shock, severe burns, or accidents. This form of peptic ulcer heals rapidly.

Chronic peptic ulcers develop slowly and for a variety of reasons. It seems likely that there is an alteration in the protective action of the mucus and its underlying cells that normally prevents digestive juices from digesting the stomach itself. Why this occurs often is not known, but it is possible that continued anxiety and stress in an individual with an inherited tendency to form ulcers can cause a peptic ulcer. The condition is made worse by certain drugs.

Q: *Can peptic ulcers occur in places other than the stomach and duodenum?*

A: Yes. Acid-secreting cells in a Meckel's diverticulum can become active, sometimes producing a peptic ulcer. Peptic ulceration may also develop in the small intestine after a gastroenterotomy (surgery cutting into both the stomach and the intestine) has been performed for a peptic ulcer. Or an ulcer may form in the lower end of the esophagus (gullet) in a patient with a hiatus hernia. *See also* DIVERTICULUM, MECKEL'S; HIATUS HERNIA.

Q: *What are the symptoms of a peptic ulcer?*

A: Pain in the abdomen is the most common symptom of a peptic ulcer, but its frequency varies. There may be long periods when the ulcer is active and symptoms are present, followed by several months during which there are no symptoms.

The pain of peptic ulcer is usually high in the abdomen and is often described as a gnawing, deep ache accompanied by a feeling of hunger or nausea. It is relieved by taking bland food, milk, or antacid drugs, but it may be made worse by alcohol and by fried or spicy foods. *See also* ANTACID.

Pain from a duodenal ulcer typically starts about two hours after a meal and is relieved by antacids or more food. The pain commonly awakens the patient in the night, and the symptoms go on for several weeks before gradually disappearing.

A gastric ulcer may be aggravated by eating, because of the sudden production of acid in the stomach. The pain of a gastric ulcer seldom awakens the patient. Pain may be relieved by vomiting.

These are the typical symptoms, but there is a great variation. In the elderly, pain may persist without relief from food or antacids.

Q: *How is a peptic ulcer treated?*

A: Most people can be treated at home. A conventional treatment is to avoid alcohol and spicy or fried foods, which cause gastrointestinal distress. Pepper seems to be particularly aggravating. Eating frequent small meals and snacks is helpful, since this keeps the stomach filled with food that helps absorb the acid.

Coffee, tea, and cola drinks contain the stimulant drug caffeine and will frequently aggravate ulcer symptoms. If these drinks do not increase the symptoms, they may be taken by the patient; however, such drinks should be reduced to a minimum and taken only when the stomach is full.

Smoking should be prohibited. Any drugs that are known to aggravate peptic ulceration should, if possible, be stopped.

Antacids and drugs to prevent gastric secretion and reduce the speed by which the stomach empties itself are effective. Antacids often promote healing and prevent recurrence of ulcers. Cimetidine reduces gastric secretion and produces rapid relief of symptoms with healing of the ulcer. Carbenoxolone, another type of drug, rapidly improves symptoms. Sedative drugs, such as tranquilizers or a small dose of phenobarbital, are frequently used to alleviate nervous stress and tension.

Hospitalization may be necessary for patients whose pain is not relieved by bed rest and home medication. The patient's stomach can be continuously filled with an antacid through a small gastric tube. This is an excellent form of treatment for preventing pain during the night.

A surgical operation (partial gastrectomy) may be performed if the ulcer produces complications, or if it is thought that cancer has developed. *See also* GASTRECTOMY.

Q: *Can complications occur with a peptic ulcer?*

A: Yes. One complication of peptic ulcer is pyloric stenosis, an obstruction of the exit of the stomach. Pyloric stenosis results from a combination of scarring at the exit of the stomach or first part of the duodenum and inflammation produced by an active ulcer. Vomiting of large volumes of fluid, often with food from the previous day, is a common symptom. In more severe cases, a partial gastrectomy is needed. *See also* PYLORIC STENOSIS.

Bleeding is a common complication of peptic ulcer, and the patient may vomit blood (hematemesis) or produce the dark, black stools of melena. Sudden, massive blood loss causes weakness and fainting, and all patients who experience this symptom should be hospitalized. Blood transfusion, bed rest, and antacid drugs form the initial stage of treatment, but if the bleeding continues, emergency surgery may be necessary.

Another complication of a peptic ulcer is continuous pain. Pain may be constant and severe, often producing intense backache, if the ulcer penetrates through the stomach wall to involve the pancreas or liver. Surgery must often be performed.

A peptic ulcer may perforate, suddenly producing severe, intense abdominal pain, often spreading to the shoulders and sometimes accompanied by vomiting. This occurrence is a form of peritonitis and requires immediate surgery. *See also* PERITONITIS.

Ulcer, stasis (stā′sis). A stasis ulcer is a lesion on the lower leg, caused by poor blood circulation. It is usually associated with varicose veins, a condition characterized by swollen and otherwise damaged veins. Treatment of a stasis ulcer may include leg elevation to improve circulation and careful cleaning of the ulcer to prevent infection.

Ulna (ul′nə) is one of the two bones of the forearm, situated on the little finger side. The other bone is the radius. At its upper end, the ulna articulates with the radius and humerus to form the elbow joint. At its lower end, it articulates with the radius and the carpal bones of the wrist to form the wrist joint.

See also ELBOW; WRIST.

Ultrasound (ul′trə sound) is sound waves with a frequency over 20,000 vibrations per second. Because of its high, inaudible frequency, ultrasound has many diagnostic and therapeutic applications.

By using ultrasound techniques, it is possible to distinguish between different types of tissue in the body, measure the organs, and detect movement. The high-pitched sound waves are focused into a thin beam and passed into the body. When ultrasound encounters bone or air in the body, most of it is reflected, while various tissues absorb the sound to different degrees. When the ultrasound is used for diagnosis, the echo is converted into a visual image. This image is then interpreted by a specialist.

Q: *Is ultrasound dangerous?*

A: No. It seems to be entirely safe. The amount of energy in ultrasound is believed too low to cause damage.

Q: *Can ultrasound techniques be used anywhere in the body?*

A: Ultrasound recordings of parts of the body that contain air, such as lungs, are difficult to interpret.

Q: *Are there any special uses of ultrasound?*

A: Ultrasound is especially useful in investigating pregnancy because it does not harm the fetus or the mother. It may be used to measure the skull of a fetus, thereby giving an indication of the fetus's age; to detect fetal movements; to determine the position of the placenta; to detect multiple pregnancies; and to evaluate the brain and intracranial contents, especially in the premature infant.

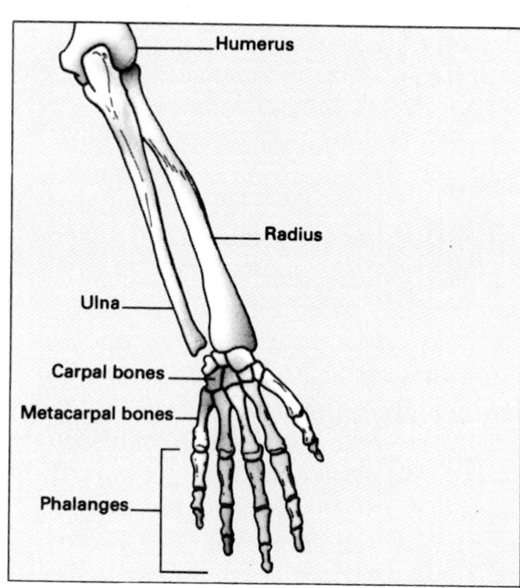

The **ulna** bone is able to twist over the radius, allowing a 180° turn of the wrist and hand.

With ultrasound techniques, pregnancy can be detected as early as five weeks after conception. Abnormalities of the mother's womb, such as placental abnormalities or a hydatidiform mole, may be revealed. Fetal abnormalities can also be detected early in pregnancy.

Ultrasound is particularly useful during amniocentesis because it can show the position of the needle inside the mother's body. *See also* AMNIOCENTESIS.

Q: *What other uses of ultrasound are there?*

A: Ultrasound may be used to distinguish between a solid tumor and a cyst, to discover the cause of liver enlargement, to investigate kidney disorders, and to aid a biopsy of the liver. It may also help to diagnose thyroid, pancreatic, and gynecological disorders and to locate devices within the body, such as an intrauterine device.

Echocardiography is a form of ultrasound technique that may be used to diagnose cardiac disorders. *See also* ECHOCARDIOGRAM.

Ultrasound techniques may also be used to detect narrowing of the arteries and alterations in the blood flow.

In the treatment of disease, a beam of ultrasound can be focused on a specific area within the body, where the energy of the beam changes into heat. This technique is used for relieving muscle and joint pains.

Umbilical cord (um bil′ə kəl) is the flexible, rope-like structure that connects the fetus with the placenta. It is usually about two feet (60cm) long and one-half inch (1.25cm) in diameter. The umbilical cord consists of two umbilical arteries and one umbilical vein, which are surrounded by a thick layer of jelly (Wharton's jelly) and a thin membrane. The umbilical vein transports oxygen and nutrients to the fetus. The umbilical arteries carry waste products from the fetus.

Soon after childbirth, the umbilical cord is tied and then cut. The part of the cord that is still in the womb is expelled with the afterbirth. The stump that remains attached to the baby shrivels and falls off after a few days, leaving a small scar called the umbilicus (navel).

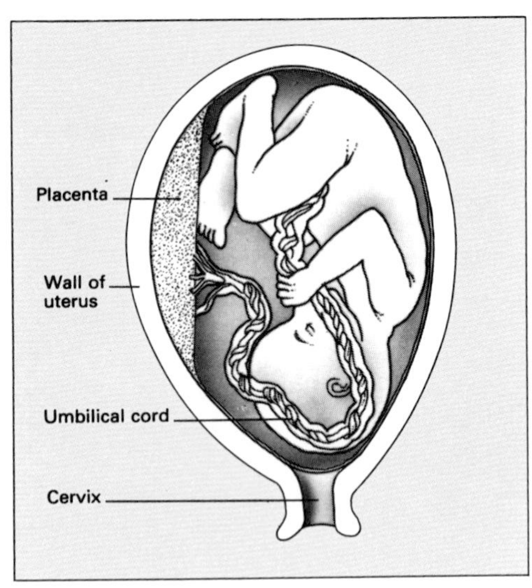

The **umbilical cord** is the rope-like structure that connects a fetus with the placenta of the mother.

See also PLACENTA.

Unconsciousness (un kon′shəs nəs) is a state of reduced awareness. It may vary in depth from a state of stupor, in which a person responds only to painful stimulation, to a state of coma, in which a person can not be roused by any form of stimulation. *See also* COMA; STUPOR; UNCONSCIOUSNESS: TREATMENT.

The term *unconscious* is also used in psychiatry to refer to the part of the psyche that is thought to operate without the individual's conscious awareness or control.

See also EGO; ID; SUPEREGO.

Unconsciousness: treatment. Unconsciousness occurs when normal brain activity is interrupted. It may progress rapidly from a state of drowsiness to a coma.

Do not give an unconscious person food or drink. *Do not* leave an unconscious person alone.

First, remove the victim from any harmful gases. Then follow the steps illustrated. If the victim has stopped breathing, give artificial respiration, following the instructions under ARTIFICIAL RESPIRATION. If the victim's heart has stopped, give external cardiac compression, using the steps under HEART ATTACK: FIRST AID. Control any bleeding, and if the victim is having an epileptic seizure, treat for convulsions. *See also* BLEEDING: FIRST AID; CONVULSION: FIRST AID. Then treat any other injuries that may have occurred.

Any person who has been unconscious should see a physician because unconsciousness may be a symptom of an underlying illness or a head injury that is not immediately obvious.

Underweight. *See* WEIGHT PROBLEM.

Undescended testicle. *See* TESTICLE, UNDESCENDED.

Undulant fever. *See* BRUCELLOSIS.

Upper respiratory tract infection. *See* RESPIRATORY TRACT INFECTION, UPPER.

Urea (yů rē′ə) is the chief end product of nitrogen metabolism in mammals. It occurs as a white, crystallizable substance primarily in the urine, but it is also found in the blood and lymph. Urea is used as a diuretic to increase urination as well as topically for various skin disorders.

See also KIDNEY DISEASE; URINE.

Uremia (yů rē′mē ə) is a toxic condition in which waste products of protein digestion, such as urea, are retained in the blood instead of being excreted in the urine. Uremia is the medical term for severe kidney failure.

Q: *What conditions can cause uremia?*

A: Uremia may be caused by any condition that reduces the flow of blood through the kidneys, such as hemorrhage, vomiting, diarrhea, or a serious illness. Kidney disease, such as nephritis, prevents the excretion of waste products that accumulate in the blood, causing uremia. Disorders of the prostate gland or bladder stones block urine flow from the bladder and cause back pressure of urine into the kidneys, resulting in kidney failure and uremia. Bacterial infections may also cause uremia. *See also* KIDNEY DISEASE.

Q: *What are the symptoms of uremia?*

A: The symptoms vary according to the underlying cause. Generally, the symptoms of acute uremia include headaches, high blood pressure, confusion, dry mouth, and reduced urination.

The symptoms of chronic uremia develop gradually. The first symptom is usually polyuria (large urine output). Later, fatigue, loss of ap-

Unconsciousness: treatment

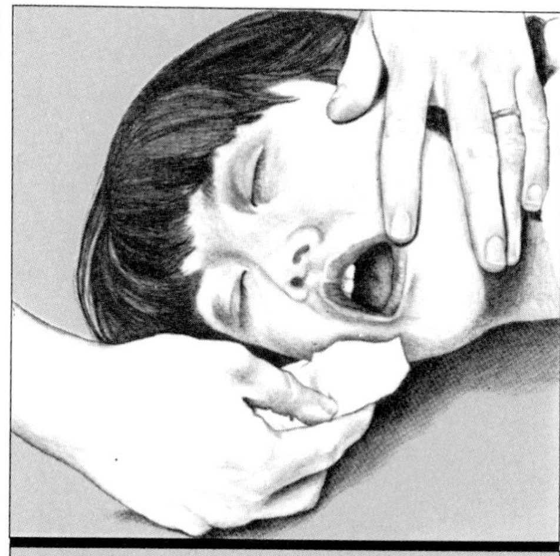

1 Ensure that the victim has a clear airway. If the airway is blocked, remove any loose dentures and clear the mouth of mucus, blood, or vomit, using a handkerchief if necessary. If the victim has difficulty breathing, the head should be pressed backward and the chin lifted just short of the jaw closing.

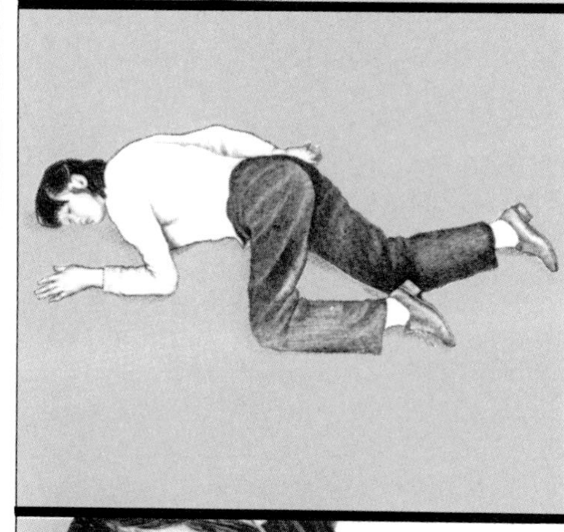

2 Place the victim in the recovery position or elevate the feet as per the instructions in FAINTING: FIRST AID. Ensure that there is plenty of fresh air. Loosen clothing around the neck and waist. Check the victim's breathing and pulse at regular intervals.

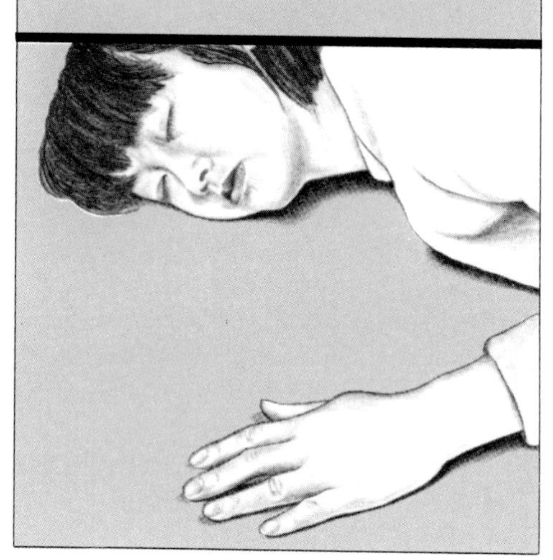

3 If the victim has no obvious injuries, look for clues as to why unconsciousness occurred. An emergency medical information tag or a syringe may indicate that unconsciousness was caused by an excess of insulin. An empty pill bottle may indicate a drug overdose. Save the bottle and any pills; these will help the physician.

petite, twitching muscles, confusion, and coma develop.

Because of the combination of illness, vomiting, and vitamin deficiency, the patient may also develop signs of malnutrition.

Q: *How is uremia treated?*

A: The treatment of uremia is directed toward the underlying cause. A physician may recommend a special diet that is low in protein, salts, and water to alleviate the symptoms. Patients with high blood pressure may require special treatment to prevent heart failure.

If kidney failure is severe, a specialist may advise kidney dialysis or, in suitable cases, a kidney transplant. *See also* KIDNEY DIALYSIS.

Q: *Can uremia cause complications?*

A: Yes. Uremia may cause heart failure, disturbance of calcium metabolism, abnormal bone formation, nerve damage, and bleeding, which may occur anywhere in the body. Uremia may also affect the immune system, leaving the patient vulnerable to infection.

If the condition is not treated, the patient becomes comatose and may die.

Ureter (yu̇ rē′tər) is one of a pair of thin, muscular tubes that drain urine from each kidney into the bladder. The urine is passed down the ureter by alternate contraction and relaxation (peristalsis) of the muscles in the ureter, occurring about three times a minute.

Several disorders may affect the ureter. For example, hydronephrosis, which is accumulation of urine in the pelvis of the kidney, may be caused by obstruction of the ureter or by a failure of normal peristalsis. The ureter may also become blocked by a stone (nephrolithiasis) or a tumor.

See also KIDNEY; URINARY SYSTEM.

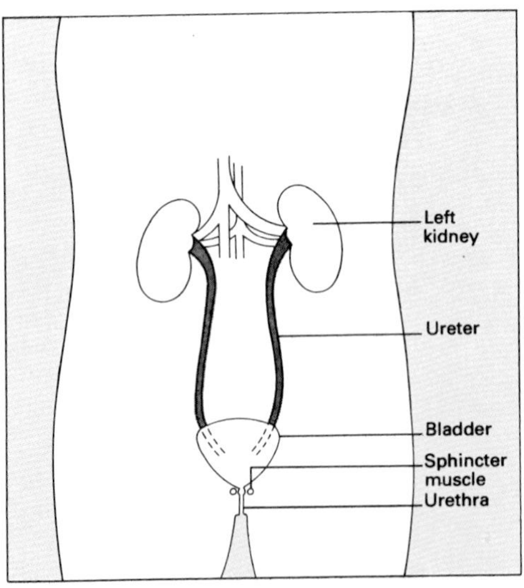

The **ureter** drains urine from a kidney to the bladder, from where it is expelled through the urethra.

Ureteritis (yu̇ rē tər ī′tis) is the inflammation of a ureter usually caused by bacterial infection. It often accompanies kidney infection.

See also URETER.

Urethra (yu̇ rē′thrə) is the tube through which urine is discharged from the bladder.

In women, the urethra is short; it opens between the vagina and clitoris. The urethra is longer in men and also serves as the passage for semen. It passes through the prostate gland, where it is joined by the sperm ducts, and opens at the end of the penis.

Various disorders may affect the urethra. It may open on the lower surface (hypospadias) or on the upper surface (epispadias) of the penis. Both these abnormalities are relatively common birth defects in boys.

The urethra may become infected and inflamed (urethritis), which may result in scarring and narrowing of the urethra in men or cystitis in women. Prostate problems may also affect the urethra, possibly leading to difficulty in urination.

See also CYSTITIS; PROSTATE DISORDERS; URETHRITIS; URETHRITIS, NONSPECIFIC.

Urethritis (yu̇r ə thrī′tis) is inflammation of the urethra, the tube through which urine passes from the bladder and out of the body. It may be caused by venereal disease, such as gonorrhea or nonspecific urethritis, or by the spread of infection from the skin.

The symptoms of urethritis include frequent urination and a painful discharge from the penis in men or from the urethra in women.

Treatment depends upon the underlying cause. Usually, antibiotics are effective.

See also GONORRHEA; URETHRITIS, NONSPECIFIC.

Urethritis, nonspecific (yu̇r ə thrī′tis). Nonspecific urethritis (NSU) is an inflammation of the urethra (the tube through which urine passes from the bladder) that is not known to be caused by a specific organism. It may be caused by various infections, including a viral infection similar to trachoma and the protozoan infection trichomoniasis. Nonspecific urethritis is a form of venereal disease and is transmitted only by sexual contact.

Q: *What are the symptoms of nonspecific urethritis?*

A: The main symptoms in men are pain on urination and a discharge from the penis that is usually worse in the morning. In severe cases, urination is extremely painful, and there may be a thick, white discharge similar to that in gonorrhea.

Most women show no symptoms. Rarely, there may be mild pain during urination, a slight vaginal discharge, and pain during sexual intercourse. In most women, the only sign of nonspecific urethritis is infection of the neck of the womb (cervicitis).

Q: *How is nonspecific urethritis treated?*

A: Nonspecific urethritis is usually treated with an antibiotic drug; tetracycline is the most effective. Treatment lasts for two or three weeks. Alcohol should not be drunk for at least two weeks after the start of treatment, and sexual intercourse should be avoided until a physician considers that the patient is cured.

Q: *Can nonspecific urethritis cause any complications?*

A: Yes. A relapse may occur before the patient is cured. This is especially likely if the patient has had sexual intercourse or has drunk alcohol during treatment. Nonspecific urethritis may also cause epididymitis, prostatitis, or salpingitis. The most serious possible complication is Reiter's disease, which may cause inflammation of the conjunctiva (conjunctivitis) and swelling of the joints (arthritis). *See also* EPIDIDYMITIS; PROSTATITIS; REITER'S DISEASE; SALPINGITIS.

See also SEXUALLY TRANSMITTED DISEASE; URETHRITIS.

Uric acid (yůr′ik) is one of the waste products of the metabolism of certain proteins and is usually excreted in the urine. Uric acid crystallizes in the tissues when it is present in excessive amounts, resulting in gout.

Other conditions that increase the production of uric acid include blood disorders, psoriasis, and disorders of the parathyroid glands. Excessive uric acid in the body does not always result in gout, but the greater the excess, the greater the likelihood of developing gout.

Too much uric acid in the urine may result in the development of kidney stones.

See also GOUT; PSORIASIS; URICOSURIC AGENT.

Uricosuric agent (yůr ə kō sůr′ik) is any drug that reduces the amount of uric acid in the body by increasing the excretion of uric acid in the urine. Such drugs are generally used in the treatment of gout. Probenecid is one well-known uricosuric agent.

Not all drugs used to treat gout are uricosuric agents, however. Another drug, called allopurinol, works by preventing the excessive formation of uric acid. Allopurinol is often used in the treatment of gout because its use presents less danger of kidney damage.

Most uricosuric agents should be used with caution during an acute attack of gout. They may temporarily aggravate the condition by causing crystals of uric acid in the body tissue to dissolve in the blood.

See also GOUT; URIC ACID.

Urinalysis (yůr ə nal′ə sis) is the detailed analysis of urine. It may be performed to detect alterations in the composition of the urine. Such detection can help in the diagnosis of many disorders, particularly those of the kidney and urinary tract.

Q: *What tests may be performed in a urinalysis?*

A: Various chemical tests may be performed on the urine to detect abnormal substances. For example, the presence of glucose is a typical, but not conclusive, sign of diabetes mellitus.

The urine may also be tested for acidity and the presence of ketones to confirm a preliminary diagnosis of diabetes mellitus. Protein in the urine (proteinuria) may indicate nephritis, myeloma, or other diseases. Bilirubin in the urine may be a sign of jaundice. The presence of blood in the urine (hematuria) may be caused by a urinary tract infection, a stone, a polyp, cancer, or some other abnormality.

The specific gravity, concentration, and volume of urine produced in 24 hours may be measured to assess kidney function.

Most of these tests can be performed in a physician's office. Special tests may require laboratory analysis of the urine to detect hormones and the concentration of various other chemicals.

See also BILIRUBIN; GLUCOSE; HEMATURIA; KETONE; NEPHRITIS.

Urinary acidifier (yůr′ə ner ē ə sid′ə fī ər) is any drug or chemical, such as ammonium chloride or ascorbic acid, that makes urine acidic. Such a chemical may be used to increase the effectiveness of certain drugs or to increase the rate at which the kidneys eliminate some drugs from the body.

Urinary disorders are disorders of various parts of the urinary system. They are usually accompanied by one or more signs or symptoms. The following table lists some urinary disorders and the urinary symptoms associated with each. For more information, see the individual entry for each symptom.

Disorder	*Symptoms*
Bladder disorders	Dysuria (painful urination)
	Hematuria (blood in the urine)
	Incontinence
	Polyuria (excessive production of urine)
Cystitis	Dysuria
	Hematuria
	Nocturia (urination at night)
	Polyuria
Kidney disease	Anuria (lack of urine)
	Glycosuria (sugar in the urine)
	Hematuria
	Hemoglobinuria (hemoglobin in the urine)
	Nocturia
	Oliguria (reduced production of urine)
	Polyuria
	Proteinuria (excessive proteins in the urine)
	Retention (inability to urinate)
Urinary tract infection (e.g., pyelonephritis, ureteritis, urethritis)	Bed-wetting
	Dysuria
	Hematuria
	Nocturia
	Polyuria

Urinary system, or urinary tract, comprises all the organs involved in the production and discharge of urine. The urinary system filters soluble waste products from the blood. It consists of two kidneys, two ureters, the urinary bladder, and the urethra. The kidneys are about 4.5 inches (11cm) long and about 2.5 inches (6cm) wide. They lie in the upper part of the abdomen at the back. The ureters are tubes about 10 inches (25cm) long that drain urine from the core of the kidneys, the renal pelvis, to the bladder. The bladder lies in the lower abdomen at the front of the body. The urethra is the tube through which urine is passed to the outside.

The renal pelvis is funnel-shaped; its widest part is in the center of the kidney. As the renal pelvis narrows, it projects from the kidney and becomes the top of the ureter. The widest part of the renal pelvis is surrounded by the renal medulla, which is in turn surrounded by the renal cortex. The renal cortex is covered by tough fibrous tissue that forms the protective outer layer of each kidney.

Blood is brought to the kidneys by the renal arteries and, after filtration, is returned to circulation through the renal veins. The blood vessels join the kidneys close to each renal pelvis.

The functional units of each kidney are microscopic filters. The renal cortex contains about one million of these filters. Each consists of a cup-shaped capsule (Bowman's capsule) that encloses a knot (glomerulus) of blood capillaries. Blood from the renal artery is pumped into the glomerulus by blood pressure. Water, sugar, salts, urea (a waste product of the breakdown of pro-

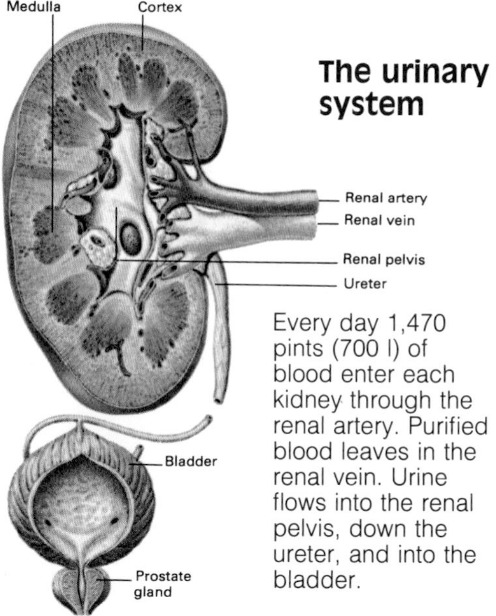

The urinary system

Every day 1,470 pints (700 l) of blood enter each kidney through the renal artery. Purified blood leaves in the renal vein. Urine flows into the renal pelvis, down the ureter, and into the bladder.

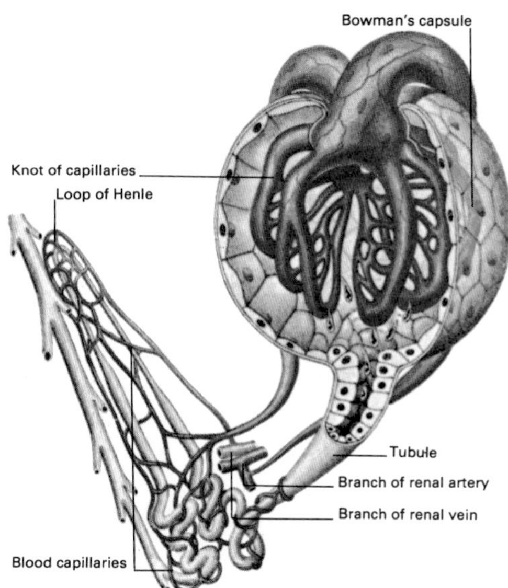

Each filtering unit, or nephron (above), starts with a cup-shaped capsule surrounding a knot of capillaries. Filtered substances pass down a tubule and through the loop of Henle, where essentials are reabsorbed into the blood.

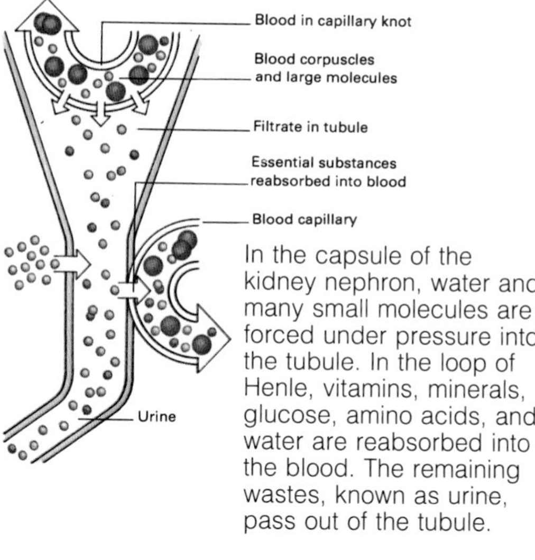

In the capsule of the kidney nephron, water and many small molecules are forced under pressure into the tubule. In the loop of Henle, vitamins, minerals, glucose, amino acids, and water are reabsorbed into the blood. The remaining wastes, known as urine, pass out of the tubule.

teins), and other small molecules pass through the capillary walls into the Bowman's capsule. Blood cells and large molecules, such as whole proteins and fats, remain in the blood.

Filtered fluids pass from the Bowman's capsule into a coiled tube, the nephron, that leads through the renal medulla to the renal pelvis. Each nephron has a U-shaped loop (the loop of Henle) halfway along its length. The whole tube is closely surrounded by blood capillaries. As the filtered fluid passes through the tube, substances that the body needs, especially water, essential salts, and sugar, are reabsorbed from the fluid in the tube into the surrounding blood capillaries.

The concentrated fluid (urine) that results from the filtration and reabsorption processes collects in the renal pelvis before passing through the ureter to the bladder. A circular ring of muscle at the top of the urethra keeps urine in the bladder until voluntarily relaxed.

See also BLADDER; KIDNEY; URETER; URETHRA.

Urinary tract infection is an infection of one or more parts of the urinary system caused primarily by bacteria. Obstructions such as stones or tumors can foster susceptibility to infection. Urinary tract infections are more common in women than in men. Symptoms include frequency of urination, painful urination (dysuria), and in severe cases blood and pus in the urine (hematuria). *See also* DYSURIA; HEMATURIA.

A physical examination of the patient and a detailed urinalysis are necessary to determine the cause and location of the infection. Treatment with antibacterial drugs is usually effective; in the case of pyelonephritis, hospitalization may be necessary. Obstructions may require surgery.

See also CYSTITIS; PYELONEPHRITIS; URETERITIS; URETHRITIS.

Urine (yůr′ən) is a fluid that is produced by the kidneys, carried to the bladder by the ureters, and transported out of the body through the urethra. Urine consists mainly of water, but it also contains waste products that are filtered from the blood by the kidneys. The elimination of waste products in the urine helps keep the body fluids at the optimum concentration.

The principal waste products are urea, uric acid, creatine, and other nitrogen compounds that are produced by various metabolic processes, mainly by the digestion of proteins. Urine also contains sodium chloride and other salts, as well as a few body cells.

Normal urine is amber in color and has a faint but distinctive odor. Occasionally, urine contains abnormal substances, such as sugar, protein, bacteria, pus, or blood. Analysis of the urine can help diagnose a large number of disorders.

See also UREA; URIC ACID; URINALYSIS.

Urogenital system (yůr ə jen′ə təl) comprises the organs associated with the production and secretion of urine (the kidneys, ureters, bladder, and urethra) as well as the genital or reproductive organs. In females, these include the ovaries, the uterine or fallopian tubes, the uterus, the cervix, and the vagina. In males, these include the testes, the seminal vesicles, the seminal ducts, the prostate, and the penis. The urogenital system is also called the genitourinary system.

See also REPRODUCTION, HUMAN; URINARY SYSTEM.

Urology (yů rol′ə jē) is the branch of medicine that is concerned with the male and female urinary tract and the male genital organs.

Urticaria (ėr tə kãr′ē ə), also known as hives or nettle rash, is a skin condition that is characterized by the eruption of welts and itching. It is usually the result of an allergic reaction to a food or drug.

See also HIVES.

Uterus (yü′tər əs), or womb, is a thick, pear-shaped organ located in the abdominal cavity of females. It is lined with layers of cells (endometrium) that respond to the varying hormonal stimulation of the menstrual cycle. During pregnancy, the uterus is the organ that holds and nourishes the developing fetus. During childbirth, the muscles of the uterus contract and force the infant out of the mother's body.

The neck of the uterus (cervix) leads into the vagina. The uterus is supported in part by a combination of ligaments that stretch from the side of the cervix to the pelvic bones.

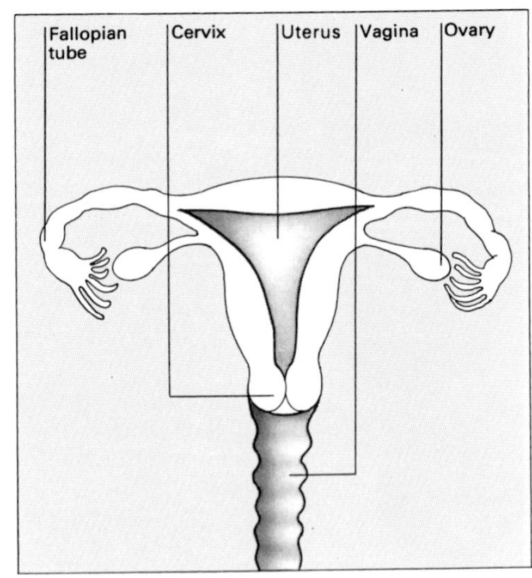

The **uterus** is the organ that contains and nourishes the fetus during pregnancy.

See also CERVICITIS; ENDOMETRITIS; FIBROID; GYNECOLOGICAL DISORDERS; HYSTERECTOMY; MENSTRUAL PROBLEMS; POLYP; PROLAPSE.

Utricle (yü′trə kəl) is the larger of the two membranous sacs in the labyrinth of the inner ear. These two sacs together with the semicircular canals form the ear's organs of balance.

See also EAR; SACCULE.

Uveitis (yü vē ī′tis) is inflammation of the uveal tract, which is the part of the eye that comprises the iris, the ciliary body, and the choroid. It can be caused by allergy, infection, trauma, diabetes, collagen disease, and skin diseases. The symptoms differ according to whether the front or the back of the eye is affected. Uveitis that affects the front of the eye causes iritis; uveitis that affects the back of the eye causes choroiditis.

See also CHOROIDITIS; EYE; IRITIS.

Uvula (yü′vyə lə) is a small, fleshy mass of tissue. The term usually refers to the structure that hangs from the soft palate at the back of the mouth. This is called the palatine uvula.

See also TONSIL.

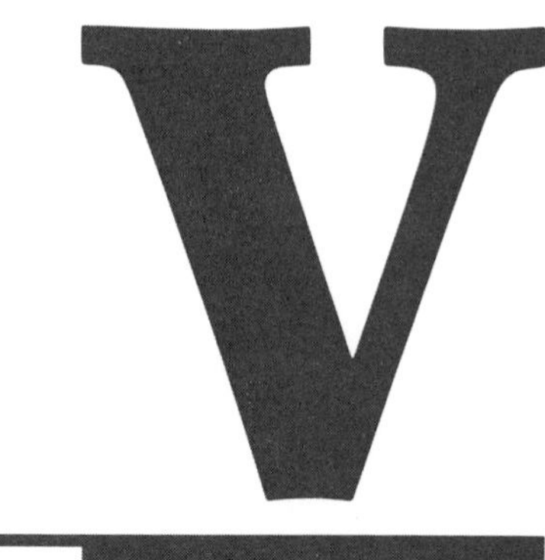

Vaccination (vak sə nā'shən) is an inoculation with infectious microorganisms or some part of them (a vaccine) in order to give immunity against a specific disease.

See also IMMUNIZATION; VACCINE.

Vaccine (vak'sēn) is a preparation of disease-producing (pathogenic) microorganisms, or some part of them, that is given to induce immunity. There are three main types of vaccine: those that contain specially treated living organisms, such as measles vaccine; those that contain dead organisms, such as whooping cough vaccine; and those that contain specially prepared toxins, such as diphtheria vaccine.

See also IMMUNIZATION.

Vaccinia (vak sin'ē ə) is a bovine virus used for human immunization against smallpox. In 1796, Edward Jenner took vaccinia virus from the sores of cows (cowpox) and injected it into humans as a protection against smallpox. This incident was the first use of an immunization, or vaccination. Today, vaccinia shots are no longer recommended because of the near-eradication of smallpox.

See also SMALLPOX.

Vacuum extractor (vak'yüm ek strak'tər) is an alternative to forceps in assisting the delivery of a baby. It is a suction cup that is placed over the baby's head. The suction allows an obstetrician to gently pull the child out during delivery. It is easier to attach than forceps, and pressure is applied over a larger area of the skull. There is no evidence that this practice eliminates the chances of brain damage to the baby, but damage is less likely to the mother and the baby than with the use of forceps.

See also FORCEPS.

Vagina (və jī'nə) is the part of a female's genital tract that extends upward and backward from the vulva to the cervix (neck of the uterus). The walls of the vagina are composed of fibrous and elastic tissue, so that it is normally a closed, flattened structure lying between the urethra in front and the rectum at the back.

A woman's vagina is about 3 inches (7.5cm) long when relaxed, but it can stretch considerably during sexual intercourse. The size of the vagina is controlled by the surrounding muscles. During intercourse and childbirth, the muscles relax and contract. The ridged skin lining the vagina (epithelium) changes with the hormonal variations that occur during the menstrual cycle. The amount of mucous secretions also varies during the cycle.

See also REPRODUCTION, HUMAN.

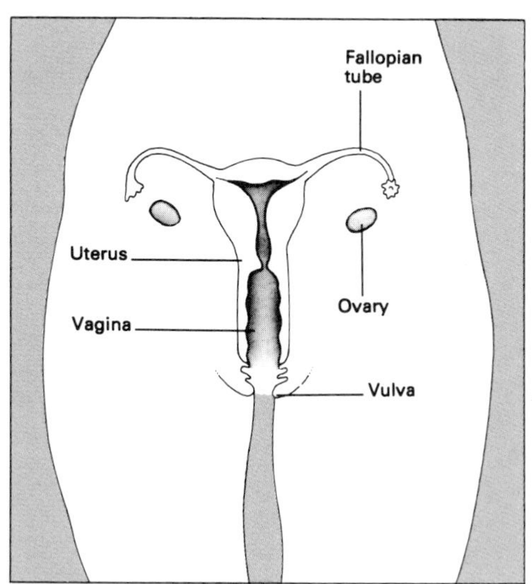

The **vagina** is the membranous passage between the uterus and the external opening, the vulva.

Vaginal discharge (vaj'ə nel), known medically as leukorrhea, is not necessarily abnormal; many women experience a slight discharge. However, it may be a symptom of vaginitis (inflammation of the vagina) or cervicitis (inflammation of the cervix). Other causes include a foreign body in the vagina, such as a bead in an infant girl or a forgotten tampon in a woman.

The discharge usually consists of secretions from the cervix (neck of the uterus) and vagina. The amount of these varies from time to time during the menstrual cycle because of the hormonal response of the cells that line the vagina and cervix. A day or two after menstruation has ended, there is a slight increase in secretions. Another noticeable increase occurs in the middle of the cycle about the time of ovulation.

Sexual stimulation, either physical or psychological, also causes an increase in secretions.

Newborn females usually have a swollen vulva and a slight vaginal discharge because of the presence of maternal hormones in their bloodstream.

See also CERVICITIS; OVULATION; VAGINITIS.

Vaginismus (vaj ə niz'məs) is an extreme spasm of the muscles surrounding the lower end of the vagina, which causes pain and makes sexual intercourse extremely difficult (dyspareunia).

Q: *What causes vaginismus?*

A: The cause is usually of psychological origin, often fear. Other causes include inflammation of the vagina.

Q: *How is vaginismus treated?*

A: A gynecologist checks for any physical cause of pain before psychiatric treatment is recommended. Overcoming fear of intercourse may take a long time.

See also SEXUAL PROBLEMS.

Vaginitis (vaj ə nī'tis) is an inflammation of the vagina. It produces an irritating vaginal discharge.

Q: *What causes vaginitis?*

A: Many women have infectious organisms in the vagina that can cause inflammation, but only a sudden change in environment triggers them into action. Such infection may be stimulated by such diverse factors as the use of antibiotics, the contraceptive pill, vaginal douching, or sexual intercourse. The common microorganisms that infect the vagina are *Candida albicans* and *Trichomonas vaginalis*. *See also* CANDIDIASIS; TRICHOMONAS VAGINALIS.

Q: *What are the symptoms of vaginitis?*

A: Vaginitis causes soreness and a discharge. Typically, candidiasis (sometimes called moniliasis) causes an intense itching, soreness, and a thick, white discharge; whereas trichomoniasis produces a foul-smelling, greenish, watery discharge that may be uncomfortable and even painful, but not usually itchy.

Q: *How is vaginitis treated?*

A: Candidiasis is treated with suppositories or creams inserted into the vagina. It is more common in women who are pregnant or who are taking contraceptive pills (because of the pills' hormonal effect on the vaginal cells), but it is seldom necessary to stop taking the pills. Patients who develop candidiasis because they are taking antibiotics for some other condition usually improve rapidly once the appropriate treatment is given.

Trichomoniasis is treated with pills taken orally; the patient's sexual partner should also be treated. Other forms of vaginitis, such as nonspecific bacterial vaginitis, can be treated with a combination of suppositories, creams, or appropriate antibiotic drugs by mouth.

Q: *Is vaginitis sexually transmitted?*

A: In a few cases, candidiasis may be sexually transmitted. If the woman has recurrent attacks, it is often advisable for the man to use a cream to be applied to the end of the penis at night.

In cases of trichomoniasis, the man usually has the infection without any symptoms, and he should be given treatment at the same time as the woman.

See also CERVICITIS; SALPINGITIS; VAGINAL DISCHARGE; VULVITIS.

Vagotomy (və got'ə mē) is an operation to cut the vagus nerve. Usually, both branches of the nerve are cut at a point adjacent to the esophagus where they pass through the diaphragm muscle. This cut greatly reduces the secretion of hydrochloric acid by the stomach. The operation is frequently done at the same time as a partial gastrectomy, used to treat a peptic ulcer, or a pyloroplasty, used to repair the pylorus in the stomach.

See also NERVE; ULCER, PEPTIC.

Vagus nerve. *See* NERVE.

Valgus (val'gəs) is any deformity in which part of the body is bent outward from the midline. For example, talipes valgus is a form of clubfoot in which the heel is turned outward. A person who is knock-kneed has a valgus deformity because the ankles turn out.

See also VARUS.

Valium® (val'ē əm) is a brand-name preparation of diazepam, a benzodiazepine compound. It is used for a variety of medical reasons. Intravenously, it is used for the acute control of seizures. In the oral form, it is used for muscle spasms and for the short-term control of anxiety.

See also TRANQUILIZER.

Valley fever, also known as San Joaquin Valley fever or coccidioidomycosis, is an infectious disease that is caused by the fungus *Coccidioides immitis.* Infection results from inhalation of the spores of the fungus. Valley fever occurs mainly in the southwest United States and most commonly affects men between 20 and 50 years old.

Valley fever usually produces relatively mild symptoms that are similar to those of a feverish cold or acute bronchitis. Rarely, it may cause a form of pneumonia in which the brain may also be affected, producing a form of meningitis.

Treatment of the mild form of valley fever is usually not necessary because most patients recover spontaneously. The severe form of the disease is treated with the antifungal drug amphotericin, but even with treatment the mortality rate is high in severe cases.

Valve (valv) is a fold of tissue within a tube in the body that prevents the backflow of fluid. Valves are present in the heart, veins, lymphatic vessels and other areas of the body. The ileocecal valve, for example, is situated between the cecum and the small intestine. It helps prevent digested food from moving backward in the intestine.

Valvotomy (val vot'ə mē) is a surgical operation in which a valve is cut. It is most commonly performed to repair a heart valve that has become deformed because of scarring.

Valvular disease (val'vyə lər) is a relatively common disorder of the heart in which there is deformity of the heart valves, lack of the usual number of flaps that form the valves, or reduction in the size of the opening.

Rheumatic fever causes scarring of the valves and may lead to narrowing (stenosis) or dilation of the passages. It usually affects the mitral valve between the left atrium and left ventricle of the heart, but other valves, such as the tricuspid, aortic, and pulmonary valves, may also be damaged. Sometimes, more than one valve is affected.

Valvular disease causes additional strain on the heart muscle and frequently leads to heart failure later in life. Special diagnostic techniques, such as echocardiography and angiocardiography, may be necessary.

Apart from heart failure, the major complication of valvular disease is infection of the damaged valves resulting in subacute bacterial endocarditis.

In most cases, the deformed valves can be corrected surgically, either by a valvotomy to remove the scarred tissue or by replacement of the defective valve.

See also ENDOCARDITIS; HEART DISEASE; MITRAL VALVE DISEASE; VALVOTOMY.

Vaporizer (vā'pə rī zər) is a device that converts a fluid into a vapor spray. A vaporizer is an effective method of administering medication for disorders of the lungs and bronchial tubes, such as asthma, bronchitis, and croup.

See also INHALATION THERAPY.

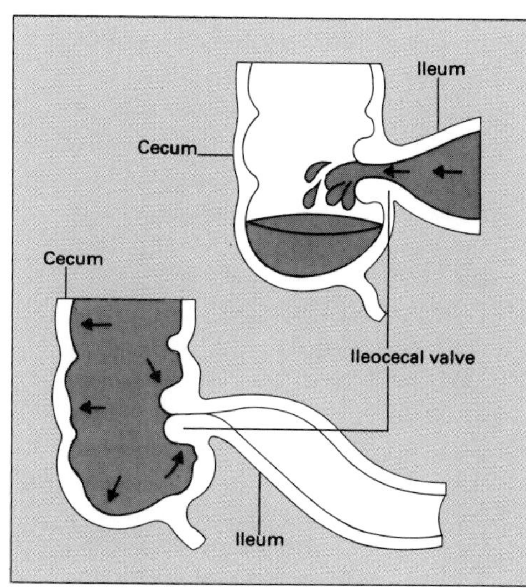

The **valve** between the ileum and the cecum prevents food from reversing out of the large intestine back into the small intestine.

Varicella (var ə sel′ə) is the medical name for chickenpox.

See also CHICKENPOX.

Varicocele (var′ə kō sēl) is varicose veins around the testes. The enlargement of the veins of the spermatic cord, which causes varicocele, is more common on the left side than the right in adolescent males. It seldom causes more than a slight ache that can be relieved, if necessary, by a scrotal support.

The increased blood flow and warmth in a varicocele occasionally may be a factor in reducing sperm production, leading to sterility in a man. In rare cases, a varicocele may occur in a woman's vulva and may cause infertility.

See also TESTIS.

Varicose vein (var′ə kōs) is a vein that is abnormally swollen and twisted. Varicose veins result from increased blood pressure in the veins and damage or absence of the normal valves.

Damage to the valves may be caused by venous thrombosis. Absence of the normal valves may be due to a congenital defect. Increased blood pressure may result from an abdominal tumor, a fibroid in the womb, an ovarian cyst, pregnancy, or obesity. Varicose veins are more common in women than men. The condition also occurs in some families more than others; that fact suggests a hereditary factor. *See also* THROMBOSIS, VENOUS.

Q: *Where do varicose veins occur?*

A: Varicose veins usually occur in the legs, but they may also occur around the anus, causing piles (hemorrhoids), around the testes (varicocele), or in the vulva of a pregnant woman. *See also* HEMORRHOID; VARICOCELE.

The veins at the lower end of the esophagus may also become enlarged as a result of cirrhosis of the liver, when there is an increase in venous pressure in the hepatic portal vein. *See also* CIRRHOSIS.

Q: *What are the symptoms of varicose veins?*

A: The most obvious symptom is the appearance of the affected veins. Varicose veins are blue and snakelike. They occur near the skin in the legs and may stand out from the legs. The legs may also ache and the ankles may swell at the end of the day.

Q: *How are varicose veins treated?*

A: In the early stages, or for those who are elderly or unfit, an elastic stocking may relieve the aching and swelling. But it does not cure the condition.

Varicose veins may also be treated by injecting a fluid that inflames the vein wall. The leg is then bandaged tightly for about six weeks to keep the walls of the veins close together. The resultant scarring causes the walls of the vein to stick together.

Surgical treatment involves cutting and tying the varicose veins, passing a wire instrument down the length of the vein, and then removing the vein by pulling on the wire. This technique is known as stripping.

Q: *What complications occur with varicose veins?*

A: The most common complication is phlebitis, which has the same inflammatory effect on the vein as injection treatment. The vein becomes tender and eventually scarred, resulting in a nodule under the skin. Severe phlebitis may require antibiotics and tight bandaging. Rarely, anticoagulants may be necessary if a deep vein has been affected by a blood clot.

See also PHLEBITIS.

Variola (və rī′ə lə) is the medical name for smallpox.

See also SMALLPOX.

Varus (vār′əs) is a deformity in which a part of the body bends inward from the midline. A person who is bowlegged has a varus deformity because the heels are turned in.

See also VALGUS.

Vascular system (vas′kyə lər) is the network of vessels that carry blood, lymph, and other fluids throughout the body.

See also CARDIOVASCULAR SYSTEM; LYMPHATIC SYSTEM.

Vas deferens (vas def′ə renz), or sperm duct, is the tube that carries the sperm from the epididymis of the testes to the seminal vesicles (alongside the prostate gland), where sperm are stored.

See also TESTIS; VASECTOMY.

Vasectomy (va sek′tə mē) is a form of sterilization for men in which a section of each of the two sperm ducts (vas

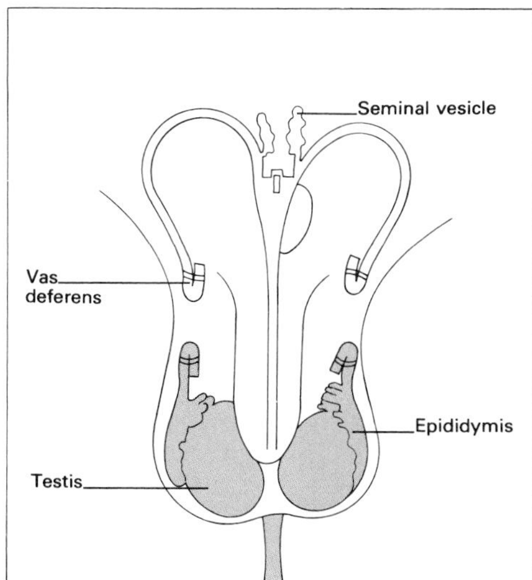

A **vasectomy** is the surgical removal of all or part of the vas deferens. It is performed for the purpose of sterilization.

deferens) is removed surgically. This operation prevents sperm from reaching the urethra. *See also* VAS DEFERENS.

Q: *How is a vasectomy performed?*

A: The operation can usually be done under a local anesthetic as an outpatient procedure. An incision is made at a site that overlies the point at which each sperm duct leaves the scrotum. The two sperm ducts are cut, and the ends are tied firmly with a material that does not dissolve, such as silk. The two incisions are then closed with one or two stitches.

Q: *How soon after a vasectomy does a man become sterile?*

A: The man is fertile for about two or three months after the operation until sperm that were in the seminal vesicles when the operation was performed have either died or been ejaculated.

Q: *Are there any immediate problems with a vasectomy?*

A: There may be slight local discomfort over the groin wounds for two or three days, but this should not interfere with normal activities. Sexual intercourse may be uncomfortable, so it is advisable to abstain until the stitches are removed or are absorbed by the body, which normally takes about four or five days.

Q: *Can a vasectomy cause long-term problems?*

A: Long-term problems are extremely rare. There may be a dull ache in the testes for several weeks after the operation, but this slowly disappears.

The most common long-term problems are usually psychological in origin. The only difference a vasectomy makes is to stop the production of sperm. A man's sex drive (libido) is usually undiminished after the operation; it may even increase because the fear of an unwanted pregnancy is removed. A vasectomy does not reduce the production of sex hormones, nor should it affect a man's feelings of masculinity.

Q: *Can a vasectomy be reversed?*

A: It is technically possible to reunite the vas deferens. This, however, may not restore fertility, and in actual practice, very few vasectomies can be successfully reversed.

See also STERILIZATION.

Vasoconstrictor (vas ō kən strik′tər) is any agent that causes constriction of the blood vessels. This effect is usually brought about by drugs, but it may also be the result of nervous stimulation.

See also VASOPRESSOR.

Vasodilator (vas ō dī lā′tər) is any agent that causes blood vessels to dilate. It is usually a drug, but dilation may also be the result of nervous stimulation.

Vasomotor rhinitis (vas ō mō′tər rī nī′tis) is a condition affecting the mucous membranes that line the nose. It causes symptoms of runny nose, sneezing, postnasal drip, and occasionally, headache. The symptoms are similar to those of hay fever, but no allergic cause can be found.

Q: *What causes vasomotor rhinitis?*

A: In most cases, there is no obvious cause. Sometimes, anxiety, changes in room temperature, or hormonal changes associated with adolescence, menstruation, or menopause may be factors.

Occasionally, a similar condition occurs in a person who has been overusing nasal sprays or drops.

Q: *How is vasomotor rhinitis treated?*

A: Treatment is difficult. The symptoms are thought to be caused partly by overactivity of the parasympathetic nervous system, so loss of weight, regular exercise, and the stopping of smoking may all help. Treatment with corticosteroid nasal sprays is effective in some cases.

See also NERVOUS SYSTEM, PARASYMPATHETIC.

Vasomotor system (vas ō mō′tər) is the section of the nervous system that regulates the size of the blood vessels and, therefore, governs circulation.

Vasopressin (vas ō pres′in), also known as antidiuretic hormone (ADH), is a hormone stored in the pituitary gland. It reduces the excretion of urine by the kidneys. A synthetic form of this hormone is used as an antidiuretic in the treatment of diabetes insipidus. Although it constricts small blood vessels, even large doses elevate the blood pressure only slightly and for a brief period in conscious patients.

See also DIABETES INSIPIDUS.

Vasopressor (vas ō pres′ər) is anything that stimulates the contraction of blood vessels, causing an increase in blood pressure.

See also VASOCONSTRICTOR.

Vasovagal syncope (vas ō vā′gəl sing′kə pē) is the medical name for fainting induced by the sudden dilatation of the blood vessels (vasodilatation). This can happen because of nervous stimulation or a fall in heart rate.

See also FAINTING.

VD is the abbreviation for venereal disease.

See also SEXUALLY TRANSMITTED DISEASE.

Vector (vek′tər) is an agent that carries an infection from one person to another or from an infected animal to a person. A vector may be a person or an animal, but it is usually an insect. For example, mosquitoes may be vectors of malaria and yellow fever.

See also FLEA; MITE; MOSQUITO; TICK.

Vein is a thin-walled blood vessel that carries blood from the body tissues back to the heart. All veins, except the pulmonary veins and the umbilical vein, carry blood with a low concentration of oxygen and a high concentration of carbon dioxide.

Like the arteries, the walls of the veins consist of three layers, but the muscle and middle layers are thinner than in the arteries and can not keep the vein open if the blood pressure is low. Many of the veins have valves to prevent the backflow of blood.

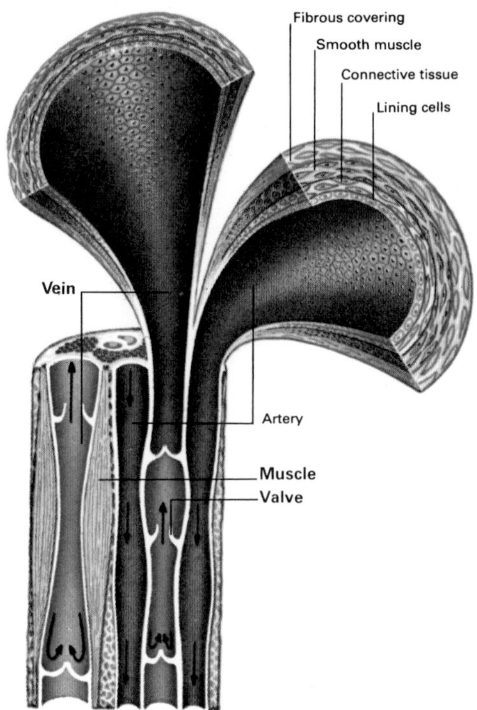

The flow of blood in a **vein** is assisted by the action of special muscles that run alongside the vein.

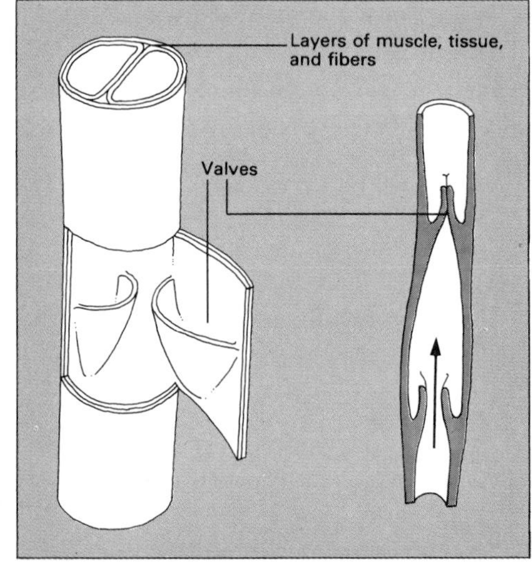

A **vein** frequently contains valves that prevent the backward flow of blood.

Veins start as capillaries within the body tissues. The capillaries unite to form venules, which then connect with larger veins, which themselves ultimately join to form two major veins (the venae cavae) that drain into the heart. The four pulmonary veins drain directly into the left atrium of the heart.

There are two veins that begin and end in capillaries. These are known as portal veins. The hepatic portal vein drains blood from the gastrointestinal tract to the liver. The hypophyseoportal vein connects the hypothalamus in the brain to the pituitary gland and conveys hormones that stimulate the production of pituitary hormones.

See also CARDIOVASCULAR SYSTEM; THROMBOSIS, VENOUS; VARICOSE VEIN; VENA CAVA.

Velopharyngeal insufficiency (vel ō fə rin'jē əl in sə fish'ən sē) is a condition caused by a congenital flaw characterized by an opening in the oral cavity below the nasal passage (similar to a cleft palate). Surgical closure is the usual treatment.

See also CLEFT PALATE.

Vena cava (vē nə kā'və) is one of the two veins (superior vena cava and inferior vena cava) that drain blood from all parts of the body (except the heart) into the right atrium of the heart. The superior vena cava returns blood from the head, neck, and arms to the heart. The inferior vena cava returns blood from the chest, abdomen, and legs to the heart.

See also CARDIOVASCULAR SYSTEM; VEIN.

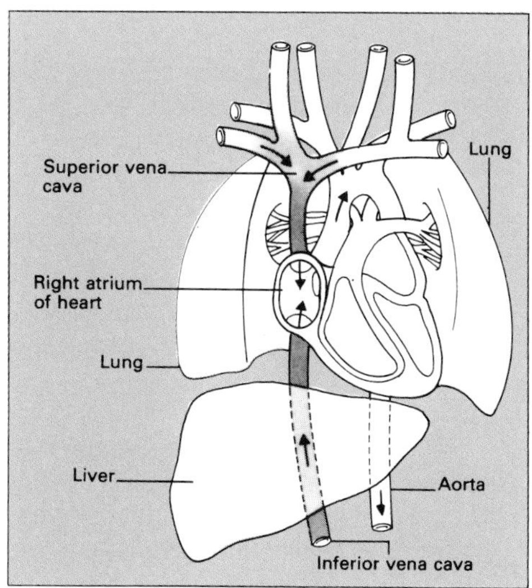

The **vena cava** is either of two veins that empty blood from the upper and lower portions of the body into the heart.

Venereal disease. *See* SEXUALLY TRANSMITTED DISEASE.

Venereal wart. *See* WART, VENEREAL.

Venereology (və nir ē ol'ə jē) is the specialty of medicine concerned with the diagnosis and treatment of venereal diseases. The physician who practices this specialty is called a venereologist.

See also SEXUALLY TRANSMITTED DISEASE.

Venipuncture (ven ə pungk'chər) is the act of puncturing a vein with a needle. It may be done to obtain a sample of blood for testing or to insert an IV (intravenous infusion), for which the needle is left in the vein.

Venogram (vē'nə gram) is a procedure in which a dye is injected into a vein so that an X-ray photograph will reveal the shape, size, and extent of the vein.

See also ANGIOGRAM.

Venom (ven'əm) is a poisonous substance from a snake, insect, or other animal that can be injected through the skin by a bite or sting. It contains a variety of poisons and toxic enzymes.

See also ANTIVENIN; BITES AND STINGS: FIRST AID.

Venous thrombosis. *See* THROMBOSIS, VENOUS.

Ventilator (ven'tə lā tər) is any of several pieces of equipment used in respiratory therapy to aid breathing.

See also RESPIRATOR.

Ventral (ven'trəl) refers to the front (abdominal) surface of the body, also called the anterior surface, as opposed to the dorsal, or posterior, surface.

Ventricle (ven'trə kəl) is either of the two lower chambers of the heart that receive blood from the atria and force it into the arteries.

See also HEART.

Venule (ven'yül) is any of the small veins that begin at the capillaries and connect with the larger veins.

See also VEIN.

Vermiform appendix (vėr'mə fôrm ə pen'diks) is the full anatomical name for the appendix. The term refers to the worm-like shape of the appendix.

See also APPENDIX.

Verruca (ve rü'kə) is another name for a wart. Verruca vulgaris, or common wart, is the most frequent type. A wart on the sole of the foot is called a plantar wart.

See also WART.

Vertebra (vėr'tə brə) is any of the 33 bones of the spinal column. The flexible part of the spinal column consists of 7 cervical vertebrae in the neck; 12 thoracic vertebrae at the back of the chest; and 5 lumbar vertebrae in the small of the back. The 5 vertebrae below the lumbar vertebrae are fused to form the sacrum. The lowest 4 vertebrae form the coccyx.

The **vertebrae** are separated by intervertebral disks, which allow the spine to bend.

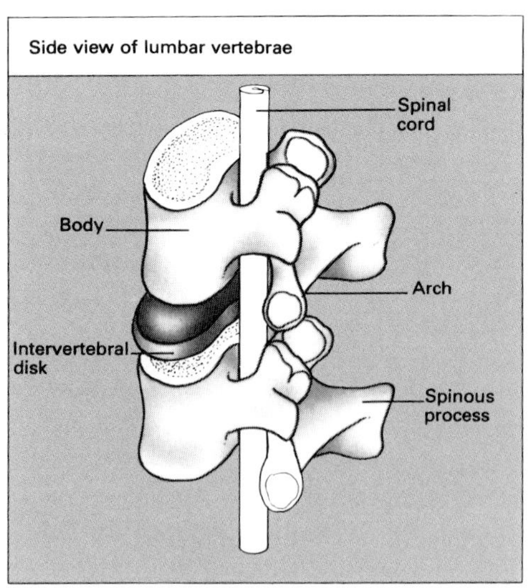

A typical vertebra consists of two main parts, an inner, ventral part called the body and an outer, dorsal part called the vertebral arch. These two parts surround a central space through which the spinal cord passes.

The body of a vertebra is roughly cylindrical in shape, with flattened upper and lower surfaces. The bodies of adjacent vertebrae are separated by tough disks of fibrocartilage (intervertebral disks). The vertebral bodies increase in size down the length of the spine.

See also DISK, HERNIATED; NECK, STIFF; SPINE.

Vertigo (vėr′tə gō) is a disorder of balance that gives a person the sensation of spinning around in space when at rest. Alternatively, objects may appear to be spinning around the person.

Q: *What causes vertigo?*

A: Any disorder that affects the ear, the auditory nerve, or the center in the brain concerned with balance may be responsible. Other causes include toxic compounds, such as drugs, alcohol, or food poisoning, and sudden disturbances of eye function.

Q: *What ear disorders cause vertigo?*

A: Infections of the middle ear and inner ear, such as otitis media and labyrinthitis, or involvement by other disorders, such as otosclerosis and Ménière's disease, may cause vertigo. Other causes are blockage of the Eustachian tube and wax in the external ear. *See also* LABYRINTHITIS; MÉNIÈRE'S DISEASE; OTITIS; OTOSCLEROSIS.

Q: *How does the auditory nerve become involved?*

A: Vestibular neuronitis infections, in which the nerve cells become inflamed, are the most common cause. A tumor of the auditory nerve may produce vertigo as well as increasing deafness.

Q: *What conditions affecting the brain cause vertigo?*

A: The centers that coordinate balance are in the brain stem and have connections with the cerebellum and the temporal lobes of the cerebral hemispheres. These may be disturbed by a stroke or arteriosclerosis, particularly in the elderly. Disorders such as multiple sclerosis, epilepsy, and a brain tumor result in vertigo. *See also* ARTERIOSCLEROSIS; EPILEPSY; MULTIPLE SCLEROSIS; STROKE; TUMOR.

Q: *What is benign paroxysmal positional vertigo?*

A: Symptoms of vertigo may occur when the head is moved quickly or placed in certain positions, but they last for only a few seconds. This type of vertigo is thought to be a minor disturbance of the organ of balance and often spontaneously improves after several months.

Q: *Are there any other symptoms that may accompany vertigo?*

A: Yes. Nausea and vomiting commonly accompany vertigo, and walking may be difficult, with a tendency to fall over sideways. The eyes may flicker (nystagmus), there may be buzzing in the ears (tinnitus), and there may be hearing loss.

Q: *How is vertigo treated?*

A: The immediate treatment is to have the person lie down in a comfortable position with the eyes closed. A physician should be consulted because antinauseant drugs can be prescribed to help control the symptoms until a diagnosis is made and the appropriate treatment given. Anti-vertiginous (anti-vertigo) drugs may be effective in a number of patients.

Vesicle (ves′ə kəl) is either (1) a bladder or sac containing fluid, such as the gall bladder or urinary bladder; or (2) a blister on the skin containing serous

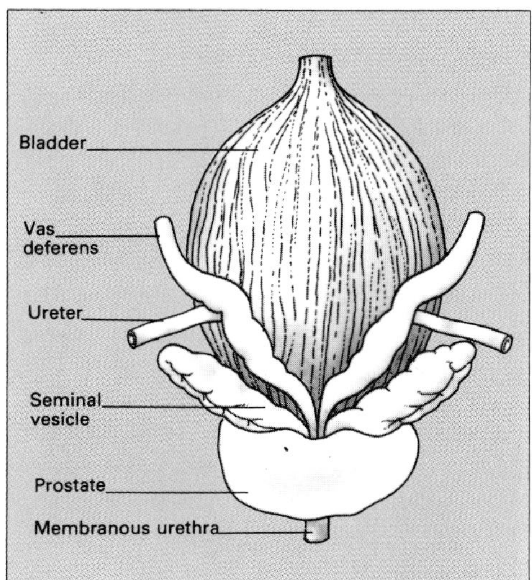

A **vesicle** is a pouch-like sac or bladder the contains fluid, such as the urinary bladder or the seminal vesicle.

fluid, as occurs in chickenpox and shingles.

See also BLADDER; BLISTER.

Veterans Administration, also called the VA, is an organization that administers services to about 30 million former members of the United States armed forces. The VA also provides benefits and services for certain eligible family members of veterans.

There are 172 veterans' hospitals, located in all states except Alaska and Hawaii.

Viable (vī′ə bəl) refers to things that are living or capable of living. A fetus is considered to be viable when it has reached a stage at which it can be kept alive outside the uterus, usually when the fetus is at least 28 weeks old. Viable tissue is, for example, tissue in a burn that is still alive and capable of surviving with proper treatment.

Vibrio (vib′rē ō) is a genus of moving, rod-shaped bacteria. There are more than 30 different species of *Vibrio;* three cause disease. *Vibrio cholerae* causes cholera. There are two strains of this species; the normal strain and a more resistant strain known as El Tor. *Vibrio fetus* and *Vibrio parahemolyticus* rarely cause disease. However, infection with *Vibrio fetus* may cause blood poisoning, abortion, pneumonia, or an illness that is similar to brucellosis. Infection with *Vibrio parahemolyticus* may cause a relatively mild form of food poisoning.

See also BRUCELLOSIS; CHOLERA.

Villi (vil′ī) are small, finger-like protrusions from the surface of a membrane in the body. The lining of the small intestine is covered with millions of villi that provide a large surface area for the secretion of intestinal enzymes and the absorption of digested food.

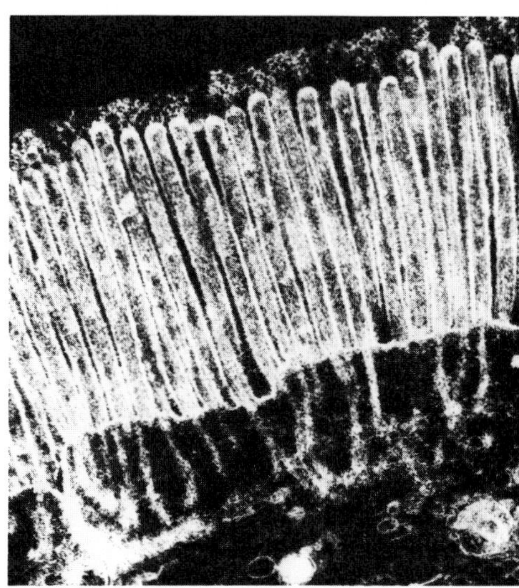

Villi, short, finger-like projections, greatly increase the absorbing surface of the small intestine.

Vincent's infection (vin′sənts), also known as trench mouth, is a form of stomatitis (inflammation of the mouth). It is caused by bacteria that infect the gums, mucous membranes, tonsils, and pharynx. This disorder may develop when oral hygiene is neglected, nutrition is poor, or some serious illness such as leukemia is present.

Q: *What are the symptoms of Vincent's infection?*

A: The chief symptom is a sudden onset of painful, bleeding gums (gingivitis), with ulceration inside the cheeks and on the tongue. The patient has foul-smelling breath and sometimes develops a fever.

Q: *How is Vincent's infection treated?*

A: Antiseptic mouthwashes and dental care produce a rapid improvement. A physician may prescribe an antibiotic drug and, if necessary, extra vitamins. Smoking should be avoided.

Virilism (vir′ə liz əm) is the development of masculine characteristics in women or children. In boys, it is associated with the bodily changes of puberty. The early development of male secondary sex characteristics is caused by excessive secretion of the male sex hormone testosterone by the adrenal glands.

Q: *What symptoms may occur in a woman?*

A: Male-type distribution of body hair develops, with deepening voice and the onset of baldness. Acne may appear, and the woman's periods may become irregular or cease (amenorrhea). There is usually an increase in sex drive (libido).

Q: *How is the condition diagnosed and treated?*

A: A diagnosis is made after the patient's urine has been examined for breakdown products of testosterone and X rays have been taken to detect the presence of an adrenal gland tumor. Corticosteroid drugs will reduce the adrenal gland activity in mild cases, but an operation is usually necessary to remove a part of the adrenal glands or a tumor.

Virulent (vir'yə lənt) means extremely toxic. The term is applied to any infection that causes a rapid onset of severe or life-threatening symptoms.

Virus (vī'rəs) is one of a group of infectious organisms that are visible only under an electron microscope. They are much smaller than bacteria. Viruses consist only of a strand of either DNA or RNA, which are complex proteins that carry genetic information, and an outer coat of protein. Viruses can not provide their own energy, nor can they replicate themselves outside living cells. They survive by altering the function of the cells they infect so that these cells supply the viruses with energy and with the means of replicating themselves.

Q: *Do viruses infect all the body tissues?*

A: Yes, but individual viruses show a preference for particular types of tissues. For example, the poliomyelitis virus infects only part of the nervous system, the rabies virus infects the brain, and the chickenpox virus infects the skin. Any viral infection may cause generalized symptoms of muscle aching and fever.

Not all viruses cause disease. Some remain within the body cells without disordering them, but they can be activated by an alteration in the body.

Q: *What diseases do viruses cause?*

A: Many common diseases are caused by viruses: for example, chickenpox, influenza, measles, mumps, rubella, and most respiratory diseases. Other viral diseases include dengue fever, encephalitis, shingles, smallpox, and yellow fever. At least 30 different viruses can cause the symptoms of the common cold.

Some diseases are caused by slow viruses that remain in the body for several years before producing any symptoms. Multiple sclerosis may be caused by an al-

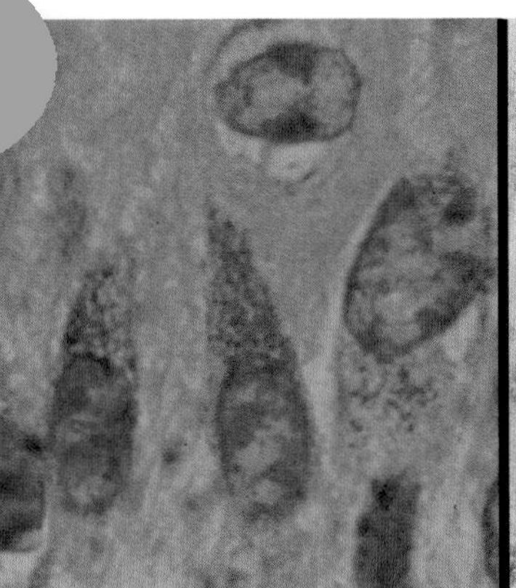

The chicken pox virus affects mostly children, but belongs to the same group of viruses causing shingles in adults.

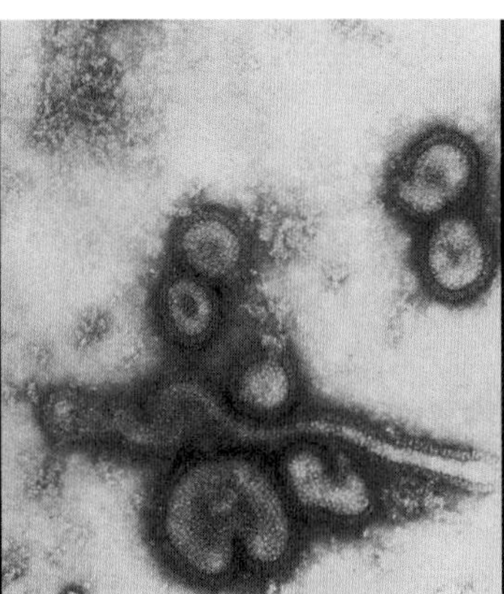

The influenza virus causes a respiratory infection, which can strike any age group.

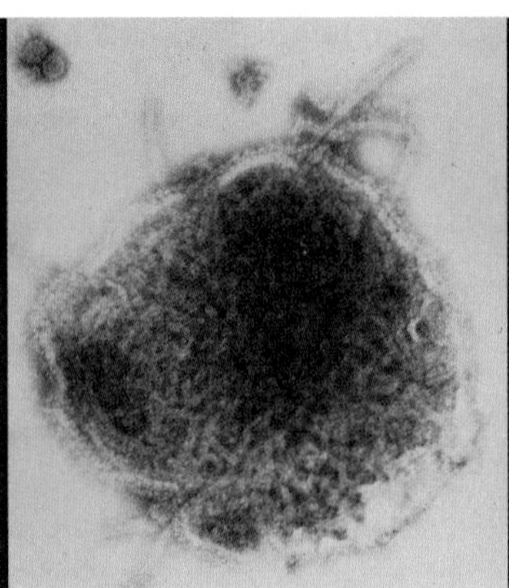

The rubella virus causes German measles, which is particularly dangerous for an unborn fetus, whose mother is infected.

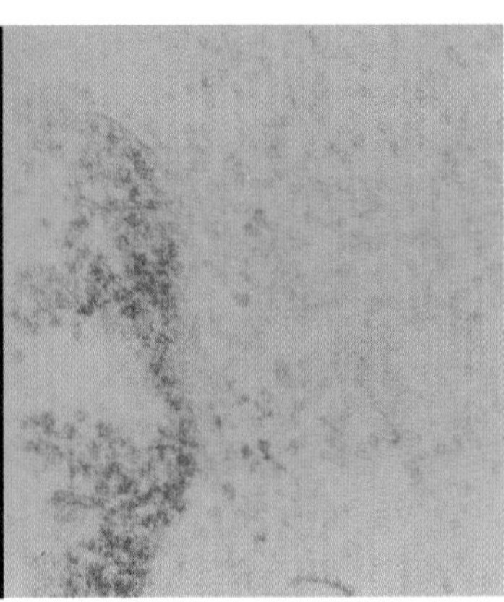

The mumps virus causes a painful swelling of the salivary glands, in particular, the parotid gland.

teration in a person's immunity to a slow virus.

Q: *How does the body react to viral infections?*

A: At the onset of a viral infection, the body has little resistance to the virus, apart from the presence of lymphocytes, which are a type of white blood cell that produces antibodies, and a small amount of interferon, which is a substance that helps destroy viruses. Within a few days of infection, the body's immune system is stimulated by the viruses to produce antibodies and greater amounts of interferon. *See also* ANTIBODY; INTERFERON.

Q: *Is it possible to prevent viral infections?*

A: Yes. Vaccines have been produced against some of the common viral infections. Vaccines to combat mumps, measles, rubella, and poliomyelitis are usually given routinely in early childhood. It is also possible to vaccinate against influenza, rabies, smallpox, typhus, and yellow fever.

Antibiotics are ineffective against most viral infections, but new drugs are available to help combat smallpox and shingles.

Q: *Can viruses cause tumors?*

A: Yes. Viruses may cause benign (noncancerous) growths, such as warts and the tumors that occur with the skin disease molluscum contagiosum.

See also IMMUNITY; IMMUNIZATION.

Virus, human immunodeficiency (i myü nō di fish'ən sē). Human immunodeficiency virus (HIV) is the virus that causes acquired immune deficiency syndrome (AIDS) and AIDS-related complex (ARC).

HIV is a virus that has no DNA, only RNA. DNA and RNA are proteins that carry genetic information. A body cell proceeds from DNA through RNA to duplication of itself. Because it has no DNA, the virus must reverse the normal sequence of duplication. RNA from the virus uses the host cell's DNA to produce its own viral DNA. Then the normal duplication process begins.

Once inside a host body, HIV homes in directly on a T cell, a major component of the immune system. The virus takes over the reproductive machinery and reproduces itself. The cell weakens and eventually dies, releasing the newly-made viruses into the bloodstream. Other white blood cells are invaded and die. The body is left vulnerable to diseases, to which it succumbs usually within two to three years. However, there are some patients who are still alive seven years after the original diagnosis of AIDS.

Q: *Given the long incubation period for AIDS, why doesn't the body have enough time to produce antibodies to ward off the disease?*

A: HIV mutates at such a fast rate that by the time an antibody is produced, the virus has changed its appearance and the antibody is unable to recognize its target. The virus also escapes detection by hiding inside a host cell's DNA or by moving directly from cell to cell, by-passing the bloodstream. In the latter case, even if there is a specific antibody against the virus, the two will never come in contact, since antibodies circulate in the blood.

See also ACQUIRED IMMUNE DEFICIENCY SYNDROME; BLOOD CELL, WHITE; DEOXYRIBONUCLEIC ACID; IMMUNITY; RIBONUCLEIC ACID; VIRUS.

Virus, respiratory syncytial (res'pər ə tôr ē sin sish'əl). Respiratory syncytial virus (RSV) is a virus that is usually spread by respiratory secretions from an infected person. RSV commonly causes bronchopneumonia, acute bronchiolitis, colds in children, and mild upper respiratory infections in adults. Symptoms of RSV include cough, extreme malaise, and fever. Treatment consists of acetaminophen, nasal decongestants, and rest.

See also VIRUS.

Virus, slow. A slow virus is a virus that may remain dormant in the body of an infected individual for most of his or her life. It is believed to be a cause of many chronic diseases. Recent evidence has indicated that some neurological disorders, such as multiple sclerosis and polyneuritis, may be caused by slow viruses.

See also VIRUS.

Viscera (vis'ər ə) is a general term for the internal organs in the abdominal and chest cavities. The viscera include the heart, lungs, liver, spleen, kidneys, gastrointestinal tract, and bladder.

Viscera is a collective term for the internal organs of the chest and abdomen.

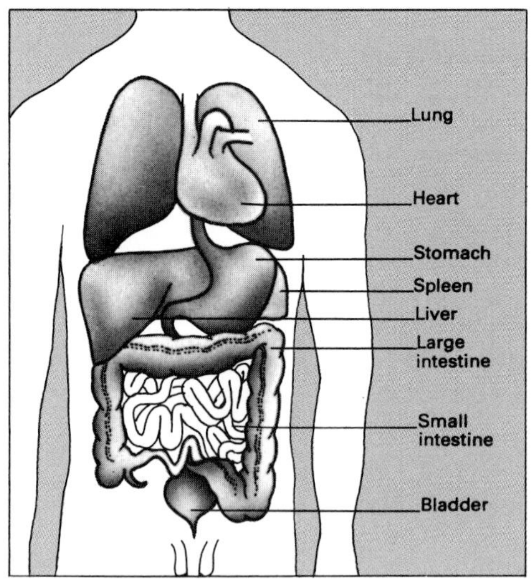

Vision. *See* EYE.

Vision, blurred. Blurred vision is a common eye disorder. Frequently, it is caused by farsightedness, nearsightedness, or astigmatism, all of which can be corrected by eyeglasses or contact lenses. In the elderly, the gradual onset of blurred vision can be caused by a cloudiness in the eye lens (cataract) or degeneration of the retina at the back of the eye. *See also* ASTIGMATISM; CATARACT.

Q: *What causes sudden blurred vision?*

A: There are several possibilities, all of which should be considered by an ophthalmologist. Conjunctivitis is one of the most common. There are other more serious possible causes, including glaucoma, in which there is abnormally high fluid pressure inside the eyeball. Some drugs, including alcohol, may also cause the occurrence of blurred vision.

Any case of persistent blurred vision should be discussed with an ophthalmologist.

Vision, double. Double vision, known medically as diplopia, is the perception of two images of a single object. Diplopia is a symptom rather than a disorder. The most common cause of double vision is a sudden imbalance in the power of the eye muscles. It may also result from astigmatism or several disorders that affect nerves and muscles.

See also ASTIGMATISM; STRABISMUS.

Vitamin (vī'tə min) is a chemical substance essential for the normal working of the human body. Vitamins are effective in extremely small amounts and act mainly as regulators of the body's metabolic processes. Most vitamins must be obtained from food, but some, such as biotin and vitamin K, can be synthesized in the body by intestinal bacteria. Vitamin D can be synthesized directly by the body from the action of sunlight on the skin.

Vitamins are classified as either fat-soluble or water-soluble. The fat-soluble vitamins are vitamin A (retinol), vitamin D (calciferol), vitamin E (tocopherol), and vitamin K (menadione). The water-soluble vitamins are vitamin C (ascorbic acid) and the vitamin B group: vitamin B_1 (thiamine), vitamin B_2 (riboflavin), vitamin B_6 (pyridoxine), vitamin B_{12} (cobalamin), biotin, folic acid, and pantothenic acid.

Q: *Is a daily intake of vitamins essential?*

A: No. A helpful method of determining adequate vitamin intake is to record intake over a period of five to eight days. If the average daily intake of each vitamin is close to the recommended dietary allowance for age, sex, and physical activity, then vitamin intake is considered adequate. Growing children need proportionately more vitamins than inactive adults. Vitamin requirements are also increased during illness, pregnancy, and breast-feeding. *See also* APPENDIX IV.

The body can store some vitamins when consumed in excess, but storage varies greatly depending on the vitamin. In general, fat-soluble vitamins can be stored, whereas water-soluble vitamins can not.

Q: *What are the effects of excessive vitamins in the diet?*

A: Vitamins A and D may produce adverse effects if excessive amounts are taken continually for a long period. An overdose of vitamin A may cause hair loss, peeling of the skin, joint pains, and liver damage. Excessive vitamin D may cause kidney damage and the formation of calcium deposits in the body tissues.

Q: *What are the effects of insufficient vitamins in the diet?*

A: Prolonged vitamin dificiency leads to depletion of the vitamin stores in the body, This, in turn, results in various deficiency diseases.

Q: *Are vitamin supplements necessary?*

A: Additional vitamins are unnecessary if a person is healthy and eats a balanced diet. Certain vitamins, particularly the fat-soluble ones, may be harmful if taken in excessive amounts.

Additional vitamins may be needed during an illness or following a surgical operation. Those with disorders in which there is insufficient absorption of vitamins in the intestine may require vitamin supplements until the underlying disorder has been cured. Other disorders that increase the metabolic activity of the body's cells, such as an overactive thyroid gland, may increase the body's vitamin needs. A physician will recommend vitamin supplements if they are necessary.

Q: *Are vitamins affected by cooking and storing?*

A: Yes. Some vitamins are unstable substances and can easily be destroyed by incorrect storing or cooking of food.

The fat-soluble vitamins can withstand normal cooking, but vitamins A and E are gradually destroyed by exposure to the air.

The amount of water-soluble vitamins is greatly reduced by boiling food because the vitamins dissolve in the water. Vitamin B_1, vitamin B_6, folic acid, and pantothenic acid are destroyed by heat; vitamin B_2 is destroyed by light; and vitamin C is destroyed by heat, light, and air. For these reasons, food should be used when fresh and should not be overcooked.

Certain food preservatives also destroy the vitamins in food. This may affect the vitamin content of canned foods.

Vitamins: sources and function

Name	*Source*	*Function*	*Effect of deficiency*	*Additional information*
Vitamin A (retinol)	Fish-liver oils, eggs, butter, milk, cheese, liver, apricots, broccoli, cabbage, carrots	Essential for night vision, healthy skin, and mucous membranes	Night blindness, dry eyes (xerophthalmia), dry skin	Excessive intake may cause hair loss, peeling of the skin, joint pains, and liver damage.
Vitamin B_1 (thiamine)	Yeast, whole grains, pork, liver, nuts, legumes, potatoes	Essential for normal functioning of nerve cells, heart muscle, and carbohydrate metabolism	Beriberi	Increased amount is needed during growth, pregnancy, and breast-feeding.
Vitamin B_2 (riboflavin)	Yeast, eggs, milk, cheese, liver, kidney, green vegetables	Essential for normal protein and carbohydrate metabolism and for maintaining mucous membranes	Cracked lips (cheilosis), skin rashes, dim vision	Increased amount is needed during growth, pregnancy and breast-feeding.
Vitamin B_6 (pyridoxine)	Yeast, whole grains, fish, liver, legumes	Essential for general functioning of body cells and amino acid metabolism	Convulsions in infants, anemia, nerve disorders	Increased amount is needed during growth, pregnancy, and breast-feeding and when taking the contraceptive pill.

Name	*Source*	*Function*	*Effect of deficiency*	*Additional information*
Vitamin B_{12} (cobalamin)	Eggs, milk, cheese, butter, liver, beef, pork	Essential for growth of red blood cells and normal functioning of nerve cells	Pernicious anemia, dim vision, peripheral neuritis	Deficiency is especially likely in total vegetarians (vegans), in persons with sprue, or following a total gastrectomy.
Biotin	Present in all common foods	Essential for energy production from fats and carbohydrates and for formation of hormones	Deficiency does not occur naturally	Biotin can be produced by bacteria in the intestine.
Folic acid	Yeast, liver, kidney, leafy green vegetables, fruit	Essential for growth of red blood cells	Anemia and peripheral neuritis	Increased amount is needed during growth, pregnancy, and breast-feeding. Deficiency is particularly likely in persons with sprue.
Pantothenic acid	Whole grains, eggs, liver, kidney, peanuts, cabbage	Essential for normal functioning of enzymes inside the body cells	Deficiency does not occur naturally	Pantothenic acid can be produced by bacteria in the intestine.
Vitamin C (ascorbic acid)	Citrus fruits, tomatoes, potatoes, green vegetables	Essential for normal tissue growth and repair and normal functioning of blood vessels	Scurvy	Vitamin C is easily destroyed by cooking.
Vitamin D (calciferol)	Fish-liver oils, eggs, butter, liver, yeast	Essential for normal absorption of calcium and phosphorus and for normal bone formation	Rickets in children, osteomalacia in adults	Vitamin D is also formed by the action of sunlight on the skin. Increased amount is needed during growth, pregnancy, and breast-feeding. Excessive intake may cause kidney damage and calcium deposits in the body tissue.
Vitamin E (tocopherol)	Eggs, vegetable oils, wheat germ, green vegetables	Essential for stability of cell membranes	Decreased resistance to rupture of red blood cells	Vitamin E may also play a part in fertility.

Name	Source	Function	Effect of deficiency	Additional information
Vitamin K (menadione)	Vegetable oils, pork, liver, leafy vegetables	Essential for normal blood clotting	Bleeding, particularly in premature babies	Vitamin K can be produced by intestinal bacteria. Deficiency is rare in adults.
Niacin (nicotinic acid)	Liver, yeast, lean meats, whole-grain and enriched breads and cereals	Essential for cell metabolism and absorption of carbohydrates, helps maintain healthy skin	Pellagra	The body does not store niacin; any excess is excreted.

Vitiligo (vit ə lī′gō) is a relatively common skin disorder that affects about 1 percent of the population. It involves the loss of normal skin pigment in irregular patches because melanin (the chemical that produces pigment) fails to be produced. About 10 percent of those affected recover spontaneously.

The condition may start at any age, but it commonly appears before the age of 20. It is generally thought to be an inherited condition.

Vitiligo is more common in patients with some form of autoimmune disorder, such as pernicious anemia, diabetes mellitus, and alopecia areata. *See also* AUTOIMMUNE DISEASE.

Q: *How is vitiligo treated?*

A: There are few drugs available to aid patients with vitiligo. Treatment with methoxsalen, a pigmentation agent, followed by exposure of the skin to sunlight, has been found to help recoloring of the skin. Persons with small patches of vitiligo can use special makeup to camouflage the area.

Vitreous humor (vit′rē əs) is the jellylike substance that fills the part of the eye behind the lens.

See also EYE; HUMOR.

Vocal cord (vō′kəl) is either of the two membranes in the throat used to make sounds.

See also LARYNX.

Vocal cord nodule (noj′ül), also called corditis, is the inflamed growth that develops on the vocal chords of individuals who repeatedly overuse their voices.

Voice box is the common name for the larynx.

See also LARYNX.

Volvulus (vol′vyə ləs) is a twisting of the intestine around itself. This condition not only creates an intestinal obstruction but also blocks the blood vessels that serve the intestine. A volvulus most commonly occurs in the small intestine, the cecum, or the sigmoid colon.

Q: *Why does a volvulus occur?*

A: A volvulus may be the result of an anomaly present at birth. One loop of bowel is larger than usual, and there is a longer membranous fold (mesentery). Another cause may be the looping of part of the intestine around an adhesion, a scar left by inflammation or surgery.

Q: *What are the symptoms of a volvulus?*

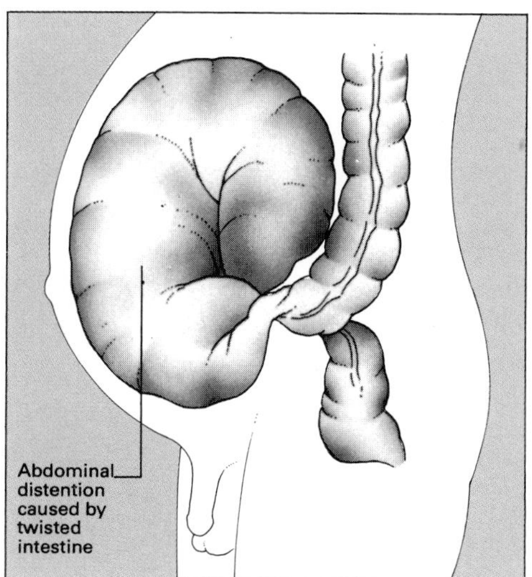

Volvulus occurs when the intestine twists over itself, causing abdominal distention.

A: The symptoms are similar to the symptoms of intestinal obstruction, abdominal pain and vomiting. A volvulus of the large intestine produces vomiting and involves complete constipation and abdominal pain, with swelling of the abdomen.

Q: *How is a volvulus treated?*

A: In most cases, an abdominal operation is needed to untwist the volvulus and, if the intestine has become gangrenous, to remove the damaged part of the intestine. It is often necessary to have a temporary colostomy while the intestine returns to normal.

See also COLOSTOMY; INTESTINAL OBSTRUCTION; INTESTINE.

Vomiting (vom′it ing), known medically as emesis, is the forceful throwing up of some or all of the stomach contents by reversal of peristalsis, the normal muscular contractions of the stomach.

Vomiting may be a symptom of various disorders, some local to the stomach and some more generalized. It is usually preceded by a loss of appetite and nausea.

Q: *What are the local causes of vomiting?*

A: The most common cause of vomiting is acute or chronic gastritis (inflammation of the stomach). Vomiting sometimes occurs with a peptic ulcer, particularly if there is pyloric stenosis (narrowing of the stomach exit). Vomiting is also a symptom of any form of intestinal obstruction. *See also* GASTRITIS; INTESTINAL OBSTRUCTION; PYLORIC STENOSIS; ULCER, PEPTIC.

Babies may vomit for a variety of reasons. Some babies vomit more easily than others, but provided there is a general weight gain and the baby is obviously well, vomiting is not a serious symptom.

Q: *What generalized disorders may cause vomiting?*

A: The onset of high fever and any condition that affects the sense of balance, such as a viral infection of the inner ear (labyrinthitis), result in vomiting.

Vomiting is a common symptom if the vomiting center in the thalamus of the brain is disturbed by a migraine or by increased brain pressure associated with a brain tumor. Disturbance takes place also with meningitis and encephalitis. Hormone changes in pregnancy alter the sensitivity of the vomiting center; this fact accounts for morning sickness and also the excessive

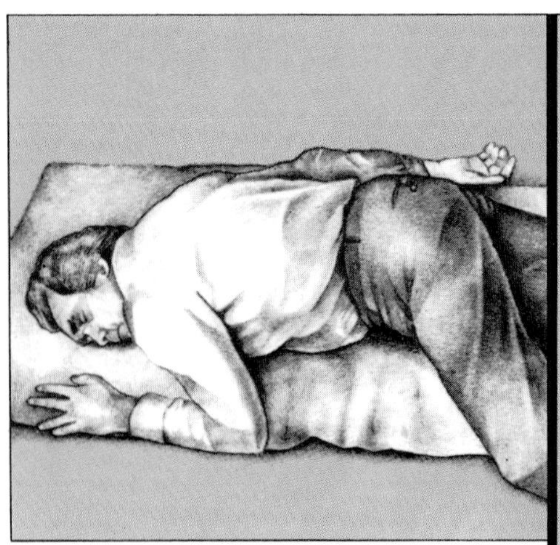

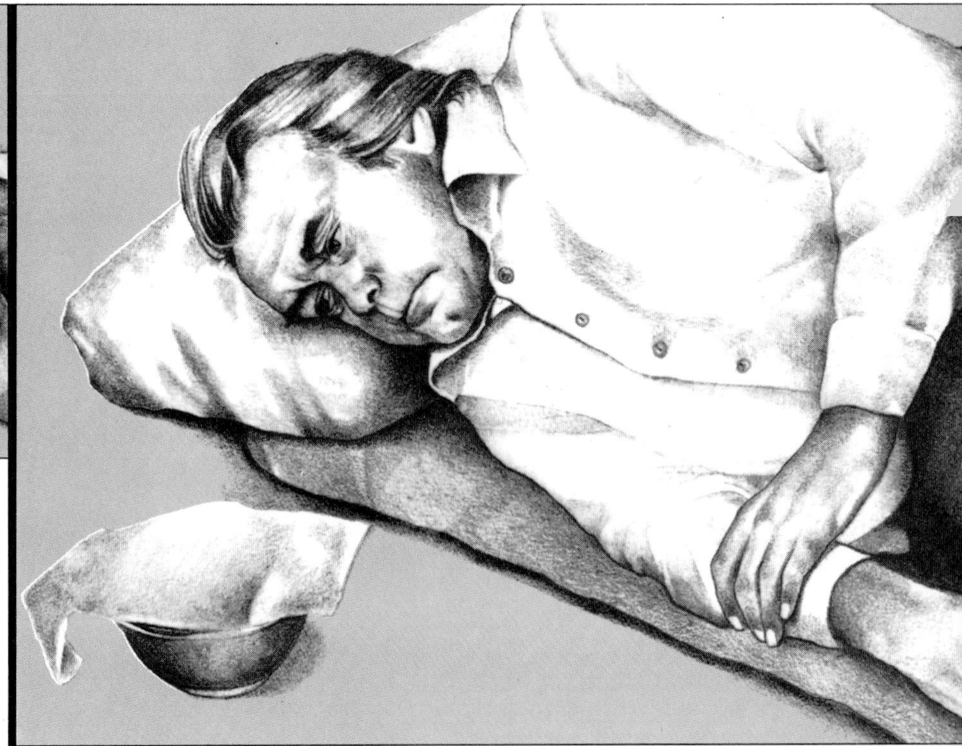

An unconscious person, *above,* should be placed in the recovery position, to prevent the inhalation of vomit (*see* FAINTING: FIRST AID). If the person has inhaled vomit and is choking, clear the airway (*see* CHOKING AND COUGHING: FIRST AID). A conscious person, *right,* should lie down on his or her side, with a basin on the same side.

vomiting that may occur with hyperemesis gravidarum. *See also* ENCEPHALITIS; HYPEREMESIS; MENINGITIS; MIGRAINE; MORNING SICKNESS; TUMOR.

Vomiting can occur for psychological reasons, such as an emotional shock or a nauseating sight or smell.

Vomiting also occurs in serious metabolic disorders, such as kidney failure and the onset of diabetic coma.

Q: *Is vomiting always a serious symptom?*

A: No. Occasional vomiting at the start of a general illness is part of that disorder. But prolonged and continual vomiting is a serious symptom because it leads to dehydration; it is also an indication of what is usually a severe underlying disorder.

Q: *How should vomiting be treated?*

A: Give the patient small sips of clear liquids, such as broth, water, or diluted fruit juices. If these sips are tolerated without vomiting, slowly increase the volume of these fluids.

Encourage the patient to lie down and relax. Once fluids are kept down consistently, foods may be slowly added.

If vomiting ceases with these simple measures and if there are no other symptoms, it may not be necessary to call a physician. If vomiting continues, however, medical care should be sought as soon as possible.

Continued vomiting is always a more serious problem in small babies than in adults because dehydration occurs more quickly in infants, especially if there is also diarrhea.

See also VOMITING: TREATMENT.

Vomiting: treatment. Vomiting is the forceful ejection of the stomach contents through the mouth. The diaphragm presses downward; the abdominal wall is drawn inward; the wave of stomach contractions moves in reverse; the sphincter leading from the stomach into the small intestine closes; the victim takes a deep breath; and the stomach muscles contract to expel the contents back up the esophagus.

Vomiting may be caused by overeating, excessive drinking of alcohol, swallowing an irritating substance, travel sickness, allergic reactions, shock, pregnancy, head injury, peptic ulcer, inflammation of certain organs, and migraine.

Action. A conscious victim should lie down in a quiet room with a basin at the bedside. *Do not* attempt to suppress vomiting. *Do not* give the victim any food. *Do not* give the victim any medicines.

Von Recklinghausen's disease (von rek'ling how zenz), named after the German pathologist Friedrich Daniel von Recklinghausen, is an inherited condition in which multiple freckle-like spots, sometimes called *café au lait* spots, appear on the skin. Nodules (fibromas) also occur and can be felt through the skin; nodules may appear on internal organs as well. The disease is also known as neurofibromatosis. The play and film *The Elephant Man* were based on the life of a man with von Recklinghausen's disease.

Q: *What are the symptoms of von Recklinghausen's disease?*

A: The nodules may be noticeable at birth or may gradually develop later. Often, the skin spots are present at birth. As the child grows, curvature of the spine (scoliosis) may develop and, occasionally, become severe.

The nodules may occur anywhere in the body and cause pressure on adjacent tissues. Therefore, a variety of symptoms may occur. Any symptoms that do develop

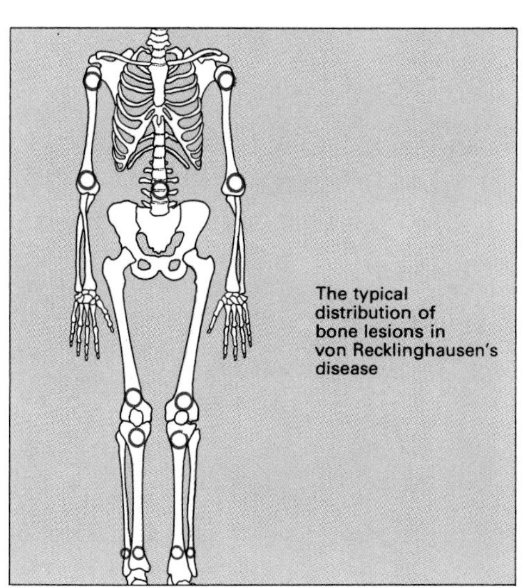
The typical distribution of bone lesions in von Recklinghausen's disease

Von Recklinghausen's disease may be associated with destructive lesions of the bones.

need careful assessment by a physician familiar with this disease.

Q: *How is von Recklinghausen's disease treated?*

A: Treatment is necessary only if the symptoms are severe. Scoliosis may need orthopedic treatment, and nodules may require surgical removal.

Vulva (vul'və) is the female external genital organ that surrounds the outside opening of the vagina and clitoris. At the front of the vulva is a soft padded area covered with hair (mons pubis); sweeping back from this area are the two large folds of the labia majora enclosing the two smaller folds of the labia minora. These folds contain lubricating glands, the largest of which (Bartholin's glands) lies at the back.

The vulva extends into the firm, fibrous tissue of the perineum, which is in front of the anus. Between the labia minora lies the fold of skin called the hymen, which partially closes the entrance to the vagina until it is broken by sexual intercourse or some other means of rupture.

Inflammation of the vulva (vulvitis) is fairly common. Other disorders are rare.

See also VULVITIS.

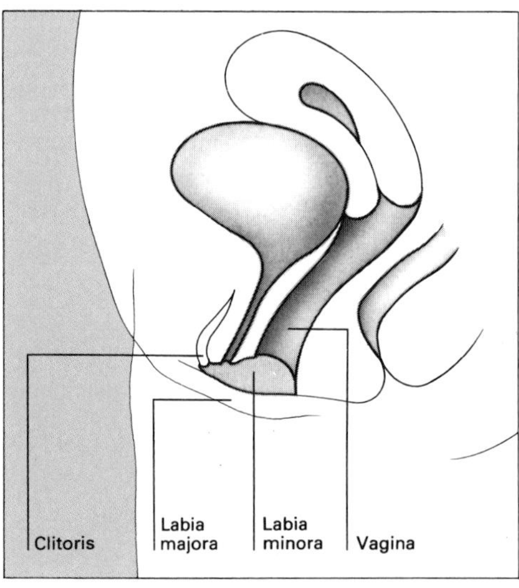

The **vulva,** the female external genital organ, includes the clitoris and the labia.

Vulvitis (vul vī'tis) is inflammation of the vulva. Its symptoms are soreness and itching.

Q: *What causes vulvitis?*

A: Any of the causes of inflammation of the vagina (vaginitis) may produce vulval itching. These commonly result from candidiasis or trichomonas vaginalis infections, but vulvitis may also occur with diabetes mellitus or general skin diseases, such as psoriasis and scabies.

In about one-third of cases of vulval irritation, there is no obvious cause, and psychological factors may be suspected. Continued scratching produces inflammation that may become infected and cause vulvitis.

Q: *What other vulval infections may occur?*

A: Other vulval infections include venereal diseases, such as syphilis, granuloma inguinale, chancroid, lymphogranuloma venereum, and a viral infection producing warts that may develop on any part of the vulva. Infection with a herpes virus may develop into painful, shallow ulcers.

Q: *How is vulvitis treated?*

A: The patient must be examined to discover the cause of the irritation. Cultures may be taken with a cotton swab to identify an infection; the appropriate treatment can then be given. Until a firm diagnosis is made and treatment is prescribed, sitz baths in warm water may be soothing to the patient.

See also BARTHOLIN'S CYST; CANDIDIASIS; LEUKOPLAKIA; SEXUALLY TRANSMITTED DISEASE; TRICHOMONAS VAGINALIS; VAGINITIS; WART, VENEREAL.

Vulvovaginitis (vul vō vaj ə nī'tis) is an inflammation of both the vulva (vulvitis) and the vagina (vaginitis). It commonly is caused by candidiasis or trichomoniasis.

See also VAGINITIS; VULVITIS.

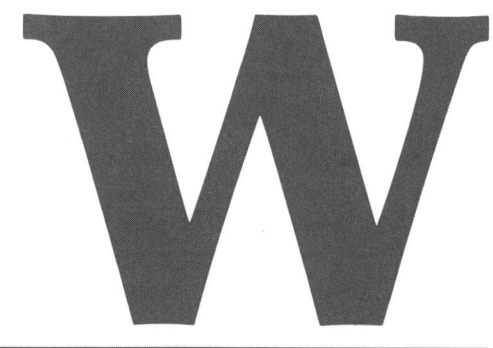

Walker. *See* WALKING AID.

Walking aid can be a cane, a walking frame, or a crutch. It is important that walking aids are the right height for the person who is using them. The use of any at the wrong height can lead to neck or shoulder tension. Long crutches should not be so high that they push upward under the patient's armpits. Most of the body's weight should be supported by the hand grips attached to each crutch, with the weight carried by the arms and hands.

A useful aid for moving material from room to room is a chair trolley. This can be made by attaching small wheels to the legs of a kitchen chair. The upright back can then be used as a support while the patient walks and pushes the chair along. The seat can be used as a tray or trolley on which to carry things. Nonslip material can be attached to the seat to provide a more secure surface.

Rails and handles fixed at strategic places around the home can be an enormous help for those who have difficulty in walking and moving independently. Where possible, a handrail should be placed on both sides of the stairs. Grab rails should be secured wherever a person has to get up or sit down, for example, next to the toilet, beside the bathtub, by an armchair in the living room, and next to the bed.

Make sure that the home has no potential hazards for the patient. Loose furniture fittings can be extremely dangerous; they should be securely attached. Check also that carpets are well tacked down. Keep a screen before an open fire, and do not position seats close to radiators. A flashlight kept at the patient's bedside may be useful at night or during a power failure.

See also WHEELCHAIR.

Walking pneumonia. *See* PNEUMONIA.

Wart (wôrt), or verruca, is a hard, rough growth on the surface of the skin. Warts vary in size and shape and may appear anywhere on the body.

Q: *What causes warts?*

A: Warts result from infection by certain viruses. The viruses live in cells on the surface layer of the skin and do not infect the underlying tissue. The thickened surface layer forms folds into which little blood vessels grow. If a wart is scratched open, the virus may spread by contact to another part of the body or to another person.
See also VIRUS.

Q: *Are there different kinds of warts?*

A: Yes. The common wart (verruca vulgaris) is a small, raised, rough lump on the skin made up of small columns of tissue arising from the base. Common warts vary in color from normal flesh tint to dark brown-black. They usually occur on the hands, elbows, knees, and less frequently on the face or eyelids. They may also appear around the edges of the nails.

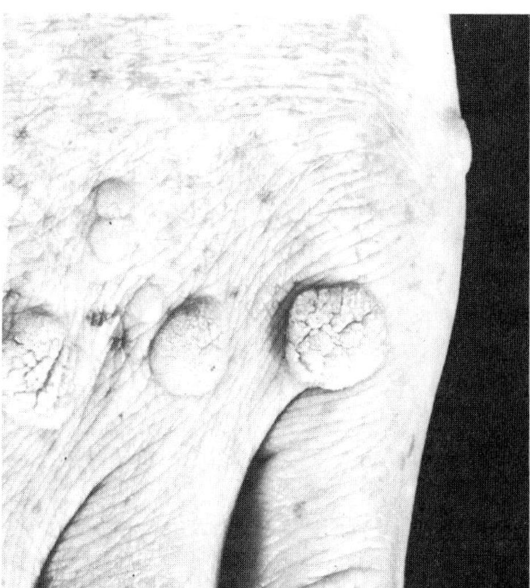

A **wart** usually begins as a small growth, but later develops into a rough, brownish lump.

Plantar warts (verrucae plantares) are the same as the common wart but are flattened by pressure because they appear on pressure-bearing areas, especially the side of the foot. They may be painful because the nodule presses into the flesh.

Venereal or genital warts (condylomata acuminata) are a typical wart infection, usually transmitted by sexual contact.

Q: *How are warts treated?*

A: Warts usually disappear spontaneously, perhaps because immunity to the virus develops. Treatment with extremely cold substances such as solid carbon dioxide (dry ice) or liquid nitrogen (cryotherapy) destroys the wart and the surrounding tissue, leaving a small blister. The various nonprescription chemical solutions that can also destroy warts should be used with care. It is advisable to remove any wart medication after one or two days and then rub away the dead tissue before reapplying the medication.

More radical methods of removing warts, such as cautery, surgery, or X rays, frequently leave a small scar and may themselves produce a small, tender nodule.

Genital warts require special treatment due to their location and possible association with other venereal diseases. *See also* WART, VENEREAL.

Wart, plantar (wôrt, plan′tər). A plantar wart is a very painful wart on the sole of the foot.

See also WART.

Wart, venereal (wôrt, və nir′ē əl). A venereal wart is a rough skin growth that flourishes in the warm and moist anal and genital regions. It is caused by a virus and may be spread via sexual contact. Although venereal warts are generally harmless, they may be a symptom of syphilis or another disease; a person with venereal warts should consult a physician.

In addition, there is medical evidence that venereal warts may increase a woman's risk of developing cancer of the uterus. For this reason, a woman with venereal warts should have a Pap smear test every 6 to 12 months.

See also PAP SMEAR TEST; SEXUALLY TRANSMITTED DISEASE; WART.

Wasp sting. *See* BITES AND STINGS: FIRST AID.

Wassermann test (wä′sər mən) is a blood test once widely used to diagnose syphilis.

See also SYPHILIS.

Wasting (wās′ting) is a gradual weakening process characterized by loss of strength and vitality, weight loss, and deterioration of body tissue. This condition may be caused by a lack of food.

See also ANOREXIA NERVOSA; ATROPHY; STARVATION.

Watering eyes. *See* EYE, WATERING.

Water on the knee. *See* KNEE, WATER ON.

Waterskiing safety. *See* WATER SPORTS SAFETY.

Water sports safety. Drowning is the third leading cause of accidental death in the United States. Only traffic mishaps and falls cause more accidental fatalities. In the U.S. about 7,000 people drown annually, many while swimming or boating. The following instructions should serve as a safety checklist for anyone, however experienced, involved with water sports.

Swimming. Learning to swim and observing basic safety rules are vital components of safe swimming. Every member of the family should learn to swim at an early age. Competent swimming instructors are available almost everywhere. The elderly or those who are sick or out of condition should consult a physician before beginning a swimming program.

There are certain times when, however good a swimmer you are, you should not go into the water. Never swim alone. Always swim with a companion and know where that person is at all times. Swim only in areas protected by lifeguards. If such an area is not available, be sure that the water bottom has no snags, trash, or weeds. Never swim immediately after eating a large meal because it might cause muscle cramps. Never swim after drinking alcohol because it dulls the senses, especially the awareness of cold. Never swim when feeling tired or cold.

Before going into the water, pay careful attention to warning signs. If you swim in the ocean or a river, you should know about tides and currents.

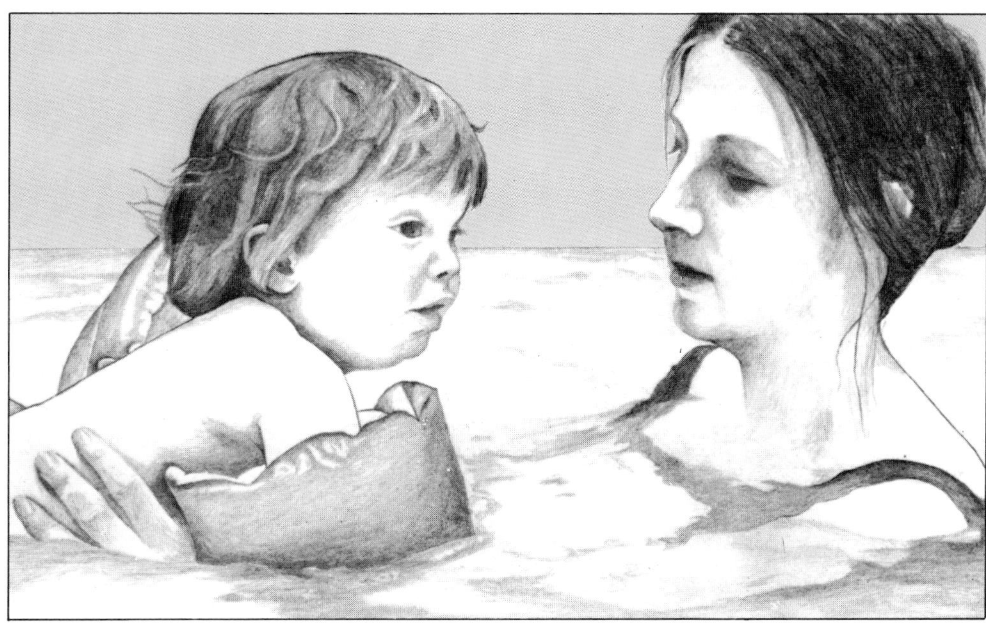

A small child should wear armband floats and always swim with an adult. Do not force a child to swim unaided, and always continue to supervise swims.

Water for diving should be deep and clear. Never dive into unfamiliar water, and always look carefully for other swimmers before you dive. When swimming, stay away from diving boards and diving platforms.

The sun can seem deceptively cool when you are in the water, and it is possible not to realize until later that you have been badly burned across the shoulders and back.

Never sunbathe on an inflatable raft or air mattress in a large lake or in the ocean. You could drift a long way from the shore and be unable to swim back.

Children should always be closely supervised around water. A child can drown in the time it takes to answer the telephone. When a child is on a boat or near water, a coastguard approved flotation vest should be worn at all times. Children should also take swimming lessons so that they are able to swim properly and safely.

Only a trained lifeguard should attempt a swimming rescue. Even a competent swimmer can be pulled under by a drowning person. However, if a person gets into trouble near the shore in an unsupervised swimming area, wade out and help him or her. Reach for the victim or try to extend a pole, tree branch, fishing rod, or oar. If the victim is beyond reach, throw something that floats, such as a spare tire or a cooler. If these attempts fail, then wade, swim, or row to the victim.

Underwater Diving. Before considering skin diving as a sport, you must be healthy. Persons with disorders such as epilepsy, diabetes, claustrophobia, and respiratory and cardiac disorders must never skin-dive. It is sensible to have regular medical checkups if you intend to take up the sport seriously.

Skin diving is not a sport you can learn casually. You should only take lessons from a qualified instructor. You must have lessons before you buy the equipment or attempt to go underwater. The best training can be obtained at a reputable diving club or school.

Always dive with a companion. Even the most experienced divers can get into trouble underwater.

Plan your trip carefully before you set out. Diving tables are available that tell you how much time you can spend at specific depths and how much time you need to resurface. You must wear an accurate timer and depth gauge.

Check the weather forecast for the area in which you are diving before going out. Always tell a responsible person where you are going to dive and how long you expect to be away. Report back to that person when you return.

Do not dive near buoys or fishing spots. Avoid fishing nets, buoys, and rocks that are covered with kelp.

Always fly a diving flag when diving, and always use a surface marker buoy as well.

Boating Safety

Each person riding aboard a smaller, open boat should wear a Coast Guard-approved flotation device. A larger boat must carry at least one wearable personal flotation device (PFD) for each person aboard and, in addition, a throwable PFD. A throwable PFD can be either a life preserver (a doughnut-shaped ring buoy) or a buoyant cushion (floating pillow). All life preservers must be ready for use and easily accessible. A small-boat user may find himself or herself in and out of the water frequently, for example, swimming or diving. In such cases, wearing a PFD is impractical. However, a child is more likely to become exhausted by swimming and must wear a flotation jacket. It should be easy to use and convenient to wear. A boat must also by law carry a fire extinguisher of the approved type. Navigation lights are also required. Closed boats must have adequate ventilation. A noise-making device, such as a horn or whistle, must be carried by motorboats over 16 feet (4.8m). Boat users should always carry plenty of spare, warm clothing for everyone aboard. Keep the clothing in waterproof bags tied firmly into the boat. In an emergency, loose equipment is dangerous. Boat users should wear sneaker-type shoes that are designed to give a good grip on wet surfaces. Never wear rain boots. Good sunglasses should be worn to prevent eye strain on sunny days.

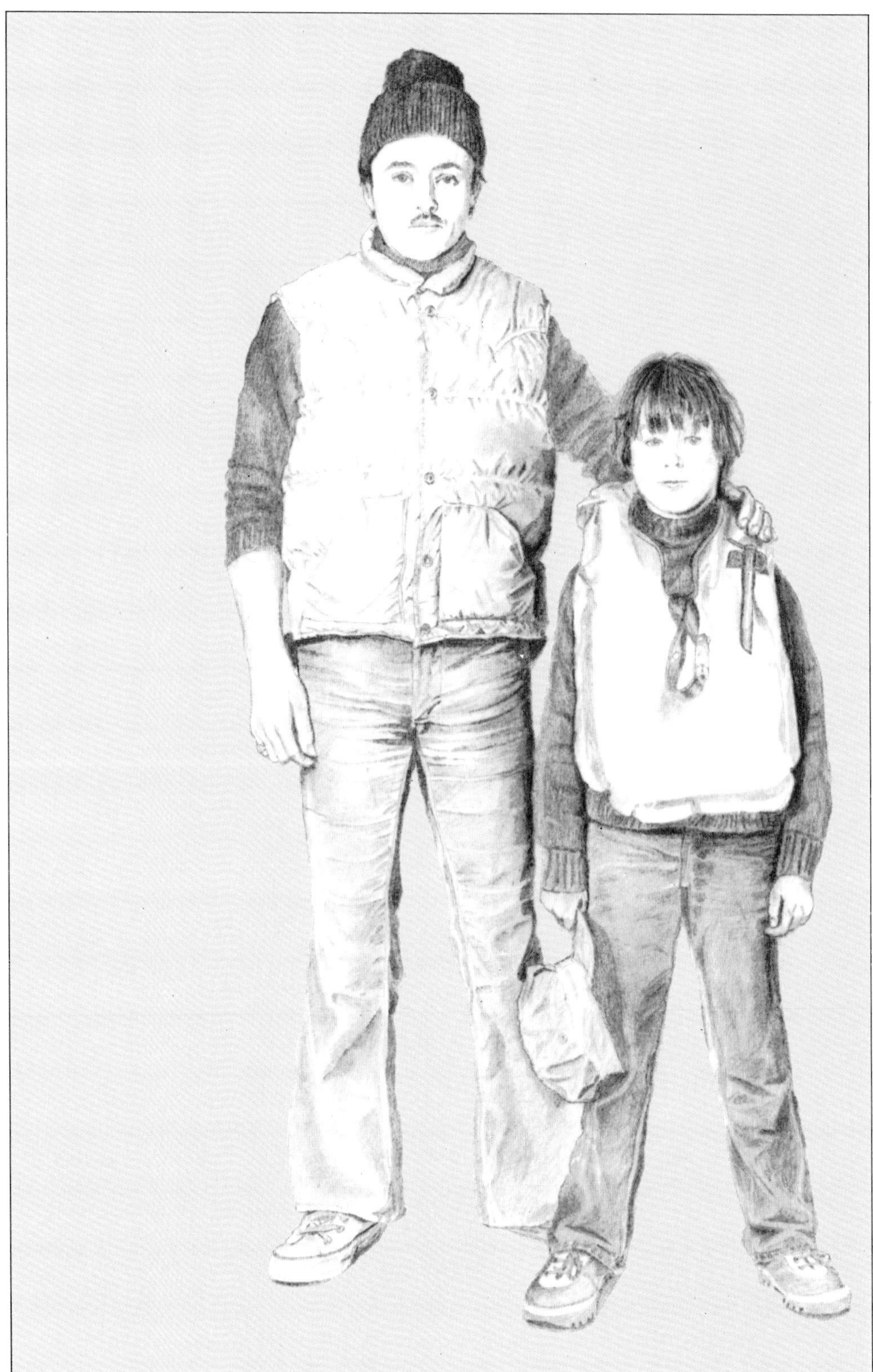

As you go down, your ears begin to hurt. This is because the pressure outside the eardrums increases with the depth. The moment you feel the pressure, you must pinch your nose and gently blow. This opens your Eustachian tubes and equalizes the pressure on each side of the eardrums. If you do not equalize the pressure, your eardrums will burst at about 30 feet. For this reason, never dive after a heavy cold or flu, as it may not be possible to clear the Eustachian tubes.

Compressed tanks contain the constituents of air, that is, 80 percent nitrogen and 20 percent oxygen. Breathing pressurized nitrogen sometimes produces a feeling of intoxication known as nitrogen narcosis. This becomes a problem when diving at depths of 75 feet (22.5m) or deeper. A diver's companion must be alert for the signs. A diver may suddenly start behaving strangely, attempt to remove the face mask, or make indistinct and fumbling communication signs. The other diver must get the person to the surface as quickly as possible without producing decompression sickness (the "bends"). Once the person has surfaced, the narcosis wears off, leaving no aftereffects. *See also* BENDS.

Decompression sickness depends on the amount of time a diver is at a certain depth as well as the depth itself. The diver experiences acute muscle cramps and breathing difficulties. He or she must be treated immediately. The only safe way of doing this is to get the diver to the nearest decompression chamber.

If you miscalculate the amount of air that you have left in your tank and consequently run out, it is extremely dangerous to hold your breath and rise to the surface. As you rise, the air in the lungs expands as it decompresses, and the lung may rupture. You must blow air out as you rise. Skilled divers sometimes share the air from one tank with their companion as they surface.

Surfing. Surfing is a physically demanding sport. The ease with which the experts do it is often misleading. You must be in good physical condition and a competent swimmer.

Before setting out to surf, wax the top of the board thoroughly to give a nonslip surface for the feet.

Check the area in which you propose to surf for any restrictions that may be in force. Surf only in areas designated for surfing.

A surfboard can be dangerous out of water. Carry it with care while on the beach. Hold it under the arm with the fin inwards. Keep clear of other people and turn carefully to prevent catching someone behind you with the board.

It is essential to be able to avoid swimmers and other surfers. Therefore, turns must be perfected at an early stage. If you realize that you and another surfer are on a collision course as you are paddling out, stay still and let the other person take evasive action.

Before taking a wave, be sure that you are well clear of other surfers. The first surfer on a wave has the right of way.

Keep well clear of all swimmers, even if they are in a surfing area. Do not keep your eyes fixed on the board or your feet. You must be on the lookout for potential hazards.

In a wipe-out, try to stay with your board. Never try to intercept a loose board, whether yours or someone else's.

Wear adequate clothing. A surfer can get cold waiting in the water for the right wave. Also, the windchill factor should be taken into account. Wear rubberized Bermuda-style shorts and a rubberized vest, or a complete wet suit.

Waterskiing. Waterskiing safety depends as much on the skiboat driver as on the skier. Often, the skier's safety depends on the driver's skill and ability to understand the skier's needs. For this reason, two people should be in the boat, one to navigate safely and one to pass on the skier's hand signals.

Operate clear of swimmers and other water users. Keep well away from rocks and buoys. If there are specially designated areas for waterskiers, use them.

Mark the take-off and landing points clearly in the water to warn swimmers.

Give the skier a steady take off. Wait for his or her signal and have the observer check that the ski tips are above the water before starting off.

Turn in wide, gradual arcs. If the skier falls, turn immediately to pick

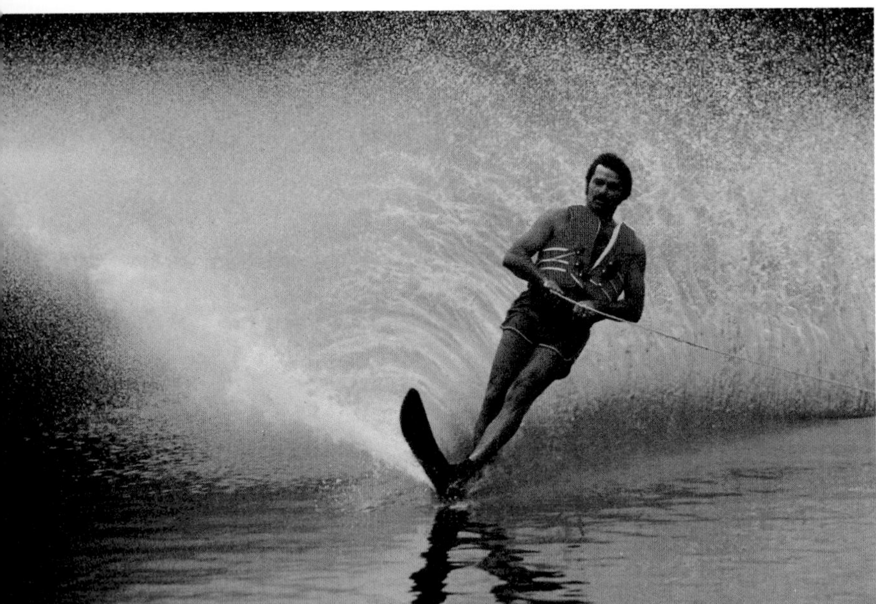

A waterskier should always wear a Coast Guard-approved flotation device, usually referred to as a life jacket.

him or her up. Cut the engine as you help the skier into the boat.

Never operate the boat while sitting on the side or behind the driving seat. Always sit in the driving seat and watch carefully for obstacles ahead.

Skiers have a responsibility to themselves and to other water users. They must make all signals to the driver clear and must signal with clarity after a fall that they are well, either by raising an arm or by raising a ski.

A waterskier must be a competent swimmer. Never go out after drinking, eating a large meal, or when tired or cold.

Before starting, check all the equipment. Look for loose bindings, splinters, sharp pieces of metal, or a frayed rope. Wait until the ski tips are up and the rope is taut before signaling to the boat to start.

Both skiers and boat passengers should wear a life jacket at all times. The boat should be equipped with spare life jackets and life buoys. Clothing should suit the weather conditions. One can suffer sunburn on a day that seems overcast or get chilled on a day that seems mild.

Watch the water ahead all the time. If you feel yourself falling, curl up into a ball to stop yourself from falling forward. Let go of the rope the moment you feel yourself going. Retrieve the skis as soon as possible. They are bouyant and can help you to float.

When coming in to land, run parallel to the shore and travel slowly. Never attempt to come directly into the shore at high speed. If in doubt, make another run.

Never wrap the rope around a hand or wrist. Hold onto the bridge at the end of the rope with the fingers; never loop it over a foot, elbow, or any other part of the body.

Ski in daylight hours only and never ski in unfamiliar or shallow water.

Canoeing. You must be a competent swimmer before taking up canoeing. Always wear a Coast Guard-approved personal flotation device (PFD), usually known as a life jacket. An approved helmet may also protect you from a head injury if you are thrown from the canoe.

Always canoe with a companion. Canoe with at least two other boats when on a fast river or in the ocean.

Before setting out on a trip, tell a responsible person where you are going and how long you expect to be away. Report your return. Check the weather forecast for that area, and make sure you know what conditions you are likely to encounter.

Learn how to deal with a capsize. In calm water it is safer to hold onto a floating, overturned canoe than to try to right it. In fast white water get away from the boat.

A canoe must be equipped with bow and stern bolts, deck lines, paddle parks, adequate buoyancy bags, and a spare split paddle secured to the stern deck.

Never carry more people than the canoe is designed to hold. Always stay seated and never change places with another person while afloat.

Keep clear of other boats. Remember that large boats are less maneuverable than you are and that a canoe can use shallower water than other craft. Keep away from fishing spots and dams.

Keep clear of rowing boats. It is often difficult for rowers to see a canoe.

Sailing. Every member of a sailing crew must be a competent swimmer and wear a personal flotation device.

Familiarize yourself thoroughly with the boat. The safest way to learn about the boat's equipment and handling is to join a class with a local boating club. Otherwise, sail with an experienced

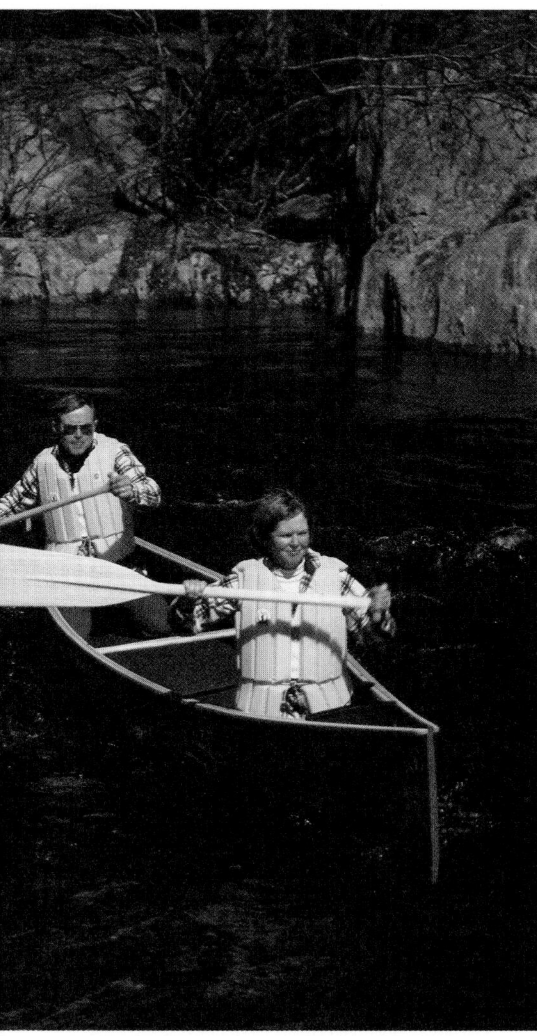

While in a canoe occupants should stay seated and wear Coast Guard-approved personal flotation devices.

colleague until he or she is confident that you can go out alone.

A dingy must have enough inbuilt buoyancy to keep afloat after a capsize. Check that the boat has a backup motor or other means of propulsion.

All sizes of boats should carry the right distress flares.

All motorized boats must carry fire extinguishers. Every member of the crew must know how to operate the equipment.

Before setting out, get the latest weather forecast. Let someone on shore know where you are going and how long you are likely to be out. Report your return.

Never overload the boat. If you have to carry fuel, keep it in a regulation container.

If a fire breaks out, head the boat into the wind and use the fire extinguisher. However, if there is a danger of an explosion, get away from the boat as quickly as possible.

Wax. *See* EARWAX.

Weakness (wēk'nes) is a sensation marked by a lack of body strength and vigor. It is a symptom of a number of conditions and disorders, and a person who continuously feels weak should consult a health professional.

Weal. *See* WHEAL.

Weaning (wēn'ing) is the period in infancy when feeding is gradually changed from being entirely milk-based to include other foods, such as cereal, fruit, and vegetables. It is also used as an expression to describe the time during which a baby is taken off the breast and given formula feeding by bottle.

The age at which weaning takes place varies widely from infant to infant and is a matter for discussion between the mother and her physician. Ideally, solid foods should not be introduced until between five and six months; many parents, however, prefer to wean the child earlier. Breast-feeding may continue for many months, even when other foods are given.

See also BABY CARE.

Weather safety. Severe weather conditions can lead to serious damage to property, to personal injury, and even to the loss of life. There are, however, many precautions that an individual can take to help minimize the danger to health and property. It is important to know what types of abnormal weather conditions (floods, hurricanes, tornadoes, etc.) are likely to affect your area; where the safety shelters are; and any appropriate safety or escape procedures. Emergency weather warnings are broadcast via radio; keep a battery radio with fresh batteries in the house.

Try to avoid any last-minute panic by preparing well in advance for any weather emergency. Preparations include making sure there is a complete stock of first-aid supplies, including adhesive bandages, antiseptic ointment, and anti-diarrheal medicines; stocking a supply of food that requires no refrigeration and little or no cooking; keeping emergency cooking, heating, and lighting equipment nearby and in good working order, with adequate fuel supplies; and keeping the automobile fueled and ready for emergency use.

General Survival Techniques. After a weather emergency, such as a tornado, if there is a smell of gas in the building, leave the building immediately and report the leakage. Never use an open flame to search a damaged building. Do not eat or drink anything that might have become contaminated by floodwater. If in doubt, boil drinking water thoroughly. Check that refrigerated food has not spoiled if there has been a power failure. Do not use any electrical appliance without first checking that it is completely dry.

Specific Survival Techniques. *Earthquakes* usually occur unexpectedly. Although the tremors can be frightening, it is essential not to panic; the main danger is from falling debris.

If you are indoors, stay there. Doorways are the strongest parts of a building's interior; the safest place for indoor safety is directly beneath a doorframe. Other safe places are against walls or beneath a table, desk, or bed. Stay away from windows or other fragile material. Douse all fires and do not use an open flame, because there may be a gas leak. If you are outdoors, move away from buildings and overhead cables. The greatest danger is from falling masonry outside doors and beneath overhanging roofs and walls. Stay out in the open until the tremors stop.

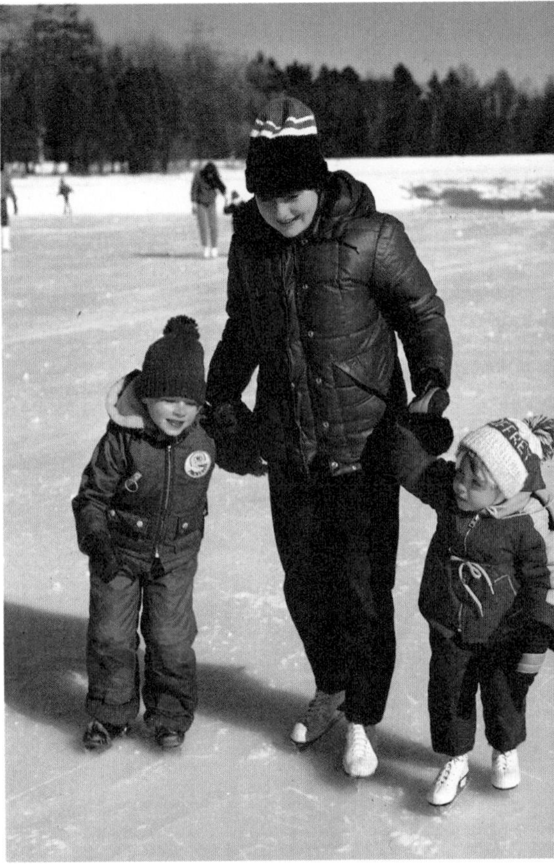
It is important for children to wear warm clothing that is both wind- and waterproof, when playing outdoors during the winter.

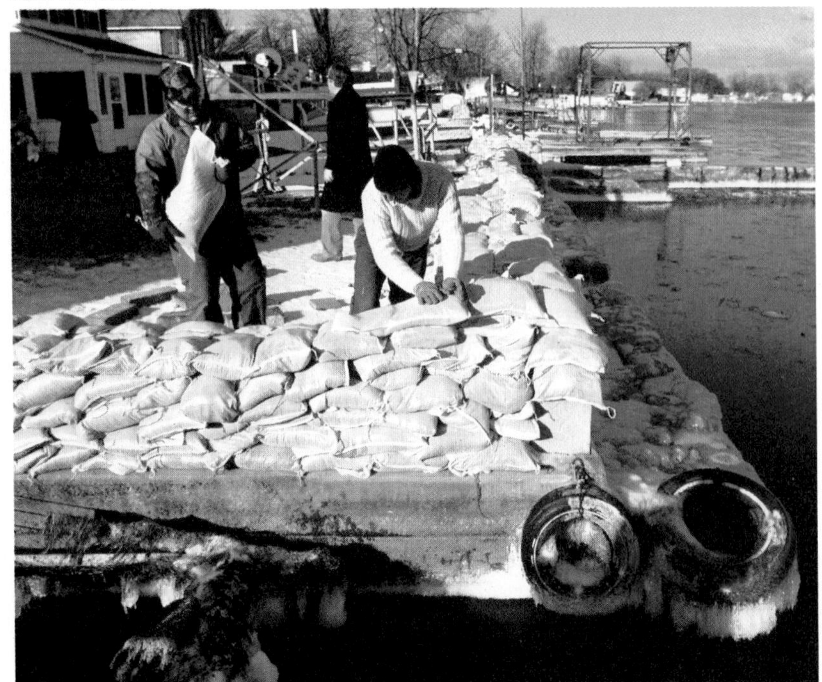
Sandbags are often used to help keep rising floodwater away from homes.

A *tidal wave*, or series of waves, may follow an earthquake in low-lying coastal regions. Anticipate this occurrence and move to higher ground, away from the coast, as soon as it is possible. Stay out of the danger zone until authorized to return.

Floods are perhaps the most common of all natural disasters. Learn the flood history of your locality and find out the elevation of the surrounding areas. In lower areas, keep sandbags, plywood, and plastic sheeting on hand. Store adequate supplies of drinking water in clean receptacles. Even the bathtub can be used as an emergency container.

After flooding, do not use gas or electric appliances; gas lines may have been ruptured and water may have seeped into burners and wiring. Do not enter a flooded area unless it is necessary. Cross a stream that is deeper than knee-level only with utmost caution. Avoid driving on flooded roads. If this is unavoidable, check the depth of the water and the road surface. Be especially cautious at night, when the dangers of floodwater are difficult to see. If the vehicle stalls, abandon it at once and move to higher ground.

Hurricanes are forecast well in advance, so stay tuned for a hurricane warning. The hurricane may not strike for 24 hours, and there should be time to move to a community shelter. If you are in your home and the house is sturdy and on high ground, remain indoors throughout the storm. Board up or shutter all windows. Stay tuned for bulletins. If the eye of the hurricane passes overhead, there will be a lull lasting for perhaps one-half hour. Stay indoors during this lull, if possible. Leave low-lying areas that may be swept by high seas. Abandon mobile homes, campers, and boats, but lash them securely. Seek refuge in a community shelter. Secure all loose outdoor objects, such as garbage cans, porch furniture, and tools.

Thunder and lightning occur during periods of strong, rising air currents. Watch for darkening skies, thunderclouds, lightning, and increasing winds. A person who is struck by lightning retains no electric current, but receives a severe electric shock and may suffer burns requiring medical treatment. A person who is knocked unconscious by lightning can often be revived by prompt artificial respiration or, if necessary, with cardiac pulmonary resuscitation. For step-by-step instruction, see ARTIFICIAL RESPIRATION; CARDIOPULMONARY RESUSCITATION.

Stay indoors, if possible. Keep away from windows, fireplaces, and all metal objects. Do not use the telephone or any electric appliance. Stay tuned to your battery radio for warnings of tornadoes or flash floods that may develop in stormy conditions.

If you are outdoors in a hard-topped automobile, stay there and keep the windows closed. If using machinery, leave it. Do not touch or go near any metal object. If in water, get out. Dock and vacate small boats. Seek shelter in a building, in a large clump of tall trees, or in a dry ditch or cave.

Where there is no shelter, keep far away from any isolated tree or other tall feature in the vicinity. If an electric charge is felt, causing the hair to stand on end, drop to the ground at once. Crouch low with hands and feet together.

Tornadoes occur seasonally. If the area has a history of tornadoes, it is wise to build a storm cellar near the home. Build it with reinforced concrete and cover the roof with three feet of dirt, sloped for drainage. The door should be heavy and open inward. Add a ventilating shaft. Slope the floor to a drainage outlet or dig a dry well. Keep a flashlight, crowbar, shovel, and pickaxe in the cellar. Seek shelter immediately after a tornado warning. If the building has neither basement nor storm cellar, take refuge in any small interior room. If there is only one large room, stay near a sturdy wall. Stay away from windows. Crouch under heavy furniture. If you are in a car or truck, park the vehicle and seek shelter. If there is an underpass or a bridge nearby, crouch behind its supports. If caught out in the open with no shelter, lie flat on the ground or in any depression such as a ditch or ravine.

Winter storms may cause weeks of isolation, and this must be kept in mind when making preparations. Stock up with adequate food, fuel, and other supplies.

During cold weather and storms stay inside as much as possible. Children must be taught that, although snow

To prepare for winter driving, a car trunk should be well stocked with emergency supplies, such as flares and jumper cables.

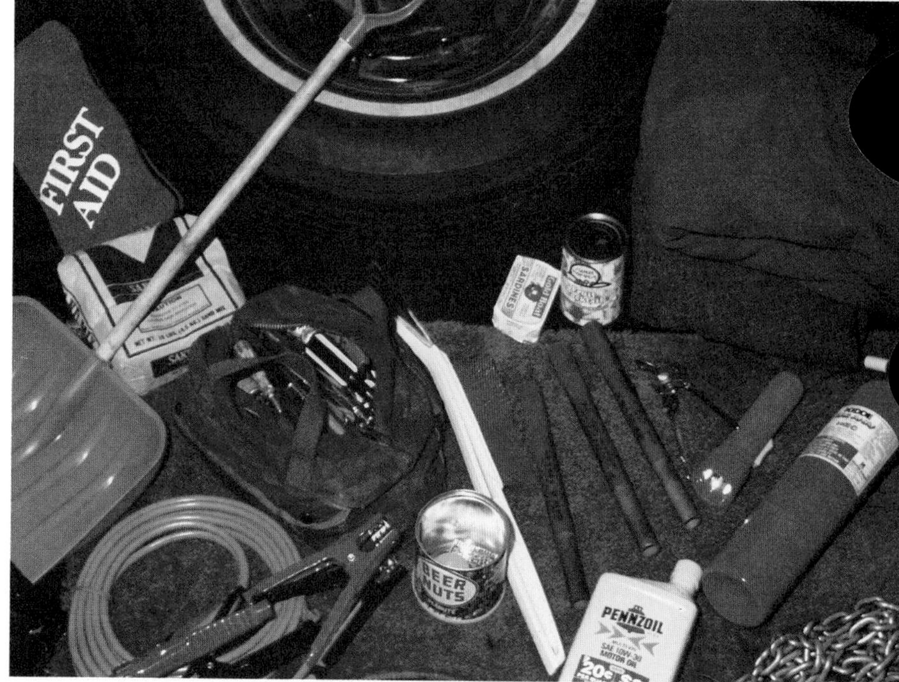

looks inviting, it can prove dangerous to play in because of deep snowdrifts. Avoid overexertion when working outside in the cold. Wear several layers of loose-fitting warm clothing and outer garments that are both waterproof and windproof. Always keep the head covered.

Weber's test (web′ərz) is a hearing test conducted by placing a vibrating tuning fork against a patient's forehead. If the sound is perceived equally in both ears, hearing is normal. If the sound is louder in one ear than the other, a disorder of the inner ear or the middle ear can then be diagnosed.

See also EAR.

Weight loss can be the result of a conscious effort to lose or avoid excessive body weight, or the loss can result from a psychiatric or medical problem. Losing weight can have important health benefits, as obesity is a major cause of high blood pressure and other serious disorders. However, weight should not be lost obsessively or as a fad; excessive weight loss can in itself entail serious health risks. In some individuals, weight loss is a reflection of a potentially serious psychiatric disorder, such as depression or anorexia nervosa. Persons suffering from anorexia nervosa can die from extreme weight loss and low body weight. *See also* ANOREXIA NERVOSA; BULIMIA; DEPRESSION.

Unless losing weight is a medical necessity, deciding when and how to lose weight is a personal decision. In all cases, however, undertaking a weight reduction program should involve planning, with care towards maintaining proper nutrition.

Diet. Although a primary factor of losing weight is eating less, it is important to maintain a balanced diet. Determining proper calorie intake also depends on body type and on how active a person is. Extreme restriction of calories is a short-term solution to a long-term problem; it is neither healthy nor very effective. *See also* DIET; DIET, SPECIAL; NUTRITION.

Exercise. A person undertaking a reducing diet should increase his or her activity level. But an obese person—even one who is otherwise healthy—should not suddenly start a program of prolonged, heavy exercise. The strain on the heart and other organs could be dangerous. An exercise program should be developed gradually. *See also* EXERCISE.

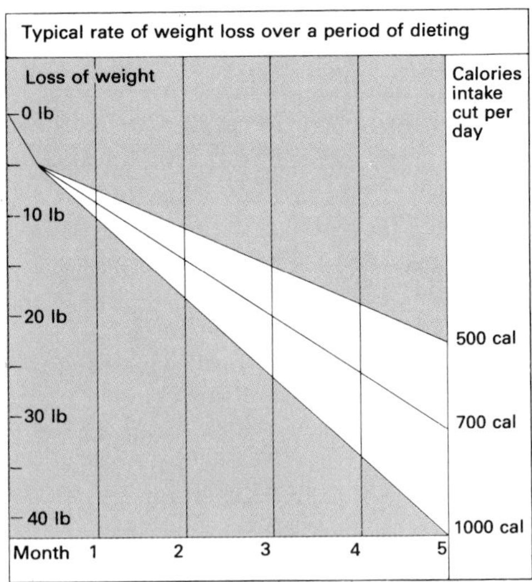

Dieting often causes a dramatic **weight loss** at first, followed by a more gradual weight reduction.

Medication. Using appetite-suppressant drugs to help reduce weight should be done with extreme caution, and only after consultation with a physician. The use of such drugs to lose weight rarely results in long-term success; patients will often regain the lost weight within one year. Taking amphetamines to reduce appetite can be very dangerous and lead to addiction. *See also* AMPHETAMINE.

In order to be successful, a weight-loss program should include long-term dietary and life style changes that allow a person to keep excess weight off. There are many support groups available which provide encouragement and motivation to lose weight.

See also WEIGHT PROBLEM.

Weight problem. Many people may think that they are overweight when, in fact, their weight may be normal for their height, age, and sex. They are concerned about their shape or figure and attribute an unsatisfactory shape to excessive weight. But very few persons are able to achieve this "ideal" shape, which may even be biologically or anatomically impossible to attain or maintain for some persons.

Apart from such shape problems, there are genuine weight problems. A person may be overweight or underweight compared to the average or de-

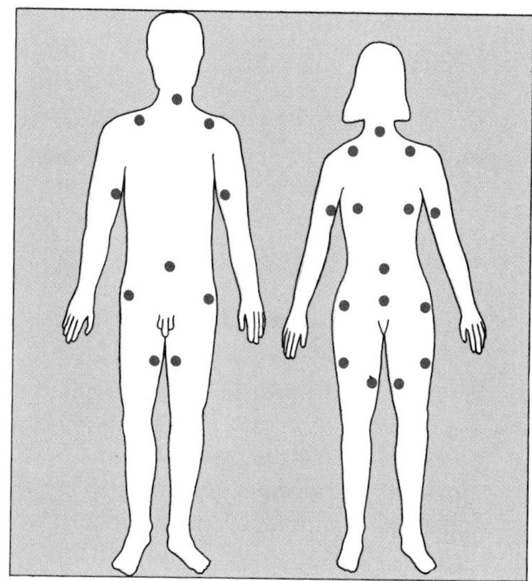

Weight problems cause excess fat to accumulate in certain areas, which differ slightly between men and women.

sirable weight. This can cause a physical disorder or anxiety.

Q: *How is average weight calculated?*

A: Weight tables are compiled by taking the weights of a large number of people and working out an average. The average weight varies because of many factors. For example, ethnic groups may vary in physical proportions; and some families are heavier than others, and their children inherit this characteristic.

Q: *How does the body normally regulate weight?*

A: Most people stay about the same weight throughout adult life or gain weight only slowly. The appetite center, in the hypothalamus of the brain, regulates the amount that is eaten. A slight overbalance results in a gradual weight gain. Even an extra slice of bread a day may cause a gain of one-half pound a month, about six pounds in a year.

Q: *When should a person consider there is a weight problem?*

A: Average expected weights should not be considered ideal weights. The correct weight varies from 10 percent below to 10 percent above the average weight. Weight well above or below this is probably abnormal.

Q: *What should be done if a person is below the normal weight?*

A: A person may decide that he or she is underweight, but this may be because of racial or inherited characteristics. If, however, there has definitely been a weight loss, a physician should be consulted and the cause found.

Q: *How do underweight people gain weight?*

A: Before a person undertakes a weight gain program, a health professional should be consulted to ensure that a medical disorder has not caused the original weight loss. Some people become dangerously underweight by starving themselves. Anorexia nervosa is an extreme form of self-starvation common in adolescent girls and needs specialized drug and psychiatric treatment. Depression, anxiety, and general fatigue are other factors in weight loss. *See also* ANOREXIA NERVOSA; BULIMIA.

Q: *Why do people become overweight?*

A: Nearly always because they consume more calories than they burn off. When people eat more than they need, the excess calories are stored as fat.

Some people may be overweight because of a physical disorder, and some gain weight because of compulsive eating, often a sign of underlying anxiety or depression. Weight gain may also follow a long illness.

Q: *Why do some people gain weight much more easily than others?*

A: The reasons for weight gain are not fully understood, but the answer may lie in an individual's metabolism. Babies who are fed excessive amounts of food become fat and often stay overweight into adulthood. There is also evidence that a tendency towards obesity may be genetically transmitted as well.

Q: *Are some foods more likely to produce obesity than others?*

A: Yes. A diet high in fat is more likely to lead to obesity than one high in carbohydrates, but excess calories, in general, should be avoided. Alcohol has a high calorie content and, apart from other damage it may cause, is a factor in obesity.

Q: *Are there any hazards in being overweight?*

A: Yes. Overweight people are at greater risk for coronary thrombosis and strokes because of arteriosclerosis. Such people are more likely to develop diabetes mellitus; hurt themselves seriously in accidents; develop osteoarthritis, particularly of the knees, hips, and ankles; and have more complications following surgery, such as venous thrombosis and chest infections.

Q: *How should an obese person lose weight?*

A: Anyone who is more than 20 percent over the expected average weight for his or her age, sex, and height should discuss weight loss and dieting with a physician. Sudden weight changes may cause extreme fatigue and exhaustion. Crash diets can be dangerous and may lead to vitamin deficiency diseases.

A gradual reduction in the amount of food eaten can result in a weight loss of 2 to 3 pounds a week, an overall loss of 10 pounds a month. The physician will probably recommend fewer carbohydrate foods, alcohol, and wheat products, and more high-protein foods and fresh salads.

Regular exercise is of value because it increases the body's metabolic rate and gives the person a sense of well-being and relative freedom from fatigue. In addition, diets usually cause equal weight loss from body fat and muscle. Exercise will increase the proportion of weight loss from body fat and will help protect the muscles.

Once a satisfactory weight has been achieved, there can be a slight relaxation in the detail of the diet so that the proper weight is maintained. It is, however, essential to keep to the same basic diet for life to avoid a return to the original eating habits that caused obesity. *See also* WEIGHT LOSS.

Q: *Can drugs help in the treatment of obesity?*

A: Yes. If obesity is caused by anxiety or depression, treatment with tranquilizers and antidepressant drugs can be a great help in reducing compulsive eating. Diuretic drugs, however, help to lose only two or three pounds of water from the body. Appetite suppressant drugs are only moderately effective and do not help the obese person to learn new ways of eating. When such drugs are stopped, the weight usually increases again.

Hormones, such as thyroid pills, have little effect unless taken in excessive amounts. Pep pills, such as amphetamines, reduce the appetite, but are dangerous, not only because of the hazard of addiction, but also because of the effect on blood pressure and mental activity.

Q: *Should vitamins be taken while dieting?*

A: No. There should be no need for supplementary vitamins if the person is in good health and keeps to a sensible, balanced new diet.

Q: *How can people help themselves if their weight is normal and they are dissatisfied with their shape?*

A: Regular exercise helps to increase muscle tone and decrease waist measurement, while also producing a slight slimming of the thighs. Weight may increase slightly due to extra muscle, but the figure will improve.

Q: *Can disorders reduce body weight?*

A: Yes. Any long-term illness, such as tuberculosis, sprue, untreated diabetes, or cancer, is accompanied by loss of weight. Fevers, operations, or accidents cause an increase in metabolic rate. Thus, the body tissues are used faster than they can be replaced, and there is a loss of weight. Another cause of increased metabolic rate is hyperthyroidism. *See also* HYPERTHYROIDISM.

Q: *Can any disorders produce an increase in weight?*

A: Yes. Heart, kidney, and liver failure are accompanied by retention of fluid in the body (edema), and this results in a weight gain. An underactive thyroid gland (hypothyroidism) is often accompanied by an increase of weight. *See also* HYPOTHYROIDISM.

Drug treatment of some mental disorders may be associated with a weight gain because of an effect on the hypothalamus.

Wen. *See* CYST.

Wet dream. *See* NOCTURNAL EMISSION.

Wheal (hwēl) is either a ridge on the skin made by a blow, as from a stick or whip, or a small swelling on the skin, as may be caused by an allergy or insect bite. In urticaria, or hives, the patient has widespread wheals.

See also URTICARIA.

Wheelchair is a mobile chair used to transport invalids or others who have difficulty walking; it can be self-propelled or propelled by another individual.

A wheelchair has large wheels and brakes. It can be specially equipped and fitted, if necessitated by long-term use. A wheelchair should be chosen with great care. When in the sitting position, the patient should be able to relax the arms comfortably on the armrests. The armrests may also be used for leverage while raising the body to a standing position. The back should be well supported, and the feet placed flat on the footrest. Sitting down for long periods of time can lead to discomfort in the pelvic area. To help prevent this, an effective cushion can be made by cutting a circular hole in a piece of foam rubber.

Moving about the home in a wheelchair is made considerably easier if steps are replaced by slopes or ramps. A short slope can be made by placing triangular wooden blocks against a step. Ramps can be bought or improvised. They consist of two tracks for the wheels of the wheelchair to run along. The ramp is placed between the upper and lower levels of a step, thus allowing the patient to move up the step under his or her own power.

See also WALKING AID.

Wheezing (hwēz′ing) is a rasping or whistling sound heard with some breathing disorders.

See also STRIDOR.

Whiplash injury (hwip′ lash) is an injury to the neck caused by a sudden jolt that snaps the head backward and then forward, as happens to a driver whose car is struck from behind. A whiplash injury causes damage to the cervical vertebrae or the muscles and ligaments that support them.

Q: *What are the symptoms of a whiplash injury?*

A: Momentary loss of consciousness is possible, usually followed by acute spasm and pain in the long muscles in the back of the neck. Almost always the victim has a stiff neck.

Sometimes, there may be a partial dislocation of one of the cervical vertebrae or an acute prolapsed intervertebral disk, also known as a herniated disk. This may cause pressure on nearby nerves, resulting in pain and weakness in the arms.

In rare cases, a fracture occurs, or a disk may press on the spinal cord and cause weakness and loss of sensation in the areas of the body below this level in the neck. Paralysis may follow.

See also DISK, HERNIATED; NECK, STIFF; PARALYSIS.

Whipworm. *See* WORM.

White blood cell. *See* BLOOD CELL, WHITE.

Whitehead (hwit′ hed), or milium, is a tiny, hard, whitish cyst within the skin, caused by the blockage of hair follicles and subsequent retention of oily (sebaceous) secretions. Whiteheads usually occur on the face, especially over the eyelids and on the forehead. They often occur in newborn infants, but disappear spontaneously. In adults, treatment may include drainage of the cyst.

See also CYST.

Whitlow. *See* PARONYCHIA.

Whooping cough. *See* PERTUSSIS.

Widal's test (ve dälz′) is a blood test performed in the investigation of typhoid fever and other salmonella infections.

See also SALMONELLA.

Wilson's disease (wil′sunz) is a rare, hereditary disorder in which there is an abnormal accumulation of copper in the body, particularly in the liver, cornea, and brain. This causes cirrhosis, anemia, and damage to the nervous system, resulting in abnormal body movements (chorea) and dementia. The chorea results from excessive deposits of copper in the basal ganglia. Wilson's disease is caused by an abnormal recessive gene that controls copper metabolism in the body. Both parents must carry the trait for a person to develop the disease. Death usually occurs unless treatment with penicillamine, a drug which increases the excretion of copper, is successful.

See also ANEMIA; CIRRHOSIS; DEMENTIA; GANGLION.

Winding: treatment (wind′ing). Winding results from a violent blow to the upper part of the abdomen, taking the breath away from a victim. The victim may gasp for air or may even lose consciousness.

Treatment. Place the victim in the recovery position, as described in FAINTING: FIRST AID. Loosen the victim's clothing around the neck, chest, and waist. If pain and difficulty in breathing persist, seek medical advice.

See also UNCONSCIOUSNESS: TREATMENT.

Wind knocked out: treatment. *See* WINDING: TREATMENT.

Windpipe. *See* TRACHEA.

Winter sports safety. In winter sports, people must protect themselves against the cold in addition to taking precautions involved with other sports. A special hazard is a condition called hypothermia, in which the body temperature falls below its normal level of 98.6°F. The symptoms of hypothermia include uncontrollable shivering, slurred speech, stumbling, and drowsiness. If left untreated, the condition may lead to death. *See also* HYPOTHERMIA: TREATMENT.

Downhill Skiing is a very popular form of recreation in the United States. Since downhill skiing involves high speeds and quick turns, it can also be a very dangerous sport, especially for the beginner. Many accidents happen on a beginners' slope at the start of a vacation. The most common injury is a muscle sprain, and this can be serious enough to keep a downhill skier off his or her feet for an entire vacation. A skier can also rupture a ligament in the knee or fracture an ankle or leg bone.

Ski instruction shortens the learning period for beginners and adds to the safety and enjoyment of the sport. All major ski areas have ski instruction available.

One of the reasons so many beginners suffer injuries is that modern resorts offer facilities to transport them to slopes beyond their skiing capability. Beginners must stay within their class and not be tempted to follow the more experienced skiers in their party.

Another factor that puts the beginner at risk is that he or she has no idea of how fast a skier can travel downhill. Skiers have been known to travel as fast as 110 miles per hour (177km/h), and a beginner could reach a speed of about 50 miles per hour (80km/h) on an advanced slope without realizing it. In addition to this, a beginner is unlikely to be able to make a high-speed stop or turn, and the results can be catastrophic. Beginners must take the advice of their instructors about which slopes to ski on.

Whatever standard a skier has reached, fatigue greatly increases the chances of an accident. Resorts report that the number of accidents rises during the afternoons. If a skier begins to take more tumbles as the day wears on, he or she should leave the slopes. The first sign of fatigue is a slight lack of concentration. As a general precaution, skiers should ensure that they eat nourishing food regularly and get at least seven hours of sleep per night in spite of "après ski" partying.

The probability of suffering from fatigue is greatly reduced if the skier has done some preseason exercising. The type of exercise program adopted is for the individual to choose. Flexibility- and endurance-type exercises to strengthen legs and ankles are traditionally recommended for skiers. If a person embarks on a skiing holiday feeling in good shape and relaxed, he or she can assume the exercises have been successful. Another wise precaution every skier should take is a quick warm-up without skis before the first run of the day. Anything helps, from touching the toes to running on the spot.

Weather conditions present a hazard to the skier. It is unwise to continue to ski if snow conditions deteriorate. For example, a slippery ice crust can form over wet snow during late afternoon. No skier should continue if visibility is reduced either by fog or by snowfall. Another weather hazard skiers must be aware of is the possibility of sunburn, particularly from the rays reflected off the snow. Sun creams must be applied underneath the chin, under the nose

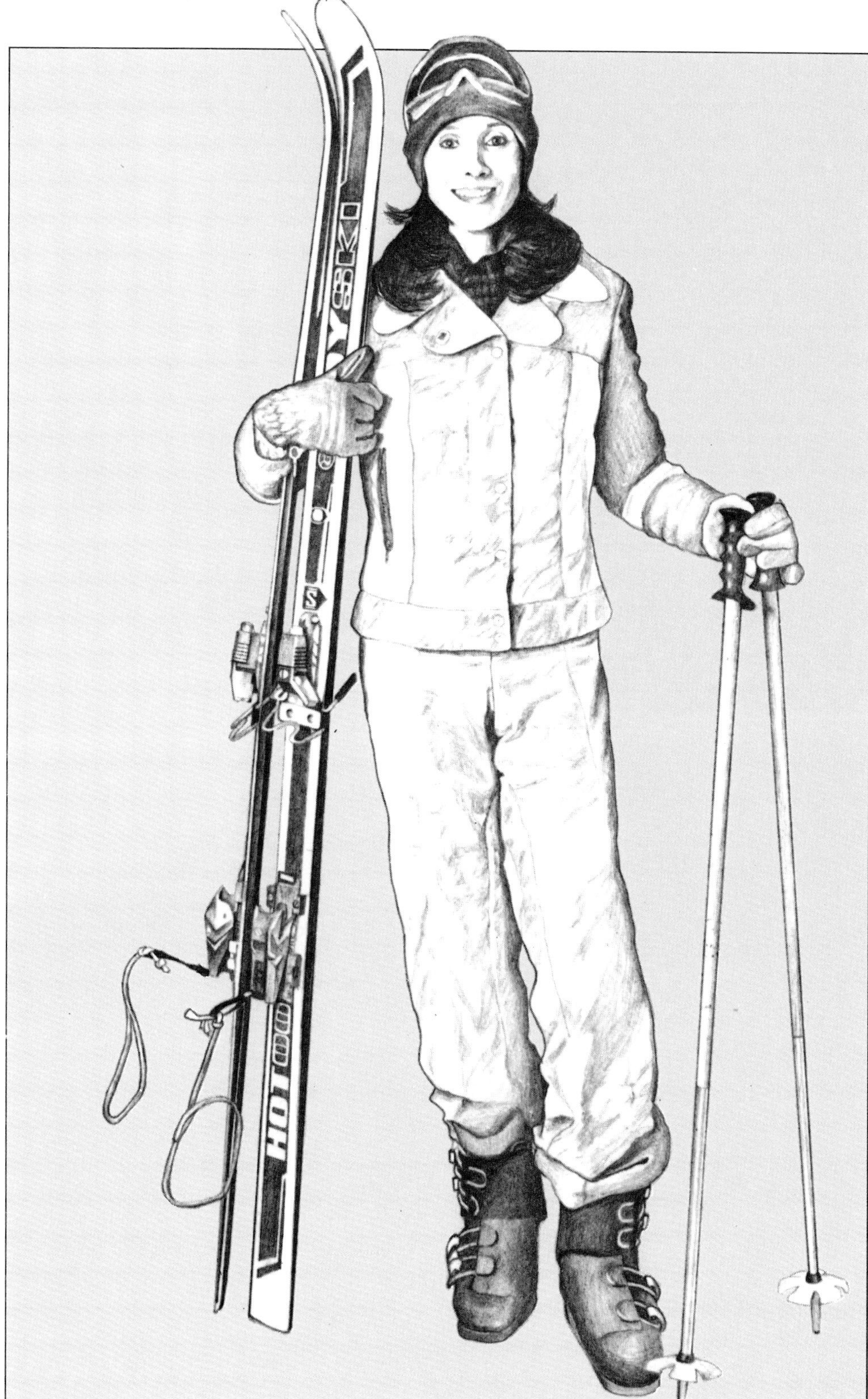

Skiing Safety

A skier must be adequately protected from extremes of weather. Hat and gloves must be warm and fit well. Tight clothing over the ears and fingers may lead to frostbite. A scarf is essential for warmth and protection from sunburn. It should always be tucked in and never allowed to flap loosely. Goggles offer more protection to the eyes than sunglasses, because they cut out the glare from the side as well as the front. They also prevent sunburn underneath the eyebrows, caused by rays reflected off the snow. Ski-jacket and pants must be made of a lightweight, water-resistant material. Woolen and rough materials get caked with snow. Clothing must be brightly colored. Socks must be well-fitting and made of a natural fiber, such as wool. A minimum of two socks should be worn on each foot. Do not pull the outer sock down over the top of the boot, because it cakes with snow, and the moisture seeps down into the boot. Boots must also be well-fitting and made of an approved design for skiing.

Release bindings are essential. Check them daily. When the bindings are correctly adjusted, do not switch the skis around. A safety strap fixed to the boot to prevent runaway skis is required in most ski areas. Even safer are ski brakes which can prevent both 'windmilling' and runaway skis.

and eyebrows (even if the skier is wearing sunglasses), and on the underside of the earlobes. Protective eyewear, such as shatterproof sunglasses or goggles, will protect eyes from the sun's ultraviolet rays and from injury, in case of a fall. Intense cold, particularly when there is a wind blowing, can lead to frostbite. Apart from the precaution of wearing the correct clothing, a skier must be aware of other potentially dangerous situations. For example, when using a chair lift without a footrest, the feet and legs must be kept on the move to maintain the circulation. The lower leg and foot may become numb and stiff, or the first signs of frostbite may develop without the skier being aware of it. *See also* FROSTBITE; FROSTBITE: FIRST AID; SNOW BLINDNESS; SUNBURN.

Good discipline on the slopes is not only courteous to other skiers, it is also safer. When skiers fall, they should flatten down any dents made in the snow. Otherwise, the next skier down the slope could catch a ski tip in the hole and fall too.

A skier must be prepared to make evasive maneuvers at all times. He or she must never assume that other skiers have the skill to get out of the way. It is every skier's duty to ski responsibly. If a skier can not maneuver out of danger, he or she is traveling too fast.

Courtesy on the ski lifts also makes for safety. A skier should sit still on a chairlift; moving about strains the cables and transmits the movement down the line.

A skier traveling on a rope tow must avoid jerking the rope, particularly when stepping off at the top of the slope. A sudden movement could flick off another skier further down the rope.

The moment a skier reaches the top of a slope, he or she must move out of the way. Having fallen from a T-bar lift, a skier must immediately get off the track and onto the side of the lift path. A fallen skier who obstructs those following causes a pile-up.

Cross-country Skiing is a form of hiking on skis over snow-covered ground that is flat or slightly hilly. It is increasing in popularity and is relatively safe and easy to learn. However, it does require a lot of physical endurance. The skis used are different in shape and length from those used in downhill skiing.

Ice Skating. Many people injure themselves skating each year. Injuries commonly occur due to skaters tripping on bumps in the ice, colliding with other skaters, or falling through thin ice. Skating areas are often crowded, and the skates themselves pose an additional hazard; the blades have sharp edges and points that are often unprotected.

A skater can quickly learn to skate forward without having first mastered maneuvering and stopping techniques. Individuals must be careful while skating to protect themselves and others against injury. Skating instructions are one method of learning safe skating techniques.

One of the most important skills a skater must learn, whether falling in a crowded area or while alone, is how to fall. A fall on ice is far less serious than a fall on solid ground, because the body tends to slide along the ice and much of the impact is absorbed. A skater must not be afraid of falling on the ice. The automatic response to loss of balance is a struggle to regain it, but a skater is safer if he or she relaxes and lets the fall take a natural course.

A skater should lean forward at the beginning of a fall. An outstretched hand slides on the ice, and the elbow can bend to absorb the jolt. Wearing gloves, a skater is unlikely to come to any harm. However, if a skater falls backward, the possibility of injury is greater. A skater might strike the back of the head on the ice; might sit down suddenly and jar the back or lower backbone; and probably most commonly, might break a wrist by stretching the arm out behind. In this position, the arm remains straight, and the wrist takes the full force of the fall.

After a fall, a skater must get up and out of the way of other skaters as quickly as possible; this will prevent injury to the skater by collision and to other skaters by falling.

A skater must keep the hands close to the body while getting up. The fingers must be tucked underneath the hand, not splayed out on the ice where they are in constant danger from skaters passing nearby.

Again, courtesy plays an important part in safe skating. A beginner should

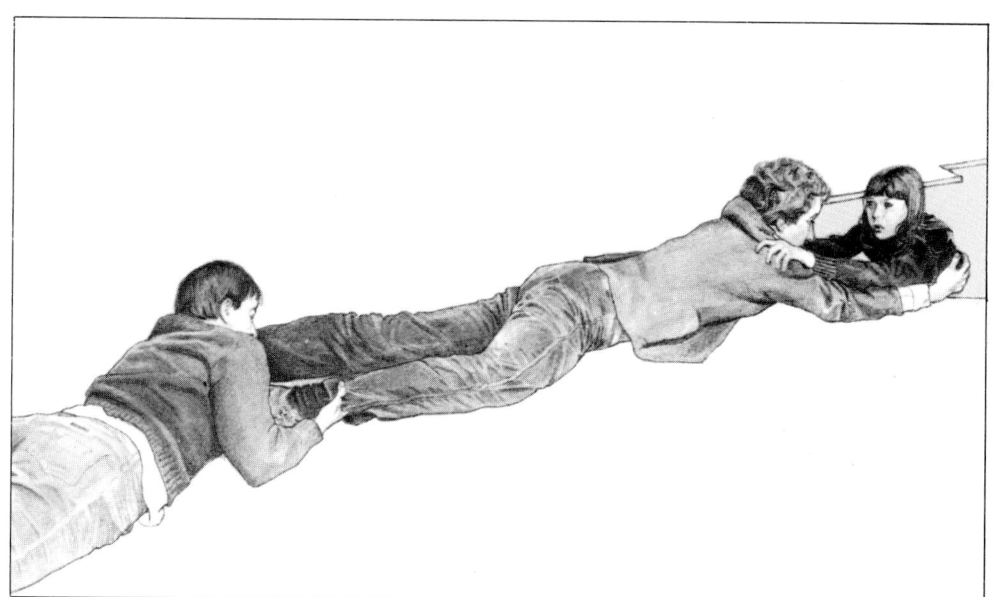

The Human Chain
A human chain is a simple, but effective method of reaching a victim on hazardous ice. The first member of the rescue party lies on the ice and wriggles gradually forward. The next person grasps firmly onto the first person's foot or skate blade. Other people then repeat the procedure, wriggling gradually forward over the ice toward the victim. The first person finally grabs hold of the victim's wrists, and the chain wriggles backward out of danger.

leave the center of a lake or iced area normally reserved for the fast and competent skaters, and should stay at the side.

A competent skater must keep a constant watch for fallen skaters or learners, particularly when skating backward.

Apart from gloves, a skater's clothing should include thick pants (they offer more protection in a fall than a skirt) and a top jacket of a slippery material, such as nylon, that helps a skater slide in the event of a fall.

Sledding. Examine your sled and repair any broken parts or split wood. Sharp edges should also be eliminated before you go sledding.

Choose your sledding area carefully. Do not sled on streets, where you might slide into the path of an oncoming automobile. Steep hills are dangerous because you might go too fast and be unable to stop. Do not go sledding on frozen ponds or lakes if the ice could break under your weight. The ideal spot for sledding is a broad, gently sloping hill that is free of trees and far from any road.

Snowmobiling is increasingly popular in many northern climates and has led to a large number of accidents. Speeding causes many snowmobile mishaps. Never go faster than the safe speed for your vehicle, and never drive too fast for the snow conditions. A snowmobile should not be operated in less than 4 inches (10cm) of snow. If possible, drive only in daylight. Approximately three of every four fatal snowmobile accidents occur after dark. Be especially careful when crossing roads and watch for such obstacles as tree stumps, fallen logs, hidden branches, and barbed wire fences.

Safety on the Ice

An ice user must be able to recognize safe ice. It is usually found on slow-flowing streams, small areas of water, such as ponds, or on small lakes. Ice is thinner at the edges of pools, under overhanging trees or bushes, and under bridges. Areas that should be avoided altogether are tidal water and fast-flowing water that has iced on the surface. Although such ice may be thick, it is constantly subjected to strain and may break up under the weight of a person. Ice of this kind should not be used if the water beneath is over 3 or 4 feet (1 to 1.3m) deep. In fact, such ice tends to be rough and uneven.

During the first freeze of winter, "black" ice forms. It is completely transparent and is usually tough and elastic. Once it has frozen to a depth of at least 5 to 6 inches (12.5cm—15.0cm) it is probably safe to use for walking, skating, and skiing. It may crack and squeak under a person's weight, but it usually does not give way.

Once ice thickens to about 6 to 8 inches (15.0cm—20.0cm), it can support snowmobile activities. By midwinter it may have attained the depth of 1 foot (30cm) and have changed color to a whitish blue. This kind of ice can support almost anything, although sometimes pressure within the ice can produce small holes that have to be avoided.

At the end of the winter, the sun and wind begin to melt the ice. Although the ice may look safe and still be a few feet in depth, it may become water-logged and break up with a slight increase of weight on the surface.

Ice accidents tend to happen in two different ways. In the first situation, the ice user breaks directly through the ice and struggles to reach hold of the edge of the ice. The body jackknifes, the ice breaks away, and the victim is drawn under the surface. The following procedure prevents this: do not attempt to climb out immediately; kick the feet up to the surface behind, as if swimming; extend the hands and arms onto the surrounding ice; using this horizontal swimming position, work carefully forward until firm ice is reached.

The other form of accident occurs when the ice splits, and the victim trips over the raised edge of ice. The automatic response is to stand up again. But this increases the pressure on a small area of already fractured ice, and the victim falls through. To prevent this from happening, the ice user must intentionally sprawl forward during the fall, then wriggle on his or her stomach or roll away from the danger area where the ice is weak.

Rescue From the Ice. If a person falls through the ice, speed is essential for a rescue. The longer a person is in icy water, the greater the chance that he or she will panic and either attempt to struggle onto the ice, breaking away more chunks of ice along the edge, or become exhausted and slip under the surface. The other great danger is cold. A person's body cools down rapidly to dangerously low temperatures when immersed in icy water. *See also* HYPOTHERMIA.

It is essential that rescuers do not rush forward to help. The area of ice around the hole is cracked and extremely dangerous. The rescue must be conducted from firm ice a few feet away, or as far away as necessary. It is important that any person approaching the victim across the ice distribute their body weight evenly by wriggling at full stretch over the ice. There should be at least one helper to pull the rescuer back to safety if the ice gives way again.

One of the best aids to rescue is a ladder that can be slid out across the ice to the victim. If more ice breaks when the victim draws himself or herself onto the ladder, the free end may rise up. The victim can then push the ladder back onto a firmer surface.

Obviously, many potentially helpful pieces of rescue equipment, such as a lifebuoy, may not be available, particularly if the accident happens on a lake in the countryside. But one item that is usually handy is a spare tire, which can be rolled out across the ice to help keep the victim afloat while rescue attempts are being organized. Alternatively, if a stronger piece of rope is also available, this can be secured to the tire, and the victim can be hauled to safety.

If rope or string is available, but no tire, attach a line to a small log and slide it out across the ice. It is more likely to reach the victim accurately than if it is free-thrown. If the victim is unable to clasp the rope with the hands, rescuers should tell him or her to wrap it around himself or herself under the arms before they attempt to haul the victim to safety.

Rescue From Under the Ice. If a victim fails to catch hold of the edge of the ice and disappears beneath it, the decision to attempt a rescue must be carefully considered to avoid a double tragedy. Some experts feel that the risk is never justifiable. Once beneath the ice, it is almost impossible to find the hole again, because visibility is poor. The only circumstance that can justify an attempt is if a very powerful swimmer goes down attached to a strong line. The rescuers must pull the swimmer up after a very short time to prevent him or her from developing hypothermia.

Wisdom teeth. *See* TOOTH, WISDOM.

Witches' milk is a common name for the small amount of rather watery milk produced for a few days after birth by the breasts of a newborn baby of either sex. This action is stimulated by maternal hormones in the baby's bloodstream.

Withdrawal (with drô'əl) is the condition of physical and psychologial distress in an addict, caused by the sudden deprivation of narcotic drugs. Withdrawal can also occur with many other substances, such as alcohol, nicotine, Valium®, and many other drugs. Symptoms of withdrawal include nausea and profuse sweating. These should not be ignored, since withdrawal may become life-threatening. *See also* DRUG ADDICTION.

The term withdrawal may also refer to an abnormal retreat from reality, as may occur in schizophrenia. It is also the term commonly used for the method of contraception more correctly known as "coitus interruptus."

See also CONTRACEPTION; SCHIZOPHRENIA.

Wolf-Parkinson-White syndrome (wůlf-park'in sun-hwīt) is a cardiac abnormality in which there is abnormal electrical conduction through the heart muscles. This may predispose the patient to symptoms of rapid heartbeat (palpitations) or the development of an irregular heartbeat (arrythmia).

See also ARRYTHMIA; PALPITATION.

Womb. *See* UTERUS.

Woolsorter's disease (wůl'sôr tərz) is an often fatal lung disorder caused by a type of anthrax.

See also ANTHRAX.

Worm (wėrm) is any of several kinds of invertebrate animals that have soft, slender bodies and no limbs. Many species of worms cause parasitic infections. Worms are classified into four main groups: flatworms (Platyhelminthes), including the tapeworm and liver fluke; roundworms (Nematoda); ribbon worms (Nemertea); and segmented worms (Annelida). *See also* FLUKE; PARASITE.

Tapeworms that infest the intestine include the beef tapeworm *(Taenia saginata)* and the fish tapeworm *(Diphyllobothrium latum)*. The most common tapeworm that infests human beings is the dog tapeworm *(Echinococcus granulosus)*, causing hydatid disease. The pork tapeworm *(Taenia solium)* can cause cysticercosis of the intestine. *See also* CYST, HYDATID; CYSTICERCOSIS; TAPEWORM.

Roundworms that infest the intestine include *Ascaris lumbricoides;* pinworms, such as *Enterobiasis vermicularis;* hookworms, such as *Ancylostoma duodenale;* threadworms, such as *Strongyloides stercoralis;* and whipworms, such as *Trichuris trichiura. See also* ANKYLOSTOMIASIS; STRONGYLOIDES; TRICHURIASIS.

Roundworms that infest the body tissues include *Wuchereria bancrofti,* which causes elephantiasis; *Loa loa,* which causes loiasis; *Onchocerca volvulus,* which causes river blindness; *Toxocara canis* and *Toxocara cati,* which causes toxocariasis; and *Trichinella spiralis,* which causes trichinosis.

See also ELEPHANTIASIS; LOA LOA; ONCHOCERCIASIS; ROUNDWORM; TOXOCARIASIS; TRICHINOSIS.

Wound (wünd) is an injury that causes damage by cutting or tearing the skin and possibly other tissue. A surgeon's incision is an aseptic (without infection) wound. A wound which penetrates the skin may cause little damage to the skin but may severely injure underlying tissue. This is especially true of puncture wounds.

See also BLEEDING: FIRST AID; CUT: TREATMENT.

Wrist (rist), known medically as the carpus, is the joint between the arm and the hand. There are eight bones in the wrist, located in two rows. The scaphoid, lunate, triquetral, and pisiform bones form a joint with the radius and ulna bones of the forearm. The trapezium, trapezoid, capitate, and hamate bones form joints with the five metacarpal bones of the hand. Each of the wrist bones forms a joint with each of the others. All of the bones are surrounded by synovial membranes and ligaments.

Wrist-drop (rist) is a condition in which the wrist remains flexed downward and is unable to be extended. It is often caused by injury to the radial nerve of the forearm or paralysis of the muscles in the hand and wrist.

Writer's cramp is pain and spasm in the muscles of the hand, often resulting from long periods of writing.

Wryneck. *See* NECK, STIFF.

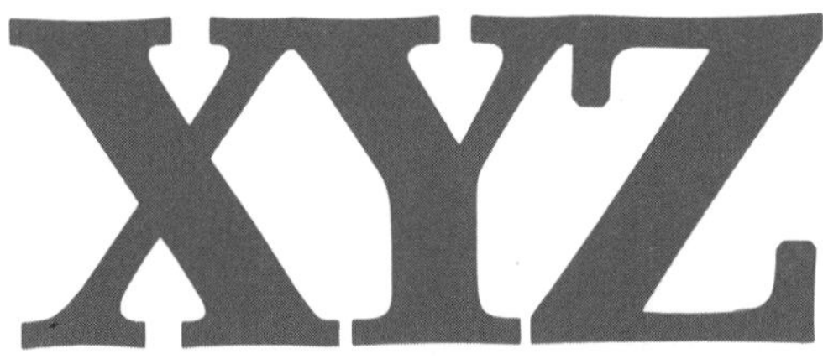

Xanthelasma (zan thə laz′mə) is a condition in which small, soft, yellow spots form on the upper and lower eyelids. It is most commonly seen in the elderly.

Q: *What causes xanthelasma?*

A: It may occur spontaneously for no obvious reason. But the condition is often associated with increased amounts of cholesterol in the blood, with lipemia, and with the appearance of a xanthoma elsewhere in the body.

Q: *What is the treatment of xanthelasma?*

A: Xanthelasma does not cause discomfort or disease, and so does not require treatment other than any that may be prescribed for lipemia. However, the spots can be removed surgically for cosmetic reasons.

See also CHOLESTEROL; LIPEMIA; XANTHOMA.

Xanthoma (zan thō′mə) is a benign deposit or lump of yellow fatty substance (lipids) in the skin and tendons. The condition is most common in the Achilles tendon and in the tendons of the hand and foot. It also occurs with lipemia, an inherited disorder in which there are excessive amounts of lipids in the blood. Xanthelasma, a yellowish tumor on the upper and lower eyelids, most common in elderly people, may also occur. Patients with xanthoma have an increased chance of developing coronary heart disease.

Q: *How is xanthoma treated?*

A: Treatment includes a low cholesterol diet (without saturated fats) and drugs that further decrease the lipids in the blood. The nodules of fatty substances sometimes ulcerate through the skin and have to be removed surgically.

See also LIPEMIA; XANTHELASMA.

X chromosome (krō′mə sōm) is one of the two types of human sex chromosomes. The other is called the Y chromosome. If two X chromosomes are present, the person is a female. If an X and a Y chromosome are present, the person is a male. The X chromosome is usually of a shape and size similar to the other 22 pairs of chromosomes present in the nucleus of every cell in the human body.

See also CHROMOSOME; GENE; HEREDITY; Y CHROMOSOME.

Xenophobia (zen ə fō′bē ə) is an abnormal fear of strangers or foreigners.

Xenopus test (zen′ə pəs) is a pregnancy test in which a female African toad (*Xenopus laevis*) is injected with urine from a woman who suspects that she is pregnant. If the woman is pregnant, the toad produces eggs within 12 hours of the injection. The xenopus test may give false results in some cases and has been replaced by more reliable tests.

See also PREGNANCY TEST.

Xeroderma (zir ə dėr′mə) is a condition in which the skin is abnormally dry and rough. It usually occurs on the lower legs of middle-aged or elderly persons, most often in cold weather, and in persons who bathe frequently.

Q: *Why does the skin become abnormally dry?*

A: The skin may become abnormally dry because of sunburn, frequent bathing, the gradual dryness that occurs with increasing age, dietary deficiencies of vitamin A or the mineral zinc, or ichthyosis, a mild type of dry skin disorder present at birth. There may also be mild to moderate itching and an associated dermatitis caused by detergents or other irritants.

Q: *How is xeroderma treated?*

A: Often, the problem is a minor one, and it is only the mild irritation that makes the patient visit a physician. The physician usually prescribes a cream to keep moisture and fat in the skin and advises against using soap. Vitamin A or zinc is prescribed only if there is evidence of deficiency.

See also ICHTHYOSIS.

Xeroderma pigmentosum (zir ə dėr′ mə pig mən tō′ səm) is a rare, genetic skin disease. Areas of pigment discoloration and scarring occur. The disease is characterized by a sensitivity to sunlight with a high rate of sun-induced skin cancers of exposed areas.

Xerophthalmia (zir of thal′mē ə) is a disorder that results in dry eyes, hazy corneas, reduced tear production, and roughness of the conjunctiva. It is often associated with night blindness.

The primary cause of xerophthalmia is vitamin A deficiency resulting from dietary deprivation or an interference with absorption, storage, or transport of Vitamin A.

Treatment involves correcting the cause and administering vitamin A in therapeutic doses.

See also VITAMIN.

X-linked dominant inheritance is a pattern of heredity in which a dominant gene on the X chromosome is transmitted, causing a trait to be passed on to the next generation. All daughters of an affected male will be affected, but none of the sons. Affected females will transmit the trait to half of their children regardless of sex. Normal children of affected parents will have normal offspring.

See also GENETIC ABNORMALITY; HEREDITY.

X-linked recessive inheritance is a pattern of heredity in which an abnormal recessive gene on the X chromosome is transmitted, resulting in a carrier state in females and conditional characteristics in males. Almost all affected persons are males, and an affected male never transmits the trait to his sons. The trait is always transmitted by the mother who appears normal. A carrier female transmits the characteristic to half of her sons. Half of her daughters will be carriers, but none will show the trait. The daughters of an affected male will all be carriers.

See also GENETIC ABNORMALITY; HEREDITY.

X ray is a short electromagnetic ray that can penetrate body tissues to varying degrees. The variation in the amount of X rays absorbed by different tissues can be projected on a screen or recorded on film to produce an X-ray photograph. X rays are used to diagnose and treat diseases and to locate broken bones or other malfunctions in the body.

See also FLUOROSCOPE; RADIATION; RADIOGRAPHY; RADIOTHERAPY.

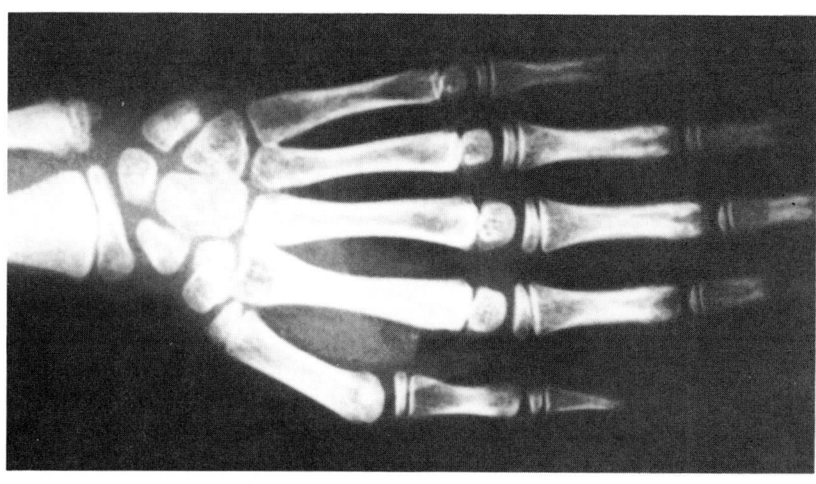

An **X-ray** photograph can be used to locate and diagnose bone disorders, such as those in the hand.

XXX syndrome is a chromosomal aberration in which affected females have three X chromosomes and two Barr bodies (inactivated sex chromosomes) instead of the normal XX chromosomes and one Barr body. This often results in some degree of mental retardation.

XXY syndrome. *See* KLINEFELTER'S SYNDROME.

XYY syndrome is a chromosomal aberration characterized by an extra Y chromosome in males. It may result in overaggressive behavior or poor mental and social development.

Yaws (yôz) is an infectious, tropical disease caused by the spiral-shaped bacterium *Treponema pertenue.* This bacterium is indistinguishable from that which causes syphilis *(Treponema pallidum)* and pinta. Yaws is spread by direct contact between the infectious swellings of a diseased person and a break in the skin of another person. The bacterium that causes yaws can not penetrate unbroken skin, nor can it pass through the placenta.

Q: *What are the symptoms of yaws?*

A: After an incubating period of three to four weeks, a swelling appears at the site of infection; this may ulcerate and then heal. While it is healing, further soft swellings appear on the lips, elbows, buttocks, and knees. They are highly infectious, but rarely produce any irritation. Occasionally, the soft swellings may affect the underlying bones, particularly in the hands and feet. This may cause a limp in children.

When the soft swellings have healed, there often is an interval of several years before any further symptoms occur. After this interval, nodules appear on the skin. They may ulcerate and often affect underlying tissues. The ulcers heal slowly, forming scars that may be greatly disfiguring. The bones may also become distorted, and there may be shortening of the ligaments in the joints.

Q: *How is yaws treated?*

A: Yaws can be cured by treatment with penicillin. Surgery may also be necessary to correct any disfigurement or bone deformity.

See also PINTA; SYPHILIS; TREPONEMA.

Y chromosome (krō′mə sōm) is one of the two chromosomes that determines sex; the other is called the X chromosome. The Y chromosome appears only in males; it is associated with the development of male sex characteristics, such as the testes.

During fertilization of the ovum, if a Y chromosome is paired with an X chromosome, the fetus will develop into a male. If two X chromosomes are paired, the fetus will develop into a female. The Y chromosome is so called because its shape is markedly different from the other 45 chromosomes, which all resemble the X chromosome.

See also CHROMOSOME; GENE; HEREDITY; X CHROMOSOME.

Yeast (yēst) is a general term for any of the single-celled fungi of the genus *Saccharomyces*, which reproduces by budding. Yeast is used for leavening bread and for brewing (brewer's yeast). Brewer's yeast is a rich source of vitamin B. Some species of yeast may cause disorders, such as candidiasis. Other species are poisonous.

See also CANDIDIASIS; FUNGAL INFECTION.

Yellow fever is a virus infection transmitted to humans by the bite of the mosquito *Aedes aegypti*. The disorder is common in tropical climates, particularly in Africa and South America. The yellow fever virus often damages many body tissues, such as the brain

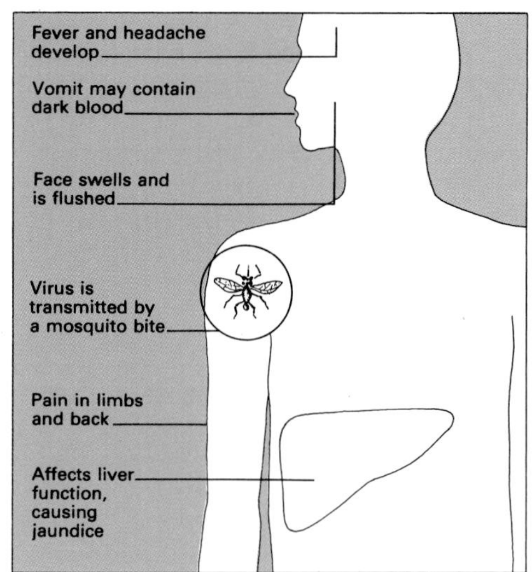

The **yellow fever** virus is transmitted via the bite of an infected mosquito. Symptoms usually take several days to develop.

and heart, but especially the liver. As a result of liver damage, yellow bile pigments gather in the skin and give the disease its name.

Q: *What are the symptoms of yellow fever?*

A: After an incubation period of three to six days, symptoms appear suddenly. They include a shivering attack (rigor), high fever, severe headache, bone pains, dizziness, and mild confusion. In many persons, the disease progresses no further, and recovery is fairly quick. But in others, the fever drops for a day or two and then rises steeply. The skin turns yellow and there is bleeding from the gums and stomach lining.

Many patients recover from this stage. Others become delirious and go into a coma. Death follows the coma in most cases. Only 2 to 5 percent of all cases of yellow fever result in death, though the figure may be higher during an epidemic. Persons who recover have a lifelong immunity to the disease.

In persons who live in the endemic areas and who have some immunity, the illness is much less severe and of shorter duration. In such people, yellow fever usually does not cause any permanent damage to the body, but full recovery may be attained only after several weeks or even months.

Q: *What is the treatment for yellow fever?*

A: There is no cure for yellow fever. The only treatment available is the administration of intravenous fluids, antinauseant drugs and, if necessary, kidney dialysis, as well as skilled medical and nursing care in the hospital.

Q: *Is there any protection against yellow fever?*

A: Yes. Immunization with an extremely mild yellow fever virus gives protection for 10 years. It should not be done within 3 weeks of a smallpox vaccination and not given to children under the age of 1 year, because there is a slight risk of causing encephalitis. It is also advisable not to immunize during pregnancy, even though fetal damage has not been detected.

An international certificate stating that a person has received immunization against yellow fever is valid for 10 years, starting 10 days after the injection. Such a certificate may be required of travelers to countries where the disease is prevalent.

Preventive measures include screening of living and working areas and mosquito control involving spraying and destruction of breeding areas. Mass immunization also helps to decrease the incidence of the disease.

Yellow jaundice. *See* JAUNDICE.

Zinc oxide (zingk ok′sīd) is a white, odorless powder that may be prepared in paste, lotion, cream, or powder form. It is used alone or combined with other substances as a soothing preparation in the treatment of eczema, varicose veins, and hemorrhoids, and around colostomies and ileostomies. It is also used as a dusting powder for prickly heat and, combined with mild antiseptics, as a cement for temporarily packing holes in the teeth (caries).

Zinc oxide is often used in preparations on special bandages that are applied to ulcerated or eczematous areas of the skin. The bandages are left in place several days to allow the underlying condition to heal.

Zoonosis (zō ə nō′sis) is any disease in animals that can be transmitted to humans, such as anthrax and rabies.

See also ANIMALS AND DISEASE; ANTHRAX; BRUCELLOSIS; CAT-SCRATCH FEVER; ENCEPHALITIS; LASSA FEVER; LYME DISEASE; PLAGUE; PSITTACOSIS; RABIES; ROCKY MOUNTAIN SPOTTED FEVER; SALMONELLA; TULAREMIA; YELLOW FEVER.

Zygote (zī′gōt) is the cell that is formed when a sperm fertilizes an egg (ovum).

See also FERTILIZATION; REPRODUCTION, HUMAN.

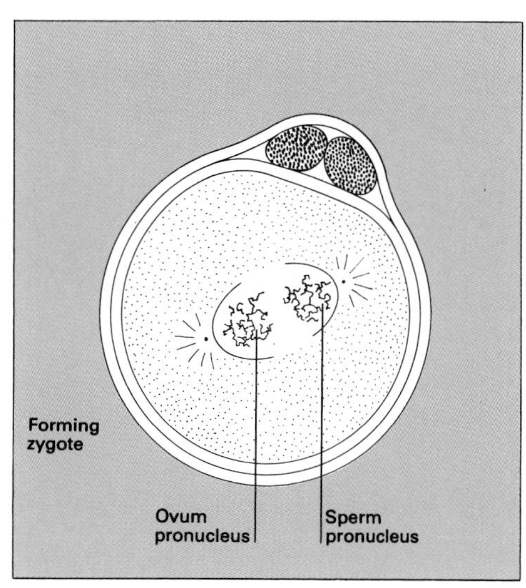

When a sperm and an ovum unite, their respective pronuclei also fuse together to form the nucleus of the new **zygote.**

Appendix: I

Charts of related symptoms

This section is most useful when two or more symptoms are present. By beginning with a symptom that is keenly felt and proceeding to less severe symptoms, a possible medical condition is suggested. This leads to a brief summary of suggested action (within the blue boxes). Finally, there is a full list of relevant articles in this encyclopedia.

The information contained in these charts is not intended to take the place of the care and attention of a physician or other medical or health care professional. On any matters related to health, always consult a physician or other appropriate health care professional.

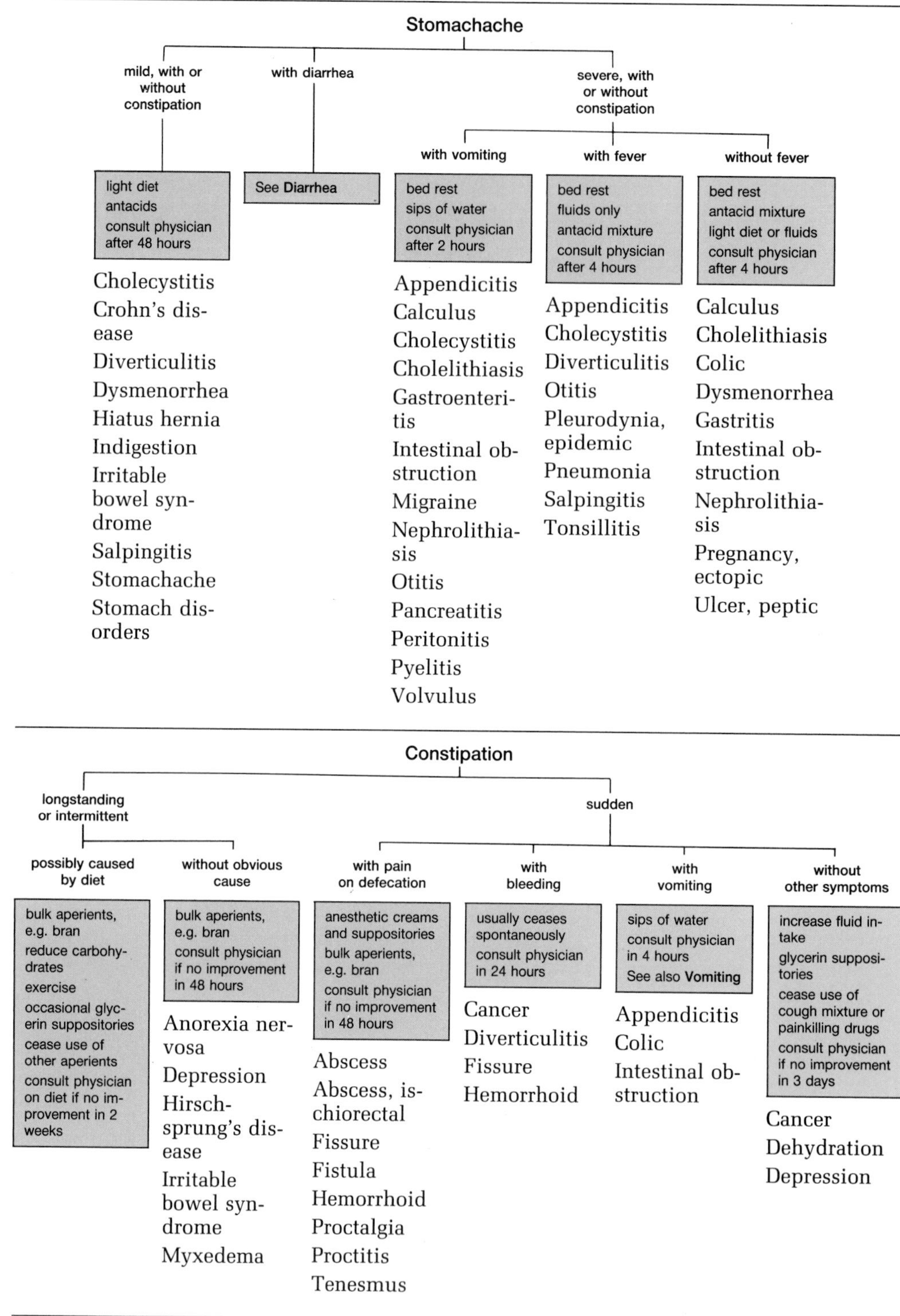
Stomachache
mild, with or without constipation
with diarrhea
severe, with or without constipation
with vomiting
with fever
without fever
light diet
antacids
consult physician after 48 hours
See Diarrhea
bed rest
sips of water
consult physician after 2 hours
bed rest
fluids only
antacid mixture
consult physician after 4 hours
bed rest
antacid mixture
light diet or fluids
consult physician after 4 hours
Cholecystitis
Crohn's disease
Diverticulitis
Dysmenorrhea
Hiatus hernia
Indigestion
Irritable bowel syndrome
Salpingitis
Stomachache
Stomach disorders
Appendicitis
Calculus
Cholecystitis
Cholelithiasis
Gastroenteritis
Intestinal obstruction
Migraine
Nephrolithiasis
Otitis
Pancreatitis
Peritonitis
Pyelitis
Volvulus
Appendicitis
Cholecystitis
Diverticulitis
Otitis
Pleurodynia, epidemic
Pneumonia
Salpingitis
Tonsillitis
Calculus
Cholelithiasis
Colic
Dysmenorrhea
Gastritis
Intestinal obstruction
Nephrolithiasis
Pregnancy, ectopic
Ulcer, peptic
Constipation
longstanding or intermittent
sudden
possibly caused by diet
without obvious cause
with pain on defecation
with bleeding
with vomiting
without other symptoms
bulk aperients, e.g. bran
reduce carbohydrates
exercise
occasional glycerin suppositories
cease use of other aperients
consult physician on diet if no improvement in 2 weeks
bulk aperients, e.g. bran
consult physician if no improvement in 48 hours
anesthetic creams and suppositories
bulk aperients, e.g. bran
consult physician if no improvement in 48 hours
usually ceases spontaneously
consult physician in 24 hours
sips of water
consult physician in 4 hours
See also Vomiting
increase fluid intake
glycerin suppositories
cease use of cough mixture or painkilling drugs
consult physician if no improvement in 3 days
Anorexia nervosa
Depression
Hirschsprung's disease
Irritable bowel syndrome
Myxedema
Abscess
Abscess, ischiorectal
Fissure
Fistula
Hemorrhoid
Proctalgia
Proctitis
Tenesmus
Cancer
Diverticulitis
Fissure
Hemorrhoid
Appendicitis
Colic
Intestinal obstruction
Cancer
Dehydration
Depression

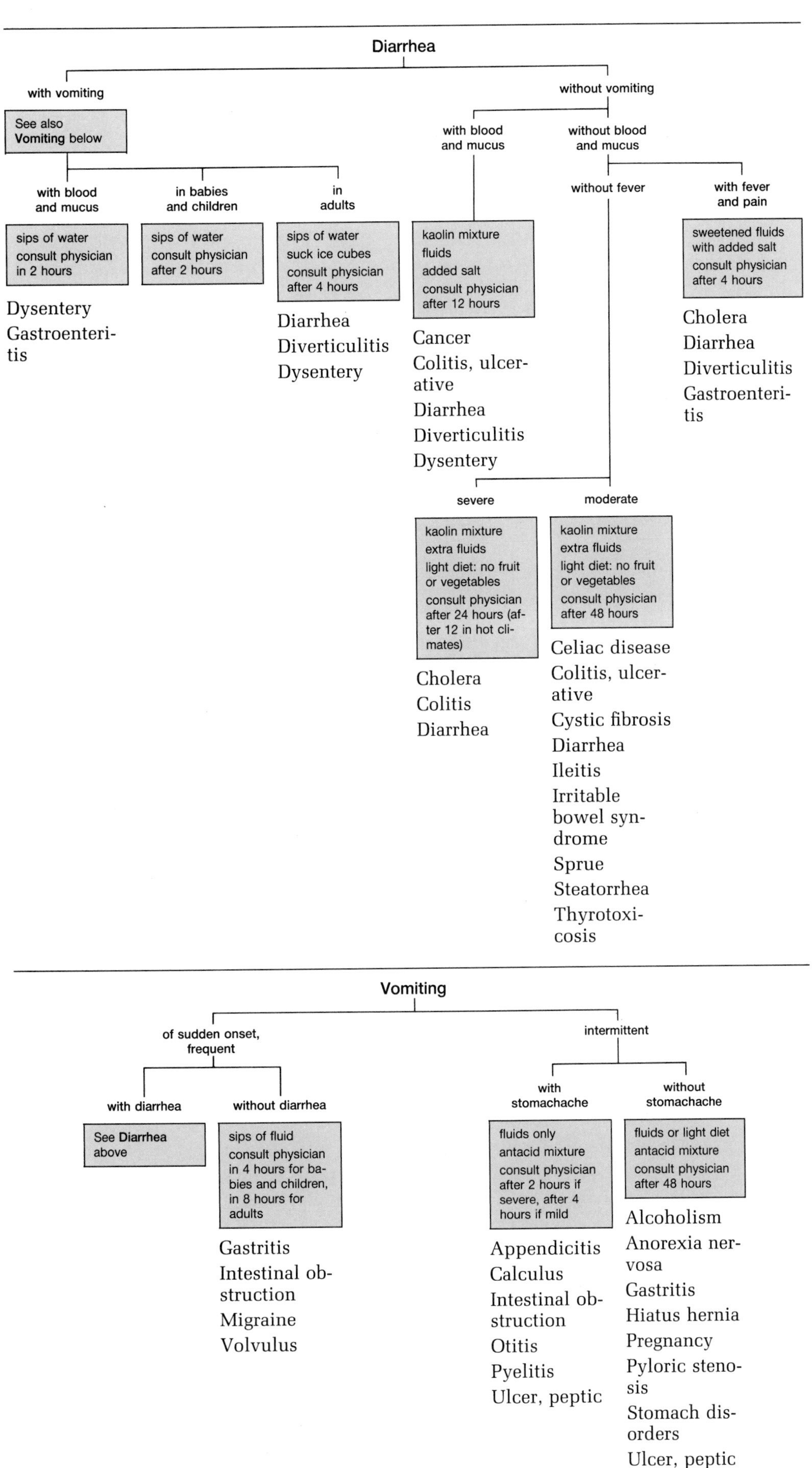

Diarrhea
with vomiting
See also Vomiting below
with blood and mucus
sips of water
consult physician in 2 hours
Dysentery
Gastroenteritis
in babies and children
sips of water
consult physician after 2 hours
in adults
sips of water
suck ice cubes
consult physician after 4 hours
Diarrhea
Diverticulitis
Dysentery
without vomiting
with blood and mucus
kaolin mixture
fluids
added salt
consult physician after 12 hours
Cancer
Colitis, ulcerative
Diarrhea
Diverticulitis
Dysentery
without blood and mucus
without fever
severe
kaolin mixture
extra fluids
light diet: no fruit or vegetables
consult physician after 24 hours (after 12 in hot climates)
Cholera
Colitis
Diarrhea
moderate
kaolin mixture
extra fluids
light diet: no fruit or vegetables
consult physician after 48 hours
Celiac disease
Colitis, ulcerative
Cystic fibrosis
Diarrhea
Ileitis
Irritable bowel syndrome
Sprue
Steatorrhea
Thyrotoxicosis
with fever and pain
sweetened fluids with added salt
consult physician after 4 hours
Cholera
Diarrhea
Diverticulitis
Gastroenteritis
Vomiting
of sudden onset, frequent
with diarrhea
See Diarrhea above
without diarrhea
sips of fluid
consult physician in 4 hours for babies and children, in 8 hours for adults
Gastritis
Intestinal obstruction
Migraine
Volvulus
intermittent
with stomachache
fluids only
antacid mixture
consult physician after 2 hours if severe, after 4 hours if mild
Appendicitis
Calculus
Intestinal obstruction
Otitis
Pyelitis
Ulcer, peptic
without stomachache
fluids or light diet
antacid mixture
consult physician after 48 hours
Alcoholism
Anorexia nervosa
Gastritis
Hiatus hernia
Pregnancy
Pyloric stenosis
Stomach disorders
Ulcer, peptic

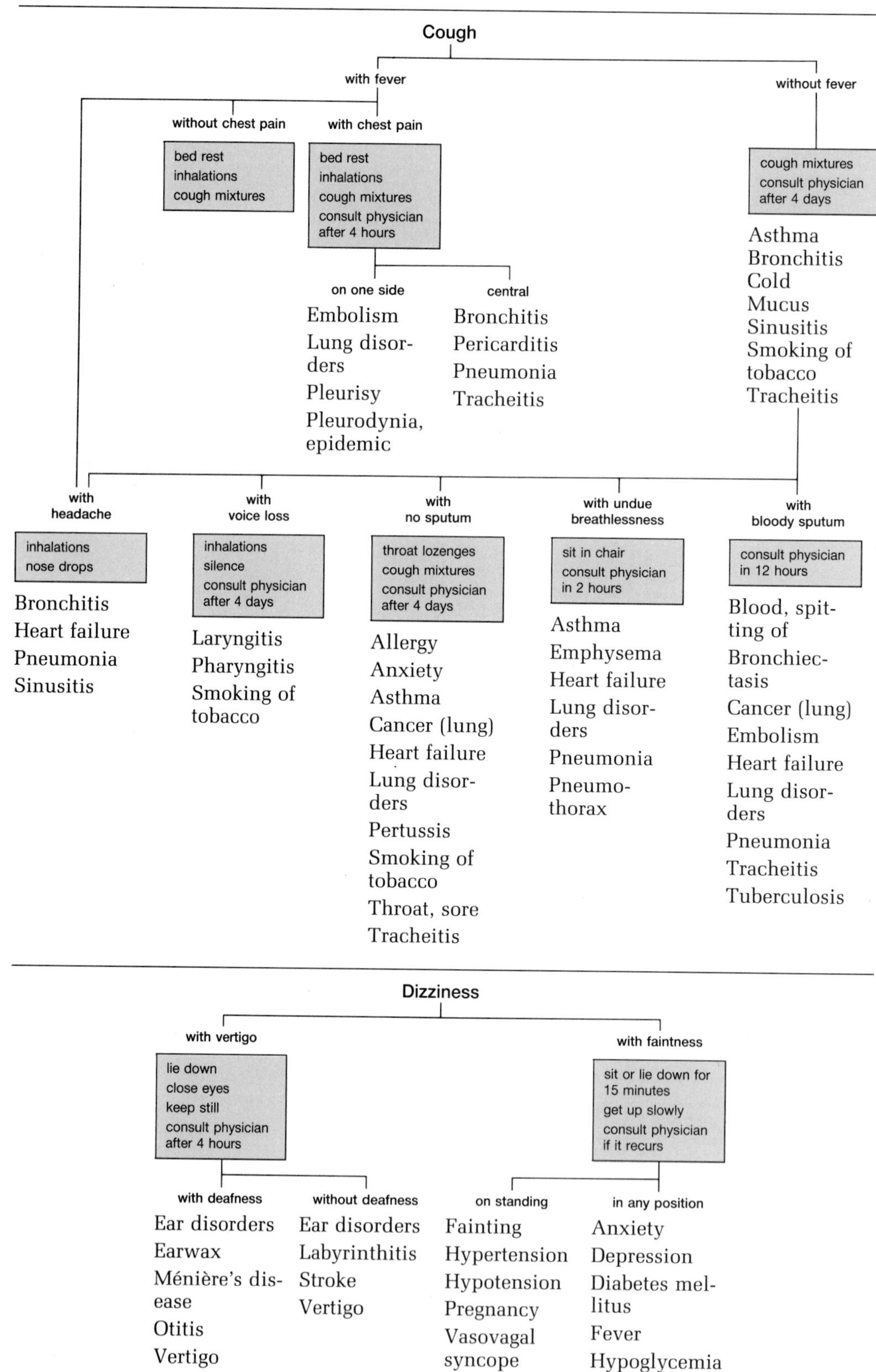
Cough
with fever
without fever
without chest pain
with chest pain
bed rest
inhalations
cough mixtures
bed rest
inhalations
cough mixtures
consult physician after 4 hours
cough mixtures
consult physician after 4 days
Asthma
Bronchitis
Cold
Mucus
Sinusitis
Smoking of tobacco
Tracheitis
on one side
central
Embolism
Lung disorders
Pleurisy
Pleurodynia, epidemic
Bronchitis
Pericarditis
Pneumonia
Tracheitis
with headache
with voice loss
with no sputum
with undue breathlessness
with bloody sputum
inhalations
nose drops
Bronchitis
Heart failure
Pneumonia
Sinusitis
inhalations
silence
consult physician after 4 days
Laryngitis
Pharyngitis
Smoking of tobacco
throat lozenges
cough mixtures
consult physician after 4 days
Allergy
Anxiety
Asthma
Cancer (lung)
Heart failure
Lung disorders
Pertussis
Smoking of tobacco
Throat, sore
Tracheitis
sit in chair
consult physician in 2 hours
Asthma
Emphysema
Heart failure
Lung disorders
Pneumonia
Pneumothorax
consult physician in 12 hours
Blood, spitting of
Bronchiectasis
Cancer (lung)
Embolism
Heart failure
Lung disorders
Pneumonia
Tracheitis
Tuberculosis
Dizziness
with vertigo
with faintness
lie down
close eyes
keep still
consult physician after 4 hours
sit or lie down for 15 minutes
get up slowly
consult physician if it recurs
with deafness
without deafness
on standing
in any position
Ear disorders
Earwax
Ménière's disease
Otitis
Vertigo
Ear disorders
Labyrinthitis
Stroke
Vertigo
Fainting
Hypertension
Hypotension
Pregnancy
Vasovagal syncope
Anxiety
Depression
Diabetes mellitus
Fever
Hypoglycemia

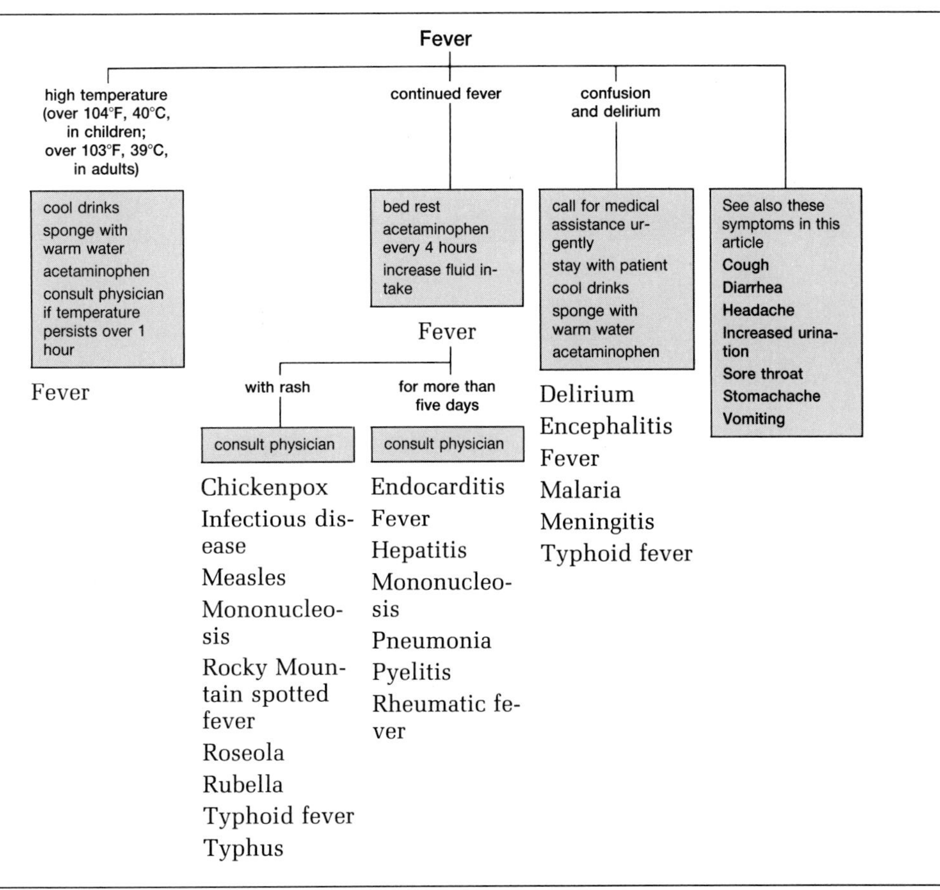
Fever
high temperature (over 104°F, 40°C, in children; over 103°F, 39°C, in adults)
cool drinks
sponge with warm water
acetaminophen
consult physician if temperature persists over 1 hour
Fever
continued fever
bed rest
acetaminophen every 4 hours
increase fluid intake
Fever
with rash
consult physician
Chickenpox
Infectious disease
Measles
Mononucleosis
Rocky Mountain spotted fever
Roseola
Rubella
Typhoid fever
Typhus
for more than five days
consult physician
Endocarditis
Fever
Hepatitis
Mononucleosis
Pneumonia
Pyelitis
Rheumatic fever
confusion and delirium
call for medical assistance urgently
stay with patient
cool drinks
sponge with warm water
acetaminophen
Delirium
Encephalitis
Fever
Malaria
Meningitis
Typhoid fever
See also these symptoms in this article
Cough
Diarrhea
Headache
Increased urination
Sore throat
Stomachache
Vomiting

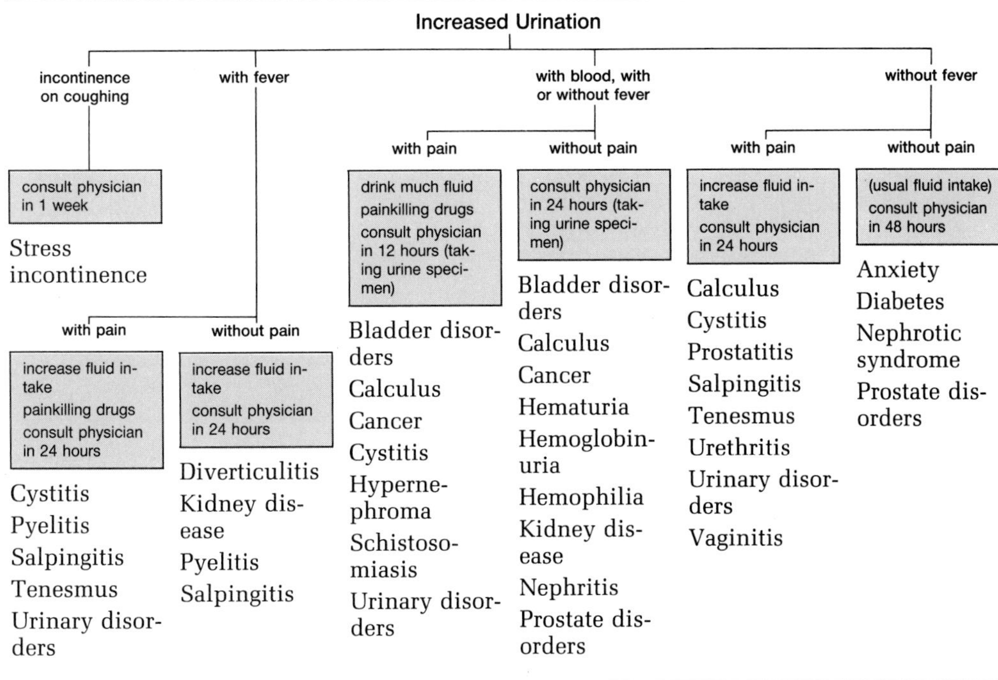
Increased Urination
incontinence on coughing
consult physician in 1 week
Stress incontinence
with fever
with pain
increase fluid intake
painkilling drugs
consult physician in 24 hours
Cystitis
Pyelitis
Salpingitis
Tenesmus
Urinary disorders
without pain
increase fluid intake
consult physician in 24 hours
Diverticulitis
Kidney disease
Pyelitis
Salpingitis
with blood, with or without fever
with pain
drink much fluid
painkilling drugs
consult physician in 12 hours (taking urine specimen)
Bladder disorders
Calculus
Cancer
Cystitis
Hypernephroma
Schistosomiasis
Urinary disorders
without pain
consult physician in 24 hours (taking urine specimen)
Bladder disorders
Calculus
Cancer
Hematuria
Hemoglobinuria
Hemophilia
Kidney disease
Nephritis
Prostate disorders
without fever
with pain
increase fluid intake
consult physician in 24 hours
Calculus
Cystitis
Prostatitis
Salpingitis
Tenesmus
Urethritis
Urinary disorders
Vaginitis
without pain
(usual fluid intake)
consult physician in 48 hours
Anxiety
Diabetes
Nephrotic syndrome
Prostate disorders

Chest Pain
any chest pain could be a heart attack and may need immediate attention
with tenderness to touch
heat or ice
mild pain relievers
consult physician if severe or persists
Anxiety
Bruise/Fracture: the spine or ribs
Fibromyalgia
Kyphosis
Neuritis
Shingles
Tietze's syndrome
with cough
cough mixtures
consult physician if persists or more ill
Asthma
Bronchitis
Lung disorders
Pneumonia
Smoking of tobacco
Tracheitis
worse with deep breath
mild pain relievers
heat or ice
if short of breath consult physician immediately
Embolism
Lung disorders
Pleurodynia, epidemic
Pneumonia
Pneumothorax
other
consult physician
Angina pectoris
Cholecystitis
Heart attack
Hiatus hernia
Pericarditis

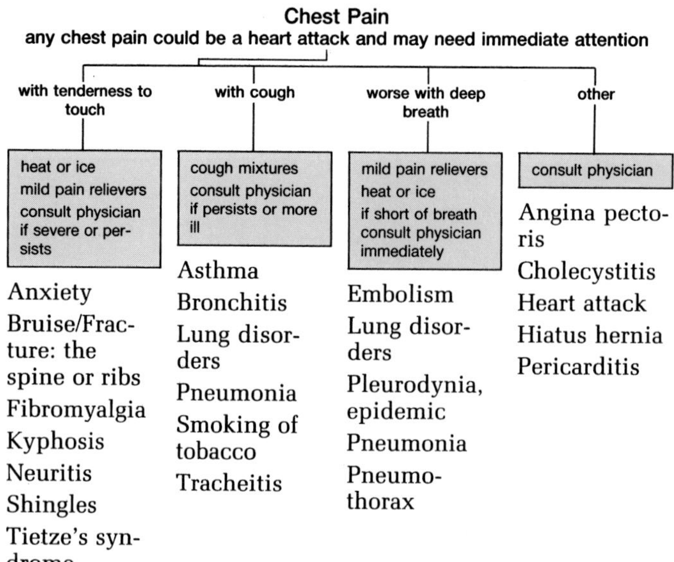

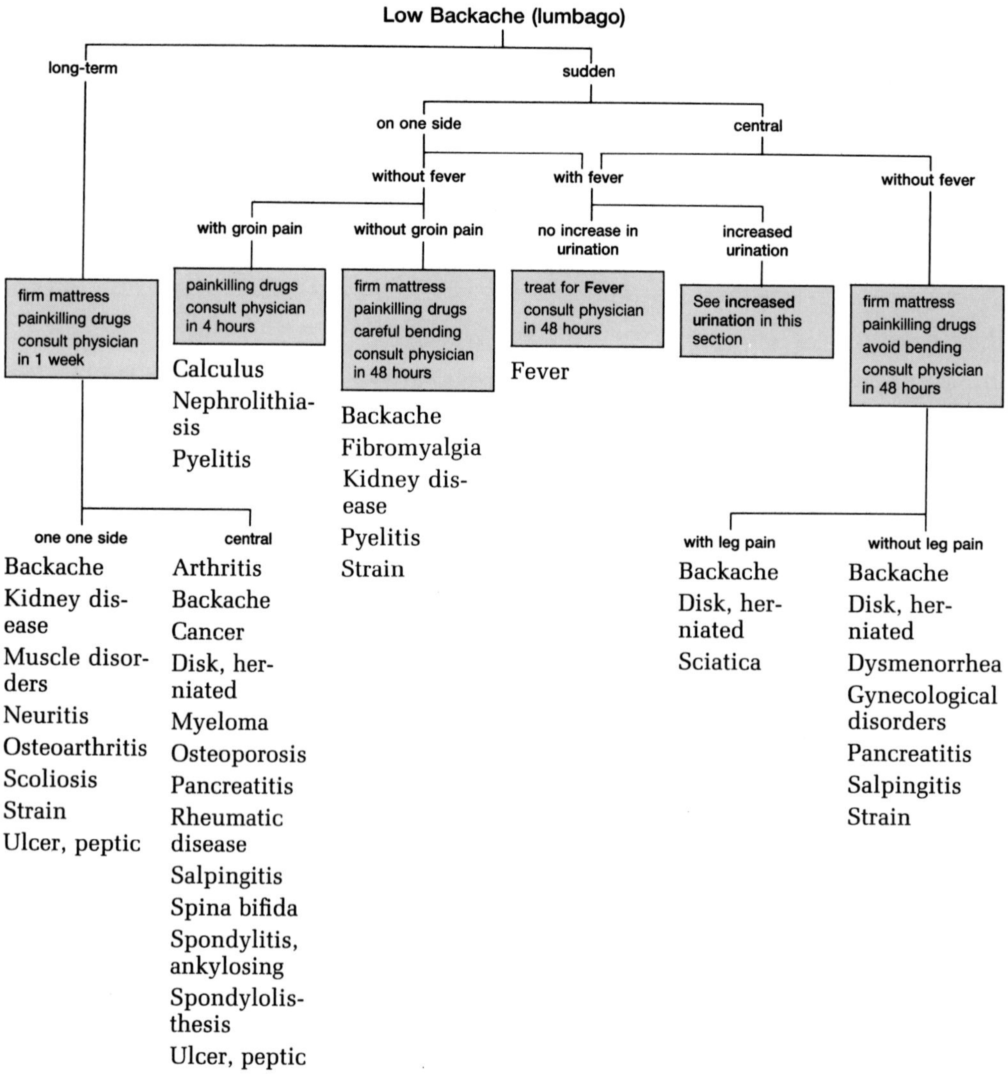

Low Backache (lumbago)
long-term
firm mattress
painkilling drugs
consult physician in 1 week
one one side
Backache
Kidney disease
Muscle disorders
Neuritis
Osteoarthritis
Scoliosis
Strain
Ulcer, peptic
central
Arthritis
Backache
Cancer
Disk, herniated
Myeloma
Osteoporosis
Pancreatitis
Rheumatic disease
Salpingitis
Spina bifida
Spondylitis, ankylosing
Spondylolisthesis
Ulcer, peptic
sudden
on one side
without fever
with groin pain
painkilling drugs
consult physician in 4 hours
Calculus
Nephrolithiasis
Pyelitis
without groin pain
firm mattress
painkilling drugs
careful bending
consult physician in 48 hours
Backache
Fibromyalgia
Kidney disease
Pyelitis
Strain
with fever
no increase in urination
treat for Fever
consult physician in 48 hours
Fever
increased urination
See increased urination in this section
central
without fever
firm mattress
painkilling drugs
avoid bending
consult physician in 48 hours
with leg pain
Backache
Disk, herniated
Sciatica
without leg pain
Backache
Disk, herniated
Dysmenorrhea
Gynecological disorders
Pancreatitis
Salpingitis
Strain

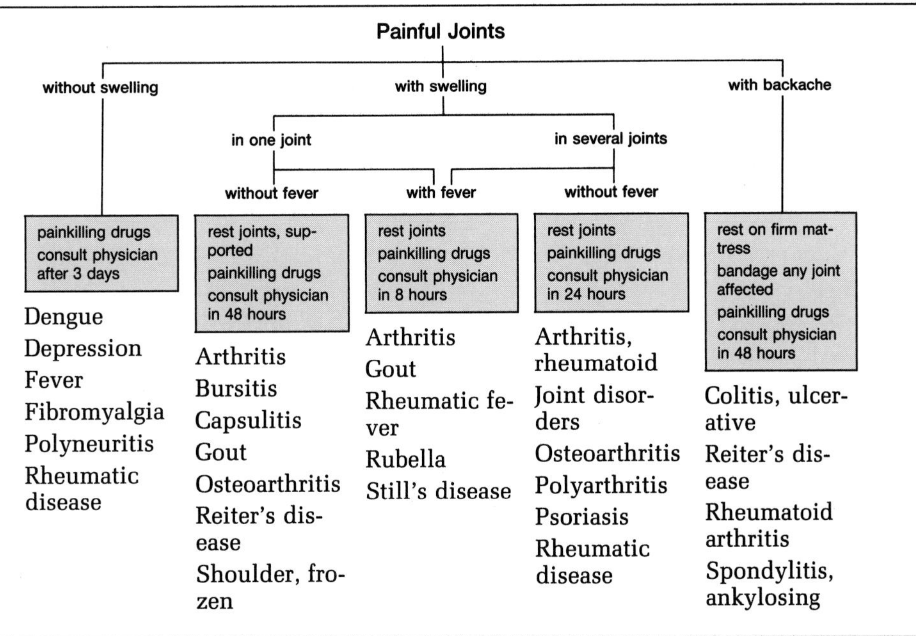

Painful Joints
without swelling
with swelling
with backache
in one joint
in several joints
without fever
with fever
without fever
painkilling drugs
consult physician after 3 days
Dengue
Depression
Fever
Fibromyalgia
Polyneuritis
Rheumatic disease
rest joints, supported
painkilling drugs
consult physician in 48 hours
Arthritis
Bursitis
Capsulitis
Gout
Osteoarthritis
Reiter's disease
Shoulder, frozen
rest joints
painkilling drugs
consult physician in 8 hours
Arthritis
Gout
Rheumatic fever
Rubella
Still's disease
rest joints
painkilling drugs
consult physician in 24 hours
Arthritis, rheumatoid
Joint disorders
Osteoarthritis
Polyarthritis
Psoriasis
Rheumatic disease
rest on firm mattress
bandage any joint affected
painkilling drugs
consult physician in 48 hours
Colitis, ulcerative
Reiter's disease
Rheumatoid arthritis
Spondylitis, ankylosing

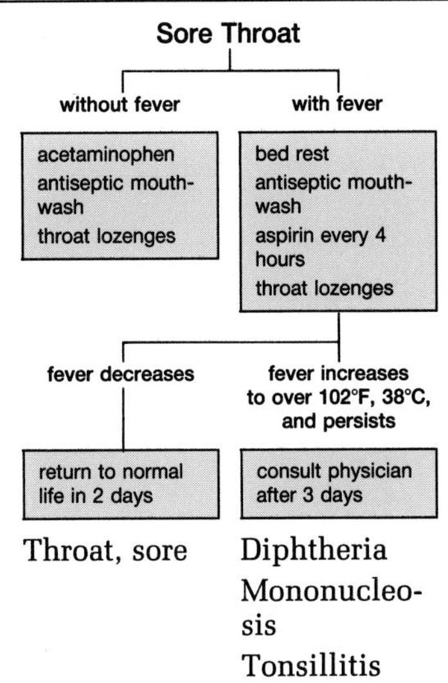

Sore Throat
without fever
with fever
acetaminophen
antiseptic mouthwash
throat lozenges
bed rest
antiseptic mouthwash
aspirin every 4 hours
throat lozenges
fever decreases
fever increases to over 102°F, 38°C, and persists
return to normal life in 2 days
consult physician after 3 days
Throat, sore
Diphtheria
Mononucleosis
Tonsillitis

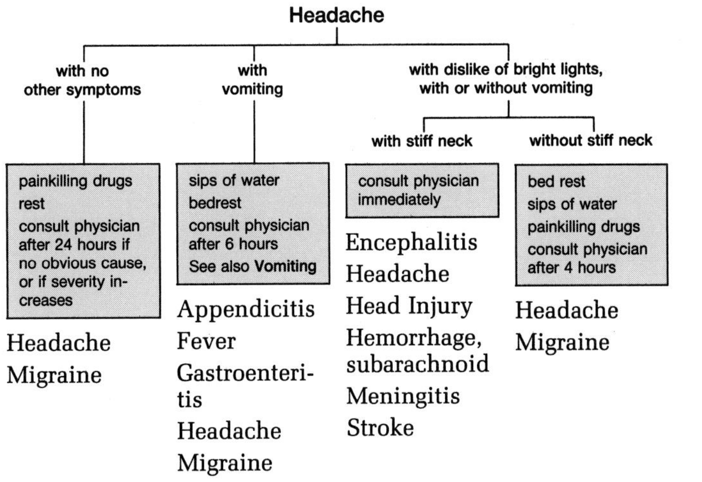

Headache
with no other symptoms
with vomiting
with dislike of bright lights, with or without vomiting
with stiff neck
without stiff neck
painkilling drugs
rest
consult physician after 24 hours if no obvious cause, or if severity increases
Headache
Migraine
sips of water
bedrest
consult physician after 6 hours
See also Vomiting
Appendicitis
Fever
Gastroenteritis
Headache
Migraine
consult physician immediately
Encephalitis
Headache
Head Injury
Hemorrhage, subarachnoid
Meningitis
Stroke
bed rest
sips of water
painkilling drugs
consult physician after 4 hours
Headache
Migraine

Appendix II

Pictorial Index of Symptoms

Each page of this pictorial index is dedicated to a specific part of the human body. Grouped around the central illustration on every page are boxes headed by an individual physical symptom. Each box contains the titles of all articles related to that symptom in the encyclopedia. The first box on each page lists general articles in the encyclopedia that give background information on the specific body part.

The eye

General articles
Blindness
Eye
Eye disorders

Blurred vision
Alcoholism
Amblyopia
Astigmatism
Cataract
Conjunctivitis
Diabetes
Eclampsia
Farsightedness
Glaucoma
Glioma
Iritis
Migraine
Multiple sclerosis
Myopia
Neuritis, retrobulbar
Retina, detached
Sarcoma

Double vision
Head injury
Multiple sclerosis
Strabismus
Vision, double

Impaired color perception
Color blindness

Intolerance of light
Conjunctivitis
Encephalitis
Hay fever
Iritis
Measles
Meningitis
Migraine

Spots in front of eyes
Hypertension
Migraine
Retina, detached
Retinitis

Squint
Strabismus

Blindness
Cataract
Diabetes
Glaucoma
Migraine
Neuritis, retrobulbar
Night blindness
Retina, detached
Snow blindness
Stroke
Trachoma
Ulcer

Watering eyes
Allergy
Blepharitis
Cold
Conjunctivitis
Dacryocystitis
Ectropion
Entropion
Hay fever
Sty
Tear

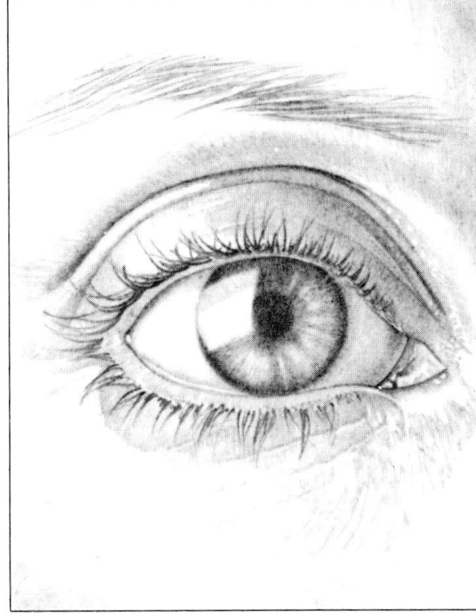

Red or pink eye
Allergy
Chemosis
Conjunctivitis
Glaucoma
Hay fever
Iritis
Marijuana
Measles
Red eye

Yellow eyes
Jaundice

Conjunctivitis
Allergy
Hay fever
Measles
Smoking of tobacco
Trachoma

Lump on lid
Carcinoma, basal cell
Chalazion
Melanoma
Mole
Papilloma
Sty
Wart
Xanthelasma

Cysts on lid
Chalazion
Sty

Gritty feeling
Allergy
Blepharitis
Chalazion
Chemosis
Conjunctivitis
Hay fever
Iritis
Sty
Ulcer
Xerophthalmia

Protruding eyes
Exophthalmos
Iritis
Proptosis
Thyrotoxicosis

Black eye
Bruise

Lids, drooping
Bell's palsy
Horner's syndrome
Myasthenia gravis
Ptosis
Stroke

Lids, sore
Allergy
Blepharitis
Chalazion
Ectropion
Entropion
Hay fever
Sty

Lids, swollen
Allergy
Angioneurotic edema
Blepharitis
Ectropion
Edema
Entropion
Hay fever
Nephritis
Sty

Lids, twitching
Anxiety

The head and face

General articles
Cranium
Headache
Salivary gland

Birthmarks
Birthmark
Hemangioma
Mole

Scalp, itching
Anxiety
Dandruff
Eczema
Nit
Ringworm
Seborrhea

Scales
Dandruff
Eczema
Psoriasis
Ringworm
Seborrhea

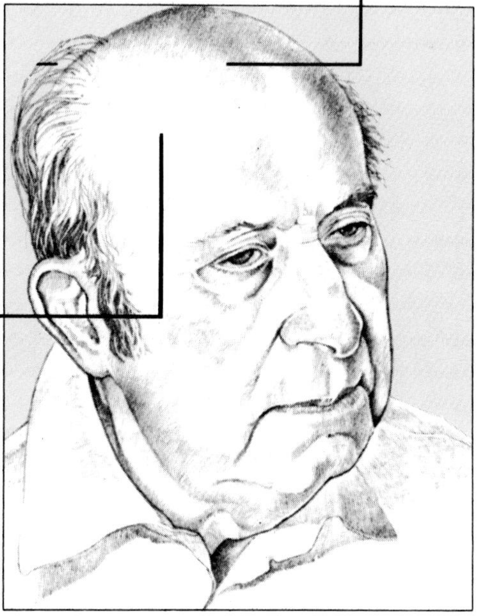

Headache
Allergy
Altitude sickness
Anxiety
Diabetes
Eye disorders
Hangover
Headache
Migraine
Sinusitis

Baldness
Alopecia
Baldness
Cyst, sebaceous
Eczema
Ringworm

Habit spasm
Anxiety
Neuralgia, trigeminal
Spasm
Tic

Pain in forehead
Headache
Herpes genitalis
Migraine
Neuralgia
Shingles
Sinusitis
Tumor

Paralysis or weakness
Bell's palsy
Mastoiditis
Motor neuron disease
Muscle disorders
Myasthenia gravis
Poliomyelitis
Polyneuritis
Stroke

Fainting
Adolescence
Arteriosclerosis
Diabetes
Epilepsy
Fainting
Menstruation
Pregnancy and childbirth

Hangover
Alcoholism
Hangover
Headache

Head, lumps
Bruise
Cyst, dermoid
Cyst, sebaceous
Head injury
Osteoma
Paget's disease of bone
Rickets
Wart

Concussion
Concussion
Headache
Head injury

Dizziness
Arteriosclerosis
Concussion
Dizziness
Ear disorders
Epilepsy
Ménière's disease
Migraine
Vertigo

See also
Ear
Eye
Mouth
Neck
Nose
Throat

Face, greasy
Acne
Rosacea
Seborrhea

Face, lumps
Abscess
Bites and stings: first aid
Boil
Bruise
Cyst, dermoid
Cyst, sebaceous
Dental disorders
Eye disorders
Hodgkin's disease
Lymph node
Mumps
Paget's disease of bone
Salivary gland
Sialolithiasis
Sinusitis
Tumor
Wart

Face, spots
Acne
Adolescence
Birthmark
Bites and stings: first aid
Blackhead
Boil
Carcinoma, basal cell
Folliculitis
Impetigo
Papule
Pimple
Pustule
Shingles
Wart

Face, rash
Allergy
Chickenpox
Measles
Roseola
Rubella
Scarlet fever
Typhoid fever

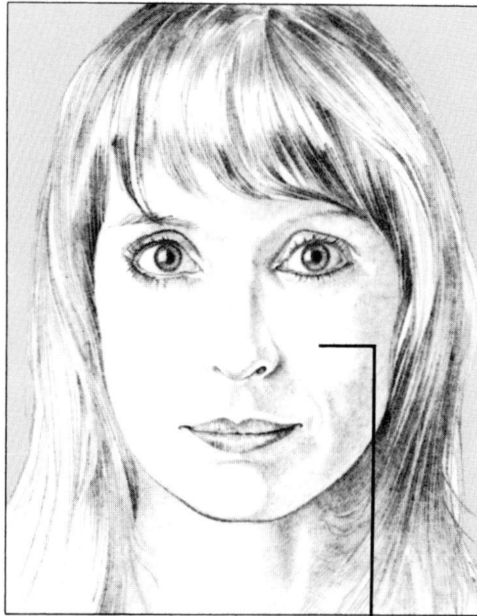

Face, swollen
Acromegaly
Allergy
Angioneurotic edema
Cushing's syndrome
Dental disorders
Eye disorders
Hydrocephalus
Mumps
Myxedema
Nephrotic syndrome
Paget's disease of bone
Pertussis

Pain in cheek
Boil
Dental disorders
Neuralgia
Shingles
Sinusitis
Tetanus
Toothache
Trigeminal neuralgia
Tumor

Skin, unusually yellow
Anemia, pernicious
Jaundice

Skin, pigment abnormalities
Freckle
Leprosy
Mole
Vitiligo

Skin, unusually brown
Addison's disease
Chloasma
Sunburn

Skin, unusually blue
Blue baby
Emphysema
Exposure
Heart disease

Skin, unusually pale
Anemia
Bleeding
Fainting
Kidney disease
Myxedema
Pallor
Shock

Skin, unusually red
Acne
Bruise
Erysipelas
Fever
Hot flash
Hypertension
Lupus erythematosus
Measles
Menopause
Polycythemia
Rosacea
Roseola
Rubella
Seborrhea

The mouth

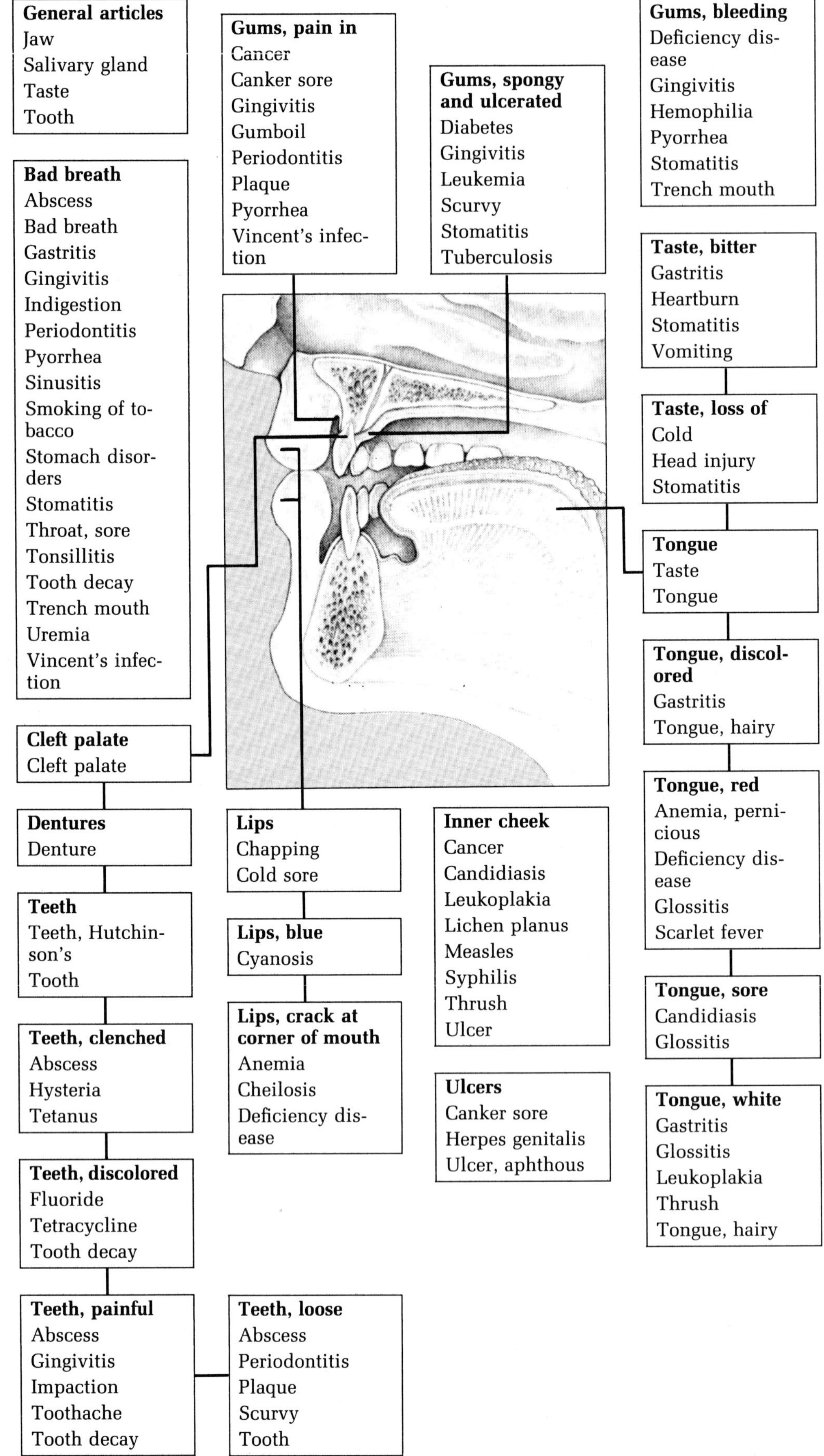
General articles
Jaw
Salivary gland
Taste
Tooth
Gums, pain in
Cancer
Canker sore
Gingivitis
Gumboil
Periodontitis
Plaque
Pyorrhea
Vincent's infection
Gums, spongy and ulcerated
Diabetes
Gingivitis
Leukemia
Scurvy
Stomatitis
Tuberculosis
Gums, bleeding
Deficiency disease
Gingivitis
Hemophilia
Pyorrhea
Stomatitis
Trench mouth
Bad breath
Abscess
Bad breath
Gastritis
Gingivitis
Indigestion
Periodontitis
Pyorrhea
Sinusitis
Smoking of tobacco
Stomach disorders
Stomatitis
Throat, sore
Tonsillitis
Tooth decay
Trench mouth
Uremia
Vincent's infection
Taste, bitter
Gastritis
Heartburn
Stomatitis
Vomiting
Taste, loss of
Cold
Head injury
Stomatitis
Tongue
Taste
Tongue
Tongue, discolored
Gastritis
Tongue, hairy
Cleft palate
Cleft palate
Dentures
Denture
Teeth
Teeth, Hutchinson's
Tooth
Teeth, clenched
Abscess
Hysteria
Tetanus
Teeth, discolored
Fluoride
Tetracycline
Tooth decay
Teeth, painful
Abscess
Gingivitis
Impaction
Toothache
Tooth decay
Lips
Chapping
Cold sore
Lips, blue
Cyanosis
Lips, crack at corner of mouth
Anemia
Cheilosis
Deficiency disease
Teeth, loose
Abscess
Periodontitis
Plaque
Scurvy
Tooth
Inner cheek
Cancer
Candidiasis
Leukoplakia
Lichen planus
Measles
Syphilis
Thrush
Ulcer
Ulcers
Canker sore
Herpes genitalis
Ulcer, aphthous
Tongue, red
Anemia, pernicious
Deficiency disease
Glossitis
Scarlet fever
Tongue, sore
Candidiasis
Glossitis
Tongue, white
Gastritis
Glossitis
Leukoplakia
Thrush
Tongue, hairy

The neck and throat

General articles
Larynx
Lymph node
Neck
Parathyroid gland
Pharynx
Swallowing
Throat
Thyroid gland
Tonsil

Adenoids
Adenoidectomy
Adenoids
Mucus
Snoring
Tonsil

Wryneck
Neck, stiff

Boils
Abscess
Boil

Lump on neck, stiff
Boil
Cyst, sebaceous
Neck, stiff
Whiplash injury

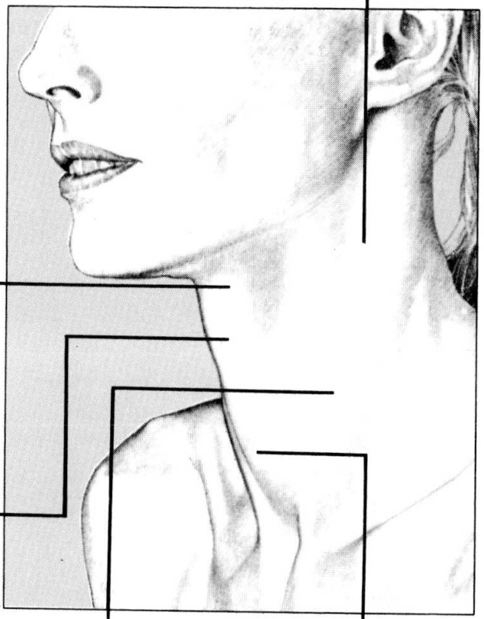

Swallowing, difficult
Achalasia
Bulbar paralysis
Esophagus
Tonsillitis

Swallowing, painful
Pharyngitis
Rheumatic fever
Tonsillitis
Throat, sore

"Lump in throat"
Globus hystericus
Goiter
Laryngitis
Lymph node
Pharyngitis

Altered voice
Laryngitis
Larynx
Muscle disorders
Neurological disorders

Cough
Cough
Laryngitis
Mucus
Pharyngitis
Sinusitis

Hoarseness
Laryngitis
Pharyngitis
Smoking
Tonsillitis

Swollen glands
Goiter
Hodgkin's disease
Leukemia
Lymph node
Lymphosarcoma
Mononucleosis
Tuberculosis

Swollen and painful glands
Lymph node
Mononucleosis
Mumps
Tonsil

Goiter
Goiter
Myxedema
Thyrotoxicosis

Neck, swollen
Goiter
Lymph node

Loss of voice
Aphasia
Aphonia
Laryngitis
Larynx
Mute

Sore throat
Abscess, peritonsillar
Mononucleosis
Pharyngitis
Throat, sore
Tonsillitis
Vincent's infection

The ear

General articles
Deafness
Ear
Ear disorders
Mastoid

Buzzing and ringing
Labyrinthitis
Ménière's disease
Otitis
Otosclerosis
Tinnitus

Deafness
Cold
Deafness
Earwax
Influenza
Ménière's disease
Mumps
Mute
Occupational hazard
Otitis
Otosclerosis
Scarlet fever

Discharge
Boil
Earwax
Mastoiditis
Otitis
Otorrhea

Dizziness
Concussion
Dizziness
Ménière's disease
Vertigo

Earache
Boil
Cold
Earache
Mastoiditis
Mumps
Occupational hazard
Otitis
Pharyngitis
Sinusitis
Tonsillitis

Itching
Chilblain
Dermatitis
Eczema
Otitis

Lumps on ear
Carcinoma, basal cell
Cyst, sebaceous
Pimple
Tumor

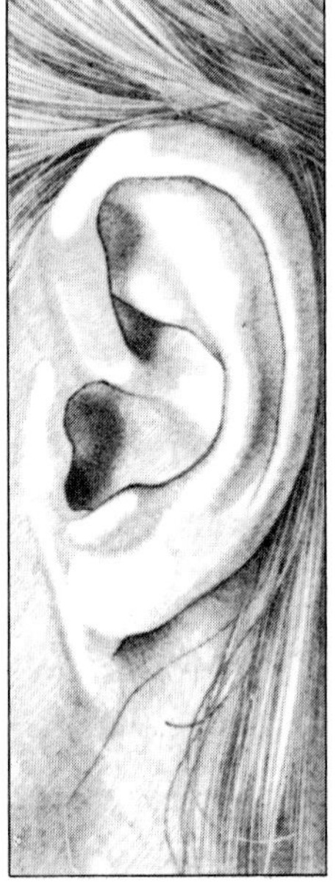

Blisters
Chilblain
Impetigo
Shingles

Boil
Boil
Carbuncle
Otitis

Mastoiditis
Mastoiditis

The nose

General articles
Nose
Smell, sense of

Red nose
Chapping
Cold
Influenza
Rhinophyma

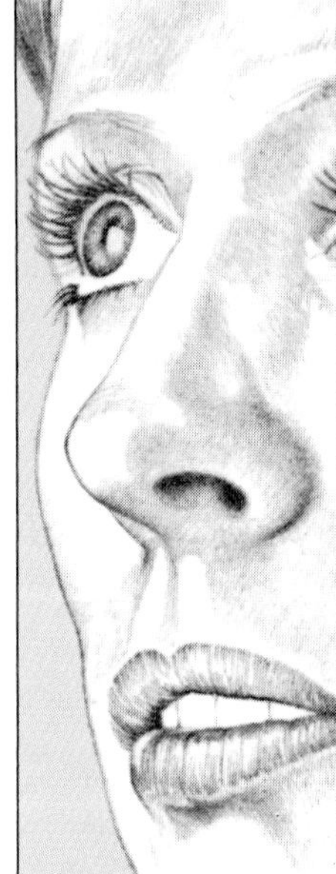

Blocked
Adenoids
Cold
Polyp
Rhinitis

Mucus
Adenoids
Allergy
Cold
Influenza
Mucus

Snoring
Adenoids
Nose, stuffy
Polyp
Septum, deviated
Snoring

Bleeding
Blood disorders
Hypertension
Nosebleed

Running nose
Allergy
Cold
Hay fever
Measles
Mucus
Nose, runny
Septum, deviated
Sneezing
Vasomotor rhinitis

Sneezing
Allergy
Cold
Influenza
Measles
Sneezing

Cold
Cold
Measles

Loss of smell
Cold
Head injury
Influenza
Mucus
Nose, stuffy
Smell, sense of

Swollen
Abscess
Boil
Cellulitis
Rhinophyma

See also
Head

Back, shoulder, arm, and hand

General articles
Armpit
Arthritis
Backache
Bone disorders
Elbow
Hand
Joint disorders
Muscle disorders
Muscle, pulled
Nail
Neurological disorders
Rheumatic disease
Scabies
Shoulder
Wrist

Shoulder
Arthritis
Dislocation
Shoulder, frozen

Sacrum
Myelocele
Sacrum
Sinus, pilonidal
Spina bifida

Back pain
Backache
Depression
Disk, herniated
Dysmenorrhea
Gall bladder
Osteoporosis
Sciatica
Spondylitis, ankylosing
Spondylolisthesis
Ulcer, peptic

Stiffness
Arthritis
Rheumatic disease
Spondylitis, ankylosing
Stiffness

Elbow
Bursitis
Capsulitis
Elbow injuries
Humerus
Osteoarthritis
Rheumatic disease
Rheumatic fever

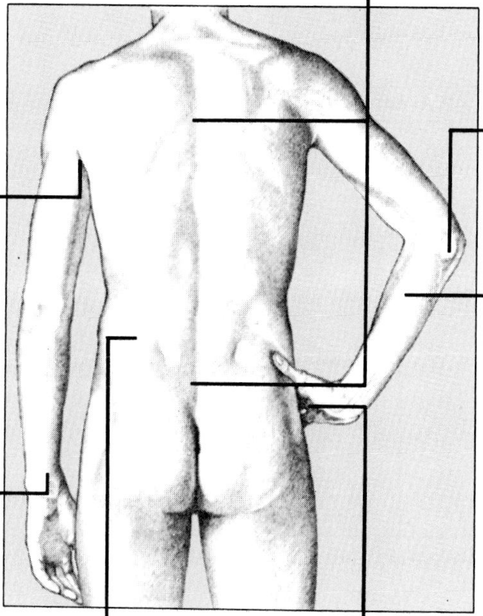

Armpit, sweating
Perspiration

Armpit, swollen
Boil
Bubo
Lymphatic system

Wrist
Colles' fracture
Wrist-drop

Arm, lumps
Bruise
Chondroma
Fibroma
Ganglion
Lipoma
Osteoma
von Recklinghausen's disease

Arm, painful
Causalgia
Fibromyalgia
Muscle, pulled
Neuralgia
Osteomyelitis
Spondylosis, cervical
Stiffness

Paralysis of the arm
Hysteria
Motor neuron disease
Muscle disorders
Neurological disorders
Poliomyelitis
Stroke

Weakness
Cerebral palsy
Muscle disorders

Finger, blistered
Allergy
Blister
Hand-foot-and-mouth disease
Pompholyx

Finger, lumps
Arthritis, rheumatoid
Heberden's node
Wart

Finger, painful
Arthritis
Arthritis, rheumatoid
Chilblain
Paronychia
Polyneuritis
Raynaud's phenomenon

Lower back pain
Back care
Kidney disease
Pancreatitis
Pyelonephritis
Shingles

Nails
Clubbing
Nail

Finger, stiff
Arthritis, rheumatoid
Capsulitis
Tenosynovitis

Hand, cramp
Carpal tunnel syndrome
Dupuytren's contracture
Scleroderma
Tetany

Hand, itching
Allergy
Dermatitis
Pompholyx
Scabies

Hand, shaking
Anxiety
Parkinson's disease
Thyrotoxicosis
Tremor

The female breast

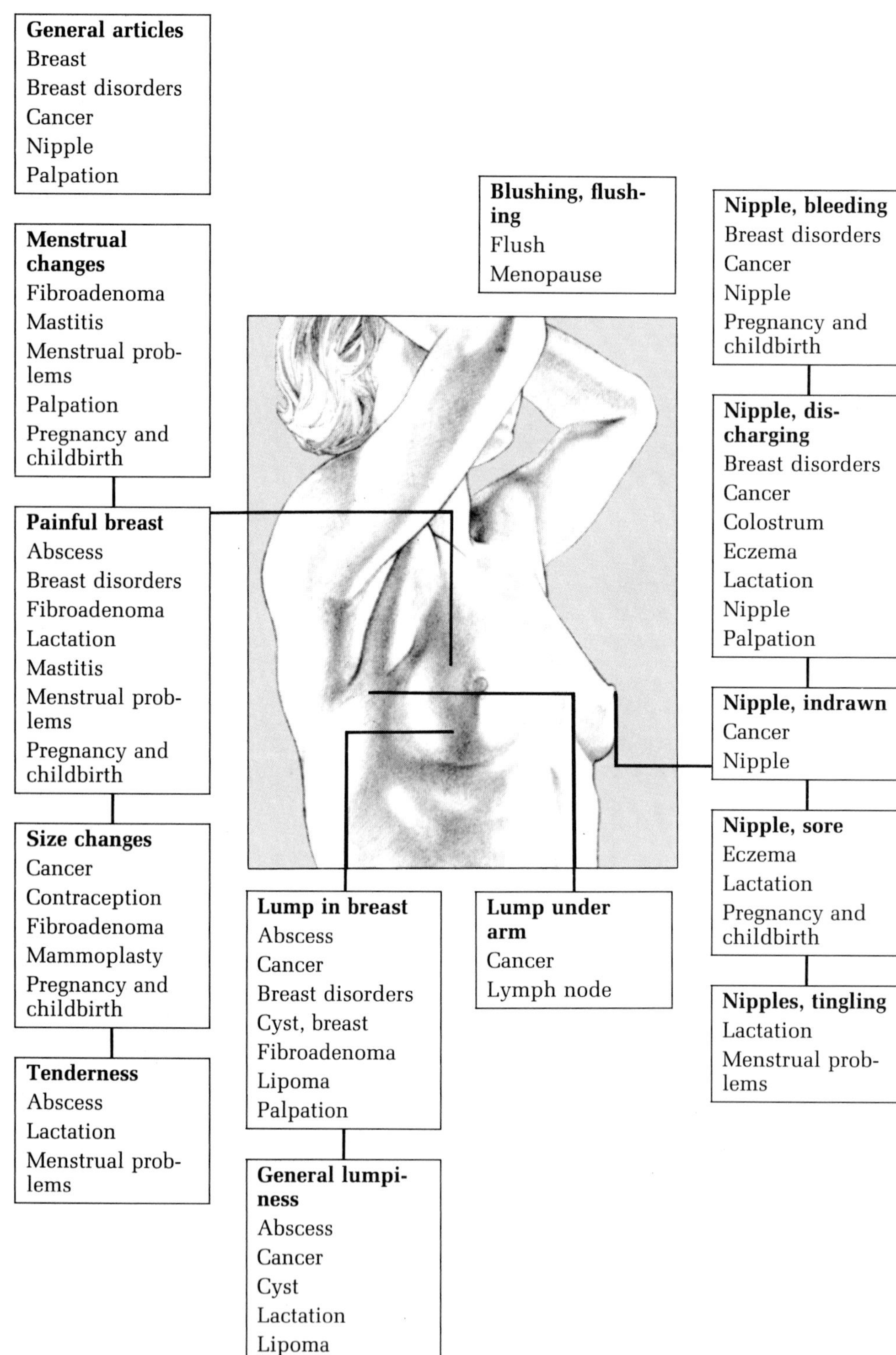

The chest

General articles
Arteriosclerosis
Heart disease
Lung disorders
Smoking of tobacco
Sternum
Valvular disease

Breathlessness
Anemia
Anxiety
Asthma
Atelectasis
Breathlessness
Emphysema
Heart failure
Hypertension
Lung disorders
Myocarditis
Obesity

Irregular breathing
Apnea
Cheyne-Stokes respiration

Pain on breathing
Embolism
Empyema
Pleurisy
Pleurodynia
Pneumonia
Tietze's syndrome
Tracheitis

Tightness in chest
Angina pectoris
Asthma
Breathlessness
Coronary heart disease
Emphysema
Heart failure
Pneumonia

Heartburn
Hiatus hernia
Indigestion

Chest pain
Abscess
Angina pectoris
Cancer
Heart disease, coronary
Hiatus hernia
Indigestion
Pericarditis
Pleurisy
Tietze's syndrome

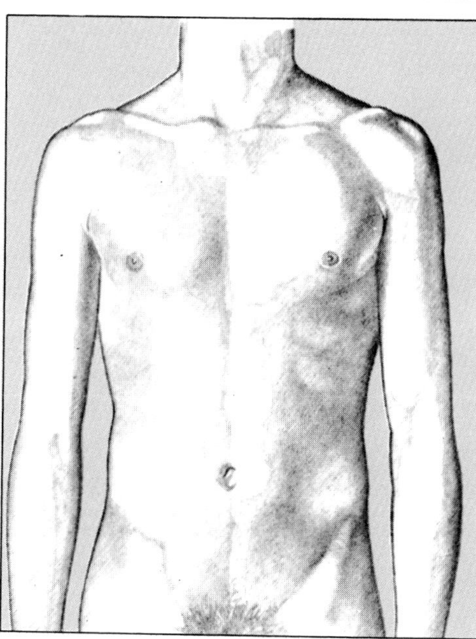

Cough
Bronchiectasis
Bronchitis
Bronchopneumonia
Cough
Croup
Laryngitis
Measles
Pertussis
Pharyngitis
Smoking of tobacco
Tracheitis
Tuberculosis

Wheezing
Asthma
Heart failure
Pneumonia

Lumps
Hernia
Lipoma
Tumor
von Recklinghausen's disease

Cyst
Cyst, sebaceous
Lipoma

Heart attack
Heart disease, coronary
Heart attack

Irregular heartbeat
Extrasystole
Palpitations
Stokes-Adams syndrome

Palpitations
Fibrillation
Indigestion
Palpitation
Tachycardia

Pain, ribs
Gallstone
Pleurodynia, epidemic

Pain, side
Colic
Shingles
Urinary tract infection

The abdomen

General articles
Abdominal pain
Colon
Gall bladder
Liver
Stomach
Stomach disorders

Liver
Cirrhosis
Hepatitis
Jaundice
Liver

Gall bladder
Colic, biliary
Gall bladder
Gallstone

Pain, top right and middle
Abdominal pain
Appendicitis
Cholecystitis
Gall bladder
Gallstone
Gastritis
Pancreatitis
Ulcer, peptic

Pain, abdominal
Aneurysm
Colic
Colitis
Crohn's disease
Food poisoning
Gastroenteritis
Intestinal obstruction
Intussusception
Pancreatitis
Peritonitis
Pleurisy
Stomachache
Stomach disorders
Urinary tract infection
Volvulus
Vomiting

Gas
Belching
Flatus
Gall bladder
Gastritis
Hiatus hernia

Hiccup
Hiatus hernia
Hiccup
Uremia

Indigestion
Cirrhosis
Gastritis
Heartburn
Hiatus hernia
Indigestion
Ulcer, peptic

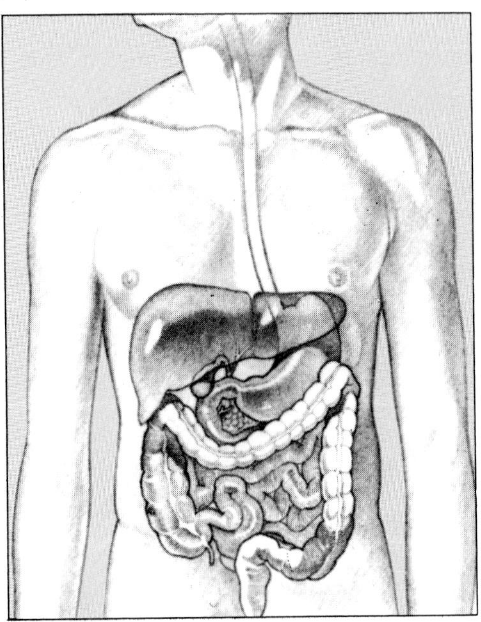

Pain, low
Appendicitis
Colitis
Diverticulitis
Diverticulosis
Dysmenorrhea
Labor pain, false
Pregnancy and childbirth
Pregnancy, ectopic
Salpingitis

Colon
Celiac disease
Colitis
Colon
Colostomy
Digestive system
Diverticulitis
Diverticulosis
Hernia

Internal parasites
Worm

See also
Anus
Heart
Rectum
Urinary system

Stomach
Cancer
Diet
Digestive system
Stomach disorders
Ulcer, peptic

Vomiting
Acidosis
Altitude sickness
Anxiety
Appendicitis
Cancer
Diabetes
Food poisoning
Gall bladder
Gallstone
Gastroenteritis
Hepatitis
Kidney disease
Ménière's disease
Meningitis
Migraine
Motion sickness
Pertussis
Poisoning
Pregnancy and childbirth
Ulcer, peptic
Vomiting

Vomiting, black
Blood, vomiting of

Vomiting, blood
Blood, vomiting of
Gastritis
Nosebleed

Vomiting, after food
Anorexia nervosa
Ulcer, peptic
Pyloric stenosis
Pylorospasm

Vomiting, at night
Hiatus hernia
Ulcer, peptic

The urinary system

General articles
Bladder
Bladder disorders
Cystitis
Kidney
Kidney disease
Urinary disorders
Urine

Urine flow, dribble
Bladder disorders
Incontinence
Prostate disorders
Urinary disorders

Urine flow, frequent
Alcohol
Anxiety
Bladder disorders
Cystitis
Diabetes mellitus
Kidney disease
Nephritis
Nephrotic syndrome
Nocturia
Polyuria
Pregnancy and childbirth
Prostate disorders
Pyelitis
Urinary disorders

Urine flow, hesitant
Anxiety
Bladder disorders
Prostate disorders

Stone
Calculus
Colic
Dysuria

Loin ache or pain
Abscess
Backache
Calculus
Kidney disease

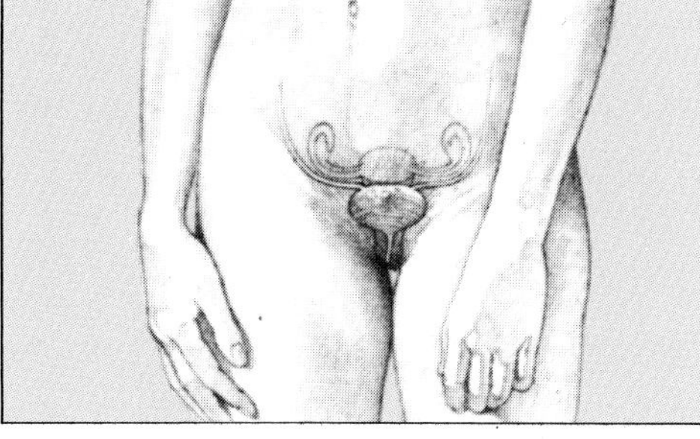

Urine flow, infrequent
Dehydration
Fever
Kidney disease
Oliguria
Preeclampsia

Urine flow, incontinent
Enuresis
Epilepsy
Incontinence
Neurological disorders
Stress incontinence
Stroke

Urine flow, with pain
Bladder disorders
Calculus
Cystitis
Dysuria
Prostate disorders
Pyelitis
Pyelonephritis
Sexually transmitted disease
Tenesmus

Inability to pass urine
Anuria
Anxiety
Pregnancy and childbirth
Prolapse
Prostate disorders
Retention
Tenesmus

Urine, blood in
Bladder disorders
Calculus
Cystitis
Hematuria
Hemoglobinuria
Kidney disease
Nephritis
Prostate disorders
Schistosomiasis
Urethritis
Urinary disorders

Urine, dark
Bladder disorders
Cystitis
Hemoglobinuria
Hepatitis
Jaundice
Oliguria
Porphyria
Urinary disorders

Urine, smoky
Calculus
Cystitis
Hematuria
Kidney disease
Pyelitis
Urinary disorders

See also
Reproduction, human

The female reproductive system

General articles
Gynecological disorders
Herpes genitalis
Menopause
Menstrual problems
Pregnancy and childbirth
Premenstrual syndrome
Sexual problems
Uterus
Vagina
Vulva

Fertility
Fertility
Infertility
Pregnancy and childbirth
Sterility

Ovary
Corpus luteum
Fertilization
Graafian follicle
Oophoritis
Ovulation
Ovum

Sexually transmitted disease
Gonorrhea
Sexually transmitted disease
Syphilis
Urethritis

Vulva
Clitoris
Labium
Vulva

Vulva, sore
Dyspareunia
Vulvitis

Vulva, swollen
Bartholin's cyst
Menstruation
Prolapse

Cervix
Cervical cancer
Cervical erosion
Cervical smear
Cervicitis
Contraception
Pregnancy and childbirth

Fallopian tube
Fallopian tube
Fertilization
Ovulation
Ovum
Pregnancy, ectopic
Salpingitis
Sterilization

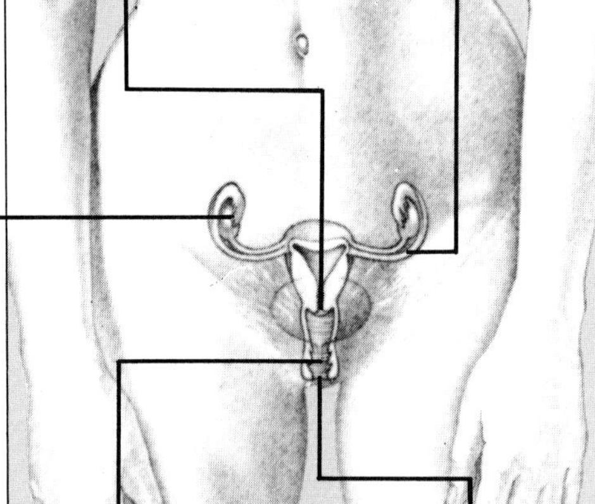

Intercourse, pain
Dyspareunia
Hymen
Sexual problems
Vaginismus

Vagina
Contraception
Pregnancy and childbirth

Vaginal itching and irritation
Candidiasis
Gonorrhea
Sexually transmitted disease
Trichomonas vaginalis
Urethritis
Vaginitis
Vulvitis

Vaginal discharge
Adolescence
Cervical cancer
Cervical erosion
Cervicitis
Endometritis
Gonorrhea
Lochia
Ovulation
Salpingitis
Candidiasis
Sexually transmitted disease
Urethritis
Vaginitis

Uterus
Contraception
Menstruation
Pregnancy and childbirth
Uterus

Bleeding after menopause
Cervical cancer
Cervical erosion
Cervicitis
Menopause

Pain in midcycle
Menstrual problems
Ovulation

Periods, flooding or heavy
Adolescence
Abortion
Endometritis
Fibroid
Menorrhagia
Menstrual problems

Periods, irregular
Adolescence
Anxiety
Menopause
Menstrual problems

Periods, nonexistent
Hematocolpos
Infertility
Menarche

Periods, painful
Dysmenorrhea
Endometriosis
Intrauterine device
Salpingitis

Periods, stopped
Adolescence
Amenorrhea
Anorexia nervosa
Contraception
Menopause
Pregnancy and childbirth
Pregnancy, false

See also
Abdomen
Urinary system

The male reproductive system

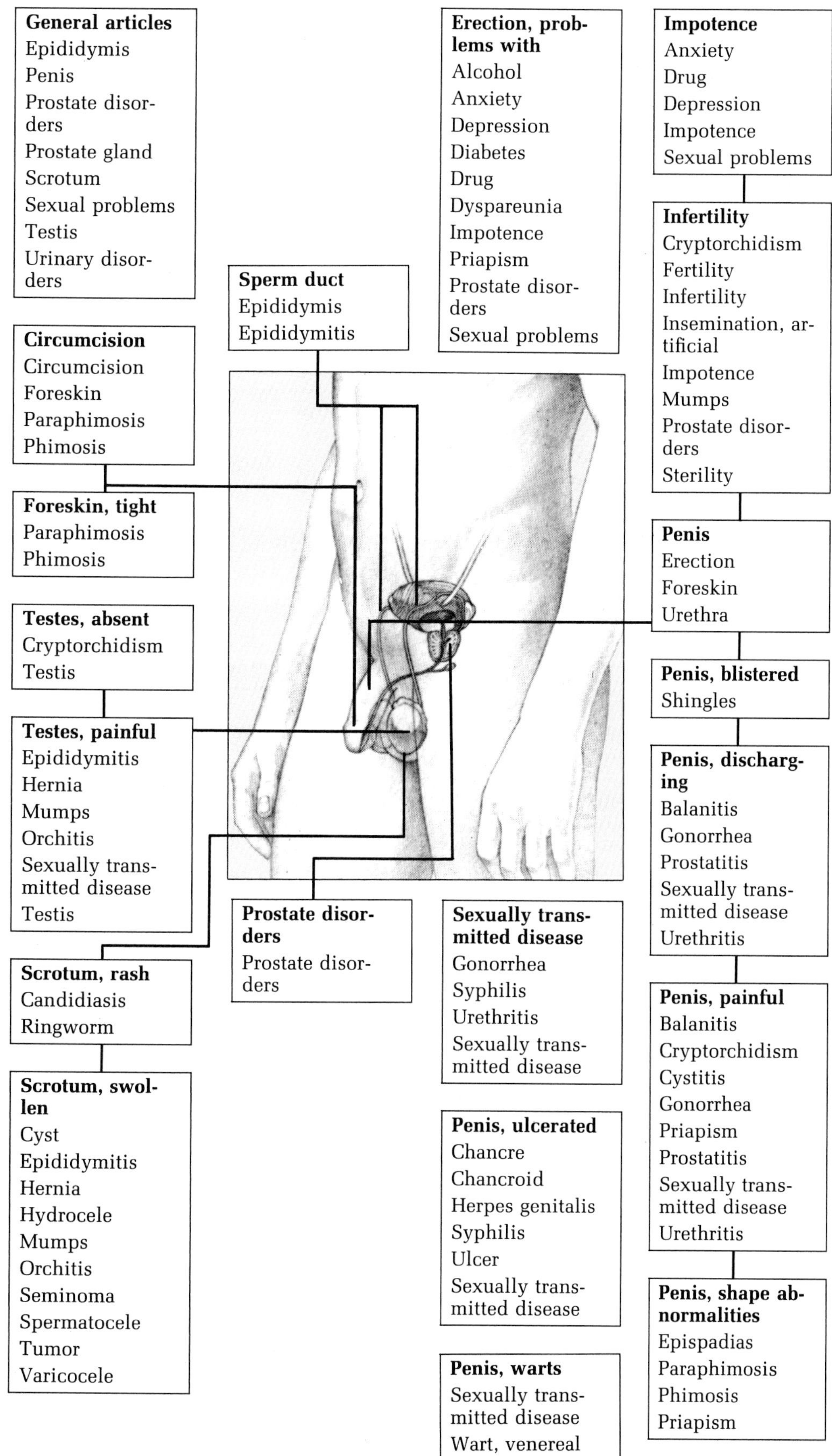

See also Abdomen and Urinary system

The anus and the rectum

General articles
Anus
Constipation
Diarrhea
Hemorrhoid
Rectum
Skin disorders

Feces
Constipation
Diarrhea
Feces

Feces, black
Cancer
Melena
Ulcer, peptic

Feces, greasy
Celiac disease
Crohn's disease
Gall bladder
Hepatitis
Sprue

Feces, red
Cancer
Diverticulitis
Diverticulosis
Dysentery
Hemorrhoid
Intussusception

Feces, white
Celiac disease
Jaundice
Steatorrhea

Pain at base of back
Abscess
Abscess, ischio-rectal
Bedsore
Coccyx
Pregnancy and childbirth
Sinus, pilonidal

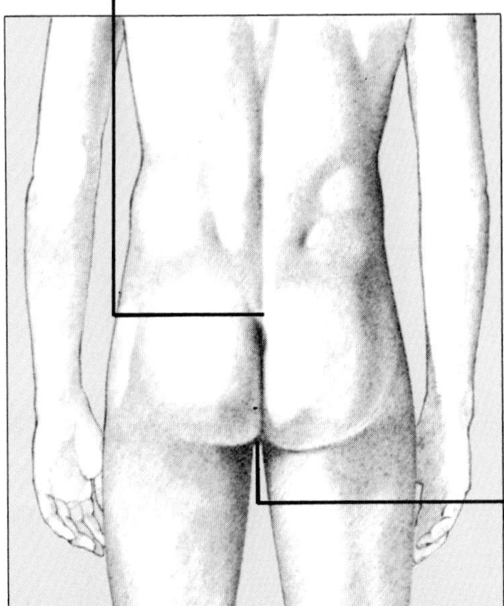

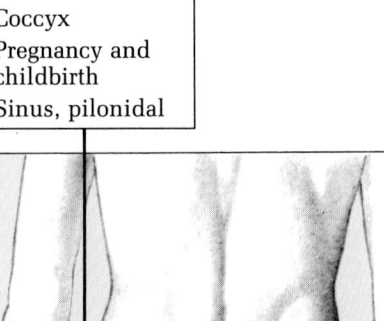

Diarrhea
Celiac disease
Cholera
Colitis
Cystic fibrosis
Diarrhea
Diverticulitis
Diverticulosis
Dysentery
Food poisoning
Gastroenteritis
Hepatitis
Ileitis
Sprue
Steatorrhea
Thyrotoxicosis
Typhoid fever

Constipation
Anxiety
Cancer
Constipation
Diverticulitis
Diverticulosis
Hemorrhoid
Hirschsprung's disease
Intestinal obstruction
Myxedema
Pregnancy and childbirth

Bleeding
Colitis
Diverticulitis
Diverticulosis
Dysentery
Fissure
Hemorrhoid
Polyp
Schistosomiasis
Sinus, pilonidal

Itching
Candidiasis
Hemorrhoid
Scabies
Worms

Pain in anus
Abscess
Cancer
Fissure
Fistula
Hemorrhoid
Proctalgia
Proctitis
Tenesmus

Piles
Cirrhosis
Constipation
Hemorrhoid
Pregnancy and childbirth

Protrusion from anus
Hemorrhoid
Intussusception
Polyp
Prolapse
Wart

Lump
Hemorrhoid
Intussusception
Polyp
Rectum
Sinus, pilonidal

Worms
Worm

See also
Abdomen

Leg, hip, knee, and foot

General articles
Ankle
Arthritis
Foot
Heel
Joint disorders
Knee
Muscle disorders
Muscle, pulled
Nail
Neurological disorders
Rheumatic disease

Paralysis
Hysteria
Neurological disorders
Poliomyelitis
Stroke

Weakness
Cerebral palsy
Muscle disorders
Weakness

Achilles tendon
Tendinitis
Tendon

Ankle, painful
Arthritis
Gout
Joint disorders
Pott's fracture
Rheumatic disease
Sprain

Ankle, swollen
Ankle
Edema
Kidney disease
Pregnancy and childbirth
Thrombophlebitis

Sciatica
Back pain, lower
Disk, herniated
Sciatica

Hip, painful
Arthritis
Perthes' disease
Rheumatic disease

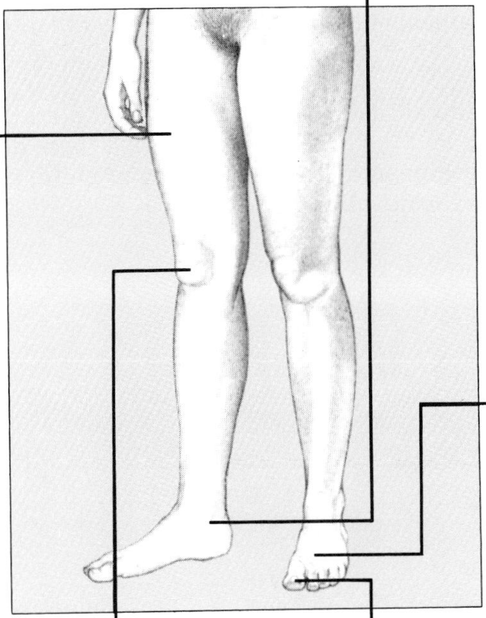

Unsteadiness
Ataxia
Neurological disorders
Parkinson's disease

Limping
Claudication
Perthes' disease

Lumps
Bruise
Chondroma
Erythema nodosum
Fibroma
Melanoma
Osteoma
Varicose vein
von Recklinghausen's disease

Pain in calf or thigh
Buerger's disease
Causalgia
Claudication
Cramp
Osteomyelitis
Phlebitis
Sciatica
Tabes dorsalis
Tenosynovitis
Thrombophlebitis

Knee, locked
Cartilage
Chondromalacia
Osteochondritis

Knee, painful
Arthritis
Chondromalacia
Rheumatic disease
Sprain

Knee, swollen
Arthritis
Bursitis
Cartilage
Chondromalacia
Gout
Sprain

Toes
Chilblain
Corn
Pigeon-toed
Ringworm
Toenail, ingrown

Foot, ulcerated
Diabetes
Ulcer

Foot, tingling
Chilblain
Polyneuritis

Foot, blistered
Allergy
Blister
Chilblain
Foot, immersion
Hand-foot-and-mouth disease
Pompholyx
Verruca

Foot, itching
Athlete's foot
Candidiasis
Hyperhidrosis
Pompholyx
Ringworm

Foot, lumps
Bunion
Corn
Hammertoe
Wart

Foot, painful
Arthritis
Buerger's disease
Callus
Chilblain
Foot disorders
Pregnancy and childbirth

Appendix III

Age-by-age charts

This age-by-age appendix is divided into nine sections, five of which pertain to childhood (at birth, infant, preschool child, elementary school child, and adolescent), and four of which pertain to adulthood (young adult, mature adult, middle-aged, and senior citizen).

Each section contains alphabetical listings of disorders that may occur in that age range, with descriptions of their symptoms, treatment, and additional comments relating to that disorder.

Additionally, the childhood sections contain charts of normal physical, emotional, and mental development, and the average age at which these developments occur. Because there is no such thing as an "average" baby or child, parents are advised to use these charts as approximate guidelines.

Section 1

At birth: introduction

In most cases a newborn child is normal and healthy. Prenatal checkups are an important part of health care during pregnancy and can do much to make the birth trouble-free.

Furthermore, with modern prenatal care, if a baby is not developing normally, this can be detected before the birth so that appropriate action can be taken to ensure the baby survives with neonatal care. Certain fetal health conditions can be altered prior to birth using procedures such as a fetal blood transfusion performed in utero. Early detection of certain fetal health problems enables the parents to consider terminating the pregnancy.

Examination of the mother's blood, to detect the presence of alpha fetoprotein, may indicate deformities such as spina bifida or anencephaly (absence of the brain and spinal cord) in the fetus. Examination of the fluid that surrounds the fetus during pregnancy (amniocentesis) may be used to check for abnormal cells or chemicals.

A relatively new technique for discovering certain congenital anomalies that can be used during the first trimester of pregnancy is the CVB, or chorionic villus biopsy, in which ultrasound guides the physician's instrument toward the placenta, from which sample tissue is taken for biopsy.

Congenital anomalies are found in about two-and-a-half percent of all babies. They arise from the faulty development of a fetus, caused either by genetic disorders or other factors, such as maternal alcohol abuse. These include bone disorders, cataract, cleft palate, hypothyroidism, Down's syndrome, endocrine gland disorders, heart disease, hemophilia, joint disorders, pyloric stenosis (a stomach deformity) and spina bifida. Often more than one anomaly is present.

The chances of giving birth to an abnormal child may be minimized by taking certain precautions before and during pregnancy. Because some congenital anomalies are caused by chromosomal abnormalities, genetic counseling may be undertaken to advise parents about the likelihood of transmitting hereditary disorders or of bearing a deformed child. Infections, such as rubella, may cause abnormalities, and therefore, the mother should be immunized against rubella at least three months before conceiving. Drugs that are potentially harmful should not be taken during pregnancy, and a pregnant woman, or a woman who suspects she is pregnant, should not undergo X-ray examination unless absolutely necessary.

A poor diet and consumption of alcohol during pregnancy are both thought to be significant causes of congenital illness. Physical deformities may occur to a fetus that grows in an awkward position in the uterus; damage may also occur if an object, such as a contraceptive intrauterine device (IUD), remains in the uterus as the fetus is developing.

Finally, some anomalies may be inherited. These may be obvious at birth, as in the case of a cleft palate, or appear only later in childhood, as in the case of Tay-Sachs disease.

The birth process

The table below summarizes the process of childbirth, from the onset of labor to the delivery of the baby. Cross-references are within this section unless otherwise specified.

Stage	*Symptoms*	*Duration*
Onset of labor This is usually identified by one of three events. (1) The "show," which is the discharge of a bloodstreaked, jelly-like substance from the vagina, caused by loosening of the plug of mucus from the cervix. (2) "Breaking the waters," which occurs when the bag (amniotic sac) surrounding the baby and containing the waters (amniotic fluid) starts to leak. (3) Contractions of the uterus. Regular, powerful contractions occurring at 10- to 30-minute intervals.	Dragging pains in the abdomen; slight nausea; lower back pain; aching at the top of the legs.	
Stage one Labor begins with the contractions of the uterus. Contractions feel like cramp pains in the abdomen and lower back. The cervix dilates gradually with each contraction until it becomes wide enough to allow the baby to emerge. The cervix is about 4 inches (10 cm) wide when fully dilated.	Lower abdominal discomfort and pain. Contractions occur at intervals of 3 to 10 minutes.	3 to 24 hours (16 hours on average) for a first baby; 1 to 24 hours (6 hours on average) for subsequent births.
Stage two The second stage of labor begins when the cervix is fully open. The mother usually feels a strong urge to push or "bear down." The baby normally passes head first through the birth canal. When the baby's head has emerged, it is seen to rotate. Then further contractions are usually followed by the emergence of first one shoulder and then the other. When the shoulders have emerged, the rest of the baby follows easily.	Discomfort in lower pelvis; strong urge to bear down. Forceful contractions every 2 to 3 minutes, each lasting about 1 minute.	30 to 120 minutes for a first baby; less than 20 minutes for subsequent births.
Stage three The period from the delivery of the child to the delivery of the afterbirth (placenta).	Usually no discomfort. Some contractions while the afterbirth is being expelled.	5 to 15 minutes in most cases.

At birth: disorders

Symptoms and Signs	*Treatment*	*Notes*
Angioma See BIRTHMARK: ANGIOMA.		
Birthmark: angioma Swelling made up of blood vessels or lymph vessels; usually occurring in skin.	None required unless angioma presses on an important body structure; usually disappears naturally within about five years.	
Birthmark: mole Small area of pigmentation of the skin; often slightly raised; occurring anywhere on the body.	Moles present at birth have a higher risk of future malignancy and generally should be removed.	
Birthmark: Mongolian spots Area of pigmentation that may be slate gray to blue in color; usually on the lower part of the back; sometimes on the thigh.	None; usually disappears naturally within a few years.	
Birthmark: port-wine stain A flat, purple, or deep-red discoloration of an area of skin caused by abnormalities in the blood vessels.	Surgical removal, if the birthmark is small, so that removal does not cause extensive scarring; camouflage of stain for cosmetic reasons.	A port-wine stain remains the same size in proportion to the rest of the body as the child grows.

At birth: disorders *(Continued)*

Symptoms and Signs	*Treatment*	*Notes*
Birthmark: strawberry Raised area of dark-red pigmentation; usually small at birth; grows rapidly for about a year; may bleed easily if scratched or injured.	Protect from accidental damage; cover the birthmark if it is likely to be scratched or rubbed; wait for natural disappearance; surgical removal is rarely necessary.	In most cases, after a strawberry birthmark has stopped growing, it gradually decreases in size, and disappears in a few years.
Blindness Not always noticed at birth; sometimes eye lens seems opaque; iris may appear defective; in most cases, lack of response to light noticed when the baby is about one month old.	Evaluation to identify treatable causes; special education in a school for the blind; precautions for safety in the home; in all cases, consult an ophthalmologist.	A defect in the iris is often associated with other deformities, for example, a cleft palate. A child may be born with a cataract if the mother was ill with rubella during the early stages of pregnancy.
Blue baby (cyanosis) Blue color to the skin and lips; rapid breathing after slight exertion; difficulty sucking; often underweight.	Medical assessment and treatment required immediately.	This condition is usually a result of congenital heart disease. It may also be caused by respiratory distress syndrome of the newborn, in which the blood is not adequately oxygenated because the lungs do not inflate and absorb oxygen correctly.
Breathing problems See INTERMITTENT BREATHING; RESPIRATORY DISTRESS SYNDROME.		
Bruising Local swelling and discoloration, often showing where instruments, such as forceps, have been used to assist the birth; bruising on the top of the scalp common in a normal delivery.	Treatment not necessary; bruising disappears within a week.	Bruising is sometimes associated with a wryneck if a muscle in the neck has been torn during the delivery. Bleeding around the white of the eye may occur. In a breech delivery there may be bruising on the buttocks. Bruising may also occur on the legs if these have been pulled or stretched during the delivery.
"Caput" Swelling on top of newborn baby's head; disappears after a few hours.	None required	The baby's skull is squeezed as the head is forced through the birth canal. As the head is squeezed, the pressure of the fluid within the skin causes this part to bulge.
Cerebral palsy (spasticity) Rarely diagnosed until the baby is about one month old. See CEREBRAL PALSY in next section.		
Cleft palate and lip A split in the upper lip; sometimes two splits; in some cases extending back through the palate (the roof of the mouth).	Plastic surgery to close the defect; treatment starting in infancy; closure of lip possible, in some cases, soon after birth; severe cases need treatment until about the age of 12. Generally, cleft lip treated at 3 months, and cleft palate closed at a later date.	There may be problems with feeding. In most cases, feeding is accomplished by the use of a special nipple. In some cases, only tube-feeding is possible. A cleft palate and lip may be associated with other congenital anomalies. Ear infections are common. Long-term treatment involves orthodontics and speech therapy.
Clubfoot Foot bent downward and inward; may affect one or both feet; sometimes associated with spina bifida.	Consultation with a children's orthopedic specialist; gentle manipulation and splinting usually sufficient.	Clubfoot may be an inherited deformity or the result of the baby developing in a cramped position in the uterus. The condition is sometimes associated with other congenital anomalies.
Congenital anomalies See introduction to this section.		
Congenital hip dysplasia No obvious symptoms; detected by a physician after birth.	Hip joint held in place by special splints; splints required for about six months.	The cause of congenital dislocation of the hip is not known. It may occur because the muscles that relax in the month before birth become too weak to hold the hip joint in place.

At birth: disorders *(Continued)*

Symptoms and signs	*Treatment*	*Notes*
Down's syndrome Short, thick hands, often with only a single crease on palm; small, slanting eyes with eyefolds; flattened bridge of nose and back of head; general floppiness of body and limbs; developmental delay and varying degrees of mental retardation.	None; special education and home care required.	Down's syndrome is due to an abnormal number of chromosomes. This anomaly is more likely to occur in the case of a child born to an older woman. The possibility of a child being born with Down's syndrome can be anticipated if amniocentesis is used to examine the uterine fluid in early pregnancy.
Eyefolds Additional fold on inner side of eyelid, next to the nose; commonly seen at birth; tends to disappear as child grows and as the shape of the face changes.	None required.	Eyefolds are normal in Oriental people. Sometimes they occur in non-Oriental families as an inherited characteristic. Eyefolds are also a sign of Down's syndrome, but are not significant unless other signs of Down's syndrome are present as well. Consult a physician if there is any doubt.
Fingers or toes, extra (polydactyly) Additional fingers or toes; usually on the outer side of the hand or foot; often an inherited condition.	Surgical removal in early childhood.	Polydactyly may be associated with more serious conditions and other anomalies. It is advisable to consult a physician.
Finger or toes, webbed (syndactyly) Skin joining two or more fingers or toes; normal opening prevented.	Toes usually left untreated; fingers separated by surgery at about age four.	For other anomalies in the shape or function of a child's fingers or toes, consult a physician.
Fracture Local swelling; pain; sometimes obvious deformity of skull, collarbone, or limb.	Examination by a physician; splinting sometimes required; results usually excellent.	Fractures occur rarely, but are more common during a breech delivery. In some cases the injury may damage a nerve, causing temporary paralysis.
Heart disease, congenital Breathlessness; slight blueness of skin and lips, as in a blue baby; easily tired; weak sucking; in some cases there are no symptoms.	Urgently required if symptoms are obvious; in other cases, surgical treatment may be required later in life.	Heart disease may be associated with other congenital anomalies, for example, Down's syndrome.
Hemolytic disease of the newborn (Rh factor incompatibility) Anemia; increasing yellow color to the skin (jaundice); heart failure; brain damage; cerebral palsy; death may occur.	Transfusion to completely replace baby's blood; treatment with ultraviolet light to destroy yellow pigment (bilirubin); baby's eyes must be protected from the ultraviolet light.	A child whose mother's blood is Rh negative and whose father's blood is Rh positive may be born with Rh positive blood that is incompatible with that of the mother. If blood from an Rh positive fetus mixes with the mother's Rh negative blood, as occurs toward the end of pregnancy, the mother will form antibodies against Rh positive blood. These antibodies do not usually appear in time to affect the first Rh positive child but are likely to affect subsequent Rh positive babies. If these antibodies enter the baby's blood, they destroy the Rh positive red blood cells. This causes anemia and heart failure in the fetus, and jaundice in the baby. All pregnant women should be examined for Rh negative blood. If a woman is found to be Rh negative, anti-Rh serum should be given to prevent her being sensitized at the birth of her Rh positive baby. If necessary, an exchange transfusion can be done while the baby is still in the uterus. Anti-Rh serum is administered during and after each subsequent pregnancy.
Hermaphrodite See SEX UNCERTAINTY.		
Hernia (rupture) Soft, local swelling on part of the abdomen; may appear and disappear without obvious cause; usually can be temporarily pushed back into the abdomen; most frequently occurs in the groin, on one or both sides (inguinal hernia); may occur at the umbilicus (umbilical hernia).	Surgical treatment needed for an inguinal hernia; in boys, check also for an undescended testicle; an umbilical hernia usually grows for six months, then diminishes; normally disappears naturally after about four years.	

At birth: disorders *(Continued)*

Symptoms and signs	*Treatment*	*Notes*
Hypoglycemia (low blood sugar) Usually appears about 12 to 24 hours after birth; drowsiness; refusal to suck; pause in breathing for up to half a minute; sometimes convulsions.	In mild cases, frequent feeding; in more severe cases, intravenous glucose.	This condition occurs most commonly in premature babies or babies born to diabetic mothers. Feeding the baby as soon as possible after birth reduces the chances of hypoglycemia. In some cases it is associated with other disorders of sugar metabolism.
Intermittent breathing (apnea) Temporary stoppages of breathing; brief stoppages, up to 10 seconds, are not serious; longer stoppages may be serious.	Consult a physician; immediate treatment required for stoppages longer than 30 seconds. Some babies need to wear a monitor that sets off an alarm if the baby pauses too long between breaths.	A blue color to the skin and lips, vomiting, and diarrhea may be associated with this breathing problem. Prolonged breathing stoppages, known as apnea, may indicate a serious condition, such as brain hemorrhage or meningitis.
Jaundice Yellow discoloration of whites of eyes; slight yellow discoloration of skin developing a few days after birth and fading slowly. Yellow color that increases and does not fade is serious.	Not usually needed for mild jaundice; ultraviolet light sometimes used for more pronounced jaundice. Progressive jaundice needs urgent medical diagnosis and care.	Slight yellow discoloration is normal in most babies and is due to the destruction of excess red blood cells. An immature liver is unable to get rid of the yellow pigment (bilirubin) fast enough. Severe jaundice may be a result of Rh factor incompatibility (see HEMOLYTIC DISEASE OF THE NEWBORN), a blocked bile duct, prematurity, or an infection. The greatest danger of severe jaundice is that it can cause brain damage.
Mongolism See DOWN'S SYNDROME.		
Nerve injury Lack of movement in a limb or part of the body; sometimes affects one side of the face.	Treatment by a physician; results usually satisfactory in cases of facial paralysis; often less successful if the limbs are affected.	Facial paralysis is most commonly due to the position of the fetus in the uterus. Limb paralysis may be caused by pulling on the limb during the delivery, or other trauma during birth.
PKU (phenylketonuria) None at birth; later, pale skin and urine that has a putrid smell; mental retardation, convulsions, and abnormal behavior in later childhood.	Phenylketonuria (PKU) test 48 hours after first feeding; following positive blood test, treatment with diet that is low in phenylalanine.	Treatment should continue for at least five years in order to prevent brain damage. The disease is due to the failure of the body to metabolize the amino acid phenylalanine correctly. The disease is inherited. All infants should be tested for phenylketonuria in the nursery.
Premature baby Birth before expected date; small size; skin appearing red; covering of fine hair (lanugo) that disappears soon after birth; short nails; few skin creases on soles of feet.	If born more than one month early, the baby may require hospitalization in neonatal intensive care unit. Close monitoring; incubator to keep baby warm; frequent, small feedings; and additional oxygen may be needed. Observe the baby's progress carefully.	Premature babies are more likely to develop breathing problems, infections, hypoglycemia, and jaundice, so they must be treated with particular care in the days after birth. In most cases, progress is rapid and such babies catch up with the growth of children that are not premature.
Respiratory distress syndrome Rapid breathing; grunting; inability to suck; common in premature babies at birth.	Immediate treatment by a physician; treatment with mechanical ventilation and continuous positive airway pressure (CPAP); intravenous infusions; care in an oxygen tent.	This syndrome occurs because the baby's lungs do not expand normally at birth.
Rh incompatibility See HEMOLYTIC DISEASE OF THE NEWBORN.		
Sex uncertainty External sexual organs not properly formed.	Assessment by physician; chromosome examination; surgical treatment may be required.	It is important to determine the sex of the infant before the baby leaves the hospital. Failure to do so may lead to social as well as medical problems.

Symptoms and signs	*Treatment*	*Notes*
Sneezing and sniffling Difficulties in breathing through nose; nose partly blocked; nose running.	None usually required; careful clearing of the nose with a bulb syringe may make the baby's breathing more comfortable.	This is relatively common in the newborn, particularly if the nose is small. A low bridge to the nose and narrow nasal passages are usually the causes of sniffling and as these structures grow larger, sniffling usually disappears. Sneezing in the newborn is more commonly the result of sensitive nasal passages than of infection.
Spasticity *See* CEREBRAL PALSY.		
Spina bifida Failure of the lower part of the spine to close; abnormality may not be obvious if spinal opening is covered by skin; indications include dimple, lump, tuft of hair, or cyst containing clear fluid akin to a blister, over lower spine; in serious cases, a raw, open area in which spinal nerves can be seen; paralysis of lower body and limbs in severe cases.	No treatment needed if skin is not damaged; type in which there is a cyst can often be treated surgically; serious form, in which spine is uncovered, is difficult to treat; urgent surgical operation to close skin over spinal cord essential; child may live if infection can be prevented; medical care as the child grows.	Babies with severe spina bifida often have anencephaly or hydrocephalus as well. Severe spina bifida causes the spine and the spinal cord to be deformed. This may lead to paralysis of the legs and the inability to control the muscles of the bladder and anus. Infection of the cerebrospinal fluid, leading to meningitis, is a common cause of death. Genetic counseling is advisable because of the risk of a subsequent child being born with spina bifida. Certain types of spina bifida can be detected early in the pregnancy through prenatal diagnosis.
Tongue-tie Tongue unable to stick out of the mouth; ligament (frenum) beneath the tongue unusually short, restricting movement.	Usually unnecessary; if no natural improvement, surgery may be required at about age four.	There are usually no problems with sucking or with the development of speech, unless the frenum is very short. Surgical division is not usually necessary, but, if it is required, is a minor procedure.
Urethra, abnormal opening Small opening along the underneath of the penis (hypospadias); rarely, along the top (epispadias).	Surgical operation to repair defect; usually done at about age five.	The purpose of surgery is to reconstruct the urethra so that the opening is in the normal place. Part of the foreskin is commonly used to cover and close the abnormal opening.
Uvula, split Double-ended uvula; visible when the mouth is open. *See also* CLEFT PALATE AND LIP.	None required.	
Vernix Oily film (vernix caseosa) covering the baby's skin at birth; collection of this in groin and in armpits.	Wash face and groin; remove excess from creases; skin covering usually left for several days after birth, before being washed off.	The vernix is thought to provide protection against infection. It may also protect against excessive heat loss.
Vulva, swollen Swollen external genitals in a baby girl; sometimes associated with enlarged clitoris and vaginal discharge; genital area inflamed.	None required; the swelling usually disappears within one or two weeks.	This condition is often associated with swollen breasts. It is caused by the presence of maternal hormones in the baby's blood.
Wryneck Head turned to one side at birth; chin tilted downward; persistence of this deformity after birth.	Turn head gently in opposite direction to the deformity several times a day for six months; consult a physician; a minor operation may be needed to repair damaged muscle.	A wryneck is usually the result of a neck muscle being torn during childbirth. Sometimes a lump can be felt in the affected muscle. Turning the neck gently in the manner described will usually encourage the muscle to grow correctly. Consult a physician if there is any doubt or if progress seems slow. Occasionally, a wryneck is a symptom of a bone abnormality, in which case this abnormality will appear on an X ray.

Section 2

Birth to age 1½: normal development

Each section of the age-by-age charts begins with an outline of the normal achievements of a child of the age group being considered. The stages of development, in this case of a baby from birth to age eighteen months, are represented in chart form. It should be remembered that these charts can only present an outline of average development, because babies can vary enormously in the rate of their individual progress. Certain babies will be more advanced in some things and slower in others. Sometimes progress is rapid over a wide range of abilities, whereas at other times it may be held back, perhaps by illness or accident. If parents are concerned about their child's progress, they should consult a physician.

The problems and disorders that can affect a baby at birth, and in the months following birth, are described in charts that emphasize the main symptoms, how to treat them, and also show other problems that can arise.

Cross-references are within the section unless otherwise specified.

Vision

Achievements include at:

Birth:	closes eyelids to bright light
Two weeks:	momentarily looks at objects
One month:	briefly follows parent's face and may smile
Two months:	follows moving objects with eyes
Three months:	begins to focus and starts to move head as well as eyes
Four months:	looks at own hands and focuses easily on nearby objects
Five months:	looks at surroundings and searches for lost toy
Six months:	looks at objects
Nine months:	looks at small objects
One year:	interested in simple shapes
Fifteen months:	recognizes simple pictures

Hearing

Achievements include at:

One month:	responds by reflex to loud noise (startle reflex)
Four months:	opens or widens eyelids in response to loud noise
Five months:	turns head to right or left toward sound
Nine months:	locates noises to one side of, or below, head
One year:	turns head toward sounds from any direction

Speech

Achievements include at:

Three months:	laughs
Seven to eight months:	says "Da" and "Ma," "Da-da" and "Ma-ma"
Ten months:	has one word with a particular meaning
One year:	uses a few words correctly (for example, "dog")
One year to eighteen months:	develops own language mixed with many normal words; often understood by family and enjoys experimenting with new sounds; some children speak well (for example, may describe events accurately)

Physical movement

Achievements include at:

Birth:	can just lift head when lying on stomach; head lags behind when pulled to sitting position and needs to be supported
One month:	may hold head up for a moment when held in sitting position
Two months:	raises head when lying on stomach but constantly drops it when held in sitting position; head needs to be supported
Three months:	"push up" with forearms; only slight head lag when pulled to sitting position
Four months:	looks around when in sitting position with only slight head wobble; slight support from legs when held in standing position
Five months:	head steady when looking around; no "lag" when pulled to sitting position; starts to drool a great deal
Six months:	holds out hands to be lifted up; able to support most of own weight when standing; sits in chair, if supported; rolls from stomach onto back
Seven months:	supports self on legs while holding onto mother's hands; rolls from back onto stomach; chews
Eight months:	can sit unaided, and can stand up holding a support; begins to crawl
Ten to twelve months:	begins to walk by holding onto a person's hands or onto furniture; drooling stops
Twelve to fifteen months:	stands alone and then takes first few steps with feet widely spaced; often falls over; crawls up stairs
Fifteen to eighteen months:	begins to walk normally and may run; may begin jumping; able to get onto chair; walks up stairs holding handrail; throws ball without falling over

Use of hands

Achievements include at:

Birth to three months:	holds objects by reflex
Three months:	pulls at clothing; momentarily grasps toy; clasps hands together
Four months:	shakes rattle; plays with hands
Five months:	takes toy that is offered; holds bottle

Achievements include at:

Six months:	drops one toy when another is offered; puts toes in mouth
Eight months:	picks up small objects using finger and thumb
Nine months:	uses index finger to pull toys and will deliberately let them drop; puts toys into parent's hand
Ten months:	plays games by dropping toy for parent to pick up and then dropping it again
Eleven months:	plays games by giving someone a toy and insisting on taking it back; plays with ball
Twelve to fifteen months:	makes marks with crayons; takes off shoes; plays with blocks
Eighteen months:	builds small tower with three or four blocks; manages spoon; scribbles; turns pages of a book

Understanding

Achievements include at:

One month:	looks at parent's face
Two months:	smiles when parent talks
Three months:	laughs when spoken to
Four months:	enjoys toys and is excited when fed; likes to sit up; holds onto toy when it is pulled
Five months:	looks toward sound; smiles at faces in mirror; looks for, and finds, lost toys
Six to seven months:	puts food into mouth; shy with strangers; plays "peek-a-boo" with adults; attracts attention by making noise
Eight months;	tries to prevent face being wiped; excited seeing favorite food; understands "no"
Nine months:	waves goodbye; tugs parent's clothing; helps when being dressed (for example, puts arm out for sleeve)

Achievements include at:

Ten months:	makes deliberate actions (for example, puts toys into a box); understands simple question like "where is the dog?"
Eleven months:	likes pictures in a book; likes simple nursery rhymes and remembers the way they are told
One year:	enjoys kisses; understands questions like "where is your sock?"
One year to fifteen months:	manages cup and feeding; asks for things by pointing; kisses pictures of things that are recognized; sometimes refuses to do things
Fifteen to eighteen months:	able to point to ear, eye, or nose, and to pictures of dog, or car; will fetch objects on request; helps when being undressed; shows anger when parent stops playing; starts to take a long time with meals

Teeth

Developments include at:

Birth:	in rare cases a child may be born with one or more teeth
Six months:	lower middle incisors
Seven months:	lower outer incisors
Seven to nine months:	four upper incisors
One year:	lower first molars
Twelve to fourteen months:	upper first molars
Fifteen to eighteen months:	upper and lower eye teeth

Disease prevention and health care

Immunization

Suggested schedule:

Two months:	diphtheria, tetanus and whooping cough (triple) injection; oral polio vaccine
Four months:	diphtheria, tetanus and whooping cough (triple) injection; oral polio vaccine
Six months:	diphtheria, tetanus and whooping cough (triple) injection

Suggested schedule:

Twelve months:	skin test for tuberculosis
Fifteen months:	measles, mumps and rubella (triple) injection
Eighteen months:	diphtheria, tetanus and whooping cough (triple) injection; oral polio vaccine (may be given at 15 months); Hemophilus influenzae B injection (HiB vaccine)

Immunization programs must begin soon after birth because infectious diseases can be more serious in babies than in adults.

Whooping cough vaccination is not recommended if the baby has had a very high fever or a convulsion, or if there is any sign of a progressing brain disorder. If in doubt, consult the child's physician.

Health care

Weight, length, and head circumference measured on each visit. Developmental progress of the infant is monitored at each visit. Suggested schedule:

At birth:	physician's examination; PKU test; blood test, if required for legal or medical reason, for example blood group, Rhesus factor, syphilis, anemia, jaundice factor; test for hypothyroidism and other congenital diseases; circumcision, if desired, usually at two or three days after birth
One to two weeks:	physician's examination; vision check
One month:	physician's examination
Two months:	physician's examination; vision check; hearing check
Four months:	physician's examination
Six months:	physician's examination; vision check; hearing check
Nine months:	physician's examination
Twelve months:	physician's examination; anemia test, if recommended; urinalysis
Fifteen months:	physician's examination
Eighteen months:	physician's examination

Birth to age 1½: disorders

Symptoms and signs	Treatment	Notes
Allergy to cows' milk May include skin rash, breathing difficulties, running nose, diarrhea, vomiting after feeding, weight loss.	Consult a physician; avoid cows' milk in the diet.	Cows' milk is a common cause of allergy in babies, particularly if this milk is given in the first month of life. Babies under one year should be fed breast milk or formula.
Anal bleeding Blood in the feces; evidence of pain (screaming) on defecation; constipation.	Consult a physician; give the child plenty of fluids to prevent constipation; suppositories or lubricants inserted with a gloved finger may be required.	Anal bleeding is often the result of constipation. Hard feces sometimes tear the mucosa lining the rectum, causing an anal fissure. Anal bleeding may also be due to an intussusception or a rectal prolapse, which are serious, so consult a physician immediately if the pain or bleeding is severe.
Anal swelling Swelling at anus; red tissue protruding through anus; sometimes colic and vomiting.	Consult a physician immediately.	A prolapse of the rectum is the most likely cause of anal swelling, but swelling may also be a symptom of an intussusception.
Anemia Pale skin; lethargic behavior; often breathlessness when crying.	Consult a physician; diagnosis from blood test; full investigation to detect deficiency of iron if deficient; small quantities of iron in liquid form added to the diet; vitamin C given, in form of orange juice, to increase iron absorption; screening for lead exposure or congenital causes such as sickle cell disease.	Blood tests should be repeated even when the condition appears to be cured. Iron deficiency anemia is the most common type of anemia, particularly in premature babies or in those that have been fed solely on milk for more than six months. In some cases anemia may be a symptom of a more serious disease. Consult a physician if there is any doubt.
Bowlegs A gap between knees when feet are placed together; generally a normal occurrence in children when they start walking.	Consult a physician; normally no treatment necessary unless other conditions are present; condition normally corrects itself, from about age two years.	If the condition persists, an orthopedic specialist should be consulted, particularly if bowlegs are associated with clubfoot. A child may appear to have bowlegs because of the normal bulge of the outer sides of the calves, when compared to the inner side. Bowlegs are diagnosed by the separation of the knees.
Bronchitis Cough; fever; rapid breathing.	Consult a physician for diagnosis; keep child in warm, humid room; hospitalization for serious cases; physician may prescribe antibiotics or cough mixture.	Bronchitis may develop after a cold and is sometimes accompanied by vomiting or diarrhea. Bronchiolitis, commonly called "wheezy" bronchitis, is the most common variety and may be an indication that asthma will develop later in childhood.
Cerebral palsy (spasticity) Lack of movement; differences in movements of either side of the body; child seeming to be too quiet; muscles feel stiff; child failing to suck normally; one hand, or both, remaining closed.	Assessment by a physician; repeated examinations over time required for complete diagnosis; deformities prevented by moving limbs gently, several times each day; limbs moved through normal range to teach correct position and use, and to relax muscles.	Cerebral palsy may occur if the baby is premature, if the baby has severe jaundice at birth, if the mother had diabetes during pregnancy, or as the result of a birth injury. Many cases do not have an obvious cause.
Chest deformities Funnel breast, a depression of the breastbone resembling a funnel; pigeon breast, a protuberance of the chest in front; altered shapes of the normal chest.	Surgical treatment seldom needed but may be given for cosmetic reasons, of if normal breathing is not possible.	Funnel breast is rarely associated with underlying disorders, but pigeon breast may be associated with congenital heart disease, asthma, or rickets. In some cases, funnel breast may be an inherited condition.
Cold Fever; running nose with nasal mucus and cough; sometimes diarrhea.	Give plenty of fluids; consult a physician who may give drugs to dry nasal secretions; pediatric nose drops may be used for few days, particularly before feeding, because sucking is difficult with a blocked nose.	A young baby may still have some protection against colds because of immunity transferred from the mother. Nevertheless, older children with colds should not go near the baby, and the mother should wear a mask if she is developing a cold.
Colic Screaming and drawing up of knees in small baby. *See also* COLIC, INFANTILE.	Further "burping" of child after feeding; sips of sweetened water; cuddling; a quiet calm environment; a change of diaper; carrying in a cloth carrier on parent's chest.	Serious causes of abdominal pain include intestinal obstruction and intussusception. It is also associated with some infections, particularly ear infections. Colic generally starts to improve by three months of age.

Symptoms and signs	*Treatment*	*Notes*
Colic, infantile (three-month colic) One to two hours of recurring colic; taking place most evenings in one- to three-month old baby.	If simple measures fail (*see* COLIC), consult a physician; antispasm medicine before baby's meal.	The colic may be due to abdominal discomfort and pain after crying, because the crying causes air to be swallowed. The baby may cry because it is bored, or because it has been fed in a hurry. Feed the baby slowly with small amounts of solids, and keep the baby sitting up for a short time after feeding.
Conjunctivitis Red eye with sticky discharge.	Keep eye clean by bathing with warm, weak saline solution two or three times a day; antibiotic eyedrops may be necessary; hand washing helps to avoid spread of infection.	Conjunctivitis commonly occurs with a cold, or other viral illness. If the discharge is increasing, discuss the condition with a physician.
Constipation Occasional passing of hard feces; may accompany a fever; sometimes occurs after diarrhea or vomiting.	Usually does not require treatment; if necessary, increase fluids by mouth; in older babies more fruit and vegetables produce a larger stool; children's suppositories may help facilitate in extreme cases.	Constipation is commonly due to insufficient fluid in the diet. Constipation and anal bleeding may be due to a painful crack in the anal skin, whereas constipation and colic may indicate an intestinal obstruction. Prolonged constipation, from birth, may be due to Hirschsprung's disease or cretinism. Breast-fed babies may have a normal stool only about once or twice a week.
Convulsion Sudden body rigidity and loss of consciousness; sometimes followed by generalized shaking that lasts between 15 and 60 seconds; convulsion may be followed by continued unconsciousness for several minutes before return to normal color and consciousness.	Hold baby on side with head down to allow any vomit to leave mouth and to prevent inhalation of vomit into lungs; do not try to force anything into mouth; consult a physician immediately.	Convulsions are most commonly caused by high fever, brain damage at birth, epilepsy, or infections such as meningitis. If the convulsion occurs with a high fever, sponge the baby down at once with lukewarm water and keep temperature below 102°F(39°C) with repeated sponging and pediatric acetaminophen.
Cough See BRONCHITIS; COLD; CROUP; NASAL MUCUS.		
"Cradle cap" Brown, flaking skin on scalp; flakes become thick if not treated. This is a normal and common occurrence.	Rub regularly with baby oil or olive oil; shampoo regularly and carefully; comb and brush flaking skin away. If scalp becomes red or looks sore, consult a physician.	This is a normal occurence. "Cradle cap" improves naturally as the baby grows and usually disappears by age one.
Crib death See SUDDEN INFANT DEATH SYNDROME.		
Croup See CROUP in next section.		
Crying Persistent crying without noticeable cause; as babies get older, mother can usually tell one cry from another.	Consult a physician if anxious; give child something to drink; change diaper; cuddle to reassure. Persistent crying may be due to pain from an ear infection, especially if fever is present.	The child may be hungry, thirsty, be too hot or too cold, have a wet diaper, be lonely or bored, or have pain due to a colic condition; crying may also be a reaction to the mother's anxiety or a way of attracting the mother. Some babies naturally cry much more than others.
Cystic fibrosis Intestinal obstruction by thick feces; usually occurring three to four days after birth; intestinal obstruction is least common but most severe symptom; other symptoms are of varying severity; baby fails to grow normally despite good appetite; frequent foul-smelling diarrhea; swollen abdomen; recurrent infections.	Physician makes diagnosis by means of a "sweat test", which measures the salt content of the baby's sweat; X-ray examination of chest and lungs; mother must be taught how to hold baby to encourage drainage of mucus from lungs; nutritious diet; vitamins and pancreatic enzymes are usually prescribed.	All body secretions of a child with cystic fibrosis are abnormally thick, and this contributes to the child's susceptibility to chronic chest infections, pancreatic failure, and sometimes liver disease. A person with cystic fibrosis requires lifelong specialized care.
Dandruff Dry, white scales on the scalp.	Shampoo scalp frequently; if condition persists, consult a physician.	Dandruff is a common occurrence at about three to nine months and is associated with "cradle cap". The condition may be severe in babies with eczema or very dry skin.

Birth to age $1\frac{1}{2}$: disorders *(Continued)*

Symptoms and signs	*Treatment*	*Notes*
Deafness Child may have made sounds until approximately four months of age and then becomes strangely silent. Child does not respond to sound and appears to lack awareness of surroundings; hearing and speech do not seem to develop normally.	Consult a physician; examination of ears for wax or foreign body; antibiotics to treat middle ear infection. Do not push anything into the ears when trying to clean them.	Because it is difficult to test the hearing of an infant, and because the symptoms of deafness may resemble the symptoms of other conditions, parents who are in any doubt about their child's hearing should consult the child's physician immediately. Generally, deafness and pain in the ear are caused by middle ear infections that need prompt treatment. In some cases a mild, chronic infection may be painless, but in need of treatment nevertheless.
Dehydration Glazed appearance in eyes; sunken eyes, that feel soft; fontanel, in the cranium, appears sunken; reduced urine output; dry mouth; flabby skin; weak cry; sometimes slight fever and constipation after a period of diarrhea, a common cause of dehydration.	Serious condition; severe dehydration can occur rapidly in a small baby; consult a physician immediately; if baby unable to drink or keep down clear fluids, intravenous fluid replacement may be necessary.	Dehydration may occur with fever, vomiting, or diarrhea. The condition may also be caused by heavy sweating, as a result of the baby's being left in a hot room or having on too many clothes, as well as by any illness in which fluid consumption is reduced.
Diaper rash Red, sore buttocks; diapers smell strongly of ammonia.	Wash buttocks area gently with soap and water; rinse and dry carefully; leave exposed to the air whenever possible; change diaper frequently; avoid plastic pants; apply creams or ointments for protection; use soft, clean diaper washed with soap, not detergent.	"Ammonia rash" may be helped by rinsing diaper in a special preparation or in vinegar. "Thrush" (candidiasis, moniliasis) forms red areas and needs to be treated with special creams. Babies with excessive dandruff or eczema are particularly likely to develop diaper rash. Some babies are allergic to disposable diapers. In this case, the baby's rash should improve with the use of cloth diapers.
Diarrhea Liquid stools; often occurring without illness; fever, blood in feces, or cramping pain are more serious symptoms; severe diarrhea, or diarrhea with vomiting may cause dehydration.	Avoid high-fiber foods until diarrhea subsides; give plenty of fluids to avoid dehydration; consult physician if diarrhea persists for more than two hours; more than five diarrheal stools in a small baby can cause rapid dehydration.	Dehydration is dangerous and a physician must be consulted as soon as possible if signs of dehydration appear. Celiac disease and cystic fibrosis are serious causes but diarrhea may occur with almost any respiratory or other infection, for example cold, ear infection, or bronchitis, and may also be caused by antibiotics. *See also* GREEN FECES.
Dry skin Dry, scale-like appearance of areas of skin; surface of skin flaking off.	Consult a physician; use creams to keep skin moist; use mild soaps for bathing.	Dry skin, in its most severe form, is a congenital abnormality. In hot climates, sweating may aggravate the problem.
Ear disorders: discharging ear A flow of waxy secretion or pus from the ear.	Consult a physician immediately for treatment and antibiotics.	A discharging ear sometimes occurs after a prolonged period of crying in a child who has a cold. This may be a sign of an infected middle ear and of a burst eardrum. Continued discharge may cause soreness on the side of the neck and cheek. Check for deafness when the ear seems better.
Ear disorders: ear pain Crying; restlessness; holding ears.	Earache is a sign of infection or inflammation of the ear; consult a physician for antibiotics or other appropriate treatment.	A baby over age 10 months may indicate that an ear is hurting by crying, by holding the ear, or refusing to allow anyone to touch the ear. Ear pain often occurs with a cold or a throat infection. Vomiting and diarrhea may occur. Recurrent ear pain may be due to swollen adenoids blocking the eustachian (auditory) tube. Check for deafness.
Eczema Red, roughened patches on the skin causing irritation and scratching.	Discuss with a physician; careful use of hydrocortisone creams and antihistamine drugs under physician's supervision; use of mild skin cleansers in place of common soap when washing; avoidance of wool clothing and, occasionally, certain foods. Gloves worn at night will help prevent scratching.	In babies, eczema generally starts on the scalp or face, but in older children it develops most commonly in the creases of the elbows, and behind the knees and ears. Bleeding and infection may occur from scratching. The condition seldom develops before the age of three months and usually improves after age three years.

Symptoms and signs	*Treatment*	*Notes*
Eye disorders: blindness See BLINDNESS in first section.		
Eye disorders: blocked tear duct Persistent flow of tears from one or both eyes.	Consult a physician; if condition persists, it can be relieved by passing a small probe down the duct to clear it.	A blocked tear duct in a baby is a tear duct that was not fully opened at birth. Sometimes blockage is caused by conjunctivitis, or by a cold if the infection has spread to the tear ducts.
Eye disorders: cataract Eyes with opaque lens; appearance of a gray spot, seen through the iris; clouding of lens may or may not interfere with vision.	Consult ophthalmologist; severely opaque lens should be surgically treated when the child is six months old.	A cataract in a baby is a congenital abnormality that is sometimes caused by the mother's having contracted rubella during pregnancy. *See also* BLINDNESS in first section.
Eye disorders: squint (strabismus) Eyes look in different directions; one eye that appears to wander, independently of the other, from object at which child is looking; symptoms may be noticed as early as age six or eight weeks.	Examination by ophthalmologist to ensure both eyes are healthy and that one is not merely nearsighted and "lazy"; treatment required if squint persists or is present at age six months; cover normal eye to allow weak eye to develop; early surgery, at about age one, produces good results if squint is due to lack of muscle balance.	There is often a family history of squint. The sudden onset of squint at any age needs thorough investigation.
"Fat baby" Baby is overweight and lethargic; late walking; appearing to be behind expected physical achievements.	Discuss diet with physician; reduce sugar and carbohydrate intake; avoid sweetened drinks between meals; increase fresh fruit and vegetables in diet; do not overdo dieting as growth may be delayed by dietary deficiency.	The condition is rarely, if ever, due to disease. Obese parents tend to have obese children. Overweight babies usually grow into overweight adults, partly because of the family eating habits, and partly because parents consider the obese shape to be a healthy one. In some cases obesity results from medical disorders that must be identified and treated.
Feeding problems: food jags Refusal to eat many different kinds of food; perference for one or two particular foods.	Parents should be firm and prepare a normal nutritious meal; end meal by leaving baby hungry if baby will not eat food that has been refused; give all the originally intended foods; repeat the next meal until baby starts eating disliked food; minimize sugary snacks; avoid snacks for two hours before mealtime; do not force feed.	Food jags are usually associated with feeding problems, such as food refusal, that have not been controlled. In general, there is no harm in selecting foods for which the child has shown a preference. At this age, children do not try to manipulate the parents, and choice of foods usually represents parental behavior towards certain foods.
Feeding problems: food refusal Refusal to feed; particularly when a new food is introduced.	Baby may have eaten enough or may want to drink; try some other item of food before trying the unwanted food again; further refusal may be ignored at the first meal but try again the next day and be prepared to stop meal if baby will not eat it; if baby refuses broccoli, for example, but eats green beans with enthusiasm, serve the beans, as they are equally nutritious.	It is normal for a baby's appetite to diminish after about 12 months because the growth rate also slows down. Refusal of a food that has been previously eaten is usually a sign that the baby wants to assert himself or herself. A gradual approach allows the parent to be sure the baby is not becoming sick, vomiting, or experiencing diarrhea. Once the baby has been able to refuse one food, it may refuse more as a way of defeating the parent. Every baby and child should be allowed one or two dislikes. Equally nutritious foods that the baby does like should be offered at the next meal.
Fever Baby who appears hot, fussy, flushed, or lethargic; chills and shivering; baby thirsty but refusing food; feeling cold at onset, but then feeling hot; fever confirmed by taking temperature.	Give plenty to drink; give pediatric acetaminophen mixture to reduce fever; if fever is over 104°F (40°C), consult a physician as soon as possible; sponge baby with lukewarm water or put in lukewarm bath; call a physician if other symptoms occur or if you are anxious.	Fever is often the first symptom of illness, for example, a cold, and is sometimes associated with diarrhea, or vomiting. A fever usually disappears in 24 hours if treated sensibly. Recurring fevers, with no obvious cause, must be assessed by a physician.

Birth to age $1\frac{1}{2}$: disorders *(Continued)*

Symptoms and signs	*Treatment*	*Notes*
Green feces Green feces being passed; occurring with diarrhea.	In young babies, give clear fluids if diarrhea occurs; treat as diarrhea; feces will return to normal color when diarrhea stops.	Green feces occur with diarrhea and are caused by unchanged bile salts leaving the intestine. The condition is commonly a sign of underfeeding in young babies. Look for the underlying causes of the diarrhea. Green feces may also occur when the baby is given fruit juice for the first time.
Hiatus hernia Upper abdominal pain, causing crying and extreme discomfort; vomiting, particularly when lying down; moderately large amounts of food regurgitated, with mucus and flecks of blood.	Diagnosis made by X ray after swallowing barium; food should be thickened with cereal; keep baby propped upright day and night; antacids given to reduce stomach acidity.	A hiatus hernia is caused by a weakness in the diaphragm at the point where the esophagus passes through. This allows food to flow back into the esophagus, particularly when a person is lying down, rather than to be held in the stomach. Frequent vomiting may cause loss of weight and failure to thrive. The condition usually improves in the first year but, if scarring and narrowing of the esophagus are caused by stomach acids, an operation may be needed.
Hiccups Sharp intake of breath; rarely lasting more than a few minutes; occurring particularly after feeding.	Not usually necessary; holding baby upright may help; give small amounts of boiled water to drink.	Hiccups are caused by contraction of the diaphragm muscle and are relatively common. They do not indicate that there is anything wrong with the baby's feeding. Sometimes a little regurgitation may occur, but this is normal.
Hirschsprung's disease Constipation from birth; 90 percent of babies with this condition fail to pass normal meconium (dark green-brown stool) within 24 hours of being born; abdomen becomes swollen and gas is passed; episodes of swelling and severe vomiting, relieved by passing gas; child usually grows slowly despite eating well.	Once diagnosis is made, physician may recommend saline enemas to empty intestine until child is old enough for surgical removal of abnormal section of large intestine.	Hirschsprung's disease is about four times more common in boys than in girls. It is a congenital abnormality in which a segment of large intestine develops without a nerve supply. This prevents feces passing through so that the intestine behind becomes distended with feces and gas. The pain is seldom severe during episodes of swelling or distention. Removal of the abnormal segment alleviates the condition. Episodes of fever, diarrhea, and acute illness may occur due to infection.
Hives See URTICARIA in next section.		
Intussusception Vomiting; sudden onset of severe colic; short periods of normal behavior and sleep before further colic; diarrhea at onset, with bloody stools that look like red jelly, then constipation.	Diagnosis by physician who may feel lump in abdomen; barium enema may not only confirm the condition but will often relieve it; urgent surgical correction may be required.	The intestine squeezes part of its own internal surface, causing it to fold into itself and so to form a blockage. Rarely, a soft lump sticks out from the anus. The condition may occur in healthy babies aged 3 to 24 months.
Jaundice See JAUNDICE in first section.		
Meningitis High-pitched cry; fever; irritability; sometimes vomiting; staring eyes; lethargy; stiff neck; skin rash like small bruises.	Immediate examination by a physician; spinal tap in hospital and antibiotic treatment; blood cultures also taken.	The baby's neck is seldom stiff but the fontanel, the soft spot on the scalp, may be bulging. Treatment must start as soon as possible, in order to prevent death. The condition can lead to hydrocephalus, deafness, nerve paralysis, convulsions, or mental handicap.
Nasal mucus Blocked nose; difficulty breathing; cough; thick mucus running from nose; cough worse at night; sometimes vomiting in the morning.	Increase environmental humidity; antibiotics rarely helpful; avoid using irritant nose drops. If simple measures do not work, consult a physician. A thick yellow or green drainage may be due to sinus infection which requires antibiotic therapy.	Recurrent minor respiratory infections or allergy cause excess nasal mucus production, leading to blockage of the narrow nasal passages of a young child. This may be troublesome, particularly at night. If the child swallows mucus during the night, vomiting is likely to occur in the morning. As the baby grows, the nasal passages widen and immunity develops.

Symptoms and signs	Treatment	Notes
Nightmare Waking at night screaming; staring into space; usually occurring at age 9 to 18 months when too young to explain fear; nightmares may occur more than once.	Seldom necessary to make special visit to physician; reassure baby until sleep resumes.	There should be a natural improvement within a few weeks. Do not be surprised if the baby stands and shakes the bars of the crib. Nightmares may be due to an overactive imagination or to a temporary feeling of insecurity.
Pyloric stenosis Persistent forceful vomiting after food is given; excessive drooling; voracious appetite; from the age of three weeks, vomiting may increase in frequency and force; constipation or green feces; weight loss, despite good appetite.	Physician may feel lump in abdomen while baby eats; barium meal may be given to baby (barium sulphate mixture, which is X-rayed as it passes through the stomach and intestines) to confirm diagnosis; operation to cut stomach muscle at site of spasm; normal feeding usually possible days after operations.	The condition is due to a spasm of muscle at the exit of the stomach. The content of the vomit brought up in a case of pyloric stenosis is usually curdled milk without bile. Pyloric stenosis is a congenital abnormality that is much more common in boys than in girls.
Rash: diaper rash *See* DIAPER RASH.		
Rash: milia Small white pinhead spots on nose and cheeks.	No treatment necessary.	The condition is normal in newborn babies and disappears gradually after a few weeks.
Rash: red skin, diffuse Vague mottled rashes; occurring in many minor illnesses, particularly colds; also occurring in hot conditions.	Consult a physician, particularly if other symptoms are present; rash is often a symptom of a more serious illness.	A diffuse rash in a baby usually indicates a raised temperature, and this may be a sign of illness. A rash may also be a sign of an allergic reaction, although this is relatively uncommon in children of this age. *See also* ECZEMA; SPOTTY FACE.
Rash: urticaria (hives) *See* URTICARIA in next section.		
Rectal prolapse Red lump protruding from anus in healthy baby; particularly in one who has been constipated; most likely to occur after straining.	Keep child comfortable; place warm, wet cloth over rectum until a physician can see child.	A baby usually recovers from a prolapse of the rectum without treatment, but in some cases an operation is required to fix the tissue in place.
Regurgitation (spitting up) Burping up of small amounts of food, usually milk, just after feeding.	None necessary; bib or piece of cloth to protect clothing; sit baby upright after feeding; burp baby frequently to avoid excessive air in stomach.	Regurgitation of food is common in many babies, and often accompanies burping after feeding. It is a normal occurrence, and bears no relation to the amount eaten, or to the health of the child.
Rickets Bony lumps on skull; swelling of wrists and ankles; swollen abdomen; bowlegs; slow in learning to crawl and walk.	Diagnosis made by a physician; additional vitamin D and plenty of milk in diet.	Rickets is due to a dietary lack of vitamin D or to lack of sunlight (which encourages vitamin D formation in the skin). Infant formula and commercially available milk are fortified with adequate amounts of vitamin D.
Skin problems *See* DRY SKIN; ECZEMA; SPOTTY FACE.		
Sleep problems *See* CRYING in this section; SLEEP DISORDERS in next section; SLEEP WALKING in fourth section.		
"Slow baby" Baby that is unusually quiet and obedient; sleeps well but physically inactive; may not grow fast and may be obese; sometimes constipated.	Discuss with physician if concerned about baby's progress.	Normal rates of development vary considerably among children. A thorough medical examination may suggest if problems exist. *See also* FAILURE TO THRIVE; FEEDING PROBLEMS.
Spasticity *See* CEREBRAL PALSY.		
Squint *See* EYE DISORDERS: SQUINT.		

Birth to age 1½: disorders *(Continued)*

Symptoms and signs	Treatment	Notes
Sudden infant death syndrome (SIDS) Baby found dead in crib; no warning or indications of illness.	It is the parents who need treatment for unexpected death of baby; seek help from physician; discuss with other parents who have lost a child in this way. A postmortem examination should be performed to determine if any underlying illness was present.	Sudden infant death may be due to prolonged stopping of breathing, catastrophic infection, or accidental smothering by a pillow. It is important that the parents discuss their feelings, which may include a sense of guilt or failure, with a physician and with other parents who have lost a child to SIDS.
Teething Increase in drooling; restlessness; rubbing of gums; thumb-sucking.	Give baby teething ring to chew; rub gums gently with warm washcloth; give comfort and reassurance when baby is miserable; a physician may prescribe mild painkilling drug, such as acetaminophen (pediatric dose).	If other symptoms, such as fever, diarrhea, or rash occur during teething, a separate cause should be looked for. Teething powders and cutting of gums are not necessary treatment in this normal, although uncomfortable, stage of development. Pediatric acetaminophen may be used to relieve pain.
Testis, undescended Testicle moves in and out of the scrotum, often not in correct position; in some cases, impossible to push testicle into scrotum.	Consult a physician; "retractile" testicles will eventually descend into correct position; treatment required at once if condition is associated with an inguinal hernia; otherwise, treatment may be delayed until child is 12 to 18 months of age.	It is sometimes difficult to decide on the best treatment for this condition. If testicles remain undescended after about one year, surgery is usually recommended.
Umbilicus, infected Discharge from umbilicus; inflammation.	Consult physician urgently; keep umbilicus clean and dry with rubbing alcohol and powder; antibiotics may be required.	A slight discharge from the umbilicus is normal for about 24 hours after the cord falls off, but it should not last longer than this. If untreated, umbilical infection can lead to liver infection.
Vomiting Small amounts of milk vomited after eating food is common in most babies (see REGURGITATION); repeated vomiting of large amounts may be serious.	Discuss with a physician; repeated vomiting in small baby must be reported within two or three hours, because of danger of dehydration.	Vomiting is associated with many conditions, including infections, fever, intestinal obstruction, pyloric stenosis and hiatus hernia. It may also occur with diarrhea. The combination of vomiting and diarrhea is particularly serious because of the risk of dehydration.

Section 3

Age 1½ to age 5: normal development

This section concerns children between the ages of eighteen months and five years. This age group is described in terms of normal development and health care, and then in terms of the more common problems and disorders that may occur. It should be remembered that these charts can only present average development, because children can vary enormously in the rate of their individual progress.

All cross-references are within this section unless otherwise specified.

Vision

Achievements include at:	
Fifteen to eighteen months:	looks at pictures
Eighteen months:	begins to judge distance, but with difficulty
Two years:	judges distances well
Four years:	able to look at objects near to face and at a distance, and to judge their relationship
Five years:	color vision fully developed

Speech

Achievements include at:	
One year to eighteen months:	develops own language mixed with many normal words; enjoys experimenting with new sounds; some children speak well
Twenty-one months:	joins words together; asks for food or toys
Two years:	uses "I" and "You"
Two-and-a-half years:	uses plurals; forms simple sentences; gives full name; knows simple colors
Three years:	talks all the time; size of vocabulary influenced by parents; may also be a measure of intelligence

Physical movement

Achievements include at:

Fifteen to eighteen months:	begins to walk normally and may run; able to get into chair; throws ball without falling over; begins to have bladder control during day
Twenty-one months:	kicks ball; throws overarm; can walk backward
Two years:	climbs stairs, two feet on each step
Two-and-a-half years:	walks on tiptoe or stands on one leg for a few seconds; pedals tricycle
Three years:	climbs stairs, one foot on each step; stands on one leg for longer periods of time
Three-and-a-half years:	skill in more delicate movements; takes off shoes, or coat
Four-and-a-half years:	runs and turns easily; gets completely dressed or undressed but may have difficulty tying shoelaces

Use of hands

Achievements include at:

Eighteen months:	builds small tower with several blocks; manages spoon; scribbles
Two years:	tower of taller blocks; opens doors by use of knob; washes hands
Two-and-a-half years:	holds pencil normally; threads large beads; uses both hands equally well
Three years:	able to cope with large buttons when dressing and undressing; feeds self; copies drawn circle
Four to five years:	copies drawn square; shows evidence of left- or right-handedness; can catch ball

Sphincter control

Achievements include at:

Eighteen months:	tells parents when pants are wet
Two years:	only the occasional loss of control
Two-and-a-half years:	dry nights when placed on toilet late in evening
Three years:	complete control of all actions except wiping of anus

Understanding

Achievements include at:

Fifteen to eighteen months:	able to point to ear, eye, nose, and pictures of common objects; fetches things
Two years:	most children can identify parts of the body and common objects by name; names simple pictures on cards and can usually identify correct card if asked; shows interest in sexual organs
Three years:	counts to four; asks questions all the time; knows own gender; enjoys playing games with other people; can dress and undress a doll; draws simple pictures
Four years:	able to select one object from a pile of six objects; counts to ten and understands simple abstract questions (for example, "What do you want to do?"); draws pictures of people; knows nursery rhymes
Five years:	knows days of week; may know alphabet and be able to read simple words

Teeth

Development includes at:

Fifteen to eighteen months:	upper and lower eyeteeth
Two years:	second molars, giving a full set of twenty baby teeth; second molars are the last baby teeth to erupt
Five years:	permanent teeth do not usually start to appear until age six or seven, but occasionally may start earlier with appearance of molars in upper jaw or loss of front baby teeth

Disease prevention and health care

Immunization

Suggested schedule:

Eighteen months:	Hemophilus influenzae B injection (HiB vaccine); preschools may require tuberculosis skin test prior to enrollment
Five years (school entry):	diphtheria, pertussis, and tetanus booster injection; oral polio vaccine

Health care

Weight and height measured each visit. Suggested schedule:

Eighteen months:	physician's examination
Two years:	physician's examination; dental visit
Three years:	physician's examination; dental visit; vision test
Four years:	physician's examination; dental visit; vision and hearing tests
Five years:	physician's examination; dental visit; color vision, general vision, and hearing tests

Age 1½ to age 5: disorders

Symptoms and signs	*Treatment*	*Notes*
Abdominal pain Varies from dull ache to acute pain; located anywhere in abdominal region; may accompany diarrhea or vomiting, or both.	Consult physician if pain is severe or continues for more than four hours; never administer laxatives to a young child yourself.	Young children are often unable to describe accurately where a pain is or what the pain feels like. Abdominal pain may be a symptom of an infection in another part of the body, such as an acute throat infection, or the onset of flu. Acute pain and continued vomiting are serious symptoms. A physician should investigate the possibility of appendicitis or intestinal obstruction.
Allergy Running nose; wheezing; irritating red patches on face and creases; itching, raised welts; breathing problems.	Assessment by physician; removal of cause; possible treatment with antihistamine or desensitizing injections.	A physician may be able to find the cause of the allergy from skin or blood tests, or the parents may notice that a particular food or environment produces the allergy. *See also* ASTHMA; HAY FEVER; URTICARIA; *also* ECZEMA in previous section.
Appendicitis Pain around the navel moving to lower right abdomen; vomiting; fever; usually constipation, but sometimes diarrhea; loss of appetite.	Consult physician if symptoms continue for more than two hours; urgent appendectomy if appendicitis is acute.	It is often not possible to make a definite diagnosis of appendicitis in a child, but if the surgeon advises an appendectomy, accept the advice. The child usually remains in the hospital until the clips or stitches from the operation are removed. He or she can return to school within two or three weeks, and will be back to normal after a month.
Asthma Wheezing, and difficulty in breathing; dry cough; anxiety due to difficulties in breathing normally; attack sometimes preceded by clear discharge from nose, or sneezing.	No restrictions on child's activities are usually needed when child is not experiencing an attack. Careful, ongoing medical care is needed since asthma is a chronic illness. Drugs to relax spasm; fluids to prevent dehydration; antibiotics if infections occur. Some children have asthma which is precipitated by exercise; medication can be given prior to such activities to prevent attack.	Children who have suffered from infantile eczema sometimes also develop asthma. An asthma attack may have a physical cause, for example, an allergy to animals, house mites, or dust. It may be triggered by exercise or by emotional stress or it may be the result of an infection, usually one of viral origin.
Bed-wetting Child over age four shows no signs of being dry at night; or child who has been dry at night suddenly begins to wet the bed.	Discuss problem with physician who can eliminate the possibility of urinary infection or epilepsy as causes of the return of bed-wetting; praise child for dry night; do not punish for wet ones.	At age 4, 60 percent of boys are dry, and 90 percent of girls. At age 5, 75 percent of boys are dry and nearly 100 percent of girls. An electric bell that rings when the child urinates may help, as may an incentive chart. Bed-wetting eventually stops. Only 2 to 3 percent of boys wet the bed after the age of 12. Bed-wetting may be a sign of emotional stress, for example, jealousy about the arrival of a new baby in the family. Indulge the child's need for attention if this is the reason.
Breath-holding Child takes deep breath as if to give loud yell, but does not breathe out; face goes dark red, then blue; child may fall to ground.	The moment child begins to hold breath, before the teeth are clenched, hook finger in child's mouth and pull tongue forward; this causes child to take reflex breath; consult a physician if attacks persist.	Although the child needs an audience for breath-holding, it is a subconscious reaction to frustration, and not necessarily an attention-seeking device. It is impossible to prevent a child meeting some frustrations, but if possible it is better to distract him or her from aggravating situations. Children usually stop having breath-holding attacks by about age three. Attacks are alarming but usually not dangerous.
Bronchitis Cough with production of phlegm; wheezy breathing; fever.	Consult a physician; deep breathing to clear bronchi of mucus; antispasmodic drugs; antibiotics may be needed; increased intake of fluids; humidifiers and inhalations helpful.	The child may be more comfortable sleeping with the head and shoulders raised. Keep the room warm and humid. A physiotherapist can show the parents how to tip the child's head down and tap the chest to relieve the mucus-congested breathing tubes, but this is seldom necessary except in the case of a child with cystic fibrosis. Bronchitis is more common in families in which someone smokes.

Symptoms and signs	Treatment	Notes
Croup High-pitched hoarse noise when breathing; shortness of breath; fever; rasping cough; symptoms made worse by crying.	If child shows breathing difficulties, contact a physician; meanwhile, hot, steamy room produces rapid improvement; sit child up; cuddle and comfort child; hospitalization if croup is severe.	Croup usually occurs at night. The parents are often more anxious than the child about the coughing. Hot, dry air, as in a centrally-heated room, aggravates the condition. To increase the humidity of the room use a cool mist humidifier.
Deafness Increasing evidence that child is partly deaf; continued deafness after attack of otitis media; poor speech development; inattention.	Assessment by physician; treatment will depend upon cause; repeated ear infections may require prolonged antibiotic use and/or insertion of small plastic or steel tubes (grommets) into the eardrum to allow drainage.	A child may seem to be backward or to have a speech problem because of undiscovered deafness. "Glue" ear is caused by a build-up of sticky glue-like mucus in the middle ear. There is often no accompanying earache. While grommets are in place, keep the ear dry. The grommets eventually ease themselves out on their own. Water must not get into the ears of a child wearing grommets, earplugs can be useful while bathing; hair must be washed carefully, and underwater swimming avoided. *See also* DEAFNESS in first section; OTITIS EXTERNA; OTITIS MEDIA; WAXY EAR in this section.
Discharging ear See OTITIS EXTERNA; OTITIS MEDIA; WAXY EAR.		
Fracture Circumstances of injury; sharp pain in limb, or pain becoming progressively worse; limb obviously misshapen; swelling; child unwilling to use limb.	Assessment by physician; X-ray photograph; treatment either by splinting, casting, traction, or surgery, according to severity and type of fracture.	Children's bones are fairly soft. It is common for only one side of a bone to crack while the other side bends. This is called a "greenstick" fracture. The orthopedic surgeon may need only to splint the limb. If the fractured bone is out of position, it has to be set straight and held in a plaster of Paris or fiberglass cast. This can be frightening for a young child, who may need to be reassured that the limb is definitely inside the cast, and not missing. In an open fracture, part of a broken bone tears the surface of the skin. The risk of infection is very high. Immobilize the limb and take the child to a hospital. Do not give the child any food, drink, or medicines because a general anesthetic may be needed.
Hair, pulling out Child pulls and sucks hair; occasionally causes thinning; child anxious or bored.	Entertain and distract child; if symptoms persist, consult physician.	Hair pulling is sometimes due to scalp irritation caused by eczema, ringworm, or lice. If a bald patch appears on the child's head, consult a physician. It may be due to a condition called alopecia areata or to infection.
Hay fever (seasonal allergic rhinitis) Summer sneezing; running nose; red eyes; eyes oversensitive to light.	Assessment by physician; antihistamine tablets; desensitizing injections.	Perennial allergic rhinitis may be caused by fur, food, or dust, and the symptoms are present all the year round. Skin tests can often identify the specific causes.
Head banging Child sways or bangs head rhythmically; usually occurs when going to sleep.	Cuddle and comfort child; consult physician.	Do not scold or restrain the child. The habit is rarely harmful, but it is wise to pad the head of the crib, and to secure it to the floor to prevent the crib from moving.
Hives See URTICARIA.		
Impetigo Red watery spots; large brown-yellow scabs that spread around lips, nose, and cheeks.	Visit physician promptly; prescription antibiotic creams or oral medication; isolate hair and hand-washing materials used by the sufferers from those used by the rest of the family.	Impetigo can affect previously healthy skin, but often appears with another skin disease, for example, eczema. It is highly infectious, and can be transmitted to other family members. Impetigo tends to occur on moist, dirty skin, and can be spread by direct contact. If dirty fingernails are allowed to pick at the scabs, the infection may spread to other parts of the body.

Age $1\frac{1}{2}$ to age 5: disorders *(Continued)*

Symptoms and signs	*Treatment*	*Notes*
Laryngitis Hoarse voice, commonly occurring after cold; cough. *See also* CROUP.	Steam inhalations; avoid talking to rest larynx; keep child in humid atmosphere using cool mist vaporizer.	Laryngitis occurs more commonly in children whose parents smoke. With careful attention the condition improves in one or two days. Acute laryngo-tracheo-bronchitis (croup) and acute epiglottitis may be serious forms in young children.
Masturbation Child rocks backward and forward; possibly handles genitals; looks preoccupied; stares and puffs; finally relaxes.	Do not punish child; distract and entertain him or her, but never appear disapproving.	Masturbation is a normal stage of development. Compulsive masturbation may imply that a child is bored or undergoing emotional distress, and the problem needs discussion with a physician. Masturbation usually continues into early childhood, then ceases for a few years before recurring in adolescence.
Nightmares *See* SLEEP DISORDERS: NIGHTMARE.		
Otitis externa (inflammation of outer canal of ear) Inflammation of the outer ear; moving ear causes pain; canal may look red; ear may be discharging.	Consult physician without delay.	This disorder may be due to swimming, or from poking a foreign body into the ear canal. Boils are sometimes associated with otitis externa in which case it may be necessary to surgically drain the boil.
Otitis media (inflammation of middle ear) Severe earache, particularly following a cold; fever; sometimes vomiting, diarrhea, and abdominal pain.	Consult physician who can see if eardrum is inflamed; antibiotics; painkilling drugs, if needed.	A child may show all the symptoms but still not be able to tell the parents that it is the ear that is causing pain. A child with otitis media may not have a fever, or feel ill. Only a physician can make an accurate diagnosis by looking at the eardrum.
Paraphimosis End of penis swollen and painful; tight foreskin rolled back constricting end of penis.	Apply cold compress for a few minutes; gently attempt to roll foreskin forward; if this fails, visit physician or hospital quickly.	This may happen if the foreskin has been forced back for washing before the fine fibers attaching it to the end of the penis have separated naturally. A physician may decide to circumcise the child to prevent paraphimosis recurring.
Pica Unusual desire to ingest earth, wood, paper, coal, hair, and even feces.	Parents should give child opportunity of playing with safe things to chew. If child is anemic, physician can treat anemia with iron supplements.	The chief danger is the risk of poisoning. A parent should be particularly careful to lock away dangerous household chemicals, and never paint crib or wall with lead-based paints. Perfectly healthy children can develop the habit.
Pigeon toes *See* WALKING PROBLEMS: PIGEON TOES.		
Pneumonia Rapid breathing; painful cough; coughing brings up sputum with streaks of blood; usually high fever; sometimes stiff neck; slight blue color to lips (cyanosis); use of shoulder and chest muscles to help breathing.	Immediate assessment by physician; chest X ray; treatment of bacterial pneumonia with antibiotics; symptom treatment for viral pneumonia; high fluid intake to prevent dehydration; complete bed rest; oxygen therapy may be needed in severe cases.	Pneumonia often attacks a child recovering from another illness such as gastroenteritis, measles, or whooping cough. The child will be more comfortable propped up in bed during the illness.
Roseola infantum (exanthema subitum; sixth disease) High fever for two to three days; red, blotchy rash appears on face when temperature falls; recovery begins after three or four days.	Keep temperature down with acetaminophen; sponging with tepid water if necessary; give plenty of fluids.	Roseola infantum seldom affects children over the age of three. It is only mildly infectious. It has an incubation period of 10 to 14 days. There are no complications associated with this disease, but the child may suffer from convulsions brought on by a high temperature. Immunization is not available.
Sleep disorders: early morning waking Child wakes two or three hours before family; playfulness makes further sleep impossible.	Blinds or heavy curtains over window to reduce morning light; sufficient toys within reach to provide entertainment.	Unfortunately for the rest of the family, this is normal between the ages of two and six. If you have to get out of bed to change the child's diaper, do not encourage playing.

Symptoms and signs	*Treatment*	*Notes*
Sleep disorders: fear of the dark Child unreasonably frightened at night; unable to sleep; more frightened in strange surroundings or when ill.	Nursery night light; an open bedroom door; normal sounds of family within earshot; a favorite toy or blanket.	Night fears are normal and relatively common. Reassure the child that although there is nothing to be afraid of, the fears are not unusual.
Sleep disorders: nightmare Child wakes up in night terrified; screams; cries; sometimes able to relate content of dream.	Reassurance; cuddles; staying until child sleeps; leaving light on.	A nightmare may be caused by frightening experience, a television program, or the onset of illness. Some children feel better the moment they wake up, others need time to recover from the dream. Nightmares seldom occur before age four. They are normal, but if they occur as often as two or three times a week, talk to a physician.
Sleep disorders: sleep refusal Child refuses to go to bed; refuses to go to sleep; stays awake for two or three hours.	Stop afternoon nap; start bedtime ritual that encourages child to relax, such as a story or warm bath; do not encourage stimulating or active play at bedtime.	A child who refuses to go to sleep may be afraid of the dark or feel insecure. Sleep requirements vary from child to child. Do not insist on a rigid "lights out" discipline if child is afraid. Do not disturb a child who is quiet.
Sleep disorders: sleep rituals Excessive time-wasting rituals before child settles to sleep.	Make sure child is not afraid of the dark; break ritual gradually with something equally enjoyable; stop new rituals from developing.	Most children need some kind of ritual, such as stories or lullabies before going to sleep. Only if the rituals are too long or complicated may they become a problem.
Sleep disorders: sleepwalking *See* SLEEPWALKING in next section.		
Sleep disorders: snoring Noisy breathing through mouth when asleep.	None necessary, unless there is an obstruction, such as adenoids, or a foreign body in the nose.	Some children snore whenever they sleep. Others develop the habit after a cold, or as a result of enlarged adenoids. If you are worried about the snoring, talk to a physician.
Talking, delayed Child over two years old shows no signs of talking.	Assessment by a physician; hearing tests; spend more time talking and reading to child.	Many children use their own language, but nevertheless understand all that is being said around them. Such children will speak normally if adults speak with them. *See also* CEREBRAL PALSY; DEAFNESS, in previous section.
Temper tantrum Two- to-four-year-old expresses immense anger; throws toys; screams and yells; goes red in face; usually ends in tears.	Stay calm; leave door open, and go into another room; do not try to stop tantrum by shouting back; remove objects on which child may injure himself or herself.	A child in a tantrum can not stop, so shouting back does not help. The child needs an audience. He or she is more likely to calm down if left alone. Avoid trouble as much as possible by distracting the child. Children usually grow out of temper tantrums by about age four. *See also* BREATH-HOLDING.
Throat infections *See* CROUP; LARYNGITIS; TONSILLITIS.		
Tonsillitis Inflamed tonsils; sore throat; sometimes earache; headache; fever; neck stiffness in some cases.	Assessment by physician; antibiotics; painkilling drugs; bed rest.	Repeated attacks of tonsillitis scar and reduce the size of the tonsils. Large tonsils, even if they seem to meet at the back of the throat, hardly ever cause an obstruction to breathing, and are usually functioning well. The decision to remove the tonsils may be made by the physician. It is rarely done before the age of four.
Urinary tract infections Frequent urination; painful urination; bloodstained urine; cloudy urine; possible loss of appetite; vomiting; fever; bed-wetting.	Assessment by physician; urine tests; investigation by X ray or ultrasound; appropriate antibiotic drugs.	Urinary infections are more common in girls because the urethra is shorter than in boys. Occasionally, congenital abnormalities of the kidneys and bladder make urine infections more likely. X-ray or ultrasound examinations can reveal if there are any congenital abnormalities.

Age $1\frac{1}{2}$ to age 5: disorders *(Continued)*

Symptoms and signs	*Treatment*	*Notes*
Urine, red Painless, red urine.	Assessment by physician.	Red dye in candies, or beetroot, often stain the urine red. Blood makes the urine cloudy. Large quantities of blood in the urine make it red or brown. If it is caused by urinary infection, nephritis, or a kidney tumor, other symptoms are usually also present.
Urticaria (hives) Rash of small white hives or welts; reddened skin; severe itching; welts join to make large, raised, white areas; then disappear.	Antihistamine; injection of adrenaline sometimes given if symptoms severe; attempt to identify cause.	If urticaria recurs regularly, it may be a reaction to a particular food, drug, or insect bite. Urticaria is unpleasant, and can be dangerous if it involves the throat.
Walking problems: bowlegs Conspicuous gap between knees when ankles are touching.	None necessary, but avoid bulky diapers.	Bowlegs are normal in the first two years; a thick layer of diaper between the legs may increase a child's bowlegged appearance. Most children need no treatment. Vitamin D deficiency can cause bowlegs (see RICKETS in previous section).
Walking problems: flat feet Complete undersurface of foot in contact with ground when standing.	None; assessment by a physician if parents are worried; remedial exercises seldom necessary; inserts in shoes may be prescribed to relieve foot pain and fatigue.	Feet vary from family to family. The fact that a foot works well is more important than the way it looks. In many children, the arch only appears when the foot is being used, for running, walking, or standing on tiptoe. All babies have flat feet at first.
Walking problems: knock-knees Knees turn inward when child stands; when knees touch, feet remain apart.	None, condition usually corrects itself by the age of six or seven.	Although knock-knees may be caused by rickets, they are usually a normal part of development and most obvious between the ages of two and three. If you are anxious, discuss the problem with the child's physician.
Walking problems: late walking Child makes no attempt to walk by the age of 18 months.	Assessment by a physician; treatment will depend on cause.	The age at which walking starts varies greatly from child to child. If development is steady and normal in other fields, the parents have no reason to worry. However, walking delayed beyond 18 months is cause for concern. *See also* CONGENITAL HIP DYSPLASIA in first section; RICKETS in previous section.
Walking problems: limping See CONGENITAL HIP DYSPLASIA in first section; FRACTURE in this section; RHEUMATIC FEVER in next section.		
Walking problems: pigeon toes (toeing-in) Toes point in when child stands; sometimes accompanied by bowlegs.	None usually necessary. Sitting with legs in a frog-leg position should be avoided.	This is a normal condition for children between one and a half and four years old. It improves naturally. Sometimes toeing-in makes a child walk on tip toe.
Walking problems: splayfoot (toeing-out) Child walks with feet turned outwards.	None usually necessary.	It is normal for a toddler to begin walking with toes pointing outwards. As balance improves, the child's feet become more parallel. A child who begins walking with parallel feet often ends up toeing-in to maintain balance.
Waxy ear Yellow, greasy discharge from ear.	Consult a physician if at all doubtful that discharge is wax; wipe wax from outer ear, not canal; physician may gently wash out the wax with warm water if the ear canal is blocked.	Wax is a natural secretion that keeps the canal of the outer ear clean. Cotton swabs tend to pack wax back down the canal. Pushing things into the ear to clean it is dangerous, and encourages the child to do the same. It is also dangerous to use an ear syringe to clear wax from the ears of young children as this may damage the eardrum.

Section 4

Age 5 to age 11: normal development

This section of the age-by age charts deals with a time of great physical and intellectual change, beginning with the school age child, and ending with the child who is on the threshold of adolescence.

Intellectual ability varies enormously from one child to another, and is determined by heredity and the home environment as well as by the child's education. Development occurs in spurts so that a child who seems to be doing less well than the rest of the class at one time may suddenly catch up and, six months later, appear to be in advance of the rest, both physically and intellectually. This variation is seen most clearly in the height of children at this age. A child whose growth starts early may be, for a time, as much as a foot taller than a child of the same age whose growth starts late.

Parents who are anxious about their child's achievements should discuss the situation with a teacher and with a physician. Parental worry may be making the child anxious and inhibiting his or her work. Alternatively, a child may be more than usually tired because of the energy spent in a growth spurt.

The first part of this section emphasizes growth characteristics that are considered normal for the age group and so outlines the general patterns of development of children at this age.

All cross-references are in this section unless otherwise specified.

Physical development

Achievements include at:	
Five years:	runs and turns easily; gets completely dressed and undressed but may have difficulty tying shoelaces; catches a ball; able to copy a square; helps parents with housework, such as washing dishes, or gardening
Six years:	draws simple pictures with considerable detail; writes own name
Seven years:	many children can ride a bicycle safely; good coordination in playing with a ball; difficulty with bat or tennis racket
Ten years:	begins to play tennis or ping-pong successfully
Eleven to thirteen years:	rapid increase in strength and skill; able to compete successfully with adults; onset of puberty with associated physical changes such as menstruation; breast development may be noticed between the ages of ten and eleven, and menstruation between ten and sixteen; pubic hair development may occur between the ages of eleven and fourteen; voice changes in boys occur between age twelve and fifteen

Understanding

Achievements include at:	
Five years:	knows days of week; may know alphabet and be able to read simple words; able to answer complicated questions; enjoys singing
Six years:	reads simple messages; recognizes traffic signs; counts and may do simple addition; talks about television programs; knows left from right hand
Seven years:	begins to learn to tell the time; writes name, age, and address; able to explain words (for example "A ball is a round toy")
Eight years:	reads simple books; writes simple arithmetic; can explain simple concepts (for example "An apple is a kind of fruit")
Nine years:	reading more complicated sentences reading alone; writing improving; begins to understand rules of spelling; enjoys pretending to buy and sell; runs errands effectively; shops for mother
Ten years:	understands the idea of historical time; also has a concept of future and has ideas about a career
Ten to thirteen years:	immense differences in achievements due to differences in intelligence, ability to concentrate, parental influences, and schooling

Disease prevention and health care

Immunization

Health steps to be taken at:	
Five years (school entry):	diphtheria, tetanus, whooping cough (triple) injection and oral polio vaccine; other injections such as cholera, typhoid, typhus, or yellow fever, should be given in advance of traveling to areas of risk
Ten to twelve years	measles, mumps, and rubella booster injection
Fourteen years (high school entry):	tetanus/diphtheria injection

Health care

Semi-annual visit to dentist and at least every two years to physician; annual vision and hearing test; regular measurement of height and weight.

Age 5 to age 11: disorders

Symptoms and Signs	*Treatment*	*Notes*
Boil Small, red, painful lump; sometimes fever; boil develops a head within three days; boil bursts, releasing pus; pain subsides.	Antibiotics; warm compress to bring boil to a head. If red streaks appear radiating from boil, if a lymph gland becomes tender, or if boils recur, consult a physician.	Single boils may occur at any time, but recurring boils appear most commonly on the buttocks and at the back of the neck, especially in boys between ages eight and ten, and in the armpits in puberty. Recurring boils are not caused by poor hygiene, but frequent showers help to clean the skin. The physician may also recommend antiseptic soaps and creams, and antibiotic lotions. Recurring boils are sometimes associated with the development of diabetes, and a test of the child's urine is advisable to exclude this possibility. In general, boils heal themselves.
Cerebral palsy (spasticity) See CEREBRAL PALSY in second section.		
Dental disorders: decay Pain in tooth or ear; broken tooth; sometimes bad breath.	Immediate dental attention.	Prevention is better than cure. Primary teeth need as much care as permanent teeth. Discourage candy and sugar consumption. Prevent children from sucking candy between meals. Encourage tooth brushing at least twice a day, three times a day if possible. The novelty of an electric toothbrush is often enough to encourage a lazy child. Adults must not assume that the loss of a primary tooth does not matter because it is not meant to be permanent. A child should be taken to the dentist regularly even when there is no obvious sign of tooth decay. The visits accustom the child to the idea of going to the dentist, and the dentist can detect a problem before it becomes severe.
Dental disorders problems: loose primary teeth Primary tooth loose in socket.	Consult the dentist if the tooth was injured.	The first teeth of children are known as primary, baby, or milk teeth. These are replaced naturally as the second, or permanent, teeth develop. Primary teeth loosen naturally and fall out from the age of six years onward. Sometimes months elapse before the permanent teeth come through. If a toddler falls and knocks out a tooth that was not loose before, wash it carefully and hold it firmly in the socket for a few minutes. If this is done quickly, the tooth will "take." It is important to do this because if a primary tooth falls out prematurely, the surrounding teeth may grow incorrectly. The permanent teeth may then emerge out of position.
Dental disorders: overcrowding Permanent teeth emerge cramped and crooked.	Orthodontic care.	An orthodontist is a specialist trained to deal with crooked and overcrowded teeth. Occasionally some teeth are removed to make room for the others, but usually braces are fitted and tightened from time to time to correct the position of the teeth. Braces may be uncomfortable at first.
Diabetes Persistent thirst; frequent urination; weight loss; sometimes drowsiness and loss of consciousness; vomiting.	Admission to hospital for urgent care; intravenous fluids; injections of insulin.	Diabetes in early childhood is relatively rare, but when it occurs it develops suddenly. Careful control with insulin injections is necessary for the rest of the person's life; nevertheless the outlook for a successful and productive life is good. It is important that the child learn to test the blood sugar and administer the injections independently. Parents must try to make the child feel as normal as possible. Infections in a diabetic are often more serious and must be treated as quickly as possible.

Symptoms and Signs	Treatment	Notes
Epilepsy: tonic-clonic seizures		
Unconsciousness; rigid body; jerking movements of arms and legs; clenching of teeth; grunting noises; in many cases incontinence; may be confused and frightened one or two minutes after attack; then gradual recovery, often sleep. Seizures sometimes preceded by characteristic warning sensations known as "aura."	Stay with child and move dangerous objects away; if vomiting starts, turn head to side to avoid choking; do not restrain limbs; do not push anything into mouth; when convulsion is over, get medical assistance. Modern drug therapy allows an epileptic to lead a normal life but, nevertheless, working with dangerous machinery should be avoided; blood levels of medication must be periodically measured to ensure that child is receiving an adequate dosage of medication.	The physician assesses the cause of the seizure by observing the electrical activity of the brain with an EEG (electroencephalogram). Epilepsy may occur as a result of brain damage at birth, a meningitis infection, severe head injury, or it may occur spontaneously. It is sometimes associated with cerebral palsy. Epileptic children should be encouraged to lead a normal, active life, while taking certain precautions, such as avoiding heights.
Epilepsy: absence seizures		
Momentary loss of awareness; blank look; staring eyes; then return to normal.	Treatment with appropriate drugs prevents attacks; sometimes spontaneous improvement occurs.	In some cases a child suffering an absence seizure may appear to be daydreaming. But the difference between daydreaming and an absence seizure is that nothing can attract the child's attention for the few seconds that the seizure lasts. Absence seizures can occur very frequently, several times an hour in some cases, and this may interfere with a child's education. Even in mild cases, medical treatment is advisable, because momentary unconsciousness may be dangerous. Most children stop having attacks after several years. *See also* CONVULSION in second section.
Fainting (syncope)		
Dry mouth; hot, then cold feeling; noises sound distant; vision becomes gray; possible nausea; loss of consciousness; sometimes vomiting during recovery; weakness and lethargy for half an hour after attack.	At onset of symptoms, lie down; or sit down with head between knees; retain position for at least five minutes.	Fainting commonly occurs when a child is tired, hungry, or standing for a long time. It may also be brought on by the shock of seeing something unpleasant or by pain.
"Growing" pains		
Vague aches and pains in limbs; no obvious cause; muscle aches (myalgia) may occur with viral infections.	None; acetaminophen, reassurance, and understanding in severe cases; massage the limb.	"Growing" pains may occur because of fatigue, or as a result of a minor knock when the child is playing. The pains usually occur in the muscles, not the joints, and are not caused by rheumatic fever. If the child is eager to run out to play, the parents can assume that the pain is not too serious. However, whatever the reason for the pain, it is real to the child, and should not be dismissed as unimportant.
Hair ball (trichobezoar)		
Habit of eating hair; noticeable hair loss; vomiting; abdominal pain, child often emotionally disturbed.	Consult a physician; diagnosis by barium meal; surgical removal of hair ball.	Because the habit of hair-chewing must be stopped, the cause must be investigated, Usually the child needs psychiatric help. Sometimes a hair ball is discovered long after the habit of chewing hair has stopped.
Hay fever		
See HAY FEVER in previous section.		
Headaches, recurrent		
Pain anywhere in head; variable intensity and duration; possibly nausea.	Assessment by a physician; painkilling drugs.	Headaches, without other symptoms, often affect older children. They are usually caused by tension and stress. The parents and physician must try to find the cause of the anxiety. The child needs reassurance and understanding. Recurrent headaches are seldom due to eye strain. *See also* MIGRAINE in next section.
Infectious diseases: chickenpox (varicella)		
Two to three days of fever; red spots on trunk; after a few hours, spots turn to clear blisters; new spots appear during first three days on face, inside mouth, and in ears; numerous spots cause severe irritation.	Dab calamine lotion on spots; cut nails to prevent scratching; cool light clothing; antihistamines reduce itching. Aspirin should *never* be used to treat fever; use only acetaminophen in children with chickenpox.	Chickenpox is one of the most infectious childhood diseases. It has an incubation period of up to 21 days, but usually develops in 15 days. The child is infectious from 1 day before the outbreak of spots, to 6 days afterwards, when all of the blisters have dried. Complications are rare in chickenpox, but are more common in older children or adults. Immunization is routinely not available. In some cases, chickenpox causes shingles (herpes zoster) in adults.

Age 5 to age 11: disorders *(Continued)*

Symptoms and Signs	*Treatment*	*Notes*
Infectious diseases: erythema infectiosum (fifth disease)		
Sudden onset of rash; bright red cheeks; faint irregular rash on limbs; rash more obvious when warm or in bath.	Keep patient cool; sponging with tepid water if temperature rises; nourishing fluids when appetite is poor.	The incubation for erythema infectiosum is 6 to 14 days. The child is infectious from the onset of the illness until about 5 to 7 days after the fever subsides. There are usually no complications and immunization is not available.
Infectious diseases: influenza (flu)		
Sudden onset of shivering; high fever; sweating; aching muscles; headache; eye pain; sore throat; cough; symptoms last four to six days; fatigue lasts one to two weeks.	Keep temperature down with acetaminophen and sponging with tepid water; nourishing fluids when appetite is poor; throat lozenges to soothe throat; avoid aspirin.	Children tend to suffer less than adults during an attack of flu. Complications may develop in the form of bronchitis, pneumonia, or sinusitis. The child is infectious for 12 hours before the fever starts until the end of the fever. Vaccination against the specific influenza virus protects most people in a severe epidemic.
Infectious diseases: measles (rubeola; morbilli)		
Fever; dry cough; sore throat; runny nose; red eyes; tiny white spots (Koplik's spots) inside mouth; then red spots developing into a pinkish red rash behind ears; rash spreads over face, onto limbs and trunk; lasts three to five days.	Keep temperature down with acetaminophen; sponging with tepid water if necessary; nourishing fluids until appetite returns; antihistamines to reduce nasal congestion; wash eyes if crusted; nurse in a quiet, darkened room.	Measles is highly infectious. It has an incubation period of up to 14 days, although it usually develops in 10 days. The child is infectious from the onset of fever until 5 days after the rash first appears. Complications, should they occur, may be serious. They include chest infections, sinusitis, middle ear infections, and encephalitis, an inflammation of the brain. The latter needs urgent hospital treatment. Measles vaccination is given at the age of 15 months, and provides nearly complete protection against the disease. Even the rare cases that are not fully protected by the vaccine suffer only a mild form of the disease. Older children who have not been immunized should be given measles vaccine. A booster dose at 10 to 12 years of age is recommended.
Infectious diseases: meningitis		
Sometimes cold-like symptoms for two days; then severe headache; vomiting; convulsions; in some cases, red rash on skin and inside mouth; stiff neck; dislike of light.	Urgent medical attention; isolation in hospital; study of cerebrospinal fluid to confirm diagnosis; rapid antibiotic treatment necessary to prevent progression of the disease; nourishing diet with plenty of fluids.	Meningitis is caused by bacteria such as meningococcus. There is a slight chance that other members of the family will become infected. This is prevented if all contacts take appropriate antibiotics. The child stops being infectious two days after antibiotic treatment begins. Complications can include arthritis, nerve paralysis, deafness, abscess inside the skull that presses on the brain, and collapse culminating in death.
Infectious diseases: mumps		
Fever; headache; salivary glands in front of ears and under jaw swell and become painful after two to three days; swelling remains for up to ten days; eating and swallowing may be painful.	Keep temperature down; sponging with tepid water if necessary; give plenty of fluids; avoid acidic foods as they cause pain in the salivary glands; nourishing diet with soft food; frequent cool drinks; painkilling drugs; ice packs held against glands may give some relief.	Mumps is usually mild in childhood, and not as infectious as other childhood diseases. It has an incubation period of 12 to 28 days, but usually develops within 18 days. The child is infectious for 2 days before the onset of symptoms until 10 days later, or until 2 days after the swelling has subsided, whichever is longer. Complications include deafness, encephalitis, meningitis, and inflammation of the pancreas or thyroid gland. Inflammation of one or both testes is fairly common after puberty. Similar inflammation of ovaries is rare. Vaccination should be carried out when a child is 15 months old. A booster injection is recommended at 10 to 12 years of age.

Symptoms and Signs	*Treatment*	*Notes*
Infectious diseases: rubella (German measles)		
Mild fever; sore throat for one or two days; pink rash behind ears, spreading over face, then body; rash lasts two or three days; tender swollen glands at back of head and joint pains may last longer.	Keep temperature down; nourishing fluids when appetite is poor. Avoid exposure to pregnant women.	Rubella is a mild childhood disease, but specific diagnosis is essential in case the child has come into contact with a woman who is in the early stages of pregnancy. If this is the case, the pregnant woman must consult her physician since the fetus may be damaged by exposure to rubella. Rubella has an incubation period of up to 21 days after last contact, but usually develops within 14 days. The child is infectious for 7 days before the rash appears until 5 days after the rash appears. Immunization is offered to boys and girls, usually at 15 months of age. A booster dose is recommended at 10 to 12 years of age.
Infectious diseases: scarlet fever		
High fever; sore throat; headache; vomiting; stomachache; fine, red rash beginning around neck and on chest, spreading over body; area around mouth remains pale; skin peels on and after seventh day; tongue is white initially, then bright red spots appear; exhaustion.	Keep temperature down; sponging with tepid water if necessary; nourishing fluids by mouth when appetite is poor; antibiotic drugs to overcome the associated strep throat infection.	Scarlet fever is a streptococcal infection that affects the throat, and also causes a rash. Contacts sometimes get the same throat infection without the rash. Children seldom complain of a sore throat during the illness. It has an incubation period of one to three days. A child who has come in contact with the disease should be treated promptly with antibiotics if sore throat or rash develops. Complications include rheumatic fever, acute nephritis, hair loss, and ear infection, but complications are reduced by early antibiotic treatment. There is no immunization available.
Infectious diseases: whooping cough (pertussis)		
Mild fever; runny nose; slight cough that becomes severe; bout of coughing ending in a "whoop"as air is inhaled; distress; vomiting; increased weakness; difficult sleeping; gradual improvement after six weeks.	Antibiotics at early stage; cough suppressives seldom helpful; nourishing fluids and light food; hold a distressed child firmly and securely during bout of coughing.	Whooping cough is one of the most serious of the childhood infectious diseases. It may have an incubation period of up to 21 days, but usually develops within 10. The child is infectious for about three weeks from the onset of symptoms. Complications include middle ear infections, bronchopneumonia, and sinusitis. Encephalitis may also occur. Children can be immunized against whooping cough at an early age beginning at two months. Although the vaccine occasionally causes severe side effects, it is much safer than contracting the disease.
Learning Problems		
See DOWN'S SYNDROME in first section; CEREBRAL PALSY and DEAFNESS in second section; EPILEPSY: ABSENCE SEIZURES, and OVERACTIVE CHILD in this section; DEPRESSION in next section.		
Leukemia		
Pallor; fatigue; malaise; fever; bruising of skin; sometimes persistent sore throat and illness at onset; often pain in limbs.	Chemotherapy.	Leukemia used to be fatal within four months, but with modern treatment the life expectancy is much greater. The physician makes the diagnosis from a special tissue sample taken from the bone marrow. Leukemia is the most common form of cancer among children, but it must be remembered that it is still a rare disease. Children with Down's syndrome have a greater chance of developing leukemia.
Lice (pediculosis)		
Itching scalp; itching skin around hair; possible secondary infection; tiny white dots (the eggs, called nits) sticking to hairs.	Speak to a physician; shampoo hair with anti-louse preparation; treat entire family; wash clothes and bedding. Certain medications should not be used on young children or pregnant women—consult physician.	If the parents discover a child has lice, they must tell the school teacher who can make sure the lice do not spread. Lice are extremely contagious and can spread to the cleanest heads. They are becoming an increasing problem because insecticide-resistant strains are developing. *See also* NIT.

Age 5 to age 11: disorders *(Continued)*

Symptoms and Signs	*Treatment*	*Notes*
Lisp Inability to pronounce "s" sound correctly.	Assessment by a physician if severe, or if lisping continues over a long period of time.	Lisping is a normal part of speech development. It tends to recur when the child loses the primary teeth at the front of the mouth. However, continued lisping and mispronunciation may occasionally be due to partial deafness. If the physician recommends speech therapy to correct the lisp, it is wise to begin the therapy before the child attends school regularly.
Meningitis See INFECTIOUS DISEASES: MENINGITIS.		
Mental handicap See DOWN'S SYNDROME in first section.		
Nail-biting Child chews and nibbles nails; nails excessively short; cuticles sometimes ragged and bleeding.	Discussion with child to find underlying reason for nail-biting; habit is not harmful but is unsightly; gloves worn at night may help; bitter-tasting nail polish useful only if child wishes to cooperate.	Nail-biting is an extremely common habit in children over the age of five. They find the habit soothing. Painting the nails with bitter-tasting substances only helps a child who has already decided to stop. Drawing attention to the habit usually makes the child defiant. The parents should try to appeal to the child's sense of vanity, and point out that it makes the hands look ugly. Nail polish often helps girls to stop. Compulsive nail-biting that causes bleeding may require medical assessment.
Nit Tiny white dots along shafts of hair.	Wash hair with anti-louse shampoo following the instructions exactly; treat entire family. Certain medications should not be used on very young children or pregnant women—consult physician.	Nits are the eggs of the head louse. They are anchored so firmly to shaft of hair that nothing can pull them off. In addition to using special shampoo, the hair can be combed with a nit comb. *See also* LICE.
Nosebleed Sudden bleeding from one nostril; usually due to injury; onset of influenza; something pushed up nose.	Sit down; bend head forward to prevent blood running into throat; mouth breathing and pressure over bleeding nostril for at least 10 minutes. If bleeding does not stop after 20 minutes, seek medical advice.	A smelly, bloodstained discharge from the nose often means that the child has put a bead or some other small object up the nostril. This needs medical attention. Some children have a tendency to have frequent and alarming nosebleeds. This is usually caused by dilated blood vessels inside the nose. A physician can verify and advise on this problem. Nosebleeds are a symptom of certain blood disorders, but are rarely a symptom of leukemia. Some children suffer from nosebleeds at the onset of puberty and at the time of menstrual periods.
Overactive child (hyperkinesis; attention deficit disorder) Restlessness; inability to sit still in class; short concentration time; poor academic and personal performance at school; slow reading and writing; requires little sleep.	Discuss with physician and school staff; specialized schooling; sometimes special drugs to aid concentration; family counseling may be needed to help manage the problem.	This condition is more common in boys than girls. The symptoms are sometimes noticed in the first few months of life, but seldom cause a problem until the child begins school. On investigation, a physician may discover that problems such as hearing or vision impairment or minimal brain damage at birth are the cause, but in most cases no specific cause is identified.
Pneumonia See PNEUMONIA in third section.		
Psoriasis Small red spots on skin; developing into dry, scaling disks; commonly on knees, behind elbows, or elsewhere on skin.	Discuss problem with a physician; drugs and creams to control condition.	Psoriasis is a familial skin disease. It is not curable, but can be controlled. Patience and understanding from the rest of the family is needed to help the child to come to terms with the condition. It is seldom itchy and may suddenly improve, particularly in sunlight.

Symptoms and Signs	Treatment	Notes
Rheumatic fever About two weeks after throat infection; fever; sweating; joints inflamed and feel hot; swollen and painful joints; pain may move from one joint to another; skin rash; nodules under skin on back of head, elbows and knees.	Diagnosis by a physician; hospitalization and complete bed rest; penicillin and aspirin-like drugs in large doses; careful regular assessment and drug therapy with penicillin for many years to prevent another attack.	Heart inflammation commonly occurs with rheumatic fever and heals to form scar tissue. Complete bed rest reduces the severity of the valve damage, but should heart symptoms occur later in life, cardiac surgery may be required. Rheumatic fever is caused by the body's reaction to the bacteria, streptococci, which cause throat infections. *See also* INFECTIOUS DISEASES: SCARLET FEVER.
Ringworm (tinea capitis) Ring of blisters, growing outward; bald patches, if scalp affected; skin on patch dry, gray, and scaly; stumps of hair visible on patch.	Antifungal medication prescribed by a physician; wash brushes, combs, and towels separately; other members of family must not use anything that has come in contact with infected parts of the patient's body.	Ringworm is a fungal infection that occurs in various forms, each type affecting a different part of the body. It is highly contagious. Prompt treatment usually clears the child's scalp of the infection within three weeks, but the hair may take more time to cover the patch. The child must be kept away from school and the family must be careful to prevent the infection spreading.
Scabies Red rash; severe itching; small gray burrows under skin may be visible; usually occurs on webs of fingers and toes, in pubic area, and sometimes on buttocks.	Consult a physician promptly; hot bath; rub body firmly with rough flannel to expose burrows; paint body with prescribed lotion and use as directed; launder all bedding, towels and clothes at high temperature.	Scabies is caused by a mite that is just visible to the naked eye. It is highly contagious, although it can live for only 24 hours away from the body. All members of the family must be checked for suspected scabies. The itching is worse at night when the mites are active. Additional skin infection, such as impetigo, may be caused by the scratching. The body's allergic reaction to the mite takes about a month to develop. Should the child be infected for a second time, the symptoms start at once.
School phobia Tears; tantrums; headaches; stomach pain; nausea; sometimes vomiting as the time for school approaches; truancy.	Discuss with teacher to exclude possibility of bullying or teasing at school; discuss with physician; give child help and reassurance.	Although school phobia may stem from a fear of teasing or bullying, it is often a reaction against parents who constantly push their children to achieve better grades. Sometimes school phobia has nothing to do with school at all, and is caused by emotional problems in the family. A child who refuses to eat breakfast, or vomits after breakfast, should not be forced to eat. A fruit drink, toast, or nothing at all, is better than a battle before school. The child makes up for a lost breakfast at lunchtime. A child who has been happy at school before, and suddenly develops a violent phobia, needs special assessment by a physician. The goal of treatment is to return child to school and treat any underlying emotional problems.
Sleepwalking Child wandering about at night unaware of surroundings; seldom knocks into things; may be able to answer questions during episode; has no recollection of incident the next day.	Lead child back to bed; do not wake; but if child is in middle of a nightmare, it may be sensible to wake. Lock doors to the outside and to those rooms that may be dangerous for the sleepwalker; remove anything that may cause child to trip or fall.	Sleepwalking is most common between the ages of 7 and 15. It may be due to anxiety about exams or some other worry. Once the cause has resolved itself, the sleepwalking usually stops. Consult a physician if sleepwalking occurs regularly.
Sore throat Pain on swallowing; pain in throat; often fever.	Acetaminophen; throat lozenges; for severe sore throat, assessment by a physician; throat swabs; prescribed antibiotics.	A small child often has difficulty in describing exactly where a pain is. Even when the throat is inflamed, or possibly ulcerated, the child may still be complaining of other symptoms, for instance stomach pain, or headache. Sore throats occur with tonsillitis, colds, and influenza, as well as the more serious diseases such as infectious mononucleosis, diphtheria, and scarlet fever. Severe sore throats must be investigated by a physician because they may be caused by streptococcal bacteria. This can lead to acute nephritis, rheumatic fever or scarlet fever.

Age 5 to age 11: disorders *(Continued)*

Symptoms and Signs	*Treatment*	*Notes*
Stuttering and stammering		
Hesitation over words; sometimes contortion of face, mouth, and tongue in effort to get word out.	In minor cases, ignore stutter; persistent stutter needs speech therapy.	Stuttering is more common in boys than girls. It tends to run in families, but is not genetic. The reason for this is probably that a family with a stutterer overreacts to the normal stage of hesitant speech that children go through. Speech therapy aims to restore the child's confidence in the ability to produce fluent speech. More than half the children are cured, and the rest make good improvement.
Testis, torsion of		
Sudden, severe pain and swelling of scrotum; severe abdominal pain; often intermittent pain; sometimes vomiting and fever.	Seek urgent medical assistance; surgery required to prevent permanent damage to testis; testis is untwisted and repositioned during the operation.	Torsion occurs when the testis twists the spermatic cord, thus obstructing the blood supply. The testis swells and causes pain. If the condition is left untreated, the testis will be destroyed in a matter of hours. If one testis is involved the other may be in danger, and so the surgeon often secures the position of the other at the same operation. Torsion of the testis is thought to be caused by a congenital defect.
Thumb-sucking		
Child sucks thumb when tired, when worried, or for comfort.	Appeal to child's sense of vanity; do not use physical restraints.	Thumb-sucking is a harmless habit until it begins to affect the position of the permanent teeth. Explain to the child that the habit is pushing the teeth forward, and that to correct the position, the child may have to wear braces in the future. Wearing a glove at night, or painting the thumb with a bitter substance may help to remind a child who has decided to stop the habit anyway. The thumb may become painful because of moisture or because of friction from sucking. In such cases the child usually changes to suck the other thumb.
Tic (habit spasm)		
Rapid, repeated movement of face or body; twitch worse when child concentrates; part of body affected works normally when required; blinking and grimacing commonest forms; twitch disappears during sleep.	None; discover reason for possible anxiety; do not try to stop child twitching; do not mention twitch.	A tic may result from a habit that used to have a useful purpose, for example, flicking hair out of the eyes. The habit continues even when the hair is cut. If the parents constantly nag the child to stop, another tic of a different nature is likely to develop. Tics are most common between the ages of 8 and 12, and tend to improve as the child gets older.
Tonsil and adenoid problems		
Inflamed tonsils; sore throat; blocked nose; snoring; earache; sometimes deafness.	Acute infections treated with antibiotics; consult a physician who can assess need for surgical removal.	Tonsils and adenoids build immunity and are important parts of the body's resistance to respiratory disease. If scarring occurs as a result of repeated infections, their usefulness is reduced and it may be necessary to remove them. Children of school age encounter many infections, and at this age the tonsils and adenoids are proportionally at their largest.
Wart (verruca)		
Small nodules, usually on hands and fingers. Warts on sole of foot (plantar wart) may be painful.	Assessment by a physician; removal by means of liquid nitrogen, dry ice, acid, foot soak, or electric cautery (burning); most disappear without treatment.	Warts are thought to be caused by a viral infection. They are not usually uncomfortable unless they appear on the foot, where the pressure of walking on them hurts the foot. Verrucas are mildly infectious, so a child with plantar warts should not be permitted to go barefoot. Sometimes "seedling" warts appear around the site of a wart that has been removed. In many cases warts disappear naturally after a few months.
Worms		
In many cases symptoms are not apparent; in others, worms may be visible in feces; sometimes intermittent diarrhea; flatulence; abdominal distension; anal itching, particularly at night.	Assessment by a physician; treatment with appropriate antiworm medicine.	Worms that infect the human intestine include hookworms, pinworms, roundworms, tapeworms, or whipworms.

Section 5

Age 11 to age 18: normal development

Normal development of children between the ages of 11 and 18 is extremely varied. This section of the age-by-age charts gives general indications of the normal changes that parents and their children can expect. A list of the most common problems and disorders encountered at this age follows this outline.

Adolescent development is closely related to situations at home, in school, and in the community. These circumstances affect mental and emotional development particularly. An understanding of this process will help parents to appreciate what their child is going through in the crucial, and sometimes difficult, transition from child to adult.

Physical growth

Developments include at:

Eleven to sixteen years:	in girls most rapid growth occurs between age eleven and fourteen; in boys it occurs between age twelve and sixteen; height increases, on average, by six to twelve inches; weight by between fifteen and sixty pounds; legs grow first; then hips, chest, and shoulders develop; and finally the trunk increases, giving depth to the chest
Sixteen to eighteen years:	growth complete in girls; in boys it usually continues, slowly, for a year or two more; in some cases there is "delayed adolescence," in which a growth spurt occurs at this age

Female sexual development

Developments include at:

Eleven to fourteen years:	development of hips may be noticeable since age nine; early breast development evident from age ten; breast swelling rapidly from age twelve, with nipple pigmentation; size of vulva increases; hair grows in pubic region and in armpits; onset of menstruation between age ten and sixteen
Fourteen to sixteen years:	breasts fully grown; slight vaginal secretion; armpit and pubic hair fully developed; sexual maturation complete.

Male sexual development

Developments include at:

Twelve to sixteen years:	increase in size of penis and testicles; spontaneous erections; appearance of pubic hair; temporary breast swelling occurs in ten percent of boys; voice beginning to deepen
Fourteen to sixteen years:	full development of pubic hair; appearance of armpit and facial hair; nocturnal emission of sperm; deep voice
Sixteen to eighteen years:	starts to shave; normal adult sexual interests and abilities

Emotional understanding

Developments include at:

Twelve to fourteen years:	friends tend to be of own sex; interests mainly concern school, sports, and home; particular interest in factual information
Fourteen to sixteen years:	interest in opposite sex with "dating"; tendency to stay in groups; steady friend or companion often changes every few weeks; bursts of great enthusiasm often fail to last; admiration of "cult" or public figures, often of same sex; transient homosexual phase; ability for abstract thought now fully developed
Sixteen to eighteen years:	deeply involved with opposite sex; rejection often causes considerable sense of hurt; wanting to be accepted as mature and adult; rebellious against authority; sexual anxieties and problems sometimes conflict with other interests and schooling; friends tend to be of similar intelligence and are usually at a similar stage of rebellion against authority; most adolescents are interested in politics, and particularly in ideas that are antiestablishment

Disease prevention and health care

Immunization

Health steps to be taken at:

Ten to twelve years	measles, mumps, and rubella booster injection
Fourteen years:	tetanus/diphtheria booster injection

Health care

Health steps to be taken at:

Twelve to fourteen years:	annual medical and semi-annual dental checkups; discussion about emotional, physical and sexual changes that are taking place; importance of personal morality and ethical values must be stressed by parents; contraception should be explained; check girls for scoliosis
Fourteen to eighteen years:	annual routine medical and semi-annual dental checkups; informal discussion of sexual matters; explanation of sexually transmitted disease; encourage the child to visit physician or dentist alone

Age 11 to age 18: disorders

Symptoms and Signs	*Treatment*	*Notes*
Acne Pustules and blackheads on face and neck; particularly affecting forehead, cheeks, and chin; also chest, back, and shoulders; severe cases result in scarring.	Keep hair and skin clean; creams that cause skin to peel sometimes applied to expose blocked pores; antibiotics; supervised ultraviolet light treatment helps in severe cases.	Acne is a disfiguring disorder occurring at an age when physical appearance is important. In most cases, the problem gradually disappears after about age 20. Parents should be sympathetic and help to maintain the child's self-confidence. In girls, acne is often worse just before menstruation. Some types of skin are more likely than others to develop acne.
Anorexia nervosa Loss of weight; often extreme emaciation; failure to eat; sometimes self-induced vomiting after meals; monthly periods cease; skin sometimes becomes covered with fine hair; denial that there is a problem.	Persuade patient to see physician; psychiatric care; drug therapy; in severe cases intravenous feeding is necessary. Family therapy is frequently needed.	Anorexia nervosa is much more common in adolescent girls than boys. The girl usually denies that anything is wrong. She is often convinced that she is obese, despite evidence to the contrary. This is a psychological illness. One interpretation is that the girl is trying to stop herself becoming an adult, thus avoiding social and sexual responsibilities. It is a sign of underlying insecurity and depression. A milder type of anorexia nervosa may occur when the girl alternates between periods of weight loss and periods of excessive eating and weight gain. Both eating disorders are different from "crash" dieting and slimming crazes, and should not be confused.
Anxiety Irritability; agitation; nail-biting; inability to sleep well; inability to concentrate.	Attempt to discover underlying worry: physician or school counselor may help.	Anxiety is a common problem during adolescence. The child may be worried about examinations, about school activities, or about making friends, particularly with the opposite sex. The parents should try to be interested and helpful without forcing the child to tell them about the problem. If it is a sexual problem, the child may find difficulty in talking about it. If the symptoms continue, suggest a visit to the physician.
Appendicitis *See* APPENDICITIS in next section.		
Cystitis Frequent and painful urination; cloudy urine; sometimes fever; in some cases, blood in urine.	Consult physician; urine tests; antibiotics; frequent emptying of the bladder.	Cystitis (an infection of the bladder) is more common in girls than boys because the female urethra is shorter, and infecting organisms from outside the body can reach the bladder more easily. It may occur for no apparent reason, and is sometimes caused by sexual intercourse or by the use of internal tampons during periods. Holding the urine for prolonged periods may also cause infections in some girls. Recurring attacks need careful investigation because they may be associated with a more serious disorder.
Depression Moodiness; persistent lack of enthusiasm; feelings of failure; sleep difficulties; feelings of isolation and loneliness; anxiety; agitation; drop in quality of school work; overeating; anorexia nervosa; thoughts of suicide.	Keep adolescent involved in family affairs; show friendship and affection; discuss realistic worries; seek the advice of a physician if condition continues; drug therapy may help; immediate medical attention if suicidal thoughts are present.	Adolescence is a difficult time in which many social and personal adjustments must be made. The adolescent has to cope with increasing academic responsibility, sexual issues, and the realization that social pressures and conflicts commonly suppress individual interest. Teachers at school often notice a change in the standard of the child's work. *See also* ANXIETY.

Symptoms and Signs	*Treatment*	*Notes*
Drug abuse Abnormal behavior, including sudden changes in habits or appearance; extreme lethargy; unusual enthusiasm; extraordinary statements; confusion; moodiness; lack of concern for personal appearance; weight loss; in some cases, scratch marks, or persistent sniffing and nasal irritation.	Seek expert advice; avoid violent confrontations; maintain secure, friendly family situation. Hospital treatment and psychiatric care may be required.	Adolescents often experiment with drugs, and in some cases, experimentation leads to active rebellion against the authority of their parents. In many cases, however, spying on a teenager's activities only increases the urge to rebel. If parents suspect that their child is experimenting with drugs, it is important to consult a physician. In many cases, a teenager finds it easier to talk the problem over with a physician, who can then advise parents on how to handle the problem. Most teenagers come into contact with drugs. They may find them discussed, or used, by friends. In most cases, however, a teenager from a happy, stable, and caring family is reasonably well-equipped to get through the difficulties of adolescence, without feeling the need for drugs of any kind.
Gonorrhea Discharge from penis or vagina; pain on passing urine; painful erection; in girls symptoms mild or absent, but sometimes low abdominal pain; may result in severe systemic infection and in sterility.	Immediate assessment by physician; antibiotics; abstinence from sexual intercourse until treatment completed; treatment of sexual partner(s); discussion of "safe sex" and prevention of sexually transmitted disease.	Gonorrhea is a highly contagious sexually transmitted disease. By the time a child has reached adolescence, the parents should have discussed the risks of sexually transmitted disease in an open and frank manner. If this has been the rule in the family, the teenager is less likely to contract the disease, and will also be able to ask the parents for advice if symptoms of it appear.
Migraine Vision disturbances that may include flashing lights, abnormal vision, and diminished field of vision; followed by severe headache, often on only one side of head; nausea; vomiting; dislike of bright lights, noise, or movement.	Immediate doses of acetaminophen; antimigraine (ergotamine) drugs; injections or suppositories needed in rare cases to control vomiting; frequent attacks may require daily treatment with drugs; evaluation by physician to rule out other causes of headaches.	Migraine headaches may occur occasionally or as often as two to three times a week. They commonly occur before or during menstruation, at times of mental stress, or just after a period of tension, when the patient finally relaxes. There is often a family history of migraine. Vomiting attacks in childhood may develop into true migraine headaches at the onset of puberty. Occasionally, migraine is associated with a certain type of food. *See also* HEADACHES, RECURRENT in fourth section.
Mononucleosis, infectious One to two weeks of lethargy; general ill health; headaches, followed by fever; other symptoms may include severe sore throat, difficulty in swallowing, swollen neck caused by enlarged lymph nodes, enlarged lymph nodes felt in armpits and groin, faint rash, jaundice; physician may detect enlarged spleen.	Consult physician; diagnosis from blood tests; painkilling drugs; antibiotics if there is a secondary bacterial infection; rest and avoidance of contact sports until recovered; immediate medical care if unable to maintain fluid intake or difficulty breathing.	Symptoms of mononucleosis vary considerably in severity, and may appear only as a low grade fever with minimal sore throat. The worst phase of the illness lasts about seven or ten days, and is followed by a gradual but steady improvement over several weeks. During the acute phase, the patient may be able to eat only soft foods, such as jello and ice cream. It is essential that the fluid intake is kept high. During convalescence extra rest is necessary, because excessive activity can cause a relapse.
Obesity Excessive weight for height and bone structure; in severe cases, knock-knees; backache and recurrent respiratory diseases.	Reduce food intake; exercise; avoid "starvation" diets or diets deficient in required nutrients.	Overfeeding may have started at birth. Parents who tend to overeat encourage similar eating habits in the children. An increase of weight at puberty is natural, due to the hormone changes occurring at this time. A child should eat high quality protein with plenty of fresh fruit and vegetables. Parents should approach the problem with understanding and sympathy, because an obese teenager is often eager to cooperate in an effort to lose weight, whereas parental rejection can lead to secret overeating.

Age 11 to age 18: disorders *(Continued)*

Symptoms and Signs	*Treatment*	*Notes*
Periods, failure to start Girls not menstruating by age 16.	Discuss with physician; physical assessment; sometimes assessment of hormone levels; in rare cases, hormone treatment.	The age that menstruation begins depends on the heredity, race, and health of the individual. The menarche (onset of menstruation) usually begins between the ages of 11 and 14, but is occasionally delayed until the age of 15 or 16. Breast and pubic hair development occur first. See *also* ANOREXIA NERVOSA.
Periods, heavy Exessive bleeding; prolonged bleeding; often accompanied by abdominal pain; loss of clots of blood.	Assessment by a physician; examination to investigate possibility of infection; drugs to control blood flow, pain, and irregularity of periods.	Occasionally, the first period is heavy and prolonged, and periods tend to be heavy until they become regular. Emotional stress often makes the problem worse. Frequent, heavy periods can cause anemia, and a physician should be consulted in case dietary iron supplements are required.
Periods, irregular Intervals of up to three months between periods; variable severity of periods.	Usually none necessary; consult physician if worried.	It is normal after the first period for subsequent ones to be irregular. A second period may not occur for three months, but the intervals lessen, and regularity is usually achieved within the first year, although some girls never become regular. This may cause problems in the future, particularly when estimating the delivery date of a baby, or if trying to use the rhythm method of contraception. Sometimes, irregular periods are caused by anxiety or nervous disorders such as anorexia nervosa.
Periods, painful Low, abdominal, colicky pain for first day or two of menstruation; low backache; pain down outside of thighs; sometimes vomiting; sometimes fainting.	Assessment by physician; regular doses of anti-inflammatory drugs; in severe cases, three to four months of hormone treatment.	About 10 percent of girls between the ages of 14 and 18 have periods that are sufficiently painful to prevent them attending school. Periods are often more painful during times of anxiety and stress.
Premenstrual syndrome Irritability; depression; headache; feeling of "heaviness"; breast tenderness for a few days before the onset of a period; some girls show antisocial behavior and poor school performance before the onset of menstruation.	Consult physician; occasionally drug therapy to reduce excess body fluid; sometimes hormone therapy; avoid salt.	Mild premenstrual symptoms are normal, but if they occur frequently and severely, seek the advice of a physician.
Sexually transmitted disease See ACQUIRED IMMUNE DEFICIENCY SYNDROME in next section; GONORRHEA; SYPHILIS.		
Sexual problems Anxiety about sexual appeal and ability; ignorance about sex; fears of homosexuality.	Parents, school counselors, and a physician should answer questions frankly and openly; informal talks in small groups, with an adviser who is experienced in dealing with adolescent sexual problems.	Anxiety and depression are often a direct result of sexual worries. Parents should answer questions truthfully and respect the adolescent's need for privacy. They should encourage discussion and try not to be disturbed by differences between their children's and their own moral codes and views. Adolescents need to make up their own minds without feeling that they have failed to keep up with their parents' standards. Most anxieties about sex are due to ignorance and to the stories spread at school about sex. Teenagers commonly feel physically inadequate and they need to know that transient bisexual attractions are normal.
Suicidal tendency Talk or threat of suicide; commonly a result of depression.	Stay near teenager; contact a physician; try to give reassurance; lock away sleeping pills and potentially dangerous drugs; take away keys until assistance arrives.	Talk of suicide should always be taken seriously, because talk of suicide or attempted suicide is commonly a cry for help. If the ideas persist, or if an attempt is made, a physician must be consulted.

Symptoms and Signs	Treatment	Notes
Syphilis Firm, painless ulcer (chancre), usually on genitals, sometimes on other parts of body, for example, lip; scar forms after about three months.	Immediate assessment by specialist; drugs; avoidance of all sexual contact.	Syphilis is usually diagnosed in the primary stage, when the chancre appears. Secondary syphilis may develop, with fever and a rash lasting for about 10 days, about 2 months after the chancre has formed a scar. Syphilis is potentially an extremely serious disease; anyone who is in doubt about it should consult a specialist.
Tinea Itching, irritation, and inflamed patches of skin; often with blisters, can affect feet, groin, scalp, and nails.	Antifungal preparations from drugstore; if infection persists, consult physician; keep area clean and dry; use medication twice daily, or as directed.	Tinea is commonly referred to as "Athlete's foot" when it affects the feet. It is caused by a fungal infection, which can spread from person to person, by walking barefoot in public places, or by borrowing shoes or clothing. *See also* RINGWORM in fourth section.
Vaginal discharge Discharge from the vagina; a pale, milky discharge is normal; a colored, smelly, irritating, or painful discharge is not normal.	Usually none necessary. For irritating or offensive discharge, assessment by a gynecologist; test for infection; appropriate drug therapy.	Many healthy women have a slight discharge. Over-enthusiastic washing and douching only aggravates the condition. It is normal for a girl to have a pale, milky discharge for up to two years before the onset of menstruation. A similar discharge may occur a day or two before and after menstruation, and at the time of ovulation in the middle of the month. However, if the discharge is colored or offensive, there may be an an infection.

Section 6

Young adults (age 18–35): introduction

The 18 to 35 age group is at a stage of physical and psychological development that should be full of enthusiasm and vitality, characteristic of young adult life.

It is also a time in which the individual should begin to think in terms of preventive medicine, and of having regular checkups and discussions with a physician, especially when symptoms occur, however trivial. If a physician is fully informed about an individual's general health and previous medical history, then he or she can be alert to signs of impending disorder and disease.

Problems in sexual and emotional relationships sometimes give rise to physical, psychosomatic, or psychological symptoms. These underlying problems, as well as the specific disorder about which the patient complains, have to be diagnosed and treated if the patient is to feel and remain basically healthy.

Psychologically based diseases and disorders are not deliberately made up by the patient, but are unconscious expressions of a need to avoid conflict in situations that may be otherwise impossible. For this reason, such patients require prompt medical diagnosis and careful management. It may be necessary for the physician or therapist to give the patient psychological support until he or she can solve the problem alone. When a solution is achieved, the symptoms usually disappear.

The only neurological problem that may be common in young adults is migraine. Psychological problems that develop may be partly biochemical, such as schizophrenia. More commonly, they are social, for example, drug abuse, alcoholism, and smoking.

Dental hygiene is an important part of general health care, and this is most easily achieved by annual visits to a dentist, who will check for decay. Such examinations may also reveal crowding of the teeth, because of a small jaw or because of the slow emergence of wisdom teeth.

Many young adults take part in energetic and sometimes dangerous sports and, as a result, are particularly likely to suffer sports injuries. Common among these are injuries to the knee, such as a torn cartilage, and injuries to the wrist and elbow, for example, fracture of the scaphoid bone in the wrist or the development of tennis elbow. Exercise, such as long-distance running, can result in orthopedic problems, such as stress fractures or heel pain. The onset of some diseases and disorders that may last for life is sometimes seen at this age. Examples include psoriasis, Raynaud's phenomenon, and vitiligo, as well as excessive sweating (hyperhidrosis) caused by anxiety or stress.

Some people suffer from a persistent backache that may be due to ankylosing spondylitis, but can also be caused by gynecological problems, such as painful periods.

The development of the early signs of pregnancy, for example an absence of periods, causes all women some concern. If the pregnancy is welcomed, the woman will be pleased, but if a child is not wanted, the mother is more likely to be anxious.

Circulation problems, apart from fainting, are rare in this age group. The first signs of chest problems are usually attacks of acute bronchitis. In some cases, the recurrent coughing results in the condition known as pneumothorax. Childhood asthma and hay fever tend to improve between the ages of 20 and 30.

Sexual intercourse is important to many young adults, and there is some likelihood that psychological problems will arise. Disorders related to sexual activity are also relatively common. Among the disorders that may occur in women are salpingitis and vaginitis, both of which may cause sexual intercourse to be painful. Infections that may be passed on by sexual contact include epididymitis in a man; urinary tract problems, such as cystitis, which usually affects women; and the sexually transmitted diseases, including AIDS.

Gastrointestinal problems affecting this age group include appendicitis, Crohn's disease, and ulcerative colitis. Usually, only the first symptoms of Crohn's disease and ulcerative colitis occur early in adult life. Infectious hepatitis may develop, and occurs most commonly in local epidemics. Cancer in any form is rare.

Increasing deafness is most likely to be due to otosclerosis, but it may also be due to recurring infections, such as otitis media (secondary to respiratory infection), or otitis externa. Eye problems, other than those requiring glasses, are uncommon.

Recurrent boils on the lower part of the back may occur, and if these develop in the cleft between the buttocks, they may be a symptom of a pilonidal sinus. Such boils are painful, but not serious if correctly treated.

Although regular health care is not usually as important at this age as it is in childhood and later in life, any symptoms of ill health should be discussed with a physician. Women should have an annual pelvic examination and regular cervical smear tests. Self-examination is very important for both men and women. Men should perform monthly exams of their testes for any lumps, which may represent testicular cancer. Women should perform a breast self-examination every month, after the completion of their period.

Developing the habits of regular exercise and avoiding an excessive intake of food or alcohol will do much to maintain good health. Even more important is the need to not smoke or stop smoking, because it is at this age that regular smoking is most likely to become a habit.

Accidents and trauma are all too frequent causes of death among young adults. Use of seat belts and the avoidance of driving after drinking alcohol are important in reducing health risks.

All cross-references are within this section unless otherwise specified.

Health care checklist

Regular checkups by a physician are sensible precautions against the development of diseases and disorders. At the same time, the following questions are useful to alert each person to danger signals. Use this checklist to assess your state of health, and try to do this regularly, for instance, at the beginning of each month.

Some of the questions apply only to women and some only to men. If the answer to all of the questions is "No", then almost certainly you are in good health. But, if the answer to any of the questions is "Yes", then a physician should be consulted for an expert medical opinion.

Q: Skin of face affected by pimples or blackheads? Skin rash on any other part of body?

Q: Chest pain when exercising?

Q: Frequent sniffing and sneezing? Cough? If cough, blood in cough? Hoarseness? Chest problems? Shortness of breath?

Q: Persistent pain and stiffness in spine, joints, limbs, or any other part of body?

Q: Weight loss that is not caused by dieting? Vomiting? Appetite loss? Indigestion? Nausea? Sudden weight gain?

Q: Change in bowel habits? Diarrhea? Constipation? Abdominal and stomach pain? Blood in feces?

Q: Change in urinary habits? Pain when urinating? Blood in urine? Pain in anal or genital region?

Q: Painful periods? Lack of menstrual blood flow? Pain on intercourse? Vaginal discharge? Unexpected vaginal bleeding? Irritation? Sexual difficulties? Anxiety?

Q: Sore on penis? Lumps on testes that will not go away?

Q: Excessive use of alcohol, heavy smoking, or habit of taking drugs?

Q: Fainting, hot flashes, or sudden feeling of weakness?

Q: Fever, with or without vomiting?

Q: Recurrent severe headaches?

Q: Hearing problems? Itching and painful discharge from ear? Deafness and earache?

Q: Vision problems? Sore eyes? Pain or irritation around eyes?

Q: Lump that will not go away in breast or other part of body?

Q: Sore that will not heal?

Q: Change in shape, color, or size of any skin mark or wart?

Q: Nervousness, irritability or depression?

Q: Apathy or lethargy?

Q: Weeping without obvious reason? Feeling of persecution? Hearing voices?

Q: Overwhelming sadness or despair? Feeling unable to cope? Feeling of being rundown or unduly fatigued? Difficulty sleeping? Insomnia?

Q: Pain and swelling around teeth? Sore, coated tongue and sore gums? Lump or sore on tongue or gums? Bleeding gums?

Q: Persistent cold sores around mouth or lips?

Q: Scalp irritated and itchy, flaking skin? Sudden loss of hair? Persistent sores on scalp?

Young adults (age 18-35): disorders

Symptoms and Signs	*Treatment*	*Notes*
Abortion See MISCARRIAGE.		
Acne See ACNE in previous section.		
Acquired immune deficiency syndrome (AIDS) Unexplained weight loss, swollen glands, cough, diarrhea, blotches on the skin, resembling bruises which grow progressively harder.	Immediate testing for AIDS antibodies; abstinence from sexual intercourse and sharing of needles in intravenous drug use. At this time, there is no known cure for AIDS. Treatment consists of treating the symptoms, psychiatric counseling, painkilling drugs, and eventual hospitalization or hospice care for the dying AIDS patient.	As the illness progresses and the AIDS patient's autoimmune system fails, the patient becomes susceptible to other diseases, such as meningitis, pneumonia, and Kaposi's sarcoma, a rare form of cancer. AIDS is believed to be transmitted during the exchange of bodily fluids in sexual intercourse or by sharing needles in drug use. It is spreading into the general population after initially being restricted to homosexuals and intravenous drug users. The threat of AIDS is being met by educational programs advocating sexual abstinence or the use of condoms, constant research for a possible vaccine, as well as for drugs to cure it. At present, AZT (Azidothymidine) and the anti-herpes drug, Acyclovir, are being used experimentally.
Allergy See ALLERGY and HAY FEVER in third section; ASTHMA in eighth section.		

Symptoms and Signs	Treatment	Notes
Amenorrhea No menstrual periods; primary amenorrhea: periods never start at puberty; secondary amenorrhea: periods cease.	Assessment by a physician; pregnancy test; hormone therapy sometimes required if pregnancy test is negative.	The most common cause of amenorrhea in this age group is pregnancy. Other causes include ending a regular course of the contraceptive pill, a serious illness, prolonged anxiety, early onset of menopause, which sometimes affects older women in this age group, and also anorexia nervosa, which is more likely to affect younger women. *See also* PERIODS, FAILURE TO START in fifth section.
Ankylosing spondylitis (bamboo spine) Increasing pain and stiffness in lower spine; symptoms worse in the morning; periods without pain; increasing rigidity of spine over several years.	X ray of spine; blood tests; aspirin-like drugs; antirheumatic drugs; regular physiotherapy; breathing exercises.	In some cases, other joints become swollen and painful or the eyes become red and sore. Physiotherapy helps to maintain normal back movement and posture.
Anorexia nervosa *See* ANOREXIA NERVOSA in fifth section.		
Appendicitis Initially slight nausea and vague central abdominal pain; pain gradually increases and moves to right lower abdomen; slight fever, gradually increasing in severity; headache; in most cases, constipation; vomiting; abdomen tender to touch.	If pain continues for two hours, consult a physician; urgent hospitalization for surgical removal of appendix (appendectomy); eat and drink nothing until hospitalized; do not take laxatives for constipation.	An appendectomy is done through a cut in the lower abdomen that leaves only a small scar. The patient stays in the hospital for about five days. If the appendix is not removed quickly, it is liable to burst, causing peritonitis, a serious infection of the internal abdominal surface. If peritonitis develops, prolonged treatment with antibiotics may be necessary.
Bronchitis, acute Cough; thick sputum; central chest pain during coughing bouts; fever; general feeling of illness.	Steam inhalation; sedative cough mixtures; if necessary, antibiotics prescribed by physician.	The infection often develops after a cold, influenza (flu), or other respiratory illness. It is also associated with asthma. The condition is aggravated by smoking, a dusty atmosphere, or a cold, damp environment, and can develop into pneumonia. Repeated attacks of acute bronchitis damage the bronchi and can lead to chronic bronchitis.
Crohn's disease Abdominal pain; diarrhea two or three times a day; loss of appetite; loss of weight; mild fever; weakness or fatigue; severity of symptoms may vary over many years.	Diagnosis from history of illness and from barium meal or enema, and X ray of gastrointestinal tract; symptoms usually controlled with drugs; sometimes operation is necessary.	The cause of Crohn's disease is not known. Parts of the gastrointestinal tract become inflamed. In most cases, the end of the small intestine and the beginning of the large intestine are the places affected. The acute form is often mistaken for appendicitis. The chronic form may lead to intestinal obstruction, or abscesses, that, in rare cases, may involve adjacent organs, for instance, the bladder or the skin.
Cystitis *See* CYSTITIS in fifth section.		
Dandruff White, scaling skin from scalp; sometimes with itching; rarely, inflammation.	Wash hair with medicated shampoo two or three times a week; brush hair regularly and vigorously.	Dandruff is the normal shedding of dead skin cells from the scalp. Dandruff is more noticeable in persons with congenital dry skin, or eczema. A diseased condition, seborrheic dermatitis of the scalp, produces larger scales that are yellow-brown and greasy.
Drug abuse *See* DRUG ABUSE: HARD DRUGS; DRUG ABUSE: SOFT DRUGS in fifth section.		
Dyspareunia (Painful intercourse) Pain during sexual intercourse; vaginal discharge; irritation; anxiety.	Consult physician; tests for sexually transmitted disease; gynecological examination, counseling.	Expert medical assessment can exclude possible physical reasons for this common complaint. It is often due to anxiety, but may be caused by poor sexual technique; by gynecological problems, such as a tight hymen, vaginitis, or salpingitis; or by disorders such as urethritis or sexually transmitted disease.

Young adults (age 18-35): disorders *(Continued)*

Symptoms and Signs	*Treatment*	*Notes*
Epididymitis Pain in the groin; swollen, tender testicle; sometimes fever; pain when urinating.	Consult physician; antibiotics; bed rest; support for scrotum; painkilling drugs.	Epididymitis is an inflammation of the epididymis (beginning of the seminal tube) in the scrotum. It is sometimes associated with prostate problems, and also with sexually transmitted diseases, particularly gonorrhea.
Fainting Dry mouth; cold perspiration; nausea; vertigo; disturbed vision; buzzing in ears; loss of consiousness; collapse.	At first signs of fainting, lie down; alternatively, sit with head between knees; avoid standing or sitting upright.	Fainting is caused by a sudden reduction in the blood supply to the brain. It sometimes affects pregnant women, but may also occur after standing in a hot room when tired, after a sudden shock, or as a result of a sudden change in posture from lying to standing.
Fracture, stress Pain, usually in a limb or in a foot; associated with repeated minor injuries; most commonly caused by long-distance running or walking.	Consult orthopedic specialist; plaster cast may be required.	Repeated minor strains on any bone may produce a fracture. Runners suffer from stress fractures of the foot (march fracture) or leg; occasionally, javelin throwers or weight lifters suffer stress fractures of the forearm. After treatment, care must be taken not to repeat the injury.
Hay fever See HAY FEVER in third section.		
Heel pain Pain in heel, aggravated by walking and running; tenderness deep under heel; sometimes tenderness behind heel.	Consult physician; sponge rubber pad in shoe; injection of corticosteroid drug may help; in some cases, plaster cast necessary; rarely, an operation.	Heel pain is most likely to develop in active young adults. X-ray examination may show a "spur" of new bone forming in the ligaments of the sole of the foot. Heel pain can also be caused by the tearing of ligaments in the sole of the foot, or by bursitis on the Achilles' tendon.
Ingrown toenail Pain on side of affected toenail; infection commonly occurs; inflammation; swelling of toe; thickening of skin.	Cut nail straight across corner; lift and clean carefully under edge with soft brush; wipe with gauze soaked in rubbing alcohol; if there is repeated infection, consult physician; antibiotics, or operation to remove side of nail may be required.	Ingrown toenails occur when the sharp edge of the nail cuts into the skin. This wound is easily infected. Any infection is made worse by tight shoes and by sweaty, dirty feet. Cutting nails straight across, rather than on a curve, usually prevents this problem.
Knee, torn cartilage Inability to straighten knee after twisting injury; swelling; pain for two weeks; followed by recurrent "locking" when knee sticks in one position; or "giving way", when knee fails to support body.	Immediate medical attention; bandaging of knee in straight position; later, operation to remove torn cartilage (meniscectomy) may be necessary.	Osteoarthritis may develop if the cartilage is not removed. Even after the knee operation, this condition may develop. A torn cartilage is a common injury among athletes, particularly football players.
Migraine See MIGRAINE in fifth section.		
Miscarriage Usually in first three months of pregnancy; heavy vaginal bleeding; abdominal pain; loss of fetus.	Contact physician immediately; lie down; painkilling drugs sometimes given; hospitalization for dilatation and curettage may be necessary if bleeding persists.	Sometimes, bleeding occurs in early pregnancy without loss of fetus. This is known as a threatened miscarriage, and the patient should rest in bed for at least two days after the bleeding has stopped. Hospitalization is sometimes recommended. At least ten percent of pregnancies miscarry before the fourteenth week. This is usually due to fetal abnormality. Occasionally, it is due to hormone imbalance. If the problem recurs, a physician should perform an evaluation to determine the cause.
Mitral valve prolapse Chest pains; palpitations; anxiety attacks; fatigue; shortness of breath.	Diagnosis confirmed by physician; usually only reassurance needed; medication may help reduce palpitations and other symptoms.	Mitral valve prolapse is more common in women than in men, and may be found in as many as 15 percent of women. In most cases, there are no symptoms, but when symptoms do arise they can be troubling to the patient. Serious complications are rare.

Symptoms and Signs	*Treatment*	*Notes*
Mononucleosis (glandular fever) See MONONUCLEOSIS, INFECTIOUS in fifth section.		
Pneumothorax Sudden chest pain; shortness of breath; pain in shoulder; dry cough; sometimes extreme shock.	Consult physician; X ray of chest; for slight symptoms, no treatment; for severe symptoms, hospitalization; mechanical removal of air from chest.	A pneumothorax is caused by air or gas entering the chest cavity. This causes part of the lung to collapse. Air enters the cavity either from a chest injury or from a local emphysema (air-filled blister) on the internal surface of the lung. An operation is necessary to treat a recurrent mild pneumothorax.
Psoriasis Clearly defined patches of red skin; silver-gray scaling; can occur anywhere on body.	Consult dermatologist; corticosteroid cream under plastic dressing; drug therapy followed by ultraviolet light often helpful in severe cases.	Although psoriasis patches appear and disappear, the condition is usually mild but persistent. One type affects the nails in particular, and another type is associated with a form of arthritis. The cause of psoriasis is not known, It is more common in women, and usually appears for the first time between the age of 10 and 25.
Salpingitis Acute: thick vaginal discharge; lower abdominal pain; fever; pain when urinating. Chronic: menstrual problems; pain during sexual intercourse; painful periods; dull lower abdominal ache; vaginal discharge.	Assessment by physician; long course of antibiotics; heat treatment; avoid sexual intercourse; sometimes surgical procedure needed.	Salpingitis is an infection of the fallopian tube. The condition can lead to sterility or, in some cases, can cause subsequent pregnancy to be ectopic (inside the fallopian tube instead of the uterus).
Schizophrenia Sudden or gradual onset of disorganized and bizarre thinking; feelings of persecution; irrational behavior; auditory hallucinations.	Consult psychiatrist; drug therapy; often, hospitalization; antipsychotic drugs, often by injection, to prevent relapse.	Schizophrenia is a complicated mental disorder, in which hereditary factors may be significant. A person with a tendency toward schizophrenia may be unable to cope with adolescent anxiety or depression and is particularly likely to be affected adversely by soft or hard drugs.
Sexually transmitted disease See ACQUIRED IMMUNE DEFICIENCY SYNDROME in this section; GONORRHEA and SYPHILIS in fifth section.		
Sexual problems See SEXUAL PROBLEMS in fifth section.		
Sprain Pain at a joint following injury; swelling; limited movement.	Rest joint; support wrist or arm in sling; support ankle with firm bandage.	A sprained joint is one that has had a ligament damaged by an injury. If only a few fibers of a ligament have been torn, the sprain will heal naturally with rest. Rarely, if a ligament is completely ruptured, surgical repair may be required.
Sweating, excessive (hyperhidrosis) Excessive production of sweat; particularly from armpits, palm of hands, and sole of feet.	Consult physician if worried; mild tranquilizing drug; special skin preparations; sometimes removal of area of skin from armpit or operation on nerves in neck.	Sweating is the body's normal way of controlling temperature. Sometimes the sweat glands are overactive, and the most common causes of this include anxiety and stimulating drugs. The condition can produce strong body odor and may lead to skin problems, such as mild rashes or infections.
Tennis elbow Pain and tenderness on outer side of elbow; weakness of forearm muscles.	Rest; antirheumatic drugs; injection of corticosteroid and local anesthetic drugs sometimes helpful.	Tennis elbow is caused by repeated rotating movements of the forearm, such as in playing tennis or in performing a manual task, such as using a screwdriver particularly after a long period of muscular inactivity. Rarely, an operation needed to cure the condition.
Tinea See TINEA in fifth section.		

Young adults (age 18-35): disorders *(Continued)*

Symptoms and Signs	*Treatment*	*Notes*
Toxic shock syndrome (TSS) High fever; severe vomiting; explosive diarrhea; vivid skin rash on the palms and the soles of the feet. In severe cases, loss of body fluids produces a sudden drop in blood pressure, causing shock.	Antibiotics and the administering of large amounts of fluids intravenously. The earlier the condition is treated, the better the chance of recovery.	Toxic shock syndrome is caused by the toxin-producing bacteria, *Staphylococcus aureus*, and can range in severity from mild to fatal. The cause is not fully understood. Although it has occurred in children, men, and post-menopausal women, the majority of cases of toxic shock syndrome have occurred in menstruating women, one percent of whom carry the bacteria in their vaginas during menstruation. Researchers have found a link between TSS and the use of superabsorbent tampons. Avoiding the use of these tampons, and changing regular tampons frequently, lessens the likelihood of contracting TSS.
Vaginitis Vaginal discharge, irritation; soreness.	Assessment by a physician; appropriate treatment, depending on the cause.	Vaginitis may be caused by the organism that causes thrush (candidiasis) or by the parasitic protozoa that causes trichomoniasis. In both these infections, the woman's sexual partner may also be infected. Candidiasis is relatively common during pregnancy, when taking the contraceptive pill, or after a course of antibiotics.
Wisdom tooth, impacted Pain; swelling at back of jaw; sometimes earache; sore throat.	Dental extraction; sometimes under general anesthetic.	In many persons, the jaw is not large enough for the third molar (wisdom) tooth. As the third molar emerges, pressure is exerted on the second molars and sometimes on other teeth in the jaw, causing pain and swelling. Dental extraction solves the problem, although post-operative pain and swelling may last for three to five days. Occasionally, extraction is followed by pain that appears to be in the ear. The pain begins on the third day after the extraction, and continues for several weeks. This is known as a "dry socket". It is not caused by an infection, but must be treated with frequent anesthetic dressings.

Section 7

Mature adults (age 35–50): introduction

Many people in this age group tend to eat and drink too much and also fail to get enough regular exercise. As a result, many are overweight, if not actually obese. Those who smoke or take drugs, including alcohol, to excess usually do so despite knowledge of the harm being done to their body.

The physical functions and responses of the person in early middle age are gradually slowing down. At this age it is more important than ever to safeguard health if the later years of life are to be enjoyable and not a burden because of illness. A major step toward better health is learning how to control eating and drinking habits.

At this age, it is particularly important to understand the relationship between the emotions, the mind, and physical health or illness. This is necessary to help prevent certain diseases and disorders from occurring or, if they do develop, from progressing to more serious conditions. Health care should emphasize preventive medicine. A physician can help each individual to avoid many of the problems of aging and to detect others as soon as they occur.

People who have become obese sometimes try to regain their youthful vigor by playing sports too energetically or too often. In most cases, such sudden bursts of activity do more harm than good. Strained joints and ligaments are among the least serious problems such exercises can cause. Bursitis and frozen shoulder are common in this age group and an Achilles' tendon rupture can be the result of a strenuous game of tennis. A herniated disk commonly results from lifting a weight that is too heavy or form moving awkwardly in some activity that the person is not used to.

Breathing problems may be associated with obesity, or may also be due to a deviated nasal septum, causing a blocked nose and recurrent attacks of sinusitis. Occasionally breathlessness is due to problems such as heart valve disease, which prevents the heart from functioning properly, or to hypertension (high blood pressure), which may be diagnosed on routine examination by a physician.

The low-fiber, high carbohydrate diet of many people is a significant factor in some of the gastrointestinal problems that develop. Diet also affects disorders such as colitis and peptic ulcer, which are often associated with stress and anxiety.

Psychological problems that affect this age group are commonly a product of competitiveness, artificially raised expectations (particularly of material achievement), and the related fear of failure. These ambitions are particularly dangerous if they reflect other people's expectations more than the person's own hopes.

A psychological problem that frequently affects people of this age is depression. This may be precipitated by an approaching crisis or by anxiety about a marriage at the same time as trying to achieve career promotion and social prestige. Depression is particularly likely to affect those who tend to suffer significant changes of mood. The condition is sometimes experienced by those who seem to be the most successful. Typically, such people alternate between an overactive stage, like a mild form of mania, and a depressed state.

Visible signs of aging include conditions such as baldness and the cosmetically unpleasant signs of rosacea (a chronic form of acne). Rosacea may affect women at the time when gynecological problems are beginning. Early symptoms of uterine or breast cancer may be detected. Possible gynecological problems include premenstrual syndrome, menstrual disorders, and fibroids, all of which are often associated with menopause. Many of these conditions develop as a result of hormonal changes, with which other endocrine gland problems, such as thyrotoxicosis, may be associated.

In this age group, regular dental care is particularly important. Smoking stains the teeth and can also cause inflammation of the mouth, which may result in gingivitis.

People in this age group are still young enough to correct the effects of physical deterioration due to an inactive, overindulgent life style. A balance between work and relaxation reduces the effects of stress in a competitive lifestyle. Regular exercises should be done daily for 10 to 15 minutes. Such exercises, combined with a diet that is low in animal fat, high in vegetable fiber, and with only a moderate carbohydrate intake, may do much to prevent heart and circulation problems. In particular, the chances of developing heart disease and arteriosclerosis will be reduced. In addition, gentle exercise will also minimize the dangers of sudden stresses and strains on joints.

Smoking is a major causative factor in heart and lung disease as well as in the development of arteriosclerosis, some forms of urinary cancer, and cancer of the throat. If it can be stopped in middle age, the individual's life will be longer and healthier. In the next stage of life, many of the diseases people suffer are partly the result of lack of care when younger. Sensible health care at age 30 or 40 is directly related to a person's comfort and convenience at age fifty or sixty. Regular assessment by a physician will help maintain good health and the physician's advice may help you identify potential causes of illness before they become dangerous. See Health care checklist at the beginning of the sixth section for a list of questions regarding danger signals of possible illnesses.

All cross-references are within this section unless otherwise specified.

Mature adults (age 35-50): disorders

Symptoms and Signs	*Treatment*	*Notes*
Achilles' tendon rupture Sudden severe pain behind calf; inability to stand on toes of affected leg; most likely to occur after jumping or running.	Operation to repair tendon by direct suture; plaster cast for a month; then intensive physiotherapy.	If an operation is delayed for more than two months, the tendon heals, but remains slightly longer than before. This makes it less efficient. The injury is more common in people who are not accustomed to physical exercise.
Alcoholism Gradual change in personality; forgetfulness; unkempt appearance; vitamin deficiency; cirrhosis of the liver; trembling hands; delirium tremens.	Attendance at Alcoholics Anonymous (AA) or other support group; psychotherapy; "drying out" in a hospital or clinic; drug Antabuse® sometimes helpful.	An alcoholic often denies excessive drinking despite being found drinking in secret. This is a complicated addiction. Effective treatment can be given only if the patient cooperates. Attendance at group therapy sessions, such as those organized by Alcoholics Anonymous frequently helpful. Delirium tremens is a potentially life-threatening condition that occurs as a result of a sudden withdrawal from alcohol. Sometimes, heavy drinking is associated with depression or other psychiatric illnesses.
Anal fissure Severe pain when defecating; bleeding on defecation.	Local anesthetic ointments and creams; if symptoms continue, surgical stretching of muscle and excision of fissure under general anesthetic.	An anal fissure is a tear in the skin lining the anus. Each time a bowel movement is passed, the tear is reopened. It may be a result of chronic constipation, but it may also occur during childbirth or as a complication of Crohn's disease.
Angina pectoris See ANGINA PECTORIS in next section.		
Arteriosclerosis See ARTERIOSCLEROSIS in next section.		
Arthritis, rheumatoid Painful swelling of joints; most commonly affects finger, wrist, foot, or ankle joints; gradual onset of pain; stiffness, particularly in the morning; general feeling of ill health; fatigue; weakness; increasing deformity of affected parts.	Consult physician; drug therapy including aspirin, antirheumatic drugs, gold salts, and corticosteroids; physiotherapy; special shoes and splints to prevent deformity; heat treatment for inflamed phase; surgery sometimes necessary.	The word arthritis means inflammation of a joint. Rheumatoid arthritis is a chronic form of unknown origin that may lead to crippling deformities. It is more common in women than in men, and often causes depression and considerable problems.
Baldness Gradual loss of hair; particularly from crown of scalp and sides of temples.	None. The effects of hair loss may be countered by transplants or by wearing a wig (toupee).	Baldness is a genetically inherited characteristic that is associated with male hormones. Gradual hair loss also occurs in women after the menopause, but is seldom severe enough to cause concern. However, sudden hair loss in either sex needs medical assessment. It sometimes follows scarlet fever infections of the scalp, lice, or ringworm.

Mature adults (age 35-50): disorders *(Continued)*

Symptoms and Signs	*Treatment*	*Notes*
Blood pressure, high (hypertension) Often none; occasionally morning headache; slight blurring of vision; breathlessness.	Assessment by physician with electrocardiogram (EKG); blood tests; urine tests; kidney X ray; drug therapy; diuretics (fluid-removing drugs); weight loss.	Hypertension is usually discovered during a routine medical examination. If the blood pressure is only slightly above normal, the patient is kept under observation but not treated. High blood pressure increases the risk of stroke, coronary thrombosis, or heart failure.
Bronchitis, acute See BRONCHITIS, ACUTE in sixth section.		
Bronchitis, chronic See BRONCHITIS, CHRONIC in next section.		
Bursitis Swelling; sharp pain; localized tenderness in elbow, shoulder, hip, knee, heel, or other joint; movement may be limited.	Rest is most important; sometimes support in splint or sling; painkilling drugs; injection of corticosteroid drugs or local anesthetics often helpful.	Bursitis may present itself as "miner's elbow," "housemaid's knee," or "typist's shoulder." The condition is due to friction or inflammation of a bursa, a sac of liquid near a joint cavity which cushions and lubricates joint movement.
Cancer, breast Early symptoms: discovery of painless, firm lump in breast which can be felt with flat of hand.	Immediate examination by physician; if necessary, surgical removal of lump and microscopic examination (biopsy) to confirm or disprove diagnosis; in certain cases, biopsy performed with a needle, particularly if the surgeon considers that the lump is a cyst.	Any lump in the breast must be examined by a physician as soon as possible to determine whether it is benign, malignant, or cystic. Additional symptoms may include a puckering of the overlying skin, bleeding from the nipple, or inflammation of the pigmented area around the nipple. Further treatment depends on the extent of spread. Possible treatments include removal of the breast, removal of only the lump, deep X-ray treatment of local glands, cancer-killing drug therapy, or a combination of these treatments.
Cancer, gynecological Early symptoms: vaginal bleeding after menopause; bleeding between periods; bleeding on intercourse; vaginal discharge; all may occur without pain.	Cervical smear test to detect presence of precancerous cells; full gynecological examination; dilatation and curettage of uterus to examine tissues of the uterine lining.	Because some forms of gynecological cancer may have no symptoms in the early stages, it is important for a woman to have a regular, routine examination, and an annual cervical smear (Pap) test. If cancer is discovered, further treatment may require operative removal of the uterus (hysterectomy) and ovaries. Early cancer of the cervix can be treated with local surgical removal, chemotherapy, radiotherapy, or laser beam therapy.
Cancer, intestinal See CANCER, INTESTINAL in next section.		
Cancer, lung See CANCER, LUNG in next section.		
Carpal tunnel syndrome Waking at night with tingling and pain in thumb, index and middle fingers of one or both hands; symptoms often relieved by shaking hands vigorously.	Consult physician; splinting wrist at night or corticosteroid injection into front of wrist gives relief in some cases; if this fails, minor operation to relieve compressed nerve may be effective.	Carpal tunnel syndrome is more common in women than in men. It is usually worse during pregnancy or before a menstrual period, and is sometimes associated with rheumatoid arthritis or with an underactive thyroid gland. The condition is caused by the ligaments in the wrist swelling and compressing the median nerve that passes through them.
Cholecystitis, acute Fever; vomiting; severe pain in upper right abdomen; sometimes jaundice; dark urine.	Consult physician; hospitalization; diagnosis with X ray and cholecystogram; antibiotics; painkilling drugs; intravenous fluids; occasionally, immediate operation to remove gall bladder (cholecystectomy).	When the acute attack has lessened and the patient has recovered, a gall bladder X ray is performed and then, if necessary, the gall bladder is removed. The condition is often associated with gallstones.
Coronary thrombosis See THROMBOSIS, CORONARY in next section.		
Cystitis See CYSTITIS in fifth section.		

Symptoms and Signs	*Treatment*	*Notes*
Deafness See EAR DISORDERS: DEAFNESS in ninth section.		
Depression Early morning waking; general unhappiness; difficulty making decisions; loss of sex drive; anxiety; tendency to avoid people; worse early in day.	Discuss with physician; appropriate antidepressant drugs may help; psychotherapy may be needed.	A severe state of depression can lead to suicidal thoughts or to an attempt to commit suicide. If so, there may be a need for hospitalization for further treatment. Depression is particularly likely to follow traumatic events, such as the death of a relative or the birth of a baby.
Deviated nasal septum Difficulty breathing through one nostril; recurrent attacks of sinusitis; snoring; nasal mucus.	Diagnosis made by physician; operation to break and straighten septum between nasal cavities, with partial removal of septum.	The symptoms of deviated nasal septum are usually at their worst during a common cold or during an attack of hay fever. The deviated nasal septum may have been bent since birth or it may be the result of a nose injury.
Diabetes mellitus See DIABETES MELLITUS in next section.		
Epididymitis See EPIDIDYMITIS in sixth section.		
Fibroid Often no symptoms: possible heavy periods, which may cause anemia (iron deficiency in blood); sometimes frequent but painless urination; infertility.	No need for treatment unless symptoms are severe; fibroids may be removed in order to treat infertility, but this can be difficult; rarely, removal of uterus.	Fibroids are benign swellings of the normal uterine muscle. They slowly increase in size until menopause because of hormonal stimulus. After menopause, fibroids usually shrink and rarely become malignant. The condition is more common in women who have never been pregnant.
Frozen shoulder Painful limitation of movement of shoulder that gradually increases in severity; pain then ceases, leaving joint stiff; slow improvement over 6 to 12 months.	Consult physician; rest arm in sling; painkilling and antirheumatic drugs; gentle exercises and heat treatment; sometimes injection of corticosteroid drugs may help.	Often, an X ray of the shoulder does not reveal anything abnormal. The patient may not have a history of injury and the pain may start spontaneously for no obvious reason. Frozen shoulder sometimes develops following coronary thrombosis.
Gingivitis Soreness and bleeding from gums, which may lead to loosening of teeth.	Regular brushing of teeth; use of dental floss to remove bacterial formation (plaque) from teeth; regular visits to dentist; consult physician if condition persists.	A lack of dental care allows infection to reach the bone under the teeth. Gingivitis is relatively common in diabetes, pregnancy, or during drug treatment for epilepsy, and often develops as a result of a lack of vitamin C. In the United States, gingivitis has become a more common cause of lost teeth than dental caries (cavities).
Heart valve disease Gradually increasing breathlessness when exercising; sometimes palpitations (abnormally rapid heart beat); "heart murmur"; ankle swelling; fainting.	Physician's assessment with X rays and specialized heart investigation; treatment with diuretics, digoxin, and rhythm-controlling drugs; heart valve replacement surgery if medical treatment ineffective.	Sometimes, more than one heart valve is diseased, and heart failure may develop with atrial flutter. Most patients know that they have a "heart murmur", and from this a specialist can detect which valve is involved. The disorder may be due to a congenital abnormality or it may be due to damage following rheumatic fever. Most heart murmurs are benign and are not caused by valve disease.
Hemorrhoids (piles) Irritation, soreness, and sometimes pain in anal region with bleeding on defecation; often a small lump can be felt; symptoms vary in intensity; in some cases no symptoms.	Anesthetic creams and suppositories under direction of physician; if symptoms persist, consult physician again; injection or operation may be needed; include bulk such as bran and vegetable fiber in diet; avoid constipation.	Hemorrhoids, which can be external to the anus or internal, are masses of swollen, inflamed veins in the rectum. The characteristic irritation is due to inflammation of the overlying skin. Hemorrhoids are commonly caused by constipation or pregnancy. Sometimes, hemorrhoids can be very painful and may swell because of a thrombosis. Relief may be gained by applying an ice bag to the affected area, taking painkilling drugs, and resting in bed.

Mature adults (age 35-50): disorders *(Continued)*

Symptoms and Signs	*Treatment*	*Notes*
Herniated disk Acute pain in lower back spreading to leg or pain at back of neck spreading through arms to fingers; usually occurs after strain of lifting heavy object; weakness and loss of sensation in area supplied by the nerve; may be very painful to walk.	Consult physician immediately; X rays to confirm diagnosis; painkilling and anti-rheumatic drugs; immobilization of neck or back in collar or corset; physiotherapy and manipulation sometimes relieve symptoms; removal of disk necessary in some cases.	A herniated disk develops because of a rupture of one of the pads of cartilage that act as shock absorbers between the spinal vertebrae.The soft center of the ruptured disk slips out of place and presses on a nerve. The condition has a tendency to improve and then relapse after a new strain, so the best method to prevent recurrence is to learn how to lift or carry heavy objects, or not to lift them at all.
Irritable bowel syndrome (colitis, mucous) Alternating episodes of constipation and diarrhea, often with mucus; lower abdominal colicky pain and vague malaise.	Consult physician; sigmoidoscopy; barium enema; anti-spasmodic drugs; increased fiber and bran in diet.	The patient is often anxious, tense, and at times depressed. He or she may experience diarrhea early in the day or after meals. The sigmoidoscope examination and the X ray allow the physician to observe the state of the internal surface of the bowel and to determine whether the bowel is diseased.
Menopause (climacteric) Irregular periods of varying length; hot flashes, sweats, and mild depression; premenstrual syndrome; periods sometimes cease, although these other symptoms continue; may last several months or years; there may be no symptoms.	Consult physician; gynecological examination necessary; drugs or hormones may stop hot flashes and regulate periods.	Menopause is the end of menstruation. The climacteric is the period of time when hormonal changes cause the symptoms of flashes, palpitations, and sometimes depression, which may be accompanied by a loss of interest in sex. Hormone replacement therapy is a temporary help for the years during which the body adjusts to the new hormone levels.
Menstrual disorders Irregular periods with heavy clots; periods that occur too frequently, or infrequently; painful periods.	Consult gynecologist; investigations of cause and then appropriate treatment; sometimes curettage of lining of uterus.	Menstrual disorders may require hormones to regulate menstruation if the trouble is hormonal in origin. The condition may also be a result of fibroids, menopause, or salpingitis. It is also sometimes caused by thyroid disorders.
Multiple sclerosis Double vision; weakness or tingling in limbs; dizziness or bladder problems; blindness; symptoms likely to disappear, then return, leading to increasingly abnormal gait, muscle weakness, and finally paralysis.	Consult physician; diagnosis made from history of recurring symptoms; physical examination and lumbar puncture to examine spinal fluid; sometimes corticosteroid drugs help during an acute attack; physiotherapy and rehabilitation may also help.	Multiple sclerosis is more common in women than in men and rarely starts after age 45. In many patients it does not develop as far as paralysis. The cause is not known but it may be due to a chronic virus infection of the nervous system.
Obesity Weight 20 percent above normal average for height, age, and sex; breathlessness; sweating; painful joints; increased fatigue; sometimes anxiety or depression.	Consult physician; appetite-reducing drugs may be prescribed in early stages; increase exercise gradually; reduce alcohol and carbohydrate intake; develop healthy diet.	Obesity increases the chances of developing diabetes mellitus, osteoarthritis, hypertension (high blood pressure), arteriosclerosis, heart disease, and bronchitis. Obesity is usually the result of dietary customs, particularly excessive carbohydrate and alcohol intake, as well as lack of exercise.
Premenstrual syndrome Irritability; depression; headaches; constipation; breast tenderness; increase in weight in the 10 days before menstruation.	Consult physician; fluid removing drugs (diuretics), mild antidepressants, or hormones may help to relieve symptoms if taken during the 10 days before menstruation.	Premenstrual syndrome is sometimes associated with menstrual disorders and painful periods. Some patients also suffer from migraine. The condition usually develops because of hormonal imbalance, and this is why the administration of hormones is often beneficial.
Rosacea Patchy, red thickening of skin on face, nose, and sometimes neck; accentuated by flushing; severity varies greatly from time to time.	Consult physician; avoid things that cause flushing, such as hot drinks, alcohol, hot fires; small doses of antibiotics by mouth; sulfur and corticosteroid creams applied to face.	This skin condition is more common in men than in women, and may be associated with anxiety, particularly in people who have an inherited tendency to develop sebaceous gland disorders. Rhinophyma (swollen red nose) may occasionally occur, and this can be treated by cosmetic surgery.

Symptoms and Signs	Treatment	Notes
Sexually transmitted disease See ACQUIRED IMMUNE DEFICIENCY SYNDROME in sixth section; GONORRHEA and SYPHILIS in fifth section.		
Sinusitis Nasal mucus; face pain; pain in teeth or jaw; often fever in an acute attack; headaches; frequently associated with a cold contracted after swimming.	Consult physician; X rays may be needed to confirm diagnosis; drugs, nose drops, and inhalations increase sinus drainage; antibiotics often needed; painkilling drugs when required; repeated attacks may need local heat treatment or surgery.	The discomfort is mainly felt in the cheek bone, sometimes above the eyes, and infrequently in the interior sinuses. Sinusitis may produce a toothache, a constant cough from postnasal "drip," and a husky voice. The condition is aggravated by smoking.
Thrombosis, venous See THROMBOSIS, VENOUS in next section.		
Thyrotoxicosis May include: irritability; anxiety; sweating; restlessness; weight loss despite increased appetite; protruding eyes; palpitations (rapid throbbing or fluttering of heart); trembling hands; sometimes diarrhea; swelling in neck may be noticed.	Consult physician; diagnosis confirmed by examination and blood tests; treatment with antithyroid drugs, radioactive iodine, or surgery (thyroidectomy).	In most cases, thyrotoxicosis is caused by the presence of an antibody that overstimulates the activity of the thyroid gland. Heart problems, such as heart failure and atrial flutter, are often associated with thyrotoxicosis in the elderly. Treatment, particularly with radioactive iodine, is sometimes followed by myxedema.
Toxic shock syndrome See TOXIC SHOCK SYNDROME in sixth section.		
Ulcer, peptic Pain often occurs before eating, and is reduced by ingestion of antacids; symptoms aggravated by alcohol and fried food; sometimes, patients wake in middle of night because of pain.	Consult physician; barium meal and gastroscopy confirm diagnosis; medical treatment with mild and alkali mixtures to relieve pain; bed rest; stopping alcohol intake and smoking; various drugs may be effective.	There may be long periods of freedom from pain, followed by several more weeks of symptoms. Recurrent ulceration may cause perforation, hemorrhage, or obstruction. Ulceration may also continue because of the failure of drug therapy and will then require surgery. Peptic ulcers are aggravated by stress, anxiety, alcohol, tobacco, and some drugs, such as aspirin and antirheumatics. If the patient wakes in the night it is more likely to be because of a duodenal ulcer, whereas pain on eating is more typically a symptom of a gastric ulcer.
Varicose vein See VARICOSE VEIN in next section		
Vertigo See VERTIGO in next section.		

Section 8

The middle-aged (age 50-65): introduction

Men and women between the ages of 50 and 65 go through a series of changes in their lifestyle as they prepare for retirement. The changes may be major, but given good health care, these should be pleasant years. No one at this age, however, can expect to have the same healthy body he or she had as a young adult.

A person of 50 or 60 will usually have a slower reaction time and may take longer to make decisions. He or she will probably function as usual during normal conditions, but may find it harder to respond quickly to changes or to physical or emotional stress. Unfortunately, as the individual ages, minor disorders become more serious, and the body is unable to compensate for some of the physical changes that may occur.

Foot problems, such as pain from bunions or metatarsalgia, are common, and orthopedic difficulties, such as arthritis, rheumatism, or gout, may develop. A major problem is the loss of some or all of the teeth. Most people adjust to the use of false teeth (dentures). If dentures are fitted correctly, they should allow food to be chewed as thoroughly as with natural teeth.

Diet is probably the most common cause of gastrointestinal problems. A diet that has too much animal fat can lead to cholecystitis; drinking too much alcohol can cause cirrhosis; and overeating often leads to obesity.

An incorrect diet, especially in someone who is overweight, can precipitate diabetes mellitus. Diet is also associated with heart and circulation problems, such as arteriosclerosis, which is aggravated by smoking. This arterial disease may cause angina pectoris, coronary thrombosis, and disorders of the heart rate (atrial flutter), and may also cause heart failure. Heart failure may also occur as a result of heart valve disease, coronary thrombosis, or endocrine gland disorders, such as thyrotoxicosis or myxedema. Heart failure may also be associated with emphysema or severe lung disease. All heart and circulation problems are aggravated by obesity and smoking. The development of varicose veins or venous thrombosis is partly due to an inherited tendency. However, it may also be associated with any condition, such as obesity or an abdominal tumor that increases abdominal pressure.

At this age, a person's vitality may diminish, and in most people there is reduced sex drive. In women, the gynecological problems of menopause are over, but the reduced level of hormone production may cause weakening of the pelvic tissue, which could cause prolapse of the uterus. Male problems are usually minor. Apart from an increasingly frequent need to urinate caused by the increasing size of the prostate gland, the most likely disorder is swelling of one side of the scrotum. Other urinary problems, such as kidney stone and pyelonephritis may occur.

Recurrent attacks of acute bronchitis may develop into chronic bronchitis. Chronic bronchitis is also likely to develop as a result of smoking or of years of work in a dusty atmosphere. The late onset of asthma is distressing and, unlike asthma in the young, is rarely caused by an allergy. Pleurisy is not only painful but is more serious in those who smoke.

At this stage of life, psychological problems associated with divorce, business worries, or elderly parents may cause insomnia as well as anxiety and mild depression.

Fortunately, neurological disorders are rare. The severe, unexpected face pain of trigeminal neuralgia is alarming and may be difficult to treat. Epilepsy may develop at this age and, if it does, it often has a cause which can be identified by appropriate tests.

Eye problems may be caused by the altering elasticity of the lens, causing farsightedness and making it necessary to wear glasses. A detached retina may also occur. Regular eye testing is needed to ensure that the first signs of glaucoma are not missed, because this causes a gradual loss of vision and may lead to blindness if not treated. Retinitis can also produce a painless, gradual deterioration in vision.

Ear problems may arise because of variable fluid pressure in the inner ear. Ménière's disease, causing severe attacks of nausea, variable deafness, and vertigo, may also occur at this age.

The main causes of anxiety about health in this age group are heart problems and cancer. Any swelling, change in normal bowel habit, or persistent cough may be suspected as an early symptom of cancer and must be checked. Often the symptom is indicative of a less serious disorder. For example, blood in the feces is as likely to be due to diverticulitis as to cancer of the intestine; blood in the urine may indicate an infection, although it may also indicate cancer of the urinary tract.

Any alteration in size, shape, or color of a skin mole or marking must be discussed with a physician immediately, because of the possibility of cancer of the skin. Another cause of lumps in the skin includes the very slow, painless swelling of a sebaceous cyst.

Prevention of arteriosclerosis can begin in childhood by avoiding animal fats in the diet. In early adult life, smoking should be avoided, not only to prevent lung cancer, arteriosclerosis, and cancer of the urinary tract, but also to protect the lungs from chronic bronchitis, emphysema, and other disorders of the respiratory system. Equally important is regular exercise. This should be more than a weekly game of golf or a swim. Daily exercise improves the condition of the heart and exercises the lungs. In this way, full use is made of the heart and lungs for a few minutes each day. A side effect of this is a sense of mental well-being.

Regular assessment by a physician will help the individual to maintain good health and may detect early signs of disease. But even if such checkups are routine, it is essential not to ignore any symptoms that last longer than a few days without consulting a physician. See Health care checklist at the beginning of the sixth section for a list of questions regarding danger signals of possible illnesses.

All cross-references are within this section unless otherwise specified.

The middle-aged (age 50–65): disorders

Symptoms and Signs	*Treatment*	*Notes*
Alzheimer's disease See ALZHEIMER'S DISEASE in next section.		
Angina pectoris Mid-chest pain often extending into one or both arms, also to neck, jaw, and sometimes abdomen; pain occurring after exercise; may also occur in cold weather, after large meals, or following extreme emotion; slight breathlessness occurs frequently; condition improves after a few minutes.	Consult physician; examination using electrocardiograph; general treatment resembles that for arteriosclerosis and includes weight loss, giving up smoking, low cholesterol diet, and medical treatment to reduce blood pressure; use of drugs to prevent attacks and to relieve pain.	The pain is caused by the narrowing of the coronary arteries that supply heart muscle, so that there is an oxygen deficiency in the muscles. Hiatus hernia, peptic ulcer, and cholecystitis may all cause similar pain. Surgery is considered only if other treatment fails.
Arteriosclerosis Symptoms caused by narrowing of arteries; if affecting heart arteries, may lead to angina pectoris, coronary thrombosis, or heart failure; if affecting arteries that supply the brain, may cause episodes of momentary weakness, difficulty in speaking, blindness, or stroke; if affecting other arteries, may cause limping when walking, due to calf pain, or gangrene of the toes.	Discuss with physician; stop smoking; reduce blood pressure; lose weight; eat low cholesterol diet; check for diabetes and thyrotoxicosis; in some cases, cholesterol-reducing drugs and anticoagulants are prescribed.	Arteriosclerosis is often associated with an increase of cholesterol and other fatty substances in the blood. Early discovery of this and early treatment may prevent the development of arteriosclerosis. Arteriosclerosis is also a potential complication of hypertension (high blood pressure), diabetes, smoking, and lack of exercise.
Arthritis, osteo- See OSTEOARTHRITIS in next section.		
Arthritis, rheumatoid See ARTHRITIS, RHEUMATOID in seventh section.		
Asthma Episodes of wheezing and breathlessness; sometimes associated with coughing; often started by contact with allergic substance or by infection; late-onset asthma, after age 50, seldom due to allergy; main symptoms include dry, persistent cough and breathlessness without wheezing.	Discuss with physician; treatment with antispasmodic drugs and sprays to relieve attack; regular use of a corticosteroid or cromolyn sodium (Intal) spray may prevent further attacks; if infection is present, causing acute bronchitis, immediate use of antibiotics needed; breathing exercises help prevent attacks.	If a person has suffered from asthma since early childhood, the symptoms usually improve as the person grows older. However, recurrence of asthma in a severe form may lead to complications that include dehydration, exhaustion, and respiratory distress. Recurrent asthma may cause lung damage and emphysema.

Symptoms and Signs	*Treatment*	*Notes*
Atrial fibrillation Rapid heartbeat; irregularities in rhythm and in rate; usually occurring periodically, but may be permanent; feeling of vague chest discomfort; slight breathlessness.	Consult physician; electrocardiogram confirms diagnosis; treatment with digoxin to normalize heart rhythm; rarely, electric shock (cardioversion) may be done in a hospital.	Atrial fibrillation is more commonly caused by heart valve disease in younger patients and by arteriosclerosis or thyrotoxicosis in older patients.
Blood pressure, high (hypertension) See BLOOD PRESSURE, HIGH (HYPERTENSION) in seventh section.		
Bronchitis, acute See BRONCHITIS, ACUTE in sixth section.		
Bronchitis, chronic Cough, particularly in the morning, producing clear sputum; sometimes shortness of breath; tendency to suffer attacks of acute bronchitis; coughing during day.	Any worsening of symptoms must be treated immediately; antibiotics; daily breathing exercises; stopping smoking; if necessary, moving to cleaner, warmer climate.	Chronic bronchitis causes lung damage (scarring), emphysema, and may eventually lead to heart failure. The chronic condition often develops in people working in a dusty environment, for example, in mining and in other industries where the atmosphere is dusty, cold, and damp.
Bunion Painful swelling on side of joint behind big toe; usually accompanied by deformity of toe (hallux valgus), in which toe points toward the other toes on foot.	Relieve pressure on bunion with pads and by cutting an opening in shoe; wear low-heeled shoes; consult a specialist; in severe cases, an operation to remove bunion.	Bunions are more common in women than in men, primarily because women tend to wear tight-fitting or high-heeled shoes. The bunion may become infected if the friction of the shoe causes inflammation of the sac of fluid over the joint. *See also* BURSITIS in seventh section.
Cancer, breast See CANCER, BREAST in seventh section.		
Cancer, esophagus See CANCER, ESOPHAGUS in next section.		
Cancer, gynecological See CANCER, GYNECOLOGICAL in seventh section		
Cancer, intestinal Early symptoms: alteration of normal bowel habit; alternating constipation and diarrhea (with mucus and blood); pain; hemorrhoids may also occur.	Consult physician; investigation with barium meal, sigmoidoscopy, or colonoscopy; blood and cancer cells may be found in feces; surgery to remove affected part; drug therapy.	In some cases, obstruction of the intestine is the first symptom of cancer, and this may be accompanied by abdominal pain and distention as well as vomiting and constipation. Annual stool testing for blood and sigmoidoscopy will often detect cancer before symptoms develop, allowing for a better prognosis.
Cancer, lung Early symptoms: cough, with blood-stained sputum, occurring without obvious cause; symptoms resemble acute bronchitis.	Consult physician; chest X-ray; sputum examination for cancer cells and bronchoscopy (a tube passed down the trachea under ageneral anesthetic) to confirm diagnosis.	If cancer appears operable, the surgeon may remove part or all of the lung (pneumonectomy). Radiotherapy and cancer-killing drugs are often effective in prolonging the lives of those who cannot be treated surgically. Lung cancer is 20 times more common in cigarette smokers than in nonsmokers, and also occurs more frequently in those who have inhaled asbestos, radioactive materials, or some other industrial pollutants regularly in the course of their occupations.
Cancer, prostate See CANCER, PROSTATE in next section.		
Cancer, skin Early symptoms: any mole or pigmented area of skin that grows larger, changes color, ulcerates, or bleeds.	Consult physician; removal of part of area (biopsy), for miroscopic examination to confirm diagnosis; surgery, drug therapy, or radiotherapy may be successful.	Basal cell carcinomas and squamous cell cancer commonly occur in fair-skinned people who have been exposed to intensive sunlight for long periods of time. Local removal usually cures the lesion. A dark mole (melanoma) may be malignant and need to be treated by the removal of a large area of skin and by skin grafting. Melanomas occur most commonly on the legs (particularly of women) and on the trunk (particularly of men), and spread rapidly if not treated.

The middle-aged (age 50–65): disorders *(Continued)*

Symptoms and Signs	*Treatment*	*Notes*
Cancer, stomach Early symptoms: loss of appetite; loss of weight; vomiting; black stools (melena); sometimes vague indigestion.	Consult physician; investigation with barium meal and gastroscopy; biopsy of part of ulcerated area will confirm diagnosis; difficult to treat as diagnosis is usually made late in the course of disease; drug therapy effective in some cases; complete removal of stomach (total gastrectomy) may be required; this may also be done to reduce later symptoms of bleeding and pain.	Several other disorders have symptoms that resemble those of stomach cancer. The most common disorder with such symptoms is a peptic ulcer. Gallstones (cholelithiasis), pancreatitis, and coronary artery disease also produce similar symptoms.
Cancer, urinary tract Early symptoms of cancer of bladder or ureter: painless bleeding into urine; pain may occur when clots of blood are passed; frequent urination may or may not be a symptom; if kidney swelling can be felt, this is a sign of kidney involvement.	Consult physician; investigation of kidneys by intravenous pyelogram; examination of bladder; examination of urine for cancer cells; cancer of the kidney treated by surgical removal of kidney; cancer of bladder treated by local removal or by radiotherapy.	Renal, ureter, and bladder cancer can all occur independently. The incidence of cancer of the bladder is increased in some industrial occupations. Cancer of the bladder is most likely to be caused by industrial dyes or by tars that pass through the kidneys of smokers.
Cirrhosis Often no symptoms until late in course of disease; loss of appetite; vague malaise; loss of sex drive; abdominal swelling may occur because of retention of fluid in abdominal cavity.	Stop all alcohol; protein diet with extra vitamins; these measures may halt progress of disease; treatment with corticosteroids, and sometimes a dietary supplement of multivitamins may be helpful.	Cirrhosis is most commonly due to excessive alcohol intake and is only rarely due to an infection of the bile ducts or to infectious hepatitis. Complications include jaundice, which may occur late in the disease, and rupture of a vein in the esophagus, which will cause massive hemorrhage.
Diabetes mellitus Often no symptoms; condition commonly discovered at routine urine examination; weight loss, despite increased appetite; in some cases, diabetes is indicated by recurrent boils, infection, lethargy, thirst, and genital candidiasis.	Diagnosis confirmed by test of urine for sugar, blood test, and glucose tolerance test; treatment with special diet to reduce weight and to control intake of sugar; in some cases, pills to stimulate insulin production; less frequently, insulin injections.	The complications of diabetes mellitus may include arteriosclerosis, gangrene, retinitis, polyneuritis, recurrent infections, kidney disease, and coma due to excess insulin or excess sugar in the blood. A sudden onset of diabetes is more common in young people, and this usually needs urgent treatment with insulin. The likelihood of developing diabetes is increased by alcoholism, obesity, pregnancy, and some thyroid gland disorders. Diabetes is also a condition that tends to run in families.
Dupuytren's contracture Nodule in palm of hand; painless, rigid flexion of ring or little fingers that develops gradually; both hands may be affected. Rarely, feet also affected.	Consult physician; injection of corticosteroids may be helpful in early stages; gradual contraction can be treated only by surgical means.	Dupuytren's contracture affects men more commonly than women. The right hand is affected more than the left. About 50 percent of the cases have relatives who have the disorder. The condition is caused by thickening and contraction of the tough membrane in the palm that surrounds finger tendons.
Ear problems: Ménière's disease Buzzing in ear may last months or years before sudden onset of dizziness, nausea, and vomiting; temporary deafness; several attacks close together, followed by long period without attacks; increasing deafness.	Consult physician; antinausea drugs during an attack; various drugs may help between attacks; surgery is effective, but may cause deafness.	The condition is due to an intermittent increase of fluid pressure in the organ of balance of the inner ear. The cause is unknown. The second ear becomes involved in 15 percent of patients. A feeling of pressure is often noticed in the ear before an attack starts.
Epilepsy Periodic, recurrent seizures; symptoms of the various forms of epilepsy include: brief periods of impaired awareness; fainting; jerky spasms of one muscle group; generalized, severe convulsions; and loss of consciousness; in some cases attacks are preceded by disturbances of smell or hearing (aura).	Consult a physician: diagnosis based on the person's medical history and on electroencephalogram (EEG) studies of the brain's electrical activity; special drug therapy is used to control the symptoms of each particular type of epilepsy.	There are several forms of epilepsy, some of them mild. The form known as absence seizures is a brief lapse of consciousness that may last between 5 and 30 seconds. After a more serious attack involving fainting or convulsions, the person may have a headache or want to sleep. Epilepsy may develop at any age but most cases are diagnosed in people younger than 18. In most cases, epilepsy can not be cured, although the symptoms can be controlled; epilepsy is therefore a lifelong disorder.

Symptoms and Signs	*Treatment*	*Notes*
Eye disorders: detached retina Flashes of light; dark spots; a "veil" across vision; partial loss of sight.	Special techniques, using laser beam surgery or freezing, to reattach retina.	The condition is more common in those who are nearsighted or have a family history of retinal detachment. It may also develop following an injury to the eye. The sooner treatment is given, the better the result.
Eye disorders: farsightedness (presbyopia) Difficulty in reading print, or in seeing near objects.	Vision corrected by wearing bifocal or multifocal eyeglasses, which help correct both near and far vision.	Farsightedness is due to the loss of the elasticity of the lens. Hyperopia, which is farsightedness in a younger age group, is a condition that develops because of the shape of the eye.
Eye disorders: glaucoma Intermittent attacks of dimness of vision, and the appearance of halos around lights; sometimes very severe eye and face pain; partial loss of vision; white of eye becomes inflamed; in some cases, no symptoms.	Examination by ophthalmologist, to detect raised pressure in eyeball; mild cases can be treated successfully with eye drops prescribed by a physician; in severe cases, operation with careful follow-up.	There are two main forms of glaucoma. The first causes symptoms in one eye only and is usually cured by an operation. The second form causes gradual loss of vision, which is usually not noticed at first, and involves both eyes. Untreated glaucoma causes blindness. People who are farsighted and who have a family history of glaucoma need to be checked annually, as do all persons over the age of 60.
Eye disorders: retinitis Gradual loss of vision; sometimes intolerance of light.	Examination of eye by ophthalmologist; protect eyes from light; consult physician for diagnosis and treatment of underlying cause.	Retinitis may be associated with arteriosclerosis, hypertension (high blood pressure), diabetes, kidney disease, or infection.
Foot problems: metatarsalgia Pain in sole of foot at front; thickening of skin and tenderness in this part.	Consult physician; muscle strengthening exercises; arch supports not recommended; operation rarely required.	Metatarsalgia may be associated with flat foot, with wearing high heels, or with rheumatoid arthritis. The condition develops when the heads of the metatarsal bones lose their arch and touch the ground. As a result, there is greater pressure on the heads of the metatarsals, and this causes pain.
Gout Attacks of acute pain in joints; often lasting several days; usually beginning in the knee and also affecting big toe but any joint can be affected; joint becomes swollen and red.	Consult physician; diagnosis from appearance of joint and blood test; immediate treatment with antirheumatics, painkilling drugs, or colchicine; long-term treatment with drugs to reduce uric acid in body.	Gout is caused by an increase in the level of uric acid in the blood, which is a result of an inability to excrete uric acid from the body. It is often an inherited disease. Prolonged gout can cause arthritis and kidney failure. Sometimes, nodules (tophi) of uric acid are found on the ears or the hands.
Heart failure Ankle swelling; shortness of breath on exercise; often slight cough; breathlessness at night, or when lying down.	Consult physician immediately in order that the underlying cause can be discovered and correct treatment given; diagnosis by means of chest X ray and electrocardiograph; treatment with diuretics; digoxin used to strengthen heartbeat; bed rest, in sitting position; light, low-salt diet; adequate sedation at night until recovery.	Heart failure is the inability of the heart to pump adequate amounts of blood through the body. Because of this, fluid retention occurs. The onset of acute heart failure with severe breathlessness (pulmonary edema) needs urgent treatment and hospitalization. Sometimes, the patient has bluish lips and hands (cyanosis) caused by an excess of carbon dioxide in the blood. In the elderly, confusion and restlessness commonly occur because of poor cerebral circulation. The condition may be caused by atrial fibrillation, coronary thrombosis, heart valve disease, hypertension (high blood pressure), scarring in the lungs due to emphysema, chronic bronchitis, or other chest infections.
Hernia (rupture) Swelling, usually in groin or at umbilicus; may be painful if it occurs suddenly, as a result of a strain; swelling often obvious only when standing or when coughing or straining; swelling can usually be pushed flat with gentle pressure unless a herniated strangulation occurs.	Consult physician; surgery is only way of curing the condition; hernias in groin can be held in place with a special rupture belt (truss); surgical repair requires hospitalization for one week, then caution for about two months; avoid lifting heavy objects.	A rupture is due to local weakness in the muscle wall, allowing abdominal contents, intestine, and fat to push through under the skin. The disorder is more common in obese patients. Sometimes, it is impossible to push back the swelling, or the intestines twist inside causing an intestinal obstruction, which leads to local pain and vomiting, and requires immediate treatment.

The middle-aged (age 50–65): disorders *(Continued)*

Symptoms and Signs	*Treatment*	*Notes*
Hiatus hernia Heartburn; acid taste in mouth; chest pain particularly when lying down, bending forward, or kneeling; pain made worse by alcohol or large meals; mild cases may have no symptoms.	Consult physician; barium meal and X ray, with head tilted down, confirms diagnosis; sleep propped up on pillows; antacid mixtures also help.	Hiatus hernia is due to part of the stomach being pushed through a weak point in the diaphragm muscle. It may be congenital and frequently occurs without symptoms. The disorder often occurs with obesity and usually improves with dieting. Major surgery is occasionally required to repair the hernia if symptoms are severe.
Kidney stone (calculus) Often no symptoms until stone moves out of kidney; then, severe pain in back, radiating to groin (renal colic); vomiting; blood in urine.	Consult physician; diagnosis from examination of urine for blood; strong painkilling drugs; rarely, surgery. A new technique, called extracorporeal lithotripsy, shatters kidney stones with high frequency sound waves without surgical intervention.	Kidney stones are caused by calcium abnormalities, parathyroid gland overactivity, deposits of uric acid, or congenital abnormalities of cystine and oxalic acid metabolism. Further stones can be prevented from forming by increasing the intake of fluid and by adapting the diet. A kidney stone may cause inflammation, and ultimately lead to infection, at the point of blockage.
Leukemia See LEUKEMIA in next section.		
Prolapse of uterus Often no symptoms; sometimes incontinence of urine, particularly when laughing, coughing, or straining; feeling of weight or discomfort in vagina.	Consult a physician; operation to tighten ligaments and muscles that support the uterus; as a temporary measure, the prolapse can also be held in place with a pessary.	With a prolapsed uterus, if the patient is too old or weak, a plastic ring can be inserted into the vagina to hold the uterus in place. This ring has to be changed at intervals recommended by the physician. The disorder is usually the result of the ligaments and muscles supporting the uterus being stretched during childbirth or because of excessive obesity.
Prostate disorders See PROSTATE DISORDERS in next section.		
Pyelonephritis (kidney disease) Frequent urination; back pain; fever, sometimes shivering attacks and vomiting.	Consult physician; urine specimen for culture of bacteria; antibiotics for two weeks; further urological investigations may be necessary.	Inadequate treatment causes damage to the kidneys, which may lead to kidney failure. Infection is more common in patients whose kidneys have congenital abnormalities or a kidney stone and in patients with prostate disorders. Infection usually enters through the urinary tract in women, but is carried by the blood in men.
Stroke See STROKE in next section.		
Teeth, loss of Loss of some or all teeth through dental disease.	Consult dentist for advice about kinds of dentures available; regular checkups help to reduce decay and loss of teeth.	Great care should be taken in choosing artificial teeth, because dentures that are fitted badly are not only painful but may also damage the mouth. Take care of dentures by regular cleaning. Rest the gums by taking the dentures out of the mouth each night.
Thrombosis, coronary (heart attack) Onset of severe mid-chest pain, often with distribution like angina pectoris; sweating; shortness of breath and anxiety; sometimes symptoms are only slight. Duration of symptoms is usually 15 minutes or longer.	Call physician immediately; lie quietly; hospitalization in coronary care unit for three to four days and then mainly bed rest for four more days before gradual movement; regular use of anticoagulants may be required.	A coronary thrombosis may follow angina pectoris but can also occur without a history of heart problems or chest pain. The patient usually feels overtired, in a state of stress, and feeling vaguely unwell for a few weeks before the attack. About 50 percent of deaths take place before the patient has reached the hospital. Other heart conditions, such as atrial fibrillation and heart failure, may occur at the same time. On recovery, an appropriate diet and careful exercise are essential parts of a regimen to prevent recurrence of the condition. Obesity, smoking, and arteriosclerosis are contributing factors to coronary thrombosis.

Symptoms and Signs	Treatment	Notes
Thrombosis, venous Superficial venous thrombosis: pain, tenderness, and slight swelling over line of superficial vein in one area of leg. Deep venous thrombosis may produce only calf pain and ankle swelling.	Consult physician; firm bandaging; painkilling and antirheumatic drugs; exercise; anticoagulant drugs may be necessary for a deep venous thrombosis.	A superficial venous thrombosis is not serious and usually improves without complications. A deep venous thrombosis may cause problems if the blood clot (embolus) is released. If an embolus reaches the lungs, it may cause the death of lung tissue, leading to pleurisy and, in severe cases, death. A superficial venous thrombosis can occur as a result of an injury, varicose veins, or ulceration of the leg.
Varicose vein Irregular, swollen vein visible in one or both legs; often slight ankle swelling; aching pain in lower part of leg.	Consult physician; elastic stockings prevent swelling and aching in legs; large veins can be removed surgically; smaller veins treated by cutting, or by injections; legs bandaged for six weeks.	Varicose veins develop because of weakness or absence of valves in the veins of the leg. This may occur after a venous thrombosis, after valves are damaged by back pressure as may occur during pregnancy, or as a result of a congenital defect. Varicose veins are cosmetically disfiguring in the early stages, and there is a tendency for varicose veins to recur. Eczema of the lower legs, hemorrhage, or ulceration may also occur, particularly in the elderly.
Vertigo Spinning sensation; may be accompanied by nausea and vomiting; unsteady gait brought on by moving head; no deafness.	Consult physician; antinausea drugs may help; avoid any movement that is known to cause vertigo.	Benign positional vertigo is of unknown origin but seldom improves. Vertigo may be caused by vestibular neuronitis, an infection of the nerve of balance that is severe at first, but usually improves. The condition may also occur because of wax in the ear or arteriosclerosis. *See also* EAR PROBLEMS: MÉNIÈRE'S DISEASE.

Section 9

Senior citizens (age 65+): introduction

The gradual changes of late middle age can cause a rigidity of mental attitude despite minimal or no deterioration in intellectual function. The physical alterations in the body are partly due to the wear and tear of a lifetime of activity, partly to disease, and partly to a natural slowing in the nervous and muscular reactions.

Senior citizens who remain in good physical and psychological health have active and useful lives. They may have accidents of any kind, but falls are most common, and fractures of the wrist and hip occur.

Such fractures may be complicated by the orthopedic problems of osteoarthritis and by loss of calcium from the bones, osteoporosis, which may lead to curvature of the spine and difficulty in standing straight. Fingers may become deformed by Heberden's nodes.

Prostate enlargement is a common male problem in this age group and is characterized by an urgency to urinate. This condition may be complicated by other ailments of the elderly, such as difficulty in walking because of an arthritic hip, which can make going to the toilet a problem.

Social isolation, particularly as experienced by those living alone, can be intensified by ear problems that cause deafness as well as by eye problems, such as blindness and cataract. The cycle of events following minor illness may result in skin problems. Reduced resistance may allow tuberculosis and shingles to develop, and the use of antibiotics may lead to the development of candidiasis in moist areas of skin. The gradual onset of chronic forms of leukemia may cause fatigue, weakness, and malaise, and may reduce a person's resistance to infections.

In those who smoke, or who have chronic bronchitis, chest problems that arise from emphysema will be intensified. In such people, pneumonia may follow any respiratory infection.

An active, elderly person who eats well should have few problems with constipation, but the condition is a common complaint in those who are inactive and who eat foods that are high in carbohydrates and low in fiber. Constipation may lead to a partial blockage of the intestine, and a type of diarrhea in which liquid feces bypass the harder mass. These symptoms may also indicate cancer or diverticular disease. Constipation may be a symptom of the glandular disorder myxedema (hypothyroidism). It is also common in immobile arthritic patients who are being treated with painkilling drugs.

The combination of myxedema, arteriosclerosis, and diabetes commonly results in arterial damage, which may cause a coronary thrombosis, gangrene, or a stroke.

It is essential for the elderly person to maintain an active routine. The diet of a person aged 65 or over must contain adequate protein as well as fresh fruit and vegetables to provide bulk and vitamin C, particularly during the winter months. Vitamin deficiency is a common result of a bland diet of cheap, processed foods, which are easy to prepare, but are of only slight nutritional value. A combination of poor diet, inadequate heating of the home, and poor health may cause confusion and death due to lowered body temperature (hypothermia).

Psychological problems of the elderly are made worse by a sense of loneliness and isolation, by the onset of depression following the deaths of close relatives or friends, and by loss of memory, leading to confusion. This confusion may be intensified by any disorder, such as deafness or blindness, by diseases such as pneumonia or leukemia, as well as by the common problem of failing to understand the correct dosage of drugs, which may cause the elderly to take an excessive number of tranquilizers. Sleep may be disturbed by prostate problems, the discomfort of arthritis, pain from cramp in the leg, breathlessness from heart failure, or coughing from bronchitis and emphysema.

These are only some of the problems of the elderly. Such problems can be overcome by encouraging a healthy attitude towards the years of retirement before psychological problems present difficulties. A strong interest in life and the world in general can make the difference between a long life of health and happiness, and a short life plagued by physical and psychological problems. Planning for retirement is particularly important. The senior citizen who does community work, attends classes in subjects of interest, or who has an absorbing hobby is usually healthier than the person who does very little or nothing with his or her time.

For those who are less active there are in most cities and small towns social clubs for the elderly as well as special centers for their use during the day. Those who have lost relatives or friends through death can find companionship in such centers, which often have a resident nurse. This is particularly valuable for people who are ill or crippled.

A common fear of people as they grow older is that they will succumb to senile dementia, lose their independence, and become confused and baby-like. Dementia affects about 10 percent of persons over the age of 65. If the condition develops, early medical care is necessary to determine if there is a correctable cause and to prevent complications. Seeing that this medical care is given is the responsibility of relatives and friends.

If a person's physical or mental deterioration is accelerating, there may be no alternative but to put the patient into a nursing home or other institution, where there are special facilities. Increasingly, however, services are available in most communities to help the family care for the patient with dementia. The emphasis must be on early diagnosis and treatment. Because a person suffering from dementia usually has no awareness of his or her condition, it is up to an alert observer to notice the onset of the disease. See the Health care checklist in the sixth section for a list of questions regarding danger signals of possible illnesses.

All cross-references are within this section unless otherwise specified.

Senior citizens (age 65+): disorders

Symptoms and Signs	*Treatment*	*Notes*
Alzheimer's disease Initially, mild forgetfullness; this can progress over a period of months and years to marked confusion, with wandering, disorientation, language problems, and emotional agitation. Occasionally, incontinence; paranoia. Ultimately the patient may become completely dependent for all aspects of care.	No known cure. A careful evaluation by a physician is necessary to assure that a correct diagnosis has been made. Studies suggest that a healthy diet may slow the progression of the disease. Many Alzheimer's patients require admission to nursing homes or other institutions, since family members find it difficult to provide the constant care necessary.	Alzheimer's disease is the most common cause of dementia, affecting 20 to 30 percent of senior citizens over 85 years of age. Researchers have found physical abnormalities in the nerve cells of the brains of Alzheimer's patients, which suggests the possibility of it being hereditary. Other suspected causes include a virus; a chemical deficiency; and an excess accumulation of aluminum deposits in the body.
Arthritis, osteo- See OSTEOARTHRITIS.		
Blood pressure, high (hypertension) See BLOOD PRESSURE, HIGH in seventh section.		
Bronchial pneumonia High fever; cough with sputum; shortness of breath; chest pain.	Consult physician; treatment with antibiotics, breathing exercises, and steam inhalations; X ray confirms diagnosis.	Bronchial pneumonia is an infection of the air passages (bronchi) in the lung. It usually occurs as a complication of bronchitis, influenza, or lung cancer. Sometimes, it develops after an operation, and is a potential danger in any illness that affects an old person. A pneumonia vaccine is available that is given just once, and will protect against one of the bacterium that causes pneumonia.
Cancer, esophagus Early symptoms: feeling that food sticks in throat or behind breastbone when swallowing; heartburn, in some cases.	Consult physician; investigation with barium meal and esophagoscopy; difficult to treat but removal of tumor may be possible; otherwise, surgical operation to shorten esophagus after removing affected part; radiotherapy; in some cases, a plastic or metal tube is inserted to prevent tumor from blocking esophagus.	Cancer of the esophagus is most commonly associated with excessive intake of alcohol. A muscular disorder (achalasia) that affects the junction between the esophagus and the stomach may also lead to the development of cancer.
Cancer, prostate Early symptoms: frequent and difficult urination; blood in urine; in some cases, the first symptoms, caused by secondary deposits, are bone pain that may be associated with backache or with spontaneous fracture of lower leg or thigh.	Consult physician; examination of prostate may detect irregular, hard enlargement; biopsy of prostate confirms presence of cancer; treatment with hormones frequently causes prostate cancer to decrease in size, and may prevent growth for many years; if cancer has not spread, removal of prostate gland may be curative; if X ray confirms presence of cancer in bones, radiotherapy to bone stops local pain.	Cancer of the prostate is often discovered only when the patient undergoes surgery for prostate disorders. Although prostate cancer is the most common form of cancer in men over 65, in many cases it has no effect on life expectancy, because it is relatively easy to control. An annual rectal exam can help detect prostate cancer in its early, more treatable stages.

Symptoms and Signs	*Treatment*	*Notes*
Candidiasis (moniliasis) Sore, slightly irritating skin infection; occurring in moist skin folds; mouth, armpit, groin, vagina, and skin under breasts commonly affected.	Consult physician; keep area clean, dry, and powdered; treatment with antifungal preparations.	Candidiasis is caused by a fungal organism that normally lives in the intestine. The fungus can spread to the skin in certain circumstances. A warm and moist environment, such as the interior of the body, is favorable if the organisms have been killed through antibiotic treatment. Other factors favoring development of candidiasis include lowered resistance due to diabetes mellitus and the effects of cortisone treatment.
Cataract See EYE DISORDERS: CATARACT.		
Corns Tender, thickened skin over or between toes, due to friction from rubbing shoes.	Consult physician; protection with special pads; removal of thickened skin with softening solutions or plasters.	Corns may be sufficiently painful to prevent normal walking. It is important that the feet of the elderly should have regular attention, so that the person is not prevented from getting enough exercise. Wearing comfortable, well-fitting shoes is also important.
Cramp in calf and foot Severe, spontaneous muscle cramps; usually occurring during night; occasionally when resting during day.	Consult physician; massage muscle and pull foot so as to stretch calf muscle; recurring cramps may be prevented with medication prescribed by physician; exercises before patient goes to bed, to move limb through full range of movement, may also help; cradle over feet in bed to relieve leg from weight of blankets.	The cause of this type of cramp is not known, so treatment is difficult. Cramps that affect the calf and foot at rest are not due to a poor arterial blood supply and do not cause pain in the calf muscle when the person is walking. Pain in the calf when walking (intermittent claudication) is usually a symptom of arteriosclerosis.
Diverticular disease Diarrhea or constipation; lower abdominal pain; rectal bleeding; in severe cases, fever; in chronic cases, symptoms occur intermittently.	Consult physician; antispasmodic pills; high-fiber diet; antibiotics if necessary; diagnosis made with barium enema and sigmoidoscopy; thorough examination necessary to exclude possibility of cancer	As people age, they tend to develop diverticulosis, a condition in which diverticula, or pouches, form in the wall of the colon. Poor diet is suspected as a primary cause of this condition, which has few symptoms except for occasional rectal bleeding. If the diverticula become inflammed or infected (diverticulitis), this may lead to an abscess formation, infection of the abdominal cavity, or intestinal obstruction. These disorders may need surgery.
Ear disorders: deafness Gradual or sudden loss of hearing.	Assessment by physician; special hearing tests to diagnose type of deafness; hearing aid may be suggested before deafness becomes extreme.	In the elderly, deafness may be due not only to wax in the ear but also to Ménière's disease, or to otosclerosis, a condition affecting the bones in the middle ear. The gradual deafness of old age may be accelerated by having worked with noisy machinery. Sudden deafness may be due to wax in the outer ear or to a hemorrhage into the inner ear. Deafness is also a social problem because it can cause the deaf person to feel isolated.
Ear disorders: wax Deafness and sometimes irritation in ear.	Examination of ear by physician; softening of wax with warm oil; syringing ear with warm water removes softened wax.	The problem of wax in the ear is more common in people with ear infections. Some people form wax more easily than others and should have regular ear examinations to prevent hard wax from causing irritation.
Emphysema Gradual and increasing breathlessness; difficulty expanding chest; often slight cough; recurrent attacks of bronchitis, frequently accompanied by wheezing.	Condition confirmed by special breathing tests and chest X rays; stop smoking; bronchitis treated with antibiotics; lose weight if obese; breathing exercises and drainage of secretions from lungs are helpful.	Emphysema is caused by a breakdown of lung tissue that leads to a reduction of the surface area and the elasticity of the lungs. The condition is more common in people with chronic bronchitis and those who smoke. Heart failure may occur because of lung damage, which prevents a normal flow of blood.
Epilepsy See EPILEPSY in eighth section.		

Senior citizens (age 65+): disorders *(Continued)*

Symptoms and Signs	*Treatment*	*Notes*
Eye disorders: blindness Sudden or momentary blindness in one or both eyes or gradual loss of vision.	Consult physician and ophthalmologist; treatment depends on the cause of blindness.	Sudden blindness in both eyes is very rare, but may be caused by a stroke. Sudden blindness in one eye is usually caused by a disorder such as a detached retina, arteriosclerosis, or multiple sclerosis. Gradual loss of vision is most commonly caused by a cataract, glaucoma, or retinitis. Gradual blindness may also be a result of chronic infections of the conjunctiva or pressure on the optic nerve from a tumor in the brain.
Eye disorders: cataract Gradually increasing mistiness of vision; cloudy appearance in the pupil; distortion or loss of vision; no pain.	Surgical removal of lens; this is usually done when useful vision is lost in worst eye. Lens may be replaced by plastic implant.	Cataract, a gradual loss of lens transparency, may be associated with diabetes, but it may also occur following eye injury or infection. The condition is usually due to deterioration with age, although it also occurs as a congenital defect in some infants.
Eye disorders: lid disorders Inflammation of lids; irritation; redness; thickening of eyelid.	Consult physician; blepharitis is treated with antibiotics and corticosteroids; a cyst may be treated by incision under local anesthetic; if the edge of the lid is turned inward (entropion) or outward (ectropion), or if the lid appears to droop (ptosis), a minor operation may be required.	Blepharitis, an inflammation of the eyelid margins, is often associated with seborrhea or irritation from dust or tobacco smoke. A cyst on the eyelid is due to a blockage of a gland. Entropion and ectropion are usually due to aging or scar formation. Drooping of the eyelid is usually a result of muscle weakness.
False teeth See TEETH, LOSS OF in eighth section.		
Fissure-in-ano See ANAL FISSURE in seventh section.		
Fracture, Colles' (wrist) Painful, swollen wrist; wrist twisted backward and outward; occurring after a fall on an outstretched hand.	Consult physician or go to a hospital immediately; injury repaired under general anesthetic; plaster cast for six weeks; recovery aided by physiotherapy.	Colles' fracture is the most common kind of fracture in people over age 50. Complete repair of the fracture may be difficult and, in some cases, weakness, stiffness, and slight deformity of the wrist persists. Occasionally, the tendon that controls the thumb is damaged after the plaster cast is removed. This requires a surgical procedure to repair it.
Fracture, hip Inability to stand; pain in hip; one foot turned outward; occurring most commonly after a fall.	Immediate hospitalization; treatment depends on point of fracture; operation to pin broken parts of bone together; sometimes necessary to replace head of femur; recovery is usually rapid, and most patients leave the hospital after two weeks.	Hip fractures are common in the elderly. Successful treatment depends on the patient's swift return to normal activity. Encouraging the patient's confidence, which may have been shaken by the accident, is particularly important because the muscles of an older person weaken rapidly if they are not exercised.
Frozen shoulder See FROZEN SHOULDER in seventh section.		
Gangrene Gradual darkening of tissue; fingers or toes particularly affected by "dry" gangrene, in which skin appears to shrivel; if area swells, becomes painful, and discharges, this indicates infection ("moist" gangrene).	Consult physician immediately; keep area cool; cover with light, dry dressing; "moist" gangrene treated with antibiotics; amputation of foot or leg may be necessary.	Gangrene occurs because the blood supply to the affected tissue is inadequate or lacking altogether, causing the tissue to die. Gangrene is more common in people with diabetes or with arteriosclerosis, but may also occur with frostbite or following an accident. The elderly must take great care with foot hygiene and the treatment of corns.
Glaucoma See EYE DISORDERS: GLAUCOMA in eighth section.		
Heart failure See HEART FAILURE in eighth section.		

Symptoms and Signs	*Treatment*	*Notes*
Heberden's nodes Swellings, sometimes tender and slightly reddened, on the end joint of the fingers; occurring particularly in elderly people.	Consult physician; injections of corticosteroids; wax baths may reduce tenderness; no treatment required in many cases.	Heberden's nodes are associated with minor underlying osteoarthritis of the joint. The disorder is a result of an inherited tendency to produce a thickening of fibrous tissue, usually from repeated movement, over the roughened edge of the joint cartilage.
Hemorrhoids (piles) See HEMORRHOIDS in seventh section.		
Hernia (rupture) See HERNIA (RUPTURE) in eighth section.		
Hiatus hernia See HIATUS HERNIA in eighth section.		
Hypothermia Mild confusion; slurred speech; staggering when moving; lethargy; may lead to coma and death; occurring when the body is too cold.	Cover with blankets; give warm drinks, but not alcohol; hospitalize as soon as possible.	Hypothermia occurs because the body is unable to produce sufficient heat to maintain the correct body temperature. This may occur either because of excessive loss of heat or because of failure of the body to produce the proper amount of heat. It is a particular hazard in the elderly, in whom it may be associated with heart failure or malnutrition.
Hypothyroidism See MYXEDEMA.		
Influenza Initially, sudden onset of fever, headache, malaise, and chills; later, dry cough, chest pain, and sore throat.	Antibiotics are not effective. Bed rest, fluids, aspirin or acetaminophen, and cough suppressant are all helpful. Care must be taken to prevent dehydration and pneumonia.	There are many influenza viruses; the types change from year to year. Because severe complications of influenza are common in the elderly, the best treatment is prevention. Persons over the age of 65 should get a "flu shot" in the autumn of every year.
Leukemia Gradually increasing fatigue and weight loss; bleeding from gums; spontaneous bruising; malaise; liable to recurrent infections; in some cases, sudden onset of high fever; bronchial pneumonia.	Consult physician; diagnosis made from examination of blood and bone marrow; various treatments with drugs and radiotherapy; results often excellent; sometimes blood transfusion required if anemia is severe.	The disease affects bone marrow and may cause swelling of the spleen and lymph nodes. There are various forms of leukemia. The acute condition is more common in childhood.
Memory, loss of Inability to remember names and recent events; tends to increase in severity in the elderly; sometimes accompanied by loss of physical skills.	Consult physician; treatment depends on whether cause of it can be found; additional vitamins and certain drugs may help.	Loss of memory may be due to the gradual death of brain cells as an individual ages. The condition can occur prematurely, however, as in Alzheimer's disease, and may be aggravated by arteriosclerosis, hypothyroidism, stroke, brain tumor, alcoholism or drug abuse.
Myxedema (hypothyroidism) Gradual development of lethargy and drowsiness; thickening of skin of face; slight loss of hair; deepening voice; constipation; feeling the cold.	Consult physician; condition hard to detect in early stages; blood test confirms diagnosis; treatment with thyroid hormone effective, but must be continued for life.	In myxedema, some circulation problems may result from a raised cholesterol level. Myxedema can cause menstrual disorders if it develops in people of a younger age group.
Osteoarthritis Stiffness, pain, and swelling of joints; usually affecting joints in legs, where use has damaged joint surfaces; also common in hands; pain and swelling aggravated by movement and improved by rest.	Discuss with physician; X ray to confirm diagnosis; use of aspirin and antirheumatic drugs helps; weight loss if obese; exercises to strengthen surrounding muscles; sometimes injections of corticosteroid drugs produce improvement; in severe cases, surgical treatment with joint fixation (arthrodesis) or joint replacement, particularly in hips and knees, may stop pain and allow normal movement.	Osteoarthritis is most likely to occur in joints that have been damaged or overused, for example, in a knee that has had its cartilage removed, in the hips of athletes, and in the hands of manual workers. Early treatment with physiotherapy prevents stiffness and deformity, and also helps to maintain mobility in an elderly patient.

Senior citizens (age 65 +): disorders *(Continued)*

Symptoms and Signs	*Treatment*	*Notes*
Osteoporosis Gradual loss in height with curvature of spine; in elderly, often occurs without pain; sometimes backache which may become severe after a slight accident.	Consult physician; occasionally cause can be found; X ray of spine necessary to exclude other causes of back pain; treatment with painkilling drugs; orthopedic corset and exercises prevent immobility.	Osteoporosis is more common in women than in men, and often occurs after menopause. A course of treatment with hormones, calcium, and vitamin D, along with regular exercise, may prevent the condition from getting worse.
Parkinson's disease Slowly progressive trembling; usually starting in one hand and then spreading through both arms; walking with shuffling gait; expressionless, immobile face; staring eyes.	Treatment may control, but does not cure; atropine-like drugs may be used at first; then L-dopa or amantadine may be used, often with great success.	The condition is commonly associated with aging and with arteriosclerosis.
Prolapse of uterus See PROLAPSE OF UTERUS in eighth section.		
Prostate disorders Poor urine stream when urinating, and difficulty starting and stopping; hesitation and dribbling when urinating; need to urinate during night; frequency of urination during day gradually increases.	Consult physician; examination of urine; kidney X ray; may require operation to remove prostate gland; cancer of prostate treated with hormones; infection treated with antibiotics.	In some cases, infection of the prostate (prostatitis) causes the painful, frequent urination. Blood may be found in urine. A sudden blockage of urine flow rarely occurs. The size of the prostate gland normally increases with age (prostatic hypertrophy), but this size increase may also occur because of cancer of the prostate.
Shingles (herpes zoster) Dull ache in one area of body followed in few days by mild fever and red rash that forms blisters, pustules, and then scabs.	Consult physician; painkilling drugs; calamine lotion and vitamin injections may help; antiviral skin solution may lead to rapid improvement, if condition is treated early.	Shingles is caused by the same virus that causes chickenpox. The shingles virus infects the nerve endings in the body. If a person has had chickenpox in childhood, the virus remains dormant for decades in the body's nerve endings. Any weakening of the person's immune system can cause the virus to become active again, and cause shingles.
Spinal curvature Back bent sideways and forward; onset may be gradual and painless, or fairly rapid and accompanied by pain.	Consult physician; X rays and blood tests confirm diagnosis; physiotherapy; antirheumatic drugs; occasionally spinal support may be needed.	Spinal curvature is usually due to the gradual compression of a vertebra as a result of osteoporosis, but sometimes it develops because of a herniated disk or a sudden collapse of a vertebra from bone disease. The condition may be associated with nerve pain in the arms and in the legs, where the pain resembles sciatica.
Stroke Sudden onset of weakness or paralysis of one side of face and body; may be followed by slow recovery, with some weakness remaining for a few months; or may lead to coma and death.	In early stages, hospitalization; nursing and medical care; physiotherapy; in some cases, use of anticoagulants; rarely, operation needed.	Incontinence is a problem in the early days after a stroke. There may also be speech problems if the right side of the body is involved in a right-handed person. In some cases, a major stroke is preceded by a series of "warning" strokes, from which the patient recovers completely.
Thrombosis, coronary See THROMBOSIS, CORONARY in eighth section.		
Thrombosis, venous See THROMBOSIS, VENOUS in eighth section.		
Tuberculosis Usually lung infection with cough; sometimes with blood-stained sputum; loss of weight; night sweats.	Consult physician; chest X ray and sputum tests confirm infection; treatment with at least two antituberculin drugs for at least one year; may need bed rest; nutritious diet; isolation to prevent spread of infection.	Tuberculosis may spread to involve bone, kidneys, or lymph nodes. Rarely, it may cause a form of meningitis. In many cases, the patient is reasonably fit. People who have come into contact with tuberculosis patients need careful follow-up examinations, as well as skin tests to assess their immunity.
Varicose vein See VARICOSE VEIN in eighth section.		
Vertigo See VERTIGO in eighth section.		

Appendix: IV

Health maintenance: nutrition and exercise

Health is more than just the absence of disease, it is a state of physical, mental, and social well-being. Having good health enables us to enjoy life and have the opportunity to achieve many of the goals we have set for ourselves.

Nutrition and exercise are two factors that have been proven to help maintain health and help fight disease. Eating the right foods increases resistance to disease and raises the level of vitality. Proper exercise, among its other benefits, establishes and maintains muscle tone, aids digestion, deepens respiration, and helps prevent weight gain.

This section has information about nutrition and exercise. It contains diagrams and charts that are useful in choosing the right foods and exercise program.

Dietary guidelines

What foods should a person eat to stay healthy? Different answers to this question appear every day. Books and magazine articles are forever being written on the subject. And new foods constantly hit the grocery shelves with claims of total nutrition. The abundance of information is confusing and, as a result, many people decide to ignore the question altogether.

The confusion surrounding nutrition exists because there really is no "ideal diet." Each person has different nutritional needs. Age, sex, body size, physical activity, and other conditions such as pregnancy or illness all play a role in determining what a person needs to stay healthy. And these conditions may change from day to day.

So what advice should a person follow? What can a person do to feel comfortable that he or she is choosing and preparing the best possible foods to stay healthy? The United States Department of Agriculture and the Department of Health and Human Services has set forth seven dietary guidelines for Americans—those who are already healthy. People who need special diets because of disease or conditions that interfere with normal nutritional requirements may need special dietary instructions from a nutritionist, in consultation with their physician.

Of course, no guidelines can guarantee health or well-being. Health is determined by a number of things aside from nutrition including heredity, lifestyle, personality traits, mental health, and environment. Food alone does not make a person healthy. However, good eating habits can help maintain health and may even improve it.

On these two pages the seven dietary guidelines are given and suggestions for following them are offered.

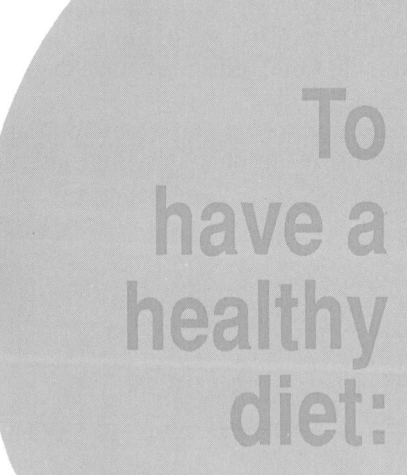

Eat food with adequate starch and fiber

- Choose foods that are good sources of fiber and starch, such as whole-grain breads and cereals, fruits, vegetables, and dry beans and peas
- Substitute starchy foods for those that have large amounts of fats and sugars

Eat a variety of foods

Eat a variety of foods daily in adequate amounts, including selections of:

- Fruits
- Vegetables
- Whole-grain and enriched breads, cereals, and other products made from grains
- Milk, cheese, yogurt, and other products made from milk
- Meats, poultry, fish, eggs, and dry beans and peas

Avoid too much sugar

- Use less of all sugars and foods containing large amounts of sugars, including white sugar, brown sugar, raw sugar, honey, and syrups
- Avoid eating sweets between meals
- Read food labels for clues on sugar content. If the word sugar, sucrose, glucose, maltose, dextrose, lactose, fructose, or syrups appears first, then there is a large amount of sugar
- Select fresh fruits or fruits processed without syrup or with light, rather than heavy syrup

Avoid too much fat, saturated fat, and cholesterol

- Choose lean meat, fish, poultry, and dry beans and peas as protein sources
- Use skim or low-fat milk and milk products
- Moderate use of egg yolks and organ meats
- Limit intake of fats and oils, especially those high in saturated fat, such as butter, cream, lard, heavily hydrogenated fats (some margarines), shortenings, and foods containing palm and coconut oils
- Trim fat off meats
- Broil, bake, or boil rather than fry
- Moderate use of foods that contain fat, such as breaded and deep-fried foods
- Read food labels carefully to determine both amount and type of fat present in foods

Avoid too much sodium

- Learn to enjoy the flavors of unsalted foods
- Cook without salt or with only small amounts of added salt
- Flavor foods with herbs, spices, and lemon juice
- Add little or no salt to food at the table
- Limit intake of salty foods such as potato chips, pretzels, salted nuts and popcorn, condiments (soy sauce, steak sauce, garlic salt), pickled foods, cured meats, some cheeses, and some canned vegetables and soups
- Read food labels carefully to determine amount of sodium
- Use lower sodium products, when available, to replace those that have higher sodium content

Maintain desirable weight

To help control overeating:

- Eat slowly
- Take smaller portions
- Avoid "seconds"

To lose weight:

- Eat a variety of foods that are low in calories and high in nutrients
  —Eat more fruits, vegetables, and whole grains
  —Eat less fat and fatty foods
  —Eat less sugar and sweets
  —Drink less alcoholic beverages
- Increase physical activity

If you drink alcoholic beverages, do so in moderation

- Don't drink and drive
- Avoid alcohol while pregnant

Understanding food labels

In order to practice the seven dietary guidelines outlined on pages 1020-1021, it is helpful to know how to find out what is in the foods you eat. Where can you find this information? In your kitchen cabinets.

Food labels are required, by law, on all packaged foods. The amount of information varies, but all labels must contain (1) the name of the product; (2) the net contents or net weight, which includes the liquid in canned foods; (3) the name and place of business of the manufacturer, packer, or distributor. In addition, nutrition information is required on those foods that have had nutrients added to them or on foods that have nutrition claims made about them (i.e., "low sodium").

There are about 300 foods, including mayonnaise, ice cream, milk, jelly, peanut butter, and cheese, for which ingredients need not be listed. A standard of identity, set by the Food and Drug Administration (FDA), describes the ingredients these foods must contain and any optional ingredients. Only the optional ingredients are required by law to be identified on the label. Other products that resemble a standard food but do not conform to the standard, cannot be called by the same name; they are "imitation." For example, a product resembling peanut butter cannot be called peanut butter unless it contains 90 percent peanuts.

Today, in answer to the public's desire to know more about what they are eating, many food manufacturers are offering information beyond the requirements. This trend has led to the possibility of stricter food labeling regulations. The FDA wants to be sure that manufacturers do not mislead the public into thinking a food is more nutritious than it really is.

Food labels offer a wealth of information. They aren't always easy to read or understand, however. The diagram here is a made-up food label. It has been made to show the variety of information that can appear on any given label. Each item is accompanied by an explanation of what it means. Knowing how to read food labels will allow you to better evaluate the foods you choose.

Light or lite: These words imply that a food is lower in calories, unless another meaning is specified or obvious. A "lite" product produced for the purpose of helping reduce body weight or calorie intake must meet FDA requirements for low- or reduced-calorie foods and provide full nutrition labeling information.

If a label says . . .
"Low-calorie": The food must contain no more than 40 calories a serving.
"Reduced-calorie": The food must be at least one-third lower in calorie content than the food to which it is compared.

Nutrition information: Manufacturers are not required to provide nutrition information unless a nutrient is added to the food or a nutritional claim is made, such as "no cholesterol." The nutrition information, if shown, must appear in the order shown here. Calories must be rounded off to the nearest 10.

Cholesterol: Manufacturers are not required to give cholesterol content, but some choose to do so. When cholesterol content is given, it must be shown in two ways—as "milligrams of cholesterol per serving" and as "milligrams per 100 grams of food."

Percentage of Recommended Daily Allowances (U.S. RDA): Information is provided on the amount of protein and the first seven vitamins and minerals listed here. The other 12 essential nutrients may also be included if they contribute at least two percent of the U.S. RDA.

The percentages represent how much one serving of the food adds to the amount recommended per day. The recommendations are, for the most part, based on the amount needed by young adult males. Therefore, many healthy people do not necessarily need 100 percent of the U.S. RDA of a given nutrient.

Ingredients: Packaged foods that have two or more ingredients must list them by their common or usual names. The ingredient that is present in the largest amount, by weight, must be listed first. Other ingredients follow in descending order.

Natural: A term that appears on many products to convey the message that a food is "good for you." It often has little meaning, however. For example, a food that contains artificial sweeteners can still be labeled as "natural."

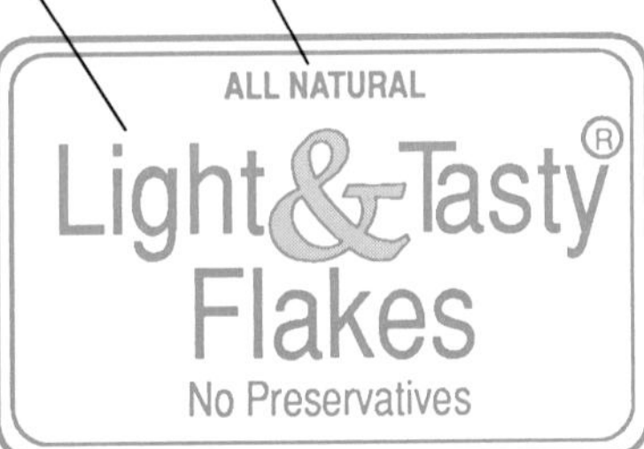

NUTRITION INFORMATION
PER SERVING

SERVING SIZE: 1 OZ. (28g, ABOUT 1/2 CUP)
SERVINGS PER PACKAGE: 16

	CEREAL	WITH 1/2 CUP VITAMINS A & D SKIM MILK
CALORIES	40	90
PROTEIN	2 g	6 g
CARBOHYDRATE	24 g	30 g
FAT	0 g	0 g
CHOLESTEROL	0 mg	0 mg
	(0 g per 100 g)	
SODIUM	0 mg	65 mg
POTASSIUM	90 mg	290 mg

PERCENTAGE OF U.S. RECOMMENDED DAILY ALLOWANCES (U.S. RDAs)

PROTEIN	4	15
VITAMIN A	25	30
VITAMIN C	25	30
THIAMINE	25	30
RIBOFLAVIN	25	35
NIACIN	25	25
CALCIUM	*	15
IRON	10	10
VITAMIN B_6	25	25

*CONTAINS LESS THAN 2% OF THE U.S. RDA OF THIS NUTRIENT.

INGREDIENTS: ENRICHED WHOLE WHEAT.

MADE BY CEREAL MANUFACTURERS, INC.
ANYTOWN, ANYSTATE U.S.A.

Enriched: This term refers to the addition of four nutrients (iron, thiamine, riboflavin, and niacin) to refined grain, from which they have been lost in processing.

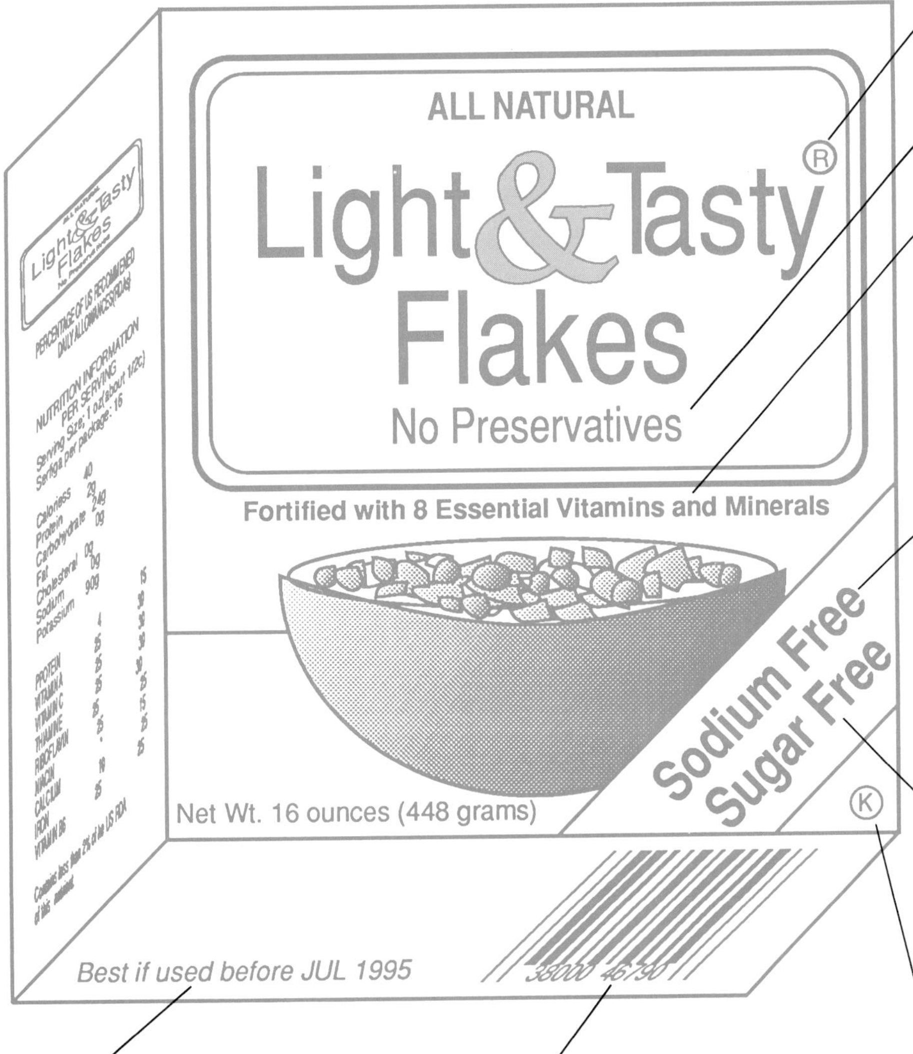

R: Shows that the trademark used is registered with the U.S. Patent Office.

Preservatives: These are substances that keep foods from spoiling.

Fortified: Refers to the addition of any nutrient to a food, even a nutrient that was not there originally, and it may involve adding nutrients in amounts well above those found naturally in foods.

Sodium: Because of the health concerns (especially hypertension) surrounding sodium, manufacturers have been making claims about the sodium content of their foods. The FDA has set terms for these claims.

If a label says . . .

"Sodium free": The food must have less than 5 milligrams of sodium in a serving.

"Very low sodium": The food must have 35 milligrams or less in a serving.

"Reduced sodium": This is used on foods in which the usual level of sodium has been reduced by at least 75 percent.

"Unsalted" or "no salt added": Can be used when a food that was once processed with salt is no longer. However, this food may contain other forms of sodium.

Sugar-free or sugarless: Calorie-containing sweeteners used in foods include common table sugar (sucrose), fructose, and corn syrup. A food can be labeled sugar-free and still contain calories from sugar alcohols, provided the label explains the claim. Aspartame (NutraSweet®) has the same calories as sugar, but is so much sweeter that only small amounts are needed to provide the desired sweetness in a product.

Date: The date gives consumers an idea of how long a product will remain fresh and safe.

Universal Product Code (UPC): This is included on most food products. Each product has its own code that may be used with computerized grocery store checkout equipment. The UPC is not a requirement.

K inside O: Indicates that the food is Kosher, i.e., it complies with Jewish dietary laws and has been processed under the direction of a rabbi.

Tips for reading food labels:

Read the ingredients. If sugar or a sugar-type ingredient is listed first, then sugar is the most prevalent ingredient. This is a clue that the food should probably be avoided.

Look for the fat content. If fat makes up more than one-third of the calories in a serving, this is probably a food to avoid.

There is a way to determine the percentage of the calories that come from fat. The important thing to remember is that each gram of fat has nine calories (kcal). This is the formula:

$$\text{\% of fat} = 100 \times \frac{\text{calories from fat}}{\text{calories per serving}}$$

As an example, let's say there are 16 grams of fat in one serving of peanut butter, and a serving has 190 calories.

$$\text{calories from fat} = 16 \text{ gm} \times 9 \text{ kcal/gm} = 144 \text{ kcal}$$

$$\text{\% of fat} = 100 \times \frac{144 \text{ kcal}}{190 \text{ kcal}} = 76\%$$

In this example, 76 percent of the 190 calories in a serving comes from fat.

Foods that are high in fiber do not necessarily help reduce the risk of some types of cancer. Medical evidence has pointed to the possibility that a diet high in fiber *and* low in fat may reduce the risk of cancer. Therefore, there is no evidence that a high-fiber muffin loaded with fat may reduce the risk of cancer.

Look for the sodium content. A healthy person should have no more than 2,000 mg of sodium per day.

A long list of ingredients can indicate the use of many artificial ingredients and preservatives, which you may not want.

Be aware that low cholesterol does not necessarily mean low fat. Foods that claim low or no cholesterol can still have high fat and saturated fat content, which can raise blood cholesterol levels.

"Hydrogenated oil" and "partially hydrogenated oil" are terms you will often see on labels. They describe the process of adding hydrogen to an unsaturated fat to make it saturated. Oils may be hydrogenated to various degrees to make them suitable for use in products such as margarine. The more an oil is hydrogenated, the more fatty acids it contains.

Eating out

A significant portion of the American diet comes from restaurants. Because today's families are so busy it seems the days of sitting down together to eat a home-cooked meal are a thing of the past. The problem with this trend is that much restaurant food is high in calories and fat and low in nutrients. Fortunately, in light of the growing concern for a healthy diet, restaurants are offering more nutritious choices. And, even in those restaurants that don't offer such choices, it is possible to find a healthy meal.

Below are some guidelines for eating healthy while eating out.

- Many restaurants offer a bread basket. Choose the breadsticks, hard rolls, wafers, and toast. Avoid butter rolls. And, skip the butter.
- When choosing an appetizer, go for the fruits, vegetables, juices, and seafood cocktails.
- Salad is a good choice—if you avoid too much salad dressing. Ask for the dressing on the side and avoid creamy and cheese dressings.
- Choose soups with clear broth. Avoid cheese soups, cream soups, egg soups, and onion soup.
- Have small portions or share portions.
- If a baked potato is your choice, leave off the butter and sour cream. Low-fat cottage cheese and plain yogurt are tasty alternatives.
- When ordering fish, choose those that are broiled or grilled. Avoid fried fish and the tartar sauce that usually accompanies it.
- Chicken, turkey, and cornish hens are always good choices—if they aren't fried or smothered in cream sauces or gravies. Avoid goose and duck for they are quite fatty.
- When choosing red meats, go with veal or lean hindquarters of beef, lamb, and pork. Avoid prime cuts and ground beef.
- Choose plain vegetables without sauce.
- Have fruit for dessert or no dessert at all.

The following charts provide nutritional information about the foods offered at popular restaurants. The * indicates that the food contains less than 2 percent of the U.S. RDA of those nutrients.

Kentucky Fried Chicken®

Food item	*size (g)*	*calories*	*protein (g)*	*carbohydrates (g)*	*fat (g)*
Original Recipe® Center Breast	115	283	28	9	15
Original Recipe® Drumstick	57	146	13	4	9
Extra Tasty Crispy™ Center Breast	135	342	33	12	20
Extra Tasty Crispy™ Drumstick	69	204	14	6	14
Kentucky Nuggets® (one) without sauce	16	46	3	2	3
Chicken Littles™ Sandwich	47	169	6	14	10
Buttermilk Biscuit (one)	65	235	5	28	12
Mashed Potatoes and Gravy	98	71	2	12	2

Pizza Hut®

Food item (2 slices of medium pizza)	*size (g)*	*calories*	*protein (g)*	*carbohydrates (g)*	*fat (g)*
Pan Pizza					
Cheese	205	492	30	57	18
Pepperoni	211	540	29	62	22
Supreme	255	589	32	53	30
Thin 'n Crispy® Pizza					
Cheese	148	398	28	37	17
Pepperoni	146	413	26	36	20
Supreme	200	459	28	41	22
Hand-Tossed					
Cheese	220	518	34	55	20
Pepperoni	197	500	28	50	23
Supreme	239	540	32	50	26
Personal Pan Pizza® (whole)					
Pepperoni	256	675	37	76	29
Supreme	264	647	33	76	28

Taco Bell®

Food item	*size (g)*	*calories*	*protein (g)*	*carbohydrates (g)*	*fat (g)*
Double Beef Burrito Supreme with Green Sauce	255	451	23	40	22
Tostada with Red Sauce	156	243	10	27	11
Nachos BellGrande®	287	649	22	61	35
Taco	78	183	10	11	11
Taco Light	170	410	19	18	29
Taco Salad with shell	595	941	36	63	61
Bean Burrito with Green Sauce	191	351	13	53	10
Cinnamon Crispas®	47	259	3	28	15

cholesterol (mg)	sodium (mg)	% U.S. RDA protein	% U.S. RDA vit. A	% U.S. RDA vit. C	% U.S. RDA thiamine	% U.S. RDA riboflavin	% U.S. RDA niacin	% U.S. RDA calcium	% U.S. RDA iron
93	672	61	*	*	6	10	58	4	5
67	275	29	*	*	3	7	16	2	6
114	790	74	*	*	7	8	65	3	5
71	324	30	*	*	4	7	19	1	4
12	140	6	*	*	*	*	5	*	*
18	331	13	*	*	11	7	11	2	10
1	655	7	*	*	16	11	13	10	9
race	339	4	*	*	*	2	6	2	2

Source: "Nutritional Facts About Kentucky Fried Chicken®," Kentucky Fried Chicken® Corporation, Louisville, Kentucky, 1990.

cholesterol (mg)	sodium (mg)	% U.S. RDA protein	% U.S. RDA vit. A	% U.S. RDA vit. C	% U.S. RDA thiamine	% U.S. RDA riboflavin	% U.S. RDA niacin	% U.S. RDA calcium	% U.S. RDA iron
34	940	54	9	12	37	35	26	63	30
42	1127	52	10	14	42	29	27	52	35
48	1363	57	12	16	54	47	30	50	28
33	867	50	7	8	26	23	24	66	18
46	986	46	7	10	28	25	26	45	18
42	1328	50	10	16	40	29	27	43	33
55	1276	61	10	16	32	29	27	75	30
50	1267	50	10	12	36	31	28	44	28
55	1470	57	11	20	46	31	36	48	45
53	1335	66	12	17	37	39	41	73	32
49	1313	59	12	18	39	39	40	52	37

Source: Pizza Hut®, Inc., Wichita, Kansas, 1989.

cholesterol (mg)	sodium (mg)	% U.S. RDA protein	% U.S. RDA vit. A	% U.S. RDA vit. C	% U.S. RDA thiamine	% U.S. RDA riboflavin	% U.S. RDA niacin	% U.S. RDA calcium	% U.S. RDA iron
57	929	36	16	13	29	129	19	13	22
16	596	15	13	75	4	10	3	18	9
36	997	33	23	96	7	20	11	30	19
32	276	16	7	2	3	8	6	8	6
56	594	29	13	8	13	19	13	16	14
80	1662	55	59	128	34	44	24	40	39
9	763	20	4	87	25	119	11	14	19
trace	127	4	*	1	9	5	5	4	7

Source: "Taco Bell® Nutritional Information," Taco Bell® Corporation, Irvine, California, 1990.

Burger King®

Food item	size (g)	calories	protein (g)	carbohydrates (g)	fat (g)
Whopper® Sandwich	270	614	27	45	36
Whopper® with Cheese Sandwich	294	706	32	47	44
Cheeseburger	121	318	17	28	15
Bacon Double Cheeseburger	160	515	32	26	31
BK Broiler Chicken Sandwich	168	379	24	31	18
Chicken Tenders™ (six)	90	236	16	14	13
Garden Salad without dressing	223	95	6	8	5
French Fries (medium, salted)	111	341	4	36	20
Chocolate Shake (syrup added)	312	409	10	68	11
Croissan'wich™ with egg and cheese	110	315	13	19	20

McDonald's®

Food item	size (g)	calories	protein (g)	carbohydrates (g)	fat (g)
Egg McMuffin®	138	290	18	28	11
Hamburger	102	260	12	31	10
Cheeseburger	116	310	15	31	14
Quarter Pounder® with Cheese	194	520	29	35	29
Big Mac®	215	560	25	43	32
Filet-O-Fish®	142	440	14	38	26
Mc D.L.T.®	234	580	26	36	37
Chicken McNuggets® (six) without sauce	113	290	19	17	16
Garden Salad without dressing	213	110	7	6	7
French Fries (medium)	97	320	4	36	17
Hot Fudge Sundae	169	240	7	51	3
Apple Pie	83	260	2	30	15

Wendy's®

Food item	size (g)	calories	protein (g)	carbohydrates (g)	fat (g)
Single Hamburger with everything	234	420	25	35	21
Single Cheeseburger with everything	252	490	29	35	27
Wendy's® Big Classic	277	570	27	46	33
Chicken Sandwich	219	430	26	41	19
Broccoli and Cheese Baked Potato	377	400	9	59	16
French Fries (small, in vegetable oil)	3.2 oz.	250	3	33	12
Frosty Dairy Dessert (small)	243	400	8	59	14

cholesterol (mg)	sodium (mg)	% U.S. RDA protein	% U.S. RDA vit. A	% U.S. RDA vit. C	% U.S. RDA thiamine	% U.S. RDA riboflavin	% U.S. RDA niacin	% U.S. RDA calcium	% U.S. RDA iron
90	865	41	11	20	24	24	34	8	27
115	1177	49	19	20	24	28	34	22	27
50	661	27	7	5	15	17	19	11	15
105	748	50	8	*	20	25	31	18	21
53	764	37	7	9	30	13	51	6	13
46	541	25	*	*	7	5	40	*	4
15	125	9	100	58	5	6	4	15	6
0	241	6	*	26	10	27	11	2	4
33	248	15	*	*	7	35	*	31	*
222	607	20	10	*	16	22	8	14	10

Source: "Your Guide to Nutrition at Burger King®," Burger King® Corporation, Miami, Florida, 1990.

cholesterol (mg)	sodium (mg)	% U.S. RDA protein	% U.S. RDA vit. A	% U.S. RDA vit. C	% U.S. RDA thiamine	% U.S. RDA riboflavin	% U.S. RDA niacin	% U.S. RDA calcium	% U.S. RDA iron
226	740	30	10	*	30	20	20	25	15
37	500	20	4	4	20	10	20	10	15
53	750	25	8	4	20	15	20	20	15
118	1150	45	15	6	25	20	35	30	20
103	950	40	8	2	30	25	35	25	20
50	1030	20	2	*	20	8	15	15	10
109	990	40	15	10	25	20	35	25	20
65	520	30	*	*	8	8	45	*	6
83	160	10	80	20	6	10	2	15	6
12	150	6	*	20	15	*	15	*	4
6	170	10	4	*	6	20	*	25	2
6	240	4	*	20	4	*	*	*	4

Source: "McDonald's® Food: The Facts," McDonald's® Corporation, Oak Brook, Illinois, 1990.

cholesterol (mg)	sodium (mg)	% U.S. RDA protein	% U.S. RDA vit. A	% U.S. RDA vit. C	% U.S. RDA thiamine	% U.S. RDA riboflavin	% U.S. RDA niacin	% U.S. RDA calcium	% U.S. RDA iron
70	865	60	15	25	25	15	30	10	30
90	1155	60	15	25	25	80	30	10	30
85	1075	60	20	25	30	15	30	15	30
60	705	60	10	15	30	20	70	10	80
trace	470	20	50	110	20	15	20	15	20
trace	145	8	*	10	10	2	10	*	4
50	220	20	10	*	8	30	*	30	6

Source: "Quality is Our Recipe®," Wendy's® International, Inc., Dublin, Ohio, 1986 and 1990.

Dietary fiber content of selected foods

Fiber provides bulk in the diet. It is derived from such plant sources as cereal grain products, vegetables, fruits, seeds, and nuts. "Dietary fiber" is the amount of fiber left after digestion.

Nutritionists recommend a consumption of 20 to 35 grams of dietary fiber per day. The chart on this page offers the approximate amount of dietary fiber in selected foods. For more information on dietary fiber, *see* page 648.

Fiber in selected foods

Food	*Portion size*	*Dietary fiber (g)*
Breads and crackers		
White bread	1 slice	0.6
Whole-wheat bread	1 slice	1.8
Matzoh	1 piece	1.2
Cereals		
All-Bran	½ c	7.5
Cornflakes	¾ c	2.1
Grapenuts	1 oz	2.0
Rice Krispies	1 c	1.3
Puffed Wheat	1 c	2.2
Shredded Wheat	1 biscuit	3.1
Fruits		
Apples	1 small	2.0
Bananas	½ small	1.0
Cherries	10 large	0.8
Grapefruit	1 c	1.1
Peaches	1 medium	2.3
Pears	1 small	3.0
Plums	2 medium	1.2
Strawberries	¾ c	2.4
Legumes and nuts		
Baked beans, canned	½ c	5.5
Peas, canned	½ c	6.0
Peanut butter	2 tbsp	2.4
Peanuts	1 tbsp	0.8
Brazil nuts	6-8 large	2.2
Vegetables		
Broccoli, cooked pieces	1 c	6.4
Brussels sprouts, cooked	1 c	4.4
Cabbage, cooked	1 c	4.1
Carrots, cooked	1 c	5.7
Cauliflower, cooked	1 c	2.3
Corn, cooked	1 c kernels	8.6
Lettuce, raw pieces	1 c	0.8
Onions, raw chopped	1 c	3.6
Peppers, green, cooked	1 c	1.5
Potatoes, cooked	1 potato	3.9
Tomatoes, canned	1 c	2.0
Tomatoes, fresh	1 tomato	1.9
Miscellaneous		
Bran, wheat	1 tbsp	4.0
Dill pickle, 3¾ × 1¼ in	1 pickle	1.0
Marmalade	1 tbsp	0.1
Strawberry jam	1 tbsp	0.2

Source: Table C-1: "Approximate Dietary Fiber Contents of Selected Foods," from *Journal of Human Nutrition-30*, by D. A. T. Southgate, B. Bailey, E. Collinson, and A. F. Walker.

Cholesterol content of selected foods

Cholesterol is a fatlike substance essential to body functions. It is found in foods of animal origin such as meat, poultry, and dairy products. Cholesterol does not exist in foods from plants.

Nutritionists recommend a cholesterol intake of 300 milligrams or less per day. The chart on this page offers the approximate amount of cholesterol in selected foods. For more information about cholesterol, *see* page 647.

Cholesterol in selected foods

Food	*Serving size*	*Cholesterol (mg)*
Meat, fish, poultry		
Beef, cooked, lean, trimmed of separable fat	3 oz	77
Lamb, lean, cooked	3 oz	83
Pork, cooked, lean, trimmed	3 oz	77
Veal, cooked, lean	3 oz	86
Chicken, dark meat	3 oz	76
Chicken, light meat	3 oz	54
Turkey, dark meat	3 oz	86
Turkey, light meat	3 oz	65
Rabbit, domestic	3 oz	52
Liver (beef, calf, lamb), cooked	3 oz	372
Chicken liver	3 oz	480
Heart	3 oz	274
Sweetbreads	3 oz	396
Brain	3 oz	1,810
Kidney	3 oz	690
Cod	3 oz	72
Haddock	3 oz	51
Halibut	3 oz	51
Flounder	3 oz	43
Herring	3 oz	83
Salmon, cooked	3 oz	40
Trout	3 oz	47
Tuna, packed in oil	3 oz	56
Sardines	1 can (3¾ oz)	109
Abalone	3 oz	120
Crab	3 oz	85
Clams	3 oz	55
Lobster	½ c	57
Oysters	3 oz	40
Scallops	½ c (scant)	45
Shrimp	3 oz	96
Eggs		
Yolk	1 medium	240
White		0
Dairy products		
Milk, whole	1 c (8 oz)	34
Milk, low-fat (2%)	1 c	22
Milk, nonfat (skim)	1 c	5
Buttermilk	1 c	14
Yogurt, low-fat plain	1 c	17
Yogurt, low-fat flavored	1 c	14
Sour cream	1 tbsp	8
Whipped cream	1 tbsp	20
Half and half	1 tbsp	6
Ice milk	1 c	26
Ice cream	1 c	56
Butter	1 tsp	12
American cheese	1 oz	26
Blue cheese or roquefort	1 oz	25
Cheddar cheese, mild or sharp	1 oz	28
Cottage cheese, creamed (4% fat)	1 c	48
Cottage cheese, uncreamed	1 c	13
Cream cheese	1 tbsp	16
Mozzarella, low moisture, part skim	1 oz	18
Muenster cheese	1 oz	25
Parmesan cheese	1 oz	27
Ricotta, part skim	1 oz	14
Swiss cheese	1 oz	28
Nondairy fats		
Lard or other animal fat	1 tsp	5
Margarine, all vegetable		0
Margarine, ⅔ animal fat, ⅓ vegetable fat	1 tsp	3

Source: Adapted from "Consumers Guide to Fat: Cholesterol-Controlled Food Products," by the Greater Los Angeles Affiliate of the American Heart Association, © 1978; and *Understanding Nutrition*, 1st ed., West Publishing Company, Minnesota, © 1977, pp. 537-538. Reprinted with permission.

Recommended Dietary Allowances

The Recommended Dietary Allowances for Americans (RDAs) are determined by a group of scientists who report their findings to the government. The government then publishes the recommendations. The group meets about every five years to review and update their findings.

The RDAs are not *requirements* and they are not *minimum requirements*. They are based on the idea that there is a range in which most healthy persons' intake of nutrients probably should fall. It should always be remembered that individual needs differ and medical problems can alter nutrient needs.

The Recommended Nutrient Intakes for Canadians (RNIs), like the RDAs for Americans, are taken as the level of dietary intake thought to be sufficiently high to meet the requirements of almost all individuals in a group with specified characteristics (age, sex, body size, physical activity, etc.). It follows that an intake below the recommended amount does not mean that the individual has failed to meet his or her requirement. However, the lower the intake in relation to the RNI, the greater the risk that the individual has not met his or her requirement. For more information about the RNI, contact the Canadian Department of National Health and Welfare.

Note: Recommended intakes of certain nutrients are not listed in this table because of the nature of the variables upon which they are based. For nutrients not shown, the following amounts are recommended: thiamine, 0.4 mg/1,000 kcal (0.48/5,000 kJ); riboflavin, 0.5mg/1,000 kcal (0.6 mg/5,000 kJ); niacin, 7.2 NE/1,000 kcal (8.6 NE/5,000 kJ); vitamin B_6, 15 μg (as pyridoxine)/g protein; phosphorus, same as calcium.

Recommended intakes during periods of growth are taken as appropriate for individuals representative of the midpoint in each age group. All recommended intakes are designed to cover individual variations in essentially all of a healthy population subsisting upon a variety of common foods available in Canada.

Source: Recommended Nutrient Intakes for Canadians, Health and Welfare Canada (Ottawa: Canadian Government Publishing Centre, 1983), Table II.1, pp. 22–23 and Table X.1, pp. 179–180.

Recommended Dietary Allowances,[a] revised 1989

		Weight		Height[b]			Fat-soluble vitamins			
Category	**Age (years) or condition**	**(kg)**	**(lb)**	**(cm)**	**(in)**	**Protein (g)**	**Vitamin A (μ RE)[c]**	**Vitamin D (μg)[d]**	**Vitamin E (mg α-TE)[e]**	**Vitamin K (μg)**
Infants	0.0-0.5	6	13	60	24	13	375	7.5	3	5
	0.5-1.0	9	20	71	28	14	375	10	4	10
Children	1-3	13	29	90	35	16	400	10	6	15
	4-6	20	44	112	44	24	500	10	7	20
	7-10	28	62	132	52	28	700	10	7	30
Males	11-14	45	99	157	62	45	1,000	10	10	45
	15-18	66	145	176	69	59	1,000	10	10	65
	19-24	72	160	177	70	58	1,000	10	10	70
	25-50	79	174	176	70	63	1,000	5	10	80
	51+	77	170	173	68	63	1,000	5	10	80
Females	11-14	46	101	157	62	46	800	10	8	45
	15-18	55	120	163	64	44	800	10	8	55
	19-24	58	128	164	65	46	800	10	8	60
	25-50	63	138	163	64	50	800	5	8	65
	51+	65	143	160	63	50	800	5	8	65
Pregnant						60	800	10	10	65
Lactating	1st 6 months					65	1,300	10	12	65
	2nd 6 months					62	1,200	10	11	65

[a]The allowances, expressed as average daily intakes over time, are intended to provide for individual variations among most normal persons as they live in the United States under usual environmental stresses. Diets should be based on a variety of common foods in order to provide other nutrients for which human requirements have been less well defined.

[b]Weights and heights of reference adults are actual medians for the U.S. population of the designated age, as reported by NHANES II. The median weights and heights of those under 19 years of age were taken from Hamill et al. (1979). The use of these figures does not imply that the height-to-weight ratios are ideal.

Recommended Nutrient Intakes for Canadians,[a] 1983

				Average energy requirements					
Age	**Sex**	**Average height (cm)**	**Average weight (kg)**	**kcal/kg[b]**	**MJ/kg[b]**	**kcal/day**	**MJ/day**	**kcal/cm**	**MJ/cm**
Months									
0–2	Both	55	4.5	120–100	0.50–0.42	500	2.0	9.0	0.04
3–5	Both	63	7.0	100– 95	0.42–0.40	700	2.8	11.0	0.05
6–8	Both	69	8.5	95– 97	0.40–0.41	800	3.4	11.5	0.05
9–11	Both	73	9.5	97– 99	0.41	950	3.8	12.5	0.05
Years									
1	Both	82	11	101	0.42	1,100	4.8	13.5	0.06
2–3	Both	95	14	94	0.39	1,300	5.6	13.5	0.06
4–6	Both	107	18	100	0.42	1,800	7.6	17.0	0.07
7–9	M	126	25	88	0.37	2,200	9.2	17.5	0.07
	F	125	25	76	0.32	1,900	8.0	15.0	0.06
10–12	M	141	34	73	0.30	2,500	10.4	17.5	0.07
	F	143	36	61	0.25	2,200	9.2	15.5	0.06
13–15	M	159	50	57	0.24	2,800	12.0	17.5	0.07
	F	157	48	46	0.19	2,200	9.2	14.0	0.06
16–18	M	172	62	51	0.21	3,200	13.2	18.5	0.08
	F	160	53	40	0.17	2,100	8.8	13.0	0.05
19–24	M	175	71	42	0.18	3,000	12.4		
	F	160	58	36	0.15	2,100	8.8		
25–49	M	172	74	36	0.15	2,700	11.2		
	F	160	59	32	0.13	1,900	8.0		
50–74	M	170	73	31	0.13	2,300	9.6		
	F	158	63	29	0.12	1,800	7.6		
75+	M	168	69	29	0.12	2,000	8.4		
	F	155	64	23	0.10	1,500	6.0		
Pregnancy (Additional)									
1st Trimester									
2nd Trimester									
3rd Trimester									
Lactation (Additional)									

[a]Requirements can be expected to vary within a range of ±30%.

[b]First and last figures are averages at the beginning and at the end of the 3-month period.

[c]The primary units are g/kg of body weight. The figures shown here are examples.

[d]One retinol equivalent (RE) corresponds to the biological activity of 1μg of retinol, 6 μg of β-carotene or 12 μg of other carotenes.

Water-soluble vitamins							Minerals						
Vitamin C (mg)	Thiamine (mg)	Riboflavin (mg)	Niacin (mg NE)[f]	Vitamin B_6 (mg)	Folate (µg)	Vitamin B_{12} (µg)	Calcium (mg)	Phosphorus (mg)	Magnesium (mg)	Iron (mg)	Zinc (mg)	Iodine (µg)	Selenium (µg)
30	0.3	0.4	5	0.3	25	0.3	400	300	40	6	5	40	10
35	0.4	0.5	6	0.6	35	0.5	600	500	60	10	5	50	15
40	0.7	0.8	9	1.0	50	0.7	800	800	80	10	10	70	20
45	0.9	1.1	12	1.1	75	1.0	800	800	120	10	10	90	20
45	1.0	1.2	13	1.4	100	1.4	800	800	170	10	10	120	30
50	1.3	1.5	17	1.7	150	2.0	1,200	1,200	270	12	15	150	40
60	1.5	1.8	20	2.0	200	2.0	1,200	1,200	400	12	15	150	50
60	1.5	1.7	19	2.0	200	2.0	1,200	1,200	350	10	15	150	70
60	1.5	1.7	19	2.0	200	2.0	800	800	350	10	15	150	70
60	1.2	1.4	15	2.0	200	2.0	800	800	350	10	15	150	70
50	1.1	1.3	15	1.4	150	2.0	1,200	1,200	280	15	12	150	45
60	1.1	1.3	15	1.5	180	2.0	1,200	1,200	300	15	12	150	50
60	1.1	1.3	15	1.6	180	2.0	1,200	1,200	280	15	12	150	55
60	1.1	1.3	15	1.6	180	2.0	800	800	280	15	12	150	55
60	1.0	1.2	13	1.6	180	2.0	800	800	280	10	12	150	55
70	1.5	1.6	17	2.2	400	2.2	1,200	1,200	320	30	15	175	65
95	1.6	1.8	20	2.1	280	2.6	1,200	1,200	355	15	19	200	75
90	1.6	1.7	20	2.1	260	2.6	1,200	1,200	340	15	16	200	75

[c] Retinol equivalents. 1 retinol equivalent = 1 µg retinol or 6 µg β-carotene. µg = microgram, or one millionth of a gram.

[d] As cholecalciferol. 10 µg cholecalciferol = 400 IU of vitamin D.

[e] α-Tocopherol equivalents. 1 mg d-α tocopherol = 1 α-TE.

[f] 1 NE (niacin equivalent) is equal to 1 mg of niacin or 60 mg of dietary tryptophan.
Source: Food and Nutrition Board, National Academy of Sciences—National Research Council.

	Fat-soluble vitamins			Water-soluble vitamins			Minerals				
Protein (g/day)[c]	Vitamin A (RE/day)[d]	Vitamin D (µg/day)[e]	Vitamin E (mg/day)[f]	Vitamin C (mg/day)	Folacin (µg/day)[g]	Vitamin B_{12} (µg/day)	Calcium (mg/day)	Magnesium (mg/day)	Iron (mg/day)	Iodine (µg/day)	Zinc (mg/day)
11[h]	400	10	3	20	50	0.3	350	30	0.4[i]	25	2[j]
14[h]	400	10	3	20	50	0.3	350	40	5	35	3
16[h]	400	10	3	20	50	0.3	400	45	7	40	3
18	400	10	3	20	55	0.3	400	50	7	45	3
18	400	10	3	20	65	0.3	500	55	6	55	4
20	400	5	4	20	80	0.4	500	65	6	65	4
25	500	5	5	25	90	0.5	600	90	6	85	5
31	700	2.5	7	35	125	0.8	700	110	7	110	6
29	700	2.5	6	30	125	0.8	700	110	7	95	6
38	800	2.5	8	40	170	1.0	900	150	10	125	7
39	800	2.5	7	40	170	1.0	1,000	160	10	110	7
49	900	2.5	9	50	160	1.5	1,100	220	12	160	9
43	800	2.5	7	45	160	1.5	800	190	13	160	8
54	1,000	2.5	10	55	190	1.9	900	240	10	160	9
47	800	2.5	7	45	160	1.9	700	220	14	160	8
57	1,000	2.5	10	60	210	2.0	800	240	8	160	9
41	800	2.5	7	45	165	2.0	700	190	14	160	8
57	1,000	2.5	9	60	210	2.0	800	240	8	160	9
41	800	2.5	6	45	165	2.0	700	190	14[k]	160	8
57	1,000	2.5	7	60	210	2.0	800	240	8	160	9
41	800	2.5	6	45	165	2.0	800	190	7	160	8
57	1,000	2.5	6	60	210	2.0	800	240	8	160	9
41	800	2.5	5	45	165	2.0	800	190	7	160	8
15	100	2.5	2	0	305	1.0	500	15	6	25	0
20	100	2.5	2	20	305	1.0	500	20	6	25	1
25	100	2.5	2	20	305	1.0	500	25	6	25	2
20	400	2.5	3	30	120	0.5	500	80	0	50	6

[e] Expressed as cholecalciferol or ergocalciferol.

[f] Expressed as d-α-tocopherol equivalents, relative to which β- and γ-tocopherol and α-tocotrienol have activities of 0.5, 0.1, and 0.3 respectively.

[g] Expressed as total folate.

[h] Assumption is made that the protein is from breast milk or is of the same biological value as that of breast milk.

[i] It is assumed that breast milk is the source of iron up to 2 months of age.

[j] Based on the assumption that breast milk is the source of zinc for the first 2 months.

[k] After the menopause the recommended intake is 7 mg/day.

Exercise and fitness

This section is about getting fit. Physical fitness is a function of muscle strength, flexibility, and endurance, and is enhanced by certain kinds of exercise. After learning about the benefits of exercise, you will learn how to evaluate your own level of fitness, get started on an exercise program, and how to make exercise part of your life from here on out.

If you carefully follow the advice in this section, you should be able to improve your level of physical fitness safely. Several precautions are necessary, however. Your age, your risks for heart disease, your personal medical history, and/or your current physical condition may have an effect on your risk of illness or injury from exercise. The table below lists those risk factors and conditions for which you should consult your physician prior to beginning any exercise program.

Reasons you should consult your physician before beginning an exercise program

- History of high blood pressure
- High serum cholesterol
- Cigarette smoking
- Family history of arterial disease before age 50 (heart attack, stroke, angina, etc.)
- Diabetes mellitus
- Obesity
- Symptoms of chest pain, palpitations, dizziness, fainting spells, or unusual shortness of breath
- Bone or joint problems such as arthritis or low back pain
- Unaccustomed to exercise
- Physical handicap
- Taking medication
- Recent onset of new physical symptoms
- Any medical condition that might interfere with ability to exercise or that might be aggravated by exercise
- Any questions about exercise and your health

The benefits of exercise

Research, observation, and common sense tell us that exercise improves the quality and extends the length of life. You do not have to be an exercise fanatic to obtain substantial health benefits from being physically active. Research has shown that people who get enough mild exertion—for example, by walking, gardening, and doing household chores—are 30 percent less likely to die of a heart attack than people who do not exert themselves much at all. Thus, people do not even have to break a sweat to experience the benefits of exercise. They merely need to maintain a sufficiently physically active life style. For most people, sufficiently active means the equivalent of walking an average of 2½ to 3 miles (4 to 4.8 kilometers) a day.

With exercise, your muscle cells increase in number and in their ability to use oxygen. This increases your strength and endurance. Stretching exercises can help improve flexibility. Participation in various sports and recreational activities helps maintain and improve strength, endurance, flexibility, and agility. Regular and sensible use of your muscles will help you maintain these abilities into your later years, and will help you remain productive and independent.

The benefits of exercise are even greater for those who regularly engage in activities that raise the heart rate high enough to improve muscle oxygen use. This ability to make use of greater amounts of oxygen is referred to as aerobic power. Aerobic training involves repetitive motion of major muscle groups, as in running, cycling, or swimming, so it is typically associated with sweating, heavier breathing, and other signs of vigorous exertion.

Aerobic exercise has been shown to reverse or retard many factors associated with premature death and illness—that is, death or illness before reaching a predicted life span of roughly 70 to 80 years of age. Heart attack, cancer, and stroke are three of the top causes of adult death in the United States today. Aerobic exercise reduces a number of risks for these diseases, including risks from high blood pressure, high cholesterol, smoking, obesity, and diabetes. In addition, aerobic exercise has been shown to decrease one's risk of colon cancer, breast cancer, brain cancer, prostate cancer, and leukemia. Regular exercise can also decrease symptoms of arthritis, irritable bowel, anxiety, and depression.

People who exercise regularly can eat more without gaining weight. Research has shown that exercise actually suppresses the appetite. Thus weight loss, if desired, is easier to achieve if you exercise. Life insurance ideal body weight tables (*see* page 399) suggest that low body weights are strongly associated with having minimized one's risk of dying of any and all causes for a period of 20 years. That is to say, for your sex, height, and frame size, there is a body weight range associated with a minimized 20-year mortality risk. Only about 10 percent of adults in the United States are at a life insurance ideal body weight, and almost every one of them gets regular exercise.

Thirty percent of U.S. adults are obese, or are 20 percent beyond the midpoint of their life insurance ideal body weight. Obesity is a significant risk factor for high blood pressure, diabetes, high cholesterol, and weight-bearing joint problems. Obesity can also aggravate a number of medical conditions, and raises the likelihood of complications with surgery or pregnancy. The body fat percentage of today's children is significantly higher than it was in children 20 years ago. Lack of exercise is partially to blame for most of these weight-related problems. This trend will be hard to reverse. One study found that U.S. adults spend less than one hour per week exercising with their children.

If regular exercise is to become a lifelong routine, it should begin in childhood. Eighty percent of obese adults had obese parents. Parents are in an ideal position to serve as role models regarding exercise and good nutrition. Where obesity is a problem, beginning an exercise program often benefits the whole family.

The risks of exercise are minimal when appropriate precautions are observed. Proper warmup, exercising at proper intensities for reasonable durations, and special attention to injury prevention will go far to insuring your ability to exercise safely over your lifetime. For those who have not exercised hard or regularly for some time, especially those who smoke or who are physically debilitated, it is important to avoid taking on too much too soon. Sometimes motivation pushes people to unreasonable extremes, and sore muscles, painful breathing, or joint injuries can quickly turn exercise into an unpleasant experience. If you have not exercised in a long time but are planning to change, be fair to yourself. Start at mild intensities and advance slowly. Consider getting expert assistance from your physician or a qualified fitness professional.

Many health clubs today offer a personal training service at an additional cost.

Exercise, by improving stamina and endurance, helps to improve productivity and self-image. Exercise not only maintains physical and mental fitness, it enhances self-esteem and reduces your chances of death or illness at an early age. Regular exercise can substantially improve the quality and extend the length of your life.

How fit are you?

Fitness is not just a matter of maintaining an ideal weight. It has to do with all aspects of your life style. It includes your attitude, your outlook, and how you treat yourself.

Most people know when they are unfit. The signs are obvious: you get tired easily; you find that you can't do all the things you used to do; you feel out of breath after climbing a flight of stairs; you catch colds and other minor infections easily; you don't make the time to relax; you don't watch what you eat; you have no organized exercise program. Many people are unwilling to acknowledge to themselves how unfit they are.

Fear of the work involved in getting fit is both unnecessary and dangerous. It is unnecessary, because the effort involved in getting fit need not be great, especially since it is largely a matter of self-discipline. And it is dangerous, because if you allow your physical condition to deteriorate, you increase the risk of suffering from heart disease or some other physical disorder.

Finding out how unfit you really are is not a cause for despair, but the first step in improving the whole quality of your life. If you are between the ages of 15 and 60, you can get a general idea of how fit you are with seven simple tests:

(1) Stand in front of a mirror. Look for areas of loose or flabby skin. Are you satisfied with what you see? This is a gauge of your general physical appearance and muscle tone. It also measures your satisfaction with yourself. If you are pleased with how your body looks, you are either already physically fit or well on your way.

(2) Pinch your body at the waist, or at a point at the back of your arm between the shoulder and the elbow. Is the fold of skin less than 1 inch (2.5 centimeters) thick? This is a test for the first signs of obesity.

(3) Can you hold your breath for more than 45 seconds? This tests the condition of your lungs.

(4) Stand up straight, with your eyes closed and your arms at your sides, and raise one knee. Can you stand like this for 15 seconds without losing your balance? This tests your balance and muscular coordination.

(5) Do you sit up straight with your stomach tight? This is a check of your posture, which has an effect on your respiration.

(6) Check the pulse rate of your heart. (Find your pulse on your neck just above and to the right or left of your Adam's apple; pressing lightly, count the beats for 15 seconds; multiply that number by four. This is your heart rate for one minute.) Next, run in place or step up and down on a footstool for three minutes. Is your pulse rate now under 120 beats a minute? And does it take less than one minute to return to its original rate? This evaluates the condition of the heart and the circulation.

(7) Do you know if you're getting enough vitamins or eating too much fat? This tests your attitude toward and awareness of nutrition. If you are not aware of what foods are good for you, chances are you aren't eating enough of them.

If your answer to any of these questions is no, you're probably not as fit as you could be.

Fitness day by day

The process of getting fit and keeping fit is more a matter of common sense and self-discipline than hard work. The rewards of fitness can be attained by any reasonably healthy person who is committed to improving his or her physical condition. For some people, this commitment may involve regular physical exercise; sensible, weight-loss diets; and sports. For others, less willing or able to alter their daily routine, many less disruptive ways of getting exercise can be equally important and beneficial.

Keep active as much as possible, whatever your occupation. The less active you are, the less your body is exercised and the weaker it gets. Anyone who has been ill in bed for even as little as a week knows how difficult it is to get straight back into working life. This is because there has been little demand on the muscles, heart, lungs, and circulation during the time spent in bed, and their efficiency has correspondingly decreased. Research has shown that people who have desk jobs or who do only light physical work are far more likely to suffer from coronary heart disease than people whose job involves a high level of physical activity.

Keeping active for long periods may not be easy, especially for the urban office worker who rides the bus, train, or car to work each day; goes up to his or her office in the elevator; sits at a desk most of the working day; and returns home at night to sit in front of the television before finally going to bed. But even a person with this life style can adapt his or her daily routine so that it has a more beneficial effect on physical health. Park the car or leave the bus a few blocks from the office and walk; use the stairs, not the elevator; walk around as much as possible in the office; and try to pursue some more active form of entertainment in the evening—even a short walk after dinner will have noticeable benefits.

Getting started on an exercise program

Beginning an organized exercise program should not be intimidating or difficult. Left to your own devices, you should be able to accomplish plenty. But it should be emphasized again that if you are at risk from exercising because of age, risk of heart disease, medical history, or current physical conditions, consult your physician for special guidelines.

In some situations, your physician will recommend exercise testing. Exercise testing is usually accomplished on a treadmill or stationary bicycle. Maximal exercise testing evaluates the circulation's response to full exertion and requires physician supervision. Submaximal exercise testing stops at less than full exertion and, therefore, may be performed without physician supervision. The decision to have maximal versus submaximal exercise testing depends on your health risks and your fitness objectives. A maximal exercise test generates more accurate information about your current aerobic power than a submaximal test. Persons with highly specific or complicated fitness objectives may benefit from more comprehensive, detailed exercise testing.

Generally speaking, a physician will recommend a maximal treadmill stress test for one or both of two reasons. First, the test is a noninvasive way to assess whether coronary arteries are narrowed. This condition might increase the risk of heart attack when exercising. Performing the test for this reason is most helpful in persons who are at increased risk of coronary artery disease. If such a test suggests a problem, additional testing or treatment may be necessary before beginning an exercise program. Second, the test helps determine whether the heart rate and blood pressure response to exertion are normal, and will also determine aerobic power. This information can be used to devise an exercise program that will be safe, effective, and enjoyable.

For aerobic exercise to be effective, the heart rate must be elevated. To determine the heart rate range at which you will experience benefits, you can use the following formula: (1) subtract your age from 220; (2) multiply this number first by .65 and again by .85.

As an example, consider a 30-year-old smoker who wants to begin an aerobic exercise program. To determine a training heart rate range for this person, we subtract 30 from 220 to obtain 190. This multiplied by .65 equals 123.5. And, multiplied times .85 equals 161.5. This person's training heart rate range is roughly 120 to 160 bpm. Because this person is a smoker who has not exercised for a while, it would be wise to begin exercising at milder intensities—that is, closer to the 120-bpm end of the range. The more fit you are already, the more you should exercise at the higher end of your training heart rate range. Competitive athletes routinely exercise at the highest end of their range.

Most physical fitness experts recommend that beginners, those who are new to exercise or out of shape, exercise in the lower end of their training heart rate range for a minimum of 20 minutes three times a week. Experienced exercisers—those who are in improved physical condition—should engage in aerobic activity four to five times a week, gradually moving up in their training heart rate range, for a minimum of 30 minutes per session.

A complete workout lasts 45 to 60 minutes. It begins with a warm-up routine of stretching exercises and light activity to begin warming your muscles (see pages 1040-1041 for suggested warm-up exercises). The workout then mixes strength-building routines, using calisthenics, free weights, or weight resistance machines with aerobic, endurance-building routines, such as jogging, cycling, stair-climbing, or swimming. Every workout should conclude with a cool-down period of stretching and light activity.

If you have questions about how to approach a personal physical fitness program, you may find it worthwhile to consult an exercise physiologist. They are uniquely qualified to tailor an exercise program to meet your specific needs and tastes.

How to calculate and monitor a training heart rate range

1. Subtract age from 220
   (220 − age = X)
2. Multiply X by .65
   X times .65 = lower range in beats per minute (bpm) = X_l
3. Multiply X by .85
   X times .85 = upper range in bpm = X_u
4. Divide X_l and X_u by 4
   $X_l \div 4$ = lower range in bpm for 15-second count
   $X_u \div 4$ = upper range in bpm for 15-second count

To determine if you are exercising at a level sufficient to improve your aerobic power, check your pulse for 15 seconds while exercising. If the number of beats is between your lower and upper ranges for a 15-second count, you are exercising at an appropriate intensity. If it is above your upper range, you are working too hard and should slow down. If it is below your lower range, you should work a little harder and check it again. Anytime you feel chest pain, light-headedness, unusual shortness of breath, or any other form of unusual discomfort, you should immediately stop exercise.

Guidelines for exercise testing

	Apparently healthy		Higher risk			With disease
	Below 45	*45 and Above*	*Below 35 No Symptoms*	*35 and Above No Symptoms*	*Symptoms*	*Any Age*
Maximal exercise test recommended prior to an exercise program	No	Yes	No	Yes	Yes	Yes
Physician attendance recommended for maximal testing	No (under 35)	Yes	Yes	Yes	Yes	Yes
Physician attendance recommended for submaximal testing	No	No	No	Yes	Yes	Yes

Source: Guidelines for Exercise Testing and Prescription by the American College of Sports Medicine.

Choosing an exercise

Almost one half of all people who begin an organized exercise program will drop out within six months to a year. Ideally, exercise should last a lifetime. The most important element associated with sticking to an exercise program is choosing activities that you enjoy. If you decide to run, and you hate running, you'll never stick with your program.

It's important to remember when choosing an exercise that in order to achieve the optimum benefits, you must exercise somewhere in your training heart rate range. Choose an activity that will provide continuous exertion on the heart. Exercises that meet this requirement include:

walking*
racewalking*
aerobic movement (classes or a video)
running
cycling
swimming*
cross-country skiing*
rowing*
stair-climbing

*Indicates an exercise with a low injury rate.

The best approach to exercise may be to switch off or combine activities—also known as cross-training. Cross-training offers a number of benefits. First of all it provides variety—the key to motivation. Doing the same activity time after time becomes monotonous. If you're bored with your exercise program, you're likely to drop out. Second, cross-training lowers the risk of injury. When you switch off activities, you aren't putting too much strain on any one muscle or joint. For example, if you switch off between running and swimming, your knees get a rest when you swim. When you run, your arms get a rest. A final benefit is that your body becomes well rounded. Instead of building up the muscles just in your legs, which can happen with cycling or running, you can switch off with rowing or swimming and build those in your arms, back, and chest as well.

A thing to keep in mind when beginning a cross-training program is that building up endurance in one activity does not necessarily mean that you can begin another activity at the same intensity. For example, say you have been exercising for a couple of months and are able to run 30 minutes for a good workout. Now you decide to take up swimming. If you haven't already been swimming, don't expect to be able to swim for 30 minutes. Just as with your running, you will have to begin slowly and work your way up to 30 minutes. Every activity has different demands on the body. Your body needs time to adjust to a new activity.

Whatever form of physical exercise you decide on, go easy at the beginning. Exercise for short periods and at a gentle pace at first, and build up gradually as your muscles become stronger. Do not attempt vigorous or demanding exercises until your body is strong enough to perform them without suffering undue strain. If you are a heavy smoker, are seriously overweight, or are suffering from any form of physical disorder, consult your physician before committing yourself to any program of exercise.

Health clubs

Those who can afford the time and expense involved may wish to take advantage of the facilities offered by health clubs. The equipment and other facilities provided by clubs are not strictly necessary to the process of getting fit, but they can add interest and variety to your exercise routine. Many clubs offer equipment that would be too costly for an individual to purchase. Health clubs also offer the opportunity to indulge in a cross-training exercise program. Two other advantages of good clubs are supervision, which enables you to exercise with safety and confidence, and a congenial atmosphere. Exercising with people who share a common purpose can provide enjoyment and incentive.

Health clubs vary widely in quality. When choosing one for yourself, you should check that it is staffed by qualified and responsible instructors. You may feel flattered to be attended by a sports celebrity, but professionally trained exercise physiologists and physical education instructors can be equally, if not more, beneficial to an unfit person. You should expect to be asked details of your medical history before being allowed to use all the facilities. If you have not exercised for some time, you may even be advised to have a medical checkup. You will probably be asked to perform some simple exercises that are designed to raise your pulse rate to around 110 beats per minute. If your pulse rate rises excessively, this may be an indication of some physical disorder.

Types of exercise

The accessories provided in health clubs to help you exercise range from simple weights and benches to more sophisticated equipment such as pulleys and rowing machines. These accessories are appropriate for different kinds of exercises.

Isometric exercises, the simplest type, involve applying muscular strength by pulling or pushing immovable objects. The muscles are tensed and this tension is sustained for short periods of time. Because little movement is involved in these exercises, they develop static rather than dynamic strength.

Isotonic exercises involve pulling or lifting an object to a certain position and then returning it to its original position. They cause the muscles to contract as you move, but, because the weight or force employed is constant, they do not exert your muscles to the same degree throughout the exercise. The weight or force used can only be the greatest amount that you can lift or pull at the weakest point in the range of motion involved. At other points your muscles are not sufficiently strained to develop in strength. For example, when you lift weights to help strengthen your biceps (the muscle in the inside of your arm between your elbow and shoulder), it is harder for your muscle to lift the weight than it is to bring it down. Therefore, the muscle is not sufficiently exerted during the motion of bringing the weight down.

The third type of exercise, known as isokinetic, requires more sophisticated equipment. When using this equipment, your muscles are made to work at their maximum capacity throughout the exercise. The resistance of the object against which you pull or push varies according to the effort you employ, so that the resistance is equal to the muscular force exerted throughout the exercise. The equipment itself automatically controls both the resistance and the speed at which you perform the exercise.

Isokinetic exercises can be designed for particular needs. For example, a person who is training for a particular sport can do exercises that simulate exactly the demands of this sport, and so develop precisely the muscles he or she most needs. In terms of the speed with which muscular power is developed, research has shown that isokinetic exercises are the most efficient of the three different types. They are also the safest, as the effort involved is automatically regulated.

Massage

Massage is used in physical therapy as a means of rehabilitating patients who are suffering from certain physical pains, ailments, or injuries. As a means of getting or keeping fit, however, its value is limited. It stimulates the circulation, relaxes the muscles, and can relieve local pains. But massage itself cannot increase muscular strength or reduce the amount of fat on the body.

Sauna baths

Sauna baths may be attached to health clubs or may exist as separate establishments. They have an invigorating effect on the whole body and aid physical and mental relaxation, but their effects are temporary rather than long term.

On entering a sauna, you first take a warm shower to wash off the superficial dirt. You then enter the dry heat room, and sit or lie on benches while perspiring in temperatures of up to 248°F. (120°C). The heat is created by stoves or by electric heaters. Your body temperature rises by about 3.6°F. (2°C), and your blood vessels dilate. This causes your heart to beat faster, in order to circulate more blood to the outside of your body. Your skin pores open, and the perspiration washes out particles of dirt, dead skin, and cosmetics. These are then rinsed off in a cold shower. Alternating periods in the heat room with cold showers has an especially invigorating effect.

Sauna baths provide a healthy and enjoyable means of relaxation, but the sudden rise in pulse rate can be dangerous for anyone with a weak heart. People with any heart disorder, pregnant women, and people with high or low blood pressure should avoid them.

Choosing an exercise

	Equipment	*Advantages*	*Disadvantages*
Running	a good pair of shoes	• efficient conditioning activity • can be done almost anywhere • community races available in some areas provide incentive as well as social opportunity	• may be too strenuous for some people • stress injuries are common • good shoes can be costly
Walking	a good pair of shoes	• a good activity for all ages and fitness levels, especially the beginner • community races available in some areas provide incentive as well as social opportunity • very low injury rate • can be done almost anywhere	• shoes can be costly • may take longer to achieve desired aerobic benefits than with other activities because the heart rate is not elevated as easily
Aerobic classes/videos	classes—membership to health club or registration in a class; good aerobic shoes video—a video; a video recorder; a television; good shoes; a mat or suitable floor (hardwood, not cement)	• an efficient conditioner • able to work all body parts at the same time • music makes more enjoyable • a wide variety of classes or videos usually available, i.e. low-impact or high-impact, etc.	• high injury rate • may be too strenuous for some people • with low-impact aerobics, harder to elevate heart rate • shoes may be expensive
Cycling	a stationary bike for indoor cycling; a sturdy bike and helmet for outdoor cycling	• good workout for the lower body • pleasant scenery and the possibility of changing route for variety	• equipment can be expensive • if living in a cold climate, outdoor cycling not easily done year round
Swimming	access to a pool or other body of water; swimming suit; goggles	• works entire body at the same time if done strenuously • low injury rate • easy on the joints • good for all fitness levels and ages	• access to water may not be easy • potential for eye and ear ailments • lessons usually necessary to get full benefits—may be costly
Rowing	stationary rowing maching for indoor use; boat with oars, access to a body of water, and boat storage for outdoor use	• works entire body if done correctly and strenuously • low injury rate	• equipment is costly • must live near water for outdoor rowing
Cross-country skiing	stationary machine for indoor use; skis, poles, and access to snowy surfaces for outdoor use	• works entire body if done correctly and strenuously • low injury rate	• equipment is costly • outdoor skiing is not available year round for most
Stair-climbing	stationary machine for indoor use; a well-ventilated stairwell for indoor or outdoor use	• effective, efficient conditioning activity • works entire body if done correctly and strenuously	• machines can be costly • may cause knee stress injury

Sticking with your program

Making exercise part of your life can be difficult at first, but it's important to make fitness a lifetime commitment. Below are some suggestions for helping you stick with your exercise program.

(1) Set realistic goals. Do not expect to make monumental progress in a week. Begin slowly and increase difficulty and duration of exercise periods as you go.

(2) Do not overdo it too soon. If you overexert yourself, you will increase the likelihood for injury and you will have sore muscles. These unpleasant experiences may discourage you from continuing.

(3) Work out a time that best suits your body. Some people can exercise in the morning with no problem—it helps them get a "jump start." Others prefer the evening as a way of releasing the tension of the day.

(4) Write down your activities and time spent exercising. Keeping track of your progress allows you to see your improvements, which will motivate you to continue.

(5) Do not depend on a scale. Too often, beginning exercisers use the scale as a means to measure progress. This can quickly become discouraging as many people may gain weight from fluid retention at the onset of an exercise program. Weigh yourself no more than once a week and always use the same scale when you do.

(6) Vary your routine. Run, walk, or cycle a different route each time you go out. If you belong to a health club that has a few different locations, visit a new one every once in a while. Combine activities: Run to your health club and then swim once you get there.

(7) Get the support of others or exercise with a friend. Family members can be especially helpful in motivating you to stay on your program. Exercising with a group also helps motivate.

(8) Don't let lapses get you down. If you miss an exercise session or two, don't dwell on it. Just get back into your program as soon as you can.

A lifetime of fitness

In old age, a certain amount of physical decline is inevitable. As the body ages, the arteries gradually harden, the capacity of the lungs diminishes, the muscles deteriorate, the bones become thinner and more brittle, and there is a reduction in both height and weight. Specialized cells in certain organs of the body die and are not replaced, thus reducing the efficiency of these organs. None of these changes, however, need reduce an older person's capacity to enjoy life, and physical exercise remains important.

Many of the advantages of regular exercise taken early in life become apparent only as you grow older. However, it is never too late to start.

Simple flexibility exercises are especially suitable for older people. Many of these exercises can be performed while you are sitting in a chair. For neck flexibility, let the head fall gently forward or to one side, and then lift it up. For flexibility of the spine and trunk, sit with your arms outstretched and move the whole of your upper body from side to side. For flexibility of the hip joints, sit with the legs outstretched and raise one knee, bending your head gently down toward it as you do so. All these movements can be repeated a number of times, but never strain yourself or force your body to make a movement that causes pain. Remember that the aim of these exercises is flexibility, not muscular strength or endurance.

Other factors related to physical fitness in old age are diet and recreational interests. Many aches and pains, as well as anemia and other ailments, are caused by diets lacking in essential vitamins, proteins, and nutrients, especially calcium and iron. The diet of elderly people should contain plenty of milk, as well as fruit and fresh vegetables. It is dangerous to assume that older people need less nutritious food than younger people.

Although older people should avoid exercise that demands sudden or prolonged effort, physical activity of some kind can be very beneficial. Short but regular walks will exercise the joints and stimulate the circulation. Gardening also provides good exercise, and by planning a garden carefully and using appropriate tools you can eliminate most of the heavy work. Once you have attained a certain degree of physical fitness, you may be able to take up swimming, running, or cycling, and surprise yourself with your own achievements.

Exercise for mind and body

There are a wide variety of physical exercises that are more effective as aids to mental relaxation than in developing physical fitness. They may improve physical balance, coordination, and flexibility, but usually have little effect on strength or stamina. Their value is often more psychological than physical or medical.

Eurhythmics are exercises involving the coordination of physical movements with rhythmical musical sounds. They emphasize the aesthetic qualities of harmonious bodily movement, and are used as a form of musical education and in the training of modern dancers. They have had considerable influence on the development of choreography in the 1900's.

Yoga, originally a school of ancient Hindu philosophy, emphasizes the unity of mind and body. The form of yoga that is usually practiced in Western countries is hatha-yoga, which consists of a system of postures and breathing exercises that aid physical and mental relaxation. They develop suppleness and mobility, especially in hip joints. It is claimed that they develop the inner resources of the body, and that they can lead eventually to complete knowledge and mastery of mind and body. Further stages of yoga involve techniques of concentration and meditation.

Various techniques of meditation itself have become popular in Western countries as aids to physical and mental relaxation. Many of these techniques are derived from Eastern religions, and include breathing and relaxation exercises. Transcendental Meditation, or TM, involves profound concentration for two periods each day on a specific mantra, which is a word or formula that, when spoken repetitively, can aid concentration.

For more information on these and other forms of meditation and relaxation techniques, consult a bookstore or library.

Warming up and cooling down

Before beginning an exercise session, it is important to warm up the muscles. Warming up reduces muscle stiffness, protects the muscles and joints from injury, and makes exercise more enjoyable.

For a long time it was believed that doing a few stretches before beginning a routine was plenty. However, it has become apparent that stretching cold muscles is not as efficient as stretching warm muscles. Stretching a cold muscle may even cause injury. The best way to warm up before exercise is to engage in the activity or an activity similar to the one you plan on doing, but at a lighter pace for three or four minutes. For example, if you plan on running a couple of miles for your workout, warm up by walking swiftly for a few blocks. Light exercise increases the blood flow to the muscles and tendons, which, in turn, increases their flexibility. This type of warmup also prepares the heart to meet the muscles' increased demand for blood during strenuous exercise.

The warmup should be followed by stretching exercises. The exercises on these two pages cover all the body parts you will use in any form of strenuous activity. Stretching the muscles may help avoid cramps and prepares them for strenuous exercise. Be sure to follow the directions given for the exercises.

Equally, if not more important, is cooling down the muscles after an exercise session. If you stop abruptly after engaging in a strenuous activity such as running, you run the risk of putting too much stress on the heart. A drop in blood pressure may occur. The best way to cool down is to repeat your warmup. Follow a hard workout of running with a swift five-minute walk or swim a few laps at a leisurely pace after half an hour of strenuous swimming. This type of cooldown allows your heart to slowly return to its resting rate. It's usually a good idea to continue at a slow pace until your breathing returns to normal and your heart rate is under 100.

Follow your cooldown with the stretching exercises pictured here. Stretching at this point may help avoid cramping and ensures that your heart fully returns to its resting rate.

How to perform these exercises:

Hold stretches 15 to 30 seconds.

Never bounce.

Be sure to breathe while stretching.

Always keep your knees slightly bent—never lock them.

Stop an exercise if you feel pain.

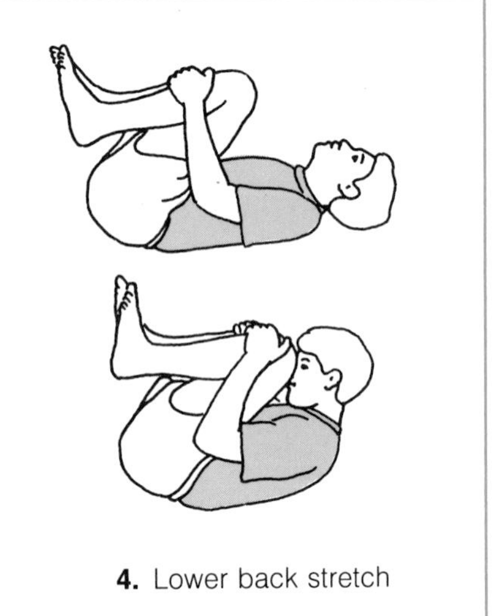

4. Lower back stretch

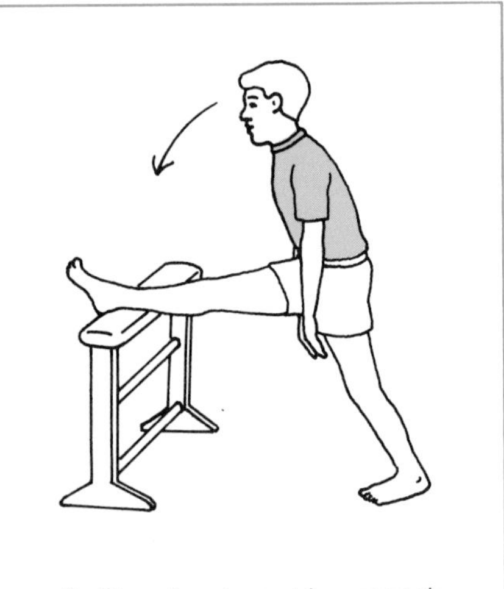

8. Standing hamstring stretch

Warm-up and cool-down exercises

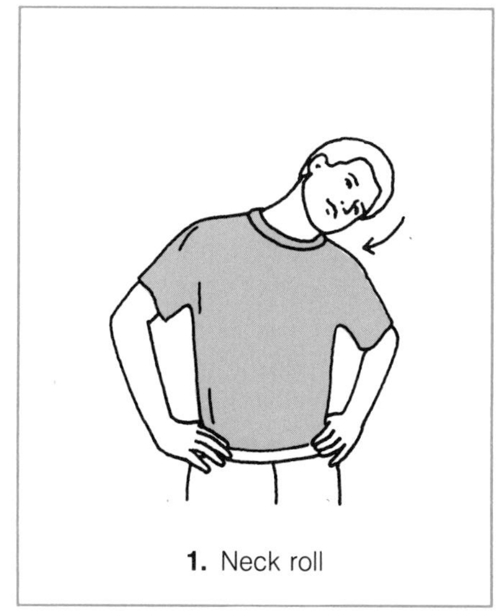
1. Neck roll

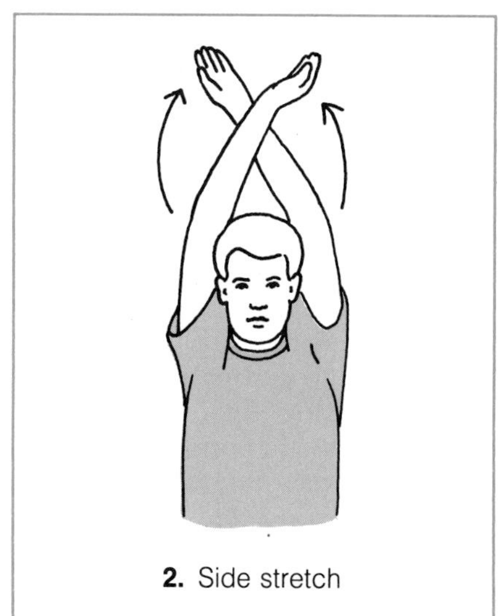
2. Side stretch

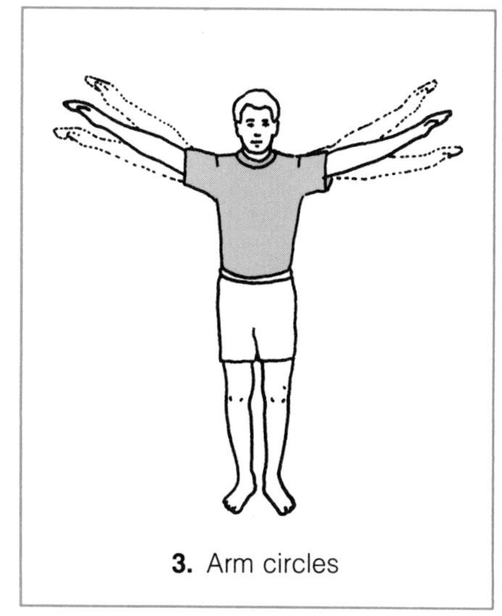
3. Arm circles

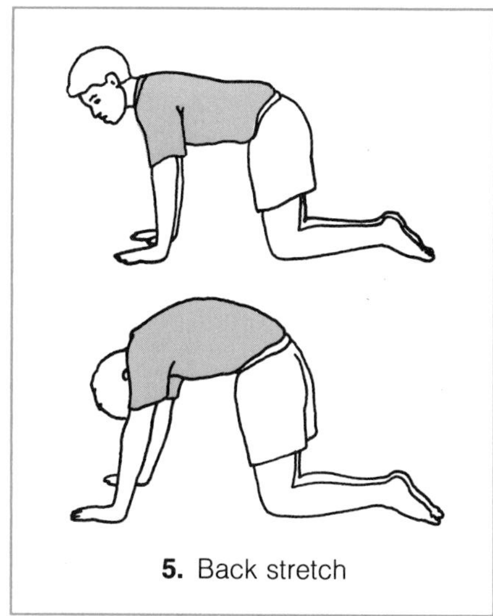
5. Back stretch

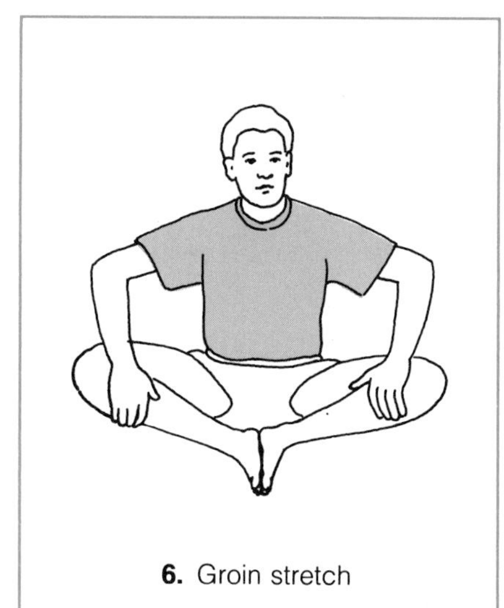
6. Groin stretch

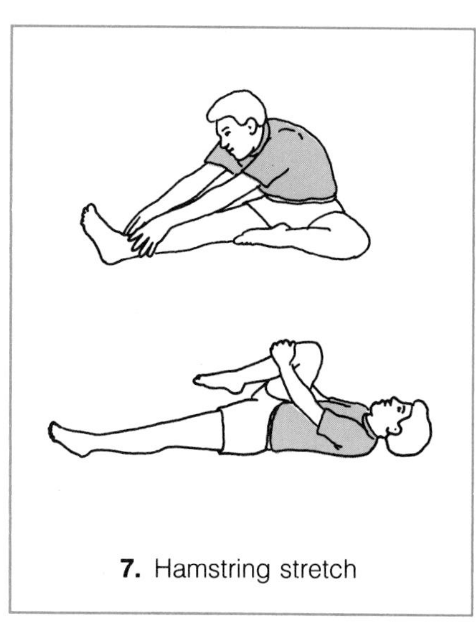
7. Hamstring stretch

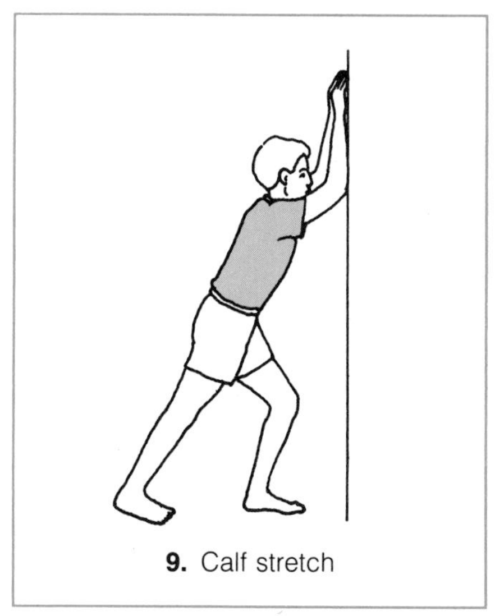
9. Calf stretch

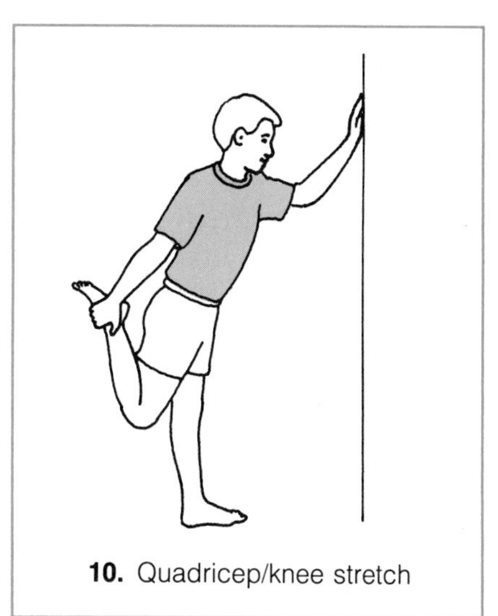
10. Quadricep/knee stretch

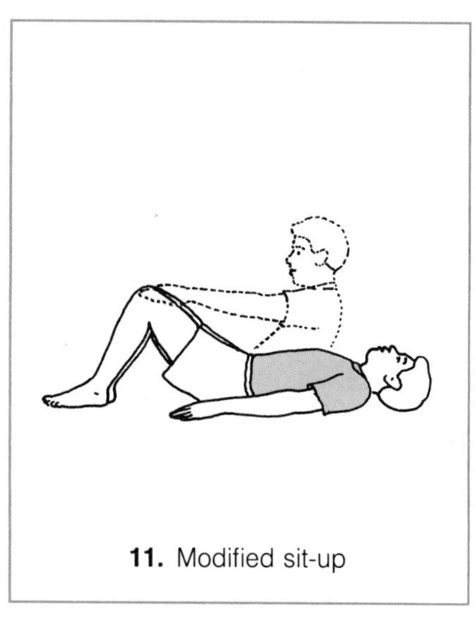
11. Modified sit-up

Appendix: V

Growing older

The population of the United States is getting older. From the late 1940's to the mid-1960's, there was what is referred to as "the baby boom." Today the first "baby boomers" are in their 40's and getting older. In 15 to 25 years these people will comprise the elderly population, thus making this population the biggest and fastest-growing segment of the entire population.

This section contains information about aging: how we age and why we age. It also has information on choosing "eldercare"—one of the biggest concerns many people and their families will have to face in the years to come. Finally, this section ends with a list of agencies set up to help the elderly and their friends and family.

Why we age

Aging is a normal process of human development. It occurs on several levels: biological, psychological, and social. Although it is not known for sure what causes aging, most gerontologists (scientists who study aging) would agree that aging is the result of a combination of processes, both internal and external. Here are some of the more widely held theories about why we age:

The *wear-and-tear theory* compares the human body to a machine that, over time, wears down from use. According to this theory, bodily systems receive cumulative damage from both external forces, such as stress, the environment, diet, and life style; and internal forces, such as toxins released as a result of metabolism. Cells become damaged and increasingly fail to reproduce or repair themselves. They die off in larger numbers as we age.

The *theory of planned obsolescence* holds that aging is genetically programmed into each of our cells. The existence of such a hereditary mechanism would explain why there are characteristic life spans, or maximum age limits for different species.

A combination of the above two theories is increasingly suggested by geriatric researchers. Many, however, believe the theory of planned obsolescence is more predominant in the combination. This "combination theory" explains that although individuals can prolong life by modifying such outside influences as stress and diet, each person is born with a genetically predetermined life expectancy that cannot be exceeded. This interaction of external factors and internal programming would account for individual variations in life span.

Two other popular theories of aging focus on the cells' activity. The *error theory* proposes that as cells divide and multiply, random errors in DNA-guided protein synthesis occur, leading eventually to failure of the entire organism.

The *free radical theory* holds that in the presence of certain types of oxygen, metabolizing cells produce chemical toxins that destroy proteins and fats vital to cell functioning.

According to yet another theory, the *autoimmune theory*, the body's immune system gradually breaks down. Antibodies once directed at detecting and destroying foreign microorganisms turn against the body, allowing cancer and other diseases to invade.

The mystery surrounding why we age is still a topic of numerous ongoing studies. Perhaps one day we will truly know why we age. Then the question "Can we slow or stop the aging process?" will become even more important.

The stages of aging

In past decades, when fewer people than today reached their 70's there was greater agreement as to when an individual entered old age. But improvements in medicine, nutrition, sanitation, and living habits have enabled more and more people to live well into their 70's, 80's, and beyond. This increase in the number of older people has changed the composition of the elderly population and has forced a reevaluation of the concept of "old."

Today, social researchers recognize "elderhood" as a continually changing, dynamic process that can be broken down into stages that reflect the variations among the old.

The *young-old*, roughly aged 65 to 75, typically are healthy, active, and independent. Although many members of this group have retired from the work force, they generally suffer few major physical impairments. They lead active social and sexual lives and participate in recreational, political, and educational activities. More than half remain married, not yet having lost a spouse through death, and only 1½ percent live in nursing homes. As "baby boomers" enter this stage, the young-old will be increasingly better educated and more affluent than they are today.

The *middle-old*, aged 76 to 85, constitute the group that are often referred to as the "frail elderly." Members of this group are more likely than the young-old to experience major physical impairments and may have at least one chronic illness that interferes with their daily functioning. These are changes traditionally associated with "old age." In a sense, this group makes up what was once believed to have been the entire elderly population.

The middle-old are more likely than the young-old to have lost a spouse, be poor, be female, and have fewer social supports (e.g., friends). Less than 10 percent of this group needs institutional care. Some of these conditions may soon change as the number of people in this group and their educational levels increase.

The *old-old*, aged 86 and older, are the most likely to suffer major losses in functioning on all levels—social, psychological, and physical. Often poor, alone, and unable to care for themselves, members of this group typically have one or more chronic medical problems. They have approximately 75 percent more hospitalizations than the middle-old and are very limited in mobility, thus requiring physical assistance. Of all the elderly people living in nursing homes, the old-old make up the greatest proportion—nearly 25 percent. In addition, a decline in mental functioning occurs mostly among the old-old. However, since individuals age at different rates, some people in the old-old stage remain vibrant and continue to grow and enjoy life despite some inevitable physical decline.

Although the aged share certain traits, it is not accurate to group them together as they have been for many years. Most of the young-old remain capable, competent, productive citizens. Limits placed on this group are generally imposed by society, not by any incapacity. As individuals advance into old age, however, they are more likely to suffer debilitating illnesses and increasing dependency. But as a rule, the elderly are highly adaptable and strive to live independently while maintaining family and other social ties.

How the body ages

What happens to the human body as it ages? Almost everyone experiences the same internal and external changes. However, the rate and degree of these changes will be different from person to person. The information offered here is a general guide to what can occur between the ages of 20 and 90.

Skin: loses its elasticity; sags and wrinkles; becomes thinner; becomes discolored in areas; bruises more easily; wounds heal more slowly; nails become thin, brittle, and ridged, and their rate of growth slows; fat beneath the skin begins to decrease.

Hair: turns gray or white; thins and/or falls out.

Muscles: lose bulk; night cramps become more frequent; decline in muscular strength; range and speed of motion becomes limited.

Eyes/vision: eyes may have a sunken appearance; reduction of tear production; color vision less acute; adaptation to darkness slows; lens of eye focuses less easily on close objects, causing farsightedness; diameter of pupil decreases, causing greater need for illumination or light.

Ear/hearing: wax accumulates faster, which may cause hearing difficulty; loss of hearing at high frequencies; ability to discriminate pitch decreases.

Taste and smell: become less acute due to progressive loss of taste buds and nerve fibers.

Brain/spinal cord: weight of brain declines; rate of new learning slows, but the capacity to learn persists; perception may become impaired; short-term memory begins to fail; senses of pain, touch, hot, and cold impaired.

Gait/balance: increasing unsteadiness; loss in confidence; slower gait; posture may be more stooped.

Bones: become lighter, more brittle, and break more easily; possible frequent backaches; loss of height.

Newborn

This is when the aging process really begins. Babies are usually born after 40 weeks of gestation. Most are normal and healthy. They are completely dependent upon their caregiver.

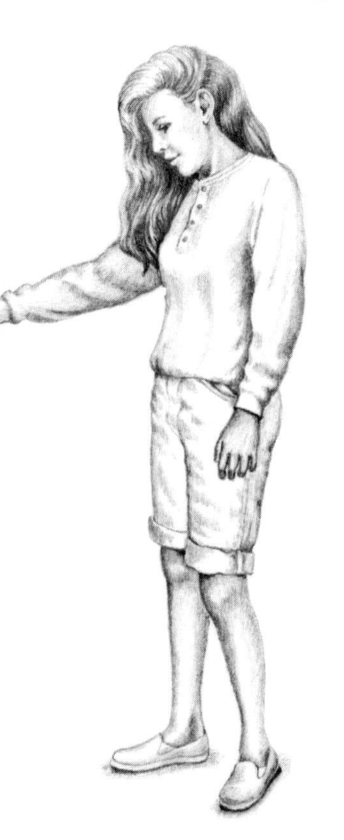

1-20

Women reach sexual maturity around age 13. Men reach sexual maturity around age 16. This is a time of rapid growth.

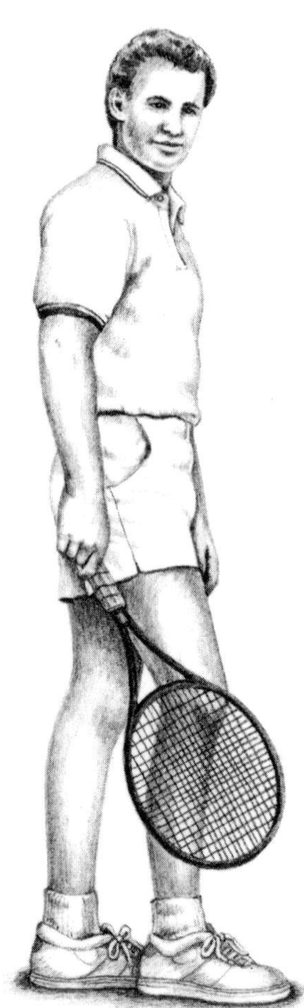

20-40

For most, the 20's are the prime of life. Muscular strength is at its greatest. Hair is at its thickest. However, some signs of "typical" aging appear. Height may be decreasing and the immune system may begin to decline in effectiveness. Atherosclerosis, or hardening of the arteries, may begin even before the age of 20. At 30, the heart muscle begins to thicken, causing it to have to work harder to circulate blood. Hearing becomes less acute. Skin begins losing its elasticity. The vertebral column (backbone) begins to deteriorate causing the disks to move closer together.

Joints: become less extensible and more rigid, leading to increased stiffness in the body; wear on hip and knee joints reduces mobility; aches and pains more apparent.

Stomach and intestines: metabolism slows; secretion of stomach decreases, making food harder to digest; constipation becomes more frequent; preference develops for smaller meals.

Liver: becomes smaller and less efficient in processing toxic substances in the blood.

Pancreas: less able to remove blood sugars due to decrease in production of the enzymes trypsin and insulin, making diabetes more likely.

Heart: becomes less efficient at pumping blood; muscle and valves thicken; rate of response to stress decreases; enlarges.

Circulation/blood pressure: blood vessels lose elasticity and harden, causing poor circulation of blood and higher blood pressure; cholesterol and calcium levels increase; advantages of some kind of exercise are more apparent as aging continues because it aids in circulation.

Kidneys: efficiency declines; ability to excrete fluids diminishes.

Respiratory system: breathing is less efficient due to loss of elasticity in lungs; decrease in oxygen consumption; cough reflex of lungs decreases.

Immune system: declines in effectiveness, causing greater susceptibility to infections; infections strike more often and last longer.

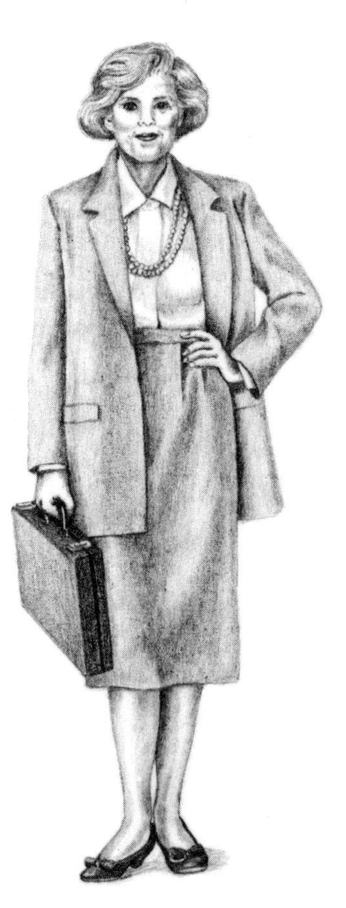

40-60

The immune system declines in effectiveness more rapidly. The hair thins and grays. Eyesight deteriorates. Many people in this age group are about ⅛″ shorter than at age 20. By 50, wrinkles become more apparent. Most women have begun menopause by the early 50's and, as a result, their bones may become lighter, more brittle, and break more easily (all conditions associated with osteoporosis—loss of bone mass). Sense of taste becomes less acute. Later in the 50's, metabolism slows. Muscles continue to deteriorate and body weight decreases as a result of this deterioration.

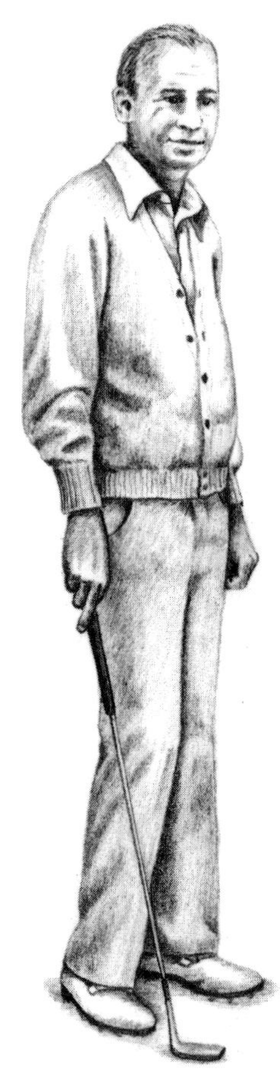

60-70

On average, height is decreased by ¾″. Muscle strength declines, often because of decreased use. Capacity of the lungs decreases by half as compared to age 20.

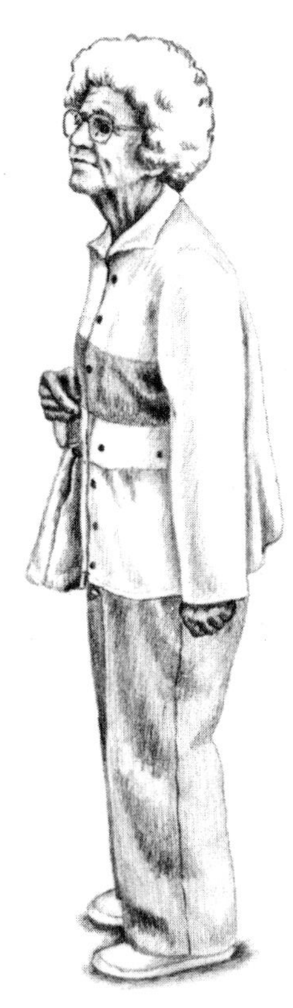

70 and beyond

Total loss in height is about one inch. Nose, ears, and earlobes are longer. External and internal signs of aging are very apparent.

Choosing eldercare

As the population of the United States grows older, many people will have to make a decision about how to care for themselves. Their families, too, will be faced with the responsibility of helping make this decision, or, in some cases, determining what is best for an aging relative.

Choosing eldercare is not easy. If you or a loved one is in need of assistance with daily living—because of a chronic illness, for example—should you care for yourself or your loved one in your home? Or should you entrust a health care facility with the responsibility of care? While both of these options have certain advantages, they represent extremes along a continuum of available care. Fortunately, as the proportion of the aged in the United States population continues to grow, more and better resources are becoming available.

Currently, only 5 percent of elderly people live in nursing homes or other long-term care facilities. And, of this group, experts estimate that half are equally or better served by alternative sources of care that allow older persons to continue living independently. Therefore, it is wise and necessary to explore the wide variety of choices that exist before deciding on a program of care for yourself or your aging family member.

The following discussion examines the advantages and disadvantages of the most popular forms of eldercare and offers some guidelines on selecting suitable care. Not all of the services and facilities described here may be available in your community. Also keep in mind that some may be too costly for you or your elderly relative's resources. In addition, needs may change over time, so there should be some degree of flexibility in whatever choice you and/or your aging relative make.

Choosing eldercare will be a long and stressful decision-making process. It is important to remember that although you may feel alone in your search, you aren't. See pages 1049-1050 for a list of agencies set up and available to help you and your family through this important time.

Home health care

This type of care varies with the older person's medical needs and covers a wide range of services: part-time skilled nursing care; restorative care, such as physical, occupational, or speech therapy; nutritional counseling; and medical equipment and supplies. These services are brought to the home of the ill or disabled senior and are individually tailored to meet his or her needs. Often less expensive than institutional care, home health care services nevertheless can become costly, even exceeding nursing-home fees, especially if intensive rehabilitation or skilled nursing care is needed for a long period of time. Moreover, private insurance plans and government assistance programs, such as Medicaid and Medicare, often will not cover the full costs of home health care services, especially if such care is required for any length of time.

Personal-care assistance

This nonmedical form of care is usually provided by a home-health aide or companion, either live-in or come-and-go, and can be arranged through a home-health service agency. This type of care may be especially appropriate for the elderly person who does not have any major health problems, but just needs help keeping up with day-to-day chores. The older person with moderate or severe dementia would also benefit from personal-care assistance, as it allows the person to remain in a familiar environment. The aide assists impaired or frail seniors with meal preparation and eating, bathing, dressing, grooming, walking, and other personal functions.

Unfortunately, the supply of such workers is limited, and costs, often fairly expensive, are typically not reimbursed by private insurance or by government assistance programs.

Protective services

Elderly persons who are unable to manage their own legal and/or financial affairs can have a conservator appointed to act on their behalf and protect them from exploitation.

Homemaker-chore services

These services focus on household maintenance, usually performed by a housekeeper, and may include personal care as well. As with personal-care assistance, it is ideal for independent elderly persons with no major health problems. The housekeeper generally shops, cooks, runs errands, does laundry, and performs other light housekeeping chores. Additional assistance may be provided with heavy cleaning, yard work, and other physically demanding chores.

Home-delivered meals

Popularly referred to as "meals on wheels," this program is offered by hospitals, church groups, social-service agencies, and various other community-service groups. Seniors who cannot prepare their own meals have nutritious, fully cooked meals delivered to their homes five days a week, and sometimes also on weekends.

Telephone-reassurance programs

For seniors who live alone and who may have a chronic illness, these programs ensure that all is well. Each day at a prearranged time, either an operator from a central switchboard calls the elderly individual, or he or she calls in to the switchboard. If the call is not answered or received, the police or neighbors are sent to check on the older person's well-being. In many communities, a device is available that allows the senior to call for help simply by pushing a button. Once activated the device sends an emergency signal, often to a hospital, indicating the need for assistance. The hospital, in turn, notifies paramedics or the family to the emergency.

Escort and transportation services

Seniors who cannot drive or use public transportation, or who need physical assistance, can turn to these services, which are usually staffed by volunteer drivers. Thus, seniors can maintain outside activities, keep medical appointments, and so on despite limited mobility.

Senior centers

These social centers, located in most communities, provide recreational and educational programs and activities for the elderly, and may also serve as informational clearinghouses on topics of interest to seniors. Many also serve free hot lunches. They are run by private groups or local government agencies.

Respite care

Various programs have been developed to give family members and friends a break, or respite, from the responsibility of caring for an elderly person full time. (Family and friends provide roughly 90 percent of all eldercare.) These programs also offer mental and social stimulation to the elderly, and may provide health-care services as well.

Adult day-care centers

These centers provide a structured, supervised program of social, therapeutic, and health activities designed to help restore or maintain impaired seniors' mental and physical functioning. Such programs can be used on a short-term basis as a bridge between institutional care and independent living, or on a long-term basis as an alternative to a nursing home, as long as intensive medical care is not needed. Many adult day-care centers also fulfill a social/recreational function, provide transportation to and from the center, and offer meals and snacks.

Participants attend the center for a scheduled number of days per week, six to eight hours a day, with any required medical or nursing care available on-site or through nearby community health centers. Costs vary depending on the degree of care and level of services the senior needs, but sliding-scale fees are usually charged. Some state or local health and social-service agencies may also offer financial assistance. Costs are generally not covered by private insurance.

Visiting volunteers

For homebound older persons who are isolated from neighbors or relatives, volunteers from church groups or social-service agencies make weekly in-home visits to ease seniors' loneliness and fears.

Short-term care

Some nursing homes and other residential centers provide temporary care—short-term holiday care, one-week or weekend stays, and even once- or twice-weekly stays. This form of respite care eases the burden on families who care for elderly members full time yet can't afford more extensive programs. Although some private insurance plans may reimburse part of these costs, these services are usually out-of-pocket expenses for the patient or family.

Group living arrangements

As with in-home care, group living offers a range of services that vary with the individual's needs and the setting. Benefits of group living are the availability of off-site care, including, in some cases, health/medical supervision, and the social stimulation that comes from living among one's peers.

Congregate housing

Now commonplace and geared toward the elderly who need some assistance yet can live independently, congregate housing blends apartment and dormitory-style living. Seniors live in specially designed apartment complexes offering meals in a common dining room, a variety of recreational programs, and some supportive services, such as transportation, housekeeping, and health care. The surroundings are usually quite pleasant. Specially equipped apartments for handicapped and wheelchair-bound residents are usually available. Residents pay a monthly rental fee, which includes meals and other amenities, based on the facility and types of services used. Some facilities may be government subsidized or charge a sliding-scale fee for low-income elderly. Most are run like rental apartments and require a refundable security deposit.

Shared housing

Under this arrangement, seniors unable to live entirely on their own, yet who are in reasonably good health, share a house or apartment with one or several other elderly persons. Each contributes to household tasks based on his or her abilities. By pooling expenses, the group can often afford services, such as cleaning, and luxuries that a single elderly person's budget could not accommodate. The built-in companionship of shared housing carries an added benefit—help in time of emergency.

Continuing-care or "life-care" communities

These retirement communities combine several types of living arrangements and citylike features within a single setting: townhomes/cottages, apartments, shops, on-site medical facilities, a central dining room, game rooms, a library, exercise rooms and pool, and an auditorium are just some of those that may be available under such an arrangement. Continuing-care communities are growing in numbers and popularity as more and more seniors remain healthy and are able to afford their expensive entrance fees (ranging anywhere from $30,000 to $100,000 or more, often paid with proceeds from the sale of the family home) and monthly rent. These centers appeal to still-active seniors desiring an attractive, relaxed, safe, centralized community offering plentiful social, cultural, and recreational opportunities within a homelike setting without the physical demands of household upkeep. Also, since these communities are aimed at providing lifetime care, they offer a complete range of personal and medical supportive services to assist the elderly as their health declines. Their costliness and often extensive lists of regulations, however, make these centers important to investigate, including a lawyer's contract review, before making a commitment.

Nursing homes

Also called long-term care facilities or institutional care, nursing homes typically provide comprehensive, around-the-clock care and close medical supervision to very infirm seniors in need of intensive care. It's estimated that almost one-quarter of the elderly will spend some time in a nursing home, if only temporarily, while recovering from an illness or surgery. Because there is such a high demand, nursing homes, especially those with favorable reputations, often have long waiting lists—it is therefore wise to plan ahead and shop around.

Nursing homes vary widely in quality and size, serving anywhere from a dozen to several hundred residents. They also differ in the kinds, or levels, of care provided. Homes can range from short-term convalescent care to skilled nursing and multilevel care. Some even have specialized units, such as for Alzheimer's patients, with specially trained staff providing individualized programs and close supervision.

Most nursing homes are privately owned and operated. Not all accept or are licensed to accept Medicaid or Medicare patients. (Check ahead; even if you do not plan to use Medicaid initially, you may choose to do so later and thus can avoid a disruptive move by using at the outset a home that accepts government assistance.) Costs for nursing homes average several hundred to several thousand dollars a month, depending on their level of care. Medicare does not, at this time, provide permanent nursing-home care under any circumstances. Medicare covers only rehabilitation or restorative care in a nursing home. For these reasons, Medicare will only cover a limited number of days in a nursing home, and then only if the person has been in the hospital in the past month.

For help in evaluating and choosing a nursing home, consult the nearest public library (dozens of books on the subject are available), a community information and referral service, or your local health department, local social-service agency, or area agency on the aging (a list of agencies is provided on pages 1049-1050). Or ask your friends, clergy, or family physician for a referral. Some local groups and organizations, such as the Alzheimer's Association, publish free informational booklets on how to select a long-term care facility and even provide lists ranking local nursing homes on their quality and level of care.

Hospice care

A relatively recent development, hospice programs provide 24-hour, 7-day-a-week supportive care to terminally ill patients either at home or in an independent facility having a homelike environment. Hospice care aims to relieve pain and provide comfort, both emotional and physical. Hospice programs work closely with a patient's physician in devising a program of care. They also typically offer emotional support, through counseling and related services, to family members. Costs, which average $40 or more a day, may be partially reimbursed by a private insurer. Medicare or a special fund established by the hospice program also may cover some expenses.

Remember, today there are a variety of community-based and privately run services that you and your aging family member can choose from—and even combine—to tailor-make a program of eldercare that suits everyone's needs and budget. Structuring such a program is bound to be complicated, time-consuming, and, admittedly, frustrating. However, the effort can help promote the elderly person's independence and increase his or her satisfaction. As the senior's needs change, so too should the types of facilities and levels of services used.

If alternative services prove to be impractical, and intensive nursing or medical attention and personal care are required, a long-term care facility such as a nursing home can be the best option if chosen with care. No matter what route you take to ensuring your loved one's well-being, always keep in mind his or her preferences. Most health-care experts agree that seniors do best in their own community so that they can maintain their ties with the people and places that have grown to be familiar and important to them. Also seek out the advice and recommendations of the professionals you trust.

For your information

These two pages contain addresses of agencies set up to help the elderly and their families. Categories, such as "housing" and "health care," are given. However, many agencies are designed to offer a number of services. It is a good idea to read the whole list when looking for an address for help with a certain matter.

General

American Senior Citizens Association
P.O. Box 41
Fayetteville, NC 28302

American Society on Aging
833 Market St., Suite 512
San Francisco, CA 94103

Association of Informed Senior Citizens
460 Spring Park Pl., Suite 1000
Herndon, VA 22070

Center for the Study of Aging
706 Madison Ave.
Albany, NY 12208

Daughters of the Elderly Bridging the Unknown Together
c/o Pat Meier
710 Concord St.
Ellettsville, IN 47429

Gray Panthers
311 S. Juniper St., Suite 601
Philadelphia, PA 19107

International Federation on Aging
1909 K St., N.W.
Washington, DC 20049

International Senior Citizens Association
1102 S. Crenshaw Blvd.
Los Angeles, CA 90019

Little Brothers—Friends of the Elderly
1658 W. Belmont Ave.
Chicago, IL 60657

Mature Outlook
1500 W. Shure Dr.
Arlington Heights, IL 60004

National Association of State Units on Aging
2033 K St., N.W.
Washington, DC 20006

National Alliance of Senior Citizens
2525 Wilson Blvd.
Arlington, VA 22201

National Association for Human Development
P.O. Box 100
Washington, DC 20044

National Association of Area Agencies on Aging
c/o National Council on the Aging
600 Maryland Ave., S.W., W. Wing
Suite 100
Washington, DC 20024

National Council of Senior Citizens
925 15th St., N.W.
Washington, DC 20005

National Geriatrics Society
212 W. Wisconsin Ave., 3rd Fl.
Milwaukee, WI 53203

National Interfaith Coalition on Aging
P.O. Box 1924
298 S. Hull St.
Athens, GA 30603

New Age
1212 Roosevelt
Ann Arbor, MI 48104

Senior Security Network
1411 K St., N.W., Suite 1010
Washington, DC 20005

Health

Alzheimer's Disease and Related Disorders Association
360 N. Michigan Ave., Rm 1102
Chicago, IL 60610

American Cancer Society
1599 Clifton Rd.
Atlanta, GA 30329

American Council of the Blind
1010 Vermont Ave., N.W., Suite 1100
Washington, DC 20005

American Dental Association
211 E. Chicago Ave.
Chicago, IL 60611

American Diabetes Association
National Service Center
P.O. Box 25757
1660 Duke St.
Alexandria, VA 22313

American Dietetic Association
216 W. Jackson Blvd., Suite 800
Chicago, IL 60606

American Heart Association
7320 Greenville Ave.
Dallas, TX 75231

American Lung Association
1740 Broadway
New York, NY 10019

American Parkinson Disease Association
116 John St., Suite 417
New York, NY 10038

American Red Cross
17th and D Sts., N.W.
Washington, DC 20006

American Speech-Language-Hearing Association
10801 Rockville Pike
Rockville, MD 20852

Arthritis Foundation
1314 Spring St., N.W.
Atlanta, GA 30309

National Association of the Deaf
814 Thayer Ave.
Silver Spring, MD 20910

National Center for Health Promotion and Aging
c/o National Council on the Aging
600 Maryland Ave., S.W., W. Wing
Suite 100
Washington, DC 20024

National Kidney Foundation
Two Park Ave.
New York, NY 10003

National Mental Health Association
1021 Prince St.
Alexandria, VA 22314

National Osteoporosis Foundation
1625 Eye St., N.W., Suite 822
Washington, DC 20006

Parkinson Support Groups of America
11376 Cherry Hill Rd., #204
Beltsville, MD. 20705

Women's Association for Research in Menopause
128 E. 56th St.
New York, NY 10022

Health care

American College of Health Care Administrators
325 S. Patrick St.
Alexandria, VA 22314

American Health Care Association
1201 L St., N.W.
Washington, DC 20005

Foundation for Hospice and Homecare
519 C St., N.E.
Stanton Park
Washington, DC 20002

Hospice Association of America
519 C St., N.E.
Washington, DC 20002

Hospice Education Institute
Five Essex Sq., Suite 3-B
Essex, CT 06426

National Association for Home Care
519 C St., N.E.
Washington, DC 20002

National Association of Rehabilitation Facilities
P.O. Box 17675
Washington, DC 20041

National Committee to Preserve Social Security and Medicare
2000 K St., N.W.
Washington, DC 20006

National Council of Community Mental Health Centers
12300 Twinbrook Pkwy., No. 320
Rockville, MD 20852

National Hospice Organization
1901 N. Moore St., Suite 901
Arlington, VA 22209

National Institute on Adult Daycare
c/o National Council on the Aging
600 Maryland Ave., S.W., W. Wing
Suite 100
Washington, DC 20024

National Institute on Community-Based Long-Term Care
c/o National Council on the Aging
600 Maryland Ave., S.W., W. Wing
Suite 100
Washington, DC 20024

PRIDE Foundation—Promote Real Independence for the Disabled and Elderly
71 Plaza Ct.
Groton, CT 06340

Save Our Security
1201 16th St., N.W.
Washington, DC 20036

Social Security Administration (Health and Human Services)
6401 Security Blvd.
Baltimore, MD 21235

Housing

American Association of Homes for the Aging
1129 20th St., N.W., Suite 400
Washington, DC 20036

National Association for Independent Living
c/o Rehabilitation Services
878 Peachtree St., N.E., Suite 718
Atlanta, GA 30309

National Institute of Senior Centers
c/o National Council on the Aging
600 Maryland Ave., S.W., W. Wing
Suite 100
Washington, DC 20024

National Voluntary Organizations for Independent Living for the Aging
c/o National Council on the Aging
600 Maryland Ave., S.W., W. Wing
Suite 100
Washington, DC 20024

North American Association of Jewish Homes and Housing for the Aging
2525 Centerville Rd.
Dallas, TX 75228

Legal

Legal Council for the Elderly
1909 K St., N.W.
Washington, DC 20049

Legal Services for the Elderly
132 W. 43rd St., 3rd Fl.
New York, NY 10036

National Senior Citizens Law Center
1052 W. Sixth St., Suite 700
Los Angeles, CA 90017

Special interest

American Association of Retired Persons
1909 K St., N.W.
Washington, DC 20049

Children of Ageing Parents
2761 Trenton Rd.
Levittown, PA 19056

Concerned Relatives of Nursing Home Patients
P.O. Box 18820
Cleveland, OH 44118

Elder Craftsmen
135 E. 65th St.
New York, NY 10021

Episcopal Society for Ministry on Aging
Sayre Hall
317 Wyandotte St.
Bethlehem, PA 18015

Foundation for Grandparenting
P.O. Box 31
Lake Placid, NY 12946

Grandparents Anonymous
1024 Beverly
Sylvan Lake, MI 48053

Inter-National Association for Widowed People
P.O. Box 3564
Springfield, IL 62708

Jewish Association for Services for the Aged
40 W. 68th St.
New York, NY 10023

National Alliance for the Advancement of the Black Aged
1101 Gratiot
Detroit, MI 48207

National Association of Nutrition and Aging Services Programs
2663 44th St., S.W., Suite 205
Wyoming, MI 49509

National Caucus and Center on Black Aged
1424 K St., N.W., Suite 500
Washington, DC 20005

National Center on Arts and the Aging
c/o National Council on the Aging
600 Maryland Ave., S.W., W. Wing
Suite 100
Washington, DC 20024

National Center on Rural Aging
c/o National Council on the Aging
600 Maryland Ave., S.W., W. Wing
Suite 100
Washington, DC 20024

National Citizen's Coalition for Nursing Home Reform
1424 16th St., N.W.
Washington, DC 20036

National Council on Black Aging
Box 51275
Durham, NC 27717

National Hispanic Council on Aging
2713 Ontario Rd., N.W.
Washington, DC 20024

National Indian Council on Aging
P.O. Box 2088
Albuquerque, NM 87103

National Pacific/Asian Resource Center on Aging
2033 6th Ave., Suite 410
Seattle, WA 98121

Index

A

B

D

E

F

H

I

JK

L

M

N

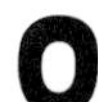

QR

S

T

UV

WXYZ